Muller & Kirk's
SMALL ANIMAL DERMATOLOGY

Muller & Kirk's
SMALL ANIMAL DERMATOLOGY

6th Edition

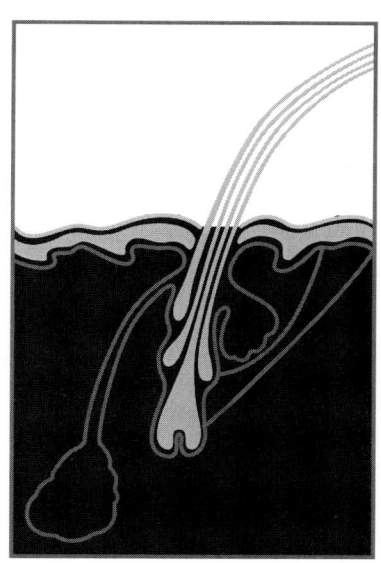

Danny W. Scott, D.V.M.
Professor of Medicine
College of Veterinary Medicine
Cornell University
Ithaca, New York

William H. Miller, Jr., V.M.D.
Professor of Medicine
College of Veterinary Medicine
Cornell University
Ithaca, New York

Craig E. Griffin, D.V.M.
Animal Dermatology Clinic
San Diego, California

W.B. SAUNDERS COMPANY
A Harcourt Health Sciences Company
Philadelphia   London   New York   St. Louis   Sydney   Toronto

W.B. SAUNDERS COMPANY
A Harcourt Health Sciences Company

The Curtis Center
Independence Square West
Philadelphia, Pennsylvania 19106

Library of Congress Cataloging-in-Publication Data

Muller, George H.
　[Small animal dermatology]
　Muller & Kirk's small animal dermatology.—6th ed./Danny W. Scott, William H. Miller, Jr., Craig E. Griffin.
　　　p. cm.
　ISBN 0-7216-7618-9
　1. Dogs—Diseases.　2. Cats—Diseases.　3. Pets—Diseases.
　4. Veterinary dermatology.　I. Kirk, Robert Warren, 1922–　II. Scott, Danny W.　III. Miller, William H. (William Howard), 1948–　IV. Griffin, Craig E.　V. Title.

SF992.S55 M85 2001　　636.089′65—dc21
　　　　　　　　　　　　　　　　　　　　　　　　00-030093

Acquisitions Editor: Ray Kersey
Book Designer: Jonel Sofian
Production Manager: Norman Stellander
Manuscript Editor: Carol DiBerardino
Illustration Specialist: Lisa Lambert

MULLER & KIRK'S SMALL ANIMAL DERMATOLOGY　　　ISBN 0-7216-7618-9

Copyright © 2001, 1995, 1989, 1983, 1976, 1969 by W.B. Saunders Company.

All rights reserved. No part of this publication may be reproduced or transmitted in any form or by any means, electronic or mechanical, including photocopy, recording, or any information storage and retrieval system, without permission in writing from the publisher.

Printed in the United States of America.

Last digit is the print number:　9　8　7　6　5　4　3　2　1

Preface and Acknowledgments

Each time we gear up to do another edition of *Small Animal Dermatology*, we optimistically—yet with the trepidation born of familiarity—tell ourselves that this rewrite will be less involved, less time consuming, less intimidating than the last. After all . . . we just did a total rewrite for the previous edition . . . so this one couldn't possibly be as extensive . . . could it?

Well, once again we have found the task daunting . . . just shy of stifling. In fact, for the first time in the history of the book, we came in 6 months late. Oof! One convenient explanation for our struggles and tardiness—one that admittedly attempts to deflect some portion of the blame from where it clearly should land, right smack-dab on our fidgeting selves—is the staggering amount of new information that has surfaced in the last 5 years in the field of veterinary dermatology. Good examples of this prodigious proliferation include the more than 70 "new" conditions described herein, and the numerous veterinary dermatology textbooks published during this time span (see Chap. 22).

In veterinary medicine, very little information is available concerning the demographics of canine and feline skin disorders. It has been estimated that between 20% and 75% of the small animals seen in the average practice have skin problems as a chief or concurrent owner complaint.[1–5] A 1978 Ralston Purina Company survey indicated that 25% of all small animal practice activity was involved with the diagnosis and treatment of problems with the skin and haircoat.[6] A nationwide survey by the Alpo Company in 1985 of 2540 small animal practitioners in the United States revealed that skin disorders were the most common reason for patient visits to the veterinarian's office.[7] Dermatologic disorders accounted for 18.8% of the dogs and 15.2% of the cats examined at a university teaching hospital.[8]

Using data gathered from 17 North American veterinary teaching hospitals for the year 1983, Sischo and associates reported that the 10 most commonly diagnosed canine skin disorders were, in decreasing order of frequency, flea bite hypersensitivity, skin cancer, bacterial pyoderma, seborrhea, allergy, demodicosis, scabies, immune-mediated dermatoses, endocrine dermatoses, and acral lick dermatitis.[9] Significant differences were noted in the frequency of those skin diseases in the various geographic regions studied. A survey conducted in 1981 by the American Academy of Veterinary Dermatology revealed the most common feline dermatologic disorders to be, in decreasing order of frequency, parasitic dermatoses, miliary dermatitis, eosinophilic granuloma complex, endocrinologic disorders, fungal diseases, hypersensitivity reactions, bacterial diseases, psychogenic dermatoses, seborrheic conditions, neoplastic tumors, and autoimmune dermatoses.[10]

During a 1-year period at a university teaching hospital,[8] the most common dermatoses in dogs and cats were as follows:

Dogs—bacterial folliculitis and furunculosis (25.3% of the cases), atopy (12.7%), food hypersensitivity (4.7%), flea bite hypersensitivity (3.4%), hyperadrenocorticism (3.4%), and hypothyroidism (2.7%).
Cats—abscesses (18.5%), otodectic mange (12.9%), cheyletiellosis (8.1%), flea bite hypersensitivity (6.5%), atopy (5.6%), flea infestation (4.9%), neoplasia (4.9%), and food hypersensitivity (4%).

Clearly, dermatology is a "big ticket item" in small animal practice; bacterial infections, ectoparasitisms, allergies, fungal infections, and neoplasia are common problems.

We cannot overstate our appreciation for those who have contributed to this sixth edition of *Small Animal Dermatology*. We couldn't have done it without you! Held up for special praise and recognition are those who have given so much in terms of love, patience, and support during this production: Kris, Travis, and Tracy (DWS); Kathy, Steven, Julia, and Andrew (WHM); and Laura, Trevor, Kyle, and Taylor (CEG). And last, but not least, we sincerely thank the whole crew at W.B. Saunders Company—especially Ray Kersey—for their patience, support, and terrific effort.

And now . . . it's time to open up our labor of love for your scrutiny. In the words of Bob Seger (and the Silver Bullet Band, of course), we invite you to "Turn the Page."

• REFERENCES

1. Schwartzman RM, Orkin M: A Comparative Study of Skin Diseases of Dog and Man. Charles C Thomas, Springfield, CT, 1962.
2. Ihrke PJ, Franti CE: Breed as a risk factor associated with skin diseases in dogs seen in northern California. Calif Vet 39:13, 1985.
3. Nesbitt GH: Canine and Feline Dermatology: A Systematic Approach. Lea & Febiger, Philadelphia, 1983.
4. Wilkinson GT: Color Atlas of Small Animal Dermatology. Williams & Wilkins, Baltimore, 1985.
5. Grant DI: Skin Diseases in the Dog and Cat. Blackwell Scientific Publications, Oxford, 1986.
6. Ralston Purina Company. An Introduction to the Nutrition of Dogs and Cats. Veterinary Learning Systems, Trenton, NJ, 1989.
7. Alpo Veterinary Panel. Dermatological problems head problem list. DVM Magazine, August, 1985.
8. Scott DW, Paradis M: A survey of canine and feline skin disorders seen in a university practice: Small Animal Clinic, University of Montréal, Saint-Hyacinthe, Québec (1987–1988). Can Vet J 31:830, 1990.
9. Sischo WM, et al: Regional distribution of 10 common skin diseases in dogs. J Am Vet Med Assoc 195:752, 1989.
10. Nesbitt GH: Incidence of feline skin disease: a survey. Proc Am Acad Vet Dermatol, Las Vegas, 1982.

D. W. Scott
W. H. Miller, Jr.
C. E. Griffin

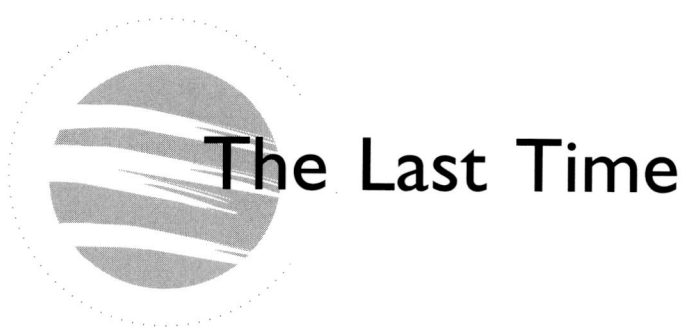

The Last Time

The greatest professional honor I have ever received was being asked to join "the book." Yo! George Muller . . . the legendary father of "the book" . . . and Bob Kirk . . . the most famous veterinarian on the planet. I mean . . . I had contributed bits and pieces to the second edition . . . but now I was coauthor of "the bible."

I have always taken "the book" very seriously: as a clinical dermatologist and educator, I could do no less. "The book" is an enormous commitment, an awesome responsibility. When it is to be "reborn," it demands your all: all your knowledge, all your experience, all your sifting and analysis of our vast literature, all your energy. Getting "the book" ready for its next viewing is all about enthusiasm, conviction, dedication, perseverance, several very short or sleepless nights, curtailed family time, a number of "Advil moments" and, when it is done, a feeling of having given all you had . . . of numbness.

I no longer have what it takes to do "the book" the way it needs to be done . . . and I love this book too much to do anything less than give it the very best there is. So, this will be my last edition. It has been a great ride, a true honor and blessing to be associated with "the book." And Ray Kersey with W.B. Saunders and my wife, Kris, have been with me for the whole 25 years. As much as it aches to say good-bye . . . it is time. I am comforted in the knowledge that—in Bill and Craig—*Small Animal Dermatology* will be left in knowledgeable, experienced, dedicated, and loving hands.

And now I am reminded of a great old song by Mick and the boys, which I have often found myself humming as I worked on this sixth edition!

The Last Time

(Mick Jagger and Keith Richard, 1965)

Thanks, George. Thanks, Bob. Thanks, Ray. Thanks, Kris. Thanks, Bill. Thanks, Craig. Thanks to everyone out there. May "the book" be with you!

Danny
Ithaca, New York—2000

NOTICE

Companion animal practice is an ever-changing field. Standard safety precautions must be followed, but as new research and clinical experience grow, changes in treatment and drug therapy become necessary or appropriate. The authors and editors of this work have carefully checked the generic and trade drug names and verified drug dosages to ensure that dosage information is precise and in accord with standards accepted at the time of publication. Readers are advised, however, to check the product information currently provided by the manufacturer of each drug to be administered to be certain that changes have not been made in the recommended dose or in the contraindications for administration. This is of particular importance in regard to new or infrequently used drugs. Recommended dosages for animals are sometimes based on adjustments in the dosage that would be suitable for humans. Some of the drugs mentioned here have been given experimentally by the authors. Others have been used in dosages greater than those recommended by the manufacturer. In these kinds of cases, the authors have reported on their own considerable experience. It is the responsibility of those administering a drug, relying on their professional skill and experience, to determine the dosages, the best treatment for the patient, and whether the benefits of giving a drug justify the attendant risk. The editors cannot be responsible for misuse or misapplication of the material in this work.

THE PUBLISHER

Contents

1	Structure and Function of the Skin	1
2	Diagnostic Methods	71
3	Dermatologic Therapy	207
4	Bacterial Skin Diseases	274
5	Fungal Skin Diseases	336
6	Parasitic Skin Diseases	423
7	Viral, Rickettsial, and Protozoal Skin Diseases	517
8	Skin Immune System and Allergic Skin Diseases	543
9	Immune-Mediated Disorders	667
10	Endocrine and Metabolic Diseases	780
11	Acquired Alopecias	887
12	Congenital and Hereditary Defects	913
13	Pigmentary Abnormalities	1005
14	Keratinization Defects	1025
15	Psychogenic Skin Diseases	1055
16	Environmental Skin Diseases	1073
17	Nutritional Skin Diseases	1112
18	Miscellaneous Skin Diseases	1125
19	Diseases of Eyelids, Claws, Anal Sacs, and Ears	1185
20	Neoplastic and Non-Neoplastic Tumors	1236
21	Dermatoses of Pet Rodents, Rabbits, and Ferrets	1415
22	Chronology of Veterinary Dermatology (1900–2000)	1459
	Index	1465

Chapter 1

Structure and Function of the Skin

What a glorious organ it is! The skin is the largest and most visible organ of the body and the anatomic and physiologic barrier between animal and environment. It provides protection from physical, chemical, and microbiologic injury, and its sensory components perceive heat, cold, pain, pruritus, touch, and pressure. In addition, the skin is synergistic with internal organ systems and thus reflects pathologic processes that are either primary elsewhere or shared with other tissues. Not only is the skin an organ with its own reaction patterns; it is also a mirror reflecting the *milieu interieur* and, at the same time, the capricious world to which it is exposed. The skin, hair, and subcutis of a newborn puppy represent 24% of its body weight.[180]

By the time of maturity, these structures constitute only 12% of body weight.

• GENERAL FUNCTIONS AND PROPERTIES OF THE SKIN

The general functions and properties of animal skin are as follows*:

1. Enclosing barrier. The most important function of skin is to make possible an internal environment for all other organs by maintaining an effective barrier to the loss of water, electrolytes, and macromolecules.
2. Environmental protection. A corollary function is the exclusion of external injurious agents—chemical, physical, and microbiologic—from entrance into the internal environment.
3. Motion and shape. The flexibility, elasticity, and toughness of the skin allow motion and provide shape and form.
4. Adnexa production. Skin produces keratinized structures such as hair, claws, and the horny layer of the epidermis.
5. Temperature regulation. Skin plays a role in the regulation of body temperature through its support of the hair coat, regulation of cutaneous blood supply, and sweat gland function.
6. Storage. The skin is a reservoir of electrolytes, water, vitamins, fat, carbohydrates, proteins, and other materials.
7. Indicator. The skin may be an important indicator of general health, internal disease, and the effects of substances applied topically or taken internally. It contributes to physical and sexual identity.
8. Immunoregulation. Keratinocytes, Langerhans' cells, and lymphocytes together provide the skin with an immunosurveillance capability that effectively protects against the development of cutaneous neoplasms and persistent infections.
9. Pigmentation. Processes in the skin (melanin formation, vascularity, and keratinization) help determine the color of the coat and skin. Pigmentation of the skin helps prevent damage from solar radiation.
10. Antimicrobial action. The skin surface has antibacterial and antifungal properties.

---

*See references 57, 65, 102, 150, 166, 172, 180, 187, and 196.

11. Sensory perception. Skin is a primary sense organ for touch, pressure, pain, itch, heat, and cold.
12. Secretion. Skin is a secretory organ by virtue of its epitrichial (apocrine), atrichial (eccrine), and sebaceous glands.
13. Excretion. The skin functions in a limited way as an excretory organ.
14. Vitamin D production. Vitamin D is produced in the skin through stimulation by solar radiation. In the epidermis, vitamin D_3 (cholecalciferol) is formed from provitamin D_3 (7-dehydrocholesterol), via previtamin D_3, on exposure to sunlight.[65] The vitamin D–binding protein in plasma translocates vitamin D_3 from the skin to the circulation. Vitamin D_3 is then hydroxylated in the liver to 25-hydroxyvitamin D_3 and again hydroxylated in the kidney to form 1,25-dihydroxyvitamin D_3, which is important in the regulation of epidermal proliferation and differentiation.[65, 96]

● ONTOGENY

Skin is a complex multicellular organ in which endoderm, neural crest, and ectoderm contribute to form a three-dimensional unit in a spatially and temporally defined manner. Skin morphogenesis involves the action of multiple genes in a coordinated fashion. Homeobox genes are a gene family that encode information critical for normal embryologic development and that likely play a very important role in the development of skin adnexa, pigment system, and stratified epithelium during embryogenesis.[181]

Epithelial-mesenchymal interactions regulate tissue homeostasis, the balanced regulation of proliferation and differentiation maintaining normal tissue architecture and function.[110] Multiple circuits of reciprocal permissive and instructive effects exist between epithelial and mesenchymal cells and extracellular matrices.

Initially, the embryonic skin consists of a single layer of ectodermal cells and a dermis containing loosely arranged mesenchymal cells embedded in an interstitial ground substance. The ectodermal covering progressively develops into two layers (the basal cell layer, or *stratum germinativum*, and the outer *periderm*), three layers (the stratum intermedium forms between the other two layers), and then into an adult-like structure.[57, 65, 166, 180] Melanocytes (neural crest origin) and Langerhans' cells (bone marrow origin) become identifiable during this period of ectodermal maturation.

Dermal development is characterized by an increase in the thickness and number of fibers, a decrease in ground substance, and the transition of mesenchymal cells to fibroblasts. This process of building a fiber-rich matrix has been referred to as a *ripening* of the dermis. Elastin fibers appear later than do collagen fibers. Histiocytes, Schwann cells, and dermal melanocytes also become recognizable. Fetal skin contains a large percentage of Type III collagen compared with the skin of an adult, which contains a large proportion of Type I collagen.[65] Lipocytes (adipocytes, fat cells) begin to develop into the subcutis from spindle-shaped mesenchymal precursor cells *(prelipoblasts)* in the second half of gestation.

The embryonal stratum germinativum differentiates into hair germs (primary epithelial germs), which give rise to hair follicles, sebaceous glands, and epitrichial (apocrine) sweat glands.[4, 10, 177] Hair germs initially consist of an area of crowding of deeply basophilic cells in the basal layer of the epidermis. Subsequently, the areas of crowding become buds that protrude into the dermis. Beneath each bud lies a group of mesenchymal cells, from which the dermal hair papilla is later formed.

As the hair peg lengthens and develops into a hair follicle and hair, three bulges appear. The lowest (deepest) of the bulges develops into the attachment for the arrector pili muscle; the middle bulge differentiates into the sebaceous gland; and the uppermost bulge evolves into the epitrichial sweat gland. These appendages develop on the ental side of primary hair follicles; secondary hair follicles develop on the extal side. In general, the first hairs to appear on the fetus are vibrissae and tactile or sinus hairs that develop on the chin, eyebrows, and upper lip as white, slightly raised dots on otherwise smooth, bare skin.[166, 177] The general body hair appears first on the head and gradually progresses caudally.

Atrichial (eccrine) sweat gland germs also begin as areas of crowding of deeply basophilic cells in the basal layer of the epidermis. They initially differ from hair germs only slightly by being narrower and by showing fewer mesenchymal cells at their base.

Cell interaction plays a central role in the formation of skin appendages.[110] Morphogens are substances that control the development of the hair follicle.[4, 50] In addition, several new adhesion molecule families that mediate cell-to-cell and cell-to-substrate adhesion have been identified: (1) neural cell adhesion molecules (N-CAM), which belong to the immunoglobulin (IgG) gene superfamily; (2) cadherins, which mediate adhesion in the presence of calcium; (3) tenascin, which is a unique matrix molecule similar to the epidermal cell growth factor (EGF); (4) fibronectin, fibrinogen, and syndecan; and (5) integrins, which serve as cellular receptors for fibronectin, collagen, and other extracellular matrix molecules.[36, 50, 65, 110] Thus, in each step of the morphogenesis of skin appendages, different adhesion molecules are expressed and are involved in different functions: induction, mesenchymal condensation, epithelial folding, and cell death.

All vessels in fetal skin develop first as capillaries.[9, 65] They have been suggested to organize in situ from dermal mesenchymal cells into single-layered endothelial tubes. Branches from large subcutaneous nerve trunks extend into the dermis and organize into deep and superficial plexuses related to the vascular plexus.

• GROSS ANATOMY AND PHYSIOLOGY

At each body orifice, the skin is continuous with the mucous membrane located there (digestive, respiratory, ocular, urogenital). The skin and haircoat vary in quantity and quality among species, among breeds within a species, and among individuals within a breed; they also vary from one area to another on the body, and in accordance with age and sex.

In general, skin thickness decreases dorsally to ventrally on the trunk and proximally to distally on the limbs.[166, 172, 180, 188, 202] The skin is thickest on the forehead, dorsal neck, dorsal thorax, rump, and base of the tail. It is thinnest on the pinnae and on the axillary, inguinal, and perianal areas. The reported average thickness of the general body skin of cats is 0.4 to 2.0 mm[172, 188]; of dogs, it is 0.5 to 5.0 mm.[102, 180] The haircoat is usually thickest over the dorsolateral aspects of the body and thinnest ventrally, on the lateral surface of the pinnae, and on the undersurface of the tail.

The skin surfaces of haired mammals are, in general, acidic. The pH of normal feline and canine skin has been reported to range from about 5.5 to 7.5.[49, 102, 132, 157, 158, 172] In a dynamic study of skin surface pH in dogs,[158] the following observations were made: pH values varied at different sites on the skin and varied from day to day; males had significantly higher pH values than females on all sites; spayed females had significantly higher pH values at all sites than intact females; black Labrador retrievers had significantly higher pH values than yellow Labrador retrievers, and Labrador retrievers and miniature schnauzers were significantly different from English springer spaniels and Yorkshire terriers. Clearly, skin surface pH appears to vary with site, day, coat color, sex, gonadal status, and breed. In addition, it has been reported that the skin surface pH of an excited dog can increase by greater than 1 unit within 1 minute.[132]

The metabolism of the skin is not well understood. All of the enzymes of the glycolytic pathway and those of the tricarboxylic acid cycle have been demonstrated in skin, but actual glucose metabolism seems to be anomalous.[19, 65, 72, 98, 180] Glucose is preferentially metabolized to lactate, rather than fully oxidized to CO_2. The skin is an active site of fatty acid metabolism (see Chap. 3).

Studies of the surface markings of the muzzle and nose have shown that there are individual, genetically determined differences similar to those of human fingerprints.[166] It has been suggested that imprints ("fingerprints") of these special skin areas (termed *labiograms* or *nasolabiograms*) could be used for the identification of animals.

Hair

Hair, which is characteristic of mammals, is important in thermal insulation and sensory perception and as a barrier against chemical, physical, and microbial injury to the skin.[65, 119, 177, 187] Hair is photoprotective. The ability of a haircoat to regulate body temperature correlates closely with its length, thickness, and density per unit area, and with the medullation of individual hair fibers. In general, haircoats composed of long, fine, poorly medullated fibers, with the coat depth increased by piloerection, are the most efficient for thermal insulation at low environmental temperatures. Coat color is also of some importance in thermal regulation; light-colored coats are more efficient in hot, sunny weather. The glossiness of the haircoat is important in reflecting sunlight. Transglutaminase is a marker of early anagen hair follicles, and it is important in the protein cross-linking that contributes to the shape and remarkable physical strength of hair.[65, 112] The diameter of the hair shaft is largely determined by the volume of the hair matrix epithelium, and the final length of the hair shaft is determined by both the rate of hair growth and the duration of anagen.

Both primary (outercoat, guard) and secondary (undercoat) hairs are medullated in dogs and cats; thus, the term *lanugo*, meaning nonmedulated, is incorrect when applied to nonfetal dogs and cats. In cats, secondary hairs are far more numerous than primary hairs (10:1 dorsally, 24:1 ventrally).[172] The hairs of the cat have been divided into three types based on gross appearance: (1) guard hairs (thickest, straight, evenly tapered to a fine tip), (2) awn hairs (thinner, possessing subapical swelling below the hair tip), and (3) down hairs (thinnest, evenly crimped or undulating).[155, 174, 177] In general, the shape of the hair fiber is determined by the shape of the hair follicle, with straight follicles producing straight hairs and curly follicles producing curly hairs.[166, 177]

In general, no new hair follicles are formed after birth. Puppies do not actually "lose" their puppy coat; rather, they *gain* an adult coat. Puppies have simple hair follicles that produce secondary hairs for the first 12 weeks of life.[50] All hair follicles grow obliquely (30 to 60 degrees) in relation to the epidermis. The direction of the slope of the hairs, which varies from one region of the body to another, gives rise to the *hair tracts*.[177] The study of hair tract patterns is called *trichoglyphics*. The true significance and the origin of hair tracts are unknown. With the hair slope generally running caudally and ventrally, benefits include minimal impediment to forward motion and the ability of water to flow off the body to the ground without soaking the haircoat, which would reduce its thermal-insulating properties.

Adult shorthaired cats produced a yearly amount of hair growth of 32.7g/kg.[75] Dogs produced 60 to 180 g/kg, depending on the breed.[137]

Hair Cycle

Analysis of the factors controlling or influencing hair growth is complicated by evolutionary history.[65] The pelage changes as a mammal grows, and that of the adult often differs markedly from that of the juvenile, reflecting different requirements for heat regulation, camouflage, and sexual and social communication. In addition, the cyclic activity of the hair follicles and the periodic molting of hairs have provided a mechanism by which the pelage can be adapted to seasonal changes in ambient temperature or environmental background. This mechanism is influenced by changes in the photoperiod, which acts through the hypothalamus, hypophysis, and pineal gland, altering levels of various hormones (including melatonin, prolactin, and those of gonadal, thyroidal, and adrenocortical origin) and modifying the inherent rhythms of the hair follicle.

Hair growth cycles involve the repeated induction of hair follicle anlagen and their concurrent downward growth and invasion through the dermis.[25, 203] Signals controlling hair follicle induction, development, regression, and reactivation have not been identified; however, multiple growth factors or their receptors (e.g., EGF, transforming growth factor [TGF]-β1, TGF-β2, neurotrophin-3) have been localized to hair follicles and the surrounding mesenchyme. These growth factors control cellular proliferation and collagenase release from cultured hair follicles. In addition, an interplay between class I major histocompatibility complex (MHC) expression, chondroitin proteoglycans, and activated macrophages is involved in the regulation of hair growth, especially during the catagen phase.[4, 62]

Neural mechanisms of hair growth control in mice have revealed that the sensory and autonomic innervation of hair follicles, the substance P content of skin, and the cutaneous nerve–mast cell contacts show changes during the hair cycle.[147] The hair follicle is a source and a target of neurotrophins, and neuropharmacologic manipulations alter hair cycling. The trophic effects of cutaneous nerves on follicular growth are exerted via regulation of vascular tone (nutrient and oxygen supply), neuropeptide stimulation of receptors on follicular keratinocytes and dermal papilla fibroblasts, and modulation of macrophage and mast cell activities. In dogs, hair growth retardation (follicular atrophy) has occurred after experimental sectioning of peripheral nerves and dorsal roots.[100] However, peripheral nerve damage can also induce increased hair growth, as seen in the unilateral hypertrichosis ("hemitrichosis") following major unilateral thoracic surgery in dogs.[100]

Hairs do not grow continuously but rather in cycles (Fig. 1–1). Each cycle consists of a growing period *(anagen)*, during which the follicle is actively producing hair, and a resting period (telogen), during which the hair is retained in the follicle as a dead (or club) hair that is subsequently lost. There is also a transitional period *(catagen)* between these two stages. It is often stated that certain breeds of dogs, such as poodles, Old English sheepdogs, and schnauzers, have continuously growing hair coats,[180] but there has been no scientific investigation that would substantiate such a statement. The relative duration of the phases of the cycle varies with the age of the individual, the region of the body, the breed, and the sex, and it can be modified by a variety of physiologic and pathologic factors.

The hair cycle, and thus the haircoat, are controlled by photoperiod, ambient temperature, nutrition, hormones, general state of health, genetics, and poorly understood intrinsic factors.[2–4, 17, 28, 65, 68, 70, 75, 119, 166, 167, 177, 180, 196] Intrinsic factors include growth factors and cytokines produced by the follicle, the dermal papilla, and other cells (lymphocytes,

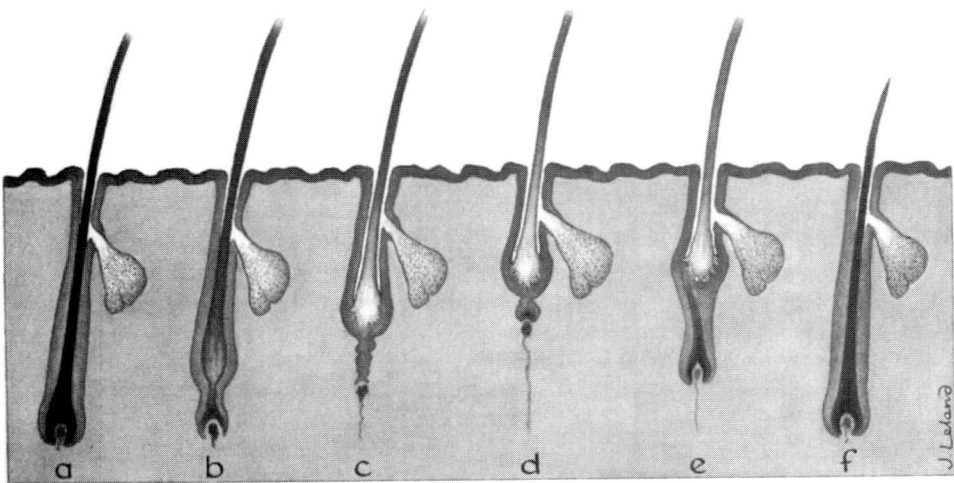

FIGURE 1–1. The hair cycle. a, Anagen: During this growing stage, hair is produced by mitosis in cells of the dermal papilla. b, Early catagen: In this transitional stage, a constriction occurs at the hair bulb. The hair above this will become a "club." c, Catagen: The distal follicle becomes thick and corrugated and pushes the hair outward. d, Telogen: This is the resting stage. The dermal papilla separates and an epithelial strand shortens to form a secondary germ. e, Early anagen: The secondary germ grows down to enclose the dermal papilla and a new hair bulb forms. The old "club" is lost. f, Anagen: The hair elongates as growth continues.

macrophages, fibroblasts, mast cells) in the immediate environment. In cats, there was no effect of repeated clipping on hair growth.[75]

Hair replacement in dogs and cats is mosaic in pattern because neighboring hair follicles are in different stages of the hair cycle at any one time. Replacement is unaffected by castration; it responds predominantly to photoperiod and, to a lesser extent, to ambient temperature. Dogs and cats in temperate latitudes such as the northern United States and Canada may shed noticeably in the spring and fall. Hair follicle activity, and thus hair growth rate, are maximal in summer and minimal in winter. For example, up to 50% of hair follicles may be in telogen in the summer, but this proportion may increase to 90% in the winter. Maximum hair follicle inactivity is reached earlier in female cats than in male cats.[75] Catagen hairs always constitute a small proportion of the total number of hairs, usually accounting for 4% to 7% of the total.[3, 180] Many dogs and cats exposed to several hours of artificial light (e.g., animals housed indoors) shed, sometimes profusely, throughout the year.[172, 180] Sinus hairs are *not* subject to a seasonal shedding, and are shed continuously as single hairs.[171]

Hair grows until it attains its preordained length, which varies according to body region and is genetically determined; it then enters the resting phase, which may last for a considerable amount of time. Each region of the body has its own ultimate length of hair beyond which no further growth occurs. This phenomenon is responsible for the distinctive coat lengths of various breeds and is genetically determined. In mongrel dogs, it was shown that hair growth rates varied at different sites and that the speed of growth was related to the ultimate length of the hair in each particular site.[68] For example, in the shoulder region, where ultimate hair length was about 30 mm, the average rate of hair growth was 6.7 mm/wk, whereas in the forehead region, which had ultimate hair length of about 16 mm, the growth rate was 2.8 mm/wk. Other investigators have reported daily hair growth rates in dogs of 0.04 to 0.18 mm (Greyhound)[28, 39] and 0.34 to 0.40 mm (beagle).[2] In the cat, daily hair growth rate has been reported to be 0.25 to 0.30 mm[17] or 62 to 289 $\mu g/cm^2$.[75]

Because hair is predominantly protein, nutrition has a profound effect on its quantity and quality (see Chap. 17). Poor nutrition may produce a dull, dry, brittle, or thin haircoat with or without pigmentary disturbances.

Under conditions of ill health or generalized disease, anagen may be considerably shortened; accordingly, a large percentage of body hairs may be in telogen at one time. Because telogen hairs tend to be more easily lost, the animal may shed excessively. Disease states may also lead to faulty formation of hair cuticle, which results in a dull, lusterless hair coat. Severe illness or systemic stress may cause many hair follicles to enter synchronously and precipitously into telogen. Shedding of these hairs (telogen defluxion; see Chap. 11) thus occurs simultaneously, often resulting in visible thinning of the coat or actual alopecia.

The hair cycle and haircoat are also affected by hormonal changes.[28, 65, 70, 119] In general, anagen is initiated and advanced and hair growth rate is accelerated by thyroid hormones and growth hormone. Conversely, excessive amounts of glucocorticoids or estrogens inhibit anagen and suppress hair growth rate. Dermal papilla cells, which are a mesenchymal component of the hair bulb, are considered to play a fundamental role in the induction of epithelial differentiation. These cells are morphologically and functionally differentiated from dermal fibroblasts and are thought to be the primary target cells that respond to hormones and mediate growth-stimulating signals to the follicular epithelial cells.[4, 84]

Obviously, the details of the regulation of hair follicle cycling and growth are extraordinarily complex and still poorly understood. The factors that control the hair follicle cycle are, in general, different from the factors that control hair follicle structure. Alterations in factors (e.g., hormones) controlling the hair follicle cycle result in *follicular atrophy*. Alterations in factors (e.g., morphogens) that control hair follicle structure result in *follicular dysplasia*.

Hair growth is a confusing subject that needs much research. It should be remembered that the haircoat of pet animals is a cosmetic or ornamental feature. Every effort should be made to minimize procedures (clipping and shaving) that may affect the animal's appearance for many weeks. Although generalizations can be misleading, normal or short coats usually take about 3 to 4 months to regrow after shaving and long coats may take as long as 18 months.[180] Occasionally, an unexplained and extremely frustrating failure to regrow hair in an area of skin occurs, usually following clipping and surgical scrubbing.[180] The skin in affected areas appears grossly normal, but biopsy reveals catagenization, or occasionally telogenization, of the hair follicles. This frustrating *follicular arrest* disappears spontaneously in 6 months to 2 years after clipping (see Chap. 11).

Attention has been focused on the usefulness of hair analysis as a diagnostic tool.[184, 216] It is well recognized by most dermatologists and nutritionists in human medicine that mineral and trace element analysis of hair samples is not a clinically useful tool in the assessment of nutritional status. The reasons for variability and unreliability include environmental effects (topical agents, geographic location, occupational exposures), differing hair growth rates (health, drugs, age, sex), and lack of standardization in analysis techniques. Until and unless adequate scientific documentation of the validity of such multielement analysis is performed, it is necessary for both health professionals and the public to be aware of the very limited value of hair analysis and of the potential to be confused and misled by it. Scientifically oriented nutritionists do not use hair analysis as a primary method of detecting nutritional problems. Cautious consumers and health professionals should regard practitioners who rely solely on this test with suspicion.[216]

Small (0.16 to 0.42 mm in diameter), hairless, knoblike structures are present in the haired skin of cats and dogs.[169, 172, 180] These tylotrich pads serve as slow-adapting mechanoreceptors.

Cell proliferation kinetic values have been established for the hair follicle epithelium of normal beagles and Cocker spaniels.[106] These values were established by intradermal pulse-labeling injections of tritiated thymidine, examination of skin biopsies, and autoradiographs. The basal cell labeling index was $1.46 \pm 0.78\%$ in beagles and $1.07 \pm 0.42\%$ in Cocker spaniels.

Hair Colors and Types

DOG

Although hair types in dogs are extremely diverse, various authors have attempted to classify them on the basis of color, length, type of bristle, and characteristics of the medulla and cortex.[180] Hair types among dogs can be divided into normal (intermediate length), short, and long coats.

Normal Coat

The normal coat is typified by that seen in the German shepherd, the Welsh corgi, and wild dogs such as wolves and coyotes. It is composed of primary hairs (coarse guard hairs or bristles) and secondary hairs (fine hairs or undercoat). A high proportion of the hairs, by number but not by weight, are secondary hairs.

The next two classes of hair coats are also made up of primary and secondary hairs, but the relative sizes of the hairs and their numbers vary markedly from those of the normal coat.

Short Coat

The short coat can be classified as coarse or fine. The coarse short coat is typified by the Rottweiler and many of the terriers. This type of coat has a strong growth of primary hairs and a much lesser growth of secondary hairs. The total weight of hair is lower, and the secondary hairs, especially, weigh less and are fewer in number than those in the normal coat. The fine short coat is exemplified by boxers, dachshunds, and miniature pinschers. This type of coat has the largest number of hairs per unit area. The secondary hairs are numerous and well developed, and the primary hairs are reduced in size as compared with those of the normal coat.

Long Coat

The long coat can also be arranged into two subdivisions: the fine long coat and the woolly or coarse long coat. The fine long coat is found in the Cocker spaniel, the Pomeranian, and the Chow Chow. This coat has a greater weight of hair per unit area than does the normal coat, except in the toy breeds (in which the weight of the hair may be less because it is finer). The woolly or coarse long coat is found in the poodle and in the Bedlington terrier and the Kerry blue terrier. Secondary hairs make up 70% of the total weight of these coats and 80% of the number of hairs; compared with other secondary-type hairs, these are relatively coarse. The three breeds mentioned have less tendency to shed hair than do many breeds.

The genetic aspects of coat color in dogs constitute a complex subject.[115, 180] Pigmentation in individual hairs may be uniform throughout the length of the shaft, or it may vary. In the agouti-type hair (German shepherd, Norwegian elkhound), the tip is white or light, the heavy body is pigmented brown or black, and the base is a light yellow or red-brown. Pigment cells in the bulb of the hair deposit pigment in or between the cortical and medullary hair cells. The amount of pigment deposited in the hair and its location there produce different optical effects; however, there are only two types of pigment. The black-brown pigment is called *eumelanin,* and the yellow-red pigment is called *pheomelanin.* In addition, the melanocytes of the follicle may or may not produce pigment throughout the period of growth. In black hair, pigment production obviously remains active throughout the period.

CAT

The colors and types of hair coat in cats have been studied in some detail.[152, 155, 213] A self (solid) cat is a single color throughout. No patterning, shading, ticking, or other variation of color is observed, although it is common for kittens to have slightly tabby markings and scattered white hairs that disappear with maturity. Whatever their coloring, all cats are genetically tabbies, possessing the Abyssinian, mackerel, or blotched tabby genes, or a combination of two of these types. Solid white is dominant over all colors but may be associated with various abnormalities; for example, white cats with blue eyes often have cochlear degeneration and deafness.

The tabby is the basic type of cat, the wild type from which all others evolved. The complex tabby coloration arises from two component patterns governed by two separate sets of genes. The underlying pattern is agouti, which is characterized by hairs with a bluish base and black tip separated by yellow banding. The tabby genes determine whether a cat has narrow, vertical, gently curving stripes (mackerel), larger patches (blotch), or an Abyssinian pattern.

Tipped hair coats are characterized by hairs that have colored tips (e.g., blue, red, black) overlying a paler color. Differences in the degree of tipping are great, with the greatest in the smokes and least in the chinchillas (silver). Pointed hair coats are characterized by pale-colored hair on the body with darker hairs on the extremities or points (nose, ears, feet, tail). Points arise through a temperature-dependent mechanism present in breeds such as Siamese, Himalayan, Balinese, and Birman. In these breeds, the dark hair color (acromelanism) is due to a temperature-dependent enzyme that converts melanin precursors into melanin by a process of oxidation.[146] With higher temperatures, the hair is light colored; with low temperatures, it is darker. Thus, kittens are light at birth, and cats kept indoors or in tropical climates are lighter than those kept outdoors or in cold climates. Inflammation and hyperemia result in more lightly colored new hair. The poor peripheral circulation that accompanies senility and shaving to remove hair often result in more darkly colored new hair.

Multicolored coats include the tortoiseshell and piebald spotting patterns. The archetypal tortoiseshell is a patchwork of black and orange, but there is range of color variation among torties. The hair may be chocolate (chestnut), cinnamon, blue, or lilac (lavender) in the nonorange areas. The tortoiseshell pattern occurs in females or in males with two X chromosomes. White spotting in piebald cats varies in degree from white gloves on the feet, a nose smudge, or a white bib, to extensive white over most of the body.

The *Maltese dilution,* which dilutes black to blue (gray), orange to cream, and seal-point (Siamese) to blue-point, is inherited as an autosomal recessive trait.[151] In non-Maltese cats, small melanin granules of uniform shape and size are scattered uniformly throughout the cortex and medulla of the hair shaft, hair follicle epithelium, and epidermis. In the skin and hair from Maltese dilution cats, a nonuniform distribution of very large, irregularly sized and shaped melanin granules results from the clumping of small granules.

In a typical shorthaired cat, the longest primary hairs average about 4.5 cm in length. By contrast, the silky coat of a good show cat has primary hairs that may exceed 12.5 cm in length. The shorthair is the fundamental wild type and is dominant to the others. Various mutant hair coat types have occurred that have been perpetuated as a breed characteristic. The rex mutant is characterized by curly hairs and occurs in two major breeds, the Devon rex and the Cornish (German) rex. The Cornish rex lacks primary hairs, and the Devon rex has primary hairs that resemble secondary hairs. Cornish rex whiskers are often short and curly, but Devon rex whiskers are often absent or stubbled. In some Devon rexes, the coat is completely absent on the chest, belly, and shoulders, a fault many breeders try to eliminate. Cornish and Devon rexes may partially or completely molt, especially during estrus or pregnancy, resulting in a symmetric alopecia that may be mistaken for an endocrine dermatosis.[54] These breeds are occasionally recommended as hypoallergenic cats to humans with animal dander hypersensitivities, but there appears to be no scientific documentation for this claim.

The wire-hair mutation, seen in the American wirehair, is characterized by a coat that looks and feels wiry because it is coarse, crimped, and springy. All hairs are curled in an irregular fashion, and the awn hairs resemble a shepherd's crook.

One survey attempted to relate feline coat color to personality.[153] Results suggested that cats with solid black, black and white, or gray tabby coats tended to have good personalities, to handle stress well, and to make excellent pets. By contrast, calicos were most likely to be aggressive and to have litter pan problems.

There are a number of cutaneous patterns or lines that are evoked to explain certain distributions of skin lesions encountered clinically.[91] *Voight's lines* are the boundaries of the areas of distribution of the main cutaneous nerve stems. *Langer's lines* reflect the course of blood vessels or lymphatics. *Blaschko's lines* form the pattern assumed by many different nevoid and acquired skin diseases. Blaschko's lines reflect a mosaic condition deriving either from a single mutated clone of cells originating from a postzygotic mutation or from an X-linked mutation made evident by lyonization.[154] These lines follow a V-shape over the spine, an S-shape on the abdomen, an axial distribution on the limbs, and a wavy pattern down the forehead, over and below the eyes, over the upper lip, and behind the ear. *Tension lines* are determined by muscle action, connective tissue fiber orientation and traction, and gravity.[82]

Footpads

The canine and feline footpad is a specialized area of integument.[131, 166, 180] The thick epidermis protects against mechanical trauma, and the large fat deposits provide shock-absorbing elasticity. A copious nerve supply provides an important sensory function. Numerous atrichial sweat glands produce a secretion that may improve traction during running and climbing and may also be important in scent marking.

● MICROSCOPIC ANATOMY AND PHYSIOLOGY

The microscopic anatomy and physiology of the skin of dogs and cats have been the subjects of numerous studies.*

---

*See references 77, 102, 117, 119, 135, 156, 166, 168, 170, 172, 180, 187, 188, 202, and 215.

Epidermis

The outer layer of the skin, or epidermis, is composed of multiple layers of cells defined by position, shape, polarity, morphology and state of differentiation of the keratinocytes (Figs. 1–2, 1–3A, 1–4, 1–5, and 1–6; see also Fig. 1–16). There are four distinct cell types within the epidermis: keratinocytes (about 85% of the epidermal cells), melanocytes (about 5%), Langerhans' cells (3% to 8%), and Merkel's cells (about 2%), which are associated with tylotrich pads.[65, 180, 206] For purposes of identification, certain areas of the epidermis are classified as layers and are named, from inner to outer, as follows: basal layer (stratum basale), spinous layer (stratum spinosum), granular layer (stratum granulosum), clear layer (stratum lucidum), and horny layer (stratum corneum). In general, the epidermis of cats and dogs is thin (two to three nucleated cell layers, not counting the horny layer) in haired skin, ranging from 0.1 to 0.5 mm in thickness or in depth.[116, 172, 180, 188, 202] The thickest epidermis is found on the footpads (see Fig. 1–4) and nasal planum (see Fig. 1–5), where it may measure 1.5 mm. The surface of the footpad epidermis is smooth in cats but papillated and irregular in dogs. Rete ridges (projections

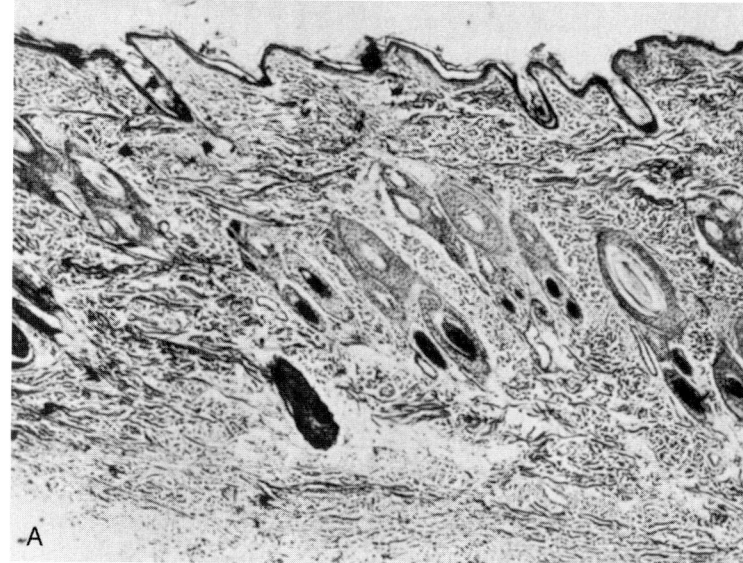
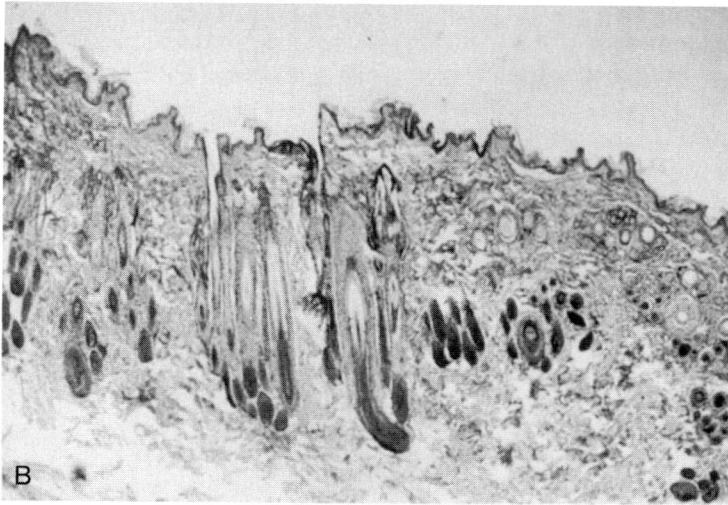

FIGURE 1–2. *A*, Normal canine skin. *B*, Normal feline skin. Note the thin epidermis and compound hair follicle arrangement of both species.

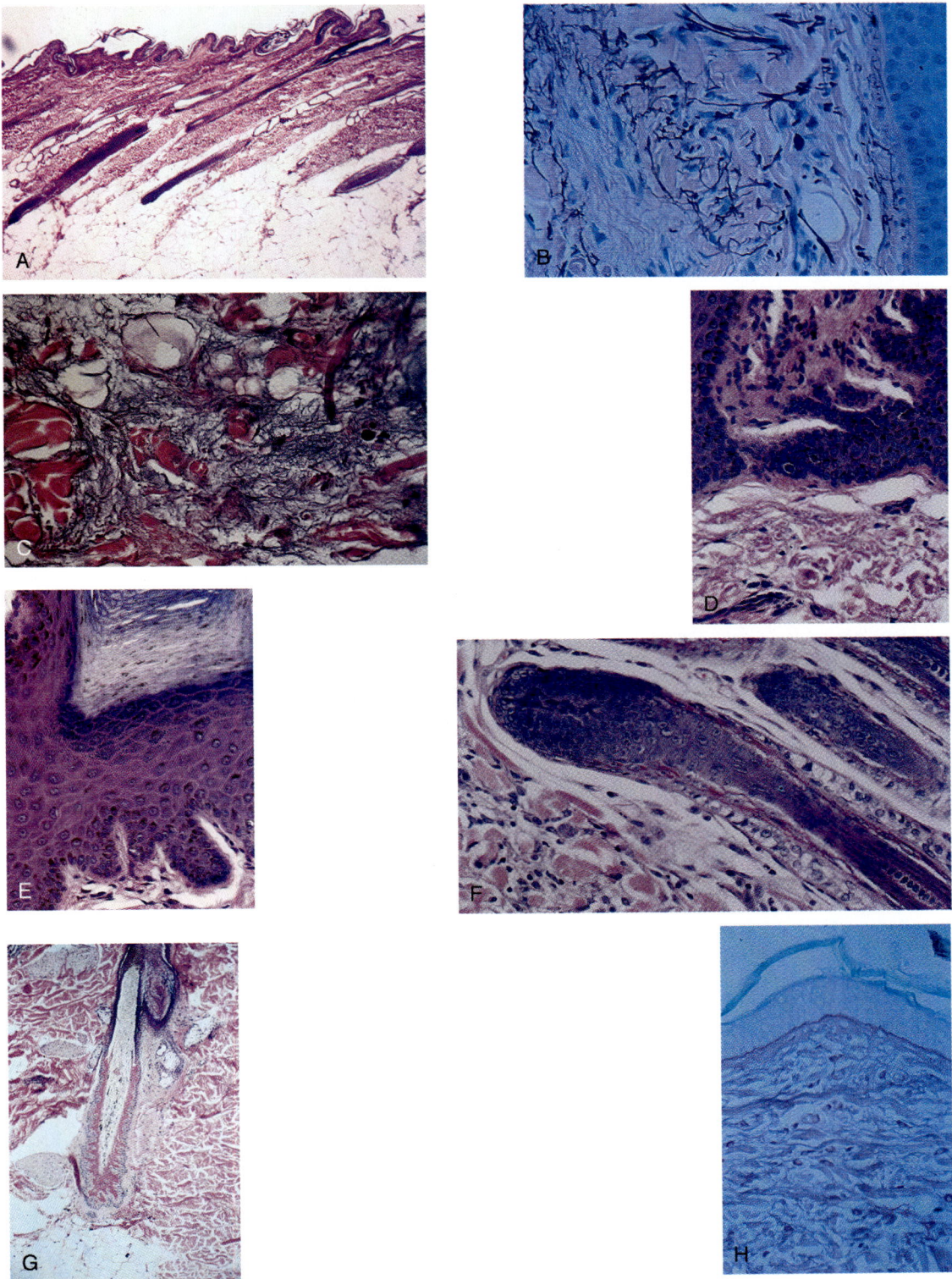

FIGURE 1–3. *A*, Normal canine skin (H & E stain). *B*, Elastin (black) and collagen (pink) fibers (AOG stain). *C*, Mucin (blue) separating dermal collagen bundles (pink) (H & E stain). *D*, Melanin granules (black) in keratinocytes and melanocytes ("clear cells") (H & E stain). *E*, Keratohyalin granules (dark blue) below stratum corneum (H & E stain). *F*, Trichohyalin granules (red) in the inner root sheath of a hair follicle (H & E stain). Note vacuolated (glycogen) appearance of outer root sheath keratinocytes. *G*, Trichilemmal keratinization (red) of central hair follicle (H & E stain). *H*, Basement membrane zone (violet) (PAS stain).

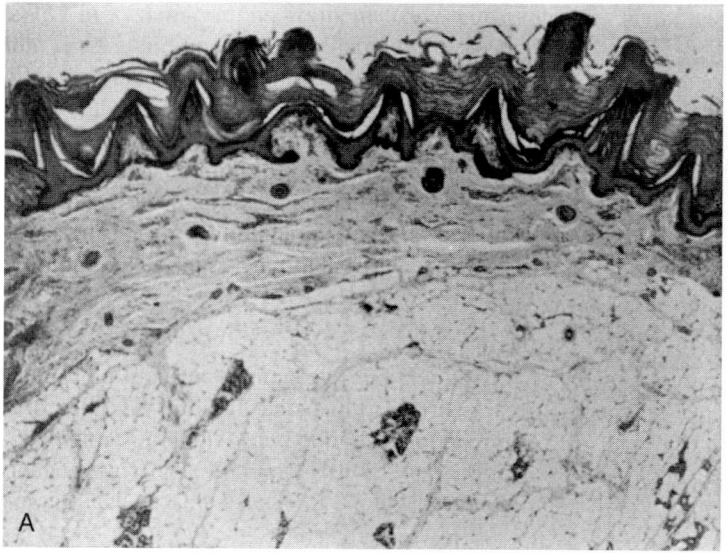

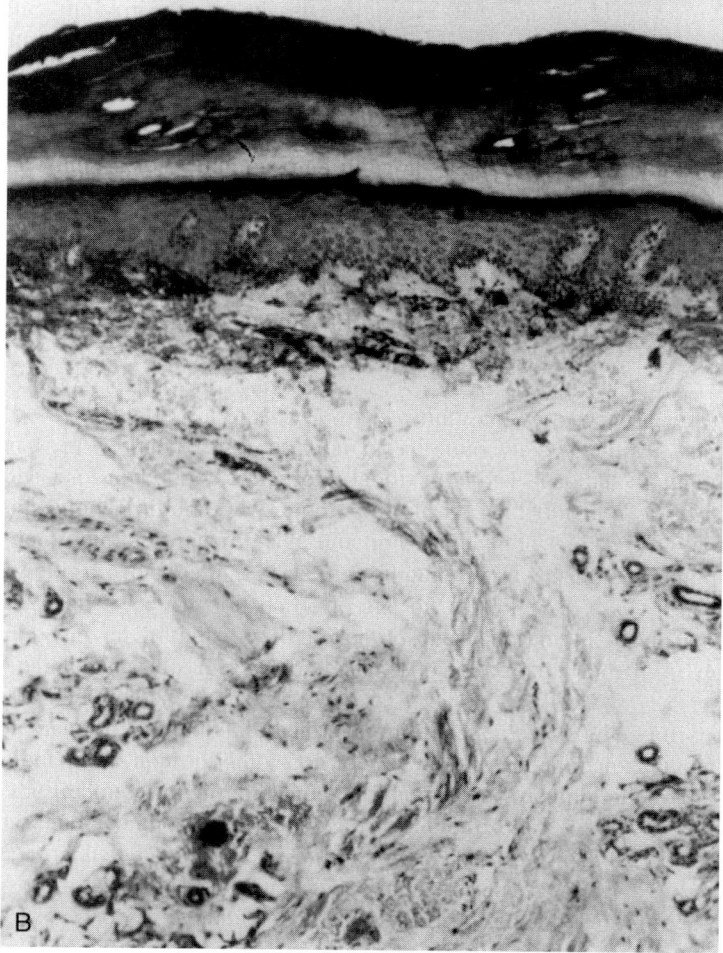

FIGURE 1–4. *A*, Histologic section of canine footpad. Note papillated surface. *B*, Histologic section of feline footpad. Note smooth surface.

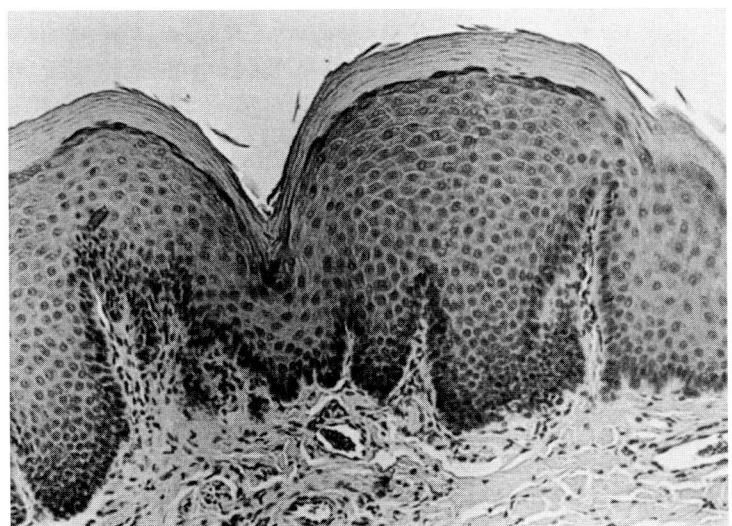

FIGURE 1–5. Histologic section of the nasal planum. Note the thick epidermis, dense stratum corneum, and rete ridges.

of the epidermis into the underlying dermis) are not found in the normal hair-bearing skin of cats and dogs. Rete ridges, however, may be found in normal footpad and nasal planum epidermis and in the lightly haired scrotum (see Fig. 1–6).

BASAL LAYER

The stratum basale is a single row of columnar to cuboidal cells resting on the basement membrane zone that separates the epidermis from the dermis (see Figs. 1–5, 1–7, and 1–10).[65, 163, 180] Most of these cells are keratinocytes, which are constantly reproducing and pushing upward to replenish the epidermal cells above. The daughter cells move into the outer layers of the epidermis and are ultimately shed as dead horny cells. Mitotic figures and apoptotic keratinocytes are occasionally seen, especially in areas of skin with thicker epidermis (e.g., nasal planum, footpad, mucocutaneous junction). There is morphologic and functional heterogenicity in basal keratinocytes[65]; some populations serve primarily to anchor the epidermis, and others serve a proliferative and reparative (stem cell) function. The tips of the deep epidermal rete ridges (in glabrous skin) and the bulge (Wulst) region of the hair follicle (site of attachment of the arrector pili muscle) are the presumed sites of the epidermal and hair follicle stem cells in humans and rodents.[65, 108, 109] Dogs and cats do not have a hair follicle bulge.[45, 50]

Hemidesmosomes are junctional complexes distributed along the inner aspect of basal keratinocytes, whose major role is epidermal-dermal adhesion.[65, 150] The linkage of the keratin intermediate filament (cytokeratin) network to the hemidesmosome and the basal keratinocyte plasma membrane involves several components, including the plaque proteins bullous pemphigoid antigen I (BPAG I or BP 230) and plectin, the transmembrane proteins $\alpha_6\beta_4$ integrin and BPAG II (collagen XVII), and laminin 5.[110, 128, 193] Various inherited defects in the hemidesmosome-anchoring filament components are known to produce various forms of epidermolysis bullosa, pemphigoid, and bullous systemic lupus erythematosus.[24a, 128]

Integrins are a large family of cell surface adhesive receptors.[110, 193] These cell surface glycoproteins are important in cell-cell and cell-matrix interactions, and also act as signal transducers through which extracellular and intracellular compartments can influence and modify each other. Each integrin consists of a heterodimer of an α and a β subunit, which are noncovalently associated. In the epidermis, integrin expression is normally confined to the basal layer. The integrin subunits that are most abundant in the epidermis are α_2, α_3, β_1, α_6 and β_4. Examples of keratinocyte integrin functions include: $\alpha_5\beta_1$, which

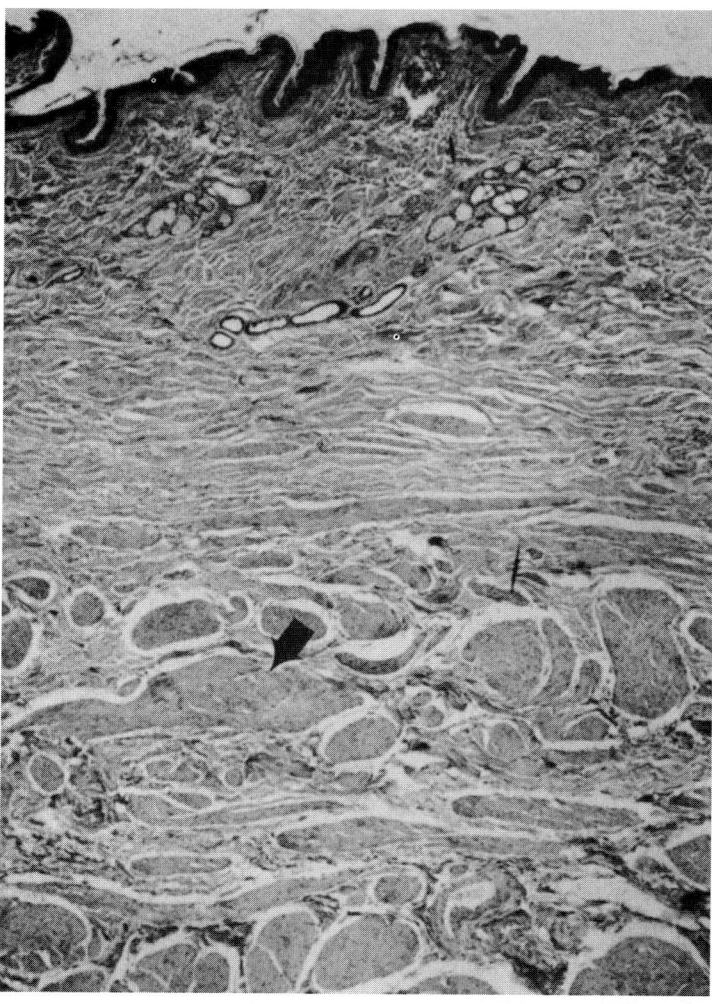

FIGURE 1–6. Histologic section of canine scrotal skin. Note muscle bundles (*arrow*).

mediates keratinocyte adhesion to fibronectin; $\alpha_2\beta_1$, which mediates keratinocyte adhesion to collagens type I and IV and laminin; $\alpha_3\beta_1$, which is a receptor for epiligrin and is involved in adhesion to laminin; $\alpha_1\beta_5$, which mediates keratinocyte adhesion to vitronectin; and $\alpha_6\beta_4$, which mediates keratinocyte adhesion to laminin (see Table 1–2).[110]

MELANOCYTES AND MELANOGENESIS

Melanocytes, the second type of cell found in the basal layer of the epidermis, are also found in the outer root sheath and hair matrix of hair follicles, in the ducts of sebaceous and sweat glands, and to a lesser extent in the superficial dermis.* Traditionally, melanocytes are divided structurally and functionally into two compartments: epidermal and follicular.[65, 67, 111, 150] Because melanocytes do not stain readily with hematoxylin and eosin (H & E) and because they undergo artifactual cytoplasmic shrinkage during tissue processing, they appear as clear cells (see Fig. 1–7B). In general, there is one melanocyte per 10 to 20 keratinocytes in the basal cell layer. They are derived from the neural crest and migrate into the epidermis in early fetal life. Although melanocytes are of nondescript appearance, with special stains, they can be shown to have long cytoplasmic extensions

---

*See references 51, 65, 77, 111, 150, 172, 180, and 206.

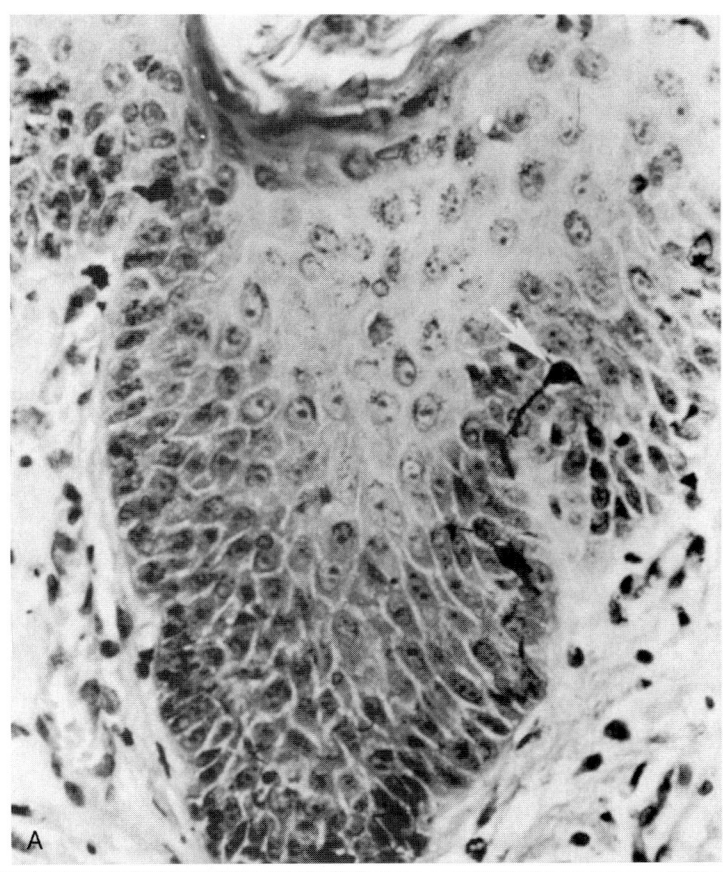
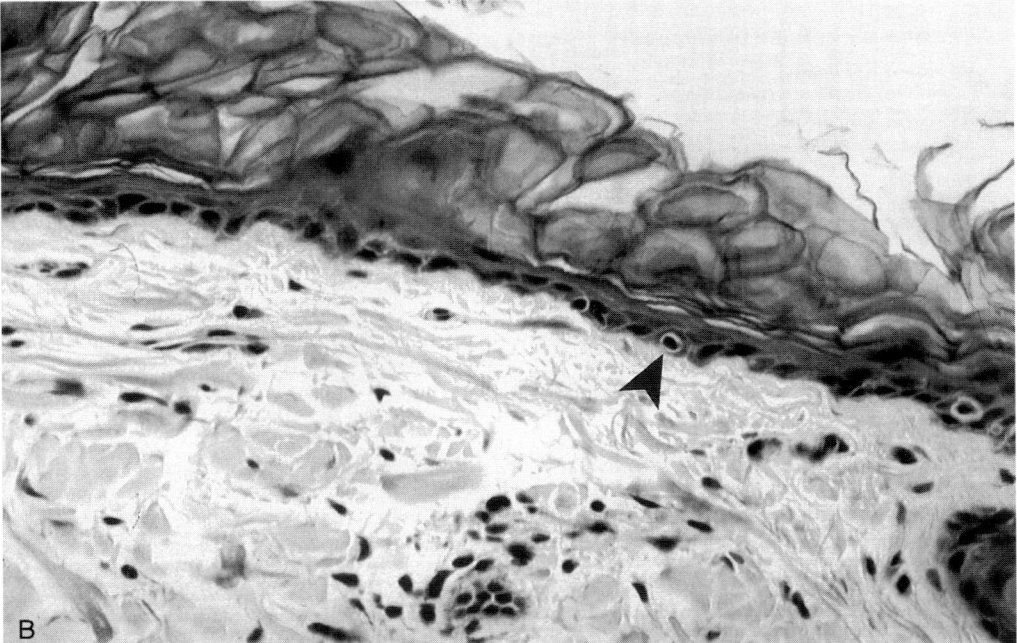

FIGURE 1-7. *A*, Dendritic melanocytes *(arrow)* in the basal layer of the epidermis. *B*, Melanocytes ("clear cells") *(arrowhead)* in the stratum basale.

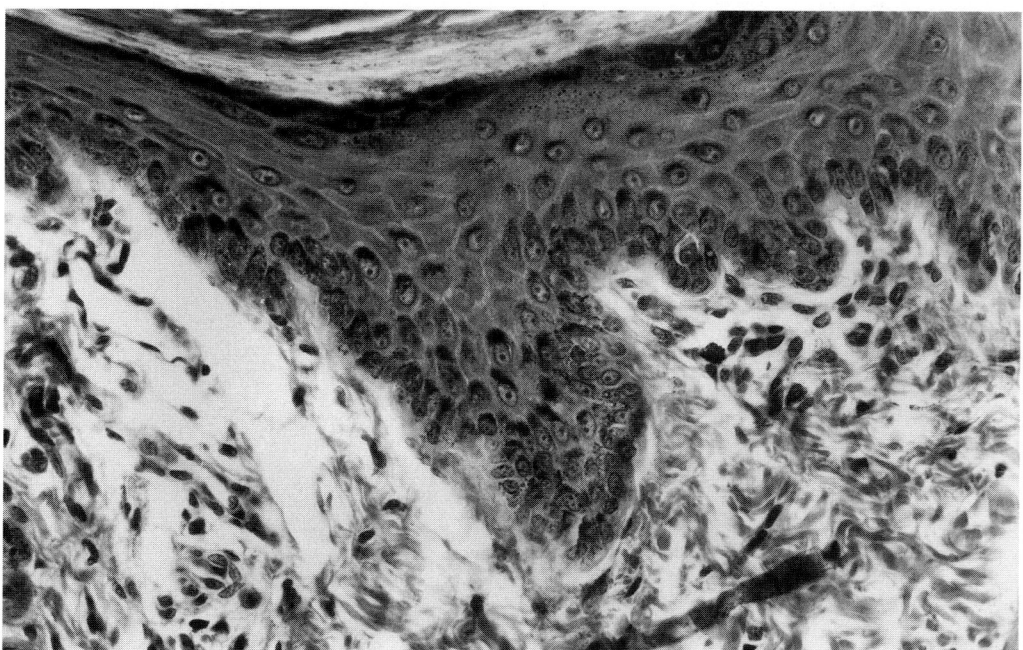

FIGURE 1–8. Pigmented epithelium from nasal planum. Note how melanin granules are often clustered in "caps" dorsal to keratinocyte nuclei.

(dendrites) (see Fig. 1–7A) that weave among the keratinocytes. There is an intimate relationship between melanocytes and keratinocytes in which both cells interact and exist as epidermal symbionts in a functional and structural unit called the epidermal melanin unit.[65, 111, 150, 196] Ultrastructurally, melanocytes are characterized by typical intracytoplasmic melanosomes and premelanosomes and a cell membrane–associated basal layer lamina (see Fig. 1–9). Most of the melanin pigment in skin is located in the basal layer of the epidermis, but in dark-skinned animals, melanin may be found throughout the entire epidermis as well as within superficial dermal melanocytes (see Fig. 1–3D). Melanin granules are often clustered as "caps" dorsal to keratinocyte nuclei (Fig. 1–8), presumably a photoprotective localization.

Although the melanocyte accounts for only a small proportion of the epidermal cells, it has a variety of important functions: (1) a cosmetic entity, participating in protective coloration and in sexual attraction; (2) a barrier against ionizing radiation, especially important in protection against ultraviolet light (UVL); (3) a scavenger of cytotoxic radicals and intermediates; and (4) a participant in developmental and inflammatory processes.[65, 111, 150] Although melanin absorbs UVL over a broad spectrum, including UVA and UVB, it is not a particularly efficient absorber of UVL. It probably photoprotects in other ways, possibly as a quencher of free radicals generated in response to UVL.

Melanin pigments are chiefly responsible for the coloration of skin and hair. Skin pigmentation is considered to consist of two components. *Constitutive* pigmentation is the pigmentation that is genetically determined in the absence of stimulatory influences. *Facultative* pigmentation is that which occurs with various stimuli (e.g., UVL, inflammation, hormones).

Melanins embrace a wide range of pigments, including the brown-black eumelanins, yellow or red-brown pheomelanins, and other pigments whose physicochemical natures are intermediate between the two. Pheomelanins differ from eumelanins by containing a high proportion of sulfur. Despite the different properties of the various melanins, they all arise from a common metabolic pathway in which dopaquinone is the key intermediate.[57, 65, 67]

Melanogenesis takes place exclusively within melanocytes and on the specialized organelle, the melanosome.[65, 111, 150] Here, the specific enzyme, tyrosinase, catalyzes the conversion of tyrosine to dopa. Tyrosinase is the rate-limiting enzyme in the melanin pathway. It is a copper-containing enzyme, is found exclusively in melanocytes, and is thus a good specific marker for these cells. Tyrosinase is an unusual enzyme in that it has three distinct catalytic activities. The most critical is its tyrosine hydroxylase activity, converting tyrosine to dopa. However, it is also able to use dopa or 5,6-dihyroxyindole (DHI) as substrates for oxidase activities. Mutations in the tyrosine structural gene are responsible for several types of albinism.[111]

Once dopa is formed, it can spontaneously autooxidize to dopaquinone without tyrosinase (though at slower rates), and continue through the melanin pathway to dopachrome, 5,6-dihydroxyindole-2-carboxylic acid (DHICA), DHI, and indole-5,6-quinone.[65, 111, 150] Another melanocyte-specific enzyme is dopachrome tautomerase, which converts dopachrome to DHICA.[111, 150] This conversion requires the presence of iron.

The determination to produce eumelanins or pheomelanins is under genetic control.[27, 65, 111, 150] If sulfhydryl groups are available, pheomelanins are produced. It has been proposed that the "switching" of melanin synthesis is mainly controlled by the levels of tyrosinase, with high levels producing eumelanins and low levels producing pheomelanins.[111]

Mammalian pigmentation is regulated at many different developmental, cellular, and subcellular levels, and is influenced by many genes.[65, 110, 111, 150] Although melanocytes in the skin have characteristic basal levels of function that are particular to each individual, they are highly responsive cells that continually sample their environment and modulate their levels of proliferation and melanogenesis. Classically, melanin production was thought to be under the control of genetics and melanocyte-stimulating hormone (MSH) from the pituitary gland.[57, 65, 67, 180, 196] The main pigmenting hormones from the pituitary gland include α-MSH (α-melanocortin), adrenal cortical stimulating hormone (corticotropin), and β-lipotropic hormone (β-lipotropin).[111, 150] These hormones are derived from a larger precursor molecule, proopiomelanocortin. However, the role of these hypophyseal origin hormones in physiologic and pathologic pigmentation in mammals is largely unknown. At present, interest focuses on the theory that melanogenesis and melanocyte proliferation and differentiation are mostly regulated locally in paracrine and autocrine fashion.

Melanocytes express a number of cell surface receptors (e.g., intercellular adhesion molecule 1 [ICAM-1]) that allow interaction with other cells in their environment, including keratinocytes, Langerhans' cells, fibroblasts, lymphocytes, and macrophages.[111, 150, 206] They express receptors for and respond to (modifying their proliferation, differentiation, and melanogenesis) growth factor (e.g., β fibroblast growth factor) hormones, interferons, interleukins, eicosanoids, retinoic acid, vitamin D_3, and a host of other cytokines. In fact, melanocytes are able to produce some of these themselves, thus acting in an autocrine manner. Melanocytes themselves secrete several cytokines (e.g., interleukin-8 [IL-8]) and participate in inflammatory and immunologic reactions. Many of the precursors and intermediates of the melanin biosynthetic pathway are cytotoxic and could contribute to cellular injury and inflammation. It can be appreciated that a highly complex interaction exists between the cellular components of the epidermis, their respective immune cytokines, and the inflammatory mediators released in response to injury.

α-MSH is a neuroimmunomodulatory and anti-inflammatory peptide that is synthesized and released by keratinocytes, Langerhans' cells, fibroblasts, and endothelial cells, as well as melanocytes themselves.[111, 118, 150] α-MSH cell surface receptors can also be identified on these cells. α-MSH can, hence, modulate keratinocyte proliferation and differentiation, and endothelial cell and fibroblast cytokine and collagenase production. It also downregulates the production of proinflammatory cytokines and accessory molecules on antigen-presenting cells (monocytes and macrophages). α-MSH is an antagonist of IL-1, an important cytokine in the cutaneous immune response. Thus, α-MSH is part of a mediator network that modulates cutaneous inflammation and hyperproliferative skin diseases. This may be far more important than any effect it has on skin pigmentation.

Melanogenesis takes place in membrane-bound organelles called melanosomes,[51, 65, 196] designated stages I through IV according to maturation (Fig. 1–9). It is often stated that the ultrastructural hallmark of the melanocyte is the melanosome. However, it is more accurate to say that stage I melanosomes are melanocyte specific, because later stage melanosomes may be found in keratinocytes and other phagocytic cells.[111] Melanosomes

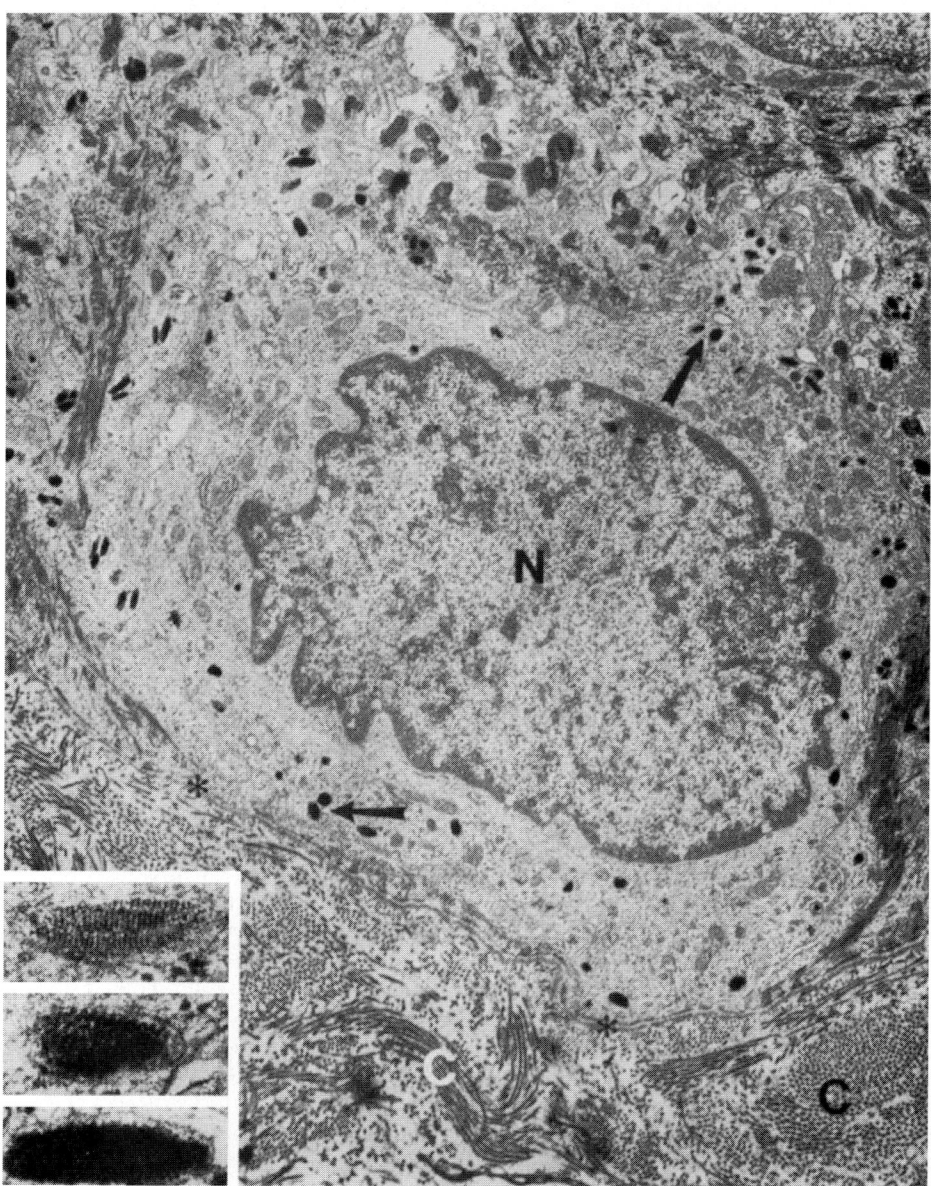

FIGURE 1–9. Melanocyte. N, nucleus of melanocyte; arrows, melanosomes; C, collagen in the dermis; asterisk, basal lamina (×10,000). Insets: Melanosomes in different stages of development: upper inset, Stage II; middle inset, Stage III; lower inset, Stage IV (×75,000). (From Lever WF, Schaumburg-Lever G: Histopathology of the Skin, 7th ed. J.B. Lippincott Co, Philadelphia, 1990, p 861.)

originate from the Golgi apparatus, where the tyrosinase enzyme is formed. Stage I melanosomes contain no melanin and are electron lucent. As melanin is progressively laid down on protein matrices, melanosomes become increasingly electron dense. At the same time, they migrate to the periphery of the dendrites, where transfer of melanin to adjacent epidermal cells takes place. Transfer involves the endocytosis of the dendrite tips of the incorporated Stage IV melanosomes by the adjacent keratinocytes. Melanocytes eject melanosomes into keratinocytes by a unique biologic transfer process called cytocrinia.[65] Dermal melanocytes are often referred to as continent melanocytes, because they do not transfer melanosomes as do the epidermal or secretory melanocytes. Skin color is determined mainly by the number, size, type, and distribution of melanosomes.

At present, there are no histochemical stains that can be performed on routinely processed skin biopsy specimens that exclusively stain melanin.[111] *Argentaffin* stains rely on the ability of melanin to reduce silver from a silver solution (e.g., silver nitrate). Examples of argentaffin stains include Fontana-Masson and Gomori's methenamine silver. These agents also stain neurosecretory granules and formalin pigment. *Argyrophil* stains are similar to argentaffin stains, but use an external silver reducer to produce elemental silver. An example of an argyrophil stain is Grimelius' stain. Argyrophil stains also stain nerves, reticulum, and elastic fibers.

MERKEL'S CELLS

Merkel's cells are dendritic epidermal clear cells confined to the basal cell layer, or just below, and occur predominently in tylotrich pads and hair follicle epithelium.* These specialized cells (slow-adapting mechanoreceptors) contain a large cytoplasmic vacuole that displaces the cell nucleus dorsally, and their long axis is usually parallel to the skin surface (Fig. 1–10). They possess desmosomes and characteristic dense-core cytoplasmic granules and paranuclear whorls on electron microscopic examination (Fig. 1–11). Merkel's cells also contain cytokeratin, neurofilaments, and neuron-specific enolase, suggesting a dual epithelial and neural differentiation. Current evidence suggests that Merkel's cells are derived from a primitive epidermal stem cell.[65, 110, 159] Merkel's cells may have other functions, such as influencing cutaneous blood flow and sweat production (via the release of vasoactive intestinal peptide), coordinating keratinocyte proliferation, and maintaining and stimulating the stem cell population of the hair follicle (hence controlling the hair cycle).[65, 206]

SPINOUS LAYER

The stratum spinosum (prickle cell layer) is composed of the daughter cells of the stratum basale.[65, 170, 172, 188, 202] In haired skin, this layer is one or two cells thick. The stratum spinosum becomes much thicker at the footpads, nasal planum, and mucocutaneous junctions, where it may occasionally approach 20 cell layers. The cells are lightly basophilic to eosinophilic, nucleated, and polyhedral to flattened cuboidal in shape. The keratinocytes of the stratum spinosum appear to be connected by intercellular bridges (prickles), which are more prominent in nonhaired skin (Fig. 1–12).

Keratinocyte adhesion is mediated by four major types of adhesive and communicative structures: desmosomes, hemidesmosomes, adherens junctions, and focal adhesions (Table 1–1).[110, 193] Hemidesmosomes and focal adhesions are located on the basal surface of basal cells and mediate adhesion to the underlying extracellular matrix, whereas desmosomes and adherens junctions mediate adhesion between keratinocytes in all epidermal layers. *Gap junctions* serve primarily as intercellular routes of chemical communication.[110]

Because of the research efforts directed at defining the pathomechanism of pemphigus, much has been learned concerning the structure and chemical composition of epidermal desmosomes.[65, 110] Desmosomes are presently known to consist of keratin intermediate

---

*See references 65, 69, 77, 110, 169, 170, 172, 173, 180, and 206.

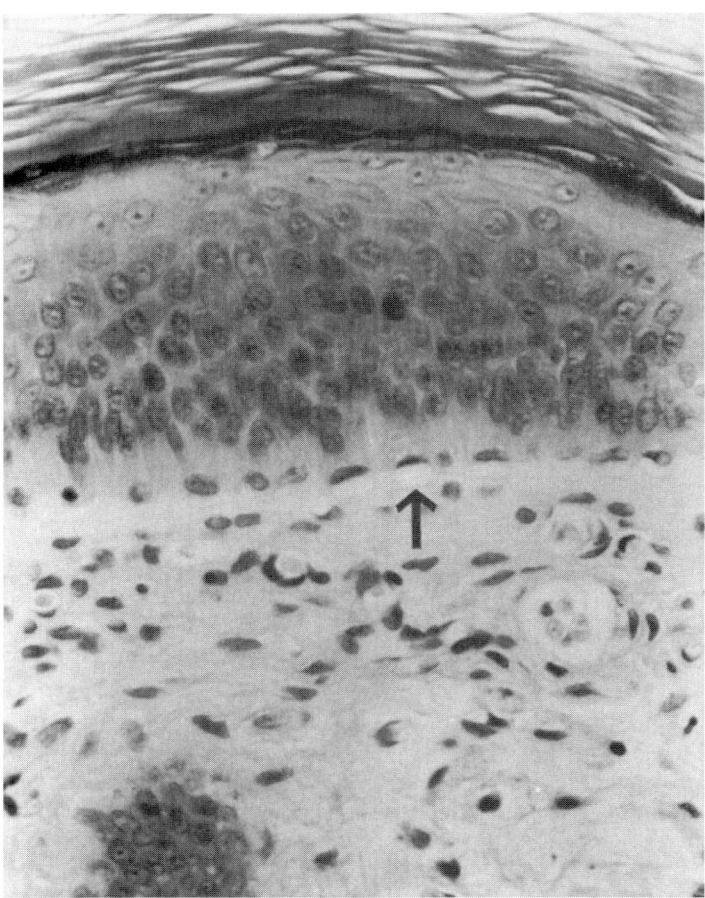

FIGURE 1–10. Merkel's cells *(arrow)* in a tylotrich pad.

filaments and their attachment plaques, the keratinocyte plasma membrane, and the desmosomal core (desmoglea), which is interposed between two adjacent keratinocyte plasma membranes. Numerous desmosomal plaque proteins (desmoplakins I and II, plakoglobin, plakophilin) and desmosomal core glycoproteins (desmogleins I, II, III and desmocollins I, II, III) have been characterized. The immunohistochemical staining pattern seen with human pemphigus foliaceus antibody is identical to that seen with an antibody directed at desmoglein I (desmosomal core glycoprotein).

Proteins of the plakoglobin (plakoglobin, β-catenin), vinculin (vinculin, α-catenin), and ezrin (talin, radixin) families are found at desmosomal and adherens junction attachments.[110]

The keratinocyte cytoskeleton consists of three types of cytoplasmic filaments: cytokeratin, actin, and microtubules (tubulin).[110] These filaments function in the orientation, polarization, organelle sorting, motility, shape change, signal transduction, and structural resilience of keratinocytes.

Ultrastructurally, keratinocytes are characterized by keratin intermediate filaments (cytokeratin, tonofilaments) and desmosomes (Fig. 1–13).[51, 65, 110] Calcium and calmodulin are crucial for desmosome and hemidesmosome formation. At least three keratinocyte-derived calmodulin-binding proteins participate in a flip-flop regulation (calcium concentration-dependent) of calcium-calmodulin interactions: caldesmon, desmocalmin, and spectrin.[65] Immunohistochemically, keratinocytes are characterized by the presence of cytokeratins.[65] All epithelia express a keratin pair: one keratin chain from the acidic subfamily (Type I keratins, cytokeratins 9–20) and one chain from the neutral-basic sub-

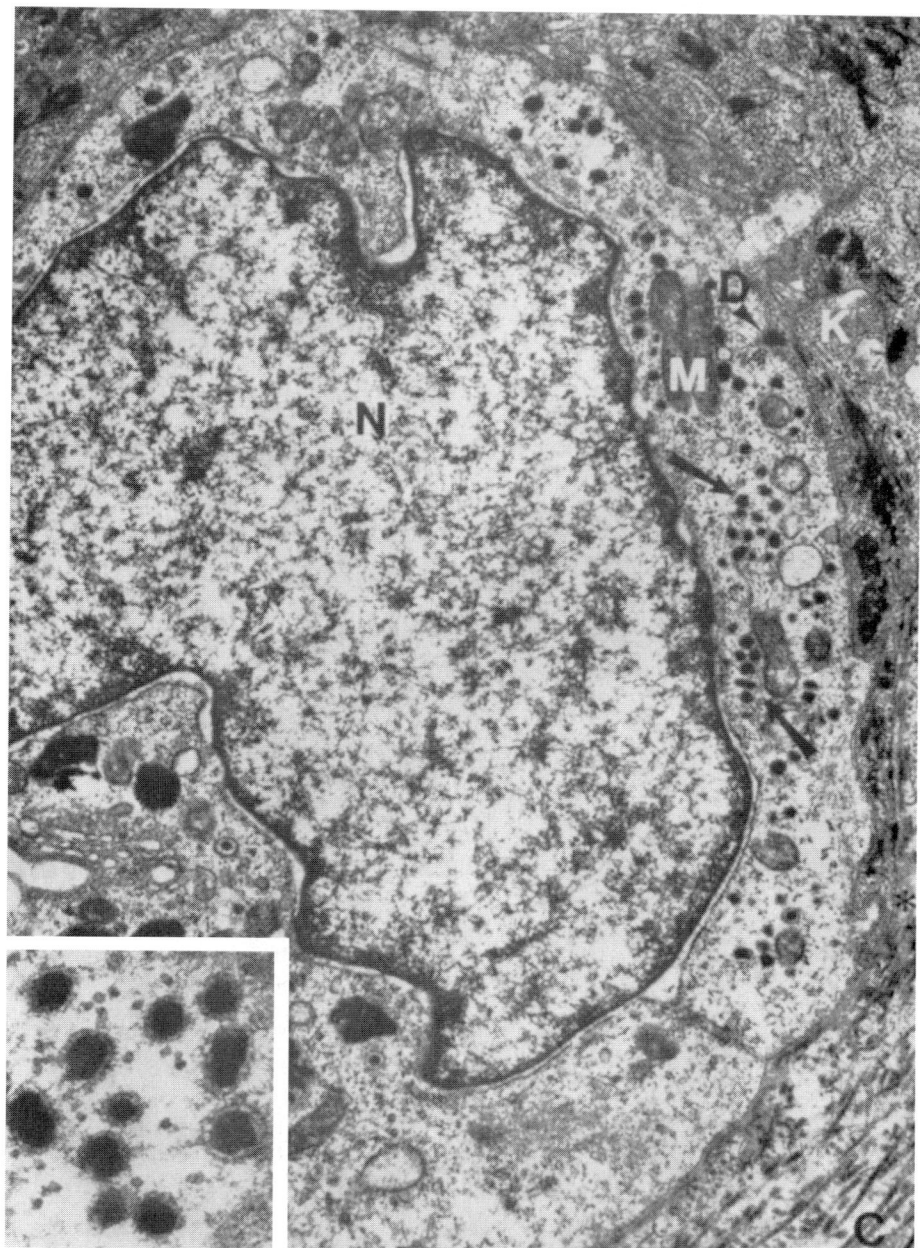

FIGURE 1–11. Merkel's cell. N, nucleus of a Merkel's cell; asterisk indicates basal lamina; M, mitochondria; arrows indicate specific granules of the Merkel's cell; D with pointer, desmosome between the Merkel cell and a keratinocyte (K); C, collagen with cross-striation (×20,000). Inset: specific membrane-bound granules at higher magnification (×75,000). (From Lever WF, Schaumburg-Lever G: Histopathology of the Skin, 7th ed. J.B. Lippincott Co, Philadelphia, 1990, p. 863.)

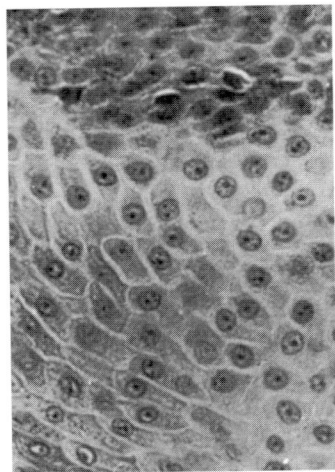

FIGURE 1–12. Prickle cells from footpad showing intercellular bridges (high power).

family (Type II keratins, cytokeratins 1–8).* The keratin pairs change with different epithelia and in the same epithelia at various stages of differentiation or proliferation. Expression of a subset of these 20 different cytokeratins is more or less tissue specific. A number of workers have published electrophoretic patterns of proteins isolated from the keratins of a variety of animals and, on the basis of observed differences in banding patterns, have suggested that the technique might be useful as an aid to taxonomy, animal classification, and identification.[65] The keratinocytes of the stratum spinosum synthesize lamellar granules (keratinosomes, membrane-coating granules, Odlund bodies), which are important in the barrier function of the epidermis (see Epidermopoiesis and Keratogenesis in this chapter).[65, 110]

Keratinocytes are phagocytic (erythrocytes, melanin, melanosomes, cellular fragments, latex beads, inorganic substances).[24]

LANGERHANS' CELLS

Langerhans' cells are mononuclear, dendritic, antigen-presenting cells located basally or suprabasally (Fig. 1–14).[65, 123, 124, 126, 136, 206] They are epidermal clear cells that, like

---

*See references 24a, 56, 85, 110, 148, 185, and 190–193.

● Table 1–1 **COMPONENTS OF ADHESION STRUCTURES**

ADHESION STRUCTURE	TRANSMEMBRANE PROTEINS	PLAQUE PROTEINS	CYTOSKELETON FILAMENTS	FUNCTION AND LOCATION
Hemidesmosome	$\alpha 6 \beta 4$ integrin BPAGII (collagen Type XVII)	Plectin, BPAGI	Cytokeratin	Cell-substrate adhesion; basal cells and basal membrane
Focal adhesion	β_1 integrins ($\alpha 2\beta_1$, $\alpha 3\beta_1$, $\alpha 5\beta_1$)	Talin, vinculin, α-actinin, paxillin, zykin	Actin	Cell-substrate, basal cells
Desmosome	Desmosomal cadherins Dsg I, II, III Dsc I, II, III	Plakoglobin; desmoplakin I, II, IV; desmocalmin; plakophilin	Cytokeratin	Cell-cell adhesion; all keratinocytes
Adherens junction	Classic cadherins (E- and P-cadherins)	Plakoglobin, α- and β-catenin, α-actin, vinculin	Actin	Cell-cell adhesion; all keratinocytes (p-cadherin in basal cells only)

BPAG, bullous pemphigoid antigen; Dsg = desmoglein; Dsc = desmocollin.

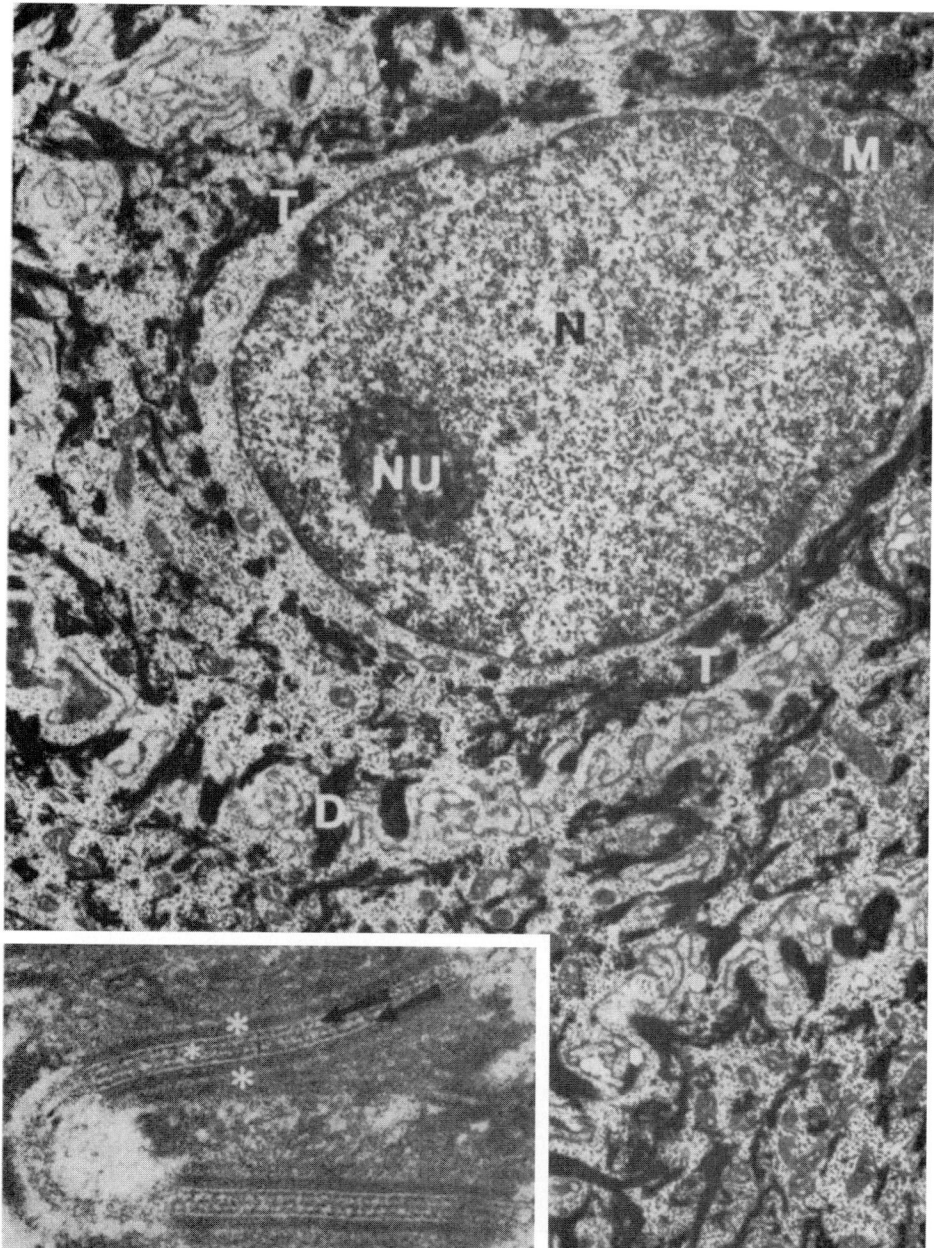

FIGURE 1-13. Squamous cell. N, nucleus; NU, nucleolus; T, tonofilaments; D, desmosome; M, mitochondria (×12,500). Inset: Desmosomes at higher magnification (×100,000). A desmosome connecting two adjoining keratinocytes consists of nine lines: five electron-dense lines and four electron-lucid lines. The two peripheral dense, thick lines *(large asterisks)* are the attachment plaques. The single electron-dense line in the center of the desmosome *(small asterisk)* is the intercellular contact layer. The two electron-dense lines between the intercellular contact layer and the two attachment plaques represent the cell surface coat together with the outer leaflet of the trilaminar plasma membrane of each keratinocyte (arrows). The two inner electron-lucid lines adjacent to the intercellular contact layer represent intercellular cement. The two outer electron-lucid lines are the central lamina of the trilaminar plasma membrane. (From Lever WF, Schaumberg-Lever G: Histopathology of the Skin, 7th ed. J.B. Lippincott Co, Philadelphia, 1990, p. 858.)

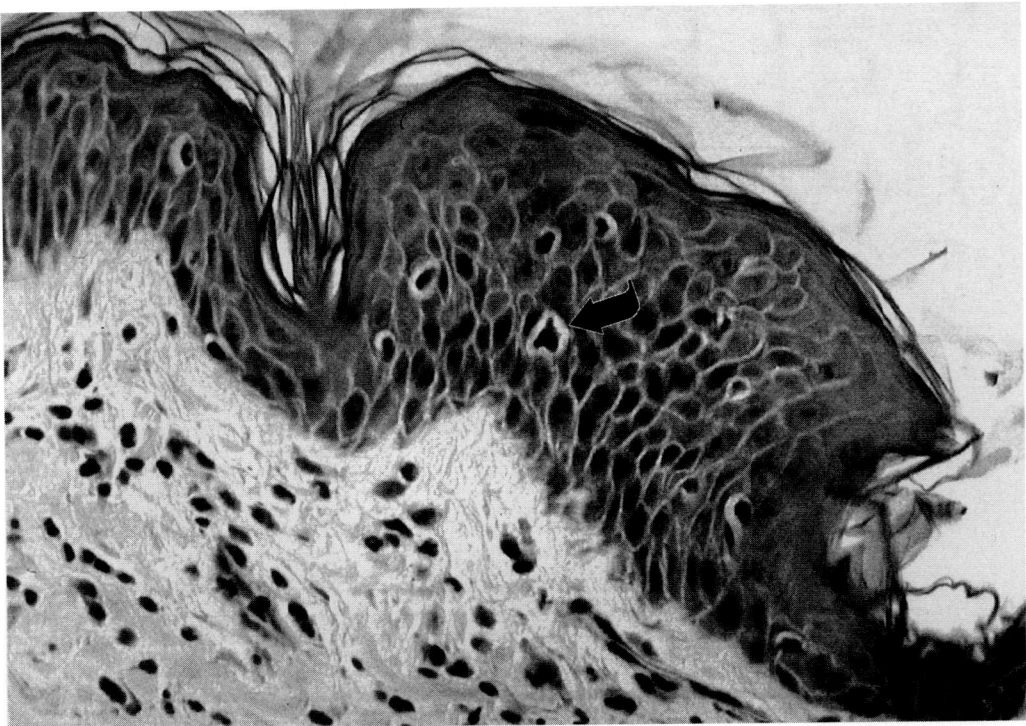

FIGURE 1–14. Epidermal Langerhans' cells. They appear as suprabasilar epidermal "clear cells" *(arrow)* in this biopsy from an atopic dog.

Merkel's cells, do not stain for melanin with dopa. The histochemical and immunophenotype of Langerhans' cells vary with species.[206] Langerhans' cells in many species—including cats and humans—have characteristic intracytoplasmic organelles (Birbeck's or Langerhans' granules), which are observed by means of electron microscopy (Fig. 1–15).[65, 126] However, the Langerhans' cells studied in dogs have inconsistently contained these granules.[123, 136, 215] Birbeck granules are variously described as being zipper, rod, flask, or tennis racket like in appearance. They form by invagination of the plasma membrane and bound antigen, thus providing the morphologic description of the mechanism by which Langerhans' cells internalize surface-bound antigen for processing and representation at the surface.[110] Langerhans' cells are aureophilic (i.e., they stain with gold chloride). Unlike Langherhans' cells in humans, those in dogs and cats are S-100 protein and ATPase negative. They have Fc fragment (Fc)-IgG and complement 3 (C3) receptors, high affinity receptors for IgE, and they synthesize and express antigens associated with the immune response gene. In the dog, Langerhans' cells are CD1a,b,c, CD11a,c, CD18, CD45, ICAM-1, MHC class II, and vimentin positive.[1, 124, 136] They are CD4 and CD90 (Thy-1) negative, which distinguishes them from dermal dendrocytes. In the cat, Langerhans' cells are CD1a, CD4, CD18, and MHC class II positive.[126] These cells are of bone marrow origin, of monocyte-histiocyte lineage, and serve antigen-processing and alloantigen-stimulating functions. Following ultraviolet light exposure, epidermal Langerhans' cells are decreased in density and altered morphologically, resulting in an immunosuppressive environment and antigen-specific tolerance.[63] Topical or systemic glucocorticoids are known to depress Langerhans' cell numbers and function as well as other cutaneous and systemic immune responses.[65] The areas of photoimmunology and photocarcinogenesis are receiving much attention, especially because they are relevant to the pathogenesis of skin cancer.[65] Studies in humans, dogs, and cats have shown that the number of Langerhans' cells per unit of skin varies from one area of skin to another in the same individual,

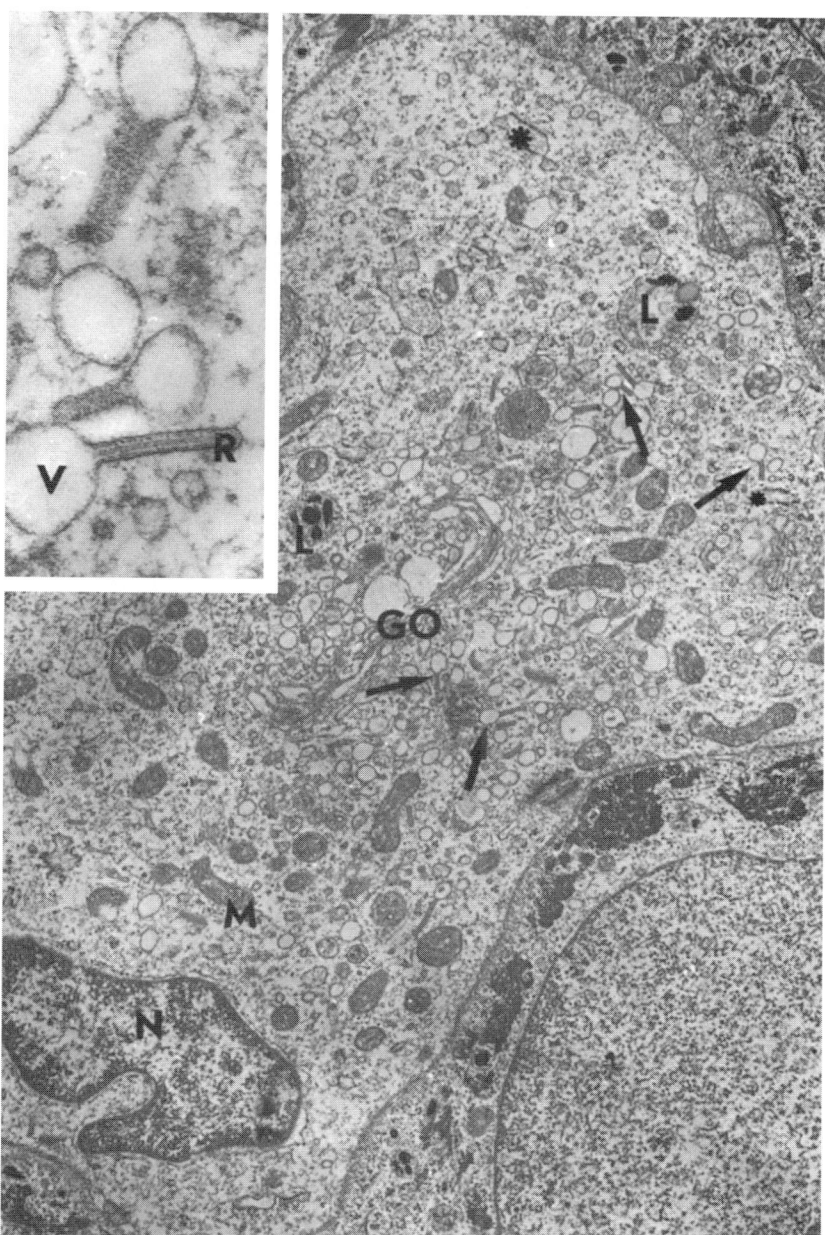

FIGURE 1-15. Electron micrograph of an epidermal Langerhans' cell. (From Elder D, et al: Lever's Histopathology of the Skin, 8th ed. Lippincott-Raven, Philadelphia, 1998, p 1021.)

emphasizing the need to use adjacent normal skin as a control when counting Langerhans' cells in skin lesions.[65, 123, 125, 126]

THE SKIN AS AN IMMUNOLOGIC ORGAN

The epidermis functions as the most peripheral outpost of the immune system (see Chap. 8). Langerhans' cells, keratinocytes, epidermotropic T lymphocytes, and draining periph-

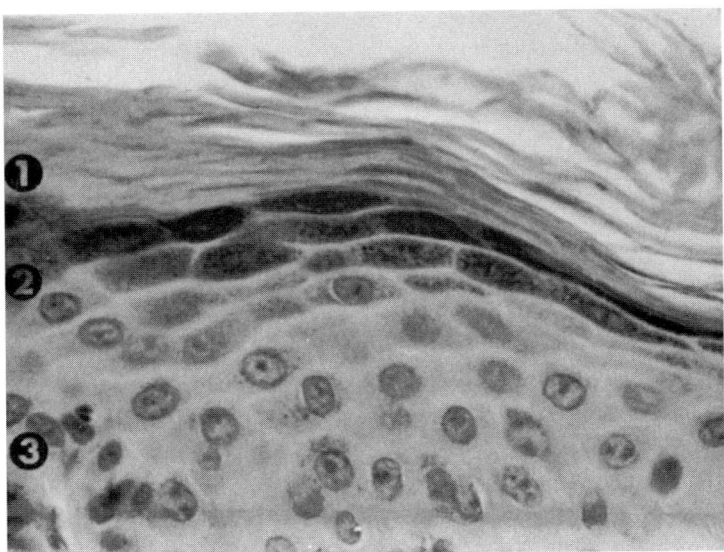

FIGURE 1–16. Horny layer (1), granular layer (2), and prickle cell layer (3) from the nasal planum (high power).

eral lymph nodes are thought to form collectively an integrated system of *skin-associated lymphoid tissue* that mediates cutaneous immunosurveillance.[65, 196] *Langerhans' cells* (see previous discussion) stimulate the proliferation of relevant helper T lymphocytes by the presentation of antigen; they also induce cytotoxic T lymphocytes directed to allogeneic and modified self-determinants, produce IL-1 and other cytokines, contain numerous enzymes, and are phagocytic.[65, 110, 196]

The *keratinocyte* also plays an active role in epidermal immunity.[65, 110, 196] Keratinocytes (1) produce IL-1, (2) produce various cytokines (e.g., IL-3, prostaglandins, leukotrienes, and interferon), (3) are phagocytic, and (4) can express antigens associated with the immune response gene in a variety of lymphocyte-mediated skin diseases (presumably as a result of interferon-γ secretion by activated lymphocytes).[65, 110, 196]

Gamma and delta T lymphocytes are rare in normal canine skin but common in various immune-mediated and inflammatory dermatoses.[29]

GRANULAR LAYER

The stratum granulosum is variably present in haired skin; it ranges from one to two cells thick in areas where it occurs.[170, 172, 188, 202] In nonhaired skin or at the infundibulum of hair follicles, the stratum granulosum may be four to eight cells thick (Fig. 1–16). Cells in this layer are flattened and basophilic, and they contain shrunken nuclei and large, deeply basophilic keratohyalin granules in their cytoplasm (see Fig. 1–3E). Keratohyalin granules are not true granules; they lack a membrane and are more accurately described as insoluble aggregates. Keratohyalin granules are the morphologic equivalents of the structural protein profilaggrin, which is the precursor of filaggrin[65] and is synthesized in the stratum granulosum. The function of keratohyalin granules is incompletely understood, but it is thought to be concerned with keratinization and barrier function. The sulfur-rich component of keratohyalin granules has been implicated as a precursor to the cornified cell envelope. Filaggrin has at least two functions. First, it aggregates, packs, and aligns keratin filaments and produces the matrix between the keratin filaments in the corneocytes. Second, it is a source of free amino acids, which are important for the normal hydration of the stratum corneum.

Loricrin is synthesized in the stratum granulosum in association with keratohyalin granules and is involved in the binding of keratin filaments together in the corneocyte and

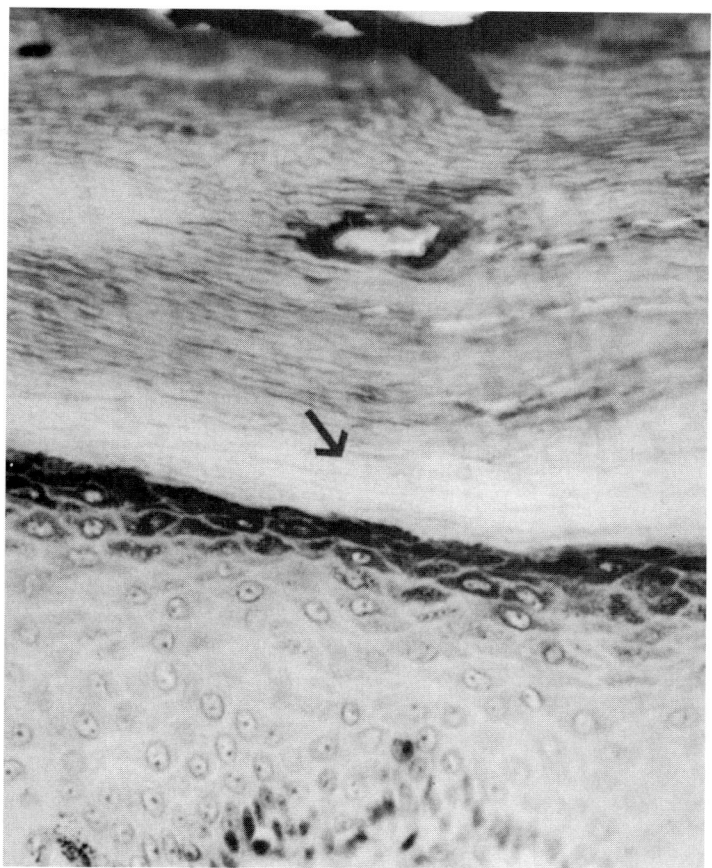

FIGURE 1–17. Stratum lucidum (*arrow*) in footpad epithelium.

in anchoring them to the cross-linked envelope.[150] Another ultrastructural feature that characterizes granular cells are clustered lamellar granules at the margins of the cells.

In rodents, two morphologic forms of keratohyalin granules occur.[110] The P-F granule is irregularly shaped and contains profilaggrin, whereas the L-granule is smaller, rounded, and contains loricrin.

CLEAR LAYER

The stratum lucidum is a fully keratinized, compact, thin layer of dead cells.[170, 172, 188, 202] This layer is anuclear, homogeneous, and hyaline like, and it contains refractile droplets and a semifluid substance called eleidin (Fig. 1–17). It differs histochemically from the stratum corneum by being rich in protein-bound lipids. The stratum lucidum is best developed in the footpads; it is less developed in the nasal planum and is absent from all other areas of normal skin. The stratum lucidum has also been called the *stratum conjunctum*.

HORNY LAYER

The stratum corneum is the outer layer of terminally differentiated keratinocytes that is constantly being shed.[107, 170, 172, 188, 202] It is a multilayered zone of corneocytes suspended in an extracellular lipid matrix, often likened to a series of bricks (corneocytes) bonded by mortar (lipids).[110] This layer, which consists of flattened, anuclear eosinophilic cells (corneocytes), is thicker in lightly haired or glabrous skin (see Figs. 1–4, 1–5, 1–7B, and 1–16). Its gradual desquamation is normally balanced by proliferation of the basal cells, which maintains a constant epidermal thickness. Corneocytes contain a variety of humectants and natural sunscreens that are synthesized from proteins.[150]

The terminally differentiated corneocyte has a highly specialized structure in the cell periphery, the *cell envelope,* which assumes protective functions.[65, 107, 150] It develops beneath the plasma membrane of stratified epidermal cells, cells of the inner root sheath and medulla of the hair follicle, and the cuticle of the claw. The corneocyte has no true cell membrane because it contains no phospholipids. Cell envelope formation is associated with the increased activity of calcium-dependent epidermal or hair follicle transglutaminases that catalyze the cross-linking of soluble and particulate protein precursors into large, insoluble polymers. Major cytoplasmic protein precursors of the cell envelope synthesized in the stratum spinosum include involucrin, keratolinin, pancornulin, cornifin, and loricrin.[65, 103, 107, 110, 150, 185] The impermeable cornified envelope provides structural support to the cell and resists invasion by microorganisms and deleterious environmental agents. The stratum corneum has also been called the *stratum dysjunctum.*

In routinely processed sections, the stratum corneum varies in thickness from 3 to 35 μm in cats and from 5 to 1500 μm in dogs. However, clipping and histologic preparation involving fixation, dehydration, and paraffin embedding result in the loss of about one half of the stratum corneum. The stratum corneum of canine truncal skin, when measured in cryostat sections, was found to have a mean thickness of 47 cell layers that measured 13.3 μm.[116] The loose, basketweave appearance of the stratum corneum is an artifact of fixation and processing.[51, 116, 127]

Transglutaminases are a superfamily of enzymes that are important in apoptosis, keratinization, and hair follicle formation.[78] Two members of the superfamily—keratinocyte transglutaminase and epidermal transglutaminase—mediate the sequential cross-linking of the cornified cell envelope precursor proteins, such as involucrin, cytostan A, elafin, and loricrin. Transglutaminases are chiefly expressed in the stratum granulosum and upper stratum spinosum, and require catalytic amino acids and calcium. Faulty keratinocyte transglutaminase expression is one cause of ichthyosis in humans.[78]

Topographic studies have shown that the epidermal surface varies from gently undulating on the densely haired skin of the back to heavily folded on the skin of the abdomen.[116, 170] The hairs arise from the follicle infundibula, which are seen as pits in the skin. At their bases, the hairs tend to be joined by amorphous material that can also be seen around the squames adhering to hairs. The surface of the stratum corneum is uneven, especially in the hairy areas (see Fig. 1–19). It is covered with a homogeneous film that tends to conceal the structure of the squames and their intercellular junctions. Globular masses that are partially concealed by this film can be seen. On closer examination, the surface can be seen to be composed of hexagonal cells and an amorphous substance that appears to be oozing to the surface of the margins of the cells. The bases of the hair follicle infundibula are sealed by an amorphous substance (sebaceous and cutaneous lipids) and squames. No evidence was found to suggest that sebum flows from the hair pore to the interfollicular region, which suggested that rubbing and grooming were important in spreading this emulsion over the skin. Hair growth may be important in "pushing" the sebum out of the pilar canal. Recent microautoradiographic studies of the disposition of topical fipronil in dogs have shown that sebum does, indeed, move over the epidermal surface.[38] It has been suggested that the thinner, more compact canine stratum corneum with less intercellular lipid material—compared with other species—may partially explain the higher incidence of bacterial pyoderma in dogs in comparison with other species.

Lipids play an important role in the differentiation, structure, and function of the epidermis.[37, 52, 65, 107] Epidermal lipid composition changes dramatically during keratinization, beginning with large amounts of phospholipids and ending with predominantly ceramides, cholesterol, and fatty acids. Epidermal surface lipids originate from maturing corneocytes, which contain about six times the amount of intracellular lipid as keratinocytes in the stratum basale. Skin surface lipids of cats and dogs were studied by thin-layer chromatography and found to contain more sterol esters, free cholesterol, cholesterol esters, and diester waxes but fewer triglycerides, monoglycerides, free fatty acids, monester waxes, and squalene than those of humans. It was suggested that the surface lipids of cats and dogs are mainly of epidermal origin, whereas those of humans are mainly of sebaceous gland origin. Skin surface lipids can be studied qualitatively by various extraction techniques (e.g., sebutape) or quantitatively using the lipometer or sebumeter.*

The stratum corneum contains antigenic or superantigenic material normally sequestered from the immune system that induces T lymphocyte activation when released following wounding and in disease.[71] This T lymphocyte activation and resultant inflammatory response may play a role in a range of skin pathologies.

EPIDERMOPOIESIS AND KERATOGENESIS

Normal epidermal homeostasis requires a finely tuned balance between growth and differentiation of keratinocytes. This balance must be greatly shifted in the direction of proliferation in response to injury and then must return to a state of homeostasis with healing. In addition, epidermal keratinocytes have important functions as regulators of cutaneous immunity and inflammation.

The most important product of the epidermis is keratin (from the Greek *keratos*, meaning "horn"), a highly stable, disulfide bond–containing fibrous protein. This substance is the major barrier between animal and environment, the so-called miracle wrap of the body. Prekeratin, the fibrous protein synthesized in the keratinocytes of the stratum basale and stratum spinosum, appears to be the precursor of the fully differentiated stratum corneum proteins.[65, 196] Keratins have classically been divided into *soft* keratins (skin) and *hard* keratins (hair, claw) and α-keratins (skin, hair) and β-keratins (scale, feather).[150]

The epidermis is ectodermal in origin and normally undergoes an orderly pattern of proliferation, differentiation, and keratinization.[65] The factors controlling this orderly epidermal pattern are incompletely understood, but the protein kinase C/phospholipase C second messenger system, the calcium/calmodulin second messenger system, the receptor-linked tyrosine kinases, and the adenylate cyclase/cAMP-dependent protein kinases are important in coupling extracellular signals to essential biological processes such as the immune response, inflammation, differentiation, and proliferation.[65] Among the intrinsic factors known to play a modulating role in these processes are the dermis, EGF, fibroblast growth factors, insulin-like growth factors, colony-stimulating factors, platelet-derived growth factor, TGFs, neuropeptides, interleukins, tumor necrosis factor, epidermal chalone, epibolin, interferons, acid hydrolases, arachidonic acid metabolites, proteolytic enzymes (endopeptidases and exopeptidases or peptidases), and various hormones (particularly epinephrine, vitamin D_3, and cortisol).[65, 149, 180] In addition, there appears to be a host of hormones and enzymes that can induce, increase, or both induce and increase the activity of the enzyme ornithine decarboxylase.[57] This enzyme is essential for the biosynthesis of polyamines (putrescine, spermidine, and spermine), which encourage epidermal proliferation. Numerous nutritional factors are also known to be important for normal keratinization, including protein, fatty acids, zinc, copper, vitamin A, and the B vitamins.[65]

There are four distinct cellular events in the process of cornification[65]: (1) keratinization (synthesis of the principal fibrous proteins of the keratinocyte); (2) keratohyalin synthesis (including the histidine-rich protein filaggrin); (3) the formation of the highly cross-linked, insoluble stratum corneum cornified cell envelope (including the structural protein involucrin); and (4) the generation of neutral, lipid-enriched intercellular domains, resulting from the secretion of distinctive lamellar granules. The lamellar granules are synthesized primarily within the keratinocytes of the stratum spinosum and are then displaced to the apex and periphery of the cell as it reaches the stratum granulosum (Fig. 1–18). They fuse with the plasma membrane and secrete their contents (phospholipid,

---

*See references 37, 65, 114, 139, 140, 142, 183, and 205.

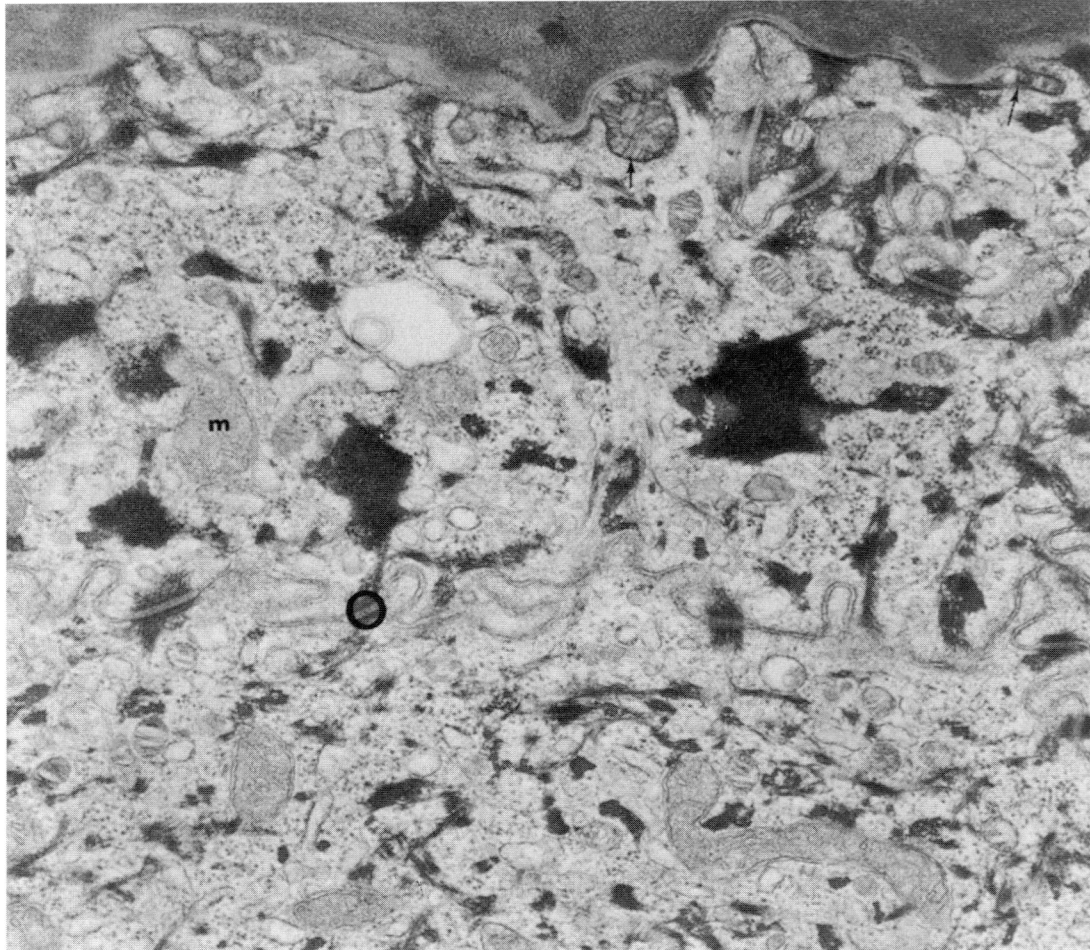

FIGURE 1–18. Lamellar granules. (From Goldsmith LA, ed: Physiology, Biochemistry, and Molecular Biology of the Skin, 2nd ed. Oxford University Press, New York, 1991. Courtesy of K. Holbrook.)

ceramides, free fatty acids, hydrolytic enzymes, and sterols). Intercellular lipids then undergo substantial alterations and assume an integral role in the regulation of stratum corneum barrier function and desquamation.

Epidermal lipids directly or indirectly influence the proliferative and biochemical events in normal and diseased skin and mediate interactions between the "dead" stratum corneum and the "living" nucleated epidermal layers.[65, 107, 150] Dynamic transformations in lipid composition and structure occur as cells migrate through the epidermis. Ceramides are the most important lipid component for lamellar arrangement in the stratum corneum and in barrier function. Polyunsaturated fatty acids are important because they are incorporated into the ceramides. Arachidonic acid is bound to the phospholipid in cell membranes and is the important precursor of eicosanoids. The eicosanoids are vital for epidermal homeostasis and the pathogenesis of inflammatory dermatoses. Lipids are important in barrier function, stratum corneum water-holding, cohesion and desquamation of corneocytes, and control of epidermal proliferation and differentiation.

The main changes in epidermal lipid composition are the replacement of phospholipids by ceramides, an increase in free sterols, and a large increase in free fatty acids at the expense of triglyceride and phospholipid.[107, 150] This transformation of lipid provides the outer epidermal layers with a much more stable, waxy, impermeable lipid barrier. Ceramides play a crucial role in plasticizing the horny layer to allow stretching and bending by fluidizing the barrier lipids.

The clinical importance of epidermal lipids in disorders of keratinization is illustrated by the following examples: (1) the scaling and poor barrier function due to abnormal lamellar granules, defective ceramides, and deranged eicosanoid production associated with essential fatty acid deficiency; (2) the scaling and poor barrier function due to the loss of ceramides, cholesterol, fatty acids, waxes, and sterols associated with exposure to solvents and detergents; (3) the poor desquamation due to the steroid sulfatase defect and resultant increased accumulation of cholesterol sulfate associated with recessive X-linked ichthyosis of humans; (4) the scaling and abnormal lipid packing due to a defect in phytanic acid oxidase production in Refsum disease humans; (5) the hyperkeratosis and defective lamellar granules in Harlequin ichthyosis of humans; and (6) the scaling and poor barrier function due to the inhibition of epidermal cholesterol synthesis seen with the administration of hypocholesterolemic agents in humans.[107, 150]

Tritiated thymidine labeling techniques have shown that the turnover (cell renewal) time for the viable epidermis (stratum basale to stratum granulosum) of dogs is approximately 22 days.[13] Clipping the hair shortened the epidermal turnover time to approximately 15 days.[14] Surgically induced wounds in the skin of normal dogs greatly increased epidermal mitotic activity.[212] Epidermal turnover time in seborrheic Cocker spaniels and Irish setters was approximately 7 days.[15]

The growth characteristics, differentiation, cell surface markers, and morphology of canine keratinocytes grown in vitro have been reported.[189–192, 208–210] Cultured canine keratinocytes express pemphigus vulgaris, pemphigus foliaceus, and bullous pemphigoid antigens, and deposit laminin and Type IV collagen.[210] The use of cultured canine keratinocytes should provide a useful model for in vitro studies of epidermal kinetics, the pathogenesis of various dermatologic diseases, and the cutaneous effects of various pharmacologic agents.

CUTANEOUS ECOLOGY

The skin forms a protective barrier without which life would be impossible. This defense has three components: physical, chemical, and microbial.[65] Hair forms the first physical line of defense to prevent contact of pathogens with the skin and to minimize external physical or chemical insult to the skin. Hair may also harbor microorganisms.

The stratum corneum forms the basic physical defense barrier. Its thick, tightly packed keratinized cells are permeated by an emulsion of sebum, sweat, and epidermal lipids that is concentrated in the outer layers of keratin, where it also functions as a physical barrier. In addition to its physical properties, the emulsion provides a chemical barrier to potential pathogens. Water-soluble substances in the emulsion include inorganic salts and proteins that inhibit microorganisms. Sodium chloride and the antiviral glycoprotein interferon, albumin, transferrin, complement, glucocorticoid, and immunoglobulins are in the emulsion.[65, 116, 180] Skin surface lipids are not constant in quantity or composition, and sebum is constantly being decomposed by resident flora into free fatty acids, some of which kill bacteria and fungi.[35] In the normal skin of dogs, (1) IgG and IgM are found in the interstitial spaces in the dermis, in dermal blood vessels, and in hair papillae; (2) IgM is found at the basement membrane zone of the epidermis (Fig. 1–19), hair follicles, and sebaceous glands; (3) IgA is found in the epitrichial sweat glands (suggesting that it functions as a cutaneous secretory immunoglobulin); and (4) C3 is found in the stratum corneum and in the dermal interstitial spaces.[60, 61, 175, 176] In the cat, IgM has been detected at the basement membrane zone of the nasal planum.[95] The polymeric immunoglobulin receptor, secretory component, is expressed and synthesized by keratinocytes and the secretory and ductal epithelium of sweat glands.[80] This receptor can interact with IgA and IgM; this interaction may be a mechanism for protecting the skin from microbial agents and foreign antigens.

A relationship exists between the acidity of the skin surface ("acid mantle" of the skin surface) and its antimicrobial activity.[35] The buffer capacity of the skin surface against anal, nasal, and oral mucocutaneous regions are also important sites of *S. intermedius* carriage.[164, 180] In fact, it has been suggested that, perhaps, *S. intermedius* is a resident of mucosae and is spread to skin and hair coat by grooming activity.[164] *Propionibacterium acnes* can also be found on the skin surface and in the hair follicles of dogs in sufficient numbers to be considered part of the normal canine flora.[164] In addition, it is well known that many saprophytic fungi—including *M. pachydermatis, Alternaria* spp., *Aspergillus* spp., and *Penicillium* spp.—can be cultured from the skin and hair of normal dogs and cats (see Chap. 5).[180]

Recent studies in normal dogs revealed the following: (1) the highest population sites for *Micrococcus* spp. and coagulase-negative staphylococci were at the skin surface, and these organisms could be considered to be residents; (2) *Clostridium* spp. were present on the skin surface and in hair follicles, and could be considered to be residents; and (3) gram-negative aerobes were present on the skin surface, in hair follicles, and at higher counts on proximal hair shafts, indicating that they could be residents.[164] Interestingly, *S. intermedius* was present in higher numbers on distal versus proximal hair shafts, but the organism was also present in higher numbers in the hair follicle versus the skin surface.[164] This suggests the possibility of two populations of *S. intermedius*.

EPIDERMAL HISTOCHEMISTRY

Histochemical studies of normal cat and dog epidermis have demonstrated distinct oxidative enzyme activity in all layers except the stratum corneum.[92, 129, 130, 180] In addition, strong reactions to nonspecific esterases were demonstrated, especially in the stratum granulosum. Oxidative enzymes that were demonstrated included cytochrome oxidase, succinate dehydrogenase, malate dehydrogenase, isocitrate dehydrogenase, lactate dehydrogenase, glucose-6-phosphate dehydrogenase, nicotinamide-adenine dinucleotide phosphate, nicotinamide-adenine dinucleotide, and monoamine oxidase. Hydrolytic enzymes that were demonstrated included acid phosphatase, arylsulfatase, β-glucuronidase, and leucine aminopeptidase. Positive reactions for cholinesterases were not observed. Thus, the enzyme pattern of normal cat and dog epidermis shows only limited similarities to that of humans, especially regarding esterase distribution.

BASEMENT MEMBRANE ZONE

Basement membrane zones are dynamic structures that undergo constant remodeling and are the physicochemical interface between the epidermis and other skin structures (appendages, neural, vascular, smooth muscle) and the underlying or adjacent connective tissue (dermis).[56, 65, 150, 193, 196] This zone is important in (1) anchoring the epidermis to the dermis, (2) maintaining a functional and proliferative epidermis, (3) maintaining tissue architecture, (4) wound healing, (5) functioning as a barrier, and (6) regulating nutritional transport between epithelium and connective tissue. Basement membranes influence many aspects of cell and tissue behavior, including adhesion, cytoskeletal organization, migration, and differentiation. The basement membrane zone is often poorly differentiated in H & E preparations, but it stains nicely with periodic acid–Schiff stain (see Fig. 1–3 H).[170, 172, 188, 203] It is most prominent in nonhaired areas of the skin and at mucocutaneous junctions. As observed by light microscopy, the basement membrane zone comprises only the fibrous zone of the sublamina densa area and is about 20 times thicker than the actual basal lamina.

Ultrastructurally, the basement membrane zone can be divided into the following four components, proceeding from epidermis to dermis (Fig. 1–20): (1) the basal cell plasma membrane, (2) the lamina lucida (lamina rara), (3) the lamina densa (basal lamina), and (4) the sublamina densa area (lamina fibroreticularis), which includes the anchoring fibrils and the dermal microfibril bundles. The first three components appear to be primarily of epidermal origin. The epidermal basement membrane is composed of a wide variety of glycoproteins and other macromolecules. Presently recognized basement membrane zone components, their localization, and their presumed functions are listed in

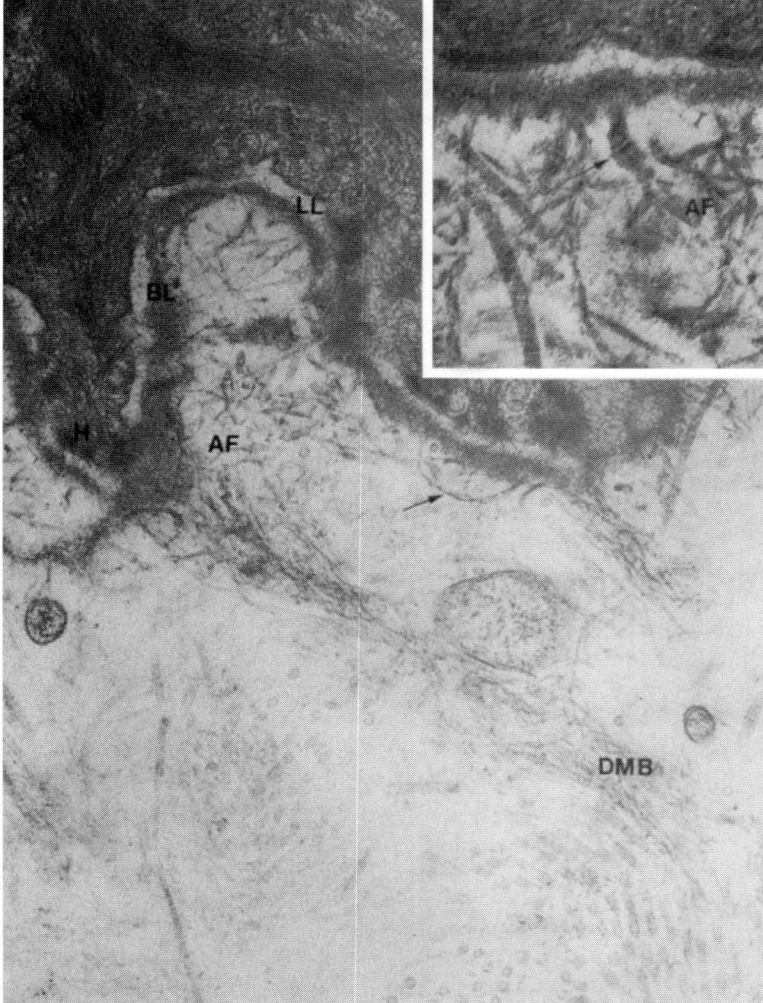

FIGURE 1–20. Epidermal-dermal junction. H, hemidesmosome; LL, lamina lucida. Anchoring fibrils (AF) form a meshwork beneath the lamina densa. A dermal macrofibril bundle (DMB) extends from the basal lamina (BL) into the dermis (×49,700). Inset: Sub-basal lamina fibrous components of the epidermal-dermal junction. Anchoring fibrils *(arrow)* with a central, asymmetric, cross-banded section. AF, interlocking meshwork of anchoring fibrils (×86,000). (From Briggaman R, Wheeler CE Jr: The epidermal-dermal junction. J Invest Dermatol 65:71–84, 1975.)

Table 1–2.[56, 65, 89, 90, 150, 193] It can be appreciated that the basement membrane is a veritable "soup" of interactive molecules with focal and regional variation that probably reflects functional differences. The involvement of the basement membrane zone in many important dermatologic disorders (pemphigoid, epidermolysis bullosa, and lupus erythematosus) and wound healing has prompted most of the current research interest.

Dermis

The dermis (corium) is an integral part of the body's connective tissue system and is of mesodermal origin.[65, 150] It is a composite system of insoluble fibers and soluble polymers that takes the stresses of movement and maintains shape. The insoluble fibers are collagens and elastin, and the major soluble macromolecules are proteoglycans and hyaluronan. The fibrous components resist tensile forces, whereas the soluble macromolecules resist or dissipate compressive forces.

In areas of thick-haired skin, the dermis accounts for most of the depth, whereas the epidermis is thin. In very thin skin, the decreased thickness results from the thinness of the dermis. The dermis is composed of fibers, ground substance, and cells (Fig. 1–21). It

Table 1-2 CHARACTERISTICS OF BASEMENT MEMBRANE ZONE COMPONENTS

COMPONENT	LOCALIZATION	FUNCTION
Bullous pemphigoid antigens	Basal cell hemidesmosome and lamina lucida	Adherence
Cicatricial pemphigoid antigen	Lamina lucida	Adherence
Laminin I	Lamina lucida (partly lamina densa)	Adherence, promote keratinocyte proliferation and differentiation
Laminin 5 (nicein/kalinin/epiligrin)	Basal cell hemidesmosome and lamina lucida	Adherence
Laminin 6	Lamina lucida	Adherence
Nidogen (entactin)	Lamina lucida (partly lamina densa)	Adherence (link laminin and type IV collagen)
Type IV collagen	Lamina densa and anchoring plaques	Adherence, networking
Type V collagen	Lamina densa (partly lamina lucida)	?
Heparan sulfate	Lamina densa	Networking, filtration
Chondroitin-6-sulfate	Lamina densa	Networking, filtration
Fibronectin	Lamina densa and lamina lucida	Networking
Epidermolysis bullosa acquisita antigen	Sublamina densa (partly lamina densa)	Adherence
Type VI collagen	Sublamina densa	Stabilization of connective tissue
Linkin	Sublamina densa	Stabilization of connective tissue
Fibrillin	Sublamina densa	Stabilization of connective tissue
Tenascin	Sublamina densa	Stabilization of connective tissue
Type VII collagen	Anchoring fibrils	Anchorage
AF1	Anchoring fibrils	Anchorage
AF2	Anchoring fibrils	Anchorage

also contains the epidermal appendages, arrector pili muscles, blood and lymph vessels, and nerves. Because the normal haired skin of cats and dogs does not have epidermal rete ridges, dermal papillae are not usually seen. Thus, a true papillary and reticular dermis, as described for humans, is not present in cats and dogs. The terms *superficial* and *deep* dermis are preferred. The dermis accounts for most of the tensile strength and elasticity of the skin; it is involved in the regulation of cell growth, proliferation, adhesion, migration, and differentiation, and it modulates wound healing and the structure and function of the epidermis.[65, 150] The dermis of scrotal skin is unique in that it contains numerous large smooth muscle bundles (see Fig. 1–6). Most of the dermal extracellular matrix (fibers and ground substance) is synthesized by fibroblasts, which respond to a variety of stimuli such as growth factors elaborated by keratinocytes, inflammatory cells, and fibroblasts themselves.[23, 150]

DERMAL FIBERS

The dermal fibers are formed by fibroblasts and are collagenous, reticular, and elastic. *Collagenous fibers* (collagen) have great tensile strength and are the largest and most numerous fibers (accounting for approximately 90% of all dermal fibers and 80% of the dermal extracellular matrix) (see Figs. 1–3B and 1–26). They are thick bands composed of multiple protein fibrils and are differentially stained by Masson's trichrome. Collagen is a family of related molecules whose diverse biological roles include morphogenesis, tissue repair, cellular adhesion, cellular migration, chemotaxis, and platelet aggregation.[65] Collagen contains two unusual amino acids—hydroxylysine and 4-hydroxyproline—whose levels in urine have been used as indices of collagen turnover. *Reticular fibers* (reticulin) are fine, branching structures that closely approximate collagen with age. They can be detected best with special silver stains. *Elastin fibers* are composed of single fine branches that possess great elasticity and account for about 4% of the dermal extracellular matrix.

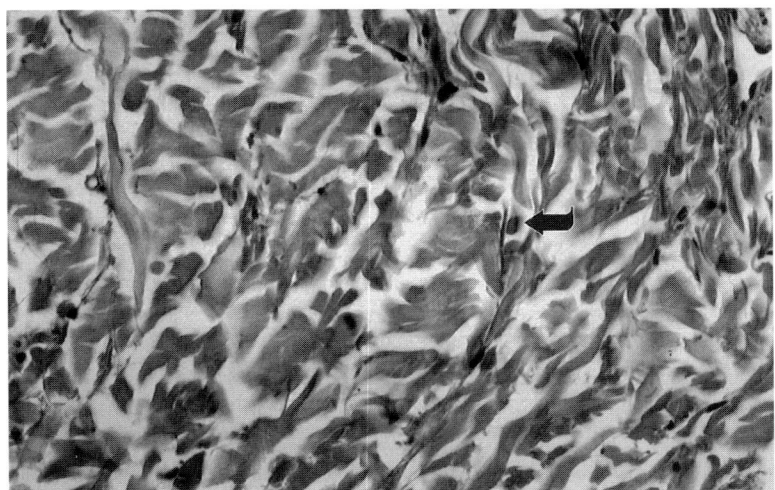

FIGURE 1–21. Normal dermis. Collagen bundles and occasional fibroblasts (arrow).

They are well visualized by Verhoeff's and van Gieson's elastin stains (see Fig. 1–3B). The two components of elastic fibers are amorphous elastin, which contains two unique cross-linked amino acids (desmosine and isodesmosine) that are not found in other mammalian proteins,[65] and microfibrils, which are composed of fibrillin and type VI collagen.[65, 150] The remarkable strength of elastic fibers is derived from the unusual cross-linking of desmosine and isodesmosine. The precursor to elastin is tropoelastin.

There are numerous (at least 17) genetically and structurally different types of collagen molecules.[65, 150] Only three collagen types are fibrillar: types I, III, and V collagen predominate in the dermis and account for approximately 87%, 10%, and 3%, respectively, of the dermal collagen. Type VI collagen is present as microfibrils and has presumed structural and communication functions. Types I, III, V, and VI collagen appear to be distributed uniformly throughout the dermis. Types III and V collagen are also concentrated around blood vessels. Types IV (lamina densa) and V (lamina lucida) collagen are found in the basement membrane zone, and Type VII collagen is found in the anchoring fibrils of the basement membrane zone. Types XII and XIV collagen are called fibril-associated collagens with interrupted triple helices (FACIT), and at present, their function is unclear. The biosynthesis of collagen is a complex process of gene transposition and translation, intracellular modifications, packaging and secretion, extracellular modifications, and fibril assembly and cross-linking. Collagen abnormalities may result from genetic defects; from deficiencies of vitamin C, iron, and copper; and from β-aminopropionitrile poisoning (lathyrism). Collagen synthesis is stimulated by ascorbic acid (vitamin C), TGF-β, IL-1, insulin-like growth factor 1 (somatomedin C), insulin-like growth factor 2, superoxide generating systems, and bleomycin.[65] Collagen synthesis is inhibited by glucocorticoids, retinoids, vitamin D_3, parathormone, prostaglandin E_2, interferon-γ, D-penicillamine, and minoxidil.

Collagenases occupy a crucial position in both the normal and pathologic remodeling of collagen.[65, 150] In the skin, a number of cell types contribute to connective tissue destruction by their capacity to synthesize and release collagenase. Dermal fibroblasts are the major source of skin collagenase under normal conditions of remodeling as well as in many pathologic conditions. However, under certain conditions, keratinocytes, neutrophils, eosinophils, and macrophages can release a variety of proteolytic enzymes, including collagenase, and contribute to local connective tissue destruction in disease. Other degradative enzymes produced by fibroblasts, polymorphonuclear leukocytes, and macrophages include gelatinase (gelatin), stromelysins, and lysosomal hydrolases (fibronectin, proteoglycans, and glycosaminoglycans).

In general, the superficial dermis contains fine, loosely arranged collagen fibers that are irregularly distributed and a network of fine elastin fibers. The deep dermis contains thick, densely arranged collagen fibers that tend to parallel the skin surface and elastin fibers that are thicker and less numerous than those in the superficial dermis. In the superficial dermis, elastic fibers, known as elaunin fibers, are organized in an arcade-like arrangement.[65] From these fibers, still thinner elastic fibers, called oxytalan fibers, ascend almost vertically to terminate at the dermoepidermal junction and anchor to the basement membrane. Elaunin and oxytalan fibers are composed of microfibrils/elastin and microfibrils, respectively.[150] Elastases are proteolytic enzymes capable of degrading elastic fibers, and a variety of tissues and cells (including fibroblasts) are capable of producing elastolytic enzymes. The elastases (serine proteinases) that are present in neutrophils and eosinophils are the most potent, and they readily degrade elastic fibers in disease states.

Multiple subsets of dendritic cells are present within the dermis.[73, 138] These *dermal dendrocytes* are mostly bone marrow derived; express CD45, MHC class II, various adhesion molecules (LFA-1, ICAM-1); and are antigen-presenting cells. They are phagocytic, variably factor XIIIa- and CD34-positive, and show immunophenotypic variation depending on their location (subepidermal, perivascular, periadnexal, superficial versus deep dermal, and so forth). In dogs, dermal dendrocytes are CD1, factor XIIIa, MHC class II, and Thy-1 positive.[136]

DERMAL GROUND SUBSTANCE

The ground (interstitial) substance is a viscoelastic gel-sol of fibroblast origin composed of glycosaminoglycans (formerly called mucopolysaccharides) that are usually linked in vivo to proteins (proteoglycans). These substances play vital roles in the epidermis, basement membrane, dermis, and hair follicle development and cycling.[23, 65, 150] The *major proteoglycans* and glycosaminoglycans include hyaluronate and heparin sulfate in the epidermis (synthesized by keratinocytes); heparin sulfate and chondroitin-6-sulfate in the basement membrane; and hyaluronic acid, dermatan sulfate, chondroitin-6-sulfate, chondroitin-4-sulfate, versican, syndecan, decorin, glypican, and serglycin in the dermis.

The ground substance fills the spaces and surrounds other structures of the dermis but allows electrolytes, nutrients, and cells to traverse it in passing from the dermal vessels to the avascular epidermis. The proteoglycans and glycosaminoglycans are extracellular and membrane-associated macromolecules that function in water storage and homeostasis; in the selective screening of substances; in the support of dermal structure (resist compression); in lubrication; and in collagen fibrillogenesis, orientation, growth, and differentiation. Although glycosaminoglycans and proteoglycans account for only about 0.1% of the dry weight of skin, they can bind over 100 times their own weight in water.

Fibronectins are widespread extracellular matrix and body fluid glycoproteins capable of multiple interactions with cell surfaces and other matrix components.[42, 43] They are produced by many cells, including keratinocytes, fibroblasts, endothelial cells, and histiocytes. The fibronectins moderate cell-to-cell interaction and cell adhesion to the substrate, and they modulate microvascular integrity, vascular permeability, basement membrane assembly, and wound healing. Fibronectin has been implicated in a variety of cell functions, including cell adhesion and morphology, opsonization, cytoskeletal organization, oncogenic transformation, cell migration, phagocytosis, hemostasis, and embryonic differentiation. Fibronectins are present in the dermis, especially perivascularly and perineurally, and within the lamina lucida and lamina densa of the basement membrane.

Tenascin is a large glycoprotein that is prominently expressed at epithelial-mesenchymal interfaces.[113] It plays a significant role in epithelial morphogenesis and proliferation and wound healing.

Small amounts of *mucin* (a blue-staining, granular- to stringy-appearing substance with H & E stain) are often seen in normal feline and canine skin, especially around appendages and blood vessels (see Fig. 1–3C). In the Chinese Shar pei, however, large amounts of mucin are normally found throughout the dermis, which could be confused with pathologic mucinosis (myxedema) in other breeds and species.

DERMAL CELLULAR ELEMENTS

The dermis is usually sparsely populated with cells.[65, 77, 138, 170, 172, 202] *Fibroblasts* (see Fig. 1–21) and *dermal dendrocytes* are present throughout. Dermal dendrocytes are predominantly perivascular antigen-presenting cells. In dogs, they are CD1, CD11, CD18, CD45, ICAM-1, and MHC class II positive.[1] They are also CD4 and CD90 (Thy-1) positive, which distinguishes them from Langerhans' cells. *Melanocytes* may be seen near superficial dermal blood vessels, especially in dark-skinned dogs. They may also be seen around the hair bulbs in darkly colored dogs, especially Doberman pinschers and black Labrador retrievers.

Mast cells (Fig. 1–22) are most abundant around superficial dermal blood vessels and appendages. In dogs and cats, many mast cells are easily recognized with routine H & E stain. The method of fixation greatly influences the number of mast cells seen, with routine formalin fixation resulting in 33% less mast cells stained as compared to Carnoy's or Mota's solutions.[18a, 57a, 203a] In cats, the cells have a fried-egg appearance, with the lightly stained intracytoplasmic granules giving the cytoplasm a stippled appearance. In both species, the mast cells are more easily recognized with special stains such as toluidine blue and acid orcein–Giemsa. In general, normal cat skin contains 4 to 20 mast cells per high-power microscopic field around superficial dermal blood vessels; normal dog skin contains 4 to 12 cells per high-power microscopic field.[172, 180, 207] In both the dog[47b] and cat,[57a] mast cell numbers may be higher in skin from the pinna. The number of canine cutaneous mast cells yielded per gram of skin was about 2.3×10^5, and the total histamine content per cell was about 4.9 pg.[47b] In frozen fixed skin from normal cats and dogs, special stains revealed about 60 to 81 mast cells/mm^2,[18] and 200 mast cells/mm^2, respectively.[203a] Toluidine blue stain detected significantly fewer mast cells than stains for tryptase or chymase. Three mast cell subtypes are distinguished in normal canine skin based on their content of mast cell–specific proteases: those that contain tryptase (T-mast cells), those that contain chymase (C-mast cells), and those that contain both (TC-mast cells).[102a, 203a]

Other cells that are occasionally seen in very small numbers in normal feline and canine skin include *neutrophils, eosinophils, lymphocytes, histiocytes,* and *plasma cells.* In dogs, lymphocytes in normal skin are T cells (CD3+) and more commonly α/β receptor positive than γ/δ receptor positive.[29]

Hair Follicles

Hair follicle morphogenesis is a complex process that occurs during the development of the skin, as part of the hair cycle, when skin repairs superficial wounds, and in response to certain pharmacologic agents.[4, 50, 65, 79] It is a complex, multistage process in which the epithelial cells of the hair follicle and the associated mesenchymal cells undergo a number of collaborative interactions. At each stage, the participating cells have different phenotypic properties and produce different products.

The hair shaft is divided into medulla, cortex, and cuticle (Fig. 1–23).* The medulla, the innermost region of the hair, is composed of longitudinal rows of cuboidal cells, or cells flattened from top to bottom. The cells are solid near the hair root, but the rest of the hair shaft contains air and glycogen vacuoles. The *cortex,* the middle layer, consists of completely cornified, spindle-shaped cells, whose long axis is parallel to the hair shaft. These cells contain the pigment that gives the hair its color. Pigment may also be present in the medulla, but there it has little influence on the color of the hair shaft. In general, the cortex accounts for one-sixth to one-third of the width of the hair shaft, and it contributes the most to the mechanical properties of hair fibers. The *cuticle,* the outermost layer of the hair, is formed by flat, cornified, anuclear cells arranged like slate on a roof, with the free edge of each cell facing the tip of the hair. Secondary ("down") hairs

---

*See references 4, 51, 65, 167, 170, 172, and 177.

42 • Structure and Function of the Skin

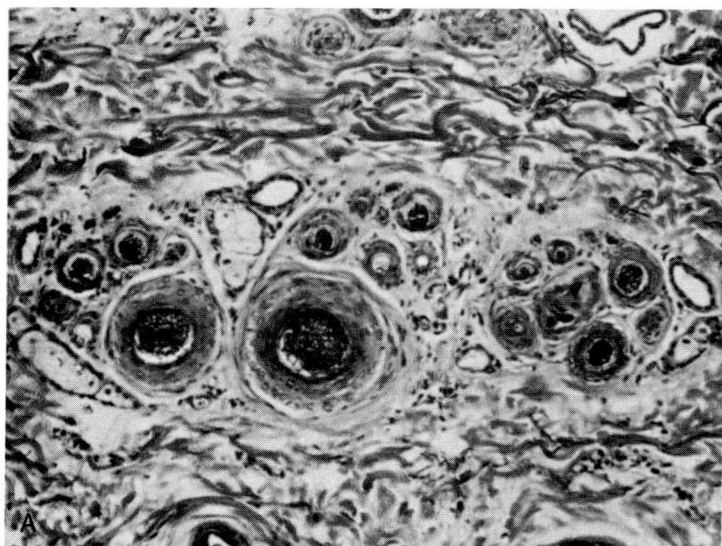

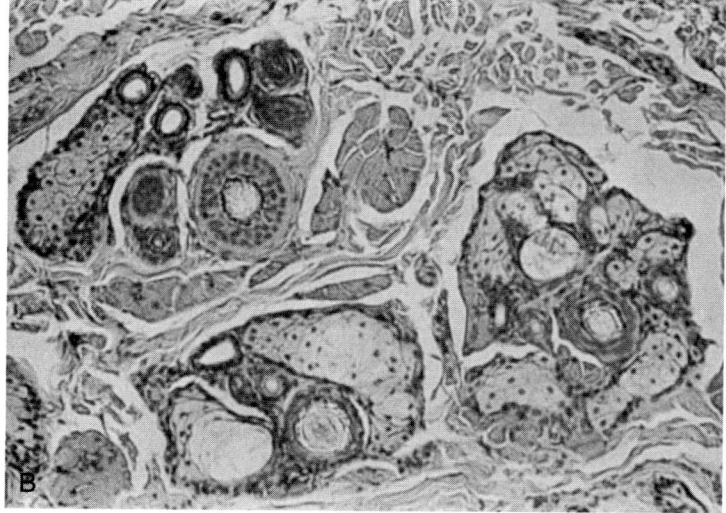

FIGURE 1-24. *A,* Three multiple hair follicle units (high power). *B,* Three apopilosebaceous complexes, each showing primary and secondary hairs, sebaceous and epitrichial glands, and arrector pili muscles (high power).

The inner root sheath (Fig. 1–26) is composed of three concentric layers (see Fig. 1–26); from inside to outside these layers include (1) the *inner root sheath cuticle* (a flattened, single layer of overlapping cells that point toward the hair bulb and interlock with the cells of the hair cuticle), (2) the *Huxley layer* (one to three nucleated cells thick), and (3) the *Henle layer* (a single layer of non-nucleated cells). These layers contain eosinophilic cytoplasmic granules called *trichohyalin granules* (see Fig. 1–1*f*). Trichohyalin is a major protein component of these granules, which are morphologic hallmarks of the inner root sheath and medullary cells of the hair follicle. Trichohyalin functions as a keratin-associated protein that promotes the lateral alignment and aggregation of parallel bundles of intermediate filaments in inner root sheath cells.[65, 144] The expression of trichohyalin is not unique to the hair follicle; it is found to occur normally in a number of other epithelial tissues, where it is closely associated with the expression of filaggrin, the major keratohyalin granule protein. The inner root sheath keratinizes and disintegrates when it reaches the level of the isthmus of the hair follicle. The prime function of the inner root sheath is to mold the hair within it, which it accomplishes by hardening in

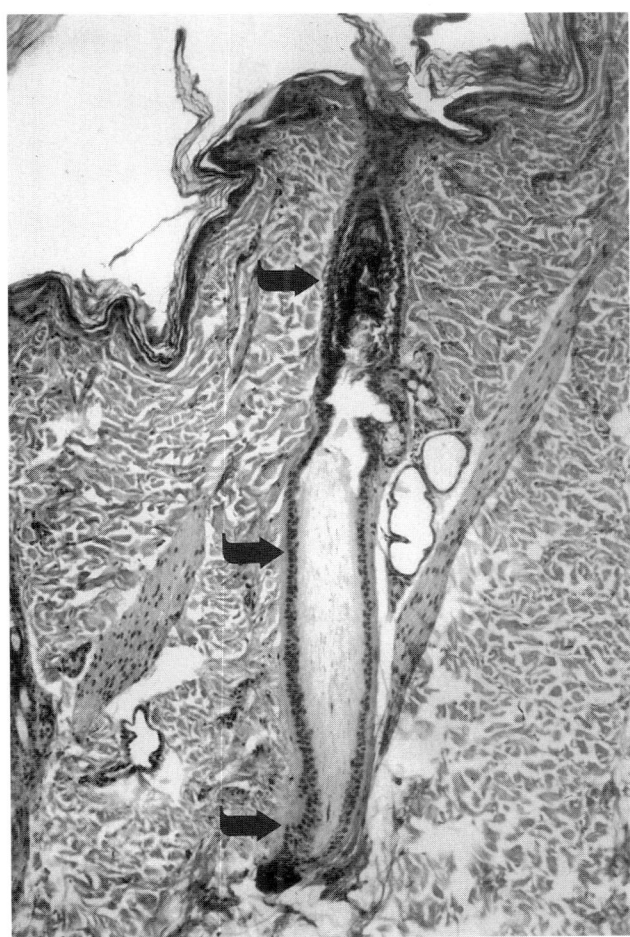

FIGURE 1-25. Anatomy of hair follicle. Dog. The infundibulum *(upper arrow)* goes from the skin surface to the entry of the sebaceous gland duct. The isthmus *(middle arrow)* goes from the sebaceous gland duct to the attachment of the arrector pili muscle. The inferior segment *(lower arrow)* goes from the attachment of the arrector pili muscle to the bulb.

advance of the hair. The amino acid citrulline occurs in high concentrations in hair and trichohyalin granules; it has been used as a marker for hair follicle differentiation. The telogen hair follicle contains no inner root sheath nor inferior segment.

The outer root sheath (see Fig. 1–26) is thickest near the epidermis and gradually decreases in thickness toward the hair bulb. In its lower portion (from the isthmus of the hair follicle downward), the outer root sheath is covered by the inner root sheath. It does not undergo keratinization, and its cells have a clear, vacuolated cytoplasm (glycogen). In the middle portion of the hair follicle (isthmus), the outer root sheath is no longer covered by the inner root sheath, and it does undergo trichilemmal keratinization (keratohyalin granules are not formed) (see Fig. 1–1g). In the upper portion of the hair follicle (infundibulum), the outer root sheath undergoes keratinization in the same fashion as occurs in the surface epidermis. The innermost cell layer of the outer root sheath is a special single-cell layer, located just outside of Henle's layer, whose pattern of cell differentiation and keratinization is ultrastructurally and immunohistochemically different from that of the main layer of the outer root sheath.[195] The cells are distinctly flattened and lack lamellar bodies.

The outer root sheath is surrounded by two other prominent structures: a basement membrane zone, or glassy membrane (a downward reflection of the epidermal basement membrane zone), and a fibrous root sheath (a layer of dense connective tissue). Perifollicular mineralization of the basement membrane zone has been described in healthy toy poodles and Bedlington terriers.[180, 182] This may also occur as a senile change in other

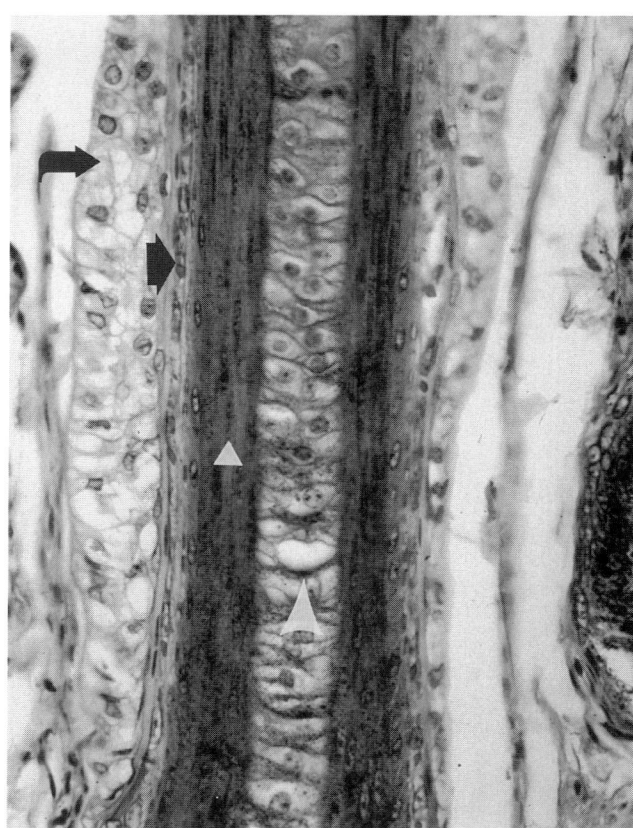

FIGURE 1–26. Hair follicle and hair shaft layers. Dog. Vacuolated (glycogen) outer root sheath *(long black arrow)*. Inner root sheath *(short black arrow)*. Cortex of hair shaft *(small white triangle)*. Central medulla of hair shaft *(large white triangle)*.

breeds of dogs and must be differentiated from the perifollicular mineralization seen in dogs with naturally occurring or iatrogenic Cushing's syndrome.

The dermal hair papilla is continuous with the dermal connective tissue and is covered by a thin continuation of the basement membrane. The inner root sheath and hair grow from a layer of plump, nucleated epithelial cells that cover the papilla. These cells regularly show mitosis and are called the *hair matrix*. The importance of the papilla in the embryogenesis and subsequent cycling of hair follicles is well known.[4, 42, 65] Additionally, the morphology of the dermal papilla changes throughout the hair growth cycle, being maximal in volume in mature anagen and minimal at telogen. This is mostly a result of changes in the amount of extracellular matrix within the papilla. In the anagen hair follicle, dermal papilla volume is proportional to the volume of the hair. Just below the dermal papilla is a fibroelastic cushion (Aaro-Perkins corpuscle).

The hair follicles of animals with straight hair are straight, and those of animals with curly hair tend to be spiral in configuration. Follicular folds have been described in the hair follicles of animals. These structures represent multiple (1 to 23) corrugations of the inner root sheath, which project into the pilar canal immediately below the sebaceous duct opening. These folds are believed to be artifacts of fixation and processing because they are not seen in unprocessed sections cut by hand.[172, 177]

Two specialized types of tactile hairs are found in mammalian skin: sinus hairs and tylotrich hairs.[65, 172, 177, 180] *Sinus hairs* (vibrissae, whiskers) are found on the muzzle, lip, eyelid, face, and throat, and on the palmar aspect of the carpus of cats (pili carpalis, carpal gland). These hairs are thick, stiff, and tapered distally. Sinus hairs are characterized by an endothelium-lined blood sinus interposed between the external root sheath of the follicle and an outer connective tissue capsule (Fig. 1–27). The sinus is divided into a superior, nontrabecular ring (or annular) sinus and an inferior, cavernous (or trabecular)

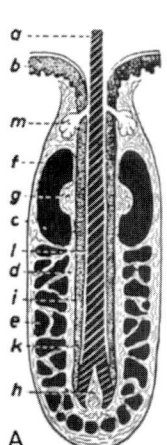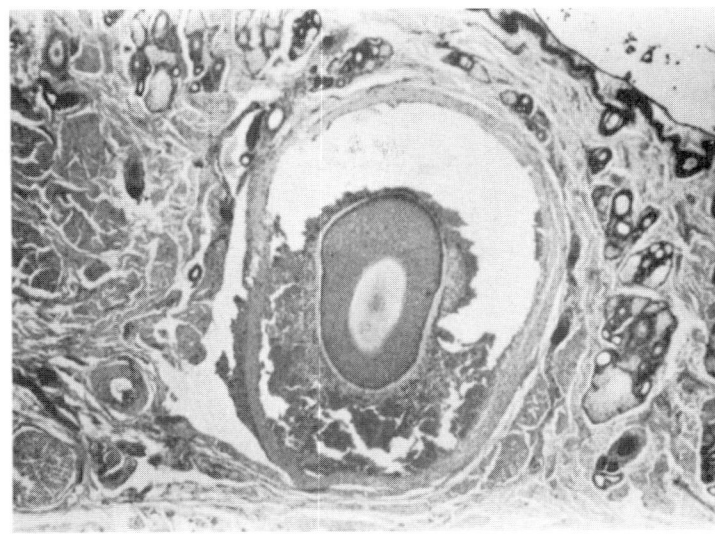

FIGURE 1–27. *A,* Hair follicle of sinus hair of cat in longitudinal section, semidiagrammatic (×150): a hair; b, epidermis; c, outer; d, inner layer of the dermal follicle; e, the blood sinus (this sinus has been differentiated into a nontrabecular annular sinus f, into which projects the sinus pad g); h, hair papilla; i, glassy membrane of the follicle; k, outer root sheath; l, inner root sheath; m, sebaceous glands. *B,* Tactile hair from upper lip of dog showing blood sinus (high power). (A, from Trautmann A, Fiebiger J: Fundamentals of the Histology of Domestic Animals. Cornell University Press, Ithaca, NY, 1952, p 342.)

sinus. A cushion-like thickening of mesenchyme *(sinus pad)* projects into the annular sinus. The cavernous sinuses are traversed by trabeculae containing many nerve fibers. Skeletal muscle fibers attach to the outer layer of the follicle. Pacinian corpuscles are situated close to the sinus hair follicles. Sinus hairs are thought to function as slow-adapting mechanoreceptors.

Tylotrich hairs are scattered among ordinary body hairs. The hair follicles are larger than surrounding follicles and contain a single stout hair and an annular complex of neurovascular tissue that surrounds the follicle at the level of the sebaceous glands. Tylotrich hairs are thought to function as rapid-adapting mechanoreceptors. Each tylotrich follicle is associated with a tylotrich pad (haarscheiben, touch corpuscle, touch dome, hair disk, tactile hair disk, tactile pad, hederiform ending, or Pinkus corpuscle, Iggo dome, Iggo-Pinkus dome, or Eimer's organ) (see Figs. 1–10 and 1–28). Tylotrich pads are

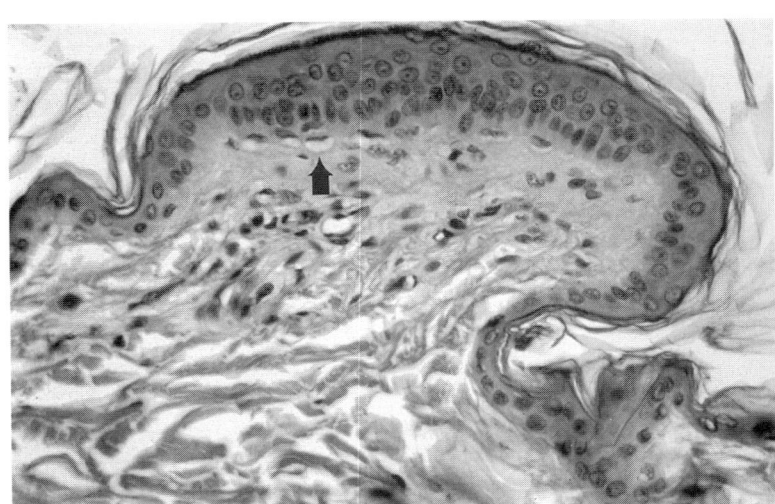

FIGURE 1–28. Tylotrich pad in cat skin. Merkel's cells *(arrow)* at basement membrane zone.

composed of a thickened and distinctive epidermis underlaid by a convex area of fine connective tissue that is highly vascularized and well innervated. Unmyelinated nerve fibers end as flat plaques in association with Merkel's cells, which serve as slow-adapting touch receptors.

The histologic appearance of hair follicles varies with the stage of the hair follicle cycle.[3, 51, 65] The *anagen* hair follicle is characterized by a well-developed, spindle-shaped dermal papilla, which is capped by the hair matrix (the ball-and-claw appearance) to form the hair follicle bulb (Fig. 1–29). Hair matrix cells are often heavily melanized and show mitotic activity. The anagen hair follicle extends into the deep dermis and often into the subcutis. Anagen has been divided into six stages: Stages I through IV, referred to as *proanagen* (differentiation); Stage V, referred to as *mesanagen* (transition to rapid growth); and Stage VI, referred to as metanagen (posteruptive hair elongation).[4, 177]

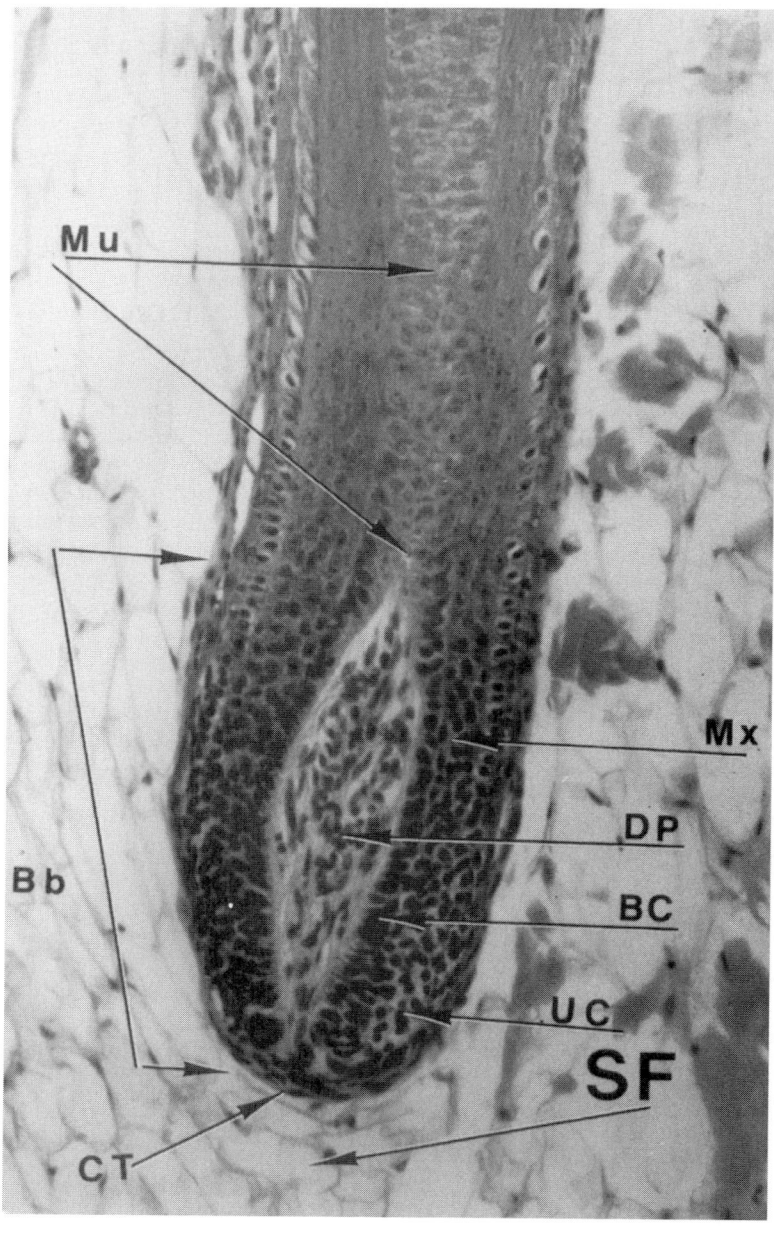

FIGURE 1–29. Anagen hair follicle. Longitudinal section of a secondary hair follicle at anagen stage, from the saddle region of a 28-month-old beagle. The bulb (Bb) extends into the subcutaneous fat (SF). The spindle-shaped dermal papilla (DP) extends toward the medulla of the hair (Mu); the base of the dermal papilla is continuous with the connective tissue (CT) of the hair follicle. The dermal papilla is surrounded by the matrix cells (Mx) of the bulb (Bb). The basal cells of the matrix are columnar (BC). The lower part of the bulb contains undifferentiated matrix cells (UC) (×350, H & E). (From Al-Bagdadi FK, Titkemeyer CW, Lovell JE: Histology of the hair cycle in male beagle dogs. Am J Vet Res 40:1734, 1979.)

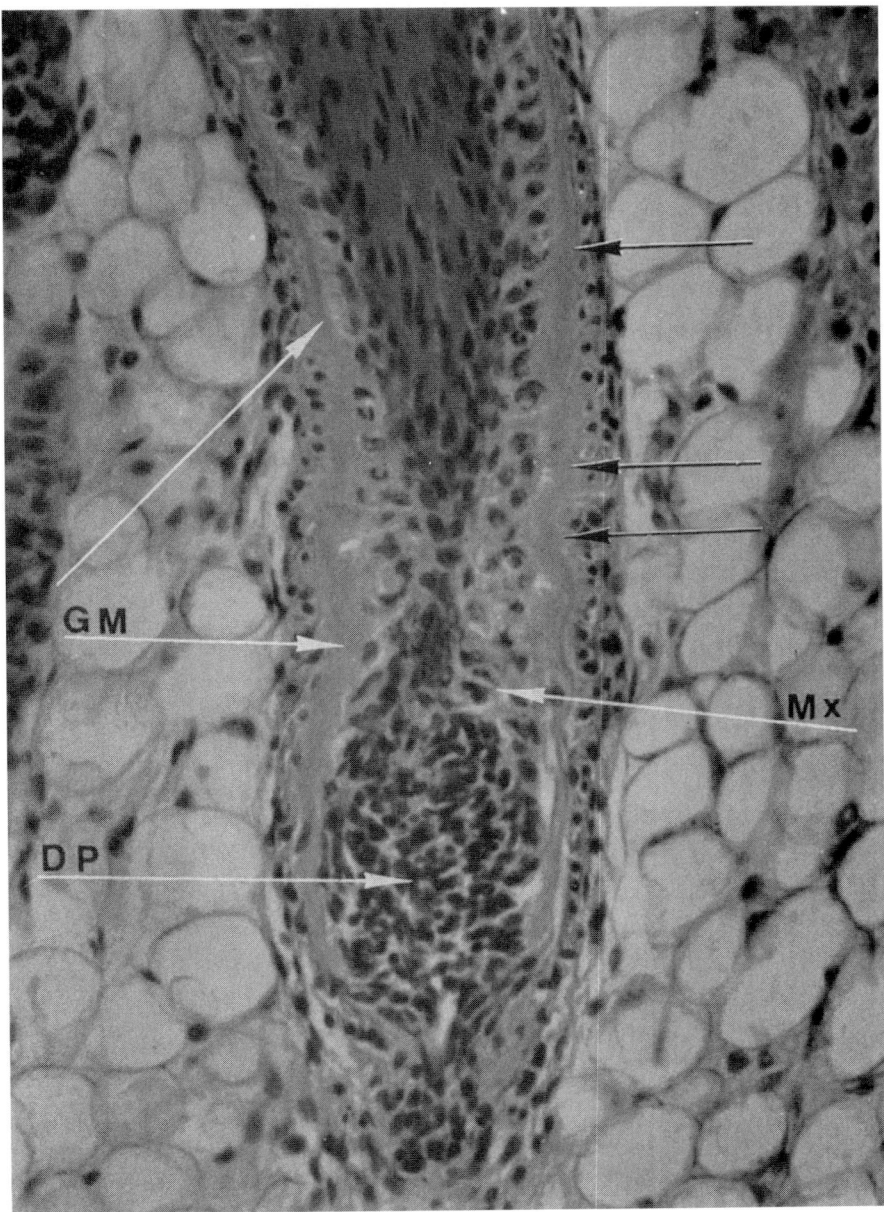

FIGURE 1-30. Catagen. Longitudinal section of a hair follicle at catagen stage from the saddle region of a 2-week-old beagle. The dermal papilla (DP) is oval in shape. The nuclei are crowded and the matrix cells (Mx) that border the dermal papilla have lost their orientation. The glassy membrane (GM) is thick and straight at the upper part of the hair follicle (single black unlabeled *arrow* in the upper part of the picture), while above the bulb, the glassy membrane is undulating (two black unlabeled *arrows* in the lower part of the picture) (×395, H & E). (From Al-Bagdadi FK, Titkemeyer CW, Lovell JE: Histology of the hair cycle in male beagle dogs. Am J Vet Res 40:1734, 1979.)

The *catagen* hair follicle is characterized by retraction toward the surface; a thickened, irregular, undulating basement membrane zone; an increased number of apoptotic keratinocytes; a thickened basement membrane zone between the hair matrix and the dermal papilla; a smaller bulb; and an ovoid or round dermal papilla (Fig. 1–30). The catagen follicle epithelium is shortened in length and reduced in volume—lost from the position of the hair bulb to just below the entry of the sebaceous duct—the volume reduction accomplished largely by the process of apoptosis. The TGF-β pathway is involved in the induction of catagen, and caspases play essential roles in the execution of apoptosis.[186] The best morphologic feature of the catagen hair follicle may be the partial replacement of the inner root sheath by trichilemmal keratinization.[50] Melanogenesis ceases, the proximal hair shaft is depigmented, and mitotic activity stops. As the follicular epithelium is lost, the adventitial collagen and neurovascular network of the follicle condenses along the tract of the pre-existing anagen follicle. This specialized adventitial structure, the *follicular stile*, is probably required to direct precisely the downward growth of the new follicular epithelium as the follicle reenters anagen.

The *telogen* hair follicle is reduced to about one third of its former length and is characterized by the small dermal papilla that is separated from the matrix cells, no hair bulb, the lack of melanin and mitotic activity, and the absence of the inner root sheath and the presence of club (brushlike) hair (Figs. 1–31 and 1–32).

Hair follicles show four morphological patterns of keratinization[4, 50]: (1) infundibular (like epidermis, with basketweave orthokeratosis and keratohyalin granules), (2) trichilemmal (a serrated, more closely packed, eosinophilic keratin with scant or no keratohyalin granules), (3) hair matrix or trichogenic (as cortex of hair shaft, characterized by retention of nuclear outlines [ghost cells]), (4) inner root sheath and hair shaft medullary (compact and opaque keratin with blue-gray to eosinophilic color and red trichohyalin granules, as in Henle's and Huxley's layers).

A hair plucked in anagen shows a larger expanded root that is moist and glistening, often pigmented, and square at the end (see Chap. 2). A hair plucked in telogen shows a tapered club root, with little or no pigment.

Langerhan's cells are present in the hair follicle outer root sheath and have been shown to migrate to the epidermis within 72 hours following ultraviolet radiation.[63] Thus, the hair follicle is a specialized immunologic compartment of the skin that serves as a reservoir to repopulate the epidermis. This follicular reservoir paradigm is also seen following thermal injury and in vitiligo, in which follicular keratinocytes and melanocytes replenish epidermal cell populations.

Sebaceous Glands

Sebaceous (holocrine) glands are simple or branched alveolar glands distributed throughout all haired skin.[65, 94, 141, 170, 172, 180] The glands usually open through a duct into the pilary canal in the infundibulum (pilosebaceous follicle). Sebaceous glands are largest and most numerous near mucocutaneous junctions, in the interdigital spaces, on the dorsal neck and rump, on the chin (submental organ), and on the dorsal tail (tail gland, supracaudal organ, preen gland). The submental organ (chin gland) also contains large nerve fibers, so it may serve tactile and scent-marking functions.[166] Sebaceous glands are not found in the footpads and nasal planum.

Sebaceous lobules are bordered by a basement membrane zone, on which there sits a single layer of deeply basophilic basal cells (called *reserve cells*) (Fig. 1–33). These cells become progressively more lipidized and eventually disintegrate to form sebum toward the center of the lobule. Sebaceous ducts are lined with squamous epithelium.

The oily secretion (sebum) produced by the sebaceous glands tends to keep the skin soft and pliable by forming a surface emulsion that spreads over the surface of the stratum corneum to retain moisture and thus maintain proper hydration. The oil film also spreads over the hair shafts and gives them a glossy sheen. During periods of illness or malnutrition, the haircoat may become dull and dry as a result of inadequate sebaceous gland function. In addition to its action as a physical barrier, the sebum-sweat emulsion forms a chemical barrier against potential pathogens (see Cutaneous Ecology in this

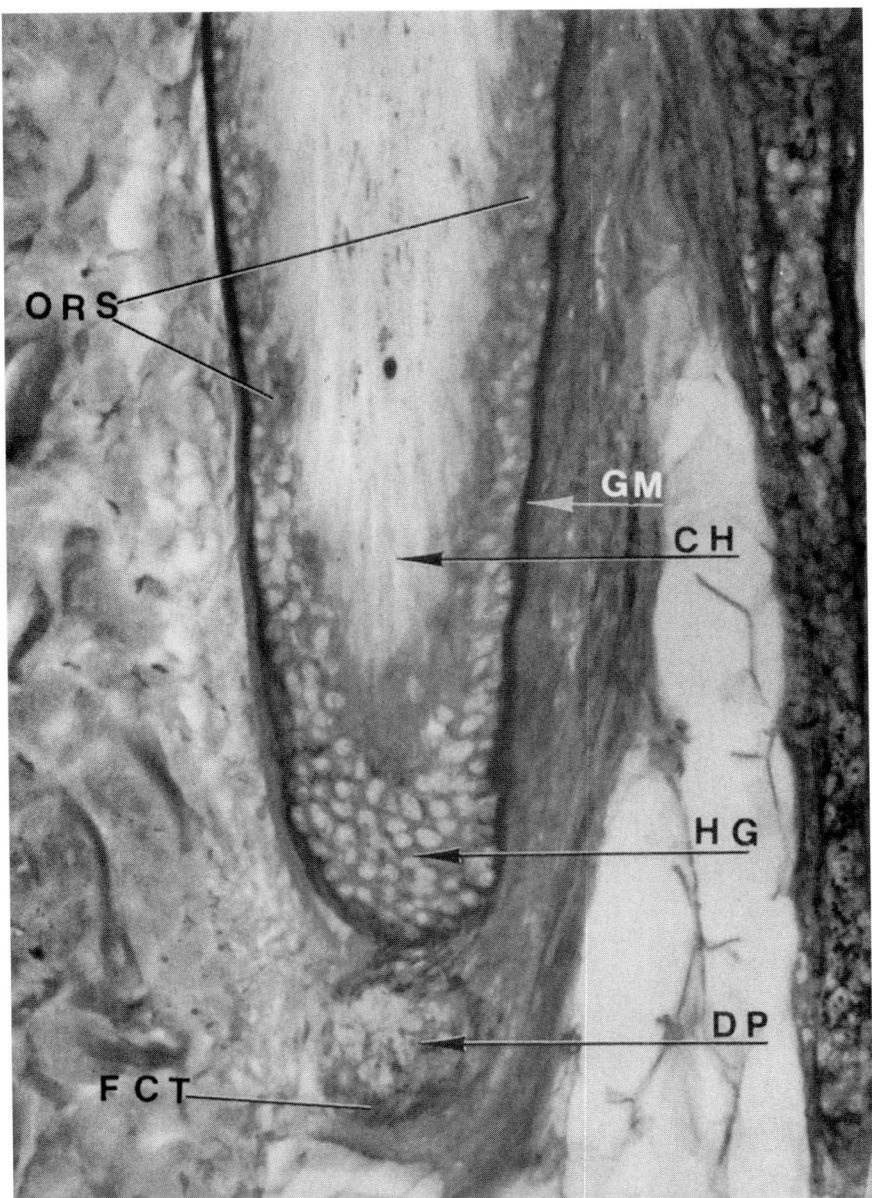

FIGURE 1-31. Telogen. Longitudinal section of a main hair follicle at telogen stage from the saddle region of a 3-month-old beagle. The dermal papilla (DP) is separated from the matrix cells of the hair follicle. It is surrounded by fibrous connective tissue (FCT) and appears to contact the base of the follicle at one point. The hair germ cells (HG) are located at the base of the club hair (CH). The cells of the outer root sheath (ORS) lack glycogen granules. The glassy membrane (GM) is thick and PAS positive. The hair follicle at this stage is surrounded by connective tissue that separates the follicle from the adipose tissue (×400). (From Al-Bagdadi FK, Titkemeyer CW, Lovell, JE: Histology of the hair cycle in male beagle dogs. Am J Vet Res 40:1734, 1979.)

50 • Structure and Function of the Skin

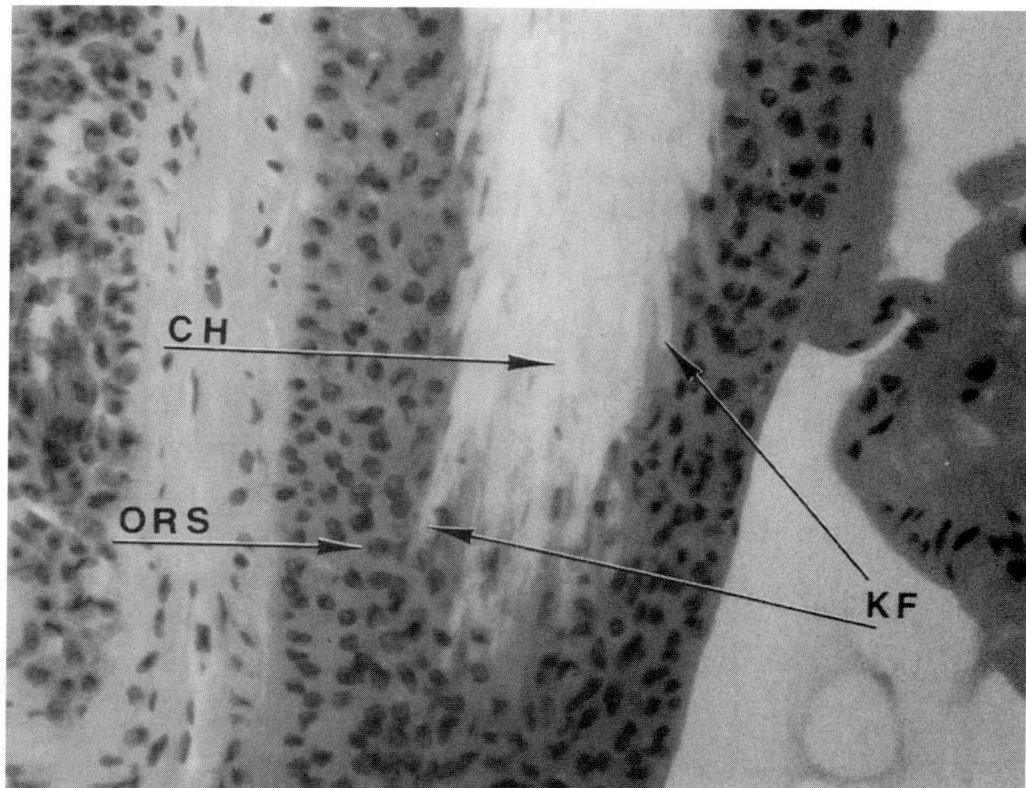

FIGURE 1-32. Club hair of telogen. Longitudinal section of a main hair follicle at telogen stage from the saddle region of a 24-month-old beagle. The club hair (CH) has many keratinized fibers (KF) that extend between the cells of the outer root sheath (ORS). These keratinized fibers give the club hair a brushlike appearance (×465, H & E). (From Al-Bagdadi FK, Titkemeyer CW, Lovell JE: Histology of the hair cycle in male beagle dogs. Am J Vet Res 40:1734, 1979.)

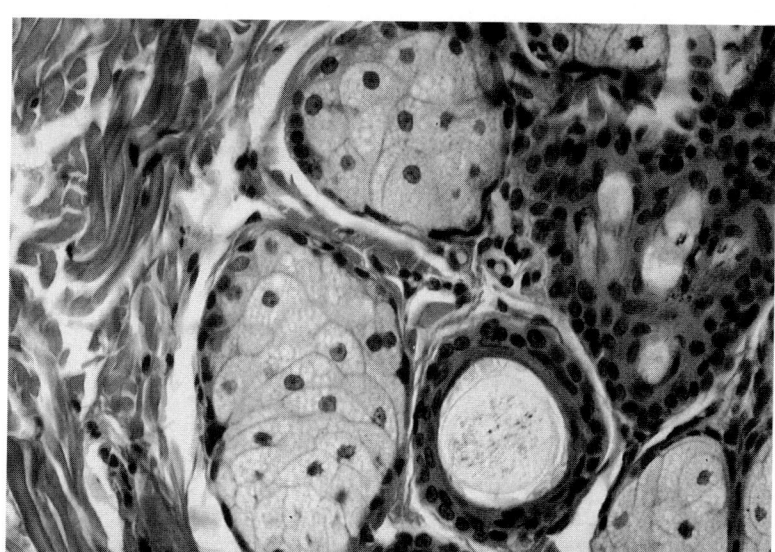

FIGURE 1-33. Canine sebaceous gland lobules.

chapter). Freshly liberated sebum contains predominantly triglycerides and wax esters.[37] In the hair follicle infundibulum, sebum becomes contaminated with lipase-producing bacteria (*Propionibacterium* spp., *Staphylococcus* spp.), which results in the production of fatty acids. Many of sebum's fatty acid constituents (linoleic, myristic, oleic, and palmitic acids) are known to have antimicrobial actions. Sebum may also have pheromonal properties.[94]

Sebaceous glands have an abundant blood supply and appear to be innervated. Their secretion is thought to be under hormonal control, with androgens causing hypertrophy and hyperplasia, and estrogens and glucocorticoids causing involution. The skin surface lipids of cats and dogs have been studied in some detail and are different from those of humans (see Horny Layer in this chapter). Enzyme histochemical studies have indicated that all mammalian sebaceous glands contain succinate acid dehydrogenase, cytochrome oxidase, and a few esterases.[135]

Sweat Glands

Because of investigations into the physiology and ultrastructural aspects of sweat production by sweat glands, it has been suggested that the *apocrine* and *eccrine* sweat glands are more accurately called the *epitrichial* and *atrichial* sweat glands, respectively.[94] We have adopted the suggested terminology for this book.

EPITRICHIAL SWEAT GLANDS

Epitrichial sweat glands are generally coiled and saccular or tubular and are distributed throughout all haired skin.* They are not present in footpads or nasal planum. These glands are located below the sebaceous glands, and they usually open through a duct into the pilary canal in the infundibulum, above the sebaceous duct opening. Epitrichial sweat glands tend to be larger in areas where hair follicle density is lower. They are largest and most numerous near mucocutaneous junctions, in interdigital spaces, and over the dorsal neck and rump. The secretory portions of epitrichial sweat glands consist of a single row of flattened to columnar epithelial (secretory) cells and a single layer of fusiform myoepithelial cells (Figs. 1–34 and 1–35). The epitrichial sweat gland excretory duct is lined by two cuboidal to flattened epithelial cell layers and a luminal cuticle but no myoepithelial cells.[88] In general, epitrichial sweat glands do not appear to be innervated. Epitrichial sweat probably has pheromonal and antimicrobial properties (IgA content).[94]

---

*See references 65, 93, 94, 141, 170, 172, 180, and 188.

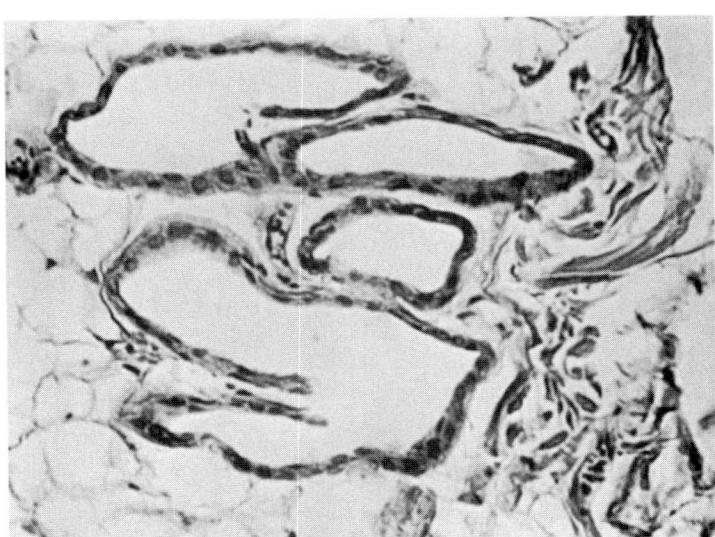

FIGURE 1–34. Section through coiled portion of epitrichial sweat gland (high power).

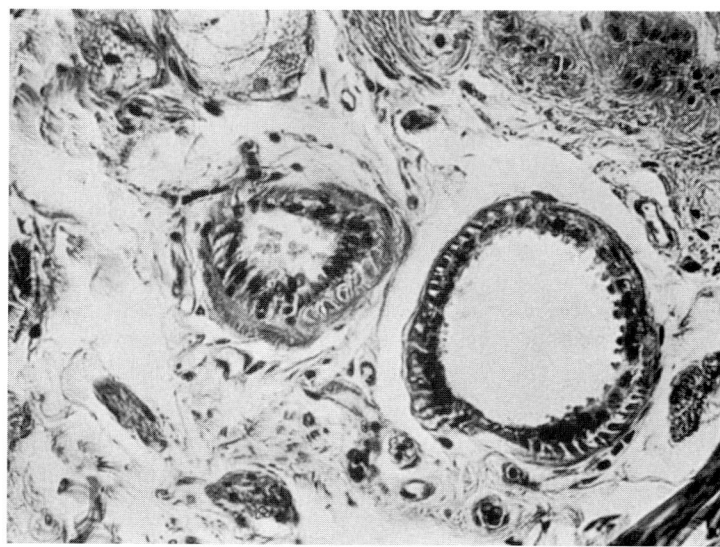

FIGURE 1–35. Epitrichial gland showing secretory epithelium (high power).

Enzyme histochemical studies have demonstrated alkaline phosphatase and acid phosphatase in epitrichial sweat gland secretory epithelium.[87, 120, 135] Immunohistochemical studies show that the acini and ducts of canine epitrichial sweat glands are positive for cytokeratin; associated myoepithelial cells are positive for both cytokeratin and S-100 protein.[55]

Recent studies in swine have shown that the sweat gland apparatus is capable of re-epithelializing the skin surface, although the resulting epidermis is not entirely normal.[134]

ATRICHIAL SWEAT GLANDS

Atrichial (merocrine) sweat glands are found only in the footpads.[172, 180, 188, 202] These glands are small and tightly coiled, and they are located in the deep dermis and subcutis of the footpads. Secretory coils consist of a single layer of cuboidal to columnar epithelial cells and a single layer of fusiform myoepithelial cells (Fig. 1–36). The intradermal

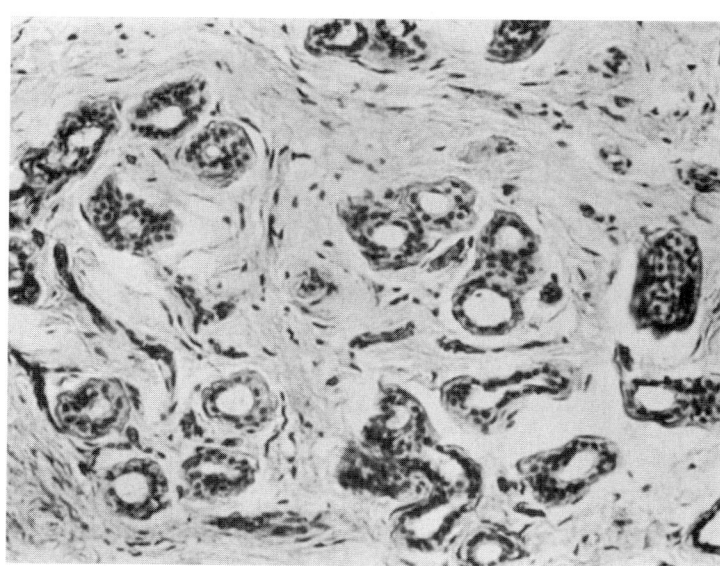

FIGURE 1–36. Atrichial sweat glands from canine footpad (high power).

portion of the excretory duct consists of a double row of cuboidal epithelial cells. The excretory duct opens directly to the footpad surface.

Enzyme histochemical studies have demonstrated cytochrome oxidase, succinate and other dehydrogenases, phosphorylases, and alkaline phosphatase in atrichial sweat glands.[135] They are richly supplied with cholinesterase-positive nerves.[135, 172, 180, 211]

SWEATING AND THERMOREGULATION

The skin of cats and dogs does not possess the extensive superficial arteriovenous shunts of humans and swine that are designed to disseminate heat in hot weather. Carnivores also lack atrichial sweat glands in the hairy skin.

The frequency of sweating and the circumstances under which sweating occurs in cats and dogs are unclear. Some authors have stated that the dog shows great variation in the degree of epitrichial sweating that takes place and that some breeds (especially German shepherds, Labrador retrievers, and other large breeds) may show visible sweating in the axillae, groin, and ventral abdomen.[180] Other authors have noted that epitrichial sweating is occasionally seen in certain febrile and excited dogs.[141] Still others have reported the absence of epitrichial sweating in dogs subjected to severe generalized temperature stress and in dogs that were struggling violently.[41] Atrichial sweating may be seen on the footpads of excited or agitated cats and dogs.[180]

In dogs, localized epitrichial sweating can be produced by local heat applications and by the intradermal injection of various sympathomimetic (epinephrine, norepinephrine) and parasympathomimetic (acetylcholine, pilocarpine) drugs.[6, 7, 40, 86, 141] Because responses to all of these can be blocked by atropine, the final physiologic stimulus appears to be cholinergic. It has also been reported that asphyxiation or the intravenous injection of epinephrine or norepinephrine has produced generalized epitrichial sweating in dogs.[86] Because these responses could not be blocked by adrenal medullectomy but were blocked by sympathetic denervation of skin, it was concluded that canine epitrichial sweating is primarily regulated by neural mechanisms and that humoral mechanisms play a subsidiary role. One group of researchers concluded—on the basis of available local and systemic pharmacologic data, local and generalized thermal responses, hypothalamic stimulation, and electron microscopic examinations—that canine epitrichial sweat glands were not directly innervated and had little, if any, thermoregulatory importance.[20, 41] It was also suggested that because the only physiologic stimulus noted to produce epitrichial sweating consistently in dogs was copulation, epitrichial sweating in dogs served a predominantly pheromonal function.[41]

Atrichial sweating from the footpads of cats and dogs can be provoked by cholinergic stimuli and, less so, by adrenergic stimuli.[172, 180, 194] Atropine blocks glandular responses to these agents. Feline atrichial sweat contains lactate, glucose, sodium, potassium, chloride, and bicarbonate, and it differs from that of humans in that it is hypertonic and alkaline and contains much higher concentrations of sodium, potassium, and chloride.[26, 58, 188]

Mechanisms to Conserve Heat

When the environmental temperature falls, the body attempts to reduce heat loss by vasoconstriction in the skin and erection of the hairs to improve the insulating qualities of the skin and coat. The external temperature at which the heat-retaining mechanisms are no longer able to maintain a constant body temperature and at which heat production has to be increased is known as the critical temperature. Normal dogs with intact pelage have a critical temperature of 14°C (57°F); when their coats are shaved off, however, they have a critical temperature of 25°C (77°F).[180] Thick subcutaneous fat also acts as efficient insulating material. Nonfasting animals have a lower critical temperature than fasting individuals; therefore, the former are better able to tolerate a low environmental temperature. When the aforementioned mechanisms of heat conservation are no longer effective in preventing a fall in body temperature, an increase in heat production begins. A rapid increase in heat production is accomplished mainly by shivering. In normal dogs, shivering begins when the rectal temperature falls 1°C.

Mechanisms to Dissipate Heat

Heat is regularly lost from the body by radiation, conduction, and convection; vaporization of water from the skin and respiratory passages; and excretion of urine and feces. The excretory losses are relatively unimportant in heat dissipation. Ordinarily, 75% of the heat loss is attributable to radiation, conduction, and convection. The efficiency of these mechanisms varies with the external temperature and humidity, and it is modified further by the animal's vasomotor and pilomotor responses. These responses become ineffective at higher temperatures, when heat loss by vaporization of water from the skin and lungs becomes more influential. Because they do not produce an abundance of atrichial sweat, dogs and cats have developed the ability to vaporize large volumes of water from their respiratory passages. In dogs, as the environmental temperature rises above 27° to 29°C (81° to 84°F), the rate of breathing also rises, but the depth of breathing (tidal volume) is markedly reduced. This helps prevent excess carbon dioxide blowoff and severe blood gas changes. At a rectal temperature of 40.5°C (105°F), the dog is in danger of thermal imbalance; at 43°C, collapse is imminent.

The rectal temperature of the cat begins to rise at an environmental temperature of 32°C (90°F), but as the respiratory rate increases, the tidal volume is only slightly reduced. As a result, the cat is more susceptible to a lowering of its blood CO_2 level (i.e., to respiratory alkalosis). The cat possesses an additional compensatory mechanism; a hot environment, or sympathetic stimulation, produces a copious flow of watery saliva from the submaxillary gland. The cat spreads this on its coat for additional water vaporization, and cooling results. Similar stimulation in dogs produces only a scanty secretion of thick saliva that cannot help the cooling process.[180]

The problem of temperature regulation in dogs and cats is often complicated by the physical condition of the coat and by the environmental temperature. Breeds with heavy coats intended for cold climates sometimes suffer when they are moved to regions of high temperatures. The problem is greatly accentuated by a matted, unkempt coat that stifles air circulation through the hair. Proper grooming greatly increases the comfort of these animals.

Specialized Glands

Specialized glands include the circumanal (perianal) glands, the glands of the external auditory canal (see Chap. 19), and the anal sacs (see Chap. 19), as well as the tail gland.

The circumanal (perianal) glands are present at birth and develop from ducts that originate from the inner and outer perianal sides of the external root sheath of hair follicles.[83, 121] These glands are also found in the skin of the prepuce and dorsal and ventral aspects of the tail. These glands are positive for cytokeratin.[199, 200]

The *tail gland* (supracaudal gland, preen gland) of the dog is an oval-shaped area located on the dorsal surface of the tail over the fifth to seventh coccygeal vertebrae, about 5 cm distal to the anus.[101, 180] This gland is consistently present in wild Canidae; it is regarded as an atavism in dogs, however, because it is somewhat different in structure, is lacking in function, and is clearly visible in only about 5% of all normal male dogs. The gland is present histologically in most dogs. The haircoat of the region is characterized by stiff, coarse hairs, each of which emerges singly from its follicle. The surface of the skin may be yellow and waxy from the abundant secretion of the numerous large glands in the area. This secretion may aid in olfactory species recognition. This area of the tail may be severely affected in seborrheic skin diseases and may also develop hyperplasia, cystic degeneration, infection, adenoma, and adenocarcinoma.

Histologically, the canine tail gland is composed predominantly of *hepatoid cells*, which are identical to those in the hepatoid (perianal, circumanal) glands. The glandular ducts empty into hair follicles. The tail gland and the circumanal glands are dependent on testosterone and form a topographic-ethnologic unit.

The tail gland (supracaudal organ) of the cat consists of numerous large sebaceous glands that run the entire length of the dorsal surface of the tail.[172, 188] Excess accumulation of glandular secretion in this area is called stud tail.

Arrector Pili Muscles

Arrector pili muscles are of mesenchymal origin and consist of smooth muscle with intracellular and extracellular vacuoles.[65, 172, 180, 188, 202] They are present in all haired skin and are largest in the dorsal neck and rump. Arrector pili muscles originate in the superficial dermis and insert approximately perpendicularly on the primary hair follicles (see Figs. 1-25 and 1-37). Branching of these muscles is often seen in the superficial dermis. Arrector pili muscles are about one fourth to one half the diameter of central primary hair follicles in most haired skin areas but are of equal diameter in the dorsal lumbar, dorsal sacral, and dorsal tail areas.

These muscles receive cholinergic innervation and contract in response to epinephrine and norepinephrine, producing piloerection. Arrector pili muscles probably function in thermoregulation and in the emptying of sebaceous glands.

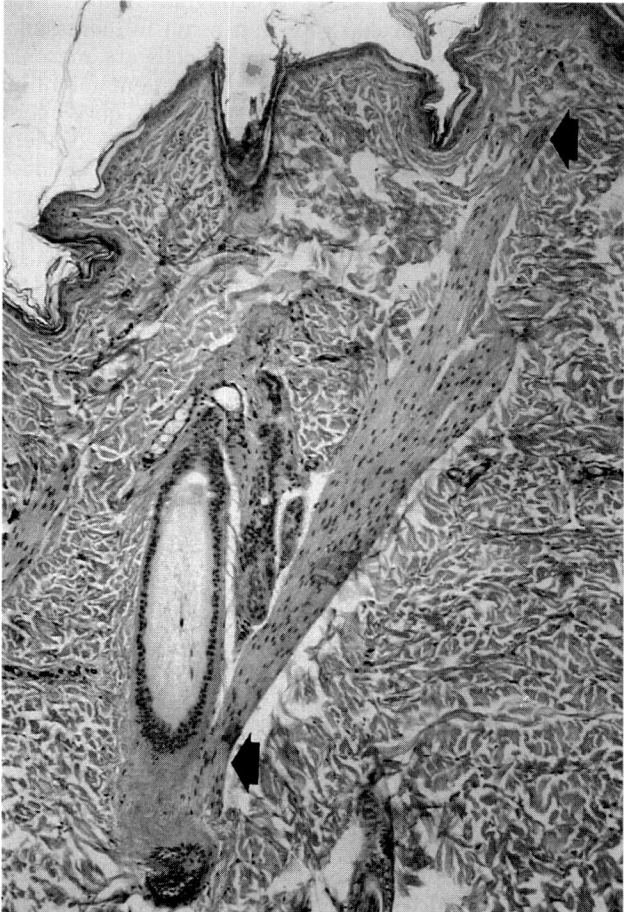

FIGURE 1-37. Arrector pili. Dog. Arrector pili muscle originates in superficial dermis *(upper arrow)* and inserts on the hair follicle *(lower arrow).*

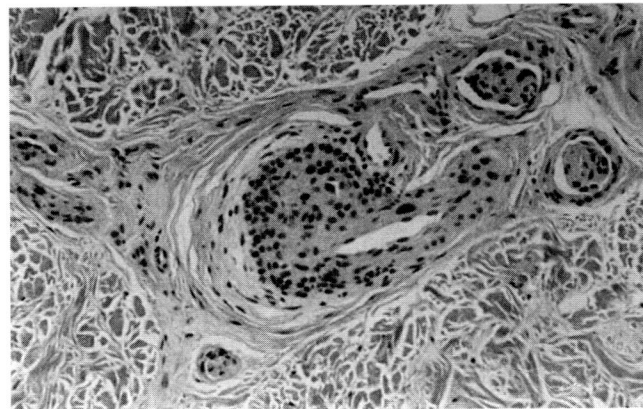

FIGURE 1-40. Glomus. (From Elder D, ed: Lever's Histopathology of the Skin, 8th ed. Lippincott-Raven, 1998, Philadelphia.)

measurement of blood flow, the pathophysiology of various skin diseases can be verified and certain treatments can be partially monitored.

Lymph Vessels

The skin is confronted by a specialized set of pathogenic organisms and environmental chemicals that represent a distinctive spectrum of antigenic specificities. It has a unique collection of lymphatics and lymphoid and dendritic cells to deal with these special demands.

Lymphatics arise from capillary networks that lie in the superficial dermis and surround the adnexa.[51, 65, 166] The vessels arising from these networks drain into a subcutaneous lymphatic plexus. Lymph vessels are not usually seen above the middle dermis in routine histologic preparations of normal skin.

The lymphatics are essential for nutrition because they control the true microcirculation of the skin, the movement of interstitial tissue fluid.[161] The supply, permeation, and removal of tissue fluid are important for proper function. The lymphatics are the drains that take away the debris and excess matter that result from daily wear and tear in the skin. They are essential channels for the return of protein and cells from the tissues to the blood stream and for linking the skin and regional lymph nodes in an immunoregulatory capacity. In skin, lymphatics carry material that has penetrated the epidermis and dermis, such as solvents, topical medicaments, injected vaccines and drugs, and products of inflammation.

Skin has a noncontractile initial lymphatic collector system that drains into contractile collector lymphatics.[161] Initial lymphatics have an attenuated endothelial layer, discontinuous basement membrane, and noncontiguous cell junctions. Lymph formation depends on the periodic expansion of the initial lymphatics, whereas compression leads to the emptying of the initial lymphatics into the contractile collector lymphatics, which have smooth muscle, exhibit peristalsis, and carry lymph toward the lymph nodes. Expansion and compression of collecting lymphatics is achieved by periodic tissue motions such as pressure, pulsations, arteriolar vasomotion, skin massage, and muscle motion.[145, 161]

In general, lymph vessels are distinguished from blood capillaries by (1) possessing wider and more angular lumina, (2) having flatter and more attenuated endothelial cells, (3) having no pericytes, and (4) containing no blood (Fig. 1–41). However, even the slightest injury disrupts the wall of a lymphatic or blood vessel or the intervening connective tissue. Consequently, traumatic fistulae are commonplace. These account for the common observation of blood flow in the lymphatics in inflamed skin.

Nerves

Cutaneous nerve fibers have sensory functions, control the vasomotor tonus, and regulate the secretory activities of glands. They also exert a number of important effector func-

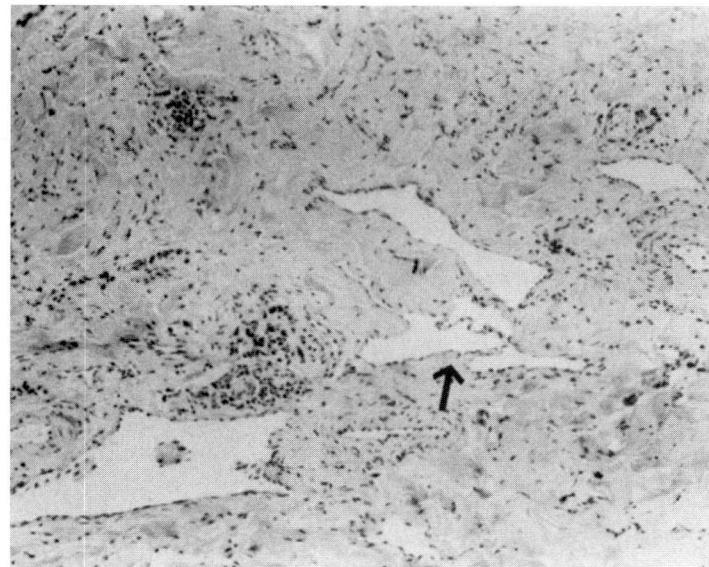

FIGURE 1–41. Lymphatic vessels (arrow). Note angular outline and absence of intravascular blood cells.

tions, including the modulation of multiple inflammatory, proliferative, and reparative cutaneous processes.[5, 77, 147, 201] Cutaneous nerves are in close contact with dermal vessels, mast cells, fibroblasts, keratinocytes, and Langerhan's cells. Neuropeptides released by cutaneous nerves can activate a number of target cells such as keratinocytes (inducing release of cytokines such as IL-1), mast cells (producing potent proinflammatory cytokines such as TNF-α), and endothelial cells (upregulating VCAM-1 expression and causing secretion of IL-8). Such neuropeptides include substance P, neurokinin A, calcitonin gene–related peptide, vasoactive intestinal peptide, neuropeptide Y, somatostatin, and pituitary adenylate cyclase activity peptide. In addition, skin epithelium can generate neurotrophins, thus influencing the development, sprouting, and survival of nerve fibers.

In general, cutaneous nerve fibers are associated with blood vessels (dual autonomic innervation of arteries) (Fig. 1–42), various cutaneous end organs (tylotrich pad [see Figs. 1–10 and 1–43], Pacini's corpuscle [Fig. 1–44], Meissner's corpuscle), sebaceous glands, hair follicles, and arrector pili muscles. The fibers occur as a subepidermal plexus (see Fig. 1–43).[65] Free nerve endings even penetrate the epidermis. The motor innervation of skin is attributable to sympathetic fibers of the autonomic nervous system. Although they are ordinarily considered somatic sensory nerves, the cutaneous nerve trunks carry myelinated postganglionic sympathetic fibers. Under the light microscope, small cutaneous nerves and free nerve endings can be demonstrated satisfactorily only by methylene blue staining, metallic impregnation, or histochemical techniques.

In addition to the important function of sensory perception (touch, heat, cold, pressure, pain, and itch), the dermal nerves promote the survival and proper functioning of the epidermis (i.e., the so-called trophic influences).

The area of skin supplied by the branches of one spinal nerve is known as its dermatome. Dermatomes have been mapped out for the cat[74, 104] and dog.[11, 12, 99, 204]

OVERVIEW OF CUTANEOUS SENSATION

The skin is a major sensory surface. Signals about external events and about the internal state of the skin are sent to the central nervous system by an array of receptor endings. *Thermoreceptors* fall into two categories: cold units, which are excited by falling skin temperatures, and warm units, which are excited by rising skin temperatures.[65] Cold units have C axons and A axons. Cold unit nerve terminals are branches of a small myelinated

60 • Structure and Function of the Skin

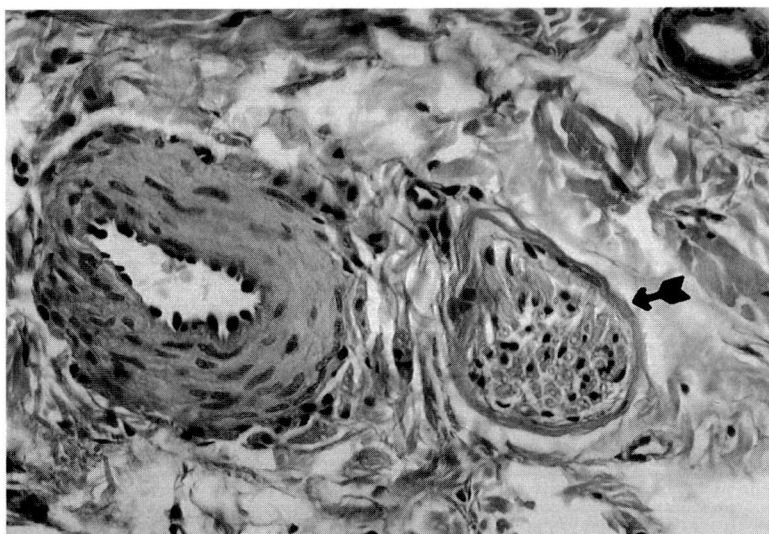

FIGURE 1–42. Dog skin. Large nerve fiber *(arrow)* to the right of a deep dermal arteriole.

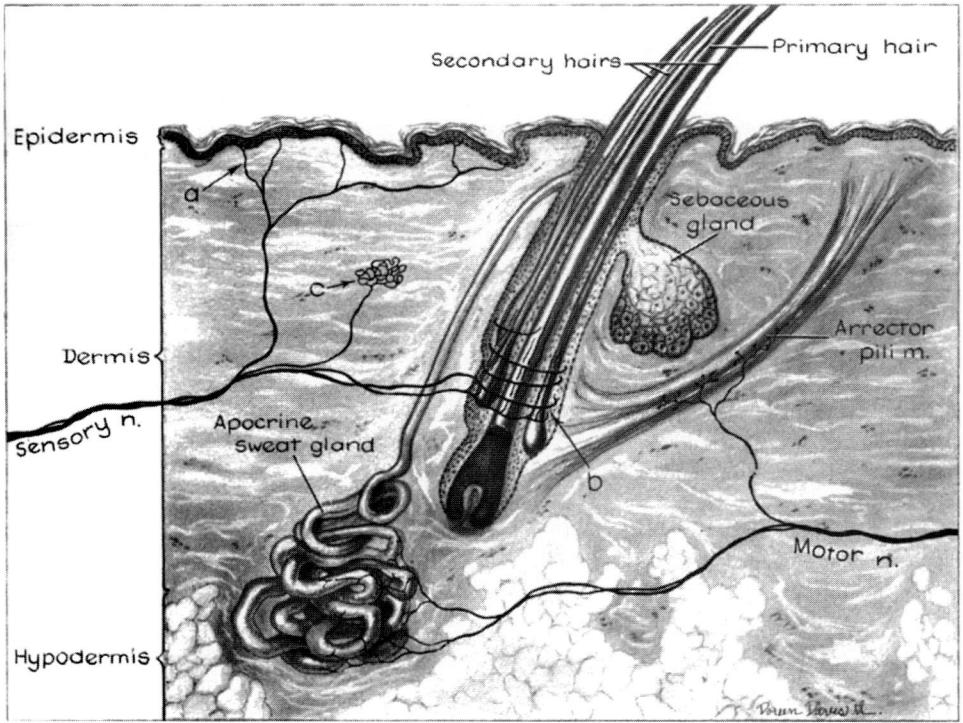

FIGURE 1–43. Nerve supply of the canine skin. a, dermal nerve network; b, hair follicle network; c, specialized end organs.

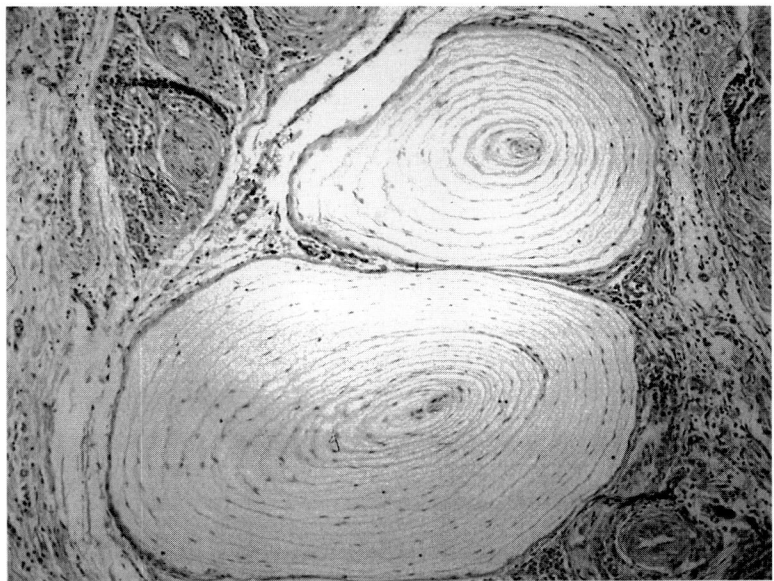

FIGURE 1-44. Cat skin. Two Pacini's corpuscles. Note typical "onion skin" appearance.

axon, ending in a small invagination in the basal cells of the epidermis.[65, 76, 180] Warm units also have C axons and A axons, but no morphologic nerve terminal has been identified.

Four types of sensitive *mechanoreceptor* units with A axons are present in most skin regions.[65] Pacinian corpuscle units are extremely sensitive to small high-frequency vibrations, deep pressure, and very rapid transients.[65, 180] Rapidly adapting units, which arise from Meissner (Wagner-Meissner corpuscle, Dogiel's end-bulb, or Ruffini's end-bulb) or Ruffini corpuscles, are primarily sensitive to the velocity of skin movement and touch.[65, 77, 180] In hairy skin, there are many afferent units that are excited by hair movement and have both A β and A δ axons. These axons provide the major tactile input from such regions. Guard and down hairs receive many nerve terminations of the lanceolate type. Such units can be subdivided into two major classes: (1) those excited only by movement of large guard or tylotrich hairs (G and T hair units), and (2) those excited by movement of all hairs, but especially by the fine down hairs (D hair units).[65, 180] The units driven from large hairs nearly always have A β axons; those driven from down hairs have A δ axons. G and T hair units are activated by rapid hair movements, and D hair units respond to slow movements. An additional class of units activated by static deflection of hairs is associated with large sinus hairs such as vibrissae.[65, 66] Finally, a characteristic class of unit with an unmyelinated axon, the C mechanoreceptor, is frequently encountered in cat haired skin.[65, 180] Slowly adapting Type I endings from Merkel's cell complexes signal about steady pressure.[65, 81, 180] Slowly adapting Type II units, which are associated with Ruffini endings,[30, 65] show directional sensitivity in response to skin stretch and may play a proprioceptive role.

Most *nociceptor* units fall into two categories: A δ high-threshold mechanoreceptor units with A δ axons, and polymodal nociceptor units with C axons.[65] The latter afferents are classic pain receptors, responding to intense mechanical and thermal stimuli and to irritant chemicals. C-polymodal nociceptor units are involved with hyperalgesia and itch. They are responsible, through the local release of vasoactive agents, for the flare around skin injuries.[65, 180, 197]

PRURITUS

Pruritus, or itching, is an unpleasant sensation that provokes the desire to scratch.[65, 180, 196] It is the most common symptom in dermatology and may be due to specific dermatologic diseases or may be generalized without clinically evident skin disease. Pruritus may be sharp and well localized (epicritic), or it may be poorly localized and have a burning quality (protopathic).

The skin is richly endowed by a network of sensory nerves and receptors (see Fig. 1–43). The sensory nerves subserve hair follicles as well as encapsulated structures such as Pacini's, Meissner's, and Ruffini's corpuscles.[65] In addition, sensory nerves may end as free nerve endings, referred to as *penicillate* nerve endings. The penicillate endings arise from the terminal Schwann cell in the dermis as tuftlike structures and give rise to an arborizing network of fine nerves, and they terminate either subepidermally or intraepidermally. These unmyelinated penicillate nerve endings are limited to the skin, mucous membranes, and cornea.

Although several morphologically distinct end organs have been described, a specific end organ for pruritus has not been found. There is a clear association between C-polymodal nociceptor activation and itch that appears to involve a subpopulation of specific itch afferent fibers.[65, 197]

On the basis of the properties of afferent units, somatosensory activity can be subdivided into mechanoreceptors, thermoreceptors, and nociceptors.[65] The nociceptors are involved in itch and pain. Nociceptors are supplied by A δ and C fibers. The A δ fibers (myelinated) conduct at about 10 to 20 m/sec and carry signals for spontaneous (physiologic), well-localized, pricking itch (epicritic itch). The C fibers (nonmyelinated) conduct more slowly (2 m/sec) and subserve unpleasant, diffuse burning (pathologic) itch (protopathic itch). Both fibers enter the dorsal root of the spinal cord, ascend in the dorsal column, and cross to the lateral spinothalamic tract. From there, they ascend to the thalamus and, via the internal capsule, to the sensory cortex. There, the itch sensation may be modified by emotional factors and competing cutaneous sensations.

At present, it has not been possible to isolate a universal mediator to explain pruritus, but a host of chemical mediators have been implicated (Table 1–3).[65, 178, 179] However, the pathophysiology of pruritus is complicated and poorly understood for most diseases in most species. The relative importance of these putative mediators and modulators of pruritus in any given species, disease, or individual is rarely known.

For years it has been stated, on the basis of studies performed in humans, that proteolytic enzymes are the most important mediators of pruritus in dogs and cats, and that histamine is relatively unimportant. Although there is no evidence to support the importance of proteolytic enzymes in dogs and cats, clinical studies have suggested that histamine and leukotrienes are important, and more so in cats than in dogs (see Chap. 8).[178, 179]

Central factors such as anxiety, boredom, or competing cutaneous sensations (e.g., pain, touch, heat, and cold) can magnify or reduce the sensation of pruritus by selectively acting on the gate-control system.[65] For instance, pruritus is often worse at night because other sensory input is low. Although the mechanisms involved here are not clear, it has been suggested that stressful conditions may potentiate pruritus through the release of various opioid peptides (central opinergic pruritus).[65] Various neuropeptides, such as en-

● Table 1–3 **MEDIATORS AND MODULATORS OF PRURITUS**

HISTAMINE	PROTEASES	PEPTIDES
Eicosanoids	Kallikrein	Bradykinin
Leukotrienes	Cathepsins	Neuropeptides (opioids)
Prostaglandins	Trypsin	Substance P
Serotonin	Chymotrypsin	Vasoactive intestinal peptide
Platelet-activating factor	Fibrinolysin	
	Leukopeptidases	
	Plasmin	
	Microbial proteases	

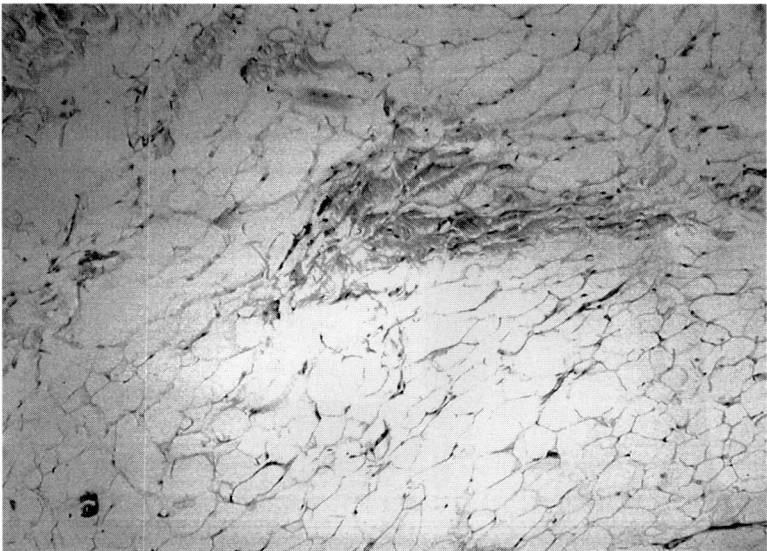

FIGURE 1-45. Dog skin. Normal adipose tissue.

kephalins, endorphins, and substance P, have been demonstrated to participate in the regulation of such cutaneous reactions as pruritus, pain, flushing, pigmentary changes, and inflammation.[65]

Subcutis

The subcutis (hypodermis) is of mesenchymal origin and is the deepest and usually thickest layer of the skin.* However, there is no subcutis in some areas for functional reasons (e.g., lip, cheek, eyelid, external ear, and anus); in these areas, the dermis is in direct contact with musculature and fascia. Fibrous bands that are continuous with the fibrous structures of the dermis penetrate and lobulate the subcutaneous fat into lobules of lipocytes (adipocytes, or fat cells) (Fig. 1-45) and form attachments of the skin to underlying fibrous skeletal components such as fascial sheets and periosteum. The superficial portion of the subcutis projects into the overlying dermis as papillae adiposae (Fig. 1-46); these structures surround hair follicles, sweat glands, and vasculature to assist in protecting these structures from pressure and shearing forces. The subcutis is about 90% triglyceride by weight, and it functions (1) as an energy reserve, (2) in thermogenesis and insulation, (3) as a protective padding and support, and (4) in maintaining surface contours. It is also important as a steroid reservoir and as the site of steroid metabolism and estrogen production. The mature lipocyte is dominated by a large lipid droplet that leaves only a thin cytoplasmic rim and pushes the nucleus to one side.

The walls of arterial and venous capillaries present in fat are much thinner than those present in the dermis, and veil cells are not always present.[22] In addition, there are no lymphatics present in fat lobules.[162] The thickness of the subcutis is inversely proportional to blood flow, with slow circulation promoting lipogenesis and fast circulation promoting lipolysis.[162] As a result of these factors, fat is particularly susceptible to disease processes and, with even minor injury, damage occurs in the absence of an efficient system for removing the damaged tissue.

---

*See references 160, 162, 166, 170, 172, 180, 188, and 202.

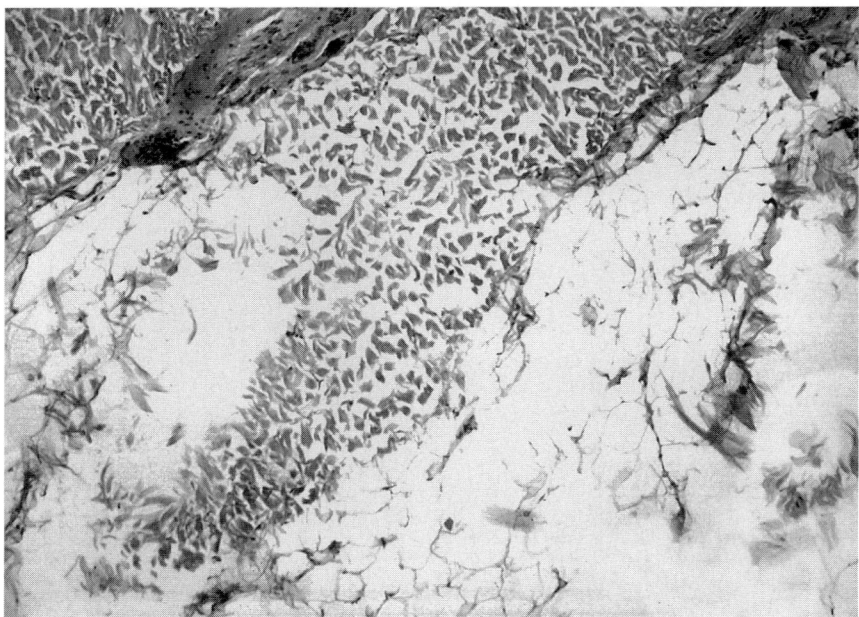

FIGURE 1–46. Dog skin. Papillae adiposae project upward into dermis toward the adnexae.

INTERMEDIATE FILAMENTS

Intermediate filaments are major cytoskeletal proteins. Immunohistochemical studies of tissues from normal dogs and cats have demonstrated typical mammalian staining patterns for cytokeratin, vimentin, desmin, and neurofilament.[46, 47, 165, 198]

Senility

Mechanistically, aging appears to result, in part, from genetically predetermined programs, and in part, from endogenous and exogenous wear and tear, with both processes expressed at the cellular and molecular levels.[214]

Senile changes have been reported in the skin of aged dogs[16] and cats.[172] The hair of some dogs was dull and lusterless, with areas of alopecia and callus formation over pressure points. An increase in the number of white hairs on the muzzle and body was often seen. The footpads and noses of some dogs were hyperkeratotic, and claws tended to become malformed and brittle.

Histologically, one may see orthokeratotic hyperkeratosis of the epidermis and hair follicles, the latter often being atrophic and containing no hairs. Atrophy of the epidermis may be manifested as a single layer of flattened keratinocytes with pyknotic nuclei. Dermal changes may include decreased cellularity, fragmentation and granular degeneration of collagen bundles, and occasional diminution and fragmentation of elastic fibers. The solar elastosis (basophilic degeneration of elastic fibers) that characterizes aging human skin is not usually seen in aged dogs and cats. It is probable that the dense haircoat of dogs and cats protects them from the damaging effects of ultraviolet light.

Variable changes may be seen in the glands of the skin, including cystic dilatation of epitrichial sweat glands and large, yellow, refractile granules in the secretory cells of the epitrichial sweat glands. Arrector pili muscles become more eosinophilic, fragmented, and vacuolated (Fig. 1–47).

Extensive studies in humans have demonstrated the following changes in senile skin: (1) epidermal atrophy, decreased adherence of corneocytes, and flattening of the dermo-epidermal junction; (2) decreased numbers of melanocytes and Langerhans' cells; (3)

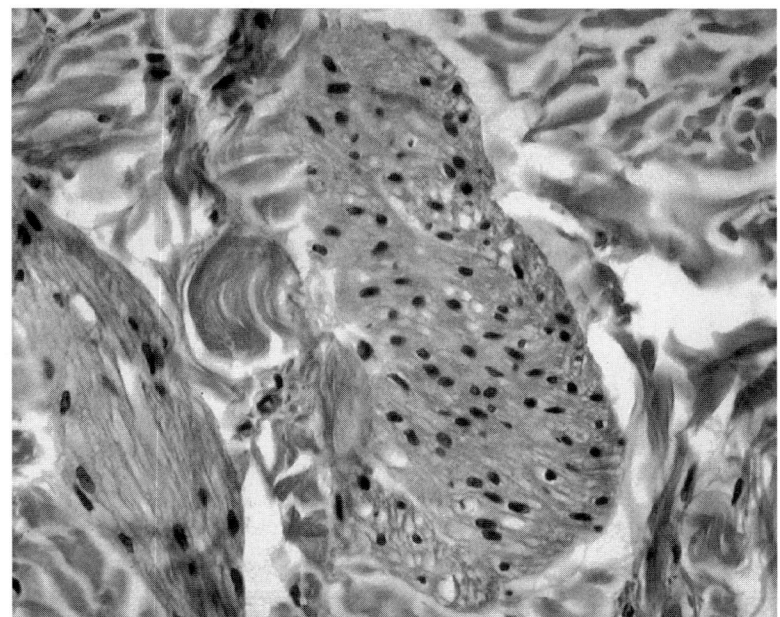

FIGURE 1–47. Arrector pili in normal skin from 9-year-old dog. Note numerous, variably sized, randomly scattered clear vacuoles within muscle section.

dermal atrophy (relatively acellular and avascular) and altered dermal collagen, elastin, and glycosaminoglycans; (4) atrophy of the subcutis; (5) attenuation of the eccrine and apocrine glands and decreased sebaceous gland secretion; (6) reduction of hair follicle density; (7) thinning, ridging, and lusterless nail plates; (8) decreased growth rate of the epidermis, hair, and nails; (9) delayed wound healing; (10) reduced dermal clearance of fluids and foreign materials; (11) compromised vascular responsiveness; (12) diminished eccrine and apocrine secretions; (13) reduced sensory perception; (14) reduced vitamin D production; (15) and impairment of the cutaneous immune and inflammatory responses.[65] Clinical correlates in humans of these intrinsic aging changes of the skin include alopecia, pallor, xerosis (dry skin), increased incidence of benign and malignant neoplasms, increased susceptibility to blister formation, predisposition to injury of the dermis and underlying tissues, increased risk of wound infections, and thermoregulatory disturbances.[65] Wounds in aged beagles and boxers healed less rapidly than in young dogs.[146]

Heterozygosity

Loss of heterozygosity is a genetic mechanism by which a heterozygous somatic cell becomes either homozygous or hemizygous because the corresponding wild-type allele is lost.[73a] Loss of heterozygosity has been documented or postulated to be causative in various neoplasms (basal cell carcinoma, melanoma, squamous cell carcinoma), benign nevi (hamartomas), and a variety of dermatoses characterized by pronounced segmental occurrences.

• REFERENCES

1. Affolter VK, Moore PF: Canine histiocytic proliferative disease. Proc Annu Memb Meet Am Acad Vet Dermatol Am Coll Vet Dermatol 15:79, 1999.
2. Al-Bagdadi FA, et al: Hair follicle cycle and shedding in male beagle dogs. Am J Vet Res 38:611, 1977.
3. Al-Bagdadi FA, et al: Histology of the hair cycle in male beagle dogs. Am J Vet Res 40:1734, 1979.
4. Alhaidari Z, von Tscharner C: Anatomie et physiologie du follicule pileux chez les carnivores domestiques. Prat Méd Chir Anim Comp 32:181, 1997.
5. Ansel JC, et al: Interactions of the skin and nervous system. J Invest Dermatol Symp Proc 2:23, 1997.
6. Aoki T: Stimulation of the sweat glands in the hairy skin of dogs by adrenaline, noradrenaline, acetylcho-

line, mecholyl and pilocarpine. J Invest Dermatol 24: 545, 1955.
7. Aoki T, Wada M: Functional activity of the sweat glands in the hairy skin of the dog. Science 114:123, 1951.
8. Arbiser JL: Angiogenesis and the skin: A primer. J Am Acad Dermatol 34:486, 1996.
9. Badawi H, et al: Morphogenesis of the cutaneous vasculature in fetal dogs. Assiut Vet Med J 18:30, 1987.
10. Badawi H, et al: Histogenesis of the pilosebaceous apparatus in dogs. Assiut Vet Med J 18:38, 1987.
11. Bailey CS, et al: Cutaneous innervation of the thorax and abdomen of the dog. Am J Vet Res 45:1689, 1984.
12. Bailey CS, et al: Spinal nerve root origins of the cutaneous nerves of the canine pelvic limb. Am J Vet Res 49:115, 1988.
13. Baker BB, et al: Epidermal cell renewal in the dog. Am J Vet Res 34:93, 1973.
14. Baker BB, et al: Epidermal cell renewal in dogs after clipping of the hair. Am J Vet Res 35:445, 1974.
15. Baker BB, Maibach HI: Epidermal cell renewal in seborrheic skin of dogs. Am J Vet Res 48:726, 1987.
16. Baker KP: Senile changes of dog skin. J Small Anim Pract 8:49, 1967.
17. Baker KP: Hair growth and replacement in the cat. Br Vet J 130:327, 1974.
18. Beadleston DL, et al: Chymase and tryptase staining of normal feline skin and of feline cutaneous mast cell tumors. Vet Allergy Clin Immunol 5:54, 1997.
18a. Becker AB, et al: Mast cell heterogeneity in dog skin. Anat Rec 213:477, 1985.
19. Bell RL, et al: Oxidative metabolism in perfused surviving dog skin. J Invest Dermatol 31:13, 1958.
20. Bell M, Montagna W: Innervation of sweat glands in horses and dogs. Br J Dermatol 86:160, 1972.
21. Berardesca E, Borroni G: Instrumental evaluation of cutaneous hydration. Clin Dermatol 13:323, 1995.
22. Berardesca E, et al: Bioengineering of the Skin: Cutaneous Blood Flow and Erythema. CRC Press, Boca Raton, FL, 1995.
23. Bernstein EF, Uitto J: The effect of photodamage in dermal extracellular matrix. Clin Dermatol 14:143, 1996.
24. Boiron G, et al. Phagocytosis of erythrocytes by human and animal epidermis. Dermatologica 165:158, 1982.
24a. Borradori L, Sonnenberg A: Structure and function of hemidesmosomes: More than simple adhesion complexes. J Invest Dermatol 112:411, 1999.
25. Botchkarev VA, et al: Neurotrophin-3 involvement in the regulation of hair follicle morphogenesis. J Invest Dermatol 111:279, 1998.
26. Brusilow SW, Munger B: Comparative physiology of sweat. Proc Soc Exp Biol Med 110:317, 1962.
27. Burchill SA: Regulation of tyrosinase in hair follicular melanocytes of the mouse during the synthesis of eumelanin and phaeomelanin. Ann NY Acad Sci 642: 396, 1991.
28. Butler WF, Wright AI: Hair growth in the greyhound. J Small Anim Pract 22:655, 1981.
29. Cannon AG, et al: Gamma delta T cells in normal and diseased canine skin. In: Kwochka KW, et al (eds). Advances in Veterinary Dermatology III. Butterworth-Heinnemann, Boston, 1998, p 137.
30. Chambers MR, et al: The structure and function of the slowly adapting type II mechanoreceptor in hairy skin. Q J Exp Physiol 57:417, 1972.
31. Chesney CJ: Water: its form, function and importance in the skin of domestic animals. J Small Anim Pract 34:65, 1993.
32. Chesney CJ: Measurement of skin hydration in normal dogs and in dogs with atopy or a scaling dermatosis. J Small Anim Pract 36:305, 1995.
33. Chesney CJ: Mapping the canine skin: a study of coat relative humidity in Newfoundland dogs. Vet Dermatol 7:35, 1996.
34. Chesney CJ: The microclimate of the canine coat: The effects of heating on coat and skin temperature and relative humidity. Vet Dermatol 8:183, 1997.
35. Chikakane K, Takahashi H: Measurement of skin pH and its significance in cutaneous disases. Clin Dermatol 13:299, 1995.
36. Chuong CM, et al: Adhesion molecules in skin development: Morphogenesis of feather and hair. Ann NY Acad Sci 642:263, 1991.
37. Clarys P, Barel A: Quantitative evaluation of skin surface lipids. Clin Dermatol 13:307, 1995.
38. Cochet P, et al: Skin distribution of fipronil by microautoradiography following topical administration to the beagle dog. Eur J Drug Metab Pharmacokinet 22: 211, 1997.
39. Comben N: Observations on the mode of growth of the hair of the dog. Br Vet J 107:231, 1951.
40. Cotton DWK, van Hasselt P: Sweating on the hairy surface of the beagle. J Invest Dermatol 59:313, 1972.
41. Cotton DWK, et al: Nature of the sweat glands in the hairy skin of the Beagle. Dermatologica 150:75, 1975.
42. Couchman JR, et al: Proteoglycans and glycoproteins in hair follicle development and cycling. Ann NY Acad Sci 642:243, 1991.
43. Couchman JR, et al: Fibronectin-cell interactions. J Invest Dermatol 94:7S, 1990.
44. Cox HU, et al: Distribution of staphylococcal species on clinically healthy cats. Am J Vet Res 46:1824, 1985.
45. Credille KM, et al: The use of hair plucking to assess canine hair follicle regeneration: Implications for the bulge activation hypothesis. Proc Annu Memb Meet Am Acad Vet Dermatol Am Coll Vet Dermatol 14: 119, 1998.
46. De Las Mulas JM, et al: Immunohistochemical distribution of vimentin, desmin, glial fibrillary acidic protein and neurofilament proteins in feline tissues. J Vet Med A 41:1, 1994.
47. De Las Mulas JM, et al: Immunohistochemical distribution of keratin proteins in feline tissues. J Vet Med A 41:283, 1994.
47a. De Los Monteros AE, et al: Coordinate expression of cytokeratins 7 and 20 in feline and canine carcinomas. Vet Pathol 36:179, 1999.
47b. DeMora F, et al: Canine cutaneous mast cell dispersion and histamine secretory characterization. Vet Immunol Immunopathol 39:421, 1993.
48. Devriese LA, et al: Identification and characterization of staphylococci isolated from cats. Vet Microbiol 9: 279, 1984.
49. Draize HH: The determination of the pH of the skin of man and common laboratory animals. J Invest Dermatol 5:77, 1942.
50. Dunstan RW: A pathomechanistic approach to diseases of the hair follicle. Br Vet Dermatol Study Grp 17:37, 1995.
51. Elder D, et al: Lever's Histopathology of the Skin VIII. Lippincott-Raven Publishers, Philadelphia, 1997.
52. Elsner P, et al: Bioengineering of the Skin: Water

and the Stratum Corneum. CRC Press, Boca Raton, FL, 1994.
52a. Emerson JL, Cross RF: The distribution of mast cells in normal canine skin. Am J Vet Res 26:1379, 1965.
53. Eun HC: Evaluation of skin blood flow by laser Doppler flowmetry. Clin Dermtol 13:337, 1995.
54. Feinman JM: The Rex cat: A mutation for the masses. Vet Med (SAC) 78:1717, 1983.
55. Ferrer L, et al: Immunocytochemical demonstration of intermediate filament proteins, S-100 protein and CEA in apocrine sweat glands and apocrine gland derived lesions of the dog. J Vet Med A 37:569, 1990.
56. Fine JD: Structure and antigenicity of the skin basement membrane zone. J Cutan Pathol 18:401, 1991.
57. Fitzpatrick TB, et al: Dermatology in General Medicine, 3rd ed. McGraw-Hill Book Co., New York, 1993.
57a. Foster AP: A study of the number and distribution of cutaneous mast cells in cats with disease not affecting the skin. Vet Dermatol 5:17, 1994.
58. Foster KA: Composition of the secretion from the eccrine sweat glands of the cat's foot pad. J Physiol 184:66, 1966.
59. Gallo RL, Huttner KM: Antimicrobial peptides: An emerging concept in cutaneous biology. J Invest Dermatol 111: 739, 1998.
60. Garrot C: Les techniques peroxydase-antiperoxydase et immunofluorescence directe appliquée à la détection d'immunoglobulines et de complément C3 dans la peau saine du chien. Proc GEDAC 7:14, 1991.
61. Garthwaite G, et al: Location of immunoglobulins and complement (C3) at the surface and within the skin of dogs. J Comp Pathol 93:185, 1983.
62. Gibson WT, et al: Immunology of the hair follicle. Ann NY Acad Sci 642:291, 1991.
63. Gillian AC, et al: The human hair follicle: A reservoir of CD40+ B7-deficient Langerhans cells that repopulate epidermis after UVB exposure. J Invest Dermatol 110:422, 1998.
64. Goebeler M, et al: The chemokine repertoire of human dermal microvascular endothelial cells and its regulation by inflammatory cytokines. J Invest Dermatol 108:445, 1997.
65. Goldsmith LA (ed): Physiology, Biochemistry, and Molecular Biology of the Skin, 2nd ed. Oxford University Press, New York, 1991.
66. Gottschaldt KM, et al: Functional characteristics of mechanoreceptors in sinus hair follicles of the cat. J Physiol 235:287, 1973.
67. Guaguère E, et al: Troubles de la pigmentation mélanique des carnivores Ire partie: Éléments de physiopathologie. Point Vét 17:549, 1985.
68. Gunaratnam P, Wilkinson GT: A study of normal hair growth in the dog. J Small Anim Pract 24:445, 1983.
69. Halata Z: Postnatale Entwicklung sensibler Nervenendigungen in der Unbehaarten Nasenhaut der Katze. Bibl Anat 19:210, 1981.
70. Hale PA: Periodic hair shedding by a normal bitch. J Small Anim Pract 23:345, 1982.
71. Hales JM, Camp RD: Potent T cell stimulatory material with antigenic properties in stratum corneum of normal human skin. J Invest Dermatol 110:725, 1998.
72. Halprin KM, Chow DC: Metabolic pathways in perfused dog skin. J Invest Dermatol 36:431, 1961.
73. Headington JT, Cerio R: Dendritic cells and the dermis: 1990. Am J Dermatopathol 12:217, 1990.
73a. Happle R: Loss of heterozygosity in human skin. J Am Acad Dermatol 41:143, 1999.
74. Hekmatpanah J: Organization of tactile dermatomes, C1 through L4 in cat. J Neurophysiol 24:129, 1961.
75. Hendriks WH, et al: Seasonal hair growth in the adult domestic cat (Felis catus). Comp Biochem Physiol 116A:29, 1997.
76. Hensel H: Thermoreception and Temperature Regulation. Academic Press, New York, 1981.
77. Hobson DW: Dermal and Ocular Toxicology. Fundamentals and Methods. CRC Press, Boca Raton, FL, 1991.
78. Hohl D, et al: In vitro and rapid in situ transglutaminase assays for congenital ichthyoses—a comparative study. J Invest Dermatol 110:268, 1998.
79. Holbrook KA, Minami SI: Hair follicle embryogenesis in the human. Characterization of events in vivo and in vitro. Ann NY Acad Sci 642:167, 1991.
80. Huff JC: Epithelial polymeric immunoglobulin receptors. J Invest Dermatol 94:74S, 1990.
81. Iggo A, Muir AR: The structure and function of a slowly adapting touch corpuscle in hairy skin. J Physiol 200:763, 1969.
82. Irwin DHG: Tension lines in the skin of the dog. J Small Anim Pract 7:593, 1966.
83. Isitor GN, Weinman DE: Origin and early development of canine circumanal glands. Am J Vet Res 40: 487, 1979.
84. Itum S, et al: Mechanism of action of androgen in dermal papilla cells. Ann NY Acad Sci 642:385, 1991.
85. Ivanyi D, et al: Patterns of expression of feline cytokeratins in healthy epithelia and mammary carcinoma cells. Am J Vet Res 53:304, 1992.
86. Iwabuchi T: General sweating on the hairy skin of the dog and its mechanism. J Invest Dermatol 49:61, 1967.
87. Iwasaki T: An electron microscopic study on secretory process in canine apocrine sweat gland. Jpn J Vet Sci 43:733, 1981.
88. Iwasaki T: Electron microscopy of the canine apocrine sweat duct. Jpn J Vet Sci 45:739, 1983.
89. Iwasaki T, et al: Expression of basement membrane macromolecules and integrin receptors by keratinocytes during canine wound healing. In: Kwochka KW, et al (eds): Advances in Veterinary Dermatology III. Butterworth-Heinemann, Boston, 1998, p 339.
90. Iwaskai T, et al: Immunomapping of basement membrane zone macromolecules in canine salt-split skin. J Vet Med Sci 59:391, 1997.
91. Jackson R: The lines of Blashko: A review and reconsideration. Br J Dermatol 95:349, 1976.
92. Jenkinson DM, Blackburn PA: The distribution of nerves, monoamine oxidase and cholinesterase in the skin of the dog and cat. Res Vet Sci 9:521, 1968.
93. Jenkinson DM: Myoepithelial cells of the sweat glands of domestic animals. Res Vet Sci 12:152, 1971.
94. Jenkinson DM: Sweat and sebaceous glands and their function in domestic animals. In: von Tscharner C, Halliwell REW (eds): Advances in Veterinary Dermatology 1. Baillière Tindall, Philadelphia, 1990, p 229.
95. Kalaher KM, et al: Direct immunofluorescence testing of normal feline nasal planum and footpad. Cornell Vet 80:105, 1990.
96. Kang S, et al: Pharmacology and molecular action of retinoids and vitamin D in skin. J Invest Dermatol Symp Proc 1:15, 1996.
97. Karasek MA: Mechanisms of angiogenesis in normal and diseased skin. Int J Dermatol 30:831, 1991.
98. Kealey T, et al: Intermediary metabolism of the human hair follicle. Ann NY Acad. Sci 642:301, 1991.
99. Kitchell RL, et al: Electrophysiologic studies of the

cutaneous nerves of the thoracic limb of the dog. Am J Vet Res 41:61, 1980.
100. Kobayashi S, et al: Experimental studies on the hemitrichosis and the nervous influences on the hair growth. Acta Neuroreg 18:169, 1958.
101. Konig M, et al: Micromorphology of the circumanal glands and the tail gland area of dogs. Vlaams Diergeneesk Tijdschr 54:278, 1985.
102. Kral F, Schwartzman RM: Veterinary and Comparative Dermatology. J.B. Lippincott Co, Philadelphia, 1964.
102a. Kube P, et al: Distribution, density, and heterogeneity of canine mast cell depending on fixation techniques. Histochem Cell Biol 110:129, 1998.
103. Kubilus J, et al: Involucrin-like proteins in non-primates. J Invest Dermatol 94:210, 1990.
104. Kuhn RA: Organization of tactile dermatomes in cat and monkey. J Neurophysiol 16:169, 1953.
105. Kwochka KW: Differential diagnosis of feline miliary dermatitis. In Kirk RW (ed): Current Veterinary Therapy, 9th ed. W.B. Saunders Co., Philadelphia, 1986, p. 538.
106. Kwochka KW, Rademakers AM: Cell proliferation of epidermis, hair follicles, and sebaceous glands of beagles and cocker spaniels with healthy skin. Am J Vet Res 50:587, 1989.
107. Kwochka KW: The structure and function of epidermal lipids. Vet Dermatol 4:151, 1993.
108. Lane EB, et al: Stem cells in hair follicles. Cytoskeletal studies. Ann NY Acad Sci 642:197, 1991.
109. Lavker RM, et al: Hair follicle stem cells: Their location, role in hair cycle, and involvement in skin tumor formation. J Invest Dermatol 101:16s, 1993.
110. Leigh IM, et al: The Keratinocyte Handbook. Cambridge University Press, New York, 1994.
111. Levine N: Pigmentation and Pigmentary Disorders. CRC Press, Boca Raton, FL, 1993.
112. Lichti U: Hair follicle transglutaminases. Ann NY Acad Sci 642:82, 1991.
113. Lighnter VA: Tenascin: does it play a role in epidermal morphogenesis and homeostasis? J Invest Dermatol 102:273, 1994.
114. Lindholm JS, et al: Variation of skin surface lipid composition among mammals. Comp Biochem Physiol [B]. 69:75, 1981.
115. Little CC: The Inheritance of Coat Color in Dogs. Comstock Publishing Associates, Ithaca, NY, 1957.
116. Lloyd DH, Garthwaite G: Epidermal structure and surface topography of canine skin. Res Vet Sci 33:99, 1982.
117. Lovell JE, Getty R: The hair follicle, epidermis, dermis, and skin glands of the dog. Am J Vet Res 18:873, 1957.
118. Luger TA, et al: The role of α-melanocyte-stimulating hormone in cutaneous biology. J Invest Dermatol Symp Proc 2:87, 1997.
119. Lyne AG, Short BF: Biology of the Skin and Hair Growth. American Elsevier Publishing Co., New York, 1965.
120. Machida H, et al: Histochemical and pharmacological properties of the sweat glands of the dog. Am J Vet Res 117:566, 1966.
121. Maita K, Ishida K: Structure and development of the perianal gland of the dog. Jpn J Vet Sci 37:349, 1975.
122. Manning TO, et al: Cutaneous laser-Doppler velocimetry in nine animal species. Am J Vet Res 52:1960, 1991.
123. Marchal T, et al: CD18 Birbeck granule containing dendritic cells present in dog epidermis are equivalent of human epidermal Langerhans cells. Eur J Dermatol 3:148, 1993.
124. Marchal T, et al: Immunophenotypic and ultrastructural evidence of Langerhans cell origin of the canine cutaneous histiocytoma. Acta Anat 153:189, 1995.
125. Marchal T, et al: Quantitative assessment of feline epidermal Langerhans cells. Br J Dermatol 136:961, 1997.
126. Marchal ISA, et al: Immunophenotypic characterization of feline Langerhans cells. Vet Immunol Immunopathol 58:1, 1997.
127. Mason IS, Lloyd DH: Scanning electron microscopical studies of the living epidermis and stratum corneum in dogs. In: Ihrke PJ, et al (eds): Advances in Veterinary Dermatology II. Pergamon Press, Oxford, 1993, p 131.
128. McMillan JR, et al: Hemidesmosomes show abnormal association with the keratin filament network in junctional forms of epidermolysis bullosa. J Invest Dermatol 110:132, 1998.
129. Meyer W, Neurand K: The distribution of enzymes in the epidermis of the domestic cat. Arch Dermatol Res 260:29, 1977.
130. Meyer W, Neurand K: Zur Leuzinaminopeptidaseaktivitat in normaler und geschadigter Katzenhaut. Zentrabl Vetarinarmed [B] 24:601, 1977.
131. Meyer W, et al: Zur Struktur und Funkten der Fussballen der Katze. Kleintierpraxis 35:67, 1990.
132. Meyer W, Neurand K: Comparison of skin pH in domesticated and laboratory mammals. Arch Dermatol Res 283:16, 1991.
133. Meyer W, et al: A computer-assisted method for the determination of hair cuticula patterns in mammals. Berl Munch Tierärztl Wochenschr 110:81, 1997.
134. Miller SJ, et al: Re-epithelialization of porcine skin by the sweat apparatus. J Invest Dermatol 110:13, 1998.
135. Montagna W: Comparative anatomy and physiology of the skin. Arch Dermatol 96:357, 1967.
136. Moore PF, et al: The use of immunological reagents in defining the pathogenesis of canine skin diseases involving proliferation of leukocytes. In: Kwochka KW, et al (eds). Advances in Veterinary Dermatology III. Butterworth-Heinemann, Boston, 1998, p 77.
137. Mundt HC, Stafforst C: Production and composition of dog hair. In: Edney ATB (ed): Nutrition, Malnutrition and Dietetics on the Dog and Cat. British Veterinary Association and Waltham Centre for Pet Nutrition, London, 1987, p 62.
138. Nestle FO, Nicoloff BJ: A fresh morphological and functional look at dermal dendritic cells. J Cutan Pathol 22:385, 1995.
139. Nicolaides N, et al: The skin surface lipids of man compared with those of eighteen species of animals. J Invest Dermatol 51:83, 1968.
140. Nicolaides N, et al: Diesterwaxes in surface lipids of animal skin. Lipids 5:299, 1970.
141. Neilsen SW: Glands of the canine skin—morphology and distribution. Am J Vet Res 14:448, 1953.
142. Nikkari T: Comparative chemistry of sebum. J Invest Dermatol 62:257, 1974.
143. Noble WC: The Skin Microflora and Microbial Skin Disease. Cambridge University Press, Cambridge, England, 1993.
144. O'Guin WM, Manabe M: The role of trichohyalin in hair follicle differentiation and its expression in nonfollicular epithelia. Ann NY Acad Sci 642:51, 1991.
145. Ohashi T, et al: Effects of vibratory stimulation and

145. mechanical massage on micro- and lymph-circulation in the acupuncture points between the paw pads of anesthetized dogs. Recent Advances in Cardiovascular Diseases. Osaka National Cardiovascular Center, Osaka, 1991, p 125.
146. Orentreich N, Selmanowitz VJ: Levels of biological functions with aging. Trans NY Acad Sci 31:992, 1969.
147. Paus R, et al: Neural mechanisms of hair growth control. J Invest Dermatol Symp. Proc 2:61, 1997.
148. Peaston AE, et al: Evaluation of commercially available antibodies to cytokeratin. Intermediate filaments and laminin in normal cat pinna. J Vet Diagn Invest 4:306, 1992.
149. Pittelkow MR: Growth factors in cutaneous biology and disease. Adv Dermatol 7:55, 1992.
150. Priestley GC: Molecular Aspects of Dermatology. John Wiley and Sons, New York, 1993.
151. Prieur DJ, Collier LL: The Maltese dilution of cats. Feline Pract 14:23, 1984.
152. Queinnec B: Nomenclatures des robes du chat. Rev Méd Vét 134:349, 1983.
153. Rach J: Coat color and personality. Cat Fancy, July 1988, p 58.
154. Restano L, et al: Blashko lines of the face: A step closer to completing the map. J Am Acad Dermatol 39:1028, 1998.
155. Robinson R: Genetics for Cat Breeders. Pergamon Press, Oxford, England, 1977.
156. Rook AJ, Walton GS: Comparative Physiology and Pathology of the Skin. Blackwell Scientific Publications, Oxford, England, 1965.
157. Roy WE: Role of the sweat gland in eczema in dogs. J Am Vet Med Assoc 124:51, 1954.
158. Ruedisueli FL, et al: The measurement of skin pH in normal dogs of different breeds. In: Kwochka KW, et al (eds): Advances in Veterinary Dermatology III. Butterworth-Heinemann, Boston, 1998, p 521.
159. Rutner D, et al: Merkel cell carcinoma. J Am Acad Dermatol 29:143, 1993.
160. Ryan TJ, Curri SB: The structure of fat. Clin Dermatol 7:37, 1989.
161. Ryan TJ, Mortimer PS: Cutaneous lymphatic system. Clin Dermatol 13:417, 1995.
162. Ryan TJ: Lymphatics and adipose tissue. Clin Dermatol 13:493, 1995.
163. Ryder ML: Seasonal changes in the coat of the cat. Res Vet Sci 21:280, 1976.
164. Saijonmaa-Koulumiès LE, Lloyd DH: Colonization of the canine skin with bacteria. Vet Dermatol 7:153, 1996.
165. Sandusky GE, et al: Immunocytochemical study of tissue from clinically normal dogs and of neoplasms using keratin monoclonal anitbodies. Am J Vet Res 52:613, 1991.
166. Schummer A, et al: The Circulatory System, the Skin, and the Cutaneous Organs of the Domestic Mammals. Verlag Paul Parey, Berlin, 1981.
167. Schwarz R: Haarwachstum und Haarwechsel—eine Zusätzliche funktonelle Beanspruchung der Haut—am Beispiel markhaltiger Primärhaarfollikel. Kleintierpraxis 37:67, 1992.
168. Schwarz R, et al: Die gesunde Haut von Hund und Katze. Kleintierpraxis 37:67, 1992.
169. Schwarz R, et al: Die gesunde Haut von Hund und Katze. Kleintierpraxis 26:395, 1981.
170. Schwarz R, et al: Micromorphology of the skin (epidermis, dermis, subcutis) of the dog. Onderstepoort J Vet Res 46:105, 1979.
171. Schwarz R, et al: Sinus haarwechsel ist nicht gleich Fellhaarwechsel Histologische Untersuchungen am Sinushaarfollikel der Katze. Kleintierpraxis 42:517, 1997.
172. Scott DW: Feline dermatology 1900–1978: A monograph. J Am Anim Hosp Assoc 16:331, 1980.
173. Scott SW: Feline dermatology 1979–1982: Introspective retrospections. J Am Anim Hosp Assoc 20:537, 1984.
174. Scott DW: Feline dermatology 1983–1985: "The secret sits." J Am Anim Hosp Assoc 20:537, 1984.
175. Scott DW, et al: Pitfalls in immunofluorescence testing in canine dermatology. Cornell Vet 73:131, 1983.
176. Scott DW, et al: Pitfalls in immunofluorescence testing in dermatology. II. Pemphigus-like antibodies in the cat, and direct immunofluorescence testing of normal dog nose and lip. Cornell Vet 73:275, 1983.
177. Scott DW: The biology of hair growth and its disturbances. In: von Tscharner C, Halliwell REW (eds): Advances in Veterinary Dermatology 1. Baillière Tindall, Philadelphia, 1990, p 3.
178. Scott DW, Miller WH Jr: Nonsteroidal anti-inflammatory agents in the management of canine allergic pruritus. J S Afr Vet Assoc 64:52, 1993.
179. Scott DW, Miller WH Jr: Medical management of allergic pruritus in the cat, with emphasis on feline atopy. J S Afr Vet Assoc 64:103, 1993.
180. Scott DW, et al: Muller and Kirk's Small Animal Dermatology V. W.B. Saunders, Philadelphia, 1995.
181. Scott GA, Goldsmith LA. Homeobox genes and skin development: A review. J Invest Dermatol 101:3, 1993.
182. Seaman WJ, Chang SH: Dermal perifollicular mineralization of toy poodle bitches. Vet Pathol 21:122, 1984.
183. Sharaf DM, et al: Skin surface lipids of the dog. Lipids 12:786, 1977.
184. Sheretz EC: Misuse of hair analysis as a diagnostic tool. Arch Dermatol 121:1504, 1985.
185. Smack DP, et al: Keratin and keratinization. J Am Acad Dermatol 30:85, 1994.
186. Soma T, et al: Analysis of apoptotic cell death in human hair follicles in vivo and in vitro. J Invest Dermatol 111:948, 1998.
187. Spearman RIC: The Integument. Cambridge University Press, London, England, 1973.
188. Strickland JH, Calhoun ML: The integumentary system of the cat. Am J Vet Res 24:1018, 1963.
189. Suter MM, et al: Extracellular ATP and some of its analogs induce transient rises in cytosolic free calcium in individual canine keratinocytes. J Invest Dermatol 97:223, 1991.
190. Suter MM, et al: Monoclonal antibodies: Cell surface markers for canine keratinocytes. Am J Vet Res 40:1367, 1987.
191. Suter MM, et al: Keratinocyte differentiation in the dog. In: von Tscharner C, Halliwell REW (eds): Advances in Veterinary Dermatology 1. Baillière Tindall, Philadelphia, 1990, p 252.
192. Suter MM, et al: Comparison of growth and differentiation of normal and neoplastic canine keratinocyte cultures. Vet Pathol 28:131, 1991.
193. Suter MM, et al: Keratinocyte biology and pathology. Vet Dermatol 8:67, 1997.
194. Takahashi Y: Functional activity of the eccrine sweat

glands in the toe-pads of the dog. Tohoku J Exp Med 83:205, 1964.
195. Tanaka T, et al: The innermost cells of the outer root sheath in human anagen hair follicles undergo specialized keratinization mediated by apoptosis. J Cutan Pathol 25:316, 1998.
196. Thoday AJ, Friedmann PS: Scientific Basis of Dermatology. A Physiological Approach. Churchill Livingstone, New York, 1986.
197. Tuckett RP, Wei JY: Response to an itch-producing substance in the cat. II. Cutaneous receptor populations with unmyelinated axons. Brain Res 413:95, 1987.
198. Vos JH, et al: An immunohistochemical study of canine tissues with vimentin, desmin, glial fibrillary acidic protein, and neurofilament antisera. Zentralbl Veterinarmed [A] 36:561, 1989.
199. Vos JH, et al: The keratin and vimentin distribution patterns in the epithelial structures of the canine anal region. Anat Rec 234:391, 1992.
200. Vos, JH, et al: The expression of keratins, vimentin, neurofilament proteins, smooth muscle actin, neuron-specific enolase, and synaptophysin in tumors of the specific glands in the canine anal region. Vet Pathol 30:352, 1993.
201. Wallengren J: Vasoactive peptides in the skin. J Invest Dermatol Symp Proc 2:87, 1997.
202. Webb AJ, Calhoun ML: The microscopic anatomy of the skin of mongrel dogs. Am J Vet Res 15:274, 1954.
203. Weinberg WC, et al: Modulation of hair follicle cell proliferation and collagenolytic activity by specific growth factors. Ann NY Acad Sci 642:281, 1991.
203a. Welle M, at al: Distribution, density and heterogeneity of canine and bovine skin mast cells depending on fixation techniques. In: Kwochka KW, et al (eds): Advances in Veterinary Dermatology III, Butterworth-Heinemann, Boston, 1998, p 488.
204. Whalen LR, Kitchell RL: Electrophysiologic studies of the cutaneous nerves of the head of the dog. Am J Vet Res 44:615, 1983.
205. Wheatley VR, Sher DW: Studies of the lipids of dog skin. I. The chemical composition of dog skin lipids. J Invest Dermatol 36:169, 1961.
206. White SD, Yager JA: Resident dendritic cells in the epidermis: Langerhans cells, Merkel cells and melanocytes. Vet Dermatol 6:1, 1995.
207. Wilkie JSN, et al: Morphometric analyses of the skin of dogs with atopic dermatitis and correlations with cutaneous and plasma histamine and total serum IgE. Vet Pathol 27:179, 1990.
208. Wilkinson JE, et al: Long-term cultivation of canine keratinocytes. J Invest Dermatol 88:202, 1987.
209. Wilkinson JE, et al: Ultrastructure of cultured canine oral keratinocytes. Am J Vet Res 50:1161, 1989.
210. Wilkinson JE, et al: Antigen expression in cultured oral keratinocytes from dogs. Am J Vet Res 52:445, 1991.
211. Winkelmann RK, Schmit RW: Cholinesterase in the skin of the rat, dog, cat, guinea pig and rabbit. J Invest Dermatol 33:185, 1959.
212. Winstanley EW: The rate of mitotic division in regenerating epithelium in the dog. Res Vet Sci 18:144, 1975.
213. Wright M, Walter S: The Book of the Cat. Summit Books, New York, 1980.
214. Yaar M: Molecular mechanisms of skin aging. Adv Dermatol 10:63, 1995.
215. Yager JA, Scott DW: The skin and appendages. In: Jubb KVF, et al (eds): Pathology of Domestic Animals, 4th ed, Vol 1. Academic Press, New York, 1993, p 531.
216. Zlotkin SH: Hair analysis. A useful tool or a waste of money? Int J Dermatol 24:161, 1985.

Chapter 2
Diagnostic Methods

• THE SYSTEMATIC APPROACH

Skin diseases are unique in medicine because the lesions and the symptoms are external and potentially visible to the owner and practitioner. This difference offers several unique opportunities for the practitioner. The progression of skin lesions and diseases can often be determined with a good history. Incomplete histories may eventually be amended because the chronic, recurrent nature of many diseases allows the practitioner to instruct clients in what observations they should try to make. The educated client may then add relevant information about the course of the disease. The physical examination reveals the gross pathologic lesions that are present for direct examination. With no other organ system is this great amount of information so readily available.

To benefit optimally from these opportunities, the clinician uses a systematic approach; this greatly increases the probability of determining the correct diagnosis in the most cost-effective manner. Ideally, a thorough examination and appropriate diagnostic procedures are accomplished the first time that the patient is seen and before any masking treatment has been initiated. However, in practice, many clients are reluctant to spend money on diagnostic tests, particularly for the initial occurrence of a problem. This makes a thorough history and physical examination even more important, because they often are the only tools available for arriving at a differential diagnosis.

At the first visit, it is important to establish the client's reliability as a historian and observer. The least expensive tool available to the practitioner is the education of the client about signs and symptoms to look for. The clinician can develop a better relationship with clients and gain valuable information by training clients in what they should observe and watch for, especially if there is a poor response to treatment or a recurrence. Spending some time educating the client in the value of this information often leads to better acceptance of the costs associated with future treatment.

A rational approach to the accurate diagnosis of dermatologic diseases is presented in Table 2–1.

• RECORDS

Recording historical facts, physical examination findings, and laboratory data in a systematic way is particularly important for patients with skin disease. Many dermatoses are chronic, and skin lesions may be slow to change. For this reason, many practitioners use outline sketches of the patient, which enable the clinician to draw the location and the extent of lesions.

Figure 2–1 is a record form for noting physical examination and laboratory findings for dermatology cases. Most important, the form leads the clinician to consider the case in a systematic manner. It also enables one to apply pertinent descriptive terms, saves time, and ensures that no important information is omitted. This form details only dermatologic data and should be used as a supplement to the general history and physical examination record. A special dermatologic history form is also useful, especially for patients with allergies and chronic diseases (Fig. 2–2).

Table 2-1 STEPS TO A DERMATOLOGIC DIAGNOSIS

MAJOR STEP	KEY POINTS TO DETERMINE OR QUESTIONS TO ANSWER
Chief complaint	Why is the client seeking veterinary care?
Signalment	Record the animal's age, breed, sex, and weight
Dermatologic history	Obtain data about the original lesion's location, appearance, onset, and rate of progression. Also determine the degree of pruritus, contagion to other animals or people, and possible seasonal incidence. Relationship to diet and environmental factors and the response to previous medications are also important
Previous medical history	Medical history that does not directly seem to relate should also be reviewed
Client credibility	Determine what the clients initially noticed that indicated a problem. Repeat questions and ask in a different way to determine how certain the clients are and whether they understand the questions
Physical examination	Determine the distribution pattern and the regional location of lesions. Certain patterns are diagnostically significant
	Closely examine the skin to identify primary and secondary lesions
	Determine skin and hair quality (e.g., thin, thick, turgid, elastic, dull, oily, or dry)
	Observe the configurations of specific skin lesions and their relationship to each other
Differential diagnosis	Differential diagnosis is developed on the basis of the preceding data. The most likely diagnoses are recorded in order of probability
Diagnostic or therapeutic plan	A plan is presented to the client. The client and the clinician together then agree on a plan
Diagnostic and laboratory aids	Simple and inexpensive office diagnostic procedures that confirm or rule out any of the most likely (first three or four) differential diagnostic possibilities should be done
	More complex or expensive diagnostic tests or procedures are then recommended
	Clients may elect to forgo these tests and pursue less likely differential diagnostic possibilities in attempts to save money. Often, this approach is not cost effective when the expense of inefficient medications and repeated examination is considered
Trial therapy	Clients may elect to pursue a therapeutic trial instead of diagnostic procedures. Trial therapies should be selected so that further diagnostic information is obtained. Generally, glucocorticoids and progestational drugs are not acceptable because little diagnostic information is obtained
Narrowing the differential diagnosis	Plan additional tests, observations of therapeutic trials, and re-evaluations of signs and symptoms to narrow the list and provide a definitive diagnosis

The disadvantage of the forms is that many chronic cases have tremendous variations in the type of lesions and their distribution, making a map confusing. For example, how would one draw the following alopecia lesion? A 10-cm plaque in the flank fold has a central (8-cm) zone of lichenification, hyperpigmentation, alopecia, and crusts. The outer (2-cm) margin is alopecic and has a papular dermatitis with mild hyperpigmentation of lattice configuration. Peripheral to the plaque are occasional papules and pustules. Representing several different lesions on a small diagram is difficult or, if done, is often unreadable. This can make a diagram unsatisfactory to use. Therefore, the authors have found that brief written descriptions of lesions in various body regions are preferable to diagrams in complicated cases.

● HISTORY

General Concepts

The pet's disease is like an unsolved mystery in which the client is the witness to what has occurred and the veterinarian is the detective who must ascertain what the client ob-

College of Veterinary Medicine, Cornell University, Ithaca, New York 14853
Dermatology

DISTRIBUTION OF LESIONS

Weight: _____

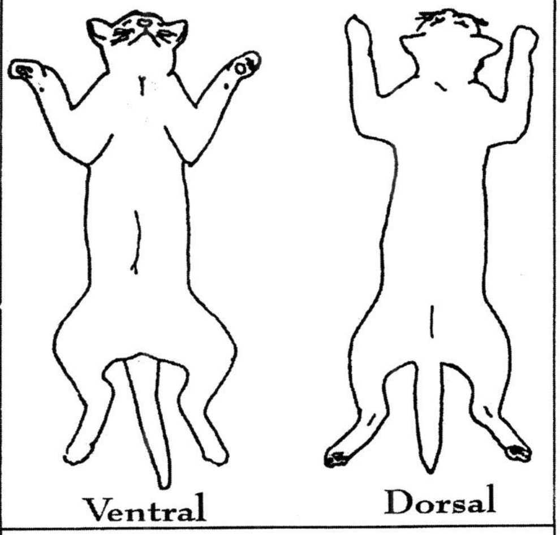

Ventral   Dorsal

PRIMARY LESIONS (Check)

___ Macule   ___ Patch   ___ Purpura   ___ Wheal
___ Papule   ___ Nodule   ___ Plaque   ___ Tumor
___ Pustule   ___ Vesicle   ___ Bullae   ___ Cyst
___ Abscess

SECONDARY LESIONS (Check)

___ Scale   ___ Crust   ___ Alopecia   ___ Erythema
___ Erosion   ___ Ulcer   ___ Fissure   ___ Scar
___ Excoriation   ___ Collarettes   ___ Nikolsky
___ Hyperpigmentation   ___ Hypopigmentation   ___ Callus
___ Hyperkeratosis   ___ Lichenification   ___ Comedo
___ Sinus   ___ Hyperhidrosis   ___ Necrosis

SKIN CHANGES (Check)

___ Normal   ___ Thick   ___ Thin   ___ Fragile
___ Hypotonic   ___ Hyperextensible   ___ Increased Laxity

HAIR COAT CHANGES (Check)

___ Alopecia   ___ Hypotrichosis   ___ Hypertrichosis
___ Dry Coat   ___ Brittle Coat   ___ Oily Coat
___ Easy Epilation: ___ Primary Hairs   ___ Secondary Hairs
                      ___ Both
___ Hair Casts   ___ Color Associated Hair Loss

CONFIGURATION OF LESIONS (Check)

___ Linear   ___ Follicular   ___ Grouped
___ Annular
___ Other: _____

CUTANEOUS PAIN (Check)

___ Absent   ___ Mild   ___ Moderate   ___ Severe

PARASITES (Check)

___ Fleas   ___ Flea Dirt   ___ Lice   ___ Ticks
___ Ear Mites   ___ Other: _____

OTHER FINDINGS

Pinnal-Pedal Reflex _____
Lymph Nodes _____
Ears L _____
     R _____
Oral _____
Anogenital _____
Footpads _____
Claws _____
Other: _____

LABORATORY

Scrape _____
Scotch Tape _____
Fungal Culture _____
Wood's Light _____
Hair Examination _____
Cytology:
1. _____
2. _____
3. _____
4. _____

DIAGNOSIS/DIFFERENTIAL

FIGURE 2–1. Dermatology examination sheet.

PATIENT HISTORY

Client Name: _____ Pet's Name: _____
Chief Complaint: _____
Age of pet when acquired: _____ Age of pet now: _____
How long has your pet had this problem? _____
Is there a time when the problem is less severe or the itching is less intense? _____
_____

What was the problem like initially and where did it start?
  ____Normal skin, just itchy   ____Rash   ____Redness   ____Hair Loss   ____Pimples
  ____Nose   ____Neck   ____Tail   ____Back legs
  ____Around eyes   ____Back   ____Front legs ____Back paws
  ____Ears   ____Rump   ____Front paws ____Chest
  ____Abdomen   ____Groin
Has it spread? ____Yes ____No If so, to what sites: _____

Does your pet scratch, chew, lick, or rub any of the following areas? Please check all that apply:
  ____Nose   ____Neck   ____Tail   ____Back legs
  ____Around eyes   ____Back   ____Front legs ____Back paws
  ____Ears   ____Rump   ____Front paws ____Chest
  ____Abdomen   ____Groin
Comments: _____

Other pets in environment? State how many: _____
  ____Dogs   ____Cats   ____Birds   ____Rabbits
  ____Rodents   ____Large/farm animals - what type? _____
Do any other pets have skin problems? Describe: _____

Do any people in the household have skin problems? ____Yes ____No
Describe: _____
Amount of time pet spends: ____% indoors   ____% outdoors
Are symptoms any worse?   ____indoors   ____outdoors   ____morning   ____night
Do any relatives of your pet have skin problems that you are aware of? ____Yes ____No
Describe: _____
Do you use routine flea control? ____Yes ____No
What types of products to you use? Brand: _____
  ____Powders   ____Dips   ____Sprays   ____Collars   ____Baths
Do you use insecticides in your home? ____Yes ____No
Please list any medications/injections your pet has had for this problem? _____
_____
Did they seem to help? If so, which one(s)? _____
What is your pet's regular diet? _____
What vitamins, supplements, or treats are given? _____
Does your pet do any of the following?
  ____Cough   ____Sneeze   ____Runny eyes   ____Vomit   ____Diarrhea   ____Limp
  ____Drink excessively   ____Urinate excessively
Has your pet ever had an ear infection? ____Yes ____No
Is your pet's appetite normal?   ____Yes ____No
Has it changed recently?   ____Yes ____No
Additional Comments: _____

FIGURE 2–2. Dermatology history sheet.

served. As this information is extracted, the veterinarian becomes the lawyer to determine whether the client is a credible or qualified witness. Obtaining a thorough history and being attentive to clues from the client are skills that must be practiced and developed by the clinician in order to develop a tentative diagnosis. A comprehensive history in conjunction with a thorough dermatologic examination is helpful for another practical reason: This is often when the veterinarian initially establishes her or his credibility as a professional with the client. In veterinary dermatology, the client-veterinarian relationship is often important for a successful outcome. Because many chronic diseases necessitate lifelong control and can be frustrating for client and veterinarian alike, it is critical for the client-veterinarian relationship to start well. If the veterinarian is thorough and obtains the most information possible from the history and the dermatologic examination, the client is more likely to recognize the effort and expertise of the veterinarian. These clients are often more agreeable to pursuing diagnostic tests or trial therapies if the information from the initial exhaustive examination is not sufficient for a diagnosis. Cursory examinations leave a sense of insecurity in some clients, making them reluctant to follow recommendations based on such examinations.

Owner's Chief Complaint

The owner's chief complaint, or chief cause of concern, is often one of the major signs initially used in establishing a differential diagnosis. Addressing the client's chief complaint is an important step in achieving satisfaction of clients and obtaining their confidence and often initiates a favorable client-veterinarian relationship. Other findings not directly related to the chief complaint may be uncovered. Although these additional findings are important to discuss, the client's chief complaint must always be addressed.

Age

Some dermatologic disorders are age related, so age is important in the dermatologic history.[5-8] For example, demodicosis usually begins in young dogs before sexual maturity. Allergies tend to appear in more mature animals, probably because repeated exposure to the antigen must occur and the immune response has to occur before clinical signs develop. Reactivity to intradermal testing in cats has also been correlated with age.[4a] Hormonal disorders tend to occur more frequently in animals between 6 and 10 years of age, and most neoplasms develop in mature to older patients. Most of the ages listed in Table 2-2 refer to the usual age at the beginning of the disease, not necessarily the age at which the animal presents.

Breed

Breed predilection determines the incidence of some skin disorders (Table 2-3).[9, 10] For example, primary seborrhea is common in Cocker spaniels; acanthosis nigricans usually occurs in dachshunds; adult-onset hyposomatotropism occurs in Keeshonds; hypogonadism in intact males is found in Chow Chows; adrenal sex hormone imbalances occur in Pomeranians; dermatomyositis is found in Shetland sheepdogs (shelties) and collies; zinc-responsive dermatosis occurs in Siberian huskies and Alaskan malamutes; and many of the wire-coated terrier breeds (Scottish, Cairn, Sealyham, West Highland White, Irish, and Welsh) seem to be particularly predisposed to allergic skin disease. See Chapter 20 for a review of breed predilections for cutaneous neoplasms.

In a study of dogs in northern California conducted at the University of California at Davis, 31 breeds were found to be at elevated risk for skin diseases, including Doberman pinscher, Irish setter, Dalmatian, Dachshund, Golden retriever, various terrier breeds, Shar pei, Chow Chow, and Akita.[9] In the same study, decreased risk of skin disease was found for dogs of mixed breeding and for 12 purebred breeds, including St. Bernard, standard Poodle, beagle, Basset hound, German shorthaired pointer, Afghan hound, and Australian shepherd.

Table 2-2. SKIN DISEASE WITH FREQUENT AGE-RELATED ONSET (STRONG CLINICAL IMPRESSION)

AGE	DISEASE
Younger than 6 months	Alopecia universalis
	Black hair follicle dysplasia
	Canine muzzle furunculosis
	Cutaneous asthenia
	Demodicosis
	Dermatomyositis
	Dermatophytosis
	Ectodermal defect
	Epidermolysis bullosa
	Hypotrichosis
	Ichthyosis
	Impetigo
	Juvenile cellulitis
	Lymphedema
	Other congenital hereditary defects
	Pituitary dwarfism
	Tyrosinemia
	Viral papillomatosis (oral)
1 to 3 years	Allergic diseases, especially atopy
	Adrenal hyperplasia syndrome
	Color dilution alopecia
	Hyposomatotropism in the mature dog
	Primary idiopathic seborrhea
Older than 6 years	Cushing's disease
	Feminization with testicular tumor
	Neoplasms
Senile dogs	Alopecia
	Decubital ulcer
	Necrolytic migratory erythema
	Thin, fragile skin

Sex

The sex of the patient affects the incidence of certain problems. Obviously, male feminization with testicular tumors occurs only in male animals. Other sex-related problems occur (e.g., circumanal adenomas are seen almost exclusively in male dogs). In addition, sex-related behaviors may affect the incidence of certain diseases, such as abscesses in fighting tomcats. One should determine whether the patient is sexually intact; in intact females, it should be determined whether the skin problem bears any relationship to the estrous cycle.

Color

The color of an animal may also be related to certain problems—most notable is the association of solar dermatitis and squamous cell carcinoma of the pinna in white-eared cats. In addition, solar dermatitis, actinic keratoses, solar-related hemangioma, hemangiosarcoma, and squamous cell carcinoma occur in white-skinned, thinly haired regions of dogs, particularly in white bull terriers, Staffordshire bull terriers (pit bull terriers), boxers, Dalmatians, beagles, Whippets, and Great Danes.

Coat color may also relate to disease, as in color dilution alopecia. Although it is most commonly described in Doberman pinschers, this hair disorder occurs in any breed that has diluted coat colors and may occur in piebald breeds as well.[16a] The color of the eyes and coat may be helpful in diagnosis, as in yellow-eyed, "smoky" Persian cats with the Chédiak-Higashi syndrome. Also, an association between positive intradermal skin test results and coat colors was observed in normal cats.[4a]

Text continued on page 82

Table 2–3. BREED PREDILECTION FOR NON-NEOPLASTIC SKIN DISEASES (STRONG CLINICAL IMPRESSION)

BREED	DISEASE
Abyssinian cat	Follicular dysplasia
	Idiopathic ceruminous otitis externa
	Psychogenic dermatitis or alopecia
Afghan hound	Hypothyroidism
Airedale	Adult-onset demodicosis
	Atopy
	Demodicosis
	Follicular dysplasia, flank
Akita	Pemphigus foliaceus
	Sebaceous adenitis
	Uveodermatologic syndrome
Basenji	Immunoproliferative enteropathy
Basset hound	Atopy
	Malassezia dermatitis
	Seborrhea, primary
	Skin fold intertrigo
Beagle	Atopy
	Demodicosis
	Immunoglobulin A (IgA) deficiency
Belgian sheepdog (Belgian Tervuren)	Sebaceous adenitis
	Vitiligo
Berger de Beauce	Epidermolysis bullosa
Borzoi	Hypothyroidism
Boston terrier	Atopy
	Demodicosis
	Facial fold intertrigo
	Hyperadrenocorticism
	Patterned alopecia
	Tail fold intertrigo
Boxer	Atopy
	Demodicosis
	Food hypersensitivity
	Follicular dysplasia (flank)
	Hyperadrenocorticism
	Hypothyroidism
	Muzzle furunculosis, bacterial
	Pedal furunculosis, bacterial
	Sertoli cell syndrome
	Solar dermatitis (white dogs)
	Sterile pyogranuloma syndrome
	Sternal callus
Brittany spaniel	Complement deficiency
	Discoid lupus erythematosus
	Hypothyroidism
Bullmastiff and Mastiff	Folliculitis and furunculosis, bacterial
Bull terrier	Atopy
	Furunculosis, scarring and bacterial
	Lethal acrodermatitis
	Solar dermatitis
	Zinc-responsive dermatosis
Cavalier King Charles spaniel	Syringohydromelia
Chesapeake Bay retriever	Atopy
	Folliculitis and furunculosis, bacterial
Chihuahua	Demodicosis
	Pinnal thrombovascular necrosis
Chow Chow	Adrenal sex hormone abnormalities
	Pemphigus foliaceus
	Color dilution alopecia
	Demodicosis
	Hyposomatotropism
	Hypothyroidism
	Uveodermatologic syndrome

Table continued on following page

Table 2–3 BREED PREDILECTION FOR NON-NEOPLASTIC SKIN DISEASES (STRONG CLINICAL IMPRESSION) Continued

BREED	DISEASE
Collie	Bullous pemphigoid
	Dermatomyositis
	Discoid lupus erythematosus
	Nasal furunculosis, bacterial
	Pemphigus erythematosus
	Pyotraumatic dermatitis
	Sertoli cell syndrome
	Systemic lupus erythematosus
	Vesicular cutaneous lupus erythematosus
Curly-coated retrievers	Follicular dysplasia
Dachshund	Acanthosis nigricans
	Alopecia areata
	Color dilution alopecia
	Demodicosis
	Folliculitis and pedal furunculosis, bacterial
	Hyperadrenocorticism
	Hypothyroidism
	Idiopathic onychodystrophy
	Juvenile cellulitis
	Linear IgA pustular dermatosis
	Malassezia dermatitis
	Nodular panniculitis (sterile)
	Pattern alopecia (ears)
	Pattern alopecia (ventral)
	Pemphigus foliaceus
	Sterile pyogranuloma syndrome
	Sternal callus
	Vasculitis (idiopathic)
Dalmatian	Atopy
	Demodicosis
	Drug reactions
	Folliculitis and furunculosis, bacterial
	Solar dermatitis
Doberman pinscher	Acral furunculosis, bacterial
	Acral lick dermatitis
	Color dilution alopecia
	Demodicosis
	Drug reaction (sulfas)
	Flank sucking
	Follicular dysplasia
	Folliculitis and pedal furunculosis, bacterial
	Hypothyroidism
	Muzzle furunculosis, bacterial
	Vitiligo
Dogue de Bordeaux	Hereditary footpad hyperkeratosis
	Sterile pyogranuloma syndrome
English bulldog	Atopy
	Demodicosis
	Facial fold intertrigo
	Folliculitis and pedal furunculosis, bacterial
	Follicular dysplasia (flank)
	Hypothyroidism
	Malassezia dermatitis
	Muzzle furunculosis, bacterial
	Sterile pyogranuloma syndrome
	Tail fold intertrigo
German shepherd	Atopy
	Cellulitis (folliculitis and furunculosis), bacterial
	Collagen disorder of footpads
	Contact hypersensitivity
	Discoid lupus erythematosus

Table 2–3 BREED PREDILECTION FOR NON-NEOPLASTIC SKIN DISEASES (STRONG CLINICAL IMPRESSION) Continued

BREED	DISEASE
German shepherd *Continued*	Erythema multiforme
	Familial vasculopathy
	Flea bite hypersensitivity
	Fly dermatitis of ear tips
	Food hypersensitivity
	Lupoid onychodystrophy
	Insect- or arachnid-related eosinophilic furunculosis (face)
	Medullary trichomalacia
	Metatarsal fistulae
	Mucocutaneous bacterial pyoderma
	Nasal furunculosis, bacterial
	Otitis externa
	Pemphigus erythematosus
	Pituitary dwarfism
	Pythiosis
	Seborrhea, primary
	Systemic lupus erythematosus
	Vitiligo
Golden retriever	Acral furunculosis, bacterial
	Acral lick dermatitis
	Atopy
	Folliculitis and furunculosis, bacterial
	Hypothyroidism
	Juvenile cellulitis
	Nasal hypopigmentation
	Pyotraumatic dermatitis
	Pyotraumatic folliculitis and furunculosis, bacterial
	Sterile pyogranuloma syndrome
	Trichoptilosis
Gordon setter	Atopy
	Hypothyroidism
	Juvenile cellulitis
Great Dane	Acral furunculosis, bacterial
	Acral lick dermatitis
	Callus formation, hygroma
	Demodicosis
	Hypothyroidism
	Muzzle furunculosis, bacterial
	Pedal furunculosis, bacterial
	Solar dermatosis in Harlequin
	Sterile pyogranuloma syndrome
Great Pyrenees	Demodicosis
	Pyotraumatic dermatitis
Greyhound	Drug reactions
	Vasculopathy
Himalayan cat	Cheyletiellosis
	Dermatophytosis (*Microsporum canis*)
	Idiopathic facial dermatitis
	Primary seborrhea
Irish setter	Acral furunculosis, bacterial
	Atopy
	Acral lick dermatitis
	Color dilution alopecia
	Folliculitis and furunculosis, bacterial
	Granulocytopathy
	Hypothyroidism
	Seborrhea, primary
Irish water spaniel	Follicular dysplasia
	Idiopathic onychodystrophy
Irish wolfhound	Elbow hygroma
	Hypothyroidism

Table continued on following page

● Table 2–3 **BREED PREDILECTION FOR NON-NEOPLASTIC SKIN DISEASES (STRONG CLINICAL IMPRESSION)** Continued

BREED	DISEASE
Keeshond	Adrenal hyperplasia syndrome
	Hypogonadism of intact male
	Hyposomatotropism
	Hypothyroidism
Labrador retriever	Acral furunculosis, bacterial
	Acral lick dermatitis
	Atopy
	Familial nasal hyperkeratosis
	Folliculitis and furunculosis, bacterial
	Food hypersensitivity
	Pyotraumatic dermatitis
	Seborrhea, primary
	Waterline disease (*Malassezia* dermatitis?)
Lhasa apso	Atopy
	Injection reaction
	Malassezia dermatitis
Malamute	Demodicosis
	Hypothyroidism
	Zinc-responsive dermatosis
Newfoundland	Folliculitis and furunculosis, bacterial
	Hypothyroidism
	Pemphigus foliaceus
	Pyotraumatic dermatitis
Old English sheepdog	Atopy
	Demodicosis
	Drug reactions
	Pedal furunculosis, bacterial
Pekingese	Facial fold intertrigo
	Injection reactions
	Sertoli cell syndrome
Persian cat	Cheyletiellosis
	Dermatophytosis
	Facial fold intertrigo
	Hair mats
	Idiopathic facial dermatitis
	Seborrhea, primary
Pointers	Acral mutilation
	Demodicosis
	Epidermolysis bullosa
	Exfoliative cutaneous lupus erythematosus
	Follicular dysplasia (flank)
	Nasal and muzzle folliculitis
Pomeranians	Adrenal sex hormone abnormalities
	Hyposomatotropism
	Injection reactions
Poodle	Ectodermal defect
	Epiphora
	Hyperadrenocorticism
	Hyposomatotropism
	Hypothyroidism
	Injection reactions
	Otitis externa
	Sebaceous adenitis (standard)
Portuguese water dog	Follicular dysplasia
Pug	Atopy
	Facial fold and tail fold intertrigo
Rex cat	Hypotrichosis
Rhodesian Ridgeback	Dermoid sinus in midline of back
Rottweiler	Folliculitis and furunculosis, bacterial
	Follicular lipidosis
	Follicular parakeratosis
	Idiopathic vasculitis
	Vitiligo

Table 2–3 BREED PREDILECTION FOR NON-NEOPLASTIC SKIN DISEASES (STRONG CLINICAL IMPRESSION) Continued

BREED	DISEASE
Samoyed	Adrenal hyperplasia syndrome
	Hyposomatotropism
	Sebaceous adenitis
	Uveodermatologic syndrome
Schipperke	Pemphigus foliaceus
Shar pei	Atopy
	Demodicosis
	Fold intertrigo
	Folliculitis, bacterial
	Food hypersensitivity
	Hypothyroidism
	Idiopathic mucinosis
	IgA deficiency
Schnauzer, miniature	Atopy
	Aurotrichia
	Drug reactions
	Follicular dysplasia (flank)
	Hypothyroidism
	Pseudohermaphroditism
	Schnauzer comedo syndrome
	Subcorneal pustular dematosis
	Superficial suppurative necrolytic dermatitis
Shetland sheepdog	Dermatomyositis
	Discoid lupus erythematosus
	Drug reactions
	Folliculitis, bacterial
	Sertoli cell syndrome
	Systemic lupus erythematosus
	Vesicular cutaneous lupus erythematosus
Shih tzu	Atopy
	Malassezia dermatitis
Siamese cat	Food hypersensitivity
	Hypotrichosis
	Periocular leukotrichia
	Psychogenic dermatitis or alopecia
	Vitiligo
Siberian husky	Discoid lupus erythematosus
	Eosinophilic granuloma
	Follicular dysplasia
	Hypogonadism in intact male
	Idiopathic onychodystrophy
	Uveodermatologic syndrome
	Zinc-responsive dermatosis
Spaniels (Cocker and Springer)	Acral mutilation (English Springer)
	Atopy (American Cocker)
	Cutaneous asthenia (English Springer)
	Food hypersensitivity
	Hypothyroidism
	Idiopathic onychodystrophy (Springer)
	Lip fold intertrigo
	Malassezia dermatitis
	Otitis externa (especially proliferative)
	Psoriasiform-lichenoid dermatosis (English Springer)
	Seborrhea, primary
	Vitamin A–responsive dermatosis (Cocker)
St. Bernard	Acral lick dermatitis
	Follicultis and furunculosis, bacterial
	Pyotraumatic dermatitis
Terriers	
Cairn	Atopy, Sertoli cell syndrome
Irish	Hereditary footpad hyperkeratosis

Table continued on following page

Table 2–3 BREED PREDILECTION FOR NON-NEOPLASTIC SKIN DISEASES (STRONG CLINICAL IMPRESSION) Continued

BREED	DISEASE
Jack Russell	Atopy
	Demodicosis
	Dermatophytosis (*Trichophyton mentagrophytes*, var. *erinacei*)
	Vasculitis
Kerry blue	Footpad keratoses (corns)
	Otitis externa
	Spiculosis
Scottish	Atopy
	Demodicosis
	Folliculitis and furunculosis, bacterial
	Hereditary nasal pyogranuloma and vasculitis
West Highland white	Atopy
	Demodicosis
	Epidermal dysplasia
	Ichthyosis
	Malassezia dermatitis
	Seborrhea, primary
Wire-haired fox	Atopy
Yorkshire	Color dilution alopecia
	Dermatophytosis (*M. canis*)
	Injection reactions
	Melanoderma and alopecia
	Traction alopecia
Vizsla	Sebaceous adenitis
Weimeraner	Demodicosis
	Muzzle furunculosis
	Sertoli cell syndrome
	Sterile pyogranuloma syndrome
Whippet	Idiopathic onychodystrophy

Medical History

The clinician should obtain a complete medical history in all cases.[3] In practice, two levels of history are taken. The first level includes those questions that are always asked, and this level is often helped by having the client fill out a history questionnaire before the examination (see Fig. 2–2). Often, the answers on these forms will change if the client is questioned directly, so these form answers should be reviewed and not relied on as initially answered. The first level should initially include questions about previous illnesses and problems. The second level in history taking relates to more specific questions that relate to specific diseases. These more pertinent questions are usually asked once the practitioner has examined the animal and is developing a differential diagnosis or has at least established what some of the problems are. However, it is vital to use a systematic, detailed method of examination and history taking so that important information is not overlooked. A complete history takes a lot of time to obtain and usually is a major component of the initial examination period. In practice, most practitioners do not take the time to collect a thorough history for the problem. Learning which historical questions are most important for specific problems and being certain to collect this information becomes critical. For example, the number of normal bowel movements per day is helpful if assessing the possibility of food hypersensitivity and is an important question to ask in perennially pruritic dogs but not for dogs with nonpruritic, endocrine appearing alopecia. Often, the history is completed during the examination and once the initial differential diagnosis is determined.

The clinician who can draw out a complete history in an unbiased form has a valuable skill. It is important that the questions presented to the client do not suggest answers or tend to shut off discussion. Some owners purposely or unconsciously withhold pertinent facts, especially about neglect, diet, previous medication, or other procedures they think may not be well received by the examining veterinarian. Other pertinent information may be left out because some owners are not aware of what is normal. They may not know how much licking or chewing it takes to consider a dog's behavior abnormal. Therefore, they may not supply valuable information because they do not perceive the information to be significant or abnormal. In other cases, they may recognize something as abnormal but attribute the observation to some other, unrelated cause (e.g., paw licking that the client interprets as behavior to obtain attention and does not list as a problem in the history).

The clinician must become skillful at extracting all the relevant history and observations, regardless of the client's perception of their importance. The skillful clinician is ever tuned to listen for side comments by the client or by the children. These may be veritable "pearls" of information in a mass of trivia. They also help to establish the client's accuracy and credibility.

Next, the following information about the skin lesions should be obtained from the owner: the date and age at onset, the original locations, the initial appearance, the tendency to progression or regression, factors affecting the course, and previous treatment (home, proprietary, or pet shop remedies used, as well as veterinary treatment). In addition, treatments of other problems should be determined and recorded. The relationships between all treatments and the onset of or changes in the disease should be recorded and a possible drug reaction considered. Drug reactions are diagnosed only when they are suspected, and because they may mimic any disease, the history aids in arriving at this diagnosis.

Almost all animals with skin disorders have been bathed, dipped, sprayed, or treated with one or more medications, and the owner may be reluctant or unable to disclose a complete list of previous treatments. It is important that the types of medication and the dates of application are completely divulged, because a modification of pertinent signs may have resulted.

Although the patient cannot relate subjective findings (symptoms such as itching, burning sensation, and pain), it is possible to determine the degree of pruritus reasonably well. The presence and severity of pain may also be evaluated in some cases by the patient's response to stimuli: Exhibiting shyness, pulling away, exhibiting skin twitching, and responding with aggressiveness may be manifested when pain is provoked.

Pruritus is one of the most common presenting complaints and, in many cases, is a hallmark of allergy. The presence, location, and degree of itching are important criteria in the differential diagnosis of many skin diseases. The owner's idea of the intensity of itching, however, may vary considerably from that of the veterinarian. Consequently, it is helpful to ask questions, "How many times daily do you see your dog scratch?" "Does it itch in many sites, or just a few?" "Does it shake its head?" "Does it lick its paws?" "Does it lick the front legs or other areas?" "Does it roll on its back or rub its chin, ears, or body against things?" It is often helpful to have the client initially grade the itching on a scale of 1 to 10, because many diseases associated with pruritus are chronic. The range is categorized as follows: Zero is no itching at all, 1 being very mild, and 10 as bad as the pet has ever itched. This level can be recorded and asked again as therapies or diagnostic procedures are tried to help determine how the pet's problem changes over time. Also, by having the answers to the previous questions asked about the pruritus, there is a record of how severe the problem is and the symptoms seen when the owner indicates a level of itching. Over time, the client's perceptions may change, and this approach allows that change to be determined and documented. It is also very helpful to determine, when possible, whether the pruritus involves initially normal-appearing skin (an itch that rashes, typical of allergy), or whether skin lesions precede or appear at the same time as the pruritus (a rash that itches).

Many times, owners disassociate other problems that their pet is having. For example, a dog is presented for paw licking and groin pruritus. The dog has also had multiple ear infections during the past few years but has only recently had pruritus of the paws and groin. The owners may not mention the ear problems, the itching, or treatments for the ears unless they are specifically asked about them because they assume it is not important or it is an unrelated problem.

The same types of specific questions are helpful when discussing diets, because the owner often states the typical feedings and leaves out treats and supplements. A more representative answer is often secured if one asks, "What did your pet eat yesterday, or during the past 48 hours?" Also: "What treats does your pet receive and what supplements do you add to its diet?" Specifically, the clinician asks whether any vitamins or flavored chewable medications are given. The clinician also asks about rawhide chew toys or other edible toys.

Because contact irritants or allergens are important contributors to or causes of skin disease, it is necessary to inquire about the animal's environment. Does it live in an apartment or is it outdoors in the fields and forests? Does it sleep in a doghouse or in the owner's house? If it sleeps in the house, in what room does it sleep and is there carpeting? If it sleeps in a person's bedroom, does it sleep on the floor or on the bed? Are there feather pillows or comforters or wool blankets? If the pet sleeps in a doghouse, in a garage, or outside, does the bedding consist of straw, wool blankets, or some other material? Are symptoms worse when the pet first awakens, sometimes suggesting exposure throughout the night?

If the pet is boarded or hospitalized, do the symptoms improve? If the pet travels, do the symptoms improve while traveling or while in other homes? Symptoms that resolve in a different environment are highly suggestive of a reaction to an environmental allergen or irritant. Questions regarding sexual behavior may also reveal important information, particularly when endocrine disorders are suspected. Other more organ-specific questions may also be asked, depending on the clinical suspicions of possible diseases. Questions regarding changes in water consumption, appetite, weight, and urination or defecation habits should be included in history taking.

In determining contagion, one should inquire about the skin health of other animals on the premises. The presence of skin disease in the people living with the patient may also be highly significant in some disorders (scabies, cheyletiellosis, and dermatophytosis).

At this point, the clinician usually has a general idea of the problem and is ready to proceed with a careful physical examination. In some cases, the clinician may want to come back to the medical history if further examinations indicate a more serious or underlying systemic disease.

• PHYSICAL EXAMINATION

General Observations

A good examination necessitates adequate lighting. Normal daylight without glare is best, but any artificial light of adequate candlepower is sufficient if it produces bright, non–color-changing, uniform lighting. The lamp should be adjustable to illuminate all body areas. A combination loupe and light provides magnification of the field as well as good illumination.

Before the clinician concentrates on the individual lesions, the entire animal should always be observed from a distance of a couple of meters to obtain a general impression of abnormalities and to observe distribution patterns.

Does the pet appear to be in good health? Is it fat or thin, unkempt or well groomed? Is the problem generalized or localized? What is the distribution and configuration of the lesions? Are they bilaterally symmetric or unilaterally irregular (Fig. 2–3)? Is the hair coat shiny or dull, and if it is dull, what is the pattern of those changes? Is it an appropriate color and pattern of colors for its breed? Are coat changes in quality or color lifelong, or did they develop before or after the symptoms for which the pet is presented?

To answer some of these questions, the clinician must examine the patient more closely. The dorsal aspect of the body should be inspected by viewing it from the rear, as

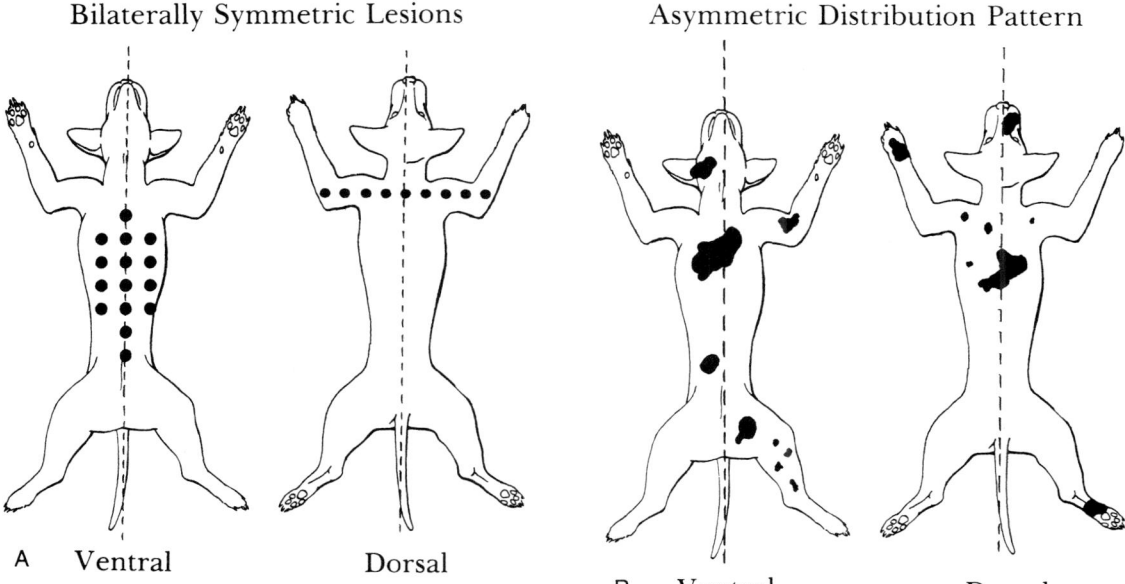

FIGURE 2–3. *A*, When a line is drawn from the tip of the nose to the end of the tail and the distribution of the lesions is relatively the same on the right and left sides, the pattern is called bilaterally symmetric. Most such skin disorders have an internal cause, and the skin reflects internal disease. Examples are hypothyroidism, hyperadrenocorticism, Sertoli's cell tumor, and autoimmune diseases such as pemphigus foliaceus. Allergies may also present symmetric lesions. *B*, When a line is drawn from the tip of the nose to the end of the tail and the lesions on one side are not identical to those on the other side, the distribution pattern is asymmetric. External environmental causes, such as ectoparasites, fungi, or contact allergens, are examples of disorders that cause asymmetric lesions.

elevated hairs and patchy alopecia may be more obvious from that angle. Then, the head, the lateral trunk, and the extremities should be observed. Next, the clinician should complete a thorough dermatologic examination.

Dermatologic Examination

After an impression is obtained from a distance, the skin should be examined more closely and palpated.[3] It is important to examine every centimeter of skin and visible mucous membranes. Many subtle clues are located where the client is unaware of problems. The authors have seen many cases in which ventrally located lesions and interdigital, paronychial, and oral lesions went unobserved by a veterinarian. These lesions may add valuable diagnostic information. It is difficult to complete a dermatologic examination without rolling animals on their sides or back. All the paws must be picked up or handled so that the ventral interdigital skin is also examined.

Many observations need to be made. What is the texture of the hair? Is it coarse or fine, dry or oily? Does it epilate easily? A change in the amount of hair is often a dramatic finding, although subtle thinning of the hair coat should also be noted. Alopecia is a partial or complete lack of hair in areas where it is normally present. Hypotrichosis implies partial hair loss and is a form of alopecia. Is the thinning diffuse, or are there numerous small focal areas of alopecia (the latter being often seen with folliculitis)? Hypertrichosis is excessive hair, and although the condition is rare in animals, it usually has hormonal or developmental causes.

The texture, elasticity, and thickness of the skin should be determined and impressions of heat or coolness recorded. It is easier to find skin lesions in some breeds than in others, depending on the thickness of the coat. Additionally, there is variation in an animal's coat density in different body areas, with skin lesions often being discerned more readily in sparsely haired regions. Therefore, the clinician must part or clip the hair in heavily haired areas to observe and palpate lesions that are present but obscured.

When abnormalities are discovered, it is important to establish their morphologic features, configuration, and general distribution. The clinician should try to appreciate the different lesions and their patterns. Together, they often represent the natural history of the skin disease.

Morphology of Skin Lesions

The morphologic characteristics of skin lesions, together with their history, are an essential feature of dermatologic diagnosis.[1, 3] Morphologic features and the medical and dermatologic history are often the only guidelines if laboratory procedures cannot be performed or do not yield useful information. The clinician must learn to recognize primary and secondary lesions. A primary lesion is the initial eruption that develops spontaneously as a direct reflection of underlying disease. Secondary lesions evolve from primary lesions or are artifacts induced by the patients or by external factors such as trauma and medications. Primary lesions (pustules, vesicles, papules) may appear quickly and then disappear rapidly. However, they may leave behind secondary lesions (such as focal alopecia, epidermal collarettes, scaling, hyperpigmentation, and crusts), which may be more chronic and give clues about the presence of previous primary lesions. Therefore, the identification and the characterization of both primary and secondary lesions are important.

Careful inspection of the diseased skin frequently reveals a primary lesion, which may suggest a limited differential diagnosis. For example, pustules most commonly represent a bacterial pyoderma, whereas sterile pustular diseases occur infrequently. Close inspection of primary lesions may also reveal elusive differences. In assessing the subtle morphologic features of lesions, the clinician may find it helpful to focus on individual lesions and examine them minutely with good light and a hand-held lens or a head loupe with 4- to 6-power magnification. This may allow better identification (e.g., whether pustules are follicular or nonfollicular).

A primary lesion may vary slightly from its initial appearance to its full development. Later, through regression, degeneration, or traumatization, it may change in form and become a secondary lesion. Although classic descriptions and textbooks refer to lesions as primary or secondary, some lesions can be either (e.g., alopecia can be primary [from endocrine disorders] or secondary [from chewing because of pruritus]). Follicular casts, scales, pigment changes, crusts, and comedones may also be primary or secondary. In some conditions, such as primary seborrhea and zinc-responsive dermatosis with secondary bacterial pyoderma, crusts may appear in the same animal as both primary and secondary lesions.

Secondary lesions may also be informative. A ring of orthokeratotic scaling usually follows a point source of inflammation, either a papule or a pustule. This is also true of small focal circular areas of alopecia. Hyperpigmentation that has a lattice-like or lacelike configuration generally reflects an area of previous inflammation such as erythematous macules, papules, and pustules. Yellow- to honey-colored crusts usually follow the rupture and drying of pustules. In many cases, however, the significant lesion must be differentiated from the mass of secondary debris. Variations of lesions and their configurations are common, because early and advanced stages coexist in most skin diseases. The ability to discover a characteristic lesion and understand its significance is an important aspect of mastering dermatologic diagnoses.

The following illustrations can help the clinician identify primary and secondary lesions. Also, the character of the lesions may vary, implying a different pathogenesis or cause. The definitions and examples in Figures 2–4 to 2–24 explain the relationship of skin lesions to canine and feline dermatoses.

- *Primary lesions*
    Macule or patch (Fig. 2–4)
    Papule or plaque (Fig. 2–5)

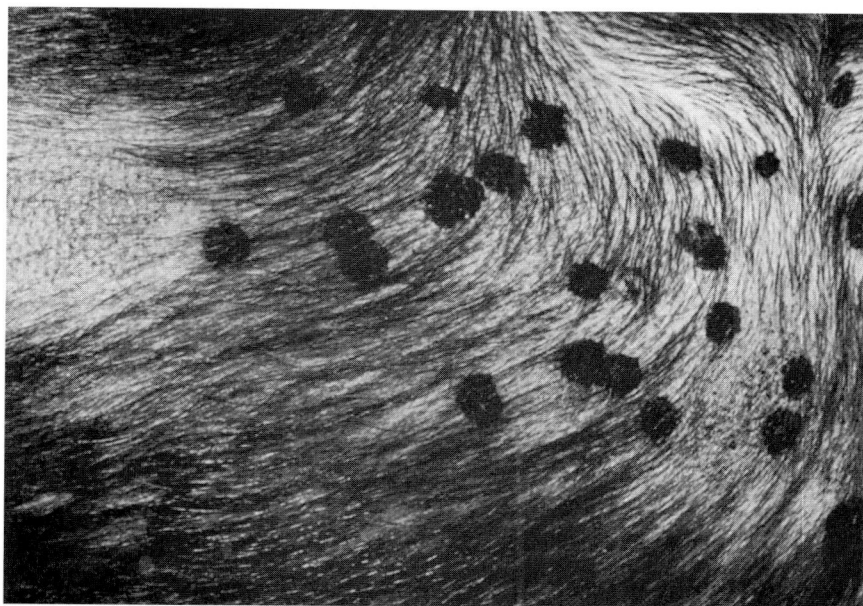

FIGURE 2–4. Macule—a circumscribed, nonpalpable spot up to 1 cm in diameter and characterized by a change in the color of the skin. Patch—a macule larger than 1 cm in size. The discoloration can result from several processes: an increase in melanin pigmentation, depigmentation, and erythema or local hemorrhage. Examples are the hyperpigmentation patches in endocrine or postinflammatory hyperpigmentation, hypopigmentation, and vitiligo. Discoloration also occurs after inflammation of the erythematous macules in many types of acute dermatitis, lentigo, and pigmented nevi. (The photograph illustrates lentigo.) Types of macules are as follows: purpura—bleeding into the skin (these are usually dark red but change to purple as absorption proceeds); petechiae—pinpoint macules that are much smaller than 1 cm in diameter and are caused by hemorrhage; and ecchymoses—patches larger than 1 cm in diameter that are caused by hemorrhage.

    Pustule (Fig. 2–6)
    Vesicle or bulla (Fig. 2–7)
    Wheal (Fig. 2–8)
    Nodule (Fig. 2–9)
    Tumor or cyst (Fig. 2–10)
- *Lesions that may be primary or secondary*
    Alopecia (Fig. 2–11)
    Scale (Fig. 2–12)
    Crust (Fig. 2–13)
    Follicular casts (Fig. 2–14)
    Comedo (Fig. 2–15)
    Pigmentary abnormalities (Figs. 2–16 and 2–17)
- *Secondary lesions*
    Epidermal collarette (Fig. 2–18)
    Scar (Fig. 2–19)
    Excoriation (Fig. 2–20)
    Erosion or ulcer (Fig. 2–21)
    Fissure (Fig. 2–22)
    Lichenification (Fig. 2–23)
    Callus (Fig. 2–24)

Two special techniques of close examination of the skin, although infrequently used, are noteworthy:

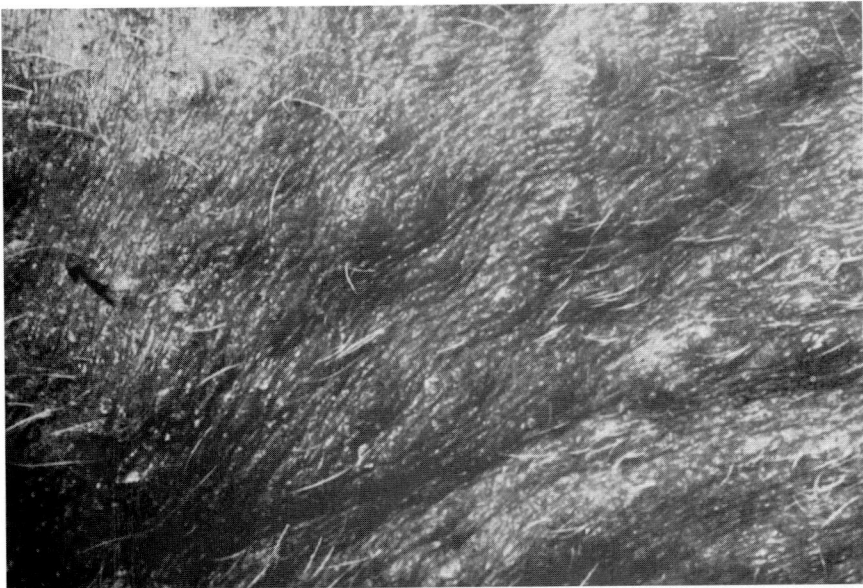

FIGURE 2-5. Papule—a small, solid elevation of the skin up to 1 cm in diameter that can always be palpated as a solid mass. Many papules are pink or red swellings produced by tissue infiltration of inflammatory cells in the dermis, by intraepidermal and subepidermal edema, or by epidermal hypertrophy. They may or may not involve hair follicles. Examples are the erythematous papules seen in scabies and flea bite hypersensitivity. In the dog, another common cause of papules is superficial bacterial folliculitis. (Photograph illustrates contact hypersensitivity.) Plaque—a larger, flat-topped elevation formed by the extension or coalition of papules. A plaque that is made up of closely packed, projecting elevations often covered by crusts is called a vegetation.

1. Diascopy is performed by pressing a clear piece of plastic or glass over an erythematous lesion. If the lesion blanches on pressure, the reddish color is due to vascular engorgement. If it does not, there is hemorrhage into the skin (petechia or ecchymosis) (Fig. 2–25A and B).
2. Nikolsky's sign is elicited by applying pressure on a vesicle or at the edge of an ulcer or erosion or even on normal skin.[18a] It is positive when the outer layer of the skin is easily rubbed off or pushed away. It indicates poor cellular cohesion, as found in the pemphigus complex, toxic epidermal necrolysis (Fig. 2–26), and erythema multiforme major.

Configuration of Lesions

The configuration of skin lesions may be helpful in establishing a differential diagnosis (Fig. 2–27).[3] Some diseases often have lesions present in certain configurations, and although exceptions exist, recognizing the pattern of lesions adds information for decision making. Lesions may be single, such as the solitary dermatophytosis lesion and a foreign-body reaction. Multiple lesions are most commonly seen in skin diseases of dogs and cats.

When lesions are linear, external forces such as scratching, being scratched by something, and having something applied to the skin are often responsible. In other cases, linear lesions may reflect the involvement of a blood or lymphatic vessel, a dermatome, or a congenital malformation. Diffuse areas of involvement tend to suggest a metabolic or systemic reaction, such as endocrine disorders, keratinization, and immunologic or hypersensitivity disorders. Annular lesions are often associated with peripheral spreading of a disease. Common examples of annular lesions are superficial spreading bacterial folliculitis

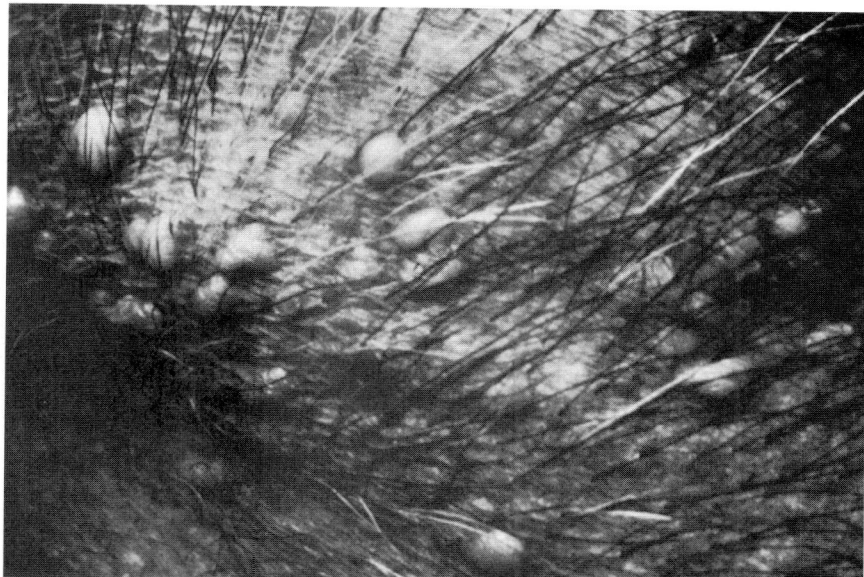

FIGURE 2-6. Pustule—a small, circumscribed elevation of the epidermis that is filled with pus. Pustules may be intraepidermal, subepidermal, or follicular in location. Their color is usually yellow but may be green or red. Most commonly, pustules primarily contain neutrophils and are infectious in origin; however, eosinophils may predominate (especially in parasitic or allergic disorders) and may be sterile (subcorneal pustular dermatosis, pemphigus foliaceus, sterile eosinophilic pustulosis). Size and color may be clues to the cause of the condition. Larger flaccid pustules (bullous impetigo) are more often associated with Cushing's disease, iatrogenic Cushing's disease, immune-suppressed cases, or pemphigus foliaceus. Larger green pustules imply gram-negative infections or marked toxic changes. Examples are acne, folliculitis, and the pustules found on the abdomen of puppies with impetigo. (Photograph illustrates nonfollicular pustules from subcorneal pustular dermatosis.) Abscess—a demarcated fluctuant lesion resulting from a dermal or subcutaneous accumulation of pus. The pus is not visible on the surface of the skin until it drains to the surface. Abscesses are larger and deeper than pustules.

and dermatophytosis. Coalescing lesions occur when multiple lesions are present and spread so that they overlap.

Different Stages

A skin disease and its individual lesions progress from its earliest appearance to a fully developed state and, in many cases, to a chronic or resolved stage. The distribution, the configuration, and the histologic appearance of lesions change. The evolution of lesions should be determined either by obtaining the history or by finding different stages of lesions on the patient. Papules often develop into vesicles and pustules, which may rupture to leave erosions or ulcers and finally crusts. An understanding of these progressions helps in the diagnostic process.

As lesions develop in specific patterns, they also involute in characteristic ways. The lesions change, along with their histologic appearance. For example, a macule may develop into a pustule and then a crust or crusted erosion. It may then spread peripherally, occurring as a ring of lesions; the lesion then appears as a circular patch with multiple pustules or crusts on the margins and central alopecia. The fully developed lesions could appear as a large alopecic patch with a central area of hyperpigmentation and multifocal erythematous macules, pustules, or crusts intermittently along the leading margin; this lesion could then appear arciform. Scaling may also occur at the leading margins of

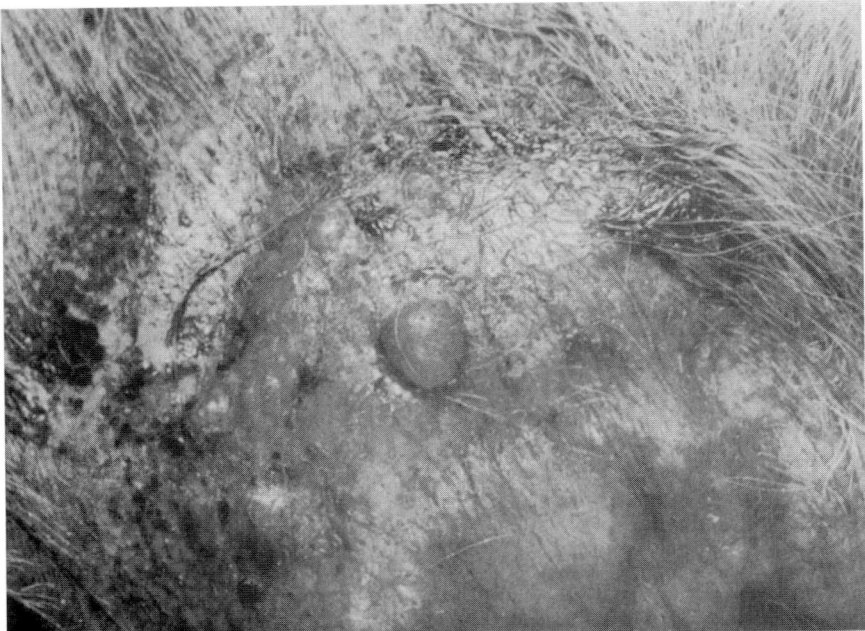

FIGURE 2–7. Vesicle—a sharply circumscribed elevation of the epidermis filled with clear fluid. It can be intraepidermal or subepidermal. Vesicles are rarely seen in dogs and cats because they are fragile and transient. They occur in viral or autoimmune dermatoses, or in dermatitis caused by irritants. Vesicles are lesions up to 1 cm in diameter; those with a diameter greater than 1 cm are called bullae. (Photograph illustrates several vesicles caused by a chemical irritant.)

inflammation. The healing phase of a chronic lesion may appear as a patch of alopecia and hyperpigmentation with no other primary or secondary lesions because they have spontaneously resolved or responded to therapy.

Because diseases and their lesions are evolutionary, the clinician must attempt to learn about all of the stages. The recognition of the different stages as well as the lesions becomes important when selecting areas to sample for diagnostic tests.

Distribution Patterns of Skin Lesions

The areas of skin involved with lesions or affected by symptoms of the disease help in determining the differential diagnosis because most skin diseases have a typical distribution.[3] It is important to emphasize that the accurate determination of the distribution necessitates detection of all changes in the haircoat or the skin, the location of symptoms related to the disease, and the location of all primary and secondary lesions. An adequate determination of the distribution pattern can be achieved only by a thorough history and dermatologic examination; cursory examinations are often incomplete.

The study of skin diseases involves understanding the primary lesions that occur as well as the typical distribution patterns. Diseases less commonly present with atypical patterns. The combination of the type of lesions present and their distribution is the basis for developing a differential diagnosis. The distribution pattern may be very helpful by allowing clinicians to establish the differential diagnosis based on the region involved when animals have lesions and symptoms confined to certain regions (Table 2–4). In some instances, this regional pattern is such a major feature that it is a required aspect of the disease. The best examples are otitis externa, pododermatitis, and nasal dermatitis. Actually, these terms refer to skin disease of a specific region, give little more information, and certainly are not specific diagnoses.

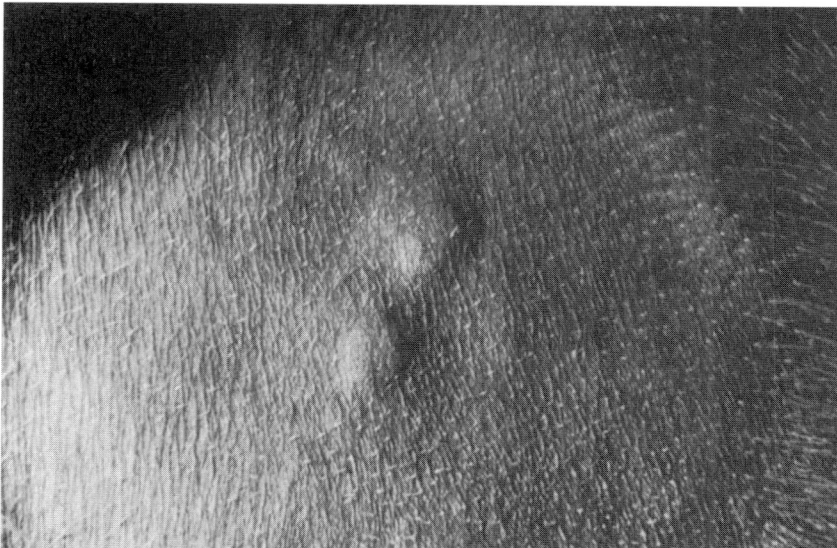

FIGURE 2–8. Wheal—a sharply circumscribed, raised lesion consisting of edema that usually appears and disappears within minutes or hours. Wheals usually produce no changes in the appearance of the overlying skin and haircoat. Wheals are characteristically white to pink elevated ridges or round edematous swellings that only rarely have pseudopods at their periphery. They blanch on diascopy (viewing the skin through a glass slide that is pressed firmly against the lesion). A huge hive of a distensible region such as the lips or eyelids is called angioedema. Examples of wheals are urticaria, insect bites, and positive reactions to allergy skin tests. (Photograph illustrates urticaria.)

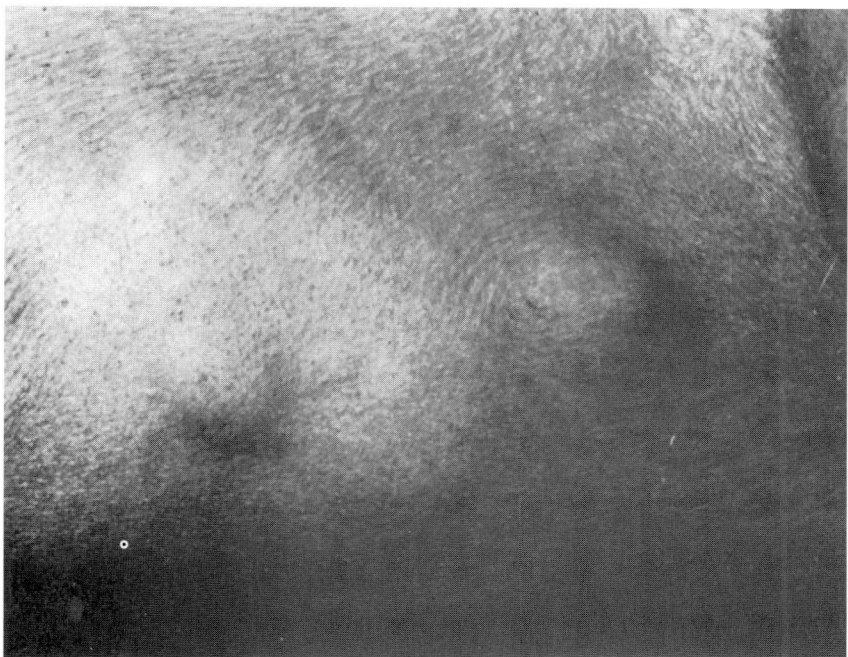

FIGURE 2–9. Nodule—a circumscribed, solid elevation greater than 1 cm in diameter that usually extends into the deeper layers of the skin. Nodules usually result from massive infiltration of inflammatory or neoplastic cells into the dermis or subcutis. Deposition of fibrin or crystalline material also produces nodules. (Photograph illustrates panniculitis.)

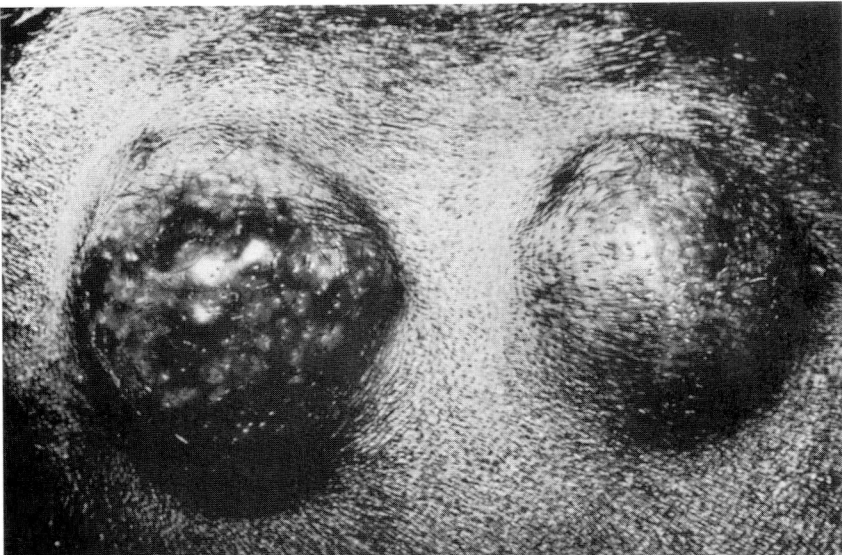

FIGURE 2–10. Tumor—a large mass that may involve any structure of the skin or subcutaneous tissue. Most tumors are neoplastic or granulomatous in origin. (Photograph illustrates pilomatrixoma.) Cyst—an epithelium-lined cavity containing fluid or a solid material. It is a smooth, well-circumscribed, fluctuant to solid mass. Skin cysts are usually lined by adnexal epithelium (hair follicle, sebaceous, or epitrichial) and filled with cornified cellular debris or sebaceous or epitrichial secretions.

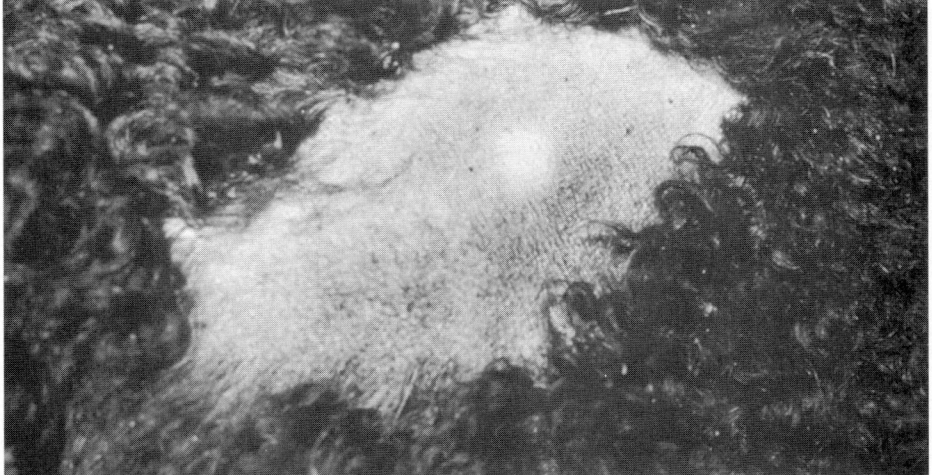

FIGURE 2–11. Alopecia is loss of hair and may vary from partial to complete. It may be primary, such as alopecia with endocrine disorders and follicular dysplasias, or it can occur secondary to trauma or inflammation. (Photograph illustrates alopecia from an injection reaction.)

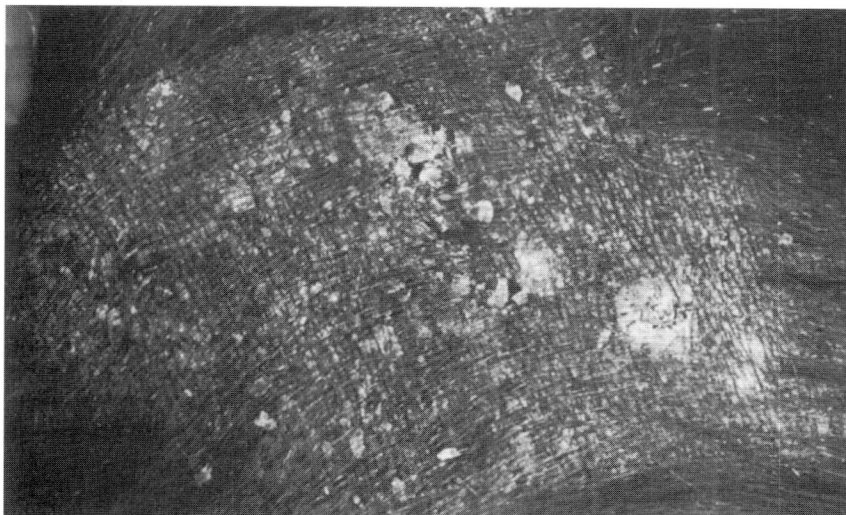

FIGURE 2–12. Scale—an accumulation of loose fragments of the horny layer of the skin (cornified cells). The corneocyte is the final product of epidermal keratinization. Normal loss occurs as individual cells or small clusters not visible to the naked eye. Abnormal scaling is the loss in larger flakes. Flakes vary greatly in consistency; they can appear branny, fine, powdery, flaky, platelike, greasy, dry, loose, adhering, or nitlike. The color varies from white, silver, yellow, or brown to gray. (Photograph illustrates seborrhea.) Scales may be the primary lesions in some cases of color dilution alopecia, follicular dysplasia, primary idiopathic seborrhea, and ichthyosis. They are common secondary lesions in chronic inflammation.

Table 2–4 lists areas or parts of the body along with the common skin diseases that are most frequently localized or especially severe in those areas. The chart is useful in the differential diagnosis. However, the clinician must also be aware that other diseases may occur in these regions and that diseases that often affect a certain region can also occur elsewhere and not involve the typical region. Therefore, regional evaluations aid in ranking differential diagnostic possibilities: they do not determine the diagnosis.

In many instances, the patterning that skin diseases take is unexplained. Recently, homeobox genes have received much attention.[16b] These genes are a family of regulatory proteins that influence pattern formation at many levels and may be fundamental to the development of the many patterns used to diagnose skin diseases.

Differential Diagnosis

A differential diagnosis is developed on the basis of a compilation of the preceding information. The possible diagnoses should be considered in their proposed likely order of occurrence. This point is important as the first step in developing a cost-effective plan.

Developing a Diagnostic or Therapeutic Plan

Laboratory tests or therapies can be recommended on the basis of tentative diagnosis and differential diagnosis. If a strong tentative diagnosis is not determined from the history and the physical examination, the approach should be directed at the two or three most likely diagnoses. Client-veterinarian interaction is critical at this point. The client decides what is going to be done, but his or her decision is based on the clinician's recommendations. Therefore, the client needs to know the tentative or possible diagnoses, as well as expected costs and anticipated results of the diagnostic or therapeutic options proposed.

Diagnostic tests and laboratory procedures are useful whenever a definitive diagnosis

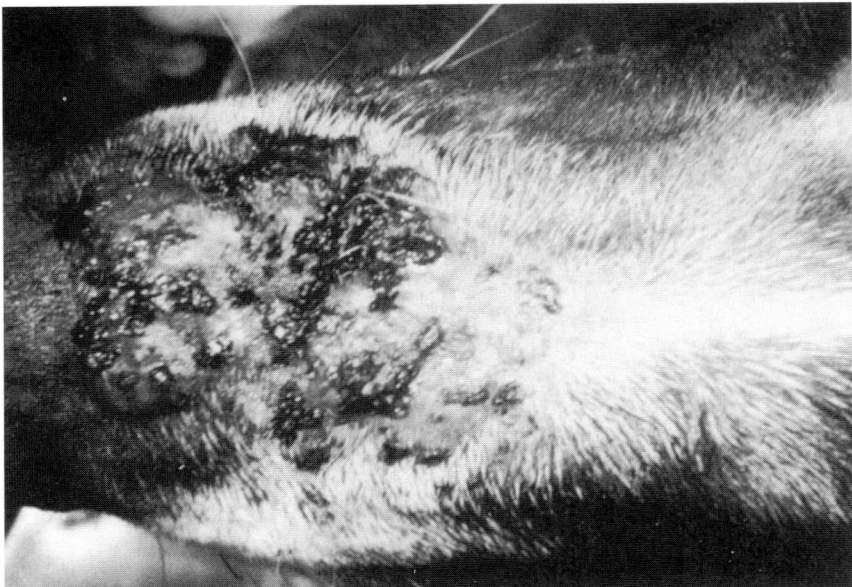

FIGURE 2–13. Crust is formed when dried exudate, serum, pus, blood, cells, scales, or medications adhere to the surface. Unusually thick crusts are found in hairy areas because the dried material tends to adhere more tightly than in glabrous skin. Crust may be primary as in primary seborrhea and zinc-responsive dermatosis, or secondary as in pyoderma, fly strike, or pruritus. Hemorrhagic crusts in pyoderma are brown or dark red; yellowish green crusts appear in some cases of pyoderma; tan, lightly adhering crusts are found in impetigo. Vegetations—heaped-up crusts seen in pemphigus vegetans. (Photograph illustrates nasal furunculosis.) Dark crusts imply deeper tissue damage or hemorrhage and may be seen more with traumatic wounds, furunculosis, fly strike dermatitis, and vasculitis. Honey-colored crusts are more commonly infectious in nature; thicker dry yellow crusts are more typical of scabies and zinc-responsive dermatosis. Tightly adherent crusts are typical in zinc-responsive dermatosis and necrolytic migratory erythema, and they also occur in some cases of seborrhea.

cannot be made from the case history and clinical examination alone.[4] Laboratory procedures may confirm many clinical diagnoses and provide a logical basis for successful therapeutic management. They should be recommended on the basis of the most likely diagnosis and should not be randomly suggested or recommended just to be comprehensive. The cost effectiveness of each test should also be considered. In practice, it is often unacceptable to recommend numerous tests to screen for the long list of possible diagnoses in any given case. Instead, the results of recommended tests should confirm or rule out the diagnoses that the clinician deems most likely.

• LABORATORY PROCEDURES

Surface Sampling

The lesions and pathologic changes of a skin disease are often readily available for study, and a variety of laboratory tests are based on this easy access to the skin's surface. A great deal of information may be obtained by studying microscopically materials collected from the hair and skin. Skin scraping, obtaining an acetate tape impression, and flea combing are all techniques to find microscopic ectoparasites. Hairs may be removed, and exudates may be collected and examined microscopically. Most of these techniques may be done in general clinical practice and rapidly add valuable information to a case work-up. However, practice and study may be necessary to maximize the benefits of many tests. The effort to

Text continued on page 101

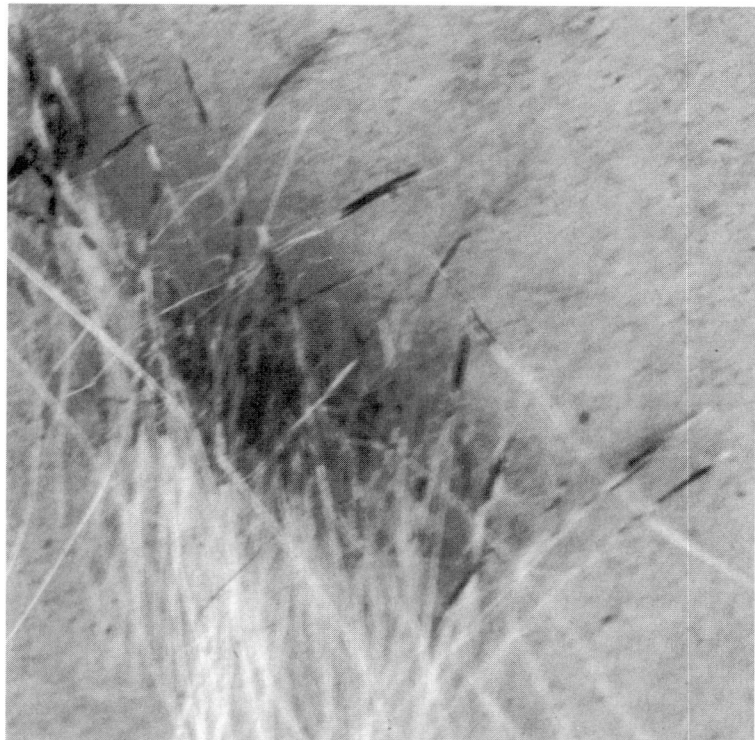

FIGURE 2–14. Follicular cast—an accumulation of keratin and follicular material that adheres to the hair shaft extending above the surface of the follicular ostia. It is a primary lesion in vitamin A–responsive dermatoses, primary seborrhea, and sebaceous adenitis. (Photograph illustrates hair epilated from a dog with sebaceous adenitis; the clumps of material at the base of multiple hairs are the casts.) Follicular casts may be secondary lesions in demodectic mange and dermatophytosis.

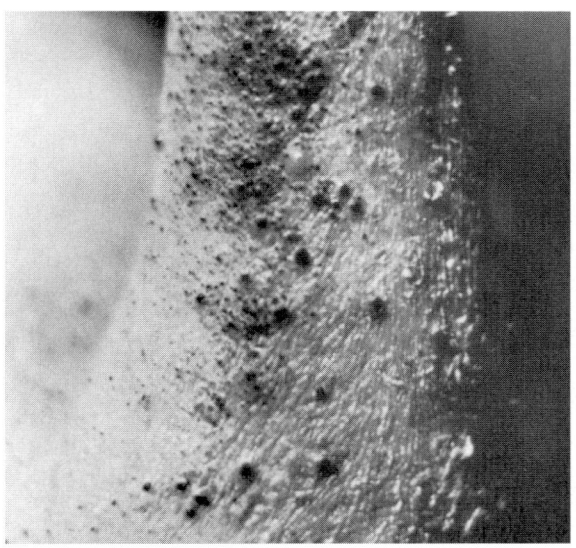

FIGURE 2–15. Comedo—a dilated hair follicle filled with cornified cells and sebaceous material. It is the initial lesion of feline acne and may predispose the skin to bacterial folliculitis. A comedo may be produced secondary to seborrheic skin disease, to occlusion with greasy medications, or to the administration of systemic or topical corticosteroids. (Photograph illustrates comedones of the skin on the tail of a dog.) When comedones are present, diseases of the hair follicle should be considered such as infection with Demodex and dermatophytosis. Comedones may be primary lesions in feline acne, vitamin A–responsive dermatosis, Schnauzer comedo syndrome, Cushing's disease, sex hormone dermatoses, and some idiopathic seborrhea disorders.

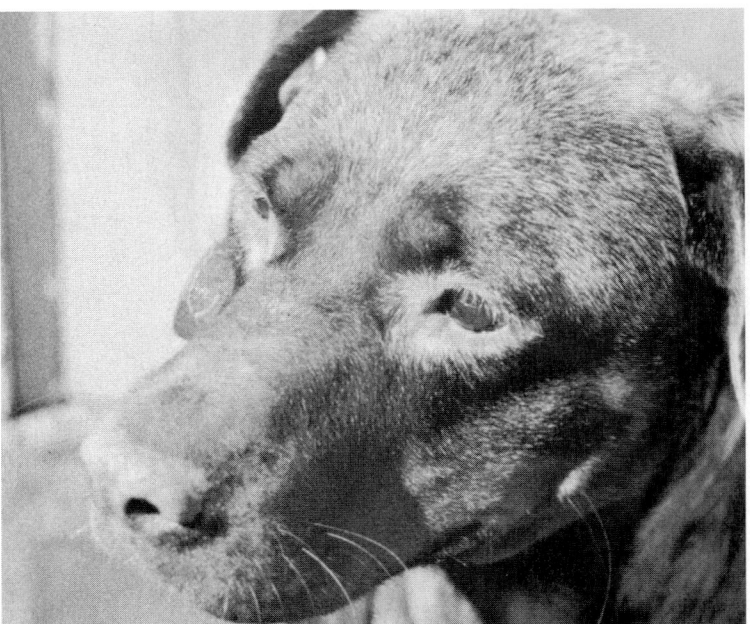

FIGURE 2–16. Abnormal pigmentation—skin coloration caused by a variety of pigments but most commonly melanin, which is responsible for many skin colors: black—melanin present throughout the epidermis (lentigo); blue—melanin within melanocytes and melanophages in the middle and deep dermis (dermal melanocytoma); gray—diffuse dermal melanosis or superficial dermal melanosis from pigment incontinence; tan, brown, black—various shades of normal skin color in breeds are due to melanin; brown—hemochromatosis is due primarily to melanin, not hemosiderin. Other pigments are as follows: red, purple—hemorrhage in the skin is red at first, becoming dark purple with time (bruises); yellow-green—accumulations of bile pigments (icterus). In hypopigmentation (hypomelanosis), loss of epidermal melanin may be primary, as with vitiligo-like disease, or secondary, as in postinflammatory change. (Photograph demonstrates Rottweiler with leukoderma and leukotrichia.) Leukoderma is a general term for white skin, whereas vitiligo refers to a specific disease. Lack of pigment in hair is called leukotrichia or achromotrichia.

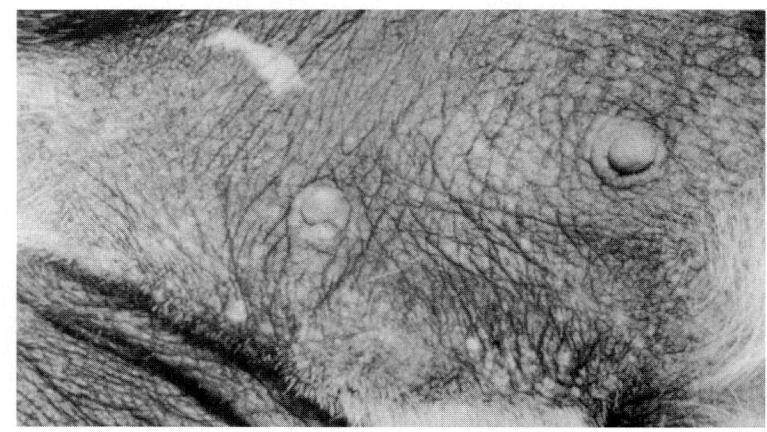

FIGURE 2–17. Hyperpigmentation (hypermelanosis, melanoderma)—increased epidermal and, occasionally, dermal melanin. Melanophages may be found in the superficial dermis. (Postinflammatory, chronic, traumatic, and endocrine skin lesions.) Excess pigment in hair is called melanotrichia. (Photograph illustrates postinflammatory hyperpigmentation.) The pattern of hyperpigmentation is helpful in determining the etiology. Endocrine hyperpigmentation tends to be diffuse, whereas postinflammatory hyperpigmentation has a latticework appearance.

Diagnostic Methods • **97**

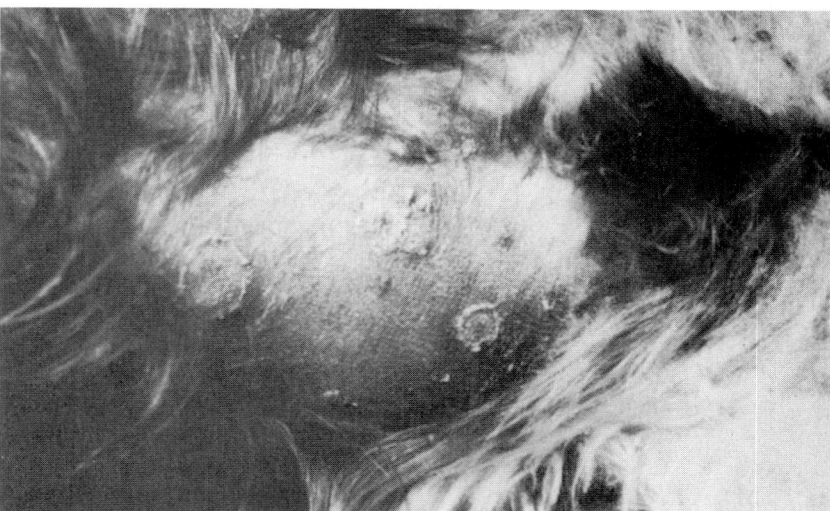

FIGURE 2–18. Epidermal collarette—a special type of scale arranged in a circular rim of loose keratin flakes or peeling keratin. It represents the remnants of the roof of a vesicle, bulla, pustule, or papule, or the hyperkeratosis caused by a point source of inflammation as seen with papules and pustules. (Photograph illustrates a healing pustule of staphylococcal folliculitis.)

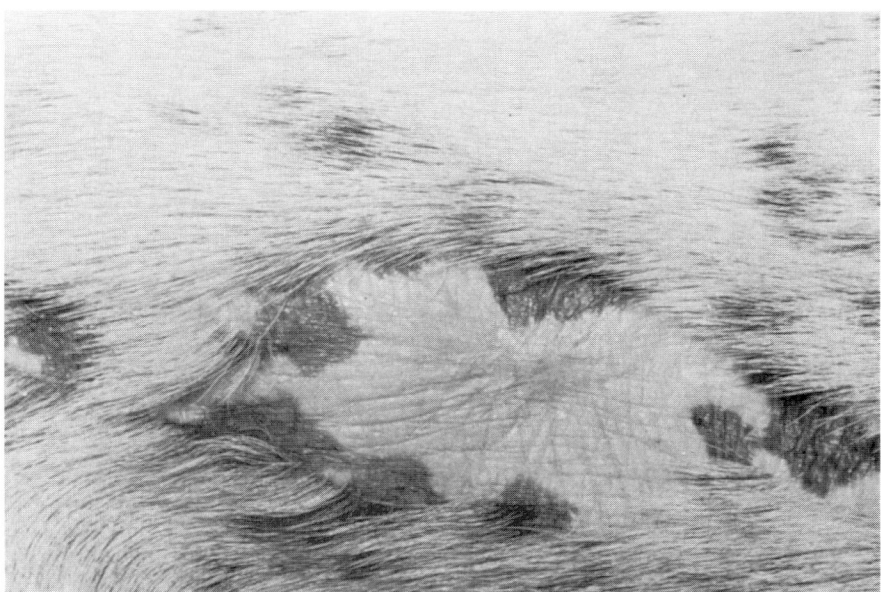

FIGURE 2–19. Scar—an area of fibrous tissue that has replaced the damaged dermis or subcutaneous tissue. Scars are the remnants of trauma or dermatologic lesions. Most scars in dogs and cats are alopecic, atrophic, and depigmented. Proliferative scars do occur, and in dark-skinned dogs scars can be alopecic and hyperpigmented. Scars are observed following severe burns and in deep pyoderma. (Photograph illustrates burn scarring.)

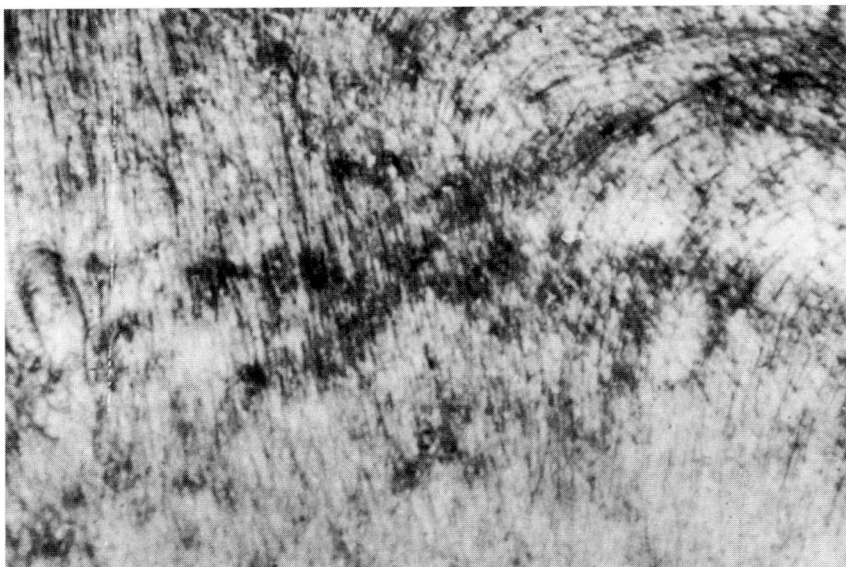

FIGURE 2–20. Excoriation—erosions or ulcers caused by scratching, biting, or rubbing. Excoriations are self-produced and usually result from pruritus; they invite secondary bacterial infection. They are often partly recognized by their linear pattern. (Photograph illustrates linear excoriations on the side of a dog with scabies.)

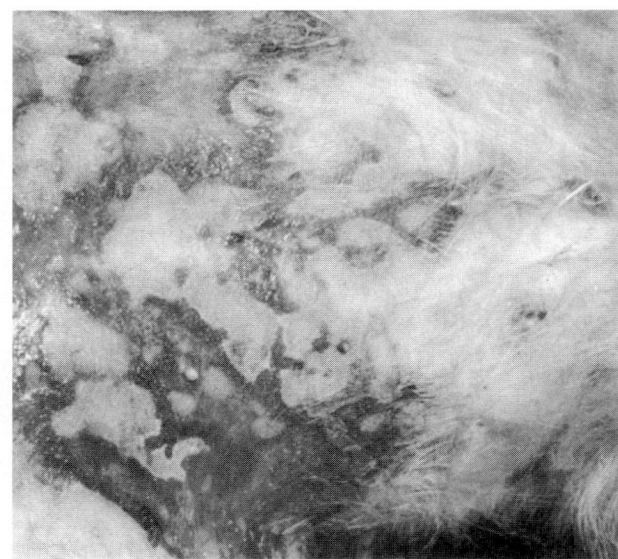

FIGURE 2–21. Erosion—a shallow epidermal defect that does not penetrate the basal laminar zone and consequently heals without scarring; it generally results from epidermal diseases and self-inflicted trauma. Ulcer—there is a break in the continuity of the epidermis, with exposure of the underlying dermis. A deep pathologic process is required for an ulcer to form. It is important to note the structure of the edge: Is it undermined, fibrotic and thickened, or necrotic (vasculitis, neoplastic, fibrosing, vascular)? The firmness of the ulcer depth and the type of exudate in the crater should also be noted. A scar is often left after an ulcer heals. Examples are feline indolent ulcer, severe deep pyoderma, and vasculitis. (Photograph illustrates vesicular cutaneous lupus erythematosus in a shelty.)

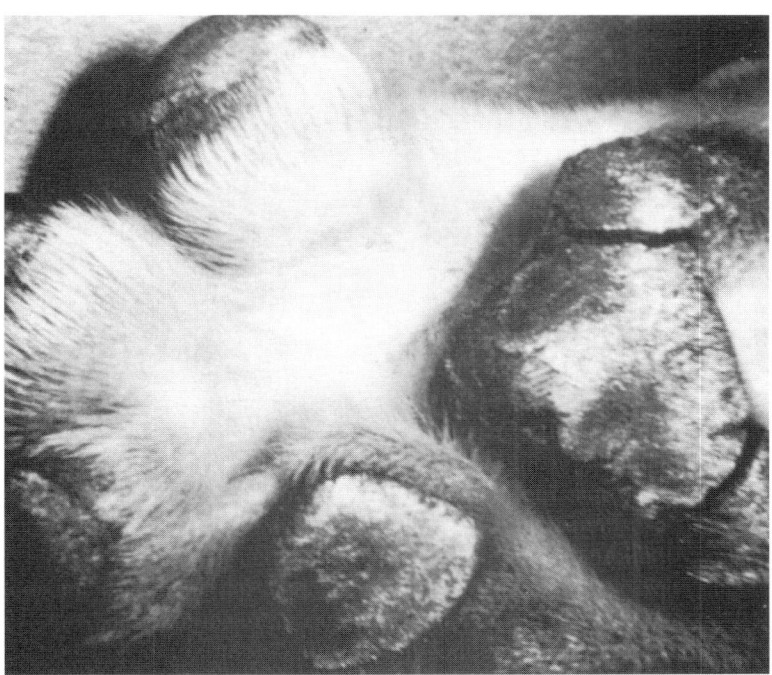

FIGURE 2–22. Fissure—a linear cleavage into the epidermis, or through the epidermis into the dermis, caused by disease or injury. Fissures may be single or multiple tiny cracks or large clefts several centimeters long. They have sharply defined margins and may be dry or moist and straight, curved, or branching. They occur when the skin is thick and inelastic and then subjected to sudden swelling from inflammation or trauma, especially in regions of frequent movement. Examples are found at ear margins, and at ocular, nasal, oral, and anal mucocutaneous borders. (Photograph illustrates two fissures in a footpad.)

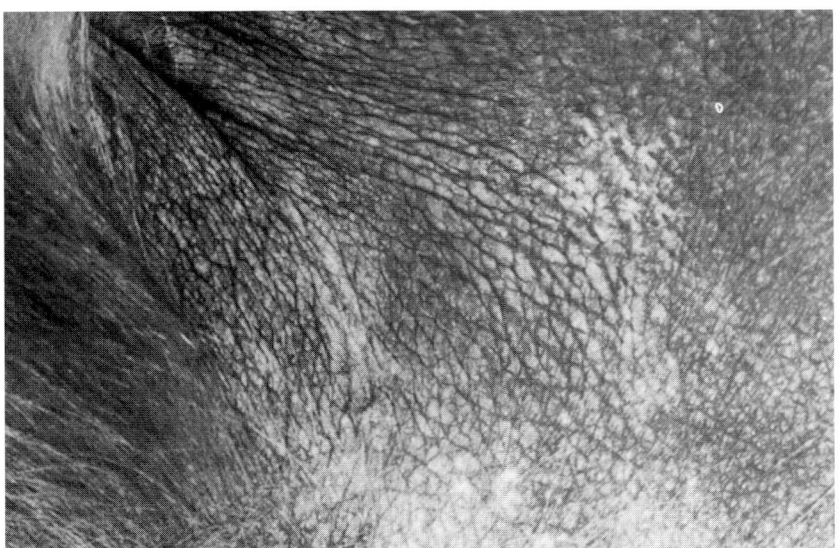

FIGURE 2–23. Lichenification—a thickening and hardening of the skin characterized by an exaggeration of the superficial skin markings. Lichenification areas often result from friction. They may be normally colored but are more often hyperpigmented. Crusted lichenified plaques usually have a bacterial component and improve with antibiotic therapy. Occasionally, *Malassezia* are found with these lesions. Examples are the axillae in acanthosis nigricans. (Photograph illustrates the axilla of a dog with chronic atopic dermatitis. The lichenification here is a result of rubbing.)

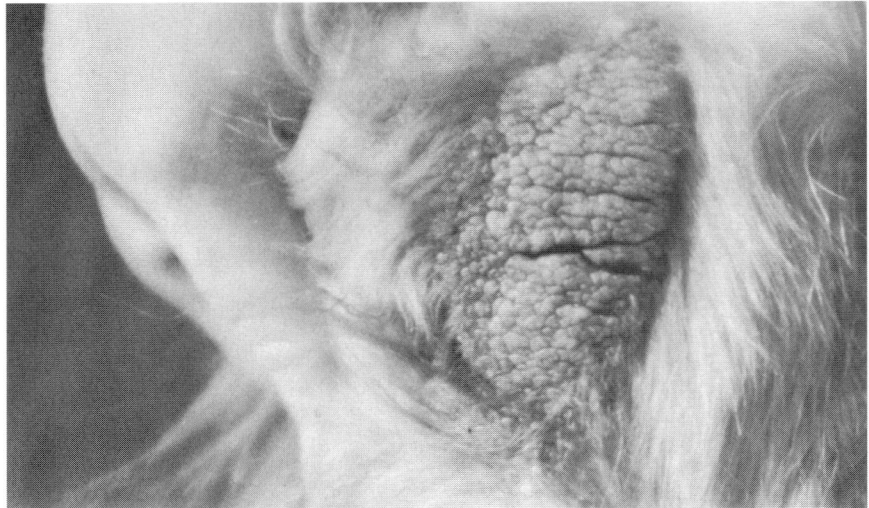

FIGURE 2–24. Callus—a thickened, rough, hyperkeratotic, alopecic, often lichenified plaque that develops on the skin. Most commonly, calluses occur over bony prominences and result from pressure and chronic low-grade friction. (Photograph illustrates an elbow callus.)

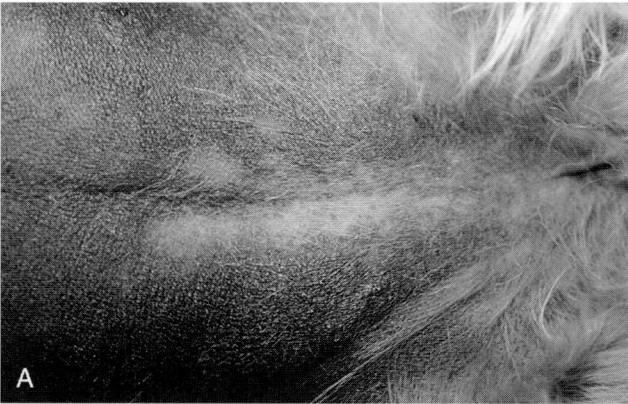

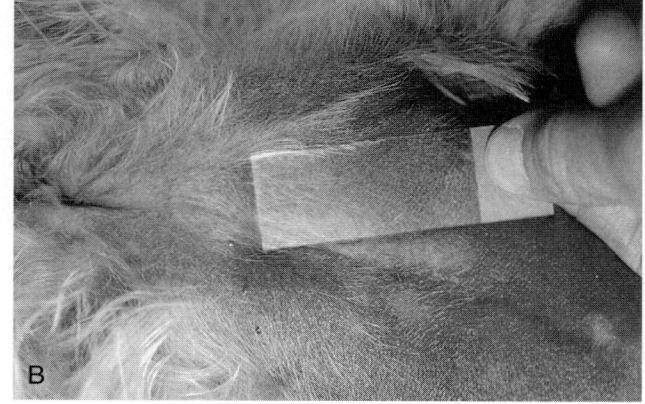

FIGURE 2–25. *A*, Abdomen of dog with drug-induced vasculitis and purpura. *B*, Erythema fails to blanch with diascopy, confirming dermal hemorrhage.

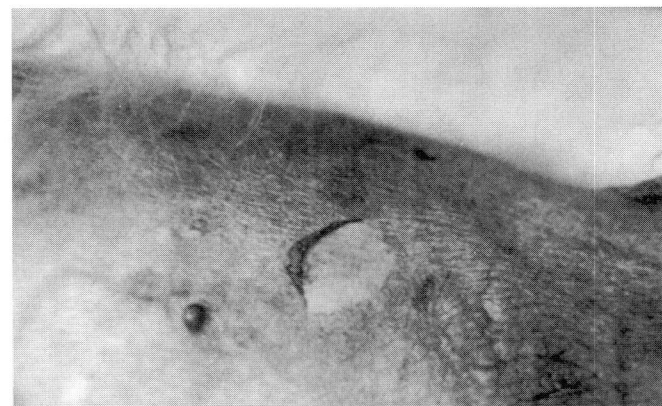

FIGURE 2–26. Photograph illustrates a case of toxic epidermal necrolysis (drug-induced) and the presence of Nikolsky's sign.

learn these techniques is well worth the time. The alternatives are not to obtain this information, to do other more expensive and time-consuming tests, or to send samples to a laboratory, which adds cost and time delays.

SKIN SCRAPING

Skin scraping is one of the most frequently used tests in veterinary dermatology and is recommended anytime the differential diagnosis includes microscopic ectoparasitic diseases. Its purpose is to enable the clinician to find and to identify small and microscopic ectoparasites. It is important to realize that, although testing may accurately confirm diseases, its sensitivity for ruling out a diagnosis depends on the disease and the aggressiveness of sampling. Skin scraping is most commonly used to verify or rule out the diagnosis of demodectic mange. It is also commonly used to try to establish the diagnosis of sarcoptic mange, *Cheyletiella* infestation, and some other ectoparasitic diseases, although it does not effectively rule out these diagnoses. The equipment needed to perform a skin scraping is mineral oil, a scalpel blade (with or without a handle) or a curet, microscope slides, coverslips, and a microscope.

Not all skin scrapings are made in the same way. Success in finding parasites is enhanced if the technique of scraping is adapted to the specific parasite that the clinician expects to find. The method of scraping for demodectic mites is different from that used for sarcoptic mites. *Cheyletiella, Dermanyssus,* cat fur mites, and ear mites each necessitate a slightly different scraping technique.

No matter which type of scraping is made, a consistent, orderly examination of the collected material should be done until a diagnosis is made or all the collected material has been examined. It is easiest to start the examination at one end of the scraped material mixed with oil and move the microscope stage straight across the slide in either a horizontal or a vertical direction. At the end of the slide, the examination moves over one field of vision and goes back in the opposite direction. This is continued back and forth until all of the scraped material on the slide has been examined.

The following discussions elaborate on the special techniques needed to enhance the effectiveness of scraping for specific parasites.

Examination for Parasites

- **Demodectic Mites.** Generally, multiple scrapings from new lesions should be obtained. The affected skin should be squeezed between the thumb and the forefinger to extrude the mites from the hair follicles. The obtained material is scraped up and placed on a microscope slide. It is helpful to apply a drop of mineral oil to the skin site being scraped, or to the scalpel blade or curet, to facilitate the adherence of material to the blade. Then, additional material is obtained by scraping the skin more deeply until

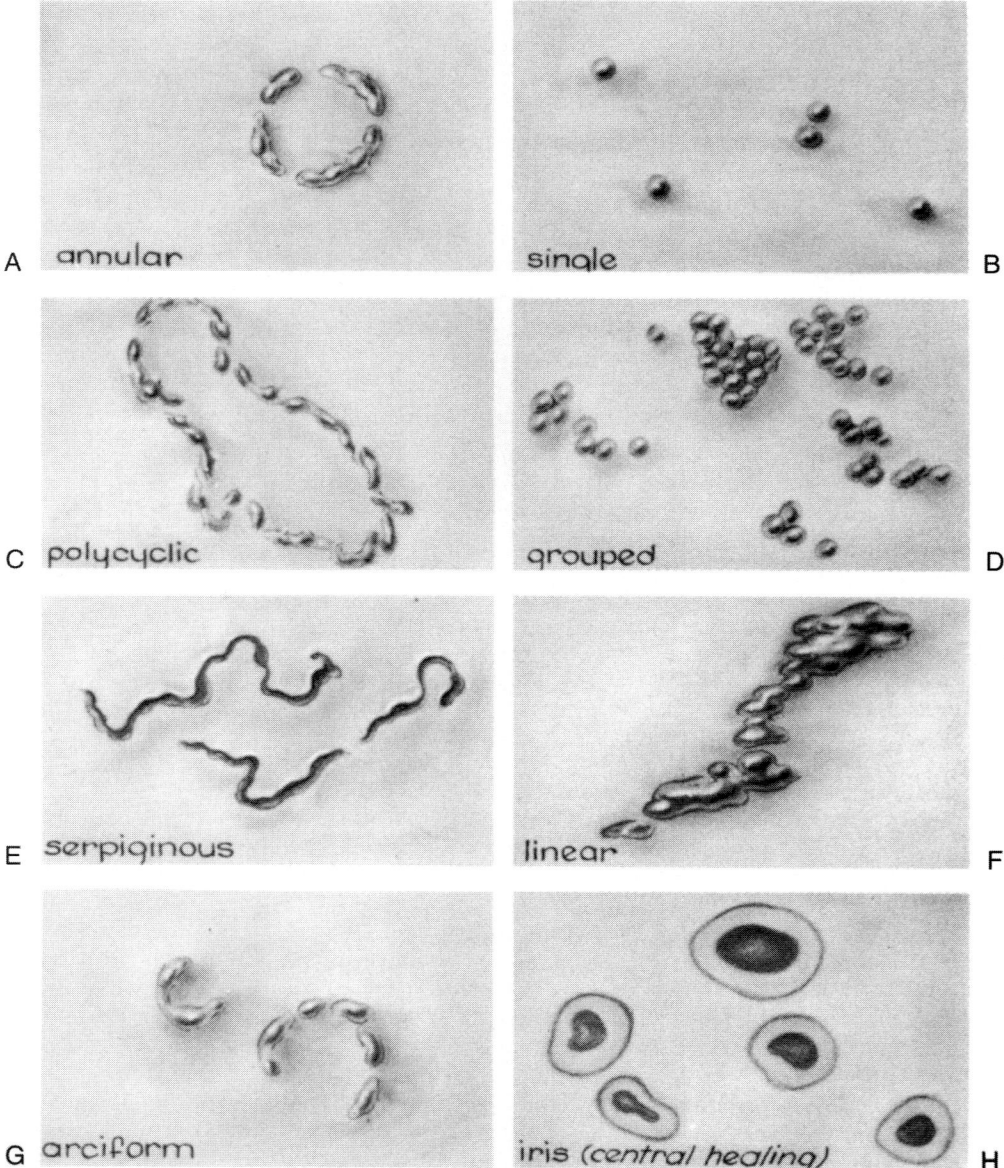

FIGURE 2-27. Configuration of skin lesions. *A,* The annular configuration has a clear or less involved center and is found in superficial spreading bacterial folliculitis, local seborrhea, demodicosis, and dermatophytosis. *B,* Single lesions are typified by feline acne, acral lick dermatitis, cysts, and many tumors. *C,* Polycyclic configurations often result from the confluence of lesions or a spreading process. Examples are superficial spreading bacterial folliculitis, demodicosis, or pyotraumatic dermatitis. *D,* Grouped lesions are clusters, often the result of new foci developing around an old lesion. They are seen in folliculitis, insect bites, contact dermatitis, and calcinosis cutis. *E,* Serpiginous lesions develop as a result of spreading, such as in canine scabies or demodicosis. They may also occur as a result of the confluence and partial resolution of polycyclic lesions. *F,* Linear configurations are best typified by the linear form of eosinophilic granuloma of cats or by contact with irritant materials streaked along the skin. *G,* Arciform lesions usually result from the partial resolution of polycyclic lesions such as spreading folliculitis, but they may result from spreading, as in canine scabies and demodicosis. *H,* Central-healing (target) configurations are produced when the skin heals behind an advancing front of a disease process. It is typical of certain dermatophytoses, demodicosis, and bacterial folliculitis.

Table 2-4 REGIONAL DIAGNOSIS OF NON-NEOPLASTIC DERMATOSES

REGION	COMMON DISEASE	LESS COMMON DISEASE
Head	Atopy Demodicosis Dermatophytosis Facial fold intertrigo Feline food hypersensitivity Folliculitis, bacterial Scabies, feline	Feline leprosy Juvenile cellulitis Pemphigus erythematosus Pemphigus foliaceus Sporotrichosis Sterile pyogranuloma syndrome Systemic lupus erythematosus Vasculitis Zinc-responsive dermatosis
Ear	Atopy Food hypersensitivity Demodicosis Dermatomyositis Dermatophytosis Fly dermatitis Otitis externa (see Chap. 19) Otodectic mange Scabies, feline and canine Seborrhea, marginal (pinna)	Alopecia, pattern Cold agglutinin disease Frostbite Melanoderma and alopecia of Yorkshire terriers Pinnal thrombovascular necrosis Solar dermatitis, feline Sterile eosinophilic pinnal folliculitis Trombiculiasis Vasculitis and vasculopathy
Eyelid	Chalazion Demodicosis Dermatophytosis Distichiasis Entropion Folliculitis, bacterial Hordeolum Seborrheic blepharitis Trichiasis	Lupus erythematosus Dermatomyositis
Nasal planum	Discoid lupus erythematosus Drug eruption Erythema multiforme Nasodigital hyperkeratosis Pemphigus erythematosus Pemphigus foliaceus	Contact dermatitis Dermatophytosis (*Microsporum persicolor*) Hereditary nasal pyogranuloma and vasculitis (Scottish terriers) Sporotrichosis Sterile pyogranuloma syndrome Uveodermatologic syndrome Vitiligo
Lip	Demodicosis Indolent ulcer, feline Lip fold intertrigo Lupus erythematosus Muzzle furunculosis, bacterial Oral papillomatosis, canine Uveodermatologic syndrome Vitiligo-like lesions	Candidiasis Contact dermatitis (plastic, rubber) Juvenile cellulitis Mucocutaneous bacterial pyoderma
Oral cavity (mucosal lesions)	Discoid lupus erythematosus Eosinophilic granuloma, canine and feline Eosinophilic plaque, feline Erosions, chemical Erosions, viral, feline Erythema multiforme Fusospirochetal stomatitis Gingival hypertrophy Indolent ulcer, feline Marginal gingivitis, ulcerative, dental Plasma cell stomatitis Vegetative glossitis (foreign body)	Bullous pemphigoid Candidiasis Pemphigus vulgaris Systemic lupus erythematosus Thallotoxicosis
Mucocutaneous junctions	Epitheliotropic lymphoma Erythema multiforme Mucocutaneous pyoderma Systemic lupus erythematosus	Bullous pemphigoid Candidiasis Pemphigus vulgaris Phaeohyphomycosis

Table continued on following page

Table 2-4 REGIONAL DIAGNOSIS OF NON-NEOPLASTIC DERMATOSES Continued

REGION	COMMON DISEASE	LESS COMMON DISEASE
Mucocutaneous junctions *Continued*	Vitiligo	Thallotoxicosis Toxic epidermal necrolysis Vesicular cutaneous lupus erythematosus (collie and Shetland sheepdog)
Chin	Demodicosis Eosinophilic granuloma, feline Furunculosis, bacterial Juvenile cellulitis	Dermatophytosis *Malassezia* dermatitis
Neck	Atopy, feline Dermoid sinus Flea bite hypersensitivity, feline Injection reactions Food hypersensitivity, feline *Malassezia* dermatitis	Contact dermatitis (collars) Ulcerative dermatitis with linear subepidermal fibrosis, feline
Lower chest	Folliculitis, bacterial Sternal callus	Contact dermatitis *Pelodera* dermatitis
Axilla	Acanthosis nigricans Atopy Folliculitis, bacterial Food hypersensitivity *Malassezia* dermatitis	Bullous pemphigoid Contact dermatitis Erythema multiforme Pemphigus vulgaris Vesicular cutaneous lupus erythematosus (collie and Shetland sheepdog)
Back	Atopy Comedo syndrome, Schnauzers Flea bite hypersensitivity Folliculitis, bacterial Food hypersensitivity Hypothyroidism Psychogenic dermatitis or alopecia, feline Seborrhea, primary	Calcinosis cutis Cheyletiellosis Pediculosis
Trunk	Demodicosis, generalized Folliculitis, bacterial Hyperadrenocorticism Hypothyroidism Sebaceous adenitis	Hyperestrogenism, female Hyposomatotropism Panniculitis, sterile Sterile eosinophilic pustulosis Subcorneal pustular dermatosis Vitamin A–responsive dermatosis
Abdomen	Atopy, feline Eosinophilic plaque, feline Feline symmetric alopecia Folliculitis, bacterial Food hypersensitivity, feline Hyperadrenocorticism Impetigo Linear prepucial erythema Panniculitis, sterile Psychogenic alopecia and dermatitis, feline Solar dermatitis, dog Trombiculiasis	Bullous pemphigoid Calcinosis cutis Contact dermatitis (ventral abdomen) Erythema multiforme Hookworm dermatitis Mycobacteriosis, atypical, feline *Pelodera* dermatitis Vesicular cutaneous lupus erythematosus (collie and Shetland sheepdog)
Tail	Feline symmetric alopecia Flea bite hypersensitivity Hyperplasia of tail gland, stud tail Mechanical irritation (tail suckers) Psychogenic dermatitis or alopecia, feline	Cold agglutinin disease Dermatomyositis Frostbite Vasculitis

● Table 2–4   **REGIONAL DIAGNOSIS OF NON-NEOPLASTIC DERMATOSES** *Continued*

REGION	COMMON DISEASE	LESS COMMON DISEASE
Tail *Continued*	Pyotraumatic dermatitis	
	Tip of tail trauma	
Anus	Anal sac disease	Bullous pemphigoid
	Malassezia dermatitis	Food hypersensitivity
		Pemphigus vulgaris
		Perianal gland hyperplasia
Legs	Acral furunculosis, bacterial	Decubital ulcers
	Acral lick dermatitis	Feline leprosy
	Contact dermatitis	Lymphangitis, bacterial, fungal
	Demodicosis	Lymphedema
	Dermatophytosis	*Pelodera* dermatitis
	Elbow callus	
	Elbow callus pyoderma	
	Eosinophilic granuloma, feline	
	Hygroma	
	Metatarsal fistulae, German shepherd	
	Scabies, canine	
Paws	Atopy	Acral mutilation
	Demodicosis	Collagen disease of German shepherd footpads
	Dermatophytosis	Contact dermatitis
	Digital pad hyperkeratosis	Hookworm dermatitis
	Food hypersensitivity	Leishmaniasis
	Interdigital foreign bodies	Mycetoma
	Malassezia dermatitis	Necrolytic migratory erythema
	Pemphigus foliaceus	*Pelodera* dermatitis
	Plasma cell pododermatitis, feline	Phaeohyphomycosis
	Sterile pyogranuloma syndrome	Tyrosinemia
	Trauma	Vitiligo (pads)
	Trombiculiasis	Zinc-responsive dermatosis
Claws	Hyperthyroidism, feline	Arteriovenous fistula
	Lupoid onychodystrophy	Bullous pemphigoid
	Paronychia	Leishmaniasis
	Bacterial	Onychomycosis
	Feline leukemia	Pemphigus foliaceus
	Traumatic	Pemphigus vulgaris
	Trauma	Systemic lupus erythematosus
		Vasculitis
		Vitiligo

capillary bleeding is produced. It is important that true capillary bleeding is obtained and not blood from laceration. This is especially true when scraping the paw or the interdigital area in cases of pododermatitis. Please note that the Chinese Shar pei breed presents an unusual situation in which mites may be confined to the deep follicle, and even with good scrapes characterized by capillary bleeding, false-negative results may occur. In addition, skin scrapings may be negative in dogs with chronic demodectic pododermatitis, wherein the paws are swollen, fibrotic, and granulomatous. Hair pluckings may reveal mites in some of these cases and should be attempted before skin biopsy. Only skin biopsies are diagnostic in some cases.

Generally, two or three drops of mineral oil are added to the usual amount of scraped material on the microscope slide. The oil is mixed with the scraped material to obtain an even consistency. Placing a coverslip on the material to be examined ensures a uniform layer that is more readily examined. Lowering the condenser or closing the iris diaphragm causes more light diffraction and contrast, resulting in easier recognition of the mites.

Diagnosis is made by demonstrating multiple adult mites, finding adult mites from multiple sites, or finding immature forms of mites (ova, larvae, and nymphs). When dogs are fractious or sites are difficult to scrape, another technique may be used. Hairs from the affected area can be plucked, placed in mineral oil on a slide, and examined. When the findings are positive, this technique precludes the need for deep skin scrapes. However, negative results of hair pluck examinations should not rule out the presence of *Demodex.*

It seems that skin scraping is a straightforward, easy laboratory procedure; however, the authors have encountered referred demodicosis cases in which false-negative skin scraping findings led to misdiagnosis or skin scrapings were not performed. Skin scrapings are advised in most cases of canine pyoderma and scaling and follicular disorders, because generalized demodicosis may be the primary disease. Skin scrapings should be performed whenever *Demodex* infection is among the primary differential diagnostic possibilities, the clinician is not certain of the diagnosis, or the dog does not adequately respond to the initial therapy. Dogs typically harbor only one species of mite, *Demodex canis,* whereas cats have two species, *D. cati* (which resembles the canine mite) and a second species that is short and squat, *D. gatoi.*

Scrapings taken from a normal dog, especially from the face, may contain an occasional adult mite. If one or two mites are observed, repeated scrapings should be done. Multiple positive results of scrapings from different sites should be considered abnormal. Observing whether the mites are alive (mouthparts or legs moving) or dead is of prognostic value while the animal is being treated. As a case of generalized *Demodex* infestation responds to treatment, the ratio of live to dead mites decreases, as does the ratio of eggs and larvae to adults. If this is not occurring, the treatment regimen should be reevaluated.

- **Canine Scabies Mites.** Canine sarcoptic mites, *Sarcoptes scabiei* (var. *canis*), reside within the superficial epidermis. However, because small numbers of mites are usually present, it is difficult to find one. Multiple superficial scrapings are indicated, with emphasis on the pinnal margins and elbows. Skin that has not been excoriated, preferably skin with red raised papules and yellowish crusts on top, should be scraped. The more scrapings are performed, the more likely is a diagnosis. However, even with numerous scrapings, scabies cannot be ruled out because of negative results.

Extensive amounts of material should be accumulated in the scrapings and spread on microscope slides. Double-sized coverslips are sometimes useful. Alternatively, a second microscope glass slide may be used instead of a normal coverslip to compress the thick crusts. The clinician examines each field until a mite is found or all material has been examined; one mite is diagnostic. Dark brown, round or oval fecal pellets or ova from adult mites, if found, are also diagnostic. In difficult cases, it may be useful to accumulate an even larger amount of hair and keratin debris from scrapings. The material is placed in a warm solution of 10% potassium hydroxide (KOH) for 20 minutes to digest keratin, and the mixture is then stirred and centrifuged. Mites are thus concentrated and can often be picked off the surface film and identified with a microscope.

- **Feline Scabies Mites.** The feline scabies mite, *Notoedres cati*, is much easier to find than the canine mite; otherwise, the diagnostic techniques described for canine scabies are appropriate. The best place to scrape is the head, the face, or the ears, in areas with crusts and scales.

- **Cheyletiella Mites.** *Cheyletiella* mites are relatively large compared with scabies mites and may even be seen with a magnifying glass. They look like small white scales that move, which is why the disease has been called "walking" dandruff. To examine for them microscopically, the clinician may obtain superficial scrapings, which are not as accurate as acetate tape impressions or flea-combing specimens. These mites may be difficult to demonstrate in some cases, especially in cats.

- **Chigger Mites.** The most common chigger mite is *Eutrombicula alfreddugesi*. These mites can be seen with the naked eye, especially on the concave surface of the pinna. They appear as bright orange objects adhering tightly to the skin or centered in a papule. They are easily recognized by their large size, relatively intense color, and tight attachment to the skin. They are often found around the external orifice of the ear canal but are not present in the canal. They should be covered with mineral oil and picked up with a scalpel blade. A true skin scraping is not needed. However, when removed from the host for microscopic examination, they should immediately be placed in mineral oil, or they may crawl away. Only the larval form is pathogenic, and these mites have only six legs.

• **Poultry Mites.** *Dermanyssus gallinae* is a mite that attacks poultry, wild and cage birds, and dogs and cats, as well as humans. It is red when engorged with blood; otherwise, it is white, gray, or black. When the animal shows evidence of itching and the history indicates exposure to bird or poultry housing, a skin scraping for this mite is indicated. One or two mites on the dog or cat may cause severe pruritus. The best place to find the mites is at excoriated sites.

The clinician collects the debris, scales, and crusts that harbor the mites. The materials are placed on a microscope slide, and several drops of mineral oil are added. The slide is covered with another glass slide instead of a coverslip. The two slides are squeezed together firmly to crush any crusted material. The acetate tape method of collection may be used successfully.

• **Cat Fur Mites.** *Lynxacarus radovsky* are mites that attach themselves to the external aspect of the hair shafts and therefore may be demonstrated microscopically by searching for salt-and-pepper hairs. The mites are usually located along the topline. A true superficial skin scraping can be made if the mites are suspected to be on the skin, but plucking affected hairs and examining them in a mineral oil preparation is usually diagnostic. The acetate tape impression method can also be used.

• **Ear Mites.** *Otodectes cynotis* mites are usually located in the external ear canal of dogs and cats. However, they may also be found on the skin, especially around the head, the neck, the rump, and the tail. They may be found by superficial scraping or acetate tape methods, such as described for *Cheyletiella* mites, and identified by microscopic examination.

ACETATE TAPE IMPRESSION

This alternative to skin scraping has been recommended to find superficial ectoparasites such as *Cheyletiella* mites, poultry mites, and cat fur mites. Clear, pressure-sensitive acetate tape (Scotch No. 602 [3M Co.] is a good type) is pressed to the hair surface and to the skin adjacent to parted hairs or in shaved areas. Superficial scales and debris are collected when one suspects cheyletiellosis or poultry mites. The tape is then stuck with pressure on a microscope slide and examined.

FLEA COMB AND FLOTATION

The recovery of *Cheyletiella* mites is enhanced with the flea-combing method. In this technique, large areas of the body are combed and the collected scale and debris are put in a fecal flotation solution. Material and scale that fall on the table or on a sheet of paper placed under the patient during combing should also be added to the flotation solution. A coverslip is applied to the surface of the flotation solution, is allowed to stand for 10 minutes, and then is transferred to a microscope slide and examined.

Debris Examination or Flotation

During examination of a pet, scabs and debris may readily be collected on the table surface. This may be enhanced by briskly rubbing the pet's skin and hair coat while the animal is standing on the table or over a piece of paper. This material may be collected and examined directly or mixed with a fecal flotation solution. Direct examination may find otherwise undetected flea dirt, flea eggs, or rarely, mites. Suspect flea dirt may be placed on moistened white paper or cotton and will dissolve to an orange-red stain.

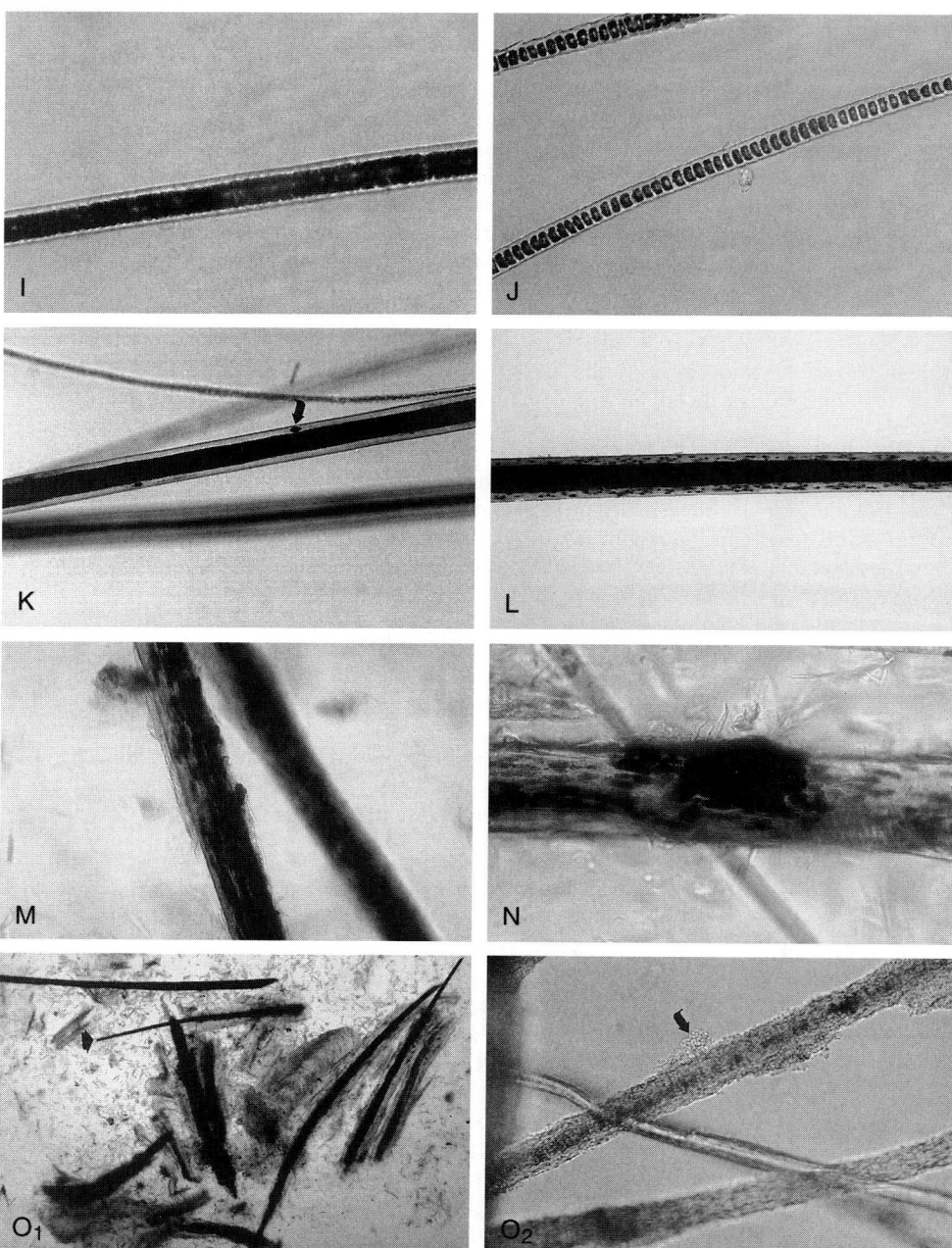

FIGURE 2–28 *Continued. I*, Primary hair shaft from a white cat. The single-layered outer cuticle covers the hair shaft in shingle-like fashion. The nonpigmented cortex is the middle layer. The largest, dark central layer is the medulla. *J*, Secondary hair shaft from same white cat; same magnification. *K*, Hair from a normal blue point Siamese cat. The Maltese dilution gene is responsible for diluting black to blue (gray) and orange to cream. It results in the irregular clumping of melanin *(arrow)*, but does not change the normal anatomy of the hair shaft. *L*, Hair from a normal color diluted dog (Weimeraner). Note that melanin clumps vary in size and shape and are dispersed irregularly. They do *not*, however, change the anatomy of the hair shaft. *M*, Hair from a dog (Doberman pinscher) with color dilution alopecia. Note how the huge, irregularly shaped, sized, and dispersed melanin clumps are associated with a loss of normal hair shaft anatomy. *N*, Close-up of another hair from dog in M. Note how the huge melanin clump has breached the surface of the hair shaft. This area is now weakened and breakage can occur at this site. O_1 and O_2, Hairs from a dog with dermatophytosis placed in mineral oil. O_2, One hair *(arrow)* is normal in appearance near the arrow, but becomes thickened and irregular (fuzzy) in outline as you follow it to the right. Also note two other infected hairs below the arrowed hair, in the center of the field. Higher magnification of such an area shows an irregular hair shaft whose anatomy has been obliterated by the presence of arthroconidia *(arrow)*.

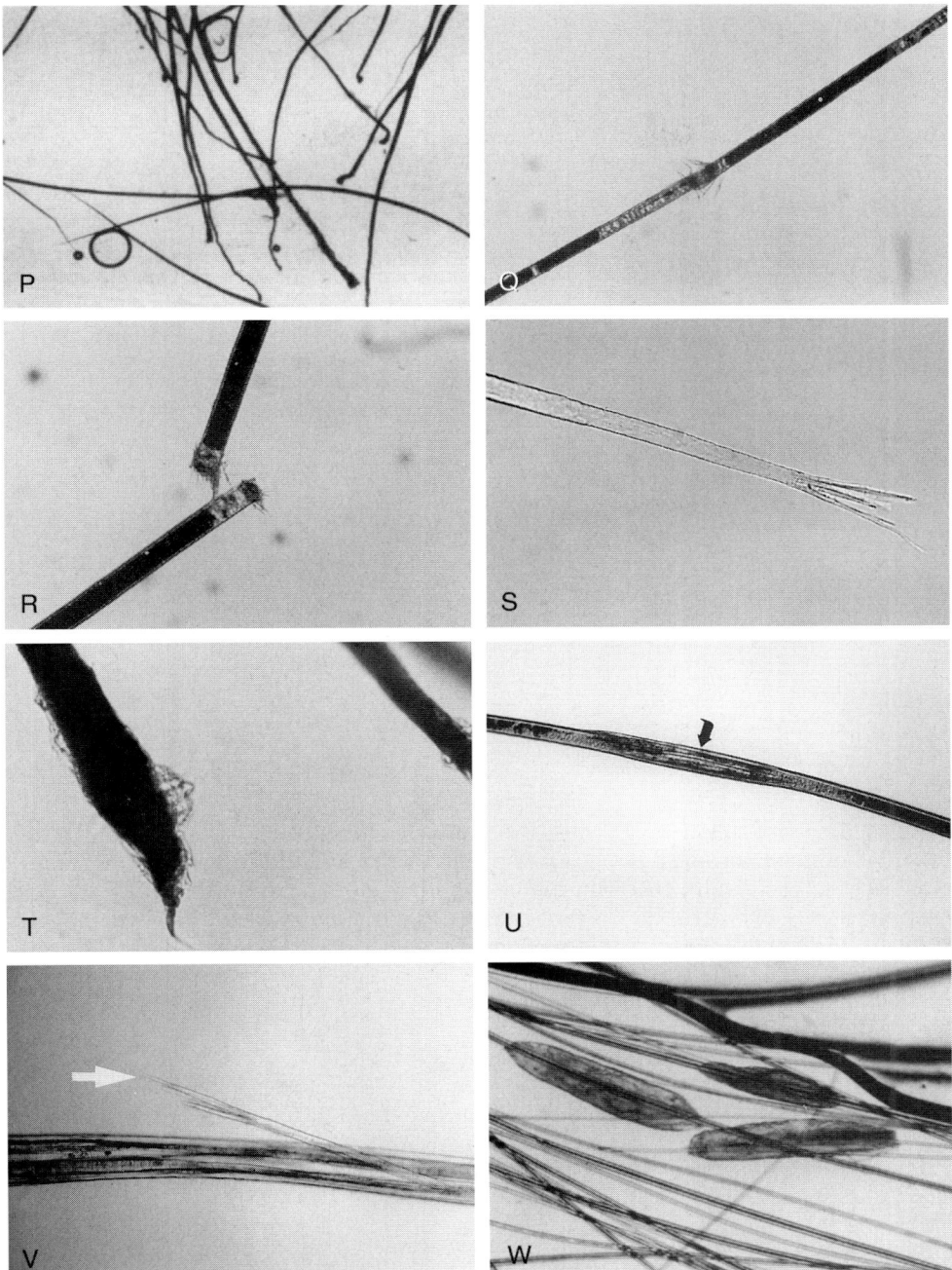

FIGURE 2-28 Continued. *P*, Nutritional deficiency. Misshapen and malformed hairs. *Q*, Trichorrhexis nodosa. Note nodular area in the center of the hair shaft where breakage will occur. *R*, Trichorrhexis nodosa. Hair has fractured at a nodule, giving the appearance of two brooms end to end. *S*, Trichoptilosis (split ends) in a dog. Note the distal end is split longitudinally through the hair shaft. *T*, "Exclamation point" hair of alopecia areata. *U*, Medullary trichomalacia in a dog. Note focal thickening of hair shaft *(arrow)* associated with a loss of medullary definition and longitudinal lamellar splitting. *V*, Another hair shaft from same dog as in *U* at higher magnification. Affected area of hair is undergoing longitudinal lamellar splitting *(arrow)*. *W*, Hair cast. Prominent casts of keratosebaceous debris surrounding numerous hair shafts.

Illustration continued on following page

112 • Diagnostic Methods

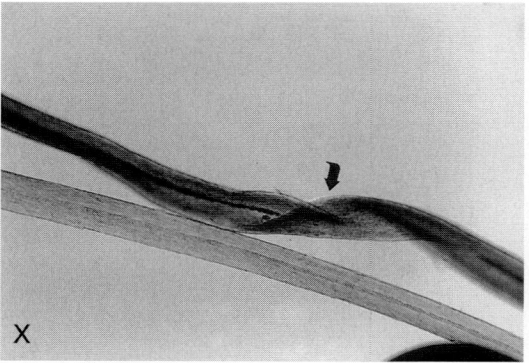
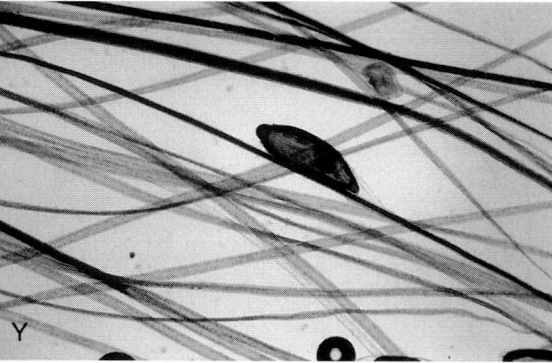
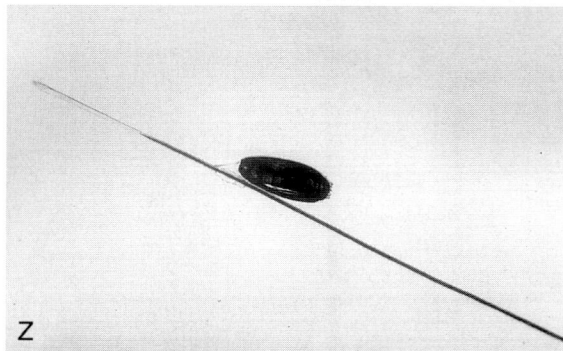

FIGURE 2–28 *Continued.* X, Pili torti. Note 360-degree twist of hair shaft on its long axis *(arrow).* Y, Louse nit. Note the nit is operculated and that most of the side of the nit is attached to the hair shaft. Z, *Cheyletiella* egg. Note that the egg is not operculated, and is only attached to the hair at one end.

Cytologic Examination

An enormous amount of vital diagnostic data can be obtained by microscopic examination of stained material, such as smears of tissues or fluids, during a clinical examination.[11] It is possible to accomplish this with minimal equipment and in less than 5 minutes. The cost is much less than that for a yeast culture, bacterial culture and susceptibility testing, or biopsy. Although the same information as obtained by these more expensive tests is not really gathered, microscopic examination often supplies sufficient data to narrow a differential diagnosis and develop a diagnostic plan.

The type of inflammatory, neoplastic, or other cellular infiltrate; the relative amount of protein or mucin; and the presence of acantholytic keratinocytes, yeasts, and bacteria can be determined by cytologic evaluation. It is the most common and most rewarding office test performed by the authors. The equipment includes a clean microscope slide, a coverslip, a stain, and a microscope.

SPECIMEN COLLECTION

Materials for cytologic examination can be gathered by a variety of techniques. Those most commonly used by the authors include direct smears, impression smears, swab smears, scrapings, and fine-needle aspiration. In most situations, clipping the hair should be the only preparation of the surface. Scrubbing and applying alcohol or disinfectants are used only in areas where a fine-needle aspirate of a mass lesion is to be done.

Direct smears are usually performed for fluid-containing lesions. A small amount of material is collected with the corner of a slide, the tip of a needle, or another sharp-edged object. The material is then smeared on the microscope slide. Smears should be made gently to minimize disruption of cells (Fig. 2–29B).

Impression smears are often obtained when lesions are moist or greasy. This technique is also used after removing crusts, expressing fluid from lesions, or gently opening

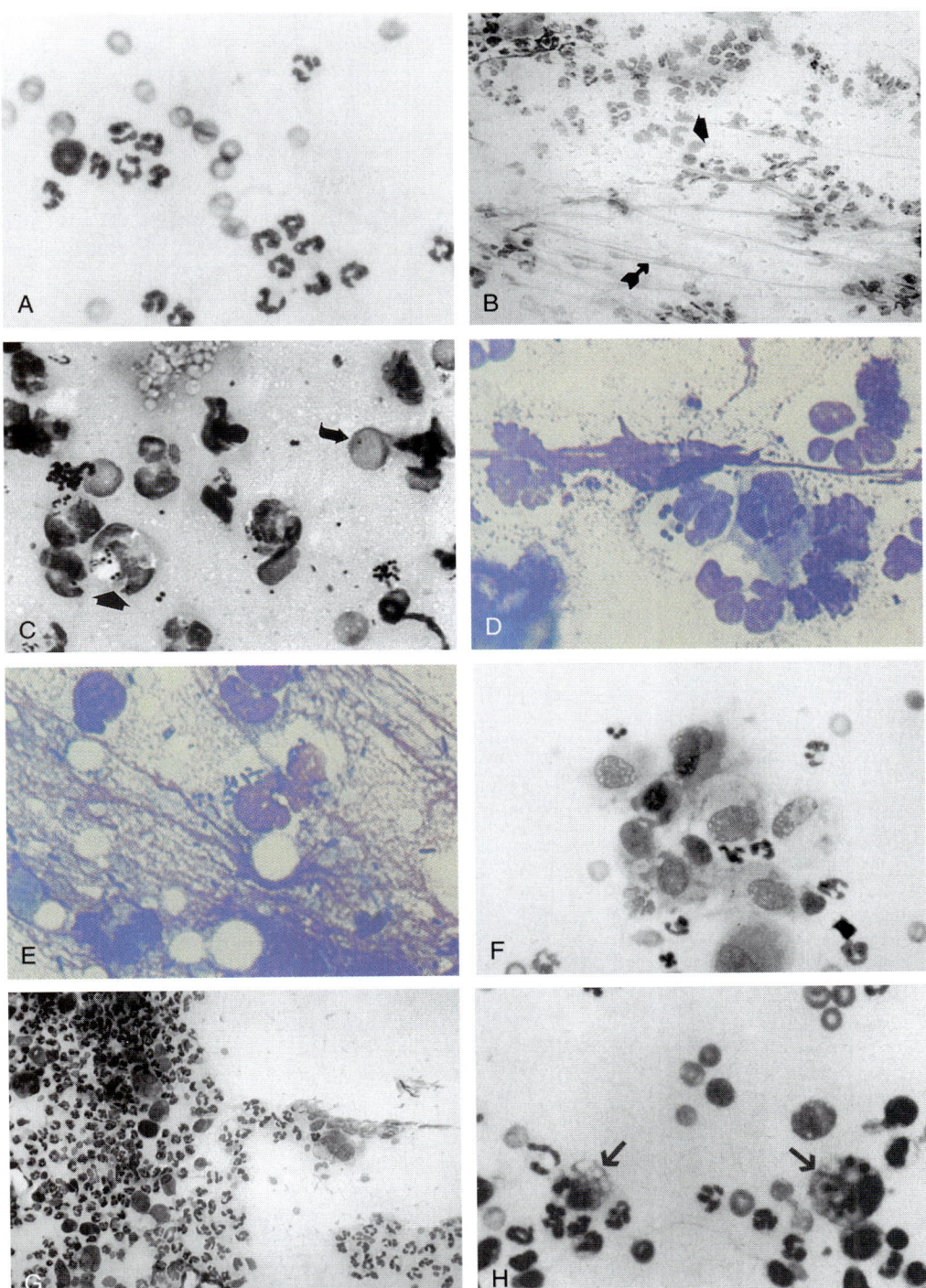

FIGURE 2–29. *A*, Nondegenerate neutrophils in sterile pus. *B*, Degenerate neutrophils and nuclear streaming in pus from a dog with staphylococcal folliculitis. Note that most neutrophil nuclei are swollen and pale-staining *(short arrow)*, and many are streamed *(long arrow)*. *C*, Close-up of another field from *B*. Most neutrophils are degenerate (nuclei lightly stained and swollen) and many contain cocci *(short arrow)*. Erythrocytes are also present *(long arrow)*. *D*, Phagocytosed cocci. *E*, Phagocytosed rods. *F*, Sterile pyogranuloma. Macrophages, nondegenerate neutrophils, and no microorganisms. *G*, Infectious pyogranuloma from a dog. Compare the smaller, well-delineated and segmented nondegenerate neutrophil nuclei at the left with the larger, swollen, lightly stained, and often streamed degenerate neutrophil nuclei to the right. *H*, Sterile pyogranuloma. Nondegenerate neutrophils, no mocroorganisms, and neutrophagocytosis *(arrows)*.

Illustration continued on following page

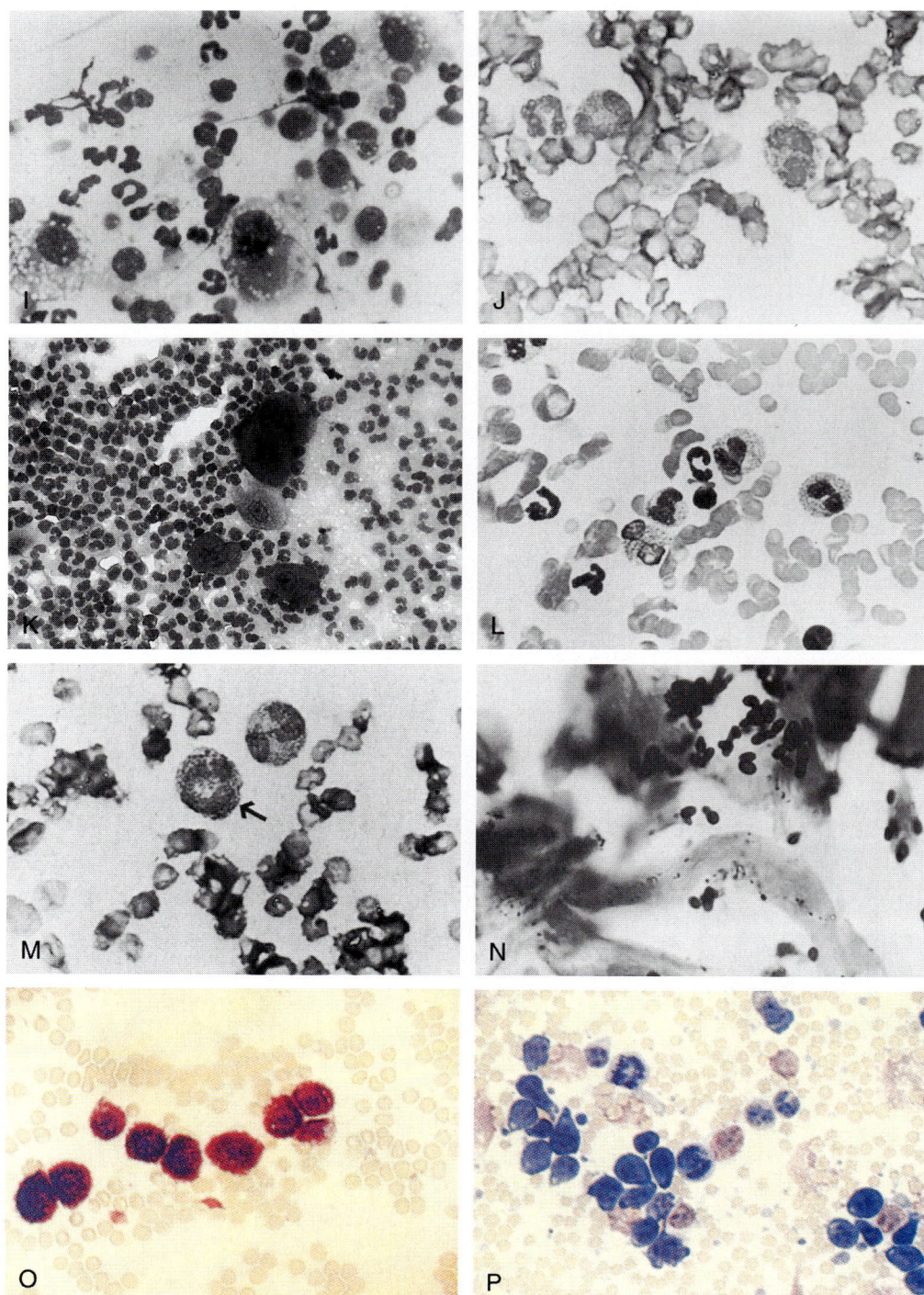

FIGURE 2–29 *Continued. I,* Sterile panniculitis. Nondegenerate neutrophils, no microorganisms, and macrophages containing numerous fat droplets. *J,* Eosinophils from a dog with sterile eosinophilic pustulosis. *K,* Pus from a cat with pemphigus erythematosus. Note the nondegenerate neutrophils and lack of nuclear streaming and microorganisms suggesting that this is a sterile inflammatory process. Note also the five acantholytic keratinocytes in the center of the field, which are very suggestive of pemphigus. *L,* Eosinophils and nondegenerate neutrophils from an atopic cat. *M,* Eosinophil and basophil *(arrow)* from a flea-hypersensitive cat. *N, Malassezia* budding yeasts. *O,* Mast cells from a canine mast cell tumor. *P,* Lymphocytes from a dog with lymphosarcoma.

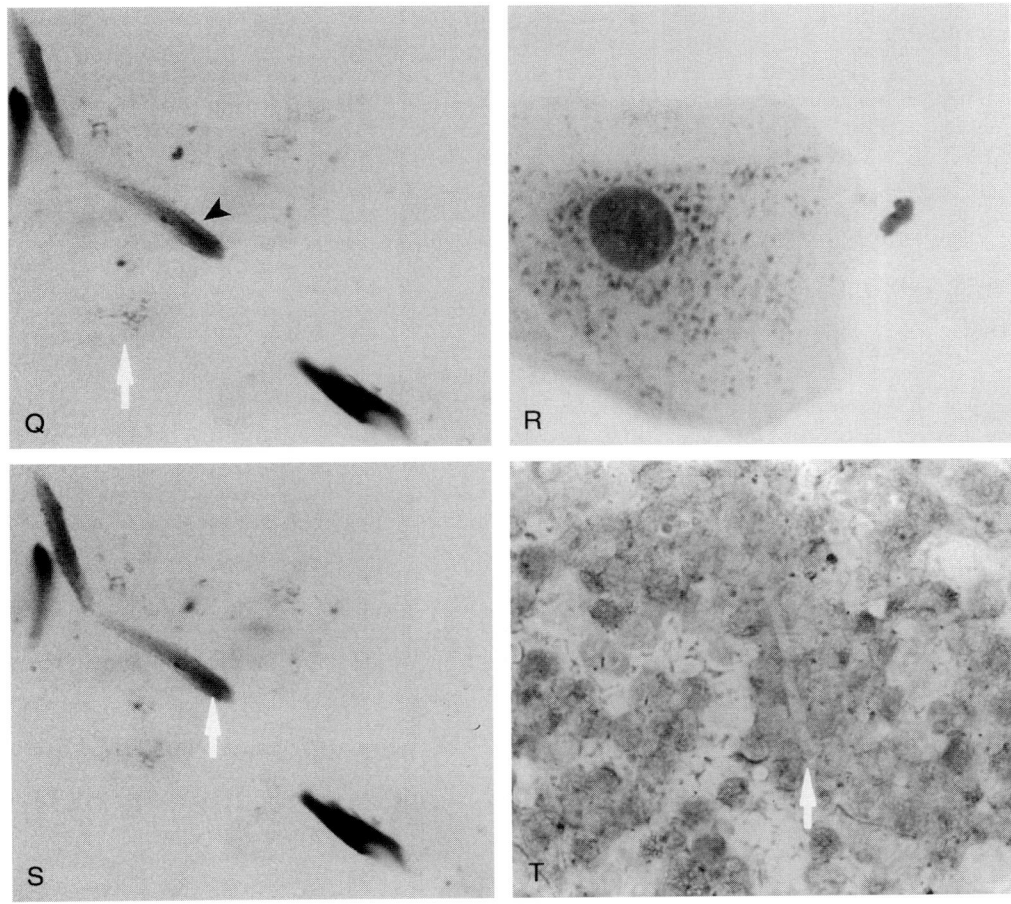

FIGURE 2-29 *Continued.* Q, Swab from normal skin. Four squames are folded or rolled *(black arrow)*. Others are faintly stained, lay flat, and contain melanin granules *(white arrow)*. R, Swab from normal skin. Nucleated keratinocyte contains numerous melanin granules. S, Same field as Q. White arrow indicates squame containing two large, dark staining keratohyalin granules. T, Swab from a dog with otitis externa. There are degenerate neutrophils, numerous rodlike bacteria, and a pseudohypha of *Candida albicans (white arrow)*.

the surface of papules, pustules, or vesicles. The microscope slide is pressed directly against the site to be examined.

Swab smears are most often used to obtain specimens from draining tracts or sinuses, ear canals and interdigital webs, and dry crusty-surfaced lesions. The cotton-tipped applicator is moistened and inserted into the tract, the sinus, or the ear canal. For dry lesions and interdigital webs, the moistened cotton tip is rubbed briskly over the skin surface. After the lesion has been sampled, the cotton tip is rolled over the surface of the microscope slide.

Scrapings are used to sample underneath crusts, vesicles, and peeling stratum corneum. They may also be used to collect more cells from the cut surface of surgically removed biopsy specimens. The skin is scraped with a scalpel blade held at a 15- to 90-degree angle to the surface. The collected material is then gently wiped onto the surface of a microscope slide.

Fine-needle aspiration is most commonly used to sample nodules, tumors, and cysts, although pustules, vesicles, or bullae may also be sampled this way. Fluid-filled lesions can be aspirated with 20- or 22-gauge needles and a 3-ml syringe. Firm lesions should be aspirated with 20-gauge needles and 6- or 10-ml syringes to obtain better suction. Fibrotic or dense masses may necessitate the use of an 18-gauge needle to get an adequate sample. The needle is introduced into the lesion, and then suction is gently applied by withdrawing the plunger of the syringe. Little withdrawing is necessary for fluid-filled lesions, and the material within the needle is sufficient. In mass lesions, the plunger is withdrawn one half to three fourths of the syringe volume. Suction is then interrupted while the needle is redirected into another area of the mass. Suction is again applied, and this procedure is repeated for a total of three or four times. Suction is then released, and the needle is withdrawn from the lesion. The syringe and the needle are then separated, air is introduced into the syringe, the needle is reattached, and the contents of the needle and hub are expelled onto the surface of a glass slide. The material is then streaked across the surface with another glass slide or the needle.

STAINS

Collected materials are allowed to dry on the slide. Oily, waxy, or dry skin samples collected by direct impression or moistened cotton applicators should always be heat-fixed before staining. After the specimens are heat-fixed and dried, the slide is stained and examined microscopically. The stains of choice in clinical practice are the modified Wright's stain (Diff Quik) and new methylene blue. Diff Quik is a quick and easy Romanovsky-type stain. It gives less nuclear detail than the supravital stains such as new methylene blue stain. However, it allows better differentiation of cytoplasmic structures and organisms. Because this is most commonly what the practitioner is interested in with non-neoplastic skin diseases, the Diff Quik stain is preferred by the authors. When a neoplasm is suspected, two slides may be made and both stains used. A Gram stain is occasionally used to acquire more information on the identity of bacteria.

CYTOLOGIC FINDINGS

The first step one takes to learn cutaneous cytology is the evaluation of normal skin. Direct impressions or swab smears should be taken from normal dogs and cats. It is valuable to sample several different cutaneous sites that are often sampled in clinical cases. The ear canals, ventral neck, axilla, and interdigital areas are good sites to select to demonstrate a variety of normal differences. These samples are dried, stained, and examined. Normal structures one will find include squames (angular, anuclear keratinocytes) (Fig. 2–29Q), occasional nucleated keratinocytes, wax and lipid from ear canals, and surface debris. Occasionally, free melanin granules may be seen, but these usually are seen within keratinocytes (see Fig. 2–29R). Melanin granules should not be mistaken for bacteria. Keratohyaline granules may also be found in keratinocytes, particularly nucleated keratinocytes that come from the stratum granulosum of the epidermis (see Fig. 2–29S). Evaluation of healthy skin sites also allows the practitioner to visualize and appreciate the incidence of normal surface bacteria and yeast.

Cytologic study is helpful in distinguishing between bacterial skin infection and bacterial colonization, to determine the relative depth of infection, to determine whether the pustule contains bacteria or is sterile, to discover yeasts and fungi, to identify various cutaneous neoplasms, or to find the acantholytic cells of the pemphigus diseases (see Fig. 2–29K).

Bacteria are a frequent finding in impression smears from skin and can be seen as basophilic-staining organisms in specimens stained with new methylene blue or Diff Quik. Although identification of the exact species of bacteria is not possible with a stain (as it is in a culture), it is possible to distinguish cocci from rods (see Fig. 2–29D and Fig. 2–29E) and often to institute appropriate and effective antibiotic therapy without performing a culture and antibiotic susceptibility testing. Generally, when cocci are seen, they are *Staphylococcus intermedius*. If no bacteria are found in the stained fluid, the clinical condition is probably not a bacterial pyoderma. If neither granulocytes nor intracellular bacteria are seen, then a pyoderma is not present. In normal dogs, the average number of cocci and rods per oil immersion field is less than two.[12] When large numbers of bacteria are found, a condition of bacterial overgrowth is present and may contribute to pruritus and disease. Although the bacteria are not a primary etiology or causing an infection, they may be clinically relevant and appropriate antibiotic therapy will help alleviate some symptoms.

It is also possible to obtain some clues as to the type of bacterial pyoderma or the underlying condition.[2] In general, deep infections have fewer bacteria present, with the vast majority being intracellular. In addition, deep infections have a mixed cellular infiltrate with large numbers of histiocytes, macrophages, lymphocytes, and plasma cells. The presence of these cells suggests that longer term antibiotic therapy is necessary. Large numbers of intracellular and extracellular cocci are seen more commonly in cases of impetigo or in dogs with bacterial infections associated with iatrogenic or natural Cushing's disease.[2]

Direct impression smears are one of the most effective methods for detecting the presence of *Malassezia* (see Fig. 2–29N). Although *Malassezia pachydermatis* is an inhabitant of the skin in most normal dogs and cats, the yeast is difficult to find by examining direct impression smears and usually only 1 or 2 yeasts (rarely more than 20) are found when 1-cm^2 sections of slide are examined (see Chap. 5).[61] In a study done on skin with lesions, the presence of more than one yeast organism per high-power microscopic field was associated with certain diseases, such as seborrhea, or with previous antibiotic therapy (see Chap. 5).[62] Although the presence of more than one or two yeast per high-power field is not diagnostic of *Malassezia* dermatitis, the authors believe that this indicates that yeasts are present in abnormally high numbers and may be contributing to the pathologic changes seen. The yeast *Candida albicans* is a dimorphic fungus with the tissue infective form developing pseudohyphae. Because this organism in the yeast form may be a contaminant and is not indicative of infection, histopathology is the preferred method of confirming infection. On direct examination of infected and not contaminated tissue, a mixture of budding yeast and pseudohyphae will be seen (see Fig. 2–29T).

Next, one looks for the cytologic response of the skin. Are there inflammatory cells (see Fig. 2–29)? Are they eosinophils (see Figs. 2–29J and 2–29L), neutrophils, or mononuclear cells? If eosinophils are present, any extracellular bacteria seen probably represent colonization—not infection—and most likely an ectoparasitic or allergic disease is the primary problem. This finding can be especially helpful when evaluating dogs with suspected atopy or food hypersensitivity, because the presence of eosinophils strongly suggests that these diseases alone are not the cause of the skin disease. Conversely, cats with allergic skin disease frequently have tissue eosinophilia and smaller numbers of basophils (see Fig. 2–29M). If large numbers of eosinophils are seen in combination with degenerate neutrophils and intracellular bacteria, furunculosis is most likely present (free keratin and hair shafts serve as endogenous foreign bodies). It must be emphasized that eosinophils may be less numerous than expected or completely absent in inflammatory exudates from animals receiving glucocorticoids.

If neutrophils are present, do they exhibit degenerative or toxic cytologic changes, which suggest infection (see Figs. 2–29A to C)? If bacteria and inflammatory cells are found in the same preparation, is there phagocytosis? Are the bacteria ingested by individual neutrophils, or are they engulfed by macrophages and multinucleate histiocytic giant cells (see Figs. 2–29F to H)? Are there many bacteria, but few or no inflammatory cells, none of which exhibit degenerative cytologic changes or phagocytosis? When macrophages containing numerous clear cytoplasmic vacuoles are present, one should consider the possibility of a lipophagic granuloma such as is seen with panniculitis and foreign-body reactions (see Fig. 2–29I).

Less commonly, cytologic examination allows the rapid recognition of unusual infections (infections due to *Actinomycetes*, mycobacteria, *Leishmania*, and subcutaneous and deep mycoses); or suggests (1) sterile pustular dermatoses (pemphigus, sterile eosinophilic pustulosis, and subcorneal pustular dermatosis); (2) autoimmune dermatoses (pemphigus) (see Fig. 2–29K); and (3) neoplastic conditions (see Fig. 2–29O and 2–29P).

A synopsis of cytologic findings and their interpretation is presented in Table 2–5. Cytomorphologic characteristics of neoplastic cells are presented in Table 2–6.

Table 2-5 CYTOLOGIC DIAGNOSIS FROM STAINED* SMEARS

FINDING	DIAGNOSTIC CONSIDERATIONS
Neutrophils	
Degenerate	Bacterial infection
Nondegenerate	Sterile inflammation (e.g., canine allergy, pemphigus, subcorneal pustular dermatosis, linear IgA pustular dermatosis), irritants, foreign-body reaction
Eosinophils	Ectoparasitism, endoparasitism, feline allergy, furunculosis, eosinophilic granuloma, feline eosinophilic plaque, mast cell tumor, pemphigus, sterile eosinophilic folliculitis, sterile eosinophilic pustulosis
Basophils	Ectoparasitism, endoparasitism, feline allergy
Mast cells	Ectoparasitism, feline allergy, mast cell tumor (poorly stained with Diff Quik)
Lymphocytes, macrophages, and plasma cells	
Granulomatous	Infectious (especially furunculosis) versus sterile (e.g., foreign body, sterile granuloma syndrome, metatarsal fistulae, and sterile panniculitis)
Pyogranulomatous (many neutrophils too)	Same as for granulomatous
Eosinophilic granulomatous	Furunculosis, ruptured keratinous cyst, eosinophilic granuloma
Plasma cells	Plasma cell pododermatitis, plasmacytoma
Acanthocytes	
Few	Any suppurative dermatosis
Many	Pemphigus, dermatophytosis
Bacteria	
Intracellular	Infection
Extracellular only	Colonization
Yeast†	
Peanut shaped	*Malassezia* or rarely *Candida* dermatitis
Fungi	
Spores, hyphae	Fungal infection
Atypical or monomorphous cell population	
Clumped and rounded	Epithelial neoplasm
Individual, rounded, and numerous	Lymphoreticular or mast cell neoplasm
Individual, rounded or elongated, and sparse	Mesenchymal neoplasm

*Diff Quik or new methylene blue.
†Commonly seen, rarely pathogenic.

Culture and Examination for Fungi

Identification of fungi that have been isolated provides important information for case management and for public health decisions (see Chap. 5). When agents causing subcutaneous or deep mycoses are suspected, the samples should be sent to a veterinary laboratory with appropriate mycology skills.[60] The propagation of many pathologic fungi, especially the agents of subcutaneous and deep mycoses, creates airborne health hazards.

Table 2-6 CYTOMORPHOLOGIC CHARACTERISTICS SUGGESTIVE OF MALIGNANCY

GENERAL FINDINGS	NUCLEAR FINDINGS	CYTOPLASMIC FINDINGS
Pleomorphism (variable cell forms)	Marked variation in size	Variable staining intensity, sometimes dark blue
Variable nucleus to cytoplasm ratios	Coarsely clumped, sometimes jagged chromatin	Discrete, punctate vacuoles
Variable staining intensity	Nuclear molding	Variable amounts
	Peripheral displacement by cytoplasmic secretions or vacuoles	
	Prominent, occasionally giant, or angular nucleoli	

Additionally, examinations of the mycelial phase should be carried out in biological safety cabinets. For these reasons, the authors recommend that, in the general practice setting, fungal assessments be limited to direct tissue microscopic examination and culturing for dermatophytes. For other suspected fungal infections, samples should be collected and sent to an appropriate laboratory.

In general, for subcutaneous and deep mycotic infections, punch biopsies from the lesion are the best way to obtain a culture specimen. Pieces from the margin and the center of lesions, as well as any different-appearing lesions, should be submitted for laboratory analysis. Tissue samples may be placed in a bacteriologic transport medium and should reach the laboratory within 12 hours, although up to 24 hours is permissible. Refrigeration may be helpful to preserve some fungi but *Aspergillus* spp. and *Zygomycetes* are sensitive to cold. When these organisms are suspected, the sample should be kept at room temperature.

Direct examination for most nondermatophyte fungal organisms is acceptable, as described under Cytologic Examination in this chapter. In general, the Diff Quik stain is suitable for many fungi, especially yeasts and *Histoplasma capsulatum*. Periodic acid–Schiff stain is useful but beyond the level of most general practice settings. India ink mixed with tissue fluid outlines the capsule of yeast and has been useful for identifying *Cryptococcus neoformans*. Clearing samples with 10% KOH as discussed for dermatophytes under Direct Examination in this chapter may help identify hyphae of other fungi. When collecting samples for hyphal examination, one should not use gauze or cotton swabs because fibers may be mistaken for hyphae.

EXAMINATION FOR DERMATOPHYTES

In contrast to the case for other mycotic diseases, suspected cases of dermatophytosis and *Malassezia* infestation can readily be tested for in a general practice situation. To ascertain the cause of a dermatophytosis, proper specimen collection and isolation and correct identification of dermatophytes are necessary.

Wood's Lamp Examination

One aid in specimen collection is the Wood's lamp examination. The Wood's lamp is an ultraviolet light with a light wave of 253.7 nm that is filtered through a cobalt or nickel filter. The Wood's lamp should be turned on and allowed to warm up for 5 to 10 minutes, because the stability of the light's wavelength and intensity is temperature dependent. The animal should be placed in a dark room and examined under the light of the Wood's lamp. When exposed to the ultraviolet light, hairs invaded by *M. canis* may result in a yellow-green fluorescence in 30% to 80% of the isolates. Hairs should be exposed for 3 to 5 minutes, because some strains are slow to show the obvious yellow-green color. The fluorescence is due to tryptophan metabolites produced by the fungus. These metabolites are produced only by fungi that have invaded actively growing hair and cannot be elicited from an in vitro infection of hair. To decrease the number of false-positive results, it is imperative that the individual hair shafts are seen to fluoresce. Fluorescence is not present in scales or crusts or in cultures of dermatophytes. Other less common dermatophytes that may fluoresce include *Microsporum distortum, M. audouinii,* and *Trichophyton schoenleinii*.

Many factors influence fluorescence. The use of medications such as iodine destroys it. Bacteria such as *Pseudomonas aeruginosa* and *Corynebacterium minutissimum* may fluoresce but not with the apple green color of a dermatophyte-infected hair. Keratin, soap, petroleum, and other medication may fluoresce and give false-positive reactions. If the short stubs of hair produce fluorescence, the proximal end of hairs extracted from the follicles should fluoresce. These fluorescing hairs should be plucked with forceps and used for inoculation of fungal medium or for microscopic examination.

Specimen Collection

Accurate specimen collection is necessary to isolate dermatophytes. Hair is most commonly collected for the isolation of dermatophytes. In rare cases of *Trichophyton* spp.

readily obtainable from the sample inoculated onto Sabouraud's dextrose agar. For this reason, a double plate containing one side of DTM and one of Sabouraud's dextrose agar has gained favor among many dermatologists. When bottles containing DTM are used, it may be difficult to get a toothbrush onto the medium surface. When bottles are used, it is also important to put the lid on loosely.

Skin scrapings, claws, and hair should be inoculated onto Sabouraud's dextrose agar and DTM. Desiccation and exposure to ultraviolet light hinder growth. Therefore, cultures should be incubated in the dark at 30°C with 30% humidity. A pan of water in the incubator usually provides enough humidity. Cultures should be incubated for 10 to 14 days and should be checked daily for fungal growth. Proper interpretation of the DTM culture necessitates recognition of the red color change simultaneously with visible mycelial growth. False-positive results occur most commonly when the cultures are not observed frequently. As a saprophyte grows, it eventually turns the media red, thus emphasizing the importance of correlating the initial mycelial growth with the color change. Figure 2–30 illustrates the gross colony morphologic patterns of some common fungi.

IDENTIFICATION OF FUNGI

If a suspected dermatophyte is grown on culture, it should be identified. This necessitates collection of macroconidia from the mycelial surface. Generally, the colony needs to grow for 7 to 10 days before macroconidia are produced. Although colonies grown on DTM may provide adequate macroconidia, in some cases the colonies on the Sabouraud's dextrose agar may need to be sampled to find them. In occasional cases, especially with *Trichophyton* spp., no macroconidia are found. Subculturing these colonies on Sabouraud's dextrose agar or potato dextrose agar may facilitate sporulation. Alternatively, the sample may be sent to a diagnostic laboratory for identification.

The macroconidia are most readily collected by gently applying the sticky side of clear acetate tape (Scotch No. 602) to the aerial surface. The tape with sample is then placed onto several drops of lactophenol cotton blue that is on the surface of a microscope slide. A coverslip is placed over the tape and sample, and this is examined by microscopy.

Salient facts useful in identifying the three major dermatophytes (Figs. 2–30 and 2–31) are briefly described in the next section.

- *Microsporum canis.* These lesions may show a yellow-green fluorescence. Hairs that fluoresce should be plucked for culture or microscopic examination. Examination of a KOH preparation may reveal arthrospores present in masses on the hair shaft.

Colony Morphology. On Sabouraud's dextrose agar, *M. canis* produces a white cottony- to woolly-appearing colony (see Figs. 2–30A and B). With age, the colony becomes more powdery, has a central depressed area, and may show radial folds. The pigment on the undersurface of the colony is yellow-orange, becoming dull orange-brown. On potato dextrose agar, the pigment is lemon yellow.

Microscopic Morphology. *M. canis* usually forms abundant spindle-shaped macroconidia with thick echinulate walls. The echinulations (spines) are more pronounced at the terminal end, which often forms a knob. The macroconidia are composed of six or more cells (see Fig. 2–31A). One-celled microconidia may be seen. Conidia develop best on rice agar medium and poorly or not at all on Sabouraud's dextrose agar.

Diagnostic Criteria. The distinctive macroconidia and the lemon yellow pigment are characteristic of *M. canis*.

- *Microsporum gypseum.* Fluorescence is rare and, if present, is dull. The arthrospores on hair shafts are larger than those of *M. canis*.

Colony Morphology. Colonies are rapid growing, with a flat to granular texture and a buff to cinnamon brown color (see Fig. 2–30C). Sterile white mycelia may develop in time. The undersurface pigmentation is pale yellow to tan.

Microscopic Morphology. Echinulate macroconidia contain up to six cells with relatively thin walls (see Fig. 2–31B). The abundant ellipsoid macroconidia lack the terminal knob present in *M. canis*. One-celled microconidia may be present.

Diagnostic Methods • 123

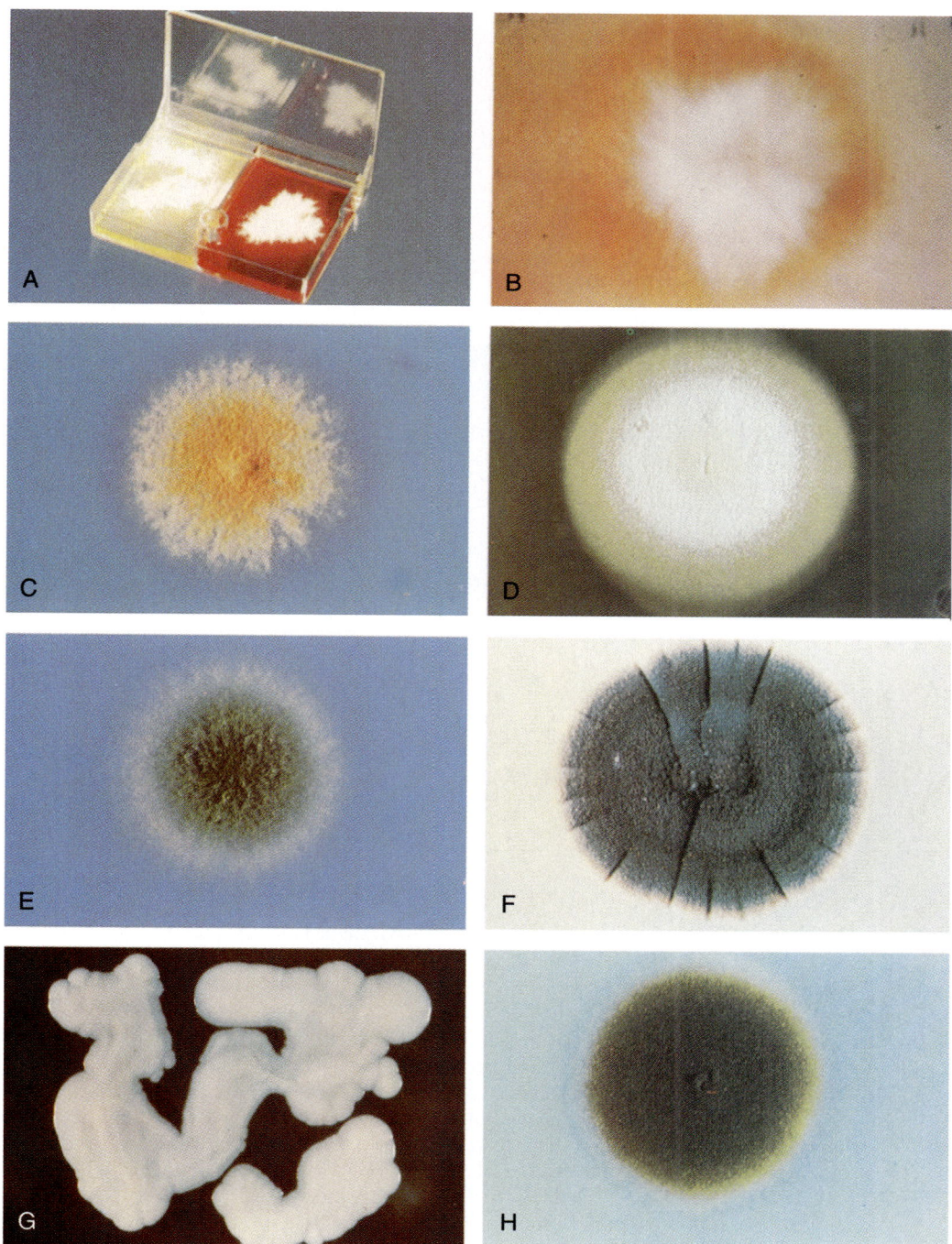

FIGURE 2–30. Fungal colonies. *A,* Seven-day culture of *M. canis.* Left side, plain Sabouraud's dextrose agar; right side, DTM medium. *B,* Gross colony of *M. canis. C,* Gross colony of *M. gypseum. D,* Gross colony of *T. mentagrophytes. E,* Gross colony of *Aspergillus. F,* Gross colony of *Penicillium. G,* Gross colony of *Candida albicans. H,* Gross colony of *Alternaria.* (*A, C, E, H,* courtesy C. Pinello. *B, D, F, G,* courtesy P. Jacobs.)

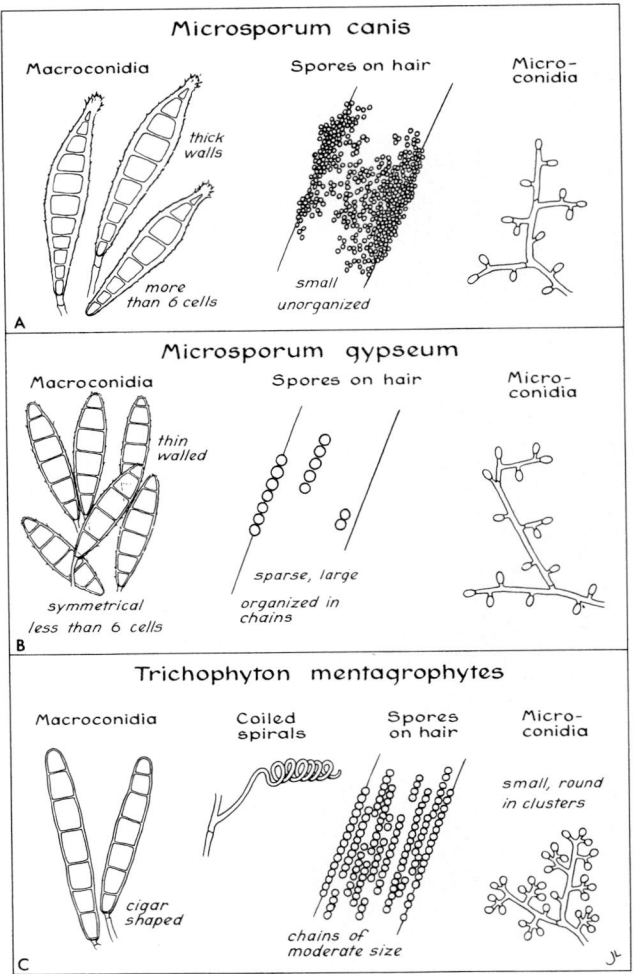

FIGURE 2–31. A, Characteristic microscopic morphology of *M. canis* B, characteristic microscopic morphology of *M. gypseum* C, characteristic microscopic morphology of *T. mentagrophytes*. The macroconidia and spirals are microscopic structures. The hair shafts are much larger.

Diagnostic Criteria. The abundant ellipsoid macroconidia and flat to granular texture of the colony are definitive features.

• *Trichophyton mentagrophytes.* No fluorescence is seen with Wood's light. Ectothrix chains of arthroconidia may be observed on hair.

Colony Morphology. Colony morphologic characteristics are variable. Most zoophilic forms produce a flat colony with a white to cream-colored powdery surface (see Fig. 2–30D). The color of the undersurface is usually brown to tan, but may be dark red. The anthropophilic form produces a colony with a white cottony surface.

Microscopic Morphology. The zoophilic form of *T. mentagrophytes* produces globose microconidia that may be arranged singly along the hyphae or in grapelike clusters. Macroconidia, if present, are cigar-shaped with thin smooth walls (see Fig. 2–31C). Some strains produce spiral hyphae, which may also be seen in other dermatophytes but are most characteristic of *Trichophyton*. Samples that show this change should be submitted to a diagnostic laboratory for identification.

Diagnostic Criteria. The colony morphologic characteristics, spiral hyphae, macroconidia, and microconidia are useful for identifying *T. mentagrophytes*. When grown on potato dextrose agar, *T. mentagrophytes* does not produce a dark red pigment like that formed by *T. rubrum*. Strains of *T. mentagrophytes* are more apt to be urease positive than is *T. rubrum*. Because *T. rubrum* may be incorrectly identified as *T. mentagrophytes*, the above-mentioned differential features are important.

Examination for Bacteria

In general practice, cytologic examination is the primary method used to identify the presence of pathogenic bacteria. Unusual lesions, nodular granulomatous lesions, and draining nodules should also be cultured. Bacterial culture and susceptibility testing are not routinely cost effective for the initial work-up of the case with a suspected bacterial pyoderma. Cytologic examination is the initial test of choice, and if intracellular cocci are seen, empirical antibiotic therapy for coagulase-positive staphylococci is warranted. When cytologic study reveals rod-shaped organisms, or when cocci are seen but appropriate empirical therapy is ineffective, bacterial culture and susceptibility testing are indicated. Veterinarians frequently take specimens for bacterial culture but infrequently grow and identify the cultures in their own practice. Specimens should be collected for culture, properly prepared, and rapidly sent to a skilled microbiologist in a laboratory equipped to provide prompt, accurate identification and antibacterial susceptibilities.

The selection of appropriate lesions for culturing is critical. Moist erosions and many crusts may be contaminated by bacteria, and cultures are not routinely recommended for these lesions. In cases with pustules, an intact pustule should be opened with a sterile needle. The pus collected on the needle should be transferred to the tip of a sterile swab. Papules may also be superficially punctured, and a relatively serous droplet of pus may be obtained. These superficial papular and pustular lesions should not be prepared at all, because negative cultures may result. With superficial cultures, a positive culture does not prove pathogenicity, and concurrent cytologic examination should be performed. If more than one type of organism is identified on cytologic examination, as is common in cases of otitis, the laboratory should be so informed. This allows documentation of the intracellular location of bacteria, which confirms their role in eliciting an inflammatory response. In cases with furuncles, needle aspirates may be taken and cultured. When plaques, nodules, and fistulous tracts are to be cultured, the surface is disinfected and samples are taken aseptically by skin biopsy. The skin sample is placed in a culture transport medium and submitted to the laboratory, where it should be ground and cultured.

When unusual bacterial diseases such as mycobacteriosis, bacterial pseudomycetoma, actinomycosis, actinobacillosis, and nocardiosis are suspected, unstained direct smears and tissue biopsy specimens should be submitted. The laboratory should be informed of the suspected disorder.

Deep lesions, cellulitis, and nodular lesions may also be cultured for anaerobic bacteria. Again, tissue biopsy is preferred, and special transport media or equipment is necessary. A good diagnostic laboratory supplies material for sample transport.

Biopsy and Dermatohistopathologic Examination

Skin biopsy is one of the most powerful tools in dermatology.[19, 23, 43, 53-55] However, maximization of the potential benefits of this tool necessitates enthusiastic, skilled teamwork between a clinician who has carefully selected, procured, and preserved the specimens and a pathologist who has carefully processed, perused, and interpreted the specimens. When the clinician and the pathologist truly work together, the skin biopsy can correctly reflect the dermatologic diagnosis in more than 90% of cases.[43] However, despite this, skin biopsies are often not performed or are done relatively late in the diagnostic work-up. In other cases, the skin biopsy findings are unrewarding because of poor specimen selection, poor technique, or both. In many dermatologic cases, the differential diagnosis primarily includes diseases that can be diagnosed only by biopsy or other nonhematologic or serum laboratory tests. Yet, the authors see numerous cases in which a variety of hematologic tests and cultures have been performed when the biopsy is the most cost-effective test to recommend to the client.

When the condition presented is not readily recognized, the skin biopsy is often the most informative test. Skin biopsy should not be regarded as merely a diagnostic aid for the difficult case or for the case that can be diagnosed only by biopsy. It is also helpful in establishing the group of diseases to consider. Even without a definitive diagnosis, a biopsy usually helps guide the clinician in the appropriate diagnostic direction. It provides a permanent record of the pathologic changes present at a particular time, and knowledge of this pathologic finding stimulates the clinician to think more deeply about the basic cellular changes underlying the disease. Symptomatic therapies may also be directed on the basis of cytologic findings.

Although biopsies are helpful, it is still important for the clinician to remember that they only add information. The diagnosis is usually made by the clinician, who correlates all the relevant findings of a case, not by the pathologist. The biopsy contributes to those findings; it does not replace a thorough history, physical examination, or other ancillary test results. Excellent textbooks on veterinary dermatopathology are now available.[24, 54, 55]

WHEN TO BIOPSY

There are no definite rules on when to perform a skin biopsy. The following suggestions are offered as general guidelines. Biopsy should be performed on (1) all obviously neoplastic or suspected neoplastic lesions; (2) all persistent ulcerations; (3) any case that is likely to have the major diseases that are most readily diagnosed by biopsy (e.g., follicular dysplasia, zinc-responsive dermatosis, sebaceous adenitis, dermatomyositis, and immune-mediated skin disease); (4) a dermatosis that is not responding to apparently rational therapy; (5) any dermatosis that, in the experience of the clinician, is unusual or appears serious; (6) vesicular dermatitis; and (7) any suspected condition for which the therapy is expensive, dangerous, or sufficiently time consuming to necessitate a definitive diagnosis before beginning treatment.

In general, skin biopsy should be performed within 3 weeks for any dermatosis that is not responding to what appears to be appropriate therapy. This early intervention (1) helps obviate the nonspecific, masking, and misleading changes due to chronicity, the administration of topical and systemic medicaments, excoriation, and secondary infection and (2) allows more rapid institution of specific therapy, thus reducing permanent disease sequelae (scarring, alopecia), the patient's suffering, and needless cost to the owner. Anti-inflammatory agents can dramatically affect the histologic appearance of many dermatoses. The administration of such agents, especially glucocorticoids, should optimally be stopped for 2 to 3 weeks before biopsy. The histopathologic changes caused by secondary bacterial pyoderma often obliterate the histopathologic features of any concurrent dermatoses. It is imperative to eliminate these secondary infections with appropriate systemic antibiotic therapy before biopsies are performed.

WHAT TO BIOPSY

The selection of appropriate biopsy sites is partly an art. Experienced clinicians often pick lesions and subtle changes that they suspect will show diagnostic changes. They are already aware of what histopathologic changes are helpful in making a diagnosis. They also know what types of changes may be expected to be found with certain clinical lesions. For example, pigmentary incontinence is a helpful histopathologic feature of lupus erythematosus. The clinician who knows this, and also knows that slate blue depigmenting lesions have that color because of dermal melanin (often from pigmentary incontinence), selects those sites for biopsy. One histologic criterion of lupus is likely to be present because the clinician knew the pathogenesis of that lesion.

If the disease is an unknown one or appears strange, a biopsy is important. If the distribution of lesions is unusual for the suspected disease, the clinician obtains biopsy specimens from the unusual areas, not just those typical of the suspected disease. It is also important to perform biopsy of areas representative of primary diseases and not just secondary complications. Many clinicians perform biopsy of secondary bacterial pyoderma lesions but not noninfected areas in cases with underlying allergy or keratinization disorders.

The histologic examination of the full spectrum of lesions present gives more information than does the examination of one lesion or stage. Therefore, the clinician should take multiple samples and obtain specimens from a variety of lesions. When primary lesions are present, a sample of at least one should be submitted to the laboratory. Fluid-filled lesions (pustules, vesicles) are often fragile and transient in canine and feline skin, and if present, should be sampled as soon as possible. If the suspected disease historically has pustules, having the patient return may allow sampling of the most appropriate lesions. In other cases, the patient may be hospitalized and be examined every 2 to 4 hours to find early intact lesions for biopsy. Most diseases that can be diagnosed by dermatopathologic examination have early, fully developed, and late changes. The greater the number of characteristic changes recognized, the more accurate the diagnoses are, and by selecting a variety of lesions, it is more likely that multiple characteristic changes are seen.

Multiple samples can document a pathologic continuum. Whenever possible, the clinician obtains biopsy specimens from the spontaneous primary lesions (macules, papules, pustules, vesicles, bullae, nodules, and tumors) and secondary lesions. Examination of crusts may sometimes add as much information as a biopsy of a papule. A greater number of biopsy specimens maximizes results. However, in practice, clinicians are usually limited to three to five samples. Most laboratories charge the same fee for one to three biopsy specimens submitted in the same container. Most important is that one learns from biopsy attempts. One should try to pay attention to what lesions are selected and what specimens give the best results. With practice, the clinician becomes more adept at selecting informative biopsy sites. Reading does not replace practice, attention to results, and experience, but it can help the clinician to achieve some proficiency in the art of maximizing the benefits of skin biopsy.

INSTRUMENTS REQUIRED

Biopsies are often performed simply and quickly with just local anesthesia. Two percent lidocaine; a selection of punch biopsies of different sizes; Adson thumb forceps; iris or small, curved scissors; formalin vials; needles and suture material; needle holders; wooden tongue depressors; and gauze pads are the equipment that is needed for most cases. Occasionally, scalpel handles, blades, and large formalin vials may also be necessary.

HOW TO BIOPSY

In general, a 6-mm biopsy punch provides an adequate specimen. Four-millimeter punches are reserved for difficult sites such as near the eye, on the pinna, and on the nasal planum and foot pads of cats and small dogs. It is imperative not to include any significant amount of normal skin margin with punch biopsy specimens. Unless the person obtaining the biopsy specimen personally supervises the processing of the specimen in the tissue block, rotation in the wrong direction may result in failure to section the pathologic portion of the specimen. In general, when a punch biopsy specimen is received at the laboratory, it is cut in half through the center. Therefore, a macule, pustule, papule, or small lesion should be centered in the biopsy specimen. If the lesion is to one side, only the normal tissue may be examined. The sample is also generally cut parallel to the growth of the hair. In many laboratories, only half of the specimen is sectioned and processed; the other half is saved in case problems occur and new sections or blocks are needed. So even with deeper cuts, if the wrong half is blocked, the lesion may not be present. The clinician must also realize that, after fixation, erythema and color changes are not detectable by the pathologist who sections the sample. Small lesions such as papules and pustules may no longer be grossly visible. The biopsy punch should be rotated in only *one* direction so as to minimize shearing artifacts.

It is important for the clinician to compare the pathologist's report with the description of the clinical lesion. If a pustule was observed clinically and the pathologist's report does not describe a pustule, it may have been missed. If a biopsied lesion is missed or the tissue is interpreted as normal, the clinician should explain this to the pathologist and obtain deeper sections to find the lesion.

It is also important for the clinician to be aware of what changes occur in the specimen after the biopsy. Autolysis starts to occur almost immediately after removal of the biopsy specimen. Therefore, it is important to place the newly acquired samples into appropriate fixatives (10% neutral phosphate buffered formalin) immediately. This should be done for each sample; one should not wait until all samples are taken before placing them in formalin. Punch biopsy specimens left under a hot surgery light have microscopically observable damage in less than 5 minutes.[19]

Secondary bacterial infections frequently complicate canine and, to a lesser extent, feline dermatoses. The histopathologic changes induced by bacterial infection can obliterate the changes associated with the underlying disease process. Thus, it is important to treat secondary infections before biopsies are performed.

Glucocorticoid therapy can drastically alter inflammatory conditions and can rapidly deplete tissue eosinophils. Thus, It is important to stop glucocorticoid therapy for 2 to 3 weeks (oral) or 6 to 8 weeks (repository injections) before biopsying.

Excisional biopsy with a scalpel is often indicated (1) for larger lesions; (2) for vesicles, bullae, and pustules (the rotary and shearing action of a punch may damage the lesion); and (3) for suspected disease of the subcutaneous fat (punches often fail to deliver diseased fat).

Skin biopsy is usually easily and rapidly accomplished using physical restraint and local anesthesia. The sites are gently clipped (if needed). Clippers should not touch the skin surface, especially when disorders of keratinization are suspected, because the surface keratin can be removed. The veterinarian is careful not to remove surface keratin, and the surface is left untouched or gently cleaned by daubing or soaking with a solution of 70% alcohol. The sites should not be prepared with other antiseptics (e.g., iodophors). Under no circumstances should biopsy sites be scrubbed. Such endeavors remove important surface pathologic changes and create iatrogenic inflammatory lesions. Sites that are being licked or scratched by the animal can have traumatic artifacts.

After the surface has air dried, the desired lesion is undermined with an appropriate amount, usually 1 to 2 ml, of local anesthetic (1% to 2% lidocaine) injected subcutaneously through a 25-gauge needle. An exception to this procedure is made when disease of the fat is suspected, in which case ring blocks, or regional or general anesthesia should be used, because injection into fat distorts the tissues. The local injection of lidocaine stings, and some animals object strenuously. The desired lesion is then punched or excised, including the underlying fat. In one study,[26] 1% lidocaine was found to be superior to 1% lidocaine with epinephrine or a prilocaine cream applied topically.

It is important to remember that lidocaine inhibits various gram-positive (including coagulase-positive *Staphylococcus*) and gram-negative (including *Pseudomonas*) bacteria, mycobacteria, and fungi.[51] Bicarbonate and epinephrine do the same.[51] Thus, if a culture is going to be obtained from the biopsy specimen, it is advisable to use a ring block, or regional or general anesthesia.

Great care should be exercised when manipulating the biopsy specimen, avoiding the use of forceps and instead using tiny mosquito hemostats, Adson thumb forceps, or the syringe needle through which the local anesthetic was injected. One cruciate (crisscross) suture effectively closes defects produced by 6-mm biopsy punches. One or two simple interrupted sutures may also be placed.

COMPLICATIONS OF SKIN BIOPSY

Complications after skin biopsy are rare. Caution should be exercised when performing biopsy on patients with bleeding disorders, including patients taking aspirin and anticoagulants. The administration of such medication should be stopped, if possible, for 1 to 2 weeks before biopsy. Problems with wound healing should be anticipated in patients with hyperadrenocorticism and hypothyroidism, in patients with various collagen defects (such as cutaneous asthenia), and in patients taking glucocorticoids or antimitotic drugs. The administration of such drugs should be stopped 2 to 3 weeks before biopsy, if possible. Wound infections are rare.

Caution should be exercised when injecting lidocaine, which may contain epinephrine, near extremities (ear tips, digits, and so forth); into patients with impaired circulation, cardiovascular disease, or hypertension; or into patients receiving phenothiazines, β-adrenergic receptor blockers, monoamine oxidase inhibitors (e.g., amitraz), or tricyclic antidepressants. Finally, one should be careful of the total amount of lidocaine injected into small kittens and puppies, because it can produce myocardial depression, muscle twitching, neurotoxicity, and death. One should not exceed a dose of 0.5 ml per kitten or puppy. Seizures have been induced when 0.5 ml of lidocaine has been injected subcutaneously on the head of small dogs or kittens.

WHAT TO DO WITH THE BIOPSY SPECIMEN

Skin biopsy specimens should be gently blotted to remove artifactual blood. In most instances, the fixative of choice is 10% neutral phosphate buffered formalin (100 ml of 40% formaldehyde, 900 ml of tap water, 4 g of acid sodium phosphate monohydrate, and 6.5 g of anhydrous disodium phosphate). It is not stable and oxidizes to formic acid, which can be seen histologically by the formation of acid hematin in blood cells. Also, the ratio of formalin to tissue is important, with a minimum of 10 parts formalin to 1 part tissue being necessary for adequate rapid fixation. Freezing should also be avoided; this sometimes occurs when samples are mailed in the winter months.[19] Freezing can be prevented by adding 95% ethyl alcohol as 10% of the fixative volume, or by allowing at least 12 hours of fixation before cold exposure.

Fixation in formalin also causes sample shrinkage, which is not a problem with 4-mm punch biopsy specimens. Larger punch biopsy specimens and elliptic excisions should be placed subcutis side down on a piece of wooden tongue depressor or cardboard to minimize the artifacts induced by shrinkage. They should be gently pressed flat for 30 to 60 seconds to facilitate adherence. Placing the specimens on a flat surface allows proper anatomic orientation and prevents potentially drastic artifacts associated with curling and folding. The specimen and its adherent splint are then immersed in fixative within 1 to 2 minutes, because artifactual changes develop rapidly in room air.

Also, formalin rapidly penetrates only about 1 cm of tissue. Samples larger than 1 cm should be partially transected at 1-cm intervals. This most commonly becomes important when large nodules and tumors are excised and submitted for histopathologic evaluation.

The last critical consideration is deciding where to send a skin biopsy specimen. Obviously, the clinician wants to send it to someone who can provide the most information. The choices should be ordered as follows: (1) a veterinary pathologist specializing in dermatopathology, (2) a veterinary dermatologist with a special interest and expertise in dermatohistopathology, (3) a general veterinary pathologist, and (4) a physician dermatopathologist with a special interest in comparative dermatopathology.

The clinician frequently does not provide adequate information concerning skin biopsy specimens. The clinician and the pathologist are a diagnostic team, and an accurate diagnosis is more likely (and the patient is best served) when both members of the team do their part. A concise description of the history, the physical examination findings, the results of laboratory examinations and therapeutic trials, and the clinician's differential diagnosis should always accompany the biopsy specimen.

TISSUE STAINS

Hematoxylin and eosin (H & E) stain is most widely used routinely for skin biopsies. In the laboratory of two of the authors (DWS and WHM), acid orcein–Giemsa (AOG) stain is also used regularly for skin biopsies. The routine use of AOG markedly reduces the need for ordering special stains (Table 2–7). Table 2–8 contains guidelines for the use of various special stains.

Table 2-7. STAINING CHARACTERISTICS OF VARIOUS CUTANEOUS COMPONENTS WITH ACID ORCEIN–GIEMSA STAIN

TEST COMPONENT	COLOR
Nuclei	Dark blue
Cytoplasm of keratinocytes	Blue-purple
Cytoplasm of smooth muscle cells	Light blue
Keratin	Blue
Collagen	Pink
Elastin	Dark brown to black
Mast cell granules	Purple
Some acid mucopolysaccharides	Purple
Melanin	Dark green to black
Hemosiderin	Yellow-brown to green
Erythrocytes	Green-orange
Eosinophil granules	Red
Cytoplasm of histiocytes, lymphocytes, and fibrocytes	Light blue
Cytoplasm of neutrophils	Clear to light blue
Cytoplasm of plasma cells	Dark blue to gray-blue
Amyloid	Sky blue to gray-blue
Hyaline	Pink
Fibrin and fibrinoid	Green-blue
Keratohyalin	Dark blue
Trichohyalin	Red
Bacteria, fungal spores, and hyphae	Dark blue
Serum	Light blue

ARTIFACTS

Even the best dermatohistopathologist cannot read an inadequate, poorly preserved, poorly fixed, or poorly processed specimen.[19, 24, 54] Numerous artifacts can be produced by errors in site selection, preparation, technique in taking and handling and fixation and processing of skin biopsy specimens. It is important that the clinician and the pathologist be cognizant of these potentially disastrous distortions.

Table 2-8. STAINING CHARACTERISTICS OF VARIOUS SUBSTANCES WITH SPECIAL STAINS

STAIN	TISSUE AND COLOR
van Gieson's	Mature collagen–red; immature collagen, keratin, muscle, and nerves–yellow
Masson trichrome	Mature collagen–blue; immature collagen, keratin, muscle, and nerves–red
Verhoeff's	Elastin and nuclei–black
Gomori's aldehyde fuchsin	Elastin, suflated acid mucopolysaccharides, and certain epithelial mucins–purple
Oil red O°	Lipids–dark red
Sudan black B°	Lipids–green-black
Scarlet red°	Lipids–red
Gomori's or Wilder's reticulin	Reticulin, melanin, and nerves–dark brown to black
Periodic acid–Schiff	Glycogen, neutral mucopolysaccharides, fungi, and tissue debris–red
Alcian blue	Acid mucopolysaccharides–blue
Hale's colloidal iron	Acid mucopolysaccharides–blue
Toluidine blue	Acid mucopolysaccharides and mast cell granules–purple
Gomori's methenamine silver	Fungi and melanin–black
Gram's or Brown-Brenn	Gram-positive bacteria–blue; Gram-negative bacteria–red
Fite's modified acid-fast	Acid-fast bacteria–red
Fontana's ammoniacal silver nitrate	Premelanin and melanin–black (hemosiderin usually positive too, but less intense)

°Require frozen sections of formalin-fixed tissue.

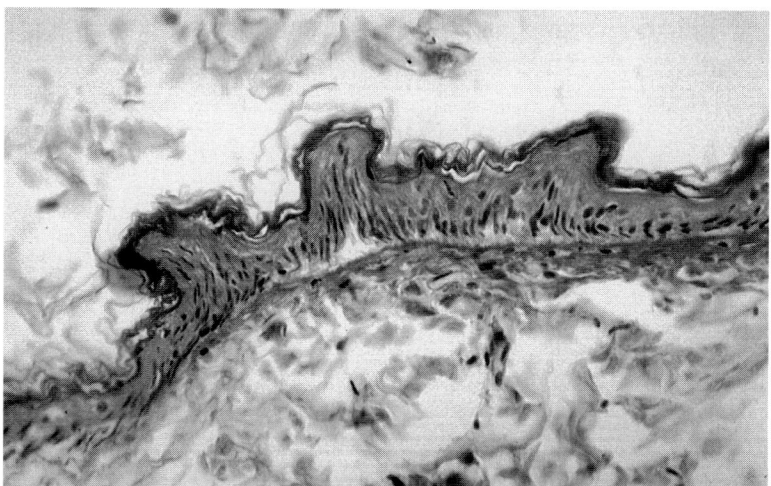

FIGURE 2–32. Electrodesiccation. Note how epidermal keratinocytes are vertically elongated, giving the appearance of standing at attention.

1. Artifacts due to improper site selection include excoriations and other physicochemical effects (e.g., maceration, inflammation, necrosis, and staining abnormalities caused by topical medicaments).
2. Artifacts due to improper preparation include inflammation, staining abnormalities, and removal of surface pathologic changes (from surgical scrubbing and the use of antiseptics), as well as collagen separation, pseudoedema, and pseudosinus formation (due to intradermal injection of local anesthetic).
3. Artifacts due to improper technique in taking and handling include pseudovesicles, pseudoclefts, and shearing (caused by a dull punch or poor technique); pseudopapillomas or pseudonodules, pseudosclerosis, pseudosinuses, pseudocysts, and lobules of sebaceous glands within hair follicles, on the skin surface, or both (squeeze artifacts due to intervention with forceps); marked dehydration, elongation, and polarization of cells and cell nuclei (due to electrodesiccation) (Fig. 2–32); and intercellular edema, clefts, and vesicles (due to friction).
4. Artifacts caused by improper fixation and processing include dermoepidermal separation, intracellular edema, and fractures (due to autolysis); shrinkage, curling, and folding (due to failure to use wooden or cardboard splints); intracellular edema, subepidermal vacuolar alteration, and multinucleate epidermal giant cells (from freezing); formalin pigment in blood vessels and extravascular phagocytes (due to the use of nonbuffered formalin); hardening, shrinkage, and loss of cellular detail (from alcohol in the fixative); poor staining and soft, easily displaced, and distorted tissue (with Bouin's solution); thick, fragmented sections (due to inadequate dehydration during tissue processing); pseudoacanthosis (in tangential sections associated with poor orientation of the specimen); and dermoepidermal separation and displacement of dermal tissues into epidermis (attributable to cutting sections from dermis to epidermis).

• THE VOCABULARY OF DERMATOHISTOPATHOLOGY

Dermatopathology is a specialty of medicine requiring many hours of training and many more of experience to master. It is beyond the scope of this book to train the student adequately in both dermatology and dermatopathology. However, because dermatopathologic examination is the single most valuable laboratory aid to the dermatologist, it is important to understand the vocabulary of the dermatopathologist.

Dermatohistopathology has a specialized vocabulary, because many of the histopathologic changes are unique to the skin. Unfortunately, as is true of most sciences, the

132 • Diagnostic Methods

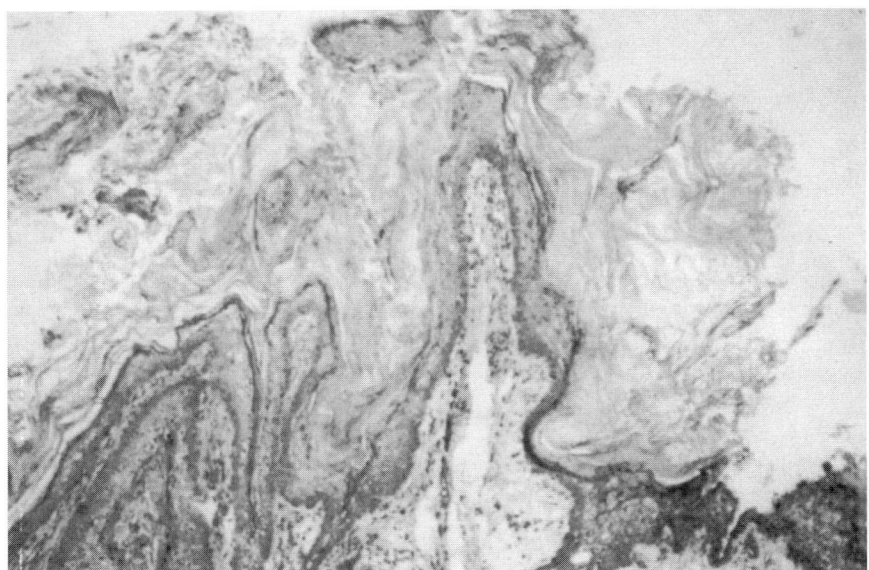

FIGURE 2–33. Marked orthokeratotic hyperkeratosis in a dog with ichthyosis.

dermatologic and general medical literatures abound with confusing and sometimes inappropriate dermatohistopathologic terms. The following discussion of terms is based on an amalgamation of such considerations as precision of definition, descriptive value, popular usage, historical precedent, and diagnostic significance in dermatohistopathology.[27, 50, 54]

Epidermal Changes

HYPERKERATOSIS

Hyperkeratosis is an increased thickness of the stratum corneum. It may be absolute (an actual increase in thickness, which is most common) or relative (an apparent increase due to thinning of the underlying epidermis, which is rare). The types of hyperkeratosis are further specified by the adjectives *orthokeratotic,* or anuclear (Fig. 2–33), and *parakeratotic,* or nucleated (Fig. 2–34). Orthokeratotic and parakeratotic hyperkeratoses are commonly, but less precisely, referred to as orthokeratosis and parakeratosis, respectively. Other adjectives commonly used to describe further the nature of hyperkeratosis include *basketweave* (e.g., dermatophytosis and endocrinopathic conditions) (Fig. 2–35A), *compact* (e.g., chronic low-grade trauma and cutaneous horns) (see Fig. 2–35B), and *laminated* (e.g., ichthyosis) (see Fig. 2–35C). Hyperkeratosis is usually found in conjunction with epidermal hyperplasia. If it occurs without epidermal hyperplasia, disorders of keratinization, corneocyte adhesion, or endocrine dermatoses should be considered.

Orthokeratotic and parakeratotic hyperkeratosis may be seen as alternating layers in the stratum corneum. This observation implies episodic changes in epidermopoiesis. If the changes are generalized, the lesions appear as horizontal layers. If the changes are focal, the lesion is a vertical defect in the stratum corneum. Orthokeratotic and parakeratotic hyperkeratosis are common, nondiagnostic findings in virtually any chronic dermatosis. They simply imply altered epidermopoiesis, whether inflammatory, hormonal, neoplastic, or developmental. However, diffuse parakeratotic hyperkeratosis suggests ectoparasitism, zinc-responsive dermatosis, lethal acrodermatitis, *Malassezia* dermatitis, some vitamin A–responsive dermatoses, thallotoxicosis, generic dog food dermatosis, necrolytic migratory erythema, hereditary nasal hyperkeratosis of Labrador retrievers, and occasionally, dermatophytosis and dermatophilosis. Parakeratotic hyperkeratosis that targets hair follicles suggests follicular inflammatory diseases and congenital follicular parakeratosis of Rottweilers and Siberian huskies. Parakeratotic hyperkeratosis associated with subjacent superficial

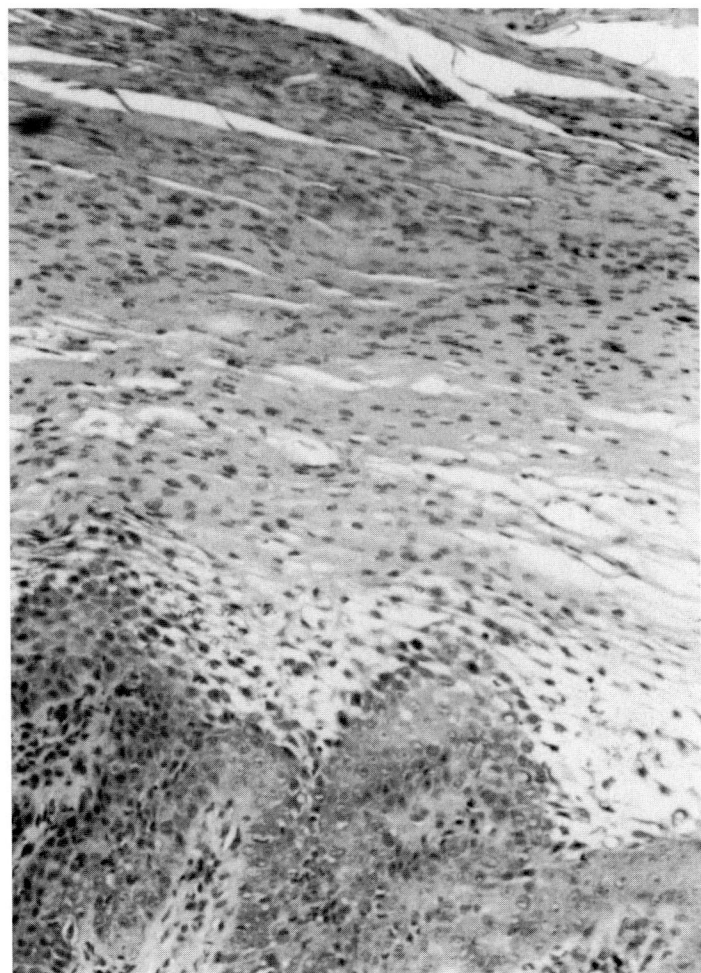

FIGURE 2–34. Marked parakeratotic hyperkeratosis in a dog with necrolytic migratory erythema.

epidermal pallor suggests zinc-responsive dermatosis, lethal acrodermatitis, thallotoxicosis, and necrolytic migratory erythema.

Focal parakeratotic hyperkeratosis overlying epidermal papillae (parakeratotic "caps") in which the subjacent dermal papillae are edematous (papillary "squirting") is seen in primary idiopathic seborrheic dermatitis and zinc-responsive dermatoses of dogs (Fig. 2–36).

Diffuse orthokeratotic hyperkeratosis suggests endocrinopathies, nutritional deficiencies, secondary seborrheas, and developmental abnormalities (ichthyosis, epidermal nevus, follicular dysplasia, and color dilution alopecia). Orthokeratotic hyperkeratosis that is disproportionately severe in hair follicles (Fig. 2–37) suggests vitamin A–responsive dermatosis, vitamin A deficiency, acne, Schnauzer comedo syndrome, follicular dysplasia, sebaceous adenitis, actinic follicular keratosis, comedo nevus, and follicular cyst.

HYPOKERATOSIS

The decreased thickness of the stratum corneum, called *hypokeratosis,* is much less common than hyperkeratosis and reflects an exceptionally rapid epidermal turnover time, decreased cohesion between cells of the stratum corneum, or both. Hypokeratosis may be found in seborrheic and other exfoliative skin disorders, and in feline paraneoplastic

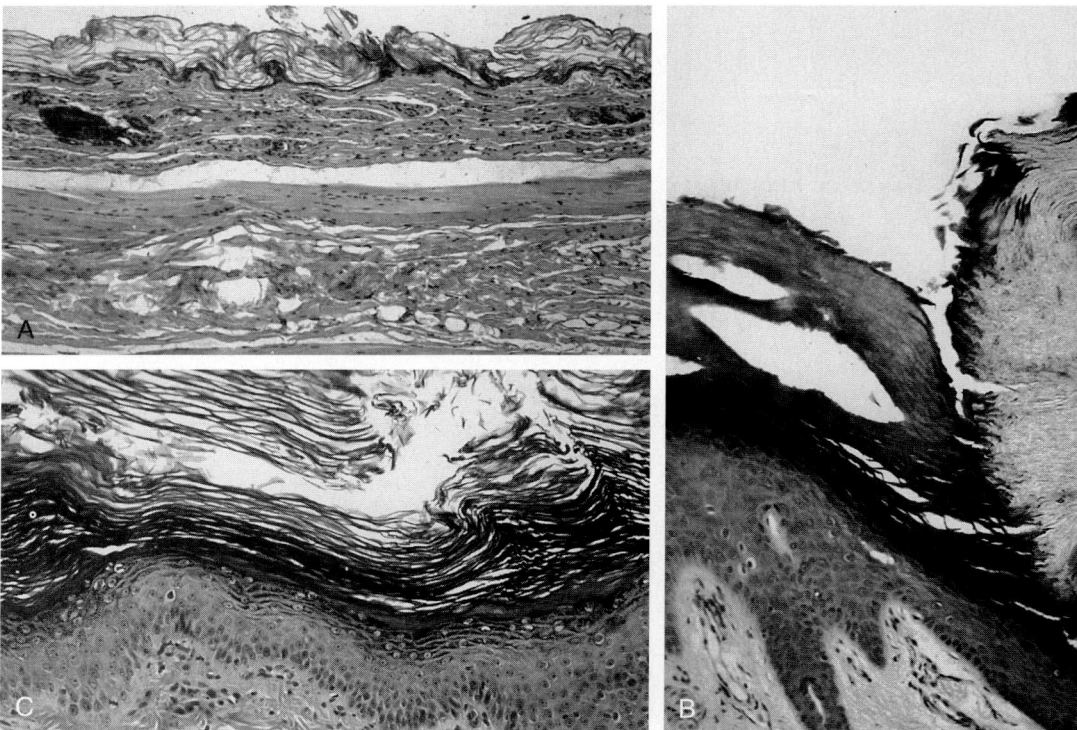

FIGURE 2–35. A, Basketweave orthokeratotic hyperkeratosis in a cushingoid cat. B, Compact orthokeratotic hyperkeratosis in a cutaneous horn form a cat. C, Laminated orthokeratotic hyperkeratosis in an ichthyotic cat.

alopecia. It may also be produced by excessive surgical preparation of the biopsy site or by friction and maceration in intertriginous areas.

HYPERGRANULOSIS AND HYPOGRANULOSIS

The terms *hypergranulosis* and *hypogranulosis* indicate, respectively, an increase and a decrease in the thickness of the stratum granulosum. Both entities are common and nondiagnostic. Hypergranulosis may be seen in any dermatosis in which there is epidermal hyperplasia and orthokeratotic hyperkeratosis (Fig. 2–38). Hypogranulosis is often seen in dermatoses in which there is parakeratotic hyperkeratosis and is most easily appreciated in the footpads and the nasal planum.

HYPERPLASIA

An increased thickness of the noncornified epidermis due to an increased number of epidermal cells is called *hyperplasia*. The term *acanthosis* is often used interchangeably with hyperplasia. However, acanthosis specifically indicates an increased thickness of the stratum spinosum and may be due to hyperplasia (true acanthosis, which is the most common) or hypertrophy (pseudoacanthosis, which is uncommon). Epidermal hyperplasia is often accompanied by rete ridge formation (irregular hyperplasia resulting in pegs of epidermis that appear to project downward into the underlying dermis). Rete ridges are not found in normal-haired skin of dogs and cats. Mitotic figures, virtually never seen in normal epidermis, are common in hyperplastic lesions.

The following adjectives further specify the types of epidermal hyperplasia: (1) *irregular*—uneven, elongated, pointed rete ridges with an obliterated or preserved rete-papilla

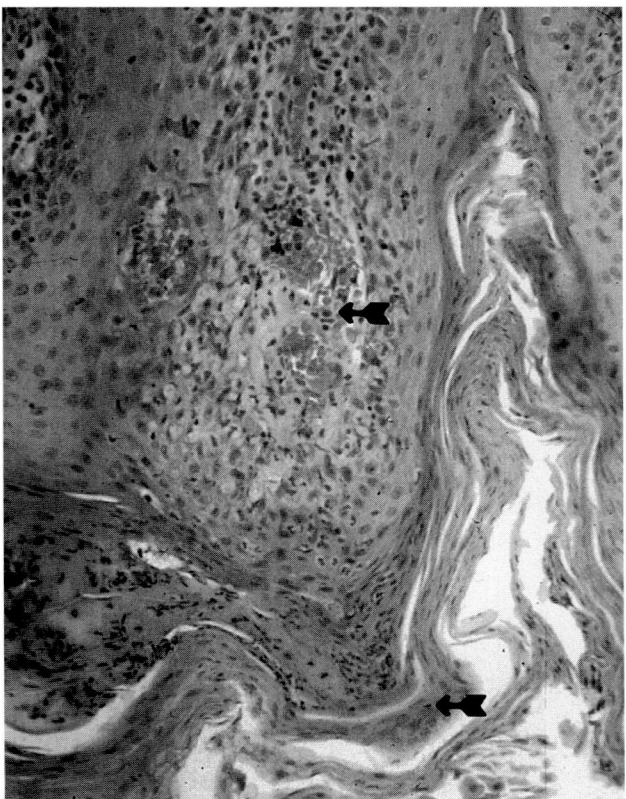

FIGURE 2-36. Zinc-responsive dermatosis in a dog. Note squirting papilla *(lower arrow)* with parakeratotic cap *(upper arrow)*.

configuration; (2) *regular*—approximately evenly thickened epidermis (Fig. 2–39); (3) *psoriasiform*—approximately evenly elongated rete ridges, which are clubbed, fused, or both at their bases (Fig. 2–40), often with thinning of the suprapillary epidermis, which may contain microabscesses and be parakeratotic; (4) *papillated*—digitate projections of the epidermis above the skin surface (Fig. 2–41); and (5) *pseudocarcinomatous* (pseudoepitheliomatous)—extreme, irregular hyperplasia, which may include increased mitoses, squamous eddies, and horn pearls, thus resembling squamous cell carcinoma; however, cellular atypia is absent, and the basement membrane zone is not breached (Fig. 2–42). These five forms of epidermal hyperplasia may be seen in various combinations in the same specimen.

Epidermal hyperplasia is a common, nondiagnostic feature of virtually any chronic inflammatory process. The five types are generally useful descriptively but have little specific diagnostic significance. Pseudocarcinomatous hyperplasia is most commonly associated with underlying dermal suppurative, granulomatous, or neoplastic processes and with chronic ulcers. Papillated hyperplasia is most commonly seen with neoplasia, callosities, epidermal nevi, primary seborrhea, and zinc-responsive dermatosis. Psoriasiform hyperplasia is most commonly seen with epitheliotropic lymphoma, psoriasiform-lichenoid dermatosis of English Springer spaniels, parapsoriasis, and chronically traumatized lesions (e.g., chronic allergy and acral lick dermatitis).

HYPOPLASIA AND ATROPHY

Hypoplasia is a decreased thickness of the noncornified epidermis due to a decrease in the number of cells. *Atrophy* is a decreased thickness of the noncornified epidermis due

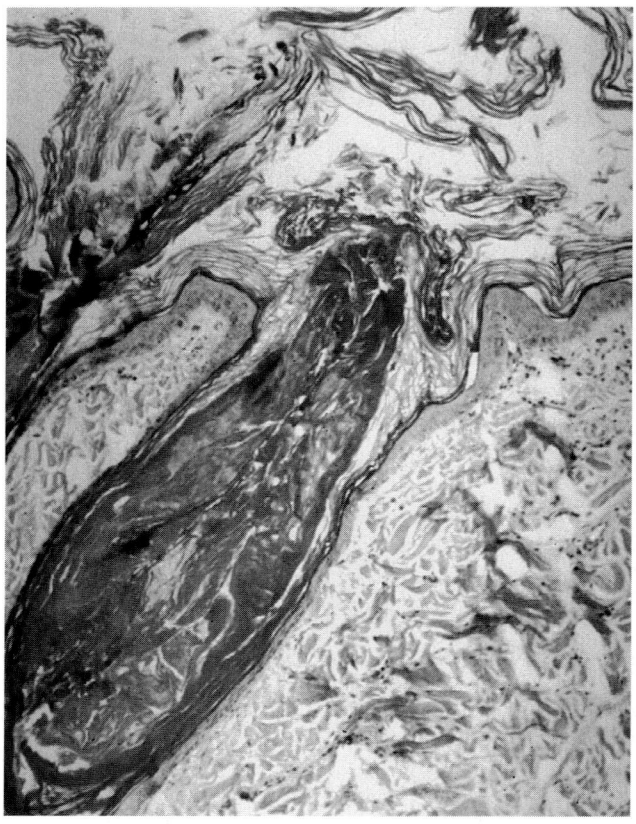

FIGURE 2–37. Disproportionate hair follicle orthokeratotic hyperkeratosis in a dog with vitamin A–responsive dermatosis.

to a decrease in the size of cells (Fig. 2–43). An early sign of epidermal hypoplasia or atrophy is the loss of the rete ridges in areas of skin where they are normally present (i.e., in the nonhaired skin of dogs and cats).

Epidermal hypoplasia and atrophy are uncommon in skin diseases of dogs and cats but are occasionally seen with hormonal (usually hyperadrenocorticism, rarely hypothyroidism), developmental (cutaneous asthenia, feline acquired skin fragility), and inflammatory (discoid lupus erythematosus, traction alopecia, dermatomyositis, vaccine-induced vasculitis) dermatoses.

NECROSIS, DYSKERATOSIS, APOPTOSIS, AND ONCOSIS

The term *necrosis* refers to the death of cells or tissues in a living organism and is judged to be present primarily on the basis of nuclear morphologic findings. The term *necrolysis* is often used synonymously with necrosis but actually implies a separation of tissue due to the death of cells (e.g., toxic epidermal necrolysis). Nuclear changes indicative of necrosis include *karyorrhexis* (nuclear fragmentation), *pyknosis* (nuclear shrinkage and consequent hyperchromatism), and *karyolysis* (nuclear ghosts). With all three necrotic nuclear changes, individual keratinocytes are characterized by loss of intercellular bridges and cytoplasmic changes of condensation, intense eosinophilia, loss of structure, and fragmentation. Necrosis is further specified by the adjectives *coagulation* (preservation of cell outlines but loss of cell detail) or *caseation* (complete loss of all structural details, the tissue being replaced by a granular material containing nuclear debris).

In fact, cell death and necrosis are different.[29, 33] Cell death—defined functionally by the point of no return—occurs long before necrosis, and is not detectable histologically.

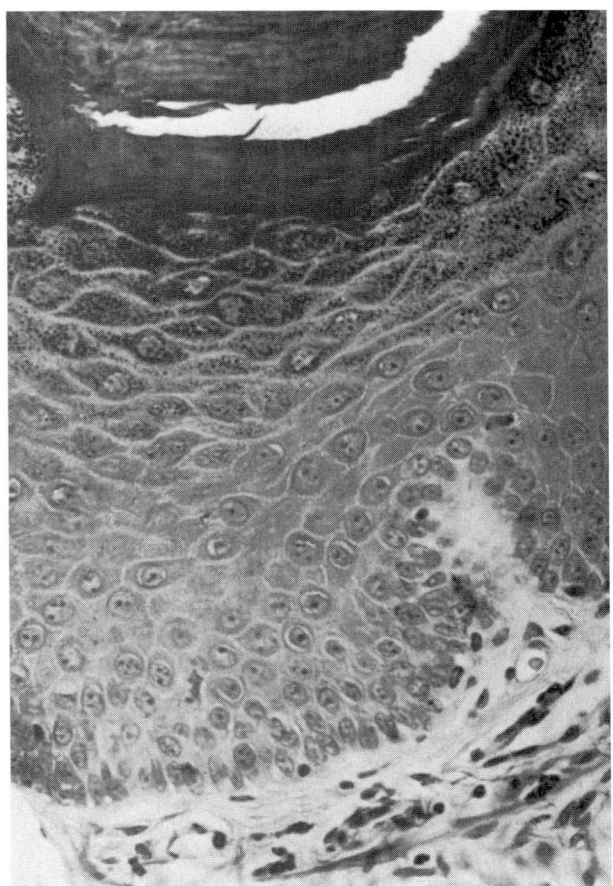

FIGURE 2–38. Hypergranulosis in a dog with ichthyosis.

Necrosis refers to changes that occur secondary to cell death by any mechanism (e.g., apoptosis, oncosis), and is histologically visible.

Epidermal necrosis may be focal as a result of cutaneous adverse drug reaction (Fig. 2–44), microbial infections, or various lichenoid dermatoses (e.g. erythema multiforme), or it may be generalized as a result of physicochemical trauma (primary irritant contact dermatitis, burns, freezing, and thallotoxicosis), interference with blood supply (vasculitis, thromboembolism, subepidermal bullae, and dense subepidermal cellular infiltrates), or an immunologic mechanism (toxic epidermal necrolysis and erythema multiforme). So-called "satellite cell necrosis" (satellitosis) is actually a misnomer.[29, 33] It is really satellite cell apoptosis. Individual apoptotic keratinocytes are seen in association with contiguous (satellite) lymphoid cells (Fig. 2–45). Satellitosis can be seen in a number of interface dermatitides, including erythema multiforme, lupus erythematosus and graft-versus-host disease.

The term *dyskeratosis* is used to indicate a premature and faulty keratinization of individual cells. The term is also used, although less commonly, to indicate a general fault in the keratinization process and thus in the state of the epidermis as a whole. Dyskeratotic cells are characterized by eosinophilic, swollen cytoplasm with normal or condensed, dark-staining nuclei. Such cells are difficult or impossible to distinguish from apoptotic or necrotic keratinocytes on light microscopic examination. The judgment usually depends on whether the rest of the epithelium is thought to be keratinizing or necrosing. No one has been able to define the term "dyskeratosis" consistently, in a way satisfactory to everyone, simply because the original concepts on which the designation was based were faulty.[49]

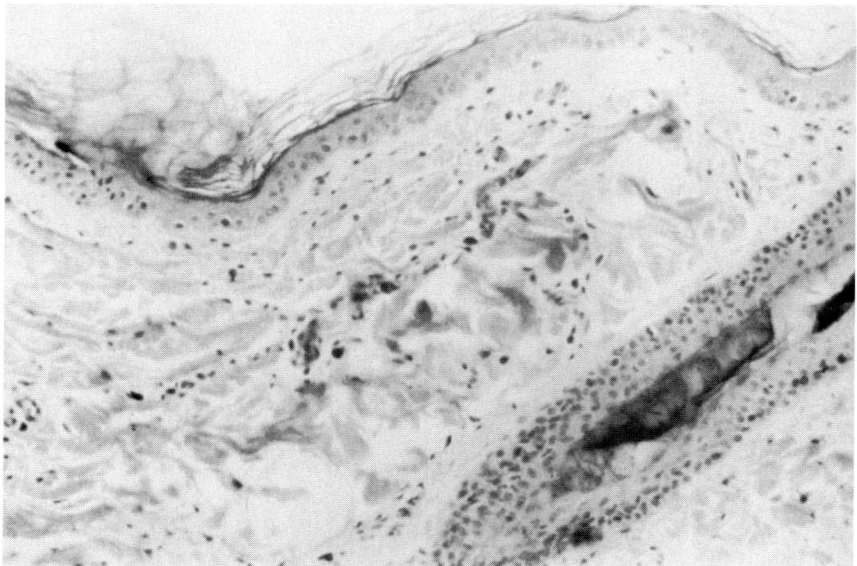

FIGURE 2–39. Regular epidermal hyperplasia in a dog with atopy.

Most of the keratinocytes previously referred to as being dyskeratotic were actually apoptotic.[19] If this term is used at all, it should be reserved for the so-called "corps ronds" (round bodies) that typify two human dermatoses—Darier's disease and transient acantholytic dermatosis (Grover's disease)—and are also seen in warty dyskeratoma, squamous cell carcinoma, and keratoacanthoma.[49]

Apoptosis is a form of intentional suicide based on a genetic mechanism.[29, 33] Programmed cell death and apoptosis are not identical, but genetic programming is involved in both. In programmed (spontaneous) cell death, there is an internal "clock" that specifies the fixed time for physiologic cell suicide. In apoptosis, genetic programming specifies

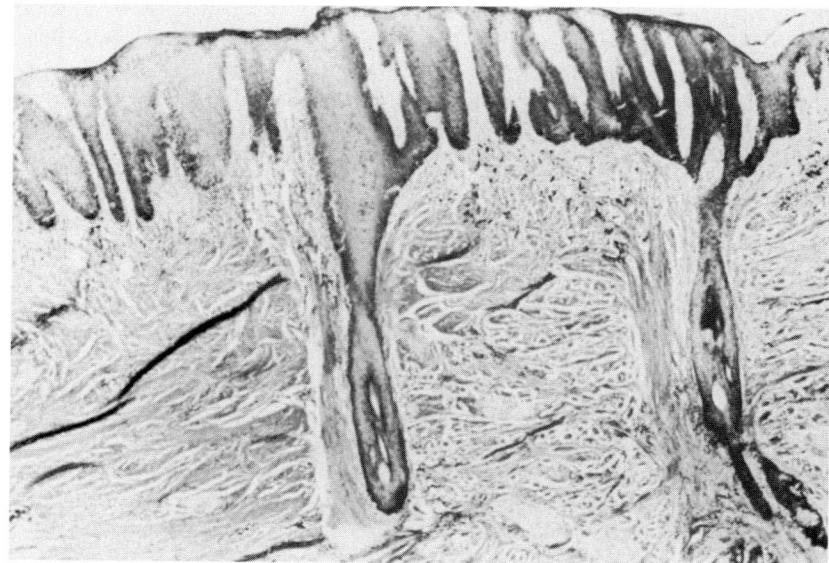

FIGURE 2–40. Psoriasiform epidermal hyperplasia in a dog with atopy.

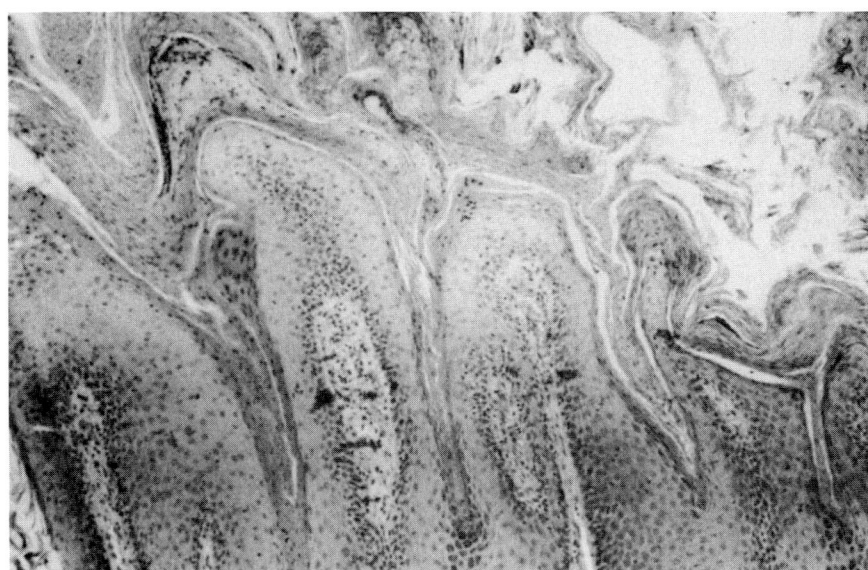

FIGURE 2–41. Papillated epidermal hyperplasia in a dog with zinc-responsive dermatosis. There is also diffuse parakeratotic hyperkeratosis.

the weapons (the means) to produce instant suicide. Apoptosis can be activated by many stimuli: growth factors, cytokines, hormones, immune system, viruses, and sublethal damage to cells. Apoptotic keratinocytes are common features of interface dermatoses (Fig. 2–46), but they may be seen in small numbers (up to six in a section through a 6-mm punch specimen) in virtually any hyperplastic epidermis. Apoptotic keratinocytes are rarely seen (one or two in a section through a 6-mm punch specimen) in normal epidermis. However,

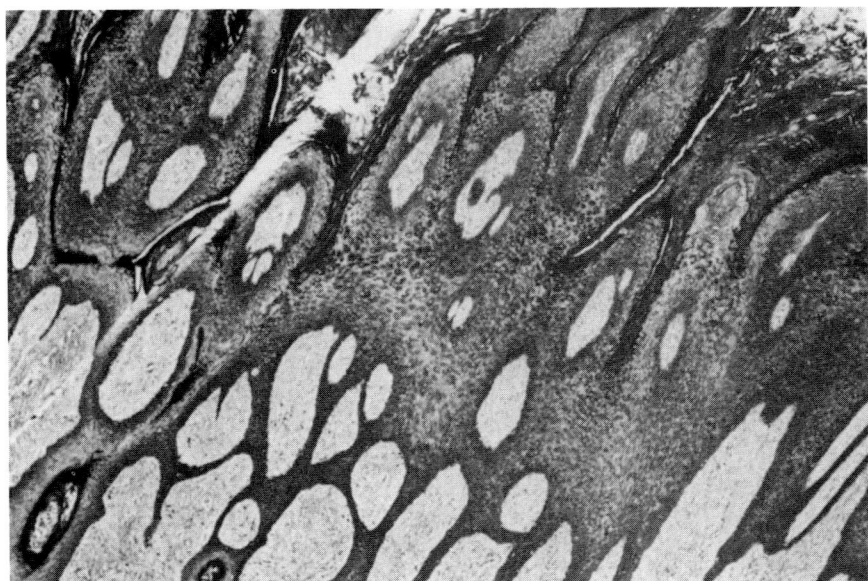

FIGURE 2–42. Pseudocarcinomatous epidermal hyperplasia in a dog with acral lick dermatitis.

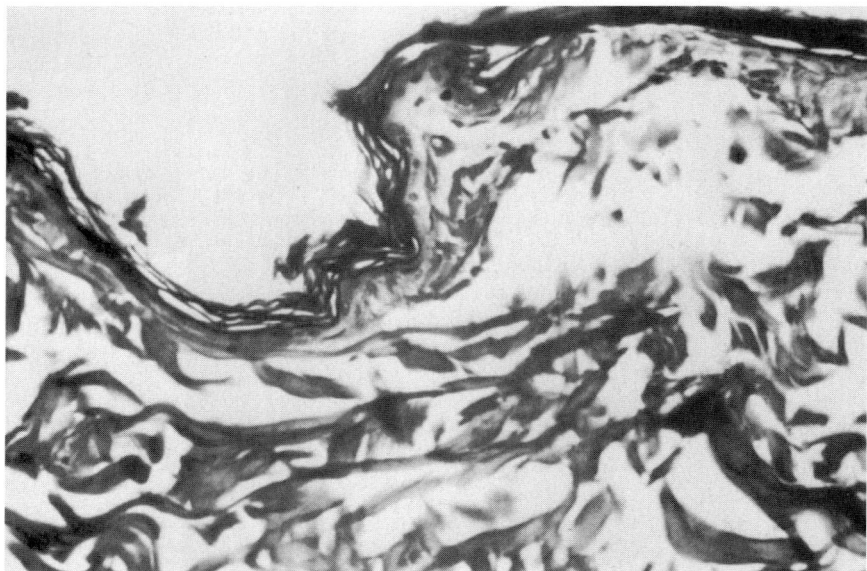
FIGURE 2–43. Epidermal atrophy in a dog with a sex hormone dermatosis.

apoptotic keratinocytes are numerous in the catagen and early telogen hair follicle epithelium. Cytotoxic drugs produce keratinocyte apoptosis, with phase-specific agents tending to target the basal cell layer, and noncycle phase-specific agents affecting all epithelial layers.

Apoptotic keratinocytes undergo a series of morphologic changes: the cell shrinks, becomes denser and more eosinophilic, and loses its normal contacts; nuclear changes include pyknosis, margination of chromatin, and karyorrhexis; the cell emits processes ("buds") that often contain nuclear fragments and organelles, and that do not swell; these buds often break off and become *apoptotic bodies*, which may be phagocytosed by macrophages or neighboring cells, or remain free. There is no swelling of mitochondria or other organelles. Synonyms for apoptotic keratinocytes include Civatte bodies (when in the stratum basale) and "sunburn cells" (when caused by ultraviolet radiation). Synonyms for apoptotic bodies include "colloid", "hyaline", "filamentous", and "ovoid" bodies. Apoptosis may be more specifically detected in routinely processed and fixed skin specimens by the terminal uridinyl transferase nick end labeling (TUNEL) method.[13]

Oncosis is cell death as a result of overwhelming damage (e.g., ischemia, toxins, chemical injury), and is characterized by cellular swelling, organelle swelling, blebbing (blister-like cell membrane structures that do not contain cell organelles, and that may swell and rupture) and increased membrane permeability.[29, 33] Oncosis and necrosis induce an inflammatory response, whereas apoptosis does not.

INTERCELLULAR EDEMA

Intercellular edema (spongiosis) of the epidermis is characterized by a widening of the intercellular spaces with accentuation of the intercellular bridges, giving the involved epidermis a spongy appearance (Fig. 2–47). Severe intercellular edema may lead to rupture of the intercellular bridges and the formation of spongiotic vesicles within the epidermis. Severe spongiotic vesicle formation may, in turn, cause blowout of the basement membrane zone in some areas, giving the appearance of subepidermal vesicles.

Intercellular edema is a common, nondiagnostic feature of any acute or subacute inflammatory dermatosis. Diffuse spongiosis, which also involves the outer root sheath of hair follicles, may be seen with feline eosinophilic plaque, feline eosinophilic granuloma,

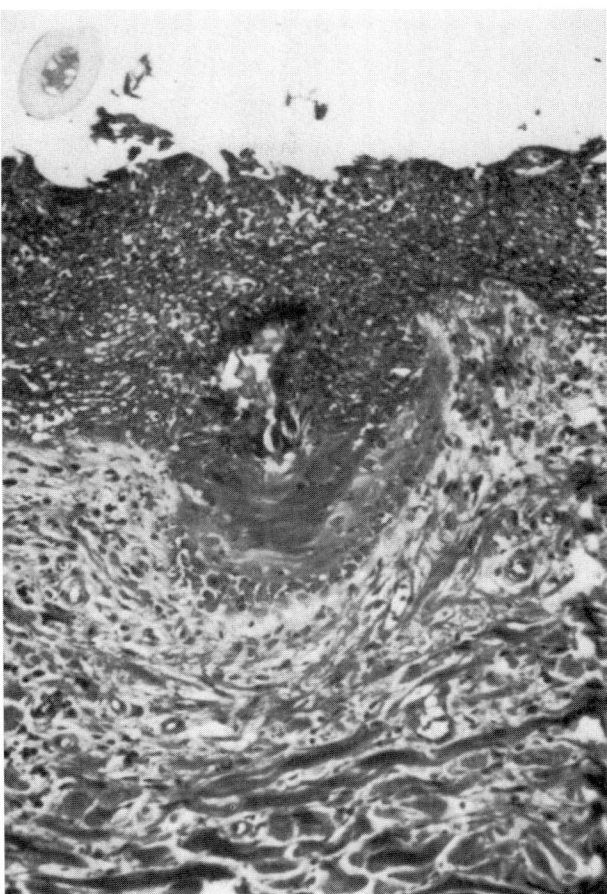

FIGURE 2–44. Full-thickness necrosis of the epidermis and outer root sheath of a hair follicle in a dog with erythema multiforme.

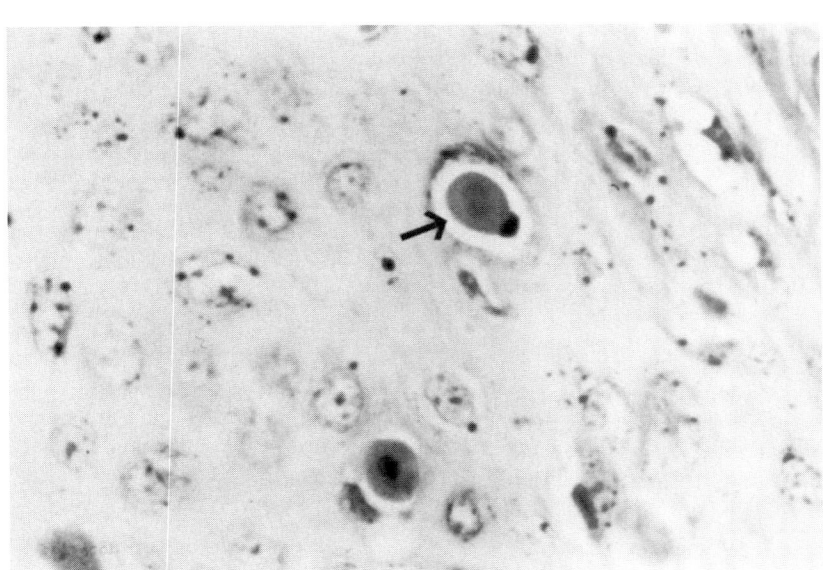

FIGURE 2–45. Satellitosis (satellite cell apoptosis) in a dog with erythema multiforme. Note the lymphocyte attached to an apoptotic keratinocyte *(arrow)*.

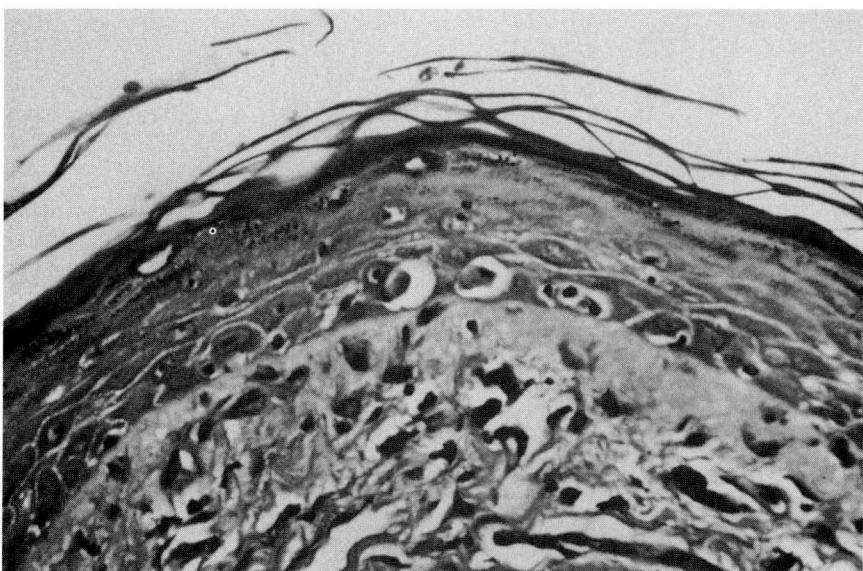

FIGURE 2–46. Two apoptotic basal epidermal cells and a thickened basement membrane zone in a dog with systemic lupus erythematosus.

seborrheic dermatitis, *Malassezia* dermatitis, zinc-responsive dermatoses, and thallotoxicosis. Spongiosis of the upper one half of the epidermis, which is overlaid by marked diffuse parakeratotic hyperkeratosis, is seen in necrolytic migratory erythema. Spongiosis of the upper half of the epidermis with superficial epidermal necrosis may be seen with contact irritant dermatitis.

INTRACELLULAR EDEMA

Intracellular edema (hydropic degeneration, vacuolar degeneration, and ballooning degeneration) of the epidermis is characterized by increased cell size, cytoplasmic pallor, and displacement of the nucleus to the periphery of affected cells (Fig. 2–48). Severe intracellular edema may result in reticular degeneration and intraepidermal vesicles.

Intracellular edema is a common, nondiagnostic feature of any acute or subacute inflammatory dermatosis. Caution must be exercised not to confuse intracellular edema with freezing artifact (Fig. 2–49), delayed fixation artifact, or the intracellular accumulation of glycogen that is seen in the outer root sheath of normal hair follicles and results from epidermal injury. In addition, one can see individual keratinocytes with condensed, pyknotic nuclei surrounded by a clear vesicular space and a rim of homogeneous cytoplasm in a number of dermatoses.[31] These epidermal "clear cells" are artifacts due to occlusion, moisture in intertriginous areas, and other unknown factors.

RETICULAR DEGENERATION

Reticular degeneration is caused by severe intracellular edema of epidermal cells in which the cells burst, resulting in multilocular intraepidermal vesicles in which septa are formed by resistant cell walls (Fig. 2–50). It may be seen with any acute or subacute inflammatory dermatosis but especially dermatophilosis and acute contact dermatitis.

BALLOONING DEGENERATION

Ballooning degeneration (koilocytosis) is a specific type of degenerative change seen in epidermal cells and characterized by swollen eosinophilic to lightly basophilic cytoplasm without vacuolization, by enlarged or condensed and occasionally multiple nuclei, and by a

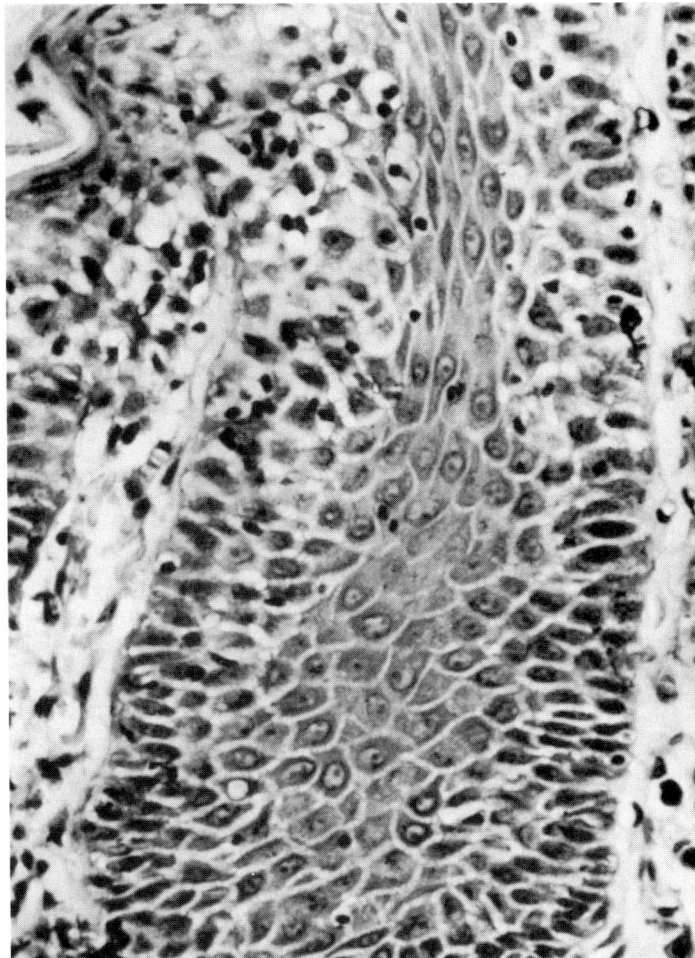

FIGURE 2–47. Spongiosis in a dog with contact dermatitis. There is also lymphocytic exocytosis.

loss of cohesion resulting in acantholysis (Fig. 2–51). Ballooning degeneration is a specific feature of viral infections.

HYDROPIC DEGENERATION

Hydropic degeneration (liquefaction degeneration or vacuolar alteration) of the basal epidermal cells describes intracellular edema restricted to cells of the stratum basale (Fig. 2–52). This process may also affect the basal cells of the outer root sheath of hair follicles. Hydropic degeneration of basal cells is usually focal but, if severe and extensive, may result in intrabasal or subepidermal clefts or vesicles owing to dermo-epidermal separation. Hydropic degeneration of basal cells is an uncommon finding and is usually associated with lupus erythematosus, idiopathic lichenoid dermatoses, adverse cutaneous drug reactions, toxic epidermal necrolysis, erythema multiforme, dermatomyositis, thymoma-associated exfoliative dermatitis of cats, various vasculopathies, and lichenoid keratoses.

ACANTHOLYSIS

A loss of cohesion between epidermal cells, resulting in intraepidermal clefts, vesicles, and bullae (Fig. 2–53), is known as acantholysis (dyshesion, dermolysis, or desmorrhexis). Free epidermal cells in the vesicles are called acantholytic keratinocytes or "acanthocytes" (Fig.

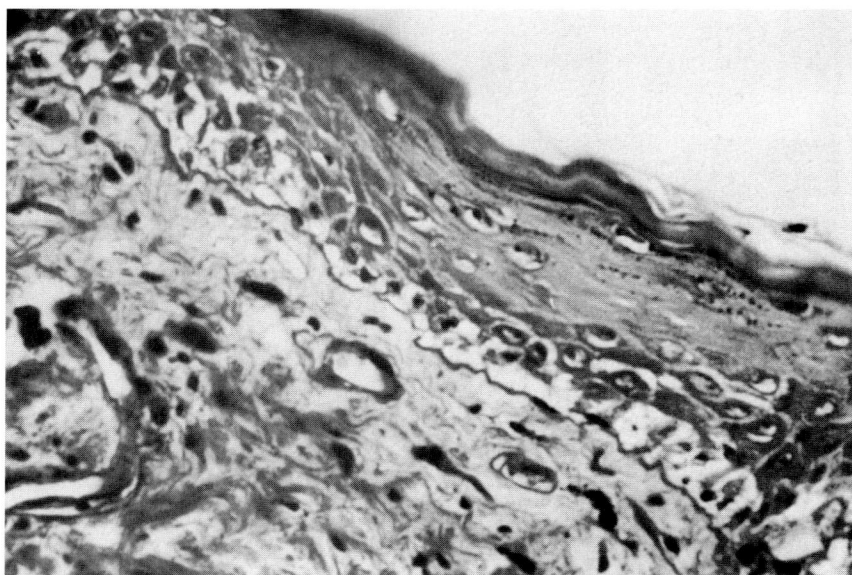

FIGURE 2–52. Hydropic degeneration of epidermal basal cells in a dog with dermatomyositis. (From Scott DW, Schultz RD: Epidermolysis bullosa simplex in the collie dog. J Am Vet Med Assoc 171:721, 1977.)

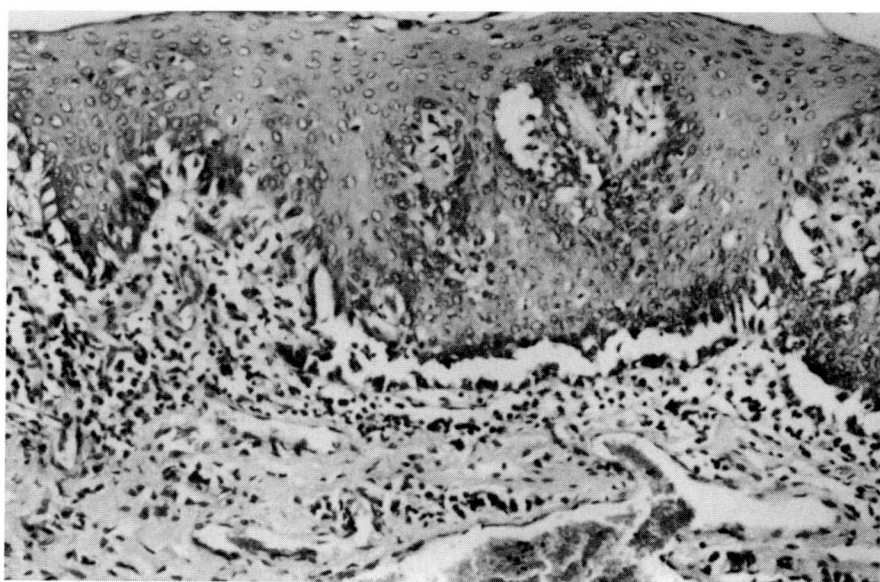

FIGURE 2–53. Suprabasilar cleft and intraepidermal vesicles containing acantholytic cells. (Courtesy A. A. Stannard.)

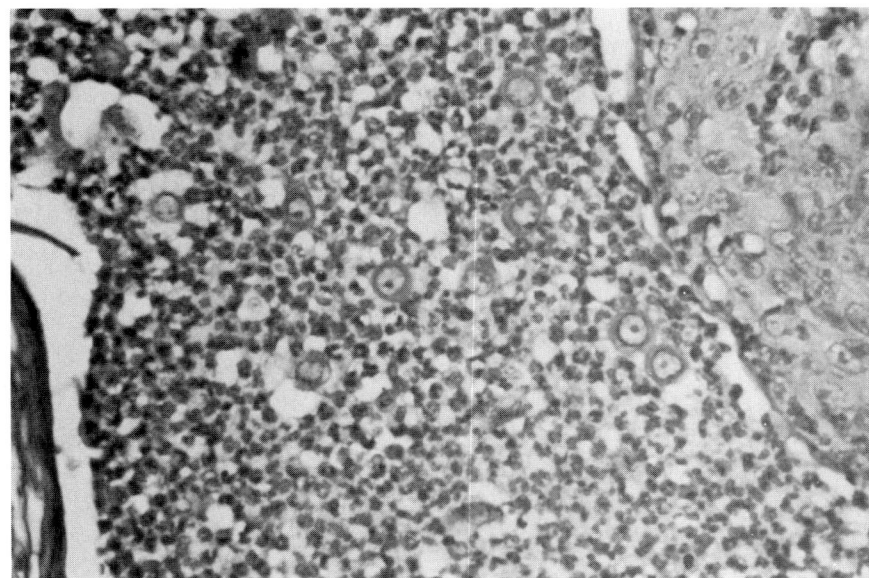

FIGURE 2–54. Acantholytic keratinocytes from a case of canine pemphigus foliaceus.

ballooning degeneration (in viral infection), proteolytic enzymes released by neutrophils (in bacterial and fungal dermatoses[32] and subcorneal pustular dermatosis) or eosinophils (in sterile eosinophilic pustulosis), developmental defects (benign familial pemphigus), and neoplastic transformation (squamous cell carcinoma, actinic keratosis, and warty dyskeratoma).

EXOCYTOSIS AND DIAPEDESIS

The term *exocytosis* refers to the migration of inflammatory cells, erythrocytes, or both through the intercellular spaces of the epidermis (Fig. 2–55). Exocytosis of inflammatory cells is a common, nondiagnostic feature of any inflammatory dermatosis. When the condition involves eosinophils in combination with spongiosis, it is often referred to as *eosinophilic spongiosis* and may be seen in ectoparasitism, pemphigus, pemphigoid, sterile eosinophilic pustulosis, eosinophilic plaque, eosinophilic granuloma, hypereosinophilic syndrome, and some cases of contact hypersensitivity. *Lymphocytic exocytosis* occurs in interface dermatoses (e.g., lupus erythematosus), *Malassezia* dermatitis, atopy, contact hypersensitivity, seborrheic disorders, and some ectoparasitisms. *Multinucleated histiocytic giant cells* are rarely seen within the epidermis (e.g., adverse cutaneous drug reaction).

Diapedesis occurs when erythrocytes are present in the intercellular spaces of the epidermis. Diapedesis of erythrocytes implies loss of vascular integrity and may be seen whenever superficial dermal inflammation and vascular dilatation and engorgement are pronounced or when vasculitis or coagulation defects occur. These intraepidermal erythrocytes can be phagocytosed by keratinocytes.[16]

CLEFTS

The slitlike spaces known as *clefts* (lacunae), which do not contain fluid, occur within the epidermis or at the dermoepidermal junction. Clefts may be caused by acantholysis or hydropic degeneration of basal cells (Max Joseph spaces; Fig. 2–56). However, they may also be caused by mechanical trauma and tissue retraction associated with obtaining, fixing, and processing biopsy specimens.

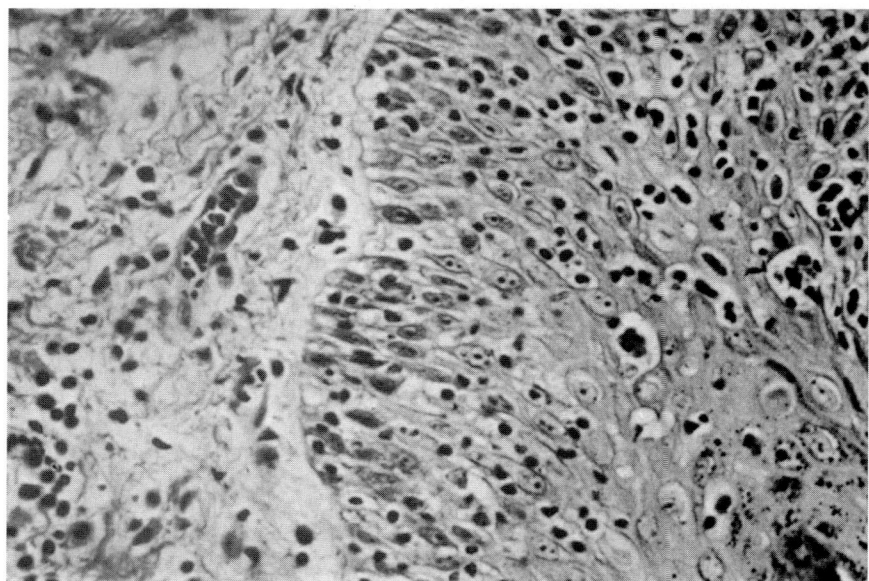

FIGURE 2-55. Exocytosis of leukocytes through the epidermis in a dog with scabies.

Artifactual dermoepidermal separation is fairly commonly observed at the margin of a biopsy specimen. In general, only tissue weakened through the dermoepidermal junction will separate in this manner during processing. Thus, this "usable artifact" may be valid evidence of basal cell or basement membrane damage. Spurious separation is characterized by clefting at different anatomic sites within the same specimen (Fig. 2-57) and evidence of tissue trauma (e.g., torn cytoplasm and fibers, bare cellular nuclei).

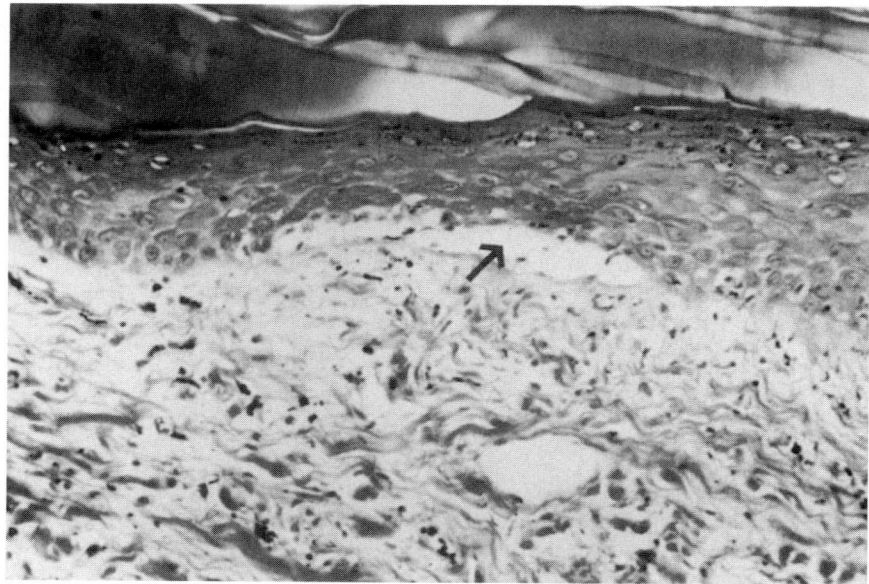

FIGURE 2-56. Intrabasal cleft (*arrow*) in a dog with dermatomyositis.

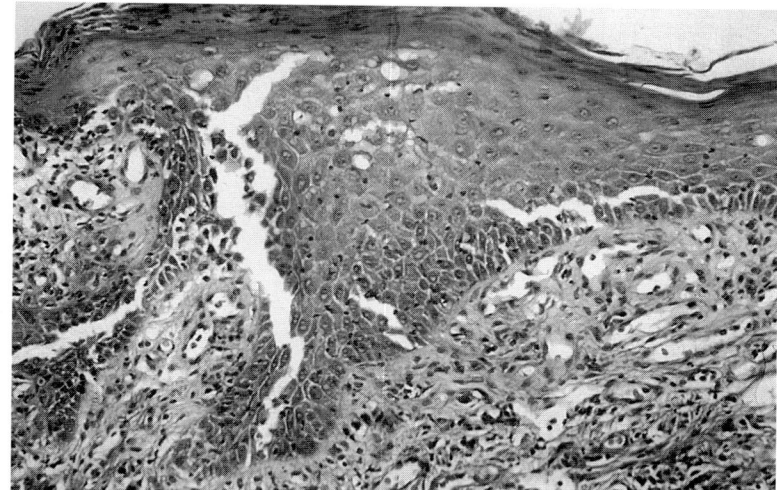

FIGURE 2–57. Artifactual clefts. Inflammatory dermatosis in a dog. Artifactual clefts occur in numerous directions (horizontally and vertically), at numerous levels (suprabasilar, intraepidermal, dermoepidermal), and are associated with ripping and tearing of cells (cytoplasmic, nuclear).

MICROVESICLES, VESICLES, AND BULLAE

Microvesicles (Fig. 2–58), vesicles, and bullae are microscopic and macroscopic, fluid-filled, relatively acellular spaces within or below the epidermis. Vesicles and bullae are often loosely referred to as *blisters*. These lesions may be caused by severe intercellular or intracellular edema, ballooning degeneration, acantholysis, hydropic degeneration of basal cells, subepidermal edema, or other factors resulting in dermoepidermal separation (e.g., the autoantibodies in bullous pemphigoid). Microvesicles, vesicles, and bullae may thus be further described by their location as subcorneal, intragranular, intraepidermal, suprabasilar, intrabasal, or subepidermal. When these lesions contain larger numbers of inflammatory cells, they are referred to as vesicopustules.

MICROABSCESSES AND PUSTULES

Microabscesses and pustules are microscopic or macroscopic intraepidermal and subepidermal cavities filled with inflammatory cells (Fig. 2–59), which can be further described on the basis of location and cell type as follows:

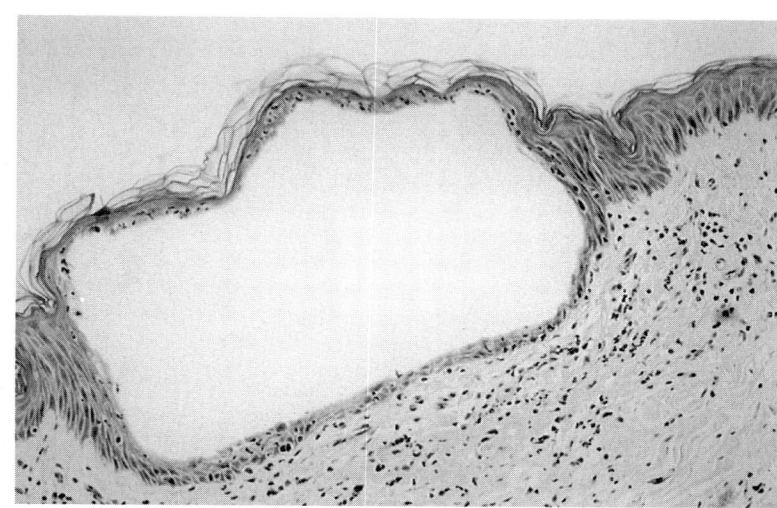

FIGURE 2–58. Intraepidermal microvesicle in a dog with food hypersensitivity.

150 • Diagnostic Methods

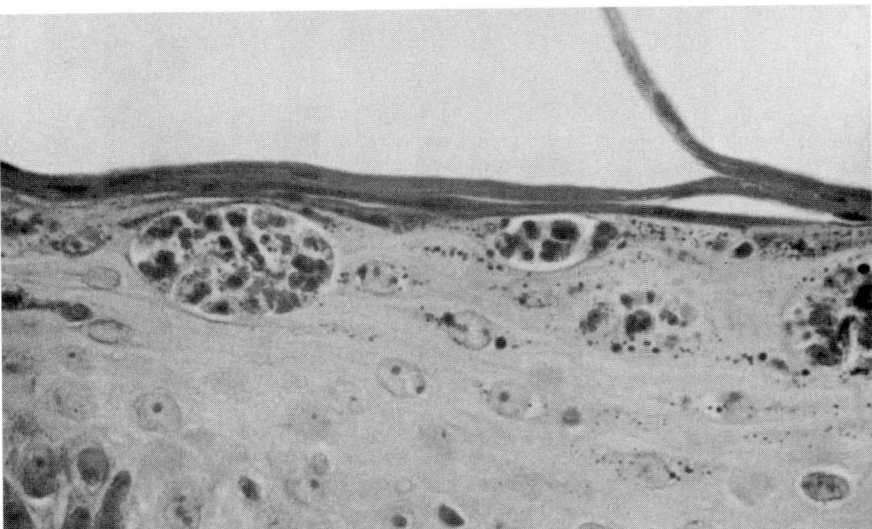

FIGURE 2–59. Microabscesses are observed in many dermatoses. This photomicrograph illustrates microabscesses containing many eosinophils located within the epidermis. (Courtesy J. D. Conroy.)

1. *Spongiform pustule (of Kogoj)* (Fig. 2–60) is a multilocular accumulation of neutrophils within and between keratinocytes, especially those of the stratum granulosum and the stratum spinosum, in which cell boundaries form a spongelike network. It is seen in microbial infections and occasionally in canine subcorneal pustular dermatosis, linear IgA pustular dermatosis, and superficial suppurative necrolytic dermatitis of Schnauzers.
2. *Munro's microabscess* (Fig. 2–61) is a small, desiccated accumulation of neutro-

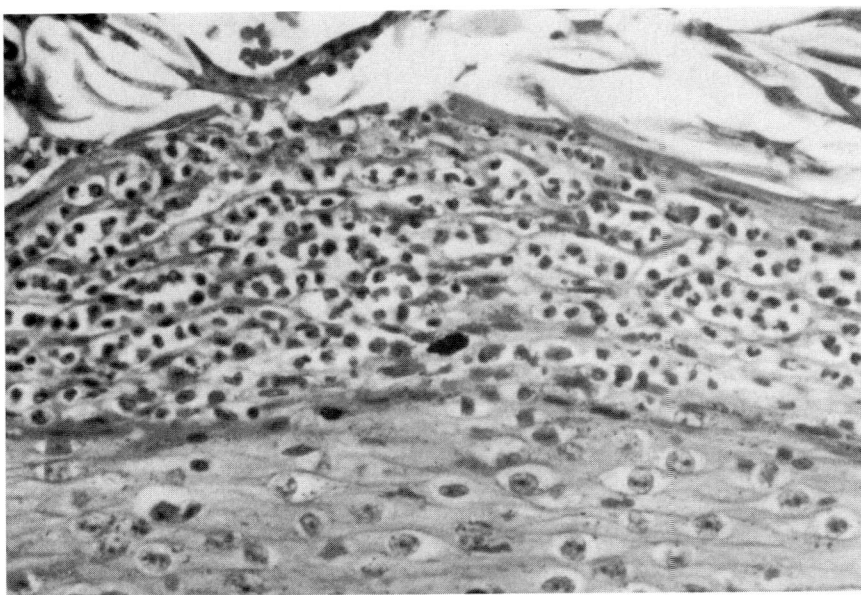

FIGURE 2–60. Spongiform microabscess in the epidermis of a dog with staphylococcal folliculitis.

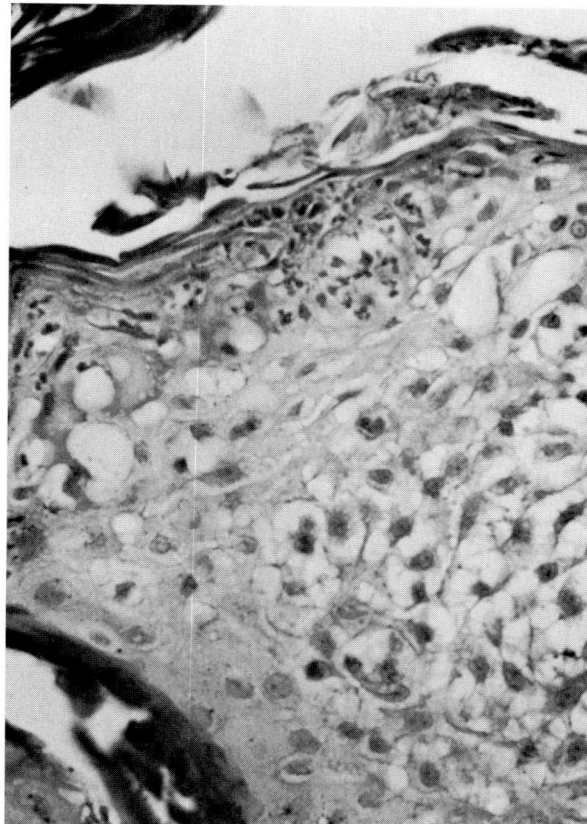

FIGURE 2–61. Munro's microabscess in the superficial epidermis of a dog with seborrheic dermatitis.

phils within or below the stratum corneum, which is seen in microbial infections, seborrheic disorders, and psoriasiform-lichenoid dermatosis of English Springer spaniels.
3. *Pautrier microabscess* (Fig. 2–62A) is a small, focal accumulation of abnormal lymphoid cells, which is seen in epitheliotropic lymphomas.
4. *Eosinophilic microabscess* (see Fig. 2–59) is a lesion seen in ectoparasitism, eosinophilic granuloma, eosinophilic plaque, eosinophilic folliculitis, sterile eosinophilic pustulosis, bullous pemphigoid, the pemphigus complex, feline allergy, canine atopy, contact hypersensitivity, and with *Malassezia* dermatitis.
5. Small spongiotic foci containing normal mononuclear cells (see Fig. 2–62B) are occasionally seen in atopy, contact hypersensitivity, and seborrheic disorders. In canine atopy, some or all of these cells may be Langerhans' cells.

HYPERPIGMENTATION

Hyperpigmentation (hypermelanosis) refers to excessive amounts of melanin deposited within the epidermis and often concurrently in dermal melanophages. Hyperpigmentation may be focal or diffuse and may be confined to the stratum basale or present throughout all epidermal layers (Fig. 2–63). It is a common, nondiagnostic finding in chronic inflammatory and hormonal dermatoses as well as in some developmental and neoplastic disorders. Postinflammatory hyperpigmentation is a common consequence of inflammatory insults. Increased melanin may be present in the epidermis (within keratinocytes) and/or dermis (within melanophages). The pathomechanism is unclear but could include epidermal injury and melanin fallout through a damaged basement membrane. Interferons

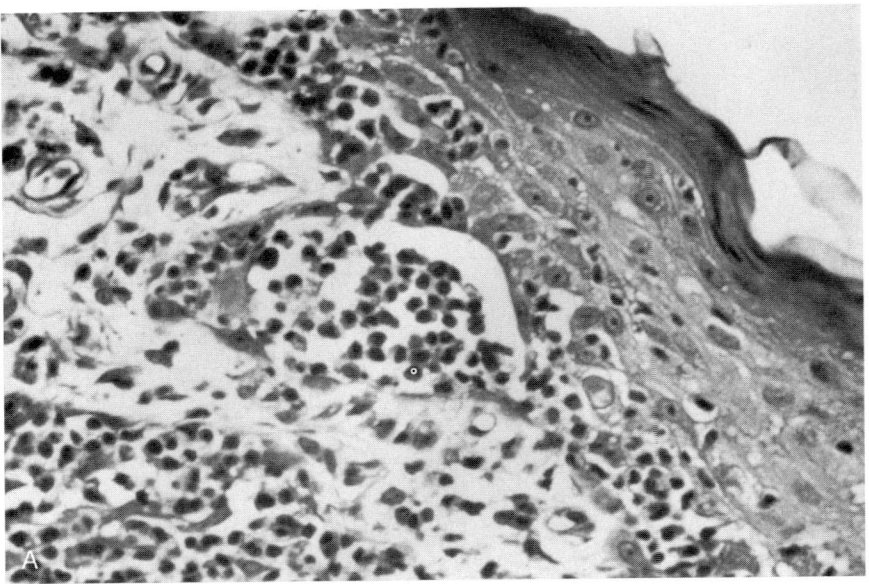
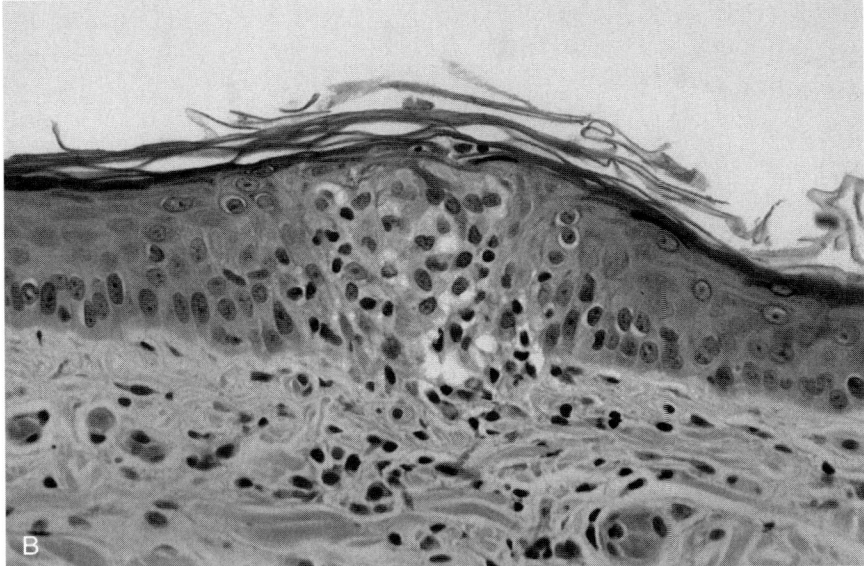

FIGURE 2–62. *A,* Pautrier microabscess in the lower epidermis of a dog with epitheliotropic lymphoma. *B,* Small intraepidermal microabscess containing lymphocytes and Langerhans' cells in an atopic dog.

stimulate melanin formation by melanocytes and may be a key mechanism in cutaneous postinflammatory hyperpigmentation. Hyperpigmentation must always be cautiously assessed with regard to the patient's normal pigmentation. Hyperpigmentation of sebaceous glands with extrusion of linear melanotic casts into hair follicle lumina is seen with follicular dysplasias or endocrinopathies (Fig. 2–64).[14]

HYPOPIGMENTATION

Hypopigmentation (hypomelanosis) refers to decreased amounts of melanin in the epidermis (Fig. 2–65). The condition may be associated with congenital or acquired idiopathic

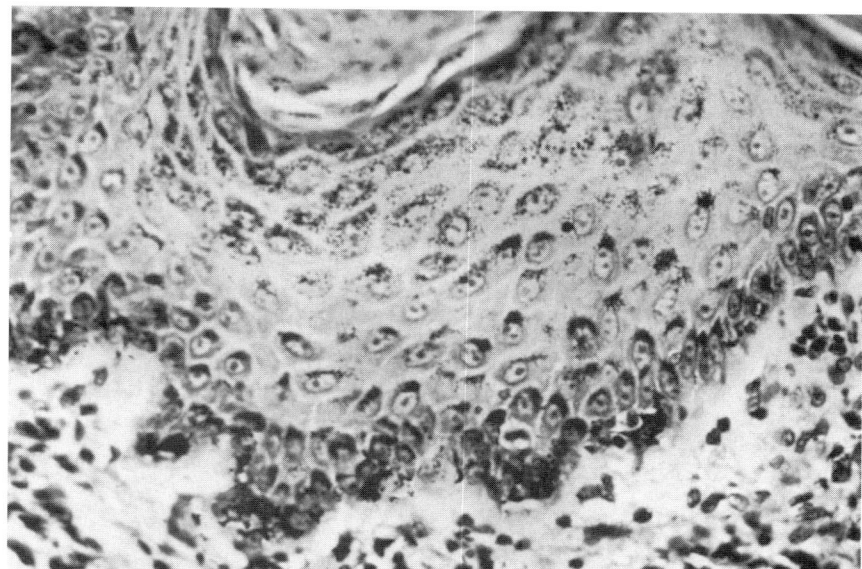

FIGURE 2-63. Epidermal melanosis (hyperpigmentation) in a dog with acanthosis nigricans.

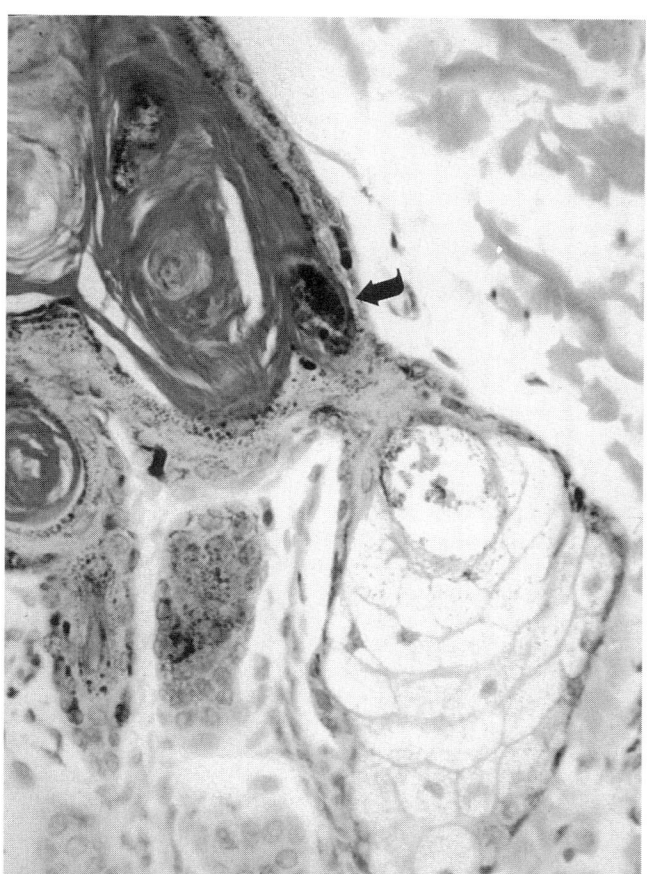

FIGURE 2-64. Sebaceous gland melanosis in a dog with cyclic follicular dysplasia. Melanin granules are concentrated into clumps in the sebaceous duct *(arrow)*.

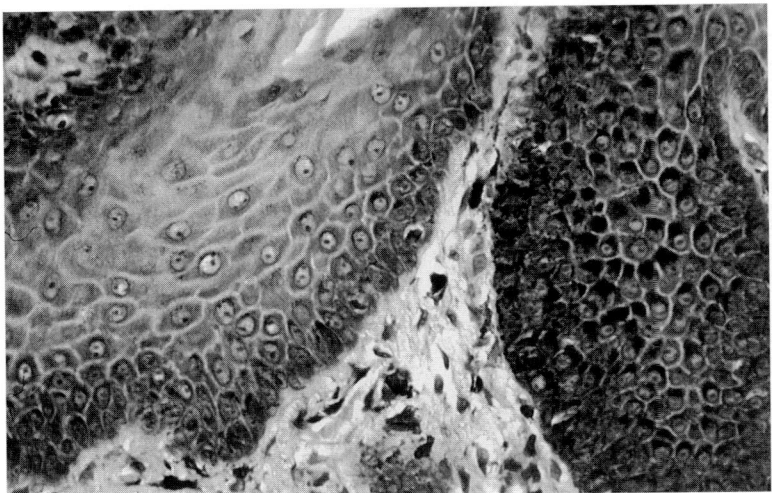

FIGURE 2–65. Epidermal hypomelanosis in a dog with vitiligo. Normal epidermis *(right)* is heavily melanized, whereas vitiliginous epidermis *(left)* is almost devoid of melanin.

defects in melaninization (e.g., leukoderma and vitiligo), the toxic effects of certain chemicals (e.g., monobenzyl ether of dihydroquinone in rubbers and plastics) on melanocytes, inflammatory disorders that affect melaninization or destroy melanocytes, hormonal disorders, and dermatoses featuring hydropic degeneration of basal cells (e.g., lupus erythematosus). In the hypopigmented dermatoses associated with hydropic degeneration of basal cells, the underlying superficial dermis usually reveals pigmentary incontinence.

CRUST

The consolidated, desiccated surface mass called *crust* is composed of varying combinations of keratin, serum, cellular debris, and often microorganisms. Crusts are further described on the basis of their composition: (1) *serous*—mostly serum, (2) *hemorrhagic*—

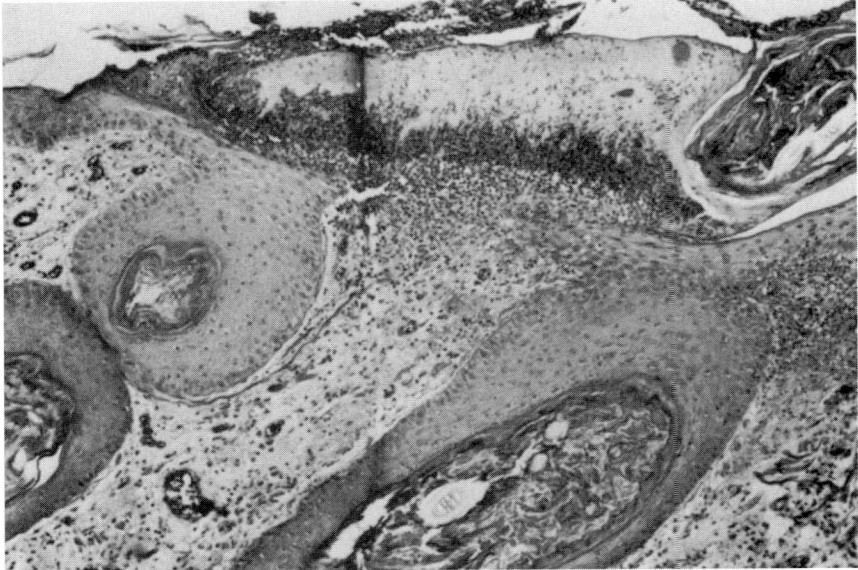

FIGURE 2–66. Serocellular crust in a cat with primary irritant contact dermatitis.

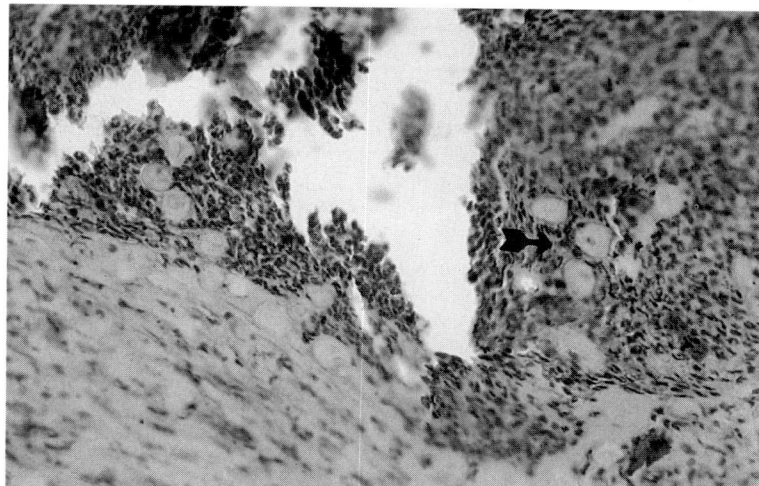

FIGURE 2–67. Acantholytic keratinocytes *(arrow)* in surface crust of a dog with pemphigus foliaceus.

mostly blood, (3) *cellular*—mostly inflammatory cells, (4) *serocellular* (exudative)—a mixture of serum and inflammatory cells (Fig. 2–66), and (5) *palisading*—alternating horizontal rows of orthokeratotic to parakeratotic hyperkeratosis and pus (e.g., in dermatophilosis and dermatophytosis).

Crusts merely indicate a prior exudative process and are rarely of diagnostic significance. However, crusts should always be closely scrutinized, because they may contain the following important diagnostic clues: (1) dermatophyte spores and hyphae, (2) the filaments and coccoid elements of *Dermatophilus congolensis,* and (3) large numbers of acantholytic keratinocytes (in pemphigus complex) (Fig. 2–67). Bacteria and bacterial colonies are common inhabitants of surface debris and are of no diagnostic significance (Fig. 2–68).

The presence of yeast in surface debris is more difficult to interpret. Yeasts *(M. pachydermatis)* are occasionally seen in surface debris and may be of no diagnostic significance.[41, 42] However, the pathologist and the clinician should always carefully consider the potential importance of yeast in contributing to dermatitis. Histopathologically, the presence of surface yeasts accompanied by subjacent epidermal parakeratotic hyper-

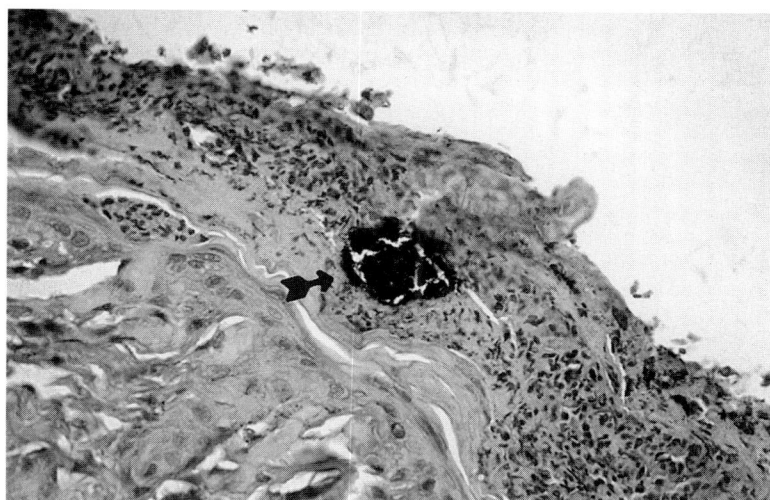

FIGURE 2–68. Microcolony of cocci *(arrow)* in a surface crust of a cat with atopy.

keratosis, spongiosis, and lymphocytic exocytosis is a reaction pattern that strongly suggests that these organisms are contributing to the clinical dermatitis.[30]

DELLS

Dells are small depressions or hollows in the surface of the epidermis. They are usually associated with focal epidermal atrophy and orthokeratotic hyperkeratosis. Dells may be seen in lichenoid dermatoses, especially in lupus erythematosus.

EPIDERMAL COLLARETTE

The term *epidermal collarette* refers to the formation of elongated, hyperplastic rete ridges at the lateral margins of a pathologic process that appear to curve inward toward the center of the lesion. Epidermal collarettes may be seen with neoplastic, granulomatous, and suppurative dermatoses.

HORN CYSTS, PSEUDOHORN CYSTS, HORN PEARLS, AND SQUAMOUS EDDIES

Horn cysts (keratin cysts) are multiple, small, circular cystic structures that are surrounded by flattened epidermal cells and that contain concentrically arranged lamellar keratin. Horn cysts are features of hair follicle neoplasms and basal cell tumors. *Pseudohorn cysts* are illusory small cystic structures formed by the irregular invagination of a hyperplastic, hyperkeratotic epidermis. They are seen in numerous hyperplastic or neoplastic epidermal dermatoses.

Horn pearls (squamous pearls) are focal, circular, concentric layers of squamous cells showing gradual keratinization toward the center, often accompanied by cellular atypia and dyskeratosis. Horn pearls are features of squamous cell carcinoma and pseudocarcinomatous hyperplasia.

Squamous eddies are whorl-like patterns of squamoid cells with no atypia, dyskeratosis, or central keratinization. Squamous eddies are features of numerous neoplastic and hyperplastic epidermal disorders.

EPIDERMOLYTIC HYPERKERATOSIS

Epidermolytic hyperkeratosis (granular degeneration) is characterized by (1) perinuclear clear spaces in the upper epidermis, (2) indistinct cell boundaries formed either by lightly staining material or by keratohyalin granules peripheral to the perinuclear clear spaces, (3) a markedly thickened stratum granulosum, and (4) orthokeratotic hyperkeratosis. It is seen in certain types of ichthyosis, epidermal nevi (Fig. 2–69), actinic keratoses, seborrheic keratoses, papillomas, keratinous cysts, and squamous cell carcinoma.

MAST CELLS IN THE EPITHELIUM AND AT THE BASEMENT MEMBRANE ZONE

Mast cells are frequently seen within the epidermis and the outer root sheath of the hair follicle in biopsy specimens from cats with inflammatory dermatoses (Fig. 2–70).[40] They are most commonly found in diseases of allergic or immune-mediated origin, especially those with tissue eosinophilia. Mast cells are often found in a linear alignment immediately below the basement membrane zone in biopsy specimens from dogs with *Malassezia* dermatitis (Fig. 2–71)[30] and rarely in other inflammatory dermatoses.[15]

Dermal Changes

COLLAGEN CHANGES

Dermal collagen is subject to a number of pathologic changes and may undergo the following: (1) *hyalinization*—a loss of fibrillar structure and amorphous change leading to

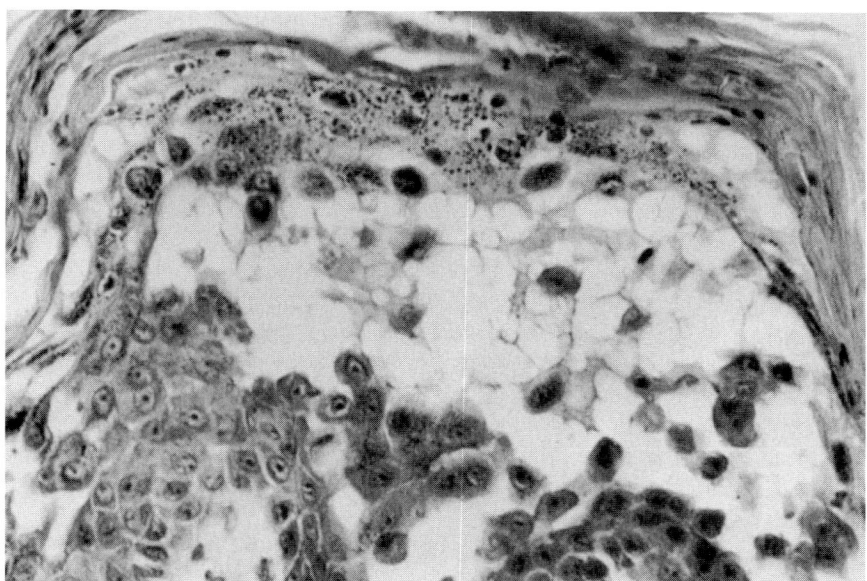

FIGURE 2–69. Epidermolytic hyperkeratosis (granular degeneration) in a dog with epidermal nevus.

confluence and an increased eosinophilic, glassy, refractile appearance, as seen in chronic inflammation, vasculopathies, and connective tissue diseases; (2) *fibrinoid degeneration*—deposition of or replacement with a brightly eosinophilic fibrillar or granular substance resembling fibrin, as seen in connective tissue diseases; (3) *lysis*—a homogeneous, eosinophilic, complete loss of structural detail, as seen in microbial infections and ischemia; (4) *degeneration*—a structural and tinctorial change characterized by slight basophilia, granular appearance, and frayed edges of collagen fibers, rarely seen in canine and feline dermatoses; (5) *dystrophic mineralization*—deposition of calcium salts as basophilic, amorphous, granular material along collagen fibers (Fig. 2–72), as seen in hyperadreno-

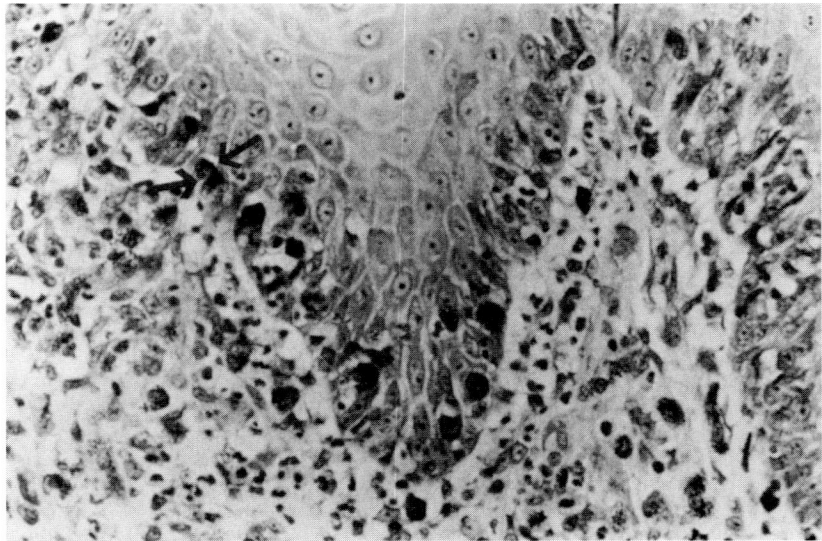

FIGURE 2–70. Epidermal mast cells *(arrows)* in a cat with flea bite hypersensitivity.

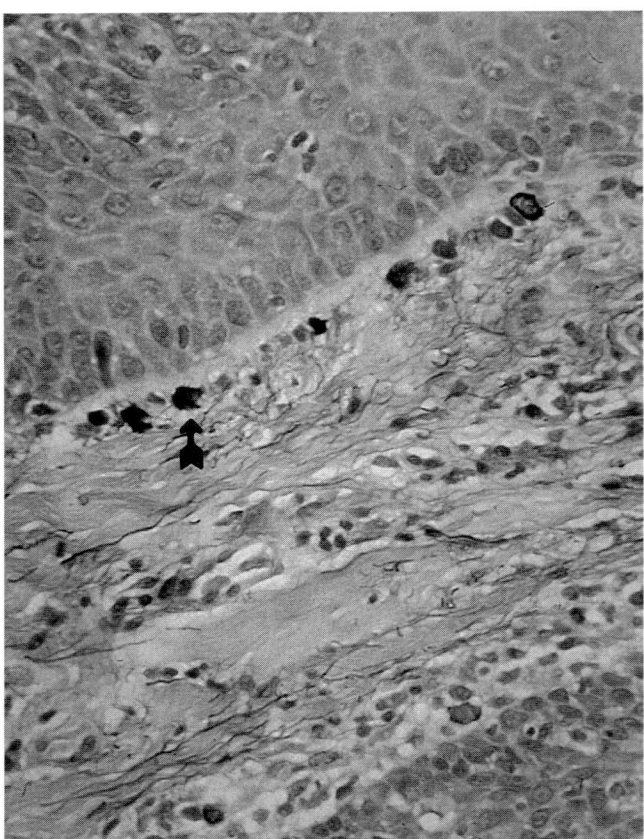

FIGURE 2-71. Linear alignment of mast cells *(arrow)* at the basement membrane zone in a dog with *Malassezia* dermatitis (AOG stain).

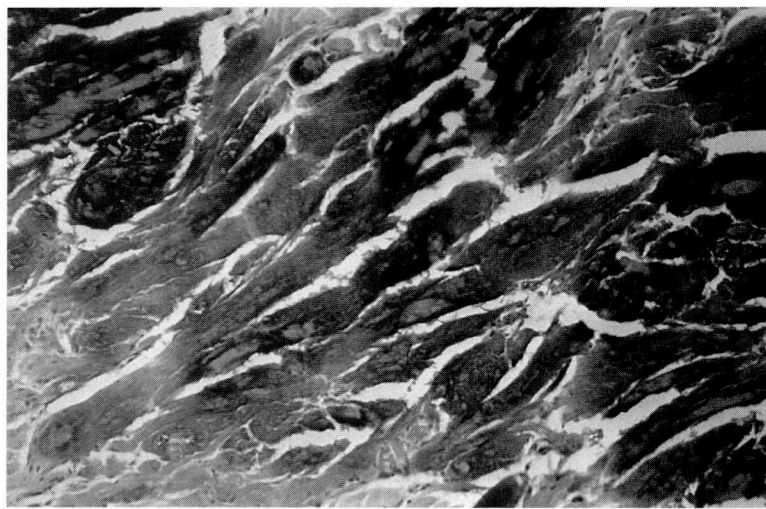

FIGURE 2-72. Dystrophic mineralization of collagen bundles in a dog with hyperadrenocorticism.

corticism; (6) *atrophy*—thin collagen fibrils and decreased fibroblasts, with a resultant decrease in dermal thickness, as seen in hormonal dermatoses; and (7) *dysplasia*—disorganization and fragmentation of collagen bundles (Fig. 2–73), as seen in cutaneous asthenia and feline acquired skin fragility.

A *flame figure* (Fig. 2–74) is an area of altered collagen surrounded by eosinophils and eosinophil granules.[21, 22, 52] Collagen fibers are surrounded totally or in part by eosinophilic material. This material is variable in shape, from annular to oval, to a radiating configuration resembling the spokes of a wheel ("starburst" appearance). Some collagen fibers within these areas appear normal, whereas others appear partially or wholly swollen, irregular or fuzzy in outline, and granular in consistency. The eosinophilic material itself varies from amorphous to granular. In the granular areas, one can see a transition from intact eosinophils, to eosinophil granules and nuclear debris, to completely amorphous material. Trichrome-stained sections show the collagen fibers to be normal in size, surface contour, and consistency.[21, 22] Thus, the irregularities, granularity, and fuzziness seen in the H & E–stained sections are due to the coating of collagen fibers with the eosinophilic material. In humans, electron microscopic studies have revealed no collagen degeneration in flame figures.[52] Immunofluorescence testing identifies eosinophil major basic protein in the amorphous material surrounding and coating collagen fibers.[52] It is likely that all feline and canine skin lesions previously described as containing "collagen degeneration," "necrobiotic collagen," or "collagenolysis" actually contained flame figures. Such conditions include feline and canine eosinophilic granuloma, insect and arthropod reactions, sterile eosinophilic pustulosis, and eosinophilic panniculitis.

ELASTIN CHANGES

Atrophy of elastin fibers is seen in dogs with pituitary dwarfism, adult-onset hyposomatotropism, and chronic hyperglucocorticoidism.

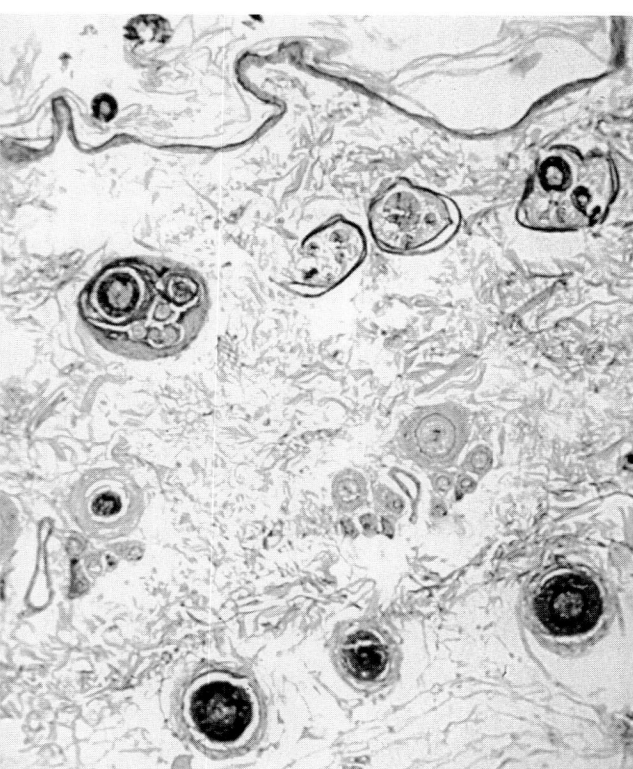

FIGURE 2–73. Collagen dysplasia in a dog with cutaneous asthenia. Note how collagen bundles vary greatly in size and appear disorganized and fragmented.

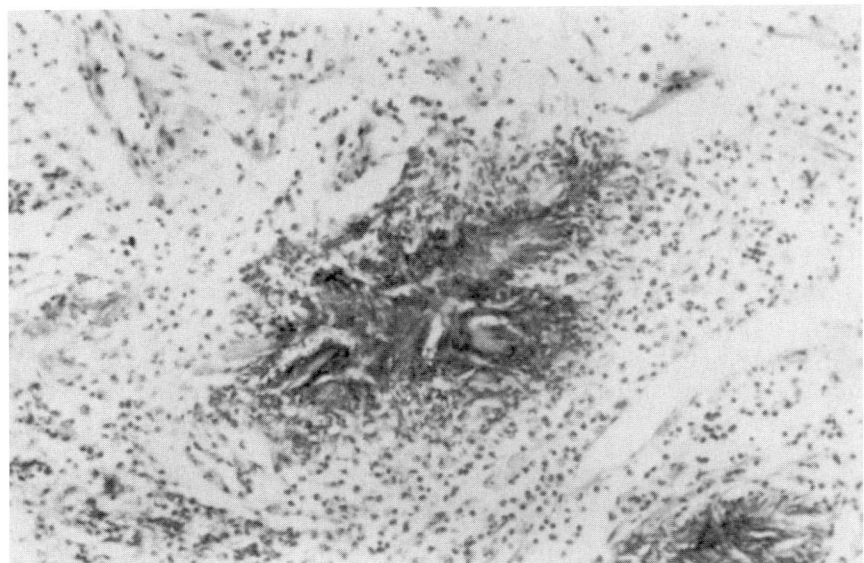

FIGURE 2–74. Flame figure. Collagen fibers are surrounded and coated by granular material from eosinophils.

Solar elastosis appears in H & E–stained sections as a tangle of indistinct amphophilic fibers, often in linear bands running approximately parallel to the surface epidermis, within the superficial dermis. With Verhoeff's or AOG stain, the tangled, thickened, elastotic material is clearly seen (Fig. 2–75). Solar elastosis is a rare manifestation of ultraviolet light–induced skin damage in dogs and cats.

DERMAL DEPOSITS

Amyloid appears in H & E–stained sections as a hyaline, amorphous, lightly eosinophilic material that tends to displace or obliterate normal structures.

Lipid deposits occur in the dermis in xanthomatosis. In H & E–stained sections, lightly eosinophilic, feathery deposits separate the collagen bundles to form small "lakes" of lipid (Fig. 2–76).

Cholesterol clefts may be seen in xanthomatosis, panniculitis, and ruptured follicular cysts. They appear as clear spaces in needle or spicule shape (Fig. 2–77).

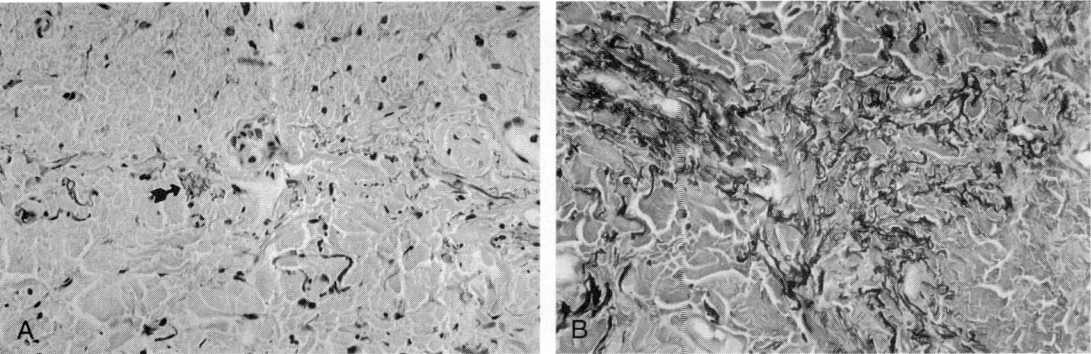

FIGURE 2–75. Solar elastosis in a dog. *A*, Tangled, elastotic material *(arrow)* is occasionally seen in H & E–stained sections. *B*, Elastotic material *(black)* is flagrant in AOG-stained sections.

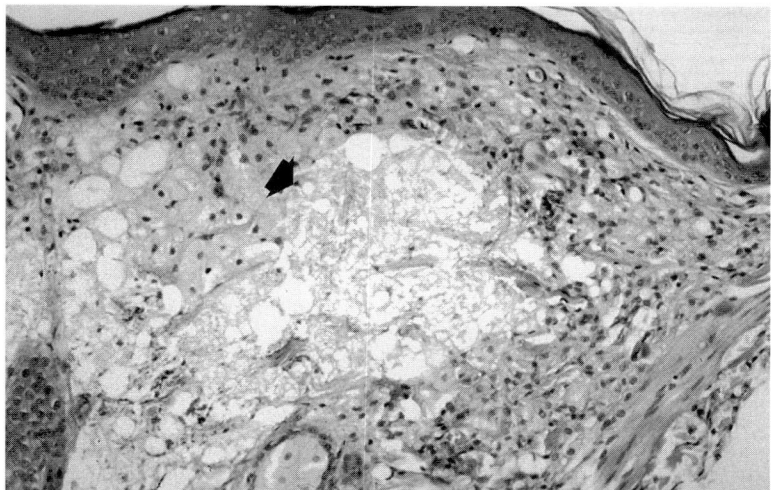

FIGURE 2–76. Lipid lakes *(arrow)* in a xanthoma from a cat.

FIBROPLASIA, DESMOPLASIA, FIBROSIS, AND SCLEROSIS

The term *fibroplasia* refers to the formation and development of fibrous tissue in increased amounts and is often used synonymously with granulation tissue. The condition is characterized by a fibrovascular proliferation in which the blood vessels with prominent endothelial cells are oriented roughly perpendicular to the surface of the skin (Fig. 2–78). The new collagen fibers, with prominent fibroblasts, are oriented roughly parallel to the surface of the skin. Edema and inflammatory cells are constant features of fibroplasia. *Desmoplasia* is the term usually used when referring to the fibroplasia induced by neoplastic processes.

Fibrosis is a later stage of fibroplasia in which increased numbers of fibroblasts and collagen fibers are the characteristic findings. Little or no inflammation is present. Alignment of collagen fibers in vertical streaks seen as elongated, thickened parallel strands of collagen in the superficial dermis, perpendicular to the epidermal surface, is found in chronically rubbed, licked, or scratched skin, such as that seen with acral lick dermatitis and hypersensitivity reactions. *Sclerosis* (scar formation) may be the end point of fibrosis,

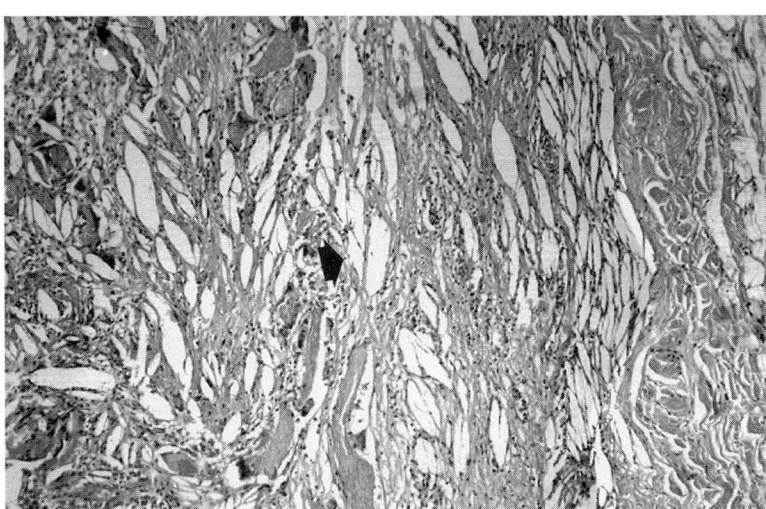

FIGURE 2–77. Cholesterol clefts *(arrow)* peripheral to a ruptured follicular cyst from a dog.

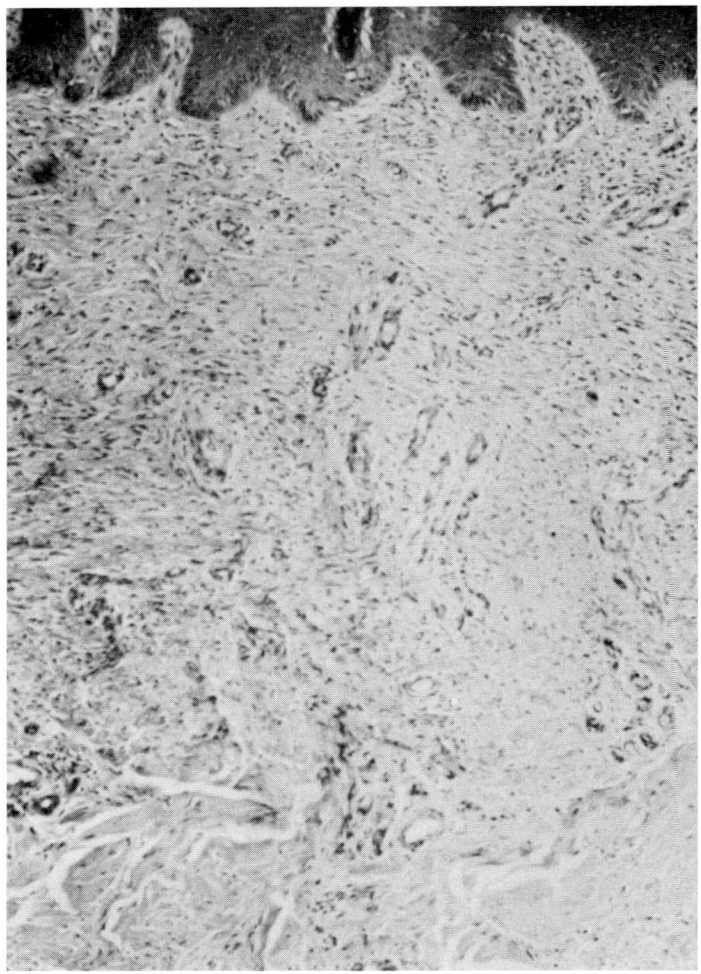

FIGURE 2–78. Fibroplasia subsequent to vascular infarct in a dog.

in which the increased numbers of collagen fibers have a thick, eosinophilic, hyalinized appearance, and the number of fibroblasts is greatly reduced.

PAPILLOMATOSIS, VILLI, AND FESTOONS

Papillomatosis refers to the projection of dermal papillae above the surface of the skin, resulting in an irregular undulating configuration of the epidermis. Often associated with epidermal hyperplasia, papillomatosis is also seen with chronic inflammatory and neoplastic dermatoses. Papillomatosis and papillate epidermal hyperplasia are often associated with primary seborrhea and zinc-responsive dermatoses.

Villi are dermal papillae, covered by one or two layers of epidermal cells (Fig. 2–79), that project into a vesicle or bulla. Villi are seen in pemphigus vulgaris and warty dyskeratoma and occasionally in actinic keratosis and squamous cell carcinoma.

Festoons are dermal papillae, devoid of attached epidermal cells, that project into the base of a vesicle or a bulla. They are seen in bullous pemphigoid, epidermolysis bullosa, and drug-induced pemphigoid.

PIGMENTARY INCONTINENCE

Pigmentary incontinence refers to the presence of melanin granules that are free within the subepidermal and perifollicular dermis and within dermal macrophages (melanopha-

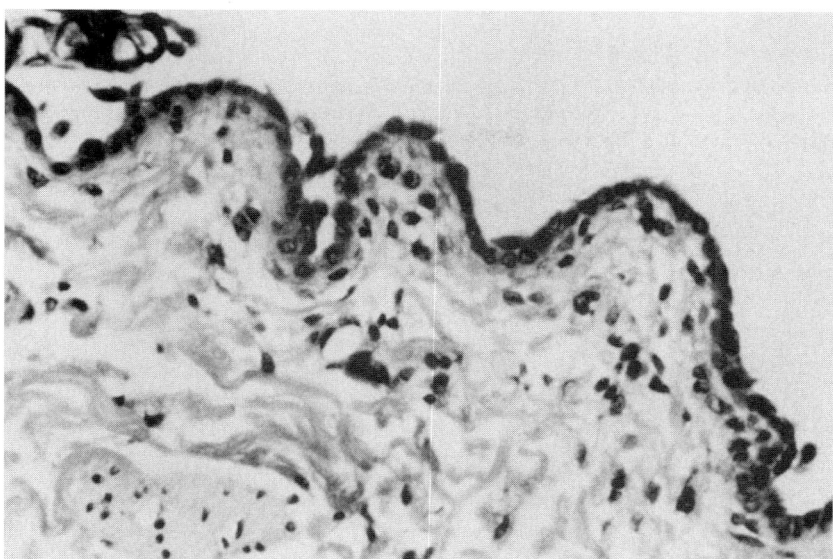

FIGURE 2–79. Villi in a cat with pemphigus vulgaris.

ges) (Fig. 2–80). Pigmentary incontinence may be seen with any process that damages the stratum basale and the basement membrane zone, especially with hydropic degeneration of basal cells (lichenoid dermatoses, lupus erythematosus, dermatomyositis, and erythema multiforme). Interestingly, it was seen in 29% of the biopsy specimens from dogs with *Malassezia* dermatitis.[30] In addition, melanophages may be seen, especially in a perivascular orientation, in chronic inflammatory conditions in which melanin production is greatly increased.

EDEMA

Dermal edema is recognized by dilated lymphatics (not visible in normal skin), widened spaces between blood vessels and perivascular collagen (perivascular edema), or widened

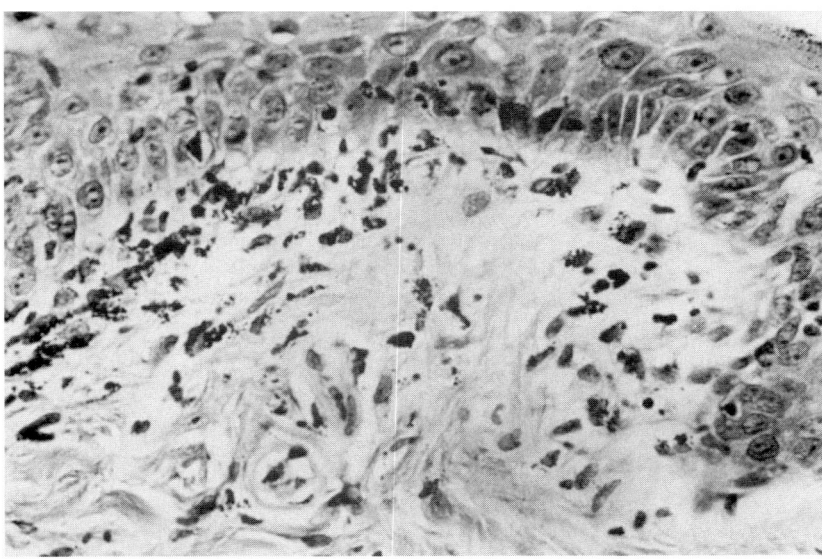

FIGURE 2–80. Pigmentary incontinence in a dog with discoid lupus erythematosus.

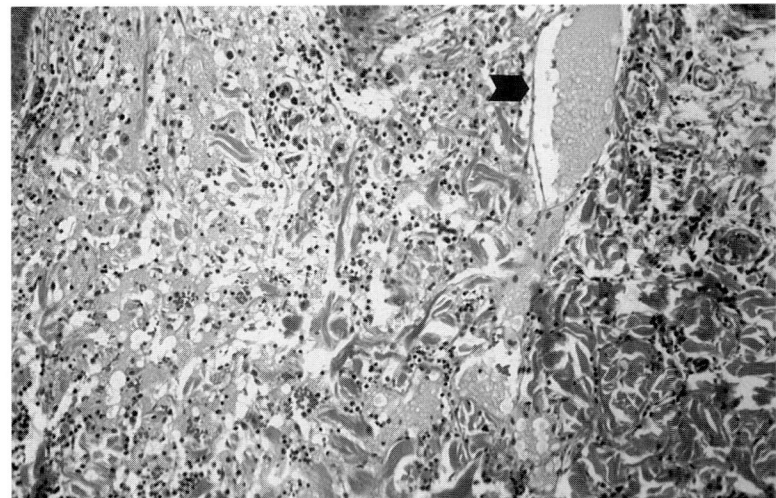

FIGURE 2–81. Dermal edema in a dog with staphylococcal folliculitis. Collagen bundles in left half of photograph are separated by interstitial edema (compare with compact collagen bundles in lower right corner), and dermal lymphatics are dilated and filled with frothy edema (arrow).

spaces between large areas of dermal collagen (interstitial edema) (Fig. 2–81). The dilated lymphatics and widened perivascular and interstitial spaces may or may not contain a lightly eosinophilic, homogeneous, frothy-appearing substance (serum). A scattering of vacuolated macrophages may be seen in the interstitium in chronic severe dermal edema.

Dermal edema is a common, nondiagnostic feature of any inflammatory dermatosis. Severe edema of the superficial dermis may result in subepidermal vesicles and bullae, necrosis of the overlying epidermis, and predisposition to artifactual dermoepidermal separation during the handling and processing of biopsy specimens. Severe edema of the superficial dermis may result in a vertical orientation and stretching of collagen fibers, producing the gossamer (weblike) collagen effect seen with erythema multiforme and severe urticaria.

MUCINOSIS

Mucinosis (myxedema, mucoid degeneration, myxoid degeneration, or mucinous degeneration) is characterized by increased amounts of an amorphous, stringy, granular, basophilic material that separates, thins, or replaces dermal collagen fibrils and surrounds blood vessels and appendages in sections stained with H & E (Fig. 2–82). Only small amounts of mucin are ever visible in normal skin, mostly around appendages and blood vessels. Mucin is more easily demonstrated with stains for acid mucopolysaccharides, such as Hale's iron and Alcian blue stains. Mucinosis may be seen as a focal (usually perivascular) change in numerous inflammatory, neoplastic, and developmental dermatoses. Diffuse mucinosis may be seen with hypothyroidism, acromegaly, lupus erythematosus, dermatomyositis, various idiopathic mucinoses, and the normal skin of the Chinese Shar pei.

Mucin may also be seen in the epidermis and hair follicle outer root sheath in cats and dogs with alopecia mucinosa, in feline dermatoses associated with numerous eosinophils (e.g., eosinophilic plaque, eosinophilic granuloma, allergies) (Fig. 2–83), and in dogs with discoid lupus erythematosus.

GRENZ ZONE

This marginal zone of relatively normal collagen separates the epidermis from an underlying dermal alteration (Fig. 2–84). A grenz zone may be seen in neoplastic and granulomatous disorders.

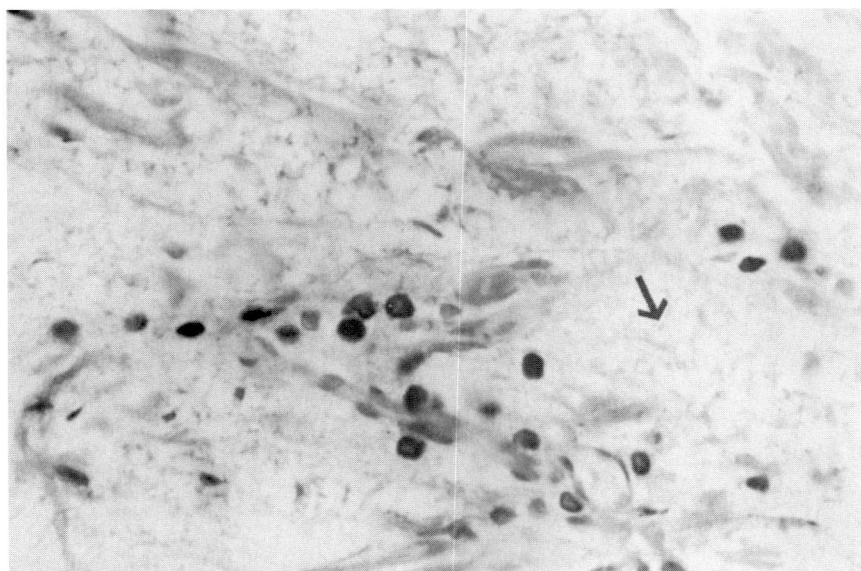

FIGURE 2–82. Dermal mucinosis *(arrow)* and scattered mast cells in a Chinese Shar pei with idiopathic mucinosis.

PAPILLARY MICROABSCESSES

Small neutrophilic microabscesses may occasionally be seen in the dermal papillae of biopsies from animals with vasculitis, bullous pemphigoid, epidermolysis bullosa acquisita, systemic lupus erythematosus, and cutaneous adverse drug reaction.

Follicular Changes

Follicular epithelium is affected by most of the histopathologic changes described for the epidermis. Follicular (poral) keratosis, plugging, and dilatation are common features of such diverse conditions as inflammatory, hormonal, and developmental dermatoses. Follicular hyperplasia and hypertrophy may be seen in chronic inflammatory dermatoses or in

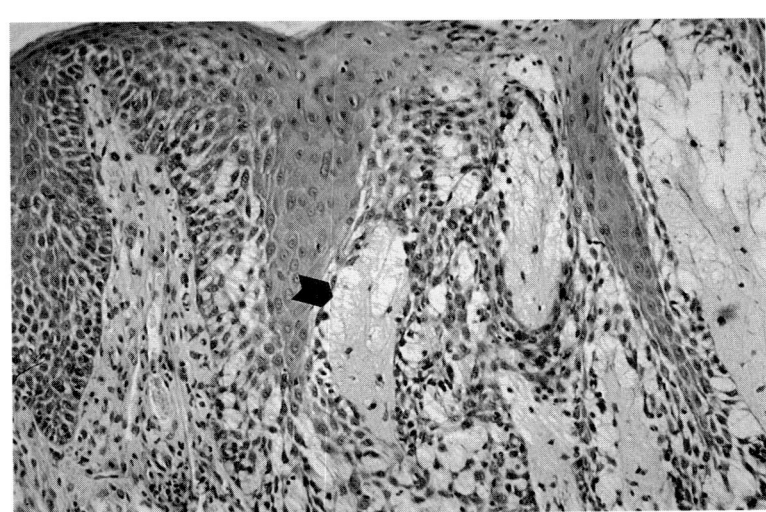

FIGURE 2–83. Lakes of epidermal mucin *(arrow)* in a cat with an eosinophilic plaque.

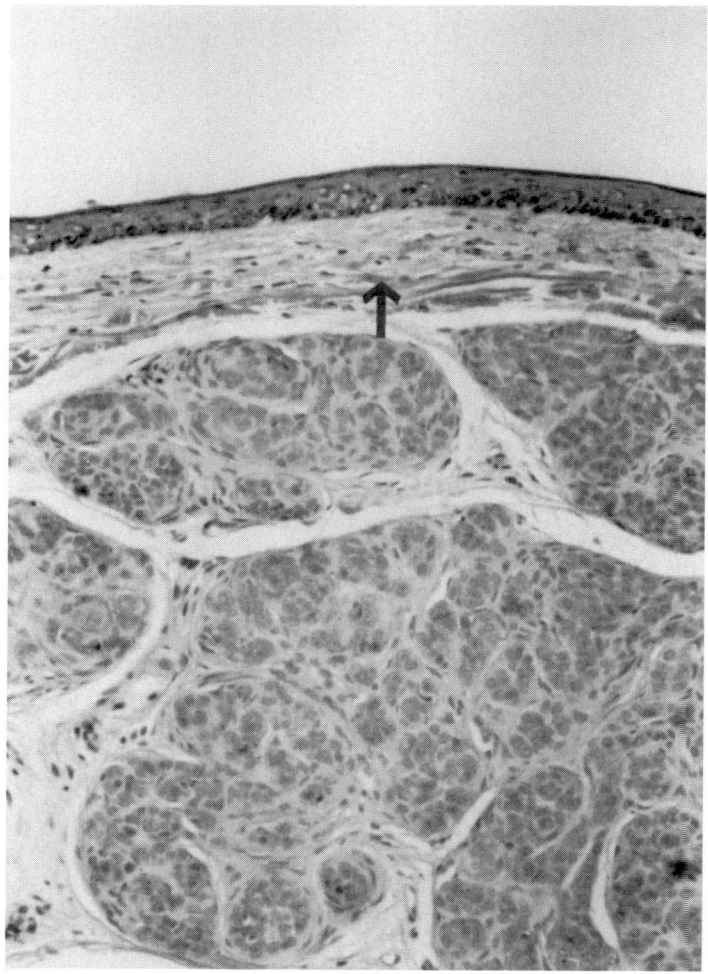

FIGURE 2–84. Grenz zone of superficial dermal collagen *(arrow)* separating epidermis from underlying neoplasia.

nevoid lesions. Excessive *trichilemmal keratinization* (flame follicles) is seen with endocrine and developmental disorders (Fig. 2–85).[39] Trichilemmal keratin is brightly eosinophilic and amorphous, and the tiered "tongues" of excessive keratin give the impression of a flickering flame. *Perifolliculitis, mural folliculitis, luminal folliculitis,* and *furunculosis* (penetrating or perforating folliculitis) refer to varying degrees of follicular inflammation. A cell-poor follicular necrosis may be seen in ischemic states and drug reactions. *Follicular atrophy* (Fig. 2–86) refers to the gradual involution, retraction, and occasionally miniaturization that are characteristic of hormonal and nutritional dermatoses.

Hair follicles should be examined closely to determine the phase of the growth cycle. *Telogenization,* a predominance of telogen hair follicles, is characteristic of hormonal dermatoses and states of telogen defluxion associated with stress, disease, and drugs. *Catagenization* ("catagen arrest") is seen with endocrinopathies, follicular dysplasias, and so-called post-clipping alopecia. *Follicular dysplasia* refers to the presence of incompletely or abnormally formed hair follicles and hair shafts, and is seen in developmental abnormalities such as follicular dysplasia, color dilution alopecia, and black hair follicle dysplasia. Dysplastic hair follicles are primary hair follicles, wherein the infundibular region is dilated and filled with concentrically arranged orthokeratotic hyperkeratosis.[20, 34, 46] One or more secondary hair follicles or sebaceous ducts are filled with orthokeratotic hyperkeratosis and extend into the subjacent dermis, giving the appearance of tentacles or toes (Fig.

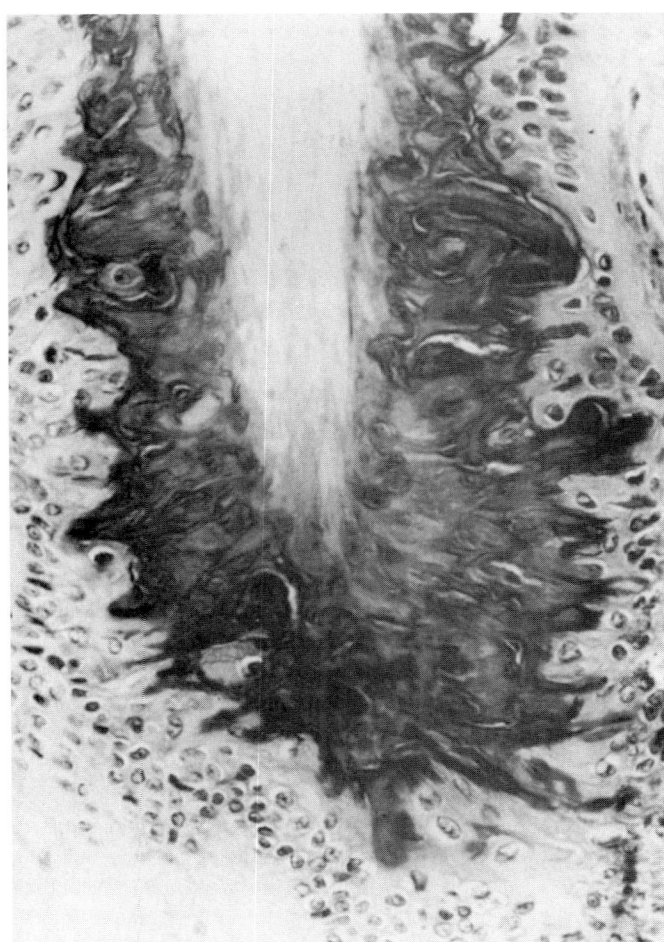

FIGURE 2–85. Flame follicle (excessive trichilemmal keratinization) in a dog with hypothyroidism.

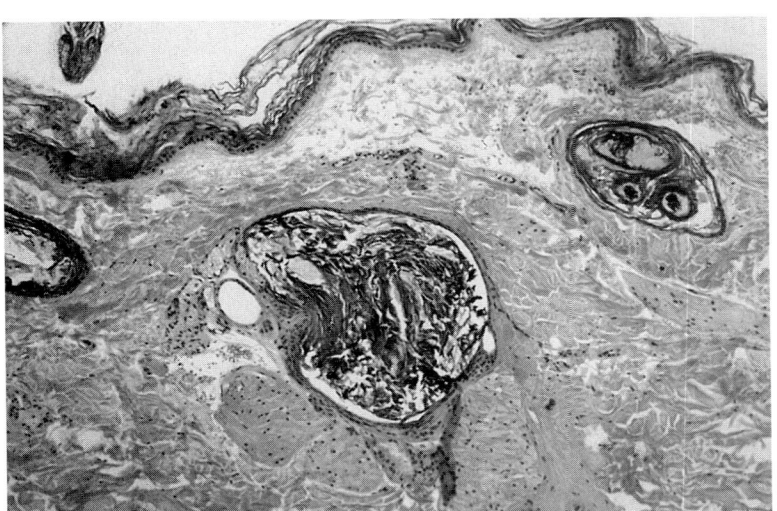

FIGURE 2–86. Follicular atrophy in a dog with hypothyroidism. Follicles are telogenized and hyperkeratotic, and have receded into the superficial dermis.

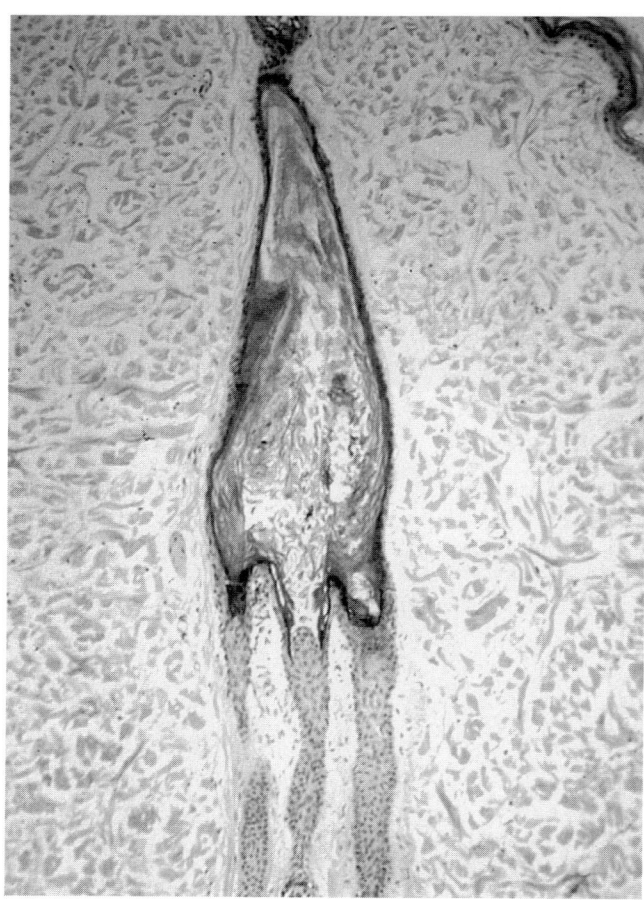

FIGURE 2–87. Dysplastic hair follicle in a dog with cyclic follicular dysplasia. Note how three secondary hair follicles dangle into the dermis below the dilated, hyperkeratotic infundibulum, resembling tentacles or toes.

2–87). *Miniaturized* hair follicles may be seen in pattern baldness, paraneoplastic alopecia of cats, sex hormone dermatoses, nutritional deficiencies, and genetic hypotrichoses.

Perifollicular melanosis (Fig. 2–88) is a common finding in canine demodicosis and follicular dysplasia.[18] *Perifollicular fibrosis* (Fig. 2–89) is seen in chronic folliculitis, canine dermatomyositis, and granulomatous sebaceous adenitis. Dystrophic mineralization of the basement membrane zone and subsequent transepithelial elimination of mineral is seen in the calcinosis cutis of hyperadrenocorticism and as a senile change in dogs, especially Poodles and Bedlington terriers.[24, 48, 55] The finding of large numbers of cocci or yeasts in noninflamed hair follicles in dogs (Fig. 2–90) almost always indicates the presence of clinically relevant bacterial or yeast infection.[41]

Glandular Changes

Sebaceous and epitrichial (apocrine) sweat glands may be affected in various dermatoses. Sebaceous glands may be involved in many suppurative and granulomatous inflammations (sebaceous adenitis). In dogs and cats, an idiopathic granulomatous sebaceous adenitis may be characterized by complete absence of sebaceous glands in the late stages. They may become atrophic (reduced in number and size, with pyknotic nuclei predominating) or cystic in hormonal (Fig. 2–91A and B) and developmental dermatoses, in occasional chronic inflammatory processes, and as a senile change. Sebaceous glands may also become hyperplastic in chronic inflammatory dermatoses, sebaceous gland nevi, and senile nodular sebaceous hyperplasia. Remarkable hyperplasia and dysplasia of sebaceous glands is

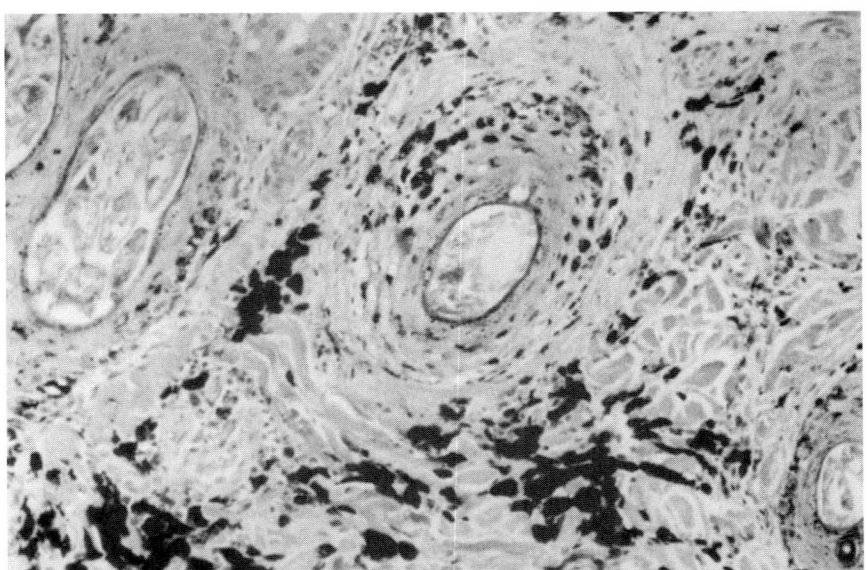

FIGURE 2-88. Perifollicular melanosis in a dog with generalized demodicosis.

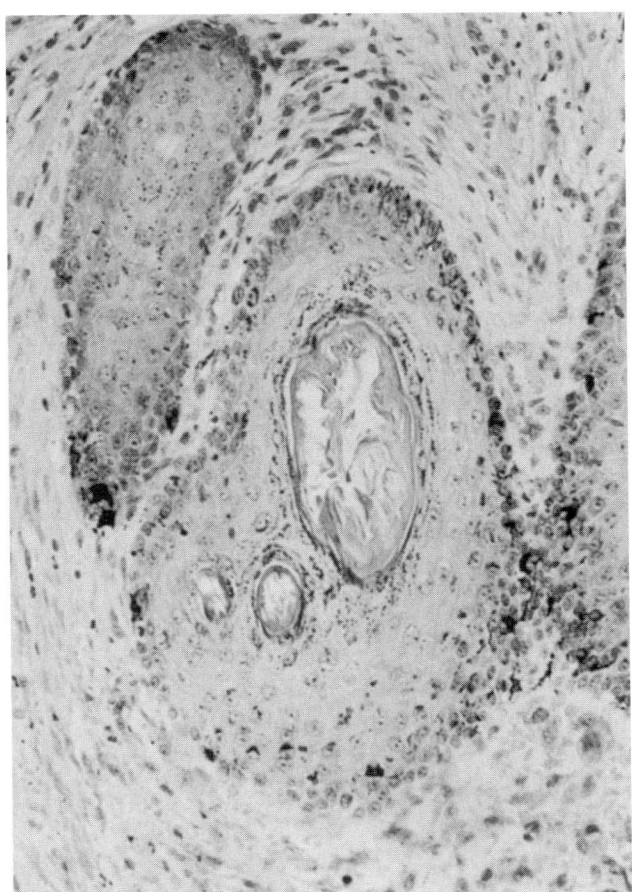

FIGURE 2-89. Perifollicular fibrosis in canine dermatomyositis.

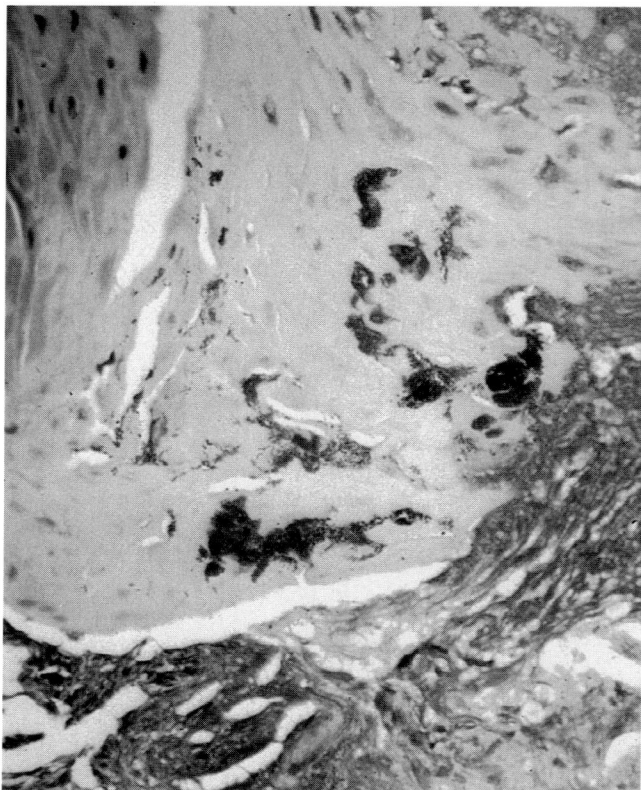

FIGURE 2–90. Microcolonies of cocci in hair follicle of a dog with staphylococcal folliculitis.

seen in dogs with a rare idiopathic greasy skin condition. Sebaceous gland atrophy and hyperplasia must always be cautiously assessed with regard to the area of the body from which the skin specimen was taken. Sebaceous gland melanosis may be seen in dogs with endocrinopathies or follicular dysplasias.

Epitrichial (apocrine) sweat glands are commonly involved in suppurative and granulomatous dermatoses (hidradenitis) (Fig. 2–92A). In one study,[44] the presence of suppurative hidradenitis in biopsy specimens from dogs was consistently associated with clinical bacterial folliculitis, furunculosis, or both, even when hair follicles in the specimens were

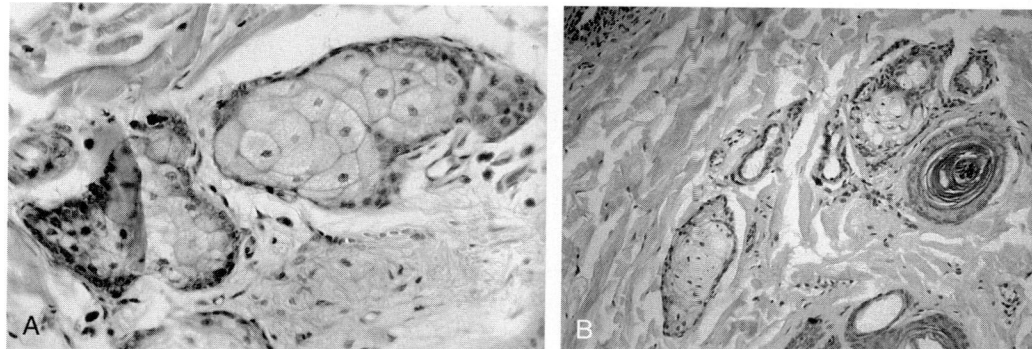

FIGURE 2–91. Normal versus atrophic canine sebaceous glands. A, Normal canine sebaceous gland. Note the sebocytes are well-lipidized and their nuclei are normal. B, Atrophic sebaceous gland in a dog with hyperadrenocorticism. Note that the sebocytes are poorly lipidized and their nuclei are pyknotic.

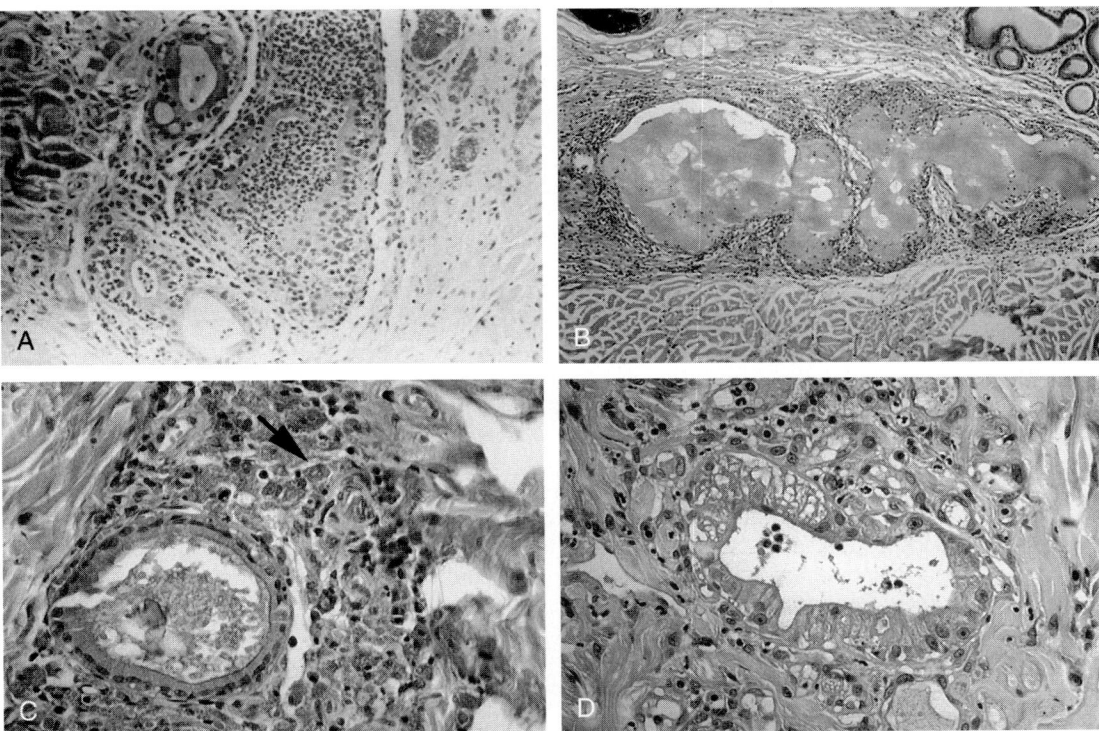

FIGURE 2-92. *A*, Suppurative hidradenitis in a dog with staphylococcal furunculosis. *B*, Epitrichial sweat glands are dilated and filled with secretion in this dog with atopy and staphylococcal folliculitis. *C*, Rupture of epitrichial sweat gland has led to the accumulation of macrophages containing brownish-green granular to globular material *(arrow)*. *D*, Epitrichial sweat gland necrosis in a cat with herpesvirus infection.

not inflamed. Periapocrine accumulation of plasma cells is commonly seen in acral lick dermatitis, chronic infections, and lichenoid dermatoses. The epitrichial sweat glands may become dilated, filled with secretion, or cystic in many inflammatory (see Fig. 2-92B), developmental, and hormonal dermatoses; in apocrine cystomatosis; and with senile changes. The light microscopic recognition of epitrichial sweat gland atrophy is moot, because dilated epitrichial secretory coils containing flattened epithelial cells are a feature of the normal postsecretory state. Damage to epitrichial sweat glands that allows leakage of secretion into the surrounding dermis is often accompanied by an accumulation of macrophages that contain a brown-green granular to globular material (see Fig. 2-92C). A cell-poor epitrichial sweat gland necrosis may be seen in drug reactions, feline herpesvirus dermatitis (see Fig. 2-92D), and in ischemic states (vasculitis, vasculopathy).

Vascular Changes

Cutaneous blood vessels exhibit a number of histologic changes, including dilatation (ectasia), endothelial swelling, endothelial necrosis, hyalinization, fibrinoid degeneration, vasculitis, thromboembolism, and extravasation (diapedesis) of erythrocytes (purpura).

Subcutaneous Fat Changes

The subcutaneous fat (panniculus adiposus or hypodermis) is subject to the connective tissue and vascular changes described earlier. It is frequently involved in suppurative and granulomatous dermatoses. In addition, subcutaneous fat may exhibit its own inflammatory changes (panniculitis or steatitis) without any significant involvement of the overlying

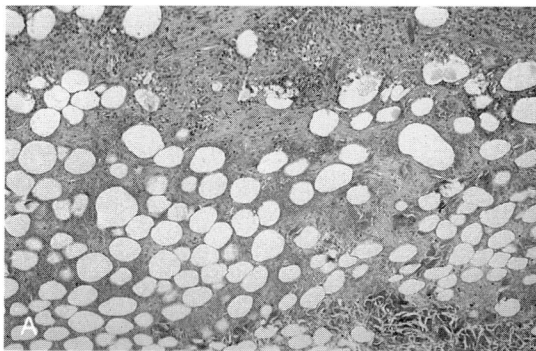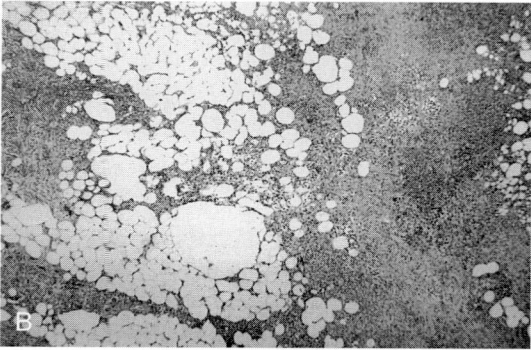

FIGURE 2–93. Fat necrosis in dogs. *A*, Fat microcysts separated by amorphous areas of necrosis. *B*, Variably sized and shaped fat microcysts in the center of a pyogranuloma.

dermis and epidermis. This occurs in sterile nodular panniculitis, feline nutritional steatitis, infectious panniculitis (especially atypical mycobacteriosis and bacterial and dermatophytic pseudomycetoma), bacterial endocarditis, subcutaneous fat sclerosis, and erythema nodosum. Subcutaneous fat may atrophy in various hormonal, inflammatory (wucher atrophy), and idiopathic dermatoses. Fat micropseudocyst formation and lipocytes containing radially arranged needle-shaped clefts are seen with subcutaneous fat sclerosis.

Fat necrosis (Fig. 2–93A) may develop whenever an inflammatory reaction involves a fat lobule. There are three different morphologic expressions of fat necrosis: (1) *microcystic fat necrosis* (see Fig. 2–93B)—the most common form, characterized by small, round microcysts that are often at the center of pyogranulomas, seen in many panniculitides; (2) *hyalinizing fat necrosis*—the lipocytes are converted into a feathery, eosinophilic amalgam trapping scattered fat microcysts, as seen in lupus erythematosus panniculitis and rabies-induced vaccine reactions; and (3) *mineralizing fat necrosis*—the deposition of irregular, granular, basophilic material, often in the peripheral cytoplasm of necrotic lipocytes, as seen in pancreatic panniculitis and some cases of traumatic panniculitis.

Miscellaneous Changes

- **Thickened Basement Membrane Zone.** Thickening of the basement membrane zone appears as focal, linear, homogeneous, eosinophilic bands below the stratum basale on light microscopic examination (Fig. 2–94). The basement membrane zone is better demonstrated with periodic acid–Schiff stain. Thickening of the basement membrane zone is a feature of lichenoid dermatoses, especially lupus erythematosus.

- **Subepidermal Vacuolar Alteration.** Subepidermal vacuolar alteration is charac-

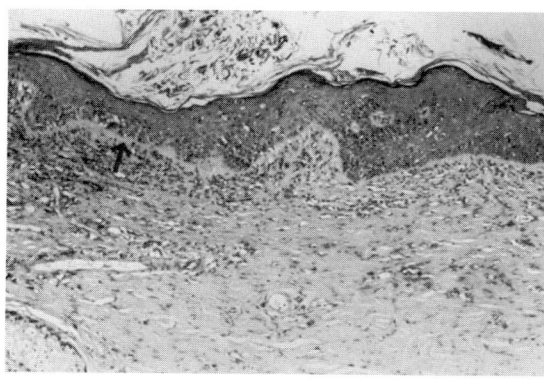

FIGURE 2–94. Focal thickening of the basement membrane zone (*arrow*) in a dog with systemic lupus erythematosus.

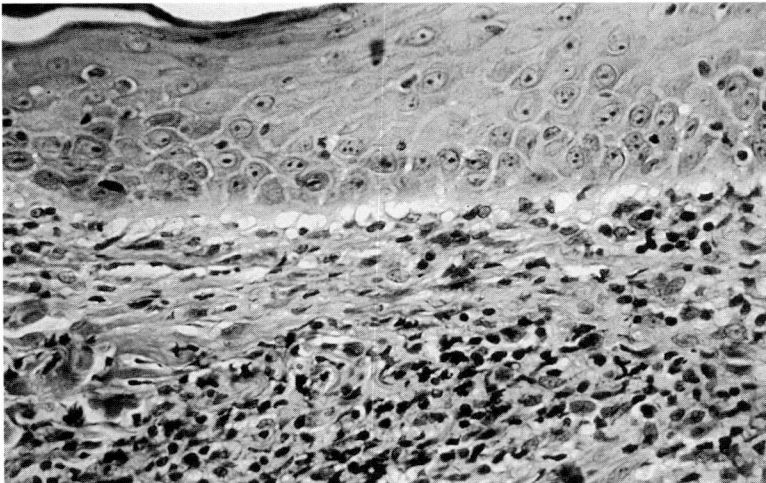

FIGURE 2–95. Subepidermal vacuolar alteration ("bubblies") in a dog with systemic lupus erythematosus.

terized by multiple small vacuoles within or immediately below the basement membrane zone, giving the appearance of subepidermal bubbles (Fig. 2–95). These "subepidermal bubblies" are seen in bullous pemphigoid, epidermolysis bullosa acquisita, lupus erythematosus, and occasionally, overlying dermal fibrosis and scar. They may also be induced by improper fixation and by freezing artifact.

- **Papillary Squirting.** Papillary squirting is present when superficial dermal papillae are edematous and contain dilated vessels and when the overlying epidermis is also edematous and often contains exocytosing leukocytes and parakeratotic scale (see Fig. 2–36). Squirting papillae are a feature of seborrheic dermatitis and zinc-responsive dermatoses.

- **Dysplasia.** The term dysplasia refers to a faulty or abnormal development of individual cells, and it is also commonly used to describe abnormal development of the epidermis (Fig. 2–96) or hair follicle as a whole. Dysplasia may be a feature of neoplastic, hyperplastic, and developmental dermatoses. Epidermal dysplasia is characterized by keratinocytes that are atypical in size, shape, and staining characteristics, and whose polarity has been disrupted.

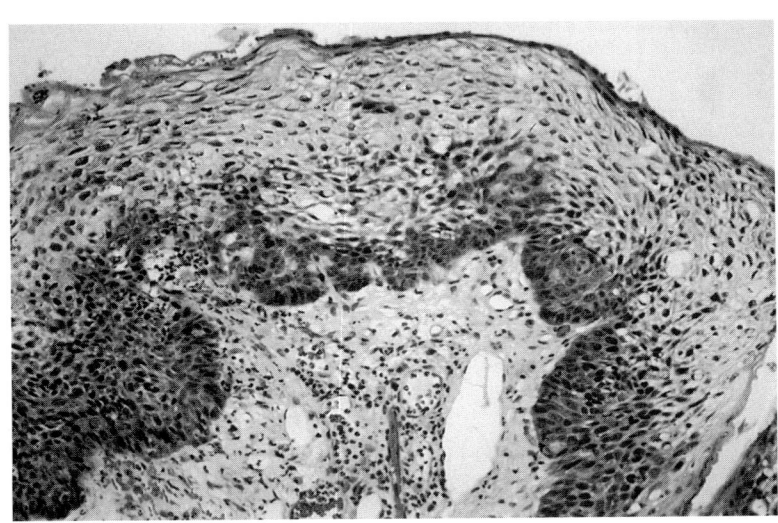

FIGURE 2–96. Epidermal dysplasia in a cat with actinic keratosis. Note how keratinocytes vary in staining intensity, size, and shape, and their polarity is totally disrupted.

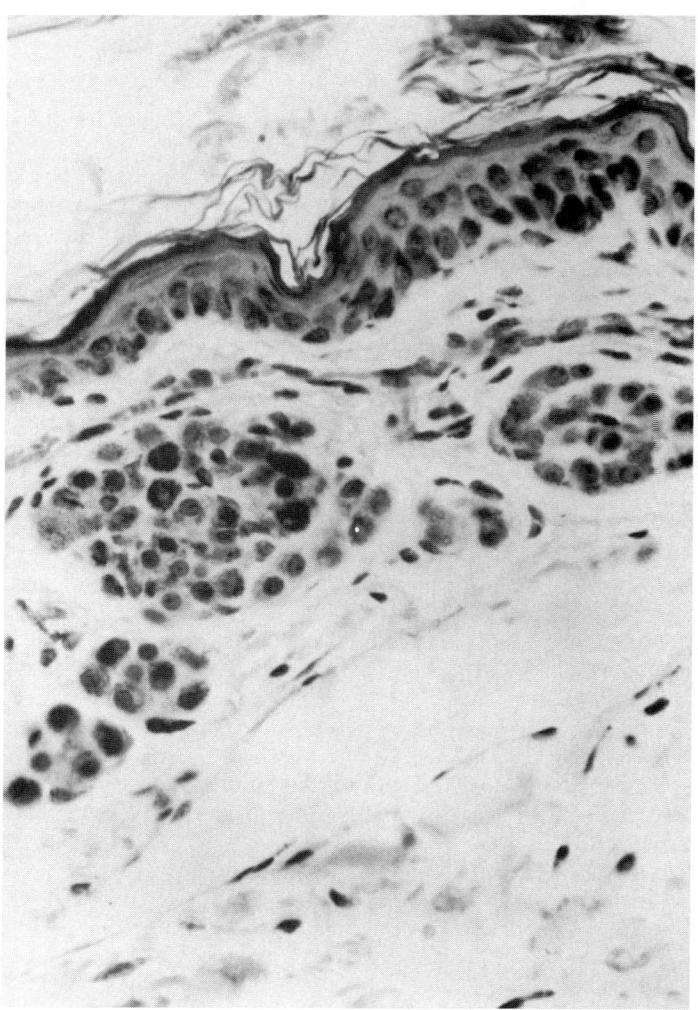

FIGURE 2–97. Nests of neoplastic melanocytes in a cat with melanocytoma.

- **Anaplasia.** Anaplasia (atypia) is a feature of neoplastic cells, in which there is a loss of normal differentiation and organization.
- **Metaplasia.** Metaplasia refers to a change in the type of mature cells in a tissue into a form that is not normal for that tissue (e.g., osseous metaplasia in the skin of a patient with hyperadrenocorticism). Through metaplasia, a given cell may exhibit epithelial, mesothelial, or mesenchymal characteristics, regardless of the tissue of origin.
- **Nests.** Nests (theques) are well-circumscribed clusters or groups of cells within the epidermis or the dermis (Fig. 2–97). Nests are seen in some neoplastic and hamartomatous dermatoses, such as melanomas and melanocytomas.
- **Lymphoid Nodules.** Lymphoid nodules are rounded, discrete masses of primarily mature lymphocytes (Fig. 2–98). They are often found perivascularly in the deep dermis, the subcutis, or both. Lymphoid nodules are most commonly recognized in association with immune-mediated dermatoses, dermatoses with tissue eosinophilia, and panniculitis.[38] They are also prominent in insect bite granuloma (pseudolymphoma), postinjection panniculitis, and some feline mast cell tumors.
- **Multinucleate Epidermal Giant Cells.** Multinucleate epidermal giant cells are found in viral infections and in a number of non-viral and non-neoplastic dermatoses characterized by epidermal hyperplasia, chronicity, or pruritus. Multinucleated keratinocy-

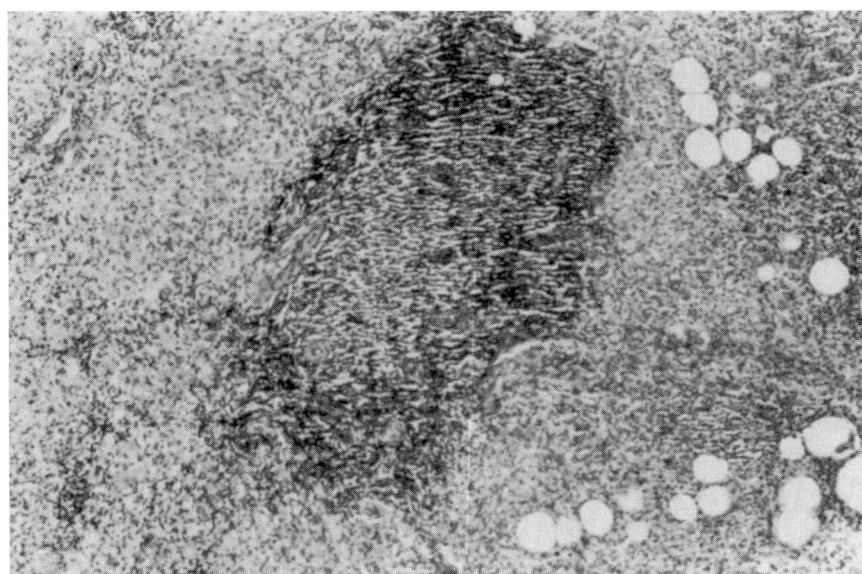

FIGURE 2-98. Lymphoid nodule in a cat with idiopathic sterile panniculitis.

tic giant cells ("syncytial" cells) are a unique feature of an FeLV-associated dermatitis in cats (Fig. 2–99).

- **Squamatization.** Squamatization refers to the replacement of the normally cuboid or columnar, slightly basophilic basal epidermal cells by polygonal or flattened, eosinophilic keratinocytes. It may be seen in lichenoid tissue reactions.
- **Transepidermal Elimination.** Transepidermal elimination is a mechanism by which foreign or altered constituents can be removed from the dermis (Fig. 2–100). The process involves unique morphologic alterations of the surface epidermis or the hair follicle's outer root sheath, which forms a channel and thereby facilitates extrusion. Transepidermal elimination may be seen in foreign-body reactions, calcinosis cutis, calcinosis circumscripta, and perforating dermatitis of cats.
- **Dunstan's Blue Line.** The overlying stratum corneum is lifted and subtended at

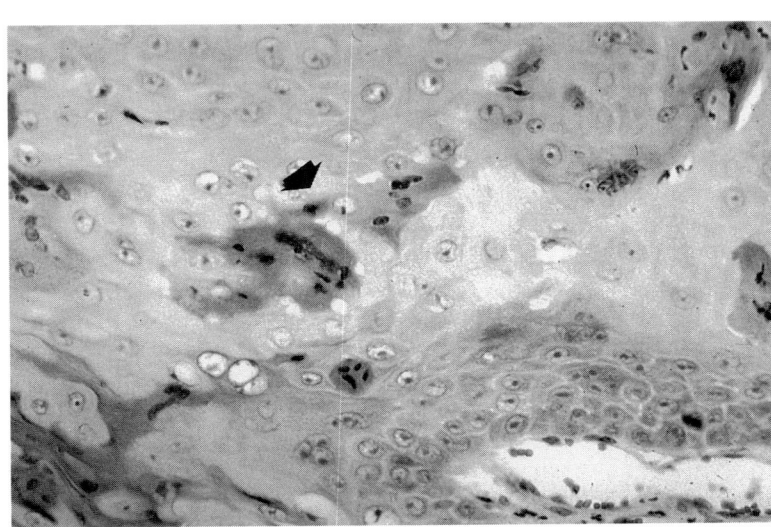

FIGURE 2-99. Multinucleated keratinocyte giant cells *(arrow)* in a cat with FeLV dermatosis.

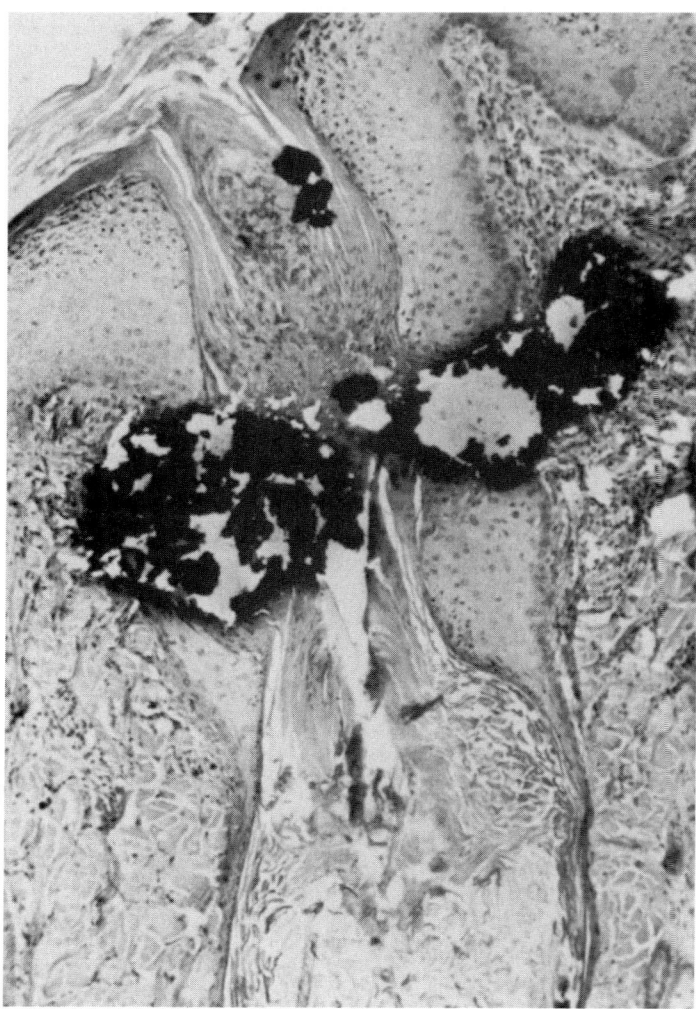

FIGURE 2-100. Transepidermal elimination of mineral through the outer root sheath of a hair follicle in a dog with spontaneous hyperadrenocorticism.

its point of attachment to the underlying epidermis by degenerate nuclear debris and staphylococci (Fig. 2–101). As such, the stratum corneum seems to be separating in the direction of a "blue line." This is most commonly seen in superficial staphylococcal infections.

Confusing Terms

NECROBIOSIS

Necrobiosis is the degeneration and death of cells or tissue, followed by replacement. Examples of necrobiosis are the constant degeneration and replacement of epidermal and hematopoietic cells. The term necrobiosis has been used in dermatohistopathology to describe various degenerative changes in collagen found in canine and feline eosinophilic granuloma and in human granuloma annulare, necrobiosis lipoidica, and rheumatoid and pseudorheumatoid nodules. The use of the term necrobiosis to describe a pathologic change is inappropriate and confusing, both histologically and etymologically, and should be discouraged. It is better to use the more specific terms described under Collagen Changes in this chapter.

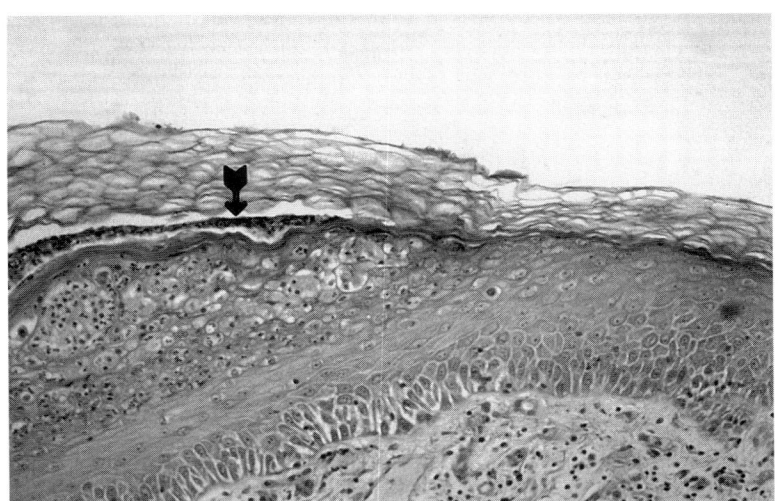

FIGURE 2–101. Dunstan's blue line. A dark line of degenerate nuclear debris and cocci *(arrow)* separates the stratum corneum from the underlying epidermis.

NEVUS AND HAMARTOMA

A nevus is a circumscribed developmental defect in the skin. Nevi may arise from any skin component or combination of components. Nevi are hyperplastic. The term nevus should never be used alone but always with a modifier such as epidermal, vascular, sebaceous, and collagenous.

Hamartoma literally means a tumor-like proliferation of normal or embryonal cells. A hamartoma is a macroscopic hyperplasia of normal tissue elements, and the term is often used synonymously with nevus. However, the term hamartoma may be applied to hyperplastic disorders in any tissue or organ system, whereas the term nevus is restricted to the skin.

Cellular Infiltrates

Dermal cellular infiltrates are described in terms of (1) the types of cells present and (2) the pattern of cellular infiltration. In general, cellular infiltrates are either monomorphous (one cell type) or polymorphous (more than one cell type). Further clarification of the predominant cells is accomplished by modifiers such as lymphocytic, histiocytic, neutrophilic, eosinophilic, and plasmacytic.

Cellular infiltrations usually have one or more of the following basic patterns: (1) perivascular (angiocentric—located around blood vessels), (2) perifollicular and periglandular (folliculocentric, appendagocentric, periappendageal, periadnexal—located around follicles and glands), (3) lichenoid (assuming a bandlike configuration that parallels the overlying epidermis and surrounds epidermal appendages), (4) nodular (occurring in basically well-defined groups or clusters at any site), and (5) interstitial or diffuse (scattered lightly or solidly throughout the dermis). The types of cells and patterns of infiltration present are important clues in the diagnosis of many dermatoses.

• DERMATOLOGIC DIAGNOSIS BY HISTOPATHOLOGIC PATTERNS

With pattern analysis, one first categorizes inflammatory dermatoses by their appearance (pattern) on the scanning objective of the light microscope and then zeroes in on a specific diagnosis, whenever possible, by the assimilation of fine details gathered by low- and high-power scrutiny. Pattern analysis has revolutionized veterinary dermatohistopathology and made the reading of skin biopsy specimens much simpler and more rewarding (for the pathologist, the clinician, and the patient).[23, 24, 43, 50, 53–55] However, as with any histologic method, pattern analysis works only when clinicians supply pathologists with adequate historical and clinical information and biopsy specimens most representative of the dermatoses being sampled.

In a retrospective study of skin biopsies from cats with inflammatory dermatoses,[43] pattern analysis was shown to be a useful technique. The specific clinical diagnosis was established in about 40% of the cases and was included in a reaction pattern–generated differential diagnosis in another 50% of the cases. A single reaction pattern was found in 75% of the cases, and mixed reaction patterns (two or three different patterns) in 25% of the cases. Mixed reaction patterns were usually caused by single etiologic factors or by a coexistence of two or three different dermatoses.

It is important to remember that many inflammatory dermatoses are characterized by a continuum of acute, subacute, and chronic pathologic changes.[45, 55] In other words, the lesions have "lives." For example, three very dissimilar lesions—cellulitis, eosinophilic plaque, and plasma cell pododermatitis—have somewhat similar developmental stages. They all begin as perivascular dermatitides, progress to interstitial dermatitides, and eventuate as diffuse dermatitides. Thus, the histopathologic pattern seen in the biopsy specimen from one of these conditions is, in part, dependent on the evolution or "age" of the lesion.

It is also important to realize that some patterns of inflammation are more important or more "powerful" than others.[45, 55] For example, perivascular dermatitis is present somewhere in virtually all inflammatory lesions: After all, the inflammatory cells usually have to exit the blood vessels in order to get to where the cutaneous action is! But, the question is: are those perivascular cells going somewhere more important, somewhere more diagnostic? Is there a more important inflammatory reaction pattern being formed? Hence, one can always find perivascular accumulations of inflammatory cells underlying an epidermal pustule, or peripheral to a dermal nodule. However, the more important or the more diagnostic patterns are those of intraepidermal pustular dermatitis and the nodular dermatitis.

Perivascular Dermatitis

In perivascular dermatitis, the predominant inflammatory reaction is centered on the superficial or deep dermal blood vessels, or both. Perivascular dermatitis is subdivided into three types on the basis of accompanying epidermal changes: (1) pure perivascular dermatitis (perivascular dermatitis without significant epidermal changes), (2) spongiotic perivascular dermatitis (perivascular dermatitis with prominent spongiosis), and (3) hyperplastic perivascular dermatitis (perivascular dermatitis with prominent epidermal hyperplasia).

Superficial perivascular dermatitis is by far the most common form of perivascular dermatitis (Fig. 2–102A). The usual causes are hypersensitivity reactions (to inhalants, dietary constituents, drugs, contact allergens, and so forth), ectoparasitisms, dermatophytosis, nutritional deficiencies, seborrheic disorders, and contact dermatitis. Deep perivascular dermatitis (see Fig. 2–102B) is less common and may be seen with systemic disorders (systemic lupus erythematosus, septicemia, hypereosinophilic syndrome, viral infections, and canine systemic histiocytosis) or severe local reactions (vasculitis, discoid lupus erythematosus, cellulitis, eosinophilic plaque, plasma cell pododermatitis, and tick bite reactions). In the cat, the most common causes of deep perivascular dermatitis are hypersensitivity disorders (inhalant, food, flea).[43]

Any perivascular dermatitis containing numerous eosinophils should first be suspected of representing ectoparasitism or endoparasitism. In the cat, tissue eosinophilia is commonly seen with hypersensitivity disorders (reactions to inhalants or dietary constituents).[43] Focal areas of epidermal edema, eosinophilic exocytosis, and necrosis (epidermal "nibbles") suggest ectoparasitism. Numerous eosinophils are also seen in the hypereosinophilic syndrome and occasionally in *Malassezia* dermatitis and zinc-responsive dermatoses.

Diffuse orthokeratotic hyperkeratosis with perivascular dermatitis suggests endocrinop-

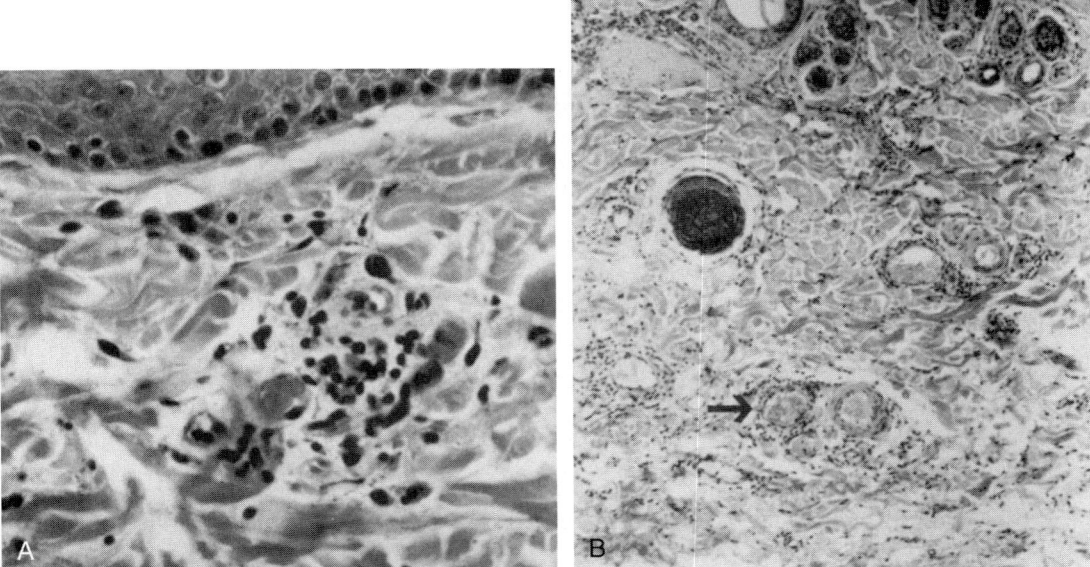

FIGURE 2–102. Perivascular dermatitis. *A,* Superficial perivascular dermatitis in a dog with atopy. *B,* Deep perivascular dermatitis *(arrow)* in a cat with atopy.

athy, nutritional deficiencies, developmental abnormalities (ichthyosis, follicular dysplasia, epidermal nevus, and color dilution alopecia), and secondary seborrheic disorders. Disproportionate follicular orthokeratotic hyperkeratosis in concert with perivascular dermatitis suggests vitamin A–responsive dermatosis, vitamin A deficiency, acne, Schnauzer comedo syndrome, follicular dysplasia, sebaceous adenitis, comedo nevus, and follicular cyst. Diffuse parakeratotic hyperkeratosis in combination with perivascular dermatitis suggests zinc-responsive dermatosis, generic dog food dermatosis, ectoparasitism, *Malassezia* dermatitis, lethal acrodermatitis, some vitamin A–responsive dermatoses, thallotoxicosis, necrolytic migratory erythema, and occasionally, dermatophytosis and dermatophilosis.

Focal parakeratotic hyperkeratosis (parakeratotic caps) may be seen with ectoparasitism, seborrheic disorders, dermatophytosis, and dermatophilosis. When parakeratotic caps are combined with papillary squirting, seborrheic dermatitis is likely. Perivascular dermatoses accompanied by vertical streaking of collagen, sebaceous gland hyperplasia, or both suggest chronic pruritus (rubbing, licking, or chewing), such as that seen with hypersensitivity reactions and acral lick dermatitis.

PURE PERIVASCULAR DERMATITIS

The most likely diagnoses include hypersensitivity reactions (to inhalants, dietary constituents, or drugs), urticaria, and dermatophytosis.

SPONGIOTIC PERIVASCULAR DERMATITIS

Spongiotic perivascular dermatitis is characterized by prominent spongiosis and spongiotic vesicle formation. Severe spongiotic vesiculation may cause blowout of the basement membrane zone, resulting in subepidermal vesicles. The epidermis frequently shows varying degrees of hyperplasia and hyperkeratosis. The most likely diagnoses include hypersensitivity reactions, contact dermatitis, ectoparasitisms, dermatophytosis, *Malassezia* dermatitis, dermatophilosis, viral infection, and eosinophilic plaque. Diffuse spongiosis, in which the outer root sheath of the hair follicle is also involved, suggests eosinophilic plaque, eosinophilic granuloma, primary seborrhea, *Malassezia* dermatitis, and zinc-responsive dermatosis. Marked spongiosis and intracellular edema of the upper one half of the epidermis with overlying diffuse parakeratotic hyperkeratosis seen with necrolytic migratory erythema.

HYPERPLASTIC PERIVASCULAR DERMATITIS

Hyperplastic perivascular dermatitis is characterized by varying degrees of epidermal hyperplasia and hyperkeratosis, with little or no spongiosis. This is a common, nondiagnostic, chronic dermatitis. It is frequently seen with hypersensitivity reactions, contact dermatitis, diseases of altered keratinization, ectoparasitisms, indolent ulcer, and acral lick dermatitis. Psoriasiform perivascular dermatoses are unusual and may represent chronic contact dermatitis, chronic hypersensitivity reactions, acral lick dermatitis, psoriasiform-lichenoid dermatosis of English Springer spaniels, necrolytic migratory erythema, and dermatophytosis. The most common cause of psoriasiform perivascular dermatitis in dogs is epitheliotropic lymphoma.

Interface Dermatitis

In interface dermatitis, the dermoepidermal junction is obscured by hydropic degeneration, lichenoid cellular infiltrate, or both (Fig. 2–103).[36] Apoptotic keratinocytes, satellite cell apoptosis and pigmentary incontinence are commonly seen. The hydropic type of interface dermatitis is seen with cutaneous adverse drug reactions (including fixed drug reaction), lupus erythematosus, toxic epidermal necrolysis, erythema multiforme, dermatomyositis, hereditary lupoid dermatosis of German shorthaired pointers (exfoliative cutaneous lupus erythematosus), idiopathic ulcerative dermatosis of collies and Shetland sheepdogs (vesicular cutaneous lupus erythematosus), graft-versus-host reactions, hereditary nasal hyperkeratosis of Labrador retrievers, and actinic dermatoses. The reactions seen with toxic epidermal necrolysis, dermatomyositis, thymoma-associated exfoliative dermatitis of cats, and various vasculitides and vasculopathies are often only mildly inflammatory ("cell-poor").

The lichenoid type is seen with drug eruptions, lupus erythematosus, pemphigus, pemphigoid, erythema multiforme, Vogt-Koyanagi-Harada–like syndrome, idiopathic lichenoid dermatoses, lichenoid keratoses, actinic keratoses, psoriasiform-lichenoid dermatosis of English Springer spaniels, contact reactions to plastic, and epitheliotropic lymphoma. The bandlike cellular infiltration of lichenoid tissue reactions consists predominantly of lymphocytes and plasma cells. If nearby ulceration or secondary infections exist, numerous neutrophils may be present. Canine mucocutaneous pyoderma often has a lichenoid inflammatory component but lacks hydropic degeneration and apoptosis, and contains numerous neutrophils and suppurative epidermitis. Uniquely, the lichenoid infiltrate of uveodermatologic syndrome has numerous large histiocytes, which contain lightly sprinkled melanin. A lichenoid tissue reaction with many eosinophils suggests an insect or arthropod bite reaction (e.g., scabies and cheyletiellosis) or a drug eruption. Small numbers of eosinophils are also a feature of psoriasiform-lichenoid dermatosis of English Springer spaniels. Focal thickening or smudging of the basement membrane zone suggests lupus erythematosus and dermatomyositis.

Vasculitis

Vasculitis is an inflammatory process in which inflammatory cells are present within and around blood vessel walls and there are concomitant signs of damage to the blood vessels (e.g., degeneration and lysis of vascular and perivascular collagen, swelling and necrosis of endothelial cells, extravasation of erythrocytes, thrombosis, effacement of vascular architecture, and fibrinoid degeneration) (Fig. 2–104). Vasculitides are usually classified on the basis of the dominant inflammatory cell within vessel walls, the types being neutrophilic, eosinophilic, and lymphocytic. This appearance, of course, can be greatly modified by duration of the lesion. Fibrinoid degeneration is rare in canine and feline cutaneous vasculitides. Biopsy specimens from animals with vasculitis sometimes do not reveal visu-

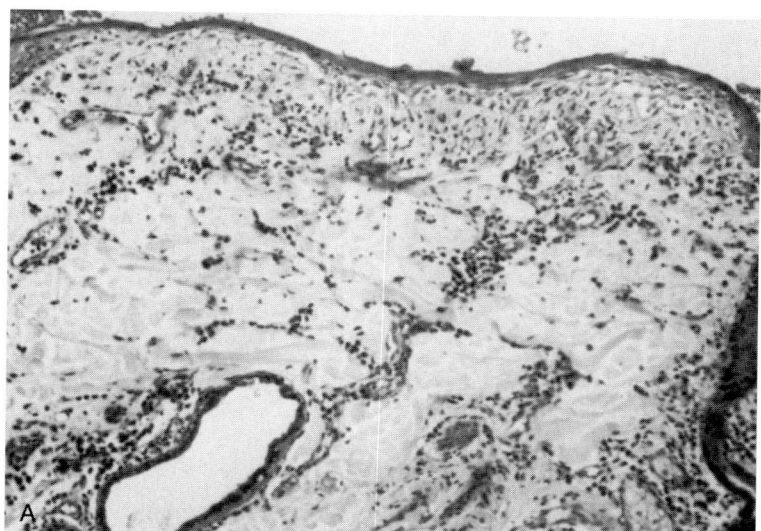
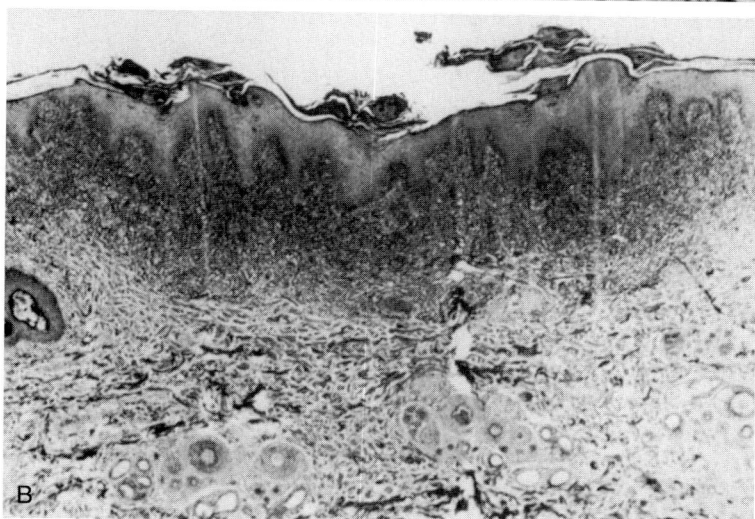

FIGURE 2–103. Interface dermatitis. *A*, Hydropic interface dermatitis in a dog with systemic lupus erythematosus. *B*, Lichenoid interface dermatitis in a dog with idiopathic lichenoid dermatitis.

ally inflamed vessels but rather some of the signposts of vasculitis (Table 2–9). Serial sections or repeated biopsy may be necessary to visualize the actual vasculitis.

Neutrophilic vasculitis, the most common type, may be leukocytoclastic (associated with karyorrhexis of neutrophils, resulting in "nuclear dust"). This pattern is seen in connective tissue disorders (lupus erythematosus, rheumatoid arthritis, and dermatomyositis), allergic reactions (adverse cutaneous drug reactions, infections, and reactions to toxins), polyarteritis nodosa, canine staphylococcal hypersensitivity, Rocky Mountain spotted fever, and canine leishmaniasis; hereditary nasal pyogranuloma and vasculitis of Scottish terriers; as an idiopathic disorder; and occasionally with plasma cell pododermatitis. Neutrophilic vasculitis may also be nonleukocytoclastic, as seen with septicemia and thrombophlebitis from intravenous catheters causing thromboembolism. Exceptions to these rules may be seen, such as in the case of allergic vasculitides, which may be leukocytoclastic or nonleukocytoclastic. Vascular thrombosis can occur in dogs receiving glucocorticoid therapy.

Lymphocytic vasculitis is rare, and may be seen in adverse cutaneous drug reactions, vaccine-induced panniculitis, lupus erythematosus, dermatomyositis, familial vasculopathy

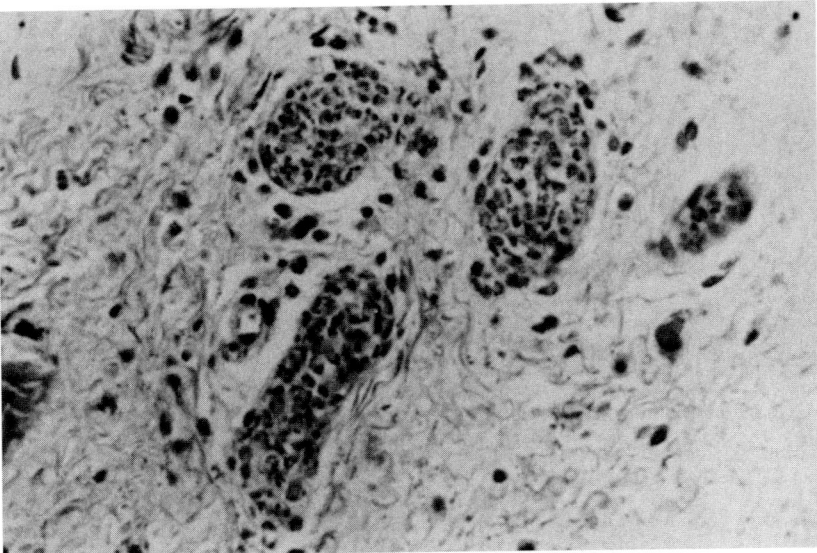

FIGURE 2–104. Vasculitis. Leukocytoclastic vasculitis in a dog with idiopathic cutaneous vasculitis.

of German shepherds, and as an idiopathic disorder. Lymphomatoid granulomatosis is characterized by vascular damage associated with atypical, pleomorphic lymphoid cells.

Eosinophilic vasculitis is very rare, and is seen with insect- and arthropod-induced lesions, feline eosinophilic granuloma, food hypersensitivity, and mast cell tumor.

By tradition, leukocytes are not found in the walls of arterioles and large venules, their presence being prima facie evidence of vasculitis. However, in a recent study,[47] eosinophils were found in the walls of large dermal and subcutaneous venules or veins in 21.4% and 38.9%, respectively, of the cats with eosinophilic granuloma and eosinophilic plaque (Fig. 2–105). In two cats with eosinophilic plaque, eosinophils were also present in the walls of deep dermal arterioles. No histologic or clinical evidence of vasculitis was present in these cats.

Interstitial Dermatitis

Interstitial dermatitis is characterized by the infiltration of cells between collagen bundles (in the interstitial spaces) of the dermis (Fig. 2–106).[45] The infiltrate is poorly circumscribed, is mild to moderate in intensity, and does not obscure the anatomic features of the skin. In dogs, most interstitial dermatoses are superficial and associated with infections or infestations, whereas those in the cat are usually superficial and deep and associated

● Table 2–9 **HISTOPATHOLOGIC SIGNPOSTS OF CUTANEOUS VASCULITIS**[40]

- Large numbers of leukocytes within the vessel wall, especially if the vessel is an arteriole or large venule.
- If the vessel is a postcapillary venule, there are disproportionately more leukocytes within the wall than in the adjacent dermis.
- Intramural or perivascular hemorrhage, intense edema, and fibrin deposition.
- The presence of leukocytoclasis within the vessel wall.
- Some evidence of damage to the vessel wall beyond edema and endothelial cell prominence.
- Evidence of cutaneous infarction.
- Atrophic changes in hair follicles, adnexal glands, and epidermis, reflecting chronic ischemia.

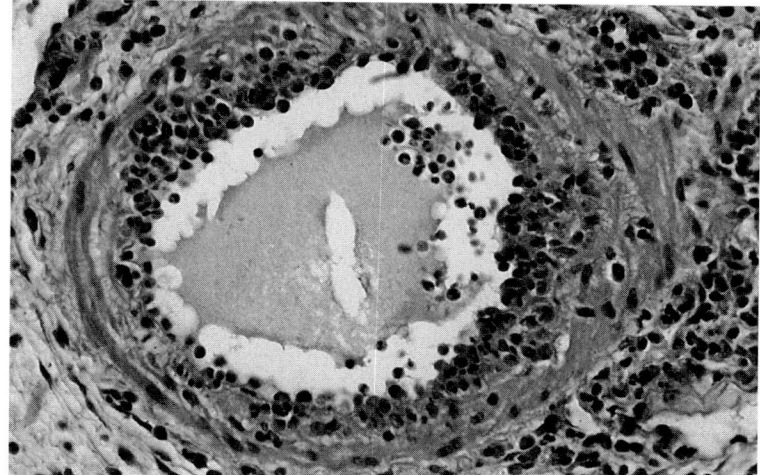

FIGURE 2–105. Numerous eosinophils in the wall of a deep dermal arteriole of a cat with an eosinophilic plaque. No vasculitis is present.

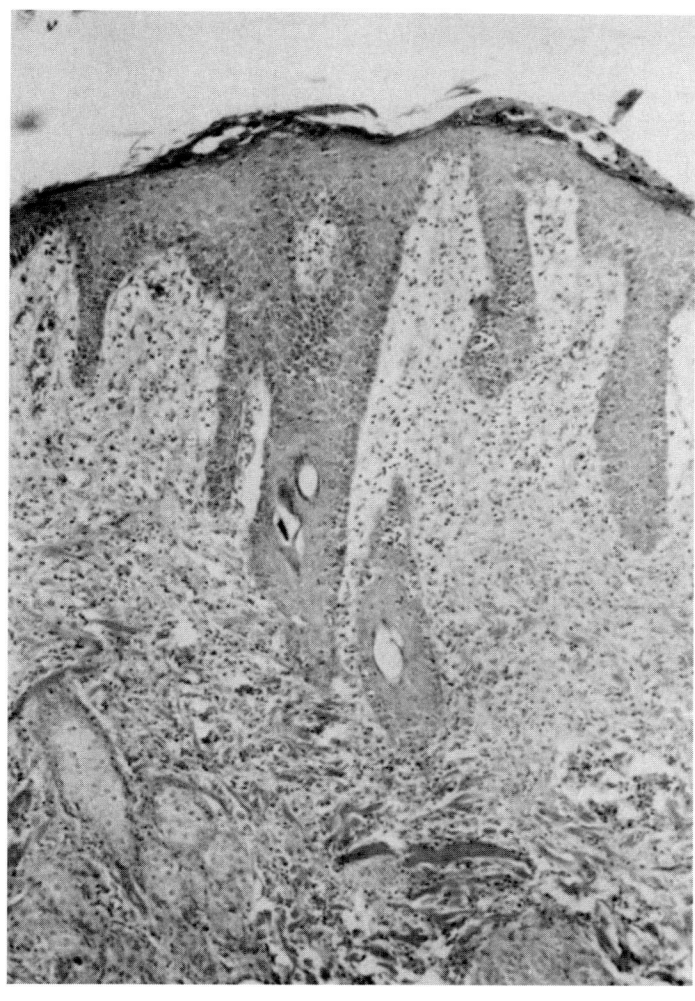

FIGURE 2–106. Interstitial dermatitis in a cat with food hypersensitivity. Note that the anatomic structures are still readily identified. There are also focal areas of mural folliculitis.

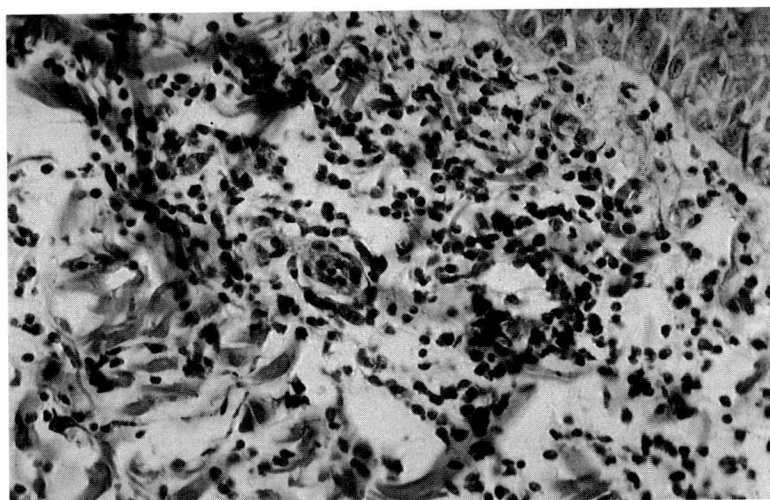

FIGURE 2–107. Interstitial dermatitis in an atopic cat. Interstitial accumulation of predominantly eosinophils and lymphocytes.

with allergies (Fig. 2–107) and ectoparasites.[45] When the superficial dermis is primarily involved and the overlying epidermis is normal, urticaria is likely. When the superficial dermis is primarily involved and the epidermis is hyperplastic, the most likely causes are staphylococcal infection (numerous neutrophils), dermatophytosis (numerous neutrophils), yeast dermatitis (numerous lymphocytes), and ectoparasitism, especially scabies and flea bite hypersensitivity (numerous eosinophils). When the superficial and deep dermis are involved, likely diagnoses include bacterial or fungal infection (numerous neutrophils, macrophages, or both), early eosinophilic plaque (numerous eosinophils), and early plasma cell pododermatitis (numerous plasma cells).

Nodular and Diffuse Dermatitis

Nodular dermatitis denotes discrete clusters of cells. Such dermal nodules are usually multiple but may occasionally be large and solitary (Fig. 2–108). In contrast, diffuse dermatitis denotes a cellular infiltrate so dense that discrete cellular aggregates are no longer easily recognized and the anatomy of the skin is no longer easily visualized (Fig. 2–109).

Granulomatous inflammation represents a heterogeneous pattern of tissue reactions in response to various stimuli. There is no simple, precise, universally accepted way to define granulomatous inflammation. A commonly proposed definition of granulomatous inflammation is as follows: a circumscribed tissue reaction that is subacute to chronic in nature and is located about one or more foci, in which the histiocyte or the macrophage is a predominant cell type. Thus, granulomatous dermatitis may be nodular or diffuse, but not all nodular and diffuse dermatoses are granulomatous. Nongranulomatous diffuse dermatoses include eosinophilic plaque, plasma cell pododermatitis, and cellulitis. Pseudolymphoma (insect or arachnid bites; drug reactions; idiopathic) is an example of a nongranulomatous nodular dermatitis. Granulomatous infiltrates that contain large numbers of neutrophils are frequently called pyogranulomatous. The most common causes of nodular pyogranulomatous dermatitis in dogs are furunculosis and ruptured keratinous cysts.

CELL TYPES

Nodular dermatitis and diffuse dermatitis are often associated with certain unusual inflammatory cell types.

Foam cells are histiocytes with elongated or oval vesicular nuclei and abundant, finely

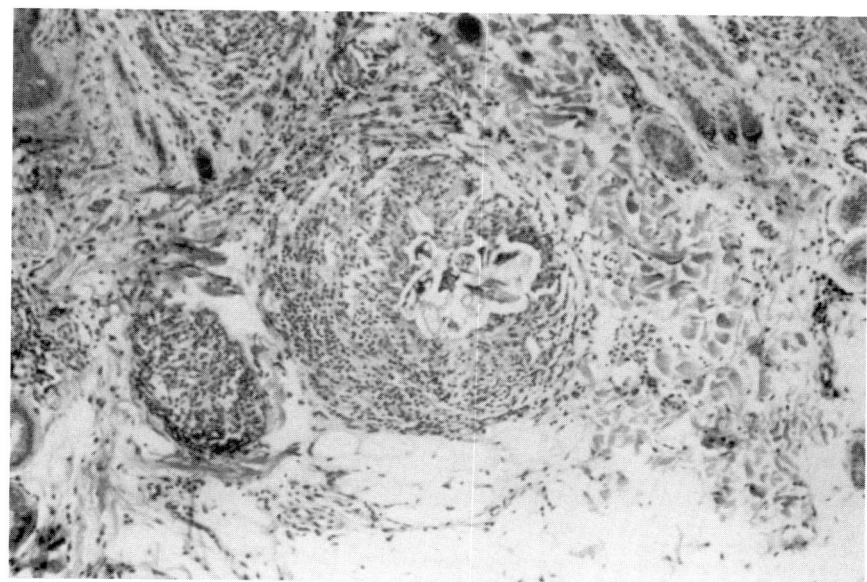

FIGURE 2-108. Nodular dermatitis. Dermal nodule with *Demodex* mites in the center in a dog with generalized demodicosis.

granular, eosinophilic cytoplasm with ill-defined cell borders. They are called *epithelioid* because they appear to cluster and adjoin like epithelial cells (Fig. 2-110).

Multinucleate histiocytic giant cells (Fig. 2-111) are histiocytic variants that assume three morphologic forms: (1) Langhans-type (nuclei form a circle or semicircle at the periphery of the cell), (2) foreign body–type (nuclei are scattered throughout the cytoplasm), and (3) Touton-type (nuclei form a wreath that surrounds a central, homogeneous, amphophilic core of cytoplasm, which is, in turn, surrounded by abundant foamy cyto-

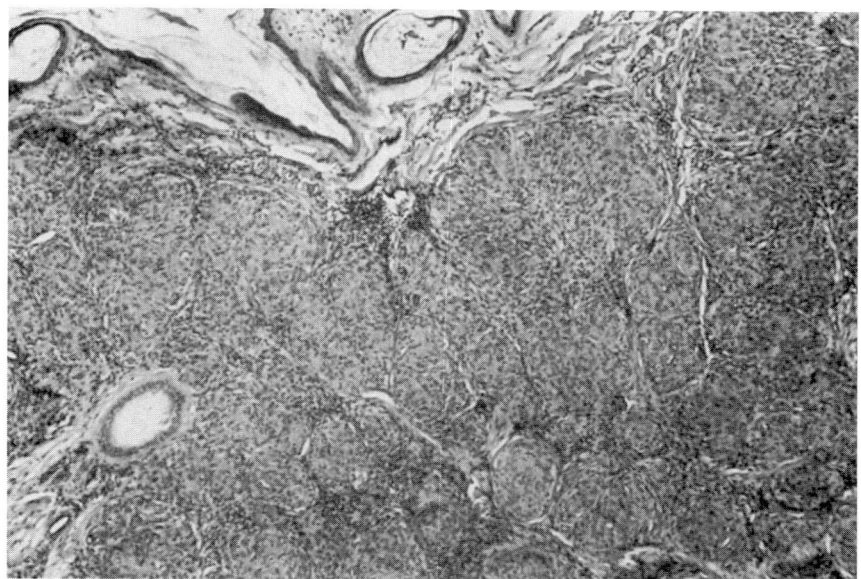

FIGURE 2-109. Diffuse dermatitis. Diffuse granulomatous dermatitis in a dog with sarcoidal idiopathic granulomas.

186 • Diagnostic Methods

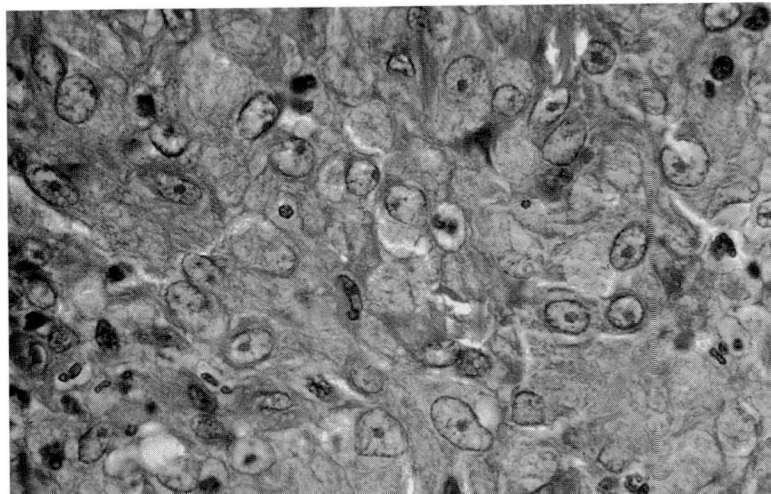

FIGURE 2–110. Dermal granuloma in a cat. Histiocytes have a voluminous, stippled cytoplasm with often ill-defined cell borders.

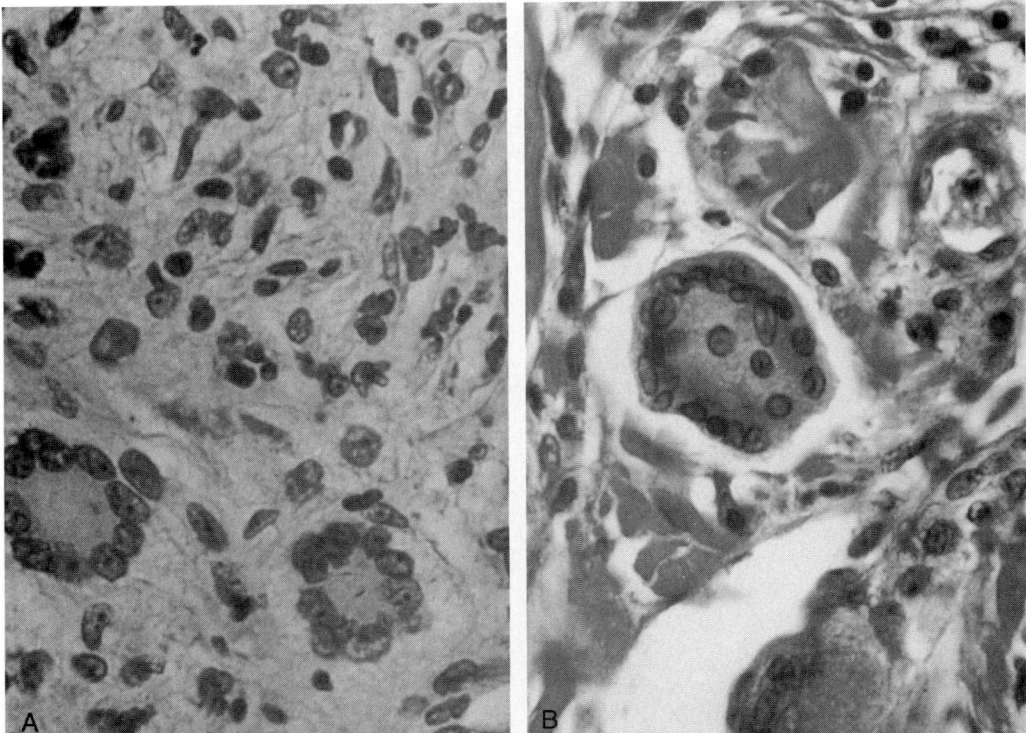

FIGURE 2–111. Multinucleate histiocytic giant cells are often present in cutaneous granulomas or chronic inflammations localized around foci of irritation. However, one should understand that identification of any one type of giant cell is not diagnostic alone. Several types may be found in a single section, and all are "foreign body" in character. Their different structure is probably related to the physiochemical nature of the foreign material. A, Touton-type giant cell. There is a complete ring of nuclei around a ground-glass center, and all are enclosed within a vacuolated cytoplasm. The photomicrograph is from a human xanthoma. (Courtesy J. D. Conroy.) B, Langhans-type giant cell. The peripheral rim of nuclei is arranged in a horseshoe fashion.

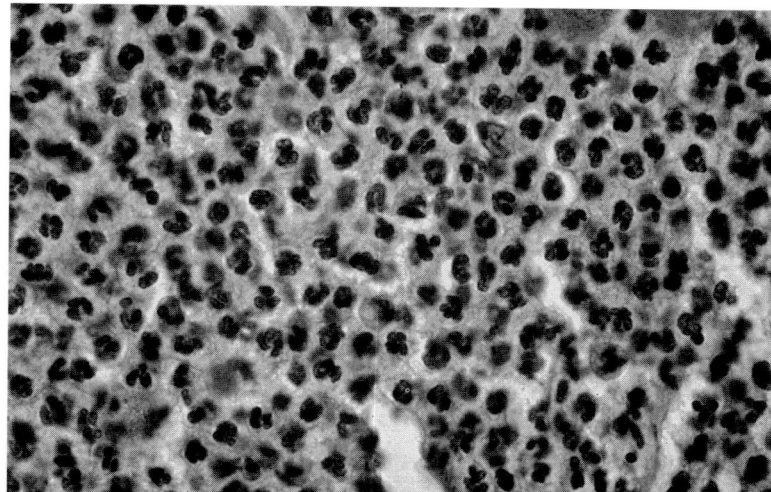

FIGURE 2–112. Dermal abscess (neutrophils) in a dog.

plasm). In general, these three forms of giant cells have no diagnostic specificity, although numerous Touton-type cells are usually seen with xanthomas.

CHARACTERIZATION

Certain general principles apply to the examination of all nodular and diffuse dermatitides. The processes that should be used are (1) polarizing foreign material, (2) staining for bacteria and fungi, and (3) culturing. In general, microorganisms are most likely to be found near areas of suppuration and necrosis.

Nodular and diffuse dermatitis may be characterized by predominantly neutrophilic, histiocytic, eosinophilic, or mixed cellular infiltrates. Neutrophils (dermal abscess) (Fig. 2–112) often predominate in dermatoses associated with bacteria, mycobacteria, actinomycetes, fungi, *Prototheca*, and foreign bodies. Histiocytes may predominate (Fig. 2–113) in

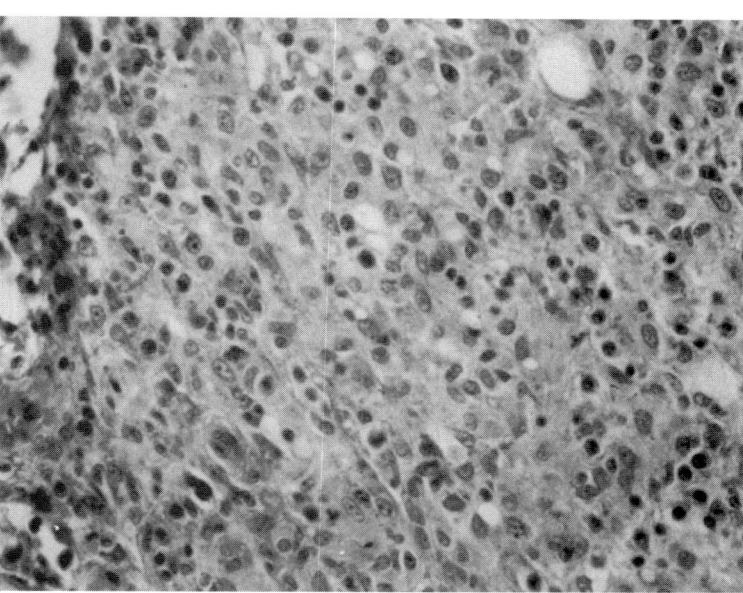

FIGURE 2–113. Granulomatous dermatitis in a dog.

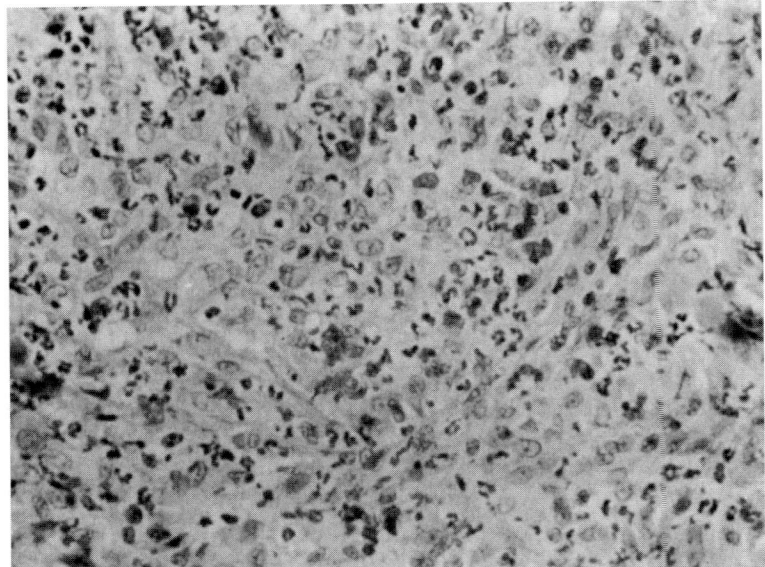

FIGURE 2–114. Pyogranulomatous dermatitis in a dog.

the chronic stage of any of the entities just listed, in xanthomas, in canine histiocytosis (cutaneous and systemic), and in the sterile pyogranuloma-granuloma syndrome. Eosinophils may predominate in feline and canine eosinophilic granuloma, in certain parasitic dermatoses (insect and arachnid bite reactions, dirofilariasis, and dracunculiasis), and in locations where hair follicles have ruptured. Mixed cellular infiltrates are most commonly neutrophils and histiocytes (in pyogranuloma) (Fig. 2–114), eosinophils and histiocytes (in eosinophilic granuloma), or a combination.

Plasma cells are common components of nodular and diffuse dermatitis (Fig. 2–115) of dogs and cats and are of no particular diagnostic significance. They are commonly seen around glands and follicles in chronic infections Periapocrine accumulations of plasma cells are also commonly seen in acral lick dermatitis and lichenoid dermatoses. Hyperactive plasma cells may contain eosinophilic intracytoplasmic inclusions (Russell bodies).

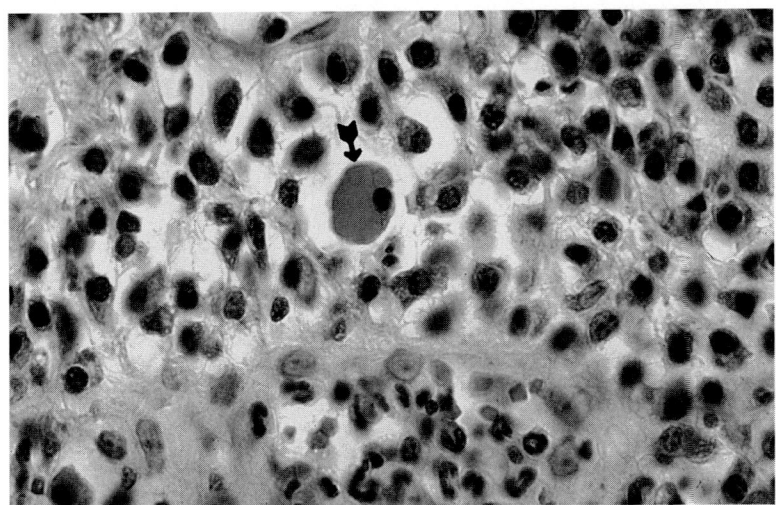

FIGURE 2–115. Plasma cells and smaller numbers of neutrophils and lymphocytes in a dog with chronic bacterial infection. One plasma cell contains large intracytoplasmic inclusions (Russell bodies) *(arrow)*.

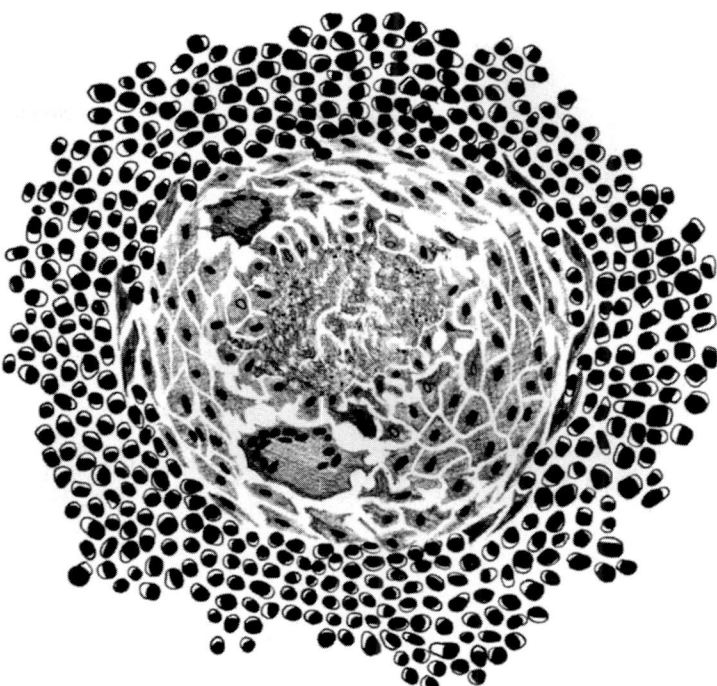

FIGURE 2–116. Tuberculoid granuloma. (From Ackerman AB: Histologic Diagnosis of Inflammatory Diseases. Lea & Febiger, Philadelphia, 1978, p 398.)

These accumulations of glycoprotein are largely globulin and may be large enough to push the cell nucleus eccentrically.

Granulomas may be subclassified as tuberculoid, sarcoidal, and palisading. Tuberculoid granulomas have a central zone of neutrophils and necrosis surrounded by histiocytes and epithelioid cells, which are, in turn, surrounded by giant cells, followed by a layer of lymphocytes, and finally an outer layer of fibroblasts. These are seen in tuberculosis, atypical mycobacteriosis, feline leprosy and, rarely, leishmaniasis and protothecosis (Fig. 2–116). Sarcoid granulomas have "naked" epithelioid cells (unaccompanied by surrounding inflammation and fibrosis), as seen in foreign body reactions, idiopathic canine sarcoidal granuloma, and histiocytosis of Bernese mountain dogs (Fig. 2–117). In palisading granulomas, the histiocytes are aligned like staves around a central focus of collagen degeneration (in canine and feline eosinophilic granuloma [Fig. 2–118]); fibrin (in rheumatoid nodule); lipids (in xanthoma); or parasite, fungus, or other foreign material (e.g., calcium, as in dystrophic calcinosis cutis and calcinosis circumscripta [Fig. 2–119]). Granulomas and pyogranulomas that track hair follicles and result in large, vertically oriented (sausage-shaped) lesions are typical of the sterile pyogranuloma-granuloma syndrome.

Reactions to ruptured hair follicles are a common cause of nodular and diffuse pyogranulomatous dermatitis, and any such dermal process should be carefully scrutinized for keratinous and epithelial debris and should be serially sectioned to rule out this possibility.

Nongranulomatous nodular and diffuse dermatitis can be a feature of infectious agents (cellulitis or abscess), feline eosinophilic plaque, feline plasma cell pododermatitis, familial vasculopathy of German shepherd dogs, pseudolymphomas (Fig. 2–120), and necrotizing dermatoses (e.g., burns, spider bites, vasculopathies).

Intraepidermal Vesicular and Pustular Dermatitis

Vesicular and pustular dermatitides show considerable microscopic and macroscopic overlap, because vesicles tend to accumulate leukocytes early and rapidly. Thus, vesicular

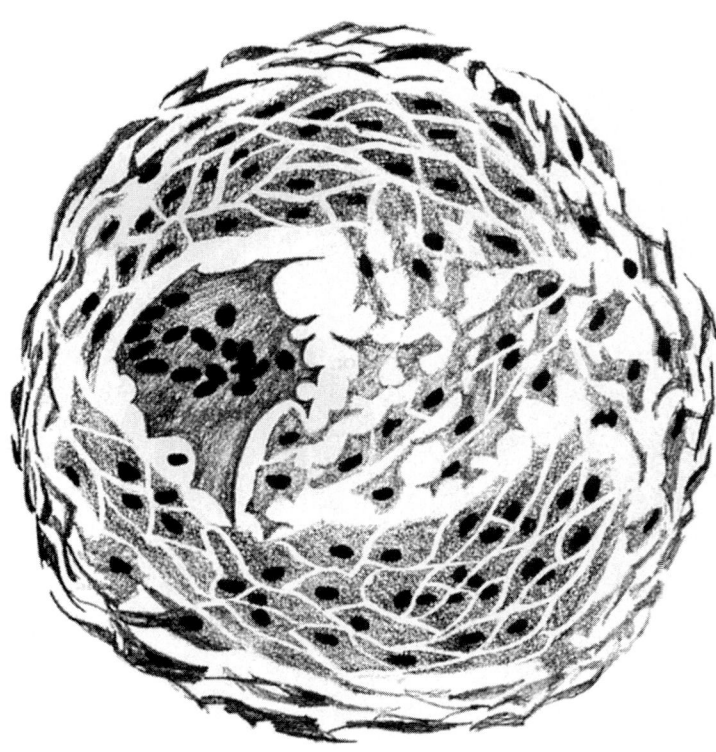

FIGURE 2–117. Sarcoidal granuloma. (From Ackerman AB: Histologic Diagnosis of Inflammatory Diseases. Lea & Febiger, Philadelphia, 1978, p 408.)

dermatitides in dogs and cats frequently appear pustular or vesicopustular, both macroscopically and microscopically.

Intraepidermal vesicles and pustules (Fig. 2–121) may be produced by intercellular or intracellular edema (in any acute to subacute dermatitis reaction), ballooning degeneration (in viral infections), acantholysis (due to the autoantibodies of pemphigus, the proteolytic enzymes from neutrophils in microbial infections and subcorneal pustular dermatosis, the proteolytic enzymes from eosinophils in sterile eosinophilic pustulosis, and substances released by some dermatophytes[32]), and hydropic degeneration of basal cells (in lupus erythematosus, erythema multiforme, toxic epidermal necrolysis, dermatomyositis, and drug eruptions). It is useful to classify intraepidermal vesicular and pustular dermatitides as to their anatomic level of occurrence within the epidermis (Table 2–10).

Subepidermal Vesicular and Pustular Dermatitis

Subepidermal vesicles and pustules (Fig. 2–122) may be formed through hydropic degeneration of basal cells (in lupus erythematosus, erythema multiforme, dermatomyositis, drug eruption, and toxic epidermal necrolysis), dermoepidermal separation (in bullous pemphigoid, drug eruption, and epidermolysis bullosa), severe subepidermal edema or cellular infiltration (especially in urticaria, cellulitis, vasculitis, ectoparasitism, and dermal erythema multiforme), and severe intercellular edema, with blowout of the basement membrane zone (in spongiotic perivascular dermatitis). Concurrent epidermal and dermal inflammatory changes are important diagnostic clues (see Table 2–10). Caution is warranted when examining older lesions, because re-epithelialization may cause subepidermal vesicles and pustules to assume an intraepidermal location. Such re-epithelialization is usually recognized as a single layer of flattened, elongated basal epidermal cells at the base of the vesicle or pustule.

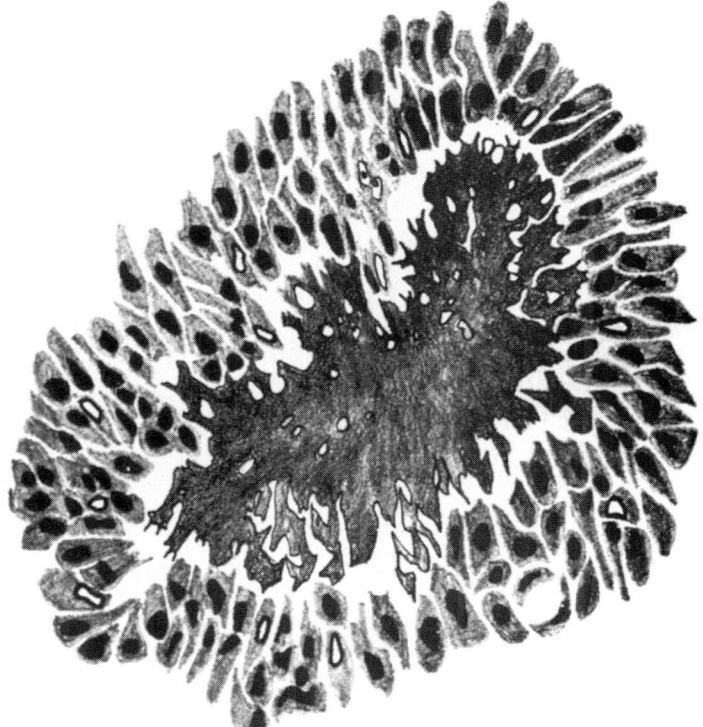

FIGURE 2–118. Palisading granuloma. (From Ackerman AB: Histologic Diagnosis of Inflammatory Diseases. Lea & Febiger, Philadelphia, 1978, p 416.)

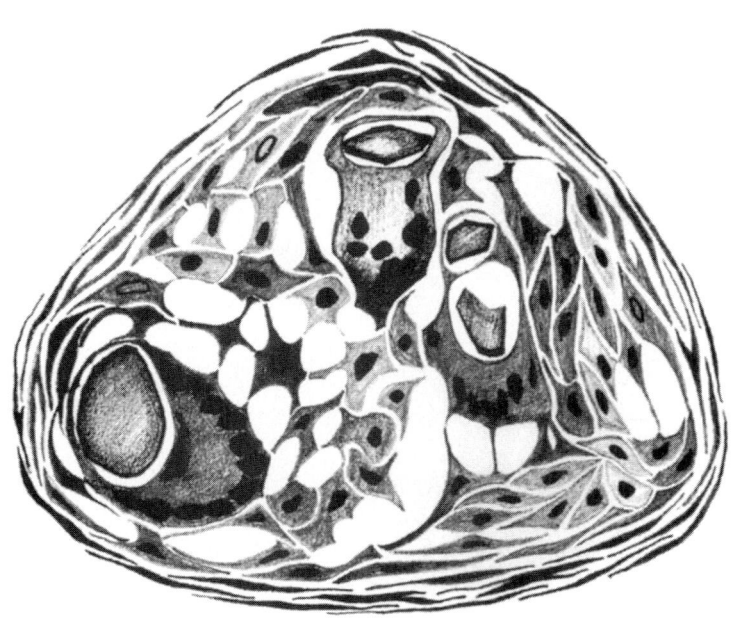

FIGURE 2–119. Foreign-body granuloma. (From Ackerman AB: Histologic Diagnosis of Inflammatory Diseases. Lea & Febiger, Philadelphia, 1978, p 436.)

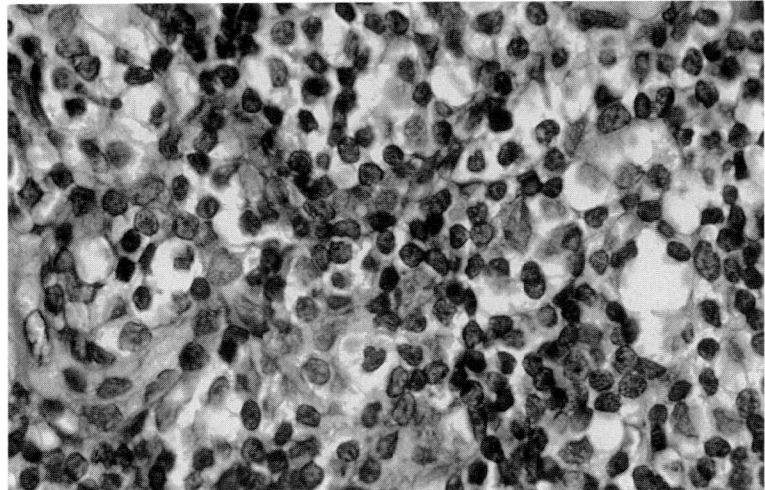

FIGURE 2–120. Lymphocytes and smaller numbers of histiocytes in a dog with insect bite pseudolymphoma.

Perifolliculitis, Folliculitis, and Furunculosis

Perifolliculitis denotes the accumulation of inflammatory cells around a hair follicle, wherein the follicular epithelium is not invaded (Fig. 2–123).[25] Dense perifolliculitis may be seen in infectious hair follicle disorders, leishmaniasis, and sebaceous adenitis.

Mural folliculitis occurs when the wall of the follicle is targeted, and the lumen is spared.[25] Four major subdivisions of mural folliculitis are recognized.

1. *Interface mural folliculitis.* As in interface dermatitis, pathologic changes (hydropic degeneration, keratinocyte apoptosis, lymphocytic exocytosis) tend to target the outermost (basal) cell layer (Fig. 2–124). Perifollicular inflammation may be cell-poor (hydropic) or cell-rich (lichenoid). Diseases to consider include lupus erythe-

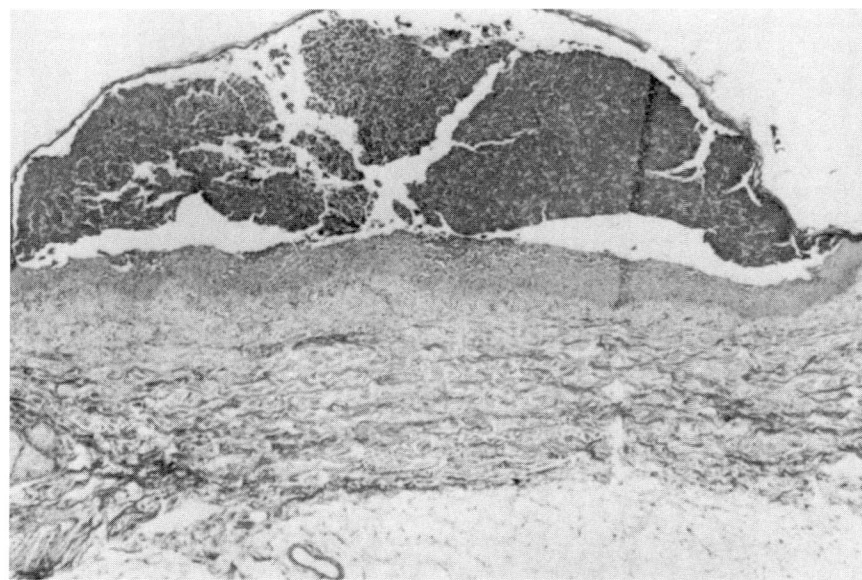

FIGURE 2–121. Intraepidermal pustular dermatitis. Large subcorneal pustule in a dog with pemphigus foliaceus.

Table 2–10 HISTOPATHOLOGIC CLASSIFICATION OF INTRAEPIDERMAL AND SUBEPIDERMAL PUSTULAR AND VESICULAR DISEASES

ANATOMIC LOCATION	OTHER HELPFUL FINDINGS
Intraepidermal	
Subcorneal	
Microbial infection	Neutrophils, microorganisms (bacteria, fungi), ± mild acantholysis, focal necrosis of epidermis, ± follicular involvement
Canine subcorneal pustular dermatosis	Neutrophils, ± moderate acantholysis
Canine sterile eosinophilic pustulosis	Eosinophils, ± follicular involvement
Pemphigus foliaceus	Marked acantholysis, neutrophils and/or eosinophils, ± follicular involvement, ± lichenoid infiltrate
Canine linear IgA pustular dermatitis	Neutrophils, ± mild acantholysis
Systemic lupus erythematosus	Neutrophils, ± mild acantholysis, interface dermatitis
Leishmaniasis	Neutrophils, ± microorganism
Superficial suppurative necrolytic dermatitis of Schnauzer	Neutrophils, epithelial necrosis
Intragranular	
Pemphigus foliaceus	Marked acantholysis, granular "cling-ons," neutrophils and/or eosinophils, ± follicular involvement
Pemphigus erythematosus	Marked acantholysis, granular "cling-ons," neutrophils and/or eosinophils, ± lichenoid infiltrate, ± follicular involvement
Intraepidermal	
Pemphigus vegetans	Marked acantholysis, eosinophils, papillomatosis
Benign familial pemphigus	Acantholysis at all levels
Epitheliotropic lymphoma	Atypical lymphoid cells, Pautrier microabscesses
Viral dermatoses	Ballooning degeneration, ± inclusion bodies, ± acantholysis
Spongiotic dermatitis	Eosinophilic spongiosis suggests ectoparasitism, pemphigus, pemphigoid, canine sterile eosinophilic pustulosis
Necrolytic migratory erythema	Diffuse parakeratosis, marked edema of upper epidermis
Suprabasilar	
Pemphigus vulgaris	Marked acantholysis, ± follicular involvement
Intrabasal	
Lupus erythematosus	Interface dermatitis, ± thickened basement membrane zone, ± dermal mucinosis
Dermatomyositis	Interface dermatitis, ± thickened basement membrane zone, ± dermal mucinosis, ± perifollicular fibrosis
Erythema multiforme	Interface dermatitis, marked single-cell apoptosis of keratinocytes at all levels of epidermis
Toxic epidermal necrolysis	Full-thickness coagulation necrosis of epidermis, little or no inflammation
Graft-versus-host disease	Interface dermatitis
Hereditary lupoid dermatosis (exfoliative cutaneous lupus erythematosus) of German shorthaired pointer	Interface dermatitis
Idiopathic ulcerative dermatitis (vesicular cutaneous lupus erythematosus) of collie and Shetland sheep dog	Interface dermatitis
Subepidermal	
Bullous pemphigoid	Subepidermal vacuolar alteration, variable inflammation, often eosinophils
Epidermolysis bullosa acquisita	Neutrophils
Canine linear IgA bullous dermatosis	Neutrophils
Mucous membrane pemphigoid	Noninflammatory
Epidermolysis bullosa	Little or no inflammation, ± hydropic degeneration
Lupus erythematosus	Interface dermatitis, ± thickened basement membrane zone, ± dermal mucinosis, ± perifollicular fibrosis
Erythema multiforme	Interface dermatitis, marked single-cell necrosis of keratinocytes

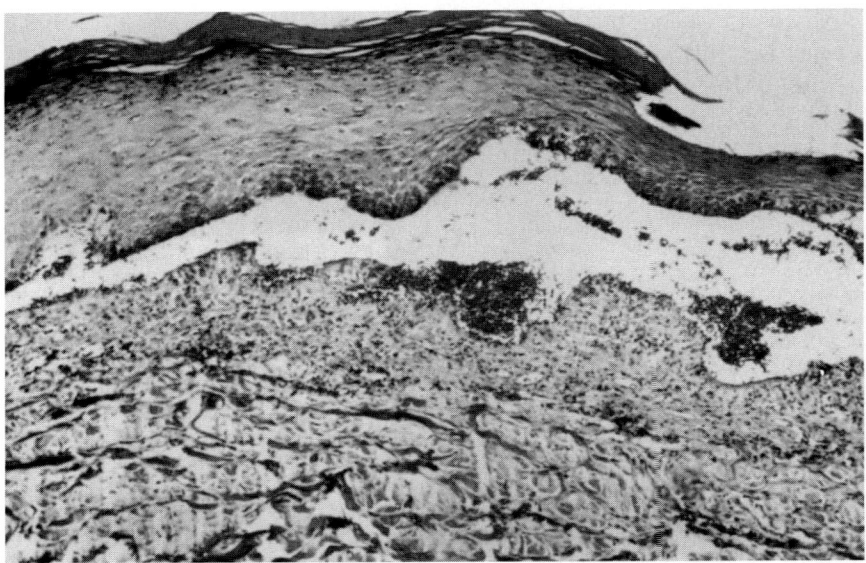

FIGURE 2–122. Subepidermal vesicular dermatitis. Subepidermal vesicle in a dog with bullous pemphigoid.

matosus, erythema multiforme, cutaneous adverse drug reaction, demodicosis, thymoma-associated exfoliative dermatitis in cats, dermatophytosis, graft-versus-host disease, and various vasculitides and vasculopathies (dermatomyositis, rabies vaccine reaction, etc.).

2. *Infiltrative mural folliculitis.* The follicle wall is infiltrated by lymphocytes and histiocytes in the absence of hydropic degeneration and apoptosis (Fig. 2–125). The differential diagnosis includes sebaceous adenitis, pseudopelade, feline idiopathic lymphocytic mural folliculitis, cutaneous adverse drug reaction, and early epitheliotropic lymphoma. Concurrent mucinosis of the outer root sheath is typical of alopecia mucinosa. In dogs, an idiopathic (possibly drug-related) granulomatous degenerative folliculopathy is characterized by massive infiltration of lymphocytes, histiocytes, and multinucleate giant cells.

3. *Necrotizing mural folliculitis.* An usually eosinophil-dominated inflammation causes explosive rupture of follicles, with hemorrhage, and severe dermal mucinosis and edema (Fig. 2–126). One often sees eosinophilic "molds" of destroyed follicle walls. The most common causes are arthropod- and insect-related damage (e.g., feline mosquito bite hypersensitivity, and canine eosinophilic folliculitis and furunculosis). A relatively cell-poor or neutrophil-dominated necrotizing mural folliculitis may be a rare manifestation of cutaneous adverse drug reaction, and may also be seen in feline herpesvirus dermatitis and ischemic states.

4. *Pustular mural folliculitis.* Microabscesses and pustules form adjacent to the follicular stratum corneum, producing subcorneal or intragranular follicular pustules (Fig. 2–127). The most common causes are pemphigus foliaceus or pemphigus erythematosus (neutrophils or eosinophils with acantholytic keratinocytes) and sterile eosinophilic pustulosis.

Luminal folliculitis implies the accumulation of inflammatory cells within the superficial or deep aspects of the lumen (Fig. 2–128). This is, by far, the most common histologic type and is usually associated with infectious agents: bacteria, dermatophytes, and *Demodex* mites. These folliculitides are dominated by neutrophils. Rare causes include *Pelodera* nematodes, sterile eosinophilic pustulosis, and sterile eosinophilic pinnal folliculitis. Focal areas of eosinophilic folliculitis may be seen in biopsy specimens from cats with atopy, food hypersensitivity, or flea bite hypersensitivity.[43]

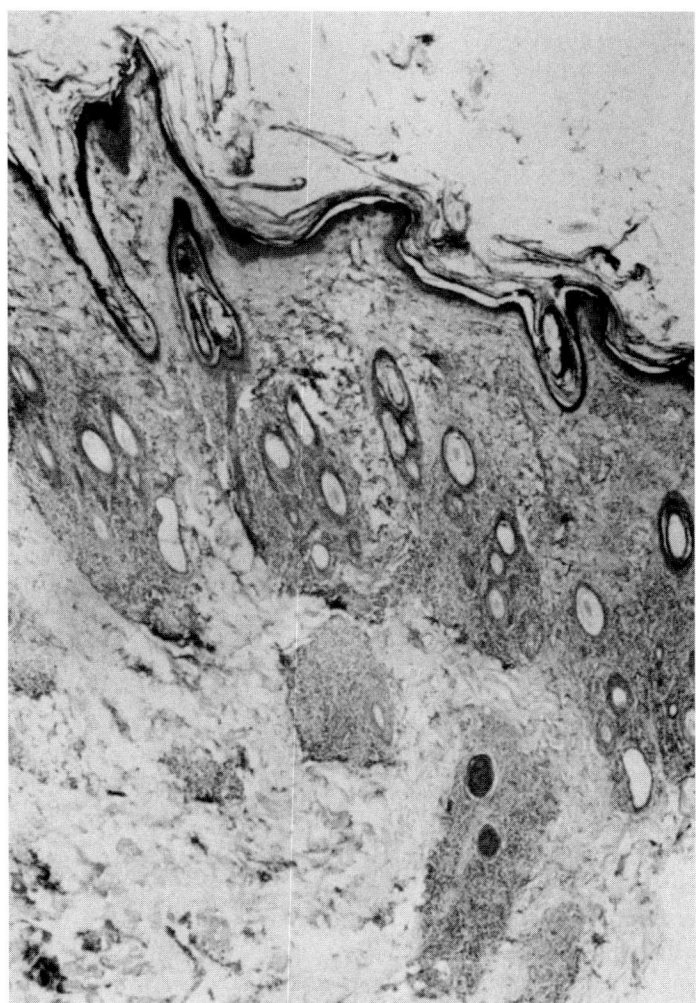

FIGURE 2–123. Perifolliculitis. Perifollicular pyogranulomas in a dog with visceral leishmaniasis.

Furunculosis (penetrating folliculitis) signifies follicular rupture (Fig. 2–129). It most commonly occurs as a result of luminal folliculitis and less commonly as a result of necrotizing mural folliculitis. Furunculosis results in pyogranulomatous inflammation of the surrounding dermis and, occasionally, subcutis. When furunculosis is seen consecutively in three or more follicles (the "domino" effect), dermatophytosis (especially kerion) is the most likely diagnosis. Furunculosis is usually associated with moderate numbers of eosinophils, presumably a foreign body–type reaction to free keratin and hair shafts. When eosinophils are the dominant cell, an antecedent necrotizing (eosinophilic) mural folliculitis is the cause.

Bulbitis indicates a targeting of the inferior segment of the follicle (Fig. 2–130). This is characteristically seen in alopecia areata. Lymphocytes surround the bulb of anagen hair follicles like "a swarm of bees." Histiocytes and eosinophils may be present in small numbers.

Perifollicular fibrosis is seen with chronic folliculitides, dermatomyositis, and chronic sebaceous adenitis. *Perifollicular melanosis* can occasionally be seen with numerous folliculitides, but is most characteristic of canine demodicosis.[18]

Follicular inflammation is a common microscopic finding, and one must always be cautious in assessing its importance. It is a common secondary complication in pruritic dermatoses (e.g., hypersensitivities and ectoparasitism), hormonal dermatoses, and disor-

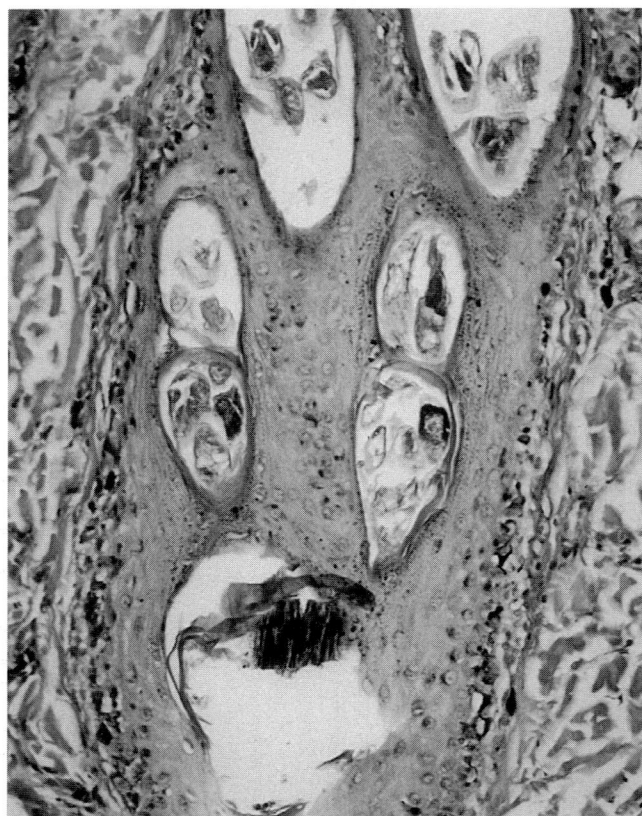

FIGURE 2–124. Interface mural folliculitis in a dog with generalized demodicosis. Hydropic degeneration and apoptosis of basal keratinocytes.

ders of keratinization. Hence, a thorough search (histologically and clinically) for underlying causes is mandatory.

Fibrosing Dermatitis

Fibrosis marks the resolving stage of an intense or insidious inflammatory process, and it occurs mainly as a consequence of collagen destruction. Fibrosis that is histologically recognizable does not necessarily produce a visible clinical scar. Ulcers that cause damage to collagen in the superficial dermis only do not usually result in scarring, whereas virtually all ulcers that extend into the deep dermis inexorably proceed to fibrosis and clinical scars.

Fibrosing dermatitis (Fig. 2–131) follows severe insults of many types to the dermis. Thus, fibrosing dermatitis alone is of minimal diagnostic value other than for its testimony to antecedent injury. The pathologist must look carefully for signs of the antecedent process, such as furunculosis, vascular disease, foreign material, lymphedema, lupus erythematosus, dermatomyositis, acral lick dermatitis, and morphea. In cats, an uncommon chronic ulcerative dermatitis is characterized by linear subepidermal fibrosis, which extends peripheral to the ulcer.

Panniculitis

The panniculus is commonly involved as an extension of dermal inflammatory processes, especially of suppurative and granulomatous dermatoses. Likewise, there is usually some deep dermal involvement in virtually all panniculitides.

Panniculitis is conveniently divided on an anatomic basis into the lobular type (pri-

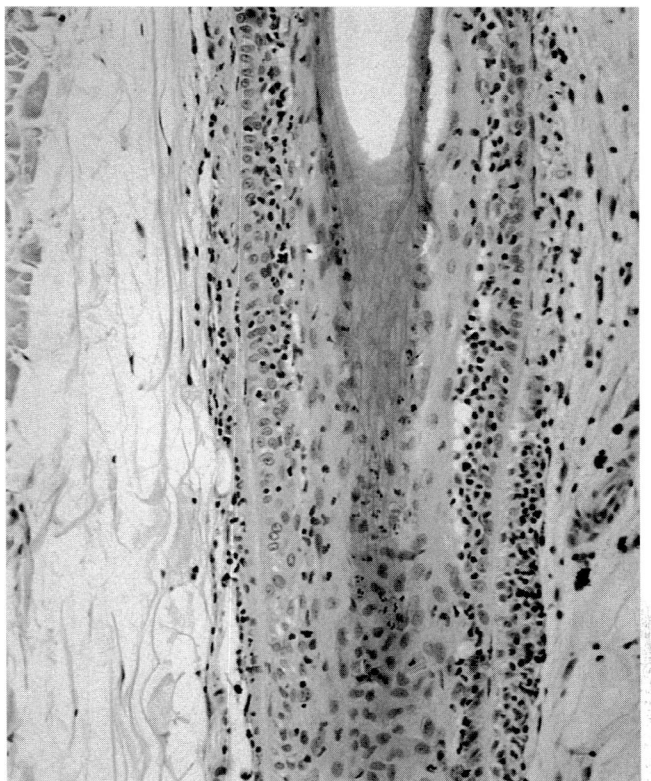

FIGURE 2–125. Infiltrative mural folliculitis in a dog with a cephalexin cutaneous adverse drug reaction. Lymphocytes infiltrate follicular outer root sheath in the absence of hydropic degeneration and apoptosis of basal keratinocytes.

marily involving fat lobules), the septal type (primarily involving interlobular connective tissue septa), and the diffuse type (both anatomic areas involved) (Fig. 2–132). Patterns of panniculitis appear to have little diagnostic or prognostic significance in dogs and cats, and all three patterns may be seen in a single lesion from the same patient.[37] Neither does the cytologic appearance (pyogranulomatous, granulomatous, suppurative, eosinophilic, lymphoplasmacytic, or fibrosing) appear to have much diagnostic or prognostic significance.[37] Most panniculitides, regardless of the cause, look histologically similar.

In dogs, diffuse panniculitis is the most common pattern, and septal panniculitis is most often found in cats. As with nodular and diffuse dermatitis, polarization, the use of special stains, and cultures are usually indicated. Septal panniculitis is seen with vasculitides and erythema nodosum. A rare form of canine panniculitis, one associated with lupus erythematosus (lupus profundus or lupus erythematosus panniculitis), is characterized by lymphoplasmacytic septal to lobular panniculitis, with septal vasculitis, numerous lymphoid nodules, mucinosis, and often an overlying interface dermatitis. Similar microscopic lesions occur at the sites of previous vaccinations (especially rabies) or drug injections. Feline subcutaneous fat sclerosis is characterized by marked septal fibrosis, fat micropseudocyst formation, and lipocytes that contain radially arranged, needle-shaped clefts.

Atrophic Dermatosis

Atrophic dermatosis is characterized by varying degrees of epithelial and connective tissue atrophy (Fig. 2–133). Disorders in this category are endocrine, nutritional, and developmental dermatoses; telogen defluxion; and postclipping follicular arrest. Endocrine dermatoses are the most common and show variable combinations of the following histopathologic changes: diffuse orthokeratotic hyperkeratosis, epidermal atrophy, follicular keratosis, follicular atrophy, telogenization or catagenization of hair follicles, excessive

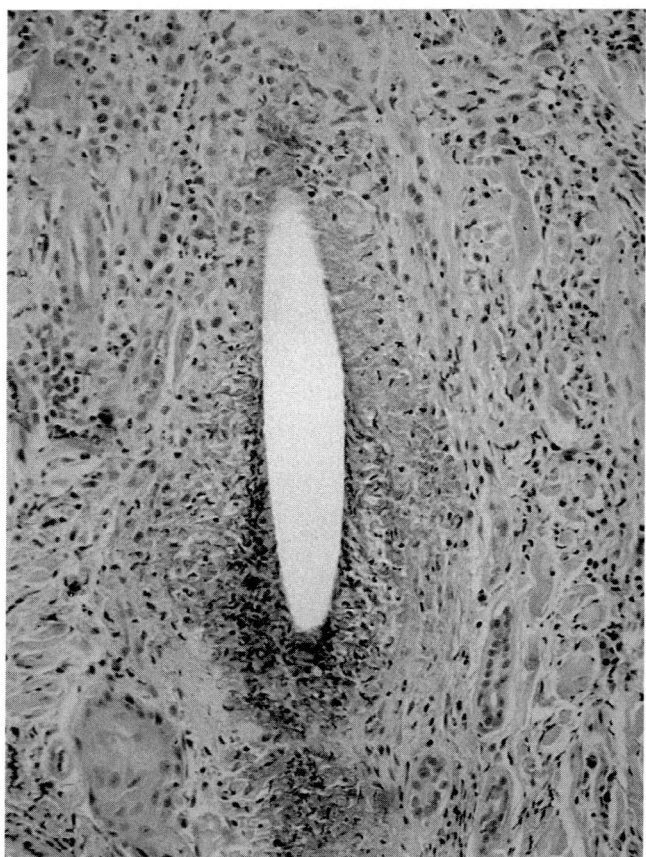

FIGURE 2–126. Necrotizing mural folliculitis in a cat with mosquito bite hypersensitivity. Necrotic follicular epithelium and eosinophils surround an empty pilar canal.

trichilemmal keratinization (flame follicles), epithelial melanosis, and sebaceous gland atrophy.[24, 35, 39, 54, 55] Inflammatory changes are frequent and potentially misleading in the atrophic dermatoses and reflect the common occurrence of secondary bacterial infection, seborrhea, or both with these disorders. Findings suggestive of specific endocrinopathies include diffuse mucinosis (hypothyroidism), dystrophic mineralization (hyperadrenocorticism), hypertrophied or vacuolated arrector pili muscles (hypothyroidism), decreased dermal elastin (hyposomatotropism and hyperadrenocorticism), dermal atrophy (hyperadrenocorticism and hyposomatotropism), and absence of arrector pili muscles (hyperadrenocorticism). Adrenal sex hormone abnormalities seem to produce a unique combination of atrophic dermatosis and follicular dysplasia.

Findings suggestive of nutritional disorders include misshapen, corkscrew hairs and small hairs. Developmental disorders such as follicular dysplasias, and color dilution alopecia are characterized by variable degrees of follicular dysplasia and anomalous deposition of melanin. The various follicular dysplasias produce dysplastic hair shafts, but endocrinopathies do not.[20, 34] Dysplastic hair shafts may also be seen in alopecia areata, anagen defluxion, and thallotoxicosis. These should not be confused with the twisted, malacic hair shafts seen in biopsy specimens from cats with allergies and psychogenic alopecia (the "twang sign" of the hair pulling cat), nor the eosinophilic, amorphous, "infarcted hairs" seen with vasculopathies. Miniaturization of hair follicles and hair shafts may be seen in nutritional disorders, genetic hypotrichoses, pattern baldness, paraneoplastic alopecia, and sex hormone dermatoses. Telogen defluxion is characterized by diffuse telogenization of hair follicles, with no other signs of cutaneous atrophy. Postclipping follicular arrest is characterized by diffuse catagenization or telogenization of hair follicles, with no other signs of cutaneous atrophy. In the chronic stage, alopecia areata may be characterized by

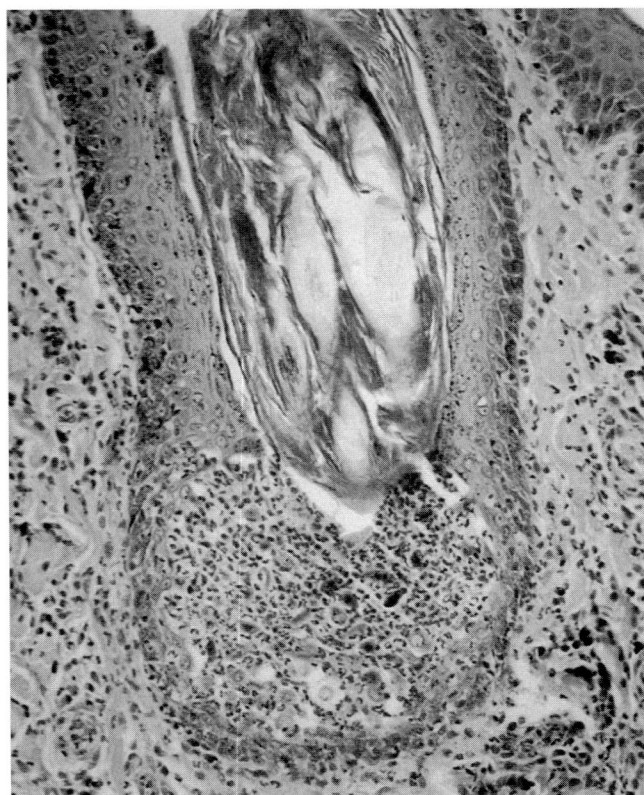

FIGURE 2–127. Pustular mural folliculitis in a dog with pemphigus foliaceus. Intramural microabscess at base of follicle is filled with neutrophils and acantholytic keratinocytes. Pilar canal is not involved.

follicular atrophy, dysplastic hair shafts, or "orphaned" cutaneous glands and arrector pili muscles. In the chronic stage, granulomatous sebaceous adenitis may have complete absence of sebaceous glands, a feature that is not seen with endocrine, nutritional, and most developmental dermatoses. The acquired skin fragility syndrome of cats is characterized by striking atrophy, attenuation, and disorganization of dermal collagen.

Mixed Reaction Patterns

Because skin diseases have a pathologic continuum, reflecting various combinations of acute, subacute, and chronic changes, and because animals can have more than one dermatosis at the same time, it is common for one or two biopsy specimens from the same animal to show two or more reaction patterns (Fig. 2–134). For instance, it is common to see an overall pattern of perivascular dermatitis (due to hypersensitivity reactions or ectoparasitism) or atrophic dermatosis (due to endocrinopathy) with a subordinate, focal pattern of folliculitis, furunculosis, or intraepidermal pustular dermatitis (due to secondary bacterial infection). Likewise, one can find multiple patterns from one or two biopsy specimens from an animal with a single disease (e.g., vasculitis, diffuse necrotizing dermatitis, and fibrosing dermatitis in a patient with necrotizing vasculitis). Mixed reaction patterns (two or three patterns) were found in about 25% of the biopsy specimens from cats with inflammatory dermatoses.[43]

Invisible Dermatoses

Generations of dermatohistopathologists have struggled with biopsy specimens from diseased skin that appear normal under the microscope. Because normal skin is rarely included in biopsy specimens in clinical practice, one must assume that some evidence of

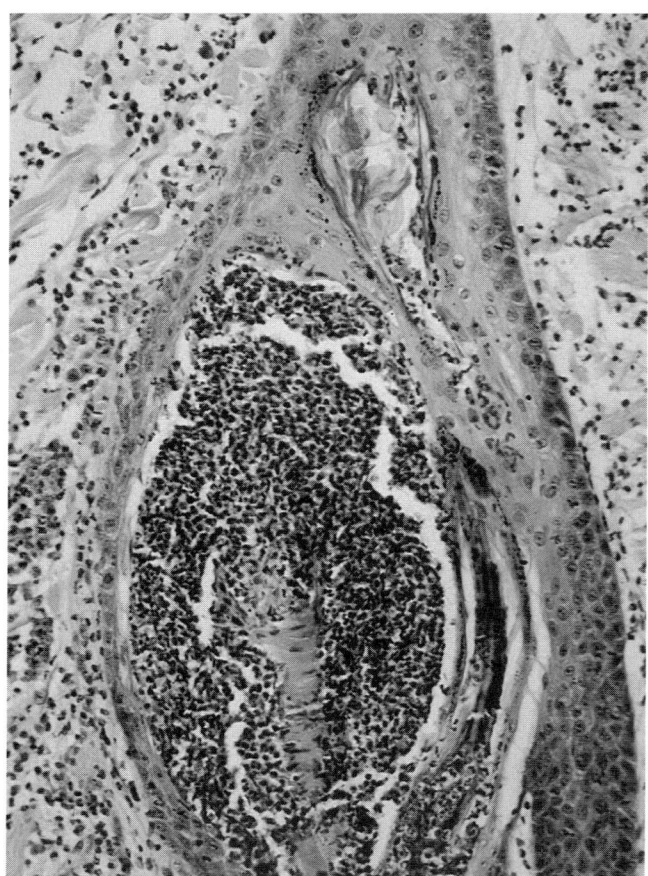

FIGURE 2–128. Luminal folliculitis in a dog with sterile eosinophilic pustulosis.

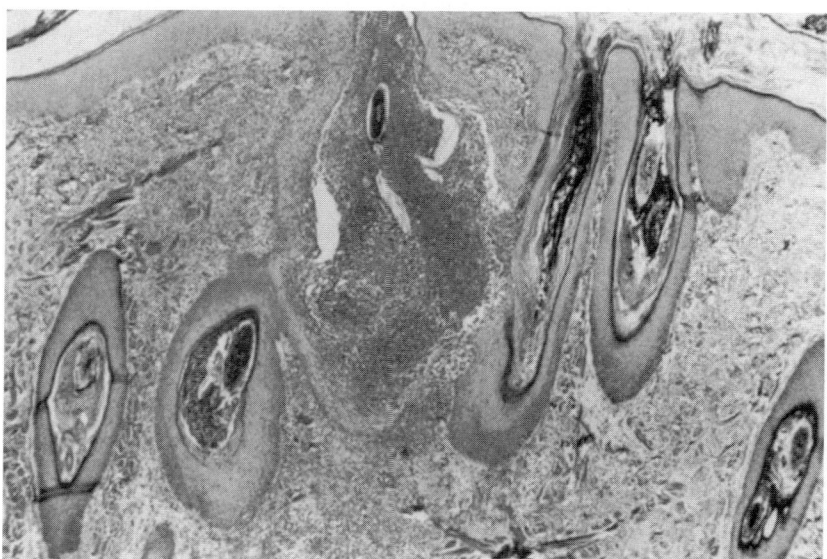

FIGURE 2–129. Furunculosis. Follicular rupture in a dog with staphylococcal furunculosis.

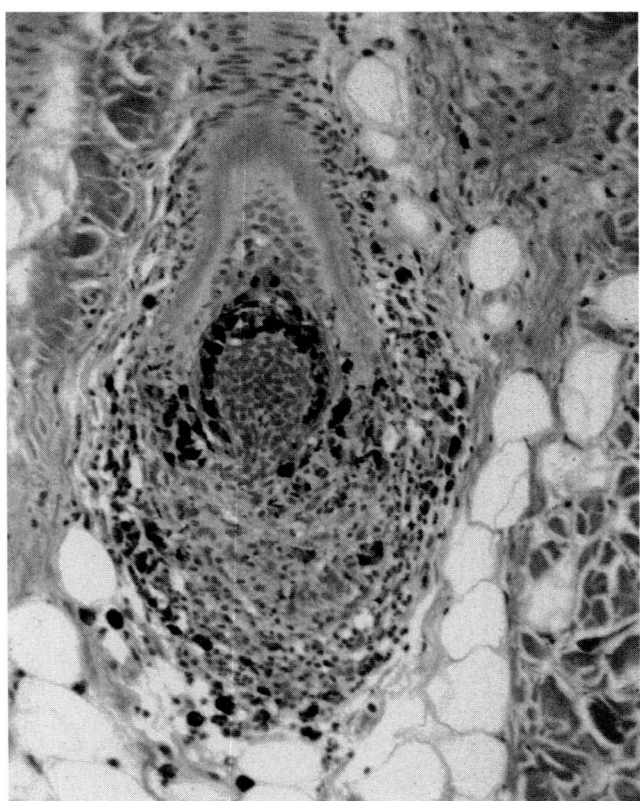

FIGURE 2–130. Bulbitis in a dog with alopecia areata.

disease is present. From the perspective of the dermatohistopathologist, the invisible dermatoses are clinically evident skin diseases that show a histologic picture resembling normal skin.[17] Technical problems must be eliminated, such as sampling errors that occur when normal skin on an edge of the biopsy specimen has been sectioned and the diseased tissue has been left in paraffin.

When confronted with an invisible dermatosis, the dermatohistopathologist should consider the following possible disorders and techniques for detecting them: dermatophytosis (special stain for fungi in keratin); ichthyosis (removal of surface keratin); psychogenic alopecia; pigmentary disturbances such as hypermelanoses and hypomelanoses, including lentigo and vitiligo; amorphous deposits in the superficial dermis (Congo red stain for amyloid deposits); urticaria; urticaria pigmentosa (toluidine blue stain for mast cells); connective tissue disorder (cutaneous asthenia); and various nevi.

Conclusion

A skin biopsy can be diagnostic, confirmatory, and helpful, or it can be inconclusive, depending on the dermatosis; the selection, handling, and processing of the specimen; and the skill of the histopathologist.

The dermatopathologist has no right to make a diagnosis of nonspecific dermatitis or inflammation. Every biopsy specimen is a sample of some specific process, but the visible changes may be noncharacteristic and may not permit a diagnosis.

The clinician should never accept the terms "nonspecific changes" and "nonspecific dermatitis." Many pathologic entities that are now well recognized were once regarded as nonspecific. Recourse to serial sections (the key pathologic changes may be focal), special stains, second opinions, and further biopsies may be necessary.

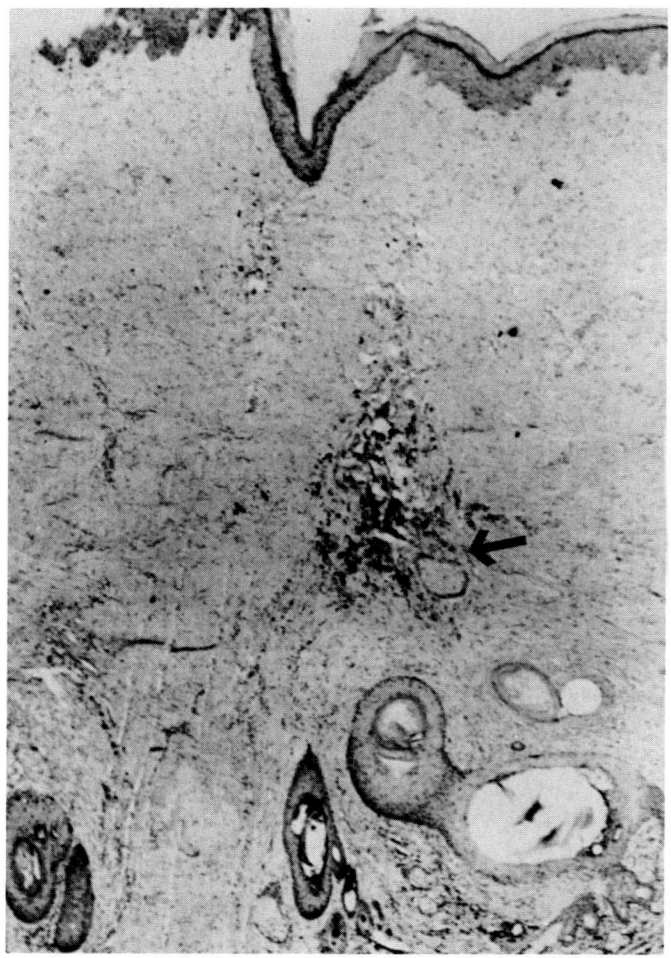

FIGURE 2–131. Fibrosing dermatitis. Dermal fibrosis after follicular rupture in a dog with staphylococcal furunculosis. Note orphaned sebaceous gland and pigmentary incontinence *(arrow)*.

A recent study in human dermatopathology assessed the utility of deeper sections and special stains.[28] Deeper sections provided diagnostic information in 37% of the cases in which they were ordered. Special stains contributed to the diagnosis in 21% of the cases for which they were ordered.

● SPECIAL PROCEDURES

In the past decade, a number of techniques have been developed for studying biopsy specimens. These techniques were usually advanced to allow the identification of special cell types. Examples of such procedures include immunofluorescence testing, electron microscopy, enzyme histochemistry, and immunocytochemistry.

Immunofluorescence testing is not routinely done in veterinary medicine (see Chap. 9). Biopsy specimens for immunofluorescence testing must be carefully selected and either snap frozen or placed in Michel's fixative. Electron microscopy is best performed on small specimens (1 to 2 mm in diameter) fixed in 3% glutaraldehyde. Enzyme histochemistry is performed on frozen sections or on tissues fixed in 2% paraformaldehyde, dehydrated in acetone, and embedded in glycol methacrylate (Table 2–11). Immunocytochemistry may be performed on formalin-fixed, routinely processed tissues (e.g., immuno-

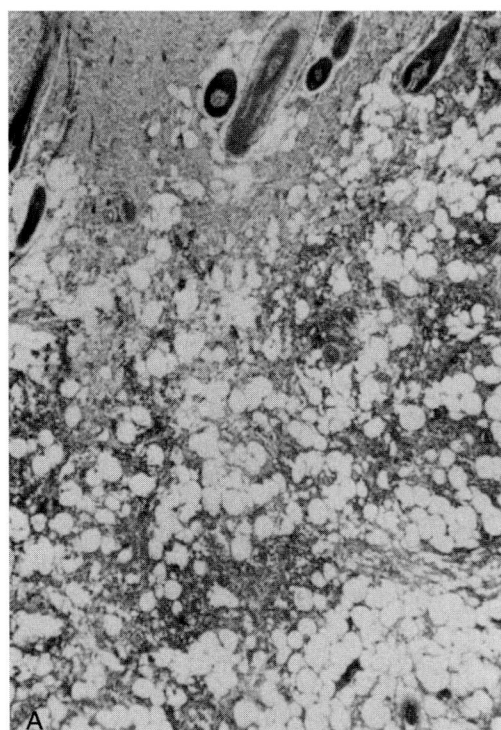
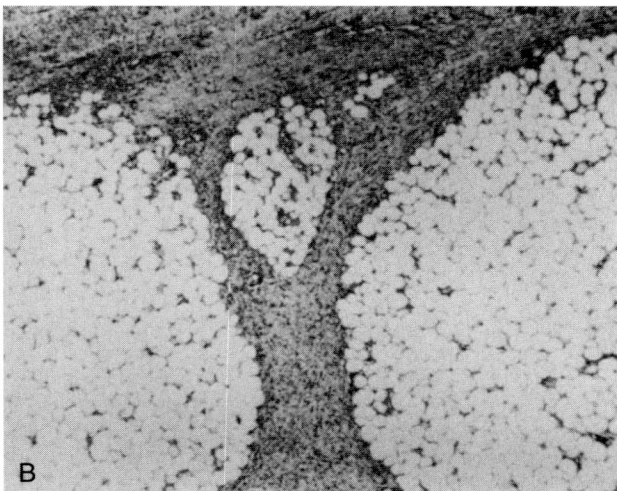

FIGURE 2–132. Panniculitis. *A*, Lobular panniculitis in a cat with idiopathic sterile panniculitis. *B*, Septal panniculitis in a cat with idiopathic sterile panniculitis.

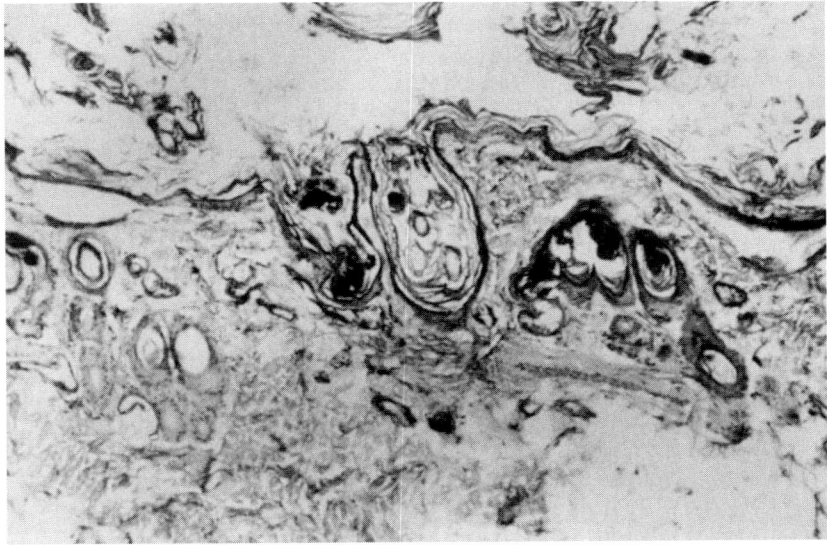

FIGURE 2–133. Atrophic dermatosis in a dog with hyposomatotropism.

● Table 2–11 **EXAMPLES OF MARKERS FOR THE IDENTIFICATION OF CELL TYPES**

MARKER	CELL TYPE
Enzyme Histochemical	
α-Naphthyl acetate esterase	Monocyte, histiocyte, Langerhans' cell, plasma cell
Chloroacetate esterase	Neutrophil, mast cell
Acid phosphatase	Monocyte, histiocyte, plasma cell
Alkaline phosphatase	Neutrophil, endothelial cell
β-Glucuronidase	Histiocyte, T lymphocyte, plasma cell
Adenosine triphosphatase	Histiocyte, plasma cell, B lymphocyte, endothelial cell
5'-Nucleotidase	Endothelial cell
Nonspecific esterase	Monocyte, histiocyte, Langerhans' cell
Lysozyme	Monocyte, histiocyte
α_1-Antitrypsin	Monocyte, histiocyte, mast cell
Chymase	Mast cell
Tryptase	Mast cell
Dipeptidyl peptidase II	Mast cell
Immunohistochemical	
Cytokeratin	Squamous and glandular epithelium, Merkel's cell
Vimentin	Fibroblast, Schwann cell, endothelial cell, myoepithelial cell, lipocyte, smooth muscle, skeletal muscle, mast cell, plasma cell, melanocyte, lymphocyte, monocyte, histiocyte, Langerhans' cell
Desmin	Skeletal muscle, smooth muscle
Neurofilament	Axon cell bodies, dendrites
S100 protein	Melanocyte, Schwann cell, myoepithelial cell, sweat gland acini and ducts, lipocyte, macrophage
Myoglobin	Skeletal muscle
Factor VIII–related antigen	Endothelial cell
Peanut agglutinin	Histiocyte
Myelin basic protein	Schwann cell
Neuron-specific enolase	Schwann cell, Merkel's cell
Collagen IV	Basement membrane
Laminin	Basement membrane
CD1a	Langerhans' cell, dendritic cells
CD1b	Dendritic cells
CD1c	Dendritic cells
CD3	T lymphocytes
CD4	Helper T lymphocytes, dendritic cells, neutrophils
CD8	Cytotoxic T lymphocytes
CD11a	All leukocytes
CD11b	Monocytes, granulocytes
CD11c	Monocytes, macrophages, granulocytes, dendritic cells
CD18	All leukocytes
CD21	B lymphocytes
CD31	Endothelial cell
CD44	Lymphocytes, monocytes, granulocytes
CD45	All leukocytes
CD49	T lymphocytes, monocytes, granulocytes
CD54	ICAM-1
CD79	B lymphocytes

peroxidase methods) or on frozen sections (e.g., lymphocyte markers), depending on the substance being studied (see Table 2–11).

Molecular biological techniques (in situ hybridization, polymerase chain reaction) are having an impact on many different aspects of medicine.[8a] In the realm of infectious agents, these nucleic acid probes are enhancing diagnostic capabilities, avoiding the need of culturing infectious agents for the purpose of diagnosis, allowing earlier detection of infection, and permitting the detection of latent infections.

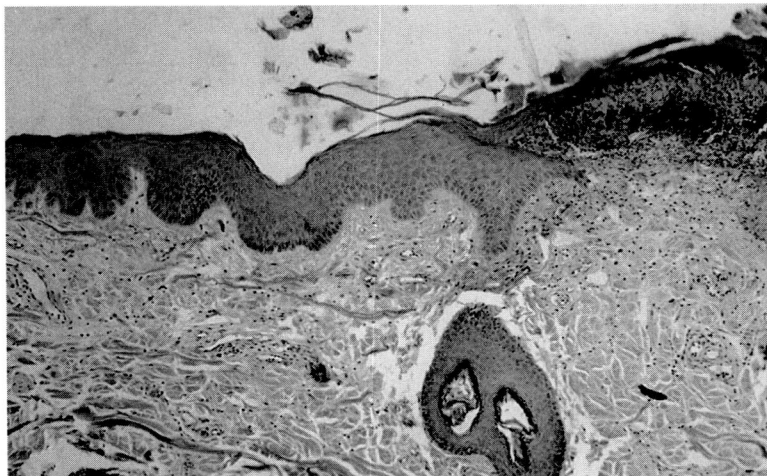

FIGURE 2–134. Mixed reaction in a dog with atopy and secondary staphylococcal dermatitis. Hyperplastic, superficial, lymphocytic perivascular dermatitis on the left (atopy) and intraepidermal neutrophilic pustular dermatitis on the right (staphylococcal infection).

• REFERENCES

General
1. Alhaidari Z: Les lésions élémentaires dermatologiques. Prat Méd Chir Anim Comp 23:101, 1988.
2. Griffin CEG: Unpublished observations.
3. Scott DW: Examination of the integumentary system. Vet Clin North Am Small Anim Pract 11:499, 1981.
4. Shearer D: Laboratory diagnosis of skin disease. In Pract 13:149, 1991.
4a. Bevier DE: The reaction of feline skin to the intradermal injection of allergenic extracts and passive cutaneous anaphylaxis using serum from skin test positive cats. In: Von Tscharner C, Halliwell REW (eds): Advances in Veterinary Dermatology, Vol. 1. Baillière Tindall, Philadelphia, 1990, p 126.

Age
5. Bourdeau P: Dermatologie du jeune carnivore. Point Vét 21:439, 1989.
6. Bourdeau P: Eléments de dermatologie du chien et du chat vieillessants. Point Vét 22:255, 1990.
7. Foil CS: The skin. In: Hoskins JD (ed): Veterinary Pediatrics. W.B. Saunders Co, Philadelphia, 1990, p 359.
8. Halliwell REW: Skin diseases of old dogs and cats. Vet Rec 126:389, 1990.
8a. Jaworsky C: The molecular diagnosis of infection. J Cutan Pathol 20:508, 1993.

Breed
9. Ihrke PJ, Franti CE: Breed as a risk factor associated with skin diseases in dogs seen in northern California. Calif Vet 39:13, 1985.
10. Scott DW, Paradis M: A survey of canine and feline skin disorders seen in a university practice: Small Animal Clinic, University of Montreal, Saint-Hyacinthe, Québec (1987–1988). Can Vet J 31:830, 1990.

Cytologic Examination
11. Perman V, et al: Cytology of the Dog and Cat. American Animal Hospital Association, South Bend, IN, 1979.
12. Columbo S: Quantitative evaluation of cutaneous bacteria in normal dogs and dogs with pyoderma by cytological evaluation. Doctoral Thesis, Faculty of Veterinary Medicine, Milan, Italy, 1997.

Biopsy and Dermatopathologic Examination; The Vocabulary of Dermatohistopathology
13. Andreoletti O, et al: Identification de l'apoptose cutanée chez le chien et le chat par méthode TUNEL: Étude préliminaire sur coupes histologiques après inclusion en paraffine. Rev Méd Vét 148:781, 1997.
14. Bagladi MS, et al: Sebaceous gland melanosis in dogs with endocrine skin disease or follicular dysplasia: A retrospective study. Vet Dermatol 7:85, 1996.
15. Beningo KE, et al: Subepidermal linear alignment of mast cells in inflammatory dermatoses of the dog. Vet Dermatol 11:13, 2000.
16. Boiron G, et al: Phagocytosis of erythrocytes by human and animal epidermis. Dermatologica 165:158, 1982.
16a. Brignac MM, et al: Microscopy of color mutant alopecia. Proc Am Acad Vet Dermatol Am Coll Vet Dermatol 4:14, 1988.
16b. Brown WM, Stenn KS: Homeobox genes and the patterning of skin diseases. J Cutan Pathol 20:289, 1993.
17. Brownstein MH, Rabinowitz AD: The invisible dermatoses. J Am Acad Dermatol 8:579, 1983.
18. Cayatte SM, et al: Perifollicular melanosis in the dog. Vet Dermatol 3:165, 1992.
18a. Doubleday DW: Who is Nikolsky and what does his sign mean. J Am Acad Dermatol 16:1054, 1987.
19. Dunstan RW: A user's guide to veterinary surgical pathology laboratories, or why do I still get a diagnosis of chronic dermatitis even when I take a perfect biopsy? Vet Clin North Am Small Anim Pract 20:1397, 1990.
20. Dunstan RW: A pathomechanistic approach to diseases of the hair follicle. Br Vet Dermatol Study Grp 17:37, 1995.
21. Fairley RA: Collagenolysis: "It ain't easy being pink." Vet Pathol 28:96, 1991.

22. Fernandez CJ, et al: Staining abnormalities of dermal collagen in eosinophil or neutrophil rich inflammatory dermatoses of horses and cats as demonstrated with Masson's trichome stain. Vet Dermatol 11:43, 2000.
23. Goldschmidt MH: Small animal dermatopathology: 'What's old, what's new, what's borrowed, what's useful.' Semin Vet Med Surg Small Anim 2:162, 1987.
24. Gross TL, et al: Veterinary Dermatopathology. A Macroscopic and Microscopic Evaluation of Canine and Feline Skin Disease. Mosby–Year Book, St. Louis, 1992.
25. Gross TL, et al: An anatomical classification of folliculitis. Vet Dermatol 8:147, 1997.
26. Henfrey JI, et al: A comparison of three local anaesthetic techniques for skin biopsy in dogs. Vet Dermatol 2:21, 1991.
26a. Jang SS, Biberstein EL: Laboratory diagnosis of fungal and algal infections. In: Greene CE (ed): Infectious Diseases of the Dog and Cat. W.B. Saunders Co, Philadelphia, 1990, p 639.
26b. Kennis RA: Quantitation and topographical analysis of *Malassezia* organisms in normal canine skin. Proc Am Acad Vet Dermatol Am Coll Vet Dermatol 9:23, 1993.
27. Leider M, Rosenblum M: A Dictionary of Dermatological Words, Terms, and Phrases. McGraw-Hill Book Co, New York, 1968.
28. Maingi CP, Helm KF: Utility of deeper sections and special stains for dermatopathology specimens. J Cutan Pathol 25:171, 1998.
29. Majno G, Joris I: Apoptosis, oncosis, and necrosis. An overview of cell death. Am J Pathol 146:3, 1995.
30. Mauldin EA, et al: *Malassezia* dermatitis in the dog: A retrospective histopathological and immunopathological study of 86 cases (1990–1995). Vet Dermatol 8:191, 1997.
31. Mehregan AH: Clear epidermal cells: An artifact. J Cutan Pathol 7:154, 1980.
32. Parker WM, Yager JA: *Trichophyton* dermatophytosis—a disease easily confused with pemphigus erythematosus. Can Vet J 38:502, 1997.
32a. Plant JD, et al: Factors associated with and prevalence of high *Malassezia pachydermatis* numbers on dog skin. J Am Vet Med Assoc 201:879, 1992.
33. Raskin CA: Apoptosis and cutaneous biology. J Am Acad Dermatol 36:885, 1997.
34. Rothstein E, et al: A retrospective study of dysplastic hair follicles and abnormal melanization in dogs with follicular dysplasia syndromes or endocrine skin disease. Vet Dermatol 9:235, 1998.
35. Scott DW: Histopathologic findings in the endocrine skin disorders of the dog. J Am Anim Hosp Assoc 18:173, 1982.
36. Scott DW: Lichenoid reaction in the skin of dogs: Clinicopathologic correlations. J Am Anim Hosp Assoc 20:305, 1984.
37. Scott DW, Anderson WI: Panniculitis in dogs and cats: A retrospective analysis of 78 cases. J Am Anim Hosp Assoc 24:551, 1988.
38. Scott DW: Lymphoid nodules in skin biopsies from dogs, cats, and horses with non-neoplastic dermatoses. Cornell Vet 79:267, 1989.
39. Scott DW: Excessive trichilemmal keratinization (flame follicles) in endocrine skin disorders of the dog. Vet Dermatol 1:37, 1990.
40. Scott DW: Epidermal mast cells in the cat. Vet Dermatol 1:65, 1990.
41. Scott DW: Bacteria and yeast on the surface and within non-inflamed hair follicles of skin biopsies from dogs with non-neoplastic dermatoses. Cornell Vet 82:371, 1992.
42. Scott DW: Bacteria and yeast on the surface and within non-inflamed hair follicles of skin biopsies from cats with non-neoplastic dermatoses. Cornell Vet 82:379, 1992.
43. Scott DW: Analyse du type de réaction histopathologique dans le diagnostic des dermatoses inflammatoires chez le chat: Étude portant sur 394 cas. Point Vét 26:57, 1994.
44. Scott DW: Suppurative inflammation of apocrine sweat glands (suppurative hidradenitis) in the dog: A retrospective clinicopathological analysis of 100 cases. Vet Dermatol 6:75, 1995.
45. Scott DW: La dermatite interstitielle chez le chien et le chat: Étude rétrospective sur la signification de cette modalité de reáction histopathologique. Méd Vét Québec 26:16, 1996.
46. Scott DW: Les agrégats de mélanine dans l'appareil pilo-sébacé: Signification en dermatohistopathologie du chat. Méd Vét Québec 28:38, 1998.
47. Scott DW: Eosinophils in the walls of large dermal and subcutaneous blood vessels in biopsy specimens from cats with eosinophilic granuloma or eosinophilic plaque. Vet Dermatol 10:77, 1999.
48. Seaman WJ, Chang SH: Dermal perifollicular mineralization of toy poodle bitches. Vet Pathol 21:122, 1984.
49. Steffen C: Dyskeratosis and the dyskeratoses. Am J Dermatopathol 10:356, 1988.
50. Teifke JP, et al: Aussagekraft und Möglichkeiten der histopahologischen Diagnostik bei rassespezifischen Hauterkrankungen. Tierärztl Prax 26:247, 1998.
51. Williams BJ, et al: Antimicrobial effects of lidocaine, bicarbonate, and epinephrine. J Am Acad Dermatol 37:662, 1997.
52. Wood C, et al: Eosinophilic infiltration with flame figures. Am J Dermatopathol 8:186, 1988.
53. Yager JA, Wilcock BP: Skin biopsy: Revelations and limitations. Can Vet J 29:969, 1988.
54. Yager JA, Scott DW: The skin and appendages. In: Jubb KVP, et al (eds): Pathology of Domestic Animals IV, Vol. 1. Academic Press, New York, 1993, p 531.
55. Yager JA, Wilcock BP: Color Atlas and Text of Surgical Pathology of the Dog and Cat. Dermatopathology and Skin Tumors. Wolfe Publishing, London, 1994.

Chapter 3

Dermatologic Therapy

• CARE OF NORMAL SKIN AND HAIRCOAT

The veterinarian is vitally concerned with the health of the patient's skin and is often consulted by clients regarding preventive care as well as optimal maintenance of the normal skin and haircoat. Most commonly, questions about the healthy pet's skin and hair relate to nutrition, skin and coat supplements, ectoparasite control (see Chap. 6), bathing, and shedding. Additionally, the veterinarian may be queried about optimal grooming. Many veterinary practices offer medicated baths and dips as well as routine bathing.

Although the skin reflects the animal's general health, many vigorous, healthy, normal pets have unkempt haircoats—mainly because of neglect or the client's lack of knowledge regarding proper grooming. Keeping the haircoat free from mats and removing the shedded undercoat allows more appropriate thermoregulation and discourages irritation and secondary bacterial infection. Therefore, it is valuable for the veterinarian to be familiar with routine grooming equipment as well as general skin and hair care.

Because most veterinarians are not groomers, questions regarding grooming and especially haircut styles are usually handled more appropriately by a qualified groomer. Styles change, and variations in clipping can enhance or mask aspects of conformation that affect the animal's appearance. These nuances of style are the province of owners, breeders, handlers, and commercial grooming establishments. However, most clients expect veterinarians to know about basic grooming and bathing. Much of the following discussion is presented as background for students or information that can be transmitted to clients.[6, 148, 172]

Basic Nutrition and the Skin

Nutritional factors that influence the skin are exceedingly complex (see Chap. 17). The skin and haircoat utilize a major part of the nutritional requirements of dogs and cats. Modifications of nutrition, therefore, may have visible effects on the skin and haircoat.

Nutritional modifications are utilized in two ways in relation to skin and haircoat. The first is the basic diet and additional supplements given to normal or diseased animals that are designed to produce a high-quality haircoat. The second is nutritional therapy or treatment wherein diets and supplements are given for a specific disease or problem. In many situations, these treatments entail high doses that most likely have metabolic or pharmacologic effects other than just meeting nutritional requirements. In most cases (other than those discussed in Chap. 17), the success of these treatments is probably not related to nutritional deficiency. The most common ingredients of the diet that seem to benefit the quality of the skin and haircoat are the protein level and fatty acids, with some effect coming from the vitamins and minerals.

The skin and hair are the organs that utilize the most protein from the diet. When there is a deficiency of protein, the haircoat is one of the first organs affected (see Chap. 17). However, protein deficiency is rare in domestic pets, particularly if a commercial food is used. Some breeders recommend supplementing diets with extra protein sources, but the need for this has not been well documented.

Fats are an important part of the diet and are valuable as a concentrated energy look forward to the day when we can make accurate statements regarding many of these newer supplements.

Routine Grooming Care

Dog and cat breeds have many different coat types, so generalization about grooming details is difficult.[116, 172] A few important principles can be emphasized—the most critical being the frequency of care. When a schedule of grooming is found to suffice for keeping the pet looking sharp, it should be followed conscientiously. It is better to spend a few minutes grooming regularly than many hours sporadically.

Excessive shedding of hair into the house environment is greatly decreased by routine grooming. Products have been marketed that claim to reduce shedding. Substantiation of these claims appears to relate more to the instructions for use than to the active ingredients. Recommended use of these products involves extensive brushing before and after each weekly bath. Properly performed brushing, 15 to 30 minutes weekly, greatly decreases the amount of hair shed into the environment, regardless of which shampoo is used.

Because the client must be motivated to perform grooming regularly, making it easy is important. If proper facilities, effective tools, and a cooperative patient are combined, the task of grooming becomes tolerable or even enjoyable. A solid, convenient table with a nonskid surface and a grooming post with a neck or body sling are helpful. Grooming is facilitated if performed in a quiet area without distractions. A grooming stand with a chair is helpful but not necessary.

The proper grooming tools should be clean and in good repair. Comb, brush, claw clipper and file, towels, cotton balls, and cotton-tipped swabs (Q-Tips) are the vital implements needed for most breeds. Shampoo, hair-conditioning rinses, ear-cleaning solution, and flea dips are also necessary. Specialized tools (discussed later) are essential for grooming and conditioning some coats.

The animal and its training can greatly affect the ease of grooming. Regular habits of good behavior during grooming, established early in life, result in cooperation. Most properly trained pets either enjoy or tolerate well their grooming care.

Prospective owners should contemplate grooming problems before purchasing a pet. If time and expense are likely to be obstacles, one should not choose a pet from a longhaired, wiry, or woolly coated breed, but instead select a short-coated animal that is easy to groom. An owner should perform simple daily or weekly grooming chores but should periodically take advantage of a professional grooming service. The grooming needs of five typical coat types are discussed later.

Cleaning the Skin

The normal skin surface film contains excretory products of skin glands and keratinocytes, corneocytes, bacteria and dirt, pollen, grains, and mold spores. Excessive amounts of these, together with altered or abnormal fatty acids, serum, red blood cells, proteinaceous exudates, degenerating inflammatory cells, and the byproducts of their degradation as well as bacterial degradation, are found in the surface film of abnormal skin. To promote health, the skin and coat should be groomed to minimize these accumulations. If proper skin and coat care is neglected, skin irritation may result or accumulations of debris may adversely affect a skin disease that is already present.

PREPARATION FOR BATHING

Before dogs are bathed, the haircoat should be brushed out and the claws should be clipped or filed to keep them short. With frequent filing, the quick recedes and the claw can be maintained properly. Also, one should check between the toes for foreign objects and remove hair under the foot between the pads. Care should be exercised when using scissors between pads. Clippers are safer because they are less apt to produce lacerations.

If the dog's coat is unkempt and severely matted, the tags and mats should be cut out before they are wet; otherwise, the mats become set and are more difficult to remove.

The anal sacs should be palpated and expressed, if necessary, before bathing so any soilage can be removed during the bath. One should place cotton over the anus and, with the thumb on one side of the anus and the fingers on the other side, press forward and together to express the sacs. A more complete expression of sac contents can be performed by inserting a gloved finger into the rectum to express each sac separately.

The ears should also receive attention and care before the animal is bathed. The ears are carefully examined as well as cleaned and dried thoroughly, if necessary (see Chap. 19). Some terriers and poodles may have large amounts of hair growing in the ear canals. Excessive hair should be plucked from the external ear canal in dogs prone to ear problems because it may allow cerumen accumulation and contribute to irritation. The process of plucking may cause irritation in normal ears and should be used only when it is deemed necessary on the basis of the history and examination of the ear canal. Antibacterial and anti-inflammatory medication should be instilled in the ear canal after the plucking is complete and the canal is clean and dry. Pledgets of cotton may be placed firmly in each ear before bathing to block the entrance of soap and water. After the bath, the cotton is removed or, if none was applied, a drying agent is put into the ear canal.

In the past, it has been recommended to apply ointments or oils to eyes as a protection against inadvertent entry of irritants. This should not be done because the oil vehicle makes rinsing an irritant from the eye more difficult. This is especially true of lipid-soluble irritants, which may cause more damage if applied to an eye pretreated with an oil or an ointment. Nothing should be applied to the eyes, and if an irritant (e.g., dip and soap) enters the eye, it should immediately be rinsed with fresh water.

HAIR CARE PRODUCTS

- **Shampoos.** Shampoos should remove external dirt, grime, and sebum and leave the hair soft, shiny, and easy to comb. To accomplish this, they should lather well, rinse freely, and leave no residue. Optimally, they would remove soil rather than natural oils, but the natural oils are removed to varying degrees. For some animals, this may require the use of oil or conditioning rinses. Some shampoos still have a soap base, but most shampoos are surfactants or detergents with a variety of additives that function as thickeners, conditioners, lime soap dispersants, protein hydrolysates, and perfumes. Dozens of products are on the market.

Many clients are familiar with pH-balanced shampoos for human use. The same promotion of pH adjusting for canine shampoos has been recommended. The canine skin is approximately neutral with a pH of 7 to 7.4, which is different from that of human skin. Therefore, human pH-adjusted shampoos are not optimal for canine use. Theoretically, pH products temporarily affect the electrostatic charges in the surface lipid bilayer and could alter the normal barrier effect. However, the clinical relevance or the documentation of alterations in barrier function related to the pH of a shampoo is lacking in veterinary medicine.

Soap shampoos work well in soft water. In hard water, they leave a dulling film of calcium and magnesium soap on the hair unless special lime-dispersing agents are added to bind calcium, magnesium, and heavy metal ions.

Detergent shampoos are synthetic surfactants or emulsifying agents, usually salts of lauryl sulfate. Sodium lauryl ether sulfate (sodium laureth sulfate) is less irritating than sodium lauryl sulfate. If dogs or cats seem to be irritated by most shampoos, trying a shampoo with sodium laureth sulfate may prove worthwhile. Such shampoos do not react with hard water, but they tend to be harsher cleaning agents than soap. This disadvantage is partially overcome by various additives.

Satisfactory detergents to use as shampoos for normal coats tend to dry the coat and contain few additives to counter the detergent effect. Conditioners should be used after detergents. Glycol, glycerol esters, lanolin derivatives, oils, and fatty alcohols are considered superfattening or emollient additives that prevent the complete removal of natural oils or tend to replace them. They also give the hair more luster and, as lubricants, make it easier to comb.

- **Conditioners.** Hair conditioners have four main purposes: (1) to reduce static electricity so that coarse hair does not snarl or become flyaway, (2) to give body to limp or thin hair, (3) to supply fatty acids or oil to coat the hair and skin, and (4) to deliver medication to the skin and hair surface in a vehicle that will not be completely rinsed away or removed. Normal hair maintains relative electric neutrality with a slight negative charge. However, if clean, dry hair is in a low-humidity environment or is brushed excessively, it picks up increased negative electric charges. Adjacent hairs that are similarly charged repel one another and produce the condition known as flyaway.

Conditioners or cream rinses are cationic (positively charged) surfactants or amphoteric materials that neutralize the charge and eliminate flyaway. They are slightly acidic, which hardens keratin and removes hard water residues. They also contain a fatty or oily component that adds a film to provide luster. Thus, these products make hair lie flat and comb easily but they do not provide the body or fluff that some coats require.

Protein conditioners, or body builders, contain oil and protein hydrolysates. Oils add luster, whereas protein hydrolysates coat the hair and make it seem thicker. This may be a slight advantage in hair with a dried, cracked, outer cuticle layer, but the effect is actually minimal. Only a thin film is added, so hair is not strengthened. If the protein is added to a shampoo rather than used separately, most of it is washed away during rinsing, further reducing the effect.

- **Oil Rinses.** Oil rinses are used after a bath to replenish and restore the natural oils removed by the shampooing. These products are emollients that add luster and improve the combability of the haircoat. They may decrease dry flaky skin and dry flakes within the haircoat. Oil rinses are primarily oils that require dilution or they will leave the haircoat too greasy, or they are oil-in-water emulsions that may be diluted or sprayed directly on the haircoat. The essential fatty acids are often incorporated into these products and are absorbed percutaneously.

BATHING

The dog is placed in a raised tub and is wet completely with warm water. A shower spray hose makes bathing easier and rinsing much faster. A bland nonmedicated, moisturizing, or hypoallergenic shampoo should be used for most dogs. The shampoo is applied to the neck and topline of the dog. More water is added, and a vigorous lather is worked up. Some owners apply excessive amounts of shampoo when the product is applied right from the bottle. This is wasteful and can lead to skin irritation because it is difficult to rinse the heavy concentration of shampoo. Predilution of the shampoo in 5 to 10 parts of water can help to eliminate this problem.

The lather should be rubbed into short-haired dogs but squeezed into long coats because rubbing may mat the long hair excessively. One can work a small rubber brush back and forth through the coat to clean the skin and remove any foreign materials from the hair. In some short-coated breeds, especially Doberman pinschers and Dalmatians, washing against the normal hair growth may induce postbathing folliculitis.

The dog's face should be washed and rinsed carefully. Gently placing a finger over the eyes keeps the eyelids closed and helps to prevent shampoo or rinse water from entering the eyes. A washcloth is also useful to control lather and keep soap from the dog's eyes.

The entire coat is rinsed thoroughly. A second lather and rinse may be needed to wash the dog until the water runs off clear. Thorough rinsing is essential. If the outer coat is rinsed but soap is left close to the skin, irritation results. This is most common in areas that tend to be overlooked or difficult to rinse, such as heavily feathered caudal thighs and axillary, groin, periscrotal, ventral tail, and interdigital areas. The haircoat should be rinsed until clear, detergent-free water runs off.

In general, except when short-coated breeds are washed or unless medicated shampoos necessitating longer contact times are used, the rinsing takes longer than the cleaning phase of bathing. The hair should squeak as it is rinsed. Vinegar, lemon, or bleaching rinses are not recommended, except for special problems. However, a small amount of dog or cat coat conditioner or oil can be added to water for the last rinse and adds gloss to the coat. Flea dips also are necessary in some cases and usually can be mixed with the conditioner.

The coat should be squeezed to eliminate water and the dog wrapped in a towel and lifted from the tub to a table. All animals should be protected from chilling and hypothermia during a bath and for several hours afterward, until thoroughly dry. Short-coated dogs can be toweled almost dry and then lightly brushed and kept confined or calm until dry.

Dogs with medium-length and long coats may be blotted with towels until only damp and then brushed. Alternatively, they may be placed in a stream of warm air and the coat can be combed, brushed, and fluffed as needed to accomplish the desired effect.

The frequency of a grooming routine depends on the breed and the individual animal's needs. In normal dogs not getting dirty, the bathing may be as infrequent as every few months. Dogs prone to normal dog odor that is noticeable to the client may require much more frequent bathing, as often as weekly. If normal dogs are bathed frequently, once monthly or more frequently, conditioners or oil rinses are advisable. The frequency of bathing needed in dogs with skin disease is generally much greater than with normal dogs.

Dry baths are sometimes used to avoid the drying influence of water baths, especially in dogs with long coats. Talc, boric acid powder, or special products available at pet stores are dusted into the coat and then thoroughly brushed out. With careful application, the coat is left relatively clean and lustrous. However, dry baths are good for only a quick cosmetic clean-up. Powder cleaners are actually inefficient: They dry the coat and increase its static electricity. They should not be used for routine cleaning because they do not replace bathing. Shampoo and water baths are still the most effective way to clean the coat thoroughly.

Special Grooming Problems

MATS

Mats can usually be teased apart and combed out if they are small. Small mats behind the ears and under the legs can be cut off. Larger mats can be slit with a scissors, a knife, or a mat and tangle splitter and then teased apart with one or two teeth of a comb. A mat and tangle splitter slices mats so they can be removed more easily, leaving some hair, as compared with clippers, which remove all hair. Some badly neglected long-coated cats or dogs may have an almost complete covering of felt matting. The only solution to some of these unfortunate cases is general anesthesia and complete, close clipping. Extreme care is necessary to avoid cutting or irritating the skin. Sometimes, the teeth of a comb can be slipped between the mat and the skin to serve as a shield so that the mat can be safely scissored away.

TAR OR PAINT

Tar or paint embedded in the coat may be difficult to remove. Small deposits should be allowed to harden and then cut off. Tar masses can be soaked in vegetable oil or an emollient oil with a surfactant for 24 hours (and bandaged if needed) to soften the tar, and then the entire mass can be washed out with soap and water. Dawn (Procter & Gamble) dish soap was found to be good for removing oil in the haircoat of otters affected by an oil spill.[80] One should never use paint removers or organic solvents such as kerosene, turpentine, and gasoline to remove tar or paint. They are irritating and toxic and may produce severe caustic burns. Ether may be used carefully for small areas. Clipping the tar or paint-coated hair is often the simplest procedure if the cosmetic appearance is not paramount.

GUM

Gum may be more easily removed if first hardened by rubbing with ice and then stripped or pulled out.[115]

ODORS

Odors about a coat usually originate from places such as the mouth, the ears, the feet, and the perineum. These areas should be checked and washed carefully. Most detergents remove the typical odors that dogs pick up. In many cases, the odor is an indication of skin disease (often, superficial bacterial pyoderma or *Malassezia* dermatitis) that may not be noted by the owner. In other cases, excessive lipid accumulation is present and degreasing agents such as benzoyl peroxide and tar may be useful.

A variety of commercial rinses may be applied, or the coat may be rinsed with a dilute chlorophyll solution or dilute sodium hypochlorite (in a white animal only). Highly scented dressings and sprays are objectionable to many people and do not reliably mask odors. Rarely, dogs are presented for severe body odor that seems to emanate from their entire body. Physical examination fails to reveal any visible abnormalities. Typically, these dogs' malodor responds transiently (24 hours) to a variety of shampoos and rinses. We have had the best results with long-term once-daily antibiotic therapy with lincomycin, erythromycin, or cephalosporins. Some dogs respond better with twice-weekly vinegar-water (equal parts of each) rinses, but the faint odor of vinegar disturbs some owners. The cause of this condition is unknown, and it is lifelong.

Skunk odor can be difficult to remove and often takes several treatments. Home remedies have described such methods as baths in soap and water followed by a rinse in a dilute ammonia-water solution (5 to 10 ml [1 to 2 tsp] of ammonia in 1 L [1 qt] of water), vinegar and water, tomato juice, and even toothpaste. We have seen all of these used with some success, though time and multiple applications may be needed. A commercial product, Skunk Odor Eliminator (The Bramton Co., Dallas, TX), has been recommended, though, again, multiple applications may be required.[115]

CLIPPING

Clipping is beneficial when topical treatment will be used. Clipping permits thorough cleaning, adequate skin contact, and a more economical application of the desired medicament. In many cases, complete removal of the coat may be preferred, but usually, clipping the local area suffices. This should be done neatly to avoid disfigurement. If the hair over the involved area is clipped closely (against the grain with a No. 40 clipper) while a border around this is clipped less closely (with the grain), the regrowth of hair more quickly blends the area into the normal coat pattern.

Clipping should always be discussed with the owner to obtain approval. This contact is especially important when treating show animals or those with long coats, such as Yorkshire terriers, Old English sheepdogs, and Afghan hounds. The corded breeds such as Pulis and Komondors take years to regrow clipped cords; therefore, clipping should be avoided unless absolutely necessary. All needless clipping should be avoided. During clipping, a vacuum cleaner can be used to remove all loose hair and debris. Shampoo therapy may be an acceptable alternative to clipping in some cases. It may remove surface lipids and clean the skin and hair enough that topical dips are able to be effectively applied to the skin surface. In other cases, the desired active ingredients may be incorporated into the shampoo formulation.

Comments on Grooming Cats

In general, the grooming implements used for dogs serve adequately for cats.[76, 146] However, special applications are outlined here. There is absolutely no substitute for routine daily grooming or for grooming every second or third day. Cats detest bathing and dematting and can be most resentful of rough treatment. Even when cats are petted, many of them slip away afterward to rearrange their haircoat thoroughly by licking and grooming themselves.

GROOMING NEEDS OF VARIOUS COAT TYPES

From the grooming standpoint, cats have three types of coats—the shorthaired, single coat; the shorthaired, double coat; and the long coat.

The shorthaired, single coat is typified by Siamese, Burmese, Havana brown, Rex, Korat, and domestic shorthaired cats. These cats can be bathed in shampoo and water, quickly dried to avoid chilling, and brushed and combed against the coat to remove dead hair. Final brushing follows the direction of natural hair growth. A fine metal comb and natural boar bristle brush are the only implements needed.

The shorthaired, double coat is typified by Abyssinian, Manx, Russian blue, and American shorthaired cats. The double coat is composed of two sets of hair. The long guard hair gives the coat its color, and the dense, short undercoat provides warmth. Both sets of hair are essential in these breeds. The basic coat care of this group is similar to that used for single coats except that caution must be employed because overgrooming can destroy the coat. Loss of the long guard hairs may give the coat a patchy or moth-eaten appearance.

The longhaired coat is typified by Persians and Himalayans. Several sizes of metal combs and a boar bristle brush are necessary for grooming these breeds. The kittens should be started with grooming at 4 weeks of age.

Older kittens and adults can be bathed with mild shampoo and water. They can be placed on a slanted window screen in a tub. Cats feel secure on the wire and stay put, yet water passes through easily. They are rinsed well and dried quickly with a towel and warm air blower. This fluffs the coat and gives it body. One should not bathe cats frequently and not within 2 weeks preceding a show. Cats almost never require bathing.

Mats tend to form behind the ears and under the chin, the legs, and the tail. The skin under the mat becomes irritated. Mats can be prevented by daily combing and brushing.

Some breeders dry-clean the coats with powder or talc sprinkled into the coat and carefully brushed out with a motion up and away from the body. This is rarely a satisfactory grooming method. If powder is left in the hair, it resembles unsightly dandruff and is highly objectionable.

The ruff or tail of a longhaired cat is never clipped. The eyes and nasal area should be cleaned to remove exudates that may accumulate.

SPECIAL FELINE GROOMING PROBLEMS

A cat's claws should be clipped only if necessary. They soon grow out again and are honed sharply.

Cats' ears are much less prone to infection than are dogs' ears, but they should always be checked and cleaned if needed. Young cats are especially predisposed to ear mite infections.

The large supracaudal organ on the dorsal surface of the tail is a mass of hyperactive sebaceous glands that may cause trouble if neglected. Breeders call the problem stud tail, although it occurs in both sexes. A waxy, unsightly accumulation builds up in the area if proper hygiene is neglected. The exudate can be removed by applying powder to soak it up, by applying a thin oil to soften it, or by sponging the area with alcohol or detergents as solvents. The oil can usually be brushed or washed off with shampoos satisfactorily. Periodic cleaning should prevent any future problem.

• CLIENT COMPLIANCE

The successful treatment of skin disorders depends to a large extent on the client. In addition to supplying the historical information needed for diagnosis, the client administers most prescribed therapies. The successful management of many dermatologic diseases necessitates long-term or lifelong therapy, often involving more than one medicament. The client must also give the medications correctly at the proper intervals and for the proper duration.

Many animals have been referred to us after the correct diagnosis was made, appropriate treatment was recommended, but treatment failed because of improper execution by the owner. Excellent diagnosticians often have poor results if they are not able to interact with clients effectively because this often leads to failure in compliance. These failures may occur for a variety of reasons. Understanding the possible reasons for poor compliance, recognizing when treatment failures occur, and developing corrective measures is an art that the successful clinician develops.

The reasons for poor client compliance include the following:

1. Failure of the client to understand the importance of giving the treatment
2. Lack of education of the client regarding the proper treatment
3. Improper frequency of or interval between medication applications
4. Faulty application, which can take multiple forms (Table 3–1)
5. Inadequate duration of therapy
6. Client's lack of time or labor-intensive treatment
7. Disagreeable cosmetic appearance or odor of treatment
8. Perceived danger of treatment
9. Premature discontinuation of treatment because of perceived lack of efficacy
10. Discontinuation of treatment because it was too difficult or not tolerated by the pet

Many of these problems are avoidable if the clinician or the veterinary assistants adequately explain the treatment plan.

It is important to make the client aware of potential problems, and these possible difficulties should be discussed before clients leave the office. We encounter numerous cases wherein the clients have unused treatments at home. This is particularly true of flea products: Because the treatment was too labor-intensive or the treatment appeared ineffective, the client discontinued it.

The successful clinician tries to prevent these treatment failures. For example, if clients do not or cannot dip their cats, a flea collar, although normally considered less effective than a properly applied dip, becomes relatively more efficacious. The best flea dip ever invented never works sitting on a shelf. Some clients may not readily admit that a treatment will be too difficult or unacceptable, and therefore alternatives may not be offered.

Another major factor influencing client compliance is the use of multiple therapeutic

● Table 3–1 **REASONS FOR IMPROPER TREATMENT APPLICATION**

REASON	EXAMPLES
Incorrect dosage	Not giving the prescribed dose
	Improperly diluting topical products
	Adding to food bowl, resulting in incomplete intake
Interactions with other substances	Giving drugs with food that should be given on an empty stomach
Incorrect frequency	Giving TID drugs with breakfast, lunch, and dinner and not closer to q8h
Improper duration	Not leaving shampoo on long enough
Failure to apply the proper site	Dipping for scabies but not treating the ears and face
Application that does not reach the skin	Failing to have dip penetrate the haircoat
	Not shaving the hair in thick-coated long-haired pets
Failure to understand the application method	Rinsing dips out of the haircoat

agents. Often, the best management of a dermatologic disease, particularly a chronic one, is a therapeutic regimen or plan that entails the use of multiple products. This makes education of the client more difficult and time-consuming as well as potentially more confusing. Despite these problems, the best long-term control is often achieved by using such a plan versus a single medicament.

Particularly with chronic skin problems, the education of the client regarding their pet's disease becomes critical. Over the life of the pet, many different therapies may be required and changes in the disease or secondary manifestations are likely. The client needs to be educated about the likely course of the disease as well as the need for follow-up and therapeutic modifications. The importance of maintenance therapy must be emphasized.

• TOPICAL THERAPY

Topical therapy has always played a large role in dermatology because of the obvious access to the affected tissue.[9, 88, 156, 158, 162, 172, 218] In the past, topical therapy was used for treating localized lesions and ectoparasite infestations. In the last 15 years, topical applications have become even more prominent and continue to flourish in treating skin disease. Undoubtedly, this growth in topical therapy reflects multiple factors, which may include (1) the development of more products, better delivery systems, and active ingredients, (2) the reduction in systemic absorption or effects and adverse reactions, and (3) the recognition of the adjunctive and synergistic effects in the overall management of numerous skin diseases. These factors are also the advantages that topical therapy offers to the clinician and the pet owner.

There are disadvantages, however. In general, topical therapy is much more time-consuming and labor-intensive than systemic therapy. Understanding the proper use and application of topical therapy is also important, and therefore client education and client compliance become harder to achieve. Localized adverse reactions not seen with systemic therapy may occur, most commonly irritant reactions.

Topical therapy is often adjunctive, and it may significantly increase the cost of the overall therapeutic plan. Some topical agents may be so costly that their use is limited to localized lesions. On the other hand, appropriate topical therapy may greatly reduce the need for systemic therapy. The clinician needs to consider the potential benefits and disadvantages, the client's preferences, and the patient's needs when deciding on the use of topical therapy.

When a clinician elects to use topical therapy, several factors must be considered. First and foremost is, What is the purpose or desired result of the topical therapy? Is this the sole therapy, or is it adjunctive to other nontopical therapies? What type of delivery system best facilitates obtaining the desired result? What active ingredients are used for this purpose? As previously discussed, patient and client considerations are paramount. Table 3–2 lists the most common delivery systems and formulations of active ingredients used in veterinary dermatology. The amount of use for each type of product relative to the others is based solely on our opinions and clinical impressions.

Factors That Influence Drug Effects on the Skin

Topical medications consist of active ingredients incorporated in a vehicle that facilitates application to the skin. In selecting a vehicle, one must consider the solubility of the drug in the vehicle, the rate of release from the vehicle, the ability of the vehicle to hydrate the stratum corneum, the stability of the active agent in the vehicle, and the interactions (chemical and physical) among the vehicle, the active agent, and the stratum corneum. The vehicle is not always inert and many have important therapeutic effects.

When topical medications are used, one basic question is whether the drug penetrates the skin and, if so, how deeply. Absorption varies highly, and most drugs penetrate only 1% to 2% after 16 to 24 hours.[8, 54] However, even in the same vehicle, similar drugs may

● Table 3–2 TOPICAL FORMULATIONS AND RELATIVE EFFICACY OF INCORPORATED ACTIVE AGENTS

TOPICAL FORMULATIONS	ASTRINGENT	EMOLLIENT	ANTISEBORRHEIC	ANTIPRURITIC	ANTIBACTERIAL	ANTIMYCOTIC	ANTIPARASITIC	ANTI-INFLAMMATORY	ULTRAVIOLET SCREEN
Shampoo	X	XX	XXX	XX	XXX	X	XX	X	—
Rinse	X	XXX	—	XX	X	XXX	XXX	X	—
Leave on conditioners	—	XXX	—	XXX	XXX	XX	—	X	—
Powder	—	—	—	X	X	?	X	X	—
Lotion	XXX	X	X	XXX	XX	XX	—	XXX	X
Spray	XX	XXX	XX	XXX	X	X	XXX	XX	XXX
Cream or ointment	—	X	X	XX	XXX	X	—	XXX	XXX
Gels	—	—	X	—	XX	X	—	—	—

Relative use based on author's opinions and clinical impressions.
— = not used; X = infrequently used or use associated with lower efficacy; XX = occasionally used; XXX = commonly used and efficacious.

vary dramatically in their absorption.[53] This was exemplified in a study with three organophosphate insecticides applied topically in three different vehicles.[70] With only one organophosphate (parathion) of the three tested, the vehicle dimethyl sulfoxide (DMSO) increased absorption from 4% to 5% up to 15% to 30%. In some cases (e.g., insecticides), the absorbability greatly influences the potential for side effects.

Clinical efficacy and absorption are not synonymous; absorption is only one factor in efficacy. Some drugs in an insoluble form in the vehicle have only a surface effect. Once absorbed, a drug must also interact with specific receptors before an action will result. The drug's affinity for the receptors as well as local factors that effect this drug-receptor interaction are also important.[35] Absorption of drugs through the skin involves many variables. There are physicochemical factors related to the topical formulation and biological factors.[9] The physicochemical factors involve the interactions between the drug and the vehicle, the drug and the skin, and the vehicle and the skin. Some of these factors are determined by the concentration of the drug, the drug's movement between the vehicle and the skin, the diffusion coefficient, and the local pH.

1. The concentration of the drug and its solubility in the vehicle affects absorption. The package label gives the percentage of drug concentration, not the percentage of solubility. In addition to concentration, the solubility of the drug and the solubilizing capacity of the vehicle affect drug absorption. In general, poor solubility and excessive solubilizing capacity decrease the rate of absorption.[9] Usually, ointment vehicles for topical corticosteroids increase solubility and drug delivery, so systemic effects after topical use are more common—and potentially dangerous.
2. The drug must move from the vehicle through the skin barrier to be effective. The solubility of the drug in the horny layer relative to its solubility in the vehicle is described by the partition coefficient. The concentration of the drug in the barrier, not in the vehicle, is what determines the diffusion force. Increased lipid solubility favors drug penetration because the stratum corneum is lipophilic.
3. The diffusion coefficient is a measure of the extent to which the barrier interferes with the drug's mobility. The stratum corneum is unsurpassed as an unfavorable environment for drug penetration. Physical disruption of the epidermal barrier by the use of lipid solvents, keratolytic agents, or cellulose-tape stripping of the top layers of cells increases the potential for absorption. In some cases, the vehicle itself may be able to diffuse through the stratum corneum and carries any dissolved drug with it. DMSO facilitates cutaneous penetration of some substances. Moisture and occlusive dressings enhance percutaneous absorption as well. Large molecular size results in poor mobility and poor absorption.
4. The pH of the drug's local environment may also affect absorption by altering the amount of drug in its unionized form. Many drugs are either weak acids or bases and occur in an ionized and unionized form. In general, the unionized form is more readily absorbed; this amount may change as the local pH is altered.[16]

The active ingredient of the drug may interact with all other components in the formulation. In practice, the addition of other ingredients or the mixing of ingredients on the skin such as ear cleanser followed by an ear treatment may alter the drug's effect. Drug effects may be altered by interactions between the drug and the new drug or its vehicle, or by interactions between the new drug or vehicle and the original vehicle. Changes that may occur include inactivation of the drug by chemical bonding or precipitation, changes in pH, allowing decomposition of the drugs by altering the stabilizing effects of the vehicle, and altering the concentration of the drug. We have seen cases in which 1% miconazole lotion is mixed in equal amounts with another ear product and fails to eliminate *Malassezia* from an ear canal. The unaltered 1% miconazole is then used alone and is effective.

Temperature and hydration of the skin can affect the interaction among the drug, the vehicle, and the skin. Hydration probably plays a greater role than temperature in affecting absorption. In general, permeability to drugs increases as the hydration of the stratum corneum increases.[8, 9]

Biological factors also affect drug absorption. The body region treated greatly influences absorption. In humans, the amount of hydrocortisone being absorbed varied tremendously, in descending order, on the scrotum, the forehead, the forearm, and the plantar foot.[54] Age is an important factor, with newborns experiencing greater absorption than adolescents, who experience greater absorption than adults. Obviously, the health and condition of the skin is important because inflamed, abraded, or otherwise damaged skin often absorbs more drug. Blood flow also affects absorption. Greater blood flow favors increased systemic absorption.

Hydrotherapy

Water is often overlooked as a therapeutic agent, especially when it is applied with a shampoo, as a rinse, or as a component of many lotions. Hydrotherapy may be used to moisten the stratum corneum, to dry out the epidermis, to cool or heat the skin, to soften surface crusts, and to clean the skin. Increased effects occur by adding other agents (topical active agents, see p. 226).

Water may be applied as a wet dressing or in baths. Frequent periodic renewal of wet dressings (15 minutes on, several hours off) prolongs the effect, but if more continuous therapy or occlusive coverings are used, the skin becomes overly moistened, the skin temperature rises, and undesirable maceration occurs. This is less likely if the wet dressings are left open.

Hydrotherapy can hydrate or dehydrate the skin, depending on how it is managed. The application of loose, damp gauze compresses for 15 minutes and then removal for 1 hour promote evaporation of water from the gauze and from the subadjacent skin surface and are drying to the underlying tissues. If water is maintained on the skin surface constantly by wet towels, soaks, or baths, the skin hydrates as water is taken up by keratin and hair. If a film of oil is applied immediately after soaking (occlusive rinses), evaporation of water (transpiration) is hindered and the skin retains moisture.

The water may be cool or above body temperature. Whirlpool baths, with or without detergents and antiseptics added, make gentle, effective cleaning possible. These treatments may be used to remove crusts and scales, to clean wounds and fistulae, to rehydrate skin, to reduce pain and pruritus, and to provide prophylaxis for patients prone to decubital problems, urine scalds, and other ills. Ten to 15 minutes of therapy once or twice daily is adequate. The patients should be toweled and placed in an air stream drier to dry. Other topical medications can be applied later, if needed.

In hydrotherapy, moisture is the specific agent, and various additives change its actions only slightly but add their own effects. Astringents, antipruritics, moisturizers, parasiticides, and antibiotics are common additives. In general, water treatment removes crusts, bacteria, and other debris and greatly reduces the possibility of secondary infection. It promotes epithelialization and allays the symptoms of pain and burning. Cool water is antipruritic. It also softens keratin. The suppleness and softness of the skin are due to its water content, not to the oils on the surface.[172] Dryness of the skin is recognized when any one of the following is present: roughness of the surface, scaliness, inflexibility of the horny layer, and fissuring with possible inflammation.

Normal skin is not a waterproof covering but is constantly losing water to the environment by transpiration. This loss depends on body temperature, environmental temperature, and relative humidity. The stratum corneum, composed of corneocytes and an intercellular matrix lipid bilayer, is the major deterrent to water loss. The lipids of this layer are derived from phospholipids and lipids secreted by the keratinocytes as they migrate to the stratum corneum and from sebum. Dry skin may result from excessive transpiration of water.

Sebum on the skin or externally applied lipid films tend to make the surface feel smoother. The flexibility of keratin is directly related to its moisture content. The amount of water that the horny layer receives from the epidermis and the transepidermal loss are major factors determining moisture content. The transepidermal loss from the stratum corneum partially depends on the environment, especially the relative humidity. Water content of the horny layer can be increased by applying occlusive dressings or agents to prevent loss, by adding water with baths or wet dressings, or by using hygroscopic medications to attract water.

Topical Formulations

Active medications may be applied to the skin by a variety of delivery systems. These different delivery systems include, but are not limited to, the following formulations: shampoos; rinses; powders; lotions; sprays; creams, emulsions, and ointments; and gels. Each type of formulation has advantages and disadvantages that the clinician should consider when selecting a topical medication. Besides incorporating active ingredients, each type of formulation contains ingredients that act as the vehicle for delivering the active agents. These vehicles may also have certain therapeutic, irritant, or cosmetic effects, making the overall formulation more or less desirable.

In general, vehicles contain ingredients to adjust the pH, stabilize the active agents, prolong the effects of the active ingredients, promote the delivery of the active agents to the skin surface or into or through the stratum corneum, and make the product cosmetically pleasing (e.g., fragrance). The selection of the topical formulation depends on a variety of factors, most notably the surface area to be treated, the need for residual activity, the presence of hair in the area to be treated, and the nature of the lesion (e.g., moist or dry).

The active ingredients are often available in a variety of different formulations and delivery systems. In general, they have the same basic activity regardless of the formulation, but their ease of use, cost, and efficacy for the desired purpose are affected by the formulation and the method of application. The following categories of active agents are used: astringents, or drying agents; emollients and moisturizers; antiseborrheics; antipruritics; antibacterials; antifungals; antiparasitics; anti-inflammatory agents; and ultraviolet screens. The following discussion describes first the different delivery systems and then the types of active ingredients.

SHAMPOOS

Medicated shampoos contain additional ingredients that enhance or add other actions to that of the shampoo.[218] With most shampoo formulations, the active drugs have a limited contact time because they are removed during the rinsing of the shampoo base. Some medicaments may have enough opportunity for effect or for limited absorption during a prolonged shampoo, and their addition may be justified (e.g., insecticides, salicylic acid, sulfur, tar, and antiseptics). Medicated shampoos are valuable in that they may be used for diseases involving large areas of the body or localized lesions.

Newer formulations of shampoos have been developed that utilize sustained-release microvesicle technology. In one, the microvesicles have an outer lipid membrane and contain water (Novasomes, EVSCO). The lipid membrane binds to hair and skin and has a long-term moisturizing effect as the microvesicles break down (Fig. 3–1A and B). This counteracts the drying that may occur with some medications and is therapeutic for dry skin. However, the active medication is not incorporated and will still be rinsed away.

The second microvesicle technology (Spherulites, Virbac) actually incorporates different ingredients, such as salicylic acid and sulfur, chlorhexidine, ethyl lactate, benzalkonium chloride, oatmeal extract, glycerin, and urea, into multiple layers of these microvesicles. Also, these microvesicles have multiple (10 to 1000) layers that slowly break down (Fig. 3–1C). With the breakdown of each layer, the active ingredients and the surfactants that make up these layers are released onto the hair and skin. The microvesicles can be made with different charges on the exterior, and by making them positively charged they bind with the negatively charged hair and skin (Fig 3–1D). Chitosanide has been used to make the microvesicles called *spherulites*. Besides supplying the outer cationic surface, chitosanide is an active moisturizing agent and is hygroscopic.

Efficacy is determined by proper use as well as active ingredients. It is imperative

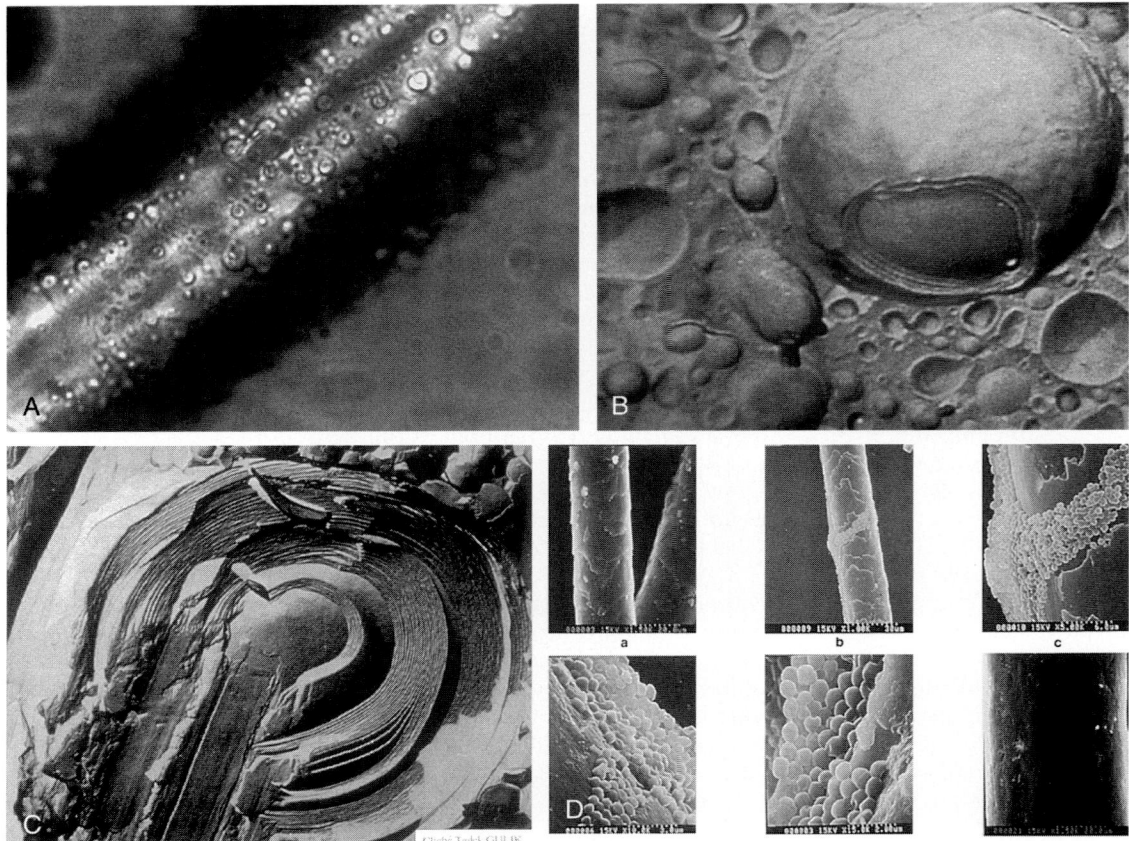

FIGURE 3–1. *A*, Novasome attached to canine hair shaft. *B*, Scanning electron micrograph of a novasome showing the multiple layers and large cargo hold. *C*, Scanning electron micrograph of a spherulite showing the multiple layers. *D*, Scanning electron micrographs showing spherulites attached to hair shafts. (Figures courtesy EVSCO and Virbac.)

that products be applied properly, left on for sufficient contact time, and then properly rinsed. Education of the client regarding their use is an important element and time well spent. The client should be instructed to use a clock to determine the correct contact time because subjective assessments are often inadequate. Contact time starts after the shampoo is applied, not when the bath begins. More severely affected regions should be the first areas to be shampooed. Sometimes, problem areas benefit from a second lathering before the final rinse.

Pharmaceutical companies provide a multitude of medicated shampoos, which often have specific indications and contraindications. It is important to become familiar with a few (perhaps one of each type) and to thoroughly understand the ingredients and their concentration and actions. Choosing the mildest or most client-pleasing shampoo that produces the desired actions often increases compliance. Strong shampoos can be harmful as well as helpful.

The clinician must evaluate the whole animal when selecting active ingredients, and some animals may benefit from the simultaneous use of different products. Although one shampoo may be recommended for the whole body, another shampoo may be applied to a more localized region. The case of an Irish setter with idiopathic seborrhea with truncal scaling, dry coat, and localized patches of comedones with pyoderma and alopecia on the ventral chest is an example. A topical antiseborrheic containing sulfur and salicylic acid may be preferred for most of the body but may not be potent enough for the ventral region. A benzoyl peroxide shampoo may be used on just the ventral thorax because of its superior antibacterial and follicular flushing effect.

Certain principles should be kept in mind when using medicated shampoos:

1. *Clipping the haircoat.* Clipping the haircoat and keeping the haircoat short may be critical to the proper use and maximal benefit of the product.
2. *Premedicated shampoo bathing.* It is often a good idea to remove grease, debris, and dirt with a nonmedicated shampoo, such as baby shampoo, or a dishwashing detergent. In this way, the medicated shampoo is better able to contact the skin, less product is used, and less expense is incurred.
3. *Contact time.* The shampoo should be allowed to remain in contact with the skin for 10 to 15 minutes. This allows the active ingredients to be effective and allows for the hydration of the stratum corneum. This time should be counted from the time lathering is finished and, for some owners, may be best measured with an actual timer.
4. *Explanation/demonstration.* It is important to explain, and perhaps demonstrate, the entire process of shampooing. This incudes application *and* removal of the product.

Medicated shampoos are often classified on the basis of their primary activity or function.

1. Emollients and moisturizers are often present in hypoallergenic shampoos and many better-quality cleansing shampoos for normal skin and haircoat. They are used when pets will be bathed frequently (weekly or more often) or for pets with slightly dry or scaly haircoats. Ingredients that moisturize are fatty acids and lipids, urea, glycerin, colloidal oatmeal, and chitosanide.
2. Antiparasitic shampoos are commonly used, but they are generally not as efficacious as antiparasitic rinses (see Chap. 6). Their main use is for quick removal of fleas in puppies, kittens, and debilitated animals. They are often ineffective for adequate long-term flea control. The most common ingredients are pyrethrins and synthetic pyrethroids.
3. Antiseborrheic shampoos usually contain salicylic acid, sulfur, tar, and selenium sulfide in various combinations and strengths. They are indicated in keratinization defects (for details, see Chap. 14). They are also indicated in any other disorder associated with excessive scaling of the skin.
4. Antibacterial shampoos contain disinfectants or antibiotics such as chlorhexidine, benzoyl peroxide, iodine, ethyl lactate, benzalkonium chloride, triclosan, and sulfur. Other ingredients with less effect include quaternary ammonium compounds and phenols (both not to be used in cats), alcohols, and parabens. These products are indicated whenever there is superficial bacterial infection (see Chap. 4 for discussions of their specific use). A common indication for long-term use is in the allergic dog that is still prone to recurrent folliculitis even though the pruritus is controlled with the allergy therapy. In these situations, nonirritating, nondrying shampoos with antibacterial agents are often beneficial if used regularly.
5. Antimycotic shampoos contain disinfectants or antifungal agents such as chlorhexidine, sulfur, selenium sulfide, miconazole, and ketoconazole (see Chap. 5). They are used mainly as adjunctive therapy for dermatophytosis (to achieve a quick decrease of contagion) and *Malassezia* dermatitis. They are not effective in treating dermatophytosis.[42] They have been recommended as sole therapy for *Malassezia* dermatitis.[110] They may be used alone, as adjunctive therapy, or as a preventive to decrease the recurrence rate. A product that combines two active ingredients (2% chlorhexidine and 2% miconazole) has been reported to have increased efficacy as a sole therapy.[111]
6. Antipruritic or anti-inflammatory agents, such as 1% hydrocortisone, 0.01% fluocinolone, 2% diphenhydramine, 1% pramoxine, colloidal oatmeal, and moisturizers, are found in a variety of shampoo formulations (see Chap. 8). In general, they are

adjunctive treatments and are not effective as the sole therapy unless they are used every 1 to 2 days. This high frequency of use is usually not acceptable to owners. The topical fluocinolone shampoos have been shown not to be systemically absorbed in the dog.[10, 191] Controlled studies of their efficacy are lacking.

RINSES

Rinses are made by mixing concentrated solutions or soluble powders with water. They are usually poured, sponged, or sprayed onto the animal's body. Similar to the case with shampoos, they may be used to treat large areas of the body. Rinses are generally a cost-effective and efficacious method to deliver topical active ingredients such as moisturizers, antipruritic agents, parasiticides, and antifungal agents.

Rinses that dry on the pet's skin leave a residual layer of active ingredients and therefore have more prolonged effects than application by shampoo therapy. Rinses are often used after a medicated or cleaning shampoo. If the active ingredient to be applied is lipid dispersed, shampooing may remove the normal surface lipids and decrease the longevity of the active ingredients. In these situations, adding a small amount of safflower oil or lipid-containing moisturizer may help to prolong the effect. This is most commonly recommended for lipid-soluble (petroleum distillate–based) parasiticidal agents.

Rinses are our preferred method of delivery for most topical medications other than antibacterials and antiseborrheics, which require whole-body coverage.

POWDERS

Powders are pulverized organic or inorganic solids that are applied to the skin in a thin film. In some cases, they are made to be added to water for use as a rinse, to liquids to form "shake lotions," or to ointments to form pastes. Some powders (talc, starch, zinc oxide) are inert and have a physical effect; other powders (sulfur) are active ingredients that have a chemical or antimicrobial effect. Powders are used to dry the skin and to cool and lubricate intertriginous areas. Most often, powders are used with parasiticidal agents (flea powders) and locally with anti-inflammatory agents (Neo-Predef powder, Pharmacia & Upjohn). Some powders may contain antimicrobials for use on localized lesions and, although not yet available in the United States, an enilconazole powder has shown promise for the treatment of dermatophytosis.

The affected skin should be cleaned and dried before the powder is applied. Powder buildup or caking should be avoided, but if it occurs, wet compresses or soaks can gently remove the excess. On long-coated animals, a fine powder is used as a retention vehicle for insecticides and fungicides. Powders dry the coat and skin and may accumulate in the environment, making them less desirable for whole-body use. Some owners find powders irritating to their own respiratory mucosa. We use powders infrequently and prefer other delivery systems.

LOTIONS

Lotions are liquids in which medicinal agents are dissolved or suspended. Some are essentially liquid powders because a thin film of powder is left on the skin when the liquid evaporates. Lotions tend to be more drying (because of their water or alcohol base) than liniments, which have an oily base. Newer lotions tend to use more propylene glycol and water with less or no alcohol. Drying, cooling lotions contain alcohol, whereas soothing, moisturizing lotions usually do not. These medications tend to be cooling, antipruritic, and drying (depending on the base).

Lotions are vehicles for active ingredients such as 1% hydrocortisone with aluminum acetate (Hydro-B 1020, Butler; Hydro-Plus, Phoenix), 0.1% betamethasone valerate (Betatrex, Savage), 1% hydrocortisone (Curticalm, DVM), 1% pramoxine (Relief, DVM), 1% diphenhydramine with calamine and camphor (Caladryl, Parke-Davis), malaleuca, and aloe vera. The liquid preparations can be applied repeatedly, but they should not be allowed to build up. In general, lotions are indicated for acute oozing dermatoses and are contraindicated in dry, chronic conditions. They are most often used to deliver localized treatment with astringents and antipruritic, anti-inflammatory, and antifungal agents. They occasionally carry ultraviolet screens and antiseborrheic agents.

SPRAYS

A variety of topical lotions are available in pump spray bottles. Most commonly, they are used when relatively larger body areas are to be treated and when the product needs to be applied to only the haircoat or small, nonhaired areas. Rinses may also be applied by pump spray bottles, but if skin contact is needed, thorough soaking through the haircoat is required. Sprays are most commonly used with emollients or moisturizers that are lightly applied and then rubbed into the coat, antiparasitic agents (particularly those with repellent activity), and antipruritic agents for local lesions. Newer sprays have antimicrobial activity such as 4% chlorhexidine.

Antipruritic sprays contain agents such as 1% hydrocortisone (Cortispray, DVM), 2% diphenhydramine (Histacalm, Virbac), 1% pramoxine (Relief, DVM; Dermal Soothe, EVSCO), hamamelis extract with menthol (Dermacool, Virbac), and tar (LyTar, DVM). Sprays are also frequently used to apply astringents and anti-inflammatory agents, such as 1% hydrocortisone with aluminum acetate. Occasionally, sprays are used for antifungal agents and the application of ultraviolet screens to the inguinal region. Sprays are valuable for local application to interdigital webs, ventral paws, and concave pinnae.

CREAMS, EMULSIONS, AND OINTMENTS

Creams and ointments lubricate and smooth skin that is roughened. They form a protective covering that reduces contact with the environment. Certain occlusive types may reduce water loss. They also transport medicinal agents into follicular orifices and keep drugs in intimate contact with the horny layer. Creams and ointments are mixtures of grease or oil and water that are emulsified with high-speed blenders. Emulsifiers, coloring agents, and perfumes are added to improve the physical characteristics of the product. Pastes are highly viscous ointments into which large amounts of powder are incorporated. Although pastes may be tolerated on slightly exudative skin (the powder takes up water), in general, creams and ointments are contraindicated in oozing areas.

A wide variation in characteristics of the products is determined by the relative amount and melting point of the oils used. This can be illustrated by comparing cold cream and vanishing cream. Cold cream is mostly oil with a little water. The oils have a low melting point, so when the water evaporates a thick, greasy film is left on the skin. A vanishing cream, on the other hand, is mostly water with oils that have a high melting point. When the water evaporates, a thin film of fat is left on the skin. This waxlike film does not feel greasy. Urea added to creams also decreases the greasy feel and, as a hygroscopic agent, helps to moisturize the stratum corneum.

Emulsions are oily or fatty substances that have been dispersed in water. As a group, they have a composition between that of lotions and ointments. Emulsions are thicker than lotions but thinner than ointments. They are similar to creams, which for the most part have replaced the use of emulsions in small animal practice. Emulsions are of two types: oil dispersed in water and water dispersed in oil. Although both types are used as vehicles, the former dilutes with water, loses water rapidly, and therefore is cooling. The latter type dilutes with oil and loses its water slowly. In both cases, after the water evaporates, the action of the vehicle on the skin is no different from that of the oil and emulsifying agent alone. Thus, the characteristics of the residual film are those of the oily phase of the vehicle.

These bases are commonly used as vehicles for other agents. They have the advantage of easy application, give mechanical protection, and are soothing, antipruritic, and softening. The more oily creams and ointments tend to be occlusive, which facilitates hydration of the stratum corneum and often increases penetration of incorporated active ingredients.

The disadvantage of their use in the hairy skin of animals is that they are occlusive, greasy, heat-retaining, and messy, and they may produce a folliculitis because of occlusion of pilosebaceous orifices. These types of medication should be applied with gentle massage several times daily to maintain a thin film on the skin. Thick films are wasteful, occlusive, and messy to surroundings. An obvious film of ointment left on the skin surface means that too much has been applied.

Water-washable ointment bases such as polyethylene glycol (Carbowax 1500) can be readily removed with water. Oily bases are not freely water washable. It is important for the clinician to understand the uses and advantages of these types of bases because the total effect on the skin is caused by the vehicle as well as its active ingredient.

Hydrophobic oils (e.g., mineral oil and sesame oil) mix poorly with water. They contain few polar groups (—OH, —COOH, and so on). These oils contact the skin, spread easily, and are often incorporated into emulsion-type vehicles. Because they are hydrophobic, it is difficult for water to pass through a film of these oils, and they are occlusive. They retain heat and water, and thick films of the more viscid forms are messy and may get on articles in contact with the pet.

Hydrophilic oils are miscible with water. They contain many polar groups, and those oils with the greatest number are most soluble in water. Although they are ointments only in terms of their physical characteristics, the polyethylene glycols are alcohols that are readily miscible with water. Polymers with a molecular weight greater than 1000 are solid at room temperature, but a slight rise in body temperature causes melting to form an oily film. (Carbowax 1500 is such a product.) It mixes with skin exudates well, is easily washed off with water, and is less occlusive than other bases.

The use of creams, emulsions, and ointments is limited to localized, relatively small lesions. Most commonly, they are used with antimicrobial, anti-inflammatory, and ultraviolet radiation–blocking agents. They are often the most efficacious delivery system for areas needing moisturization or keratolytic effects, but their application is usually limited to localized areas such as nasal planum, paws, and elbows.

GELS

Gels are topical formulations composed of combinations of propylene glycol, propylene gallate, disodiumethylenediamine tetra-acetate, and carboxypolymethylene, with additives to adjust the pH. They act as a clear, colorless, thixotropic base and are greaseless and water-miscible. The active ingredients incorporated in commercially used bases of this type are completely in solution.

Gels are being more widely used because, despite their oily appearance, they can be rubbed into the skin completely and do not leave the skin with a sticky feeling. Gels are relatively preferable to creams and ointments because they pass through the haircoat to the skin and are not messy. Most commonly, they are used for localized lesions for which antimicrobial or antiseborrheic effects are desired.

The most common ingredient is benzoyl peroxide for areas of bacterial pyoderma and follicular hyperkeratosis (such as acne) or areas of comedones. (Examples of gels used in veterinary medicine with benzoyl peroxide are OxyDex, DVM; Pyoben, Virbac). However, because they are cosmetically tolerated better than creams and ointments, their use is expanding to include virtually any ingredient that can be stabilized in a gel form. KeraSolv (DVM) is a keratolytic, humectant gel for hyperkeratotic conditions such as nasal hyperkeratosis.

Topical Active Agents

ASTRINGENTS

Astringents precipitate proteins and generally do not penetrate deeply. These agents are drying and decrease exudations. They are indicated in acute, subacute, and some chronic exudative dermatoses.

Vegetable astringents include tannins from oak trees, sumac, or blackberries. They are especially recommended for more potent action. Tan Sal (Tanni-Gel, Vet-A-Mix—4% tannic acid, 4% salicylic acid, and 1% benzocaine in 70% alcohol) is a potent astringent and should not be used more than once on the same lesion (it may cause irritation or sloughing). Witch hazel (hamamelis) contains tannins that are astringent and anti-inflammatory and that decrease bleeding.

Aluminum acetate solution (Burow's solution) is available commercially as Domeboro (Bayer). It is drying, astringent, antipruritic, acidifying, and mildly antiseptic. The solution is usually diluted 1:40 in cool water, and soaks are repeated three times daily for 30 minutes. (One packet of powder, or one tablet, is added to 0.5 L [1 pt] or 1 L [1 qt] of water.) It is tolerated better than tannins and does not stain. It tends to be used more frequently than other astringents.

Acetic acid in a 0.25% to 0.5% solution (e.g., 1 part vinegar with 9 parts water) is also an effective astringent, acidifying, and drying agent.

Silver nitrate 0.25% solution may be applied to moist, weeping, denuded areas as an antiseptic, coagulant, and stimulating agent. It should be used frequently and sparingly. It stains the skin.

Potassium permanganate 1:1000 to 1:30,000 solution (1-grain tablet or 5 ml [1 tsp] to 15 ml [1 tbsp] of crystals per 1 L [1 qt] of water) may be applied in fresh preparations for soaks or irrigations. It is astringent, antiseptic, and antimicrobial and toughens and stains the skin.

EMOLLIENTS AND MOISTURIZERS

Emollients are agents that soften, lubricate, or soothe the skin; moisturizers increase the water content of the stratum corneum. Both types of drugs are useful in hydrating and softening the skin. Demulcents are high-molecular substances in aqueous solution that coat and protect the skin (e.g., glycerin, propylene glycol).

Many of the occlusive emollients are actually oils (safflower, sesame, and mineral oil) or contain lanolin. These emollients decrease transepidermal water loss and cause moisturization. These agents work best if applied immediately after saturation of the stratum corneum with water. For maximal softening, the skin should be hydrated in wet dressings, dried, and covered with an occlusive hydrophobic oil. The barrier to water loss can be further strengthened by covering the local lesion with plastic wrap under a bandage. Nonocclusive emollients are relatively ineffective in retaining moisture.

1. Vegetable oils—olive, cottonseed, corn, and peanut oil
2. Animal oils—lard, whale oil, anhydrous lanolin (wool fat), and lanolin with 25% to 30% water (hydrous wool fat)
3. Hydrocarbons—paraffin and petrolatum (mineral oil)
4. Waxes—white wax (bleached beeswax), yellow wax (beeswax), and spermaceti

Hygroscopic agents (humectants) are moisturizers that work by being incorporated into the stratum corneum and attracting water. These agents, such as propylene glycol, glycerin, colloidal oatmeal, urea, sodium lactate, carboxylic acid, and lactic acid, may also be applied between baths. Both occlusive and hygroscopic agents are found in a variety of veterinary spray and rinse formulations, which are more effective than shampoo bases. A liposome-based humectant technology (Hydra-Pearls cream rinse, Evsco) was shown to be superior to a traditional humectant emollient (Humilac, Virbac) for the treatment of dry skin in dogs.[169]

ANTISEBORRHEICS

The seborrheic complex comprises important and somewhat common skin diseases, such as primary seborrhea (in Cocker and Springer spaniels, Irish setters, and Doberman pinschers), secondary seborrhea (accompanying atopy, scabies, and demodicosis), Schnauzer comedo syndrome, and tail gland hyperplasia.[91] Topical antiseborrheic therapy is the primary mode of treatment for these diseases. Other primary scaling disorders such as sebaceous adenitis, vitamin A-responsive dermatosis, and some follicular dysplasias may benefit from adjunctive therapy with antiseborrheics, which speed the response to the primary treatment.

Antiseborrheics can be applied as ointments, creams, gels, and lotions, but the most popular form for hairy skin is the antiseborrheic shampoo or the humectant rinse. Antiseborrheics are commercially available in various combinations. The clinician must decide which combination of drugs to use and needs to know each drug's actions and concentrations. Ideal therapeutic response depends on the correct choice, but individual patient variation does occur. For dry and scaly seborrhea (seborrhea sicca), a different preparation is needed than for oily and greasy seborrhea (seborrhea oleosa). Emollients, for instance, are useful in dry seborrhea but are not good degreasers. Benzoyl peroxide, on the other hand, degreases well but can be too keratolytic and drying for dry, brittle skin (see Chap. 14 for details).

ANTIPRURITICS

Antipruritic agents attempt to provide temporary relief from itching but are not usually satisfactory as sole therapy because of their short duration of effect. Pruritus is a symptom of many diseases, and most antipruritic topical therapies are directed at the sensation, not the cause. As such, they are still useful symptomatic treatments while waiting to alleviate the primary disease or when the cause cannot be determined. As adjunctive therapy or for small localized areas of pruritus, they can be more beneficial. Some antipruritic agents listed here have other actions and are discussed elsewhere in this chapter. Table 3-3 lists some veterinary nonsteroidal, topical, antipruritic agents. In general, antipruritics give relief from itching by means of six methods:

1. Decreasing the pruritic load by depleting, removing, or inactivating pruritic mediators. For example, astringents denature proteins and high-potency corticosteroids deplete cutaneous mast cells. Shampoos or cleaners can also remove surface irritants, bacteria, pruritogenic substances, and allergens that are on the surface of the skin waiting to be absorbed and to contribute to the pruritic load.
2. Substituting some other sensation, such as heat and cold, for the itch. This may also help by raising the pruritic threshold. Heat initially lowers the pruritic threshold, but if the heat is high enough and is applied for a sufficient duration, the increased itching or burning sensation abates and induces a short-term antipruritic effect. Cooling tends to decrease pruritus. Examples of such agents are menthol 0.12% to 1%, camphor 0.12% to 5%, thymol 0.5% to 1%, heat (warm soaks or baths), and cold (ice packs) or cool wet dressings.
3. Protecting the skin from external influences such as scratching, biting, trauma, temperature changes, humidity changes, pressure, and irritants. This can be done with bandages or any impermeable protective agents.
4. Anesthetizing the peripheral nerves by using local anesthetics such as pramoxine, benzocaine, tetracaine, lidocaine, benzoyl peroxide, and tars. These products generally have short actions, and in cases of chronic pruritus, resistance often occurs. Pramoxine has antipruritic effects that appear to be from a mechanism other than its anesthetic effect.[219] Pramoxine has also been added to hydrocortisone for additive antipruritic effects in people and in veterinary medicine is available with colloidal oatmeal (Relief shampoo and creme rinse, DVM; Dermal Soothe shampoo and cream rinse, EVSCO; Resiprox leave on lotion, Virbac).
5. Raising the pruritic threshold by cooling or moisturizing the skin. Dry skin lowers the pruritic threshold, and the effective use of emollients and moisturizing agents, such as fatty acids, glycerin, urea, and colloidal oatmeal, partially alleviates pruritus by reducing the dry skin.
6. Using specific biochemical agents, such as topical glucocorticoids, antihistamines, and moisturizers.

Table 3-3 USEFUL NONSTEROIDAL TOPICAL AGENTS FOR PRURITIC DOGS AND CATS

PRODUCT	ACTIVE INGREDIENTS OR ACTION	FORM	MANUFACTURER
Spot Application			
Caladryl	1% diphenhydramine hydrochloride, 8% calamine, camphor	Lotion	Parke-Davis
Dermacool	*Hamamelis* extract, menthol	Spray	Virbac
Domeboro	Aluminum sulfate, calcium acetate	Soak	Miles
Histacalm	2% diphenhydramine	Spray	Virbac
Ice	Water—cold	Pack	Nature!
PTD Lotion	2% benzoyl alcohol, 0.05% benzalkonium chloride, *Hamamelis* distillate	Lotion	Veterinary Prescription
Relief, Dermal Soothe, Resiprox	1% pramoxine	Spray, lotion	DVM, EVSCO, Virbac
Total Body Application			
Allergroom	Moisturizing, hypoallergenic	Shampoo	Virbac
Hy-Lyt°efa	Moisturizing, hypoallergenic	Shampoo	DVM
Epi-Soothe	Colloidal oatmeal	Shampoo	Virbac
Histacalm	2% diphenhydramine	Shampoo	Virbac
Hydra-Pearls cream rinse	Humectant, hypoallergenic	Rinse	EVSCO
Hy-Lyt°efa	Moisturizing, hypoallergenic	Rinse	DVM
Water	Water	Soak	Nature!
Aveeno	Colloidal oatmeal	Soak	Rydelle
Epi-Soothe	Colloidal oatmeal	Soak	Virbac
Relief, Dermal Soothe, Resiprox	1% pramoxine	Shampoo, rinse	DVM, EVSCO, Virbac

Most potent glucocorticoids, administered systemically and topically, are helpful because of their anti-inflammatory effect, but they are not without risk (see p. 232).[182] Hydrocortisone 0.5% to 2% is safest for topical use and could be considered an antipruritic agent because it has mild anti-inflammatory effects at these concentrations. The fluorinated corticosteroids are more potent and penetrate better but with greater risk of systemic absorption and both local or systemic adverse effects. Antihistamines administered systemically are occasionally useful, but when applied topically, they have even less efficacy. They may be helpful as a component of a combination product, such as 1% diphenhydramine with calamine and camphor (Caladryl, Parke-Davis). Some topical antihistamines were shown to cross the stratum corneum and may exert their antihistaminic effect after topical application.[12, 77]

Topical anesthetics may be partially effective, but they may be toxic (causing methemoglobinemia) or have sensitizing potentials (phenol 0.5%; tetracaine and lidocaine 0.5%).[40, 216] Also, their duration of effect is short and becomes even less when used frequently and repetitively. Veterinary products with these types of agents are Histacalm shampoo, Resihist leave on lotion, and Histacalm spray (Virbac—2% diphenhydramine); 1% pramoxine shampoos, sprays, rinses, and leave on lotions (DVM, EVSCO, and Virbac); Dermal Soothe shampoo and cream rinse (EVSCO—1% pramoxine); and Dermacool (Virbac—hamamelis extract and menthol).

Cool wet dressings are often helpful, and in general, any volatile agent provides a cooling sensation that might be palliative. This is the basis for using menthol (1%), thymol (1%), and alcohol (70%) in antipruritic medications. In addition, menthol has a specific

Table 3–5 EFFECTS OF GLUCOCORTICOIDS ON ADRENOCORTICAL FUNCTION IN DOGS

DRUG	PROTOCOL	ROUTE OF ADMINISTRATION	DURATION OF SUPPRESSION AFTER TREATMENT STOPPED
Parenteral Administration			
Dexamethasone	0.2 mg/kg once	IV	32 hr
Dexamethasone sodium phosphate	0.1 mg/kg once	IV	<24 hr
Dexamethasone alcohol	1 mg/kg once	IM	48 hr
Dexamethasone 21-isonicotinate	0.1 mg/kg once	IM	10 days
Dexamethasone 21-isonicotinate	1 mg/kg once	IM	4 wk
Methylprednisolone acetate	2.5 mg/kg once	IM	5 wk
Methylprednisolone acetate	4 mg/kg once	IM	9 wk
Methylprednisolone acetate	0.56 mg/kg once	SC	3 wk
Triamcinolone acetonide	0.22 mg/kg once	IM	4 wk
Triamcinolone acetonide	0.22 mg/kg/day for 8 days	PO	2 wk
Topical Administration			
Betamethasone valerate	1.36 mg/kg/day for 5 days	Skin ointment	4 wk
Dexamethasone	0.03 mg/kg/day for 8 wk	Ophthalmic drops	2 wk
Dexamethasone	0.31 mg/kg/day for 3 wk	Otic drops	3 wk
Fluocinonide	0.68 mg/kg/day for 5 days	Skin ointment	4 wk
Prednisolone acetate	0.75 mg/kg/day for 4 wk	Ophthalmic drops	2 wk
Triamcinolone acetonide	1.36 mg/kg/day for 5 days	Skin ointment	4 wk
Triamcinolone acetate	0.31 mg/kg/day for 3 wk	Otic drops	3 wk

IV = intravenously; IM = intramuscularly; SC = subcutaneously; PO = orally.
From Scott DW: Rational use of glucocorticoids in dermatology. In: Bonagura JD, Kirk RW (eds): *Kirk's Current Veterinary Therapy XII*, 1995, p. 578.

ketoconazole shampoo in inhibiting *Microsporum canis* growth from infected cat hairs.[215] Its parasiticidal activity is thought to be due to H_2S and polythionic acid. Lime sulfur is inexpensive and nontoxic (Lym Dyp, DVM). Side effects include occasional excessive drying and/or irritation of the skin. Cosmetic drawbacks include a disagreeable odor (rotten eggs), temporary yellow staining of light haircoats and skins, staining of clothing and other materials, and tarnishing of jewelry.

• **Vitamin A Acid.** A 0.05% concentration of retinoic acid (tretinoin [Retin-A, Roche]) is popular in human dermatology (used for treating acne, decreasing wrinkles, and treating ichthyosis). It is relatively expensive but has been used in dogs and cats for acne and some localized keratinization disorders.[90]

The effectiveness of topical tretinoin for the treatment of the effects of photoaging is well documented. The gel form at 0.01% concentration is initially used because it is less irritating than the 0.025% concentration. It increases the epidermal turnover time, reduces the cohesiveness of keratinocytes, normalizes maturation of follicular epithelium, and is comedolytic.[203] In animal models it prevents corticosteroid-induced skin atrophy.[155] Local irritation is a significant problem for many people and cats (e.g., with Retin-A). A microsphere formulation (Retin-A-MICRO) is now available that irritates much less in humans.

Synthetic retinoids are also becoming available as topical formulations. Adapalene (Differin, Galderma) is a new topical retinoid with specific receptor activity for intranuclear retinoic acid receptors and causes less irritation than retinoic acid. It also inhibits neutrophil activation and lipoxygenase enzymes.[175, 204] Tazarotene (Tazorac, Allergan) is a new topical formulation. It is a novel acetylenic retinoid that is being evaluated as a 0.1% and 0.05% gel formulation.[30] As a topical therapy it appears to have minimal systemic absorption, with no adverse systemic signs yet reported.

Tazarotene acts on retinoic acid receptors and results in downregulation of keratinocyte proliferation, differentiation, and inflammation.[45, 107] It does this by a combination of effects, including the induction and activation of new genes, downregulation of AP1 (a proinflammatory genetic factor), and antagonizing the effects of interferon-γ. It has been shown to be effective for acne and psoriasis while having no adverse systemic reactions.

- **Urea.** Urea has hygroscopic and keratolytic actions that aid in normalizing the epidermis, especially the quality of the stratum corneum.[209a] The application of urea in a cream or an ointment base has a softening and moisturizing effect on the stratum corneum and makes the vehicle feel less greasy. It acts as a humectant in concentrations of 2% to 20%; however, in concentrations above that level, it is keratolytic. That action is a result of the solubilization of prekeratin and keratin and the possible breakage of hydrogen bonds that keep the stratum corneum intact. It also promotes desquamation by dissolving the "intercellular substance."

  A hypoallergenic, moisturizing shampoo (Allergroom, Virbac) contains 5% urea free and in spherulites. Humilac (Virbac) contains both urea and lactic acid, and it can be used as a spray or rinse. To make a rinse, 5 capfuls of Humilac are added to 1 L (1 qt) of water. The mixture is rinsed over the dog's coat and allowed to dry. KeraSolv (DVM) contains 6% salicylic acid, 5% urea, and 5% sodium lactate. It is a potent keratolytic used to treat nasal hyperkeratosis, calluses, ear-margin dermatosis, and acne.[91]

- **α-Hydroxyacids 2% to 10%.** These include lactic, malic, citric, pyruvic, glutamic, glycolic, and tartaric acids. They are effective in modulating keratinization, being keratoplastic, and being able to delay terminal differentiation and to reduce the intercellular cohesion forces of the stratum corneum. Lactic acid and sodium lactate can absorb up to 30 times their weight in water.[43a]

- **Fatty Acids.** These acids are keratolytic and fungistatic. Examples are caprylic, propionic, and undecylenic acids. The best of these (although it is weak) is undecylenic acid (e.g., Desenex). Topical fatty acids are also used to treat essential fatty-acid deficiency. Topical sunflower oil, which is high in linoleic acid, decreased transepidermal water loss in seborrheic dogs.[26]

- **Propylene Glycol.** This agent is primarily used as a solvent and a vehicle.[58, 86] At higher concentrations (>75%), it occasionally causes irritation or sensitization. It is an excellent lipid solvent and defats the skin; however, its chief value is probably the ability to enhance percutaneous penetration of drugs. Propylene glycol is also a potent and reliable antibacterial agent and has antidermatophyte and anticandidal properties. For most dermatologic cases, it can be used in concentrations of 30% to 40%. Propylene glycol is a superior humectant (hygroscopic) and can induce keratolysis. Thus, higher concentrations are particularly helpful in hyperkeratotic conditions, and 75% propylene glycol spray is effective in managing sebaceous adenitis (see Chap. 18).

- **Dimethyl Sulfoxide (DMSO).** DMSO is a simple, hygroscopic, organic solvent.[20] Because it is freely miscible with lipids, organic solvents, and water, it is an excellent vehicle. When exposed to the air, concentrated solutions take in water to become hydrated at 67%. Stronger concentrations tend to cross the skin barrier better. DMSO penetrates skin (within 5 minutes), mucous membranes, and the blood-brain barrier, as well as cell, organelle, and microbial membranes. Unlike most solvents, DMSO achieves penetration without membrane damage. It facilitates absorption of many other substances across membranes, especially corticosteroids. On a cellular level, DMSO and steroids exert a synergistic effect.

  DMSO has properties of its own as a cryoprotective, radioprotective, anti-ischemic, anti-inflammatory (free-radical scavenger, decreases prostaglandin synthesis, stabilizes lysosomal membranes), and analgesic (blocks C fibers) agent. It also has variable antibacterial, antifungal, and antiviral properties, depending on the concentration (usually 5% to 50%) and the organism involved. It decreases fibroplasia.

  Although its mechanism of action is incompletely understood, the systemic toxicity and teratogenicity of this solvent in its pure form are considered low. Toxicity may be of concern, depending on the dose, the route of administration, the species, and the individual animal's reaction. Impurities or combinations with other agents may make DMSO dangerous as a result of its ability to enhance transepidermal absorption. Industrial forms of DMSO should never be used for medical purposes because the contained impurities are absorbed and may be toxic. Well-known minor side effects include a garlic-like odor, increased warmth and/or pruritus (histamine release, exothermic with water), and dehydration (too hygroscopic).

Potential uses might include topical application to cutaneous ulcers, burns, insect bites, interdigital granulomas, open wounds, and skin grafts; reduction of exuberant granulation tissue; and treatment of acral lick dermatitis. One formula shown to be safe and useful contains Burow's solution, hydrocortisone, and 90% DMSO.[172] Equal parts of 90% DMSO and Hydro-B 1020 (1% hydrocortisone and 2% Burow's solution in a water and propylene glycol base) are mixed. The formulation is applied daily to benefit patients with pyotraumatic dermatitis and acral lick dermatitis. Application of the 90% gel can hasten the resolution of calcinosis cutis (see Chap. 10).

- **Aloe Vera.** Much of the information on aloe vera is anecdotal.[7, 174] There are over 300 species of Aloe plants, and they differ in chemical composition with the species, climate, and growing conditions. The terms *aloe, aloe vera, aloin,* and *aloe extract* refer to the end products of different methods of extracting juice from Aloe plants. The result of this nonuniformity of collection or extraction is a wide difference between the contents, consistency, and appearance of different products. Likewise, interpreting and comparing various studies is often impossible.

Aloe vera contains a large number of organic compounds and inorganic elements: anthraquinones (e.g., anthracene, emodin), saccharides (e.g., glucose, cellulose, mannose), enzymes (e.g., oxidase, lipase), vitamins (e.g., niacinamide, C, E, A), amino acids, and minerals (e.g., copper, zinc). Anti-inflammatory properties include salicylic acid, bradykininase activity (reduction of pain, swelling, and erythema), magnesium lactate (reduction of histamine production), antiprostaglandin activity, and protease inhibitor activity. In vitro studies indicate that aloe vera inhibits the growth of *Staphylococcus aureus, Pseudomonas aeruginosa,* and *Trichophyton mentagrophytes*.

Anecdotal reports indicate that aloe vera is useful for the treatment of pain, pruritus, fungal infections, bacterial infections, insect bites, burns, and exuberant granulation tissue.[7, 126, 174]

- **Acetic Acid.** Acetic acid is a potent antibacterial agent: A 5% solution (e.g., vinegar) kills coagulase-positive staphylococci in 5 minutes, and a 2.5% solution (e.g., one part vinegar, one part water) kills *P. aeruginosa* in 1 minute (see Chap. 19). A 2.5% solution kills *Malassezia pachydermatis* (see Chap. 5). Acetic acid may also be used in ears (0.25% to 0.5% solution) as a ceruminolytic, astringent, and acidifier (see Chap. 19).

- **Melaleuca Oil.** Melaleuca oil ("tea tree oil") is extracted from the leaves of the "tea tree" (genus *Melaleuca*).[200] It has proven antibacterial (e.g., coagulase-positive staphylococci) and fungicidal (e.g., *Candida albicans, T. mentagrophytes*) properties. Melaleuca oil is marketed for use on dogs, cats, and ferrets in skin care products for cleaning, healing, and relieving pruritus. Claims are also made that it is a deodorizer, detangler, and external parasite repellent. The inappropriate or excessive application of melaleuca oil to the skin may result in toxicosis: hypersalivation, incoordination, weakness, hypothermia, and hepatic injury.

- **Colloidal Oatmeal.** Colloidal oatmeal is useful in the management of dry skin and pruritus by virtue of its demulcent, humectant, and antipruritic properties. It is incorporated into a number of veterinary shampoos. It may also be used as a rinse or soak by adding 1 to 2 tablespoons (15 to 30 ml) of the powder (Epi-Soothe, Virbac; Aveeno, Rydelle Laboratories) to 1 gallon (4 L) of water. Colloidal oatmeal can leave a residue in the haircoat as well as in the bathtub. The bathtub can become slippery.

- **Topical Sunscreens.** A dense haircoat protects most small animals from excessive exposure to sunlight. In some dogs, the skin is pigmented, which also protects from ultraviolet radiation damage. However, whenever nonpigmented, unhaired skin is exposed to sunlight, solar damage may occur. Predisposed areas include the ear tips in white cats, the glabrous abdomen in Dalmatians and bull terriers, and hairless areas. Some animals respond with hyperpigmentation, whereas other animals do not experience hyperpigmentation but may incur sunburn or solar dermatitis.

Protection from the sun can be attained by staying indoors from 10 AM to 4 PM, by tanning the skin (a process of building up pigmentation and mild acanthosis and hyperkeratosis), and by using topical or oral sunscreens.[133] Topical sunscreens may act physically or chemically. In chemical screens, aminobenzoic acid or benzophenone derivatives act to absorb ultraviolet rays. They are clear, cosmetically acceptable lotions or gels.

Physical sunscreens include chemicals such as zinc oxide and titanium dioxide, which reflect and scatter light by forming an opaque barrier. These barrier types are available in many colors (Bullfrog brand), including black, which some owners prefer for use on noses. They also are water-resistant and are not as easily removed by the pet. These agents are messy, especially in long haircoats. Topical sunscreens are rated for efficiency by a sun protective factor (SPF) number. Numbers 2 to 4 are mild blockers, 8 to 10 give moderate protection, and 15 or higher gives blockage. For use in animals, water-resistant sunscreens with an SPF of 15 or greater should be used. These numbers are only guides, because the frequency and thickness of application, temperature, humidity, potency of light exposure, patient's sensitivity, and many other factors modify results.

Usually, sunscreen needs to be applied three or four times a day for greatest effectiveness. Photodecomposition is a problem, and titanium dioxide or zinc oxide sunscreens tend to resist this and are preferred if repeat application is not possible.[197] A common misconception is that if the animal licks the area after application, the sunscreen is removed. Although this is true for the physical blockers (e.g., zinc oxide), it is a minimal problem with chemical blockers because these products are absorbed into the skin and pool within the stratum corneum to produce a reservoir of protection. Chemical blockers are not effective if no epithelium is present (e.g., on ulcers).

● PHYSICAL THERAPY

The use of heat, cold, light, and radiation therapy for the treatment of skin disorders is not new, but advances have made the therapies more specific and more effective. Freezing, heat, electricity, and laser light are presented as surgical techniques at the end of this chapter.

Photochemotherapy

Photochemotherapy uses light waves to excite or increase the energy of a photosensitive drug that causes a selective cytotoxic effect on tumors. The initial drug used in veterinary medicine is a hematoporphyrin derivative porfimer sodium (Photofrin-V, QLT Phototherapeutics).[187] The drug has a much greater affinity for tumor tissue than for surrounding normal cells. A newer-generation photosensitizer is chloroaluminum sulfonated phthalocyanine (Porphyrin products). It is reported to have the advantages of less cutaneous photosensitization and better light absorption for the wavelengths commonly used in this therapy.[134] Light is effective on only a few layers of surface cells, except red-range lights, which can penetrate as much as 1 to 2 cm. The light source is a laser system that produces a red laser beam that passes through low-attenuation fiberoptic tracts. These are directed through 19-gauge needles into the appropriate areas of tumor. Treatment takes about 20 minutes, and repeated exposures are no problem. Patients should be kept out of sunlight for 3 to 4 weeks as they are systemically photosensitized.

Approximately 50% of tumors respond completely, and an additional 30% show partial responses.[187] The most favorable results were obtained in patients with malignant melanoma, fibrosarcoma, mast cell tumor, adamantinoma, and synovial cell sarcoma. Mixed responses occurred in animals with squamous cell carcinoma, adenocarcinoma, leiomyosarcoma, and hemangiopericytoma.

Hyperthermia

Local current-field radiofrequency is used to produce enough heat in a local superficial area to cause tissue necrosis. Two groups have used a temperature of 50°C for 30 to 60 seconds to treat feline tumors.[63, 87] The heat was controlled to affect only the tumor and 2 to 3 mm of surrounding normal tissue. Results were much better with lesions less than 5 mm in diameter by 2 mm deep. In these cases, approximately 70% of the tumors completely regressed, and an additional 20% partially regressed. With larger tumors, the results were much poorer. Favorable responses were obtained with squamous cell carcinomas, fibrosarcomas of cats, and circumanal gland tumors of dogs. There were no serious side effects. This therapy should not be used on the pinna of the ear because it may cause necrosis and sloughing.

Hyperthermia has also been used for topical treatment of localized dermatophytosis. By using the same system and producing heat of 50°C for 30 seconds in an area 4 mm deep by 1 cm in diameter, successful results were achieved after only one treatment. For large lesions, the heat probe was moved sequentially to new areas of 1 cm in diameter until the whole lesion was treated. Fluorescence disappeared within 48 hours, and healing was complete in 2 to 6 weeks. Hyperthermia was considered the treatment of choice for localized dermatophytosis. However, this type of therapy necessitates anesthesia, is cumbersome, is impractical with widespread lesions, and has not been corroborated by other investigators.

Heat is also used in electrosurgical procedures such as fulguration to destroy tissue.

Radiation Therapy

Radiation therapy has important benefits in the treatment of skin tumors, carefully selected cases of feline indolent ulcer, and canine acral lick dermatitis. Because not all cells are equally sensitive to radiation, these rays act selectively. Cells that divide rapidly, such as carcinoma cells, basal cells of the hair papilla, and vascular endothelial cells, are damaged more easily than those of the remaining skin. X-ray beams that are filtered through aluminum or copper sheets to remove soft rays penetrate deeply into the tissues because of their short wavelengths. Radiation delivered at about 80 kV with little or no filtration (0.5 mm of aluminum) has longer wavelengths, and its energy is dissipated superficially.

Before considering radiation therapy for a patient, the clinician must be certain of the following:

1. The treatment has good potential for benefit and little potential for harm.
2. Safer forms of therapy were not effective or radiation therapy is considered a therapy of choice. For indolent ulcers and acral lick dermatitis, radiation therapy is generally a treatment of last resort.
3. Relative cost of this therapy is acceptable.
4. The number and frequency of treatments is acceptable.
5. Proper, safe equipment and facilities are available so that
   a. The exact dose can be administered.
   b. The patient can be anesthetized or restrained for therapy without exposure of personnel.
   c. Proper shielding of unaffected parts is provided.
6. Adequate records are kept for future reference.

If these points can be accomplished, radiation therapy may be considered. Such cases should be referred to a radiologist who specializes in radiation therapy.

• BROAD-SPECTRUM SYSTEMIC THERAPIES

Systemic Nonsteroidal Antipruritic or Nonsteroidal Anti-Inflammatory Agents

In practice, one is often presented with a pruritic or inflammatory dermatosis that is not microbial or parasitic. In other cases, even though a specific cause (e.g., scabies) is determined, symptomatic antipruritic or anti-inflammatory therapy may be desired.[97] Systemic glucocorticoids are most commonly prescribed. However, although glucocorticoids are highly effective in managing these cases and many hypersensitivity disorders, the frequent occurrence of side effects of variable severity stimulates continual investigations for alternative drugs or methods that will allow an avoidance or reduction in the dose of glucocorticoid.[18, 41, 119, 160, 166, 167]

Reasons for electing nonsteroidal agents include (1) unacceptable acute or chronic glucocorticoid side effects, (2) immunosuppressed patients (e.g., cats with feline leukemia virus or feline immunodeficiency virus infections), (3) patients with infectious diseases (viral, fungal, and bacterial), (4) patients with other diseases in which glucocorticoids may be contraindicated (diabetes mellitus, pancreatitis, renal disease, and neoplasia), and (5) pet owners who do not want to use glucocorticoids in their animals. A variety of unrelated nonsteroidal drugs may be used.

Scott and Buerger[163] used a supplement that contained omega-3/omega-6 fatty acids (DermCaps, DVM), three different antihistamines (chlorpheniramine, diphenhydramine, hydroxyzine), an antibiotic (erythromycin), and aspirin in an open study of nonsteroidal anti-inflammatory agents in the management of 45 cases of canine pruritus. Thirty-two dogs had atopy or flea-bite hypersensitivity, and 13 dogs had idiopathic nonseasonal pruritus. As a group, the six drugs controlled itching in 40% of the cases, and there was improvement in another 15%. However, side effects occurred in 46% of cases, being severe enough in 33% of the dogs to prompt halting of treatment with one or more of the drugs. Good to moderate improvement of pruritus was obtained for each medication (see Table 3–5).

Subsequent studies, several of which were placebo-controlled and double-blind studies, show that options other than systemic glucocorticoids are available. Other agents with reported anti-inflammatory effect have been tried with limited success on allergic dogs. The following agents were of no benefit: acetylsalicylic acid,[163] doxycycline,[164] papaverine,[164] vitamin C,[121] zinc,[118] and the combination of tetracycline and niacinamide.

The majority of work has evaluated three main classes of drugs: antihistamines, fatty acids, and psychotropic agents. Because antihistamines function primarily in allergic diseases, they are covered in Chapter 8. Psychotropic drugs, which can also be useful in managing allergic pruritus, are primarily used to treat psychogenic disease and are covered in Chapter 15.

Fatty Acids

Fatty acids, as previously discussed, are an important part of the normal diet. By controlling the relative levels of omega-6 to omega-3 in the total diet, the development of inflammatory mediators in neutrophils and other organs may be modified. Two studies utilizing these omega-6/omega-3 ratios of 5:1 showed similar results, with over 40% of atopic or allergic pruritic dogs experiencing good results.[151, 171]

The use of supplements for treating pruritic inflammatory diseases and crusting diseases in dogs and cats has been the subject of multiple open and controlled studies.[14, 15, 73–75, 100, 101, 103, 117, 119, 120, 170, 211] In general, this method has shown success for the management of pruritus and inflammation associated with a variety of diseases, though predominantly allergic.

The proposed mechanism, besides the inhibition of arachidonic acid metabolism, relates to metabolic byproducts of fatty acid metabolism. Supplements used for pruritus usually contain one or both of γ-linolenic acid and EPA. γ-Linolenic acid is found in relatively high concentrations in evening primrose, borage, and black currant oils. It is elongated to DGLA, which directly competes with arachidonic acid as a substrate for cyclooxygenase and 15-lipoxygenase. The result of DGLA metabolism is the formation of prostaglandin E1 and 15-hydroxy-8,11,13-eicosatetraenoic acid, both of which are thought to have anti-inflammatory effects.[211]

EPA, which is usually supplied by using cold water marine fish oils, also competes as a substrate for cyclooxygenase and 5- and 15-lipoxygenase. The metabolism of EPA by the lipoxygenase enzymes results in the formation of leukotriene B5 and 15-hydroxyeicosapentaenoic acid. These two products are thought to inhibit leukotriene B4, which is a potent pro-inflammatory mediator. This mechanism was reviewed by White,[211] and Figure 3–2 demonstrates the interactions of γ-linolenic acid, EPA, and arachidonic acid.

Consumption of a diet enriched in N-3 (omega-3) fatty acids reduced delayed-type hypersensitivity responses, decreased production of prostaglandin E2, and resulted in increased postvaccinal total lymphocyte count in aged Beagle dogs.[72] An omega-3 fatty acid–enriched diet had no long-term negative effect on wound healing in dogs.[148a]

Another area that still needs investigation is the importance or effect of combining the fatty acids with other elements such as vitamins and minerals and cofactors. Some manufacturers and authors[101] have claimed that the right combination of cofactors maximizes the beneficial effects. Controlled studies to determine this and what cofactors are most important have not yet been presented.

In one double-blind study, a fatty acid product containing cofactors was no more effective than products that did not contain cofactors.[170] Other formulations claim to improve fatty acid absorption by such techniques as miscillization. Again, controlled studies are needed. How long one should try a product has also not been definitively

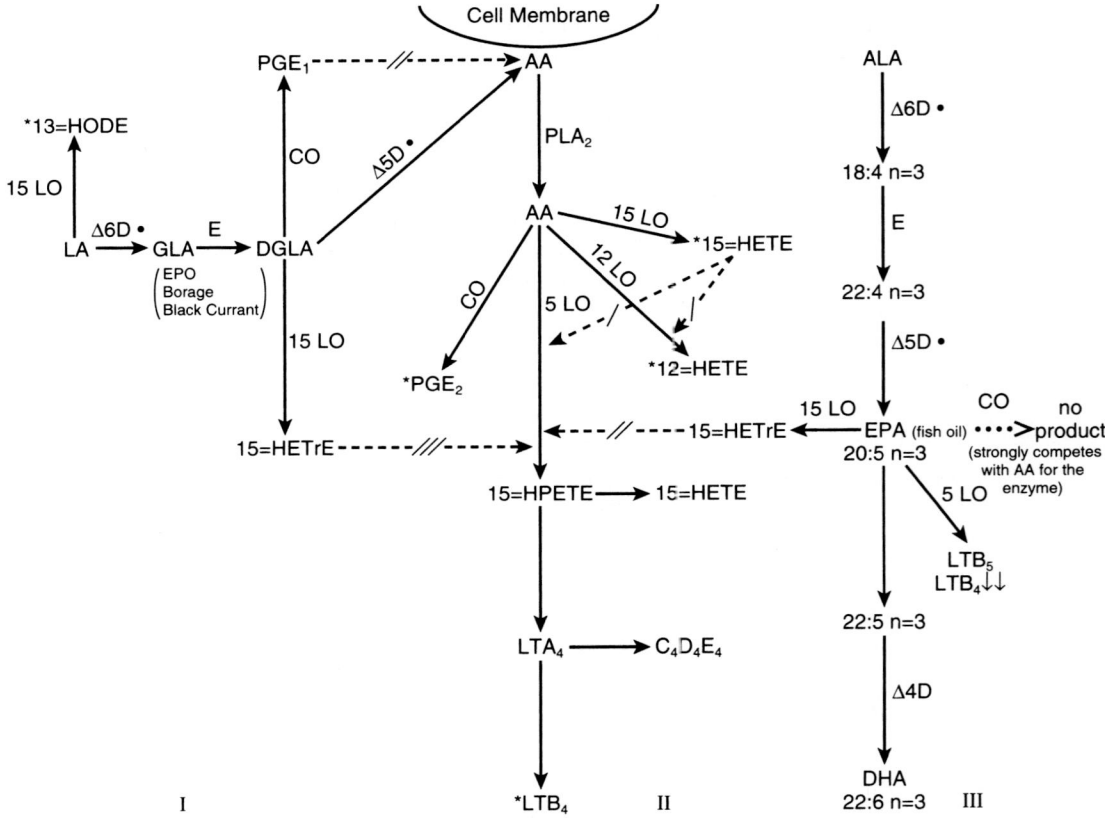

FIGURE 3–2. *I*, N-6 fatty acid metabolism with production of anti-inflammatory eicosanoids. *II*, Arachidonic acid cascade with production of proinflammatory eicosanoids. *III*, N-3 fatty acid metabolism with production of anti-inflammatory eicosanoids. 13-HODE, 13-hydroxyoctadecadienoic acid; PG, prostaglandin; E, elongase; Δ-6-D, Δ-6-desaturase; LA, linoleic acid; GLA, γ-linolenic acid; EPO, evening primrose oil; DGLA, dihomo-γ-linolenic acid; AA, arachidonic acid; ALA, α-linolenic acid; EPA, eicosapentaenoic acid; DHA, docosahexaenoic acid; DES, desaturase; PLA2, phospholipase A2; CO, cyclooxygenase; LO, lipoxygenase; HETE, hydroxyeicosatetraenoic acid; HPETE, hydroperoxyeicosatetraenoic acid; HEPE, hydroxyeicosapentaenoic acid; 15-HETrE, 15-hydroxy-8,11,13-eicosatriaenoic acid; LT, leukotriene. ★ Indicates arachidonic acid–derived eicosanoids identified in inflammatory skin disease; → indicates inhibitory or anti-inflammatory eicosanoid (number of slash lines indicates degree of inhibition). (From White P: Essential fatty acids: Use in management of canine atopy. Comp Cont Educ 15:451, 1993.)

determined. Although some dogs and cats show a favorable response within 1 to 2 weeks, an adequate therapeutic trial might necessitate 9 to 12 weeks.

The risks and side effects of fatty acid supplementation are few. The most serious, although rarely reported, side effect is pancreatitis.[64] With large doses, weight or diarrhea may also increase. With supplements containing fish oil, some clients have reported an unpleasant odor or increased eructation ("fish breath").

Pentoxifylline

Pentoxifylline (Trental, Hoechst-Roussel) is a methylxanthine derivative that produces a variety of physiologic changes at the cellular level.[147] Immunomodulatory and rheologic effects include increased leukocyte deformability and chemotaxis, decreased platelet aggregation, decreased leukocyte responsiveness to interleukin-1 (IL-1) and tumor necrosis factor (TNF)-α, decreased production of TNF-α from macrophages, decreased production of IL-1, IL-4, and IL-12, inhibition of T- and B-lymphocyte activation, and decreased natural killer cell activity. It also has been shown to inhibit T-cell adherence to keratinocytes.[24] In humans, these effects are beneficial in the treatment of peripheral vascular disease, vasculitis, and contact hypersensitivity.

Pentoxifylline also has been used for a variety of inflammatory diseases such as necrobiosis lipoidica, granuloma annulare, and brown recluse spider bites. The drug also affects wound healing and connective tissue disorders through increased production of collagenase and decreased production of collagen, fibronectin, and glycosaminoglycans. In humans, the drug has been used to treat scleroderma. Pentoxifylline has been used in veterinary medicine for the treatment of canine familial dermatomyositis[71] and allergic contact dermatitis[109] and in some atopic dogs. We have used it successfully in pinnal thrombovascular necrosis, ear-margin dermatosis, vasculitis, rabies vaccine–related alopecia, erythema multiforme, and idiopathic mucinosis of the Chinese Shar Pei. Anecdotal reports indicate that pentoxifylline may be useful in dogs with lupoid onychodystrophy, vesicular cutaneous lupus erythematosus, acral lick dermatitis, Greyhound vasculopathy, and metatarsal fistulae of German Shepherds.[173a]

Pentoxifylline is available in a 400-mg coated tablet. It is usually dosed at 10 mg/kg q8h to q24h or tablets are broken and given q12h or q48h, depending on the size of the dog. Once there is a favorable response, which may take 1 to 3 months, the dose may be tapered to q12h or q24h. Some cases require the q8h dosing to remain effective.

Side effects are minimal and usually consist of vomiting and diarrhea. There is an anecdotal report of thrombocytopenia.[143a]

Synthetic Retinoids

Retinoids refer to all the chemicals, natural or synthetic, that have vitamin A activity. Synthetic retinoids are primarily retinol, retinoic acid, or retinal derivatives or analogs. They have been developed with the intent of amplifying certain biological effects while being less toxic than their natural precursors. More than 1500 synthetic retinoids have been developed and evaluated.[90, 139] Retinoids are usually classified as being first generation (e.g., tretinoin, isotretinoin), second generation or monoaromatic (e.g., etretinate, acitretin), or third generation or polyaromatic (e.g., adapalene, tazarotene).[209a]

Different synthetic drugs, all classed as synthetic retinoids, may have profoundly different pharmacologic effects, side effects, and disease indications. The existence of different types of receptors, dimers, response elements, and intermediary proteins means that retinoid physiology is mediated by multiple pathways. Nonselective retinoids that activate multiple pathways are likely to be associated with a high incidence of adverse effects.[29] With all the retinoid research being conducted, there will undoubtedly be many new discoveries and uses in the near future. To date, the biggest deterrent to their use is expense.

Naturally occurring vitamin A is an alcohol, all-trans retinol. It is oxidized in the body to retinal and retinoic acid. Each of these compounds has variable metabolic and biological activities, although both are important in the induction and maintenance of normal growth and differentiation of keratinocytes. Only retinol has all the known functions of vitamin A.

Two compounds have been used clinically the most in veterinary dermatology: isotretinoin (13-cis-retinoic acid [Accutane, Roche]), synthesized as a natural metabolite of retinol, and etretinate (Tegison, Roche), a synthetic retinoid. Etretinate is no longer available but is mentioned because many of the studies in veterinary medicine used it. It has been replaced by acitretin, which is a carboxylic acid, metabolically active metabolite of etretinate. Acitretin is less toxic owing to a shorter terminal elimination half-life of 2 days versus etretinate's 100 days. Etretinate is stored in body fat and has been found in trace amounts up to 3 years after cessation of therapy.[135]

Retinoids function by entering cells and being transported to the nuclei, where they interact with specific gene regulatory receptors. The natural vitamin A works at the cellular level by binding first to the cell membrane then transferring through the cellular cytoplasm by specific proteins, cellular retinol binding protein, and cellular retinoic acid binding protein. There are nuclear retinoid receptor molecules that transfer the retinoids through the nucleus.

There are two main nuclear receptor families: the retinoic acid receptors and the retinoid X receptors.[106] They both have at least three members for a minimum of six different nuclear receptors. These receptors can function as heterodimers, homodimers, or in conjunction with other nuclear receptors such as those for vitamin D_3 and thyroid hormone. The nuclear receptor(s) and retinoid complex then bind with specific areas of target genes and alter gene transcription. A new class of retinoids are being investigated that may act by a unique mechanism and has been called *inverse agonists*. Another mechanism by which retinoids function is by suppression of other nuclear transcription factors, which results in less production of other proteins. This is thought to be a mechanism responsible for some of the anti-inflammatory effects.

Some of the different tissue and individual sensitivity for toxic effects may relate to the relative and absolute levels of the cellular and nuclear binding proteins present in the target cells. Once these genetic changes are made, the cells may alter their growth and differentiation by altering the expression of growth factors, keratins, and transglutaminases.[135] Another method of action relates to an anti-inflammatory effect in epithelial structures by the downregulation of nitrites and TNF-α.[11]

All retinoids have variable antiproliferative, anti-inflammatory, and immunomodulatory effects. Because of their numerous pharmacologic effects, retinoids are being used in the management of numerous diseases in humans. The long list includes such diverse diseases as acne, gram-negative folliculitis, hidradenitis suppurativa, the ichthyoses, multiple forms of psoriasis, a variety of cutaneous neoplasms, epidermal nevi, subcorneal pustular dermatosis, discoid lupus erythematosus, lichen planus, cutaneous sarcoidosis, Darier's disease, and acanthosis nigricans.[48, 135] The biological effects of retinoids are numerous, but their ability to regulate proliferation, growth, and differentiation of epithelial tissues is their major benefit in dermatology.[11] However, retinoids also affect proteases, prostaglandins, humoral and cellular immunity, and cellular adhesion and communication.[135] In general, the response of established skin cancers to retinoids is disappointing, with remissions being uncommon, incomplete, and of short duration.[96] Retinoids enhance wound healing by stimulating fibroblasts to produce various chemicals (e.g., TGF-ß).[49]

Isotretinoin is usually dosed at 1 to 3 mg/kg q24h and appears to be indicated in diseases that require alteration or normalization of adnexal structures, although some epidermal diseases may respond.[90] Diseases in which isotretinoin has been reported to be effective in veterinary dermatology include Schnauzer comedo syndrome,[90] sebaceous adenitis (particularly early in the disease in Poodles and Vizslas or shorthaired breeds),[90, 139, 180] ichthyosis,[90] feline acne,[90] epitheliotropic lymphoma,[90, 139, 213] keratoacanthoma,[90, 139, 213] and sebaceous gland hyperplasias and adenomas.[139] Isotretinoin has been ineffective for primary idiopathic seborrhea of Cocker spaniels and Basset hounds and epidermal dysplasia of West Highland white terriers.[52, 90, 139] It was also ineffective in the treatment of preneoplastic and squamous cell carcinoma lesions in cats.[50]

Isotretinoin must be administered with food or absorption is quite variable.[207] Toxicity of isotretinoin in the dog and cat appears to be less of a problem than in humans.[90, 139] In the dog, conjunctivitis, hyperactivity, pruritus, pedal and mucocutaneous junction erythema, stiffness, vomiting, diarrhea, and keratoconjunctivitis may occur. Laboratory abnormalities that are generally not associated with clinical signs include hypertriglyceridemia, hypercholesterolemia, and increased levels of alanine aminotransferase, aspartate aminotransferase, and alkaline phosphatase.[90, 139] In cats, conjunctivitis, diarrhea, anorexia, and vomiting have been the major side effects.[67, 90, 139] These side effects may be transient or self-limited with discontinuation or decrease in dose of the drug. With long-term use, skeletal abnormalities, including cortical hyperostosis, periosteal calcification, and long bone demineralization, are a concern.[48, 90, 135, 139] All retinoids are potent teratogens.

Etretinate was believed to be indicated for disorders of epithelial or follicular development or keratinization. Most commonly, etretinate was given at 1 mg/kg q24h. Etretinate was reportedly effective for primary idiopathic seborrhea of Cocker and Springer spaniels,[67, 90, 139, 140] Golden retrievers, Irish setters, and some mixed breeds. It has not been effective in West Highland white terriers, Basset hounds, or collies.[90, 139] However, one of us (C.E.G.) saw some partial responses in West Highland white terriers after secondary *Malassezia* dermatitis was controlled. Although the use is more controversial, etretinate may also be effective in sebaceous adenitis.[67, 139] One study on 30 dogs with sebaceous adenitis showed etretinate to be as effective as isotretinoin (about 50% of the cases responding), and there was no breed difference in response.[214] Some cases that fail to respond to one retinoid respond to the other.

Ichthyosis has also been reported to respond to etretinate. In dogs, solar dermatosis and squamous cell carcinoma were reported to improve.[108, 139] Follicular dysplasias such as color dilution alopecia may also respond, with less scaling and partial hair growth.[65] Keratoacanthomas may also respond, although it appears that isotretinoin is more effective.[65] In humans, acitretin is considered as efficacious as etretinate. However, this has not been documented in dogs and cats. It is more expensive than etretinate and, at this time, is being dosed the same or at one half the recommended dose of etretinate. Acitretin (Soriatane, Roche) must be given with food or absorption is highly variable.[208]

Toxicity with etretinate is similar to that with isotretinoin. In humans, etretinate is considered safer for long-term use because of a lower propensity for producing skeletal abnormalities. However, it is considered more of a teratogen and should be used only in spayed females, nonbreeding males, or female dogs that will not be used for breeding. Teratogenicity may persist even 2 years after cessation of therapy.[135, 139, 140] Monitoring for both synthetic retinoids includes pretreatment measurement of tear production, hemogram, chemistry profile, and urinalysis. This is repeated in 1 to 2 months and, if no problems are detected, repeated only as deemed necessary.[139, 140]

Because experience with increased triglyceride levels shows that they normalize when animals are receiving low-fat diets, it is suggested that dogs being given etretinate may benefit from changing to such a diet.[139, 140] Acitretin has a much shorter half-life and is not readily stored in fat; therefore, it has less potential for post-treatment teratogenicity.[135] However, in humans there is some conversion to etretinate, producing some, though probably less, risk.

Cyclosporine

Cyclosporine (Sandimmune, Novartis) is a fat-soluble cyclic polypeptide metabolite of the fungus *Tolypocladium inflatum gams*.[144, 145, 195] It is effective in preventing human organ transplantation rejection.[129] In animal models, it has been used with similar excellent results.[210] It is being used for a wide variety of dermatologic diseases in humans such as atopic dermatitis, psoriasis, lichen planus, pyoderma gangrenosum, epidermolysis bullosa acquisita, actinic dermatitis, and chronic hand eczema.[60, 98] It has also been evaluated for the treatment of immune-mediated skin diseases and epitheliotropic lymphoma in animals.[144] Anecdotal reports have suggested efficacy in atopic dermatitis in dogs and cats.[143a] Most clinicians use the microemulsified capsule or solution forms of cyclosporine (Neoral, Novartis) because these products are absorbed better and produce more stable blood levels.

Cyclosporine has low cytotoxicity relative to its immunosuppressive potency. Cyclosporine blocks IL-2 transcription and T cell responsiveness to IL-2, leading to impaired T-helper and T-cytotoxic lymphocytes.[62] It also inhibits IFN-α transcription, thus diminishing amplification signals for macrophage and monocyte activation. The production of other cytokines, including IL-3, IL-4, IL-5, TNF-α, and IFN-α may be impaired. In these ways, cyclosporine inhibits mononuclear cell function, antigen presentation, mast cell and eosinophil production, histamine and prostaglandin release from mast cells, neutrophil adherence, natural killer cell activity, and growth and differentiation of B cells. It has also been suggested that a mechanism of action in the treatment of atopic dermatitis involves the inhibition of mast cell degranulation by affecting the interaction between mast cells and nerves.[190] Cyclosporine also directly inhibits histamine release from dog mast cells.[55]

Humans experience a high incidence of nephrotoxicity and hepatic toxicity. Dogs (daily doses of 20 to 30 mg/kg) may experience gingival hyperplasia and papillomatosis, vomiting, diarrhea, bacteriuria, bacterial skin infection, anorexia, hirsutism, involuntary shaking, nephropathy, bone marrow suppression, and lymphoplasmacytoid dermatosis.[144, 145] These appear to be rare with daily doses of 5 to 10 mg/kg.[143a] Cats are reported to have only minor side effects (primarily soft feces), although they may be more susceptible to viral infections.[64, 144, 145] Cyclosporine should probably be stopped at least 4 weeks prior to intradermal skin testing.[143a]

The clinical indications for cyclosporine therapy are organ transplantation and inhibition of delayed-type hypersensitivity reactions of many immune-mediated diseases. It is used in pemphigus foliaceus and immune-mediated myasthenia gravis, thyroiditis, neuritis, uveitis, and arthritis. Initial studies in dogs and cats with immunologic dermatoses such as pemphigus foliaceus, pemphigus erythematosus, and discoid lupus erythematosus have shown cyclosporine by itself to be rarely effective.[144, 145] It has been effective in canine sebaceous adenitis (see Chap. 18). Cyclosporine has been ineffective in the treatment of canine and feline epitheliotropic lymphoma (mycosis fungoides).[144] Recent reports indicate that cyclosporine is effective for the treatment of canine perianal fistulae.[112, 113] It is being evaluated for the treatment of canine atopic dermatitis.[128]

The oral dosage for dogs and cats is 5 to 10 mg/kg daily, the dose for cats being divided and given twice daily.[93, 145] Blood concentrations achieved after a specific dose vary from patient to patient and within each patient over time. These variabilities are largely determined by differences in absorption, distribution, and metabolism. Absorption may be enhanced by administration with a fatty meal. Frequent drug monitoring is needed to maintain blood cyclosporine concentrations in an effective range yet avoid toxicities. After a response occurs, tapering to as low as 10 mg/kg every 48 hours may be effective.[144] Because this is an expensive drug, the reduction to the lowest effective levels is usually important. Additionally, the expense and marginal efficacy usually limit its use to cases of treatment failure with or adverse reaction to alternative treatments.

Drugs that inhibit cytochrome P-450 microsomal enzyme activity (e.g., ketoconazole, itraconazole, fluconazole, erythromycin, methylprednisolone, and allopurinol) potentiate cyclosporine toxicity. When ketoconazole was given to normal dogs (average dose 13.6 mg/kg/day) that had targeted blood levels of cyclosporine (average daily dose 14.5 mg/kg), the cyclosporine doses could be reduced by an average of 75%, resulting in a 57.8% savings in the cost of therapy.[39a] Clinical applications of this "synergy" are awaited.

Glucocorticoid Hormones

Glucocorticoid hormones have potent effects on the skin, and they profoundly affect immunologic and inflammatory activity.[37, 143, 152, 160, 161, 205] They directly or indirectly affect leukocyte kinetics, phagocytic defenses, cell-mediated immunity, humoral immunity, and the production of inflammatory mediators. The major effects thought to be important in counteracting allergic inflammatory reactions are presented in Table 3–6 and have been reviewed.[37, 159, 205] In addition, fibroblastic activity is reduced, synthesis of histamine is delayed, and complement is inhibited. Antibody production is not stopped but may be decreased, especially autoantibody titers.

At pharmacologic levels, glucocorticoids increase the production of lipocortin-1, which is thought to cause a reduction in the action of phospholipase A_2 on cell membranes, which results in inhibition of the arachidonic acid cycle.[38] This action is probably one of the more clinically relevant actions in decreasing inflammation. High doses of glucocorticoids may suppress antibody production.[37, 205] There is circumstantial evidence that in some allergic dogs glucocorticoids may suppress IgE production at therapeutic protocols used by some veterinarians.[38, 114]

Glucocorticoid response to inflammatory stimuli is nonspecific: It is the same whether it is a response to infection, trauma, toxin, or immune complex deposition. The drug must reach the local site of inflammation to be effective, and the degree of response and cellular protection from injury is proportionate to the concentration of glucocorticoid in the inflamed tissue. Thus, dosages and dose intervals should vary with the patient's specific needs.

Several other factors influence the tissue glucocorticoid effect. One is the relative potency of the drug. Synthetic compounds made by adding methyl or fluoride groups to the basic steroid molecule increase the potency and the duration of action. Another factor is the effect of protein binding. Only free glucocorticoid is metabolically active. Many synthetics are poorly protein-bound, which partly explains their relatively high potency at low doses.

Corticosteroid-binding globulin is a specific glycoprotein that binds glucocorticoids, but it has a relatively low binding capacity. When large doses of glucocorticoids are administered, its capacity is exceeded, and albumin becomes the protein used for binding. Animals with low serum albumin levels have a lower binding capacity, and the excessive unbound glucocorticoid becomes freely available, increasing toxicity.[66, 159] In addition, the route of administration and water solubility affect the duration of action. Oral glucocorticoids, given as the free base or as esters, are rapidly absorbed. Parenteral glucocorticoids are usually esters of acetate, diacetate, phosphate, or succinate. Acetate and diacetate are relatively insoluble, resulting in slow release and prolonged absorption. The phosphates and succinates are water-soluble and are rapidly absorbed. As a result, parenteral gluco-

● Table 3–6 **ANTI-INFLAMMATORY ACTIONS OF GLUCOCORTICOIDS**

Effects on eosinophils	Decrease formation in bone marrow
	Induce apoptosis and inhibit prolongation of eosinophil survival and function from IL-3 and IL-5
Effects on lymphocytes and monocytes	Reduce number of lymphocytes and monocytes that bear low-affinity IgE and IgG receptors
	Decrease serum immunoglobulin levels
	Decrease all lymphocyte subpopulations
	Decrease lymphocyte production of IL-1, -2, -3, -4, -5, -6, and IFN-γ
	Inhibit release of IL-1 and TNF-α from monocytes
Effects on mast cells	May decrease number of mast cells
Effects on neutrophils	Decreased chemotaxis, adherence, and enzyme secretion
Inhibition of phospholipase A_2	Decrease production of arachidonic acid metabolites
	Decrease production of platelet-activating factor
Decreased vascular permeability	Mechanism unknown
Reversal of reduced β-adrenergic responsiveness	Part of this effect is by increasing the number of β-adrenergic receptors expressed on cell surface

IL = interleukin; TNF = tumor necrosis factor; IFN = interferon.

corticoids produce continuous low levels of glucocorticoid for days (water-soluble) or weeks (water-insoluble). The effect produces significant adrenal suppression, a problem that can be diminished by giving short-acting glucocorticoids orally every other day.

Many of the desirable properties of glucocorticoids can be responsible for adverse effects if present in excess or at the wrong time. In addition, adverse effects may relate to the numerous other effects that glucocorticoids have on carbohydrate, protein, and lipid metabolism. It is imperative to make an accurate diagnosis so that the need for, type, duration, and level of glucocorticoid therapy can be determined. Except in the case of hypoadrenocorticism, glucocorticoids do not correct a primary deficiency but act symptomatically or palliatively. The anti-inflammatory and immunosuppressive actions desired for one therapeutic need may facilitate the establishment or spread of concomitant infections or parasitic diseases.

Animals treated with glucocorticoids tend to experience bacterial infections of the skin and the urinary and respiratory systems.[66, 160] Because of the profound effects of glucocorticoids on phagocytosis and cell-mediated immunity, increased susceptibility to fungal infections and intracellular pathogens is to be expected.[37]

INDICATIONS

The major indications for glucocorticoid therapy are hypersensitivity dermatoses (flea-bite hypersensitivity, atopy, and food hypersensitivity), pyotraumatic dermatitis ("hot spot"), contact dermatitis (irritant or hypersensitivity reactions), and immune-mediated dermatoses (pemphigus, pemphigoid, and lupus erythematosus). They are occasionally used in other inflammatory skin diseases such as keratinization and many diseases listed in Chapter 18. Whenever possible, their use should be short term (less than 3 months).

Glucocorticoids are usually only part of the management employed for most dermatoses, and the clinician must control or minimize other predisposing, precipitating, and complicating factors to keep the glucocorticoids in their proper perspective, which is to use them (1) as infrequently as possible, (2) at as low a dose as possible, (3) in alternate-day regimens whenever possible, and (4) only when other less hazardous forms of therapy have failed or could not be employed.[81, 83, 160, 161]

ADMINISTRATION

For dermatoses, glucocorticoids are usually administered orally, by injection (intramuscularly, subcutaneously, intralesionally, and intravenously), topically, or in some combination thereof. In any given patient, the decision as to which route or routes to employ depends on various factors.

Of the systemic routes, oral administration is preferred because (1) it can be more closely regulated (a daily dose is more precise than with a repository injection; the drug can be rapidly withdrawn if undesirable side effects occur) and (2) it is the only safe, therapeutic, physiologic way to administer glucocorticoids for more long-term therapy.[22, 31, 66, 69, 82, 124, 160, 161]

Injectable glucocorticoids are usually administered intramuscularly or subcutaneously. Although most injectable glucocorticoids are licensed for only intramuscular use, many clinicians administer them subcutaneously. The reasons purported for choosing the subcutaneous route are (1) there are few patient objections (and fewer pet-owner crises) and (2) it is clinically as effective as intramuscular administration.[160]

There is a theoretical preference for using the intramuscular route in the obese patient because subcutaneous deliveries could be sequestered in fat tissue. However, the major reason for using the intramuscular route (other than the liability or legal issue) is to decrease the occurrence of local atrophy. Although this problem may be more common in humans, it also occurs in the dog. Local areas of alopecia, pigmentary changes, and epidermal and dermal atrophy are more commonly induced by subcutaneous injection. These reactions are noninflammatory and atrophic in contrast with most other injection reactions. Yorkshire and Silky terriers, Lhasa apsos, Poodles, and Shih tzus may be predisposed to this reaction.[67]

An excellent injectable anti-inflammatory glucocorticoid is methylprednisolone acetate (Depo-Medrol, Pharmacia & Upjohn). Clinically, dogs are given doses of 1.1 mg/kg and cats are given 20 mg/cat or 5.5 mg/kg, subcutaneously or intramuscularly, and the effect may last for 1 week to 6 months. Other commonly used injectable glucocorticoids are presented in Table 3–7.

Intralesional injections of glucocorticoids are often thought of as local, intracutaneous therapy, devoid of any systemic effect. Intralesional therapy is employed for solitary or multiple cutaneous lesions, but it has systemic effects, some of which can be serious. The major indications for intralesional use are acral lick dermatitis, histiocytomas, sterile granulomas, eosinophilic granulomas, feline indolent ulcers, and proliferative otitis externa. In general, triamcinolone acetonide is the glucocorticoid of choice for intralesional therapy.

Intravenous use for dermatologic indications is primarily limited to regimens of pulse therapy for immune-mediated dermatoses. In addition to the intravenous route, high dosages are used. In a study, dogs were hospitalized and given 11 mg/kg of methylprednisolone sodium succinate intravenously in 250 ml of 5% dextrose and water during a 1-hour period for 3 consecutive days.[212] The reported advantages of glucocorticoid pulse therapy include immediate symptomatic relief, avoidance of the side effects that accompany high-dose oral administration of glucocorticoids, and the ability to lower the dosage or discontinue the use of oral glucocorticoids after the pulse therapy. The side effects occurring with intravenous pulse therapy, such as cardiac arrhythmias, pancreatitis, diabetes mellitus, and gastric or duodenal ulcers, are enough of a concern, although not routinely observed, to limit this form of therapy to animals with severe disease.[37, 78, 212]

CHOOSING A GLUCOCORTICOID

The choice of a glucocorticoid may be difficult. One cannot establish a single rule or set of rules that applies to all patients with a given glucocorticoid-responsive dermatosis. Factors that must be considered include the duration of therapy, the personality of the patient, the personality and reliability of the owner, the response of the patient to the

● Table 3–7 **INJECTABLE GLUCOCORTICOIDS FOR USE IN PRURITIC DOGS AND CATS**

AGENT	BRAND NAME	COMPANY	MANUFACTURER'S REGIMEN	
			Dose	Route
Betamethasone	Betasone	Schering-Plough	0.2–0.4 mg/kg in dog	IM
Dexamethasone	Azium	Schering-Plough	0.25–1 mg/dog	IM
			0.125–0.5 mg/cat	IM
Dexamethasone	Generic	Many	0.25–1 mg/dog	IM
			0.125–0.5 mg/cat	IM
Flumethasone	Flucort	Fort Dodge	0.06–0.25 mg/dog	IM or SC
			0.03–0.125 mg/cat	IM or SC
Methylprednisolone	Depo-Medrol	Pharmacia & Upjohn	2–40 mg/dog	IM
			10–20 mg/cat	IM
Triamcinolone	Vetalog	Fort Dodge	0.1–0.2 mg/kg in dog	IM or SC
			0.1–0.2 mg/kg in cat	IM or SC
Prednisone	Meticorten	Schering-Plough	0.5–2.2 mg/kg q24h in dog	IM
			0.5–2.2 mg/kg q24h in cat	IM
	Generic	Many	0.5 mg/kg q24h	IM

IM = intramuscular; SC = subcutaneous.

drug, the response of the patient's disease to the drug, and other considerations specific to the patient or the disease.

The personality of the patient can significantly influence the choice of glucocorticoid; witness the attempts to administer pills to the obstreperous cat that is a blur of fur, fangs, and claws. Likewise, the reliability of the owner can be the deciding factor: There are owners who cannot, or will not, give oral medicaments to their pets. However, for long-term use even in these situations, the risk of injectable glucocorticoids overrides these drawbacks.

The clinician learns, by history or personal experience, that some glucocorticoids do not seem to work as well as others in certain patients. However, the claim that injectable glucocorticoids are needed in some cases and that oral glucocorticoids are not effective is rarely accurate. In the majority of these cases, ineffective oral dosages were used or tapered too fast. A common mistake is to give an injection, then go immediately to a low alternate-day oral dose.[67, 160] In some cases, the problem probably reflects dosage, absorption, and metabolic differences.

As a corollary, the clinician notes that, in some patients, a glucocorticoid that was previously satisfactory apparently loses its effectiveness. For example, in an atopic dog that initially did well when given prednisolone, the prednisolone seemed to lose its effect. Subsequently, the dog responded well to equipotent doses of orally administered triamcinolone. In most cases, after a variable length of time, the clinician is able to return to managing the atopy successfully with prednisolone. This well-recognized but poorly understood phenomenon is called *steroid tachyphylaxis*.[46, 160] However, in most clinical cases referred to dermatology specialists for the development of steroid resistance or steroid tachyphylaxis, the real problem is the development of concurrent disorders.[64, 160] In such cases, secondary bacterial pyoderma, *Malassezia* dermatitis, increased exposure to fleas or reactions to ongoing topical therapy are often the reasons for failure of previously effective glucocorticoid regimens.

Finally, the clinician may discover, by history or personal experience, that a patient can receive certain glucocorticoids without significant adverse effects but not other glucocorticoids. Hence, a dog may experience colitis or behavioral changes with prednisolone but not with methylprednisolone, dexamethasone, or triamcinolone. In some cases, switching to methylprednisolone or triamcinolone may have a relative steroid-sparing effect. A lower dose than the prednisolone equivalent may be effective for that disease in that animal. In some cases, signs of iatrogenic Cushing's disease or marked liver enzyme activity elevations greatly improve on the alternative glucocorticoid alternate-day regimen.[64]

THERAPEUTIC DOSAGE

Optimal therapeutic doses have not been scientifically determined for any canine or feline dermatosis. Presently espoused anti-inflammatory, antipruritic, antiallergic, or immunosuppressive glucocorticoid doses have been determined through years of clinical experience. Moreover, it is imperative to remember that every patient is unique and that glucocorticoid therapy must be individualized. Recommended glucocorticoid doses are only guidelines.

The two most commonly used oral glucocorticoids are prednisolone and prednisone. For all practical purposes, these two drugs are identical (the choice of one or the other is usually based on cost). However, prednisone must be converted in the liver to prednisolone, the active form. Dosage recommendations in this text are based on prednisolone (prednisone) equivalents. Table 3–8 contains information on approximate equipotent dosages of other oral glucocorticoids.

Physiologic doses of glucocorticoids are those that approximate the daily cortisol (hydrocortisone) production by normal individuals. In dogs, daily cortisol production has been reported to be 0.2 to 1 mg/kg/day.[161] No such information is available for cats. Pharmacologic doses of glucocorticoids exceed physiologic requirements. Significantly, any

Table 3–8 RELATIVE POTENCY AND ACTIVITY OF ORAL GLUCOCORTICOIDS

DRUG	EQUIVALENT DOSE (mg)	DURATION OF EFFECT (h)	ALTERNATE-DAY THERAPY
Short-Acting			
Cortisone	25	8–12	NAS
Hydrocortisone	20	8–12	NAS
Intermediate-Acting			
Prednisone	5	24–36	P
Prednisolone	5	24–36	P
Methylprednisolone	4	24–36	P
Long-Acting			
Flumethasone	1.3	36–48	A‡
Triamcinolone	0.5†	36–48	‡
Dexamethasone	0.5	36–54	
Betamethasone	0.4	36–54	

NAS = not acceptable because of short duration; P = preferred; A = alternative selection for alternate-day therapy.
†Previous publications stated dosages often equivalent to those of methylprednisolone. No studies on clinical effects are available.
‡May be useful on every-third-day regimen.

pharmacologic dose of glucocorticoid, no matter how large or small, may suppress the hypothalamic-pituitary-adrenal axis.[160, 165, 181]

Clinicians usually talk in terms of anti-inflammatory versus immunosuppressive doses of glucocorticoids. A commonly used anti-inflammatory (as in allergic dermatoses) induction dosage of oral prednisolone in dogs is 1.1 mg/kg q24h. However, in severe allergy, such as the dog with flea bite hypersensitivity that has numerous fleas, a higher dosage of 1.75 to 2 mg/kg/day may often be needed.[64] For maintenance, the dosage should be lowered as much as possible and optimally ends up at less than 0.25 to 0.5 mg/kg every 48 hours. For immune-mediated diseases, the initial dosage is usually 2.2 mg/kg q24h. If there is no response, this may be raised to as high as 6.6 mg/kg q24h.

Many clinicians (D.W.S., W.H.M.; see also ref. 69) administer oral glucocorticoids only once daily and find no loss of clinical efficacy but a definite reduction in side effects. A commonly used immunosuppressive maintenance dosage for dogs is 1.1 mg of prednisolone per kilogram every other morning.

In general, compared with dogs, cats require about twice the dose of glucocorticoid orally for induction (anti-inflammatory: 2.2 mg/kg/d; immunosuppressive: 4.4 mg/kg/d) and maintenance therapy.[31, 159–161, 172] Resistance of cats to glucocorticoid effects may relate to their decreased number of glucocorticoid receptors.[196] It is probable that the diurnal rhythm of dogs and cats is not dramatic, and timing dosages to morning or evening hours is less important than was previously thought. It is important, however, to maintain the 24-hour alternate-day freedom from medication so that adrenal suppression and chronic side effects are minimized.

REGIMEN

Glucocorticoid regimens vary with the nature of the dermatosis, the specific glucocorticoid being administered, and the use of induction versus maintenance therapy.

In general, dermatoses necessitating anti-inflammatory doses of oral glucocorticoid need smaller doses and shorter periods of daily induction therapy to bring about remission compared with dermatoses necessitating immunosuppressive doses. Anti-inflammatory induction doses are usually given for 2 to 6 days, whereas immunosuppressive induction doses are often administered for 4 to 10 days. Initially, the doses are given every 24 hours or divided and given every 12 hours for 2 to 4 days; then, the total daily dose is given every 24 hours. This is continued until signs of disease are markedly decreased or in remission. After this point, tapering to maintenance therapy begins.

Maintenance therapy with oral glucocorticoid is best accomplished with prednisolone, prednisone, or methylprednisolone on alternate days.[32, 160, 161, 165] Oral triamcinolone is often effective in managing prednisone-responsive cases at doses of approximately 10% to 20% of the prednisone dose (on a milligram basis).[66, 160] According to the standard published glucocorticoid potency equivalency, this is a significant steroid-sparing effect. However, because triamcinolone suppresses the hypothalamic-pituitary-adrenal axis for 24 to 48 hours, it is best given every 72 hours.

With alternate-day therapy, the daily dose of glucocorticoid used for successful induction therapy is given as a single massive dose, usually every other morning for dogs and every other evening for cats. Some clinicians (D.W.S. and W.H.M.) begin alternate-day therapy as soon as remission is achieved with induction therapy.[160, 161] Other investigators gradually reduce one alternate-day dose until no drug is given, whereas the other alternate-day dose remains at the induction dose.[66] For maintenance therapy, the alternate-day dose is reduced by 50%, every 1 to 2 weeks, until the lowest satisfactory maintenance dose is achieved. This regimen does not eliminate adrenal atrophy, but the atrophy is less severe and its onset is delayed. It is the only dosage system that should be used for long-term therapy of steroid-responsive diseases in small animals.

In some animals, alternate-day glucocorticoid therapy can be extended to every third or fourth day. Rarely, anti-inflammatory alternate-day glucocorticoid therapy with the preferred prednisolone, prednisone, or methylprednisolone is not successful. In these cases, the clinician has three therapeutic options (assuming that glucocorticoid therapy is all that can be done):

1. Administer prednisolone, prednisone, or methylprednisolone daily, informing the owner of the inevitability of iatrogenic hyperglucocorticoidism.
2. Switch to a more potent oral glucocorticoid on an alternate-day basis.
3. Switch to injectable glucocorticoids.

Although the more potent oral glucocorticoids are usually satisfactory for alternate-day therapy unless given at low doses, they do not spare the hypothalamic-pituitary-adrenal axis (because of potency and duration of effect). They may occasionally be employed with few or no significant side effects, especially in cats.[64, 160] Clinically, the most satisfactory agents in this respect appear to be triamcinolone and dexamethasone. Because of factors related to the patient and the owner, not the disease, some animals may be satisfactorily managed with only injectable glucocorticoids.

Intramuscular or subcutaneous glucocorticoid therapy is usually fine for acute, short-term diseases that necessitate a single injection. Additionally, animals that need only three or four injections per year probably do not experience significant side effects. However, for dermatoses that need long-term maintenance therapy, injectable glucocorticoids are usually not satisfactory. It has been shown that a single intramuscular injection of methylprednisolone acetate (Depo-Medrol, Pharmacia & Upjohn) is capable of altering adrenocortical function in dogs for at least 5, and up to 10, weeks.[81] In other studies, a single intramuscular injection of triamcinolone acetonide (Vetalog, Fort Dodge) was capable of altering adrenocortical function in dogs for up to 4 weeks.[82, 160]

Intralesional injections of glucocorticoids are usually repeated every 7 to 10 days until the dermatosis is in remission (usually two to four treatments) and then given as needed.

SIDE EFFECTS

The side effects associated with systemic glucocorticoid therapy in dogs are numerous.[161, 165] In contrast, cats appear relatively tolerant to this therapy, although they infrequently experience iatrogenic Cushing's disease with unkempt haircoat, curling of the pinnae, alopecia, thin and easily torn skin, and diabetes mellitus. Rare cases may even involve steroid hepatopathy.[149]

Because of the diverse effects of glucocorticoids on protein, lipid, and carbohydrate metabolism; endocrine function; fluid balance; and host defense mechanisms, it is expected that glucocorticoids are associated with many side effects. Sequelae may appear with any duration or form of glucocorticoid therapy. In most cases, the side effects with short-term therapy may also occur with long-term therapy but are not generally major health problems. The exceptions are the acute sequelae of high-dose therapy. These include gastrointestinal ulceration, perforation, myopathy, and pancreatitis. These side effects most commonly occur with dosages at or greater than 2.2 mg/kg/day of prednisone (or equipotent doses of other glucocorticoids).

In a study published in 1998, 105 dogs with neurologic injury were treated with prednisolone sodium succinate at 30 mg/kg IV q6h for 36 hours.[39] In this group of dogs, none of the serious side effects was seen, suggesting that the incidence is relatively low. One third of the dogs did experience less severe complications, including diarrhea and melena in 10%, and lower percentages experienced vomiting, hematochezia, anorexia, and hematemesis. In other studies, dogs given 15 to 30 mg/kg methylprednisolone sodium succinate intravenously developed gastric hemorrhage which was not prevented by misoprostol.[143b, 143c]

The other side effects that are not related to treatment duration include polyuria, polydipsia, polyphagia (which may lead to weight gain), behavioral changes (depression, hyperactivity, and aggression), panting, and diarrhea. Most of these side effects are somewhat dose-related. However, the disease being treated may not be controllable at a dosage that does not produce the undesired results. In general, these side effects are minimized with low-dose, alternate-day therapy or may occur on only the day of treatment. Switching types of glucocorticoid may also eliminate these sequelae. About 30% of the dogs treated with anti-inflammatory doses of prednisone or prednisolone experience side effects that are sufficiently undesirable to necessitate stopping treatment. This percentage drops to about 10% when methylprednisolone is used.

Long-term therapy is associated with many more side effects, particularly side effects leading to poor health or disease. Of major concern is the increased risk of infections. A variety of bacterial infections may occur, but the most common are bacteriuria, pyoderma, septicemia, and respiratory infections. Prolonged distention of the bladder with dilute urine likely contributes to the increased incidence of urinary tract infections in dogs on long-term glucocorticoid therapy. Generalized demodicosis or *Malassezia* dermatitis may also occur. Common cutaneous and subcutaneous changes include dry poor coat, dry scaly skin, fat redistribution, and an increase in lipomas or their size. In more susceptible dogs or dogs receiving higher dosages, alopecia, thin skin, hypotonic skin, calcinosis cutis, atrophic remodeling of scars, comedones, and milia-like follicular cysts may occur alone or in combination.

Musculoskeletal abnormalities may go unrecognized as glucocorticoid side effects. Osteoporosis, muscle atrophy, and weak ligaments may result from the glucocorticoid effects of protein catabolism, fibroblast inhibition, and decreased intestinal calcium absorption. Although no studies have documented an association, it has been suggested that dogs receiving long-term glucocorticoid therapy are at higher risk for ligament damage, particularly cruciate rupture.[186] Steroid myopathy and traumatic rupture of the gastrocnemius muscle was attributed to glucocorticoid therapy in one dog.[141]

The alteration in metabolism may lead to hyperlipidemia and steroid hepatopathy. Endocrine changes induced may include adrenal gland suppressions, then atrophy, diabetes mellitus, decreased thyroid hormone synthesis, and increased parathyroid hormone levels. Significant side effects with appropriate anti-inflammatory systemic glucocorticoid regimens are uncommon in dogs, occurring in less than 10% of the animals treated. However, with immunosuppressive regimens, the frequency and the severity of glucocorticoid side effects escalate alarmingly and less than 50% of the dogs so treated can be satisfactorily managed.[160, 173]

It must be emphasized that alternate-day therapy with prednisolone is not a panacea.[22] Occasionally, some dogs cannot be successfully managed with such therapy without experiencing iatrogenic hyperglucocorticoidism.[160, 161, 173] This probably reflects differences in serum protein levels, receptor levels, or absorption, metabolism, or clearance of glucocorticoid in those individuals. Additionally, individual variation is occasionally dramatic in susceptibility to acute or chronic glucocorticoid side effects;[160, 161] therefore, (1) various degrees of iatrogenic hyperglucocorticoidism occur after as little as 3 weeks to as long as 7 years of therapy, and (2) calcinosis cutis or full-blown Cushing's syndrome may be an individual dog's only manifestation of hyperglucocorticoidism.[159–161, 165]

Although clinically effective doses of systemic glucocorticoids in cats are usually twice those needed in dogs, significant side effects are rare.[158, 160, 161] Polydipsia, polyuria, polyphagia, a tendency for weight gain, depression, and diarrhea occasionally occur. Significant iatrogenic hyperglucocorticoidism has been produced in cats only after the weekly subcutaneous administration of methylprednisolone acetate for 10 weeks. Cats rarely experience typical iatrogenic Cushing's syndrome with fewer doses.[158] Obviously, such therapy would never be either employed or indicated in clinical situations.

Significant side effects after intralesional glucocorticoid therapy have not been reported in dogs and cats. Local cutaneous atrophy and local inflammatory reactions (presumably due to crystalline material left at the injection site) are rare. These side effects, as well as panniculitis, sterile abscesses, necrosis, and pigmentary disturbances, are well recognized in humans.[57, 181, 186]

A potentially much more significant side effect of intralesional therapy is systemic hyperglucocorticoidism.[160, 172] Normal dogs given subconjunctival injections of methylprednisolone acetate had suppressed adrenocortical responses to exogenous ACTH for 9 to 20 days.[172] Additionally, dogs that received intracutaneous or subconjunctival injections of methylprednisolone or betamethasone were unresponsive to intradermal histamine and skin test allergens for up to 4 weeks. The health significance of such findings in dogs is unknown. Certainly, such medications could influence interpretation of results of hematologic, adrenal function, and intradermal allergy skin tests.

EVALUATION

Evaluation of the results during glucocorticoid therapy is important. When appropriate systemic anti-inflammatory glucocorticoid therapy is given to an otherwise healthy dog or cat, the risks are minimal. The risks associated with immunosuppressive doses are of greater concern, especially because the medication is usually prescribed for serious or life-threatening diseases, which will probably be treated for the rest of the animal's life. Significant concurrent dysfunction of major organ systems also drastically increases the risks. Some owners balk at the expense, the risk, the unpleasant side effects, or the complex therapy protocol, and they refuse treatment. Occasionally, the clinician may be forced to choose between using drugs that may not be in the animal's best long-term interest or performing euthanasia at the owner's request.

When long-term systemic therapy is started, owners should be instructed to observe their animals closely and to immediately report any significant side effects. A physical check-up is advised every 6 to 12 months. Periodic urinalysis and urine cultures may be needed to recognize urinary tract infections that are not clinically apparent. Serum chemistry screens are advised every 12 to 24 months before more medication is dispensed. The ACTH response test is useful in animals with suspected iatrogenic Cushing's disease. Marked suppression indicates that other attempts at lowering the dosage should be made because major problems are inevitable. Dogs receiving appropriate long-term, alternate-day steroid therapy usually have mildly to moderately suppressed adrenocortical responses to ACTH and elevated serum alkaline phosphatase levels but are otherwise clinically normal.

Interferons

Interferons are a family of regulatory proteins that can act on a variety of different cell types and profoundly affect a number of biological functions, including host defense mechanisms against viral and bacterial infections; cell proliferation, differentiation, and functional activation; antitumor effects; IFN-γ immunomodulation; monocyte and macrophage activation; cytotoxic T cell activation and differentiation; stimulation of MHC I and II expression; B cell antibody production; regulation of lipid metabolism, and direct and indirect activation of numerous cytokines.[145a] In humans, various recombinant products (IFN-α-2a [Roferon-A, Roche]; IFN-α-2b [Intron-A, Schering]; IFN-β-1b [Betaseron, Berlex]) are used with variable success for everything from melanomas, papillomas, and epitheliotropic lymphoma to atopy, discoid lupus erythematosus, and chronic granulomatous disease.

In dogs and cats, anecdotal reports indicate that IFN-α-2a (Roferon-A) and IFN-α-2b are being tried in a number of dermatologic conditions.[156a] These include multiple papillomas in young and old dogs and cats, herpesvirus dermatitis in cats, idiopathic facial dermatosis of Himalayan and Persian cats, epitheliotropic lymphoma in dogs, and recurrent bacterial pyoderma in dogs. Some cases of feline indolent ulcer have responded, but eosinophilic plaques and eosinophilic granulomas have not.

The standard dilution procedure is as follows: 3 million IU into 1 L of sterile saline gives a solution of 3000 IU/ml, which can be frozen for 1 year. Ten milliliters of this solution added to 1 L of sterile saline gives a solution of 30 IU/ml, which can be stored (*not* frozen) in the refrigerator for several months. This solution may be given orally or subcutaneously. Doses for dogs vary from 1 to 1.5 million IU/m^2 BSA to 1 to 3 million IU/dog/day or 3 times weekly. The dose for cats is 60 to 120 IU/cat/day. Little factual information is available on the immunologic and therapeutic effects of interferons in dogs and cats.

In humans, side effects are usually mild and reversible, with flulike symptoms being the most common.[215] Side effects are not reported in dogs and cats.

Melatonin

The hormone melatonin is synthesized in the pineal gland from L-tryptophan. It is most readily known and often studied in reptilian and amphibian species. Melatonin is involved in the neuroendocrine control of photoperiod-dependent molting and/or pelage color in many mammals. The hormone may act directly on hair follicles or within the central nervous system to alter secretion of melanocyte-stimulating hormone (MSH) and/or prolactin. Melatonin secretion is tied to the photoperiod, with the greatest production during dark hours. Greatest daily secretion occurs in the winter, when the length of daylight is shortest.[132]

When melatonin was administered orally to normal dogs, blood levels were significantly increased for 8 hours.[9a] In female dogs, there was a significant decrease in blood levels of estradiol, testosterone, and dehydroepiandrosterone. In male dogs, there was a significant decrease in blood levels of estradiol and 17-OH progesterone. Blood levels of prolactin and thyroid hormone were unaffected.

There is an inverse relation with circulating prolactin levels and the secretion of MSH.[132] Melatonin and prolactin levels may be involved in the seasonal growth of winter haircoats and spring molt in mammalian species such as mink, in which implants of melatonin have been used to artificially induce early winter coat production.

The original uses for melatonin in veterinary dermatology go back to the 1960s, when it was recommended for the treatment of acanthosis nigricans.[142] However, melatonin has recently received attention because of possible effects on a variety of canine hair growth disorders. The beneficial effects of melatonin for the treatment of chronic recurrent flank alopecia and various forms of pattern baldness have been reported.[130, 131] In canine recurrent flank alopecia, nine dogs were treated, three with two subcutaneous injections of melatonin (12.5 mg) in soybean oil at 2-week intervals and six dogs with 36 mg of melatonin subcutaneous implants. All nine dogs failed to experience the typical recurrence of alopecia.[130]

In canine pattern baldness, 11 dogs all had improved hair growth after melatonin therapy. Seven dogs received subcutaneous implants, but four dogs were treated orally with 5 mg q24h for 30 days.[131] We and others have noted varying responses to oral melatonin treatment with these diseases. In addition, cases with pinnal alopecia, suspected adrenal sex hormone imbalance, or alopecia associated with excessive trichilemmal keratinization histologically have responded to melatonin treatment.[132]

Melatonin is available in nonprescription form as a dietary supplement at most health food stores, often in 3-mg tablets. Only licensed products have guaranteed purity. Capsules can be made from melatonin crystalline powder (Sigma Chemical Company). Oral melatonin has a short half-life, and empirical protocols call for 3 to 6 mg/dog q8h. The relative efficacy of oral versus injectable or subcutaneous implant therapy still needs to be evaluated. Injectable melatonin is available from Rickards Research Foundation (Cleveland, OH). Constant-release implants with 2.5 mg or 12 mg are available from Wildlife Pharmaceuticals (Fort Collins, CO).[132] Some dogs receiving subcutaneous implants experience sterile abscesses or granulomas.

• ORAL SUNSCREENS

Oral sunscreens are chemicals such as ß-carotene and chloroquine that quench free radicals and stabilize membranes. They have not been proved to prevent sunburn in humans but have been useful in cases of light-induced dermatosis.[102, 150] A β-carotene derivative has been used in cats and dogs to reduce phototoxicity (see Chap. 16). Canthaxanthin (β,β-carotene-4,'-dione) is a red-orange pigment found in plants and other sources. The safety of this product has been challenged. Side effects include orange-brown skin, brick-red stools, crystalline gold deposits on the retinae, orange plasma, and lowered amplitudes on electroretinograms. The usual maximal dosage for humans is 25 mg/kg daily, but some companies recommend four 30-mg capsules once daily (Golden Tan, Orobronze). In toxicity studies of dogs, the long-term and short-term lethal dose is greater than 10,000 mg/kg.

• SKIN SURGERY

Skin surgery can be an important part of small animal dermatology. Many new developments have arisen, from skin biopsies for diagnosis to cryosurgery for specialized procedures. It is essential to know what equipment is needed and to be able to use the equipment properly. Cold steel surgery, cryosurgery, laser surgery, and electrosurgery are discussed in this chapter. Biopsy techniques are covered in Chapter 2.

Dermatologists recommend plastic surgery for the correction of anatomic defects causing dermatoses of facial, tail, vulva, and lip folds. Skin grafting (pinch, strip, mesh, and pedicle grafts) is useful to repair defects of skin of the extremities when tumors or lesions such as acral lick dermatitis have been removed surgically. Plastic repair of ear flaps and the external ear canal may be helpful in correcting associated dermatologic or cosmetic problems. Plastic surgery techniques are not discussed in this chapter, but information on them can be found in references.[13, 177, 183]

Cold Steel Surgery

Excision of small tumors and other lesions is a minor procedure that can often be performed on an outpatient basis but is usually better performed if the animal is held in the hospital for several hours. This enables the practitioner to use tranquilization, sedation, or general anesthesia as needed to promote control and relaxation of the patient. Cases requiring extensive surgery with plastic repair procedures and grafts need an operating room with complete aseptic routine. Even minor cases, however, must be handled with proper preparation, sterile instruments, and other measures to accomplish a scrupulously clean operation.

The dermatologist who employs surgical treatment of human diseases usually performs minor techniques on skin that is relatively hairless; therefore, the cosmetic effects are crucial. Most procedures appear complex because avoidance of scarring is a primary consideration. In veterinary dermatology, the clinician should, of course, avoid disfigurement, but because of the dense pelage, small scars are relatively unimportant.

With any surgical procedure, it is necessary to clip the hair closely, wash the unbroken skin surface carefully until it is clean using a surgical scrub solution such as 1% chlorhexidine diacetate (Nolvasan, Fort Dodge) or 0.75% povidone-iodine (Betadine, Purdue Frederick), and rinse thoroughly. The skin is defatted by wiping the surface in a circular fashion from the center outward, using sterile swabs soaked in 70% alcohol. The skin can then be sprayed or swabbed with 0.5% solution of chlorhexidine diacetate or, as a second choice, 1% solution of povidone-iodine. The surgical site is then ready to drape. If a mast cell tumor is suspected, one should avoid a rough surgical preparation, which could trigger the release of vasoactive substances.

Basic instruments needed for skin surgery are in the average emergency or spay pack. The following additional instruments are useful for the delicate work in many skin surgical procedures:

1. Bard-Parker handles and blades, Nos. 10, 11, and 15
2. Small curved mosquito hemostats
3. Allis tissue forceps
4. Skin hooks (sharp single prong)
5. Iris forceps (mouse-toothed)
6. Olsen-Hegar needle holder with suture scissors
7. Skin punches, sizes 1 to 9 mm
8. Small automatic skin retractor

The lesions should be outlined by elliptic scalpel incisions that extend through the skin. The specimen or lesion is dissected free from the underlying tissue with scissors, hemostats, or both. Healing and final results are better if the long-axis incisions are oriented parallel to the tension lines. For closure, nylon sutures such as Vetafil produce good approximation with minimal scarring. Many quality suture materials are available, and the exact selection is a matter of personal preference. Swaged-on needles can further reduce the chance of infection and result in smaller scars. In routine cases with small incisions, the sutures can be removed in 10 to 14 days.

Cryosurgery

Cryosurgery is the controlled use of freezing temperatures to destroy undesirable tissue while doing minimal damage to surrounding healthy tissue. In general, cryosurgery is the most useful for small, localized skin lesions treated on an outpatient basis. Cryosurgery does not cure where a blade does not cure, but it is sometimes more convenient.

The anal and oral areas are preferred sites for cryosurgery, and it is indicated in selected cases of acral lick dermatitis. Specific conditions in which cryosurgery may be indicated include perianal fistulae, oral tumors, rectal tumors, nasal mucosal tumors, tail gland hyperplasia, feline indolent ulcers, and acral lick dermatitis. In the nasal, oral, and rectal areas, where surgical access and hemostasis are difficult, cryosurgery has advantages. In large lesions of acral lick dermatitis that cannot be removed by cold steel surgery, cryosurgery offers a favorable alternative to skin grafting. For readers who are seriously considering using cryosurgery, excellent references are available.[177, 209]

The discussion of cryosurgery includes basic principles, freezing agents, cryosurgical units, and dermatologic indications.

BASIC PRINCIPLES

The lethal effect of subzero temperatures on cells depends on five factors:

1. Type of cell being frozen
2. Rate of freezing
3. Final temperature (must be at least $-20°C$)
4. Rate of thawing
5. Repetition of the freeze-thaw cycle

Cell damage is more severe with rapid freezing, slow thawing, and three freeze-thaw cycles. A final temperature of $-70°C$ is reached at the surface of the probe with nitrous oxide equipment so that it can cool only a limited mass of tissue below the required $-20°C$, thereby restricting its application to small, superficial lesions. A final temperature of $-185°C$ can be reached at the tissue junction using liquid nitrogen. This enables the forming of a larger ice ball of tissue and allows larger areas to be effectively frozen.

A spray of liquid nitrogen is the most effective way to freeze large tumor masses, but this technique poses the greatest potential hazard if used carelessly. One advantage is that the base or periphery of a mass can be frozen first by careful spraying around a delineated area extending 3 to 5 mm beyond the visible edge. The remaining tissues within this frozen "stockade" can be treated by spraying in ever-decreasing circles. Used with care, the spray may prevent the escape of malignant cells into the circulation, and it enables the operator to form superficial, solid frozen plaques on the surface without damaging deeper structures. In contrast, a probe must freeze a hemisphere as deep as the visible radius. It is important to use needle thermocouples at the deep margins of the tissues to be frozen to monitor the effect and to prevent excessive damage to normal tissue.

In human dermatology, it is common to apply liquid nitrogen with an ordinary cotton applicator stick, which is dipped into the container of liquid and touched to the lesion, frequently a small tumor or wart. The applicator stick is touched intermittently to the lesion until the desired area and depth are frozen. Dermatologists with experience in using this method get good results. The pain is minimal and well tolerated without local anesthesia by most patients.

Many soft tissues, especially glandular tissues, are particularly susceptible to freezing. On the other hand, bone, fascia, tendon sheath, perineurium, and the walls of large blood vessels are fairly resistant. A knowledge of relative tissue susceptibility is of great practical importance.

To ensure that no cells escape destruction, the freeze-thaw cycle should be repeated two times or more. Thawing usually takes one and a half to two times as long as freezing. Freezing is accomplished much more rapidly during the second and third freeze because circulation to the target area has been compromised.

It has been speculated that useful immunologic effects are possible with cryosurgery. When a cell mass is frozen and left to die in situ, membrane lipoprotein complexes, and hence antigen-antibody complexing and receptor sites, are inevitably disrupted or altered. They are probably not totally destroyed. The nucleus may remain relatively intact. Thus, for a short time, antigenicity may be enhanced. Enough antigen is released systemically to produce a strong specific immunologic response that may kill escaped cells of the same tumor species.

After cryosurgery of canine skin tissue, histopathologic changes occur in an orderly progression of edema, erythema, infiltration of inflammatory cells, tissue necrosis, sloughing, repair by granulation, and re-epithelialization.[25]

ADVANTAGES

Cryosurgery has the following advantages:

1. Lesions can be removed in areas where the skin is so tight or the lesion so large that closure with sutures is impossible. Large lesions of acral lick dermatitis or tumors on the lower portions of the leg are examples.
2. In cases in which conventional excision surgery would produce shock or excessive blood loss, cryosurgery results in minimal hemorrhage. This is particularly effective in old or debilitated patients. Scarring is slight, and the cosmetic effect is good.
3. Selective destruction of diseased or neoplastic skin is possible with little damage to normal tissue. Chances of tumor cells spreading from premalignant lesions are reduced.
4. Cryosurgery has a possible immunotherapeutic effect on malignant neoplasms.

DISADVANTAGES

Cryosurgery has the following disadvantages:

1. The surgeon performing cryosurgery must be experienced and needs postgraduate training. Without specialized knowledge and skill, undesirable sequelae can result.
2. The necrosis and sloughing of frozen tissue are visually unpleasant and malodorous for 2 to 3 weeks after cryosurgery.
3. Regrowth of depigmented, white hair on the surgery site sometimes leaves a cosmetic defect.
4. Vital structures surrounding the frozen lesion may be damaged. This applies especially to blood vessels, nerves, tendons, ligaments, and joint capsules. For example, in cryosurgery for multiple perianal fistulae, fecal incontinence can result if the anal sphincter is damaged. Freezing of bone can result in pathologic fractures.
5. Large blood vessels frozen during cryosurgery for tumor removal may start bleeding 30 to 60 minutes later, when postoperative attention has been relaxed, or several hours later when the animal is at home. Air embolism is possible if sprays are used on open vessels.
6. Cryosurgery is contraindicated for mast cell tumors.

FREEZING AGENTS

Liquid nitrogen and nitrous oxide are the agents of choice in veterinary medicine. Carbon dioxide and Freon have also been used, although not commonly by veterinarians.

Liquid nitrogen is the most popular freezing agent in cryosurgery. It is a clear, colorless, odorless liquid. It is not flammable and produces a temperature of $-195.8°C$ ($-320.5°F$). It can usually be obtained from the medical supply companies that sell oxygen or from welding gas suppliers. Liquid nitrogen is delivered in variously sized vacuum-insulated Dewar's flasks. It can easily be poured from the flask into the cryosurgical unit. When small quantities are sufficient, physicians keep liquid nitrogen in ordinary quart insulated (Thermos) bottles that are refilled as needed by the supplier. If not agitated, liquid nitrogen remains active in the insulated container for about 2 days. Liquid nitrogen can be kept active for a limited time. Usually, 1 month is the maximum if the original container is opened several times.

Nitrous oxide is the second most popular freezing agent and is most effective for removing small tumors (less than 3 cm) or for treating superficial skin lesions. It requires cryosurgical units specifically designed for its use. Applied with probes, it produces a temperature of $-89°C$ ($-138°F$). Although it is more expensive on a per-unit basis than liquid nitrogen, there is no waste and nitrous oxide is readily available in veterinary hospitals that use gas anesthesia (halothane, nitrous oxide, and oxygen). One large tank can be used for many months because it is usually connected directly to the unit and is not poured, as is liquid nitrogen.

CRYOSURGICAL UNITS

Cryosurgical units deliver the freezing action by spray or probe. Some units (smaller, hand-held bottles) are designed to spray the gas only. Other units have both spray and probe attachments.

Some cryosurgery units deliver gas to a probe that is held against the tissue or inserted into crevices, fistulae, or other tracts to be destroyed. Cryoprobes use the Joule-Thompson effect: Rapid expansion of the gas under pressure provides low freezing temperatures. This is the method used with nitrous oxide. A great variety of probes are available, each for a different purpose. They can be round, flat, curved, pointed, or needle sharp. A special probe has even been devised for anal sac destruction.

There is a trend toward the use of the spray units. Some units look like modified insulated (Thermos) bottles with a spraying tip at the top. A mixture of liquid and vaporized liquid nitrogen is sprayed directly on the area to be treated. Different spray devices deliver different mixtures of liquid nitrogen, vapor, and liquid. This can vary from 15% vapor and 85% liquid to 55% vapor and 45% liquid. The higher the percentage of liquid in the spray, the lower the temperature and the deeper the freeze.

DERMATOLOGIC INDICATIONS

Cryosurgery differs in many ways from cold steel surgery and electrosurgery. Although it has specific uses, it is never a total replacement for conventional surgery. Proponents of cryosurgery believe that it has an excellent place in small animal practice, but knowledge, skill, and experience are necessary for best results. Detractors may have used the technique for the wrong conditions or without proper training, consequently experiencing poor results or complications. Some clinicians were once enthusiastic about cryosurgery but now use it less frequently. As improved units are manufactured, some designed especially for veterinary surgery, the practitioner will find it easier to select the proper cryosurgical apparatus and use it effectively.

Podkonjak reported a series of dermatologic problems treated with cryosurgery. The success rate after one treatment was 86%, and after one or more treatments, 93%. Cases included melanoma, squamous cell carcinoma, fibrosarcoma, papilloma, basal cell tumor, hemangioma, histiocytoma, and trichoepithelioma. Also treated were follicular cysts, nonhealing ulcers, granulation tissue, proliferative tissue in the external ear canal, tail gland hyperplasia, perianal fistulae, and circumanal adenomas.[137]

- **Tumors.** Cryosurgery does not and should not replace conventional surgery. However, scalpel surgery is difficult or impossible to use in some situations.
- **Oral Cavity.** Access to the oral cavity by means of conventional surgical instruments may be difficult, and hemorrhage may be hard to control. Cryosurgery is a simple and more effective method of therapy. It is an alternative in treating recurrent tumors for cases in which other surgical procedures have failed, especially for malignant neoplasms. Oral cavity squamous cell carcinomas may respond well to cryosurgery. Gingival epulis can be frozen, and sloughing occurs without the need for hemostasis.
- **Anal Area.** The main advantage of cryosurgery in managing anal tumors, especially circumanal adenomas, is that it involves less risk of damaging the anal sphincter or the vital anal nerve supply. In general, though, careful cold steel surgery is still the preferred method of removing circumanal adenomas.
- **Acral Lick Dermatitis.** Cryosurgery is indicated in acral lick dermatitis when the lesion is so large that the skin cannot be stretched for suturing after surgical excision. Skin grafting has been used successfully, but only by practitioners highly skilled in plastic surgery. It is difficult to keep dogs from damaging the grafted area because it is their favorite place to lick. Freezing the large lick lesion destroys the thickened skin, which is then replaced by granulation tissue that is covered by normal epithelium from the wound margins.

Because cryosurgery temporarily deadens the sensory nerves, there is less licking and less chance of recurrence at the same site for up to 6 months. Care must be taken not to freeze the underlying bone. To have complete control of the depth of freezing, it is essential to insert thermocouples under the lesion. After the lesion heals, the resulting scar and white hair are seldom objectionable in these difficult cases. Regrettably, recurrences are the rule, usually within 6 to 12 months.

- **Multiple Perianal Fistulae.** Perianal fistulae may be difficult to treat, but the use of cyclosporine is encouraging though expensive. Alternatively, favorable results have been described using cryosurgery. This method of therapy for perianal fistulae reached a high level of popularity in the late 1970s, but some veterinary surgeons are now returning to the use of surgical excision. The number of lengthy cryosurgical procedures (two or more) and the frequent recurrences of fistulae are two reasons that cryosurgery has lost favor. In addition, the occurrence of anal strictures is high.

Anal sac removal is always recommended before cryosurgery. However, the anal sac area is usually difficult to see because of surrounding scar and granulation tissue. Every attempt must be made to avoid the complication of fecal incontinence, which can be a greater problem.

Laser Surgery

Laser surgery is highly successful in some branches of medicine[179] and is rapidly finding a place in veterinary dermatology. The word *laser* is an acronym for *l*ight *a*mplification by the *s*timulated *e*mission of *r*adiation. Laser light, in contrast with regular light, is characterized in three different ways. It is monochromatic, meaning it is a wavelength of one color. It is coherent, meaning all the light waves are traveling in the same parallel direction and in phase. It is intense, which means the number of photons delivered to a surface area is great.

Multiple types of lasers are available and usually named for the dye or mineral used to elicit the light, but only two are being reported with any frequency in the United States. The argon pumped dye laser is more versatile in the wavelength of light that may be emitted and has been used to activate the photosensitizing agents in photochemotherapy. This type of laser has limited availability at certain specialty centers. The carbon dioxide (CO_2) laser is the most widely used type of laser in medicine worldwide. The CO_2 laser is gaining acceptance in the veterinary field, and a model for veterinarians has been developed (Accuvet, Luxar). Its cost is low enough that some moderate- to high-volume practices are justifying the expense.

When a laser light is directed at a tissue it is either absorbed, reflected, scattered, or transmitted. The absorbed light is the goal, which results in transfer of energy to the molecules in the absorbing tissue. This results in the majority of uses in the creation of heat. The tissue destruction that results from the rapid and high heat formation is called *photothermolysis*. The CO_2 laser emits a beam of light at 10,600 nm, which is the wavelength that water maximally absorbs the light energy. Because water is a major component of cells, they are heated and removed layer by layer. When the temperature of the tissue rises, different effects occur. At 43° to 45°C, cells heat up and die; at 60°C, there is protein denaturation and coagulation; at 80°C, collagen denaturation and membrane permeabilization occur; at 90° to 100°C, carbonization and tissue burning occur; and at 100°C, vaporization and ablation occur.[17, 125]

In veterinary dermatology, laser therapy has been reported to be useful in removing a variety of skin tumors, particularly of the eyelid, pinna, and tail.[21] In some situations it greatly speeds the time of surgery and results in improved cosmetic effect and decreased postoperative complications (Fig. 3–3). It has been used to rapidly treat skin tumors, especially when there are multiple lesions such as sebaceous hyperplasia/adenomas.

Laser therapy has also been reported to be helpful for certain cases of feline indolent ulcer and eosinophilic granuloma, acral lick dermatitis, excessive granulation tissue, interdigital granulomas, onychectomy, ear canal ablation, fox tail removal, chronic stomatitis, and interdigital abscess removal and sterilization.[21] Multiple hemangiomas and hemangiosarcomas from solar dermatitis are readily vaporized, allowing rapid and minimally invasive surgery (Fig. 3–4).

Advantages of laser surgery are less pain (the nerve endings are sealed during the cutting), less bleeding (due to sealing of small vessels and the ability to cause coagulation by defocusing and lower power emission), and less tissue destruction. The laser light also sterilizes the surgical incision site except for viral particles, and the surgical field can be sterilized by defocusing the beam, an advantage in contaminated lesions such as foreign body removal. These advantages result in less postoperative swelling and inflammation. Disadvantages are limited to the cost of the equipment and safety requirements. The disadvantages of the safety requirements are readily overcome with training.

Electrosurgery

Just as heat cautery was replaced by electrocautery, the latter has been improved on by modern electrosurgery.[13, 177] However, electrocautery equipment is still used to destroy

Such electrodesiccation and curettage are especially useful for removing many sebaceous adenomas, circumanal adenomas, fibrovascular papillomas, nevi, actinic keratoses, seborrheic keratoses, and small basal cell tumors.

- **Coagulation.** Electrocoagulation is used to seal small blood vessels by boiling the vessels' endothelial cells with the current from the ball-like probe.

  There are two methods of applying coagulation. One is to touch the electrode (ball) directly to the small blood vessel until the vessel wall shrinks and the hemorrhage is stopped by the tissue coagulation. The other method is to grasp the small blood vessel with a hemostat, which is then touched with the electrode (a flat probe is best), and turn on the current with the foot switch. It is important to be sure that a good seal of the vessel is produced by either method because new hemorrhage results from insufficient coagulation of the vessel walls.

- **Fulguration.** Electric fulguration is the destruction of tissue by electric sparks generated by a high-frequency current. Direct fulguration occurs when the metal point of the probe is connected to the uniterminal of the high-frequency unit and a spark of electricity is directed to the tissue to be treated. Electrosurgical units capable of fulguration usually have a special probe into which the handpiece is inserted. Some units use the same handpiece, whereas others have special fulguration handpieces that cannot be plugged into cutting or coagulation plugs. Fulguration is used for destruction of superficial warts and tumors. Without the need to touch the lesion, the current dehydrates and coagulates the tissue at the same time. This tissue does not need curettage but is allowed to slough. Most fulguration probes have a sharp point.

- **Electrolysis.** Electric epilation of hair can be performed with battery-operated units or electrosurgical units that can be used at low power. The probe must be a special tiny wire of such small diameter that it can be introduced into the hair follicle. With skill and experience, and under magnification, epilation can be accomplished. A too-low current allows epilated hair to grow back, whereas a current that is too high or an application that is too long can cause scarring. This method has been used for the removal of cilia in trichiasis and distichiasis (eyelid diseases—see Chap. 19).

Radiosurgery

The next generation beyond electrosurgery is radiowave surgery or radiosurgery. This form of surgery utilizes high-frequency radiowaves around 4 million hertz (4 MHz) and does not require a grounding plate (Ellman Surgitron, Ellman). However, a passive electrode is placed beneath the patient in the area of the surgery to act as an antenna to focus the radiowaves.[2] This plate does not require skin contact to function.

Multiple settings for different types of current allow some selection in the tissue effects produced. Also, the power setting is variable and needs to be set so that there is smoothest cutting with no sparking. Tissue damage is minimized when fully rectified and fully filtered current is utilized because there is little lateral heat spread to adjacent tissue. However, for better hemostasis, only fully rectified current may be used and will cause coagulation as well as cutting. Partially rectified current is mainly used for coagulation and hemostasis.

Advantages over cold steel surgery are that cutting is accomplished without pressure being required, hemostasis with fully filtered current effectively seals vessels under 2 mm in diameter, and the incision site and electrode tip are sterilized. Radiosurgery equipment is available at lower costs than laser equipment. Practice is required to develop a technique that minimizes lateral tissue damage, but with experience the advantages of radiosurgery over cold steel surgery become obtainable.

Disadvantages of this type of surgery include the risk for combustion of volatile gasses and liquids (thus alcohol is contraindicated as a prepping solution or near the antennae), radiosurgery should not be used to cut cartilage or bone, and there is risk if this technique is used near an unshielded pacemaker—persons or pets with such devices should not be in the vicinity.[2] Smoke and an unpleasant odor may be produced, but this is minimized with the use of a vacuum smoke evacuator. Tissue burning is possible, especially if the equipment is improperly used. Adequate training and practice make this a useful surgical option.

Indications described for veterinary dermatology include cutaneous biopsy (but samples should only be taken with the fully rectified and fully filtered current) and removal of cutaneous neoplasms. For small or pedunculated tumors, a loop electrode is available that makes the procedure rapid.

• ALTERNATIVE THERAPIES

Interest in so-called alternative therapies is increasing among pet owners. Unfortunately, little in the way of scientific evaluation is available in the veterinary dermatology literature. We encourage clinicians who use these modalities to design, perform, and publish meaningful clinical trials. We have so much to learn about these "natural" remedies.

Acupuncture

Acupuncture can be defined as the insertion of very fine needles into specific, predetermined points on the body to produce physiologic responses.[5, 153, 154] In addition to needles, many other methods are used to stimulate acupuncture points, including acupressure, moxibustion, cupping, applying heat or cold, ultrasound, aquapuncture, electrostimulation, implantation, and laser use. The International Veterinary Acupuncture Society (IVAS, PO Box 2074, Nederland, CO 80466-2074) conducts courses, seminars, and international veterinary acupuncture congresses, and it is responsible for the accreditation of veterinary acupuncturists throughout the world.

In dogs, acupuncture has been reported to be useful in various dermatologic conditions, especially acral lick dermatitis and other psychodermatoses.[5, 104, 153, 154]

Holistic Medicine (Herbal Medicine, Homeopathy)

Holistic health involves the use of herbs and other natural substances.[36, 43, 136, 217] A list of holistic veterinarians can be obtained from the American Holistic Veterinary Medical Association (2214 Old Emmerton Road, Bel Air, MD 21015), which also publishes a veterinary journal. We are aware of no well-designed clinical studies using this modality in veterinary dermatology.

In Asian and some European countries, many herbal products are in routine use for various dermatoses in humans.[23, 89] Examples include Calendula (from *Calendula officinalis*, the marigold flower, which contains flavonoids and saponins that have anti-inflammatory, immunomodulatory, wound-healing properties—available in ointment or cream for burns, diaper rash, minor wounds, leg ulcers; chamomile (from *Matricaria recutita*, the daisy flower family, containing oxides, flavonoids, and matricin that inhibit cyclooxygenase, lipoxygenase, and histamine release)—available in ointment or cream for various dermatitides, including atopic dermatitis and a 10-herb product ("decoction") taken by mouth and shown to be effective for atopic dermatitis in double-blinded, placebo-controlled studies.[23, 89]

There have been a number of anecdotal reports on the use of a multiaction herbal skin gel (Phytogel, Ayuvet).[3, 176, 194] The product contains *Pongamia glabra, Cedrus deodara, Azadirachta indica,* and *Eucalyptus globus*. These are claimed to have antibacterial, antifungal, antiparasitic, anti-inflammatory, antipruritic, and wound-healing properties. The product is recommended for bacterial pyoderma, dermatophytosis, scabies, demodicosis, insect bites, acral lick dermatitis, pyotraumatic dermatitis, wounds, maggots, burns, nasal solar dermatitis, papillomatosis, and so forth. Unfortunately, published trials are not interpretable.

• GENE THERAPY

Gene therapy may someday be used to treat skin diseases in companion animals. Skin gene therapy can be defined as insertion or introduction of a desired gene into the skin in order to express the gene product.[202] The goal is to treat a specific disease process with the protein product of the introduced gene. There are potentially large numbers of diseases that could be treated in this manner, including diseases without a clear genetic basis (polygenic diseases).

Generally, there are two gene therapy approaches: (1) the in vivo approach, wherein the genes are directly introduced into the skin, and (2) the ex vivo approach, wherein target cells (e.g., keratinocytes) are cultured from biopsy specimens, the desired gene is inserted into the cultured cells, and the genetically modified cells are then grafted back onto the donor.[202] Genes may be introduced by chemical (DNA transfection), physical (microprojectiles, direct injection), or biological (retrovirus, adenovirus) techniques.

• WOUNDS

Healing

Veterinary dermatologists perform minor surgical procedures and manage ulcers and other skin defects. Therefore, a basic understanding of wound healing is essential. In addition to the discussion that follows, more in-depth information can be found in the references.[34, 47, 94, 95, 184]

Wound healing is divided into three overlapping series of events: (1) inflammation, (2) new tissue formation, and (3) matrix remodeling. These stages progress along a continuum, and they may overlap considerably. An incised wound begins to heal by 5 to 8 days, with re-establishment of epidermal continuity and a proliferation of connective tissue from the papillary layer of the dermis. Thus, healing occurs in a "dished," or inverted, configuration until the production of underlying connective tissue pushes the epithelium up into an everted position. (The major cell, matrix, and mediator components of wound healing are presented in Table 3–9.)

In the inflammatory stage, the immediate reaction to a full-thickness skin loss is for

• Table 3–9   MAJOR COMPONENTS OF WOUND HEALING

CELLS	MATRIX	ENZYME CASCADES/MEDIATORS
Inflammation		
Neutrophils	Fibrin	Hagemen factor pathways
Endothelial cells	Fibronectin	Coagulation
Mast cells		Fibrinolysis
Platelets		Complement
New Tissue Formation		
Keratinocytes	Fibrin	PDGF
Macrophages	Fibronectin	FGF
		EGF
Endothelial cells	Collagen Types I or III	TGF-α
Fibroblasts	Hyaluronic acid	TGF-β
Matrix Remodeling		
Keratinocytes	Basement membranes	TGF-β
Endothelial cells	Laminin	Collagenase
Fibroblasts	Type IV collagen	Other proteases
	Heparin sulfate	
	Type VI collagen	Glycosidases
	Chondroitin sulfate	
	Dermatan sulfate	

PDGF = platelet-derived growth factor; FGF = fibroblast growth factor; EGF = epidermal growth factor; TGF = transforming growth factor.

the normal elasticity of skin and muscle tension to enlarge and distort the defect. Vessels contract and constrict for 5 to 10 minutes to limit hemorrhage to the injured area, resulting in more widespread leakage of plasma constituents. Infiltrating neutrophils attempt to clear the area of foreign particles, especially bacteria. Peripheral blood monocytes are progressively attracted, are activated, and become macrophages. Macrophages, like platelets, produce growth factors critical for the initiation of granulation tissue formation. Blood vessel disruption leads to extravasation of blood constituents. Platelet aggregation and blood coagulation initiate the early phase of inflammation. Clot formation within vessel lumina affects hemostasis and, within the surrounding connective tissue, provides a substrate for cell migration into the wound space. Mediators released as a consequence of blood coagulation, complement pathways, and cell activation (or death) cause the influx of inflammatory leukocytes and increase the permeability of undamaged adjacent vessels.

As the inflammation progresses, the infiltrate changes from primarily neutrophils to having large numbers of macrophages. The macrophages play an important part in the late stages of inflammation to help with the phagocytosis, débridement, and initiation of the changes that promote growth and granulation tissue formation. The mechanisms dispose of microorganisms, foreign material, and devitalized tissue and set the stage for wound repair.

The new tissue formation stage proceeds quickly when clots, necrotic tissue, and other barriers to healing are removed from the wound. During this stage, the following processes occur: re-epithelialization, fibroplasia and wound contraction, and neovascularization. In simple wounds, fibroblast proliferation and capillary infiltration start by the third to the fifth day. In open wounds, evidence of these processes is recognized as granulation tissue. Fibroblasts are most active in a wound for 14 to 21 days, and they advance along lines of fibrin within a clot and along capillaries that are growing into a wound. At first, the fibrin, fibroblasts, and new collagen fibers are vertically oriented in a wound, but after about 6 days they are horizontally oriented.

The fibroblasts secrete various glycoproteins that constitute the ground substance, aligned parallel to the surface of the wound. Collagen synthesis by the fibroblasts begins on the fourth or fifth day, and the tiny fibrils bond together into larger fibers that become ever stronger and less soluble. As sufficient collagen is formed, the number of fibroblasts in the wound decreases, marking the end of the repair stage. Elastic fibers play little part in wound repair, which explains the lack of scar elasticity.

Capillary infiltration of the healing wound is important to ensure optimal oxygen supply for the fibroblasts. Without optimal oxygen tension, fibroblasts cannot adequately synthesize collagen. The capillaries are a major part of the bright-red granulation tissue that appears in open wounds 3 to 6 days after injury. In small wounds, this occurs beneath a scab and is not visible. The proliferating capillaries form loops, or "knuckles," that give the wound a granular surface. The new vessels anastomose freely and differentiate progressively into arterioles and venules. Lymphatic vessels develop in a similar manner but a little later in the healing process.

Epithelial proliferation and migration are the first obvious signs of rebuilding and repair. Re-epithelialization of the epidermal defect begins within 24 hours after injury and continues during granulation tissue formation. Peripheral epidermal and infundibular hair follicle keratinocytes participate in the repair. An intense epidermal reaction occurs up to 5 mm back from the wound edge, and the number of epidermal cell layers dramatically increases. The cells lose their firm attachment to the underlying dermis, and they flatten and extend outward and downward over the incised dermis in a leapfrog fashion.

In simple wounds with clean, close approximation of edges, the defect may be covered by epithelium in 24 hours. In larger wounds, granulation tissue must form before wound epithelialization can start and the process may take days or even weeks to complete. If hair follicles are damaged, they participate in healing because the ends of the cut follicles are deep in the dermis and closer to the depth of the wound. The new epithelium has a smooth undersurface with weak attachment to the connective tissue, so it is easily traumatized and may be knocked from a healing wound. With the passage of time, new sebaceous glands and hair follicles may regenerate by differentiation of migrating cells.

Wound contraction is the reduction in size of an open wound as a result of centripetal movement of the whole-thickness skin that surrounds the lesion. Contraction can be useful in loose skin because it decreases the size of the wound that must be covered with epithelium. Over joints and in areas of tight skin, contractures can cause deformities. Contracture takes place between 5 and 45 days after injury. It is thought to result from a pulling action by modified fibroblasts in granulation tissue that take on some of the characteristics of smooth muscle cells. These cells are called myofibroblasts, and they align themselves along the lines of contraction. They are also capable of producing collagen.

The matrix remodeling stage is a period of consolidation, strengthening, and remodeling of the wound. In a fresh wound, a lag phase occurs (4 to 5 days), during which there is little gain in wound strength. The initial strength is due to the fibrin clot, adhesive forces of epithelialization, coagulation of protein in the wound, and ingrowth of capillaries, fibroblasts, and collagen fibrils. The amount of collagen increases rapidly during the first 3 weeks of healing and then reaches a state of equilibrium. Over a long time, maturation and remodeling take place by cross-linkage and changes in the physical weave of the collagen fibers. The strength of skin and fascia increases but always remains 15% to 20% weaker than surrounding normal tissue. All repair activity is confined to an area within approximately 15 mm of the wound.

Initially, scar tissue is vascular and cellular and appears pink and raised. As maturation occurs, the scar becomes white, hard, and flattened.

The following general factors are often considered to enhance or hasten wound healing: young age, administration of anabolic steroids, administration of topical and systemic vitamin A, ambulation of the patient, warm environment, and general good health. Ultrasound therapy has been reported to benefit wound healing when connective tissue is needed.[172] Although it increases inflammation and delays epithelialization, it stimulates fibroblast and collagen production and enhances vascularization of granulation tissue.

Wound healing is stimulated by maintaining a favorable environment at the wound site. This includes the removal of toxic exudate, maintenance of a moist but bacteria-free environment, access to oxygen, and prevention of trauma. Much research clearly shows a moist environment is much superior to the dry environment often created with the old fashioned dry bandage approach to wound dressings.[79, 84, 193] In response to these observations on what creates a favorable environment, the pharmaceutical industry has developed a wide variety of new wound materials that have been called *interactive dressings*.[193] These interactive dressings come in several forms, such as polymeric films, polymeric foams, in situ foams, hydrogels, hydrocolloids, and particulate and fibrous polymers.[84, 193] In many studies with these new wound-management materials, the healing time 50 (when the wound will be 50% healed) is much faster but the long-term response is similar to that with more traditional approaches. Therefore, the additional cost would seem most appropriate in animals at greater risk for poor wound healing, such as old or debilitated dogs and cats. As the costs for these new materials decrease, they may find a place for routine use in veterinary medicine.

Factors that generally delay or are detrimental to wound healing, in addition to the poor health factors mentioned earlier, include obesity and old age, steroids and steroid-related factors, denervation, the presence of foreign bodies, infection, devitalized tissue, dead space, insulin deficiency, hypoproteinemia, anemia, hypovolemia, malnutrition, shock, increased catabolic rate, movement of the wound, neoplasia, tissue anoxia, radiation and cytotoxic drugs, seromas and hematomas, edema, cold temperatures, excessive trauma, and exposure during surgery. Nutritional deficiencies (especially of vitamins A, K, E, and C; the B complex; and zinc) are also detrimental to wound healing.

MANAGEMENT

- **Epidermal Abrasions.** Margins of an abraded area are shallow and usually involve only the epidermis. Centrally, the defect may extend into the dermis. Initially, the injury fills with a blood clot and necrotic debris that dehydrate to form a scab. The epidermal adnexa may be injured, but they remain and regenerate. In partial-thickness wounds, they are the major source for re-epithelialization. The only care needed is initial gentle cleaning, allowing the scab to form, and protection from infection and trauma while the epidermal cells slide under the scab to re-epithelialize the exposed dermis.

• **Contaminated Wounds.** The early time after a wound is called the "golden period"—an interval of about 6 hours during which prophylactic antibiotics are effective. The first aid for wounds should involve only covering the wound with moist, dry, clean, nonadhering material to control bleeding and to minimize contamination until definitive care can be provided. Nearly all topical antibiotics, except bacitracin, retard experimental wound healing.[84]

Proper care may require sedation or anesthesia, if allowed by the status of the patient. Otherwise, flushing the wound with 1% lidocaine or using regional anesthesia may be sufficient for proper wound manipulation. Prophylactic antibiotics are completely effective for only up to 3 hours after trauma; therefore, systemic agents should be given first. One of the cephalosporins and gentamicin provide broad, effective coverage. The wound can be filled with a water-soluble gel (such as K-Y jelly) to protect it from further contamination while the area is prepared for surgery. Mineral oil or petroleum jelly can be applied to clippers to cause the hair to adhere to the blades while the area is being clipped. A vacuum is used to collect and direct debris away from the wound.

The skin is prepared with chlorhexidine surgical scrub and gently cleaned with alcohol wipes. The clinician should then thoroughly irrigate the wound with large volumes of sterile saline or chlorhexidine solution 0.05% to remove the gel and all foreign particles such as hair, dirt, and clotted blood. It has been reported that 0.05% chlorhexidine can cause a retardation of experimental wound healing,[84] but the clinical significance of this in dogs and cats is unknown.

Chlorhexidine is preferred to povidone-iodine solution because it has a wide spectrum of antibacterial effectiveness, immediately reduces the bacterial flora, and has a residual effect as a result of binding to the stratum corneum so tightly that it cannot be removed with alcohol.[185] In the 0.05% dilution, it is nonirritating and does not delay healing. Systemic absorption, toxicity, and inactivation by organic matter are not a problem. However, if the tympanic membrane is ruptured, chlorhexidine solution should be used cautiously in the external ear canal because it may cause ototoxicity.

Clay is by far the most deleterious of the soil contaminants. Pressure lavage (10 psi) applied with an 18-gauge needle and 30-ml syringe, or 70-psi pulsating pressure lavage, as provided with a dental water pick, may be used to decontaminate the wound. These pressures have not been found to spread infection.

The wound can then be draped and explored for special problems. Layered débridement and sharp dissection are used to remove devitalized or severely traumatized tissue. The wound is closed with properly placed sutures to approximate skin and to obliterate dead spaces. Proper placement of drains, if needed, and bandaging as appropriate complete the initial treatment.

For treatment of wounds with impaired healing rates, the use of products containing zinc oxide and cod liver oil or hydrogel-polyurethane wound dressings have been recommended.[84]

• **Decubital Ulcers.** Debilitated, paralyzed patients have poor circulation, and their immobility allows pressure between bony prominences and their bedding to restrict circulation further to a local tissue area. The area becomes red, and a punched-out ulcer develops later. The ulcer may have a gray fibrous coating with surrounding necrotic tissue.

Prevention via frequent turning, gentle massage, flexion of muscles and joints, and placing the patient on a waterbed is most important. After it has developed, the ulcer is treated by cleaning with 0.05% chlorhexidine solution to remove necrotic tissue, pus, and debris. The ulcer should be covered with moist occlusive bandages or a nonadherent film and protected from pressure by "doughnut" rings or bandage rolls. Although mild antibacterial dressings are often useful initially, the application of a live yeast cell derivative and phenylmercuric nitrate in shark liver oil (Preparation H, Whitehall) ointment increases oxygen utilization and collagen formation in tissues, and it increases wound healing. It also lubricates and protects the ulcer. When the patient becomes mobile, the ulcers heal spontaneously.

• REFERENCES

1. Ackerman L: Nutritional supplements in canine dermatoses. Can Vet J 28:29, 1987.
2. Ackerman LJ: Dermatologic applications of radiowave surgery (radiosurgery). Comp Cont Educ 19:463, 1997.
3. Agrawal AK: Therapeutic efficacy of a herbal gel for skin affections in dogs. Indian Vet J 74:417, 1997.
4. Alpo Pet Center: Canine Nutrition and Feeding Management. Alpo Pet Foods, Inc., Allentown, 1984.
5. Altman S: Acupuncture therapy in small animal practice. Comp Cont Educ 19:1233, 1997.
6. American Kennel Club: The Complete Dog Book, 17th ed. Howell House, New York, 1985.
7. Anderson BC: Aloe vera juice: A veterinary medicament? Comp Cont Educ 5:S364, 1983.
8. Andreassi L: Bioengineering of the skin. Clin Dermatol 13:289, 1995.
9. Arndt KA, et al: The pharmacology of topical therapy. In: Fitzpatrick TB, et al (eds): Dermatology in General Medicine, 4th ed. McGraw-Hill Book Co., New York, 1993, p 2837.
9a. Ashley PF, et al: Effect of oral melatonin administration on sex hormone, prolactin, and thyroid hormone concentrations in adult dogs. J Am Vet Med Assoc 215:111, 1999.
10. Beale KM, et al: A study of long term administration of FS shampoo in dogs. Proc Annu Memb Meet Am Acad Vet Dermatol Am Coll Vet Dermatol 9:36, 1993.
11. Becheral PA, et al: CD23 mediated nitric oxide synthase pathway induction in human keratinocytes is inhibited by retinoic acid derivatives. J Invest Dermatol 106:1182, 1996.
12. Bernstein JE, et al: Inhibition of histamine induced pruritus by topical tricyclic antidepressants. J Am Acad Dermatol 5:582, 1981.
13. Bojrab MJ: Current Techniques in Small Animal Surgery, 3rd ed. Lea & Febiger, Philadelphia, 1990.
14. Bond R, Lloyd DH: A double blind comparison of olive oil and a combination of evening primrose oil and fish oil in the management of chronic atopy. Vet Rec 131:558, 1992.
15. Bond R, Lloyd DH: Randomized single-blind comparison of an evening primrose oil and fish oil combination and concentrates of these oils in the management of canine atopy. Vet Dermatol 3:215, 1992.
16. Boothe DM: Topical drugs: Component interactions, vehicles, and the consequences of alterations. Dermatol Rep 6:1, 1987.
17. Boulnois JL: Photophysical processes in recent medical laser developments: A review. Lasers in Medical Science I. Baillière Tindall, Philadelphia, 1986, p 48.
18. Bourdeau P, Paragon BM: Alternatives aux corticoides en dermatologie des carnivores. Rev Méd Vét 168:645, 1992.
19. Bourdeaux MK, et al: The effects of varying dietary n-6 to n-3 fatty acid ratios on platelet reactivity, coagulation screening assays, and antithrombin III activity in dogs. J Am Anim Hosp Assoc 33:235, 1997.
20. Brayton CF: Dimethyl sulfoxide (DMSO), a review. Cornell Vet 76:61, 1986.
21. Breen PT: Lasers in dermatology. In: Kirk RW (ed): Current Veterinary Therapy X. W.B. Saunders Co, Philadelphia, 1989, p 580.
22. Brockus CW, et al: Effect of alternate-day prednisolone administration on hypophyseal-adrenocortical activity in dogs. Am J Vet Res 60:698, 1999.
23. Brown DJ, Dattner AM: Phytotherapeutic approaches to common dermatologic conditions. Arch Dermatol 134:1401, 1998.
24. Bruynzeel I, et al: Pentoxifylline inhibits T-cell adherence to keratinocytes. J Invest Dermatol 104:1004, 1995.
25. Bushby PA, et al: Microscopic tissue alterations following cryosurgery of canine skin. J Am Vet Med Assoc 173:177, 1978.
26. Campbell KL, Kirkwood AR: Effect of topical oils on transepidermal water loss in dogs with seborrhea sicca. In: Ihrke, PJ, et al (eds): Advances in Veterinary Dermatology, Vol 2. Pergamon Press, New York, 1993, p 157.
27. Campbell KL, et al: Effects of oral sunflower oil on serum and cutaneous fatty acid concentration profiles in seborrheic dogs. Vet Dermatol 3:29, 1992.
28. Carlotti DN, Maffart P: La chlorhexidine, revue bibliographique. Prat Méd Chir Anim Comp 31:553, 1996.
29. Chandraratna RAS: Rational design of receptor-selective retinoids. J Am Acad Dermatol 39(part 2):S124, 1998.
30. Chandraratna RAS: Tazarotene: The first receptor-selective topical retinoid for the treatment of psoriasis. J Am Acad Dermatol 37(Suppl 2, Part 3):S12, 1997.
31. Chastain CB, Ganjam VK: Clinical Endocrinology of Companion Animals. Lea & Febiger, Philadelphia, 1986.
32. Chastain CB, Graham CL: Adrenocortical suppression in dogs on daily and alternate day prednisolone administration. Am J Vet Res 40:936, 1979.
33. Chew BP, et al: Importance of ß-carotene nutrition in dog and cat: Uptake and immunity. In: Reinhart GA, Carey DP (eds): Recent Advances in Canine and Feline Nutrition II. Orange Frazer Press, Wilmington, OH, 1998, p 513.
34. Clark RAF: Cutaneous wound repair. In: Goldsmith LA (ed): Physiology, Biochemistry, and Molecular Biology of the Skin II. Oxford University Press, Oxford, 1991.
35. Clark TP: Pharmacodynamics drug action and interaction. In: Dowling PM, et al (eds): Clinical Pharmacology: Principles and Practice. Western Veterinary Conference, Las Vegas, 1998, p 5.
36. Climer J: Herbal medicine. Cat Fancy, June 1990, p 36.
37. Cohn LA: Glucocorticoids as immunosuppressive agents. Semin Vet Med Surg 12:150, 1997.
38. Croxtall JD, et al: Lipocortin 1 and the control of cPLA2 activity in A459 cells: Glucocorticoids block

39. EGF stimulation of cPLA2 phosphorylation. Biochem Pharmacol 52:351, 1996.
39. Culbert LA, et al: Complications associated with high-dose prednisolone sodium succinate therapy in dogs with neurological injury. J Am Anim Hosp Assoc 34:129, 1998.
39a. Dahlinger J, et al: Effect of ketoconazole on cyclosporine dose in healthy dogs. Vet Surg 27:64, 1998.
40. Davis JA, et al: Benzocaine-induced methemoglobinemia attributed to topical application of the anesthetic in several laboratory animal species. Am J Vet Res 54:1322, 1993.
41. DeBoer DJ, et al: Inability of short-duration treatment with a 5-lipoxygenase inhibitor to reduce clinical signs of canine atopy. Vet Dermatol 5:13, 1994.
42. DeBoer DJ, Moriello KA: Inability of topical treatment to influence the course of experimental feline dermatophytosis. J Am Vet Med Assoc 207:439, 1995.
43. De-Hui S, et al: Manual of Dermatology in Chinese Medicine. Eastland Press, Seattle, 1995.
43a. Draelos ZD: New developments in cosmetics and skin care products. Adv Dermatol 12:3, 1997.
44. Drake LA, et al: Guidelines of care for the use of topical glucocorticoids. J Am Acad Dermatol 35:615, 1996.
45. Duvic M, et al: Molecular mechanisms of tazarotene action in psoriasis. J Am Acad Dermatol 37(Suppl 2, Part 3):S18, 1997.
46. duVivier A, Stoughton RB: Tachyphylaxis to the action of topically applied corticosteroids. Arch Dermatol 111:581, 1975.
47. Dyson M: Advances in wound healing physiology: The comparative perspective. Vet Dermatol 8:227, 1997.
48. Ellis CN, Voorhees JJ: Etretinate therapy. J Am Acad Dermatol 16:267, 1987.
49. Elson ML: The role of retinoids in wound healing. J Am Acad Dermatol 39(Part 3):S79, 1998.
50. Evans AG, et al: A trial of 13-cis-retinoic acid for treatment of squamous cell carcinoma and preneoplastic lesions of the head in cats. Am J Vet Res 46:2553, 1985.
51. Fadok VA: Nutritional therapy in veterinary dermatology. In: Kirk RW (ed): Current Veterinary Therapy IX. W.B. Saunders Co, Philadelphia, 1986, p 591.
52. Fadok VA: Treatment of canine idiopathic seborrhea with isotretinoin. Am J Vet Res 47:1730, 1986.
53. Fledman RJ, Maibach HI: Regional variation in percutaneous penetration of C14 cortisol in man. J Invest Dermatol 48:181, 1967.
54. Franz TJ: Kinetics of cutaneous drug penetration. Int J Dermatol 22:499, 1983.
55. Garcia G, et al: Inhibition of histamine release from dispersed canine skin mast cells by cyclosporine A, rolipram and salbutamol but not dexamethasone or sodium cromoglylate. Vet Dermatol 9:81, 1998.
56. Glaze MR, et al: Ophthalmic corticosteroid therapy: Systemic effects in the dog. J Am Vet Med Assoc 192:73, 1988.
57. Goette DK, Odom RB: Adverse effects of corticosteroids. Cutis 23:477, 1979.
58. Goldsmith LA: Propylene glycol. Int J Dermatol 17:703, 1978.
59. Goldyne ME: Leukotrienes: Clinical significance. J Am Acad Dermatol 10:659, 1984.
60. Granlund H, et al: Long-term follow-up of eczema patients treated with cyclosporine. Acta Dermatol Venereol 78:40, 1998.
61. Greene JA, Knecht CD: Electrosurgery: A review. Vet Surg 9:327, 1980.
62. Gregory CR, et al: Response to isoantigens and mitogens in the cat: Effects of cyclosporine A. Am J Vet Res 48:126, 1987.
63. Grier RL, et al: Hyperthermic treatment of superficial tumors in cats. J Am Vet Med Assoc 177:227, 1980.
64. Griffin CE: Canine atopic disease. In: Griffin CE, et al (eds): Current Veterinary Dermatology. Mosby Year Book, St. Louis, 1993, p 99.
65. Griffin CE: Open forum—Etretinate—How is it being used in veterinary dermatology? Derm Dialog Spring-Summer, 1993.
66. Griffin CE: Systemic glucocorticoid therapy in veterinary medicine. Presentation at the American Academy of Veterinary Dermatology, New Orleans, March, 1986.
67. Griffin CE: Unpublished observations.
68. Gross TL, et al: Subepidermal bullous dermatosis due to topical corticosteroid therapy in dogs. Vet Dermatol 8:127, 1997.
69. Guaguère E, et al: Efficacité clinique de la méthylprednisolone dans le traitement symptomatique des dermatoses allergiques du chien. Prat Méd Chir Anim Comp 31:171, 1996.
70. Gyrd-Hansen N, et al: Percutaneous absorption of organophosphorus insecticides in pigs—The influence of different vehicles. J Vet Pharmacol Ther 16:174, 1993.
71. Hargis AM, Mundel AC: Familial canine dermatomyositis. Comp Contin Educ 14:855, 1992.
72. Hall JA, et al: Effect of dietary n-6-to-n-3 fatty acid ratio on complete blood and total white blood cell counts, and T-cell subpopulations in aged dogs. Am J Vet Res 60:319, 1999.
73. Harvey RG: A comparison of evening primrose oil and sunflower oil for the management of papulocrustous dermatitis in cats. Vet Rec 133:571, 1993.
74. Harvey RG: Effect of varying proportions of evening primrose oil and fish oil on cats with crusting dermatosis ("miliary dermatitis"). Vet Rec 133:208, 1993.
75. Harvey RG: Management of feline miliary dermatitis by supplementing the diet with essential fatty acids. Vet Rec 128:326, 1991.
76. Helgren JA: Splish splash. Cat Fancy, May 1991, p 32.
77. Humphreys F, Shuster S: The effect of topical dimethindene maleate on wheal reactions. Br J Clin Pharmacol 23:234, 1987.
78. Jeffers JG: Diabetes mellitus induced in a dog after administration of costicosteroids and methylprednisolone pulse therapy. J Am Vet Med Assoc 199:77, 1991.
79. Kannon GA, Garrett AB: Moist wound healing with occlusive dressings: A clinical review. Dermatol Surg 21:583, 1995.
80. Kelly L: Veterinary technician in EXXON Valdez cleanup. Personal communication, 1998.
81. Kemppainen RJ, et al: Adrenocortical suppression in the dog after a single dose of methylprednisolone acetate. Am J Vet Res 42:822, 1981.
82. Kemppainen RJ, et al: Adrenocortical suppression in the dog given a single intramuscular dose of prednisone or triamcinolone acetonide. Am J Vet Res 42:204, 1982.
83. Kemppainen RJ: Principles of glucocorticoid therapy in nonendocrine disease. In: Kirk RW (ed): Current

Veterinary Therapy IX. W.B. Saunders Co, Philadelphia, 1986, p 954.
84. Kietzmann M: Improvement and retardation of wound healing: Effects of pharmacological agents in laboratory animal studies. Vet Dermatol 10:83, 1999.
85. Kietzmann M, et al: Untersuchungen Zur Verträglichkeit, Wirkung im epidermalen Stoffwechsel und Metabolisierung von Benzoylperoxid beim Hund. Kleinterpraxis 35:31, 1990.
86. Kinnunen T, Koskela M: Antibacterial and antifungal properties of propylene glycol, kexylene glycol, and 1,3-butylene glycol in vitro. Acta Dermatol Venereol 71:148, 1991.
87. Kobay MJ, and Jones BR: Local current yield radiofrequency hyperthermia for the treatment of superficial skin tumors in cats. N Z Vet J 31:173, 1983.
88. Koch HJ, Vercelli A: Workshop report 3: Shampoos and other topical therapies. In: Ihrke PJ, et al (eds): Advances in Veterinary Dermatology, Vol 2. Pergamon Press, Oxford, 1993, p 409.
89. Koo J, Arain S: Traditional Chinese medicine for the treatment of dermatologic disorders. Arch Dermatol 134:1388, 1998.
89a. Koo J, et al: Advances in psoriasis therapy. Adv Dermatol 12:47, 1997.
90. Kwochka KW: Retinoids and vitamin A therapy. In: Griffin CE, et al (eds): Current Veterinary Dermatology. Mosby Year Book, St. Louis, 1993, p 203.
91. Kwochka KW: Symptomatic topical therapy of scaling disorders. In: Griffin CE, et al (eds): Current Veterinary Dermatology. Mosby Year Book, St. Louis, 1993, p 191.
92. Kwochka KW, Kowalski JS: Prophylactic efficacy of four antibacterial shampoos against *Staphylococcus intermedius* in dogs. Am J Vet Res 52:115, 1991.
93. Latimer KS, et al: Effects of cyclosporin A administration in cats. Vet Immunol Immunopathol 11:161, 1986.
94. Lees MJ, et al: Factors influencing wound healing: Lessons from military wound management. Comp Contin Educ 11:8550, 1989.
95. Lees MJ, et al: Second-intention wound healing. Comp Contin Educ 11:857, 1989.
96. Levine N: Role of retinoids in skin cancer treatment and prevention. J Am Acad Dermatol 39(Part 3):S62, 1998.
97. Lichtenstein J, et al: Nonsteroidal anti-inflammatory drugs: Their use in dermatology. Int J Dermatol 26:80, 1987.
98. Lim KK, et al: Cyclosporine in the treatment of dermatologic disease: An update. Mayo Clin Proc 71:1183, 1996.
99. Lin AN, et al: Sulfur revisited. J Am Acad Dermatol 18:553, 1988.
100. Lloyd DH, Thomsett LR: Essential fatty acid supplementation in the treatment of canine atopy: A preliminary study. Vet Dermatol 1:41, 1989.
101. Lloyd DH: Essential fatty acids and skin disease. J Small Anim Pract 30:207, 1989.
102. Lober CW: Canthaxantin: The "tanning" pill. J Am Acad Dermatol 13:660, 1985.
103. Logas D, Kunkle GA: Double-blinded crossover study with marine oil supplementation containing high-dose eicosapentaenoic acid for the treatment of canine pruritic skin disease. Vet Dermatol 5:99, 1994.
104. Looney AL, Rothstein E: Use of acupuncture to treat psychodermatosis in the dog. Canine Pract 23(5):18, 1998.
105. Maibach HI, Stoughton RB: Topical corticosteroids. Med Clin North Am 57:1253, 1973.
106. Manglesdorf DJ, et al: The retinoid receptors. In: Span HG, et al (eds): The Retinoids: Biology, Chemistry, and Medicine. New York, Raven Press, 1994, p 319.
107. Marks R: Pharmacokinetics and safety review of tazarotene. J Am Acad Dermatol 39(Part 2):S134, 1998.
108. Marks SL, Song MD, et al: Clinical evaluation of etretinate for the treamtent of canine solar induced squamous cell carcinoma and preneoplastic lesions. J Am Acad Dermatol 27:11, 1992.
109. Marsella R, et al: Use of pentoxifylline in the treatment of allergic contact reactions to plants of the *Commelinceae* family in dogs. Vet Dermatol 8:121, 1997.
110. Mason KV: Clinical and pathophysiologic aspects of parasitic skin diseases. In: Ihrke PJ, et al (eds): Advances in Veterinary Dermatology, Vol 2. Pergamon Press, New York, 1993, p 177.
111. Mason KV, Atwell R: Clinical efficacy trials on a chlorhexidine/miconazole shampoo for the treatment of seborrheic dermatitis associated with an overgrowth of *Malassezia pachydermatis* and coccoid bacteria. Proc Eur Soc Vet Dermatol 12:222, 1995.
112. Mathews KA, et al: Cyclosporine treatment of perianal fistulas in dogs. Can Vet J 38:39, 1997.
113. Mathews KA, Sukhiani HR: Randomized controlled trial of cyclosporine for treatment of perianal fistulas in dogs. J Am Vet Med Assoc 211:1249, 1997.
114. McColl C: Oral presentation. In: Proceedings of the American Academy of Veterinary Dermatology, American College of Veterinary Dermatology, San Antonio, 1998.
115. McDonough S: Grooming. In: Kunkle GA (ed): Feline Dermatology. Vet Clin North Am Small Anim Pract 25:767, 1995.
116. Miller D: Know How to Groom Your Dog. Pet Library Ltd., New York, 1990.
117. Miller WH, Jr: Fatty acid supplements as anti-inflammatory agents. In: Kirk RW (ed): Current Veterinary Therapy X. W.B. Saunders Co, Philadelphia, 1989, p 563.
118. Miller WH Jr: Non-steroidal anti-inflammatory agents in the management of canine and feline pruritus. In: Kirk RW (ed): Current Veterinary Therapy X. W.B. Saunders Co, Philadelphia, 1989, p 566.
119. Miller WH Jr, Scott DW: Medical management of chronic pruritus. Comp Contin Educ 16:449, 1994.
120. Miller WH Jr, et al: Efficacy of DVM Derm Caps Liquid in the management of allergic and inflammatory dermatoses of the cat. J Am Anim Hosp Assoc 29:37, 1993.
121. Miller WH Jr, et al: Investigation on the antipruritic effects of ascorbic acid given alone and in combination with a fatty acid supplement to dogs with allergic skin disease. Canine Pract 17(5):11, 1992.
122. Moriello KA, et al: Adrenocortical suppression associated with topical otic administration of glucocorticoids in dogs. J Am Vet Med Assoc 193:329, 1988.
123. Mukhtar H, et al: Green tea and skin: Anticarcinogenic effects. J Invest Dermatol 102:3, 1994.
124. Mulnix JA: Corticosteroid therapy in the dog. In: Proceedings of the American Animal Hospital Association Annual Meeting, Boston, 1977.
125. Nelson JS, Berns MW: Basic laser physics and tissue interactions. Contemp Dermatol 2:3, 1998.
126. Northway RB: Experimental use of aloe vera extract

in clinical practice. Vet Med Small Anim Clin 71:196, 1975.
127. Noxon JO, et al: Minimal inhibitory concentration of silver sulfadiazine on *Pseudomonas aeruginosa* and *Staphylococcus intermedius* isolates from the ears of dogs with otitis externa. Proc Am Acad Vet Dermatol Am Coll Vet Dermatol 13:72, 1997.
128. Olivry T: Personal communication, 1999.
129. Page EH, et al: Cyclosporine A. J Am Acad Dermatol 14:785, 1986.
130. Paradis M: Canine recurrent flank alopecia: Treatment with melatonin. Proc Am Acad Vet Dermatol Am Coll Vet Dermatol 11:49, 1995.
131. Paradis M: Melatonin in the treatment of canine pattern baldness. In: Kwochka KW, et al (eds): Advances in Veterinary Dermatology III. Butterworth-Heinemann, Boston, 1998, p 511.
132. Paradis M: Melatonin therapy in canine alopecia. In: Bonagura J (ed): Kirk's Current Veterinary Therapy XIII. W.B. Saunders Co, Philadelphia, 2000, p 546.
133. Pathak MA: Sunscreens, topical and systemic approaches for protection of human skin against harmful effects of solar radiation. J Am Acad Dermatol 7:285, 1982.
134. Peaston AE, et al: Photodynamic therapy for nasal and aural squamous cell carcinoma in cats. J Am Vet Med Assoc 202:1261, 1993.
135. Peck GL, DiGiovanna JJ: The retinoids. In: Freedberg IM, et al (eds): Fitzpatrick's Dermatology in General Medicine V. McGraw-Hill, New York, 1999, p 2810.
135a. Pedersen NC: A review of immunologic diseases in the dog. Vet Immunol Immunopathol 69:251, 1999.
136. Pitcairn R: Dr. Pitcairn's Complete Guide to Natural Health for Dogs and Cats. Rodale Press, Inc, New York, 1995.
137. Podkonjak KR: Veterinary cryotherapy—2. Vet Med (Small Animal Clinician) 77:183, 1982
138. Poppenga RH, et al: Hexachlorophene toxicosis in a litter of Doberman pinschers. J Vet Diagn Invest 2:129, 1990.
139. Power HT, Ihrke PJ: Synthetic retinoids in veterinary dermatology. Vet Clin North Am Small Anim Pract 20:1525, 1990.
140. Power HT: Personal communication.
140a. Rees C: Pentoxifylline (Trental). Derm Dialogue, Winter, p 10, 1999.
141. Rewerts JM, et al: Atraumatic rupture of the gastrocnemius after corticosteroid administration in a dog. J Am Vet Med Assoc 210:655, 1997.
142. Rickards RA: A new treatment for canine melanosis. Mod Vet Pract 47:38, 1966.
143. Rinkardt NE, et al: The effects of prednisone and azathioprine on circulating immunoglobulin levels and lymphocyte subpopulations in normal dogs. Can J Vet Res 63:18, 1999.
143a. Rosenbaum M: Cyclosporine. Derm Dialogue, Summer, p 5, 1999.
143b. Rohrer CR, et al: Gastric hemorrhage in dogs given high doses of methylprednisolone sodium succinate. Am J Vet Res 60:977, 1999.
143c. Rohrer CR, et al: Efficacy of misoprostol in prevention of gastric hemorrhage in dogs treated with high doses of methylprednisolone sodium succinate. Am J Vet Res 60:982, 1999.
144. Rosenkrantz WS, et al: Clinical evaluation of cyclosporine in animal models with cutaneous immune-mediated disease and epitheliotropic lymphoma. J Am Anim Hosp Assoc 25:377, 1989.
145. Rosenkrantz W: Immunomodulating drugs in dermatology. In: Current Veterinary Therapy X: Small Animal Practice. W.B. Saunders Co, Philadelphia, 1989, p 570.
145a. Ruszczak Z, Schwartz RA: Interferons in dermatology. Adv Dermatol 13:235, 1998.
146. Salzberg K: Tools and techniques for home grooming. Cat Fancy, May 1994, p 48.
147. Samlaska CP, et al: Pentoxifylline. J Am Acad Dermatol, 30:603, 1994.
148. Saunders B: How to Trim, Groom, and Show Your Dog. Howell House, New York, 1967.
148a. Scardino MS, et al: The effects of omega-3 fatty acid diet enrichment on wound healing. Vet Dermatol 10:283, 1999.
149. Schaer M, Ginn PE: Iatrogenic Cushing's syndrome and steroid hepatopathy in a cat. J Am Anim Hosp Assoc 35:48, 1999.
150. Schauder S, Ippen H: Photodermatoses and light protection. Int J Dermatol 21:241, 1982.
151. Schick RO, et al: Efficacy of an omega-3 fatty acid adjusted diet in pruritic dogs. Proc Eur Soc Vet Dermatol 12:245, 1995.
152. Schleimer RP: Glucocorticosteroids. In: Middleton E, et al (eds): Allergy Principles and Practice. Mosby Year Book, St. Louis, 1993.
153. Schoen AM: Problems in Veterinary Medicine: Veterinary Acupuncture. J.B. Lippincott, Philadelphia, 1992.
154. Schoen AM: Veterinary Acupuncture: Ancient Art to Modern Medicine. American Veterinary Publications, Goleta, California, 1994.
155. Schwartz E, et al: *In vivo* prevention of corticosteroid-induced skin atrophy by tretinoin in the hairless mouse is accompanied by modulation of collagen, glycosaminoglycans, and fibronectin. J Invest Dermatol 102:241, 1994.
156. Schwartzman RM: Topical dermatologic therapy. In: Kirk RW (ed): Current Veterinary Therapy VI. W.B. Saunders Co, Philadelphia, 1977, p 506.
156a. Schwassman M: Uses of interferon. Derm Dialogue, Winter, p 9, 1999.
157. Scott DW: Clinical assessment of topical benzoyl peroxide in treatment of canine skin diseases. Vet Med (Small Animal Clinician) 74:808, 1979.
158. Scott DW: Feline dermatology 1900–1978. J Am Anim Hosp Assoc 16:331, 1980.
159. Scott DW: Hyperadrenocorticism. Vet Clin North Am Small Anim Pract 9:3, 1979.
160. Scott DW: Rational use of glucocorticoids in dermatology. In: Bonagura J (ed): Kirk's Current Veterinary Therapy XII. W.B. Saunders Co, Philadelphia, 1995.
161. Scott DW: Systemic glucocorticoid therapy. In: Kirk RW (ed): Current Veterinary Therapy VII. W.B. Saunders Co, Philadelphia, 1980, p 988.
162. Scott DW: Topical cutaneous medicine, or "Now what should I try?" Proc Am Anim Hosp Assoc 46:89, 1979.
163. Scott DW, Buerger RG: Nonsteroidal anti-inflammatory agents in the management of canine pruritus. J Am Anim Hosp Assoc 24:425, 1988.
164. Scott DW, Cayatte SM: Failure of papaverine hydrochloride and doxycycline hyclate as antipruritic agents in pruritic dogs: Results of an open clinical trial. Can Vet J 34:164, 1993.
165. Scott DW, Green CE: Iatrogenic secondary adreno-

There has been speculation about the means by which only a small number of a vast array of bacteria in the environment are able to colonize or infect the skin. The potent cleaning forces of dilution, washout, drying, and desquamation of surface cells prevent many organisms from colonizing the skin. It is now recognized that bacterial adhesion is a prerequisite to colonization and infection.[103, 185, 237, 240] Bacterial adhesion is a complex process influenced by both the host and the organism. Bacteria possess surface adhesion molecules, which influence their ability to bind to keratinocytes. For staphylococci, teichoic acid and protein A appear to be most important surface adhesion molecules.[124] These molecules bind to host surface receptors (e.g., fibronectin and vitronectin) to prevent the bacteria from being brushed from the skin.

Adhesion is increased with increasing time, temperature, and concentration of bacteria as well as in certain diseases.[16, 26, 27, 126] In hyperproliferative disorders (e.g., seborrhea complex), more bacteria adhere to the skin because more binding sites are available. Some atopic dogs bind more bacteria, which could increase the likelihood of infection. However, an increased binding ability does not equate with increased pathogenicity or virulence. To date, a specific virulence factor for *S. intermedius* has not been identified.[39, 195, 240, 242]

Other organisms from the transient group are pathogenic in rare cases.[57, 87, 179, 233] Gram-negative organisms tend to flourish in moist, warm areas and to predominate when medications depress the gram-positive flora.[192, 242] Cats infrequently experience pyoderma but commonly have subcutaneous abscesses. Because these are often from bite wounds, the mouth flora of the cat is an important factor. It includes *Pasteurella multocida*, β-hemolytic streptococci, *Corynebacterium* spp., *Actinomyces* spp., *Bacteroides* spp., and *Fusobacterium* spp. *Staphylococcus felis* is increasingly isolated from cats with otitis externa, subcutaneous abscesses, paronychia, and other skin infections.[4, 140]

Anaerobic bacteria are usually abundant in gastrointestinal secretions; therefore, fecal contamination is a cause of soft tissue infections due to these organisms. Anaerobic bacteria isolated from dog and cat infections include *Actinomyces* spp., *Clostridium* spp., *Peptostreptococcus* spp., *Bacteroides* spp., *Fusobacterium* spp., and *Prevotella* spp.[25, 91, 145, 181, 226] They are usually found in granulomas, cellulitis, abscesses, fistulae, and other soft tissue wounds, but they may also be cultured from more superficial pyoderma, otitis, or stomatitis cases.[90]

Antibacterial susceptibility for obligate anaerobic bacteria has been rated as follows[25, 26, 135]: Ninety percent or more are susceptible to ampicillin, amoxicillin clavulanate, carbenicillin, chloramphenicol, clindamycin, and metronidazole; 75% to 90% are sensitive to cephalosporin, lincomycin, and penicillin G (except *Bacteroides* spp., which are resistant to penicillin, ampicillin, and cephalothin); 50% to 75% are sensitive to tetracycline and erythromycin; and less than 25% are susceptible to gentamicin and the fluoroquinolones.[145]

Staphylococci are among the most resistant of the non–spore-forming organisms. They resist dehydration, are relatively heat-resistant, and tolerate antiseptic medications better than the vegetative forms of most bacteria. Their toxins may cause tissue necrosis at the point of infection. Repeated injections of heat-killed staphylococci protect rabbits against otherwise fatal doses of *S. aureus*. Bacterins may be valuable in combating chronic infections in dogs and cats.

The numbers of resident bacteria on the skin tend to vary among individuals; some animals have many organisms, whereas others have few. The number per individual may remain constant, unless disturbed by antibacterial treatment or changes in climate. More bacteria are found on the skin in warm, wet weather than in cold, dry weather.[237] Moist, intertriginous areas tend to have large numbers, and individuals with oily skin have higher counts. Total counts of aerobic organisms on normal skin ranged from 100 to 103 organisms/cm^2, and similar counts from seborrheic skin ranged from 103 to 107/cm^2.[136]

Disease states influence the species and numbers of bacteria present. In seborrheic skin, coagulase-positive staphylococci predominate.[136] This is also true in most pyodermas and in most other bacterial infections of the skin. In patients with various dermatoses (atopy, seborrheic dermatitis, and allergic and irritant contact dermatitis in humans), increased numbers of resident bacteria are found in all areas of the skin, not just in the affected areas.[158, 242] Compared with dogs that are normal, dogs with dermatoses have a more prolific growth of aerobic organisms, a greater number of sites carrying coagulase-positive staphylococci, and a higher number of gram-negative microorganisms. Thus, these animals are heavily colonized with potentially pathogenic bacteria, a fact to consider when providing basic therapy for the primary dermatosis.

Microorganisms isolated from an intact lesion such as a pustule are evidence of infection, not colonization. Colonization means that a potential pathogen is living on the skin or in a lesion but that its presence is causing no reaction in the host. The problem in evaluating a pyoderma culture is to separate secondary colonization from secondary infection. The presence of many degenerate neutrophils and phagocytosed bacteria is direct evidence of a host reaction and is compatible with infection. Infection can be determined by direct smears of lesion exudates, which may be more informative than cultures.

• SKIN INFECTIONS

The staphylococcal organisms, the primary isolates from skin infections in dogs and cats, are not particularly virulent; thus, any skin infection should be considered a sign of some underlying cutaneous, metabolic, or immunologic abnormality. Bacterial pyoderma is very common in dogs, but rare in humans. The reasons for this are not known, but could include anatomic and physiologic factors. The failure to detect differences in pathogenicity of *S. intermedius* isolates has suggested that host factors, such as poorly developed epidermal defenses, are important.[191a] Canine skin is characterized by a relatively thin, compact stratum corneum, a paucity of intercellular lipids, a lack of a lipid follicular plug, and a higher pH. Traditionally, skin infections are classified as either primary or secondary to reflect the absence or the presence of an underlying cause.

Secondary infections are by far the most common and result from some cutaneous, immunologic, or metabolic abnormality. Secondary infections may involve organisms other than staphylococci, tend to respond slowly or poorly to treatment if the underlying problem is ignored, and recur unless the cause is resolved. Virtually any skin condition described in this text can predispose to infection, but allergic, seborrheic, or follicular disorders are the most common causes of infection. Interestingly, infection appears to be relatively uncommon in the autoimmune disorders.[228] This may be due to the presence of high cutaneous levels of cytokines, which have antimicrobial properties.

Allergic dogs are especially prone to infections because of the damage they do to their skin while itching, the corticosteroids that they often receive, and possibly some immunologic abnormalities associated with their allergic predisposition.[193] When their skin becomes infected, the level of pruritus increases quickly and does not respond well to corticosteroid administration. Antibiotic treatment resolves the lesions of infection and reduces, but does not eliminate, the pruritus.

Seborrheic animals have greatly increased numbers of bacteria on their skin surface, which can colonize an epidermal or follicular defect and cause infection. They also contribute to the alteration of the surface lipid layer to one that can induce inflammation. In this situation, the patches of seborrheic dermatitis cause the animal to itch and induce true infection in these areas. Superficial infections result in significant scaling during their development and resolution. It can sometimes be difficult to decide whether the seborrhea induced the infection or vice versa. Scaling caused by infection decreases quickly with antibiotic therapy. If seborrheic signs are still pronounced after 14 to 21 days of antibiotic treatment, the animal should be evaluated for an underlying seborrheic disorder.

Follicular inflammation, obstruction, degeneration, or a combination of these predisposes the follicle to bacterial infection. Inflammatory causes are numerous, but demodicosis and dermatophytosis are most commonly implicated. Follicular obstruction occurs as part of generalized seborrhea, in focal seborrheic disorders (e.g., feline acne and Schnauzer comedo syndrome), sebaceous adenitis, follicular dysplasias and other congenital disorders of the follicle, and endocrine disorders. Follicular degeneration can be caused by all of these conditions plus alopecia areata. In cases of follicular infection, examination of skin scrapings for demodicosis and evaluations for dermatophytes (e.g., trichogram and fungal culture) are always recommended. After those tests, the skin biopsy is most useful because pathologic changes are too deep to be appreciated with the naked eye. The inflammation associated with the secondary bacterial infection can mask some of the histologic features of the predisposing disease; thus, it is best to resolve the infection first and then perform the skin biopsy.

The most common metabolic causes of skin infection are hypothyroidism and hyperadrenocorticism (iatrogenic or spontaneous), but diabetes mellitus, other endocrine skin disorders, and other systemic metabolic problems (e.g., hyperlipidemia) must also be considered. These disorders predispose to infection by their impact on the animal's immune system and the changes they induce in the hair follicle. In most instances, the number of infected follicles is small compared with the number that are visually abnormal (e.g., hyperkeratotic and hairless), so the index of suspicion for an underlying metabolic disorder should be high.

The classification of primary infection is more problematic. Primary infections are described as those that occur in otherwise healthy skin, are staphylococcal with rare exception, and are cured by appropriate antibiotic therapy. This definition overlooks the tendency for the infection to recur. It is common to examine a dog for a skin infection and find no historical or physical abnormality to explain the infection. Is this a primary infection, an infection secondary to some transient insult to the skin, or an infection secondary to some as yet undefined underlying problem? The key to the primacy of the infection is its tendency to recur. Infections that resolve with no residual skin disease and do not recur with regularity or within a reasonable period (e.g., 3 to 6 months) could be considered primary infections. If the infection recurs early, the animal has some subclinical skin disease or an immunologic abnormality.

• IMMUNODEFICIENCIES

Immunodeficiencies are classified as either primary or acquired. Primary immunodeficiencies are congenital and are usually inherited. In these animals, infections develop early in life for no apparent reason. Although German shepherd pyoderma tends to have a genetic basis, the defect is not expressed until adulthood. Infections of the respiratory, gastrointestinal, urogenital, and integumentary systems are most common. In some cases, the skin infection follows a known insult (e.g., flea bites) but is far out of proportion in severity to the insult. Depending on the nature and severity of the immunodeficiency, the infection may or may not respond to treatment as expected. If there is a response, relapse weeks to months after the discontinuation of treatment can be expected. A variety of primary immunodeficiencies have been described in dogs, and those with associated skin infection are listed in Table 4–1.

One of the most common primary immunodeficiencies diagnosed in dogs is selective IgA deficiency.[41] Caution is warranted because wide variation in serum IgA levels is seen with the use of different commercial kits.[117a] Laboratories using these kits must prepare their own reference ranges rather than rely on values found in the literature or provided by the manufacturers. If the animal is not IgA deficient, a cell-mediated deficiency is most likely.[54a]

IgA and IgG deficiencies were described in Rottweiler puppies that had bacterial pyoderma, subcutaneous abscesses, and demodicosis.[74b] In addition, these puppies had a paucity of CD3+ T cells in their secondary lymphoid tissue and irregularities in plasma cell development.

Acquired immunodeficiencies are common complications of many serious systemic illnesses.[52, 60, 68, 155, 265a] Because the immunodepression follows the underlying disease, there is no age, breed, or sex predilection for these acquired immunologic disorders. The best-known examples of acquired immunodeficiency disease are associated with viral infections, especially feline immunodeficiency virus, and leishmaniasis. In most other conditions, the signs of the primary illness predominate and precede those of the immunodepression. Examples in which the skin looks normal or nearly so before the infection include adult-onset demodicosis (see Chap. 6), hypothyroidism (see Chap. 10), and hyperadrenocorticism (see Chap. 10). Granulocyte colony-stimulating factor deficiency was de-

Table 4-1 PRIMARY IMMUNODEFICIENCIES OF DOGS

DISEASE	BREED INVOLVED	MECHANISMS OF DEFECT	REFERENCES
Phagocytic Defect			
Cyclic hematopoiesis	Collie, Pomeranian, Cocker spaniel	Blockade of bone marrow release	58
Granulocytopathy	Doberman pinscher, Irish setter, Weimaraner	Bactericidal defect in neutrophils	35, 67, 230
Granulocytopathy	Irish setter	Reduced granulocyte adherence	108, 269
Humoral Defect			
Complement deficiency	Brittany spaniel	Absence of C3	30
Transient hypogammaglobulinemia	Many	Delayed development of functioning humoral system	105
Selective IgM deficiency	Doberman pinscher	Low IgM levels	225
Selective IgA deficiency	Many	Low IgA levels	41, 75, 77, 225
Cell-Mediated Defect	Bull terrier, Weimaraner, others	T-cell dysfunction	100, 146, 204, 234
Combined Immunodeficiency	Basset hound, Cardigan Welsh corgi	B-cell and T-cell dysfunction	104, 120a, 147, 227

Ig = immunoglobulin.

scribed in a Rottweiler with chronic neutropenia and recurrent infections of the skin and ears.[166a]

• TREATMENT OF SKIN INFECTIONS

Satisfactory resolution of a skin infection necessitates that the cause of the infection be identified and corrected and that the infection receive proper treatment. If the cause of the infection persists, either the response to treatment is poor or the infection recurs shortly after treatment is discontinued. If the cause is resolved but inappropriate treatment for the infection is given, the infection persists and worsens.

Skin infections can be treated topically, systemically, surgically, or by some combination of these. Most infections of dogs and cats are too widespread or too deep to be resolved with topical treatment alone, but judicious topical therapy can make the patient more comfortable and hasten its response to antibiotics. Topical treatment can take considerable time and effort on the owner's part and can irritate the skin if the products are too harsh. Surgery alone can be useful with focal lesions or can be performed as an adjunct to other treatments. Management must be individualized.

Topical Treatment

Topical treatments are used to reduce or eliminate the bacterial population in and around an area of infection and to remove tissue debris.[113, 167, 276] Debris removal is of paramount importance because it allows direct contact of the active ingredient with the organism and promotes drainage. Agents commonly used include chlorhexidine, povidone-iodine, ethyl lactate, benzoyl peroxide, and various antibiotics, especially fusidic acid, mupirocin, and bacitracin.*

Infections restricted to the skin surface (e.g., impetigo) or intact hair follicles may be effectively treated with topical agents alone. When the number of lesions is small and they are confined to a limited area (e.g., feline acne),[282] antiseptics or antibiotics in a cream, ointment, or gel formulation may be sufficient to resolve the infection. Benzoyl peroxide gels or antibiotic formulations receive widest use. The benzoyl peroxide gels marketed to veterinarians contain 5% active ingredient, which can be irritating, especially with re-

---

*See references 14, 49, 112, 113, 164, 175, 216.

peated application. In most instances, antibiotic preparations are nonirritating. In most cases, transdermal absorption of the agent is limited, but frequent application over wide areas should be avoided.

Many potent antibacterial agents are available in topical form.[40, 81a, 239, 276, 282] The most commonly used are mupirocin, fusidic acid, neomycin, gentamicin, bacitracin, polymyxin B, and thiostrepton. Important considerations for some of these agents are as follows: (1) mupirocin and fusidic acid are more effective than other topical agents for treatment staphylococcal pyodermas, (2) mupirocin has poor activity against gram-negative infections, (3) neomycin has more potential for allergic sensitization than do most topicals, and susceptibility is variable for gram-negative organisms, and (4) polymyxin B and bacitracin in combination may be effective for gram-negative as well as gram-positive organisms; however, they are rapidly inactivated by purulent exudates and do not penetrate well. Mupirocin is particularly useful because of its ability to penetrate the skin and its very low incidence of adverse reactions. Potentiation of topical antibiotics with EDTA-Tris is currently being studied, especially in the treatment of ear disease, and is likely to increase the activity of the agent being studied.[99]

Often, topical antibiotics are formulated with other ingredients, most commonly glucocorticoids. There are numerous antibiotic-steroid combinations (Gentocin spray, Otomax, Tresaderm, and Panalog). These are occasionally indicated in chronic, dry, lichenified, secondarily infected dermatoses (seborrhea complex and allergic dermatoses) and pyotraumatic dermatitis and are commonly indicated in otitis externa. Several clinical and bacteriologic trials in humans and dogs showed that these antibiotic-steroid combinations were superior to either agent alone.

Widespread superficial infections are best treated with antibacterial shampoos.[49, 175, 216] The manipulation of the skin during its application and the vehicle of the shampoo removes tissue debris, which allows better contact between the antiseptic and the bacteria. When four commercial antibacterial shampoos were studied, none could completely sterilize the skin but all significantly reduced the bacterial population.[164] Benzoyl peroxide was the most effective, followed by chlorhexidine acetate. Another study demonstrated equal efficacy of benzoyl peroxide and ethyl lactate, with fewer adverse reactions to the latter.[14] Mixtures of acetic and boric acid are also effective.[24]

Product selection depends on the preferences of the owner and the clinician and the condition of the animal's skin. Animals with underlying hypersensitivity disorders or "sensitive" skin (e.g., Shetland sheepdogs) should be bathed with nonirritating or minimally irritating agents such as chlorhexidine or ethyl lactate. Benzoyl peroxide products should be reserved for greasy dogs or dogs with deep crusted infections. In this latter group, shampoo selection should be re-evaluated in 10 to 14 days because the skin will be much different then.

A thorough bath with a 10- to 15-minute shampoo contact time is indicated at the beginning of treatment. The timing to the next bath depends on the severity of the infection, the cause of the infection, and the speed of the animal's response to the antibiotics used. Some clinicians request that the client bathe the animal at a set interval, typically every third to seventh day, whereas other clinicians give the client guidelines for when a bath is indicated and let the client decide when to bathe. If the client is not overzealous, the latter method is most appropriate because it treats the animal on the basis of its needs.

In the case of deep draining infections, the hair in the area must be clipped to prevent the formation of a sealing crust and to allow the topical agents to contact the diseased tissues. Although shampooing is beneficial, soaks are more appropriate at the onset of treatment. Hydrotherapy loosens and removes crusts, decreases the number of surface bacteria, promotes epithelialization, and helps to lessen the discomfort associated with the lesions. With warm-water soaks, the vascular plexus opens, which may allow better distribution of the systemic antibiotic. For widespread infection, tub soaks with or without whirlpool are most appropriate. Antiseptics such as chlorhexidine and povidone-iodine are added for additional antibacterial activity. Chlorhexidine has been most effective but may retard wound healing.[167]

If there are draining lesions on a foot or distal limb, the area can be soaked in a bucket. For lesions higher up on the limb, a newborn disposable baby diaper is a useful aid. The outer plastic layer protects the house while the high absorbency pad holds the soaking solution next to the skin. For these lesions, a mildly hypertonic drawing solution of magnesium sulfate (2 tbsp/qt or 30 ml/L of warm water) can be beneficial. Because hydrotherapy hydrates the epithelium, excessively soaked skin macerates easily and may become infected more easily. As the antibiotic therapy progresses, drainage should decrease. When drainage is slight after a soak, the frequency of soaking should be decreased or stopped entirely. Typically, soaking is continued for 3 to 7 days.

Systemic Antibiotics

Systemic antibiotic agents are used for bacterial skin diseases that are not treatable with topical therapy.[32, 47, 246] Because the overwhelming majority of canine skin infections are caused by *S. intermedius*, antibiotics that affect these bacteria and concentrate in the skin are of primary interest.[34, 66, 83] Occasionally, *Proteus* spp., *Pseudomonas* spp., and *E. coli* are involved as secondary invaders in deeper soft tissue infections. In cats, the primary bacteria are *P. multocida* and β-hemolytic streptococci.[120, 248] Thus, the penicillins and ampicillins are frequently effective antibiotics for cats with nonstaphylococcal infections.

Because each antibiotic has its own unique features,[1, 2] the drugs used frequently in veterinary dermatology, namely the penicillins,[129] sulfonamides,[42] macrolides and lincosamides,[210] cephalosporins,[196] and fluoroquinolones,[144] should be studied before they are used. Proper antibiotic use necessitates that the antibiotic inhibit the specific bacteria, preferably in a bactericidal manner. Bacteriostatic drugs may also be effective as long as the host is not immunocompromised. The drug should have a narrow spectrum so that it produces little effect on organisms of the natural flora of the skin or the intestinal tract (for oral medications). The antibiotic should be inexpensive, should be easily given (orally, if it is to be prescribed for home use) and absorbed, and should have no adverse effects.

The most important factors influencing the effectiveness of antibiotics are the susceptibility of the bacteria and the distribution to the skin in effective levels of activity at the infection site. Only about 4% of the cardiac output of blood reaches the skin, compared with 33% that reaches muscle.[17] This variation is reflected in the relative distribution of antibiotics among organs. In studies of the different regions of skin, the levels of penicillin-type antibiotic in the subcutis reached about 60%, and dermal-epidermal junction levels reached about 40%, of the peak serum levels in dogs.[17] Cephalexin levels in dog skin are only 20% to 40% of those in plasma.[152]

Although the epidermis is relatively avascular, studies of skin infections showed that the systemic route of therapy is better than the topical route for all but the most superficial infections. The stratum corneum is a major permeability barrier to effective topical drug penetration. These facts led to the inescapable conclusion that the skin is one of the most difficult tissues in which to obtain high antibiotic levels. Factors that may reduce the effectiveness of a therapeutic plan are the following:

1. The organism is resistant to the antibiotic and, because most *S. intermedius* organisms produce β-lactamase, antibiotics resistant to this substance should be selected.
2. The dosage is inadequate to attain and then maintain inhibitory concentrations in the skin.
3. The organism may be surviving inside macrophages, where it is not exposed to the effect of most antibiotics.
4. The organism is within a necrotic center or protected by a foreign body such as a hair fragment.
5. The organism is walled off by dense scar tissue.
6. The duration of therapy is inadequate to eradicate the infection.

Over the years, multiple studies on the in vitro susceptibility of *S. intermedius* from dogs have been published.[19, 63, 65, 130, 134, 141, 161, 163, 174, 182, 192, 197, 207, 209, 212, 218–224, 288] In many instances, in vivo results parallel the in vitro ones, but not always. In the disparate cases, the conflicting results may be due to pharmacokinetic problems or because the wrong organism was cultured. As noted earlier, it is possible to isolate two or more different strains of S. intermedius from the same dog and each can differ in its antibiotic susceptibility. Another consideration is the pH of the skin and its influence on susceptibility data. As the pH increases from 7.2 to 8.5, the in vitro susceptibility of S. intermedius changes dramatically with resistance to most drugs at this higher pH.[223, 224] Because the in vivo and in vitro results usually correlate well regardless of the pH of the skin, this pH influence probably is of little clinical concern.

The early susceptibility studies focused on the data collected during the years of the study and often compared the susceptibility data from dogs that had or had not received previous antibiotic treatments. In general, these studies indicated that previous antibiotic use usually induced in vitro resistance to macrolides, lincosamides, and potentiated sulfa drugs. More recent studies have reported data from the same institution over many years to see if the resistance pattern changed. If S. intermedius used plasmid transfer for resistance, the organism should become more resistant with time.

Unlike the pattern of increasing resistance in human S. aureus, S. intermedius is really no different in its susceptibility now than it was in the 1980s.[19, 130, 161, 174, 192, 207, 209, 212, 218, 219, 223, 224, 288] Some variation occurs from year to year but, in general, a drug with an excellent sensitivity (see later) in 1980 is just as likely to be effective in 2000. In one study, previous antibiotic use in a dog did not increase the resistance to potentiated sulfas and lincomycin.[62] Our case material also confirms this.[255–257] With little exception,[266] canine S. intermedius has not become more resistant to antibiotics over the years, which allows the clinician to select an antibiotic on an empirical rather than cultural basis. In general, methicillin-resistant strains of S. aureus and S. intermedius are rarely isolated from dogs.[109a, 213a] An exception would be a report from Spain wherein an unparalleled 28% of S. intermedius isolates from dogs were resistant to methicillin.[223]

In most clinics worldwide, S. intermedius from dogs is almost uniformly (>95%) sensitive to the various fluoroquinolone antibiotics, amoxicillin clavulanate, oxacillin, and first-generation cephalosporins. Although each fluoroquinolone and cephalosporin has its own unique feature, in vitro susceptibility to one typically indicates susceptibility to the others.[261] Enrofloxacin may be two to four times more active against S. intermedius than difloxacin, marbofloxacin, and orbifloxacin.[224a] Azithromycin and clarithromycin probably will also give excellent results, but there are insufficient data to date.[139, 258, 271] Lincomycin, clindamycin, tylosin, erythromycin, and chloramphenicol have a very good efficacy (>75%), whereas potentiated sulfonamides are still problematic. In some studies, these drugs have excellent susceptibility while others show only 50% efficacy.[161, 174, 218, 223] In a similar fashion, there is poor sensitivity of S. intermedius in the United States to ampicillin, amoxicillin, and the tetracyclines, whereas doxycycline or ampicillin is much more effective in Australia or the United Kingdom, respectively.[29, 174] Other regional variations are also reported.

Data for cats are much more limited. Current studies on coagulate-positive staphylococci show excellent sensitivity to oxacillin, cephalosporin, chloramphenicol, enrofloxacin, erythromycin, potentiated sulfonamides, and amoxicillin clavulanate; good susceptibility to clindamycin; fair susceptibility to tetracycline; and poor susceptibility to penicillin and amoxicillin.[50, 64, 198, 199, 215, 280]

With the stability in antibiotic susceptibility of S. intermedius, the routine and regular use of the bacterial culture and susceptibility test is not indicated. If exudative cytology indicates an infection with coccoid organisms, it is safe to assume that the organism is S. intermedius with whatever pattern of susceptibility it maintains in that practice area. Multiple strains of S. intermedius with differing resistance spectra can often be found on an individual dog.[174] Thus, the value and validity of antibiotic susceptibility tests on single isolates need to be questioned. If the animal has a history of drug intolerance or allergy, has not responded to a rationally selected drug in the past, or is very large with a significant variation in the daily cost of antibiotics, culture and susceptibility testing may be indicated.

In addition to the susceptibility of the organism, various owner and animal factors enter into the equation during antibiotic selection. Antibiotics are either time-dependent or concentration-dependent in their action. Time-dependent drugs must be given at their specified interval of administration for maximal efficacy. The total dose administered is more important for the concentration-dependent drugs. It would be ill advised to dispense oxacillin, a time-dependent drug to be administered three times daily, when the dog's owner works 12-hour shifts. The owner could administer the drug three times daily, but it would not be at the 8-hour intervals needed. Macrolides tend to be gastric irritants and would be poor choices in a dog who vomits easily. Such factors as cost, taste of medication, and ease of administration all enter the picture when a drug is selected and may "force" the clinician to use a drug he or she may not ordinarily use.

The depth of the staphylococcal infection also influences drug selection. Deep infections require protracted courses of treatment, can respond less favorably to certain drugs than more superficial infections, and tend to become fibrotic. Twelve-week courses of antibiotics are not unusual in treating some infections in dogs. At the time of this writing, a 12-week course of fluoroquinolone would cost the owner about $150 more than would treatment with a generic cephalosporin. Assuming that there was no medical indication for the selection of the fluoroquinolone, the cephalosporin would be a wiser drug choice. Long courses also make the use of sulfonamide drugs more risky. These drugs, especially when used for long periods, are known to cause keratoconjunctivitis sicca,[28] can induce hypothyroidism (see Chap. 10), and are a common cause of adverse cutaneous drug reactions[268] (see Chap. 9).

Deeper infections may not respond as favorably as superficial infections. For example, in one study, doxycycline was effective in 53% of canine superficial infections and in only 14% of deep infections.[29] Finally, deep infections tend to be fibrotic and the organism may assume an intracellular location where many drugs cannot reach it. For intracellular organisms, the fluoroquinolones, lincosamides, and chloramphenicol are better choices. With significant fibrosis, antibiotic penetration can be poor. Co-administration of rifampin and a β-lactamase–resistant antibiotic may result in cure when the antibiotic alone is of little use.[5, 46] However, rifampin should not be used casually because it is expensive and can cause hepatotoxicity.

Antibiotic selection is not so straightforward when the empirically selected antibiotic is not effective or when the infection recurs shortly after treatment is discontinued. If the empirically selected antibiotic has only good susceptibility, most clinicians empirically select another drug with excellent susceptibility. If this new drug fails to be effective, one must carefully evaluate whether the owner is complying with the treatment regimen and whether the skin is truly infected. If no reason for this poor response can be found, susceptibility testing is mandatory.

More commonly, the clinician is faced with the problem of antibiotic selection in recurring infections. Most studies show that drugs with excellent susceptibility (amoxicillin clavulanate, oxacillin, cephalosporin, and fluoroquinolones) maintain their efficacy in recurrences but that the in vitro susceptibility to the other antibiotics decreases and becomes unpredictable. Some clinicians empirically select one of the excellent drugs, whereas other clinicians perform susceptibility testing in all cases. Either position can be argued, and each case should be managed on its own merits.

If cytologic study shows a mixed infection, susceptibility testing is mandatory because the sensitivity of nonstaphylococcal organisms is not always predictable. If all organisms are susceptible to a safe, reasonably inexpensive drug, that drug should be used. Occasionally, no one drug fits the susceptibility profile of all organisms or the singular drug is too toxic or expensive for long-term use. If the infection contains *S. intermedius*, as most do, the initial antibiotic selection should be aimed at that organism. Eradication of the staphylococcal component may make the microenvironment unfavorable for the growth of the other organisms. If the antistaphylococcal antibiotic improves but does not resolve the infection, alternative drugs must be used.

After an antibiotic has been selected, it should be dispensed at the correct dosage, administered at the appropriate dosage interval, and be used for a sufficient period.

Dosages for the antibiotics routinely used in treating staphylococcal infections are given in Table 4–2. Licensed veterinary drugs have detailed pharmacologic data to support the recommended dosage. In our experience, the use of the manufacturer's dosage is satisfactory in most cases, and we initiate treatment at that dosage. Others suggest higher dosages. For example, some references indicate that the dosage of amoxicillin-clavulanate should be 22 mg/kg instead of the manufacturer's dose of 13.75 mg/kg.[165] When the efficacy of these two drug dosages was compared, no statistical difference in the rate of cure could be detected.[177] Other studies have shown that the cure rate of deep infections with cephalexin is increased when the dosage is increased from 15 mg/kg every 12 hours to 30 mg/kg every 12 hours.[114, 115] We, on the other hand, do not routinely increase the dosage of cephalexin in deep infections and do not appreciate a difference in the rate of cure. Clinical experience will dictate when larger drug dosages are indicated.

The most commonly recognized cause of the inability to resolve a skin infection, or of its relapse days after the treatment is discontinued, is an insufficient course of treatment. Although textbooks and clinical experience can suggest appropriate courses of treatment, each animal responds at its own rate and must be treated until its infection is resolved. Resolution means that all lesions have healed both on the surface and in the deeper tissues. Surface healing is easy to determine by visual inspection, but deep healing is much more difficult to assess and necessitates palpation of the lesions and regional lymph nodes.

Intercurrent corticosteroid administration confounds the problem greatly. Corticosteroids decrease visual and palpable inflammation, which is the key sign in determining when an infection is resolved. An inflamed hair follicle is still infected, whereas one that looks and feels normal is probably healed. With concurrent corticosteroid use, it is impossible to

Table 4–2 ANTIBIOTIC DOSAGES

ANTIBIOTIC	DOSAGE	REFERENCES
Narrow-Spectrum Agents		
Erythromycin	15 mg/kg q8h	210
Clindamycin	5 mg/kg q12h	1, 122, 169, 210, 217, 257
	11 mg/kg q24h	
Lincomycin	15 mg/kg q8h	1, 23, 122, 210
	22 mg/kg q12h	
Tylosin	10–20 mg/kg q12h	127, 255, 256
Broad-Spectrum Agents		
Azithromycin	5–15 mg/kg q12h	139, 258
Clarithromycin	5–10 mg/kg q12h	271
Amoxicillin-clavulanate	13.75 mg/kg q12h	1, 129, 169, 177
Oxacillin	22 mg/kg q8h	129
Cefadroxil	22 mg/kg q12h (D)	1, 196
	22 mg/kg q24h (C)	
Cephalexin	22 mg/kg q8–12h	10, 45a, 107, 112, 115, 196
Chloramphenicol	50 mg/kg q8h (D)	2, 3
	50 mg/cat q12h (C)	
Difloxacin	5–10 mg/kg q12h	1, 224a
Enrofloxacin	5 mg/kg q24h	83, 144, 214, 224a, 272
Marbofloxacin	2.0 mg/kg q24h	48, 144, 224a
Orbifloxacin	2.5 mg/kg q24h	1, 144, 224a, 261
Trimethoprim-sulfadiazine	15–30 mg/kg q12h	42, 200
Trimethoprim-sulfamethoxazole	15–30 mg/kg q12h	42, 200
Ormetoprim-sulfadimethoxine	55 mg/kg (day 1)–27.5 mg/kg q24h	42, 254
Bacquiloprim-sulfadimethoxine	30 mg/kg (days 1, 2)–30 mg/kg q48h	33, 42
Miscellaneous Agents		
Doxycycline	5 mg/kg (day 1)–2.5 mg/kg q12h	29
Rifampicin	5–10 mg/kg 24h	5, 46

(D) = dog; (C) = cat.

determine whether the antibiotic resolved the inflammation, and therefore the infection, or whether the corticosteroid is masking the infection. If an individual animal requires both antibiotics and corticosteroids, the corticosteroid administration should be discontinued at least 7 days before the final evaluation of the infection.

In infections of the intact hair follicle, deep tissues rarely become inflamed enough to be detected by palpation, so infection could still be present when the surface has healed. To prevent relapses because of this inapparent infection, it is recommended that antibiotic treatment be continued for 7 days after surface healing. In deeper infections, surface healing is misleading and antibiotic treatment must be continued after the dermal inflammation is gone. Deep lesions always heal on the surface well before the deep infection is resolved. Because some small, nonpalpable nidi of infection can persist even when the tissues feel normal by palpation, antibiotic treatment should be continued for 7 to 21 days after the tissues return to apparent normalcy. The time to resolution dictates the length of postnormalcy treatment.

Ideally, the clinician should re-examine all animals to determine when true healing has occurred. This is impractical in many instances and is not absolutely necessary in the case of more superficial infections. As long as the owner is an astute observer and treats the animal after clinical normalcy is present, most infections can be resolved without re-examination. Re-examination is mandatory for animals with deep infections. Owners cannot tell when the deep infection is resolved and always underestimate the need for antibiotics. Some clinicians schedule examinations every 14 days, whereas other clinicians examine the animal only when the owner reports that the lesions have healed. The approach is individualized for best results.

Deep infections are problematic for both the client and the clinician. With follicular rupture and damage to the dermal tissues, the inflammation tends to be pyogranulomatous and endogenous foreign bodies (keratin, hair shafts, and damaged collagen) are usually found in the dermis. During the first 2 to 4 weeks of antibiotic treatment, the lesion improves dramatically and then apparently stops responding. If treatment is stopped at this point, any ground gained is lost because it is unlikely that the deep infection is resolved. The rapid initial improvement is due to the resolution of the pyogenic component of the infection, but the granulomatous component remains and responds much more slowly. As long as there is slow, steady improvement, the antibiotic administration should be continued, even if the course of treatment approaches 12 weeks or longer. With long-term treatment, most lesions resolve completely, but the healing of some lesions reaches a certain point and improves no further. In these cases, the tissues never return to palpable normalcy because of resultant fibrosis, the presence of sterile endogenous foreign bodies in the dermis, or walled-off nidi of infection.

Skin biopsies can be both helpful and misleading. If infection is apparent, the need for additional treatment is documented. If no infection is visible, the question remains as to whether some infection is present in areas that do not undergo biopsy. If the lesion does not improve at all with 2 to 3 weeks of additional antibiotic treatment, one must assume that the infection is resolved and stop treatment. If infection is present, the lesion begins to worsen again in 2 to 21 days.

Relapses are common in skin infections, either because the current infection was not treated appropriately or because the underlying cause of the infection was not identified or resolved. The timing to relapse is important. If new lesions appear within 7 days of the termination of treatment, it is likely that the infection was not resolved. More intense treatment is necessary. If the relapse occurs weeks to months after the last treatment, the animal has some underlying problem that must be resolved.

No discussion of antibiotics would be complete without mentioning some of the anti-inflammatory and immunomodulatory properties inherent to some of these agents: macrolides (inhibit leukocyte chemotaxis, IL-1, and lymphocyte blastogenesis), trimethoprim (inhibits leukocyte chemotaxis), tetracyclines (numerous effects, see Chap. 3), and fluoroquinolones (inhibit IL-1, leukotriene, and TNF-α synthesis; inhibit granulomatous inflammation).[96a, 225a, 274a] These effects can be beneficial, but may also be misleading.

Management of Chronic Recurrent Skin Infections

Despite diligent diagnostic and therapeutic measures, some dogs have recurrent or nearly constant skin infections. The infection responds to prolonged treatment but recurs within weeks of drug withdrawal. Some of these dogs have a documented immunodeficiency, whereas other dogs appear normal with the currently available tests or cannot be tested. Poorly managed or poorly responsive allergic skin diseases must also be considered. The allergic pruritus damages the skin and predisposes to infection. This is especially true if corticosteroids are being used.

Immunomodulation can be considered in dogs with an immunodeficiency. The hope is that this type of treatment will make the animal's immune responsiveness more normal. It does not make a normal immune system hyper-responsive, so it has little or no benefit when the skin infections are due to weak skin and not a weak immune system. These treatments cannot resolve any pre-existing infection, but it is hoped that they can prevent or minimize further relapses.[165, 204]

The agents are given concurrently with an appropriate antibiotic until the infection is completely resolved. If the animal has received a sufficient course of treatment with the immunomodulator by the time that the infection is resolved, the administration of the antibiotic is discontinued at that point while that of the modulator is continued. The success of treatment depends on the time to, and severity of, any relapse. If no relapses occur, treatment was a complete success. Because it is difficult to normalize the immune system completely, many animals that undergo successful treatment do have other episodes of infection, but these are widely spaced, are less severe, and respond rapidly to antibiotic therapy. In many dogs, no response to immunomodulators occurs.

Chemical modulation with levamisole or cimetidine has received attention for treatment of recurrent skin infections, but no published reports offer specific details on the efficacy of either product.[80, 165] Levamisole, when administered at 2.2 mg/kg every other day, is thought to modulate the cell-mediated immune system and may be of some benefit in approximately 10% of dogs with idiopathic recurrent infections.[141] At this dosage, side effects are rare but include adverse cutaneous drug reaction, gastrointestinal irritation (vomiting and diarrhea), and blood dyscrasias. Because histamine receptors are found on the cell surface of many mononuclear cells, histamine can affect cellular function.[290] Cimetidine, an H_2-receptor antagonist, may inhibit histamine-influenced immunosuppression. For dogs, dosages between 6 and 10 mg/kg every 8 hours are suggested and side effects are rarely reported. If either of these drugs helps to prevent relapses, it is continued for the life of the patient at the dosages indicated above. The cost of the cimetidine may be prohibitive, especially in large dogs.

Anecdotal reports indicate that human recombinant IFN-α may be useful in some dogs with recurrent bacterial pyoderma.[246a] The recommended doses are 1 to 1.5 million IU/m² BSA or 1 to 3 million IU/dog, given orally or subcutaneously, daily or twice weekly (see Chap. 3).

Various bacterial products have received wide use in dogs with recurrent pyodermas. Autogenous staphylococcal bacterins, *S. aureus* phage lysate (Staphage Lysate [SPL, Delmont Laboratories]) and *P. acnes* (Immunoregulin [Immunovet]) are the most commonly used preparations. The exact mechanism of action of these products in dogs is unknown, but it seems to focus on improving cell-mediated immunity with subsequent impact on nonspecific and humoral immunity.[79–81, 165] No studies have been published in which dogs with recurrent pyodermas have been given all three preparations on a rotating basis to determine which is most effective. Placebo-controlled studies with SPL and Immunoregulin have been conducted, but none with autogenous products has been reported.

Autogenous staphylococcal vaccines are prepared from cultures taken from the dog's skin and thus contain the specific strain of *S. intermedius* causing the infection. Most of the reports on the efficacy of autogenous bacterins involve small numbers of dogs and are self-controlled.[16, 54, 70, 204] Despite these shortcomings, the studies show that some dogs experience a good to excellent response to the bacterin. In a pilot study of 13 dogs with idiopathic recurrent pyoderma published in 1997, 9 (69%) showed a good-to-excellent response.[70] Anaphylaxis can occur with these products.

Immunoregulin is licensed for intravenous use only and can cause a necrotizing dermatitis if it is given subcutaneously or intramuscularly. It is given every third to fourth day for 2 weeks, then weekly until the condition is resolved or stabilizes. Maintenance doses are given as needed, usually once monthly. When 28 dogs with recurrent skin infections were given either Immunoregulin or a placebo for 12 weeks, the rate of cure in the Immunoregulin-treated group was much better: 80% versus 38.5%.[21] Because the dogs were given antibiotics concurrently with the immunomodulator and details on relapses were not available, it is difficult to determine the efficacy of the product.

SPL was first developed for use in humans and contains components of *S. aureus*.[78-80, 165, 234] It is licensed for use in dogs by subcutaneous injection. Dosage schedules vary, but most investigators administer 0.5 ml twice weekly for 10 to 12 weeks. If response occurs, maintenance injections are given every 7 to 14 days. If a partial response is seen to the 0.5-ml dosage, gradual increases to 1.5 ml (the maximum dosage suggested by the manufacturer) may improve the responses. When 21 dogs with recurrent superficial pyoderma were given either SPL or a placebo for 18 weeks, 10 of 13 dogs (77%) given the SPL had a good response, whereas 3 of 8 (46%) in the placebo group had a good response.[78] Responders did have subsequent infections, but they were reported to be less severe with the SPL treatment and could resolve spontaneously.

This information suggests that immunomodulation may be of some benefit in carefully selected cases. If the recurrent infections are due to skin disease and not immunodeficiency, response beyond that occurring with a placebo should not be expected. These agents are expensive and not innocuous; thus, casual use should be discouraged. Because cats rarely have recurrent skin infections other than abscesses associated with fighting, no data are available on the safety and efficacy of these products in cats. One of us (W.H.M.) has treated one cat with SPL given at 0.5 ml once weekly, and results were positive with no adverse reactions.

When the dog's recurrent pyoderma is due to an unresolvable skin disease, usually an allergic disorder, or does not respond to immunomodulation, control can usually be achieved with long-term antimicrobial therapy. Topical antibacterial shampoos are usually insufficient and may be detrimental if the shampoos irritate or macerate the skin. Antibiotics are necessary. Because the drug is given for a prolonged period, only drugs with a wide margin of safety should be used. Most cases are treated with a cephalosporin, oxacillin, amoxicillin clavulanate, or a fluoroquinolone. Macrolides and lincosamides are safe for long-term administration, but bacterial resistance usually precludes their use.

Antibiotics can be administered to these dogs on a recurrent episodic basis or continually. If the interinfection interval is 2 months or longer, episodic administration is most appropriate. At the first sign of infection, the drug is given at full therapeutic levels until the infection is resolved and then for an additional 7 to 14 days. When the infections recur shortly after the drug administration is discontinued, long-term treatment is indicated.[165] The dog is first treated with the full therapeutic dosages for 7 to 14 days after clinical remission, and then therapy is changed to a suboptimal or pulse regimen. No data suggest that one method is more effective or less likely to cause side effects, so the protocol selected should be tailored to the patient's needs. The pulse method involves the administration of full therapeutic dosages for 7 days, with none given for the next 7 days. Depending on the animal's response, the interval with no treatment could be extended to 10 to 21 days.

A variety of suboptimal protocols are used. To clarify the discussion, let us say that the full therapeutic dosage of the drug of choice for the patient is 500 mg every 12 hours. After the infection is resolved, some investigators administer 500 mg every 24 hours, whereas others administer 500 mg every 12 hours every other day and one investigator administers 500 mg q12h for 2 consecutive days each week.[22] If the patient's infection does not recur, additional reductions may be indicated. The investigators who use once-daily therapy often reduce the daily dosage to 250 mg or maintain the 500-mg dosage but administer it less often (e.g., every 48 or 72 hours). When the drug is not administered daily, the treatment interval is extended to every third or fourth day. After the lowest appearance and by documentation of the bacterial cause by direct smears and stains or by cultures of the pustular exudate. Histopathologic findings show nonfollicular subcorneal pustules (Fig. 4–2). Bacteria may or may not be visible within the pustules.

CLINICAL MANAGEMENT

Impetigo may regress spontaneously, but therapy can hasten the healing process. When the lesions are few and widely separated, topical antibiotic or antibacterial creams or water-miscible ointments, such as mupirocin and chlorhexidine, can be effective.[40] Typically, the lesions are too numerous to make this form of therapy practical, and bathing with antibacterial shampoos, such as chlorhexidine, ethyl lactate, and benzoyl peroxide, is indicated. The skin of puppies and kittens is easily irritated, and benzoyl peroxide should be used carefully. The affected areas are washed daily or on alternate days until healing occurs, typically in 7 to 10 days. Rarely are systemic antibiotics necessary, but if needed, a 10- to 14-day course is usually sufficient unless there is an intercurrent superficial folliculitis. It is desirable to check health management procedures to eliminate debilitating factors that may have influenced the onset of the disorder.

Impetigo-like lesions in unusual locations (e.g., facial) in puppies or in mature dogs necessitate more careful consideration and may carry a more guarded prognosis because immunosuppression and other serious disorders mentioned earlier may be involved in the pathogenesis. Bullous impetigo usually responds rapidly to the administration of appropriate antibiotics and treatment of the underlying disease.

Mucocutaneous Pyoderma

Mucocutaneous pyoderma occurs in dogs and affects primarily the lips and perioral skin.[142] Its etiology is unknown.

CLINICAL FEATURES

Dogs of any age, breed, or sex can be affected. German shepherd dogs and German shepherd crosses may be at greater risk. The first noticeable change is symmetric swelling and erythema of the lips (Fig. 4–3), especially at the commissures. Crusting follows and

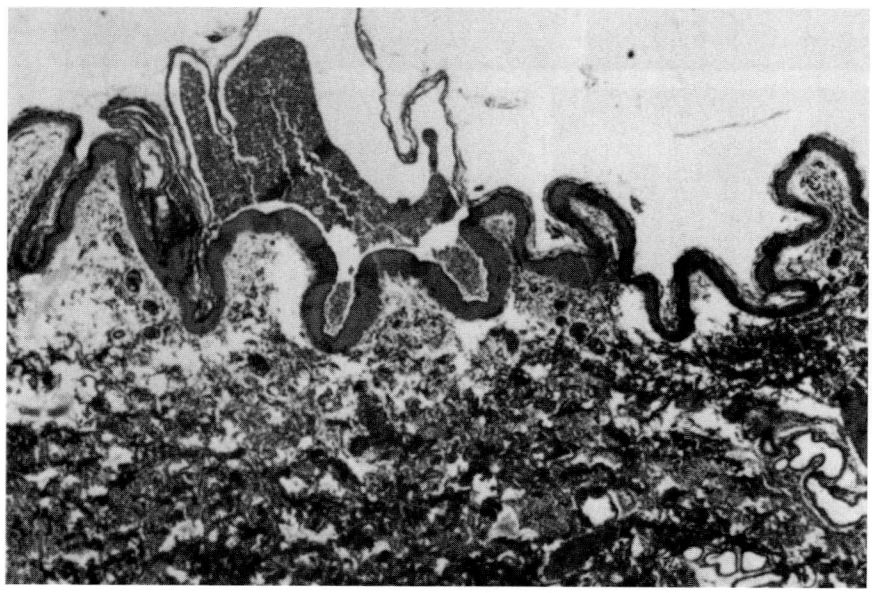

FIGURE 4–2. Staphylococcal impetigo in a dog. Note nonfollicular subcorneal pustule.

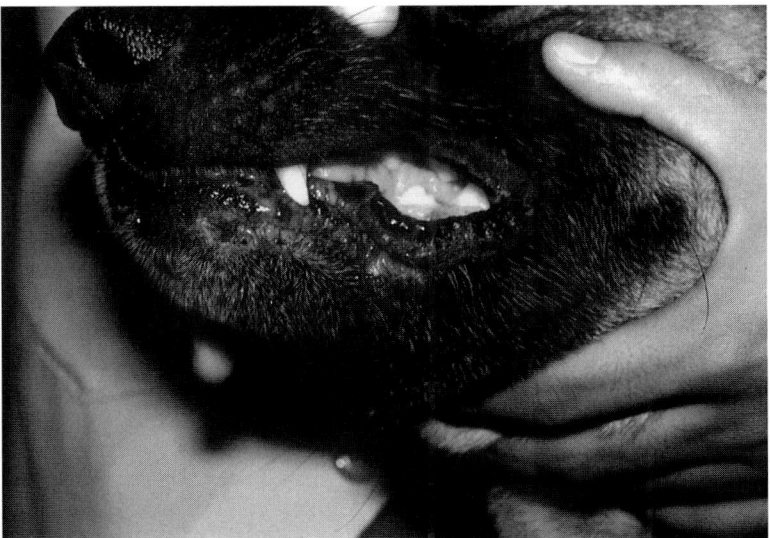

FIGURE 4–3. Mucocutaneous pyoderma. Involvement of most of the lower lip. The crusting has been removed to show the erosion and depigmentation.

can lead to fissuring and erosion (see Fig. 4–1C). Exudate may be present beneath the crusts, especially ventral to the lips. Similar lesions may be at the eyelids, the nares, the vulva, the prepuce, or the anus. Depigmentation of the lips can occur in chronic cases.

The lesions are tender, and the dogs rub the areas and resent examination and palpation of the area. Mucocutaneous pyoderma does not originate in lip folds but can coexist with lip fold dermatitis.

DIAGNOSIS

Mucocutaneous pyoderma is visually distinctive.[142] Differential diagnostic possibilities include discoid lupus erythematosus, lip fold intertrigo, zinc-responsive dermatosis, early pemphigus foliaceus or erythematosus, and adverse cutaneous drug reaction.

Diagnosis is confirmed by clinical examination and skin biopsy. Histopathologic study shows epidermal hyperplasia with superficial pustulation and crusting (Fig. 4–4). In the dermis, a dense, predominately plasmacytic, lichenoid dermatitis is visible. Neutrophils are also prominent in the inflamed dermis, and pigmentary incontinence may be striking (Fig. 4–5). However, the dermal-epidermal interface is not obscured, and hydropic degeneration is minimal to absent. Similar but milder inflammatory changes may be detectable around appendages in biopsy specimens of haired skin.

CLINICAL MANAGEMENT

The condition responds to topical or systemic antibacterial therapy. For topical treatment, the surrounding hairs should be clipped and then the areas gently washed with benzoyl peroxide or some other suitable antibacterial shampoo. After the lesions are cleaned, a light film of an antibacterial ointment is applied. Mupirocin is particularly effective. The areas are treated daily for 14 days and then once to twice weekly. In severe cases, systemic antibiotics are necessary for 3 to 4 weeks.

After the lesions have resolved, treatment can be discontinued, but relapses are common. For relapsing cases, normalcy can be maintained by an individualized topical program or, more rarely, maintenance administration of systemic antibiotics.

Superficial Bacterial Folliculitis

A common clinical presentation is infection confined to the superficial portion of the hair follicle.

292 • Bacterial Skin Diseases

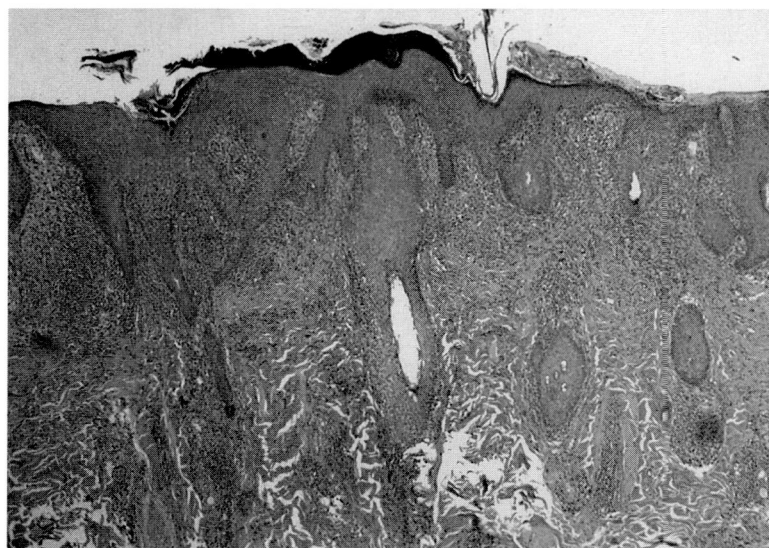

FIGURE 4–4. Mucocutaneous pyoderma. Marked epidermal hyperplasia and surface crusting.

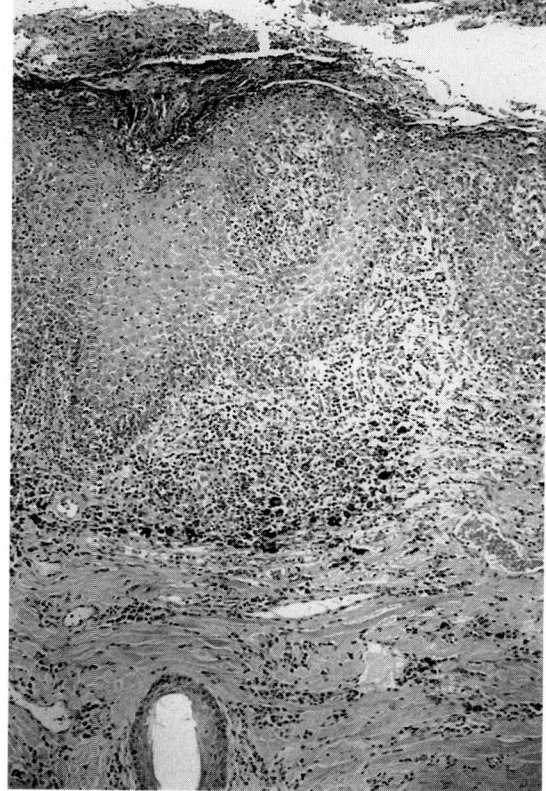

FIGURE 4–5. Mucocutaneous pyoderma. Lichenoid dermatitis with plasma cells, neutrophils, and pigmentary incontinence.

CAUSE AND PATHOGENESIS

In most cases, superficial folliculitis in dogs is caused by *S. intermedius*, although other staphylococcal species and other bacteria may be involved. Organisms may be introduced by local trauma, by bruising or scratching, or as an infection resulting from contamination due to dirty coats or poor grooming, seborrhea, parasitic infestation (especially demodicosis), hormonal factors, local irritants, or allergies. The three most common etiologic agents in canine folliculitis are staphylococci, dermatophytes, and demodectic mites. Superficial folliculitis may progress to deep folliculitis, furunculosis, and even cellulitis.

Folliculitis may or may not be pruritic, and if it is pruritic, its intensity can vary. It is not clear why these two types of folliculitis exist or even if the two syndromes (pruritic and nonpruritic) are separate dermatoses. The clinical lesions, described histopathologic findings, and levels of antistaphylococcal IgE antibodies[118] are identical for both types, the only difference between the two being the pruritus. A few cases may be due to bacterial hypersensitivity (so-called pruritic superficial pyoderma).[206] Because staphylococcal folliculitis can be pruritic, and because so many pruritic dermatoses (e.g., hypersensitivities and ectoparasitisms) are frequently complicated by secondary staphylococcal folliculitis, it is crucial and apt to ask, "Is it a rash that itches or an itch that rashes?" Often, the answer is determined only by training the client to observe the skin before and during the next recurrence.

CLINICAL FEATURES

The primary feature of folliculitis, regardless of the cause, is a tiny, inflammatory pustule with a hair shaft protruding from the center. The typical pustule may be difficult to find because pustular lesions are transient in dogs and cats, especially when the patient is pruritic. More common lesions are follicular papules (earliest lesion), which may or may not be crusted; epidermal collarettes; hyperpigmentation; excoriation; and alopecia (see Fig. 4–1D to F). Annular areas of alopecia, erythema, scaling, crusting, and hyperpigmentation—the so-called bull's eye or target lesions (see Fig. 4–1G)—are highly suggestive, but many vesicular and highly inflammatory processes that begin from a point (e.g., impetigo and pemphigus foliaceus) may produce similar circular lesions. English bulldogs have a fairly unique presentation. Infected areas are hairless and hyperkeratotic with minimal inflammation (Fig. 4–6). Dalmatians may develop bronzing of the hairs in areas of folliculitis.

Superficial folliculitis has neither a specific distribution pattern nor a characteristic clinical presentation. Because staphylococcal infections are typically secondary to external or internal skin damage, the localization of the infection depends on the predisposing cause. With external trauma (e.g., laceration, fleas), the infection is initially localized in the area of trauma. With underlying systemic disorders, truncal lesions predominate. In either case, the infection can spread to involve wider areas, especially if the lesions are pruritic. In chronic cases, most of the skin can be involved.

The clinical lesions depend on density and length of the hairs in the involved area. In relatively glabrous areas, the papulopustular lesions described above are easily seen. In haired skin, these lesions are not appreciated unless the hair is clipped away. In short-coated dogs, the first sign of superficial folliculitis is a dishevelment of the coat in the involved area, with small groups of hairs tufting together and rising above the skin's surface. These early lesions are often confused with urticaria. With time, the hairs fall out of the infected follicles and the dog is left with multiple, small areas of alopecia (see Fig. 4–1D). The exposed skin is usually inflamed, but in the Shar Pei and dogs with darkly pigmented skin, the hairless areas look nonreactive, which can lessen the suggestion of bacterial folliculitis.

With increasing chronicity, the alopecic areas enlarge to give the dog a moth-eaten look. Adjacent lesions can coalesce to form large areas of inflamed skin,[143] which can be confused with dermatophytosis and a variety of other conditions. Careful inspection of the periphery of the hairless area usually shows an inflamed epidermal collarette and more

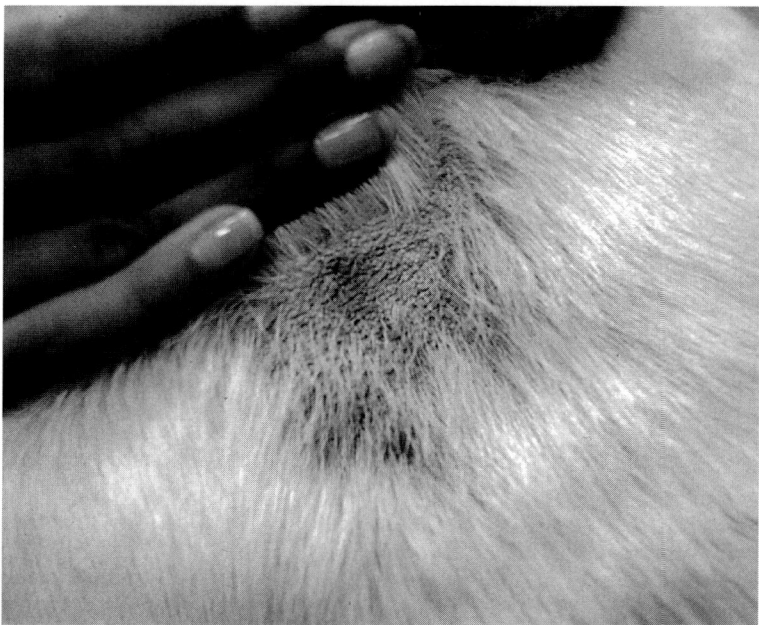

FIGURE 4–6. Superficial folliculitis. Instead of the classic papular lesions, the English bulldog often develops partial hair loss and hyperkeratosis, mimicking that seen in demodicosis, dermatophytosis, and nutritional disorders.

typical lesions of superficial folliculitis. In chronic cases, the coalescence can be so advanced that the dog looks like it has an endocrine alopecia. However, the approximately annular appearance of the alopecic areas and the discrete borders between alopecic and haired areas are highly suggestive of follicular inflammation or dysplasia.

Superficial folliculitis in long-coated dogs is much more insidious, especially when the lesions are not pruritic. The first sign is usually a loss of luster of the hairs in the involved area with increased shedding. The area may or may not be seborrheic. With time, the scaling increases or becomes apparent and the hair loss increases so that the hypotrichosis is obvious. Coincidental with the increasing hair loss is the recognition of underlying skin lesions. Collies and Shetland sheepdogs can have large, approximately symmetric areas of alopecia over the trunk resembling endocrine hair loss. Careful inspection of the margins of the alopecic areas reveals erythema, scaling, and epidermal collarettes.

Superficial folliculitis is rare in cats.[199, 215, 248–251, 280] The most common presentation is a crusted papular eruption (miliary dermatitis), which is clinically indistinguishable from the other crusted papular lesions of cats. Some cats have annular areas of alopecia, scaling, and crusting over the head and neck (see Fig. 4–1H), which is more commonly produced by dermatophytosis or demodicosis.

DIAGNOSIS

With adequate visualization of the lesions, the clinical diagnosis of superficial folliculitis is usually straightforward. The papular or pustular lesion has a follicular orientation. Because most cases of superficial folliculitis in the dog are staphylococcal in origin, it is likely that the patient being examined has a pyoderma. However, this is not absolute because follicular inflammation (folliculitis) also occurs in a number of conditions, including demodicosis, dermatophytosis, and a variety of immune-mediated skin disorders such as pemphigus foliaceus. To confuse the issue further, an inflamed hair follicle is easily infected such that secondary staphylococcal folliculitis is commonly superimposed on some other folliculopathy.

To confirm the diagnosis of bacterial superficial folliculitis, diagnostic tests must be performed. Skin scrapings and fungal techniques (hair examination and fungal culture) should be performed to rule out the other common causes of folliculitis, and exudative cytologic specimens should be evaluated. The pus should contain cocci, neutrophils in varying stages of degeneration and, most importantly, evidence of bacterial phagocytosis.

If no exudate is available or if the cytologic examination shows bacterial infection but the distribution and nature of the lesions suggests that the infection was caused by some other inflammatory folliculopathy, skin biopsies are necessary to define the problem. The histopathologic study of bacterial folliculitis shows a neutrophilic exudate within the hair follicles (suppurative luminal folliculitis) (Fig. 4–7). Bacteria may or may not be visible within the infected follicles. If a biopsy is performed on chronic nonpustular lesions, one often finds superficial, suppurative interstitial dermatitis, perifolliculitis, perifollicular fibrosis, and/or intraepidermal neutrophilic microabscesses. In the folliculitis of English bulldogs, the predominant alteration is marked follicular and surface hyperkeratosis, papillomatosis, and interstitial to periadnexal inflammation (Fig. 4–8).

Because skin infections rarely occur spontaneously in dogs and cats, the diagnostic effort should not stop at the identification of staphylococcal folliculitis. The most important question to be answered is, "Why is the skin infected?" The history and physical examination become important here. If there is any evidence of antecedent pruritus or skin disease before the pyoderma develops, the diagnostic effort needs to continue to define the underlying cause of the infection. In many cases, especially when the pyoderma is chronic and the lesions are pruritic, the history and the physical examination are of minimal use. Here, one is faced with the choice of performing other diagnostic tests (e.g., routine laboratory screening, endocrine testing, and allergy testing) or simply treating the infection appropriately.

Obviously, the specifics of the case dictate the best course of action, but if the animal has never been adequately treated for a superficial staphylococcal folliculitis, it is probably best to resolve the infection. It is not unusual for dogs with chronic widespread superficial folliculitis to return to clinical normalcy and remain normal after the infection is resolved. Obviously, the cause of the pyoderma in those cases was transient. If the animal's uninfected skin is abnormal or if the pyoderma recurs within 3 months of the cessation of treatment, the animal has some other disease that must be diagnosed and treated to prevent further relapses. Careful review of the history and the physical examination findings after antibiotic treatment directs the diagnostic effort.

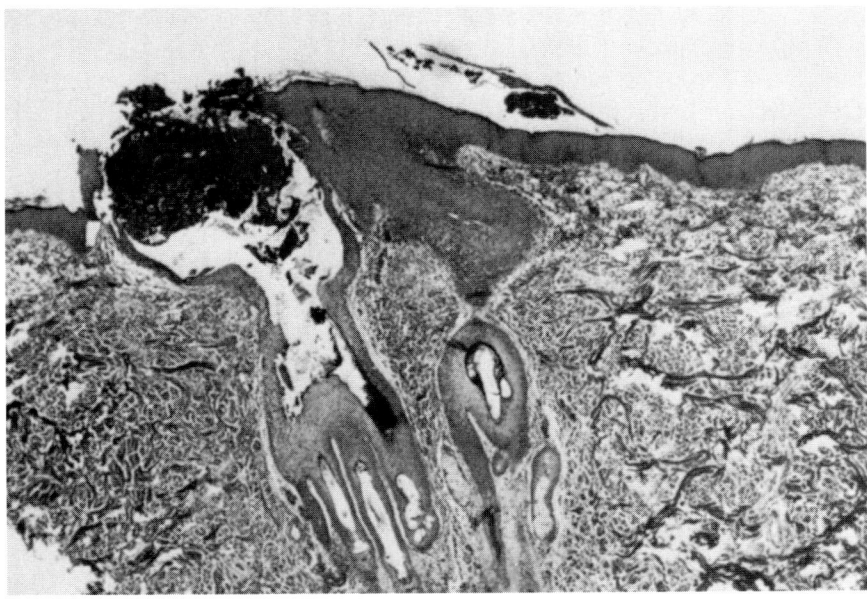

FIGURE 4–7. Staphylococcal folliculitis in a dog. Note cellular exudate within hair follicle.

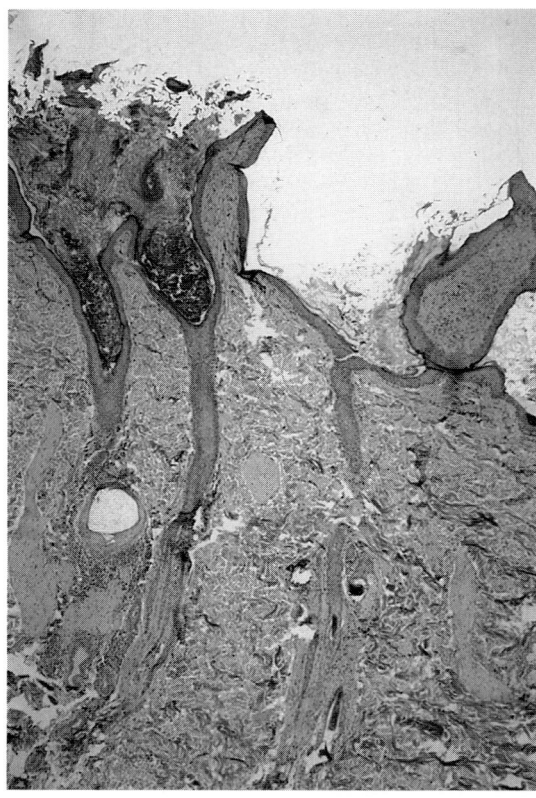

FIGURE 4–8. Superficial folliculitis in an English bulldog. Marked luminal hyperkeratosis, papillomatosis, and periadnexal inflammation.

CLINICAL MANAGEMENT

A superficial folliculitis in an immunologically normal animal heals fairly rapidly with a typical course of treatment of 21 to 28 days. In the case of recurrent infections, it is not uncommon for the lesions to heal more slowly, so longer courses of treatment can be expected.

Dermatophilosis

Dermatophilosis (cutaneous streptotrichosis) is an actinomycetic disease that produces a superficial, crusted dermatitis caused by *Dermatophilus congolensis*. It is rare in small animals.[2, 44, 55, 203]

CAUSE AND PATHOGENESIS

The organism is a gram-positive coccus that has rarely been found in the environment and therefore is thought to come from only carrier animals, usually farm animals.[9, 44, 203] The clinical disease often develops shortly after the rainy season begins and is uncommon in dry climates. Moisture that releases the infectious zoospores is an essential initiating factor. Affected animals usually have skin defects from ectoparasites, minor trauma, maceration, inflammation, or infection. Thus, the organism is usually a secondary invader that is easily found by stained smears or cultures. These are motile organisms that eventually form flagellated zoospores. That form is highly resistant and may persist in affected crusts for several years. The motile cocci are chemotropically attracted to carbon dioxide diffusing from the surface of the skin. There, they germinate to produce a filament that invades the living epidermis and proliferates within it, causing the production of typical crusts.[171]

CLINICAL FEATURES

Dermatophilosis is a rare disease in small animals, but it may be more common than is realized in moist, warm climates such as northern Australia, New Zealand, and the southeastern United States. It should be suspected in cases of acute moist dermatitis, chronic folliculitis, seborrheic dermatitis, and other crusted dermatoses in which excessive moisture is present. It has been noted to affect dogs[2, 231] and cats,[2, 44, 203, 248] and one report suggests that the fox is the only natural canine host.[231]

Lesions may involve all parts of the hairy or glabrous skin, and in cats, the organism has been isolated from soft tissue fistulae and granulomatous lesions of the lymph nodes, the mouth, and the bladder. With skin lesions, the crusts are usually concentrated on the dorsal back and over the scapula and lateral thigh. The face, the ears, and the feet may also be affected, and pain is evident because the animals appear to be unhappy and are disinclined to move around.

Local lesions may start as erythematous papules and pustules, with crusts that occasionally thicken and expand to several centimeters in diameter. They may be isolated, circular lesions or may coalesce into larger areas. The classic lesion is an exudative, purulent dermatitis below raised tufts of hair and crusts. In early lesions, these crusts and the embedded hairs are easily removed ("paintbrush" lesions) to reveal greenish pus on an oval, bleeding, ulcerated surface. The healing lesions are characterized by dry crusts, scaling, hyperpigmentation, and alopecia.

DIAGNOSIS

The purulent exudate or crushed crusts can be made into a direct smear and stained with Giemsa's, Wright's, or Gram's stain or Diff Quik. The organisms can be difficult to identify but appear as two to six parallel rows of gram-positive cocci that look like railroad tracks (Fig. 4–9).

For isolation and culture of the organisms, crusts are ground with sterile distilled water and let stand for 30 minutes. The inoculum is taken from the top of the water mixture and placed in antibiotic-enriched (polymyxin B) media. Many media, such as

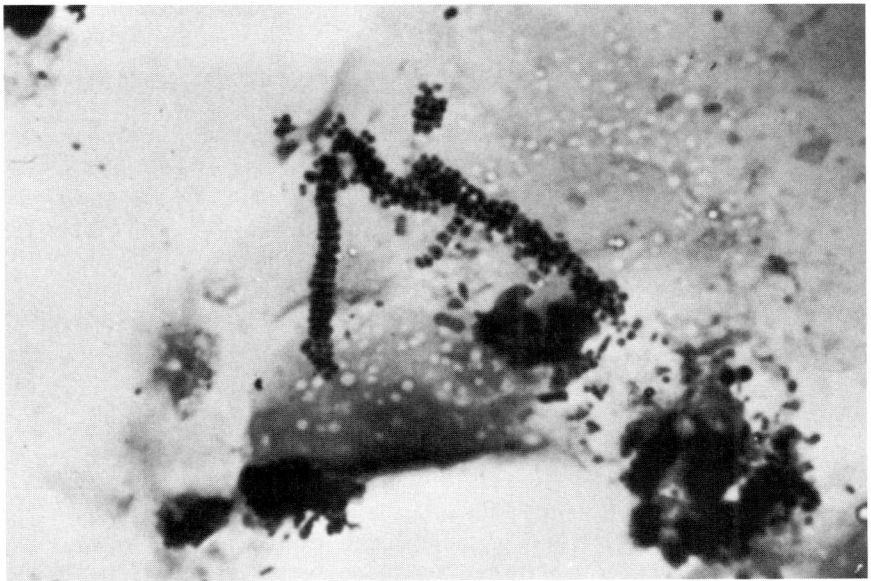

FIGURE 4–9. Dermatophilosis. Note branching chains of cocci ("railroad tracks") characteristic of *D. congolensis* in this direct smear of pus.

blood agar, are satisfactory, but Sabouraud's agar and MacConkey's agar should be avoided. Growth of a rough colony (later becoming smooth) occurs in 3 days, but organisms are small at first and may be missed in the midst of contaminants.

Skin biopsy of the affected skin is diagnostic and is especially useful in chronic cases, in which the exudative cytologic findings are often negative. Histopathologic study shows a hyperplastic superficial perivascular dermatitis or perifolliculitis-folliculitis with a palisading crust of orthokeratotic-parakeratotic hyperkeratosis and leukocytes. Organisms are usually easily demonstrated within the keratin on hematoxylin and eosin (H & E), acid orcein-Giemsa, or Brown-Brenn stains.

Differential diagnosis should include seborrheic dermatitis, pustular dermatitis (impetigo, subcorneal pustular dermatosis, and pemphigus foliaceous), acute moist dermatitis, staphylococcal folliculitis, demodicosis, dermatophytosis, and zinc-responsive dermatosis.

CLINICAL MANAGEMENT

With elimination of the primary inciting factors, many cases of dermatophilosis resolve spontaneously. This involves removing the moisture, parasites, or trauma that may be present.

The *Dermatophilus* organism should be eliminated from the skin. Because it does not thrive in an acid pH, topical therapy and good skin hygiene are useful. Crust removal and disposal are essential. Daily soaks with povidone-iodine or lime-sulfur solution given for 1 week and repeated weekly for 3 to 4 weeks are helpful. The systemic use of antibiotics is most effective and should be the primary focus of treatment. The organism is usually sensitive to ampicillin, cephalosporin, cloxacillin, lincomycin, tetracycline, tylosin, and high doses of penicillin. It is resistant to erythromycin, novobiocin, sulfonamides, polymyxin B, and low doses of penicillin. Positive cultures can often be obtained from the skin of healed animals for 7 to 8 months and up to 15 months, an important factor in recurrence of the disease.[2]

● DEEP BACTERIAL INFECTIONS (DEEP PYODERMAS)

Deep pyodermas are serious bacterial infections that involve tissues deeper than the hair follicle. They invade the dermis and often the subcutaneous tissue. They can cause systemic signs of illness and often heal with scarring.

Deep pyodermas do not occur spontaneously in normal dogs and cats. There is always a cause of the infection, and successful treatment mandates the identification of the predisposing problem. When the infection remains localized to a small area, external trauma (e.g., laceration, penetrating wound, animal bite, and foreign body) is the most likely cause. When lesions are discrete but widely disseminated over the body, involve an entire region of the body (e.g., the rump), or are generalized, the animal has some additional disease that must be identified.

Deep skin infections are generally the continuation of a superficial infection or superficial folliculitis. The infection goes deeper into the follicles and breaks through the follicular wall to produce furunculosis and infection of the dermis and subcutis. The infection follows tissue planes and may extend to the surface, producing multiple fistulae, or move deeper to invade subcutaneous and fatty tissues, producing cellulitis and panniculitis. The terminology for the condition depends on the location of the most obvious lesion, which may be called folliculitis and furunculosis, dermal fistulae, or cellulitis and panniculitis. Virtually any disease discussed in this text can be complicated by a deep staphylococcal infection.

In most instances, the infection remains confined to the hair follicle or progresses deeper at a gradual pace. In some cases, the progression is explosive. Factors that predispose to deep pyoderma include host immunoincompetence, severe follicular or dermal damage done by the primary disease (e.g., severe demodicosis), trauma (pressure, intense licking or chewing, and scratching) to the infected area, and inappropriate treatment of a superficial infection with an inefficient antibiotic, a corticosteroid, or both. In addition, many infections have distribution patterns that reflect areas of the body most subject to surface trauma. The basic pathogenesis of several common clinical syndromes is the same: deep folliculitis, furunculosis, and cellulitis; pyotraumatic folliculitis; nasal folliculitis and furunculosis; muzzle folliculitis and furunculosis; pedal folliculitis and furunculosis; German shepherd dog folliculitis, furunculosis, and cellulitis; acral lick furunculosis; anaerobic cellulitis; and subcutaneous abscesses.

Deep Folliculitis, Furunculosis, and Cellulitis

Deep folliculitis is a follicular infection that breaks through the hair follicle to produce furunculosis and cellulitis.

CAUSE AND PATHOGENESIS

Folliculitis and furunculosis start as a surface or follicular infection of bacterial, fungal, or parasitic origin. If there is a generalized distribution, one should suspect causes such as generalized demodicosis (see Chap. 6, Fig. 6–31D and E), generalized dermatophyte infection (see Chap. 5, Fig. 5–4A and B), adverse cutaneous drug reactions, endocrine abnormalities, seborrhea, and immunosuppression. Bacteria present are usually *S. intermedius*, but deep skin infections are more apt to have secondary infections from *Proteus* spp., *Pseudomonas* spp., and *E. coli*.

Histologic examination of biopsy samples may be useful in understanding the mechanism, etiology, and state of development of the folliculitis and furunculosis syndrome. Folliculitis is an exceedingly common gross and microscopic finding in dogs. Because it is often a secondary development, a thorough search for an underlying cause is mandatory. Folliculitis associated with bacteria, fungi, or parasites is usually suppurative initially. The occasional case associated with atopy, food hypersensitivity, or seborrheic dermatitis is usually spongiotic and mononuclear. Any chronic folliculitis, especially if there is furunculosis, can become granulomatous or pyogranulomatous (Fig. 4–10).

Furunculosis, regardless of cause, is usually associated with a tissue eosinophilia,

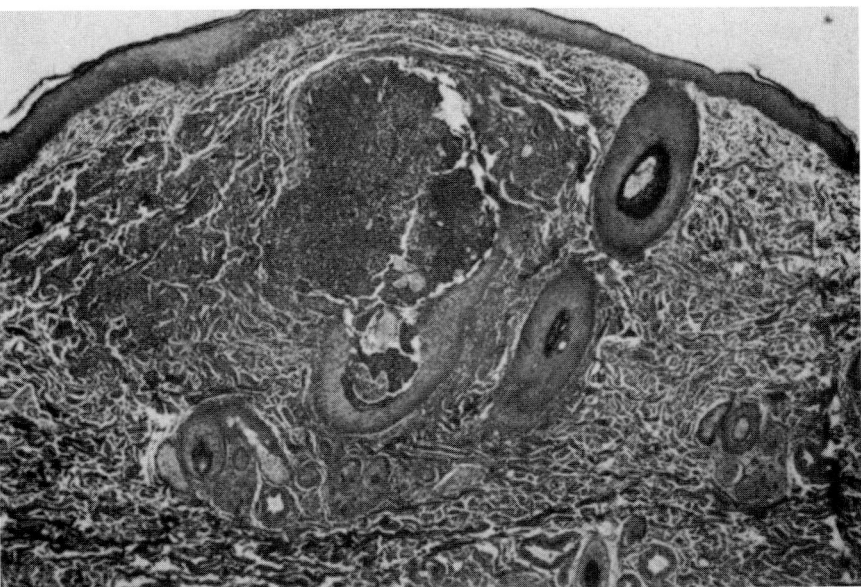

FIGURE 4–10. Staphylococcal furunculosis in a dog. Note follicular rupture with resultant pyogranulomatous dermal reaction around hair follicle.

which is assumed to suggest the presence of a foreign body (keratin or hairs). When tissue eosinophilia is secondary to infectious furunculosis, the neutrophil is the predominant intraluminal and intramural leukocyte and is present in similar numbers to the eosinophil in the perifollicular dermal inflammation. When the eosinophil is the predominant cell in all these sites, the etiology is probably *not* infectious and the likely causes are insect/arachnid-related damage or other sterile eosinophilic follicular disorders. The absence of tissue eosinophilia with furunculosis usually implies immunosuppression, especially that due to concurrent glucocorticoid therapy or demodicosis.

CLINICAL FEATURES

The nature of the initial lesions depends on the number of follicles involved in the area, the depth and severity of the follicular involvement, and various host factors, especially its immunocompetence. Infection of one or a few contiguous follicles induces discrete papular lesions of varying size, whereas simultaneous involvement of many follicles causes poorly demarcated areas of alopecia, tissue swelling, and inflammation. The severity of the infection can be estimated by the coloration and size of the lesions. Large dark red to violescent lesions are more severely involved (see Fig. 4–12D) than those that are smaller, more superficial, or more pinkish (Fig. 4–11H).

The progression of the initial lesions varies. Papular lesions soften to form deep pustules that ulcerate centrally and usually crust over. Before ulceration, hemorrhagic bullae may be present. Vibrissal follicles, which are infected, hemorrhage early in the course of infection before more classic changes occur. The larger lesions become more inflamed, become darker, and usually develop one or more fistulae that discharge exudate to the surface, where it crusts. Some of the severely infected larger areas become necrotic before fistulae develop and are irregular ulcers in the skin, which may or may not crust. If the infected area is traumatized (by pressure or pruritus), the speed and severity of progression is accelerated and the normal perilesional skin often becomes involved.

Lesions of folliculitis and furunculosis can occur wherever there are hair follicles but tend to be most common over pressure points or on the trunk. In short-coated dogs, the lesions described earlier are easily recognized. In long-coated dogs, the long hairs surrounding the infection entrap the exudate and tissue debris and encourage the development of large crusted lesions. The severity of the skin lesions in these crusted regions cannot be appreciated until the hair and crust are removed.

Bacterial folliculitis and furunculosis are rare in the cat (Fig. 4–12A). When they appear, follicular papules and pustules are usually located on the face and head (see Fig. 4–1H) or over the dorsum in a flea bite hypersensitivity pattern. Cultures from these lesions have most commonly grown staphylococci, both coagulase-positive and coagulase-negative, and occasionally β-hemolytic streptococci and *P. multocida*. Feline chin folliculitis and furunculosis may occur as a secondary infection complicating cases of feline acne (see Chap. 14).

CLINICAL MANAGEMENT

Although bacteremia and sepsis are apparently uncommon sequelae of a deep pyoderma, these serious debilitating infections necessitate careful, thorough, long-term treatment. Identification and resolution of the underlying cause is essential for a complete response. Most animals require a minimum of 4 to 6 weeks of treatment to resolve the visible lesions. Resolution of palpable lesions may necessitate treatment for 12 weeks or longer. Because of the seriousness of these infections, many investigators continue antibiotic administration for a full 21 days after clinical healing.

Pyotraumatic Folliculitis and Furunculosis

Clinicians have long recognized that not all cases of pyotraumatic dermatitis (acute moist dermatitis or hot spots) respond to therapy rapidly and completely. One study reported a

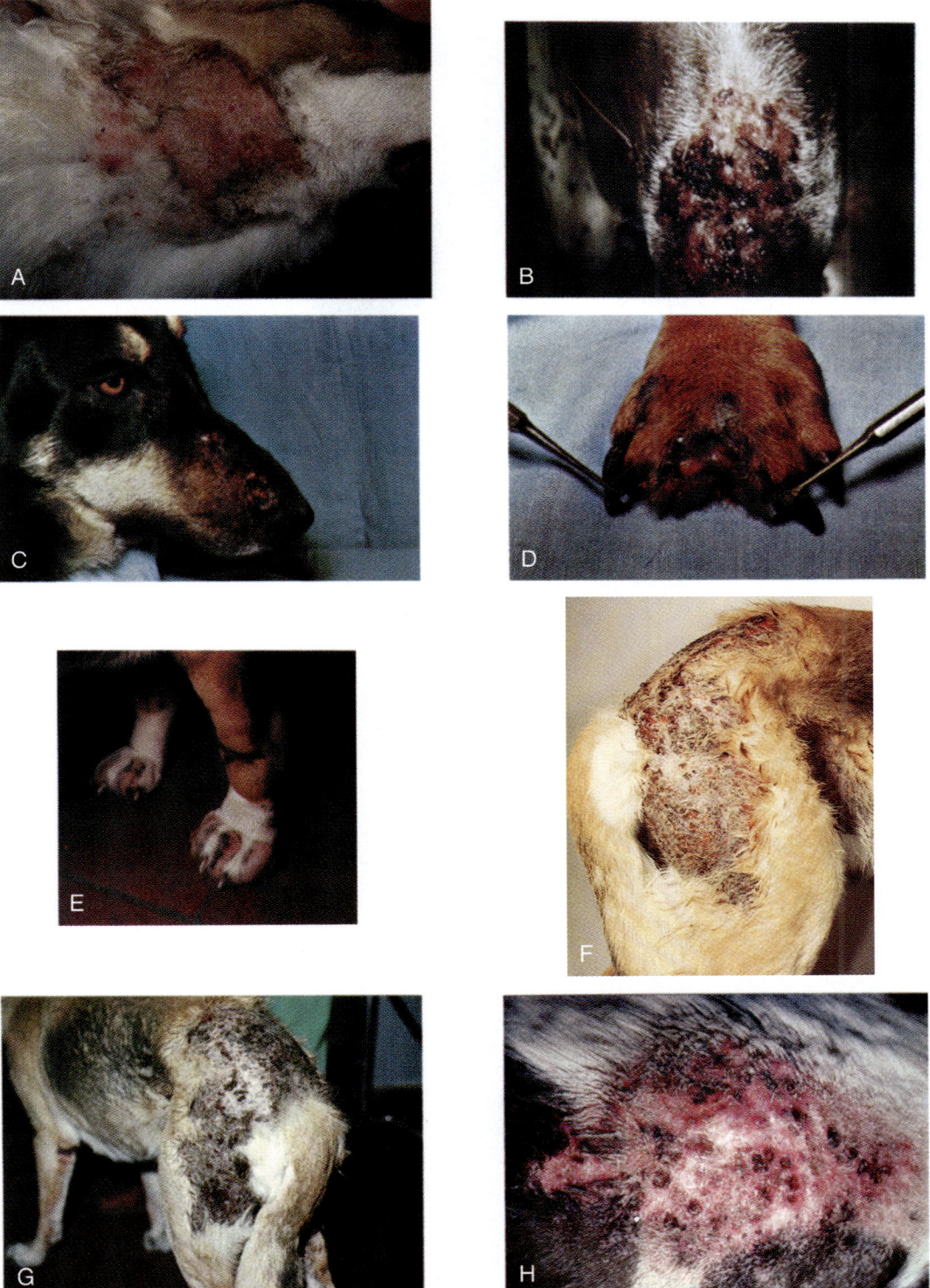

FIGURE 4–11. Folliculitis—deep pyodermas. *A*, Pyotraumatic folliculitis and furunculosis on the cheek and neck of a dog. *B*, Nasal folliculitis (pyoderma) of a Pointer's nose. Pustules and crusts are typical of painful lesions. *C*, Nasal folliculitis (pyoderma) showing pustules on dorsum of the nose. *D*, Pododermatitis (interdigital pyoderma) showing pustules and draining fistulae. *E*, Pododermatitis (interdigital pyoderma) with severe edema, cellulitis, and draining sinuses. *F*, Lateral rump and thigh of a German shepherd with furunculosis. *G*, Rump, thigh, and trunk of a German shepherd with furunculosis. Note flea bite hypersensitivity type of distribution pattern. *H*, Rump of a Springer spaniel with deep folliculitis and furunculosis.

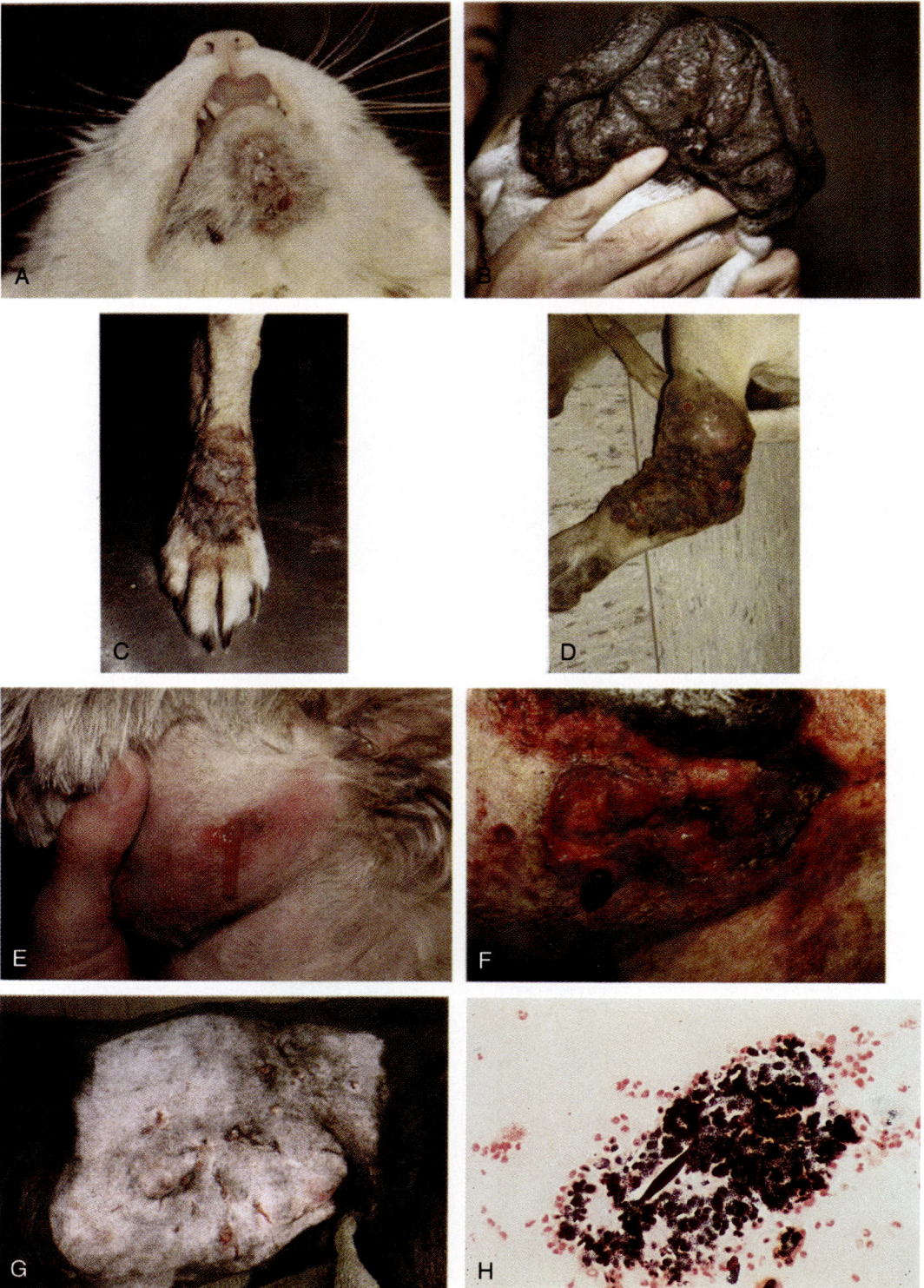

FIGURE 4–12. *A*, Furunculosis of the chin in a cat with feline acne. *B*, Muzzle furunculosis in a dog. *C*, Acral furunculosis in a dog. *D*, Severe pyogranulomatous furunculosis and fistulae on the hock of a dog. *E*, Draining abscess in the neck region of a dog (area has been clipped). *F*, Clostridial cellulitis and necrosis associated with mastitis. *G*, Bacterial pseudomycetoma (botryomycosis) on dog trunk. Area has been clipped to show nodules and draining tracts. *H*, Canine bacterial pseudomycetoma. Gram's stain of cutaneous discharge shows a tissue grain containing clumps of gram-positive cocci.

series of cases and discovered that they could be classified histologically into two groups.[229] In one group, the lesion did not have a large bacterial component. It was a superficial, ulcerated, inflammatory process of undetermined cause and pathogenesis (true pyotraumatic dermatitis or acute moist dermatitis) that responded readily to simple cleaning and corticosteroid administration (see Chap. 16, Fig. 16–17F).

The second group also had superficial ulceration but, in addition, had deep suppurative and necrotizing folliculitis and occasional furunculosis (see Fig. 4–11A). Clinically, this type of lesion is thickened, plaquelike, and surrounded by satellite papules and pustules. Lesions are especially common on the cheek and the neck. Numerous gram-positive cocci were present in the deep follicles, and panniculitis and hidradenitis with a neutrophilic infiltrate were common. The authors of this study speculated that the folliculitis was merely a complicating factor in some cases of pyotraumatic dermatitis. Alternatively, the infection could have been the primary event that induced the self-trauma. There was a strong tendency for young dogs to be affected; this pattern was observed in 70% of the Golden retrievers and St. Bernards presumed to have pyotraumatic dermatitis but in only 20% of all other breeds. Labrador retrievers and Newfoundlands are also commonly affected. These cases represent true local pyodermas.

Treatment of pyotraumatic folliculitis should include early administration of a systemic antibiotic effective against *S. intermedius*. It should be continued for 7 to 10 days beyond clinical cure. Local clipping, cleaning, and applying agents such as Burrow's solution, chlorhexidine soaks, and calamine lotion daily are often helpful. Elizabethan collars may be indicated, but chemical sedation or analgesia is rarely necessary. Glucocorticoid administration is contraindicated.

Nasal Folliculitis and Furunculosis

Bacterial nasal folliculitis and furunculosis (nasal pyoderma) is an uncommon, painful, localized deep infection of the bridge of the nose and the area around the nostrils (see Fig. 4–11B and C). It is most common in the German shepherd, Bull terrier, collie, Pointer, and hunting-type (dolichocephalic) breeds. The cause is unknown, but the disorder may start from rooting or other local trauma. The onset is rapid, and the condition is progressive until treatment is initiated. Initially, a small number of papules or pustules appear on the bridge of the nose. Because the lesions are either painful or pruritic, the animal traumatizes the area, expanding the number of lesions and area of involvement.

The differential diagnostic possibilities can be extensive, depending on the number and size of the lesions and the degree of self-trauma. With multiple, coalescent, crusted papular lesions, the primary differential diagnostic possibilities include pemphigus (foliaceus or erythematosus), lupus erythematosus, drug eruption, and dermatomyositis. When lesions are more discrete and papular to nodular, the primary differential diagnosis is nasal eosinophilic folliculitis and furunculosis. Other differentials include foreign body, other furuncular disorders (demodicosis; dermatophytosis, especially that due to *Trichophyton mentagrophytes* or *Microsporum gypseum*), sterile pyogranuloma syndrome, and early juvenile cellulitis.

Clinical management should include a careful consideration of underlying causes, especially if the examination of smears and cultures are negative for bacteria or fungi. The bacterial infections are usually secondary. Appropriate systemic antibiotics should be given in full dosage for 7 to 10 days beyond clinical cure. Gentle topical therapy with wet soaks using Burrow's solution or chlorhexidine, three times daily for 10 minutes, is excellent. This must be applied gently to prevent further trauma to the tender, inflamed tissues. The use of Elizabethan collars and sedation are rarely needed to alleviate pain and prevent self-induced trauma during the first few days of treatment.

Muzzle Folliculitis and Furunculosis

This is a chronic inflammatory disorder of the chin and lips of young dogs (canine acne) characterized by deep folliculitis and furunculosis (see Fig. 4–12B). It is almost exclusively a disorder of short-coated breeds, such as boxers, Doberman pinschers, English bulldogs, Great Danes, Weimaraners, Mastiffs, Rottweilers, and German shorthaired pointers.

The cause of this syndrome is unknown, but it is clear that bacterial involvement is secondary. The initial lesions are hairless follicular papules of varying size, which histopathologically are characterized by marked follicular keratosis, plugging, dilatation, and perifolliculitis. Bacteria cannot be seen or isolated, and there is no response to systemic antibiotics. With time, the papules enlarge, ulcerate, and may discharge a seropurulent exudate. At this stage, suppurative folliculitis or furunculosis is present and antibiotic treatment often improves but does not completely resolve the problem.

We speculate that local trauma and possibly some undetermined genetic predisposition play a central role in the development of the initial sterile lesions. Many short-coated dogs do not have muzzle folliculitis, even among the breeds predisposed to this disorder. Those who do may be more genetically susceptible to the disorder. During play, puppies frequently rub their muzzles and chins on hard, rough surfaces. Long hairs protect the underlying skin, but short hairs offer little protection and could break off below the skin's surface, inflaming the follicle and leaving the pilar canal open to bacterial invasion. Further trauma aggravates the condition and effectively seals off the pilar canal such that sterile or secondarily infected furunculosis occurs. After one infected furuncle develops, more can be expected.

Treatment depends on the severity and the chronicity of the problem. Early on, the lesions are few and are sterile. With modification of behaviors that traumatize the chin (e.g., chewing bones and chasing balls over carpeted surfaces) and frequent cleanings, the process can be arrested and the lesions heal slowly. Benzoyl peroxide products (shampoo or gel) are commonly used for cleaning because they also reduce the surface bacterial population and keep the hair follicle open. The chin is first treated daily and then as needed. These products should not be overused because they can be irritating and increase the follicular inflammation. If the gel is used, the owner should be cautioned that the product can bleach carpets, furniture, and other fabrics. In cases that continue to worsen despite these measures, corticosteroids can be beneficial. If the lesions are not too deep, a potent cream or gel (e.g., betamethasone valerate) applied three or four times daily rapidly decreases the follicular inflammation. For cases of deep lesions, we find that fluocinolone in dimethyl sulfoxide (Synotic) is beneficial. After the follicular inflammation is resolved, the use of the steroid should be gradually decreased and stopped.

Advanced cases are usually infected and necessitate a long (4- to 6-week) course of an appropriate antibiotic. Because deep infections heal with scarring, the chin is easy to traumatize, and endogenous foreign bodies (e.g., keratin and hair shafts) are typically found deep in these lesions, the antibiotic treatment does not resolve the entire condition. After the infection is resolved, the use of topical corticosteroids may be necessary to prevent new lesions.

Rarely, a dog is presented for bleeding from the muzzle. Close inspection of the area will show that the hemorrhage is coming from the vibrissal follicles. Aside from the hemorrhage, the follicles usually appear normal and documentation of the infection is difficult without a skin biopsy. Unless some other reason for the hemorrhage (e.g., cutaneous amyloidosis [see Chap. 9], bleeding dyscrasia) is apparent, treatment for infection is indicated.

Pedal Folliculitis and Furunculosis

Pododermatitis (interdigital pyoderma) is an inflammatory, multifaceted disease complex that affects the feet of dogs.[189, 247, 279]

CAUSE AND PATHOGENESIS

The cause of this disease is often unknown, but in no cases are the resulting lesions cysts. The disease is complex and may be frustrating to diagnose and treat.[189] Focal etiologic factors include foreign bodies (e.g., foxtails, awns, thorns, wood slivers, and seeds) and local trauma. When a single foot is affected, a foreign body, local injury, or neoplasia should be suspected, especially if there is only one interdigital fistula. Arteriovenous fistulae and lymphedema are rare causes of pyodermatitis. The feet are subject to great variety and intensity of trauma, the front feet more so than the rear. Hunting or field dogs commonly have bruises from stones, stubble, and briars. Animals working in sticky substances may accumulate masses of sand, stone, tar, and hair that initiate injury. Contact with irritant chemicals, fertilizers, or weed killers may also cause trouble. Clipper burns from grooming procedures, irritation from housing on wire or rough stones, and inflammation from contact, inhalant, or food hypersensitivities have all initiated pododermatitis. Any of these factors may lead to intense licking, which accentuates the irritation.

Fungal infections associated with pododermatitis include dermatophytosis, *Malassezia* dermatitis, candidiasis, mycetoma, phaeohyphomycosis, sporotrichosis, blastomycosis, and cryptococcosis. These are uncommon but should be suspected in cases that are refractory to usual antibiotic therapy. Bacterial infections are always secondary and can include a wide variety of organisms. Bacterial hypersensitivity may be a complication (see Chap. 8).

Parasitic pododermatitis is particularly common, with demodicosis being its most troublesome cause. Every case of chronic interdigital pyoderma must be evaluated carefully for demodectic mites. Biopsy may be necessary to confirm the diagnosis of parasitic pododermatitis in chronically inflamed and fibrosed feet. It is often missed by other diagnostic techniques (e.g., skin scrapings). Other parasites involved may include *Pelodera strongyloides, Ancylostoma* spp., and *Uncinaria stenocephala.* Ticks and chiggers favor the interdigital webs and may initiate inflammation.

Psychogenic dermatitis may be manifested as excessive licking of the feet by high-strung, nervous animals, especially Poodles, terriers, and German shepherds.

Sterile pyogranulomas may occur on the feet. The cause is unknown, but they are most common in smooth, short-coated breeds such as English bulldogs, Dachshunds, Great Danes, and boxers (see Chap. 18). Osteomyelitis or local neoplasms more characteristically involve a single foot.

Cases of pododermatitis that involve several feet, are recurrent or refractory to treatments, and are nonpruritic may be caused by an inherited or acquired immunodeficiency. Pododermatitis may also be the only clinical sign of hypothyroidism or demodicosis with secondary suppression of cell-mediated immunity. One report suggested that the flat foot and the scoop-shaped web of breeds such as the Pekingese and some terriers predispose the area to folliculitis and pedal dermatitis.[283]

Cases of pododermatitis with significant footpad involvement (hyperkeratosis and ulceration) may have an autoimmune basis (pemphigus, pemphigoid, or lupus erythematosus) or may be a manifestation of adverse cutaneous drug reaction, zinc-responsive dermatitis, necrolytic migratory erythema, or canine distemper.

In spite of all these possibilities, a substantial number of cases are idiopathic, recurrent bacterial infections. These can be exceedingly frustrating to manage.

CLINICAL FEATURES

Pododermatitis may affect dogs of any age, sex, or breed, but males of short-coated breeds, such as the English bulldog, Great Dane, Basset hound, Mastiff, Bull terrier, boxer, Dachshund, Dalmatian, German shorthaired pointer, and Weimaraner, are more commonly represented. Longer-coated breeds that are commonly affected include the German shepherd, Labrador retriever, Golden retriever, Irish setter, and Pekingese. The front feet are more often affected, but one or all four feet may be involved.

Affected tissue may be red and edematous with nodules, ulcers, fistulae, hemorrhagic bullae, and a serosanguineous or seropurulent exudate (see Fig. 4–11D). The feet may be grossly swollen (see Fig. 4–11E). Pitting edema of the metacarpal and metatarsal areas can be marked. The skin may be alopecic and moist from constant licking, and varying degrees of pain, pruritus, and paronychia may be present. The pain may produce lameness. In some cases, the interdigital nodules are nontender and unresponsive to treatment and may be scars from previous lesions. Although the regional lymph nodes are enlarged, other systemic signs are rare.

DIAGNOSIS

A careful history and physical examination findings provide the diagnosis of pododermatitis. Because of the complex pathogenesis, all cases for which a cause is not quickly and easily discerned should undergo multiple skin scrapings, exudative cytologic study, fungal culture, and a representative skin biopsy. The direct smear may provide early clues of the cause by establishing the presence or the absence of neutrophils or phagocytosed bacteria and their staining property or by showing large numbers of eosinophils, mycetoma or pseudomycetoma grains, yeast, or largely granulomatous cell exudate. Radiographs may also be needed to identify bony changes and opaque foreign bodies. An evaluation of the immune status is sometimes indicated and should include hemogram, serum immunoglobulin quantitation, and evaluation of the thyroid and adrenal glands.

Histopathologic studies are essential to document foreign bodies (including free hair shafts or keratin in the tissue), bacteria, parasites, fungi, and neoplasia and to evaluate the cellular response. Special stains may be needed. In general, the histologic response is that of perifolliculitis, folliculitis, or furunculosis; with the last, a nodular to diffuse pyogranulomatous inflammation is common. Contrast radiography studies are needed to document arteriovenous fistulae and lymphedema.

CLINICAL MANAGEMENT

Pododermatitis can be a frustrating problem because it is often self-perpetuating. Lesions heal with scarring, which makes the foot more susceptible to future infections. Delays in treatment of the infection and its cause increase the scarring potential, so the diagnostic and therapeutic effort should be maximal in these cases.

If the lesions are draining, foot soaks for 10 to 15 minutes twice daily are indicated until the drainage stops. Magnesium sulfate is particularly effective. Antibiotic treatment is prolonged, and 8- to 12-week courses are not unusual. Palpation is critical in monitoring these patients because the surfaces of these lesions heal weeks before the deep lesions are resolved. Lesions that are tender on palpation are likely still infected. As long as dermal lesions are present and are becoming smaller, treatment should be continued.

Cases with advanced disease at the onset of treatment have varying degrees of scarring of the digital and interdigital skin and may have sterile dermal granulomas due to endogenous foreign bodies. Protection of the foot via restricting the animal's activity or having the animal wear boots can help prevent future infections. Focal areas of scarring or individual dermal granulomas may be amenable to surgical removal.

Some cases, especially those in which the infection includes secondary gram-negative organisms, are resistant to medical treatment alone. Surgical débridement of all the devitalized tissue may make medical treatment more effective. In severe cases, fusion podoplasty in which all disease is removed and the digits are joined together can be beneficial.[265]

German Shepherd Dog Folliculitis, Furunculosis, and Cellulitis

This is a familial, immunologically mediated deep pyoderma of German shepherd dogs or German shepherd crosses.[22, 84, 157, 204, 234, 285–287] Affected dogs have deep skin infections, which resolve slowly and recur frequently. Either there is no definable cause of the infection or, if one is defined (e.g., flea infestation),[157, 234] the severity of the infection is well out of proportion to the stimulus.

CAUSE AND PATHOGENESIS

This condition has been studied extensively. Early work demonstrated a familial predisposition (possibly autosomal recessive). Affected dogs either had some underlying skin disease (e.g., allergic skin disease, hypothyroidism) or a cell-mediated immunoincompetence. Dogs with an immunodeficiency appeared to be in the minority.

Recent studies have shown convincing evidence of immunodeficiency in all dogs studied. Affected dogs have an increased number of $CD8^+$ and decreased numbers of $CD4^+$ and $CD21^+$ lymphocytes in their circulation.[53] Serum IgA levels were low in one study but because selective IgA deficiency occurs in some normal German shepherds,[23, 75, 105] the significance of this finding is unknown. Immunopathologic studies of skin biopsies from dogs with deep pyoderma have shown that all breeds had similar numbers of IgG, IgM, and IgA-bearing β-lymphocytes and plasma cells.[76] However, German shepherd dogs had markedly fewer T lymphocytes than other breeds. German shepherds with bacterial pyoderma had the same number of Langerhans' cells in skin biopsy specimens as other breeds with bacterial pyoderma.[74a]

The striking and seemingly inappropriate magnitude of inflammation seen in this condition has led some authors to speculate that the heritable defect in these dogs is associated with an exaggerated tissue response to staphylococcal bacteria, characterized by an inappropriate release of cytokines and other inflammatory mediators.[141a]

Because affected dogs do not experience infections of other organ systems and skin infection until middle age, they must have some degree of immunocompetence. With an insult to their skin (e.g., flea bite hypersensitivity) or immune system (e.g., hypothyroidism), they decompensate and experience a disproportionately severe pyoderma. Some dogs decompensate for no known reason, which suggests that the immunodeficiency can worsen with advancing age. Dogs in this latter group require lifelong treatment, whereas the other dogs may remain infection-free if the triggering disease is resolved.

CLINICAL FEATURES

The disease almost exclusively affects middle-aged German shepherd dogs and is not sex-specific or influenced by gonadal status. A familial history is occasionally given. In most dogs, the lesions are pruritic, and the pruritus usually stops after the infection is resolved. The distribution pattern is typical, with the rump, back, ventral abdomen, and thighs being affected in all cases. Some animals have more generalized lesions spreading to the chest and the neck. The front legs, the head, and the ears are usually much less involved.

Lesions are initially follicular in origin with clusters of papules, pustules, erosions, and crusts followed by ulcers, fistulae, furunculosis, alopecia, and hyperpigmentation (see Fig. 4–11F and G). Early lesions may be surrounded by strikingly erythematous halos. The lesions in haired skin are heavily crusted and the presence, depth, and severity of the infection in these areas cannot be appreciated until the crusts are removed. There may be a great deal of excoriation from the pruritus. Lesions may develop rapidly, forming confluent plaques of ulcerated, friable, necrotic skin. Some animals have secondary seborrhea, and cellulitis is evident in deeper infections. Peripheral lymphadenopathy is common. Animals with the disorder are usually in general good health, although there may be weight loss, poor appetite, and pyrexia. The lesions are usually painful, especially when the crusts are removed.

The course of the disease is long and stormy, with frequent stages of partial healing and exacerbation. This is usually produced by improper selection or inadequate dosage of antibiotics and inadequate duration of treatment, the concurrent use of corticosteroids, or failure to resolve predisposing factors.

DIAGNOSIS

The physical examination, coupled with exudative cytologic study, confirms the diagnosis of deep pyoderma but does not document this syndrome. The diagnosis of this syndrome is confirmed by the exclusion of other causes of deep pyoderma (e.g., demodicosis, allergy, ehrlichiosis), by the disproportionate severity of the infection if the dog has not received corticosteroids, or by repeated relapses.

All routine diagnostic tests are indicated in these dogs, as is an evaluation for thyroid disorders. If the lesions are pruritic and the pruritus does not stop with elimination of the infection, an evaluation for allergy should be performed. When all of these are determined to be noncontributory, an immunocompetency evaluation should be considered.

Skin biopsies are useful to determine underlying causes and to document the severity of the tissue damage. In most cases, histopathologic examination of skin biopsy tissues revealed folliculitis, furunculosis, and cellulitis as the most common findings.[157, 234] Perifollicular pyogranulomatous inflammation was common, which supports the idea of the disease being of follicular origin. Only a few biopsy specimens showed the large number of eosinophils expected in furunculosis.

CLINICAL MANAGEMENT

Because many cases have an intercurrent allergic disorder or hypothyroidism, every effort should be made to identify and resolve this triggering event. If the predisposing disease is ignored, the animal's response to treatment will be poor or the infection will recur shortly after the antibiotics are withdrawn.

Clipping and topical therapy are essential in this disease. Twice-daily soaks or the use of whirlpool baths helps to remove any crusts, improves drainage, and makes the patient more comfortable. Long-term antibiotic administration is necessary, with 6- to 10-week courses not uncommon.[22, 154] It is imperative that the drug be given at the correct dosage and frequency during and after clinical cure has occurred. Because these dogs are prone to experience disproportionately severe infection, premature termination of therapy guarantees a severe relapse. Some authors consider enrofloxacin (5 to 10 mg/kg q24h) to be the antibiotic of choice.[141a] Enrofloxacin is concentrated within inflammatory cells and is unimpeded by granulomatous inflammation, fibrosis, and purulent debris. In addition, the effectiveness of enrofloxacin may be partially explained by its anti-inflammatory properties.

With resolution of the infection and the triggering event, many of these dogs stay infection-free for long periods. The owners must be made aware that their dog is susceptible to skin infections. Any irregularities in the dog's management or grooming should be corrected, and the owners should be instructed to seek prompt attention whenever any skin lesions occur.

Some dogs experience relapse each time that antibiotics are withdrawn. These dogs probably have a cell-mediated immunodeficiency[204, 234] and may respond to immunomodulation. Chronic antibiotic therapy can maintain these dogs for long periods.[22] Anecdotal reports indicate that pentoxifylline may be a useful therapeutic adjunct, presumably due to its anti-inflammatory properties (see Chap. 3).

Acral Lick Furunculosis

Acral lick dermatitis (see Chap. 15) is well recognized in dogs and has a variety of causes. Cytologic or histologic evidence of infection is found in many cases, especially those with an ulcerated surface. What is unclear is whether the infection preceded the dog's licking of the area or was superimposed on some underlying condition.

CLINICAL FEATURES

Acral lick lesions are typically found on the distal portion of a front limb but can occur on a hind leg or on multiple limbs. The clinical appearance varies with the chronicity of the lesion and the amount of trauma to the area. Typically, the lesion is firm, raised, hairless, hyperpigmented at the periphery, and eroded or ulcerated centrally (see Fig. 4–12C). In some cases, there is significant tissue destruction with exposure of underlying tendons or bone.

DIAGNOSIS

Infection should be suspected in all acral lick lesions, especially if the surface is ulcerated. This suspicion can be confirmed by biopsy or, in many cases, by exudative cytologic examination. For correct cytologic evaluation, the surface of the lesion should be scrubbed to remove all debris and surface bacteria. After the surface has dried, the lesion is squeezed firmly between the thumb and the forefinger until drops of seropurulent or serohemorrhagic exudate appear on the surface. This material is examined cytologically. This is painful, so the dog may need to be muzzled or tranquilized.

In many cases, evidence of infection (e.g., intracellular bacteria within phagocytic cells) is found, and staphylococci are the primary organisms. In some cases, gram-negative organisms are co-infectors. If gram-negative organisms are detected, a culture should be performed, preferably from tissue taken via sterile biopsy technique. Culture of the discharge expressed by manual pressure can be misleading because it may contain contaminating but not infecting organisms.

In some cases, no bacteria are visible cytologically or no exudate can be expressed. In these cases, infection can be proved or disproved by biopsy or by a therapeutic trial with antibiotics. If the latter course is chosen, a broad-spectrum drug should be used for a minimum of 30 days before response is estimated.

CLINICAL MANAGEMENT

In acral lick furunculosis, the clinician is faced with the problem of determining the cause of the infection and the treatment of a deep, fibrosing infection. With solitary lesions, the cause of the infection is often a transient insult to the skin, which is not evident when the animal is presented for treatment. Unless the history, physical examination findings, and exudative cytologic study suggest some underlying problem, it may be best to resolve the infection first and then to determine whether the diagnostic effort should go forward. With lesions on multiple limbs, transient trauma can be discounted and a complete diagnostic evaluation should be performed, especially for allergy or hypothyroidism.

Soaks, especially with magnesium sulfate, and prolonged courses of antibiotics are necessary in acral lick furunculosis. The minimal course of treatment is 8 weeks, and some cases necessitate many months of treatment. Because of the need for long-term treatment, potentiated sulfonamide drugs should not be used. Most clients notice remarkable improvement within the first 3 weeks and then comment either that the lesion is getting no better or that the rate of improvement is much slower. Because these lesions are fibrotic at the onset of treatment, antibiotic administration should not be expected to resolve the lesion completely. Treatment is continued until no further improvement is detected by the clinician, not the client, and then for an additional 2 weeks. If, at the end of the treatment, the area is more fibrotic and hairless or if the animal continues to traumatize the area, the diagnostic effort must go forward.

The key to successful management of acral lick furunculosis is early and vigorous intervention. The more chronic the infection, the poorer the prognosis for a complete resolution. Large lesions heal incompletely and are covered by a thin, hairless, fragile epithelial layer. Because these lesions are often found over joints or in areas that are traumatized during normal activities, the area probably will be damaged in the future, which could trigger another infection. If there is significant tissue destruction at first presentation or after the infection is resolved, amputation of the limb may be indicated.

Aerobic Cellulitis

Cellulitis is a severe, deep, suppurative infection in which the areas of infection are poorly contained and spread laterally.[2] Depending on the cause of the cellulitis, there may be extensive edema and the overlying skin is often friable, darkly discolored, and devitalized.[54, 55] The weakened tissues may be sloughed.

In companion animals, most cases of focal aerobic cellulitis follow wounding and are diagnosed and treated accordingly. With more diffuse disease, deep extension of staphylococcal folliculitis and furunculosis is most likely. Rarely, one isolates an unusual (e.g., *Pseudomonas* spp.) organism.[233] In these cases, the skin lesions typically look more severe than those with staphylococci. In these cases, the question to be answered is whether the organism caused all of the damage or whether some other skin disease is present that is being secondarily infected by the bacterium. Each case must be evaluated on its own merits. Once these unusual bacteria are infecting deep tissues, aggressive antibiotic treatment are needed.

Anaerobic Cellulitis

Lesions of anaerobic cellulitis in companion animals tend to be more rapidly progressive and severe than their aerobic counterparts. Anaerobic cellulitis typically follows bite wounds, traumatic puncture wounds, or foreign body introduction but can be a sequela to surgery, trauma, burns, or malignancy.[69, 226] Poor management of indwelling catheters can predispose to *Serratia* infection.[13] In humans, diabetes mellitus, corticosteroid administration, or immunodeficiency predisposes to anaerobic infection, and these factors are probably important in animals.

Anaerobic infections are characterized by rapid progression, poor demarcation, massive tissue edema and swelling, and necrosis (see Fig. 4–12F). The wounds often, but not uniformly, have a putrid smell and are crepitant if the organism is a gas producer (*Clostridium* spp. and *Bacteroides* spp.).[90, 91, 102] Depending on the organism, toxins may be produced and cause profound systemic signs.

The presumptive diagnosis of anaerobic cellulitis can be confirmed by the presence of the clinical signs described. Exudative cytologic examination that yields neutrophilic and polybacterial findings is supportive. Anaerobes commonly isolated from dogs and cats are, in decreasing order of frequency, *Bacteroides* spp., *Peptostreptococcus* spp., *Fusobacterium* spp., *Porphyromonas* spp., *Clostridium* spp., and *Prevotella* spp.[145] With rare exception, all these anaerobes are susceptible to metronidazole, chloramphenicol, and amoxicillin clavulanate. Aside from *Bacteroides* spp., near-uniform susceptibility to ampicillin or clindamycin can be expected. Facultative anaerobes are of more concern because the susceptibility of these organisms can be limited and unpredictable.

Surgery is indicated to drain the exudate, remove necrotic tissue, and remedy tissue hypoxia. Hyperbaric oxygen treatment can be beneficial but is usually not available.[95, 222] Systemic antibiotics should be administered until the infection is resolved and then for an additional 7 to 14 days. Drugs of choice include metronidazole, chloramphenicol, and amoxicillin clavulanate.

Subcutaneous Abscesses

Subcutaneous abscesses are uncommon in dog but occur frequently in cats. In dogs, abscesses can be due to bite wounds, abscessed teeth, or foreign bodies (see Figs. 4–12E and 4–13), whereas bite wounds are most common in cats. *P. multocida* is the most common organism cultured from dog and cat bite wounds.[73, 137] Other organisms that can be involved include *S. intermedius*, β-hemolytic streptococci, and various anaerobes, including *Fusobacterium* spp., *Bacteroides* spp., *Clostridium* spp., *Peptostreptococcus* spp., and *Porphyromonas* spp.[151a, 211] Bacteria from claw or fang are injected under the skin when it is punctured during a cat fight. The wound is small and seals rapidly; a local infection develops in 2 to 4 days. Some bite wounds are handled well by the cat's normal defense mechanisms. Those that abscess are most commonly found around the tail base and the neck and shoulders.

Abscess from bite wounds is one of the most common cat diseases handled in a small animal practice. Untreated, the abscess may rupture, drain, and heal over 2 to 3 weeks. However, the treatment of choice is liberal surgical drainage and thorough flushing of the area with saline or chlorhexidine solution together with systemic antibiotics for 5 to 7

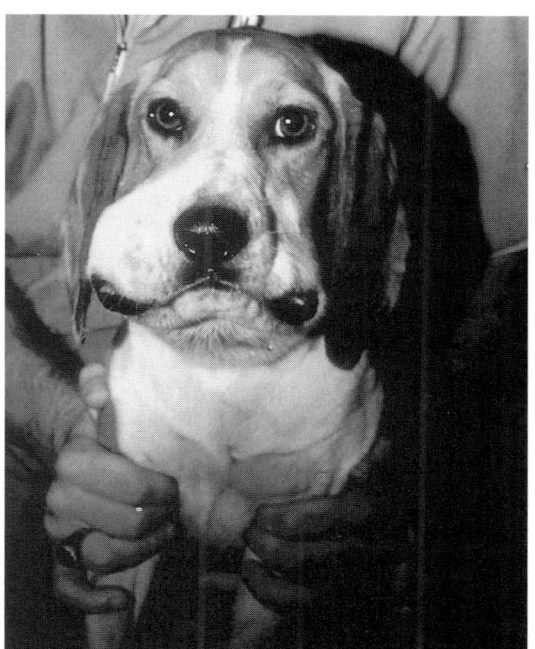

FIGURE 4–13. Facial abscess secondary to a tooth root abscess.

days. *P. multocida* with rare exception is susceptible to the penicillins (penicillin, amoxicillin, amoxicillin clavulanate), and these are the drugs of choice in known bite wounds. If there is a poor response to the initial medication or the abscess is not due to a bite wound, cytologic or cultural procedures should be taken to identify the offending organism.

Castration of intact male cats has been a helpful preventive measure, resulting in either rapid or gradual decline in fighting and roaming behavior to 80% to 90% of the cats so treated.[120] Recurrent or nonhealing feline abscesses should prompt a consideration of immunosuppression (feline leukemia virus infection or feline immunodeficiency virus infection), and other infectious agents (*Actinomyces* spp., *Nocardia* spp., *Yersinia pestis*, and mycobacteria), mycoses, or sterile panniculitis. Many anaerobic organisms can be found in feline abscesses.[137, 248–251] *Mycoplasma* and *Mycoplasma*-like organisms (discussion follows in this chapter) have been isolated from cats with chronic subcutaneous abscesses.

Rhodococcus (Corynebacterium) equi and *Corynebacterium pseudotuberculosis* have been isolated from the feet and subcutaneous abscesses in the cat.[98, 132, 159, 187] Internal organ involvement can occur with either organism, especially if the cat is immunosuppressed. Cytologically, a pyogranulomatous reaction is visible with gram-positive coccoid to coccobacillary bacteria within clear cytoplasmic spaces in macrophages.[98] Treatment is best determined by culture and susceptibility testing, but amoxicillin clavulanate is usually effective.

Bacterial Pseudomycetoma

Bacterial pseudomycetoma (cutaneous bacterial granuloma or botryomycosis) is a chronic, suppurative, granulomatous disease caused by nonbranching bacteria. They form grains of compact colonies in tissues that are surrounded by pyogranulomatous inflammation.[5, 274] Bacterial pseudomycetoma is common in many species but is rarely reported, probably because it is misdiagnosed or overlooked. The causative bacteria are usually coagulase-positive staphylococci, but in some cases other bacteria, alone or associated with staphylococci, may be responsible. There may be *Pseudomonas* spp., *Proteus* spp., *Streptococcus* spp., and *Actinobacillus* spp. In cases involving dogs and cats, multiple organisms can be found.[274]

Most cases are initiated by local trauma from bites or other wounds, and some are associated with a foreign body. There may also be muscle or bone involvement. The granuloma develops because a delicate balance exists between the virulence of the organisms and the response of the host. The host is able to isolate and contain the infection but is unable to eradicate it. This may also be a type of bacterial hypersensitivity, or the grain formation may be associated with the formation of a polysaccharide slime coating[151] produced by the bacteria or with a glycoprotein covering resulting from a localized antigen-antibody reaction on the surface of the microorganisms.

Clinically, the lesions appear as firm, solitary or multiple nodules with draining fistulae (see Fig. 4–12G). The purulent exudate may have small white granules similar to grains of sand (see Fig. 4–12H). Special bacterial and fungal stains are necessary to differentiate the granules from those found in actinomycosis, nocardiosis, or mycetomas.

Histopathologically, there is a nodular to diffuse dermatitis and/or panniculitis, with tissue granules surrounded by a granulomatous to pyogranulomatous infiltrate of histiocytes, plasma cells, lymphocytes, neutrophils, and multinucleate histiocytic giant cells (Fig. 4–14). The edges of the bacteria masses (granules) may show clubbing and may stain brightly eosinophilic with H & E (Hoeppli-Splendore material). The bacteria are best demonstrated with Gram's tissue stain or Brown-Brenn stain (Fig. 4–15).

Differential diagnosis must include actinomycosis, nocardiosis, eumycotic mycetoma, systemic mycoses, dermatophytic pseudomycetoma, foreign body reactions, and chronic bacterial abscesses. Because of the variable prognoses and therapeutic formats, a specific diagnosis is imperative.

Simple systemic antibiotic therapy is usually not adequate. Frequent relapses are the rule. Therapy for isolated lesions is complete surgical excision because the granulomatous mass is relatively impermeable to antibiotics.[5, 274] With large numbers of lesions, cotreatment with rifampin and β-lactamase-resistant antibiotic may be effective.

Mycobacterial Granulomas

Mycobacteria can be divided into three groups: obligate pathogens such as *Mycobacterium tuberculosis* and *M. lepraemurium,* which do not multiply outside vertebrate hosts; facultative pathogens, which normally exist as saprophytes in the environment but sporadically cause disease; and environmental saprophytes, which almost never cause disease.[2, 180] Mycobacteria and the disease syndromes they cause can be further classified as follows:

1. True tuberculosis mycobacteria. *M. tuberculosis,* both bovine and human types, cause small animal tuberculosis in endemic areas. They are photochromogenic and slow growers, and if injected into guinea pigs, cause death in 6 to 8 weeks; opportunistic mycobacteria do not (see discussion that follows).
2. Leprosy mycobacteria. *M. lepraemurium* causes rat leprosy, which is possibly transmitted to small animals. It is scotochromogenic and grows with great difficulty in the laboratory. Many acid-fast organisms are usually found in histologic sections (see Feline Leprosy in this chapter).
3. Opportunistic mycobacteria. These can be divided into groups according to their rate of growth and pigment production. One group of slow-growing organisms (longer than 7 days) is nonchromogenic and pathogenic only to cold-blooded animals. Another group of slow-growing mycobacteria of this group include *M. kansasii, M. marinum, M. ulcerans,* and *M. avium* and are facultative pathogens. The fast-growing (2 to 3 days, or less than 7 days) mycobacteria in the atypical, or opportunistic, group include *M. fortuitum, M. chelonei, M. thermoresistible, M. xenopi, M. phlei,* and *M. smegmatis.* Organisms may be scattered through tissues, necessitating a careful search. They are often found in small vacuoles in the granulomatous tissue (see Opportunistic Mycobacterial Granulomas in this chap-

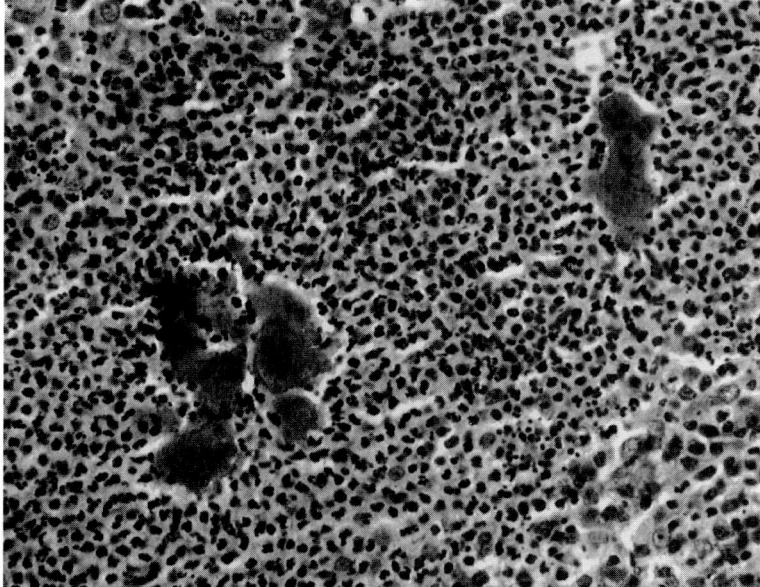

FIGURE 4–14. Bacterial pseudomycetoma. Pyogranulomatous dermatitis with multiple tissue grains.

ter). Natural water may be teaming with saprophytic mycobacteria, including some that are facultative or opportunistic pathogens. These can produce infection after contamination when predisposing factors are present. In attempts to isolate and to identify individual species, decontamination of saprophytes from cultures, differentiation by biochemical tests, and immunodiffusion analysis are difficult.[2]

In one cat with cutaneous mycobacteriosis, the histopathological findings resembled fibrosarcoma, and no granulomatous inflammation was seen.[202a]

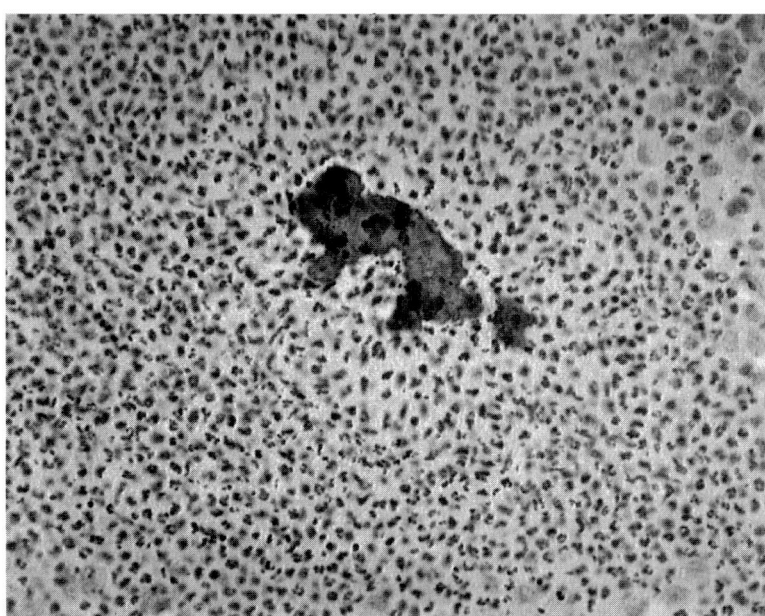

FIGURE 4–15. Bacterial pseudomycetoma. Same sample under Brown-Brenn stain. The clusters of cocci are visible.

TUBERCULOSIS: *M. TUBERCULOSIS* AND *M. BOVIS*

The incidence of "true" tuberculosis in dogs and cats decreased with the decrease of the disease in humans and cattle but may be becoming more prevalent owing to an increasing frequency in humans.[260] It is a rare disease in most parts of the world unless pets experience a high degree of exposure.[2, 50, 59, 82, 151a, 170] Animals that live where there are large numbers of people (restaurants or public places), have close contact with an infected owner (e.g., sleeping in the sick person's room), or are fed a variety of unprocessed meat or milk from areas of endemic disease have an increased chance of infection. Although both dogs and cats are susceptible to both *M. tuberculosis* and *M. bovis*, there appears to be a higher incidence of *M. bovis* infection in cats.[82] The predominant lesions in small animals are respiratory and digestive, but there can be some skin lesions. In cats, clinical signs may be insidious, and because diagnostic tests are unreliable, epidemiologic data are of questionable validity.[248, 260]

Clinical Features

Cutaneous lesions are single or multiple ulcers, abscesses, plaques, and nodules. Nodules may be in the skin or adherent to subcutaneous tissues. They fail to come to a head and may discharge a thick, yellow to green pus with an unpleasant odor. The lesions are most common on the head, the neck, and the limbs. Patients usually appear sick; they have anorexia, weight loss, fever, and lymphadenopathy.[2, 50, 59, 82]

Diagnosis

Diagnosis is by history, physical examination, radiography, biopsy, culture, bacille Calmette-Guérin (BCG) or purified protein derivative (PPD) test (in dogs),[2] serologic testing, or lymphocyte blastogenesis test (in cats).[156] Biopsy specimens may show a nodular-to-diffuse dermatitis due to pyogranulomatous inflammation (with necrosis and caseation), rare multinucleate histiocytic giant cells and mineralization, and few to many acid-fast organisms. Smears or biopsy do not differentiate between true tuberculosis and opportunistic mycobacterial granulomas. Injection of cultures into guinea pigs causes death in 6 to 8 weeks, but not if the organism is nontuberculous.

BCG or PPD (250 tuberculin units/0.1 ml) prepared for humans can be used to test dogs for tuberculosis. Intradermal injection (0.1 ml of PPD or 0.1 to 0.2 ml of BCG) is best performed on the inner surface of the pinna and is read at 48 to 72 hours (no sooner). Erythema that resorbs by that time is a negative test result. Severe erythema with central necrosis progressing to ulceration at 10 to 14 days is significant. Ulceration after 18 to 21 days may occur in normal dogs. This testing is unreliable in the cat.

TUBERCULOSIS: UNNAMED VARIANT

Multiple cases of tuberculosis caused by an organism with cultural characteristics between *M. tuberculosis* and *M. bovis* have been reported in the cat.[31, 116]

Clinical Features

Affected cats typically experience nonhealing, nodular skin lesions on the face, chest wall, legs, base of tail, or perineum.[116] Historically, many involved cats are hunters and the distribution of the lesions supports wounding as the route of inoculation. The nodules may or may not ulcerate, and the regional lymph nodes enlarge. Involvement of lungs and visceral lymph nodes is reported.[31, 116] Systemic signs of illness occur with generalized disease.

Diagnosis

Differentiation of this disorder from true tuberculosis or the other mycobacterial disorders to be discussed requires culture or polymerase chain reaction (PCR) analysis.[138]

TUBERCULOSIS: M. AVIUM

M. avium is a slow-growing environmental saprophyte. Dogs and cats were thought to be relatively resistant to infection,[50, 148, 263] but more and more cases are being reported.[93, 149, 166, 262] Clustering of cases within breeds (Basset hounds,[50] Siamese cats[148]) and within an individual family of miniature Schnauzers[93] suggests a genetic predisposition with immunologic manifestations.

Clinical Features

Affected animals may present for signs of respiratory and/or gastrointestinal disease, generalized lymphadenopathy, or nodular skin disease with regional lymphadenopathy.

Diagnosis

Because the organisms tend to be numerous, they may be visible in aspirates of masses, in white blood cells in the peripheral blood and bone marrow, and in various tissues.[166, 263] In specimens stained with Wright's stain, the organism is rod-shaped, refractile, and nonstaining. Acid-fast stains are needed to highlight the organism. Differentiation of this organism from other mycobacterial species requires culture or PCR.

Clinical Management of Tuberculosis

Dogs and cats with true tuberculosis can be a point source of infection for humans and other animals and should be destroyed. The public health significance of the unnamed variant is unknown. Because *M. avium* is abundant in the environment, treatment of infected animals is reasonable provided that all contact individuals are immunologically normal and excellent hygiene is practiced.

Most details on the treatment of *M. avium* tuberculosis are found for the cat.[116, 117] For maximum efficacy, the intercurrent use of two, preferably three, drugs is suggested for a minimum of 6 to 9 months. Classic drug combinations involve the use of rifampicin (10–20 mg/kg q12–24h), isoniazid (10–20 mg/kg q24h), and ethambutol (15 mg/kg q24h). Other potentially useful drugs include clarithromycin (5–10 mg/kg q12h), clofazimine (2–8.5 mg/kg q24h), doxycycline (10 mg/kg q12h), enrofloxacin (25 mg/kg q24h, provided *M. avium* is not being treated), and dapsone (2 mg/kg q24h). Again, two or three of these alternative drugs should be used simultaneously.

The course of treatment is long and should be continued long after all clinical signs of disease are resolved.

FELINE LEPROSY

Feline leprosy is a granulomatous, nodular, cutaneous infection with an acid-fast organism that is impossible to culture.

Cause and Pathogenesis

Since its recognition, feline leprosy has been known to be caused by a mycobacterium, but specific identification of the causative organism was delayed because of cultural difficulties. Transmission studies with fresh tissues from affected cats into rats and mice supported the role of *M. lepraemurium* as the etiologic agent.[2, 243] In 1997, PCR gene sequencing identified *M. lepraemurium* as the causative agent in four of eight cats with presumptive leprosy.[138] In one of the four remaining cases, co-infection with *M. avium* and *M. chitae* was documented. Two other cats were infected with a species that most closely resembles *M. malmoense*. If these data are substantiated in other studies, more details on such factors as the mode of transmission can be ascertained.

The disease has been reported in New Zealand, Australia, Great Britain, France, Italy, the Netherlands, the United States, and Canada. Typically, clinical disease has a long incubation period with recognition of disease during winter after exposure during summer.[184] Live *M. leprae* (leprosy bacillus of humans) has been found in mosquitos, fleas, and ticks, and these vectors may be important in the feline disease.

Clinical Features

Lesions are single or multiple cutaneous nodules, which may or may not be ulcerated. Lesions are most common on the head or extremities. There may be abscesses or fistulae that show no signs of healing (Fig. 4–16A) but do not spread. Lesions also have been found on the nasal, buccal, and lingual mucosae. Regional lymphadenopathy is common, although without local pain or systemic illness. There is no sex prevalence, but two thirds of cases occur in cats 1 to 3 years of age.

Diagnosis

Diagnosis is confirmed on the basis of history, physical examination results, and the finding of acid-fast bacilli in direct smears and biopsy specimens (Ziehl-Neelsen stain or Fite-Faraco modification). Tissue homogenates should be cultured on the surface of 1% Ogawa egg yolk medium[2] and also inoculated into guinea pigs to eliminate the diagnosis of tuberculosis. Specific identification requires PCR sequencing from tissue specimens.

Histopathologic examination may reveal two types of reactions. One is the tuberculoid response with caseous necrosis and relatively few organisms, and the organisms are often only in the areas of necrosis. These epithelioid granulomas are usually surrounded by zones of lymphocytes, which are also commonly aggregated around vessels (Fig. 4–17). The second type of reaction (lepromatous leprosy) is a granuloma composed of solid sheets of large foamy macrophages containing significant numbers of acid-fast bacilli. The organisms are clustered in globi in a parallel stacking arrangement. Multinucleate histiocytic giant cells often contain bacilli, and lymphocytes and plasma cells may surround vessels (Fig. 4–18). Many polymorphonuclear leukocytes may be present and may cause the lesion to resemble a pyogranuloma.

Differential diagnostic considerations include tuberculosis; granulomas due to opportunistic mycobacteria or foreign bodies; mycotic infections such as kerion, mycetoma, and phaeohyphomycosis; chronic bacterial infection; and neoplasms such as mast cell tumors, carcinomas, and lymphoreticular tumors.

Clinical Management

Although lesions may resolve spontaneously,[232] surgical excision is the treatment of choice when there are solitary or circumscribed lesions. When surgery fails or is impractical, chemotherapy with dapsone, rifampin, or clofazimine may or may not be successful (see discussion of opportunistic mycobacteria).

CANINE LEPROSY

In the 1970s, a nodular skin disease of dogs from Zimbabwe was reported that had many similarities to feline leprosy. Affected animals usually had lesions on their head or extremities and were healthy beyond their skin; they had easily visible mycobacterium in biopsy samples, but cultural and transmission work failed to identify the organism; and surgical treatment was curative. A study published in 1998 on 45 dogs from Australia sheds more light on the disorder.[185]

Cause and Pathogenesis

Although mycobacteria are easily visible in tissue samples, cultures are always negative. Because the true tuberculoid and opportunistic mycobacteria are easily cultured whereas those of feline leprosy are not, one or more unusual species of mycobacteria are probably causal. PCR gene sequencing is needed to identify the organism.

The data from the Australian study have many similarities to data concerning the feline disorder. The majority (84%) of affected dogs have lesions on their head and/or pinna, 93% of dogs have a short coat, and the majority of dogs experience their lesions in fall or winter. These data suggest that the organism is transmitted by biting flies.

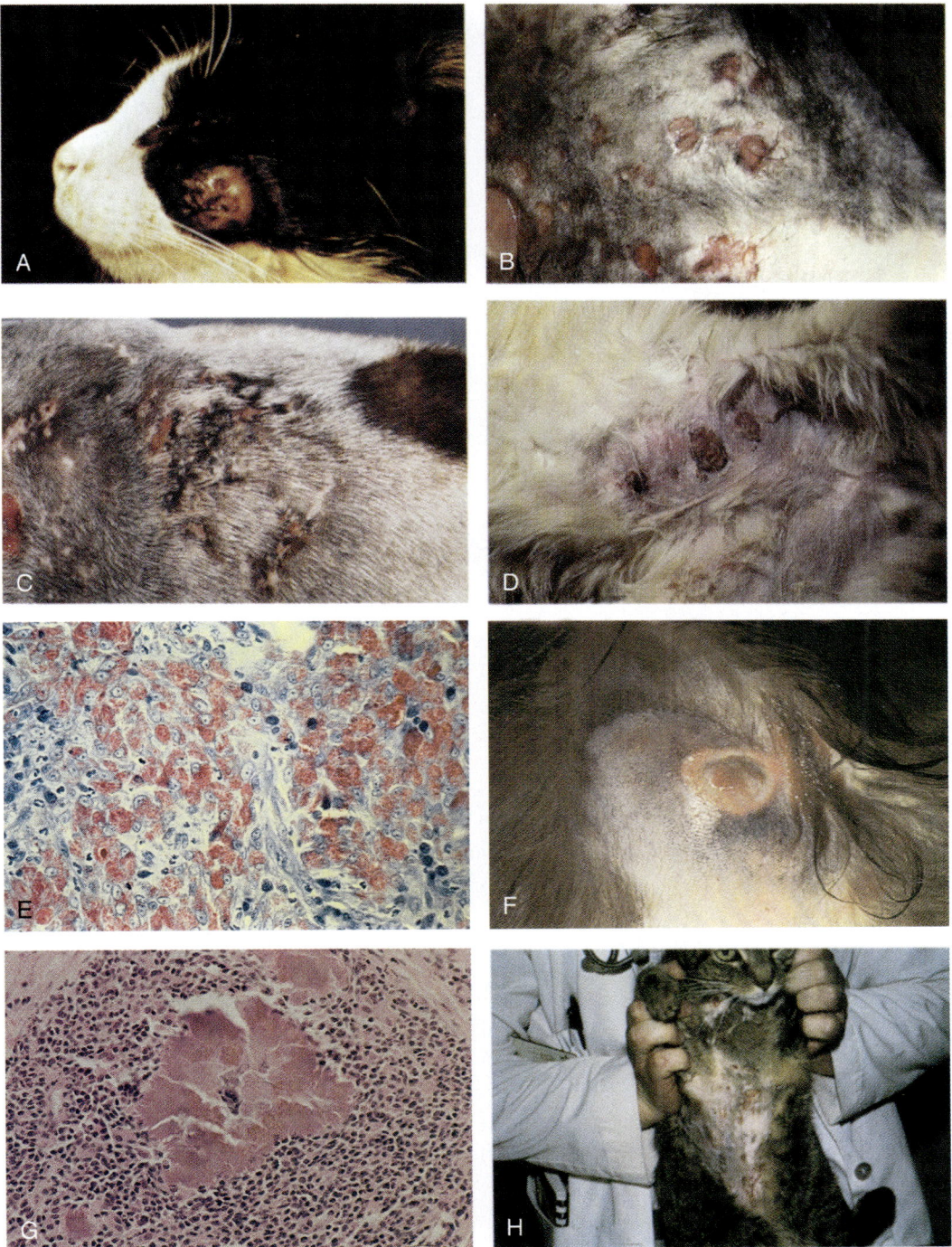

FIGURE 4–16. *A*, Ulcerated lesion of feline leprosy on the face of a cat. (Courtesy of G.T. Wilkinson.) *B*, Multiple necrotic granulomatous lesions on the body of a cat associated with *M. fortuitum* infection. *C*, Soft tissue infection with draining fistulae on the thorax of a dog with atypical mycobacterial granulomas due to *M. chelonei*. (Courtesy G.A. Kunkle.) *D*, Atypical mycobacteriosis (with panniculitis) on the abdomen of a cat. *E*, Feline atypical mycobacteriosis. Note numerous acid-fast organisms within dermal macrophages (Fite-Faraco stain). *F*, Nonhealing ulcer with suppurative discharge over the shoulder of a dog with actinomycosis. *G*, Actinomycosis. Eosinophilic (Hoeppli-Splendore phenomenon) tissue grain (sulfur granule) in pyogranulomatous dermatitis. *H*, Cutaneous nocardiosis (with panniculitis) in a cat.

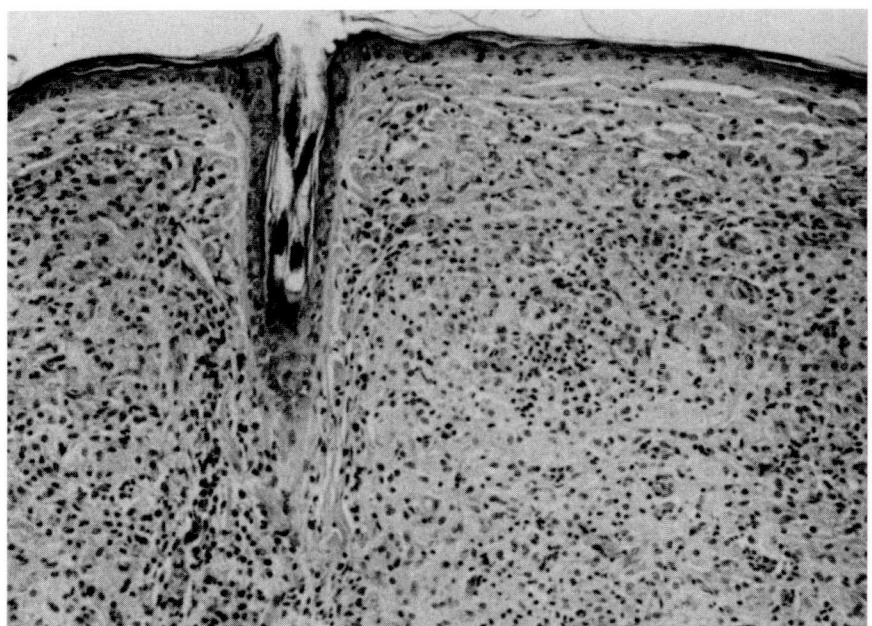

FIGURE 4–17. Granulomatous inflammation of dermis in a cat. Epidermis intact (H & E stain). (From Schiefer B, et al: A disease resembling feline leprosy in western Canada. J Am Vet Med Assoc 165:1085, 1974.)

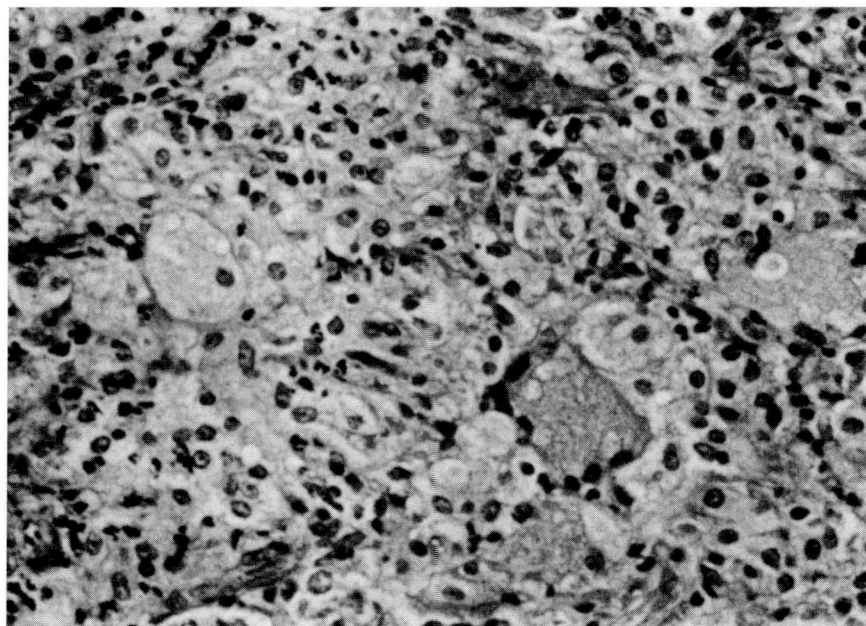

FIGURE 4–18. Histiocytes with foamy cytoplasm and giant cells (H & E stain). (From Schiefer B, et al: A disease resembling feline leprosy in western Canada. J Am Vet Med Assoc 165:1085, 1974.)

Clinical Features

Affected dogs usually are short-coated and have one or more asymptomatic nodules on their head, especially on the pinna, varying in size from several millimeters to 5 cm in diameter. Large lesions may ulcerate. Regional lymph nodes are not enlarged, and there are no systemic signs of illness.

Diagnosis

Diagnosis is confirmed on the basis of history, physical examination results, and the finding of acid-fast bacilli in direct smears and biopsy specimens. Histopathologic findings include pyogranulomatous dermatitis and panniculitis with variable numbers of multinucleated histiocytic giant cells and very few to numerous bacteria.[54b] Differential diagnosis includes the sterile pyogranuloma syndrome, granulomas due to foreign bodies or other infectious agents, and neoplasms such as mast cell tumors, histiocytic tumors, or lymphoma.

Clinical Management

Surgical excision of individual lesions is curative. Beyond surgery, treatment recommendations are difficult to make because spontaneous resolution of lesions is reported. In the Australian study, six dogs underwent self-cure whereas 13 were reported cured with either doxycycline (n = 8) or amoxicillin clavulanate (n = 5). Some of the cures attributed to the drugs may have been spontaneous remissions.

If insect vectors are important, some dogs can be expected to experience new lesions.

OPPORTUNISTIC MYCOBACTERIAL GRANULOMAS

Opportunistic mycobacterial granulomas (atypical mycobacterial granulomas) in dogs and cats can be caused by several atypical mycobacteria that are facultative pathogens. The disease is characterized by chronicity, resistance to antibiotics and antituberculosis drugs, and possible spontaneous resolution.

Cause and Pathogenesis

Organisms reported to cause cutaneous granulomas in dogs and cats include *Mycobacterium fortuitum, M. chelonei, M. phlei, M. xenopi, M. thermoresistible,* and *M. smegmatis*.* Because *M. fortuitum* and *M. chelonei* share several metabolic characteristics and are facultative pathogens that produce similar clinical signs, they may be called the *M. fortuitum-chelonei* complex. The disease has been reported most commonly in cats (perhaps because infection may be introduced through cat bite wounds), but cases in dogs have been recorded.[2, 106, 110, 111, 162, 267]

These mycobacteria are ubiquitous, free-living organisms that are usually harmless and are commonly found in nature. They are found in the soil, but they especially favor water tanks, swimming pools, and sources of natural water.[180] After injury or injection, animals can experience chronic subcutaneous abscesses and fistulae due to these organisms. The history of cases of these granulomas in humans commonly cites instances of the disease after a contaminated injection or an infected wound.

Clinical Features

After contaminated injection, infection of a wound, or other trauma, the lesion develops slowly during a period of weeks. The course is prolonged, and lesions often have been present as nonhealing wounds for several months. Chronic soft tissue abscessation occurs, with ulcers and draining fistulae (see Fig. 4–16B and C).

Lesions can occur anywhere but are most common in the cat in the caudal abdominal or inguinal region[168] (see Fig. 4–16D) or in the lumbar region. The lesions may or may not be painful, and regional lymph nodes are not always enlarged. With solitary lesions, systemic illness, such as fever and anorexia, is rarely observed, and the animal feels well.

---
*See references 2, 88, 111, 151a, 162, 186, 191, 205, 264, 267, 270, 277, 284.

If the animal is immunosuppressed,[106, 110, 137a, 205, 267] widespread skin lesions can develop or the animal may experience sepsis with its accompanying signs of illness.[105a]

One cat with a co-infection with an atypical mycobacterium and a *Nocardia* spp. had a significant hypercalcemia associated with the granulomatous tissue reaction.[196a] Although apparently rare, this case demonstrates that animals with granulomatous disorders should have a complete and thorough evaluation.

Diagnosis

Diagnosis is confirmed by finding acid-fast organisms in smears, cultures, or biopsy specimens (see Fig. 4–9*E*). The organism is often difficult to demonstrate. Smears made from fine-needle aspirates of closed lesions are more likely to contain detectable organisms than are those made from exudates or tissue samples.[264] Cultures usually grow rapidly, but may take weeks, and should be made on blood agar, Löwenstein-Jensen medium, or Stonebrink's medium at 37°C (98.6°F).[2, 151a] Because cultures and biochemical tests for positive identification may be complex, the laboratory handling the cultures should be informed that a mycobacterial infection is suspected.

Histopathologic examination may be helpful. There is nodular to diffuse dermatitis, panniculitis, or both due to pyogranulomatous inflammation. Stains such as Ziehl-Neelsen or Fite-Faraco modification should be used, and a careful search may be needed to find organisms (see Fig. 4–16*E*). They are often clumped in the center of a clear vacuole and surrounded by clusters of neutrophils within the mature granuloma[168] (Fig. 4–19). Alcohol processing in paraffin embedding may cause the acid-fast organism to stain poorly.[277] Using rapid Ziehl-Neelsen stain or snap-freezing the formalin-fixed tissues with subsequent acid-fast stain enables the bacilli to be seen.

Clinical Management

The prognosis in opportunistic mycobacterial infection is always guarded, especially when the lesions are large or multiple. Although spontaneous resolution of lesions can occur after months to years of disease, most cases need treatment. In early cases wherein the lesion is small, wide surgical excision with removal of all subjacent fat may be curative. With large lesions, multiple lesions, or a relapse after surgery, surgery alone is not likely to resolve the infection and an appropriate chemotherapeutic agent should be used long-term after surgery.

Opportunistic mycobacteria do not respond to antitubercular drugs, and susceptibility to conventional antibiotics varies among and within the various species of organisms.[2]

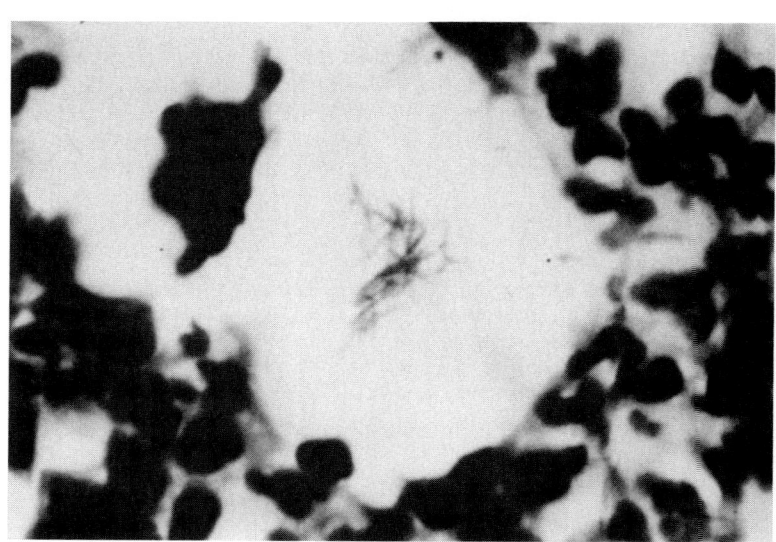

FIGURE 4–19. Atypical mycobacteriosus. Acid-fast organisms in the center of a clear vacuole in pyogranulomatous panniculitis. (Courtesy T.L. Gross.)

Drug selection for each case should be based on cultural data. In the absence of individual susceptibility data, a response to tetracyclines, clarithromycin, or enrofloxacin may occur.[2, 191, 196a, 264] The most successful antibiotics in cats appear to be doxycycline (5 mg/kg q12h) or enrofloxacin (5 to 20 mg/kg q24h).[151a] Clofazimine (2 to 8.5 mg/kg q24h PO) can be effective. Side effects to this drug are infrequent, include orange-red discoloration of the skin, corneal pigmentation, gastrointestinal distress, pruritus, seborrhea sicca, and are dose-related.[117, 151a, 191, 201, 208]

To be successful, the chemotherapeutic agent is needed for months. The drug should be administered until all clinical signs of disease are visually and palpably gone and then for an additional 4 to 6 weeks.

Actinomycosis

Actinomycosis is a rare pyogranulomatous or suppurative disease of many species caused by *Actinomyces* organisms. *A. odontolyticus*, *A. viscosus*, *A. meyeri*, and *A. hordeovulneris* have been suggested as causes.[2, 15, 36, 89, 151a] They are gram-positive, non–acid-fast, catalase-positive, filamentous anaerobic rods that are opportunistic, commensal inhabitants of the oral cavity and the bowel.[2, 37, 153, 248] Infection occurs from trauma and contamination of penetrating wounds, especially those involving foreign bodies such as awns and quills.[89, 119, 153, 291] Hunting or field dogs in southern climates are most commonly affected. It takes from months to 2 years for signs to develop after the injury; however, organisms can be found in the exudate within 2 weeks. The typical clinical lesion is a subcutaneous swelling or abscess of the head or neck, thoracic, paralumbar, or abdominal region (see Fig. 4–16*F*). The lesion is usually tender and may or may not have draining tracts. Paralumbar lesions are usually a direct extension from retroperitoneal involvement. Other forms include osteomyelitis and empyema. Draining tracts (mycetoma-like) may discharge a thick, yellowish-gray or thin, hemorrhagic, foul-smelling exudate that may or may not contain yellow sulfur granules.

Diagnosis is by anaerobic culture (may require 2 to 4 weeks), direct smears of fine-needle aspirates, and biopsy using special stains (Gram's, Brown-Brenn, or Gomori's methenamine silver). No method is completely reliable, and cytologic study appears to be most effective.[153] Histopathologic examination reveals nodular to diffuse dermatitis, panniculitis, or both due to suppurative or pyogranulomatous inflammation (Fig. 4–20). Tissue grains (sulfur granules) are present in approximately 50% of cases. The granules are basophilic and often have a clubbed, eosinophilic periphery (Hoeppli-Splendore material) (see Fig. 4–16*G*). The gram-positive, non–acid-fast, filamentous, occasionally beaded organisms (Fig. 4–21) are found within the granules, but they are not easily visible in ordinary H & E preparations. Actinomycosis must be differentiated from nocardiosis, a disease that it closely resembles.

The most successful treatment involves surgical excision or debulkment with a long course of antibiotics. High-dose penicillins (e.g., penicillin, amoxicillin, oxacillin) are the optimal empirical treatment of choice.[2, 151a] Other drugs that may or may not be effective include clindamycin, erythromycin, cephalosporins, chloramphenicol, and tetracycline.[151a, 275] The treatment must continue for at least 1 month after complete remission and usually lasts 3 to 4 months. Prognosis is guarded, with relapses reported to vary from 15% to 42%.[153]

Actinobacillosis

Actinobacillosis is a rare disease of several animal species caused by *Actinobacillus lignieresii*.[2] It resembles actinomycosis in many of its cutaneous manifestations, but the causative organism is a gram-negative, aerobic coccobacillus that does not survive for a long time outside the host animal. It is a commensal organism found in the mouth of many animals, and clinical lesions often follow bite wounds or injuries around the face and mouth. Infection develops during weeks to months, and its course is long.

Clinical features include single or multiple thick-walled abscesses of the head, neck,

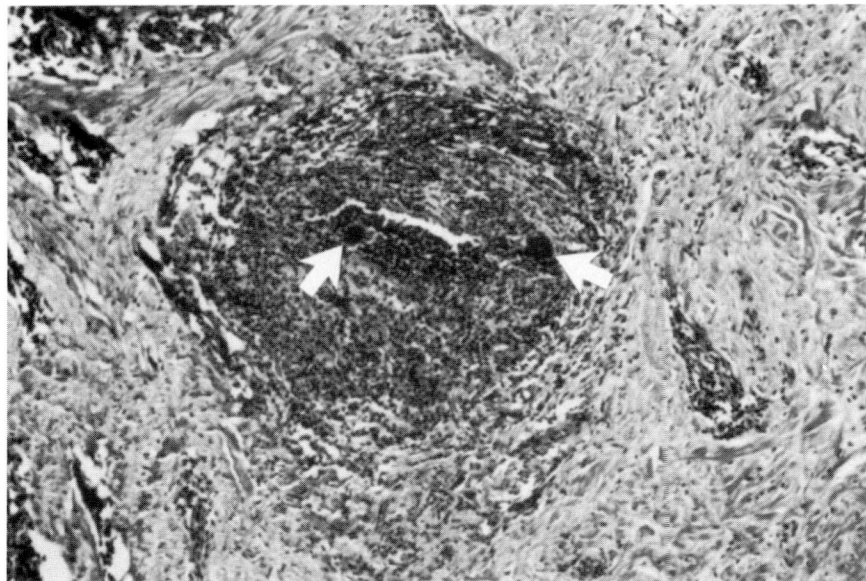

FIGURE 4–20. Actinomycosis in a dog. Note focal pyogranuloma with two tissue grains (*arrows*).

mouth, and limbs.[45] They discharge a thick, white to green, odorless pus with soft yellow granules. Diagnosis is based on aerobic cultures of pus, direct smears, or biopsy of affected tissues.

Histopathologic examination reveals a nodular to diffuse dermatitis, panniculitis, or both due to suppurative or pyogranulomatous inflammation. Tissue grains (sulfur granules) are usually present. The grains are basophilic and usually surrounded by eosinophilic Hoeppli-Splendore material. Special stains (Gram's or Brown-Brenn) are required to demonstrate the gram-negative organisms.

Clinical management includes surgical extirpation or drainage and curettage. Sodium iodide (20 mg/kg or 0.2 ml/kg of 20% solution, orally q12h) and high doses of streptomycin or sulfonamides have been suggested for therapy. The organism is also usually sensi-

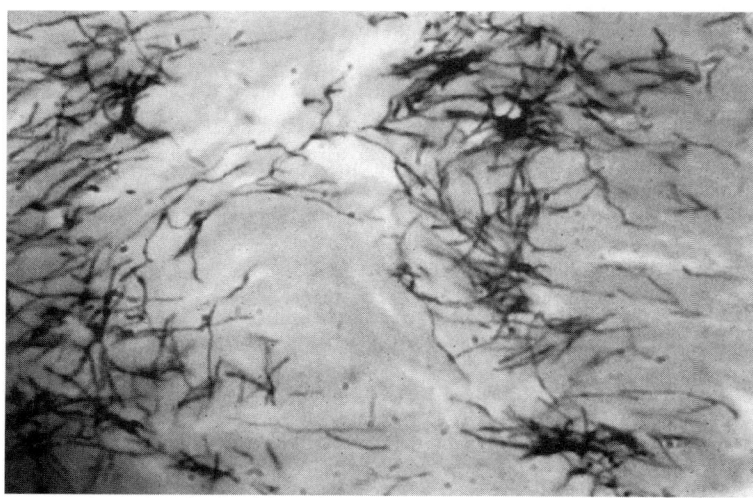

FIGURE 4–21. Actinomycosis. Gram-positive, non–acid-fast, filamentous organisms.

tive to tetracycline and chloramphenicol. The course is long, and the prognosis is guarded.[45]

Nocardiosis

Nocardiosis is a rare disease characterized by pyogranulomatous and suppurative infection of the skin or the lungs or by widespread dissemination. It is caused by *Nocardia* spp.[2, 97, 151a, 153, 190] The organisms involved, including *N. asteroides, N. brasiliensis,* and *N. caviae,* are common soil saprophytes that produce infection by wound contamination, inhalation, and ingestion, particularly in immunocompromised animals. Nocardia are gram-positive, partially acid-fast, branching filamentous aerobes. Except for *N. brasiliensis,* their geographic distribution is worldwide.

Nocardia nova was isolated in pure culture from cats with cutaneous swelling and draining tracts.[133a] *N. nova, N. asteroides,* and *N. farcinica* previously formed the *N. asteroides* complex. The distinguishing characteristics that separate these three species are the types of cell wall mycolic acids and the antimicrobial susceptibility patterns. The authors speculated that *N. nova* may be the main species affecting cats.

Clinical features are indistinguishable from those seen in actinomycosis and include cellulitis, ulcerated nodules, and abscesses that often develop draining sinuses (see Fig. 4–16H). Lesions typically occur in areas of wounding, especially on the limbs and feet, and are often accompanied by lymphadenopathy. Cats often have lesions on the ventral abdomen that resemble panniculitis or opportunistic mycobacterial infection. Pyothorax may be present along with other systemic signs, such as weakness, anorexia, fever, depression, and dyspnea, and neurologic signs may be present.[2, 71, 153, 190] Hypercalcemia may be present and influence the animal's renal function.[196a]

Diagnosis is by direct smear of fine-needle aspirates, aerobic culture, and biopsy. Histopathologic study reveals nodular to diffuse dermatitis, panniculitis, or both, with or without tissue grains (Fig. 4–22). Special stains (Gram's and Brown-Brenn) are needed to demonstrate organisms. Nocardia spp. can be distinguished from *Actinomyces* spp. because they are partially acid-fast (with modified Fite-Faraco stain) and usually branch at right angles (Fig. 4–23). When branched and beaded, the organisms appear similar to Chinese characters.

Clinical management includes surgical drainage of infected tissues, but antibacterial therapy is mandatory. Nocardial organisms show varying susceptibility to antibiotics, and the correlation between in vivo and in vitro results varies.[2, 151a, 153] For instance, *N. nova* is

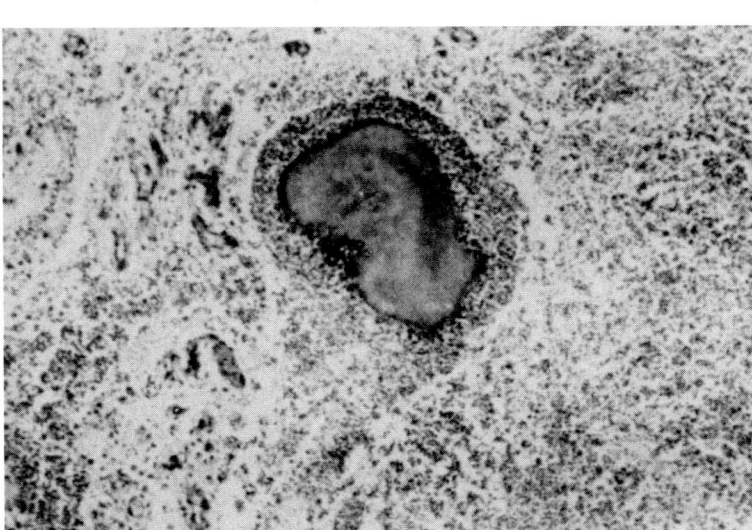

FIGURE 4–22. Nocardiosis. Tissue grain in pyogranulomatous dermatitis.

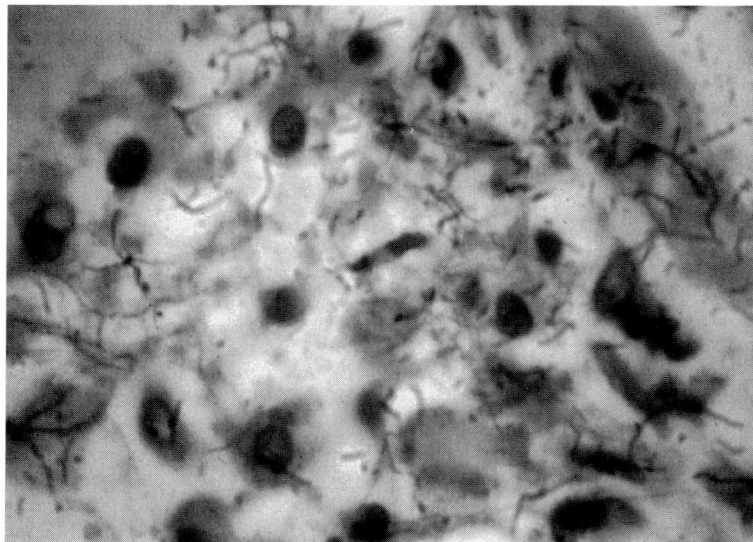

FIGURE 4–23. Nocardiosis. Partially acid-fast, filamentous organisms that tend to branch at right angles.

susceptible to the macrolides, and often to the penicillins, while *N. asteroides* is resistant to the macrolides and, often, to the penicillins.[133a] *N. nova* isolates are usually susceptible to ampicillin, but not amoxicillin clavulanate. If at all possible, susceptibility data should be developed for each case. If the organism cannot be isolated, drugs that can be effective empirically include potentiated sulfonamide drugs, enrofloxacin, amoxicillin clavulanate, ampicillin alone or in combination with erythromycin, clarithromycin, cephalosporins, chloramphenicol, tetracyclines, and various parenteral drugs.[151a] Treatment must be continued for at least 1 month after clinical remission. Prognosis is guarded.

• MISCELLANEOUS BACTERIAL INFECTIONS

Streptococcal and Staphylococcal Necrotizing Fasciitis

A streptococcal toxic shock syndrome with a rapidly progressive course has been described in seven dogs.[202] Group C streptococci, especially *S. canis*, are responsible for the disorder.[87a] Infected dogs experience rapid development of sepsis and shock or sepsis and necrotizing fasciitis. With the necrotizing fasciitis, the wound is disproportionately painful, with significant local heat and swelling. As the infected exudate travels along fascial planes, the fascia, fat, and overlying skin become necrotic.

It is unclear why the streptococci in these cases became so toxic to their host dogs. If a subset of the streptococcal population is developing virulence, additional cases will be recognized. Recent work suggests that the emergence of these syndromes is not the result of clinical expansion of one or more highly virulent strains of *S. canis*.[87a] Most strains of *S. canis* from dogs with these syndromes are positive for M protein and streptolysin O, which are probably virulence factors.[87b] The toxic shock syndrome should be suspected when a dog has a rapidly progressive, intensely painful wound with deep necrosis. After diagnostic samples are taken, treatment with a macrolide or β-lactam antibiotic should be initiated until the culture results are available. Histopathologic findings include severe necrosis and suppuration and extensive edema and hemorrhage of the dermis and subcutis. Thrombosed blood vessels, with or without vasculitis, and colonies of cocci within the necrotic exudate are visible. The area of fasciitis requires débridement. With aggressive treatment, the disorder may not be fatal.

Cellulitis and toxic shock was recently reported in a dog in association with *Staphylo-*

coccus intermedius infection.[108a] This is not surprising, given the ability of some strains of *S. intermedius* to produce one or more exotoxins similar to those that produce toxic shock in humans.[134a]

Brucellosis

Brucellosis is a systemic bacterial infection caused by *Brucella canis*.[2] Despite widespread dissemination in the body, systemic signs of illness are rare, as are skin lesions. Brucellosis may produce a secondary scrotal dermatitis (see Fig. 8–11D) resulting from the animal's licking the skin over painful epididymitis and orchitis.[244] Some cases may involve necrosis of the testis, with severe inflammation of the entire scrotum, and draining ulcers. *B. canis* has been isolated from the exudate.[244]

B. canis has also been isolated from a 15-month-old female laboratory Beagle with chronic exudative lesions that resembled acral lick dermatitis.[72] During a period of 16 months, expanding painful lesions developed on both hocks and the dorsum of the right carpus. The lesions were hyperemic, edematous, and granulomatous, with an irregularly pitted surface. A sanguinopurulent exudate was present, and the regional lymph nodes were enlarged. Histologic examination revealed dermal, subcutaneous, and tendinous edema; pronounced lymphoid nodules; a prominent infiltration of macrophages, plasma cells, and lymphocytes; and scattered neutrophils. The enlarged lymph nodes were characterized by sinusoid histiocytosis and medullary cord plasmacytosis. These findings are typical of the tissue response to *Brucella* infection.[72] Diagnosis is supported by serologic examination findings and confirmed by culture.[18]

Treatment of canine brucellosis should not be undertaken lightly because the infection can spread to humans and is not easily eradicated in the dog.[2] Affected dogs should be removed from breeding programs and neutered if possible. Although the organism shows in vitro sensitivity to tetracyclines, chloramphenicol, aminoglycosides, spectinomycin, rifampin, ampicillin, sulfonamides, and the quinolones, relapses are common when a specific drug is used individually for a single course of treatment. The highest rate of success involves the use of multiple drugs. Synergism between the tetracyclines and fluoroquinolones and the aminoglycosides and sulfonamides has been demonstrated.

Plague

Plague is an acute, febrile, infectious disease that has a high mortality rate and is caused by the gram-negative organism *Yersinia pestis*, a bipolar coccobacillus of the family Enterobacteriaceae.[2] It is a facultative anaerobic, nonmotile, non–spore-forming organism that cannot penetrate unbroken skin but can invade mucous membranes. Plague occurs in three forms: bubonic, pneumonic, and septicemic.[93, 96] The most common is bubonic plague, in which localized abscesses form near the site of infection (especially the head and neck). The septicemic and pneumonic forms are more serious because they may be undiagnosed until it is too late for effective treatment.

The incubation period is 1 to 3 days if the organism is ingested or inhaled, 2 to 6 days if the organisms enter through a flea bite, a skin wound, or a mucous membrane. The course is fulminating and can lead to death. Plague exists in every continent except Australia.[2] There have been outbreaks in all states of the United States west of the Rocky Mountains, including Hawaii. Rodents and cats are highly susceptible, dogs are less susceptible, and other domestic animals are resistant. It primarily affects rodents, especially prairie dogs, rock and ground squirrels, and rats.[2, 93]

Plague typically is transmitted by fleas or by ingestion of infected animals. *Diamanus montanus* and four less common rodent-hosted fleas are the primary vectors. The common dog and cat fleas are not normally involved.[238]

An epizootic plague can develop if susceptible rodents come in contact with the *Yersinia* organisms, causing a massive die-off in the rodent colony. The sick rodents become easy prey for cats, dogs, or other carnivores, and the fleas seek new hosts. Cats can spread the infection to humans by transmitting infected fleas mechanically, by bringing dead or affected rodents home (thus facilitating human contact with the rodent or its fleas), or by causing direct infection. The latter occurs by bites, contact with pus, or inhalation of droplets from a sneezing or salivating cat. Plague can be a most serious public health problem for people exposed to infected material from clinical cases.[235]

Animal health personnel handling supposed cat abscesses in endemic plague areas have contracted the disease. In endemic areas, all animals with abscesses should be handled carefully by personnel using disposable gloves and masks, and all animals with plague should be kept in isolation. Oral administration of medications should be avoided, as well as any unnecessary handling, to reduce exposure. Bedding, contaminated bandages, and animal carcasses should be placed in double plastic bags and should be incinerated.

Rodents and cats are highly susceptible to plague. Cats experience severe systemic signs of high fever, depression, anorexia, and lymphadenopathy with abscess formation and drainage. Mortality rates in untreated cats approach 75%. Approximately 50% of infected cats have the bubonic form and have the systemic signs plus one or more abscesses, typically on the face, the neck, or the limbs. The systemic form is next most common, and the pneumonic form occurs in approximately 10% of cases. Overlap in the three presentations occurs.[2, 93] Dogs are more resistant to infection with less dramatic signs of disease. Anorexia, lethargy, and fever with or without draining skin lesions are common findings.[213]

Diagnosis is made by culture of the exudate, by immunofluorescence of impression smears, or by serologic confirmation based on a fourfold increase in antibody titers, from acute to convalescent.[2, 93] The latter is useful only in epidemiologic investigations. It is important to be cautious about the diagnosis, because *P. multocida* is often cultured from the abscess too. Differential diagnosis should include cat abscesses, wound infections, and other pyogranulomatous diseases.

Treatment should be instituted as soon as possible, even before the results of the diagnostic tests are available. With prompt treatment, survival rates approaching 90% have been reported. Drugs of choice are gentamicin with or without rifampin, chloramphenicol, tetracycline, and the fluoroquinolones. Some clinicians reserve tetracyclines for prophylaxis, whereas other clinicians report success with it in treatment.[2, 93] Local abscesses should be opened and drained carefully and irrigated daily with an antibacterial solution. Flea control is important to prevent further spread

The use of lufenuron-impregnated feed cubes to control fleas on ground squirrels was shown to be an effective, cost-saving (compared with traditional flea control protocols, such as insecticides for burrow dusting and in bait stations), and proactive technique for controlling fleas and reducing the risk of disease transmission in plague endemic areas.[71a]

Lyme Borreliosis

Lyme borreliosis is a complex multisystemic disorder caused by the spirochete *Borrelia burgdorferi*.[2, 11, 12, 34, 61] The organism is transmitted by hard-shelled ticks of the genus *Ixodes*. Other ticks, flies, fleas, and mosquitoes have been found to harbor the organism, but the vector status of these other arthropods and insects is uncertain.

In all species, the predominant sign of Lyme borreliosis is polyarthropathic. In humans, a characteristic expanding ringlike macule or papule (erythema chronicum migrans) develops in 1 to 2 weeks at the site of the tick bite. Although lesions of erythema chronicum migrans have been reported in dogs, no histologic studies were performed to confirm that diagnosis.[11] In experimental dogs, erythema was not observed.[12] No doubt such lesions do occur but are obscured by the haircoat.

Because Lyme borreliosis is a systemic immune complex disorder, skin lesions other than erythema chronicum migrans could occur but are apparently rare. In a report of 110 seropositive dogs, 4 had skin lesions of urticaria, rash, or moist dermatitis.[61] Another investigator reported recurrent, tetracycline-responsive lesions of pyotraumatic dermatitis in seropositive dogs.[289] One of us (W.H.M.) treated a seropositive dog that had small vessel cutaneous vasculitis with tetracycline. The skin lesions resolved with treatment and did not recur, and the dog seroconverted.

The diagnosis of Lyme borreliosis is corroborated by serologic study.[20] Because not all strains of *B. burgdorferi* are arthritogenic and cross-reactivity with other spirochetes can occur, a single positive serologic finding is not diagnostic. A significant rise or fall in antibody titer is more diagnostic.

Tetracyclines and ampicillin are the drugs of choice and are typically administered for 10 to 14 days.[2] Early treatment is essential to prevent irreversible joint changes.

Trichomycosis Axillaris

Trichomycosis axillaris is a bacterial infection of the hair shafts of humans. It involves mainly axillary and pubic hair. A similar infection with *Corynebacterium* spp. has been reported in a Beagle dog.[38] The animal had diffuse, irregular, and patchy alopecia that affected the neck and flank regions. There was no dermatitis. In the involved areas, some hairs were broken off and some hair shafts displayed small, hard nodules. Masses of bacteria ensheathed the hair at those locations. Nodules developed on inoculated hair and eventually involved the whole hair. Inoculation of normal hair from other dogs produced no alopecia and no bacterial growth. This is not a fungal disease, in spite of its name, and no fungal elements were seen or isolated on culturing.

This is an uncommon and inconsequential disorder that should respond readily to clipping of the hair and frequent use of antibacterial shampoos.

Mycoplasma Infections

Mycoplasmas are part of the normal oral flora and, as such, can be introduced into bite wounds.[273] Because bite wounds usually are contaminated with various aerobic and anaerobic bacteria,[73, 74] the role of *Mycoplasma* is obscured. There are several reports of abscesses in cats in which conventional treatments failed.[273] *Mycoplasma* organisms were isolated, and response was complete with appropriate therapy. Treatment for extended periods with macrolides, lincosamides, the tetracycline group, or the fluoroquinolones should be effective.

L-Form Infections

L-forms are partially cell wall–deficient bacteria that resemble *Mycoplasma*.[2, 51, 150, 151a] Retention of some cell wall, variability in size and morphologic characteristics, and the ability to revert to the parental type with *in vitro* passage differentiate L-forms from *Mycoplasma*. L-forms cannot be cultured by routine techniques and may or may not be isolated with special L-form techniques. The organisms can be found by electron microscopy of fresh tissues.

Most reports of L-form infections in dogs or cats describe a polyarthropathic presentation.[51, 150] Some cats have abscesses and are febrile, are depressed, and have one or more draining abscesses, typically over joints. The draining exudate is nonodoriferous and contains numerous nontoxic neutrophils and macrophages. The neutrophils often contain ingested erythrocytes, vacuoles, and granules. Treatment with the antibiotics used to treat routine feline abscesses results in no improvement. Response to the administration of tetracycline is rapid. Macrolides and chloramphenicol are other treatment options. Anecdotal reports indicate that infections can be spread to attending veterinarians, and that gloves should be worn.[151a]

Listeriosis

Listeria monocytogenes is a ubiquitous saprophyte that can cause infection when it is ingested in contaminated foods.[2] Immunocompromised hosts are more susceptible. Infection in companion animals is rare, and signs typically are those of bacteremia and organ abscessation, especially of the nervous system. There is one report of an otherwise healthy dog who experienced cutaneous listeriosis.[179] Infection presumably followed the dog's rolling on a decaying carcass and was characterized by multiple nodules over the back.

55. Chastain CB, et al: Dermatophilosis in two dogs. J Am Vet Med Assoc 169:1079, 1976.
56. Chesney CJ: The microclimate of the canine coat: The effect of heating on coat and skin temperature and relative humidity. Vet Dermatol 8:183, 1997.
57. Christensen GD: Coagulase-negative staphylococci—saprophyte or parasite? Int J Dermatol 22:463, 1983.
58. Chusid MJ, et al: Defective polymorphonuclear leukocyte metabolism and function in canine cyclic neutropenia. Blood 46:921, 1975.
59. Clerex C, et al: Tuberculosis in dogs: A case report and review of the literature. J Am Anim Hosp Assoc 28:207, 1992.
60. Clercx C, et al: Nonresponsive generalized bacterial infection associated with systemic lupus erythematosus in a Beauceron. J Am Anim Hosp Assoc 35, 220, 1999.
61. Cohen ND, et al: Clinical and epizootiologic characteristics of dogs seropositive for *Borrelia burgdorferi* in Texas: 110 cases (1988). J Am Vet Med Assoc 197:893, 1990.
62. Conceicao LG, et al: Identification of bacterial flora and antimicrobial staphylococcal sensitivity from canine pyoderma in Brazil. In: Kwotchka KW, et al (eds): Advances in Veterinary Dermatology III. Butterworth Heinemann, Oxford, 1998, p 546.
63. Cox HU, et al: Antimicrobial susceptibility of coagulase positive staphylococci isolated from Louisiana dogs. Am J Vet Res 44:2039, 1984.
64. Cox HU, Hoskins JD: Distribution of staphylococcal species on clinically healthy cats. Am J Vet Res 46:1824, 1985.
65. Cox HU, et al: Species of *Staphylococcus* isolated from animal infections. Cornell Vet 74:124, 1984.
66. Cox HU, Schmeer N: Protein A in *Staphylococcus intermedius* isolates from dogs and cats. Am J Vet Res 47:1881, 1986.
67. Couto CG, et al: *In vitro* immunologic features of weimaraner dogs with neutrophil abnormalities and recurrent infections. Vet Immunol Immunopathol 23:103, 1989.
68. Couto CG: Patterns of infection associated with immunodeficiency. In: Kirk RW, Bonagura, JD (eds): Kirk's Current Veterinary Therapy XI. W.B. Saunders Co., Philadelphia, 1992, p 223.
69. Crowe DT, Kowalski JJ: Clostridial cellulitis with localized gas formation in a dog. J Am Vet Med Assoc 169:1094, 1976.
70. Curtis C, Lloyd D: Treatment of canine idiopathic recurrent pyoderma. Vet Rec 140:587, 1997.
71. Davenport DJ, Johnson GC: Cutaneous nocardiosis in a cat. J Am Vet Med Assoc 188:728, 1986.
71a. Davis RM: Use of orally administered chitin inhibitor (lufenuron) to control flea vectors of plague on ground squirrels in California. J Med Entomol 30:562, 1999.
72. Dawkins BG, et al: Pyogranulomatous dermatitis associated with Brucella canis infection in a dog. J Am Vet Med Assoc 181:1432, 1982.
73. Davidson EB: Managing bite wounds in dogs and cats: Part I. Comp Cont Ed 20:811, 1998.
74. Davidson EB: Managing bite wounds in dogs and cats: Part II. Comp Cont Ed 20:974, 1998.
74a. Day MJ: Expression of major histocompatibility complex class II molecules by dermal inflammatory cells, epidermal Langerhans' cells and keratinocytes in canine dermatological disease. J Comp Pathol 115:317, 1996.
74b. Day MJ: Possible immunodeficiency in related rottweiler dogs. J Small Anim Pract 40:561, 1999.
75. Day MJ, Penhale WJ: Serum immunoglobulin A concentrations in normal and diseased dogs. Res Vet Sci 45:36, 1988.
76. Day MJ: An immunopathological study of deep pyoderma in the dog. Res Vet Sci 56:18, 1994.
77. Day MI: Inheritance of serum autoantibody, reduced serum IgA, and autoimmune disease in a breeding colony. Vet Immunol Immunopathol 53:207, 1996.
78. DeBoer DJ, et al: Evaluation of commercial staphylococcal bacterin for management of idiopathic recurrent superficial pyoderma in dogs. Am J Vet Res 51:636, 1990.
79. DeBoer DJ, et al: Clinical and immunological responses of dogs with recurrent pyoderma to injection of staphylococcus phage lysate. In: von Tscharner C, Halliwell REW (eds): Advances in Veterinary Dermatology, Vol 1. Bailliáere-Tindall, London, 1990, p 335.
80. DeBoer DJ, Pukay BP: Recurrent pyoderma and immunostimulants. In: Ihrke PJ, Mason IS, White SD (eds): Advances in Veterinary Dermatology, Vol 2. Pergamon Press, Oxford, 1993, p 443.
81. DeBoer DJ: Management of chronic and recurrent pyoderma in the dog. In: Bonagura JD (ed): Kirk's Current Veterinary Therapy XII. W.B. Saunders Co., Philadelphia, 1995, p 611.
81a. Degim IT, et al: In vitro percutaneous absorption of fusidic acid and betamethasone-17-valerate across canine skin. J Small Anim Pract 40:515, 1999.
82. deLisle GW, et al: A report of tuberculosis in cats in New Zealand, and the examination of strains of *Mycobacterium bovis* by DNA restriction endonuclease analysis. N Z Vet J 38:10, 1990.
83. DeManuelle TC, et al: Determination of skin concentration of enrofloxacin in dogs with pyoderma. Am J Vet Res 59:1599, 1998.
84. Denerolle P, et al: German shepherd dog pyoderma: A prospective study of 23 cases. Vet Dermatol 9:243, 1998.
85. Devriese LA: Identification and characterization of staphylococci isolated from cats. Vet Microbiol 9:279, 1984.
86. Devriese LA, DePelsmaecker K: The anal region as a main carrier site of *Staphylococcus intermedius* and *Streptococcus canis* in dogs. Vet Rec 121:302, 1987.
87. Devriese LA, Haesebrouch F: *Streptococcus suis* infection in horses and cats. Vet Rec 130:300, 1992.
87a. DeWinter LM, Prescott JF: Relatedness of *Streptococcus canis* from streptococcal toxic shock syndrome and necrotizing fasciitis. Can J Vet Res 63:90, 1999.
87b. DeWinter LM, et al: Virulence of *Streptococcus canis* from canine streptococcal toxic shock syndrome and necrotizing fasciitis. Vet Microbiol 70:95, 1999.
88. Donnelly TM, et al: Diffuse cutaneous granulomatous lesions associated with acid-fast bacilli in a cat. J Small Anim Pract 23:99, 1982.
89. Donohue DE, Brightman AH: Cervicofacial *Actinomyces viscosus* infection in a Brazilian Fila: A case report and literature review. J Am Anim Hosp Assoc 31:501, 1995.
90. Dow SW, et al: Anaerobic bacterial infections and response to treatment in dogs and cats: 36 cases (1983–1985). J Am Vet Med Assoc 189:930, 1986.
91. Dow SM, Jones RL: Anaerobic infections. Part I: Pathogenesis and clinical significance. Comp Cont Educ 9:711, 1987.
92. Eggers JS, et al: Disseminated *Mycobacterium avium*

infection in three miniature schnauzer litter mates. J Vet Diag Invest 9:424, 1997.
93. Eidson M, et al: Clinical, clinicopathologic, and pathologic features of plague in cats: 119 cases (1979–1988). J Am Vet Med Assoc 199:1191, 1991.
94. Edwards VN, et al: Characterization of the canine type C enterotoxin produced by Staphylococcus intermedius pyoderma isolates. Infect Immun 65:2346, 1997.
95. Elkins AD: Hyperbaric oxygen therapy: Potential veterinary applications. Comp Cont Ed 19:607, 1997.
96. Emerson JK: Plague. Canine Pract 12:43, 1985.
96a. Esterly NB, et al: The effect of antimicrobial agents on leukocyte chemotaxis. J Invest Dermatol 70:51, 1978.
97. Fadok VA: Granulomatous dermatitis in dogs and cats. Semin Vet Med Surg Small Anim 2:186, 1987.
98. Fairley RA, Fairley NM: Rhodococcus equi infection in cats. Vet Dermatol 10:43, 1999.
99. Farca AM, et al: Potentiating effect of EDTA-Tris on the activity of antibiotics against resistant bacteria associated with otitis, dermatitis, and cystitis. J Small Anim Pract 38:243, 1998.
100. Farrow BRH, et al: Pneumocystis pneumonia in the dog. J Comp Pathol 82:447, 1972.
101. Fehrer SL, et al: Identification of protein A from Staphylococcus intermedius isolated from canine skin. Am J Vet Res 49:697, 1988.
102. Feingold DS: Gangrenous and crepitant cellulitis. J Am Acad Dermatol 6:289, 1982.
103. Feingold DS: Bacterial adherence, colonization, and pathogenicity. Arch Dermatol 122:161, 1986.
104. Felsburg PJ, et al: Canine X-linked severe combined immunodeficiency. Vet Immunol Immunopathol 69:127, 1999.
105. Felsburg PJ: Primary immunodeficiencies. In: Kirk RW, Bonagura JD (eds): Kirk's Current Veterinary Therapy XI. W.B. Saunders Co., Philadelphia, 1992, p 448.
105a. Foster SF, et al: Chronic pneumonia caused by Mycobacterium thermoresistible in a cat. J Small Anim Pract 40:433, 1999.
106. Fox LE, et al: Disseminated subcutaneous Mycobacterium fortuitum infection in a dog. J Am Vet Med Assoc 206:53, 1995.
107. Frank LA, Kunkle GA: Comparison of the efficacy of cefadroxil and generic and proprietary cephalexin in the treatment of pyoderma in dogs. J Am Vet Med Assoc 203:530, 1993.
108. Giger U, et al: Deficiency of leukocyte surface glycoproteins mo1, LFA-1 and Leu M5 in a dog with recurrent bacterial infections: An animal model. Blood 69:1622, 1987.
108a. Girard C, Higgins R: Staphylococcus intermedius cellulitis and toxic shock in a dog. Can Vet J 40:501, 1999.
109. Goodacre R, et al: An epidemiologic study of Staphylococcus intermedius strains isolated from dogs, their owners, and veterinary surgeons. J Anal Appl Pyrolysis 44:49, 1997.
109a. Gortel K, et al: Methicillin resistance among staphylococci isolated from dogs. Am J Vet Res 60:1526, 1999.
110. Grooters AM, et al: Systemic Mycobacterium smegmatis infection in a dog. J Am Vet Med Assoc 207:457, 1995.
111. Gross TL, Connelly MR: Nontuberculous mycobacterial skin infections in two dogs. Vet Pathol 20:117, 1983.
112. Guaguère E, Picard G: Utilization de la céfalexine et du lactate d'ethyle dans le traitement des pyodermites canines. Prat Méd Chir Anim Comp 25:547, 1990.
113. Guaguère E: Topical treatment of canine and feline pyoderma. Vet Dermatol 7:145, 1996.
114. Guaguère E, et al: Utilisation de la céfalexine dans le traitement des pyodermites canines: Comparaison de l'efficacité de différentes posoligies. Prat Méd Chir Anim Comp 33:237, 1998.
115. Guaguère E, et al: Cephalexin in the treatment of canine pyoderma: Comparison of two dose rates. In: Kwochka KW, et al (eds): Advances in Veterinary Dermatology III. Butterworth Heinemann, Oxford, 1998, p 547.
116. Gunn-Moore DA, et al: Feline tuberculosis: A literature review and discussion of 19 cases caused by an unusual mycobacterial variant. Vet Rec 138:53, 1996.
117. Gunn-Moore DA, Shaw S: Mycobacterial disease in the cat. In Pract 17:493, 1997.
117a. Hall JA, et al: Comparison of three commercial radial immunodiffusion kits for the measurement of canine serum immunoglobulins. J Vet Diagn Invest 7:559, 1995.
118. Halliwell REW, Gorman NT: Veterinary Clinical Immunology. W.B. Saunders Co., Philadelphia, 1989, p 253.
119. Hardie EM, Barsanti JA: Treatment of canine actinomycosis. J Am Vet Med Assoc 180:537, 1982.
120. Hart BL, Barrett RE: Effects of castration on fighting, roaming, and urine spraying in adult male cats. J Am Vet Med Assoc 163:290, 1973.
120a. Hartnett BJ, et al: Bone marrow transplantation for canine X-linked severe combined immunodeficiency. Vet Immunol Immunopathol 69:137, 1999.
121. Harvey RG, et al: Distribution of propionibacteria on dogs: A preliminary report of the findings on 11 dogs. J Small Anim Pract 34:80, 1993.
122. Harvey RG, et al: A comparison of lincomycin hydrochloride and clindamycin hydrochloride in the treatment of superficial pyoderma in dogs. Vet Rec 132:351, 1993.
123. Harvey RG, Nobel WC: Aspects of nasal, oropharyngeal and anal carriage of Staphylococcus intermedius in normal dogs and dogs with pyoderma. Vet Dermatol 9:99, 1998.
124. Harvey RG: Aspects of the interaction between the skin and staphylococci. In: Proceedings of the North American Veterinarians Conference, 1998, p 79.
125. Harvey RG, Lloyd DH: The distribution of bacteria (other than staphylococci and Propionibacterium acnes) on the hair, at the skin surface and within the hair follicles of dogs. Vet Dermatol 6:79, 1995.
126. Harvey RG, Noble WC: A temporal study comparing the carriage on Staphylococcus intermedius on normal dogs or atopic dogs in clinical remission. Vet Dermatol 5:21, 1994.
127. Harvey RG: Tylosin in the treatment of canine superficial pyoderma. Vet Rec 139:185, 1996.
128. Harvey RG, et al: Nasal carriage of Staphylococcus intermedius in humans in contact with dogs. Microb Ecol Health Dis 7:225, 1994.
129. Harvey RG, Hunter PA: The properties and use of penicillins in the veterinary field with special reference to skin infections in the dog and cat. Vet Dermatol 10:177, 1999.
130. Hesselbarth J, et al: Characterization of Staphylococ-

131. Hesselbarth J, et al: Studies on the production of an exfoliative toxin by *Staphylococcus intermedius*. J Vet Med B 41:411, 1994.
132. Higgins R, Paradis M: Abscess caused by *Corynebacterium equi* in a cat. Can Vet J 21:63, 1980.
133. Hill PB, Moriello KA: Canine pyoderma. J Am Vet Med Assoc 204:334, 1994.
133a. Hirsh DC, Jang SS: Antimicrobial susceptibility of *Nocardia nova* isolated from five cats with nocardiosis. J Am Vet Med Assoc 215:815, 1999.
134. Hinton M, et al: The antibiotic resistance of pathogenic staphylococci and streptococci isolated from dogs. J Small Anim Pract 19:229, 1978.
134a. Hirooka EY, et al: Enterotoxigenicity of *Staphylococcus intermedius* of canine origin. Int J Food Microbiol 7:185, 1988.
135. Hirsch DC, et al: Changes in prevalence and susceptibility of obligate anaerobes in clinical veterinary practice. J Am Vet Med Assoc 186:1086, 1985.
136. Horwitz L, Ihrke PJ: Canine seborrheas. In: Kirk RW (ed): Current Veterinary Therapy VI. W.B. Saunders Co., Philadelphia, 1977.
137. Hoskuyama S, et al: Isolation of obligate and facultative bacteria from subcutaneous abscesses. J Vet Med Sci 58:273, 1996.
137a. Hughes MS, et al: Disseminated *Mycobacterium genavense* infection in an FIV-positive cat. J Feline Med Surg 1:23, 1999.
138. Hughes MS, et al: Determination of the etiology of presumptive feline leprosy by 16 sRNA gene analysis. J Clin Microbiol 35:2464, 1997.
139. Hunter RP, et al: Pharmacokinetics, oral availability and tissue distribution of azithromycin in cats. J Vet Pharmacol Ther 18:38, 1995.
140. Igimi S, et al: *Staphylococcus felis*, a new species from clinical specimens from cats. Int J Syst Bacteriol 39:373, 1989.
141. Ihrke PJ: Antibacterial therapy in dermatology. In: Kirk RW (ed): Current Veterinary Therapy IX. W.B. Saunders Co., Philadelphia, 1986, p 566.
141a. Ihrke PJ, DeManuelle TC: German Shepherd dog pyoderma: An overview and antimicrobial management. Compend Cont Educ Pract Vet 21 (Suppl): 44, 1999.
142. Ihrke PJ, Gross TL: Canine mucocutaneous pyoderma. In: Bonagura JD (ed): Kirk's Current Veterinary Therapy XII. W.B. Saunders Co., Philadelphia, 1995, p 618.
143. Ihrke PJ, Gross TL: Conference in Dermatology, No. 1. Vet Dermatol 4:33, 1993.
144. Ihrke PJ, et al: The use of fluoroquinolones in veterinary dermatology. Vet Dermatol 10:193, 1999.
145. Jang SS, et al: Organisms isolated from dogs and cats with anaerobic infections and susceptibility to selected antimicrobial agents. J Am Vet Med Assoc 210:1610, 1997.
146. Jezyk PF, et al: Lethal acrodermatitis in bull terriers. J Am Vet Med Assoc 118:833, 1986.
147. Jezyk PF, et al: X-linked severe combined immunodeficiency in the dog. Clin Immunol Immunopathol 52:173, 1989.
148. Jordon HL, et al: Disseminated *Mycobacterium avium* complex infection in three Siamese cats. J Am Vet Med Assoc 204:90, 1994.
149. Kaufman AC, et al: Treatment of isolated *Mycobacterium avium* complex infection with clofazimine and doxycycline in a cat. J Am Vet Med Assoc 207:457, 1995.
150. Keane DP: Chronic abscesses in cats associated with an organism resembling mycoplasma. Can Vet J 24-289, 1983.
151. Keane KA, Taylor DJ: Slime-producing *Staphylococcus* species in canine pyoderma. Vet Rec 130:75, 1992.
151a. Kennis RA, Wolf AM: Chronic bacterial skin infections in cats. Compend Cont Educ Pract Vet 21:1108, 1999.
152. Kietzmann M, et al: Vertraglichkeif and Pharmakoknetik von Cefalexin (cefaseptin dragees) beim Hund. Kleintierpraxis 35:390, 1990.
153. Kirpensteijn J, Fingland RB: Cutaneous actinomycosis and nocardiosis in dogs: 48 cases (1980–1990). J Am Vet Med Assoc 201:917, 1992.
154. Koch HJ, Peters S: Antimicrobial therapy in German shepherd dog pyoderma (GSP): An open clinical study. Vet Dermatol 7:177, 1996.
155. Krakowaka S: Acquired immunodeficiency diseases. In: Kirk RW, Bonagura JD (eds): Kirk's Current Veterinary Therapy XI. W.B. Saunders Co., Philadelphia, 1992, p 453.
156. Kramer TT: Immunity to bacterial infections. Vet Clin North Am Small Anim Pract 8:683, 1978.
157. Krick SA, Scott DW: Bacterial folliculitis, furunculosis, and cellulitis in the German shepherd: A retrospective analysis of 17 cases. J Am Anim Hosp Assoc 25:23, 1989.
158. Kristensen S, Krogh HV: A study of skin diseases in dogs and cats. III: Microflora of the skin of dogs with chronic eczema. Nord Vet Med 30:223, 1978.
159. Kristensen F, Aalbaek B: Sårinfektian med *Rhodococcus equi* hos en kat. Dansk Vet 75:969, 1993.
160. Krogh HF, Kristensen S: A study of skin diseases in dogs and cats. Nord Vet Med 28:459, 1976.
161. Kruse H, et al: The antimicrobial susceptibility of *Staphylococcus* species isolated from canine dermatitis. Vet Res Commun 20:205, 1996.
162. Kunkle GA, et al: Rapidly growing mycobacteria as a cause of cutaneous granulomas: Report of five cases. J Am Anim Hosp Assoc 19:513, 1983.
163. Kunkle GA: New considerations for rational antibiotic therapy of cutaneous staphylococcal infection in the dog. Semin Vet Med Surg Small Anim 2:212, 1987.
164. Kwochka KW, Kowalski JJ: Prophylactic efficacy of four antibacterial shampoos against *Staphylococcus intermedius* in dogs. Am J Vet Res 52:115, 1991.
165. Kwochka KW: Recurrent pyoderma. In: Griffin CE, Kwochka KW, MacDonald JM (eds): Current Veterinary Dermatology. Mosby Year Book, St. Louis, 1993, p 3.
166. Latimer KS, et al: Disseminated *Mycobacterium avium* complex infection in a cat: Presumptive diagnosis by blood smear examination. Vet Clin Pathol 26:85, 1997.
166a. Lanevschi A, et al: Granulocyte colony-stimulating factor deficiency in a Rottweiler with chronic idiopathic neutropenia. J Vet Intern Med 13:72, 1999.
167. Lee AH, et al: Effects of chlorhexidine diacetate, providone iodine, and polyhydroxydine on wound healing in dogs. J Am Anim Hosp Assoc 24:77, 1988.
168. Lewis DT, et al: Experimental reproduction of feline *Mycobacterium fortuitum* panniculitis. Vet Dermatol 5:189, 1994.
169. Littlewood JD, et al: Clindamycin hydrochloride and

170. Liu S, et al: Canine tuberculosis. J Am Vet Med Assoc 177:164, 1980.
171. Lloyd DH, Jenkinson DM: The effect of climate on experimental infection of bovine skin with Dermatophilus congolensis. Br Vet J 136:122, 1980.
172. Lloyd DH: Skin surface immunity. Vet Dermatol News 5:10, 1980.
173. Lloyd DH: The cutaneous defense mechanisms. Vet Dermatol News 1:9, 1976.
174. Lloyd DH, et al: Sensitivity to antibiotics amongst cutaneous and mucosal isolates of canine pathogenic staphylococci in the U.K., 1980–96. Vet Dermatol 7:171, 1996.
175. Lloyd H, Reyss-Brion A: Le peroxide de benzoyle: Efficacité clinique et bacteriologique dans le traitement des pyodermites chroniques. Prat Méd Chir Anim Comp 19:445, 1984.
176. Lloyd DH, et al: Carriage of *Staphylococcus intermedius* on the ventral abdomen of clinically normal dogs and those with pyoderma. Vet Dermatol 2:161, 1991.
177. Lloyd DH, et al: Treatment of canine pyoderma with co-amoxyclav: A comparison of two dose rates. Vet Rec 141:439, 1997.
178. Lloyd DH, et al: Fluoroquinolone resistance in *Staphylococcus intermedius*. Vet Dermatol 10:248, 1999.
179. Loncarevic S, et al: A case of canine cutaneous listeriosis. Vet Dermatol 10:69, 1999.
180. Lotti T, Hartmann G: Atypical mycobacterial infections: A difficult and emerging group of infectious dermatoses. Int J Dermatol 32:499, 1993.
181. Love DN, et al: Antimicrobial susceptibility patterns of obligately anaerobic bacteria from subcutaneous abscesses and pyothorax in cats. Aust Vet Pract 10:168, 1980.
182. Love DN, et al: Characterization of strains of staphylococci from infections in dogs and cats. J Small Anim Pract 22:195, 1981.
183. McEwan NA: Bacterial adherence to canine corneocytes. In: von Tscharner C, Halliwell REW (eds): Advances in Veterinary Dermatology, Vol 1. Bailliáere-Tindall, London, 1990, p 454.
184. McIntosh DW: Feline leprosy: A review of forty-four cases from western Canada. Can Vet J 23:291, 1982.
185. Malik R, et al: Mycobacterial nodular granulomas affecting the subcutis and skin of dogs (canine leproid granuloma syndrome). Aust Vet J 76:403, 1998.
186. Malik R, et al: Diagnosis and treatment of pyogranulomatous panniculitis due to *Mycobacterium smegmatis* in cats. J Small Anim Pract 35:524, 1994.
187. Malik R, et al: Localised *Corynebacterium pseudotuberculosis* infection in a cat. Aust Vet Practit 26:27, 1996.
188. Manders SM: Toxin-mediated streptotoccal and staphylococcal disease. J Am Acad Dermatol 39:393, 1998.
189. Manning TO: Canine pododermatitis. Dermatol Rep 2:1, 1983.
190. Marino DJ, Jaggy A: Nocardiosis: A literature review with selected case reports in two dogs. J Vet Int Med 7:4, 1993.
191. Mason KV, Wilkinson GT: Results of treatment of atypical mycobacteriosis. In: von Tscharner C, Halliwell REW (eds): Advances in Veterinary Dermatology, Vol 1. Bailliére-Tindall, London, 1990, p 452.
191a. Mason IS: Pathogenesis of canine pyoderma. Proc Br Vet Dermatol Study Group, Autumn 1999, p 37.
192. Mason IS, et al: A review of the biology of canine skin with respect to the commensals *Staphylococcus intermedius, Demodex canis,* and *Malassezia pachydermatitis.* Vet Dermatol 7:119, 1996.
193. Mason IS, Lloyd DH: The role of allergy in the development of canine pyoderma. J Small Anim Pract 30:216, 1989.
194. Mason IS, Lloyd DH: Scanning electron microscopic studies of the living epidermis and stratum corneum in dogs. In: Ihrke PJ, Mason IS, White SD (eds): Advances in Veterinary Dermatology, Vol 2. Pergamon Press, Oxford, 1993, p 131.
195. Mason IS, Lloyd DH: The macroscopic and microscopic effects of intradermal injections of crude and purified staphylococcal extracts on canine skin. Vet Dermatol 6:197, 1995.
196. Mason IS, Kietzmann M: Cephalosporins—pharmacological basis of clinical use in veterinary dermatology. Vet Dermatol 10:187, 1999.
196a. Mealey K, et al: Hypercalcemia associated with granulomatous disease in a cat. J Am Vet Med Assoc 215:959, 1999.
197. Medleau L, et al: Frequency and antimicrobial susceptibility of *Staphylococcus* spp. isolated from canine pyodermas. Am J Vet Res 47:229, 1986.
198. Medleau L, Blue JL: Frequency and antimicrobial susceptibility of *Staphylococcus* spp. isolated from feline skin lesions. J Am Vet Med Assoc 193:1080, 1988.
199. Medleau LM, et al: Superficial pyoderma in the cat: Diagnosing an uncommon skin disorder. Vet Med 86:807, 1991.
200. Messinger LM, Beale KM: A blinded comparison of the efficacy of daily and twice daily trimethoprim-sulfadiazine and daily sulfamethoxine-ormetoprim therapy in the treatment of canine pyoderma. Vet Dermatol 4:13, 1993.
201. Michaud AJ: The use of clofazimine as treatment for *Mycobacterium fortuitum* in a cat. Feline Pract 22:7, 1994.
202. Miller CW, et al: Streptococcal toxic shock syndrome in dogs. J Am Vet Med Assoc 209:1427, 1996.
202a. Miller MA, et al: Inflammatory pseudotumor in a cat with cutaneous mycobacteriosis. Vet Pathol 36:161, 1999.
203. Miller RI, Ladds PW: Probable dermatophilosis in two cats. Aust Vet J 60:155, 1983.
204. Miller WH Jr: Deep pyoderma in two German shepherd dogs associated with a cell-mediated immunodeficiency. J Am Anim Hosp Assoc 27:513, 1991.
205. Monroe WE, Chickering WR: Atypical mycobacterial infections in cats. Comp Cont Educ 10:1043, 1988.
206. Morales CA, et al: Antistaphylococcal antibodies in dogs with recurrent staphylococcal pyoderma. Vet Immunol Immunopathol 42:137, 1994.
207. Muller RS, et al: Antibiotic sensitivity of *Staphylococcus intermedius* isolated from canine pyoderma. Aust Vet Practit 28:10, 1998.
208. Mundell AC: The use of clofazimine in the treatment of three cases of feline leprosy. In: von Tscharner C, Halliwell REW (eds): Advances in Veterinary Dermatology, Vol 1. Baillière-Tindall, London, 1990, p 451.
209. Noble WC, Kent LE: Antibiotic resistance in *Staphylococcus intermedius* isolated from cases with pyoderma in the dog. Vet Dermatol 3:71, 1992.

210. Noli C, Boothe D: Macrolides and lincosamides. Vet Dermatol 10:217, 1999.
211. Norris JM, Love DN: The isolation and enumeration of three feline oral *Porphyromonas* species from subcutaneous abscesses in cats. Vet Microbiol 65:115, 1999.
212. Oluoch AO, et al: Trends of bacterial infections in dogs: Characterization of *Staphylococcus intermedius* isolates (1990–1992). Canine Pract 21:12, 1996.
213. Orloski KA, Eidson M: *Yersina pestis* infection in three dogs. J Am Vet Med Assoc 207:316, 1995.
213a. Pak SI, et al: Characterization of methicillin-resistant *Staphylococcus aureus* isolated from dogs in Korea. J Vet Med Sci 61:1013, 1999.
214. Paradis M, et al: Efficacy of enrofloxacin in the treatment of canine bacterial pyoderma. Vet Dermatol 1:123, 1990.
215. Patel A, et al: Antimicrobial resistance of feline staphylococci in south-eastern England. Vet Dermatol 10:257, 1999.
216. Paul JW, Gordon MA: Efficacy of a chlorhexidine surgical scrub compared to that of hexachlorophene and providone-iodine. Vet Med 73:573, 1978.
217. Pechereau D, et al: Abces sous-cutanés et plaies infectées chez le chat: Bactériologie et efficacité clinique de la clindamycine. Prat Méd Chir Anim Comp 30:99, 1995.
218. Pellerin JL, et al: Epidemiosurveillance of antimicrobial compound resistance of *Staphylococcus intermedius* clinical isolates from canine pyodermas. Comp Immunol Microbiol Infect Dis 21:115, 1998.
219. Petersen A, et al: Frequency and antimicrobial susceptibility of *Staphylococcus intermedius* and *Pseudomonas aeruginosa* isolated from dogs over a six year period (1992–1997). Proc Annu Memb Meet Am Acad Vet Dermatol Am Coll Vet Dermatol 14–35, 1998.
220. Phillips WE, Kloos WE: Identification of coagulase-positive *Staphylococcus intermedius* and *Staphylococcus hyicus subspp. hyicus* isolated from veterinary clinical specimens. J Clin Microbiol 14:671, 1981.
221. Phillips WE, Williams BJ: Antimicrobial susceptibility patterns of canine *Staphylococcus intermedius* isolates from veterinary clinical specimens. Am J Vet Res 45:2377, 1984.
222. Pickler ME: Gaseous gangrene in a dog: Successful treatment using hyperbaric oxygen and conventional treatment. J Am Anim Hosp Assoc 18:807, 1982.
223. Piriz S, et al: *In vitro* activity of fifteen antimicrobial agents against methicillin-resistant and methicillin-susceptible *Staphylococcus intermedius*. J Vet Pharmacol Ther 19:118, 1996.
224. Piriz S, et al: Comparative *in vitro* activity of 11 beta-lactam antibiotics against 91 *Staphylococcus intermedius* strains isolated from staphylococcal dermatitis in dogs. J Vet Med B 42:293, 1995.
224a. Pirro F, et al: Bactericidal and inhibitory activity of enrofloxacin and other fluoroquinolones in small animal pathogens. Compend Cont Educ Pract Vet 21(Suppl):19, 1999.
225. Plechner AJ: IgM deficiency in two Doberman pinchers. Mod Vet Pract 60:150, 1979.
225a. Plewig G, Schopf E: Anti-inflammatory effects of antimicrobial agents: an in vivo study. J Invest Dermatol 65:532, 1975.
226. Price PM: Pyoderma caused by *Peptostreptococcus tetradius* in a pup. J Am Vet Med Assoc 198:1649, 1991.
227. Pullen RP, et al: X-linked severe combined immunodeficiency in a family of Cardigan Welsh corgis. J Am Anim Hosp Assoc 33:494, 1997.
228. Raychaudhuri SP, Raychaudhuri SK: Relationship between kinetics of lesional cytokines and secondary infection in inflammatory skin disorders: A hypothesis. Int J Dermatol 32:409, 1993.
229. Reinke SI, et al: Histopathologic features of pyotraumatic dermatitis. J Am Vet Med Assoc 190:57, 1987.
230. Renshaw HW, et al: Canine granulocytopathy syndrome. Am J Pathol 95:731, 1979.
231. Richard JL, et al: Experimentally induced canine dermatophilosis. Am J Vet Res 34:797, 1973.
232. Roccabianca P, et al: Feline leprosy: Spontaneous remission in a cat. J Am Anim Hosp Assoc 32:189, 1996.
233. Rosenkrantz WS: *Pseudomonas aeruginosa* necrotizing dermatitis, vasculitis, and panniculitis in the cat. Proc Annu Memb Meet Am Acad Vet Dermatol Am Coll Vet Dermatol 14:77, 1998.
234. Rosser EJ: German shepherd dog pyoderma: A prospective study of 12 dogs. J Am Anim Hosp Assoc 33:355, 1997.
235. Rosser WW: Bubonic plague. J Am Vet Med Assoc 191:406, 1987.
236. Roth JA, et al: Improvement in clinical condition and thymus morphologic features associated with growth hormone treatment of immunodeficient dwarf dogs. Am J Vet Res 45:1151, 1984.
237. Roth RR, James WD: Microbiology of the skin. J Am Acad Dermatol 20:369, 1989.
238. Ryan CP: Selected arthropod-borne diseases: Plague, lyme disease, babesiosis. Vet Clin North Am Small Anim Pract 17:179, 1987.
239. Saijonmaa-Koulumies LE, et al: Elimination of *Staphylococcus intermedius* in healthy dogs by topical treatment with fusidic acid. J Small Anim Pract 39:341, 1998.
240. Saijonmaa-Koulumies LE, Lloyd DH: Adherence of *Staphylococcus intermedius* to canine corenocytes *in vitro* In: Kwochka KW, et al (eds): Advances in Veterinary Dermatology III. Butterworth Heinemann, Oxford, 1998, p 540.
241. Saijonmaa-Koulumies LE, Lloyd DH: Carriage of bacterial antagonists towards *Staphylococcus intermedius* on canine skin and mucosal surfaces. Vet Dermatol 6:187, 1995.
242. Saijonmaa-Koulumies LE, Lloyd DH: Colonization of the canine skin with bacteria. Vet Dermatol 7:153, 1996.
243. Schiefer HB, Middleton DB: Experimental transmission of a feline mycobacterial skin disease (feline leprosy). Vet Pathol 20:460, 1983.
244. Schoeb TR, Morton R: Scrotal and testicular changes in canine brucellosis. J Am Vet Med Assoc 172:598, 1978.
245. Schultz RD: Basic veterinary immunology and a review. Vet Clin North Am Small Anim Pract 8:569, 1978.
246. Schwarz S, Noble WC: Aspects of bacterial resistance to antimicrobials used in veterinary dermatologic practice. Vet Dermatol 10:163, 1999.
246a. Schwassman M: Uses of interferon. Derm Dialogue, Winter 1999, p 9.
247. Scott DW: Canine pododermatitis. In: Kirk RW (ed): Current Veterinary Therapy VII. W.B. Saunders Co., Philadelphia, 1980.

248. Scott DW: Feline dermatology 1900–1980: A monograph. J Am Anim Hosp Assoc 16:331, 1980.
249. Scott DW: Feline dermatology 1979–1982: Introspective retrospections. J Am Anim Hosp Assoc 20:537, 1984.
250. Scott DW: Feline dermatology 1983–1985: The secret sits. J Am Anim Hosp Assoc 23:255, 1987.
251. Scott DW: Feline dermatology 1986 to 1988: Looking to the 1990s through the eyes of many counselors. J Am Anim Hosp Assoc 26:515, 1990.
252. Scott DW: Bacteria and yeast on the surface and within non-inflamed hair follicles of skin biopsies from dogs with non-neoplastic dermatoses. Cornell Vet 82:379, 1992.
253. Scott DW: Bacteria and yeast on the surface and within non-inflamed hair follicles of skin biopsies from cats with non-neoplastic dermatoses. Cornell Vet 82:371, 1992.
254. Scott DW, et al: The combination of ormetoprim and sulfadimethoxine in the treatment of pyoderma due to *Staphylococcus intermedius* infection in dogs. Canine Pract 10:29, 1993.
255. Scott DW, et al: Efficacy of tylosin tablets for the treatment of pyoderma due to *Staphylococcus intermedius* infection in dogs. Can Vet J 35:617, 1994.
256. Scott DW, et al: Further studies on the efficacy of tylosin tablets for the treatment of pyoderma due to *Staphylococcus intermedius* infection in dogs. Can Vet J 37:617, 1996.
257. Scott DW, et al: Efficacy of clindamycin hydrochloride capsules for the treatment of deep pyoderma due to *Staphylococcus intermedius* in dogs. Can Vet J 39:753, 1998.
258. Shepard RM, Falkner FC: Pharmacokinetics of azithromycin in rats and dogs. J Antimicrob Chemother 25:49, 1990.
259. Shimizu A, et al: Genomic DNA fingerprinting, using pulsed-field gel electrophoresis, of *Staphylococcus intermedius*, isolated from dogs. Am J Vet Res 57:1458, 1996.
260. Snider WR: Tuberculosis in canine and feline populations: Review of the literature. Am Rev Respir Dis 104:877, 1971.
261. Spring M, et al: Antibacterial activity of marbofloxacin: A new fluoroquinolone for veterinary use against canine and feline isolates. J Vet Pharmacol Ther 18:284, 1995.
262. Stevenson K, et al: Feline skin granuloma associated with *Mycobacterium avium*. Vet Rec 143:109, 1998.
263. Stewart LJ, et al: Cutaneous *Mycobacterium avium* infection in a cat. Vet Dermatol 4:87, 1993.
264. Studdert VP, Hughes KL: Treatment of opportunistic mycobacterial infections with enrofloxacin in cats. J Am Vet Med Assoc 201:1300, 1992.
265. Swaim SF, et al: Fusion podoplasty for the treatment of chronic fibrosing interdigital pyoderma in the dog. J Am Anim Hosp Assoc 27:264, 1991.
265a. Toman M, et al: Secondary immunodeficiency in dogs with enteric, dermatologic, infectious or parasitic diseases. J Vet Med B 45:321, 1998.
266. Tomlin J, et al: Methicillin-resistant *Staphylococcus aureus* infection in 11 dogs. Vet Rec 144:60, 1999.
267. Tredten HW, et al: Mycobacterium bacteremia in a dog: Diagnosis of septicemia by microscopic evaluation of blood. J Am Anim Hosp Assoc 26:359, 1990.
268. Trepanier L: Delayed hypersensitivity reactions to sulphonamides: Syndromes, pathogenesis, and management. Vet Dermatol 10:241, 1999.
269. Trowald-Wigh A, et al: Leukocyte adhesion protein deficiency in Irish setter dogs. Vet Immunol Immunopathol 32:261, 1992.
270. van Dongen AM, et al: Atypical mycobacteriosis in a cat. Vet Q 18:347, 1996.
271. Vilmanyi E, et al: Clarithromycin pharmacokinetics after oral administration with or without fasting in crossbred beagles. J Small Anim Pract 37:535, 1996.
272. Walker RD, et al: Serum and tissue cage fluid concentration of ciprofloxacin after oral administration of the drug to healthy dogs. Am J Vet Res 51:896, 1996.
273. Walker RD, et al: Recovery of two mycoplasma species from abscesses in a cat following bite wounds from a dog. J Vet Diag Invest 7:154, 1995.
274. Walton DK, et al: Cutaneous bacterial granuloma (botryomycosis) in a dog and cat. J Am Anim Hosp Assoc 19:537, 1983.
274a. Webster GF: New antibiotics: A dermatologist's guide. Adv Dermatol 11:105, 1996.
275. Welsh O, et al: Amikacin alone and in combination with trimethoprim-sulfamethoxazole in the treatment of actinomycotic mycetoma. J Am Acad Dermatol 17:443, 1987.
276. Werner AH, Russell AD: Mupirocin, fusidic acid, and bacitracin: Activity, action, and clinical uses of three topical antibiotics. Vet Dermatol 10:225, 1999.
277. White SD, et al: Cutaneous atypical mycobacteriosis in cats. J Am Vet Med Assoc 182:1218, 1983.
278. White SD, et al: Occurrence of *S. aureus* on the clinically normal canine hair coat. Am J Vet Res 44:332, 1983.
279. White SD: Pododermatitis. Vet Dermatol 1:1, 1989.
280. White SD: Pyoderma in 5 cats. J Am Anim Hosp Assoc 27:141, 1991.
281. White SD: Systemic treatment of bacterial skin infections of dogs and cats. Vet Dermatol 7:133, 1996.
282. White SD, et al: Feline acne and results of treatment with mupirocin in an open clinical trial: 25 cases. Vet Dermatol 8:157, 1997.
283. Whitney JC: Some aspects of interdigital cysts in the dog. J Small Anim Pract 11:83, 1970.
284. Willemse T, et al: *Mycobacterium thermoresistible*: Extrapulmonary infection in a cat. J Clin Microbiol 21:854, 1985.
285. Wisselink MA, et al: Immunologic aspects of German shepherd pyoderma. Vet Immunol Immunopathol 19:67, 1988.
286. Wisselink MA, et al: German shepherd pyoderma: A genetic disorder. Vet Q 11:161, 1989.
287. Wisselink MA, et al: Deep pyoderma in the German shepherd dog. J Am Anim Hosp Assoc 21:773, 1985.
288. Woldehiwet Z, Jones JJ: Species distribution of coagulase-positive staphylococci isolated from dogs. Vet Rec 126:485, 1990.
289. Von Tscharner C: Personal communication, Bad Kreuznach, Germany, 1988.
290. Yager JA: The skin as an immune organ. In: Ihrke PJ, Mason IS, White SD (eds): Advances in Veterinary Dermatology, Vol 2. Pergamon Press, Oxford, 1993, p 3.
291. Yovich JC, Read RA: Nasal actinomyces infection in a cat. Aust Vet Practit 25:114, 1995.

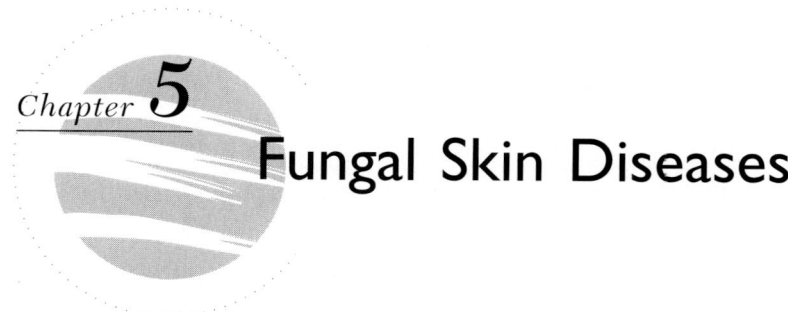

Chapter 5: Fungal Skin Diseases

• CUTANEOUS MYCOLOGY

Fungi are omnipresent in our environment. Of the thousands of different species of fungi, only a few have the ability to cause disease in animals. The great majority of fungi are either soil organisms or plant pathogens; however, more than 300 species have been reported to be animal pathogens.

A *mycosis* (pl. *mycoses*) is a disease caused by a fungus. A *dermatophytosis* is an infection of the keratinized tissues, claw, hair, and stratum corneum that is caused by a species of *Microsporum, Trichophyton,* or *Epidermophyton*. These organisms—dermatophytes—are unique fungi that are able to invade and maintain themselves in keratinized tissues. A *dermatomycosis* is a fungal infection of hair, claw, or skin that is caused by a nondermatophyte, a fungus not classified in the genera *Microsporum, Trichophyton,* or *Epidermophyton*.

Dermatophytosis and dermatomycosis are different clinical entities. Fungi, however, are not nearly as common a cause of skin disease as supposed; many dermatoses are misdiagnosed as "fungus infections" on the basis of clinical presentation. On the other hand, many true fungal infections are probably not diagnosed because of the variability of clinical presentations.

General Characteristics of Fungi

The term *fungus* includes yeasts and molds. The kingdom of Fungi is recognized as one of the five kingdoms of organisms. The other four kingdoms are Monera (bacteria and blue-green algae), Protista (protozoa), Plantae (plants), and Animalia (animals).[1-3, 9, 10] Fungi are eukaryotic achlorophyllous organisms that may grow in the form of a yeast (unicellular), a mold (multicellular-filamentous), or both. The cell walls of fungi consist of chitin, chitosan, glucan, and mannan and are used to distinguish the fungi from the Protista. Unlike plants, fungi do not have chlorophyll. The kingdom of Fungi contains five divisions: Chytridomycota, Zygomycota, Basidiomycota, Ascomycota, and Fungi Imperfecti or Deuteromycota.

Fungi have traditionally been identified and classified (1) by their method of producing conidia and spores, (2) by the size, shape, and color of the conidia, and (3) by the type of hyphae and their macroscopic appearance (e.g., by the color and texture of the colony and sometimes by physiologic characteristics). Therefore, it is important to understand the terms that describe these characteristics.

A single vegetative filament of a fungus is a *hypha*. A number of vegetative filaments are called *hyphae*, and a mass of hyphae is known as a *mycelium*. Hyphae are *septate* if they have divisions between cells or *sparsely septate* if they have many nuclei within a cell. This latter condition is known as *cenocytic*. The term *conidium* (pl. *conidia*) should be used only for an asexual *propagule* or unit that gives rise to genetically identical organisms. A *conidiophore* is a simple or branched mycelium bearing conidia or conidiogenous cells. A *conidiogenous cell* is any fungal cell that gives rise to a conidium. (Modern taxonomists also may use sexual reproduction characteristics and biochemical and immunologic methods for identification.) There are six major types of conidia: blastoconidia, arthroconidia, annelloconidia, phialoconidia, poroconidia, and aleuriconidia. More detailed information about fungal taxonomy can be found in other texts.[1-3, 9, 10]

Changes in the scientific names resulting from recent taxonomic studies have caused some confusion regarding the names of pathogenic fungi. Some disease names have been based on geographic distribution or have been created by the indiscriminate lumping together of dissimilar diseases. We attempt to name diseases on the basis of a single etiologic agent and common usage, tempered by contemporary knowledge of geographic distribution and current taxonomy. Mycotic diseases are divided into three categories: superficial, subcutaneous, and systemic. The first category contains the most common fungal diseases in veterinary dermatology.

Characterization of Pathogenic Fungi

Fungi that are pathogenic to plants are distributed throughout all divisions of fungi, but those that are pathogenic to animals are found primarily in the Fungi Imperfecti and the Ascomycota.[1-3, 9, 10]

A yeast is a unicellular budding fungus that forms blastoconidia, whereas a mold is a filamentous fungus. Some pathogenic fungi, such as *Histoplasma capsulatum, Coccidioides immitis, Sporothrix schenckii,* and *Blastomyces dermatitidis,* are *dimorphic.* Dimorphic fungi are capable of existing in two different morphologic forms. For example, at 37°C (98.6°F) in enriched media or in vivo, *B. dermatitidis* exists as a yeast, but at 30°C (86°F) it grows as a mold. *C. immitis* is unique in that at 37°C (98.6°F) or in tissue, spherules containing endospores are formed. Some fungi such as *Aspergillus* form true hyphae in tissue and are a mold at either 30°C or 37°C (86°F or 98.6°F). Another manifestation of fungal growth in tissue is the presence of granules (grains) that are organized masses of hyphae in a crystalline or amorphous matrix. These granules are characteristic of the mycotic infection mycetoma and are the result of interaction between the host tissue and the fungus.

At one time, numerous fungi were thought to be pathogens. Today, with the increased use of broad-spectrum antibiotics and immunosuppressive therapy, the presence of chronic immunosuppressive diseases (e.g., feline leukemia virus [FeLV] and feline immunodeficiency virus [FIV] infections), and improved mycologic techniques, many fungi that were considered contaminants have, in fact, been found to be pathogenic. The following criteria can be helpful in differentiating pathogenic from contaminant fungi: (1) source, (2) number of colonies isolated, (3) species, (4) whether the fungus can be repeatedly isolated, and most important (5) the presence of fungal elements in the tissue.

A fungus isolated from a normal sterile site, such as a biopsy specimen, warrants greater credence as a pathogen than that same fungus isolated from the surface of the skin, where it may be an airborne contaminant. The number of colonies isolated should influence the decision as to whether an organism is a contaminant or a pathogen. One isolated colony of *Aspergillus* may have resulted from an airborne conidium that floated into a plate, whereas a Petri dish filled with *Aspergillus fumigatus* could represent a pathogen. Colonies that are not visible on the streak line of the agar should be considered contaminants. Certain species of fungi are definitely recognized as pathogens, however, so if even only one colony is isolated, it should be reported. Such organisms include *B. dermatitidis, H. capsulatum, C. immitis,* and *Cryptococcus neoformans.* Another indication of fungal pathogenicity is that the same fungus can be repeatedly isolated from the lesion. In order to confirm that a fungus is a cause of a mycosis, the fungal structures observed in tissue or a direct smear must correlate with the fungus identified in culture.

Although gross colonies of dermatophytes are never black, brown, or green, organisms in fungal cultures are properly identified by medical laboratory clinicians who have expertise in such matters. Detailed information on the cultural growth of three common dermatophytes (*Microsporum canis, Microsporum gypseum, Trichophyton mentagrophytes*) and commonly isolated fungal contaminants is available in other texts.[1, 2, 9, 10]

Table 5–1	SAPROPHYTIC FUNGI ISOLATED FROM THE HAIRCOAT AND SKIN OF NORMAL DOGS AND CATS		
Absidia	*Cephalosporium*	*Geotrichum*	*Rhizopus*
Acremonium	*Chaetomium*	*Gliocladium*	*Rhodotorula*
Alternaria	*Chrysosporium*	*Gymnascella*	*Scopulariopsis*
Anixiopsis	*Cladosporium*	*Malassezia*	*Stemphylium*
Arthrinium	*Diheterospora*	*Malbranchea*	*Trichocladium*
Arthroderma	*Doratomyces*	*Mucor*	*Trichoderma*
Aspergillus	*Drechslera*	*Paecilomyces*	*Trichosporon*
Aureobasidium	*Epicoccum*	*Penicillium*	*Trichothecium*
Beauveria	*Fusarium*	*Pestalotia*	*Ulocladium*
Botrytis	*Geomyces*	*Phoma*	*Verticillium*
Candida			

NORMAL FUNGAL MICROFLORA

Dogs and cats harbor many saprophytic molds and yeasts on their haircoats and skin (Table 5–1). The most common of these fungi isolated from dogs are species of *Alternaria, Aspergillus, Aureobasidium, Chrysosporium, Cladosporium, Mucor, Penicillium,* and *Rhizopus*.[10a, 13, 26, 65, 68, 87–89] In cats, the most commonly isolated fungi are species of *Alternaria, Aspergillus, Chrysosporium, Cladosporium, Mucor, Penicillium, Rhodotorula,* and *Scopulariopsis*.[13, 13a, 65, 67, 88] Most of these saprophytic isolates probably represent repeated transient contamination by airborne fungi or by fungi in soil. Cats infected with FeLV and/or FIV have a greater diversity of fungi isolated from their skin and mucosal surfaces.[13a]

Dermatophytes are also isolated from the haircoats and skin of normal dogs and cats.* It is likely that dermatophytes isolated from normal dogs and cats—such as *M. gypseum, T. mentagrophytes, Trichophyton rubrum, Trichophyton terrestre*—simply represent recent contamination from the environment. For instance, it is not unheard of to isolate a geophilic dermatophyte, such as *M. gypseum,* from normal dogs or from a dog presented for a skin disease (e.g., pododermatitis) wherein these dermatophytes are playing no pathogenic role. This is particularly true in outdoor animals. Dermatophytes, especially *M. gypseum,* were isolated from the majority of soil samples in urban and rural areas of Greece.[24] In one study, anthropophilic dermatophytes were isolated from about 10% of the stray cats in various animal shelters, indicating that cats can mechanically carry human pathogens.[68] *M. canis,* however, is undeniably present as a persistent infection in many asymptomatic or inapparently infected cats.†

Culture and Examination of Fungi

Proper specimen collection, isolation, culture, and identification are necessary to determine the cause of a fungal infection. Detailed information on these important techniques is presented in Chapter 2.

• SUPERFICIAL MYCOSES

The superficial mycoses are fungal infections that involve superficial layers of the skin, hair, and claws. The organisms may be dermatophytes such as *Microsporum* and *Trichophyton,* which are able to use keratin. However, other fungi such as *Candida (Monilia),*

---

*See references 13, 15, 24, 26, 49, 65, 68, 88–90.
†See references 13, 15, 26, 43, 65, 68, 88, 90.

Malassezia (*Pityrosporum*), and *Trichosporon* (piedra) may also produce superficial mycoses.

Dermatophytosis

CAUSE AND PATHOGENESIS

The dermatophytes that most frequently infect animals are *Microsporum* and *Trichophyton*. These genera can be divided into three groups on the basis of natural habitat: geophilic, zoophilic, and anthropophilic. Geophilic dermatophytes, such as *M. gypseum*, normally inhabit soil, in which they decompose keratinous debris. Zoophilic dermatophytes, such as *M. canis, Microsporum distortum,* and *Trichophyton equinum,* have become adapted to animals and are only rarely found in soil. Anthropophilic dermatophytes, such as *Microsporum audouinii,* have become adapted to humans and do not survive in soil.

Three fungi cause the great majority of clinical cases of dermatophytosis in dogs and cats[13, 17, 43, 49, 87, 89]: *M. canis, M. gypseum,* and *T. mentagrophytes*. In general, *M. canis* is the most common cause of dermatophytosis in cats and dogs.[13, 17, 43, 49, 89] There is, however, great variation in the proportion in which these three fungi occur in different parts of the world.* The incidence and prevalence of dermatophytosis vary with the climate and natural reservoirs. In a hot, humid climate, the incidence is higher than in a cold, dry climate. In one study, there was a strong positive correlation between the frequency of isolation of *M. canis* and higher relative humidity.[88] *M. canis* was isolated from 4% of the cats in various animal shelters in the southeastern United States (Florida) but in none of the shelter cats sampled in the northern United States (Wisconsin).[68]

The frequency of isolating *M. canis* from shelter cats is significantly correlated with housing practices.[82] In Greece, *M. canis* was the only dermatophyte isolated from the hair coat of normal dogs living in urban areas, whereas *M. gypseum, T. mentagrophytes,* and *T. terrestre* were the most commonly isolated from the hair coat of normal dogs living in rural areas.[24] It has been reported that the seasonal incidence of dermatophytosis in dogs and cats in the United States varies with the species of fungus,[46, 49] but no seasonality was evident in Spain[27] or the United Kingdom.[89] The incidence may also depend on the climate and on the amount of time the animal spends outdoors and thus is more exposed to geophilic species. In New Zealand, the frequency of isolation of *M. canis* was significantly greater in the winter months.[88]

In general, the incidence for dogs in the northern hemisphere can be summarized as follows: (1) *M. canis* is high in the period from October to February and low from March to September, (2) *M. gypseum* is high in the period from July to November and low from December to June, (3) *T. mentagrophytes* is present all year, with a peak occurring in November and December. In general, the incidence for cats can be summarized as follows: (1) *M. canis* varies little all year, (2) *M. gypseum* and *T. mentagrophytes* are seldom reported in cats, but a slight increase may occur during the summer and fall months. Other fungi reported to cause dermatophytosis in cats and dogs are listed in Table 5-2. Rarely, dermatophytosis in dogs and cats is caused by simultaneous infection with two different fungi.[20, 21, 25]

Dermatophytes are transmitted by contact with infected hair and scales or fungal elements on animals, in the environment, or on fomites.[13, 43, 66] Combs, brushes, clippers, bedding, transport cages, and other paraphernalia associated with the grooming, movement, and housing of animals are all potential sources of infection and re-infection. *M. canis* can be cultured from dust, heating vents, and furnace filters.[66] Visitors to catteries and multiple-cat households may introduce organisms.[66] The source of *M. canis* infections is usually an infected cat. *Trichophyton* spp. infections are usually acquired directly or indirectly by exposure to typical reservoir hosts, which may be determined by specific

---

*See references 13, 24, 26, 27, 29, 49, 87–89.

Table 5-2 DERMATOPHYTES ISOLATED FROM DOGS AND CATS

DERMATOPHYTE	HOST*	SOURCE†
Epidermophyton floccosum	B	A
Microsporum audouinii (M. langeronii, M. rivalierii)	B	A
M. canis (M. equinum, M. felineum, M. lanosum, M. obesum)	B	Z
M. cookei	B	G
M. distortum	B	Z
M. equinum	D	Z
M. ferrugineum	D	A
M. fulvum	B	Z
M. gypseum (M. fulvum, M. duboisii, Achorion gypseum)	B	G
M. nanum	B	Z
M. persicolor	B	Z
M. vanbreuseghemii	B	G
Trichophyton ajelloi (Keratinomyces ajelloi)	B	G
T. equinum	B	Z
T. erinacei (T. mentagrophytes var. erinacei)	B	Z
T. gallinae (M. gallinae, A. gallinae)	B	Z
T. megninii	B	A
T. mentagrophytes (T. asteroides, T. caninum, T. felineum, T. granulosum, T. gypseum, T. quinckeanum)	B	Z
T. rubrum (T. multicolor, T. purpureum)	B	A
T. schoenleinii (A. schoenleinii)	B	A
T. simii	D	Z, G
T. terrestre	B	G
T. tonsurans (T. accuminatum, T. cerebriforme, T. crateriforme, T. epilans, T. fumatum, T. plicate, T. sabouraudi, T. sulfureum)	B	A
T. verrucosum (T. album, T. discoides, T. faviforme, T. ochraceum)	B	Z
T. violaceum (T. glabrum, T. kagewaense, T. vinosum)	B	A

°B = dog and cat; D = dog.
†A = anthropophilic; G = geophilic; Z = zoophilic.

identification of the fungal species or subspecies. For example, most *T. mentagrophytes* infections are associated with exposure to rodents or their immediate environment. *M. gypseum* is a geophilic dermatophyte that inhabits rich soil. Cats and dogs are usually exposed to it by digging and rooting in contaminated areas. In Greece, *M. gypseum* was isolated from 7.2% of the dogs with dermatophytosis, 4% of the clinically normal dogs (especially the paws), and 32.6% of the soil samples.[24] However, rooting did not seem to play a significant role in contamination of the bridge of the nose of dogs in Greece.[10a] *Microsporum persicolor* is a natural resident and occasional pathogen of mice and voles, and contact with these rodents (hunting, rural animals) is the source of infection.

Infections with anthropophilic species are rare; they are acquired as reverse zoonoses by contact with infected humans. Hair shafts containing infectious arthrospores may remain infectious in the environment for many months—for example, up to 18 months in the case of *M. canis*.[13, 43, 66, 90] The floors of 50 private veterinary clinics were cultured, and *M. canis*, *T. terrestre*, *M. gypseum*, and *T. mentagrophytes* were grown from 30%, 22%, 10%, and 4% of them, respectively.[53] Thus, the veterinarian's clinic could be the source of infection!

Numerous studies on the asymptomatic carriage of *M. canis* by cats have often yielded conflicting results, with positive cultures in 0% to 36% of cats attending veterinary clinics, 0% to 27% of healthy pet cats, 6% to 35% of pet cats at cat shows, and 0% to 88% of stray cats.° Such differences presumably relate to differences in environment and management. The isolation of *M. canis* from an asymptomatic cat may represent passive

---

°See references 13, 26, 27, 37, 40, 63, 68, 88, 90.

carriage of arthrospores and hyphae on the haircoat, acquired either directly from an infected cat or indirectly from a contaminated environment.

When an animal is exposed to a dermatophyte, an infection may be established. Mechanical disruption of the stratum corneum appears to be important in facilitating the penetration and invasion of anagen hair follicles.[13, 66, 74] Hair is invaded in both ectothrix and endothrix infections. The ectothrix fungi produce masses of arthrospores on the surface of hair shafts, whereas endothrix fungi do not. Fungal hyphae invade the ostium of hair follicles, proliferate on the surface of hairs, and migrate downward (proximally) to the hair bulb, during which time the fungus produces its own keratinolytic enzymes (keratinases) that allow penetration of the hair cuticle and growth within the hair shaft until the keratogenous zone (Adamson's fringe) is reached. At this point, the fungus either establishes an equilibrium between its downward growth and the production of keratin or it is expelled.

Spontaneous resolution occurs when infected hairs enter the telogen phase or if an inflammatory reaction is incited. When a hair enters telogen, keratin production slows and stops; because the dermatophyte requires actively growing hairs for survival, fungal growth also slows and stops. Infectious arthrospores may remain on the hair shaft, but re-infection of that particular hair follicle does not occur until it re-enters anagen.

In experimental models of *M. canis* infection in cats,[33, 93] the incubation period between inoculation and development of clinical lesions was 7 to 14 days. Lesions enlarged until 6 to 8 weeks post inoculation, then decreased in size and healed by 12 to 14 weeks post inoculation. Toothbrush cultures commonly remained positive until 1 to 2 weeks after clinical resolution. Hence, infection spontaneously resolved in 2½ to 3 months. Interestingly, cats who were able to groom themselves typically had lesions only on the head and pinna, whereas collared cats experienced more widespread lesions, indicating that grooming behavior can limit the development of lesions.[40] Clipping of the haircoat of infected cats sometimes leads to a worsening of clinical signs within 7 to 10 days after clipping.[71] This emphasizes the importance of skin trauma in the spread of infection.

Cutaneous inflammation is due to toxins produced in the stratum corneum that provoke a sort of biological contact dermatitis.[6, 13, 43] Host factors are poorly documented, but the host's ability to mount an inflammatory response plays a critical role in determining the type of clinical lesions produced and in terminating the infection. Dermatophyte infections in healthy dogs and cats are often self-limiting. Conversely, the relatively poor inflammatory response of most typical feline dermatophyte lesions produced by *M. canis* attests to the cat's relative tolerance of this fungus and probably accounts for the high rate of asymptomatic or subclinical carriage of this species among cats.[13, 43, 66]

It has been shown that *T. rubrum* and *T. mentagrophytes* produce substances (especially mannans) that diminish cell-mediated immune responses and indirectly inhibit stratum corneum turnover.[31] These effects could predispose the animal to persistent or recurrent infections. *M. canis* has been shown to possess multiple enzymatic properties, which can vary according to the strain of fungus.[42, 75] The keratinase from *M. canis* is an α-chymotrypsin–type serine proteinase.[42] Strains of *M. canis* with α-chymotrypsin activity may be associated with more inflammation and pruritus.[42] *Trichophyton* spp. can produce proteolytic enzymes that induce keratinocyte acantholysis in vitro and in vivo.[76]

As with many infectious diseases, young animals are predisposed to acquiring symptomatic dermatophyte infections.[43, 48, 49, 56, 89] This is partly due to a delay in development of adequate host immunity. However, differences in biochemical properties of the skin and skin secretions (especially sebum), the growth and replacement of hair, and the physiologic status of the host as related to age may also play a role. Local factors, such as the mechanical barrier of intact skin and the fungistatic activity of sebum caused by its fatty acid content, are deterrents to fungal invasion.

Natural and experimental infections have been shown to incite various forms of hypersensitivity in their hosts.[13, 43, 45, 79, 91, 93] *M. canis* contains numerous antigens, and *M. canis*–infected cats have antibodies against several of these.[92] When *M. canis* glycoprotein antigens or mycelial suspensions of *M. canis* were given by intradermal injection or skin scarification, respectively, to normal cats and cats that had recovered from *M. canis* dermatophytosis, all previously infected cats experienced immediate and delayed-type hypersensitivity reactions. By comparison, the control cats did not experience delayed-type hypersensitivity reactions and, uncommonly (20% of animals), experienced immediate hypersensitivity reactions.[32, 93]

There is no correlation between circulating antibodies and protection. Cats that had recovered from previous *M. canis* infections experienced either no clinical lesions or lesions that were more inflammatory and transient (25 days) than those in *M. canis*–naive cats.[93] It is believed that the cell-mediated immune response is the mainstay of the body against fungal infection. This is corroborated by the increased incidence of fungal infections in patients with various acquired or inherited forms of immunosuppression, such as FeLV infection, FIV infection, and cancer; poor nutrition and anti-inflammatory or immunosuppressive drug therapy (such as glucocorticoids) also lead to an increased incidence.[13, 30, 43, 57] The stress of pregnancy and lactation may increase susceptibility to fungal infection.[30, 66] The presence of ectoparasites, especially fleas and *Cheyletiella* mites, can be important in the establishment and spread of dermatophytosis in catteries and multiple-cat households.[30, 66]

Genetic influences probably play an important role in the transmission and clinical course of feline dermatophytosis.[37] The common belief that long-haired cats are more commonly affected than are shorthaired cats may reflect less efficient grooming of the haircoat or genetic breed predispositions (e.g., Persians and Himalayans).[37]

CLINICAL FINDINGS

When clinicians rely on clinical signs alone, dermatophytosis (ringworm, tinea) is greatly overdiagnosed, especially in dogs. In most studies of skin diseases in dogs and cats, the incidence of dermatophytosis is low, accounting for only 0.26% to 5.6% of all cases examined.* A striking exception was reported from the Dermatology Service at the University of Sao Paulo in Brazil, where dermatophytosis accounted for about 30% of all feline skin cases examined![48] The analysis of cultures submitted from suspected dermatophytosis cases in dogs and cats generally reveals that between 2.1% and 40% (average, 15%) are positive.[13, 17, 27, 48, 49, 88] Several other dermatoses, especially staphylococcal folliculitis and demodicosis, mimic the classic ringworm lesion. On the other hand, dermatophytosis is a diagnosis that is often missed because of the protean nature of the dermatologic findings.[13, 28, 37, 40, 43]

Because the infection is almost always follicular in dogs and cats, the most consistent clinical sign is one or many circular patches of alopecia with variable scaling.[13, 43] Some patients may experience the classic ring lesion with central healing and fine follicular papules and crusts at the periphery. However, signs and symptoms are highly variable and depend on the host-fungus interaction and, therefore, the degree of inflammation. Pruritus is usually minimal or absent; however, it is occasionally marked and suggests an ectoparasitism or allergy. This is especially true with "miliary dermatitis-like" *M. canis* infections in cats and *Trichophyton* and *M. persicolor* infections in dogs. In addition, dermatophytosis may be complicated by secondary bacterial (usually staphylococcal) infection. In vitro studies have shown that dermatophytes can produce antibiotic substances and encourage the development of penicillin-resistant staphylococci.[16, 50]

Dog

Dogs more often exhibit the classic annular areas of peripherally expanding alopecia, scale, crust, and follicular papules and pustules (Fig. 5–1A to D). However, less common syndromes are frequent enough that dermatophytosis should be considered in the differ-

---

*See references 17, 19, 28, 29, 40, 49, 56, 86.

ential diagnosis of any annular, papular, or pustular eruption. Symmetric nasal or facial folliculitis and furunculosis, mimicking autoimmune skin disease (e.g., pemphigus erythematosus or foliaceus), may be caused by a dermatophyte, especially *T. mentagrophytes* (Fig. 5–2; also see Fig. 5–1E and F) and *M. persicolor* (Fig. 5–3). *Trichophyton* infections may also present as folliculitis and furunculosis affecting one paw or one leg (see Fig. 5–1G). These infections often scar significantly.

A seborrhea-like eruption with greasy scale may occur with generalized infections. The dermatophyte kerion is a boggy, exudative, variably well-circumscribed, nodular type of furunculosis that develops multiple draining tracts. It is often associated with *M. gypseum* or *T. mentagrophytes* infections and occurs most commonly as a solitary lesion on the face or a distal limb (see Fig. 5–1H). Onychomycosis is rare[11]; it is usually associated with *T. mentagrophytes* and may present as an asymmetric (one digit or multiple digits on one paw) paronychia or onychodystrophy. Widespread collarettes, erythema, and scales without hair follicle involvement was produced by *Trichophyton ajelloi* infection in a dog.[23] Severe dermatophytosis and dermatophytic pseudomycetoma with marked lymph node involvement was reported in a young Yorkshire terrier in association with *M. canis* infection.[52]

In general, the nature of the dermatophyte cannot be determined from the clinical presentation. Dermatophyte infections are most often localized, with lesions occurring most commonly on the face, pinnae, paws, and tail.

Whereas dermatophytosis is usually a disease of young animals (<1 year old),[13, 27, 43, 49, 89] sylvatic ringworm (that acquired from wild mammals) is more common in adults.[13, 89] *M. persicolor* is an increasingly recognized cause of dermatophytosis in Europe,[18, 20, 22, 89] where it typically produces facial lesions that may be predominantly scaly or papulopustular and crusty; in addition, concurrent depigmentation of the nasal planum and nostrils may occur. Extensive dermatophytosis in older dogs may be associated with concurrent immunosuppressive diseases (e.g., cancer, hyperadrenocorticism) or inappropriate systemic glucocorticoid therapy (Fig. 5–4A and B).[13, 43, 56] Yorkshire terriers of any age seem to be susceptible to severe forms of dermatophytosis associated with *M. canis* infection. In Europe, it has been reported that dermatophytosis occurs more commonly in the Jack Russell terrier (especially sylvatic), Yorkshire terrier (especially *M. canis*), and Pekinese (especially *M. canis*).[13, 27, 89] German shorthaired pointers were predisposed to *M. gypseum* infections in one study.[29]

Cat

Feline dermatophytosis most often appears as one or more irregular or annular areas of alopecia with or without scales (see Fig. 5–4C and D).[13, 28, 37, 43] Hairs in these areas often appear broken and frayed. Follicular hyperkeratosis may result in exaggerated hair follicle openings or comedo formation. The alopecia may be severe and widespread, accompanied by little evidence of inflammation. Cats occasionally have more inflammatory areas of folliculitis characterized by alopecia, erythema, scale, crust, and follicular papules (see Fig. 5–4E and F). The so-called *miliary dermatitis*, which is characterized by an often pruritic, widespread, papulocrustous dermatitis, is an uncommon manifestation of dermatophytosis that is usually caused by *M. canis*. Recurring chin folliculitis resembling feline acne or a dermatitis of the dorsal tail resembling "stud tail" may occur.[13, 30] Onychomycosis is rare[12]; it is usually caused by *M. canis* and may present as an asymmetric (one digit, or multiple digits on one paw) paronychia or onychodystrophy (see Fig. 5–4G). Generalized seborrhea-like eruptions can be visible, wherein dry or greasy scales are prominent. The condition is usually due to *M. canis*.

Widespread, pruritic, exfoliative erythroderma occasionally occurs in association with *M. canis* (see Fig. 5–4H). Some cats groom lesions vigorously (pruritus?) and can produce very erythematous, indurated, eroded lesions within 48 hours that resemble eosinophilic plaques.[33] Dermatophyte kerion reactions occasionally occur in the cat, as do cases of otitis externa due to *M. canis*.[13] Dermatophytic pseudomycetoma has been reported only in Persian cats; it is characterized by one or more subcutaneous nodules that are often

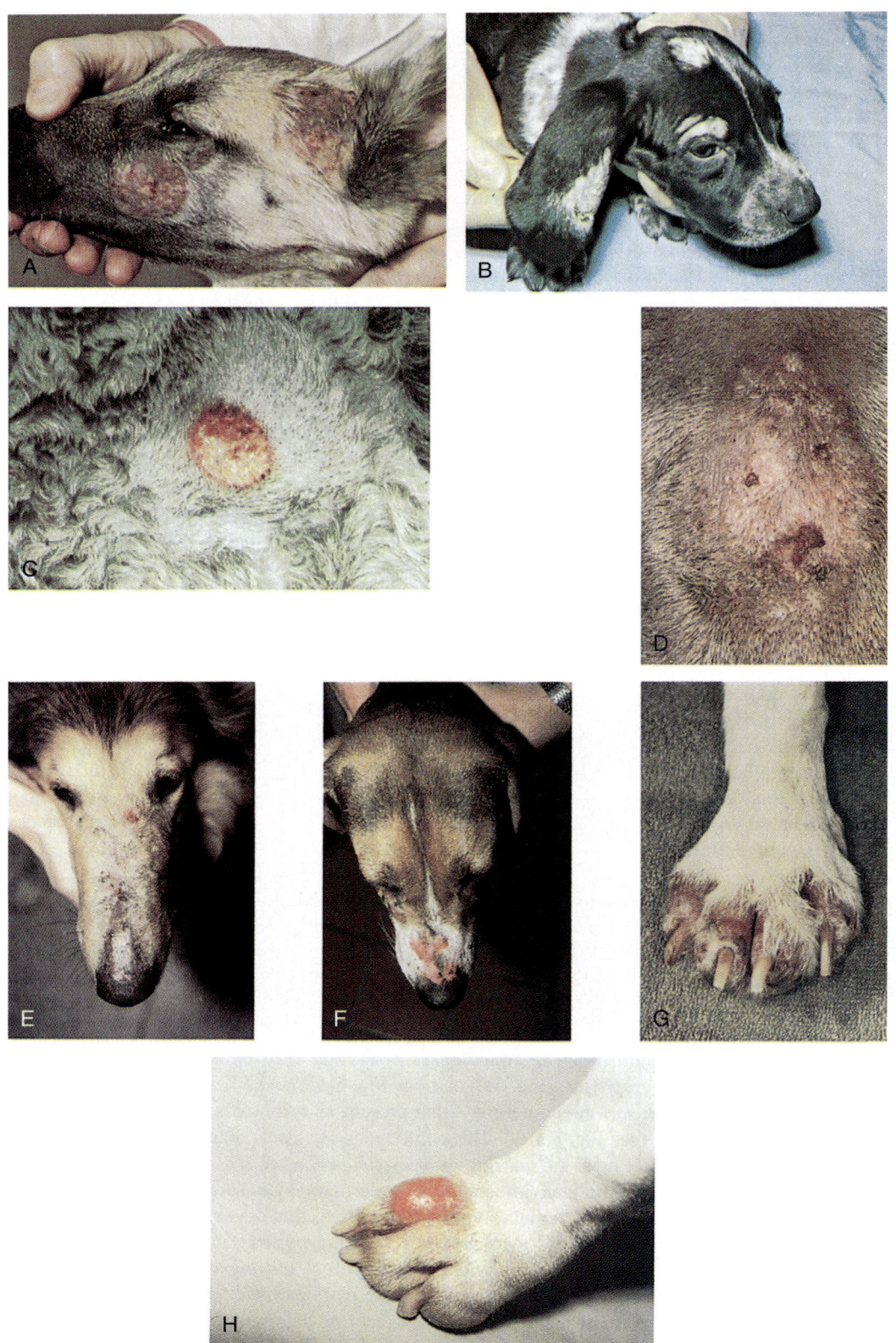

FIGURE 5–1. *See legend on opposite page*

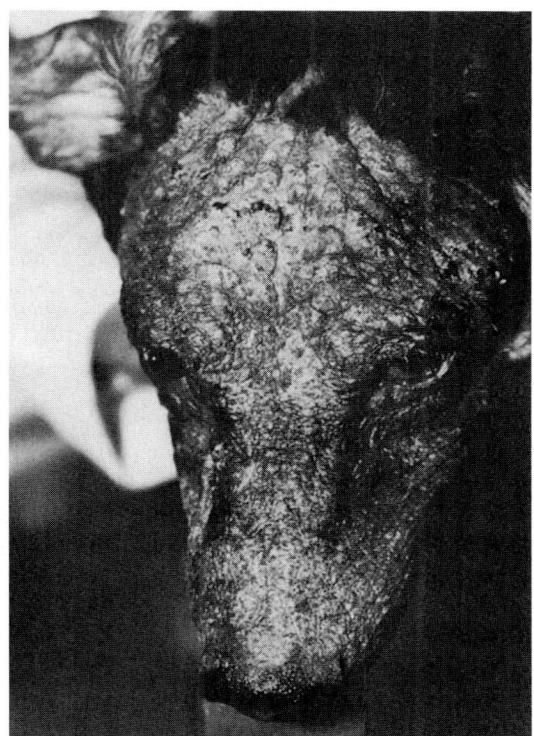

FIGURE 5–2. Extensive facial dermatitis in a dog caused by *T. mentagrophytes*.

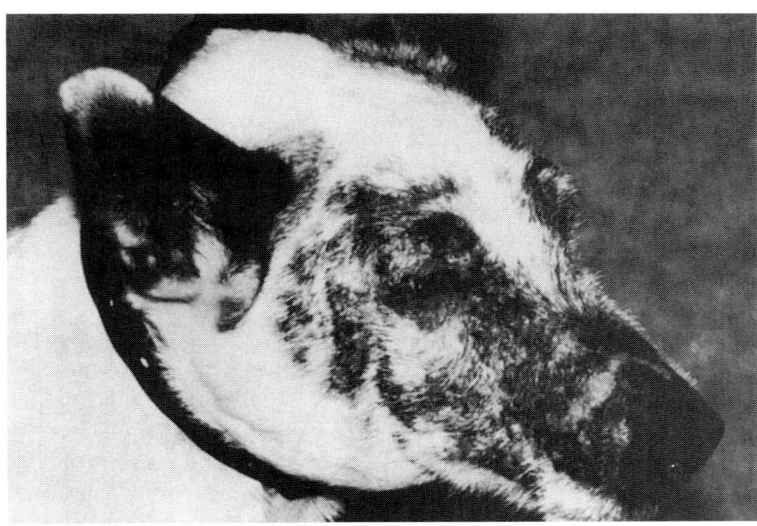

FIGURE 5–3. Chronic facial dermatitis with areas of hyperpigmentation and depigmentation in a dog caused by *M. persicolor*. (Courtesy D. Carlotti.)

FIGURE 5–1. Dermatophytosis. *A*, German shepherd puppy with annular inflammatory lesions below the eye and cranial to the pinna caused by *M. canis*. (Courtesy B. Farrow.) *B*, Pointer puppy with well-circumscribed areas of alopecia and grayish crusts above the eye and on the pinna caused by *M. canis*. *C*, Annular, erythematous, oozing, pruritic lesion resembling pyotraumatic dermatitis on a Poodle caused by *M. canis*. *D*, Crusted follicular papules and pustules on the bridge of the nose of a dog caused by *M. persicolor*. (Courtesy D. Carlotti.) *E*, Collie with a crusting, erosive, alopecic dermatitis on the bridge of the nose caused by *T. mentagrophytes*. *F*, Coonhound with a highly inflammatory nasal dermatitis caused by *T. mentagrophytes*. *G*, Severe pododermatitis in a Beagle caused by *T. mentagrophytes*. *H*, Kerion on the digit of a dog caused by *M. gypseum*. Note the pinpoint draining tracts.

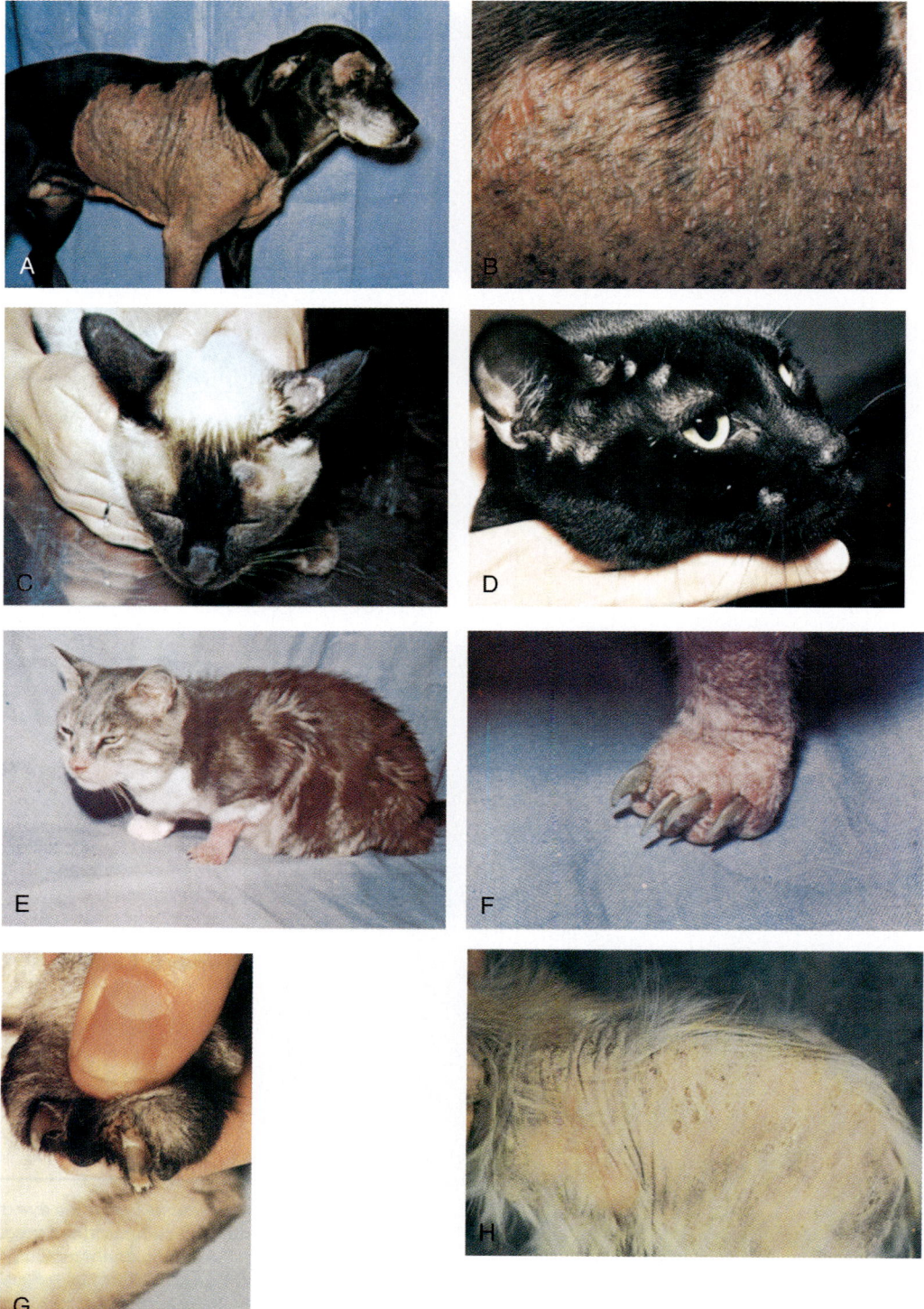

FIGURE 5–4. Dermatophytosis. *A*, Chronic widespread dermatitis in an old dog caused by *T. mentagrophytes*. Note the strikingly well-circumscribed nature of the lesions. *B*, Close-up of the dog in *A* showing the erythematous papulovesicular dermatitis. *C*, Classic "ringworm" lesions on the left pinna and dorsal to the left eye in a Siamese cat caused by *M. canis*. *D*, Multiple annular areas of alopecia and grayish crusts on the face of a cat caused by *M. canis*. *E*, Well-circumscribed areas of alopecia and erythema on the muzzle and left front paw of a cat caused by *T. mentagrophytes*. *F*, Closer view of the paw lesion in *E*. *G*, Brownish paronychial exudate, leukonychia, and onychorrhexis in a cat caused by *M. canis*. *H*, Generalized exfoliative erythroderma in a Persian cat caused by *M. canis*. (Courtesy G. Wilkinson.)

ulcerated and discharging. The nodules occur most commonly over the dorsal trunk or tail base (Fig. 5–5A and B). These cats may have more typical, superficial dermatophyte lesions on other areas of the body, or they may be clinically normal except for the nodules.[42a, 52, 56, 61, 64] Lesions of *M. canis* infections in a hypotrichotic Rex cat were characterized by annular areas where hairs were darker and longer than normal.[83]

In general, the nature of the dermatophyte cannot be determined from the clinical presentation. Lesions are most common on the head, pinnae, and paws.[12, 17, 35, 43, 46] Generalized dermatophyte infection is more common in cats than in dogs.[13, 49] As with dogs, dermatophytosis is more common in young cats (<1 year old),[13, 27, 48, 49, 89] but sylvatic ringworm is more common in adults.[13, 89] Longhaired cats, especially Persians and Himalayans, are predisposed to this infection.[27, 30, 49, 86, 89]

Zoonotic Aspects

Prior to the 1990s, about 30% of all cases of *Microsporum* infections and about 15% of all cases of dermatophytosis (tinea) in humans were reported to be caused by *M. canis*, the vast majority of these infections being acquired from cats.[13, 85] However, a 1998 report indicated that *M. canis* was isolated from only 3.3% of the cases of dermatophytosis in humans in the United States.[94] *M. canis* continues to be the most common dermatophyte isolated from humans in Italy.[62] Approximately 50% of humans exposed to symptomatic or asymptomatic infected cats acquire the infection.[13] In about 30% to 70% of all households with infected cats, at least one person in the household becomes infected.[13, 40, 85]

The cutaneous changes with animal-origin dermatophytosis in humans are variable and most commonly occur on areas of the body that contact infected animals, such as the arms, scalp, and trunk (see Fig. 5–5C).[13, 85] Other dermatophytes (*M. gypseum*, *M. persicolor*, *T. mentagrophytes*) are rarely, if ever, transmitted from dogs and cats to humans.

DIAGNOSIS

The differential diagnosis for dermatophytosis is extensive as a result of the variable clinical appearance of the disease. Because most infections are follicular, the primary differential diagnoses are staphylococcal folliculitis and demodicosis. In dogs, staphylococcal folliculitis is much more common than dermatophytosis.[13, 43, 86] In fact, the following adage is useful regarding dogs: "If it looks like ringworm, it is probably not! It is probably staphylococcal folliculitis." In cats, however, dermatophytosis is more common than demodicosis and staphylococcal folliculitis. Other causes of annular areas of alopecia, crusts, and variable inflammation include pemphigus foliaceus and erythematosus, *Pelodera* dermatitis, flea bite hypersensitivity, food hypersensitivity, seborrheic dermatitis, subcorneal pustular dermatosis, and the various sterile eosinophilic folliculitides. Although alopecia areata and pseudopelade produce annular areas of alopecia, the alopecic skin appears otherwise normal. Dermatophyte kerions may resemble other infectious or foreign-body granulomas, acral lick dermatitis, or neoplasms such as histiocytoma, mast cell tumor, and lymphoma. Dermatophytic pseudomycetoma must be differentiated from other infectious or foreign-body granulomas, sterile panniculitis, and various neoplasms.

History-taking may be of limited value unless exposure is known to have occurred; this is so because clinical dermatophytosis is so variable and the incubation period is incompletely defined (in general, 4 days to 4 weeks).[13, 28, 33] The number, types, and sources of contact animals should be determined. The source of kittens and puppies presented for examination should be ascertained because animals from some breeding establishments, pet shops, or animal shelters may have a high incidence of infection. Evidence for contagion—in other animals or human contacts—should be sought.

Fungal tests are useful in diagnosis. These tests are described in detail in Chapter 2. Wood lamp examination for fluorescence causes only certain strains of *M. canis*, *M. audouinii*, *M. distortum*, and *Trichophyton schoenleinii* to produce a positive yellow-green

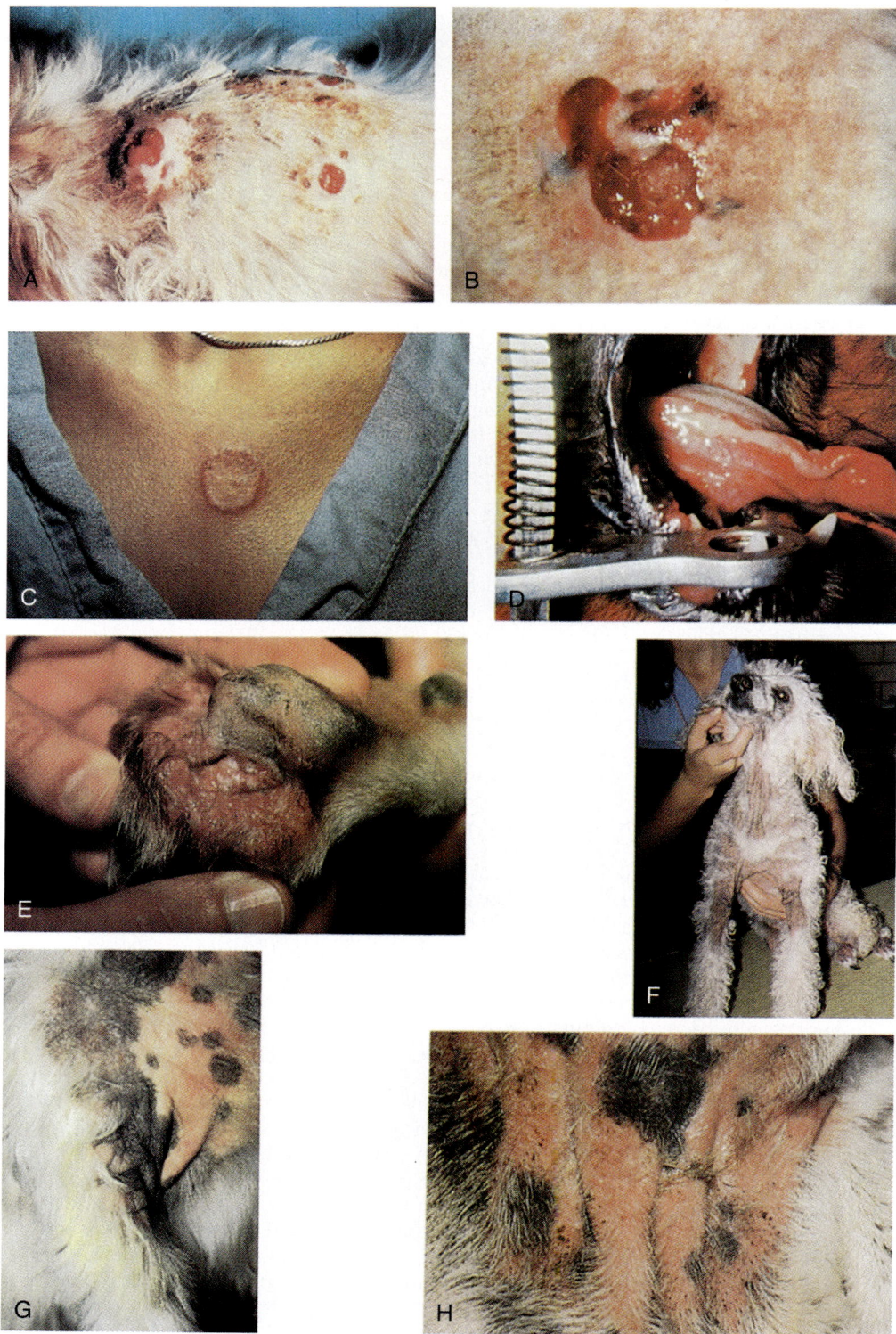

FIGURE 5–5. Dermatophytosis and yeast infections. *A*, Ulcerated nodules (dermatophytic pseudomycetoma) over the back of a cat due to *Trichophyton* sp. *B*, Close-up of lesion in *A*. *C*, Annular erythema and scaling with a slightly raised papulovesicular border in a human caused by *M. canis*. *D*, Candidiasis in a dog.

Legend continued on opposite page

color on infected hairs.[13] Only about 50% of *M. canis* infections fluoresce.* Several important pitfalls exist in the use and interpretation of the Wood lamp results (see Chap. 2).

Microscopic examination of plucked hairs and scraped scales may reveal hyphae and arthrospores in 40% to 70% of the cases, and it is definitive evidence of dermatophytosis (Fig. 5–6A) (see Chap. 2).[13, 17, 27, 28, 43, 66] *M. persicolor* and *Epidermophyton floccosum* do not invade hairs and could be called true epidermophytes.[13, 18, 20, 22]

Fungal culture of affected hair and scales is the most reliable diagnostic test and is the only way to identify the specific dermatophyte.[13, 17, 28, 43, 66] Caution is warranted here, however, because dermatophytes may be cultured from the haircoat and skin of normal cats and dogs as well as those with nonfungal skin diseases. These dermatophyte isolates may reflect a true carrier state or recent exposure to a contaminated environment (e.g., hunting dogs and *M. gypseum*).

False-positive and false-negative results are possible.[26, 27, 88, 89] Cultures may be negative when microscopic examination of hairs is positive.[89] Although dermatophyte test medium is widely used and recommended for culturing dermatophytes,[17, 43, 56, 66] some mycologists have reported it to be unreliable and inferior to Sabouraud's dextrose agar.[13, 27] In addition, some *M. canis* isolates do not produce the initial red color change on dermatophyte test medium.[27, 66, 78] Culturing asymptomatic cats and dogs requires using a brush (toothbrush, hairbrush, surgical scrub brush) or carpet square method (see Chap. 2).[13, 28, 37, 66, 67, 88] Surface keratin must be harvested in order to culture *M. persicolor*.

Biopsy findings are as variable as the clinical lesions, and they are not as sensitive as culture.[7, 13, 43] On the other hand, when the true significance of a cultural isolation is questioned, demonstration of the organism in biopsy specimens is definitive proof of true infection. Histopathologic examination is most useful in the nodular forms of dermatophytosis—the kerion and pseudomycetoma. It may be impossible to culture the organism in such cases by collecting hair and scales. The most common histopathologic patterns observed in dermatophytosis are (1) perifolliculitis, folliculitis, and furunculosis (see Figs. 5–6B, 5–7, and 5–8), (2) hyperplastic or spongiotic superficial perivascular or interstitial dermatitis with prominent parakeratotic or orthokeratotic hyperkeratosis of the epidermis and hair follicles, and (3) intraepidermal pustular dermatitis (suppurative, neutrophilic epidermitis). When hair follicles are serially damaged by necrotizing and pyogranulomatous inflammation (the "domino effect") (see Fig. 5–8), dermatophytosis is the most likely diagnosis, and every hair shaft must be inspected for the presence of fungal hyphae and arthroconidia, which are often sparse in number.

In cats, *M. canis* infections may be associated with a hydropic interface folliculitis/dermatitis pattern wherein fungal elements are few (Fig. 5–9). In *M. persicolor* infections, fungal hyphae are found only in the surface keratin (Fig. 5–10)[18, 29] Dermatophytic pseudomycetoma is characterized by nodular to diffuse, granulomatous to pyogranulomatous panniculitis and dermatitis wherein the fungus is present as broad (2.5 to 4.5 μm), hyaline, septate hyphae, chainlike pseudohyphae, and large (12 μm) chlamydospore-like cells within granules (pseudogranules) (Figs. 5–11, 5–12, and 5–13).

In dogs with *Trichophyton* spp. infection, the reaction pattern can include marked epidermal and/or follicular acantholysis with or without concurrent lichenoid interface

---

*See references 9, 13, 17, 28, 38, 56, 66, 89.

FIGURE 5–5. *Continued* Note the whitish gray plaque on the cheek and the linear lesion on the tongue. (Courtesy N. Field.) *E*, Candidiasis in a dog. Multiple whitish gray, mucoid plaques on markedly erythematous interdigital skin. *F*, *Malassezia* dermatitis. Note the symmetric, greasy, erythematous dermatitis in a Poodle. (Courtesy K. Mason.) *G*, *Malassezia* dermatitis secondary to atopy and glucocorticoid therapy in a Lhasa apso. Note erythema, alopecia, hyperpigmentation, lichenification, and yellowish crusts in the axilla and on the medial forearm. *H*, *Malassezia* dermatitis in intertriginous areas of an English bulldog. Note moist, erythematous, alopecic dermatitis of the ventral neck.

350 • Fungal Skin Diseases

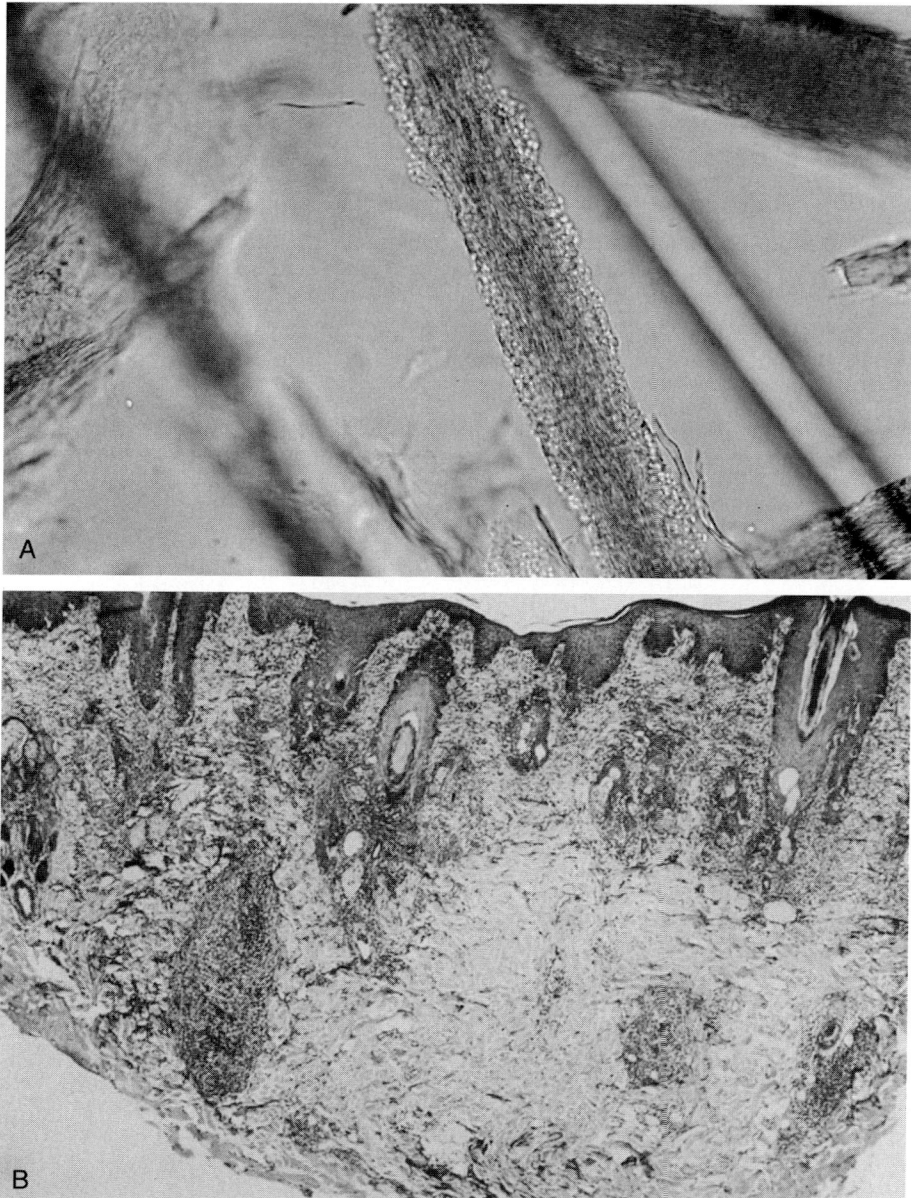

FIGURE 5–6. *A, M. canis*–infected dog hair in mineral oil. Anatomy of hair is destroyed and arthroconidia are numerous. *B,* Follicularly oriented inflammation in a cat with dermatophytosis.

dermatitis, thus being easily confused with pemphigus erythematosus or foliaceus (Fig. 5–14).[23, 76, 80] In such cases, fungal elements may only be present in surface and follicular keratin, not in hair shafts. In cats with alopecia that clinically does not appear to be inflammatory, biopsy findings often reveal enormous numbers of arthrospores and hyphae associated with infected hairs, minimal lymphohistiocytic perivascular dermatitis or no apparent inflammation, and minimal orthokeratotic hyperkeratosis. Septate fungal hyphae and spherical to ovoid arthrospores may be present in and around infected hairs, in hair follicles, and within the stratum corneum of the surface epidermis. The number of fungal

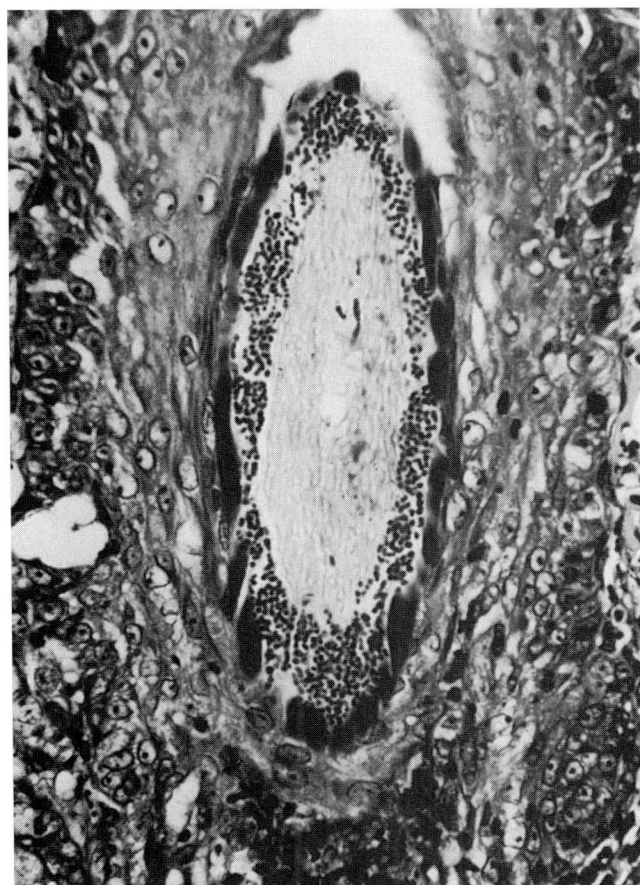

FIGURE 5–7. *M. canis* in a cat. Note arthroconidia surrounding hair shaft (AOG stain).

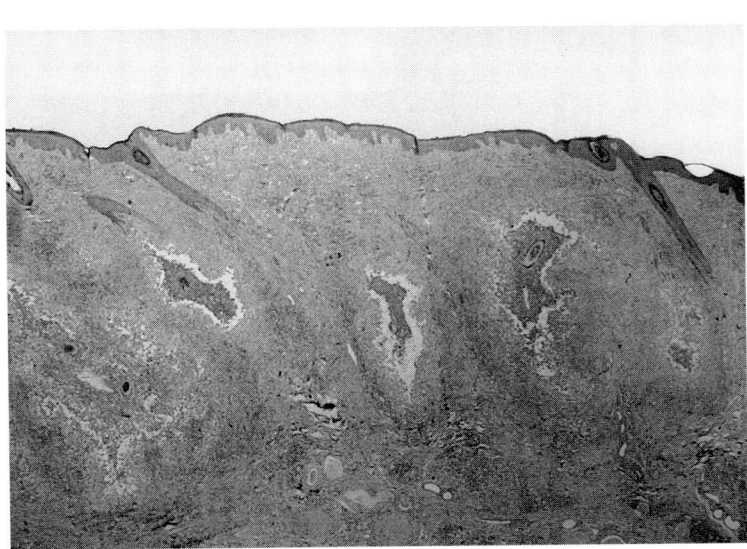

FIGURE 5–8. Kerion. Severe pyogranulomatous furunculosis. Five consecutive pilosebaceous units are severely affected (the "domino effect").

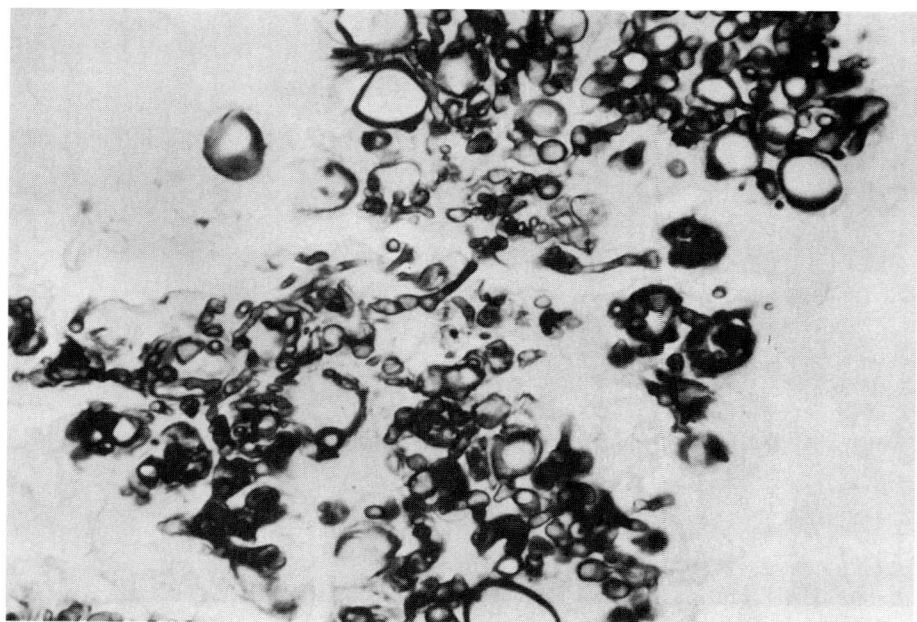

FIGURE 5-13. Subcutaneous dermatophytosis (*Trichophyton* sp.). Numerous hyphae with bulbous dilatations (GMS stain).

(but not always)[58, 60, 66] require aggressive therapy. Even longhaired cats can undergo spontaneous resolution, but it may take 1½ to 4 years.[58, 66] In general, sylvatic ringworm (especially *M. persicolor* and *Trichophyton* spp.) in dogs does not spontaneously resolve and requires aggressive therapy.[13, 18, 43] However, it has been reported that several cases of *T. mentagrophytes* infection in cats resolved spontaneously.[13]

The goals of therapy are (1) to maximize the patient's ability to respond to the dermatophyte infection (by the correction of any nutritional imbalances and concurrent disease states and by the termination of systemic anti-inflammatory and immunosuppressive drugs), (2) to reduce contagion (to the environment, other animals, and humans), and (3) to hasten resolution of the infection.[13, 28, 38] A critical feature of clinical management is the treatment of all dogs and cats in contact with the infected animal and treatment of the environment.[13, 28, 30, 38, 41, 43, 66, 71]

Topical Therapy

Every confirmed case of dermatophytosis should receive topical therapy.[13, 28, 38, 41, 43, 58] Hair is clipped from a wide margin (6 cm) surrounding all lesions.[13, 43, 47] Clipping should be gentle (using scissors or No. 10 clipper blade) so as to avoid traumatizing the skin and encouraging the spread of infection.[71] Longhaired animals should be clipped entirely.[28, 30, 43, 58, 66] Although clipping may spread the lesions, it is more important to get rid of infected hairs.[28, 38, 69, 71] Owners should be warned that the lesions may worsen 7 to 10 days after clipping.[41, 71] Clipped hair is carefully disposed of. Veterinary practices and grooming parlors are strongly advised against extensive clipping of infected animals on the premises because contamination of the room is likely.[28, 38] Owners should use clippers at home, where the environment is already contaminated. Clipping should be performed in an area of the home/cattery/shelter that is easy to disinfect.

Creams and lotions are available for use on focal lesions, and these are typically applied every 12 hours, to include a 6-cm margin of clinically normal skin, if possible. A wide variety of topical antifungals is available, and there is no particular advantage of one product over another (Table 5–3). For highly inflamed lesions, a product containing

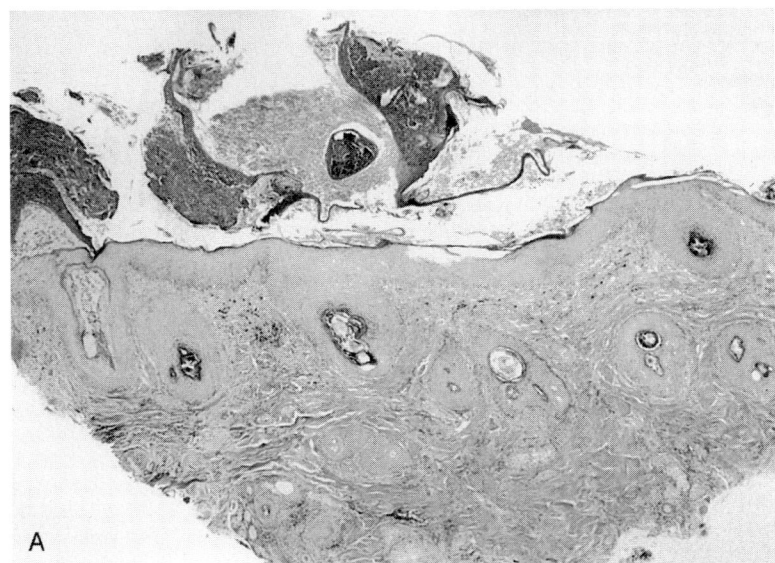
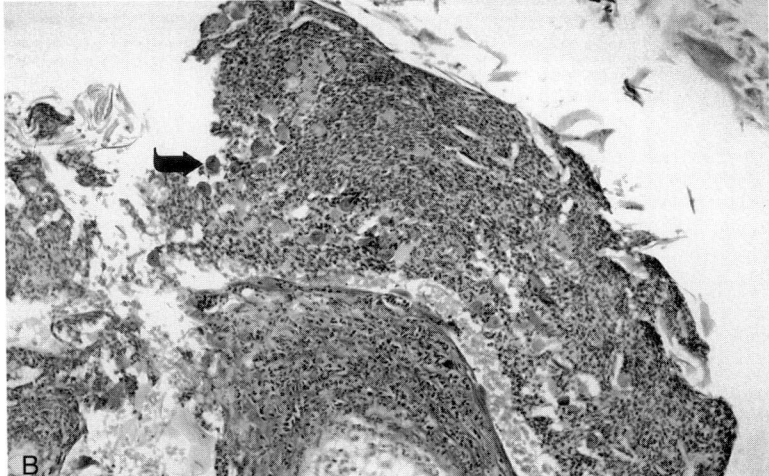
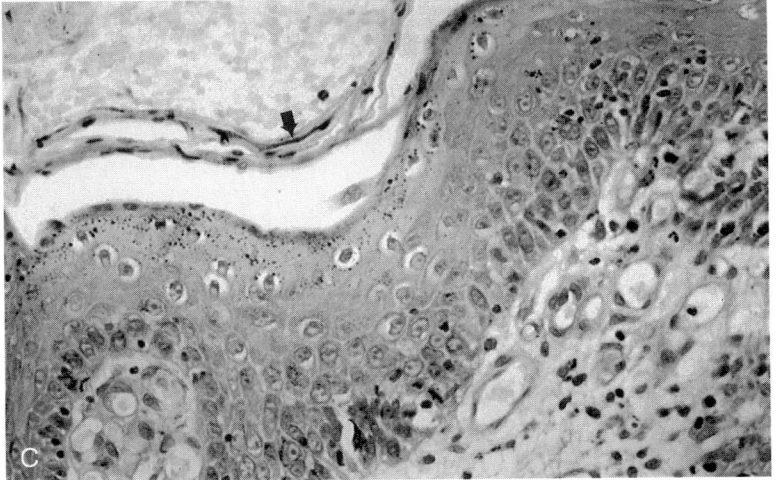

FIGURE 5–14. *T. mentagrophytes* infection in a dog. *A,* Interface dermatitis with intracorneal pus and cellular crust. *B,* Close-up of surface crust in *A*. Note numerous acantholytic keratinocytes *(arrow)*. *C,* Close-up of surface keratin. Note sparse fungal hyphae *(arrow)* (PAS stain).

Table 5–3 PRODUCTS FOR THE TOPICAL TREATMENT OF SUPERFICIAL MYCOSES

PRODUCT		INDICATION*
Spot Treatment		
Amphotericin B 3% cream, lotion	Fungizone (Apothecin)	C,M
Chlorhexidine 4% spray	ChlorhexiDerm Maximum (DVM)	C,D,M
Clotrimazole 1% cream, lotion	Lotrimin (Schering)	C,D,M
Clotrimazole 1%/betamethasone 0.1% cream	Lotrisone (Schering)	C,D,M
Clotrimazole 1%/betamethasone 0.3%/gentamicin ointment	Otomax (Schering)	C,D,M
Miconazole 2% cream, 1% lotion, 1% spray	Conofite (Mallinckrodt)	C,D,M
Miconazole 2% spray	Miconazole Spray (EVSCO)	C,D,M
Naftifine 1% cream, gel	Naftin (Allergan)	C,D
Nystatin cream	Mycostatin (Squibb)	C,M
Nystatin/triamcinolone cream, ointment	Panalog (Solvay)	C,M
Terbinafine 1% cream	Lamisil (Novartis)	C,D
Thiabendazole 4% dexamethasone	Tresaderm (Merck Ag Vet)	C,D,M
Shampoos†		
Chlorhexidine 2%	ChlorhexiDerm (DVM)	C,M
Chlorhexidine 2%	Seba-Hex (EVSCO)	C,M
Chlorhexidine 2%	Hexadere (Allerderm/Virbac)	C,M
Chlorhexidine 4%	ChlorhexiDerm Maxi (DVM)	C,M
Miconazole 2%	Dermazole (Virbac)	C,M
Miconazole 2%	Miconazole (EVSCO)	C,M
Sulfur 2%/Benzoyl peroxide 2.5%	Sulf/OxyDex (DVM)	C,M
Rinses		
Acetic acid 2.5%	(Vinegar:Water)	C,M
Enilconazole 0.2%	Imaverol (Janssen)	C,D,M
Lime sulfur 2%	LymDyp (DVM)	C,D,M

*C = candidiasis; D = dermatophytosis; M = *Malassezia* dermatitis.
†Shampooing may disperse more anthrospores into the haircoat and environment, and is *not* recommended in dermatophytosis.

glucocorticoid in combination with antifungal agents may hasten resolution of clinical disease. However, because the glucocorticoid can be absorbed systemically, it is not recommended in the treatment of very young kittens and puppies or pregnant queens and bitches. Clipping and spot-treatment of dogs with focal lesions is usually curative.[13, 29, 43, 58]

For dogs and cats with multifocal or generalized skin involvement, antifungal rinses (dips) are indicated. Cats that have focal lesions should also be given this treatment because they inevitably have or soon will have widespread to generalized infected hairs but are often asymptomatic.[43, 58, 66, 71] Rinses are preferred because the entire body surface can be treated, rubbing of the haircoat is minimized, and the antifungal agent can be allowed to dry on the skin. Rinses should be applied twice weekly. Lime sulfur 2% and enilconazole 0.2% are the most effective.[28, 29, 38, 41, 71, 95] Shampoos are less desirable because (1) they have no residual action and (2) the physical act of their application and removal may macerate fragile hairs and increase the release and dispersal of infective spores into the coat, thus increasing the likelihood of spreading the infection and of human exposure.[69, 71] Topical medications are continued until two or preferably three fungal cultures at weekly intervals are negative.[71] See page 409 for details on topical antifungal agents.

Local hyperthermia was reported to be effective therapy for focal dermatophyte lesions in dogs and cats.[51] However, such therapy is not readily accessible, it requires chemical restraint, and it is impractical for multifocal or generalized disease.

Systemic Therapy

Dogs and cats that have multifocal lesions, all longhaired animals, and those in multiple animal settings should receive systemic antifungal therapy. Animals that are not responding to topical therapy after a 2- to 4-week course of treatment should also receive

Table 5–4 PRODUCTS FOR THE SYSTEMIC TREATMENT OF SUPERFICIAL MYCOSES

PRODUCT	DOSE (mg/kg)	INTERVAL
Griseofulvin		
Microsized*	25–60	q12h
Ultramicrosized†	2.5–15	q12h
Fluconazole‡	10–20	q12h
Itraconazole§	10	q24h
	20	q48h
Ketoconazole¶	10	q24h
	20	q48h

*Fulvicin U/F (Schering).
†Gris-PEG (Herbert).
‡Diflucan (Roerig).
§Sporanox (Janssen).
¶Nizoral (Janssen).

systemic therapy (Table 5–4).[29, 43, 58] Griseofulvin is the drug of choice.* Dosage and frequency protocols vary widely. Side effects are uncommon and generally mild in dogs; they may be more common and potentially severe in cats, however. Anecdotal reports indicate that Persians, Himalayans, Siamese, and Abyssinians may be predisposed to side effects,[30, 41, 66] but we have not experienced this. Side effects are especially severe in cats with FIV infection, so griseofulvin probably should be avoided in these cats.[38, 41, 58, 66] Griseofulvin is a teratogen and must never be used during the first two thirds of pregnancy. It is advisable to not use recently treated males for breeding.[38] See page 410 for details concerning the use of griseofulvin in dogs and cats.

Ketoconazole is effective in the treatment of dermatophytoses in dogs and cats.[13, 28, 29, 43, 58, 59] However, ketoconazole is not labeled for use in dogs and cats in the United States, and most veterinarians reserve this drug for cases in which griseofulvin resistance is encountered or when the patient cannot tolerate griseofulvin.[13, 43, 58, 66] Although concern has been expressed about the efficacy of ketoconazole against *M. canis*[43] and a report has indicated that about 50% of the *M. canis* isolates from cats showed in vitro resistance to ketoconazole,[81] such concerns and in vitro findings have not been corroborated either clinically or by other in vitro studies.[13, 28, 44] See page 412 for details on the use of ketoconazole in dogs and cats.

Itraconazole is effective for the treatment of dermatophytoses of dogs and cats.[28, 54, 58, 69] However, it is not labeled for use in dogs and cats in the United States. Itraconazole may be useful when griseofulvin resistance or toxicity are encountered or when animals cannot tolerate ketoconazole. See page 413 for details concerning the use of itraconazole in dogs and cats.

It is important to remember that systemic antifungal therapy does not rapidly reduce contagion and is always to be used in conjunction with clipping and topical antifungal agents.† In addition, fungal cultures continue to be positive for at least 2 weeks and sometimes longer after clinical cure.[33, 36, 38, 69, 71] It is recommended that therapy be continued until three successive fungal cultures, performed at weekly intervals by a brush technique, are negative.[36, 71] This usually requires 4 to 20 weeks of therapy. The successful treatment of infected claws always requires systemic antifungal agents (usually for 6 to 12 months) or onychectomy.[13, 43, 58]

Dermatophytic pseudomycetoma in cats is often frustrating to treat. Lesions usually recur after wide surgical excision, and griseofulvin and ketoconazole are often ineffective or only partially effective.[13, 43, 52, 58, 64] One cat with dermatophytic pseudomycetoma was

---

*See references 28, 30, 41, 43, 58, 66, 69.
†See references 13, 28, 38, 41, 43, 58, 66.

cured after 10 months of treatment with itraconazole, and another cat's disease was controlled after 18 months.[58, 61] A young Yorkshire terrier with dermatophytic pseudomycetoma with multiple lymph node involvement associated with *M. canis* infection did not respond to griseofulvin, ketoconazole, or itraconazole.[52]

Anecdotal reports indicate that terbinafine is effective and safe for the treatment of dermatophytosis in dogs and cats (see page 415 for details).

Vaccination

Fungal vaccines (lyophilized, modified live fungus) have been successful in Europe in the management of endemic dermatophytoses in cattle and foxes.[13, 34] In 1994, a killed *M. canis* vaccine (Fel-O-Vax MC-K, Fort Dodge Laboratories) was released for the treatment and prevention of dermatophytosis in cats. To date, there is still no published scientific information on this product, and we do not recommend it. We as well as others[34] have received anecdotal reports from cat breeders that, when the commercial *M. canis* vaccine was used, cats that already were clinically infected often experienced a worsening of clinical signs and that allegedly uninfected cats in the same cattery "broke" with clinical signs. The latter observation most likely represents an augmentation of immune responsiveness producing more inflammatory lesions in cats that had subclinical infections.[34]

Moriello and associates[70] and DeBoer and colleagues[32] have conducted extensive studies with a killed *M. canis* vaccine in laboratory cats. Intradermal injections produced immediate- and delayed-type hypersensitivity reactions in cats with active *M. canis* infections and those that had recovered from *M. canis* infections but not in normal unexposed cats.[32, 70] In placebo-controlled studies, cats given the killed *M. canis* vaccine had high titers of anti–*M. canis* immunoglobulin G (IgG) (similar to those produced by natural infections) and increased lymphocyte blastogenic responses to *M. canis* antigen (lower responses than those produced by natural infections).[34, 35] However, all cats experienced dermatophytosis when inoculated with *M. canis* or when an *M. canis*–infected cat was introduced into the colony. Again, there is presently *no* good evidence to suggest that *any* killed *M. canis* vaccine has any preventive or therapeutic properties!

Chronic and recurring cases of dermatophytosis are usually associated with (1) inappropriate therapy, including wrong drug or wrong drug dosage; inadequate duration of therapy; failure to use topicals; failure to clip the haircoat; failure to treat all other animals in the house; and failure to treat the environment, (2) underlying diseases (e.g., hyperadrenocorticism, diabetes mellitus, FeLV infection, FIV infection, or cancer), (3) immunosuppressive drug therapy, or (4) the genetic background of the patient.[13, 29, 38, 41, 43, 57] A resistant strain of dermatophyte is theoretically possible but extremely rarely documented. *Trichophyton* spp. infections in dogs may be difficult to clear with griseofulvin.[76]

Management of Catteries and Multiple-Cat Households

The elimination of dermatophytosis in a cattery or other multiple-cat facility requires the separation of carriers from noncarriers, the treatment or destruction of infected animals, and the institution of measures to prevent re-infection of the premises.[28, 30, 66] Successful elimination of dermatophytosis requires aggressive systemic and topical therapy, interruption of breeding programs and show campaigns, isolation of the colony, environmental decontamination, and the testing and isolation of future cattery or household members. Such control programs are complicated by the cost of medical expenses, by the loss of revenue from the sale of cats and kittens, by the time commitment and effort required, and by the fear of permanent damage to the reputation of the cattery. This fear is often the most difficult obstacle to overcome.

M. canis is the dermatophyte involved in almost all cattery and multiple-cat household infections, especially in longhairs.[13, 38, 43, 66] However, both *M. gypseum* and *T. mentagrophytes* have been responsible for cattery dermatophytosis when the cats were housed in screened porch buildings or outdoor runs.[30] In catteries where *M. canis* infection has been present for over 60 days, the dermatophyte can be isolated from coat brushings of *all* cats, whether they have clinical lesions or not.[43, 66, 89]

Control options include three general approaches.[30, 38, 66] The first requires total depopulation of the cattery or household, decontamination of the facility, and repopulation with only animals that test negative on three consecutive brush cultures performed at 2-week intervals. Most breeders reject this because of the loss of their gene pool. The second approach requires treatment of the entire colony and facilities with appropriate topical medications, systemic therapy, and environmental clean-up. The colony is isolated, and breeding and showing are interrupted. The third option is to treat only the kittens. This is practical only for catteries, pet shops, or kitten mills that produce kittens for the pet cat market. The following recommendations have been reprinted, with slight modification, from Moriello's excellent article.[66]

Specific Recommendations for the Treatment of Infected Catteries

- **Treatment of Cats**

1. Perform toothbrush fungal cultures on all cats in the cattery and all animals in the household.
2. Isolate any animals that are found to be free of *M. canis*. These animals should be quarantined in a separate facility. Reculture these animals because they will probably be found to be infected with *M. canis* when recultured.
3. Isolate the cattery. Cats should not be sold, shown, or sent on breeding loans. New members should not be added, and breeding programs should be interrupted.
4. Clip the entire haircoat of all cats, especially those of longhaired cats. Be sure that all whiskers are clipped. Clipping should be performed in a room that is easy to decontaminate. The infected hairs should be burned or transferred to a plastic biohazard bag and autoclaved prior to disposal.[38] The individual performing the clipping should be dressed in disposable clothing to prevent infection from animal to human. Clipping should be repeated every month until the infection is eliminated.
5. Begin aggressive topical therapy with an antifungal dip (lime sulfur or enilconazole are preferred). Ideally, cats should be treated twice a week. The haircoat should be kept short.
6. Initiate oral griseofulvin therapy in all *nonpregnant* queens and kittens older than 12 weeks of age. Topical therapy should be continued. Monitoring complete blood counts and platelet counts in all cats, and especially in Persians, Himalayans, Abyssinians, and Siamese cats, is highly recommended. Many clients refuse to have precautionary blood work performed because of the cost. Be sure to warn clients clearly of the potential for toxicity.
7. The duration of treatment varies and may last from weeks to months (at least 12 to 16 weeks).[38] Continue treatment until *all* cats are culture-negative, using the toothbrush technique three times at weekly intervals. False-positive cultures can occur in cats that are clinically recovered, and cured of dermatophytosis, if they are living in a contaminated environment.[38, 71]
8. If a griseofulvin-resistant strain is suspected, confirm that the client is administering the griseofulvin correctly. If so, submit an *M. canis* culture for griseofulvin, ketoconazole, and itraconazole sensitivity testing. It may be necessary to contact the Centers for Disease Control and Prevention to locate the appropriate laboratory for performance of the testing.

- **Environmental Decontamination.** The critical role of premise disinfection in eradication of *M. canis* from an endemic cattery or household cannot be overemphasized.[38, 71] Even when a regular disinfection schedule was employed, the environment became severely contaminated (floors, walls, all inanimate objects in room).[36] This probably explains why all cats in such environments became culture-positive: They are constantly being contaminated from their environment. Whether such cats are truly infected by or only passively carrying *M. canis* is irrelevant because the presence of fungal elements on the haircoat is a potential human health hazard.

1. *M. canis* spores remain viable in the environment for up to 18 months. All nonporous surfaces should be thoroughly vacuumed and disinfected, including all floors, walls, countertops, windowsills, and transport vehicles. Sodium hypochlorite 0.5%, when added to a suspension of *M. canis* arthrospores for 5 minutes, prevented fungal growth on culture media.[84] Sodium hypochlorite 0.5%, when added to *M. canis*–infected cat hairs for 5 minutes twice weekly, prevented fungal growth only after 8 "treatments."[95] When 10 disinfectants were tested at various dilutions as single applications to a surface contaminated with *M. canis*–infected cats' hairs and spores, only undiluted bleach (5.25% sodium hypochlorite) or 1% formalin were able to inactivate infected cat hairs within 2 hours.[72] Enilconazole was effective within 8 hours.[72] When 14 disinfectants were repeatedly applied to isolated *M. canis*–infected cats' hairs, stabilized chlorine dioxide (Oxygene, Oxyfresh USA, Spokane, WA), glutaraldehyde and quaternary ammonium chloride (GPC 8, Solomon Industries, Cocoa, FL), potassium monoperoxysulfate (Virkon, S. Durvet, Blue Springs, MO), and a 0.525% sodium hypochlorite were the most effective.[72] Undiluted bleach is corrosive and irritating and cannot be safely used in homes or catteries. Because of its human health hazards, formalin solution is not recommended for routine use in disinfecting premises. Enilconazole sprays and "foggers" have been used successfully in Europe.[28, 38, 41]
2. Destroy all bedding, rugs, brushes, combs, and the like.
3. Rugs that cannot be destroyed or removed should be washed with an antifungal disinfectant. Be sure to recommend that the client test for colorfastness. Steam cleaning of carpets has been recommended as a method of decontamination. To kill fungal spores, the temperature of the water being forced into the carpets must be at least 43.3°C (110°F). Five do-it-yourself machines were tested to determine whether this was possible. To reach a temperature of 43.3°C (110°F) at the carpet level, the water chamber had to be filled with water exceeding 76.6°C (170°F). In a household situation, achieving this required boiling water to reach this temperature. Unfortunately, the temperature of the water rapidly cooled in the clean water reservoir, and within 15 minutes of filling the chamber, the temperature of the water being forced out of the nozzle was less than 37.7°C (100°F). Steam cleaning of carpets may therefore not be a reliable method of killing *M. canis* unless an antifungal disinfectant such as chlorhexidine or sodium hypochlorite is added to the water.
4. All heating and cooling vents should be vacuumed and disinfected. Furnaces should be cleaned with high-power suction equipment by a commercial company. Furnace filters should be changed weekly.
5. The cattery should be vacuumed daily, preferably twice daily. *Do not use fans.*
6. Cages should be disinfected daily.
7. Remind the cattery owner to disinfect all portable cages, automobiles, and so forth.
8. *Do not let the cats roam freely in the house or cattery.*

• **Treatment of Kittens Only.** In some situations, a cattery owner may be unable or unwilling to treat the entire cattery. If the owner is interested only in producing kittens that are not infected with *M. canis*, an alternative strategy is available. Although this strategy is not ideal, it is a reasonable alternative to depopulation and to the sale of *M. canis*–infected kittens to the public.

1. Isolate breeding and pregnant queens from the remainder of the cattery.
2. Clip the haircoat of the queens.
3. Treat the queens topically with lime sulfur or enilconazole dips twice weekly.
4. After the kittens are born, begin oral griseofulvin therapy in queens. Although griseofulvin is contraindicated in pregnant queens, some feline practitioners have routinely begun administering griseofulvin during the last week of pregnancy and have not observed any ill effects.
5. Wean the kittens as soon as possible, preferably by 4 weeks of age, and isolate

them from all other cats. Some cattery owners choose to separate the kittens from the queens at birth and to raise them in isolation.

6. When the kittens are 4 weeks of age, culture all of them with a sterile toothbrush. Pending fungal culture results, begin topical therapy. Lime sulfur and enilconazole have been reported to be safe in young kittens. If the fungal culture indicates that the kittens are infected, begin oral griseofulvin therapy. Oral griseofulvin is not recommended for use in kittens less than 12 weeks of age, although there is no specific product label contraindication to this practice; it has, however, been used in kittens as young as 6 to 8 weeks of age without any ill effects.[13, 28] The potential for griseofulvin toxicity should be thoroughly explained to the owner.

7. Kittens should not be sold until at least one, and preferably two, negative fungal cultures have been obtained.

• **Monitoring Response to Therapy.** Response to therapy in both cats and kittens is best monitored via fungal culturing. The toothbrush culturing technique is recommended. It is critical that the brushing be aggressive during this period. During treatment, the number of infective spores decreases, and if the individual sampling is not aggressive enough with combing, false-negative results could be obtained. Do not use a Wood lamp to monitor therapy because this device is much less reliable than culturing.

• **Preventive Measures.** The prevention of the introduction or re-introduction of *M. canis* into a cattery requires the isolation of any new cats, the isolation of cats returning from shows or breeding loans, and periodic culturing of the entire colony. Cats entering or re-entering the cattery should be cultured for *M. canis* and kept in isolation until the results are obtained. It is suggested that these cats be dipped or washed with one of the previously mentioned products during this isolation period to minimize contamination of the cattery in the event that they are infected. It is difficult to decontaminate the environment, and re-infection is possible. Ideally, there should be no visitors to the cattery so that introduction of the organism from clothing or other fomites can be prevented.

Cat shows present a tremendous threat to an *M. canis*–free cattery because it is extremely difficult to prevent re-infection and to prevent exposure to spores.[38] The cats should be groomed in an area free of other cats, if possible, and no grooming equipment from other exhibitors should be used. The cat carriers should be covered when cats are not being examined by the judges.

Candidiasis

CAUSE AND PATHOGENESIS

Candida spp. yeasts are normal inhabitants of the alimentary, upper respiratory, and genital mucosa of mammals.[1-3, 9, 96, 101, 102] *Candida* spp., especially *Candida albicans* and *Candida parapsilosis*, are isolated from the ears, nose, oral cavity, and anus of clinically normal dogs and dogs with candidiasis.[97-105] *Candida tropicalis*, *Candida pseudotropicalis*, *Candida krusei*, *Candida stellatoidea*, and *Candida guilliermondii* are occasionally found. *Candida* species cause opportunistic infections of skin, mucocutaneous areas, external ear canal, and claws. Factors that upset the normal endogenous microflora (prolonged antibiotic therapy) or disrupt normal cutaneous or mucosal barriers (maceration, burns, indwelling catheters) provide a pathway for *Candida* spp. to enter the body.[101, 102] Once in the body, further spread of infection correlates with cell-mediated immunocompetence and neutrophil function.[101, 102] Immunosuppressive disease states (diabetes mellitus, hyperadrenocorticism, hypothyroidism, viral infections, cancer, inherited immunologic defects) or immunosuppressive drug therapy predispose some animals to candidiasis.[101, 102] *Candida* spp. produce acid proteinases and keratinases (degrade stratum corneum) and phospholipases (penetration of tissues).[102]

Candidiasis has been reported under the following names in earlier literature: *candidosis*, *moniliasis*, and *thrush*.

CLINICAL FINDINGS

Dog

Candidiasis is a rare disease with a distinct predilection for mucous membranes (see Fig. 5–5D), mucocutaneous junctions, or areas in which moisture may persist and macerate the skin, such as the external ear canal and lateral pinnae, intertriginous areas, the clawbed, and interdigital areas (see Fig. 5–5E).[97, 100–102] Pruritus may be intense.[102] On mucous membranes, the lesions appear as foul-smelling, nonhealing ulcers covered with thick, whitish gray plaques with erythematous borders.[13, 102] On the skin, lesions are initially papular and pustular and evolve into oozing erythematous plaques and ulcers.[90, 100, 102, 104]

Candida infection should always be suspected in a dog with erythema and oozing affecting one or two paws when there has been no response to antibiotics and glucocorticoids.[99] Solitary or locally grouped lesions may resemble pyotraumatic dermatitis or staphylococcal infection.[100, 105] In two dogs, the lesions were more hyperkeratotic and crusted, affecting especially the nose, face, pinnae, genitalia, and footpads.[97, 104] One dog experienced three nodules on the neck and lateral thighs associated with *Candida zeylanoides* after injections of calcium gluconate.[103] Candidiasis isolated to the clawbeds is rare.[11] Candidiasis rarely presents as a mucocutaneous ulcerative disorder.[13]

Cat

Candidiasis involving the skin is extremely rare in cats. Lesions include erythema, erosions, ulcers, crusts, and oozing in intertriginous areas, paws, and mucocutaneous junctions.[98] Bilateral, ulcerative otitis externa has been reported.[102] One cat experienced vesicles and ulcers of the mucocutaneous areas of the nose, lips, prepuce, and anus, as well as the oral cavity, after 2 weeks of tetracycline therapy for an upper respiratory infection.[8] Nystatin therapy was curative.

DIAGNOSIS

The differential diagnosis for localized forms of candidiasis includes pyotraumatic dermatitis, staphylococcal infection, and intertrigo. Mucocutaneous candidiasis must be differentiated from immunologic diseases (e.g., pemphigus vulgaris, bullous pemphigoid, epidermolysis bullosa acquisita, systemic lupus erythematosus, erythema multiforme), drug eruptions, necrolytic migratory erythema, thallium poisoning, epitheliotropic lymphoma, and other unusual infections (leishmaniasis, protothecosis, phaeohyphomycosis). Cytologic examination of direct smears reveals suppurative inflammation and numerous yeasts (2 to 6 μm in diameter) and blastoconidia (budding cells).[1–3, 9, 10, 101, 102] Pseudohyphae may occasionally occur. In contrast with *Malassezia pachydermatis*, *Candida* spp. show narrow-based and multilateral budding.[102] Biopsy findings include suppurative epidermitis, parakeratotic hyperkeratosis, and occasionally suppurative superficial folliculitis. Numerous yeasts and blastoconidia are present in the keratin of the surface epidermis and infundibular portion of hair follicles (Fig. 5–15). Pseudohyphae and true hyphae may also occur. *Candida* species grow on Sabouraud's dextrose agar at 25° to 30°C. The API 20C system is a convenient and reliable system for identification.

CLINICAL MANAGEMENT

Correction of predisposing causes is fundamental. Excessive moisture must be avoided. For localized lesions, clipping, drying, and topical antifungal agents are usually effective. Useful topical agents include nystatin (100,000 U/g), azoles (2% miconazole, 1% clotrimazole), 3% amphotericin B, gentian violet (1:10,000 in 10% alcohol), and potassium permanganate (1:3000 in water).[13, 101, 102] These agents should be applied two to three times daily until lesions are completely healed (1 to 4 weeks).

Oral, widespread mucocutaneous, and generalized lesions require systemic antifungal therapy.[101, 102] Although intravenous amphotericin B is effective, ketoconazole or itracona-

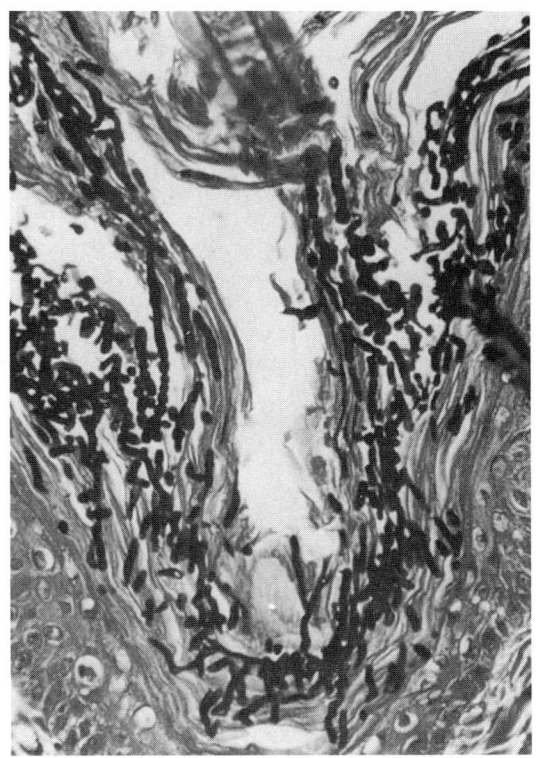

FIGURE 5–15. Candidiasis in a dog. Numerous yeasts and pseudohyphae in hair follicle. (Courtesy M. Pichler-Schick.)

zole administered orally is the drug of choice.[101, 102] Therapy should be continued for 7 to 10 days beyond clinical cure (2 to 4 weeks).

Malassezia Dermatitis

CAUSE AND PATHOGENESIS

Malassezia pachydermatis (M. canis, Pityrosporum pachydermatis, P. canis) is a lipophilic, non–lipid-dependent, nonmycelial saprophytic yeast that is commonly found on normal and abnormal skin, in normal and abnormal ear canals, on mucosal surfaces (oral, anal), and in the anal sacs and vagina of normal dogs and cats.[13, 113, 134, 135, 138, 138a, 139, 146] *M. pachydermatis* can be isolated from the skin of 3-day-old puppies.[156] It is possible that mucosal carriage plays a role in skin colonization and infection through licking and grooming. Topical treatments of Basset hounds with *Malassezia* dermatitis produced significantly reduced population sizes and frequency of isolation of *M. pachydermatis* from the skin and the oral cavity.[125] This might indicate that oral carriage reflects contamination of the mucosae by constant seeding from a reservoir of the yeast on the skin. Alternatively, reduced yeast counts in the mouth could have resulted from a direct antiyeast effect by transfer of the topical agent to the oral mucosae by licking.

Recent advances in electrophoretic karyotyping have shown that the genus *Malassezia* contains six lipid-dependent species (*M. furfur* [*P. ovale*], *M. globosa, M. obtusa, M. restricta, M. slooffiae,* and *M. sympodialis*) and one non–lipid-dependent species (*M. pachydermatis*).[106, 108, 135, 136] *Malassezia sympodialis* and *M. globosa* have been isolated from the skin and external ear canal of healthy cats.[118, 122] In one study, *Malassezia* spp were isolated more frequently from cats infected with FeLV and/or FIV.[13a]

The diversity of *M. pachydermatis* isolates from a wide variety of hosts was investigated, and seven types or strains (sequevars), Ia through Ig, were identified.[105a, 137, 138, 146a]

The predominant sequevar, type Ia, appeared to be ubiquitous, whereas type Id was exclusively recovered from dogs. None of the seven sequevars correlated with isolation from healthy skin or a particular lesion (otitis externa or dermatitis). In addition, this study indicated that the skin of a given animal may be colonized by more than one type of *M. pachydermatis*. A recent study identified a strain that was different from the seven previously described and two isolates that more closely resembled *M. furfur*.[105a]

Malassezia pachydermatis is a commensal on canine and feline skin and in the external ear canal. It is thought to have a symbiotic relationship with commensal staphylococci, wherein the organisms produce mutually beneficial growth factors and microenvironmental alterations that are mutually beneficial.[138, 146] Hence, it is not surprising that dogs with *Malassezia* have increased numbers of *S. intermedius* on their skin[112, 115] and frequent concurrent staphylococcal pyodermas.[126, 134] Trypsin-sensitive proteins or glycoproteins on yeast cell walls are important for adherence to canine corneocytes,[116] and mannosyl-bearing carbohydrate residues on canine corneocytes serve as ligands for adhesins expressed by *M. pachydermatis*.[119] There is variability among strains of the organism, however.[119, 124] Enhanced adherence of *M. pachydermatis* to corneocytes does not appear to be important in the pathogenesis of *Malassezia* dermatitis in Basset hounds.[120]

Because *M. pachydermatis* does not invade subcorneally, dermatitis is hypothesized to result from inflammatory and/or hypersensitivity reactions to yeast products and antigens.[138, 146] Virulence factors for *M. pachydermatis* have not been characterized. It has been shown that *M. pachydermatis* isolated from dogs with dermatitis and otitis externa produces proteases, lipases, lipoxygenases, phosphatases, phosphohydralases, glucosidase, galactosidase, leucine arylamidase, urease, and zymosan.[108a, 130, 138, 145, 146] These substances could contribute to the pathogenesis, inflammation, and pruritus of *Malassezia* dermatitis through proteolysis, lipolysis, alteration of local pH, eicosanoid release, and complement activation. *Malassezia* strains from healthy dogs contain significantly greater amounts of C4 esterase activity.[108a]

The protein fractions of *M. pachydermatis* isolates from dogs with *Malassezia* otitis externa or *Malassezia* dermatitis were investigated by gel electrophoresis.[128] A number of protein bands were identified, and there were no statistical differences in terms of the number of protein bands and their molecular weight values between isolates from the ear or the skin. Neither is there any clear association between the particular protein(s) expressed and the origin of the *Malassezia* strain (e.g., normal versus infected dogs).[108a] Western immunoblotting identified 14 bands of immunoreactivity, and there were significantly more bands in Basset hounds with *Malassezia* dermatitis than in healthy Basset hounds, Beagles, and Irish setters.[108a]

Histologically, *Malassezia* dermatitis is often characterized by prominent exocytosis of lymphocytes (CD3-positive) and a subepithelial accumulation of mast cells, which suggest a hypersensitivity reaction.[146] Immediate intradermal skin test reactivity to *M. pachydermatis* antigens was reported in 30% of 46 dogs with "seborrheic dermatitis"[149] and all atopic dogs with concurrent *Malassezia* dermatitis,[147, 148] whereas all normal dogs and atopic dogs without concurrent *Malassezia* dermatitis did not react. In humans, concerns have been raised over the number of in vitro cross-reactions between commercial house dust mite allergen extracts and *M. furfur*.[157] Because the substrates for house dust mite cultures usually contain human skin scales, *M. furfur* organisms might be in the mite cultures. However, cross-reactivity between *M. pachydermatis* antigens and house dust mite or mold antigens was not found.[148]

Hypersensitivity to *Malassezia* antigens is also thought to be important in atopic humans.[140, 146] The levels of *M. pachydermatis*–specific IgG (by enzyme-linked immunosorbent assay [ELISA]) were significantly greater in dogs with *Malassezia* dermatitis than in normal dogs.[123] One investigator found significantly higher levels of specific IgG (by ELISA) in atopic dogs—with or without concurrent *Malassezia* dermatitis—than in nonatopic dogs with *Malassezia* dermatitis or normal dogs.[150]

Many predisposing factors have been hypothesized to allow the commensal *M. pachydermatis* to become a pathogen.[126, 134, 138, 144, 146] Increased humidity is probably important because *Malassezia* seems to be more common in humid climates (e.g., summer) and in certain anatomic locations (e.g., ear canals, skin folds). Skin folds were thought to be the predisposing factor in 16% to 28% of the canine cases in two studies.[126, 134] Increased availability of yeast nutrients and growth factors are also probably important: hormonal alterations of the quantity and quality of sebum, "seborrheic" skin (keratinization disorders), increased populations of commensal symbiotic staphylococci.

Immunologic dysfunction—especially as concerns cell-mediated immunity and secretory IgA—could play a role in the pathogenesis of *M. pachydermatis* infection.[126, 134, 144, 146] Chronic glucocorticoid therapy could have a precipitating role here. Healthy Basset hounds and Beagles experienced significantly greater in vitro lymphocyte blastogenic response to *M. pachydermatis* antigen than did Basset hounds with *Malassezia* dermatitis.[123] Serum titers of *M. pachydermatis*–specific IgG and IgA (measured by ELISA) in Basset hounds and other breeds with *Malassezia* dermatitis exceeded those of healthy Basset hounds and Beagles, suggesting that serum antibody responses confer no protection against *Malassezia* infection.[123] Widespread *Malassezia* dermatitis in cats has been associated with concurrent FIV infection,[13, 98, 144] thymoma,[131] and pancreatic adenocarcinoma.[132] As mentioned previously, hypersensitivity to *M. pachydermatis* antigens likely plays an important role in many dogs.

Genetic predisposition would appear to be important because certain breeds—especially the West Highland white terrier, Basset hound, American Cocker spaniel, Shih Tzu, English setter, and Dachshund—are at significantly increased risk for *Malassezia* dermatitis.[115, 138, 146, 151]

It is commonly stated that *Malassezia* dermatitis in dogs is usually secondary to an ongoing skin disorder, predominantly hypersensitivity diseases (especially atopy), keratinization defects ("seborrhea"), recurrent bacterial pyodermas, and endocrine diseases (especially hypothyroidism).[13, 138, 144, 146] Indeed, 72% to 83% of the dogs with *Malassezia* dermatitis in two large studies had dermatoses that preceded the occurrence of yeast infection.[134, 146] However, the significance of these "underlying" diseases remains to be delineated.[146] In one study, the prevalence of atopy, primary keratinization defects, and endocrinopathies in dogs with *Malassezia* dermatitis was comparable with that in dogs seen for dermatologic disease, in general.[115]

It has been shown that numbers of cutaneous *M. pachydermatis* are significantly greater in the groin, interdigital spaces, ear canals, and directly under the tail base of atopic dogs than in normal dogs.[109, 110, 157] In addition, normal dogs are significantly more likely to have negative cultures for *M. pachydermatis* than atopic dogs.[155] Atopic dogs with interdigital erythema had significantly higher numbers of yeast in interdigital scrapings than did atopic dogs without interdigital erythema.[157] It is certainly possible that any dermatosis that results in disruption of the stratum corneum barrier—be that mechanical as a response to pruritus or biochemical as a result of keratinization, endocrinologic, and immunologic abnormalities—could permit the subcorneal immune system and inflammatory cascades to be exposed to *Malassezia* antigens and products.

It has been suggested that canine *Malassezia* dermatitis is often associated with prior antibiotic therapy.[13, 138, 144, 146, 151] This has not been sufficiently corroborated. In fact, unlike *Candida* spp., *Malassezia* populations are not subject to the inhibitory effects of bacteria.

CLINICAL FINDINGS

Dog

Malassezia dermatitis is common in dogs.* It occurs in dogs of any age, sex, and breed. The following breeds are predisposed: West Highland white terrier, Basset hound, American Cocker spaniel, Shih Tzu, English setter, and Dachshund.[115, 138, 146, 151] The dermatitis often begins in the summer or highly humid months, which also correspond to the allergy season (pollens, molds), and then persists into winter. Over 70% of the dogs have

---

*See references 5, 126, 129, 134, 138, 143, 144, 146.

concurrent dermatoses, especially allergies, keratinization defects, endocrinopathies, and bacterial pyodermas.[134, 146]

Pruritus is a major sign and is virtually constant. Dogs with generalized skin disease (exfoliative erythroderma) are erythematous, greasy or waxy, scaly (yellow or slate gray), and crusty. They often have an offensive, rancid, or yeasty odor (Fig. 5–16A; see Fig. 5–5F, G, and H). Chronic cases can have marked lichenification and hyperpigmentation. Regional dermatitis occurs on the ears, lips, muzzle, interdigital spaces, ventral neck, medial thighs, groin, axillae, perianal region, and intertriginous areas. Focal scaly plaques and erythematous macules and patches may coalesce into serpiginous tracts. Some dogs may have a contact dermatitis–like disease, with remarkably well-demarcated ventral distribution ("waterline disease"). Others have a papulocrustous dermatitis resembling superficial staphylococcal infection or interdigital furuncles ("cysts"). *Malassezia* paronychia and/or claw infections produce red-brown discoloration of paronychial hairs or claws (see Fig. 5–16B).[133] Occasionally, the dog is presented for so-called frenzied fits of nose and lip scratching with the front paws. Otitis externa associated with *Malassezia* infection is discussed in Chapter 19.

Remember that most dogs with *Malassezia* dermatitis have concurrent dermatoses.[126, 134, 144, 146] In addition, about 40% of the dogs with *Malassezia* dermatitis have concurrent staphylococcal pyoderma.[126, 134]

Cat

Malassezia dermatitis *(M. pachydermatis)* is rarely reported in cats; when found, it may be associated with a black and waxy otitis externa (see Chap. 19), recalcitrant feline chin acne, refractory paronychia, and a generalized erythematous, scaly to waxy dermatitis (exfoliative erythroderma) (Figs. 5–17, 5–18).[13, 98, 138, 144] Recurrent, generalized *Malassezia* dermatitis has been observed in cats with FIV infection,[98, 144] in one cat with a thymoma,[131] and in one cat with paraneoplastic alopecia associated with a pancreatic adenocarcinoma.[132] *Malassezia sympodialis* was consistently isolated from the ears of a group of cats with mild otic pruritus and mild to moderate accumulations of yellow to brown cerumen in the external ear canals.[118] Signs of inflammation were not present. *M. furfur* was isolated from the ears in one of 33 normal cats.[128a]

Zoonotic Aspects

Malassezia pachydermatis has been cultured from the blood, urine, and cerebrospinal fluid of low-birth-weight neonates that were receiving intravenous lipid emulsions in an intensive care facility.[127] An identical strain of *M. pachydermatis* was cultured from one health worker and pet dogs. These problems were terminated when handwashing procedures were enforced.

DIAGNOSIS

The differential diagnosis is extensive and includes atopy, food hypersensitivity, flea bite hypersensitivity, drug eruption, superficial staphylococcal folliculitis, demodicosis, feline acne, scabies, acanthosis nigricans, contact dermatitis, seborrheic dermatitis, and epitheliotropic lymphoma. The diagnosis can be even more perplexing for the clinician because *Malassezia* dermatitis is often associated with one or more of the potential differential diagnoses. *Malassezia* dermatitis should be considered a factor in any scaly, erythematous, greasy to waxy, pruritic dermatitis in which other differential diagnoses have been eliminated by diagnostic tests and there is a lack of response to treatment (e.g., glucocorticoids, antibiotics, antiseborrheic shampoos, insecticides, miticides).

The most useful and readily available tool for the clinician presented with a suspected case of *Malassezia* dermatitis is cytologic examination.[126, 134, 138, 144, 146] Samples of surface scale or grease are gathered by making a superficial skin scraping, vigorously rubbing a cotton swab on the skin surface, pressing a piece of clear cellophane tape onto lesional skin several times, or pressing a section of a clean glass microscope slide on the skin.[13, 134, 144, 146] It is not clear which of these methods is the best, and each has its own benefits and

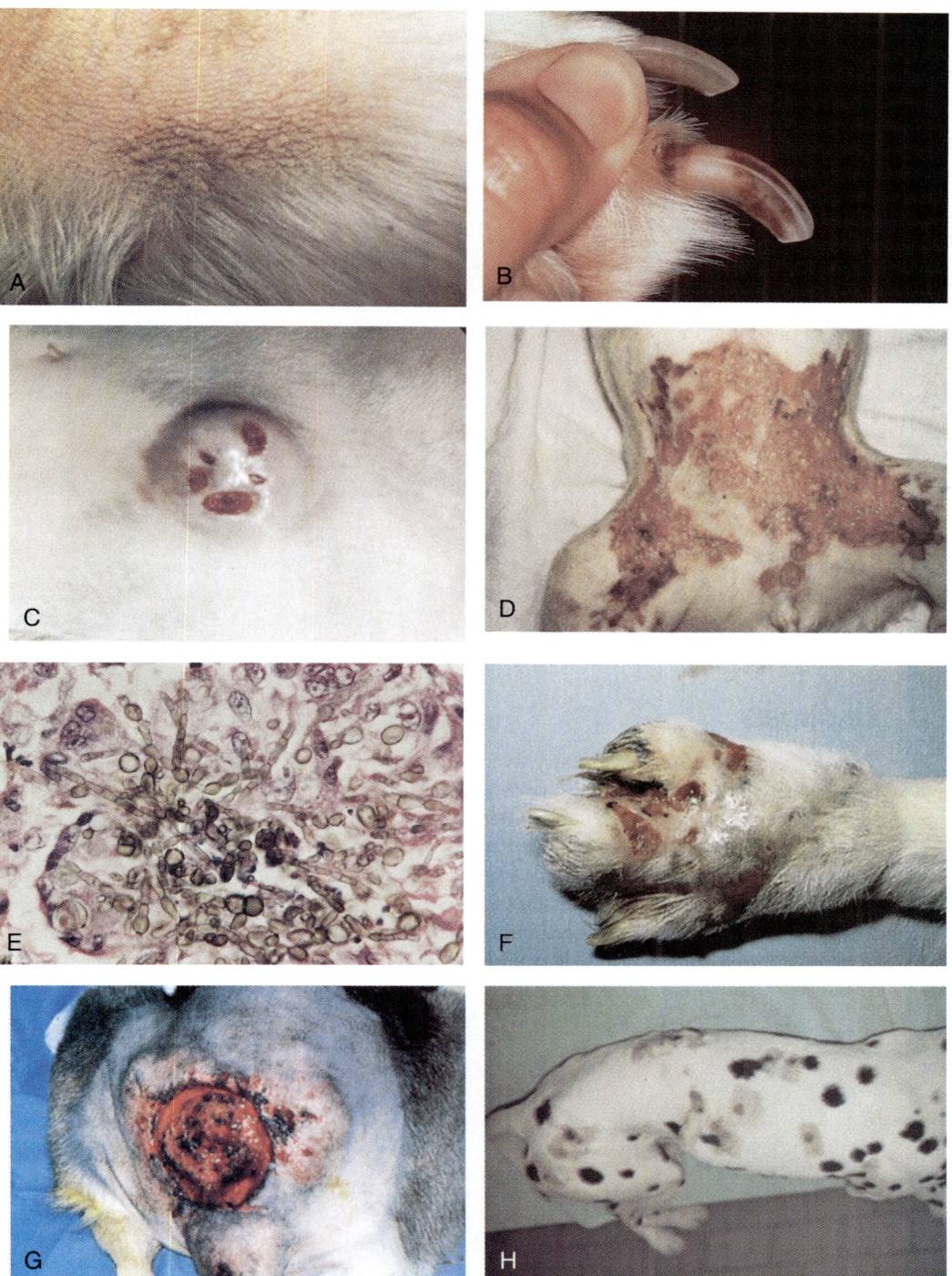

FIGURE 5-16. Miscellaneous fungal infections. *A*, *Malassezia* dermatitis in a dog. Alopecia, erythema, and yellowish brown, crumbly surface debris. *B*, *M. pachydermatis* infection of dog's claw. The red-brown discoloration of the distal and proximal claw is caused by the infection. The normal area of claw in between represents the time period when the dog was being treated with ketoconazole. *C*, Phaeohyphomycosis in a cat. Truncal nodule that is multifocally ulcerated. *D*, Phaeohyphomycosis in a dog. The ulcerative dermatitis on the ventral abdomen and medial thighs is more or less symmetric. (Courtesy K. Kwochka.) *E*, Phaeohyphomycosis in a cat. Numerous greenish brown fungal elements in granulomatous dermatitis. *F*, Pythiosis in a dog. Swollen paw with multiple areas of necrosis and ulceration. (Courtesy D. Chester.) *G*, Ulcerated nodules over the lumbosacral area of a dog with pythiosis. (Courtesy C. Foil.) *H*, Sporotrichosis in a Dalmatian. Widely scattered crusted plaques (hair has been clipped around each lesion).

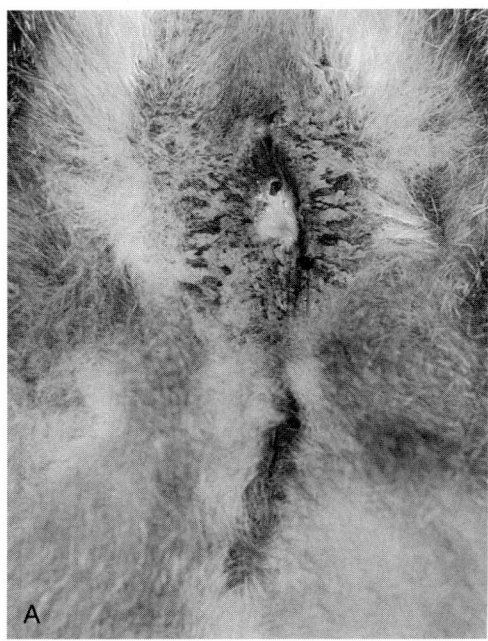
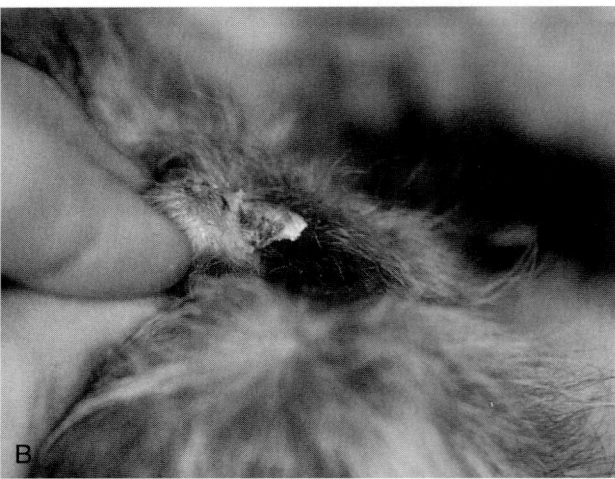

FIGURE 5–17. *Malassezia* dermatitis in a cat. *A*, Alopecia, erythema, and accumulation of dark brown waxy material in perianal region. (Courtesy D. Carlotti.) *B*, *Malassezia* paronychia in a cat. (Courtesy C. Tieghi.)

shortcomings. *Superficial scrapings* are reliable but can be difficult to perform in certain areas (interdigital spaces, facial folds). *Tape strips* are good where the skin surface is flat and not overly waxy or greasy. *Direct impression with a glass slide* is good for flat surfaces and where grease and wax are plentiful. *Cotton swab (Q-Tip) smears* are good for ears, interdigital spaces, and facial folds. In normal dogs, impression smears, skin scrapings, and swabs gave similar results.[139] Other investigators found scrapings and tape strippings to be superior to swabs.[109, 157] Still others have found tape stripping to be unsatisfactory.[134] Results of a study on dogs with *Malassezia* pododermatitis indicated no statistically significant difference between the numbers of yeasts recovered with superficial scrapings, tape strippings, and direct impressions.[107] However, swabs were significantly inferior to the other three techniques.[107]

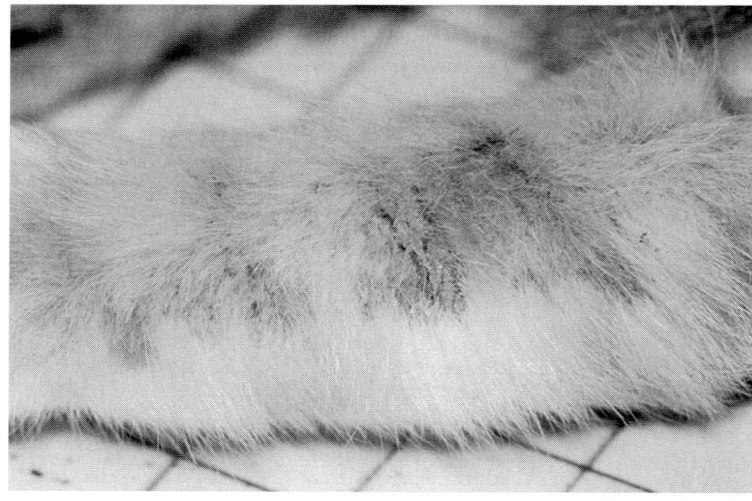

FIGURE 5–18. *Malassezia* dermatitis in a cat. Patchy alopecia, scaling, crusting, and accumulations of dark brown waxy debris on medial surface of forearm. (Courtesy D. Carlotti.)

Whichever method is used, all material is transferred to a glass slide, heat-fixed (not if cellophane tape has been used!), and stained for cytologic examination. Heat fixing can be avoided by using a direct stain such as New Methylene Blue. One looks for yeasts that are round to oval or the classic peanut shape. *Malassezia pachydermatis* is characterized by monopolar budding of daughter cells from one site on the cell wall, formation of a prominent bud scar or collar at the site of daughter cell development, a peanut shape, and a diameter of 3 to 8 μm.[138] Yeasts are often visible in clusters or adhered to keratinocytes (Fig. 5–19). *Malassezia sympodialis* has a more rounded, bulbous shape and a narrower-based monopolar budding, and it is smaller than *M. pachydermatis*.

The full diagnostic value of cytologic examination remains to be determined. An extensive study of normal dog skin sampled by impression smears, skin scrapings, and swabs revealed that most specimens contained less than 10 organisms/1.25 cm^2 (0.5 in^2) of sample (median value of one organism per sample).[139] Another study of normal and affected skin of dogs with various dermatoses, sampled by impression smears, revealed that normal skin had less than one organism/high-power field (HPF), whereas affected skin had less than one organism/HPF (80% of samples) or one to three organisms/HPF (20% of samples).[151]

Other investigators consider that *Malassezia* dermatitis is more likely when greater than 10 organisms are visible in 15 randomly chosen oil-immersion microscopic fields (1000×) using tape strip samples,[109] when an average of greater than or equal to four organisms are visible per oil-immersion microscopic field,[134] when an average of greater than or equal to one organism is visible in 10 oil-immersion microscopic fields,[126] or when greater than two organisms/HPF (400×) are found with any of the commonly used sampling techniques.[146]

Swabs taken from claw beds revealed the following: an average of 0.44 organisms/oil-immersion field in normal dogs; an average of 0.44 organisms/oil-immersion field in dogs with pedal pruritus; and an average of 7.9 organisms/oil-immersion field in dogs with atopy, pedal pruritus, and red-brown staining of claws and/or paronychial skin.[133] Further

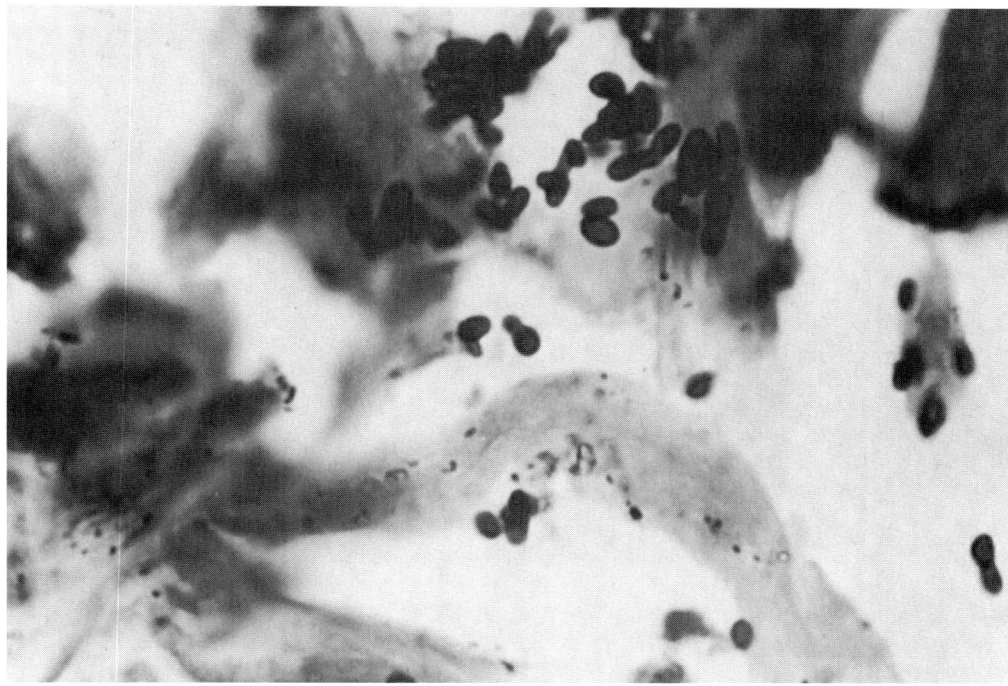

FIGURE 5–19. Superficial skin scraping from a dog with *Malassezia* dermatitis. Numerous budding yeasts among the squames.

confusion is added by the following findings: *M. pachydermatis* numbers are significantly larger (1) on healthy Basset hounds than on healthy Irish setters,[120] (2) in the ears of laboratory Beagles than in the ears of pet dogs of several breeds,[157] (3) on pet Beagles than on other pet dogs,[113] and (4) on healthy Basset hounds than on healthy mongrels.[121] In addition, population size and frequency of isolation of *M. pachydermatis* vary on different body sites.[113, 121] Clearly, there is great variability in diagnostic criteria used and significant differences between breeds and body sites.

Skin biopsy findings in dogs are characterized by a superficial perivascular-to-interstitial dermatitis with irregular hyperplasia, diffuse spongiosis, and diffuse lymphocytic exocytosis of the epidermis and follicular infundibulum (Figs. 5–20, 5–21).[134, 146] Parakeratosis is prominent (Fig. 5–22), and dermal inflammatory cells are dominated by lymphocytes, histiocytes, and plasma cells. Eosinophils, neutrophils, and mast cells are common. Yeasts are visible in surface and/or infundibular keratin in about 70% of cases (see Fig. 5–22). They are randomly distributed. Eosinophilic epidermal microabscesses may be visible in about 14% of cases, and mast cells are linearly aligned at the dermoepidermal junction in about 47% of cases (Fig. 5–23).[146] Signs of concurrent bacterial infection (suppurative epidermitis and folliculitis) are common.[134, 146]

Uncommonly, yeasts may be visible in association with suppurative folliculitis and pyogranulomatous furunculosis (especially chin and feet) (Fig. 5–24). In cats, one may see a hydropic interface dermatitis wherein lymphocytes and eosinophils are the dominant inflammatory cells. It must be remembered that yeasts are occasionally visible on the surface of biopsies from numerous canine and feline dermatoses and yet play no known role in their pathogenesis or treatment.[153, 154] Yeasts present in hair follicles, however, must always be assumed to be possibly pathogenic.

The majority of intraepithelial and dermal lymphocytes in dogs with *Malassezia* dermatitis are CD3-positive (T cells).[146] Immunofluorescence testing revealed immunoglobu-

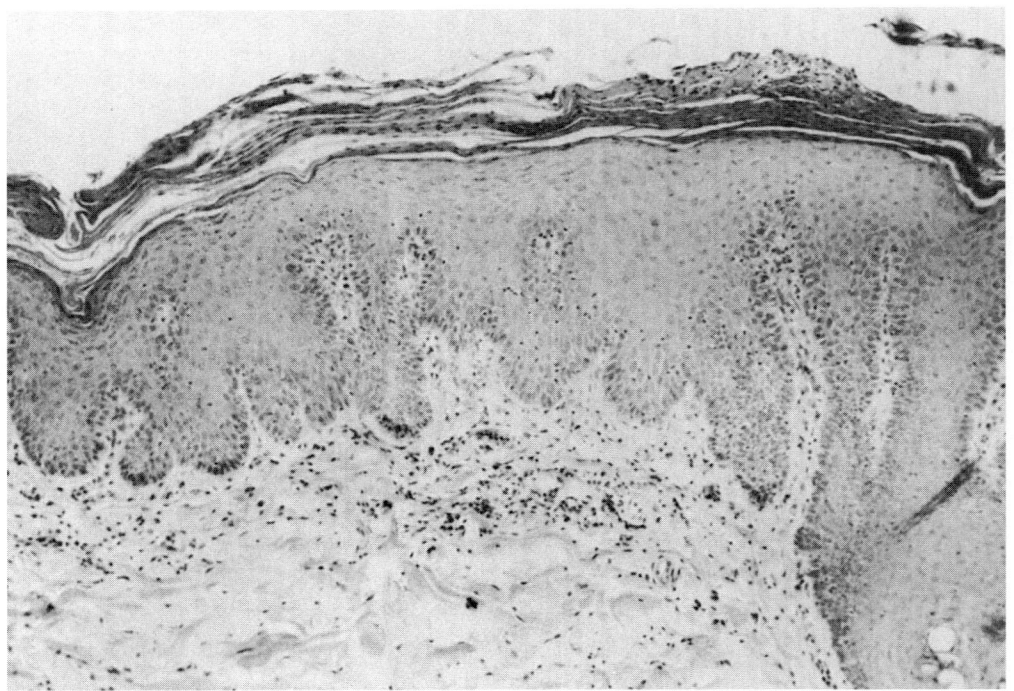

FIGURE 5–20. *Malassezia* dermatitis in a dog. Superficial interstitial dermatitis with parakeratotic hyperkeratosis, spongiosis, and lymphocytic exocytosis.

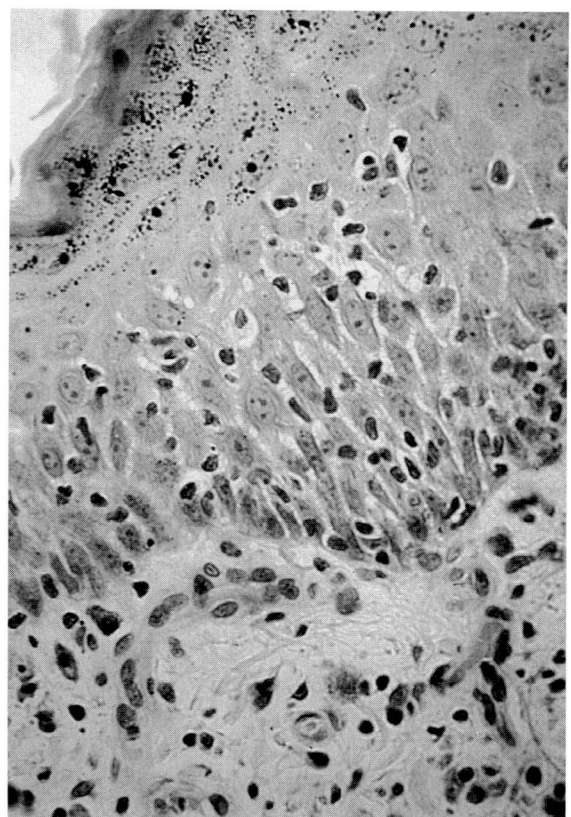

FIGURE 5–21. *Malassezia* dermatitis in a dog. Epidermal hyperplasia, spongiosis, and exocytosis of lymphocytes.

lin deposited in the intercellular spaces or basement membrane zone in 10% and 23%, respectively, of the cases examined.[146]

Malassezia pachydermatis is usually easy to culture.[110, 111, 117, 135, 138] Because it is not lipid-dependent, it grows well on routine Sabouraud's dextrose agar at 32° to 37°C. However, some strains of *M. pachydermatis* do show poor growth on unsupplemented media.[114] An atmosphere containing 5% to 10% carbon dioxide significantly increased the frequency of isolation and colony counts on Sabouraud's dextrose agar but not on modified Dixon's agar.[117] The lipid-dependent *Malassezia* spp. will not grow on Sabouraud's dextrose agar and require alternative, supplemented media.[118, 122, 138] Modified Dixon's agar grows all *Malassezia* spp.[110, 111, 118, 122, 138] Because *Malassezia* spp. are commensal organisms, their isolation in culture is of little or no practical diagnostic value.[107, 146]

Ultimately, the diagnosis of *Malassezia* dermatitis rests on the response to antiyeast treatment.[13, 107, 126, 134, 138, 144, 146] We have seen dogs with classic historical and clinical findings wherein various surface sampling techniques demonstrated little or no yeast, yet these dogs responded completely to specific treatment. These cases truly emphasize the hypersensitivity nature of this disease in some patients.

CLINICAL MANAGEMENT

The treatment of *Malassezia* dermatitis is individualized according to severity and various dog and owner considerations. Although topical therapy is often effective, this can be difficult in large dogs, in dogs with long or thick haircoats, in obstreperous dogs, or for

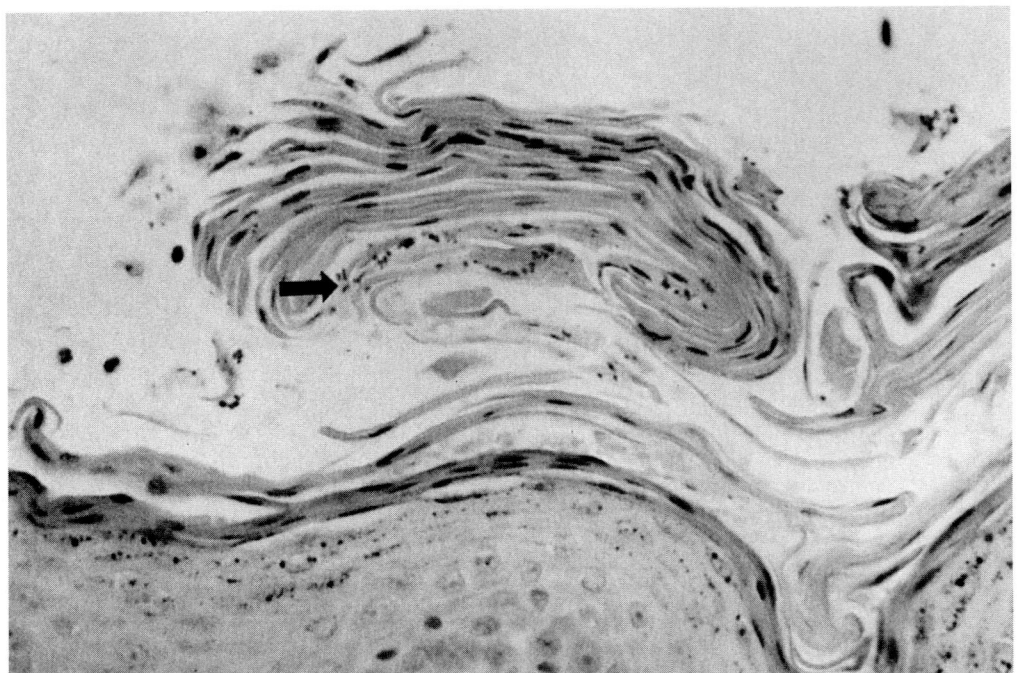

FIGURE 5–22. *Malassezia* dermatitis in a dog. Budding yeasts in surface keratin *(arrow)*.

elderly or physically challenged owners. A combination of topical and systemic therapy would be the most rapidly and totally effective.

Focal areas of *Malassezia* dermatitis (e.g., skin fold) may be easily treated with the daily spot application of an antifungal cream, ointment, lotion, or spray (see page 409).[142, 144, 146] Multifocal or more generalized cases are treated with total body applications of shampoos and/or rinses (see page 410).[112, 126, 134, 138, 141, 144, 146] Miconazole 2% (Dermazole, Miconazole Shampoo), chlorhexidine 3% (Hexadene) or 4% (Chlorhexi-Derm Maximum), and combinations of 2% miconazole and 2% chlorhexidine are excellent shampoos. If the animal is very greasy, waxy, and scaly, these shampoos should

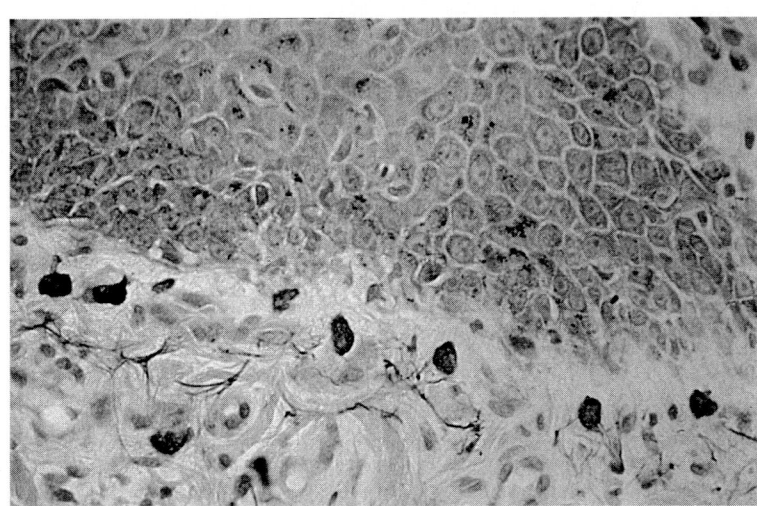

FIGURE 5–23. *Malassezia* dermatitis in a dog. Linear alignment of mast cells at the dermoepidermal junction (AOG stain).

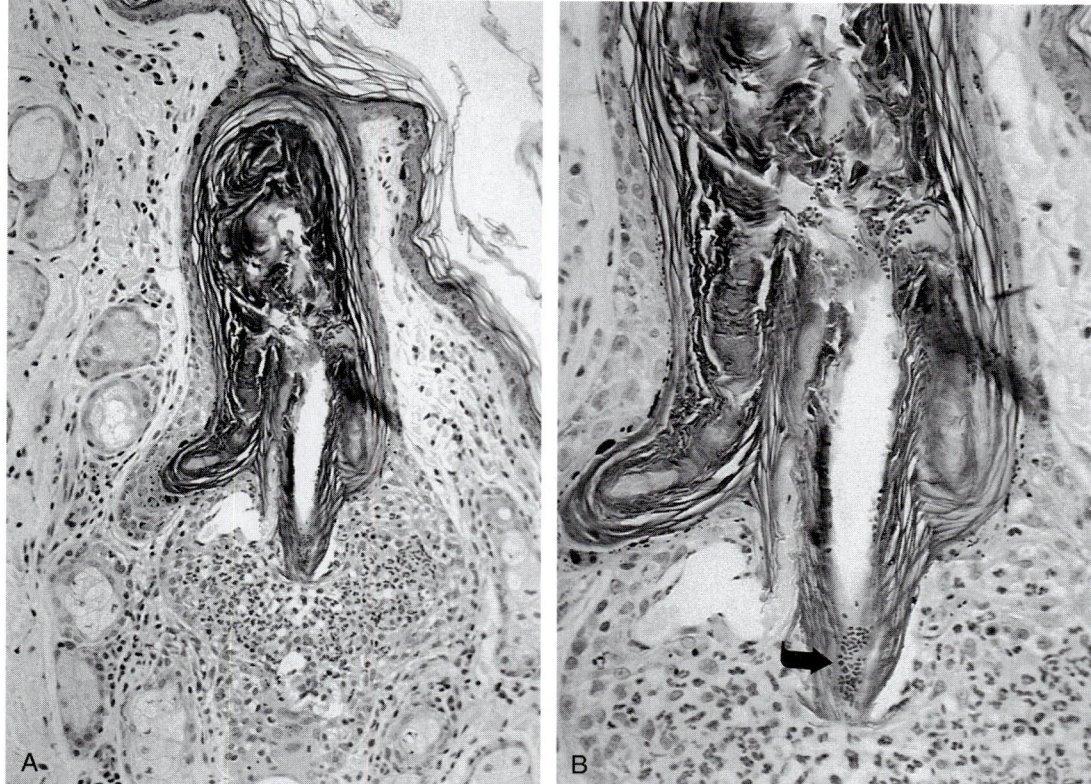

FIGURE 5–24. *A*, *Malassezia* dermatitis in a dog. Suppurative luminal folliculitis and follicular keratosis. *B*, Close-up of *A*. Note numerous yeast bodies in follicular keratin *(arrow)*.

be preceded by a keratolytic degreasing shampoo. Alternatively, selenium sulfide 1% shampoo is keratolytic, degreasing, and antiyeast all in one. For stubborn cases, twice-weekly shampoos can be followed by leave-on rinses such as lime sulfur 2% (LymDyp), acetic acid 2.5% (one part water : one part vinegar), or enilconazole 0.2% (Imaverol).[126, 134, 138, 144, 146] Enilconazole is not licensed for use in the United States.

Wherein topical therapy is unsuccessful or undesirable, the oral azoles are effective. The most commonly used drug is ketoconazole (Nizoral) at 10 mg/kg q24h PO.[13, 133, 134, 138, 146] Itraconazole and fluconazole are effective but expensive. Griseofulvin and the allylamine antifungals are not effective.

Dramatic clinical improvement occurs within 7 days with combined systemic and topical therapy, within 7 to 14 days with systemic therapy alone, and within 14 days with topical therapy alone. Therapy should be continued for 7 to 10 days beyond clinical cure. An average duration of treatment would be 4 weeks.

Because most cases of *Malassezia* dermatitis are associated with concurrent dermatoses, recognition and control of these possible predisposing factors may be critical to success and prevention of recurrent yeast infections. Additionally, concurrent staphylococcal infections are frequent and require specific antibiotic therapy.

Recurrent cases of *Malassezia* dermatitis are not uncommon. If the recurrences are infrequent, they can be treated as described earlier. Frequent recurrences may require the administration of "maintenance" topicals (shampoos and/or rinses) on a once- or twice-weekly basis or even oral ketoconazole every 3 days.

The development of ecologically based forms of therapy and prophylaxis, such as the use of inhibitors of the in vivo adherence process, are highly desirable.[124] However, given the apparent variability among strains of *M. pachydermatis*, it may prove difficult to find a universal inhibitor of adherence.[124, 138]

Atopic dogs with *Malassezia* dermatitis showed immediate skin test reactivity to *M. pachydermatis* antigens, whereas atopic dogs without *Malassezia* dermatitis had negative skin test reactions.[148] This, in conjunction with the lack of cross-reactivity with mold and house dust antigens, suggests that immunotherapy with *M. pachydermatis* antigens may be a useful therapeutic measure in the future.[148]

Surgical removal of a thymoma resulted in spontaneous remission of exfoliative dermatitis associated with *M. pachydermatis* in a cat.[131]

Piedra

CAUSE AND PATHOGENESIS

Piedra is an asymptomatic fungal infection of the extrafollicular portion of the hair shaft caused by *Piedraia hortae* ("black piedra") and *Trichosporon beigelii* ("white piedra").[4] White piedra has been described in a dog.[159] White piedra is most common in the temperate climates of South America, Europe, Asia, Japan, and the southern United States. The source of the infection is unknown, and direct transmission is thought to be rare.

CLINICAL FINDINGS

White piedra was reported in an 11-year-old black Cocker spaniel.[159] The dog had white-to-gray concretions on and encircling the hair shafts around the lips (Fig. 5–25). The "nodules" were soft to the touch. The animal was otherwise healthy.

DIAGNOSIS

The differential diagnosis includes trichorrhexis nodosa, trichomycosis axillaris, hair casts, and various developmental defects of hair shafts. Microscopic examination of affected hairs shows nodules up to a few millimeters in diameter on and encircling the hairs shafts (Fig. 5–26). These nodules may result in a weakening and breakage of infected hair shafts. Microscopic examination of infected hairs reveals extrapilar and intrapilar hyphae arranged perpendicularly to the hair surface. Septate hyphae and arthroconidia (3 to 7 μm in diameter) may be visible. *Trichosporon beigelii* (*T. cutaneum*) grows readily on Sabouraud's dextrose agar at 25°C but is inhibited by cycloheximide.

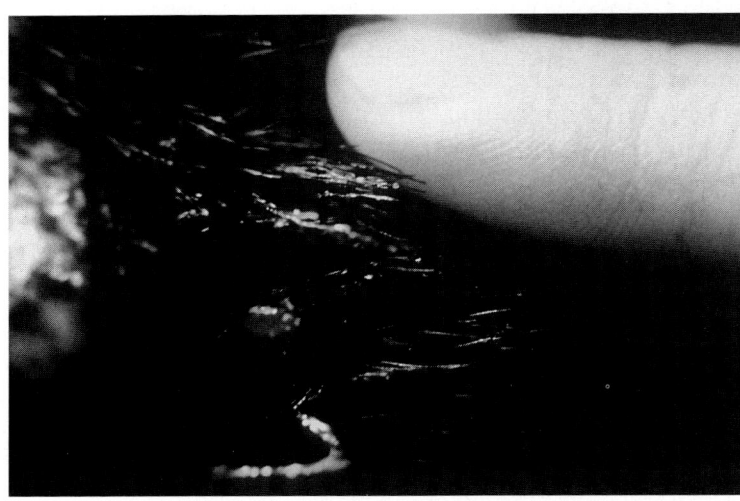

FIGURE 5–25. Piedra in a dog. White concretions on the hairs of a black Cocker spaniel. (Courtesy M. Pereiro-Miguens.)

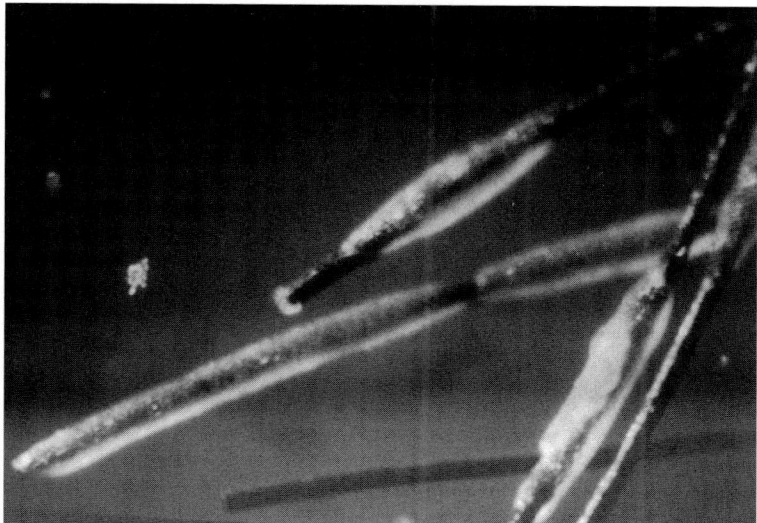

FIGURE 5–26. Piedra in a dog. White material encircling hair shafts. (Courtesy of M. Pereiro-Miguens.)

CLINICAL MANAGEMENT

In humans, the condition is cured by shaving off the hair.[4] Spontaneous remissions are common.

Rhodotorula Dermatitis

CAUSE AND PATHOGENESIS

Rhodotorula spp. are normal inhabitants of the skin, ear canal, and alimentary tract.[1, 2, 158] These yeastlike fungi are opportunistic pathogens of immunosuppressed patients.

CLINICAL FINDINGS

Rhodotorula dermatitis appears to be extremely rare. One cat had erythematous dermatitis with adherent brown-red, doughy crusts on the nasal planum, nostrils, bridge of the nose, periocular region, and one digit (Fig. 5–27).[158] *Rhodotorula mucilaginosa* was isolated in culture. The cat was positive for FeLV and FIV.

DIAGNOSIS

Biopsy revealed an interstitial dermatitis with ovoid, yeastlike organisms in the dermis.[158] *Rhodotorula* spp. grow on Sabouraud's dextrose agar.

CLINICAL MANAGEMENT

A cat treated with ketoconazole orally for 4 months was still in remission 18 months later.[158]

• SUBCUTANEOUS MYCOSES

The subcutaneous (intermediate) mycoses are fungal infections that have invaded the viable tissues of the skin.[1–6, 9, 10] These infections are usually acquired by traumatic implantation of saprophytic organisms that normally exist in soil or vegetation. The lesions are chronic and, in most cases, remain localized. The terms used to refer to the subcuta-

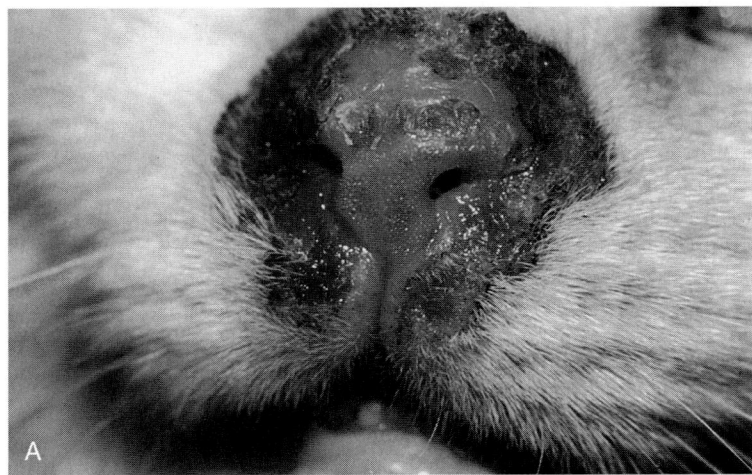
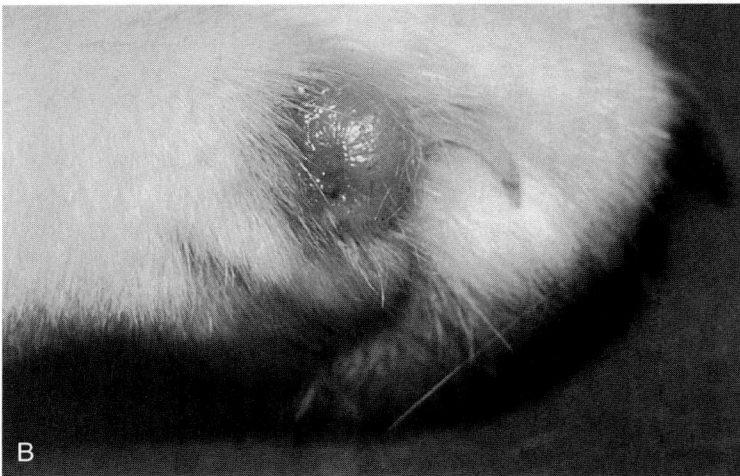

FIGURE 5–27. *Rhodotorula* dermatitis in a cat. *A*, Alopecia, erythema, and crusting on the nose and muzzle. (Courtesy P. Bourdeau.) *B*, Alopecia and erythema of digit. (Courtesy P. Bourdeau.)

neous mycoses have been contradictory, confusing, and frequently changing. The term *chromomycosis* includes subcutaneous and systemic diseases caused by fungi that develop in the host tissue in the form of dark-walled (pigmented, dematiaceous) fungal elements.[3, 5, 6, 10] Chromomycosis is separated into two forms, depending on the appearance of the fungus in tissues. In *phaeohyphomycosis*, the organism appears as septate hyphae and yeastlike cells. In *chromoblastomycosis*, the fungus is present as large (4 to 15 μm in diameter), rounded, dark-walled cells (sclerotic bodies, chromo bodies, Medlar bodies).

A *mycetoma* is a unique infection wherein the organism is present in tissues as granules or grains.[3, 5, 6, 10] Mycetomas may be *eumycotic* or *actinomycotic*. The etiologic agents of eumycotic mycetomas are fungi, whereas actinomycotic mycetomas are caused by members of the Actinomycetales order, such as *Actinomyces* and *Nocardia*, which are bacteria (see Chap. 4). Eumycotic mycetomas may be caused by dematiaceous fungi (black-grained mycetomas) or nonpigmented fungi (white-grained mycetoma). Pseudomycetomas have differences in granule formation and are caused by dermatophytes (dermatophytic pseudomycetoma) or bacteria such as *Staphylococcus* (bacterial pseudomycetoma or botryomycosis).

The term *hyalohyphomycosis* has been proposed to encompass all opportunistic infections caused by nondematiaceous fungi (at least 19 genera), the basic tissue forms of these being hyaline hyphal elements that are septate, branched or unbranched, and nonpigmented in tissues.[5, 10, 233]

Another term that creates confusion is *phycomycosis*.[3, 5, 6, 10] The class Phycomycetes no longer exists. *Pythiosis* (oömycosis) and *zygomycosis* are now the preferred terms for phycomycosis. Members of the genus *Pythium* are properly classified in the kingdom Protista and in the phylum Oömycetes. The phylum Zygomycota includes the orders Mucorales and Entomophthorales. The term *zygomycosis* is used to include both *mucormycosis* and *entomophthoromycosis*.

Eumycotic Mycetoma

CAUSE AND PATHOGENESIS

The fungi causing eumycotic mycetoma in dogs and cats are ubiquitous soil saprophytes that cause disease via wound contamination.[3, 5, 10, 164] The condition occurs most frequently near the Tropic of Cancer between the latitudes 10°S and 30°N, including Africa, South and Central America, India, and southern Asia. The disease is rare in the United States and Europe. The most commonly reported fungus causing eumycotic mycetoma in the United States is *Pseudoallescheria boydii*.

CLINICAL FINDINGS

The three cardinal features of eumycotic mycetoma (maduromycosis) are tumefaction, draining tracts, and grains (granules) in the discharge.[3, 5, 10, 164] Lesions are usually solitary and occur most commonly on the limbs and face (Fig. 5–28A and B). Early papules evolve into nodules that are often painful. As lesions enlarge, they develop draining tracts that exude a serous, purulent, or hemorrhagic discharge. As some fistulas heal, scar tissue develops and forms the hard, tumor-like mass that characterizes mycetoma. Grains present in discharge vary in color, size, shape, and texture, depending on the particular fungus involved (Fig. 5–29). Black- or dark-grain mycetomas are usually associated with *Curvularia geniculata*, occasionally with *Madurella grisea* and *Torula* sp.[161, 166] White-grain mycetomas are usually caused by *Pseudoallescheria* (*Allescheria, Petriellidium*) *boydii* and occasionally *Acremonium hyalinum*.[160, 163–165] Chronic infections can extend into underlying muscle, joint, or bone. Pyogranulomatous panniculitis in a dog was caused by *Phialemonium curvatum*.[162]

DIAGNOSIS

The differential diagnosis includes infectious and foreign-body granulomas and neoplasms. Cytologic examination of aspirates or direct smears reveals pyogranulomatous inflammation with occasional fungal elements. Fungi are easily seen by squashing and examining grains. Biopsy findings include nodular to diffuse, pyogranulomatous to granulomatous dermatitis and panniculitis. Fungal elements are present as a grain (granule, thallus) within the inflammatory reaction (Fig. 5–30). The grains (0.2 mm to several millimeters in diameter) are irregularly shaped, often taking a scalloped or scroll-like appearance, and consist of broad (2 to 6 μm in diameter), septate, branching hyphae, which often form chlamydoconidia, and a cementing substance.[3] The fungal elements may be pigmented or nonpigmented. The fungi grow on Sabouraud's dextrose agar at 25°C. Either tissue grains or punch biopsies are the preferred material for culture (see Chap. 2).

CLINICAL MANAGEMENT

Wide surgical excision is the treatment of choice.[163, 164] In some cases, amputation of an affected limb is necessary. Any attempt at antifungal chemotherapy should be based on in vitro susceptibility testing of the isolate.[4, 164] Medical therapy is often unsuccessful. Keto-

378 • Fungal Skin Diseases

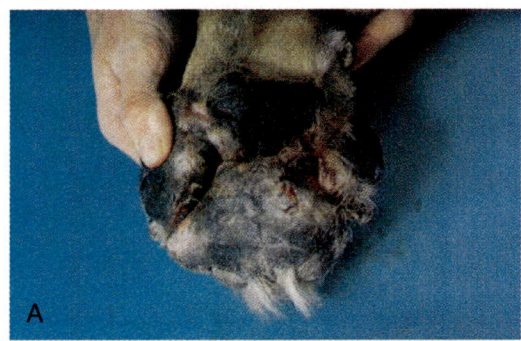

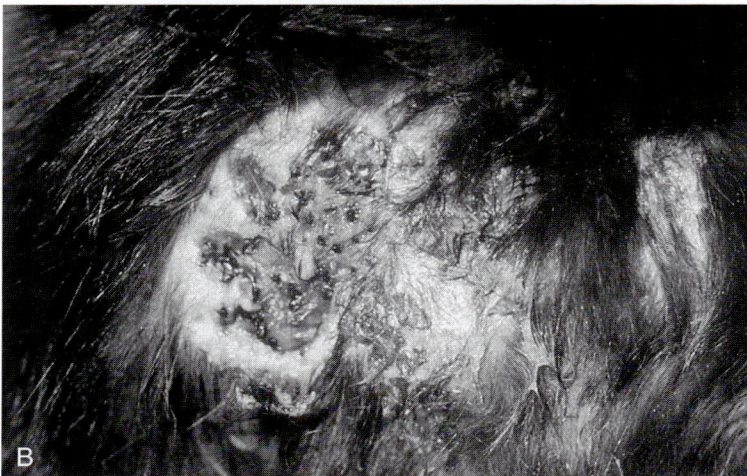

FIGURE 5–28. *A*, Mycetoma foot in a dog. (Courtesy D. Chester.) *B*, Mycetoma due to *Torula* sp. in a cat. Note multiple black tissue grains associated with draining tracts over the hip. (Courtesy K. Thoday.)

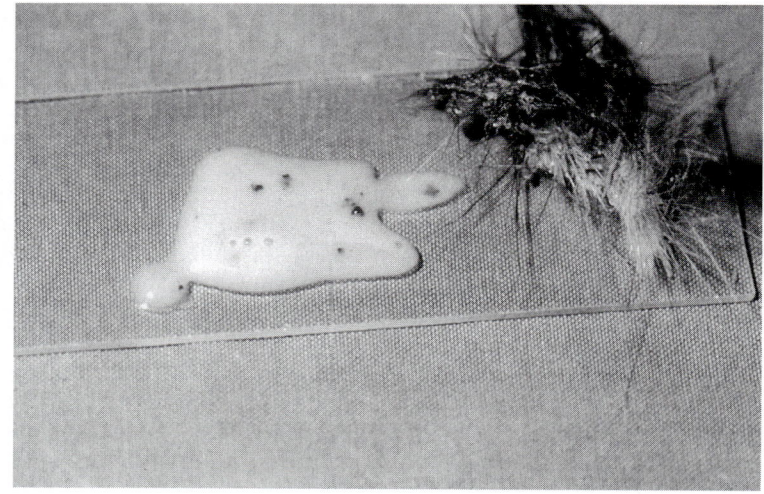

FIGURE 5–29. Mycetoma due to *Torula* sp. in a cat. Glass slide with wad of hair and crust to the right, and pus containing black tissue grains to the left. (Courtesy K. Thoday.)

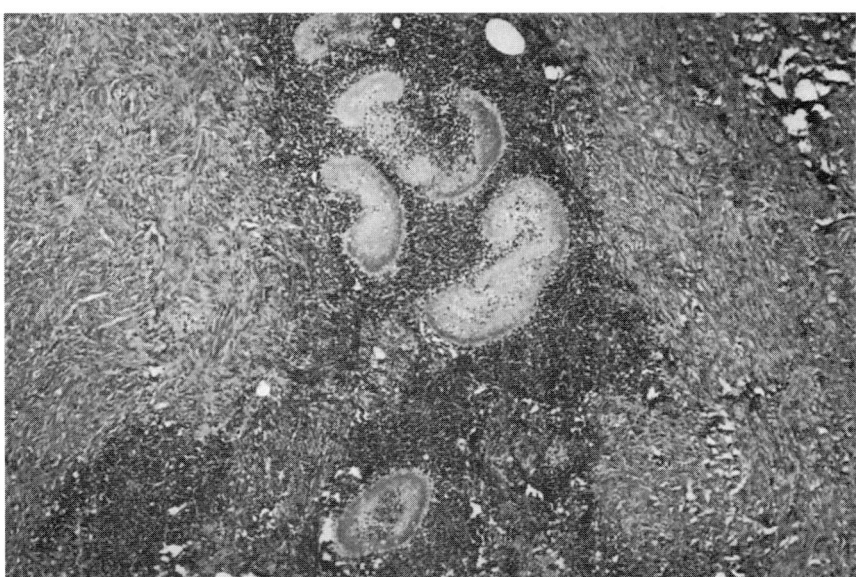
FIGURE 5–30. Mycetoma in a dog. Note numerous tissue grains within a pyogranuloma.

conazole and itraconazole have enjoyed erratic success.[4, 164] Treatment must be continued for 2 to 3 months past clinical cure.

Phaeohyphomycosis

CAUSE AND PATHOGENESIS

Phaeohyphomycosis (chromomycosis) is caused by a number of ubiquitous saprophytic fungi found in various soils and organic materials.[1, 170] Infection occurs via wound contamination. These fungi have the characteristic of forming pigmented (dematiaceous) hyphal elements (but not grains) in tissues.

CLINICAL FEATURES

Dog

Phaeohyphomycosis appears to be rare in dogs. Fungi isolated include *Bipolaris spiciferum* (*Brachycladium spiciferum*, *Drechslera spiciferum*), *Phialemonium obovatum*, *Pseudomicrodochium suttonii*, and *Xylohypha bantiana* (*Cladosporium trichoides*, *C. bantianum*).[10, 167, 170, 173, 174] Solitary subcutaneous nodules, often ulcerated, may occur occasionally, especially on extremities. However, widespread nodular or necrotizing and ulcerative lesions are also possible (see Fig. 5–16D).[173, 183] Contiguous skeletal or disseminated infections have been reported.[170, 174, 183]

Cat

Phaeohyphomycosis is uncommon in cats. Fungi isolated include *Bipolaris spiciferum* (*Brachycladium spiciferum*, *D. spiciferum*), *X. bantiana* (*C. trichoides*, *C. bantianum*), *X. emmonsii*, *Exophiala jeanselmei* (*Phialophora gougerotii*), *Exophiala spinifera*, *Moniliella suaveolens*, *Phialophora verrucosa*, *Alternaria alternata*, *Cladophialiophora* sp., *Dissitimurus exudrus*, *Scolecobasidium humicola*, and *Stemphylium* spp.[168–172, 175–182] In most cases, lesions are solitary and affect the paw, leg, head (especially the nose, cheek, and pinna), or trunk (see Fig. 5–16C). Slow-growing, firm to fluctuant, dermal to subcutaneous nodules are visible. The lesions may be blue-gray, perhaps owing to the pigmented nature of the fungi. Ulceration and draining tracts may occur. Disseminated infection is rare.[170]

DIAGNOSIS

The differential diagnosis includes infectious granulomas, sterile granulomas, foreign-body granulomas, and neoplasms. In dogs with widespread mucocutaneous and footpad lesions,[173] the differential diagnosis includes immunologic diseases (pemphigus vulgaris, bullous pemphigoid, epidermolysis bullosa acquisita, systemic lupus erythematosus, erythema multiforme), drug eruptions, necrolytic migratory erythema, thallium poisoning, epitheliotropic lymphoma, and other unusual infections (leishmaniasis, protothecosis, candidiasis).

Cytologic examination of aspirates or direct smears reveals granulomatous to pyogranulomatous inflammation. Pigmented fungal hyphae may be visible (Fig. 5–31). Biopsy findings include nodular to diffuse, granulomatous to pyogranulomatous dermatitis and panniculitis (Fig. 5–32). Numerous fungal elements are present as broad (2 to 6 μm in diameter), often irregular, pigmented, septate, branched or unbranched hyphae with occasional chlamydoconidia and numerous round to oval, pigmented yeast forms (Medlar bodies, so-called copper pennies) (see Fig. 5–16E).[3] Although *P. curvatum* is a dematiaceous fungus,[9] it was not visible in H & E–stained biopsy specimens from a dog with pyogranulomatous panniculitis.[168] The fungi grow on Sabouraud's dextrose agar at 25° to 35°C, and punch biopsies are the preferred material for culture.

CLINICAL MANAGEMENT

Wide surgical excision of solitary lesions may be curative, but recurrence at the same site or at new sites is common.[170, 172, 175, 177] Chemotherapy may be curative, depending on the agent, but the response is unpredictable. This may be due to differing susceptibilities of

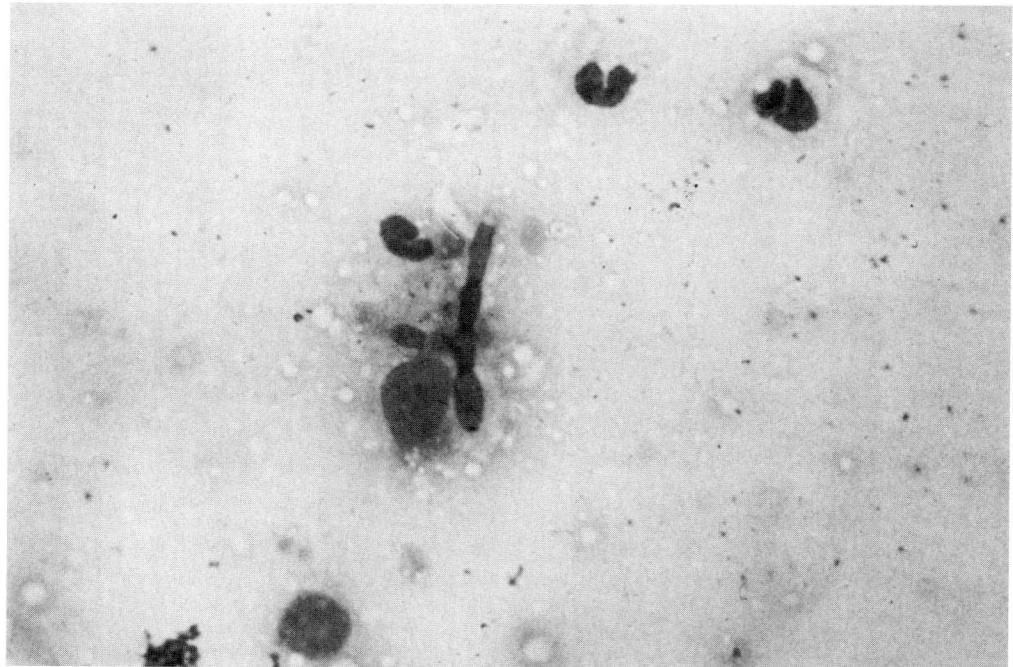

FIGURE 5–31. Direct smear from a cat with phaeohyphomycosis. Pigmented fungal hypha within a macrophage.

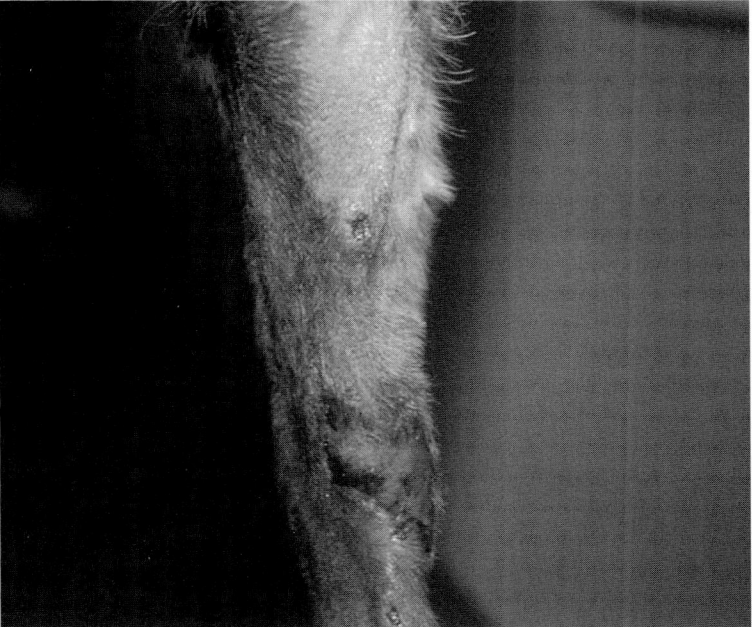

FIGURE 5–36. Zygomycosis in a dog. Ulcerated nodules on leg. (Courtesy T. Manning.)

elements stain well with GMS but variably with PAS. *Zygomycetes* grows on Sabouraud's dextrose agar at 25°C, and punch or wedge biopsies are the preferred material for culture. Biopsy specimens submitted for culture should not be ground or macerated because this may destroy the organism. Cycloheximide may inhibit fungal growth.

CLINICAL MANAGEMENT

The susceptibility of the *Zygomycetes* to antimycotic agents is variable and largely unknown.[4, 184, 189] Solitary lesions may be surgically excised. In other cases, surgical excision or debulking may be followed by chemotherapy as dictated by in vitro susceptibility tests (amphotericin B, azoles, potassium iodide).[4, 184, 189] One dog was cured with 2 months of

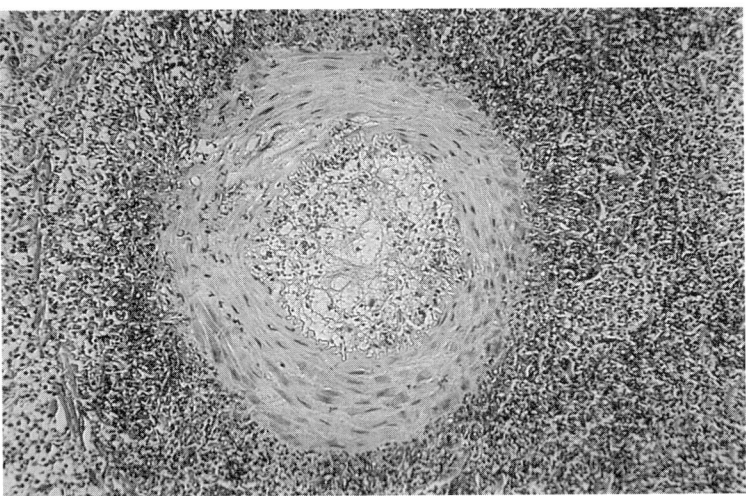

FIGURE 5–37. Zygomycosis in a dog. Fungal elements invading wall and occluding lumen of subcutaneous artery. (Courtesy T. Manning.)

itraconazole (10 mg/kg q12h),[184] whereas itraconazole (4 mg/kg q12h) produced no response in another dog.[190]

Sporotrichosis

CAUSE AND PATHOGENESIS

Sporotrichosis is caused by the ubiquitous dimorphic fungus *Sporothrix schenckii*, which exists as a saprophyte in soil and organic debris.[1, 195, 196] Infection results from wound contamination. Glucocorticoids and other immunosuppressive drugs are contraindicated in dogs or cats with sporotrichosis.[193, 195, 196] These drugs should be avoided both during and after treatment of the disease because immunosuppressive doses of glucocorticoids have been reported to cause a recurrence of clinical sporotrichosis as long as 4 to 6 months after apparent clinical cure.[195]

CLINICAL FINDINGS

Dog

Sporotrichosis is uncommon to rare. The disease is often related to puncture wounds from thorns or wood splinters.[195, 196] This is presumably why the disease is more common in hunting dogs.[195] The *cutaneous form* of sporotrichosis is the most commonly reported.[195, 196] Multiple firm nodules, ulcerated plaques with raised borders or annular crusted and alopecic areas are present, especially on the head, pinnae, and trunk (see Figs. 5–16H and 5–38A). Some lesions have a verrucous appearance. Nodules may ulcerate or develop draining tracts (see Fig. 5–38B).

Lesions are neither painful nor pruritic, and affected dogs are usually healthy otherwise. The *cutaneolymphatic form* is characterized by a nodule on the distal aspect of one limb, with subsequent ascending infection via the lymphatics.[195, 196] Secondary nodules may be firm or fluctuant; they often ulcerate and discharge a brownish red exudate, and they are associated with regional lymphadenopathy. Affected dogs are usually otherwise healthy. Ulcers and nodules affecting the nares, mucocutaneous junctions, and scrotum may be seen, as well as papulonodular otitis externa.[13] Disseminated sporotrichosis is extremely rare.[195, 196]

Cat

Sporotrichosis is uncommon. The disease is believed to be acquired by inoculation of the organism by contaminated claws or teeth from another cat.[195, 196] This may explain why the disease is usually seen in intact male cats that roam outdoors.[195, 196] Lesions are common on the head (see Fig. 5–38C), distal limbs, or tail base region.[195, 196] The cats may initially present with fight wound abscesses, draining tracts, or cellulitis. Affected areas ulcerate, drain a purulent exudate, and form crusted nodules. Large areas of necrosis may develop, with exposure of muscle and bone. The disease may be spread to other areas of the body (other limbs, face, pinnae) via autoinoculation during normal grooming behavior. Some cats may present with a history of lethargy, depression, anorexia, and fever, which suggest the potential for disseminated disease.[195, 196] Although affected cats frequently appear clinically to have only dermatologic disease, most have necropsy evidence of lymph node and lymphatic vessel involvement, and *S. schenckii* is commonly isolated in culture from numerous internal organs and feces.[195, 196]

Zoonotic Aspects

The zoonotic potential of sporotrichosis, especially in cats, must be seriously considered and respected.[85, 192, 194–196] Several reports have documented transmission of sporotrichosis to humans through contact with an ulcerated wound or the exudate from an infected cat.[85, 192, 194–196] Human infections have occurred even though there had been no known injury or penetrating wound prior to the onset of the disease.[196] Transmission from animals to humans has been limited to feline sporotrichosis, presumably because

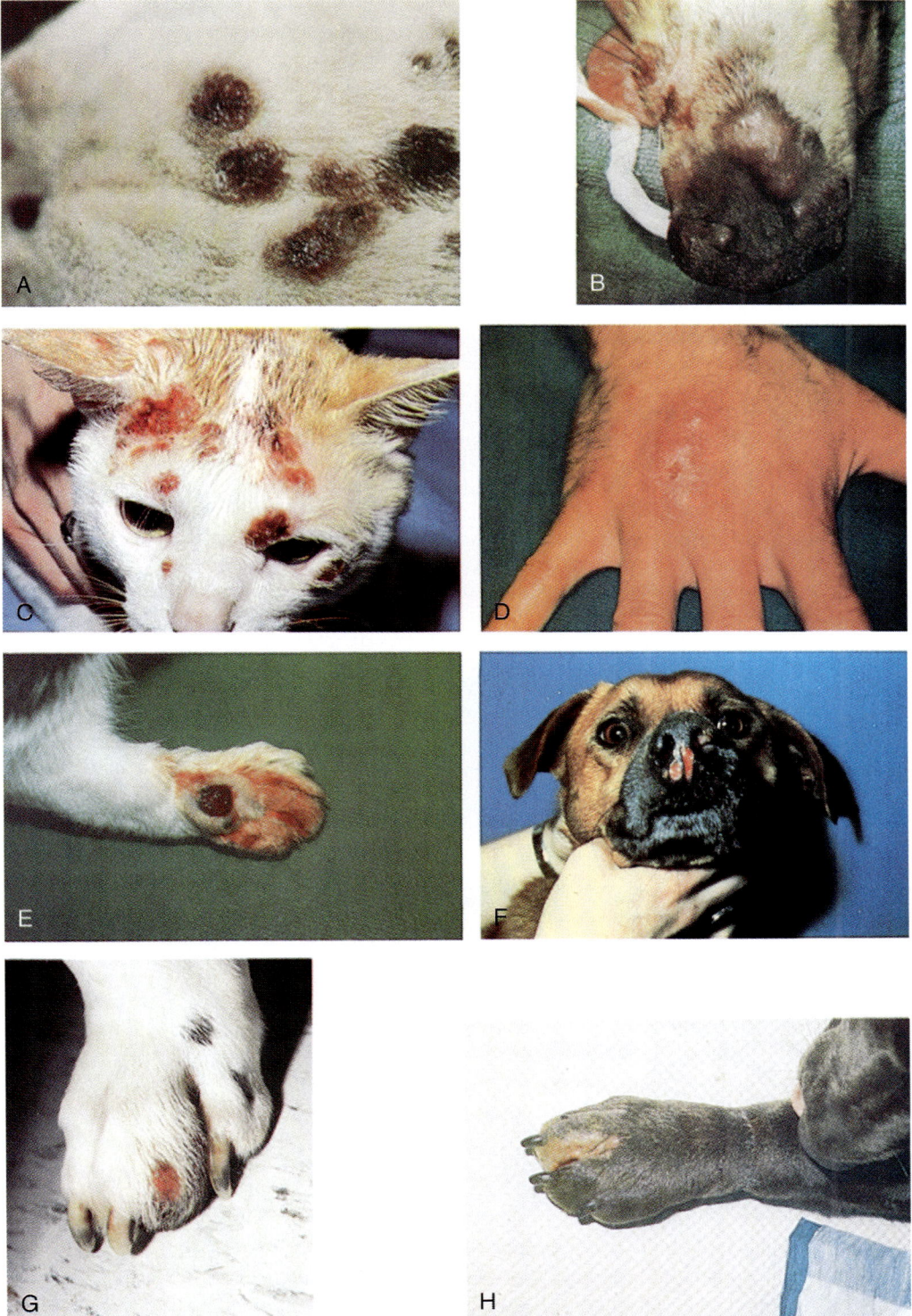

FIGURE 5-38. Miscellaneous fungal infections. *A*, Sporotrichosis. Close-up of the top of the head of a dog. Multiple crusted plaques. *B*, Sporotrichosis presenting as multiple papules and nodules on the bridge of the nose of a collie. *C*, Sporotrichosis presenting as multiple ulcers on the face of a cat. *D*, Multiple erythematous papules and a large, ulcerated nodule on the hand of a human with sporotrichosis. (Courtesy R. Goltz.) *E*, Large nodule with a central ulcer on the hind paw of a cat caused by *Alternaria* sp. *F*, Ulcerated nodules on the nose of a dog with blastomycosis. (Courtesy J. Brace.) *G*, Swollen digit with a focal ulceration in a dog with blastomycosis. *H*, Alopecic, erythematous nodule on the digit of a dog with coccidioidomycosis. (Courtesy D. Chester.)

large numbers of organisms are found in contaminated feline tissues, exudates, and feces.[192, 195, 196] Veterinarians, veterinary technicians, veterinary students, and owners of infected cats have a higher risk of infection.[85, 192, 194, 196]

The most common form of sporotrichosis in humans is cutaneolymphatic.[4, 85, 195] A primary lesion—which may be a papule, pustule, nodule, abscess, or verrucous growth—develops at the site of injury. This lesion may be painful. Most lesions are on an extremity (finger, hand, foot) (see Fig. 5–38D) or the face. Secondary lesions then ascend proximally via lymphatic vessels. The cutaneous (fixed) form is less common.

DIAGNOSIS

The differential diagnosis includes other infectious granulomas, foreign-body granulomas, and neoplasms. Sporotrichosis should always be suspected in cats with nonhealing, fight-wound abscesses. Because of the zoonotic potential of sporotrichosis, precautions must be taken. All people handling cats suspected of having sporotrichosis should wear gloves. Gloves should also be worn when samples are taken of exudates or tissues. The gloves should then be carefully removed and disposed of. Forearms, wrists, and hands should be washed in chlorhexidine or povidone-iodine.

Cytologic examination of aspirates or direct smears reveals suppurative to pyogranulomatous to granulomatous inflammation. The organism is difficult to find in the exudates of dogs but is easily found in those of cats (Fig. 5–39). *S. schenckii* is a pleomorphic yeast that is round, oval, or cigar-shaped, 2 to 10 μm in length. Biopsy findings include nodular to diffuse, suppurative to granulomatous to granulomatous dermatitis (Fig. 5–40). Fungal elements are numerous and readily found in cats but rarely in dogs (Fig. 5–41). The fungi have a refractile cell wall from which the cytoplasm may shrink, giving the impression that the organism has a capsule. When this occurs, the organisms may be confused with *Cryptococcus neoformans*. *S. schenckii* grows on Sabouraud's dextrose agar at 30°C; samples submitted for culture should include both a sample of the exudate (from deep within a draining tract) and a piece of tissue (removed surgically) for a macerated tissue culture. A fluorescent antibody test is most useful in dogs because it may be positive when cultures are negative.[13, 195]

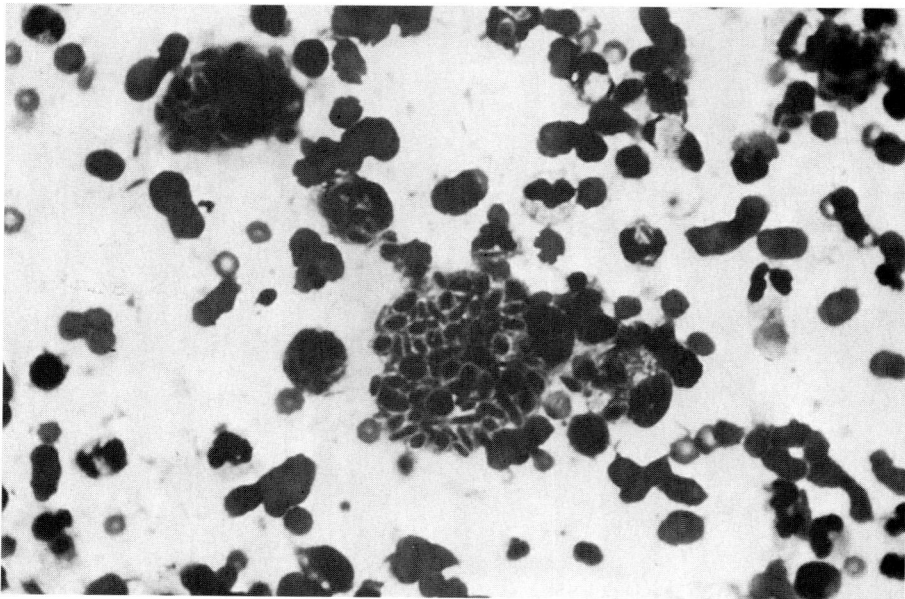

FIGURE 5–39. Feline sporotrichosis. Numerous yeast and cigar bodies in a macrophage. (Courtesy J.M. MacDonald.)

Fungal Skin Diseases • **389**

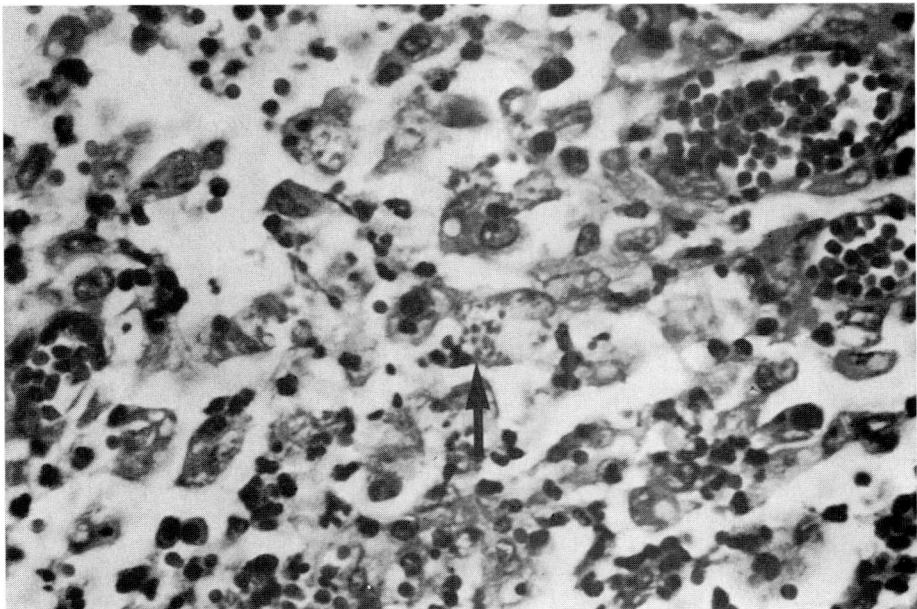

FIGURE 5-40. Feline sporotrichosis. Pyogranulomatous dermatitis with intracellular yeast and cigar bodies *(arrow)*.

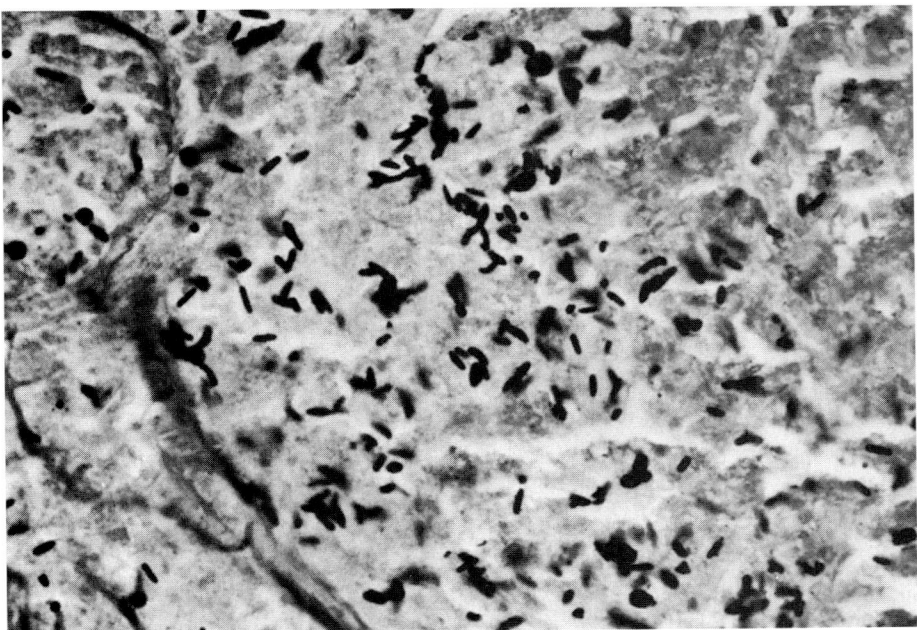

FIGURE 5-41. Canine sporotrichosis. Numerous yeast and cigar bodies (GMS stain).

CLINICAL MANAGEMENT

Dog

The treatment of choice is oral administration of a supersaturated solution of potassium iodide, 40 mg/kg q8h to q12h with food.[5, 13, 195, 196] Treatment must be continued for 30 days beyond clinical cure (4 to 8 weeks). Signs of toxicity (iodism) include ocular and nasal discharge, a dry haircoat with excessively scaling skin, vomiting, depression, and collapse.[195, 196] If iodism is observed, medication should be stopped for 1 week. The drug may then be re-instituted at the same or a lower dosage. If iodism becomes a recurrent problem or if side effects are severe, alternative treatment should be considered.

The imidazole and triazole classes of drugs may be considered for dogs that do not tolerate iodides, are refractory to them, or experience relapse after apparent clinical cure.[5, 195, 196] Ketoconazole or itraconazole may be used successfully and are continued for 30 days beyond clinical cure. Side effects are usually mild.

Cat

Increased sensitivity to the toxic side effects of iodides and ketoconazole in cats poses a greater challenge for the treatment of sporotrichosis. A supersaturated solution of potassium iodide may be administered orally at 20 mg/kg q12h to q24h with food[5, 192, 195, 196] for 30 days beyond clinical cure (4 to 8 weeks). Signs of iodism include vomiting, anorexia, depression, twitching, hypothermia, and cardiovascular failure. In animals that cannot tolerate or fail to respond to iodides, ketoconazole or itraconazole should be used.[5, 195, 196]

Rhinosporidiosis

CAUSE AND PATHOGENESIS

Rhinosporidium seeberi is a fungal organism of uncertain classification.[1, 197] Attempts to culture it using conventional fungal culture media were unsuccessful; however, the organism has been grown in tissue culture.[197] The disease is endemic in India and Argentina, but North American reports have come almost exclusively from the southern United States. It is thought that infection is acquired by mucosal contact with stagnant water or dust and that trauma is a predisposing factor.

CLINICAL FINDINGS

The disease appears to be rare, and it is reported only in dogs.[1, 197] There appears to be a predilection for large-breed, male dogs. Affected dogs typically present for wheezing, sneezing, unilateral seropurulent nasal discharge, and epistaxis. Nasal polyps may be visible in the nares or may be visualized by rhinoscopy. Single or multiple polyps varying in size from a few millimeters up to 3 cm are pink, red, or grayish and are covered with numerous pinpoint, white foci (fungal sporangia). Polyps may be sessile or pedunculated, and they may protrude out of, or involve, the mucocutaneous area of the nostril.

DIAGNOSIS

The differential diagnosis includes numerous infectious granulomas and neoplasms. Cytologic examination of nasal exudate or histologic examination of the polyp should be diagnostic. Biopsy findings include a fibrovascular polyp containing numerous sporangia (spherules) having a thick, double outer membrane. The sporangia vary from 100 to 400 μm in diameter and contain a variable number of sporangiospores (endospores).[1, 197] A variable number of lymphocytes, plasma cells, and neutrophils are often found where sporangiospores (2 to 10 μm in diameter) have been released into the surrounding connective tissue.

CLINICAL MANAGEMENT

Surgical excision is the treatment of choice, although recurrence 6 to 12 months after surgery has been reported.[197] Successes have been reported with dapsone or ketoconazole administered orally; however, the utility of medical therapy in canine rhinosporidiosis requires further evaluation.

Alternaria Dermatitis

CAUSE AND PATHOGENESIS

Alternaria spp. are ubiquitous saprophytic fungi in soil and organic debris and a common component of the flora of the canine and feline integument.[3, 9, 13] They cause opportunistic wound infections.

CLINICAL FINDINGS

Alternaria spp. are rarely reported to cause skin disease in dogs and cats. In the dog, dermatologic abnormalities attributed to *Alternaria* spp. infection include (1) poorly circumscribed areas of alopecia, erythema, and scaling, especially in intertriginous or traumatized areas of skin,[198, 230] and (2) nodular, ulcerated, depigmented inflammation of the nose (*Alternaria tenuissima*).[199] In the cat, *Alternaria* spp. have been associated with phaeohyphomycosis (*Alternaria alternata*)[169] and ulcerated nodules on the paw (see Fig. 5–38E).

DIAGNOSIS

The differential diagnosis for superficial inflammatory disease includes staphylococcal folliculitis, demodicosis, dermatophytosis, and *Malassezia* dermatitis. The differential diagnosis for nodules includes infectious and foreign-body granulomas and neoplasms. Cytologic examination of aspirates or direct smears from nodular lesions reveals pyogranulomatous inflammation and numerous fungal elements. Biopsy findings include nodular to diffuse pyogranulomatous dermatitis and panniculitis with numerous broad (3 to 6 μm in diameter), septate, branched or unbranched hyphae (Fig. 5–42). *Alternaria* spp. grow on Sabouraud's dextrose agar. Punch biopsies are the preferred culture material.

CLINICAL MANAGEMENT

Surgical excision of nodules may be curative. Antifungal chemotherapy should be based on in vitro susceptibility tests. One dog was cured after 8 weeks of oral ketoconazole.[199]

• SYSTEMIC MYCOSES

Deep mycoses are fungal infections of internal organs that may secondarily disseminate by hematogenous spread to the skin. Fungi that cause deep mycoses exist as saprophytes in soil or vegetation. These infections are usually not contagious because the animal inhales conidia from a specific ecologic niche. Skin lesions that occur via primary cutaneous inoculation are very rare, and animals with skin lesions are assumed to have systemic infection until proven otherwise. The deep mycoses are discussed only briefly here. The reader is referred to texts on mycology and infectious diseases for additional information.

Blastomycosis

CAUSE AND PATHOGENESIS

Blastomyces dermatitidis is a dimorphic saprophytic fungus.[1, 2, 9, 10, 14, 223] Four elements— moisture, soil type (sandy, acid), presence of wildlife, and soil disruption—make up

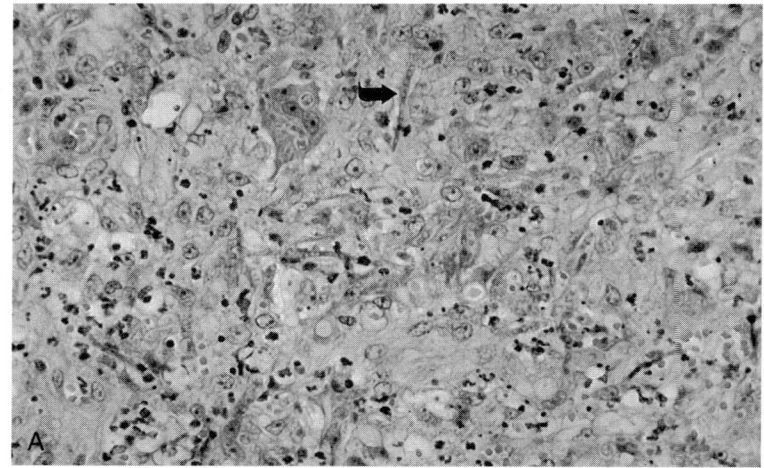
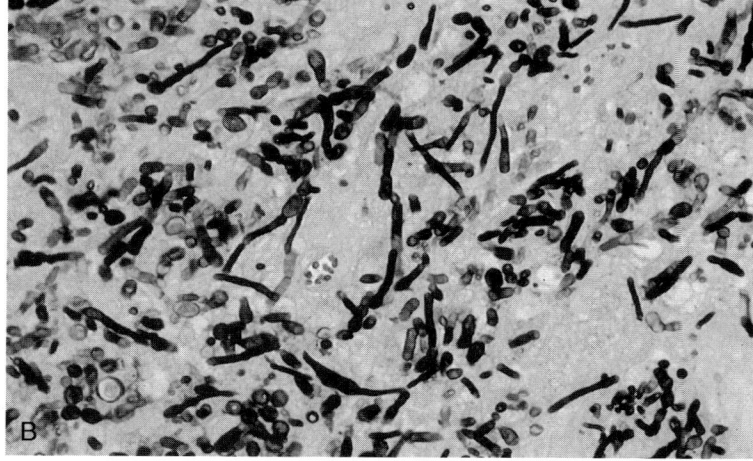

FIGURE 5–42. *Alternaria* dermatitis in a cat. *A*, Pyogranulomatous panniculitis containing numerous fungal hyphae *(arrow)*. *B*, Close-up of *A* stained with GMS. Fungal hyphae are more obvious.

the "microfocus model" that helps explain where *B. dermatitidis* is most likely to be found.[219, 220] Even within endemic areas, the fungus does not seem to be widely distributed. Rarely has the organism been successfully isolated from the environment. Most people and dogs living in such areas show no serologic or skin test evidence of exposure. A point source where the exposure occurs within an enzootic area is more likely. Blastomycosis (Gilchrist's disease, Chicago disease) is principally a disease of North America, but it has been identified in Africa and Central America. In North America, the endemic distribution of blastomycosis is well-defined and includes the Mississippi, Missouri, New York, Ohio, and St. Lawrence River Valleys and the Mid-Atlantic states.

CLINICAL FINDINGS

Dog

Blastomycosis is an uncommon disease in endemic areas. Young (2 to 4 years old) male dogs of large breeds and sporting breeds (especially Doberman pinscher, Labrador retriever, Bluetick coonhound, Treeing Walker coonhound, pointers, Weimaraners) are predisposed.[219, 223, 225] A larger number of cases occur in the fall.[219, 225] Proximity to a body of water was a significant risk factor for affected dogs.[219] Clinical signs usually include anorexia, weight loss, coughing, dyspnea, ocular disease, lameness, and skin disease.[219, 223] Up to 40% of dogs with blastomycosis have skin lesions that include firm papules, nodules, and plaques, ulcers, draining tracts, and subcutaneous abscesses.[223] Lesions are usually multiple and may be found anywhere; however, the nasal planum (see Fig. 5–38F), face, and clawbeds (see Fig. 5–38G) appear to be preferred sites. Calcinosis cutis developed in 3 dogs with systemic blastomycosis after treatment with amphotericin B had been instituted.[221a]

Cat

Blastomycosis is very rare in cats. Dyspnea, draining skin lesions (especially the digits) (see Fig. 5–51A), and weight loss are the most prominent clinical signs.[8, 223] Siamese cats may be predisposed.

DIAGNOSIS

A history of travel to an endemic area should increase the clinician's index of suspicion. Cytologic examination of aspirates or direct smears is often diagnostic, revealing suppurative to pyogranulomatous to granulomatous inflammation containing round to oval yeast-like fungi (5 to 20 μm in diameter) that show broad-based budding and have a thick, refractile, double-contoured cell wall (Fig. 5–43). Biopsy findings include nodular to diffuse, suppurative to pyogranulomatous to granulomatous dermatitis wherein the fungus is usually found easily (Fig. 5–44). Culture of cytologic specimens is not recommended for in-hospital laboratories because of the danger of infection from the mycelial form of the organisms. Only after the organisms have been searched for extensively should serologic testing (agar-gel immunodiffusion, ELISA) be used to help establish a diagnosis.[219, 223]

CLINICAL MANAGEMENT

All animals with clinical blastomycosis should be treated because spontaneous remission is rare.[14, 219, 223] Although either amphotericin B (83% response rate) or ketoconazole (62% rate) may be effective alone, the sequential administration of these two antifungal agents is preferred.[14, 219, 223] In dogs, itraconazole is the drug of choice.[219, 224] It is more effective than ketoconazole, as effective as amphotericin B, is easily administered at home, has few side effects, and is equal cost-wise to amphotericin B. A dosage of 5 mg/kg q24h has the same success rate and fewer side effects than 10 mg/kg q24h.[224] The administration of an amphotericin B lipid complex appears to produce comparable therapeutic results while reducing the toxicities inherent to traditional amphotericin B treatment protocols.[222]

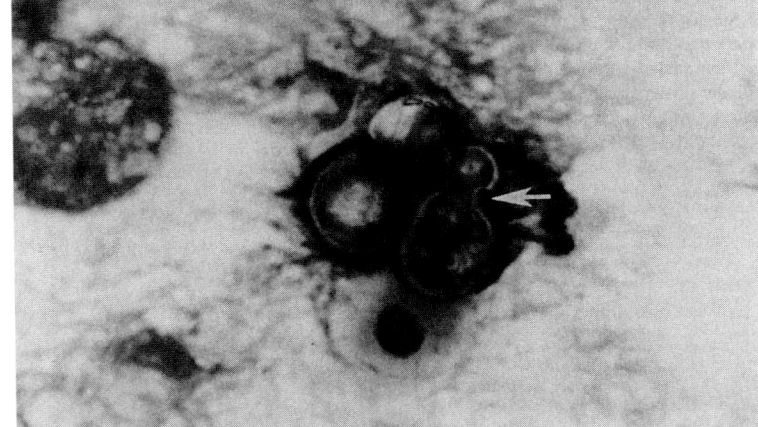

FIGURE 5–43. Direct smear from a dog with blastomycosis. Oval yeasts demonstrate broad-based budding (*arrow*). (Courtesy T. French.)

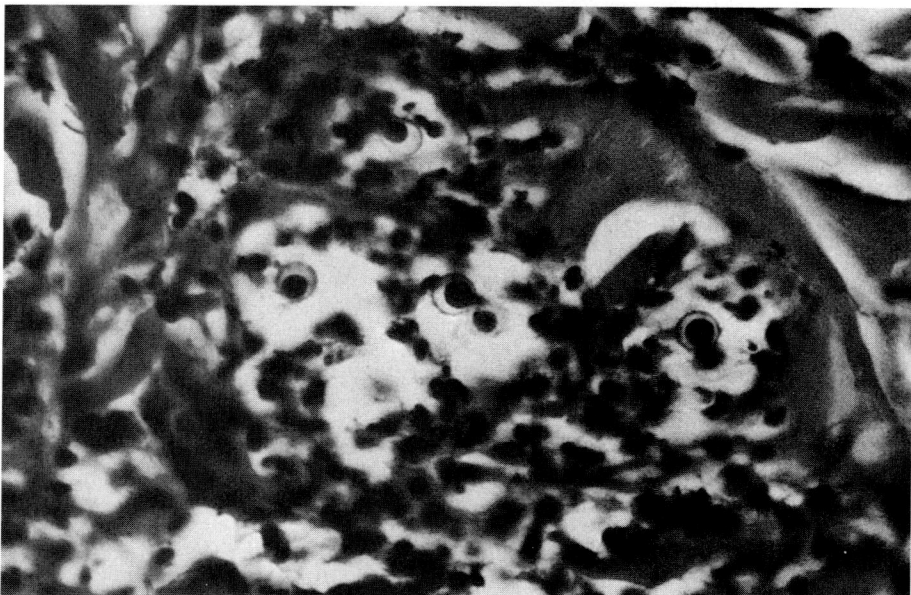

FIGURE 5–44. Canine blastomycosis. Large, round, thick-walled yeast bodies (H & E stain).

PUBLIC HEALTH CONSIDERATIONS

Dogs appear to have a tenfold increased risk for blastomycosis compared with humans and can serve as sentinels for blastomycosis in humans.[219] Penetrating wounds contaminated by the organisms have produced infections in humans.[221, 223] Care should be taken to avoid getting bitten when handling infected animals. Accidental inoculation of organisms by contaminated knives or needles should be avoided at necropsy or during fine-needle aspiration. Culturing of the organism should be limited to laboratories with proper facilities.[221]

Coccidioidomycosis

CAUSE AND PATHOGENESIS

Coccidioides immitis is a dimorphic saprophytic soil fungus.[1, 2, 9, 10, 14, 226] The ecologic niche of this fungus is characterized by sandy, alkaline soils, high environmental temperature, low rainfall, and low elevation. Geographically, this area is called the Lower Sonoran Life Zone and includes the southwestern United States, Mexico, and Central and South America. Serologic surveys indicate that most human and canine inhabitants of the endemic area become infected. Coccidioidomycosis has also been called *San Joaquin Valley Fever*.

CLINICAL FINDINGS

Dog

Coccidioidomycosis is an uncommon disease in endemic areas.[14, 226] Young (1 to 4 years old) male dogs are predisposed, and the Boxer and Doberman pinscher are predisposed to disseminated infections. Clinical signs usually include coughing, dyspnea, persistent or fluctuating fever, anorexia, weight loss, lameness, skin disease, and ocular disease.[14, 226] Skin lesions are usually multiple and include papules, nodules, abscesses, draining tracts, and ulcers. Skin lesions almost always occur over sites of infected bone (especially the distal diaphyseal, metaphyseal, and epiphyseal areas of long bones) (see Fig. 5–38*H*).

Cat

Coccidioidomycosis is rare in cats.[14, 226, 227] Clinical signs include anorexia, weight loss, cough, dyspnea, lameness, ocular disease, and skin lesions. In one study, over one half of affected cats had dermatologic signs, especially draining tracts, subcutaneous granulomas, and abscesses.[227]

DIAGNOSIS

A history of travel to an endemic area should increase the clinician's index of suspicion. Cytologic examination of aspirates or direct smears reveals suppurative to pyogranulomatous to granulomatous inflammation. Fungal elements are seldom found (Fig. 5–45B).[226] Biopsy findings include nodular to diffuse, suppurative to pyogranulomatous to granulomatous dermatitis and panniculitis. Fungal elements are usually present but may be sparse. The organisms are present in spherule (20 to 200 μm in diameter) and endospore (2 to 5 μm in diameter) forms (see Fig. 5–45A).[1, 2, 9, 226]

Attempts should not be made to culture *C. immitis* in veterinary practices because of the risk of human infection.[226] Culturing of the organism should be limited to laboratories with appropriate facilities. Serologic tests (precipitin, complement fixation) are useful for diagnosis.[226]

CLINICAL MANAGEMENT

All animals with clinical coccidioidomycosis should be treated because spontaneous remission is unlikely.[226] The current drug of choice is ketoconazole.[14, 226, 227] Treatment of animals with disseminated disease should continue for a minimum of 1 year. Amphotericin B is used to treat animals that cannot tolerate or do not respond to ketoconazole.[14, 226]

Cryptococcosis

CAUSE AND PATHOGENESIS

Cryptococcus neoformans is a ubiquitous, saprophytic, yeastlike fungus that is most frequently associated with droppings and the accumulated filth and debris of pigeon roosts.[8, 10, 211] In one study, however, 42% of affected cats lived indoors, their source of infection being undetermined.[202] Males appear to be over-represented (roaming behavior?),[202] and Abyssinians and Siamese may be at risk.[200] Currently there are four serotypes (A, B, C, D) and two varieties of *C. neoformans*: *C. neoformans* v. *neoformans* (serotype A and D), and *C. neoformans* v. *gattii* (serotypes B and C).[206, 214] *C. neoformans* v. *neoformans* is most prevalent in the United States and Europe, whereas *C. neoformans* v. *gattii* is prevalent in Australia, Southeast Asia, Africa, and South America. In humans, *C. neoformans* v. *gattii* infects immunocompetent persons and may be more difficult to treat.[214]

The establishment and spread of infection are highly dependent on host immunity; however, underlying diseases are often not detected in dogs and cats with cryptococcosis.[14, 211, 217] Both experimental and natural cases of cryptococcosis in dogs and cats are accelerated or worsened by glucocorticoid therapy.[211] In the cat, cryptococcal infection has often been associated with FeLV or FIV infections.[8, 204, 211] Cryptococcosis has also been called *European blastomycosis* and *torulosis*.

CLINICAL FINDINGS

Dog

Cryptococcosis is a rare disease.[14, 207, 211] Young (average age 3 years) large-breed dogs are predisposed. Clinical signs include various abnormalities of the central nervous system and eyes.[14, 211] Skin lesions are found in about 20% of cases; these lesions are characterized by papules, nodules, ulcers (Fig. 5–46A), abscesses, and draining tracts. The nose, lips, and clawbeds are often affected.[11, 211]

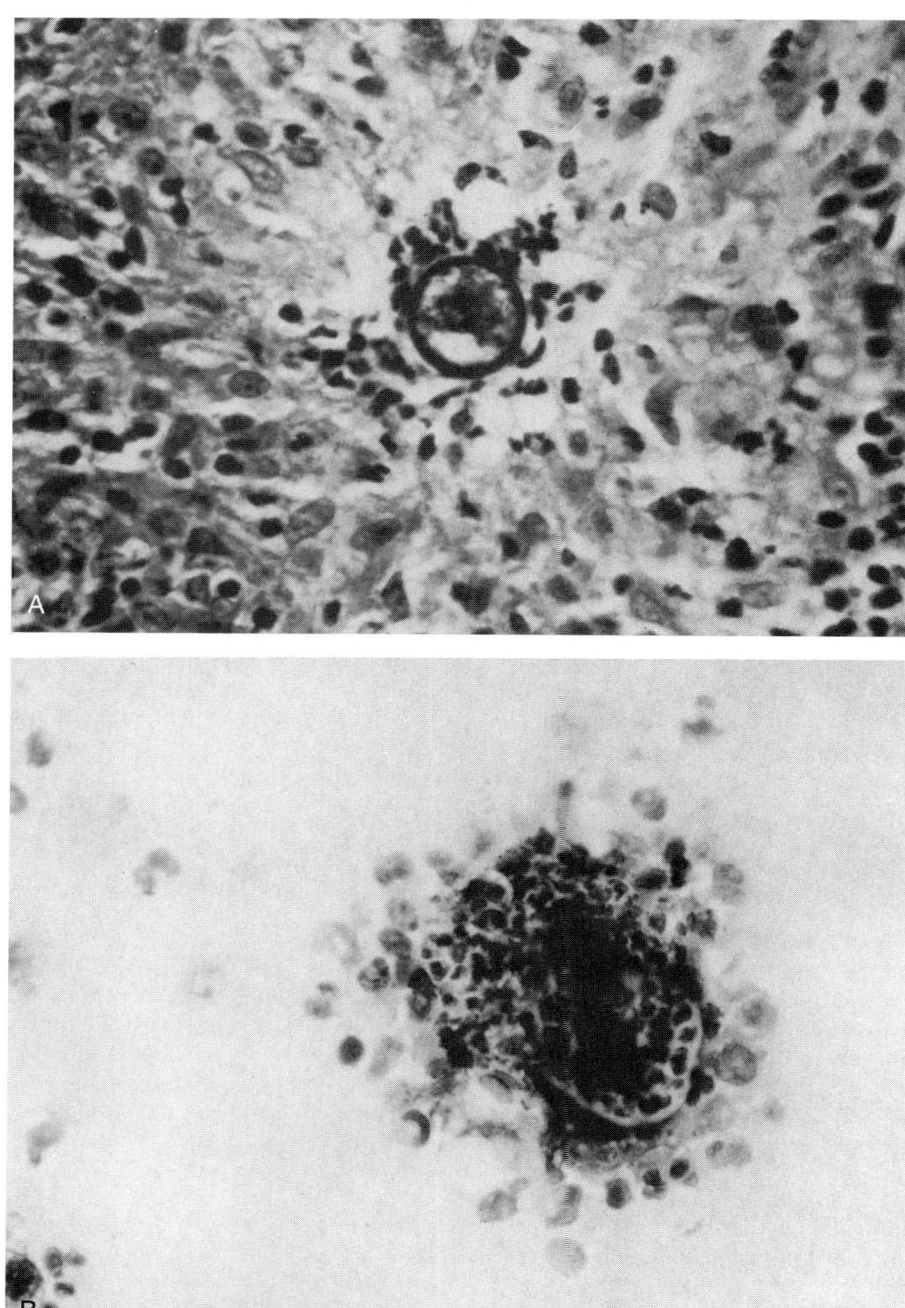

FIGURE 5–45. *A*, Canine coccidioidomycosis. *Coccidioides immitis* spherule in center of pyogranuloma (PAS stain). *B*, Direct smear from a dog with coccidioidomycosis. Ruptured spherule releasing endospores and surrounded by degenerate neutrophils. (Courtesy T. French.)

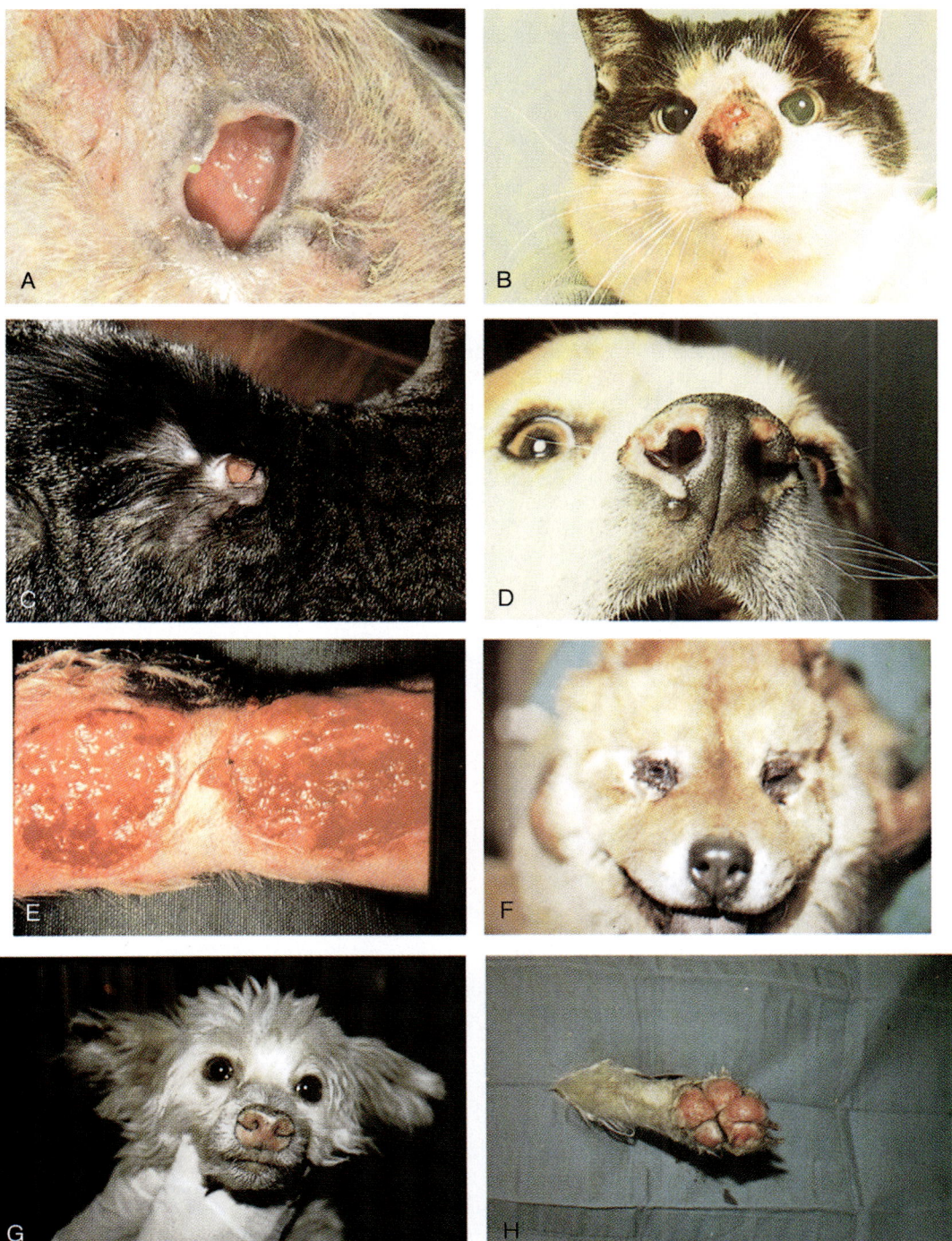

FIGURE 5–46. Miscellaneous fungal infections. *A,* Necrosis and ulceration in a dog with cryptococcosis. *B,* Granulomatous nasal dermatitis in a cat with cryptococcosis. *C,* Ulcerated nodule containing gelatinous exudate on the back of a cat with cryptococcosis. *D,* Multifocal areas of depigmentation and ulceration of the nostrils in a dog with nasal aspergillosis. *E,* Ulcers on the leg of a dog with aspergillosis. (Courtesy R. Halliwell.) *F,* Chronic blepharitis with sticky, black exudate in a Chow Chow caused by *Aspergillus niger. G,* Swollen, erythematous ulcerated nose of a dog with protothecosis. (Courtesy J. Perrier.) *H,* Swollen, ulcerated footpads of a dog with protothecosis. (Courtesy J. Perrier.)

Cat

Cryptococcosis is an uncommon disease, but it is the most common deep mycosis of the cat.[8, 14, 200, 202, 204, 211] Clinical signs occur from abnormalities of the upper respiratory, cutaneous, central nervous, and ocular systems.[8, 14, 200, 202, 211] In about 70% of cases with upper respiratory signs, a flesh-colored, polyp-like mass is visible in the nostril, or a firm to mushy subcutaneous swelling over the bridge of the nose is evident (see Fig. 5–46B). The skin or subcutaneous tissues are involved in about 40% of cases.[8, 14, 200, 201, 211] Lesions are usually multiple and include papules, nodules (see Fig. 5–46C), abscesses, ulcers, and draining tracts.[9, 208, 211, 216, 217] Skin lesions can occur anywhere but most commonly involve the face, pinnae, and paws.

DIAGNOSIS

Cytologic examination of aspirates or direct smears reveals pyogranulomatous to granulomatous inflammation with numerous pleomorphic (round to elliptical, 2 to 20 μm in diameter) yeastlike organisms. These show narrow-based budding and are surrounded by a mucinous capsule of variable thickness, which forms a clear or refractile halo (Fig. 5–47).[1–3, 9, 10, 211] Biopsy findings include a cystic degeneration or vacuolation of the dermis and subcutis that is surprisingly acellular (sometimes likened to an infusion of soap bubbles) (Figs. 5–48, 5–49) or a nodular to diffuse, pyogranulomatous to granulomatous dermatitis and panniculitis (Fig. 5–50) containing numerous organisms. Mayer's mucicarmine is a useful special stain because it stains the organism's capsule (carminophilic) red.[3, 211] The only clinically useful serologic test is a latex agglutination test that detects cryptococcal capsular antigen.[209, 211] It may, however, yield negative results in cats with disease apparently isolated to the skin.[209, 211, 217] The test may also be used to monitor response to therapy.[209, 211, 215, 217] However, serum titers to cryptococcal antigens in cats can persist, with or without clinical signs, for months to years after initial diagnosis and treatment.[201, 204]

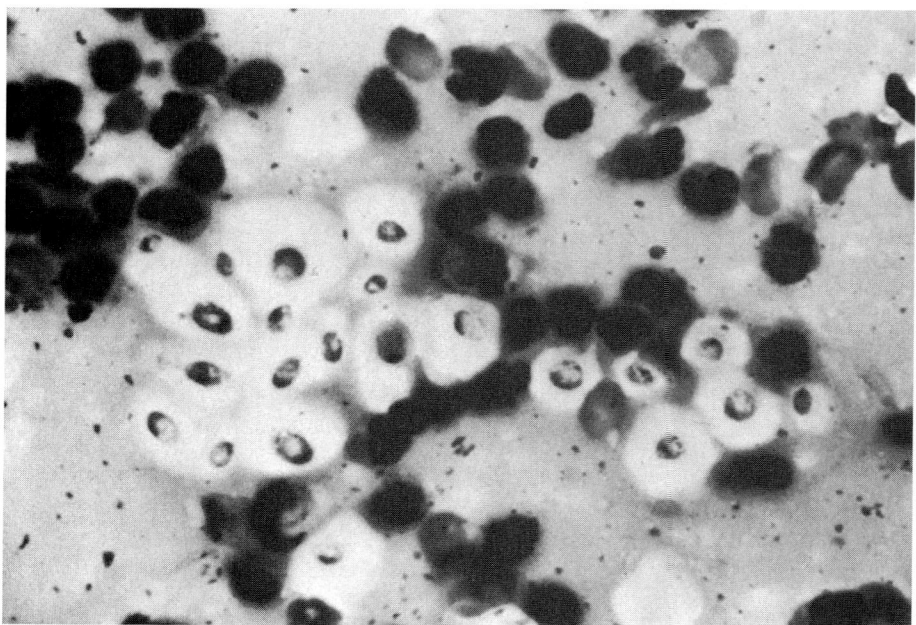

FIGURE 5–47. Canine cryptococcosis. Encapsulated yeast bodies in direct smear (NMB stain).

Fungal Skin Diseases • 399

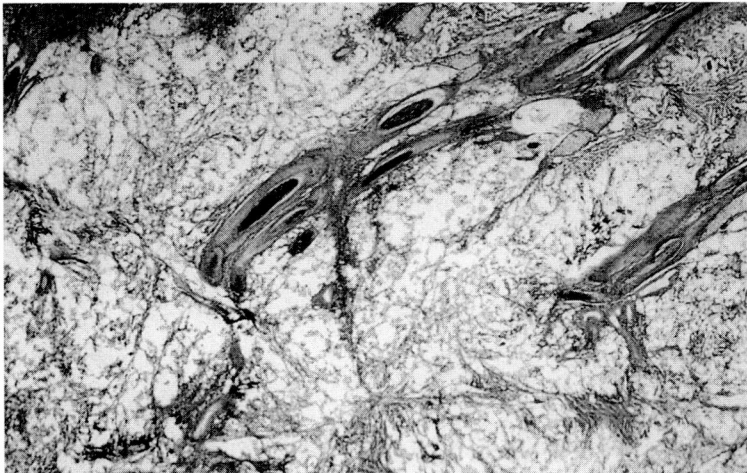

FIGURE 5–48. Canine cryptococcosis. Dermis and subcutis have a cystic or bubbly appearance. Numerous fungal organisms and very few inflammatory cells are seen on higher power (see Fig. 5–49).

CLINICAL MANAGEMENT

The drugs of choice are ketoconazole, itraconazole, and fluconazole.* Itraconazole was successful in cats in which ketoconazole had produced no response.[204, 212] Treatment outcome was not influenced by gender, location of infection, or magnitude of pretreatment serum antigen titer.[204] However, cats seropositive for FeLV or FIV had a higher

---

*See references 201, 203, 205, 208, 210–212, 215, 216.

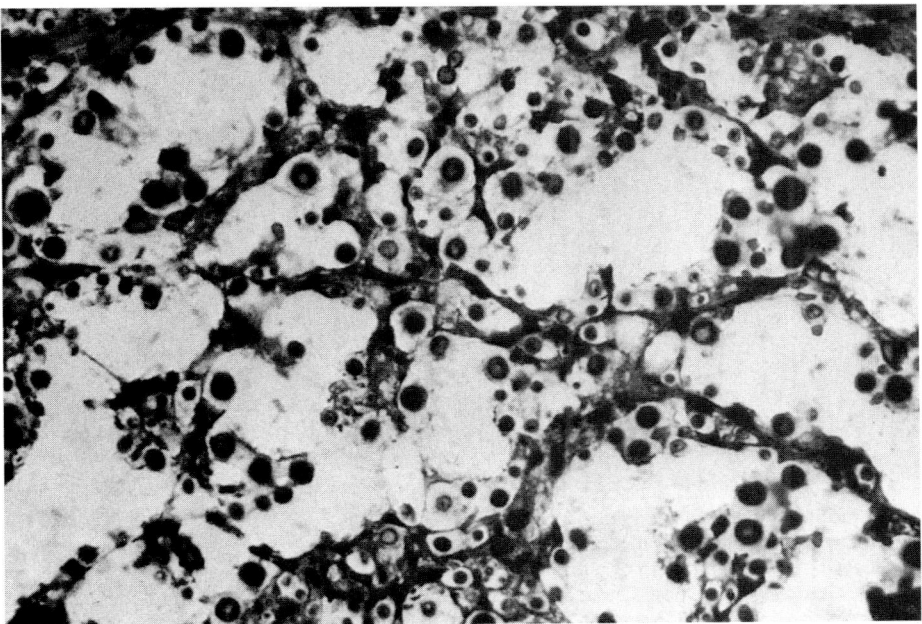

FIGURE 5–49. Feline cryptococcosis. Numerous encapsulated yeast bodies on a cystic background (mucicarmine stain).

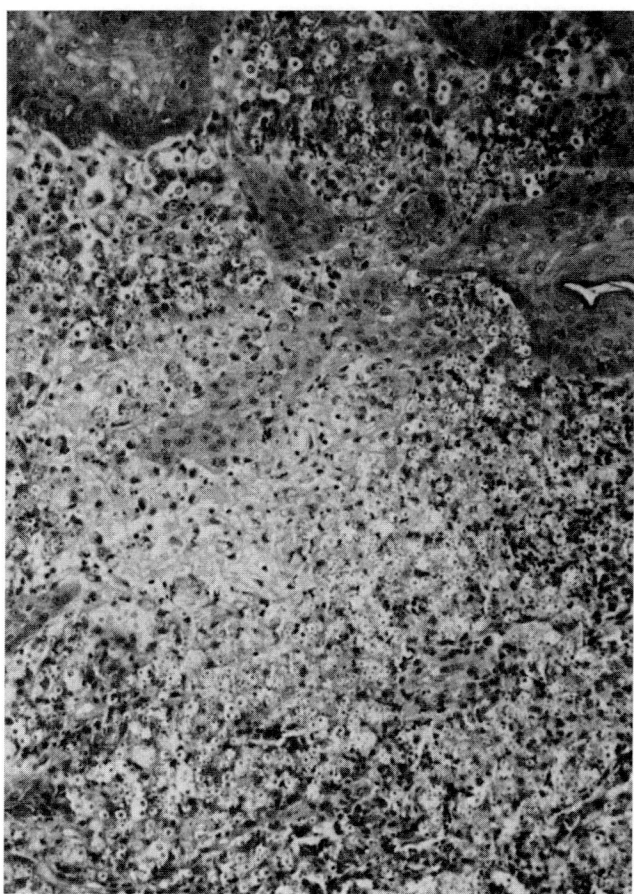

FIGURE 5–50. Feline cryptococcosis. Numerous encapsulated yeast bodies in pyogranuloma (H & E stain).

likelihood of treatment failure.[204] The combination of ketoconazole and flucytosine, with lower doses of both, may produce more rapid cures and a reduction in side effects.[213, 217] Amphotericin B, flucytosine, and the combination of both drugs have also been successfully used to treat cryptococcosis.[8, 14, 211, 218] Rarely, solitary lesions in animals with primary cutaneous cryptococcosis can be surgically excised and the animals cured.[208, 211] A preliminary report indicated that the subcutaneous administration of amphotericin B was effective and associated with less azotemia than traditional amphotericin B protocols.[206]

Histoplasmosis

CAUSE AND PATHOGENESIS

Histoplasma capsulatum is a dimorphic saprophytic soil fungus.[1, 2, 9, 10, 14, 229] The organism prefers areas with moist, humid conditions and soil containing nitrogen-rich organic matter such as bird and bat excrement. Most cases of histoplasmosis occur in the central United States in the Ohio, Missouri, and Mississippi River Valleys. Surveys indicate that most human and canine inhabitants of endemic areas become infected.

CLINICAL FINDINGS

Dog

Histoplasmosis is an uncommon disease in endemic areas.[14, 229] Young dogs (<4 years old) are usually affected, and Pointers, Weimaraners, and Brittany spaniels may be predisposed.[14, 229] Clinical signs include anorexia, weight loss, fever that is unresponsive to antibiotic therapy, coughing, dyspnea, gastrointestinal disease, ocular disease, and skin disease.[14, 229] Skin lesions are usually multiple, occur anywhere on the body, and are characterized by papules, nodules, ulcers, and draining tracts.

Cat

Histoplasmosis is an uncommon disease in endemic areas.[14, 228, 229] Most affected cats are younger than 4 years old, and most have disseminated disease. Clinical signs include depression, weight loss, fever, anorexia, dyspnea, ocular disease, and skin disease.[14, 228, 229] Skin lesions are usually multiple, occur anywhere on the body (especially the face, nose, and pinnae), and are characterized by papules, nodules, ulcers, and draining tracts (Fig. 5–51B).

DIAGNOSIS

A history of travel to an endemic area should increase the clinician's index of suspicion. Cytologic examination of aspirates or direct smears reveals pyogranulomatous to granulomatous inflammation containing numerous small (2 to 4 μm in diameter), round yeast bodies with a basophilic center and lighter halo caused by shrinkage of the yeast during staining (Fig. 5–52).[1, 2, 9, 10, 229] Biopsy findings include nodular to diffuse, pyogranuloma-

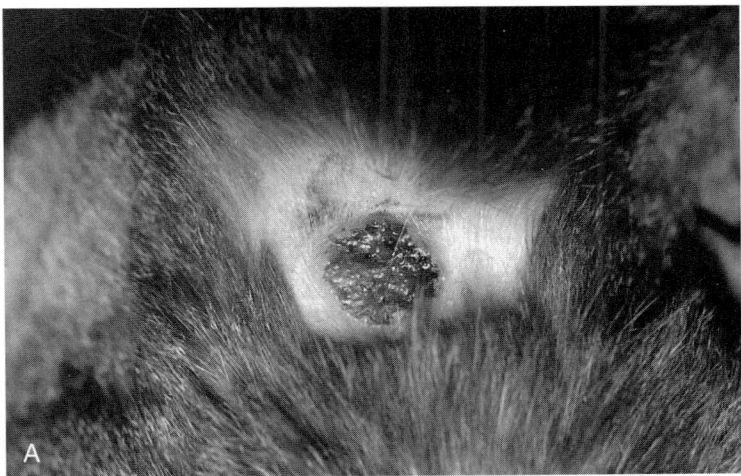
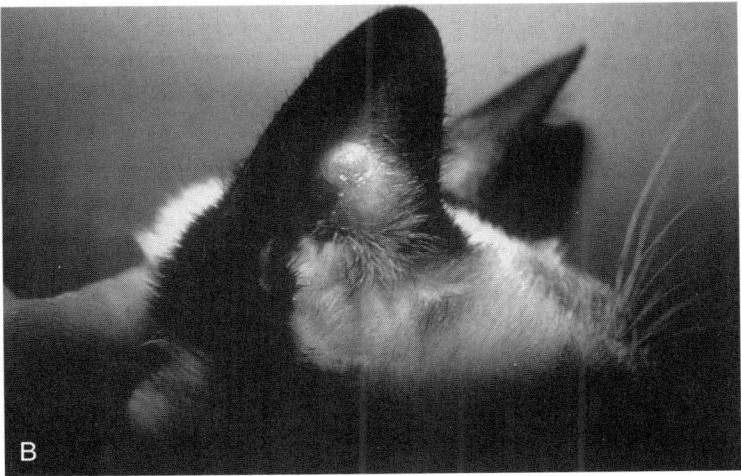

FIGURE 5–51. *A*, Feline blastomycosis. Nonhealing ulcer over lateral thorax. *B*, Feline histoplasmosis. Nodule on lateral surface of pinnae. (Courtesy J. MacDonald.)

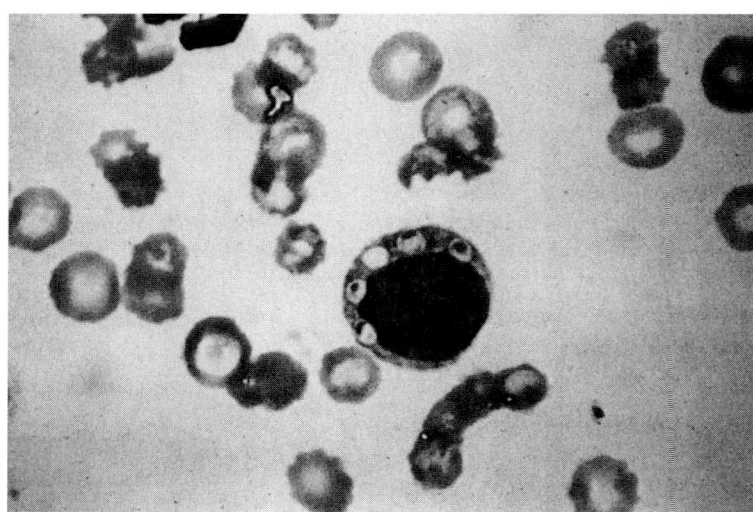

FIGURE 5–52. Direct smear from a dog with histoplasmosis. Multiple small, intracytoplasmic yeasts in a macrophage. (Courtesy T. French.)

tous to granulomatous dermatitis with numerous intracellular organisms (Fig. 5–53). At present, no reliable serologic test exists.[14, 229] Attempts to culture *H. capsulatum* in a routine practice setting are not recommended because of the pathogenic potential of this organism.[229]

CLINICAL MANAGEMENT

All animals with clinical histoplasmosis should be treated because spontaneous remission is unlikely.[229] The current drug of choice is ketoconazole.[14, 229] For severe or fulminating

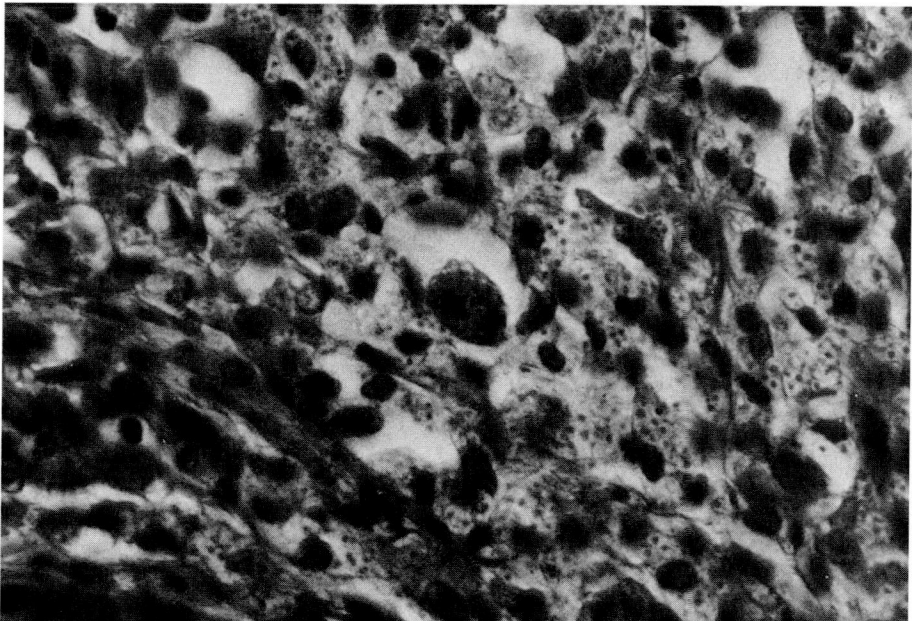

FIGURE 5–53. Canine histoplasmosis. Numerous small, intracellular yeast bodies in a granuloma (H & E stain).

cases, the combination of ketoconazole and amphotericin B is recommended.[14, 229] Itraconazole and fluconazole have shown promise in early trials.[228, 229]

• MISCELLANEOUS MYCOSES

Aspergillus Dermatitis

CAUSE AND PATHOGENESIS

Aspergillus spp. are ubiquitous fungi that exist in nature as soil and vegetation saprophytes and as a component of normal skin, haircoat, and mucosal flora in humans and animals.[13, 231] In humans, many cases of aspergillosis are associated with immunosuppression; in dogs, however, predisposing factors are not usually identified.[231] The organism is believed to produce opportunistic infections by invading mucosal or cutaneous surfaces. *A. fumigatus* is the most common species encountered in nasal aspergillosis, with *A. niger*, *A. nidulans*, and *A. flavus* being occasionally involved.[231] In disseminated aspergillosis, infection has involved, in decreasing frequency, *A. terreus*, *A. deflectus*, *A. flavipes*, and *A. fumigatus*.[231]

CLINICAL FINDINGS

To date, cutaneous and mucocutaneous *Aspergillus* infections has been reported only in dogs.[13, 230] Dolichocephalic and mesocephalic breeds are more susceptible to nasal aspergillosis, but there is no apparent age or sex predilection.[231] Inflammation, depigmentation, ulceration, and crusting of the external nares and, occasionally, the nasal planum may be visible secondary to nasal discharge (see Fig. 5–46D). Most cases of disseminated aspergillosis have occurred in German shepherds and have been reported from Australia or California.[13, 231] These dogs may have cutaneous nodules, abscesses, and draining tracts as well as oral ulcers. *Aspergillus* spp. have rarely been associated with cutaneous nodules and ulcers (see Fig. 5–46E) or blepharitis (see Fig. 5–46F) in otherwise healthy dogs.[13]

DIAGNOSIS

The differential diagnosis includes other infectious diseases, neoplastic diseases, and in the case of nasal aspergillosis, various immune-mediated disorders such as discoid and systemic lupus erythematosus, pemphigus foliaceus and erythematosus, and drug eruption. Cytologic examination of aspirates or direct smears reveals suppurative to pyogranulomatous inflammation, with fungal elements occasionally visualized. Biopsy findings include nodular to diffuse suppurative or pyogranulomatous dermatitis or necrotizing dermatitis with minimal inflammation. Organisms are usually plentiful and characterized by broad (3 to 6 μm in diameter) septate, dichotomously branched hyphae. *Aspergillus* spp. can be grown on Sabouraud's dextrose agar at 25°C.

In nasal aspergillosis, blind culture or cytologic examination of discharge is often unrewarding and can erroneously suggest that the disease is bacterial in origin.[231] Heavy growths of *Pseudomonas* spp. or other *Enterobacteriaceae* are common. In addition, *Aspergillus* or *Penicillium* spp. can be cultured from nasal swabs in up to 40% of normal dogs or dogs with nasal neoplasia.[231] Rhinoscopy allows fungal plaques (a white, yellow, or light-green mold) to be visualized and sampled directly for cytologic, histopathologic, and cultural examinations. Serologic diagnosis is possible using agar-gel immunodiffusion, counter immunoelectrophoresis, or ELISA techniques.[231]

CLINICAL MANAGEMENT

Thiabendazole (10 to 20 mg/kg q12h) or ketoconazole (5 to 10 mg/kg q12h) administered orally eliminates the disease in about 50% of the cases.[13, 231] Fluconazole (2.5 to 5 mg/kg q12h) is reported to be more effective than itraconazole (5 mg/kg q 12h), but few clinical trials have been conducted to date.[231, 255, 259] These medications must be administered for 3 to 4 weeks beyond clinical cure, so a total of 6 to 8 weeks of treatment is required. For nasal aspergillosis, the most successful therapeutic regimen is enilconazole administered topically for 7 to 10 days through tubes implanted in each nasal chamber via the frontal sinuses.[231, 255, 259] To date, no form of therapy has been successful in disseminated aspergillosis.[14]

Paecilomycosis

CAUSE AND PATHOGENESIS

Paecilomyces spp. are ubiquitous saprophytic, opportunistic yeastlike fungi that exist in nature in soil and decaying vegetation.[1, 2, 9, 10] In humans, disease occurs in immunosuppressed persons. The organism is presumed to produce opportunistic infections by invading mucosal or cutaneous surfaces. Evidence for immunosuppression has not been present for most reported cases of paecilomycosis in dogs and cats.

CLINICAL FINDINGS

Dog

The disease appears to be extremely rare. Most dogs have had disseminated infections with no skin lesions.[6, 13, 235] One dog had severe, chronic, bilateral otitis externa characterized by severe hyperplasia, ulceration, pain, and a brownish-black aural discharge.[236] Another dog had an ulcerated, crusted nodule in the region of the left caudal mammary gland.[234] Both dogs experienced disseminated disease.

Cat

The disease appears to be extremely rare.[233] One cat experienced an ulcerated, nonhealing nodule on a paw that was caused by *Paecilomyces fumosoroseus*.[232] The cat subsequently experienced other cutaneous, nasal, and disseminated lesions despite receiving ketoconazole orally at 10 to 40 mg/kg/day. Another cat had soft tissue swellings of a digit and contiguous metacarpus and an upper lip, from which *P. lilacinus* was consistently isolated.[237] Surgical excision and oral itraconazole was curative.

DIAGNOSIS

The differential diagnosis includes numerous infectious granulomas and neoplasms. Cytologic examination of aspirates or direct smears reveals pyogranulomatous inflammation and numerous pleomorphic fungal elements, including thick, branched, septate pseudohyphae and round to oval, often unipolar, broad-based budding, yeastlike structures (2 to 15 μm in diameter) (Fig. 5–54).[10, 232–234, 236] Biopsy findings include nodular to diffuse pyogranulomatous dermatitis with numerous fungal elements. *Paecilomyces* spp. grow on Sabouraud's dextrose agar at 25°C, and punch biopsy is the preferred material for culture.

CLINICAL MANAGEMENT

Paecilomyces spp. are usually resistant to amphotericin B but may be susceptible to azole compounds such as ketoconazole or itraconazole.[233, 234] Ketoconazole was of no benefit in one dog[234] and one cat[232] with paecilomycosis. Too few cases have been treated to allow detailed therapeutic and prognostic recommendations.

Prototheccosis

CAUSE AND PATHOGENESIS

Prototheca spp. are ubiquitous, saprophytic achlorophyllous algae that are found in soil, raw and treated sewage, the slime flux of trees, animal wastes, tap water, fresh water

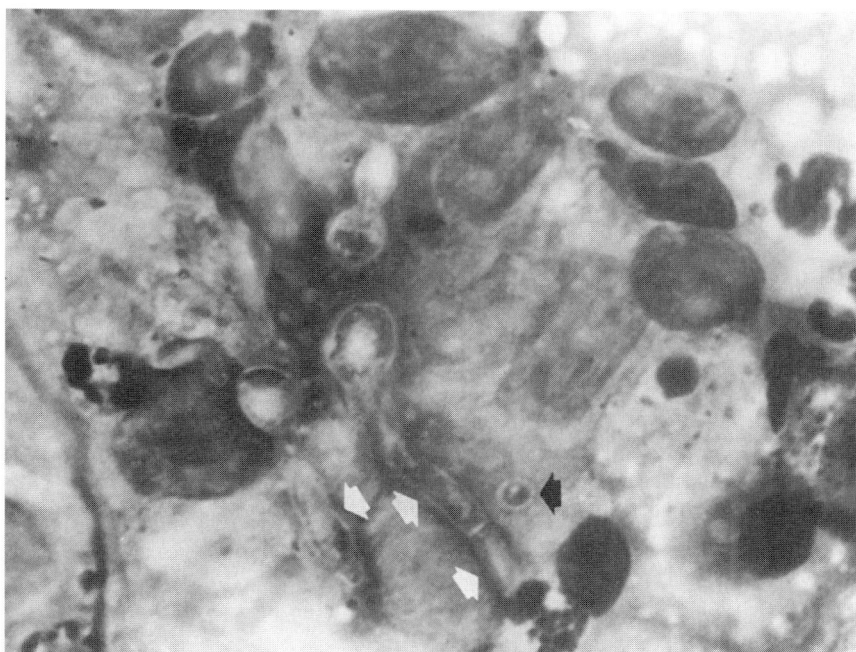

FIGURE 5–54. Paecilomycosis. Yeast-like structure (*black arrow*) and pseudohyphae (*white arrows*). (From Elliott GS, Whitney MS, Reed WM, Tuite JF: Antemortem diagnosis of paecilomycosis in a cat. JAVMA 184:93, 1984.)

streams, swimming pools, and contaminated and stagnant water.[238, 245] In North America, most cases are reported from the southern United States. The organism causes opportunistic infections, and disseminated disease is often associated with dysfunction of host immunity. The portal of entry is believed to be the colon in disseminated infections and wound contamination in cutaneous lesions. The virulence of the *Prototheca* organisms may differ; only *Prototheca wickerhamii* is isolated from cutaneous infections in dogs and cats, and *Prototheca zopfii* is nearly always isolated from disseminated infections in dogs.[245]

A 1997 immunohistochemical analysis of serial skin biopsy specimens from a dog with protothecosis, before and during treatment, revealed an inverse relation between the number of protothecal organisms and the number of infiltrating macrophages, neutrophils, T lymphocytes, and B lymphocytes.[243] These findings suggest either that protothecal organisms inhibit the migration or proliferation of cellular inflammatory infiltrate or that only dead organisms induce an effective local immune response.

CLINICAL FINDINGS

Dog

Protothecosis is a rare disease. Collies appear to be predisposed, and the majority of *Prototheca* spp. infections have occurred in females.[242, 244, 245] Dogs with disseminated protothecosis frequently have colitis and ocular and central nervous system involvement, but they rarely have skin lesions.[245] Disseminated disease is almost always associated with *P. zopfii*.

Dogs with cutaneous or mucocutaneous protothecosis usually do not have clinical signs of systemic involvement, and infection is invariably due to *P. wickerhamii*.[239, 241, 246] Dermatologic lesions may include multiple papules and nodules, often over pressure points, or nodules and ulcers involving mucocutaneous junctions (especially nostrils), scrotum, and footpads (see Fig. 5–46G and H). Depigmentation of the nasal planum may be striking (see Fig. 5–46).[239]

DIAGNOSIS

The differential diagnosis includes numerous infectious granulomas, foreign-body granulomas, and neoplasms. Cytologic examination of aspirates or direct smears reveals pyogranulomatous inflammation and numerous pleomorphic fungal elements, including septate, branching hyphae, arthroconidia (2.5 to 10.4 μm), and pleomorphic blastoconidia (2.5 to 8 μm in diameter).[247, 248] Biopsy findings include nodular to diffuse pyogranulomatous dermatitis with numerous fungal elements. Mycotic invasion of blood vessels may be visible; this often results in areas of necrosis. Trichosporon can be grown on Sabouraud's dextrose agar, and punch biopsies are the preferred material for culture.

CLINICAL MANAGEMENT

Trichosporon spp. are generally more susceptible to azole compounds than to amphotericin B or flucytosine.[248] Affected cats should be treated with oral ketoconazole or itraconazole. Not enough cases have been treated to allow detailed therapeutic and prognostic recommendations.

Geotrichum Dermatitis

CAUSE AND PATHOGENESIS

Geotrichum candidum is a ubiquitous soil saprophyte and a minor component of the normal flora of the oral cavity, gastrointestinal tract, and integument.[1, 233, 248a] The organism is believed to produce opportunistic infections by invading mucosal or cutaneous surfaces.

CLINICAL FINDINGS

Geotrichum dermatitis appears to be extremely rare. *Geotrichum* was cultured from both a cat with a nonhealing wound on its back and its owner, who had a granulomatous infection of the skin and subcutis.[8] One dog had a pinnal and periocular dermatitis that "spread" to its handler (human culture was not performed).[249] Another dog had a symmetric onychodystrophy from which *Geotrichum* was repeatedly isolated.[11] A healthy 5-month-old Rottweiler had 2 nodules, one on the head and one on the rump.[248a]

DIAGNOSIS

Cytologic examination of aspirates or direct smears reveals suppurative to pyogranulomatous inflammation with broad (3 to 6 μm in diameter), septate, infrequently branched hyphae, spherical yeastlike cells, and rectangular or cylindrical arthroconidia (4 to 10 μm wide) with rounded or squared ends.[1, 2, 8–10] Biopsy findings include nodular to diffuse, suppurative to pyogranulomatous dermatitis with numerous fungal elements. In one dog, biopsy specimens were characterized by suppurative epidermitis and folliculitis and by pyogranulomatous furunculosis, in which only a few fungal hyphae were seen, mainly adherent to follicular keratin and hair shafts.[248a] *Geotrichum* grows on Sabouraud's dextrose agar at 25°C, and punch biopsies are the preferred material for culture.

CLINICAL MANAGEMENT

Little information is available on the treatment of *Geotrichum* dermatitis. One cat and its owner were cured with amphotericin B.[8] One dog was cured with the topical application of miconazole.[249] The Rottweiler puppy described in Clinical Findings was cured after surgical excision of the two nodules.[248a]

• ANTIFUNGAL THERAPY

Topical

Topical therapy (see Table 5–3) is often curative in superficial yeast infections (*Malassezia*, *Candida*) and may be curative or adjunctive in dermatophytosis. Dermatophyte infections are difficult because the fungi are relatively protected within hair shafts and hair follicles. Topical agents tend to be more effective in short-coated animals, for localized alopecic lesions, and in long-haired animals that have been clipped. Many topical antifungal agents are of historical interest only and are not discussed in this text. Examples of such products include povidone-iodine, sodium hypochlorite, tolnaftate, Whitfield's ointment (benzoic and salicylic acids), Gentian violet, potassium permanganate, and so forth.[256] The interested reader is referred to previous editions of this book. Dermatophytosis is a difficult situation. Topical antifungal agents kill unprotected hyphae and spores rapidly, but not hyphae and spores within hairs.[38, 72]

SPOT TREATMENTS

Focal applications of topical antifungal agents are useful for the treatment of candidiasis, *Malassezia* dermatitis, and localized dermatophyte lesions in dogs and shorthaired cats.

Nystatin and *amphotericin B* 3% are polyene antibiotics that bind with ergosterol in fungal cell membranes, resulting in altered cell permeability and eventual cell death.[256] Either product may be applied every 12 hours to treat *Candida* or *Malassezia* infections, but they are *not* effective against dermatophytes. Nystatin is also available in combination with triamcinolone for highly inflammatory lesions.

Azoles inhibit the synthesis of ergosterol, triglyceride, phospholipid, chitin, and oxidative and peroxidative enzymes.[152, 256, 257] The imidazoles *clotrimazole* 1% and *miconazole* 1% or 2% may be applied every 12 hours for the treatment of dermatophytosis, candidiasis, and *Malassezia* dermatitis.[256] *Thiabendazole* 4% with dexamethasone 0.1% may be applied every 12 hours for the treatment of highly inflammatory dermatophyte lesions (kerions) or highly inflammatory *Malassezia* lesions (skin or ear).

Naftifine 1% (Naftin cream or gel) and *terbinafine* 1% (Lamisil cream) are allylamines that bind to stratum corneum and penetrate into hair follicles.[257] They inhibit ergosterol biosynthesis and squalene epoxidase and may be applied every 12 hours for the treatment of dermatophytosis and candidiasis. Naftifine also has anti-inflammatory activity and is useful for highly inflammatory dermatophyte lesions.

Chlorhexidine 4% (ChlorhexiDerm Maximum spray) is a synthetic biguanide (see Chap. 3 for details) that may be applied every 12 hours for the treatment of *Malassezia* and *Candida* infections and dermatophytosis.

SHAMPOOS

Antifungal shampoos are useful for the treatment of *Malassezia* dermatitis. However, because of their lack of demonstrated efficacy against dermatophytes and the danger of dispersing arthrospores into the haircoat and environment as a result of their application, shampoos are not recommended for the treatment of dermatophytosis. However, one study suggested that simultaneous treatment of dermatophytosis due to *M. canis* in Persian cats with oral griseofulvin and a 2% chlorhexidine/2% miconazole shampoo resulted in quicker resolution of clinical signs and less environmental contamination than with oral griseofulvin alone.[77]

Shampoos containing 2% to 4% chlorhexidine or 2% miconazole are effective for the treatment of *Malassezia* dermatitis and are the least likely to be drying or irritating. Daily application is most effective but more likely to be irritating, and it is impractical for most owners. Twice-weekly applications (every 3 days) seem to be adequate in most cases.

For animals who are particularly greasy or waxy, selenium sulfide 1% or sulfur 2%

with benzoyl peroxide 2.5% are effective. These two products can be too drying and are more likely to be irritating than chlorhexidine or miconazole.

RINSES

Antifungal rinses are the most effective topical products for the treatment of widespread superficial mycoses. They have more residual activity than shampoos. The preferred products are lime sulfur 2% (see Chap. 3 for details) or enilconazole 0.2%.[30, 36, 95] *Enilconazole* is an imidazole that is not presently approved in the United States. Although anecdotal information had suggested that enilconazole was not well-tolerated in cats,[71] a study in Persian cats indicated that no clinical, hematologic, or biochemical toxicities were observed.[39] Enilconazole is reported to be safe and effective for cats in France.[28, 255] Many people find the odor of the product to be objectionable. Enilconazole infusions are also one of the most effective methods for the treatment of nasal aspergillosis.[259]

Lime sulfur is typically applied once or twice weekly for *Malassezia* dermatitis and every 5 to 7 days for dermatophytosis (see Chap. 3 for details). Enilconazole is applied twice weekly.

Another useful rinse for the treatment of *Malassezia* dermatitis is *acetic acid* 2.5% (see Chap. 3 for details). The solution can be prepared by combining equal parts of vinegar (5% acetic acid) and water. The solution is well tolerated on the skin (*not* in the ears!) and is particularly useful as a foot soak (5 to 10 minutes daily) for *Malassezia* pododermatitis.

Systemic

The most common indication for systemic antifungal therapy (see Table 5–4) is dermatophytosis. Griseofulvin is still the systemic antifungal agent of choice in these cases.[66, 69, 71, 73] However, if it is ineffective, has caused complications, or is otherwise contraindicated, ketoconazole or itraconazole may be acceptable alternatives. For *Malassezia* infections, griseofulvin is not effective and ketoconazole is the drug of choice. Other regimens or treatments may be necessary for the less commonly encountered mycotic infections. Newer antifungals, particularly the triazole compounds and the allylamines, are available, but in general, they still have not been shown to be preferred over griseofulvin for routine use. In addition, they are not approved for use in the United States. Finally, they are expensive.

GRISEOFULVIN

Griseofulvin is a fungistatic antibiotic obtained by fermentation from several species of *Penicillium*. Its antifungal activity results from the inhibition of cell wall synthesis, nucleic acid synthesis, and mitosis. This agent is primarily active against growing cells, although dormant cells may be inhibited from reproducing.[256, 261] The drug inhibits nucleic acid synthesis and cell mitosis by arresting division at metaphase, interfering with the function of spindle microtubules, morphogenetic changes in fungal cells, and possibly antagonizing chitin synthesis in the fungal cell wall. After oral administration, the drug may be detected in the stratum corneum within 8 hours to 3 days. The highest concentrations are attained in the stratum corneum and the lowest are in the basal layers. The drug is carried to the stratum corneum by diffusion, sweating, and transepidermal fluid loss and is deposited in keratin precursor cells and remains bound during the differentiation process. Consequently, new growth of hair or claws is the first to be free from disease. Because griseofulvin is not tightly bound to keratin, tissue levels drop rapidly when therapy is stopped. Thus, it must be administered until an infected claw grows out, which takes months.

Griseofulvin is in a state of flux in the skin; consequently, a dosage administered once or twice daily is needed to maintain constant blood levels. When therapy is stopped, stratum corneum levels are gone in 2 to 3 days. This drug is indicated for only dermatophyte infections (*Microsporum* and *Trichophyton*). It is not effective against yeasts (*Candida* and *Malassezia*).

Griseofulvin is variably and incompletely absorbed from the gastrointestinal tract. Therefore, not all animals respond at the lower end of the dosage scale. If response is poor, the dosage may have to be increased. It should be given with a fatty meal to enhance absorption. Griseofulvin has a disagreeable taste, and nausea may be seen. Dividing daily doses increases absorption and reduces nausea. The particle size of the drug also affects absorption, and this influences the dosage. There are two common forms, a microsize crystal Fulvicin-U/F (Schering) given in a dosage of 25 to 60 mg/kg q12h (the most common initial dose is 25 mg/kg q12h), and ultramicrosize Gris-PEG in polyethylene glycol (Herbert) given in a dosage of 2.5 to 15 mg/kg q12h. This difference is important to recognize or toxicities may result. Idiosyncratic toxic reactions, particularly bone marrow suppression, have been reported.[260]

In problem cases, the dosage of microsize griseofulvin can be increased to at least 120 mg/kg/day with reasonable safety. One author recommended that kittens younger than 12 weeks of age not receive griseofulvin, although some clinicians use it in kittens as young as 6 weeks.[13, 25, 66] Kunkle and Meyer gave cats 110 to 145 mg/kg daily for 11 weeks without any signs of clinical, hematologic, or hepatic toxicity.[262] They concluded that abnormalities developing with the use of high-dose griseofulvin therapy may be an idiosyncratic reaction found in only a few cats. Anecdotal reports suggest that adverse reactions to griseofulvin may be more common and severe in Persians, Himalayans, Siamese, and Abyssinians, but this has not been our experience.[66]

Griseofulvin is a potent teratogen[266]; therefore, it is absolutely contraindicated in pregnant animals. However, many clinicians have administered griseofulvin to cats during the last week of pregnancy with no ill effects.[13, 261] Because griseofulvin can cause abnormalities in spermatozoa in rodents, it is advisable to avoid using recently treated male cats for breeding.[38] The most common problem is gastrointestinal upsets that resolve when the drug is discontinued. Anemia, leukopenia, depression, ataxia, and pruritus have also been reported.[13, 260] Rarely reported adverse cutaneous reactions include maculopapular or exfoliative eruptions as well as erythema multiforme or toxic epidermal necrolysis. They usually regress when the drug is withdrawn, although fatal reactions may occur. Hemograms every 2 weeks and careful observation are advisable during therapy to monitor those blood variables and the early onset of toxicity. The bone marrow reactions occur more commonly in cats with FIV infection, and screening before therapy is indicated.[267] Although produced by various species of *Penicillium*, griseofulvin, penicillins, and cephalosporins rarely exhibit cross-reactive side effects.

Griseofulvin does have anti-inflammatory and immunomodulatory properties and is known to suppress delayed-type hypersensitivity reactions and irritant reactions in the skin.[253, 263, 268] These properties can lead to important clinical misinterpretations. We have seen dogs and cats whose inflammatory skin diseases (e.g., bacterial pyoderma and pemphigus foliaceus) showed significant improvement while the animals were receiving large doses of griseofulvin for presumed dermatophytosis.

AZOLES

The systemically administered azoles include imidazole, ketoconazole, and the triazoles itraconazole and fluconazole.[256-259] They inhibit the cytochrome P-450 enzyme, lanosterol 14-demethylase, thereby inhibiting the conversion of lanosterol to ergosterol and causing the accumulation of C14 methylated sterols. Other actions include an inhibition of intracellular triglyceride and phospholipid biosynthesis, inhibition of cell wall chitin synthesis, and inhibition of oxidative and peroxidative enzymes. The potency of each azole is related to its affinity for binding the cytochrome P-450 moiety. The relative toxicity of each azole is associated with the selectivity of its action on fungal versus mammalian enzymes. Side effects occur in about 10% of dogs and 25% of cats treated with ketoconazole. Side effects are much less frequent and, in general, less severe with itraconazole and fluconazole.

Because the triazoles and allylamines are lipophilic and keratinophilic and because therapeutic levels persist in the skin and nails of humans for several days to weeks after treatment is stopped, shorter durations of treatment and pulse regimens (e.g., once-a-week dosing or 1 week of treatment per month) are feasible.[254, 256–258, 265] This has not been investigated in dogs and cats.

Drug interactions with the azoles are well-recognized.[257a] Interactions with certain antihistamines (terfenadine, astemizole), gastrointestinal motility agents (cisapride), benzodiazepines, calcium channel blockers, anticonvulsants, antimycobacterial agents, and cyclosporine are of particular concern.

Ketoconazole

Ketoconazole (Nizoral [Janssen]) is an imidazole that is active against many fungi and yeasts, including dermatophytes, *Candida*, *Malassezia*, and numerous dimorphic fungi responsible for systemic mycoses.[30, 59, 256, 259, 261] The therapeutic effect of ketoconazole is delayed for about 5 to 10 days. Consequently, in serious cases of systemic fungal disease, amphotericin B, which acts rapidly, is often used in combination with ketoconazole to compensate for this initial delay. Alternatively, one can use itraconazole or fluconazole.

Ketoconazole is insoluble in water but soluble in dilute acid solutions, and increased gastric acidity promotes absorption. When it is given with food, especially tomato juice, absorption is enhanced. Still, ketoconazole is variably absorbed, which probably accounts for the variation of doses needed in certain patients. It should not be given with gastric antacids, H_2 blockers, or anticholinergics. The major routes of delivery of ketoconazole to the stratum corneum are via sweat, sebum, and incorporation into basal keratinocytes. Ketoconazole is not approved for use in dogs and cats in the United States. A dosage of 10 mg/kg every 24 hours is effective for dermatophytosis, *Malassezia* dermatitis, and candidiasis. For systemic mycoses, higher dosages (30 to 40 mg/kg/day) are more commonly needed. Because ketoconazole does not readily enter the central nervous system, a dosage of 40 mg/kg every 24 hours is commonly necessary for life-threatening central nervous system and nasal mycoses.

About 10% of treated dogs experience side effects, including inappetence, vomiting, pruritus, alopecia, and a reversible lightening of the haircoat.[13, 259, 261] Side effects are more common with doses in excess of 10 mg/kg/day. It also enhances the effects of anticoagulants and increases the blood levels of cyclosporine and antihistamines, and its concentration may be decreased if it is given concurrently with rifampin. At dosages higher than 40 mg/kg/day, there were anorexia, nausea, and increased liver enzyme levels. Cats are more sensitive; about 25% experience side effects, including anorexia, fever, depression, vomiting, diarrhea, elevated liver enzymes, rarely icterus or neurologic abnormalities, and even death; therefore, one rarely exceeds 10 mg/kg/24 hours or 20 mg/kg/48 hours in cats. Cholangiohepatitis has also occurred in cats treated with ketoconazole.[13] Ketoconazole is embryotoxic and teratogenic in rodents, causes mummified fetuses and stillbirths in bitches, and is not recommended in pregnant animals. In dosages of 10 mg/kg/day or greater, it suppressed basal cortisol concentration and response to adrenocorticotropic hormone, suppressed serum testosterone concentrations, and increased serum progesterone concentrations in dogs.[271]

When administration of the drug is halted, a sharp rebound of testosterone levels occurs. In therapeutic use, one should be aware of the possible effect on libido and breeding effectiveness in male animals, adrenal insufficiency, the possibility of inducing or exacerbating prostate disease, and the potential for managing prostate disease, mammary carcinoma, and spontaneous hyperadrenocorticism.[13] Ketoconazole also has various immunomodulatory and anti-inflammatory effects, including suppression of neutrophil chemotaxis and lymphocyte blastogenic responses, inhibition of 5-lipoxygenase activity, and inhibition of leukotriene production.[264, 270, 272]

In veterinary medicine, ketoconazole is effective in the treatment of dermatophytosis, candidiasis, *Malassezia* dermatitis, blastomycosis, coccidioidomycosis, histoplasmosis, and cryptococcosis. In addition, it may be effective in some cases of mycetoma, phaeohyphomycosis, zygomycosis, sporotrichosis, alternariosis, aspergillosis, and protothecosis. Ketoconazole is often prescribed in combination with amphotericin B for systemic infections because the antifungal activity of both seems to be enhanced.

Itraconazole

Itraconazole (Sporanox [Janssen]) is a triazole, and, compared with ketoconazole, has increased potency, decreased toxicity, and wider spectrum of action.[55, 257, 259, 261] Susceptible organisms include dermatophytes, *Candida* spp., *Malassezia,* those causing many intermediate and deep mycoses, *Aspergillus, Sporotrichum,* and the protozoans *Leishmania* and *Trypanosoma.* The drug is given orally, with food, and concurrent antacids, H_2 blockers, and anticholinergics are contraindicated. For cats and small dogs, the capsules may be opened and the pellets mixed with food. A pediatric suspension is also available for oral administration and, because its bioavailability is greater than that of the capsules, does not need to be given with food. In cats, 10 mg/kg/day should be sufficient in most cases.[250] Some cats may require 10/mg/kg q12h. Occasional cats better tolerate 20 mg/kg q48h.

Anecdotal reports indicate that these doses of itraconazole often produce vomiting and/or anorexia in cats.[54] Lower doses of itraconazole (1.5 to 3.0 mg/kg/day) produced complete recovery (clinical and cultural) in only 8 of 15 cats with *M. canis* infection.[54] In dogs, most authors recommend 10 mg/kg/day,[13, 259] although a recent study indicated that 5 mg/kg/day was just as effective and caused less side effects.[224] The major routes of delivery to the stratum corneum are sweat, sebum, and incorporation into basal keratinocytes.

Itraconazole is lipophilic and keratinophilic, and levels in skin and claws may be 3 to 10 times higher than those in plasma. In humans, skin and nail levels persist up to 4 weeks and 6 to 9 months, respectively, after therapy is stopped.[265] Side effects are similar to those occurring with ketoconazole, but they occur much less frequently and with reduced severity. Because itraconazole is more specific for fungal than mammalian cytochrome P-450 enzymes, endocrinologic side effects are not produced.

Like ketoconazole, itraconazole also has various immunomodulatory and anti-inflammatory properties.[265, 270, 272] Toxicity studies in dogs showed that, even at a dosage of 40 mg/kg/day for 90 days, there were no reactions.[259] Although it is not recommended during pregnancy owing to teratogenic effects at high dosages, there were no detectable teratogenic effects at 10 mg/kg/day. In cats, 50 to 100 mg/kg/day produced some side effects, which appeared to be dose-dependent. Anorexia, nausea, and hepatotoxicity were the primary side effects and usually resolved after drug withdrawal. In dogs, doses of 10 mg/kg/day produce vasculitis and necroulcerative skin lesions in 7.5% of dogs treated.[224] These lesions did not occur at doses of 5 mg/kg/day. In humans, intermittant ("pulse") therapy (e.g., standard doses for 1 week each month) is effective.[265]

Fluconazole

Fluconazole (Diflucan [Roerig]) is a triazole and, compared with ketoconazole, has increased potency, decreased toxicity, and a wider spectrum of action: Susceptible organisms include dermatophytes, *Candida, Malassezia,* and those causing deep and intermediate mycoses. The drug can be given with or without food. The major routes of delivery to the stratum corneum are sweat, sebum, and incorporation into basal keratinocytes. High levels are achieved in skin, claw, and even the cerebrospinal fluid. Therapeutic levels persist in stratum corneum for 10 days after therapy is stopped. In humans, fluconazole persists in nails for 3 to 6 months post treatment.[258, 265] Because fluconazole is the most fungal enzyme–specific of the three systemic azoles, side effects are rare.[269] Only extremely high doses are embryotoxic and teratogenic, and endocrinologic side effects are not produced.

Recommended doses of fluconazole in cats and dogs vary from 10 to 20 mg/kg q12h to 10 mg/kg q8h.[205, 252, 259] The results of two pharmacokinetic studies indicate that fluconazole can effectively be administered to cats at 50 mg/cat q24h.[252, 269] In humans, intermittant therapy (e.g., every other day; once weekly) is effective.[265]

IODIDES

Iodides are given orally in daily doses of saturated solutions.[5, 13, 256, 261] They have a disagreeable taste and may cause nausea and iodism, especially in cats. Iodism may manifest as vomiting, diarrhea, depression, and anorexia. In dogs, ocular and nasal discharge, scaling, and a dry haircoat may be visible. Other signs that have been described in cats include twitching, hypothermia, and cardiovascular failure. Although iodides are widely distributed in the body, their mechanism of action is unknown because they have no efficacy against fungal organisms in vitro. Iodides do enhance the halide-peroxidase killing system of phagocytic cells. Iodides are anti-inflammatory agents by virtue of their ability to quench toxic oxygen metabolites and inhibit neutrophil chemotaxis.

Iodides are highly effective in the treatment of cutaneous and cutaneolymphatic sporotrichosis. A supersaturated solution of potassium iodide is used. Dogs are given 40 mg/kg orally q12h with food, and iodides are best tolerated when given with a fatty liquid such as cream or whole milk.[5, 261] Cats are given 10 to 20 mg/kg q12h to q24h with food. Cats may better tolerate the taste of sodium iodide over that of potassium iodide.[5, 261]

AMPHOTERICIN B

Amphotericin B (Fungizone [Squibb]) is a generally fungistatic polyene antibiotic that disrupts fungal (and bacterial) cell membranes by irreversible binding with ergosterol.[13, 256, 261] This results in altered cell permeability, leakage of intracellular constituents, and cell death. It also binds to a lesser extent to other sterols, such as cholesterol in mammalian cell membranes, and therefore is relatively toxic. Other possible mechanisms of action include oxidative membrane damage and enhanced cell-mediated immunity.

Amphotericin B stimulates lymphocyte, macrophage, and neutrophil function and induces production of tumor necrosis factor.[272] Amphotericin B is most effective for blastomycosis, histoplasmosis, coccidioidomycosis, cryptococcosis, and candidiasis: In the first three diseases when combined with ketoconazole, and in the last two when combined with flucytosine. These combination protocols are used to take advantage of the prompt action of amphotericin B and to reduce its toxicity.

Problems of therapy include nephrotoxicity (especially in dehydrated and hyponatremic animals), anemia, phlebitis, and hypokalemia.[261] One should avoid concurrent use of nephrotoxic drugs (e.g., aminoglycosides) and potassium-depleting diuretics. Amphotericin B may also be useful in the treatment of *Aspergillus, Trichosporon, Zygomycetes,* and disseminated *Sporotrichum* infections.

Organisms tend to develop resistance to the drug. Amphotericin given systemically must be given intravenously dissolved only in 5% dextrose and water. A reasonable dosage is as follows: 0.5 mg/kg on alternate days for dogs and 0.15 mg/kg for cats, which are more sensitive. Treatment with this drug is dangerous and complicated, and clinicians are advised to consult other references for specific guidelines.[6, 14, 261]

An amphotericin B lipid complex (Abelcet [The Liposome Company]) is reported to maintain therapeutic efficacy while being only one tenth as toxic as traditional amphotericin B solutions.[222, 263a] Amphotericin B was also reported to be useful when administered subcutaneously by gravity flow, but this study is difficult to interpret and needs further evaluation.[206]

FLUCYTOSINE

Flucytosine (Ancobon [Roche]) is an orally administered fluorinated pyrimidine that has been useful against *Candida, Cryptococcus, Aspergillus,* and some fungi associated with phaeohyphomycosis.[13, 256, 261] Fungal cells are susceptible if they contain the enzyme cytosine permease, which enables 5-fluorocytosine to be taken into the fungal cell, where it is deaminated by cytosine deaminase to 5–fluoro-21-deoxyuridylic acid. These substances inhibit thymidylate synthetase and subsequent DNA synthesis.

Resistant, mutant organisms emerge regularly and rapidly in the presence of the drug, which is why it is combined with amphotericin B. The oral dosage is 60 mg/kg q8h, but it is used as a second-line treatment, when more effective drugs, such as the imidazole and thiazole derivatives, are not available or are not well tolerated. As a single agent, flucytosine rarely produces side effects. Hematologic, gastrointestinal, and hepatic toxicities are reported. Fixed drug eruptions on the scrotum of dogs and toxic epidermal necrolysis have occurred.

TERBINAFINE

Terbinafine (Lamisil [Novartis]) is an allylamine that is well absorbed orally in the presence or absence of food.[257] It inhibits ergosterol biosynthesis and squalene epoxidase, resulting in fungal cell wall ergosterol deficiency and the intracellular accumulation of squalene. Terbinafine is fungistatic and fungicidal. Because it is generally not inhibitory to cytochrome P-450 systems, it is more selective than the azoles.

Terbinafine is lipophilic and keratinophilic and achieves high concentrations in stratum corneum, hair, sebum, and subcutaneous fat. The stratum corneum/plasma ratio varies from 13:1 to 73:1. The drug is delivered to the stratum corneum primarily via the sebum, then through the basal keratinocytes and to a lesser extent by diffusion through the dermis and epidermis. In humans, terbinafine persists in therapeutic levels in the skin for 2 to 3 weeks and in the nails for 2 to 3 months.

Terbinafine is active against dermatophytes, *Candida* spp., *Sporotrichum*, and *Aspergillus* spp. The major side effects are gastrointestinal. No embryonic or fetal toxicity or teratogenicity has been demonstrated.

There have been anecdotal reports of the use of terbinafine for the treatment of dogs and cats with dermatophytosis. Terbinafine (20 mg/kg q48h PO) was reported to be effective for dermatophytosis in cats, and no toxicities were noted.[255] Terbinafine (20 to 30 mg/kg q24h PO) was also reported to be effective and safe for the treatment of dermatophytosis in dogs.[251]

• REFERENCES

General Laboratory, Pathology, and Clinical Bibliography

1. Carter GR, Cole JR Jr: Diagnostic Procedures in Veterinary Bacteriology and Mycology V. Academic Press, New York, 1990.
2. Carter GR, Chengappa MM: Essentials of Veterinary Bacteriology and Mycology IV. Lea & Febiger, Philadelphia, 1991.
3. Chandler FW, Watts JC: Pathologic Diagnosis of Fungal Infections. ASCP Press, Chicago, 1987.
4. Fitzpatrick TB, et al: Dermatology in General Medicine IV. McGraw-Hill Book Co., New York, 1993.
5. Foil CS: Fungal diseases. Clin Dermatol 12:529, 1994.
6. Greene CE: Infectious Diseases of the Dog and Cat II. W.B. Saunders Co., Philadelphia, 1998.
7. Gross TL, et al: Veterinary Dermatopathology. Mosby Year Book, St. Louis, 1992.
8. Holzworth J: Mycotic diseases. In: Holzworth J (ed): Diseases of the Cat. Medicine and Surgery, Vol 1. W.B. Saunders Co., Philadelphia, 1987, p 320.
9. Kwon-Chung KJ, Bennett JE: Medical Mycology. Lea & Febiger, Philadelphia, 1992.
10. Rippon JW: Medical Mycology III. W.B. Saunders Co., Philadelphia, 1988.
10a. Saridomichelakis MN, et al: Recovery of *Microsporum gypseum* and *Malassetia pachydermatis* from the nasal bridge in various dog groups. Vet Rec 145:171, 1999.
11. Scott DW, Miller WH Jr: Disorders of the claws and clawbed in dogs. Comp Cont Educ 14:1448, 1992.
12. Scott DW, Miller WH Jr: Disorders of the claws and clawbed in cats. Comp Cont Educ 14:449, 1992.
13. Scott DW, et al: Muller and Kirk's Small Animal Dermatology V. W.B. Saunders Co., Philadelphia, 1995.
13a. Sierra P, et al: Fungal flora on cutaneous and mucosal surfaces of cats infected with feline immunodeficiency virus or feline leukemia immunodeficiency virus or feline leukemia virus. Am J Vet Res 61:158, 2000.
14. Wolf AM, Troy GC: Deep mycotic diseases. In: Ettinger SJ, Feldman EC (eds): Textbook of Internal Medicine IV. W.B. Saunders Co., Philadelphia, 1995, p 439.

Dermatophytosis

15. Antos I, et al: Nachweis von Dermatophyten bei klinisch gesunder Katzen und Hunden in Wien. Wien Tieräztl Mschr 83:199, 1996.
16. Bibel DJ, Smiljanic RJ: Interactions of *Trichophyton mentagrophytes* and micrococci in skin culture. J Invest Dermatol 72:133, 1979.
17. Blakemore JC: Dermatomycosis. In: Kirk RW (ed):

100. Dale JE: Canine dermatosis caused by *Candida parapsilosis*. Vet Med Small Anim Clin 67:548, 1972.
101. Greene CE, Chandler FW: Candidiasis. In: Greene CE (ed): Infectious Diseases of Dogs and Cats. W.B. Saunders Co., Philadelphia, 1990, p 723.
102. Guillot J, et al: Les Candidoses des carnivores domestiques: Actualisation à propos de 10 cas. Point Vét 28:51, 1996.
103. Ichijo S, et al: A canine case of cutaneous phyma caused by *Candida zeylanoides*. Jpn J Vet Med Assoc 37:773, 1984.
104. Kral F, Uscavage JP: Cutaneous candidiasis in a dog. J Am Vet Med Assoc 136:612, 1960.
105. Schwartzman RM, et al: Experimentally induced cutaneous moniliasis (*Candida albicans*) in the dog. J Small Anim Pract 6:327, 1965.

Malassezia *Dermatitis*

105a. Aizawa T, et al: Molecular heterogeneity in clinical isolates of *Malassezia pachydermatis* from dogs. Vet Microbiol 70:67, 1999.
106. Anthony RM, et al: The application of DNA typing methods to the study of the epidemiology of *Malassezia pachydermatis*. Microb Ecol Hlth Dis 7:161, 1994.
107. Bensignor E, et al: Comparaison de quatre techniques cytologiques pour la mise en évidence de *Malassezia pachydermatis* sur la peau du chien. Prat Méd Chir Anim Comp 34:33, 1999.
108. Boekhout T, Bosboom RW: Karyotyping of *Malassezia* yeasts: Taxonomic and epidemiological implications. System Appl Microbiol 7:146, 1994.
108a. Bond R: How might *Malassezia pachydermatis* cause canine skin diseases? Proc Br Vet Dermatol Study Group, Autumn 1999, p 41.
109. Bond R, Sant RE: The recovery of *Malassezia pachydermatis* from canine skin. Vet Dermatol Newsl 15:25, 1993.
110. Bond R, et al: Use of contact plates for the quantitative culture of *Malassezia pachydermatis* from canine skin. J Small Anim Pract 35:68, 1994.
111. Bond R, et al: Evaluation of a detergent scrub technique for the quantitative culture of *Malassezia pachydermatis* from canine skin. Res Vet Sci 58:133, 1995.
112. Bond R, et al: Comparison of two shampoos for treatment of *Malassezia pachydermatis*-associated seborrhoeic dermatitis in basset hounds. J Small Anim Pract 36:99, 1995.
113. Bond R, et al: Population sizes and frequency of *Malassezia pachydermatis* at skin and mucosal sites in healthy dogs. J Small Anim Pract 36:147, 1995.
114. Bond R, Anthony RM: Characterization of markedly lipid-dependent *Malassezia pachydermatis* isolates from healthy dogs. J Appl Bacteriol 78:537, 1995.
115. Bond R, et al: Factors associated with elevated cutaneous *Malassezia pachydermatis* populations in dogs with pruritic skin disease. J Small Anim Pract 37:103, 1996.
116. Bond R, Lloyd DH: Factors affecting the adherence of *Malassezia pachydermatis* to canine corneocytes in vitro. Vet Dermatol 7:49, 1996.
117. Bond R, Lloyd DH: Comparison of media and conditions of incubation for the quantitative culture of *Malassezia pachydermatis* from canine skin. Res Vet Sci 61:273, 1996.
118. Bond R, et al: Isolation of *Malassezia sympodialis* from feline skin. J Med Vet Mycol 34:145, 1996.
119. Bond R, Lloyd DH: Evidence for carbohydrate-mediated adherence of *Malassezia pachydermatis* to canine corneocytes in vitro. In: Kwochka KW, et al (eds): Advances in Veterinary Dermatology III. Butterworth-Heinemann, Boston, 1998, p 530.
120. Bond R, Lloyd DH: The relationship between population sizes of *Malassezia pachydermatis* in healthy dogs and in basset hounds with *M. pachydermatis*–associated seborrhoeic dermatitis and adherence to canine corneocytes in vitro. In: Kwochka KW, et al (eds): Advances in Veterinary Dermatology III. Butterworth-Heinemann, Boston, 1998, p 283.
121. Bond R, Lloyd DH: Skin and mucosal populations of *Malassezia pachydermatis* in healthy and seborrhoeic basset hounds. Vet Dermatol 8:101, 1997.
122. Bond R, et al: Isolation of *Malassezia sympodialis* and *Malassezia globosa* from healthy pet cats. Vet Rec 141:200, 1997.
123. Bord R, et al: Humoral and cell-mediated immune responses to *Malassezia pachydermatis* in healthy dogs and dogs with *Malassezia* dermatitis. Vet Rec 143:381, 1998.
124. Bond R, Lloyd DH: Studies on the role of carbohydrates in the adherence of *Malassezia pachydermatis* to canine corneocytes in vitro. Vet Dermatol 9:105, 1998.
125. Bond R, Lloyd DH: Effect of topical therapy of *Malassezia pachydermatis*–associated seborrheic dermatitis on oral carriage of *M. pachydermatis*. Vet Rec 142:725, 1998.
126. Carlotti DN, Laffort-Dassot C: Dermatite à *Malassezia* chez le chien: Étude bibliographique et rétrospective de 12 cas généralisés traités par des dérivés azolés. Prat Méd Chir Anim Comp 31:297, 1996.
127. Chang HJ, et al: An epidemic of *Malassezia pachydermatis* in an intensive care nursery associated with colonization of health care workers' pet dogs. N Engl J Med 338:706, 1998.
128. Coutinto SD, et al: Protein profiles of *Malassezia pachydermatis* isolated from dogs. Mycopathologia 139:129, 1997.
128a. Crespo MJ, et al: Isolation of *Malassezia furfur* from a cat. J Clin Microbiol 37:1573, 1999.
129. Dufait R: *Pityrosporum canis* as the cause of canine chronic dermatitis. Vet Med Small Anim Clin 78:1055, 1983.
130. Dworecka-Kaszak B, et al: Evaluation of selected physiological and morphological characteristics of *Pityrosporum pachydermatis* isolated from clinical cases of otitis externa and dermatitis in dogs and cats. Arch Vet Polon 34:3, 1994.
131. Forstervanhijfte MA, et al: Resolution of exfoliative dermatitis and *Malassezia* overgrowth in a cat after surgical thymoma resection. J Small Anim Pract 38:451, 1997.
132. Godfrey DR: A case of feline paraneoplastic alopecia with secondary *Malassezia*-associated dermatitis. J Small Anim Pract 39:394, 1998.
133. Griffin CE: *Malassezia* paronychia in atopic dogs. Proc Annu Memb Meet Am Acad Vet Dermatol Am Coll Vet Dermatol 12:51, 1996.
134. Guaguère E, Prélaud P: Etude rétrospective de 54 cas de dermite à *Malassezia pachydermatis* chez le chien: Résultats épidémiologiques, cliniques, cytologiques et histopathologiques. Prat Méd Chir Anim Comp 31:309, 1996.
135. Guillot J, et al: Prévalence du genre *Malassezia* chez les mammiferes. J Mycol Méd 4:72, 1994.
136. Guillot J, Guého J: The diversity of *Malassezia* yeasts

confirmed by rRNA sequence and nuclear DNA comparisons. Antonie van Leeuwenhoek 67:297, 1995.
137. Guillot J, et al: Epidemiological analysis of *Malassezia pachydermatis* isolates by partial sequencing of the large subunit ribosomal RNA. Res Vet Sci 62:22, 1997.
138. Guillot J, et al: Importance des levures du genre *Malassezia*. Point Vét 29:691, 1998.
138a. Guillot I, Bond R: *Malassezia pachydermatis*: A review. Med Mycol 37:295, 1999.
139. Kennis RA, et al: Quantity and distribution of *Malassezia* organisms on the skin of clinically normal dogs. J Am Vet Med Assoc 208:1048, 1996.
140. Kieffer M, et al: Immunological reactions to *Pityrosporum ovale* in adult patients with atopic and seborrheic dermatitis. J Am Acad Dermatol 22:739, 1990.
141. Lloyd DH, Lamport AI: Activity of chlorhexidine shampoos in vitro against *Staphylococcus intermedius*, *Pseudomonas aeruginosa*, and *Malassezia pachydermatis*. Vet Rec 144:536, 1999.
142. Lorenzini R, et al: In vitro sensitivity of *Malassezia* spp. to various antimycotics. Drugs Exp Clin Res 11:393, 1985.
143. Mason KV, Evans AG: Dermatitis associated with *Malassezia* pachydermatis in 11 dogs. J Am Anim Hosp Assoc 27:13, 1991.
144. Mason KV, Stewart LJ: *Malassezia* and canine dermatitis. In: Ihrke PJ, et al (eds). Advances in Veterinary Dermatology II. New York: Pergamon Press, 1993, p 399.
145. Mathieson I, et al: Enzymatic activity of *Malassezia pachydermatis*. In: Kwochka KW, et al (eds): Advances in Veterinary Dermatology III. Butterworth-Heinemann, Boston, 1998, p 532.
146. Mauldin EA, et al: *Malassezia* dermatitis in the dog: A retrospective histopathological and immunopathological study of 86 cases (1990–1995). Vet Dermatol 8:191, 1997.
146a. Midreuil F, et al: Genetic diversity in the yeast species *Malassezia pachydermatis* analysed by multilocus enzyme electrophoresis. Int J Syst Bacteriol 49:1287, 1999.
147. Morris DO, Rosser EJ: Immunologic aspects of *Malassezia* dermatitis in patients with canine atopic dermatitis. Proc Annu Memb Meet Am Acad Vet Dermatol Am Coll Vet Dermatol 11:16, 1995.
148. Morris DO, et al: Type-I hypersensitivity reactions to *Malassezia pachydermatis* extracts in atopic dogs. Am J Vet Res 59:836, 1998.
149. Nagata M, Ishidu T: Cutaneous reactivity to *Malassezia pachydermatis* in dogs with seborrheic dermatitis. Proc Annu Memb Meet Am Acad Vet Dermatol Am Coll Vet Dermatol 11:11, 1995.
150. Nuttall TJ: Serum specific IgG levels to cutaneous *Malassezia* in normal and atopic dogs. Proc Annu Cong Eur Soc Vet Dermatol Eur Coll Vet Dermatol 14:166, 1997.
151. Plant JD, et al: Factors associated with and prevalence of high *Malassezia pachydermatis* numbers on dog skin. J Am Vet Med Assoc 201:879, 1992.
152. Schmidt A: In vitro activity of climbzole, clotrimazole, and silver-sulfadiazine against isolates of *Malassezia pachydermatis*. J Vet Med B 44:193, 1997.
153. Scott DW: Bacteria and yeast on the surface and within noninflamed hair follicles of skin biopsies from dogs with nonneoplastic dermatoses. Cornell Vet 82:379, 1992.
154. Scott DW: Bacteria and yeast on the surface and within noninflamed hair follicles of skin biopsies from cats with nonneoplastic dermatoses. Cornell Vet 82:371, 1992.
155. Vitale C, et al: Quantification of *Malassezia pachydermatis* obtained from skin of normal and atopic dogs. Proc Annu Memb Meet Am Acad Vet Dermatol Am Coll Vet Dermatol 11:14, 1995.
156. Wagner R, Schadle S: *Malassezia* in 3 days old puppies. Proc Annu Memb Meet Am Acad Vet Dermatol Am Coll Vet Dermatol 15:45, 1999.
157. White SD, et al: Comparison via cytology and culture of carriage of *Malassezia pachydermatis* in atopic and healthy dogs. In: Kwochka KW, et al (eds): Advances in Veterinary Dermatology III. Butterworth-Heinemann, Boston, 1998, p 291.

Rhodotorula Dermatitis
158. Bourdeau P, et al: Suspicion de dermatomycose à *Rhodotorula mucilaginosa* chez un chat infecté par le FeLV et le FIV. Rec Méd Vét 168:91, 1992.

Piedra
159. Miguens MP, Ferreiros MP: Un caso de piedra blanca en un perro. Rev Ibér Micol 4:69, 1987.

Eumycotic Mycetoma
160. Allison N, et al: Eumycotic mycetoma caused by *Pseudoallescheria boydii* in a dog. J Am Vet Med Assoc 194:797, 1989.
161. Beale KM, Pinson D: Phaeohyphomycosis caused by two different species of *Curvularia* in two animals from the same household. J Am Anim Hosp Assoc 26:67, 1990.
162. Bourdeau P, et al: Pyogranulomatous panniculitis due to *Phialemonium curvatum* in the dog. In: Kwochka KW, et al (eds): Advances in Veterinary Dermatology III. Butterworth-Heinemann, Boston, 1998, p 447.
163. Coyle V, et al: Canine mycetoma: A case report and review of the literature. J Small Anim Pract 25:261, 1984.
164. Foil CS: Eumycotic mycetoma. In: Greene CE (ed): Infectious Diseases of Dogs and Cats. W.B. Saunders Co., Philadelphia, 1990, p 738.
165. Mezza LE, Harvey HJ: Osteomyelitis associated with maduromycotic mycetoma in the foot of a dog. J Am Anim Hosp Assoc 21:215, 1985.
166. van den Broek AHM, Thoday KL: *Eumycetoma* in a British cat. J Small Anim Pract 28:827, 1987.

Phaeohyphomycosis
167. Ajello L, et al: Phaeohyphomycosis in a dog caused by *Pseudomicrodochium suttonii*. Mycotaxon 12:131, 1980.
167a. Bond R: Phaeohyphomycosis in two cats, Proc Br Vet Dermatol Study Group, Autumn 1999, p 47.
168. Bostock DE, et al: Phaeohyphomycosis caused by *Exophiala jeanselmei* in a domestic cat. J Comp Pathol 92:479, 1982.
169. Dhein CR, et al: Phaeohyphomycosis caused by *Alternaria alternata* in a cat. J Am Vet Med Assoc 193:1101, 1988.
170. Foil CS: Phaeohyphomycosis. In: Greene CE (ed): Infectious Diseases of Dogs and Cats. W.B. Saunders Co., Philadelphia, 1990, p 737.
171. Jang SS, et al: Feline abscesses due to *Cladosporium trichoides*. Sabouraudia 15:115, 1977.
172. Kettlewell P, et al: Phaeohyphomycosis caused by *Exophiala spinifera* in two cats. J Med Vet Mycol 27:257, 1989.
173. Kwochka KW, et al: Canine phaeohyphomycosis

caused by *Drechslera spicifera*: A case report and literature review. J Am Anim Hosp Assoc 20:625, 1984.
174. Lomax LG, et al: Osteolytic phaeohyphomycosis in a German shepherd dog caused by *Phialemonium obovatum*. J Clin Microbiol 23:987, 1986.
175. Malik R, et al: Phaeohyphomycosis caused by *Exophiala jeanselmei* in a cat. Aust Vet Practit 24:27, 1994.
176. McKeever PJ, et al: Chromomycosis in a cat: Successful medical therapy. J Am Anim Hosp Assoc 19:533, 1983.
177. McKenzie RA, et al: Subcutaneous phaeohyphomycosis caused by *Moniliella suaveolens* in two cats. Vet Pathol 21:582, 1984.
178. Outerbridge CA, et al: Phaeohyphomycosis in a cat. Can Vet J 36:629, 1995.
179. Padhye AA, et al: *Xylohypha emmonsii* sp. nov., a new agent of phaeohyphomycosis. J Clin Microbiol 26:702, 1988.
180. Pukay BP, Dion WW: Feline phaeohyphomycosis: Treatment with ketoconazole and 5–FC. Can Vet J 25:130, 1984.
181. Sousa CA, et al: Subcutaneous phaeohyphomycosis (*Stemphyllium* sp. and *Cladosporium* sp. infections) in a cat. J Am Vet Med Assoc 185:673, 1984.
182. Van Steenhouse JL, et al: Subcutaneous phaeohyphomycosis caused by *Scolecobasidium humicola* in a cat. Mycopathologia 102:123, 1988.
183. Waurzyniak BJ, et al: Dual systemic mycosis caused by *Bipolaris spicifera* and *Torulopsis glabrata* in a dog. Vet Pathol 29:566, 1992.

Pythiosis and Zygomycosis

184. Bauer RW, et al: Oral conidiobolomycosis in a dog. Vet Dermatol 8:115, 1997.
185. Bentinck-Smith J, et al: Canine pythiosis—isolation and identification of *Pythium insidiosum*. J Vet Diagn Invest 1:295, 1989.
185a. Dykstra MJ, et al: A description of cutaneous-subcutaneous pythiosis in fifteen dogs. Med Mycol 37:427, 1999.
186. English MP, Lucke VM: Phycomycosis in a dog caused by unusual strains of *Absidia corymbifera*. Sabouraudia 8:126, 1970.
187. Foil CSO, et al: A report of subcutaneous pythiosis in five dogs and a review of the etiologic agent *Pythium* spp. J Am Anim Hosp Assoc 20:959, 1984.
188. Foil CS: Oömycosis (pythiosis). In: Greene CE (ed): Infectious Diseases of Dogs and Cats. W.B. Saunders Co., Philadelphia, 1990, p 731.
189. Foil CS: Zygomycosis. In: Greene CE (ed): Infectious Diseases of Dogs and Cats. W.B. Saunders Co., Philadelphia, 1990, p 734.
190. Hillier A, et al: Canine subcutaneous zygomycosis caused by *Conidiobolus* sp. A case report and review of *Conidiobolus* infections in other species. Vet Dermatol 5:205, 1994.
191. Thomas RC, Lewis DT: Pythiosis in dogs and cats. Compend Cont Educ 20:63, 1998.

Sporotrichosis

192. Dunstan RW, et al: Feline sporotrichosis: A report of five cases with transmission to humans. J Am Acad Dermatol 15:37, 1986.
193. Macdonald E, et al: Reappearance of *Sporothrix schenckii* lesions after administration of Solu-Medrol to infected cats. Sabouraudia 18:295, 1980.
194. Nogueira RHG, et al: Relato de esporotricose felina (*Sporothrix schenckii*) com transmissão para o homem: Aspectos clínicos, microbiológicos e anatomopatológicos. Arq Bras Med Vet Zootec 47:43, 1995.
195. Rosser EJ Jr: Sporotrichosis. In: Griffin CE, et al (eds): Current Veterinary Dermatology. Mosby-Year Book, St. Louis, 1993, p 49.
196. Werner AH, Werner BE: Sporotrichosis in man and animals. Int J Dermatol 33:692, 1994.

Rhinosporidiosis

197. Breitschwerdt E: Rhinosporidiosis. In: Griffin CE, et al (eds): Current Veterinary Dermatology. Mosby-Year Book, St. Louis, 1993, p 711.

Alternaria Dermatitis

198. Baumgärtner W, Posselt HJ: Kutane Alternariose bei Hunden mit unspezifischen Dermatitiden. Kleintierpraxis 28:353, 1983.
199. Weiss R, et al: Schimmelpilzmykose beim Hund durch *Alternaria tenuissima*. Kleintierpraxis 33:293, 1988.

Cryptococcosis

200. Davies C, Troy GC: Deep mycotic infections in cats. J Am Anim Hosp Assoc 32:38, 1996.
201. Flatland B, et al: Clinical and serologic evaluation of cats with cryptococcosis. J Am Vet Med Assoc 209:1110, 1996.
202. Gerdes-Grogan S, Dayrell-Hurt B: Feline cryptococcosis. A retrospective evaluation. J Am Anim Hosp Assoc 33:118, 1997.
203. Hansen BL: Successful treatment of severe feline cryptococcosis with long-term high doses of ketoconazole. J Am Anim Hosp Assoc 23:193, 1987.
204. Jacobs GJ, et al: Cryptococcal infection in cats: Factors influencing treatment, outcome, and the results of sequential serum antigen titers in 35 cats. J Vet Int Med 11:1, 1997.
205. Malik R, et al: Cryptococcosis in cats: Clinical and mycological assessment of 29 cases and evaluation of treatment using orally administered fluconazole. J Med Vet Mycol 30:133, 1992.
206. Malik R, et al: Combination chemotherapy of canine and feline cryptococcosis using subcutaneously administered amphotericin B. Aust Vet J 73:124, 1996.
207. Malik R, et al: Cryptococcosis in dogs: A retrospective study of 20 consecutive cases. J Med Vet Mycol 33:291, 1995.
208. Medleau L, et al: Cutaneous cryptococcosis in three cats. J Am Vet Med Assoc 187:169, 1985.
209. Medleau L, et al: Clinical evaluation of a cryptococcal antigen latex agglutination test for diagnosis of cryptococcosis in cats. J Am Vet Med Assoc 196:1470, 1990.
210. Medleau L, et al: Evaluation of ketoconazole and itraconazole for treatment of disseminated cryptococcosis in cats. Am J Vet Res 51:1454, 1990.
211. Medleau L, Barsanti JA: Cryptococcosis. In: Greene CE (ed): Infectious Diseases of Dogs and Cats. W.B. Saunders Co., Philadelphia, 1990, p 687.
212. Medleau L, et al: Itraconazole for the treatment of cryptococcosis in cats. J Vet Int Med 9:39, 1995.
213. Mikicluk MG, et al: Successful treatment of feline cryptococcosis with ketoconazole and flucytosine. J Am Anim Hosp Assoc 26:199, 1990.
214. Mitchell DH, et al: Cryptococcal disease of the CNS in immunocompetent hosts: Influence of cryptococcal variety on clinical manifestations and outcome. Clin Infect Dis 20:611, 1995.
215. Noxon JO, et al: Ketoconazole therapy in canine and

feline cryptococcosis. J Am Anim Hosp Assoc 22:179, 1986.
216. Pentlarge VW, Martin RA: Treatment of cryptococcosis in three cats using ketoconazole. J Am Vet Med Assoc 188:536, 1986.
217. Shaw SE: Successful treatment of 11 cases of feline cryptococcosis. Aust Vet Pract 18:135, 1988.
218. Wilkinson GT, et al: Successful treatment of four cases of feline cryptococcosis. J Small Anim Pract 24: 507, 1983.

Blastomycosis
219. Arceneaux KA, et al: Blastomycosis in dogs: 115 cases (1980–1995). J Am Vet Med Assoc 213:658, 1998.
220. Côté E, et al: Blastomycoses in six dogs in New York State. J Vet Med Assoc 210:502, 1997.
221. Côté E, et al: Possible transmission of *Blastomyces dermatitidis* via culture specimen. J Am Vet Med Assoc 210:479, 1997.
221a. Gortel K, et al: Calcinosis cutis associated with systemic blastomycosis in three dogs. J Am Anim Hosp Assoc 35:368, 1999.
222. Krawiec DR, et al: Use of an amphotericin B lipid complex for treatment of blastomycosis in dogs. J Am Vet Med Assoc 209:2073, 1996.
223. Legendre AM: Blastomycosis. In: Greene CE (ed): Infectious Diseases of Dogs and Cats. W.B. Saunders Co., Philadelphia, 1990, p 669.
224. Legendre AM, et al: Treatment of blastomycosis with itraconazole in 112 dogs. J Vet Int Med 10:365, 1996.
225. Rudmann DG, et al: Evaluation of risk factors for blastomycosis in dogs: 857 cases (1980–1990). J Am Vet Med Assoc 201:1754, 1992.

Coccidioidomycosis
226. Barsanti JA, Jeffery KL: Coccidioidomycosis. In: Greene CE (ed): Infectious Diseases of Dogs and Cats. W.B. Saunders Co., Philadelphia, 1990, p 696.
227. Greene RT, Troy GC: Coccidioidomycosis in 48 cats: A retrospective study (1984–1993). J Vet Int Med 9: 86, 1995.

Histoplasmosis
228. Hodges RD, et al: Itraconazole for the treatment of histoplasmosis in cats. J Vet Int Med 8:409, 1994.
229. Wolf AM: Histoplasmosis. In: Greene CE (ed): Infectious Diseases of Dogs and Cats. W.B. Saunders Co., Philadelphia, 1990, p 679.

Aspergillus Dermatitis
230. Nooruddin M, et al: Cutaneous alternariosis and aspergillosis in humans, dogs, and goats in Punjab. Indian J Vet Med 6:65, 1986.
231. Sharp, N. J. H., et al: Canine nasal aspergillosis and penicilliosis. Comp Cont Educ 13:41, 1991.

Paecilomycosis
232. Elliott GS, et al: Antemortem diagnosis of paecilomycosis in a cat. J Am Vet Med Assoc 184:93, 1984.
233. Foil CS: Hyalohyphomycosis. In: Greene CE (ed): Infectious Diseases of Dogs and Cats. W.B. Saunders Co., Philadelphia, 1990, p 735.
234. Littman MP, Goldschmidt MH: Systemic paecilomycosis in a dog. J Am Vet Med Assoc 191:445, 1987.
235. Nakagawa Y, et al: A canine case of profound granulomatosis due to *Paecilomyces* fungus. J Vet Med Sci 58:157, 1996.
236. Patterson JM, et al: A case of disseminated paecilomycosis in the dog. J Am Anim Hosp Assoc 19:569, 1983.
237. Rosser EJ: Cutaneous paecilomycosis in a cat. Proc Annu Memb Meet Am Acad Vet Dermatol Am Coll Vet Dermatol 15:37, 1999.

Protothecosis
238. Boyd AS, et al: Cutaneous manifestations of *Prototheca* infections. J Am Acad Dermatol 32:758, 1995.
239. Dechervois I, Plassiart G: Protothécose cutanéo-nasale chez un chien. Prat Méd Chir Anim Comp 33: 145, 1998.
240. Dillberger JE, et al: Protothecosis in two cats. J Am Vet Med Assoc 192:1557, 1988.
241. Ginel P, et al: Cutaneous protothecosis in a dog. Vet Rec 140:651, 1997.
242. Macartney L, et al: Cutaneous protothecosis in the dog: First confirmed case in Britain. Vet Rec 123:494, 1988.
243. Pérez J, et al: Canine cutaneous protothecosis: An immunohistochemical analysis of the inflammatory cellular infiltrate. J Comp Pathol 117:83, 1997.
244. Sudman MS, et al: Primary mucocutaneous protothecosis in a dog. J Am Vet Med Assoc 163:1372, 1973.
245. Tyler DE: Protothecosis. In: Greene CE (ed): Infectious Diseases of Dogs and Cats. W.B. Saunders Co., Philadelphia, 1990, p 742.
246. Wilkinson GT, Leong G: Protothecosis in a dog. Aust Vet Pract 18:147, 1988.

Trichosporon Dermatitis
247. Doster AR, et al: Trichosporonosis in two cats. J Am Vet Med Assoc 190:1184, 1987.
248. Greene CE, Chandler FW: Trichosporonosis. In: Greene CE (ed): Infectious Diseases of Dogs and Cats. W.B. Saunders Co., Philadelphia, 1990, p 728.

Geotrichum Dermatitis
248a. Reppas GP, Snoeck TD: Cutaneous geotrichosis in a dog. Aust Vet J 77:547, 1999.
249. Sidhu RK, et al: Cutaneous geotrichosis in a dog and its handler—a case report. Indian J Anim Hlth 32:1, 1993.

Antifungal Therapy
250. Boothe DM, et al: Itraconazole disposition after single oral and intravenous and multiple oral dosing in healthy cats. Am J Vet Res 58:872, 1997.
251. Chen C: Personal communication, 1997.
252. Craig AJ, et al: Pharmacokinetics of fluconazole in cats after intravenous and oral administration. Res Vet Sci 57:372, 1994.
253. D'Arcy P, et al: The anti-inflammatory action of griseofulvin in experimental animals. J Pharm Pharmacol 12:659, 1960.
254. deDoncker P, et al: Antifungal pulse therapy for onychomycosis. Arch Dermatol 132:34–41, 1996.
255. Guillot J, Chermette R: Le traitement des mycoses des carnivores domestiques. Point Vét 28:51, 1997.
256. Gupta AK, et al: Antifungal agents: An overview: Part I. J Am Acad Dermatol 30:677, 1994.
257. Gupta AK, et al: Antifungal agents: An overview: Part II. J Am Acad Dermatol 30:911, 1994.
257a. Gupta AK, et al: Drug interactions with intraconazole, fluconazole, and terbinafine and their management. J Am Acad Dermatol 41:237, 1999.
258. Faergemann J: Pharmacokinetics of fluconazole in skin and nails. J Am Acad Dermatol 40:S14, 1999.
259. Heit MC, Riviere JE: Antifungal therapy: Ketoconazole and other azole derivatives. Comp Cont Educ 21, 1995.
260. Helton KA, et al: Griseofulvin toxicity in cats: Litera-

ture review and report of seven cases. J Am Anim Hosp Assoc 22:453, 1986.
261. Hill PB, et al: A review of systemic antifungal agents. Vet Dermatol 6:59, 1995.
262. Kunkle GA, Meyer DJ: Toxicity of high doses of griseofulvin in cats. J Am Vet Med Assoc 191:322, 1987.
263. Mitchell F, et al: Griseofulvin: Immunosuppressive action. Proc Soc Exp Biol Med 143:165, 1973.
263a. Plotnick AN: Lipid-based formulations of amphotericin B. J Am Vet Med Assoc 216:838, 2000.
264. Rowan-Kelly B, et al: Modification of polymorphonuclear leukocytes by imidazoles. Int J Immunopharmacol 6:389, 1984.
265. Scher RK: Onychomycosis: Therapeutic update. J Am Acad Dermatol 40:S21, 1999.
266. Scott FW, et al: Teratogenesis in cats associated with griseofulvin therapy. Teratology 11:79, 1975.
267. Shelton GH, et al: Severe neutropenia associated with griseofulvin therapy in cats with feline immunodeficiency virus infection. J Vet Int Med 4:317, 1990.
268. Tamaki K, et al: Differential effect of griseofulvin on interferon-induced HLA-DR and intercellular adhesion molecule-1 expression of human keratinocytes. Br J Dermatol 127:258, 1992.
269. Vaden SL, et al: Fluconazole in cats: Pharmacokinetics following intravenous and oral administration and penetration into cerebrospinal fluid, aqueous humour, and pulmonary epithelial lining fluid. J Vet Pharmacol Therap 20:181, 1997.
270. Van Cutsem J, et al: The anti-inflammatory effects of ketoconazole. J Am Acad Dermatol 25:257, 1991.
271. Willard MD, et al: Ketoconazole-induced changes in selected canine hormone concentrations. Am J Vet Res 47:2504, 1986.
272. Yamaguchi H, et al: Immunomodulatory activity of antifungal drugs. Ann N Y Acad Sci 685:447, 1993.

Chapter 6
Parasitic Skin Disease

Animal skin is exposed to attack by many kinds of animal parasites.[1-10] Each species has a particular effect on the skin; the effect can be mild, as in the case of an isolated fly or mosquito bite, or severe, as in the case of generalized demodicosis or canine scabies. Although the reaction of the skin to the infestation may be slight, the common parasitisms must be considered here because the dermatologist is the logical consultant in such cases.

When ectoparasites are vectors or intermediate hosts of bacterial, rickettsial, or parasitic diseases, they become more important than when they produce only their own effect. A severe local or systemic reaction may result when toxins are injected into the skin (e.g., tick paralysis). The larvae of some parasites live in wounds or on macerated skin and produce a condition known as myiasis. The most serious dermatologic concern occurs when the dermatosis produced by parasites living in or on the skin produces irritation and sensitization.

Some parasites (*Cheyletiella* mites and biting lice) live on the skin, subsisting on the debris and exudates that are produced on its surface. Other parasites (fleas, sucking lice, and ticks) live on the skin but periodically penetrate its surface to draw nourishment from blood and tissue fluids. Still other parasites (demodectic and sarcoptic mites) live within the skin for at least part of their life cycle, producing more severe cutaneous effects. The reaction of the skin to these insults varies from trivial to lethal but usually includes inflammation, edema, and an attempt to localize the foreign body, toxin, or excretory products of the parasite. These secretions are often allergenic and cause itching and burning sensations.

• ANTIPARASITIC AGENTS

Over the years, dozens of pesticides have been brought to the market to treat or prevent external parasitic disorders, especially flea infestation, in companion animals. Some groups of compounds (e.g., chlorinated hydrocarbons) were so deleterious to the environment and wildlife that they virtually have disappeared from use. Other insecticides disappear or remain, depending on market pressures. In the mid-90s, two new insecticides, imidacloprid and fipronil, were introduced for flea control. These products are so effective that other agents, such as malathion, have disappeared. Environmental awareness also impacts product availability. In the early 1990s, microencapsulated chlorpyrifos (Duratrol) was used widely, whereas pyrethrin- and pyrethroid-based products were few in number. Today, the microencapsulated chlorpyrifos is not available through veterinarians and pyrethrin and pyrethroid products abound. In general, the products we use today are far safer for animals and the environment than those we used 5 years ago. Efficacy also has increased, but methods of delivery have a great deal of impact here.

Antiparasitic agents are delivered by collar, shampoo, cream rinse, powder, spray, dip or spot application vehicle. Some agents are delivered by mouth, injection, or transdermal absorption. The vehicle has a direct impact on ease of use and also can influence safety. Many antiparasitic agents would be highly toxic if applied in a vehicle that promoted absorption or in a form that enabled the animal to ingest quantities by licking the medication. Cats, because of their licking habits, are particularly susceptible to toxic reactions with chlorinated hydrocarbons, organophosphate, and pyrethroid products.

It is critical that clinicians prescribe topical and environmental antiparasitic agents within the bounds of label indications. Most insecticides are registered by the United States Environmental Protection Agency (EPA), and extralabel use, either for the species treated or in the concentration, method, or frequency of application, is illegal. Failure to follow label indications is not condoned or allowed, and the practitioner is not protected by the argument that it is a standard acceptable practice. Many of these products, if improperly used, pose environmental dangers. The Food Quality Protection Act of 1996 dramatically altered pesticide regulation. Even the disposal of insecticidal products is facing regulation, and it is possible that, as a profession, veterinarians will be severely limited in their ability to use or prescribe, or may be required to be licensed to use, these agents to ensure that safe practices are followed.

Amitraz, ivermectin, milbemycin, and selamectin are four drugs that are regulated by the United States Food and Drug Administration (FDA) and are commonly used to treat external parasitic disorders of companion animals. Amitraz is licensed for generalized demodicosis and tick control in dogs. Selamectin is licensed for prevention of heartworms and the treatment of certain intestinal parasites, fleas, and nonfollicular mites. All other uses are extralabel applications, which, by definition, are illegal. However, the FDA recognizes that extralabel drug usage is necessary in companion animal medicine and guidelines for extralabel usage have been developed by the American Veterinary Medical Association. First and foremost, a valid veterinarian, client, and patient relationship must exist. This requirement has greatest impact on the treatment of other animals at home who have been exposed to the patient being examined or treated for scabies, cheyletielliosis, or otodectic mange. Ivermectin or milbemycin, commonly used agents in these disorders, cannot legally be dispensed for animals not considered a patient of the veterinarian. Beyond the valid relationship, the guidelines indicate that if a veterinary drug exists in the proper dosage form; is labeled for the indication; and is clinically effective, that product should be used. If no licensed drug exists or one or more of the three prerequisites cannot be satisfied, extralabel drug usage is appropriate.

Topical Treatments

Topical antiparasitic therapy is primarily directed against ectoparasites that feed or live on dogs and cats. When treating the dermatosis, it is critical that the parasite; its life cycle, epidemiology, and natural behavior; and the pathogenesis of the disease that it is causing be considered. Topical therapy may be just one aspect of an overall treatment plan or the sole therapy prescribed. Proper application becomes critical if it is the sole therapy.

CHLORINATED HYDROCARBONS

Chlorinated hydrocarbons, which are dangerous insecticides, have become outdated and replaced by safer products. They persist in the environment and animal tissue for long times (for years, in some cases). Surprisingly, a lindane dip (Happy Jack Kennel Dip, Happy Jack, Inc.) and several methoxychlor flea and tick powders are still marketed. The authors suggest the use of safer alternatives.

CHOLINESTERASE INHIBITORS

Two kinds of cholinesterase inhibitors are available, carbamates and organophosphates. They were once the mainstay of insect control. However, with the advent of safer products and better alternative treatment regimens, their use on pets is decreasing. They are still valuable for environmental treatment in cases of infestation by fleas and other insects or arachnids.

Carbamates

Carbamates are typified by carbaryl and are safe for dogs and cats in 3% to 5% concentrations in powders and 0.5% to 2% concentrations in sprays and dips. Carbaryl should be avoided on pets with white hair, because long-term use may turn the coat golden yellow. Although lower concentrations may be used on kittens and puppies older than 6 weeks, it is probably safer to use only pyrethrin until these animals are several months old.

A flea colony bred from a newly collected strain of Florida fleas was compared with commercially available fleas (which had been reared away from the natural environment for the past 20 years) in susceptibility to insecticides. The Florida fleas were more tolerant to bendiocarb, malathion, and carbaryl as compared with the strain raised commercially.[13] This more susceptible commercial strain was most commonly used for flea product efficacy tests in the past. Bendiocarb is a carbamate used by exterminators for premises flea control.

Organophosphates

The most toxic insecticides in use are organophosphates. They are potent cholinesterase inhibitors, and a cumulative effect may be seen if animals are exposed to similar insecticides in another preparation or in lawn and garden applications. None of this group should be used on kittens, and most are also dangerous to adult cats. Malathion is different in some respects from the rest of the group. It provides a quick insect knockdown, and it could be used carefully on adult cats. The main use of this class is for fleas and ticks. Chlorpyrifos and phosmet are the most commonly used products.

D-LIMONENE

D-Limonene is a volatile citrus oil extract used in some botanical flea control products. Its insecticidal properties appear to be desiccant in nature because epicuticular oils are removed. Efficacy is poorly defined, and adverse reactions have been seen in dogs and cats.[38]

FIPRONIL

Fipronil is a new insecticide and acaricide in the phenylprazole class.[11] It acts as an antagonist at the insect γ-aminobutyric acid (GABA) receptor. Fipronil is marketed in a spray (Frontline, Merial) or spot application product (Frontline Top Spot, Merial) for flea control in dogs and cats. Its efficacy in nonfollicular mite and lice infestations also has been demonstrated.

FORMAMIDINES

These newly formulated acaricidal agents act by inhibition of monoamine oxidase. They are also prostaglandin synthesis inhibitors and α-adrenergic agonists. Amitraz (Mitaban, Upjohn & Pharmacia), the veterinary form, is available as a rinse and a collar for tick control. In the United States and Canada, the rinse is licensed for use only in the treatment of generalized demodicosis in the dog at a concentration of 250 ppm with an application rate of every 14 days. It is also effective in the treatment of feline demodicosis, *Cheyletiella*, *Otodectes*, *Sarcoptes*, and *Notoedres*. The drug is unstable and rapidly oxidizes on exposure to air and sunlight, so it is important not to use expired product or parts of a bottle exposed to the air for long periods. Oxidized product may have increased toxicity. The collar formulation is of no use in treating demodicosis.[162]

Its other actions include α-adrenergic agonist and prostaglandin inhibition. Side effects of treatment often include transient sedation and pruritus, hypothermia, bradycardia, hypotension, and hyperglycemia (use with caution in animals with diabetes mellitus). The vehicle, xylene, is thought to contribute to toxicity problems.[27, 45] Amitraz dips are used at different strengths and frequencies in various parts of the world.

INSECT GROWTH REGULATORS

Insect growth regulators (IGRs) can be divided into two types: (1) juvenile hormone analogs (juvenoids) and (2) chitin synthesis inhibitors. Juvenile hormones are natural chemicals in insects that control early stages of their metabolism, morphogenesis, and reproduction.[25] Final maturation and pupation of flea larvae proceed only in the presence of appropriate levels or absence of the juvenile hormone for that stage of larval growth. Methoprene, fenoxycarb, and pyriproxyfen are the available topical agents (juvenoids) with biochemical activities that mimic those of the natural juvenile hormone. Application to the premises by spray or fogger prevents maturation of pupal fleas if they are exposed to it. Duration of action depends on the agent used and its concentration, but 6- to 12-month control can be expected.[29] Methoprene is sensitive to ultraviolet light, so that it has little value outdoors. A problem with these products is the difficulty in delivering the product deep into rugs, cracks, and recessed places where the larvae are developing. Environmentally applied juvenoids do not affect the adult flea, so that complete results (flea-free outcome) are delayed for several weeks. This is corrected by simultaneous spraying or mixing with insecticides that kill adult fleas. Juvenoids can be applied directly to the environment or indirectly by on-animal applications. In the on-animal application mode, the juvenoid is incorporated into a collar, spray, or spot application product and covers the animal's body. During feeding, the flea is exposed to the agent and eggs layed are exposed to high levels before they fall off the host into the environment. These eggs do not hatch.[33, 307] Adult fleas exposed continuously to pyriproxyfen die of internal organ damage after 5 to 10 days of exposure.[33]

IMIDACLOPRID

Imidacloprid is a new insecticide of the chloronicotinyl nitroguanidine class.[264] It binds to the flea's nicotinic receptor on the postsynaptic neuron and blocks impulse transmission. It is available in a spot application product (Advantage, Bayer) for dogs and cats. Imidacloprid is also effective against lice.

PYRETHRINS

Pyrethrin is a volatile oil extract of the chrysanthemum flower. It contains six active pyrethrins that are contact poisons and have a fast knockdown action and flushing action on insects but no residual activity. It is rapidly inactivated by ultraviolet light. Pyrethrins, because of their low toxicity, rapid inactivation, and lack of tissue residue and buildup, are relatively environmentally safe, although they are still toxic to fish and bees. For clients concerned with chemicals, the use of pyrethrins may be more acceptable, because this is an organic natural insecticide.

There is no cholinesterase suppression. Pyrethrin demonstrates a rapid kill but low toxicity, and the low concentration of 0.06% to 0.4% is effective if it is synergized with 0.1% to 2% piperonyl butoxide, which forms a stable complex with cytochrome P450, thus limiting the metabolism of pyrethrins in insects. Cats may develop central nervous system (CNS) signs in response to piperonyl butoxide, but otherwise toxicity is low. Pyrethrins are effective against fleas, *Otodectes*, flies, lice, and mosquitos. Effective use for fleas usually necessitates daily application as a spray or a rinse unless microencapsulators or ultraviolet light stabilizers are added to the formulation.

PYRETHROIDS

These synthesized chemicals are modeled after pyrethrin and include D-trans-allethrin, bioallethrin, resmethrin, tetramethrin, deltamethrin, fenvalerate, and permethrin. The LD_{50} varies with the agent selected.[22] In action and toxicity, they are relatively comparable, although not identical, to pyrethrin. They produce a quick kill that is improved by the addition of a synergist and pyrethrin. Some of the early pyrethroids degrade on exposure to ultraviolet light, so there is little or no residual activity. The new pyrethroids are relatively photostable compared with pyrethrin.

One of the most popular pyrethroid agents is permethrin, which is found in numerous products with a wide variety of delivery systems. Part of permethrin's desirability is its low toxicity (except in cats, so only limited low-concentration formulas are approved in this species), relative stability on exposure to ultraviolet light, and potential for use as a repellent. As with pyrethrins, the synthetic pyrethroids are often combined with other active agents, particularly repellents.

REPELLENTS

Although these chemicals are capable of keeping insects away, they need frequent application—often, every few hours depending on temperature, humidity, the density of insects, the movement of the animal, and the drying effect of the wind. For control of fleas, some products only need daily or alternate-day application. Spray repellents are the primary form for flea control because large areas must be treated frequently. Compounds with repellent action include pyrethrin, permethrin, citronella, diethyltoluamide (DEET), ethohexadiol, dimethyl phthalate, butoxypropylene glycol, MGK-264, and ingredients in Skin-So-Soft (Avon) bath oil (some believe that the fragrance is the effective ingredient).[14, 17] Amitraz has been effective in repelling ticks and is available in a tick collar formulation.

ROTENONE

Rotenone, which is a natural organic compound, is derived from the root of the *Derris* plant. It is similar to pyrethrins in having low toxicity, rapid action, and quick degradation. It is available mixed with pyrethrin for use as a rinse or a shampoo for dogs and cats (Durakyl, DVM Pharmaceuticals) and is used in some products that are safe for puppies and kittens.

SULFUR

With the emphasis on newer, more effective drugs, it is sometimes forgotten that sulfur and its derivatives are excellent and safe parasiticides. The commercial lime sulfur solution (LymDyp, DVM Pharmaceuticals) is safe for dogs and cats; is an inexpensive effective treatment of infestations of nonfollicular mites; and is fungicidal, bactericidal, keratolytic, and antipruritic. A 28% lotion (Happy Jack Mange Medicine, Happy Jack, Inc.) and 10% sulfur ointment USP are other forms of sulfur medications. These high concentration products can be irritating.

Sulfur is a natural parasiticide that is relatively nontoxic and environmentally safe. Its major drawback is the foul odor. It also stains jewelry and temporarily discolors hair, especially white hair. It is drying but only rarely irritating when used at a 2% concentration. A 2% to 5% lime sulfur solution is effective against *Sarcoptes, Notoedres, Cheyletiella*, chiggers, fur mites, and lice. Contrary to common belief, sulfur is not an effective flea repellent, either topically or systemically.

Systemic Antiparasitic Agents

A variety of oral, topical, or parenterally given products are available that produce either blood levels or cutaneous levels of the active agents. The advantages of these products are their relative ease of administration and the certainty of their reaching the whole body. The diffuse and certain distribution make this type of product especially valuable in eliminating parasites in long-coated animals. The disadvantages are the relative risks and the use of the parasitic poisons internally to kill ectoparasite infestations. There is also the risk of additive toxicity if the pet is exposed to other topical insecticides. Another potential difficulty is the duration of the effective blood levels between treatments. Fortunately, the newer generations of systemic parasiticidal agents are not similar to the poisons of the past.

The use of systemic agents should be approached with knowledge regarding the parasite to be treated and, most importantly, the biology of the parasite. For example, feeding habits of the parasite may influence efficacy. Female fleas, because they ingest large quantities of blood, are more effectively killed by cythioate than are male fleas. Systemic agents are particularly valuable in treating obligate parasites such as *Sarcoptes*, *Notoedres*, *Cheyletiella*, and *Demodex* mites. They are valuable as adjunctive therapy for nonobligate parasites, such as fleas, because they are generally not effective as a sole therapeutic agent. The mechanism of action of the drug, the route of parasitic exposure, the duration of effective tissue or exposure levels, and the biology of the parasite must all be considered when using systemic antiparasitic agents.

SYSTEMIC ORGANOPHOSPHATES

Two organophosphates, cythioate and fenthion, received wide usage in flea control programs.[7] Cythioate was given orally twice weekly to dogs at 3 mg/kg and cats at 1.5 mg/kg (extralabel usage in the United States). Fenthion was marketed for dogs with a topical application rate of 8 mg/kg every 14 days. Although it was applied topically, the fenthion was absorbed transdermally and killed fleas when they fed on treated blood. Although both products showed some efficacy, both have been withdrawn from the market in the United States and receive little use elsewhere.

SYSTEMIC ENDECTOCIDES

These parasiticides were developed from macrocyclic lactones produced by the fermentation of various actinomycetes.[5, 7, 44] This class of drugs includes avermectins (ivermectin, doramectin, abamectin, selamectin) and milbemycins (milbemycin, moxidectin). At present, the two products used in veterinary dermatology are ivermectin and milbemycin but preliminary studies suggest that all of these products may have some efficacy. Both at least partly act by potentiating the release and effects of GABA. GABA is a peripheral neurotransmitter in susceptible nematodes, arachnids, and insects. Avermectins and milbemycins are also agonists of glutamate-gated chloride channels. In mammals, GABA is limited to the CNS. Because these drugs do not cross the blood-brain barrier in most adult animals, they are relatively safe and have a wide margin between efficacy and mammalian toxicity. In general, these drugs are effective for nematodes, microfilaria, lice, fur mites, *Otodectes*, *Sarcoptes*, *Notoedres*, *Cheyletiella*, and *Demodex*.

Ivermectin, milbemycin, and moxidectin are licensed for use orally every 30 days at 0.625 µg/kg, 0.5 mg/kg, and 3 µg/kg, respectively, for the prevention of dirofilariasis. At this dosage, no adverse side effects are seen in dogs of any breeding. In treating external parasites, ivermectin is administered at 200 to 600 µg/kg daily, weekly, or bimonthly and toxic side effects can be seen. Milbemycin is administered at 1 to 2 mg/kg daily or weekly, and toxic side effects, although rare, have been reported. Selamectin is a novel new avermectin that has been shown to be efficacious for the treatment of fleas,[314] ear mites, scabies, ticks, some intestinal nematodes, and prevention of heartworms. It is applied topically and absorbed systemically, with efficacy for fleas and heartworms shown with once-monthly dosing for both dogs and cats.

High-dose ivermectin or milbemycin can be toxic to dogs younger than 3 months of age and to adult dogs within certain breeds. Breeds widely reported to be sensitive to high-dose ivermectin include the collie, Old English sheep dog, Australian shepherd, Shetland sheepdog, and crosses thereof.[246] Individual reports of an adverse reaction in a border collie, West Highland White terrier, German shepherd dog, and Samoyed can be found.[36] Toxic side effects are neurologic in origin and include mydriasis, hypersalivation, lethargy, ataxia, tremors, coma, and death. Ivermectin-sensitive collies lack adequate quantities of P-glycoprotein necessary to successfully exclude ivermectin from the brain.[10a] In breeds very sensitive to high-dose ivermectin, for example, the collie, one dose of more than 125 µg/kg can produce coma. In less sensitive individuals, side effects may not be seen for days to weeks. To try to identify individuals sensitive to high-dose ivermectin, an increasing dosage schedule has been proposed.[36] For the first 5 days of treatment, the dog is given 50, 100, 150, 200 and 300 µg/kg of ivermectin, respectively. If the dog is highly sensitive to high-dose ivermectin, subtle neurologic signs, for example, lethargy, ataxia, should develop within 24 hours of the administration of the sensitizing dosage. If the drug is discontinued immediately, the dog should return to normal within 24 to 48 hours. Because some dogs do not develop these signs for weeks, the owner should always observe the dog carefully.

Collies sensitive to high-dose ivermectin also are sensitive to high-dose milbemycin when the dosage exceeds 5 mg/kg.[44] Cross sensitivity to doramectin and moxidectin remains untested but should be expected. High-dose milbemycin has been used to treat hundreds of dogs with demodicosis and scabies, and neurologic side effects have not been reported, even in ivermectin-sensitive breeds, with dosages below 3 mg/kg. In a recent study of 70 dogs with nasal mite infestation, milbemycin was given weekly for three consecutive weeks at dosages of 0.5 to 1.0 mg/kg.[116] Sixteen dogs had side effects. In 12, one or more episodes of vomiting or diarrhea, or both, occurred. Two dogs seemed lethargic, one was uncoordinated, and the last dog's sneezing worsened with treatment. The dosage used did not seem to influence the frequency of side effects, and a breed frequency was not reported. All dogs return to normal within 48 hours of drug withdrawal. When moxidectin was given to ivermectin-sensitive collies, no toxicity was seen with 15 µg/kg monthly.[10a] However, when it was given at 90 µg/kg, mild signs of toxicity were seen.

Ivermectin

Ivermectin (Ivomec, Merial) is a derivative of avermectin B from fermentation products of *Streptomyces avermitilis*. This drug is noted for activity against nematodes, microfilaria, and *Sarcoptes, Cheyletiella, Notoedres,* and *Otodectes* mites. Although ivermectin was not shown to be efficacious for *Demodex* with the treatment protocols that had been effective for other ectoparasites (e.g., 0.2 to 0.4 mg/kg, orally or subcutaneously, weekly for up to 8 weeks), it can be effective when it is administered orally daily. Ivermectin does not affect trematodes and cestodes, because GABA is not involved in neurotransmission in those species. Parasite paralysis is the main action of ivermectin, but it also suppresses reproduction. Ticks are not killed, but their egg production and molting are suppressed.

Ivermectin can be given parenterally, orally, or topically with good absorption. Ivermectin is rapidly absorbed orally and persists in the tissues for prolonged periods. This is important because it does not have a rapid killing effect on susceptible parasites. Dosages used to treat all nonfollicular mites range from 0.2 to 0.5 mg/kg. If given by injection or applied topically, two doses at 14-day intervals should be sufficient. Orally, the drug is given three times at weekly intervals.[6] In rare cases, additional doses may be needed.

Ivermectin also has apparent anti-inflammatory properties. The authors have seen many dogs, whose ultimate dermatologic diagnosis was atopy, food hypersensitivity, or bacterial pyoderma, that had marked reduction in pruritus or decreased visible inflammation for 3 to 7 days after receiving ivermectin. Ivermectin has been shown to have immunomodulatory effects, especially at the level of T cells, in mice but this does not appear to be true in the dog.[5, 23]

Ivermectin toxicosis is rare in cats (usually seen in kittens), develops within 1 to 12 hours after administration of the drug, and is characterized by abnormal behavior, ataxia, lethargy, weakness, recumbency, apparent blindness, coma, and death.

Milbemycin

Milbemycin (Interceptor, Novartis) is derived from fermentation products of *Streptomyces hygroscopicus*.[178, 246] It is similar to ivermectin in activity with the notable addition of efficacy in the control of various intestinal parasites. Milbemycin has been used only in dogs to treat nasal mites, scabies, or generalized demodicosis. No adverse reactions have been reported in ivermectin sensitive breeds when doses of 1 to 2 mg/kg were given so it receives widest usage in these dogs. In demodicosis, it is given daily, whereas it is given every seventh day for 3 to 5 treatments in the other disorders. In some dogs, live scabies mites can be found after three treatments, suggesting that more frequent administration might be needed in some cases.

Moxidectin

Moxidectin (Proheart, Fort Dodge) is derived from fermentation products of *Streptomyces cyaneogriseus* subsp. *noncyanogenus*.[10a] It is marketed for heartworm prevention in the United States. Moxidectin (Cydectin, Fort Dodge) is also licensed in cattle for the treatment and control of various nematodes, *Hypoderma* spp., mites, lice, and horn flies. Although it is not approved for this use, moxidectin has been given orally or subcutaneously at 0.2 to 0.4 mg/kg for the successful treatment of *Octodectes* infestations and generalized canine demodicosis.

Doramectin

Doramectin (Dectomax, Pfizer) is derived from fermentation of selected strains of *Streptomyces avermitilis*. In the United States it is marketed for the treatment and control of various nematodes, mites, and lice in cattle and swine. Although not approved for this use, doramectin has been given subcutaneously at 0.2 to 0.3 mg/kg for the successful treatment of feline and canine scabies.

Selamectin

Selamectin (Revolution, Pfizer) is the first FDA-approved topically applied product that prevents heartworm disease, kills adult fleas, and prevents their eggs from hatching and treats and controls ear mites in dogs and cats.[43a, 314] It also treats and controls canine scabies and *Dermacentor variabilis* infestations in dogs.[43a] Selamectin is a novel semisynthetic avermectin produced by a new strain of *Streptomyces avermitilis*. Following topical application, selamectin is identified in sebaceous glands, hair follicles, and basal layers of the epithelium. It is applied topically, at a dose of 6 to 12 mg/kg, at the base of the neck in front of the shoulder blades, every 30 days. When used according to the manufacturer's directions, selamectin is safe in ivermectin-sensitive dogs, in breeding animals, and in puppies and kittens 6 weeks of age or older.[43b] Occasional local reactions (inflammation, alopecia) are seen following topical application of selamectin.

INSECT DEVELOPMENT INHIBITORS

These products are basically IGRs given by mouth or injection. Fleas feeding on treated blood lay eggs that do not hatch or develop beyond the larval stage. Larvae feeding on the feces of treated fleas also will not develop. The most widely marketed product, lufenuron (Program, Novartis), is given by mouth once monthly to dogs or cats or by injection every 6 months to cats.[15, 21, 26, 43] Lufenuron is a benzyl-phenol urea compound that inhibits chitin synthesis. Chitin is a major component of the flea exoskeleton but is not found in mammals. With altered chitin synthesis, embryogenesis and hatching does not occur.

Cyromazine is another oral flea development inhibitor. It belongs to the triazine group of compounds. It does not inhibit chitin synthesis but increases its stiffness so the exoskeleton cannot expand. The internal pressure in the larvae increases and results in lethal body wall defects.[42] Because the drug must be given daily, it has not received wide usage.

NEONICOTINOIDS

These agents act at the nicotinic acetyl-choline receptor. Nitenpyram is a novel, orally administered flea adulticide.[14a] However, it is rapidly eliminated from dogs after oral administration, and is lethal to fleas only for 24 to 48 hours.

• HELMINTH PARASITES

Ancylostoma and *Uncinaria* (Hookworm) Dermatitis

The larvae of *Ancylostoma braziliense, A. caninum,* and *Uncinaria stenocephala* cause a characteristic skin lesion in humans that is called creeping eruption. The skin lesions that these larvae produce in dogs or cats are not as severe, because these animals are their specific hosts.[46] The skin lesions are often incidental to completion of the normal life cycle of the parasite, with the larvae quickly abandoning the skin and proceeding to other parts of the body. Although percutaneous entry can lead to completion of the life cycle, larvae penetrating by this route rarely mature. The larvae are present on the grass and in the soil of runs and paddocks during the spring and summer in cool climates, and animals exposed to them become infected. Thus, the disease is essentially one of kenneled dogs on grass or earth runs that have poor sanitation.

Cutaneous lesions seem to be more prevalent in areas with predominant infection with *U. stenocephala* (Ireland, parts of England, and the United States), although animals with ancylostomiasis may also have skin lesions. *U. stenocephala* produces a marked dermatitis on skin penetration but rarely completes its life cycle by this route. It is insignificant as a blood sucker compared with *A. braziliense* or *A. caninum*.[46] *A. caninun* can complete its life cycle via skin penetration.

Hookworm dermatitis has been produced by natural and experimental infestations with *U. stenocephala*. With both types of infection, similar clinical and histologic lesions were produced. The third-stage larvae enter the dog's skin on areas of the body that frequently contact the ground. They enter primarily at an area of desquamation on the skin, although a few larvae may use hair follicles. The larvae enter the horny layer parallel to the skin surface, and there is little evidence of enzymatic activity. The larvae are thought simply to exert pressure by undulating activity, the forward movement being achieved by pushing back against rigid keratinized cells. This route follows the line of least resistance through the outer layers.[47] After they penetrate the epidermis, the dermis appears to cause little hindrance to the migrating larvae. After larvae pass through tissue, the cells reunite and there is little lasting evidence of their passage.[47] Some other species of hookworm larvae cause loss of integrity of the epidermis as they penetrate it.

Clinical signs of hookworm dermatitis are initially red papules on the parts of the body in frequent contact with the ground. Later, these areas become uniformly erythematous and then thickened and alopecic. The feet are especially affected (Fig. 6–1). However, the skin of the sternum, ventral abdomen, posteromedial thighs, and tail may also be involved. Skin over the bony prominences of the elbows, hocks, and ischial tuberosities may have more obvious lesions owing to the thickened skin and hair loss. The interdigital webs may be erythematous, and the feet may be swollen, painful, and hot. The footpads become spongy and soft, especially at the pad margins, where the tissue can be readily grooved and often stripped from the underlying dermis. Chronically inflamed foot pads become variably hyperkeratotic (Fig. 6–2). The chronic inflammation causes the claws to grow rapidly and to appear deformed. The claws may be friable and may break off, leaving thick, tapered stumps. Arthritis of the interphalangeal joints may be present, too. Pruritus is a constant finding but varies in its intensity.

Histopathologic examination reveals varying degrees of perivascular dermatitis (hyperplastic or spongiotic) with eosinophils and neutrophils. The epidermis may contain recent larval migration tracts, which may occasionally be traced into the dermis as linear tracts of neutrophils and eosinophils. Larvae are rarely found but, if present, are surrounded by clusters of neutrophils, eosinophils, and mononuclear cells. Hypersensitivity has been suggested as a cause of the lesions.

Diagnosis can be made with reasonable certainty by the clinical signs, a positive fecal examination finding of hookworm eggs, and a history of poor housing and sanitation. Differential diagnosis may be complicated by a coincidental infection with hookworms. Differential diagnostic possibilities include demodectic mange, contact dermatitis, *Pelodera* dermatitis, and intradermal penetration by parasites such as *Strongyloides* and schistosomal agents.

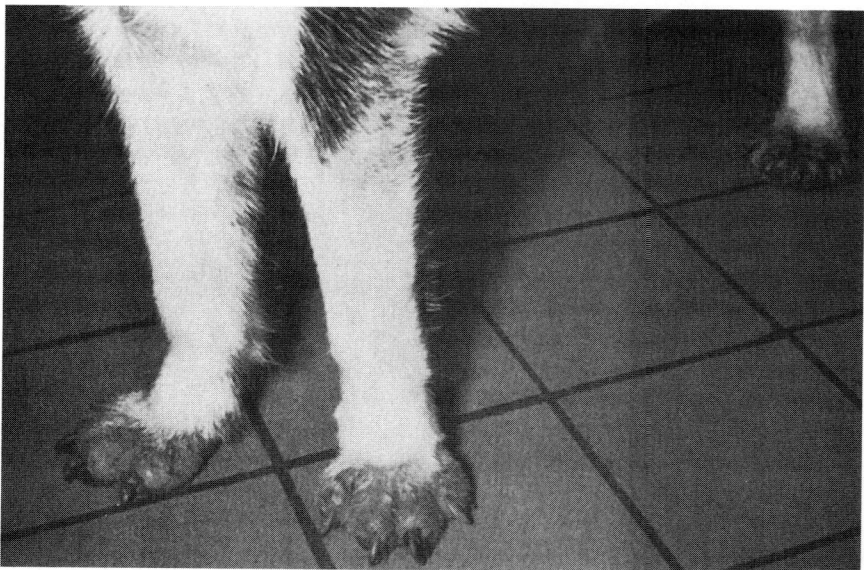

FIGURE 6-1. Hookworm dermatitis. A Siberian husky confined to a dirt-based run and affected with *A. caninum* shows lesions of chronic hookworm dermatitis on all four feet. There is alopecia, erythema, swelling, and crusting.

Treatment should emphasize cleaning of the premises, frequent removal of feces, and generally improved hygiene, combined with appropriate routine anthelmintic treatment and prophylaxis of all dogs in the kennel. Routine use of heartworm preventatives helps minimize the frequency of this disorder. Dry, paved runs, or periodic treatment of dirt or gravel runs with 4.5 kg (10 lb) of borax per 30 m² (100 ft²) of run may be helpful, but borax or salt kills vegetation. Attention to measures designed to improve foot health are important. Claws should be kept trimmed short to improve foot conformation and help to alleviate joint stress. The paws should be kept clean and dry. Exercising dogs on new clean pasture is beneficial.

Pelodera Dermatitis

Pelodera dermatitis (rhabditic dermatitis) is a local erythematous, nonseasonal pruritic dermatitis caused by a cutaneous infestation with the larvae of *Pelodera strongyloides*.[2, 10]

Under filthy conditions, the larvae of the free-living nematode *P. strongyloides* may invade the skin of dogs. The adult parasites have a direct life cycle and live in damp soil or decaying organic material, such as rice hulls, straw, and marsh hay that has been stored in contact with the ground for many months. The larvae may invade the skin of animals that comes in contact with contaminated soil or hay.[10] The larvae are about 600 μm long (Fig. 6-3) and may be found in skin scrapings from affected skin or in the associated bedding. In histologic sections, larvae and some parthenogenetic female nematodes may be found in the hair follicles where a typical folliculitis is present.

Pasyk[50] described *Pelodera* dermatitis in an 11-year-old girl who slept with a pet dog with the condition. The larvae invaded the epidermis and hair follicles, and the inflammatory infiltrate of mononuclear and eosinophilic cells surrounded necrotic hair follicles and extended to capillaries and venules of the upper dermis. It was noted that the child might have contracted the infestation from the dog, but it seems more reasonable that both individuals were infested from the same environmental source. Smith and colleagues[51] reported that human skin infections with larval nematodes can be contracted from dogs with *A. braziliense, A. caninum, U. stenocephala, Gnathostoma spinigerum,* and *Strongyloides stercoralis,* as well as *P. strongyloides*.

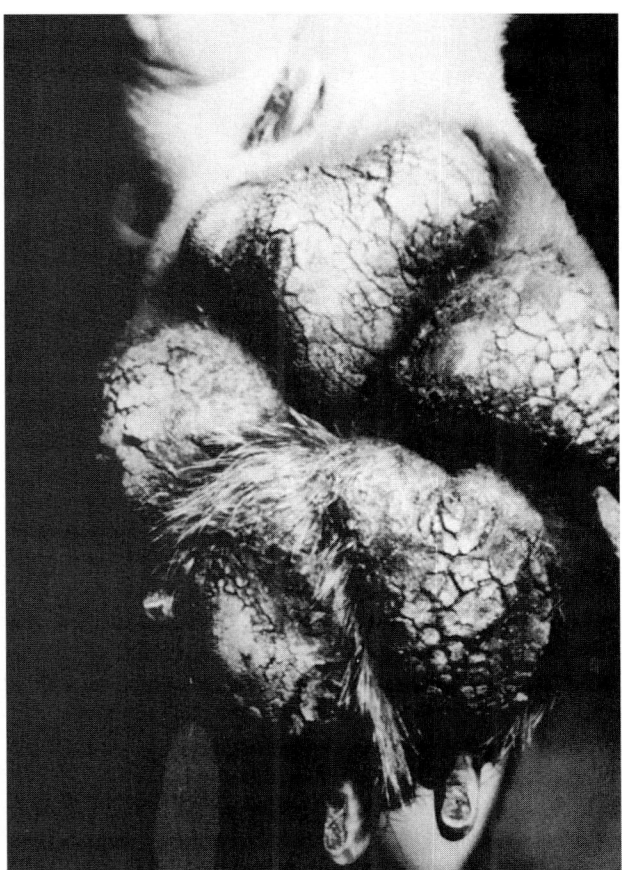

FIGURE 6–2. Digital hyperkeratosis due to hookworm *(Uncinaria stenocephala)* pododermatitis. (Courtesy K. Thoday.)

Clinical features of *Pelodera* dermatitis include a distribution of skin lesions that typically involves areas that contact the ground—feet, legs, perineum, lower abdomen and chest, and tail (Fig. 6–4A).[48, 49] The affected skin is erythematous and partially to completely alopecic. Multiple papules later develop to crusts, scales, and secondary infection from the constant scratching (see Fig. 6–4B). Pruritus varies from mild to intense.

Diagnosis is by skin scrapings, which readily reveal small, motile nematode larvae (625 to 650 μm in length). Larvae and adults can also be identified in contaminated litter by using the Baermann technique.[48] The history of contaminated bedding and pruritus, together with the skin scraping findings, should be diagnostic, but the differential diagnostic possibilities include hookworm dermatitis, dirofilariasis, and strongyloidiasis (all on the basis of the larval findings). Grossly, skin lesions may suggest contact dermatitis, bacterial folliculitis, demodicosis, or scabies.

Skin biopsy reveals varying degrees of perifolliculitis, folliculitis, and furunculosis (Fig. 6–5). Nematode segments are present within hair follicles and dermal pyogranulomas. Eosinophils are numerous.

Treatment is simple and effective. Complete removal and destruction of bedding are mandatory. Beds, kennels, or cages should be thoroughly washed and sprayed with an insecticide. The bedding should be replaced with cedar or other wood shavings, cloth, or shredded paper. The patient should be bathed with a warm water shampoo to soften and remove crusts and then with a parasiticidal dip, as for scabies. This procedure usually results in prompt relief of itching and rapid healing. Although repeated parasiticidal dips have been recommended in the past, it is highly unlikely that they are necessary.[48] Prednisolone may be given for a few days to help to stop the pruritus; systemic antibiotics

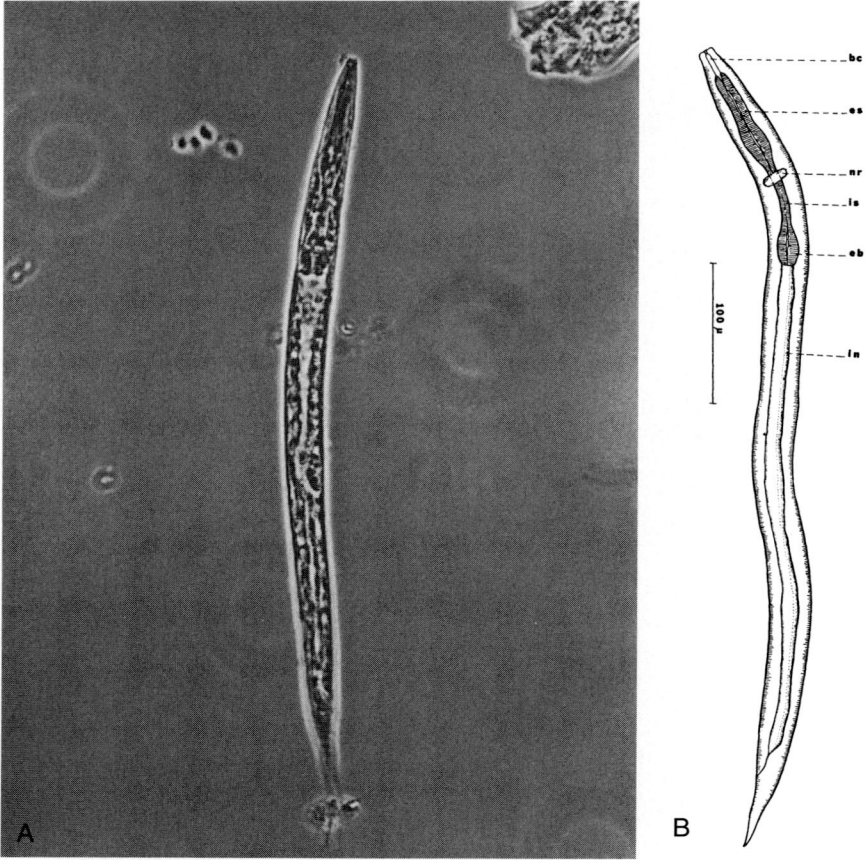

FIGURE 6–3. *A,* Larva of the free-living nematode *Pelodera strongyloides.* (Courtesy J. Georgi.) *B,* Larva of *P. strongyloides:* bc, buccal capsule; es, esophagus; nr, nerve ring; is, isthmus; eb, esophageal bulb; in, intestine. (From Willers WB: *Pelodera strongyloides* in association with canine dermatitis in Wisconsin. J Am Vet Med Assoc 156:319, 1970.)

may be indicated for any secondary pyoderma. The infestation is self-limited and resolves spontaneously after the animals are removed from the source of contamination.

Strongyloides stercoralis–like Infection

In a single report, an apparently rare cutaneous manifestation of *S. stercoralis* infection was reported in 5 of 10 Boston terriers in a kennel.[52] Three weeks after a new pup was placed in the kennel, 6-month-old puppies developed mucoid, blood-flecked feces; anemia; general lymphadenopathy; and focal dermatitis. The hair was rough, dull, and dry, and crusted lesions of 1 cm in diameter were on the tail, distal hindlegs, the ventral trunk, and other areas with ground contact. Some pups had a severe, hemorrhagic pododermatitis. The dogs were housed in outdoor pens with concrete and shaded grassy areas. Fecal samples contained large embryonated and unembryonated ova (80 by 35 μm) and first-stage larvae (200 μm). The ova were larger than those of *S. stercoralis* (normally 55 by 32 μm), and this parasite usually sheds only first-stage larvae in the feces. When feces were cultured for 18 hours, free-living adults and third-stage larvae were produced.

Treatment with thiabendazole,[52] 11.4 mg/kg once daily orally for 5 days, or ivermectin,[53] 200 to 500 μg/kg orally, can be effective, but retreatments may be necessary.

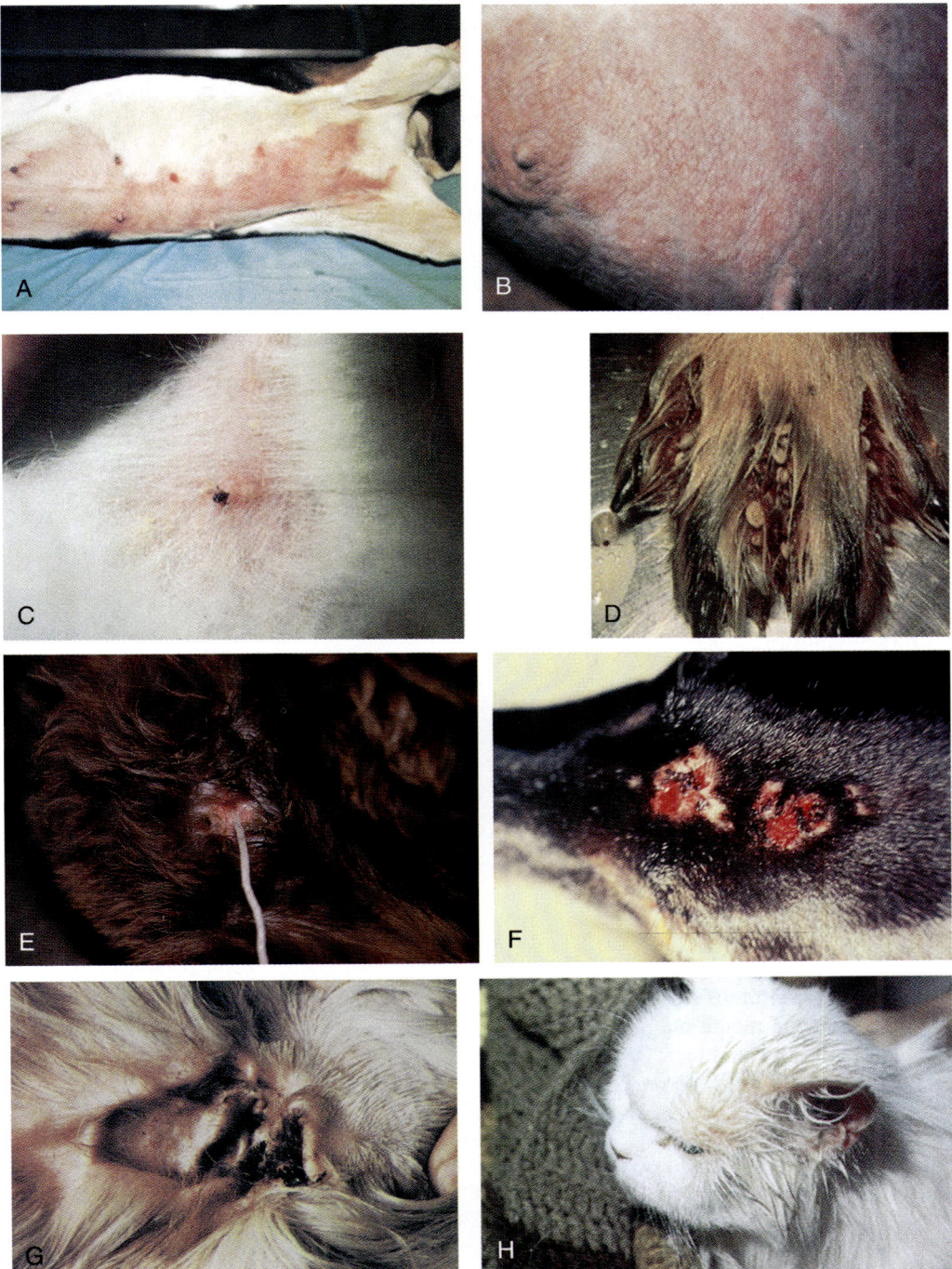

FIGURE 6–4. *A*, Ventral chest and abdomen of a beagle with *Pelodera* dermatitis. The involved areas are alopecic and erythematous. *B*, Close-up view of the skin of the patient in *A*, showing intense erythema, multiple papules, and alopecia. *C*, Tick bite. Note the erythematous nodule with a tick attached. *D*, Tick infestation. Pododermatitis in a dog with numerous interdigital ticks. *E*, Dracunculiasis. Nodular lesion in the axillary region with an emerging adult. *F*, *Acanthocheilonoma* infection. Ulcerated nodular lesions on the head. (Courtesy A. Hargis.) *G*, Dark brown, waxy exudate and crusts in the ear of a dog with *Otodectes cynotis*. (Courtesy R. L. Collinson.) *H*, Erythema and excoriation of pinna and temporal region in a cat with *O. cynotis*.

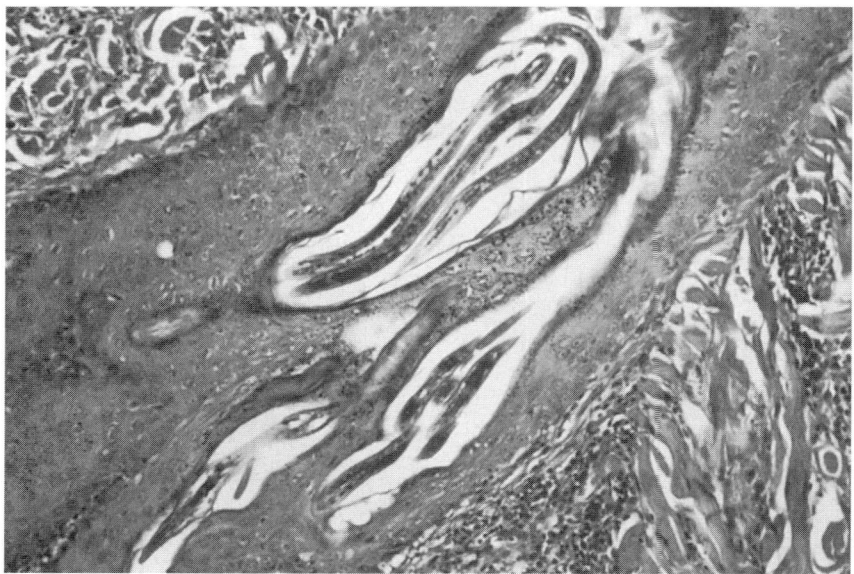

FIGURE 6–5. *Pelodera* dermatitis in a dog. Numerous nematodes within hair follicle.

Anatrichosomiasis

Anatrichosomiasis is a type of larval migrans caused by the nematode *Anatrichosoma cutaneum*, which produces blisters on the hands and feet of monkeys and humans in Africa. A case caused by an *Anatrichosoma* sp. worm was reported in a 13-year-old South African cat.[8] The cat was presented for lameness with necrosis, sloughing, and ulceration of the footpads of all four feet. Treatment was not attempted, and the cat was euthanized. Histopathologic findings included superficial perivascular dermatitis with numerous worms and bioperculate eggs located in necrotic migratory tracts within the epidermis (Fig. 6–6). Female worms averaging 42 mm in length were identified as *Anatrichosoma* sp.[8]

A female, 5-month-old Boxer was found to be passing double-operculate eggs in its feces. Similar eggs were obtained from skin scrapings taken from a raised, flaking, erythematous nodule on the dorsal midline in the lumbar region. The nodule was removed surgically, and the eggs from the scraping and the nematode segments found in histologic sections were identified as an *Anatrichosoma* sp.[54]

Schistosomiasis

Schistosoma cercariae of ducks, shore birds, voles, mice, or muskrat (natural hosts) penetrate the skin of humans, or other warm-blooded animals that are abnormal hosts, and produce a pruritic dermatitis (*Schistosoma* dermatitis).

Schistosome eggs are shed in the feces of the natural host. The miracidia hatch within 20 minutes and must either find a mollusk (snail) host within 12 hours or die. They form sporocysts in the mollusk and hatch in 4 weeks as cercaria. These are shed into water but die in 24 hours unless they reach a warm-blooded natural host. In the natural host, they go to the liver and the intestinal wall, where eggs are laid and passed in the feces.[56] These parasites are trematodes: *Trichobilharzia ocellata, T. stagnicolae,* and *T. physellae* infest waterfowl of the Great Lakes area, whereas *Austrobilharzia variglandis* affects ducks and terns in Florida and Hawaii.[55] In humans, the condition has been called swimmers' itch, clam diggers' itch, and rice paddy itch. These conditions occur because the cercariae penetrate the skin of the abnormal host and produce clinical disease. Although skin exposed to infested bodies of water from spring to fall may become infected, animals are

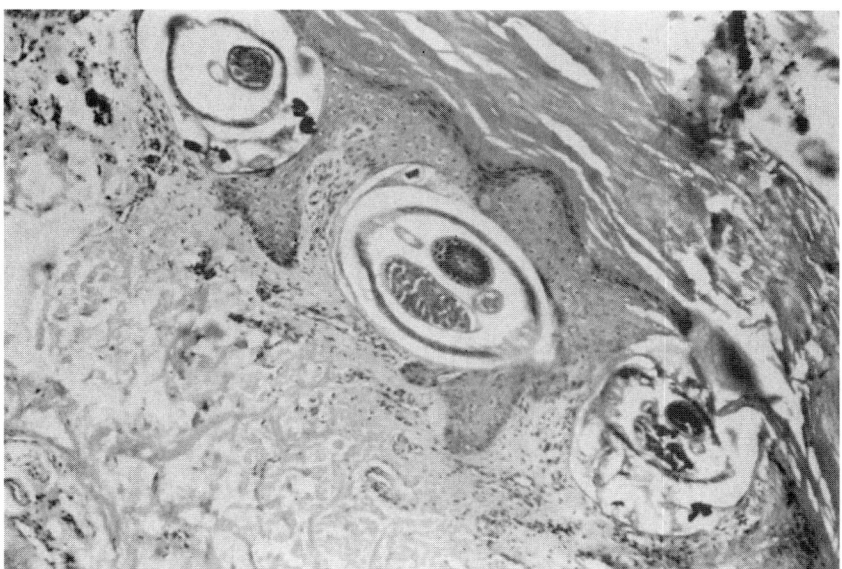

FIGURE 6–6. Anatrichosomiasis. Nematode segments within the epidermis of a cat's footpad.

more apt to be swimming and the cercariae are much more numerous in the water on bright warm days of midsummer; thus, infection is most common then.

At the time of penetration, the cercariae produce macules and wheals that last 15 to 20 hours. These later develop into papules and, after 2 to 4 days, into vesicles. These stages are intensely pruritic. They are often confused with mosquito, chigger, or flea bites. Healing takes place in 5 to 7 days, because the cercariae are walled off by an acute inflammatory reaction, with infiltration of neutrophils, lymphocytes, and eosinophils. Some humans with the condition have only one strong reaction and on subsequent exposures seem immune, but most people experience increasingly severe reactions on each re-exposure.

Local treatment of the skin is not effective, except with palliative antipruritic lotions. Control measures should primarily emphasize staying out of the water. Actions such as removing water vegetation that encourages snail populations or killing the mollusks by adding dilute copper sulfate solution to small ponds are of limited value. The authors are not aware of documented cases of canine schistosomiasis in the literature but have seen dogs that had signs and a history suggestive of the problem.

Dracunculiasis

Dracunculus insignis is a parasite of dogs and wild carnivores of North America.[58, 60] *D. medinensis* (guinea worm) affects humans, cats, and other animals in Asia and Africa.[59] *D. insignis* has been reported to affect the dog, raccoon, mink, fox, otter, and skunk.[58] The intermediate host is a *Cyclops* (a crustacean) that is ingested from contaminated water by the host. The larvae develop in the host during a period of 8 to 12 months. The adults develop in the subcutaneous tissue of the abdomen and limbs. Usually, a nodule forms, and eventually, a fistula develops (Fig. 6–7). Just before the fistula opens, the host may show urticaria, itching, and a slight fever. When the host enters cool water, the female worm is stimulated to release larvae (Fig. 6–8), which escape through the cutaneous fistula. Some larvae may enter the blood, but they can be distinguished from *Dirofilaria* and *Dipetalonema* larvae by their long tapered tails. One can also apply cold water to the fistula to stimulate the female worm and then make a smear of the exudate to identify the larvae.

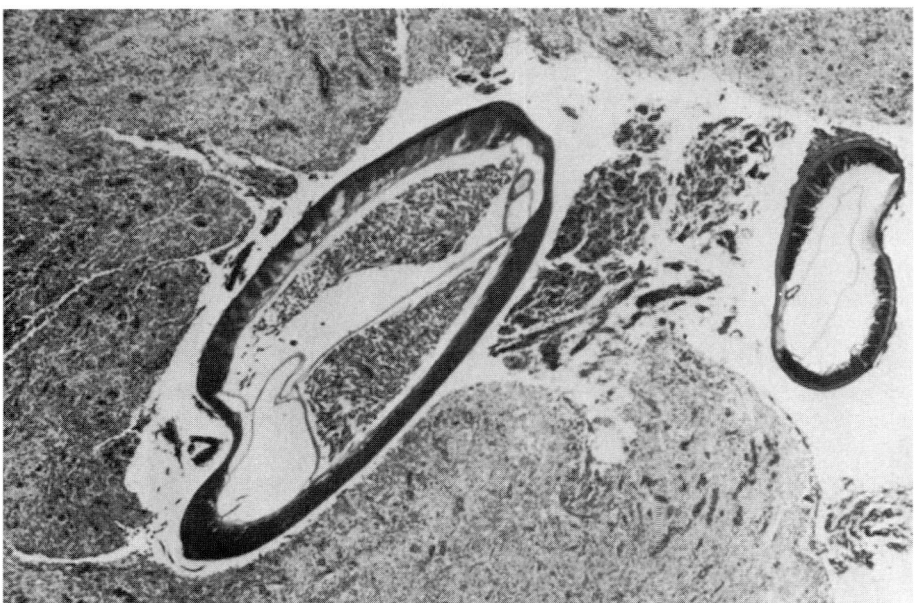

FIGURE 6–7. Dracunculiasis. Nematode segments in an abscess.

Clinical features are chronic, single to multiple nodules on the limbs, the head, or the abdomen that eventually ulcerate and do not heal (see Fig. 6–4E). The lesions are often painful and pruritic. The adult parasites (female, 1.7 mm wide by 70 cm long; male, 1.7 mm by 22 cm) may occasionally be seen in fistulae. Exfoliative cytologic study may reveal neutrophils, eosinophils, and macrophages as well as larvae (about 500 μm length). Histologic examination of an excised lesion reveals a nodular-to-diffuse dermatitis containing adult and larval nematodes surrounded by fibrosis and eosinophilic pyogranulomatous inflammation.[57, 60]

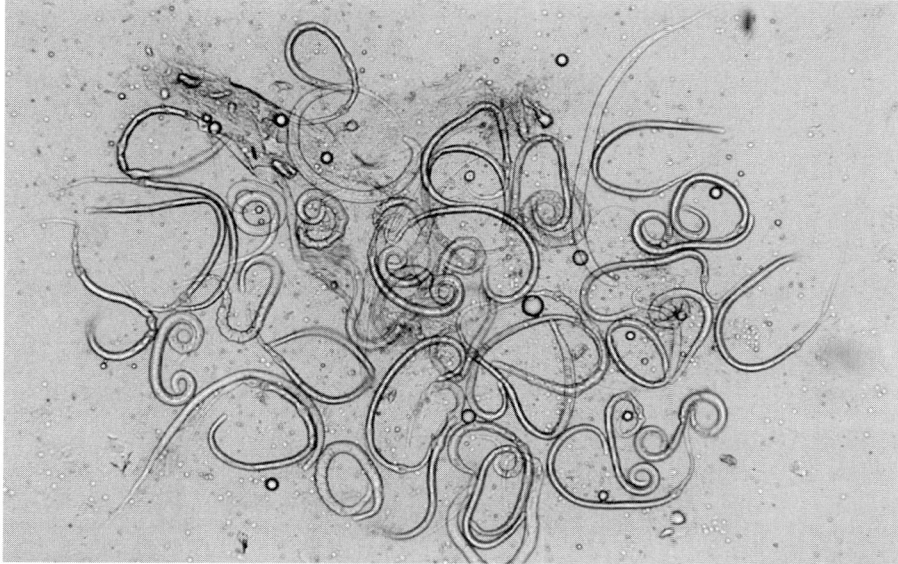

FIGURE 6–8. Dracunculiasis. Multiple larvae collected from the nodule shown in Figure 6–4E.

Individual lesions may be removed surgically, or the worm may be removed gently by *carefully* winding it up on a stick during a period of several days. With multiple lesions, treatment is more difficult and may not be effective. Although there are reports on the efficacy of diethylcarbamazine, thiabendazole, metronidazole, nitridazole, and ivermectin in the treatment of dracunculiasis, treatment is not uniformly successful.[10, 57, 60]

Control measures depend on decontaminating water supplies. With time, the incidence of disease decreases and the disease dies out. Dracunculiasis can be prevented also by drinking only water that is passed through a fine filter.

Dirofilariasis

Adults of *Dirofilaria immitis* live in the heart, and larvae are found in the blood and occasionally in the subcutaneous tissues. Adult worms can rarely be found in abscess-like lesions in the skin, especially on the legs.[8, 62, 63] The microfilaria rarely cause skin disease. Although pustular eruptions, ulcerative dermatitis, and scabies-like dermatitis have been associated with dirofilariasis,[67, 68] the cause-and-effect relationship was not well established in those cases. A pruritic papulonodular dermatitis has been proved to be associated with these larvae and probably results from a hypersensitivity to the larvae (see Chap. 8).[64–66]

Dogs with cutaneous dirofilariasis (heartworm dermatitis) typically have a chronic, pruritic dermatitis with ulcerated papules, nodules, and plaques. Lesions are most commonly found on the head or the limbs but can be seen anywhere. Response to antibiotics, topical agents, sedatives, and glucocorticoids is poor.

Peripheral eosinophilia and a positive Knott's test for microfilaria are common findings, but lesions can occur in dogs with occult filariasis.[66] Histopathologic examination revealed varying degrees of angiocentric pyogranulomatous dermatitis. Microfilarial segments were present intravascularly and extravascularly within the granulomatous dermal nodules. Eosinophils varied in number from few to numerous. Many of the blood vessels in the central areas of the lesions contained microfilariae, but none of the deep dermal or subcutaneous vessels outside the lesions showed cellular infiltrates or microfilariae. Immunohistochemical staining shows positive immunoreaction of the microfilariae with antiimmunoglobulin G (IgG) serum.[64]

With standard heartworm treatments, the lesions become nonpruritic within 2 weeks and heal completely within 8 weeks.

Other Filarial Infections

A large number of filarial nematodes are found worldwide. The adults reside in subcutaneous tissues, whereas microfilariae circulate in the blood. Typically, no disease is caused by either life stage, but the microfilariae can be confused with those of *D. immitis*. Ocular onchocerciasis has been reported in dogs from the western United States.[70] Adult worms and larvae were found within the pyogranulomatous mass and were either causal or coincidental. Nodular lesions and various nonspecific skin changes (e.g., pruritic papulocrustous dermatitis, especially over the caudal half of the body) have been associated with *Dirofilaria repens*[61, 69, 72, 344] and other filarial nematodes.[68] It is not clear whether the parasites induced the dermatitis or were a coincidental finding in some pre-existing skin disease. Because the clinical findings were similar to those seen in filarial dermatitis in other species (e.g., equine onchocerciasis), the nematode is probably causal. In addition, adulticidal (arsenical) and microfilaricidal (ivermectin) therapy cures the dermatoses associated with *D. repens*.[72a]

Ten dogs from the western United States were described with a novel filarial infection.[71] All dogs had singular or multiple, typically pruritic, papules or plaques with alopecia, scarring, erythema, ulceration, and crusting. The head (see Fig. 6–4F), neck, shoulder region, and back were most commonly affected. On biopsy, a perivascular-to-interstitial dermatitis with plasma cells and eosinophils was seen. In most dogs, dermal microgranulomas surrounding microfilariae (Fig. 6–9) are observed. In one dog, an *Acanthocheilonema* sp. adult was isolated and this nematode is suspected as the causal agent in all dogs.

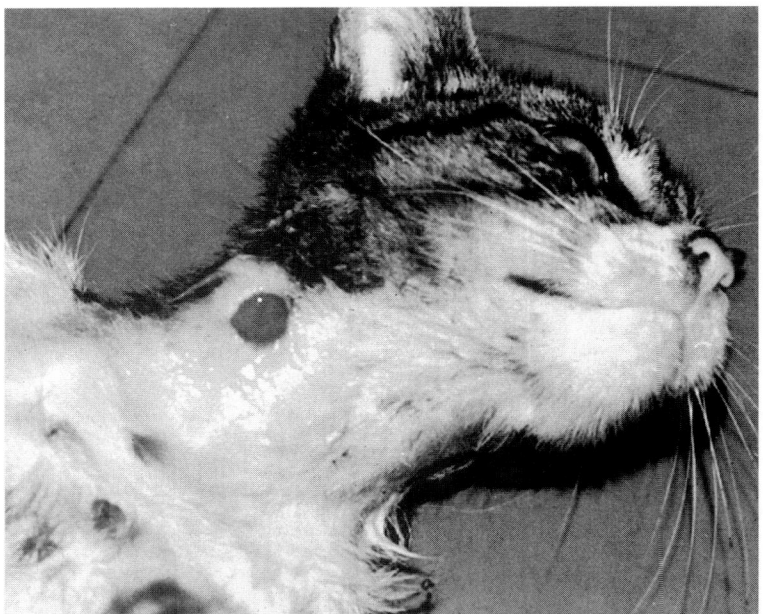

FIGURE 6–12. *Lagochilascaris major* infection. Ruptured abscess with draining tract. (Courtesy A. Dell'Porto.)

The rest of the parasite consists of fused elements of the head along with the thorax and abdomen, together called the *idiosoma*. There are separate sexes.

PARASITIC TICKS

Ticks differ from mites in their larger size, the hairless or short-haired leathery body, the exposed armed hypostoma, and the presence of a pair of spiracles near the coxae of the fourth pair of legs. Most ticks are not host specific. Ticks are divided into argasid, or soft, ticks and ixodid, or hard, ticks. The argasid ticks are more primitive and less often parasitic, produce fewer progeny, and infest the premises occupied by their hosts. Ixodid ticks are more specialized and highly parasitic, produce more progeny, and infest the open country frequented by their hosts.[4]

Argasid (Soft) Ticks

Argasid ticks are more commonly parasites of birds and are found frequently in warmer climates. In regions where they are endemic, they may infest all types of wild and domestic animals. They have no dorsal plate, the sexes are similar, the capitulum is not visible dorsally, and the spiracles lie in front of the third pair of unspurred coxae. Ticks of this class seldom travel far from their lairs and are often nocturnal feeders. Only one species is discussed.

• **Spinous Ear Tick.** *Otobius megnini* is found in the external ear canal of dogs and cats. Its range is limited to the southern and western United States. The larvae and nymphs infest the ear canal of the host, producing acute otitis externa, pain, and occasional convulsions. Asymptomatic infection also can be seen.[89] Often, the ear canals become packed with immature ticks, but in some cases, only a few are found. Adults are fiddle shaped with a constriction in the middle, but they are not spiny and do not feed because they are not parasitic. Adults can live 6 to 12 months in a protected environment and lay 500 to 600 eggs. Eggs hatch in days, and larvae typically feed immediately but can survive unfed for 2 to 4 months. The larvae, engorged on lymph from the ear canal, are yellow or pink. They are about 0.3 cm and spherical, with three pairs of minute legs. After 5 to 10 days of feeding, they develop into nymphs. The nymphs, which also inhabit the ear canal, are bluish gray with four pairs of yellow legs (Fig. 6–13). They are widest in the middle, and the skin has numerous sharp spines. The nymphs feed for 1 to 7 months before molting to adults.

Damage from spinous ear ticks results from the loss of blood and lymph. In addition, severe irritation and secondary otitis cause vigorous head shaking and scratching. Treatment involves mechanically removing ticks with forceps, spraying or dipping the coat with insecticidal materials such as pyrethroids and malathion, and treating the otitis externa. Otic treatments with an oil base may smother and kill some ticks.[89]

Reinfestation is a problem, so destruction of the lairs or nests of the ticks is important. Spraying the sheds, grounds, woodpiles, and other homesites with malathion or chlorpyrifos may be effective. An amitraz tick collar (Preventic, Virbac) may prevent reinfestation.

Ixodid (Hard) Ticks

Hard ticks possess a chitinous shield, the scutum, which covers the dorsal surface of the male and the anterior dorsal part of the female tick. The capitulum is visible dorsally at the anterior end, and its base is important taxonomically. The sexes are dissimilar, although both are bloodsuckers. It is beyond the scope of this text to identify ticks specifically, but because *Rhipicephalus sanguineus* (in comparison with *Dermacentor*) can reproduce easily in buildings and thus presents special control problems, a few key features for identifying genera are described (Fig. 6–14).

Rhipicephalus is recognized by the vase-shaped base of the capitulum, by elongated spiracles, and by triangular adanal plates in the male tick. The fourth coxae are no larger than the other three. *Dermacentor* ticks are characterized by the large fourth coxae, the rectangular base of the capitulum, and the ornate scutum.

The general life cycle of ixodid ticks is similar, although each species may vary slightly in some details. Eggs hatch in 2 to 7 weeks. Larvae feed for 3 to 12 days and then drop from the host for 6 to 90 days before molting. Nymphs also feed for a short period (3 to 10 days) before an extended, off-host rest (17 to 100 days). Adults are hardy (up to a 19-month life span) and prolific, with egg lays of 2000 to 8000. Generally, completion of the life cycle necessitates three hosts, preferably animals of varied size, for the larva, nymph, and adult, although some species pass through all stages on the same mammal. If the complicated life cycle is interrupted, the tick can survive for long periods or hibernate through the winter. Although the life cycle is usually completed in a single year, it may extend for 2 or 3 years.

While off the host, these ticks infest ground that is covered with small bushes and shrubs. They resist cold but are susceptible to strong sunlight, desiccation, and excessive rainfall. They require a moist environment.

Common Species of Ixodid Ticks Affecting Dogs and Cats

- *Rhipicephalus sanguineus.* The brown dog tick is widely distributed in North America and causes the primary tick problem in many sections of the United States. It

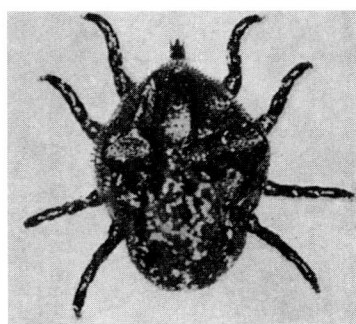

FIGURE 6–13. Nymph of *Otobius megnini,* the spinous ear tick. (From Lapage G: Monnig's Veterinary Helminthology and Entomology, 5th ed. Williams & Wilkins Co., Baltimore, 1962.)

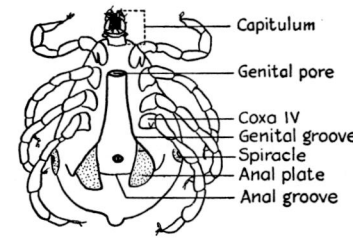
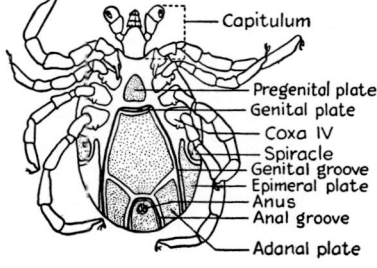
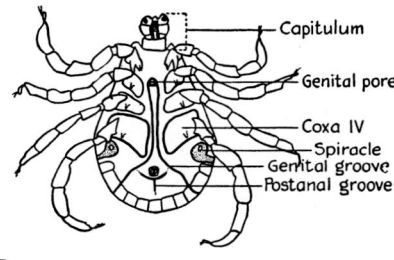

FIGURE 6-14. Ventral view of various species of male ixodid ticks, showing genital and anal grooves, coxae, and plates. Differential characteristics are indicated by heavy lines and dotted areas. (From Belding DL: Textbook of Parasitology. Appleton-Century-Crofts, New York, 1965; redrawn from Hegner, Root, Augustine, and Huff: Parasitology, Appleton-Century Company, 1938.)

can survive indoors, owing to its low moisture requirements, and can complete its life cycle with only one animal as host. Although its principal host is the dog, it is found on other canine species, cats, rabbits, horses, and humans. It requires three distinct hosts (but perhaps the same animal) in its life cycle. It can transmit babesiosis and anaplasmosis, *Ehrlichia canis* and *Francisella tularensis* infection, and can cause tick paralysis.

- *Dermacentor variabilis.* The American dog tick is also widely distributed in North America but is especially common along the Atlantic coast in areas of shrub and beach grass. The principal host of the adult tick is the dog, but humans, domestic animals, and large fur-bearing mammals may be attacked. The principal host of the immature tick is the field mouse, but other small rodents or larger mammals may be infested. It spreads Rocky Mountain spotted fever, St. Louis encephalitis, tularemia, and anaplasmosis, and causes tick paralysis.

Other Ticks That May Affect Dogs and Cats

These include *Dermacentor andersoni* (Rocky Mountain wood tick), *Dermacentor occidentalis* (Pacific or West Coast tick), *Ixodes scapularis* (black-legged tick), *Ixodes dammini* (deer tick), and *Amblyomma maculatum* (Lone Star tick).

Damage From Ticks

Ticks injure animals by causing irritation via their bites; by producing hypersensitivity reactions (see Chap. 8); by serving as vectors for bacterial, rickettsial, viral, and protozoal diseases; and by producing tick paralysis through their poisonous secretions (see Fig. 6–4C and D).

Tick paralysis has been produced by 12 ixodid species, including *D. variabilis*, and is seen in many hosts including dogs and cats.[85] The paralysis is caused by a protein toxin produced by the salivary glands of the tick. It may be elaborated by ovarian function, because it is associated with egg production. Individual ticks vary in their toxin-producing capacity, although those attached near the spine and neck seem to produce a more severe intoxication. The toxin affects the lower motor neurons of the spinal cord and cranial nerves, and produces a progressive ascending flaccid paralysis.

Treatment and Control of Ticks

In cases of tick paralysis, rapid recovery follows mechanical removal of the complete tick or ticks. When animals are infested by small numbers of ticks, manual removal from the host is simple and easy. An effective method is to soak the tick in alcohol, grasp the head parts at the surface of the skin gently with a 5-inch curved Crile mosquito hemostat, and apply firm traction. Ticks are commonly found in the ears and between the toes. The collected ticks should be soaked in alcohol or an insecticide until dead.

For heavy or recurrent infestations, dogs can be treated with fipronil or have permethrin applied as a spray, dip, or spot treatment.[14, 39, 84, 88] Frequent treatment is needed for maximum efficacy. Cats can be treated with fipronil or ivermectin.[87, 88] The amitraz tick collar for dogs is reported to be highly effective in detaching or preventing the attachment of ticks.[86] Although an amitraz-impregnated collar and a spot-on fipronil both killed ticks and inhibited attachment and feeding, the amitraz collar had a longer duration of effect and reduced egg hatchability and percentages of surviving and feeding larvae.[86a] Selamectin was effective in controlling *D. variabilis* when administered monthly.[43a]

Immunotherapy with a tick vaccine to overcome a tick-induced immunosuppression, with its subsequent larger number of ticks, has been proposed.[84a]

Infestations of *R. sanguineus* in houses and kennels can often be controlled or eliminated by repeated spraying of woodwork, crawl spaces, pipe clearances, and cracks with chlorpyrifos. For severe infestations, professional exterminators should be employed.

Outdoor control measures are usually impractical but can help limit the number of ticks. Their habitat can be destroyed by cutting and burning brush and grass, by cultivating land, and by rotating pastures. In urban areas, grass and shrubbed areas can be treated with appropriately registered pesticides. Application is done in the spring and repeated once during midsummer.

PARASITIC MITES

Mites are members of the order Acarina.[1, 10] They are smaller than ticks and do not have a leathery covering; the hypostome may be unarmed, and some mites have spiracles on the cephalothorax. Parasitic mites are chiefly ectoparasites of the skin, mucous membranes, or feathers, but a few are endoparasites. They are distributed worldwide, are found on plants and animals, cause direct injury to animals, and spread disease. Because of their prevalence and clinical importance, four parasitic mites—*Cheyletiella* spp., *Demodex* spp., *Sarcoptes scabiei* (var. *canis*), and *Notoedres cati*—and the diseases they cause are discussed in depth.

Most disorders discussed subsequently can be effectively treated with topical pesticides or oral or parenteral avermectins (ivermectin and milbemycin). At present, the avermectins are licensed in dogs and cats for monthly administration at low dosages. Their acaricidal dosages are much higher (ivermectin: 200 to 600 μg/kg; milbemycin: 1 to 2 mg/kg). Use at these doses is an extralabel drug use and should not be considered unless no licensed product exists, the licensed products cannot be used because of animal idiosyncrasies, or the licensed product is not effective. Casual use could subject the veterinarian to legal action, especially if the animal had an adverse reaction.

Dermanyssus gallinae

This mite attacks poultry (poultry mite), wild and cage birds, dogs, and cats, as well as humans. It is called the red mite, but it is red only when engorged with blood. At other times, it is white, gray, or black. The engorged adult, which is the largest form, is only 1.1 mm in size (Fig. 6–15). It lives in nests and cracks in cages or houses. After a meal of blood, it lays up to seven eggs at a time. They hatch to six-legged nymphs that do not feed. After 24 ± 12 hours, these molt to eight-legged protonymphs that feed and molt, 30 ± 15 hours later, to deutonymphs. These also feed and molt 30 ± 15 hours later to adults. The whole cycle takes only 8 days under ideal conditions, but without feeding

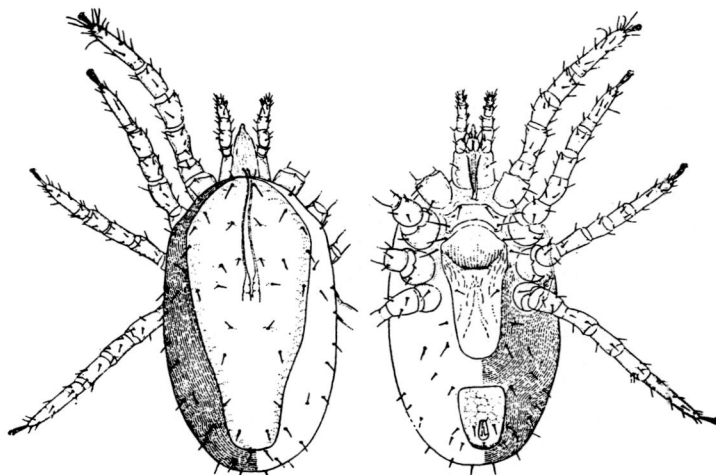

FIGURE 6–15. *Dermanyssus gallinae* (Degeer). Left, dorsal view of female; right, ventral view of female. (From Lapage G: Monnig's Veterinary Helminthology and Entomology, 5th ed. Williams & Wilkins Co., Baltimore, 1962.)

opportunities, it may last 5 months.[92] Mites survive for up to 9 months without food when kept at 5° to 25°C.[90a]

This mite affects dogs and cats only rarely and almost accidentally.[90] Wild birds nesting in the eaves of houses have mites, which may enter open windows and affect people and animals living there. Ramsay and Mason[91] found such large numbers of mites covering a dog's body that the small grayish white mites crawling on the hair resembled the "walking" dandruff of cheyletiellosis. In that case, itching was not severe. Most cases occur in pets that have access to chicken houses or live in recently converted poultry quarters. Clinical signs include erythema and papulocrustous, intensely pruritic eruptions, especially over the back and the extremities. Diagnosis is made by finding the mites in skin scrapings. Almost any insecticidal bath, dip, or spray eliminates the mites. The affected premises that initiated the infection should be treated to prevent reinfestation. Because −20°C and temperatures >45°C were lethal for *D. gallinae*, freezing, heating, or both could be advocated as alternatives to chemical sanitation.[90a]

Lynxacarus radovsky

The small cat fur mites are common in Australia, Hawaii, and Brazil[93, 96] and have been reported in Florida,[95] and Texas.[94] They have elongated bodies, 430 to 520 μm in length, and flaplike sternal extensions. These contain the first two legs, which grasp the hair of the host (Fig. 6–16). All of the legs have terminal suckers. Because all fur mites are generally alike, a competent parasitologist is needed for accurate species identification. These mites are not highly contagious and infection typically occurs by direct contact, but fomites may be important for transmission.[94] Bowman[93] reported only 1 of 14 cats in a group to be affected. Severity of clinical signs relates to the chronicity and extent of the infestation. In mild cases, there is little itching and the mites attached to the hair give a salt-and-pepper appearance to the dull and dirty coat. Because hairs epilate easily, some patchy alopecia can be seen. In severe cases, there is a generalized maculopapular to exfoliative dermatitis. Severely involved cats tend to be more pruritic. Mites usually congregate along the topline attached to the terminal parts of the hair. However, they may occasionally be found all over the body. Diagnosis is made by isolation of mites on skin scrapings or acetate tape impression. Treatment with insecticidal sprays or dips, lime sulfur dips weekly, or ivermectin is usually adequate.[95, 96]

Trombiculosis

Although 20 of about 700 species of chigger mites (harvest mites) can cause disease, only two are reported here.

Parasitic Skin Diseases • 447

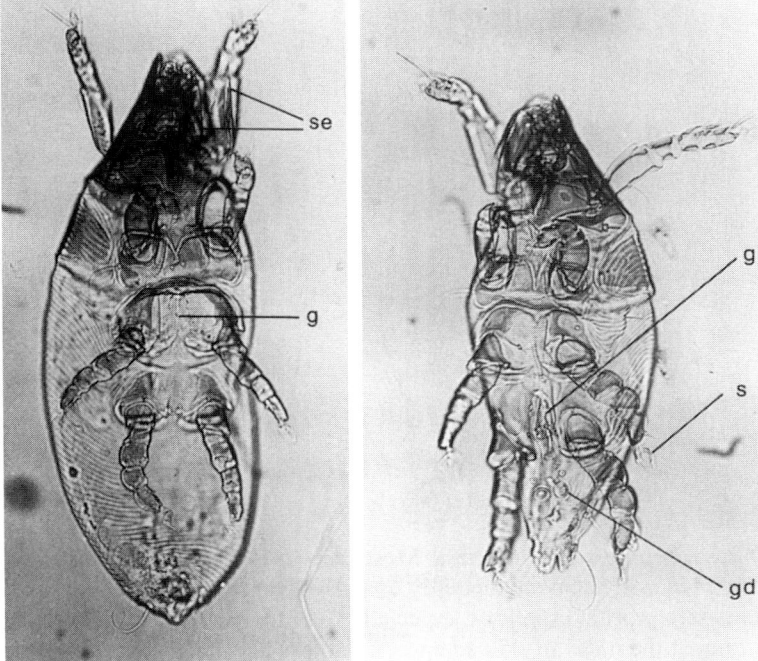

FIGURE 6–16. A, *Lynxacarus radovsky*, female in ventral view: se, sternal extensions; g, genitalia. Body length, 515 μm. B, *L. radovsky*, male in ventral view: g, genitalia; s, sucker; gd, genital disc. Body length, 430 μm. (From Bowman WL, Domrow R: The cat-fur mite in Australia. Aust Vet J 54:403, 1978. Photographs by R. Wilson.)

Eutrombicula (Trombicula) alfreddugesi (North American Chigger) and *Neotrombicula (Trombicula) autumnalis*

The adult form is a scavenger living on decaying vegetable material. It is orange red, is about the size of the head of a pin, and lives about 10 months, producing probably one generation per year. The eggs are laid in moist ground and hatch to six-legged red larvae that are parasitic and feed on animals. They drop to the ground and become nymphs, and finally adults (Figs. 6–17 and 6–18). The entire cycle is complete in 50 to 70 days, but adult female mites may live longer than a year. They are usually found in areas where the skin is in contact with the ground, such as the legs, the feet, the head, the ears, and the ventrum. Signs are variable. The bite usually produces severe irritation and an intensely pruritic papulocrustous eruption (Fig. 6–19B), but it may also cause nonpruritic papules,

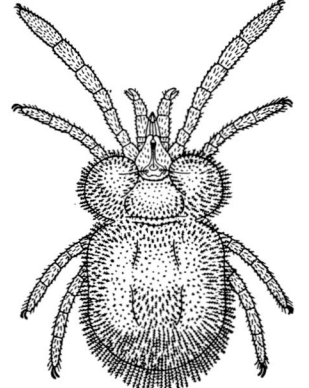
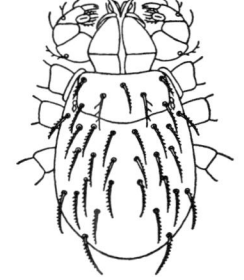

FIGURE 6–17. A, *Trombicula alfreddugesi* (North American chigger) adult; B, *T. alfreddugesi* larva, dorsal view (legs omitted). (From Belding DL: Textbook of Parasitology. Appleton-Century-Crofts, New York, 1965.)

X 20   X 100

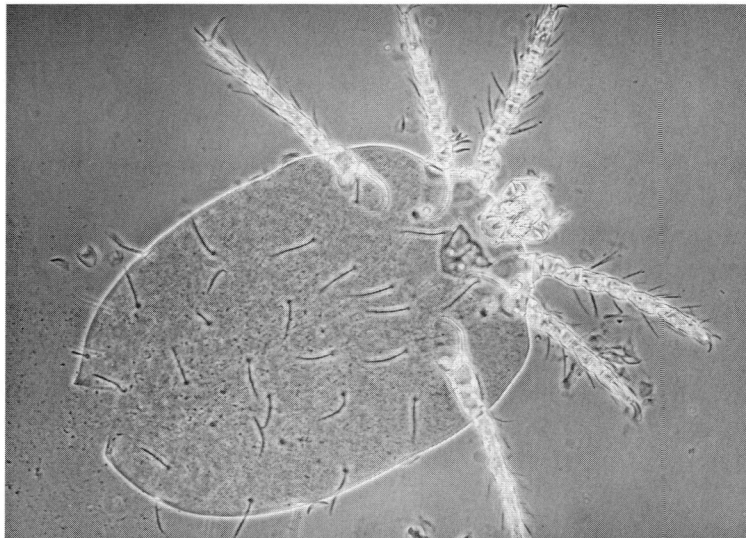

FIGURE 6–18. *Neotrombicula autumnalis.* (Courtesy J. Georgi.)

pustules, and crusts. Secondary scaling and alopecia may appear. Mites may be found in and around the ears of cats but are easily distinguished from *Otodectes* (ear mites) by their intense orange-red color (see Fig. 6–19C) and their tight adherence to the skin.[97, 98] They are about 500 μm in size. When removed from the host for microscopic examination, they should be placed in mineral oil immediately or they will escape.

Chiggers are seasonal in late summer and fall. Affected patients have a history of environmental contact in woods and fields. Skin biopsy reveals varying degrees of superficial perivascular dermatitis (spongiotic or hyperplastic) in which eosinophils are numerous.

Treatment is successful with one or two parasiticidal dips or topical otic preparations containing a parasiticide (Tresaderm, Merck AgVet).[98] Systemic corticosteroids administered for 2 to 3 days help relieve the itching, if present. Unless rural animals are prevented from roaming, reinfestation can be expected. In one study, the application of a 0.25% fipronil spray blocked reinfestation in 15 of the 18 treated dogs.[100] The three treated cats were reinfested within 7 to 10 days. Others have also had success with the topical application of fipronil.[96a]

Walchia americana

This chigger mite (Fig. 6–20) has been reported to be common in squirrels and small rodents in the southwestern and eastern United States and has been reported in the cat.[99] The larvae live on the surface of the skin. Their salivary secretions allow them to feed on tissue liquids of the host. A walled-off channel is formed on the skin surface as a host reaction that attempts to isolate the parasite. The larvae detach and enter decaying wood for a quiet period. Active nymphs emerge and forage, become quiet again as they pass through the imagochrysalis stage, and then emerge as adults. These feed principally on the Collembolla insect (spring tail). The adults lay many eggs, which hatch to parasitic larvae. Some chiggers have a special liking for certain body locations on the host. The mite prefers the ventrum but is also found on the ears and the back.

In the cat reported by Lowenstine and colleagues,[99] the lesions were on the ventral trunk, the medial surface of the legs, and the interdigital spaces. Lesions could be palpated, but the hair needed to be parted carefully to see them easily. There was nodular thickened skin, and the surface was cracked and scaly, with moist, serous yellow exudate. The paws were swollen, and the claws were cracked. The cat shook its feet as if it had stepped into something noxious. Close inspection revealed nonpruritic papules (0.1 to 0.3

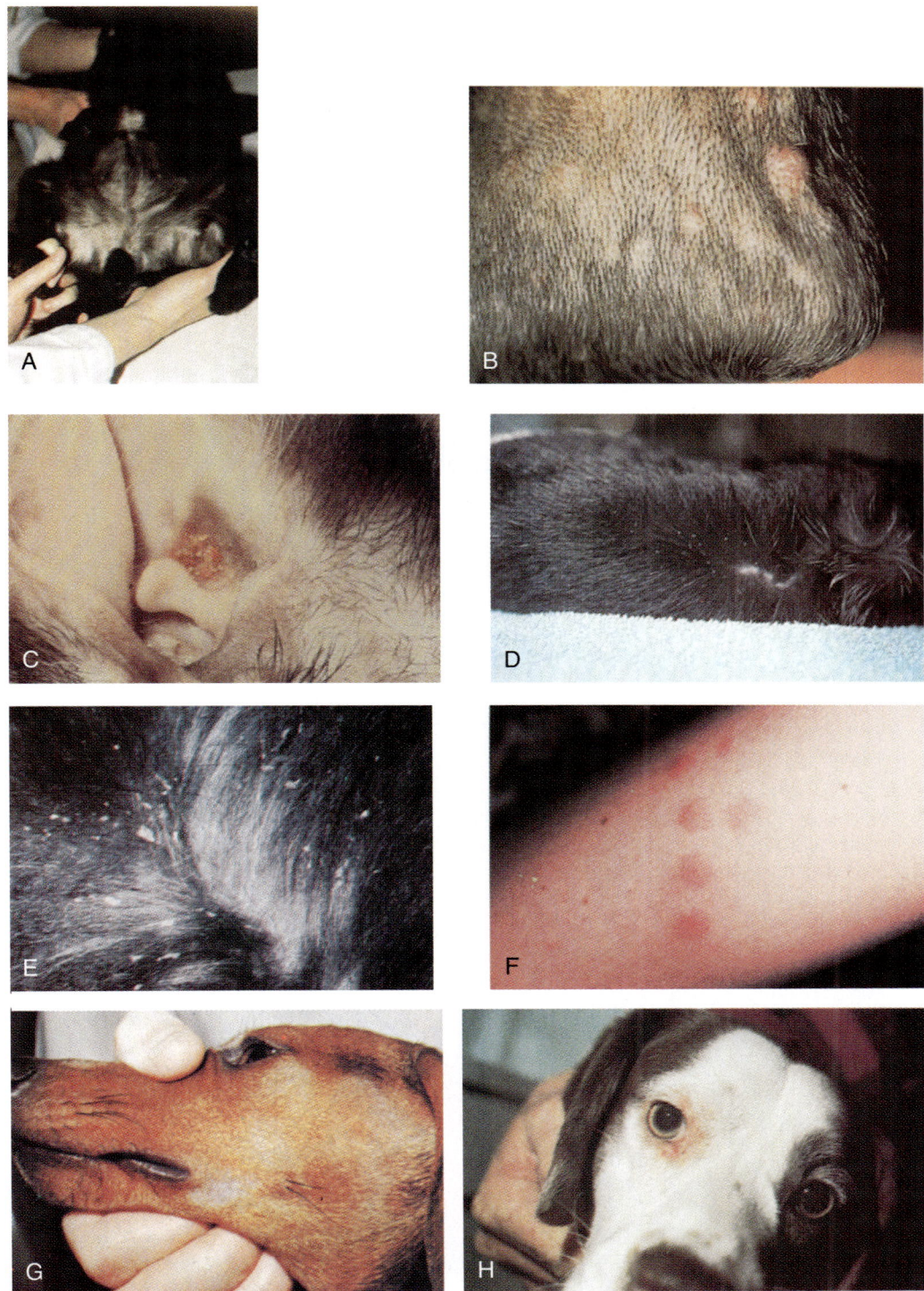

FIGURE 6–19. *A*, Self-induced hypotrichosis in a cat with *Otodectes cynotis*. *B*, Papules on the medial elbow of a dog due to chigger bites. *C*, Orange chigger mites on a crust in the temporal region of a cat. (Courtesy T. Manning.) *D*, Scaling over the dorsum of a cat with cheyletiellosis. (Cat is lying on its side on a green towel.) *E*, *Cheyletiella* infestation in dog. The white specks are walking dandruff. *F*, Papular urticaria of human skin due to *Cheyletiella blakei* bites. *G*, Localized demodicosis. A single alopecic patch at the commissure of the lips. *H*, Periocular alopecia and erythema in a dog with localized demodicosis.

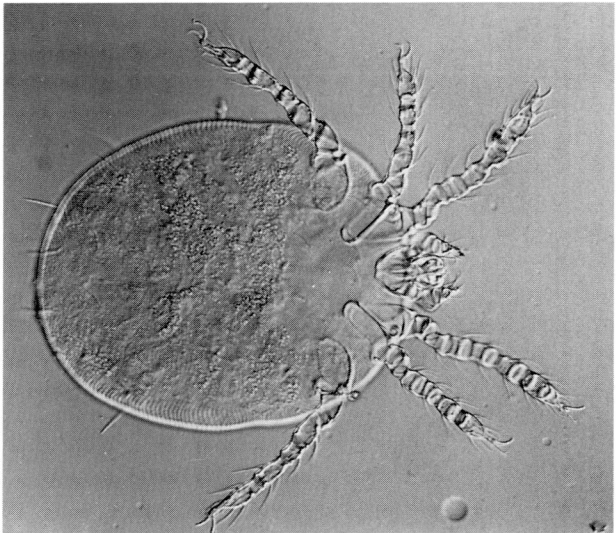

FIGURE 6–20. *Walchia americana.* (Courtesy J. Georgi.)

cm) with a few wheals and flares. Skin scrapes produced few mites, but a skin biopsy specimen contained many mites.

Histopathologic examination reveals varying degrees of intraepidermal pustular to vesicular dermatitis. Hyperkeratosis is marked, and mite segments are seen within the epidermis (Fig. 6–21). Eosinophils and mast cells are numerous.

Treatment with insecticidal products for the mites and broad-spectrum antibiotics for the secondary infection produces a good response in 10 days.

Otodectes cynotis

O. cynotis (ear mite) is a psoroptid mite that does not burrow but lives on the surface of the skin. Adult mites are large and white and move freely. The anus is terminal, they have four pairs of legs, and all except the rudimentary fourth pair of the female mite extend beyond the body margin. All legs of the male mite bear short, unjointed stalks (pedicles) with suckers, which are also present on the first two pairs of legs of the females.

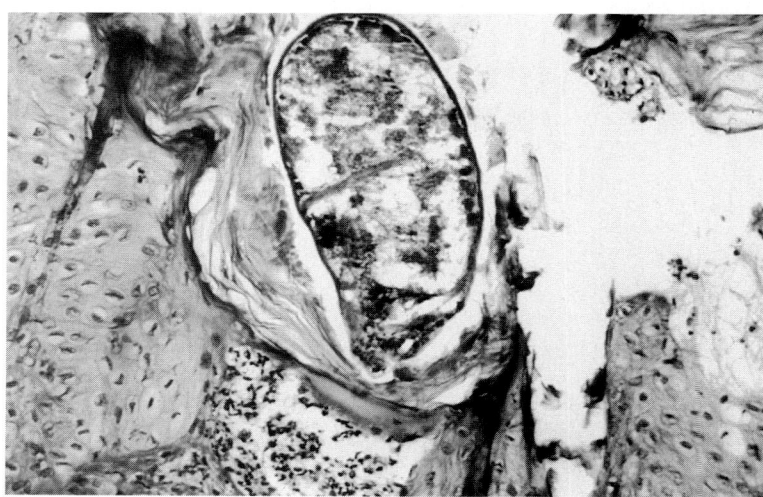

FIGURE 6–21. *Walchia americana* larva buried in the epidermis of a cat.

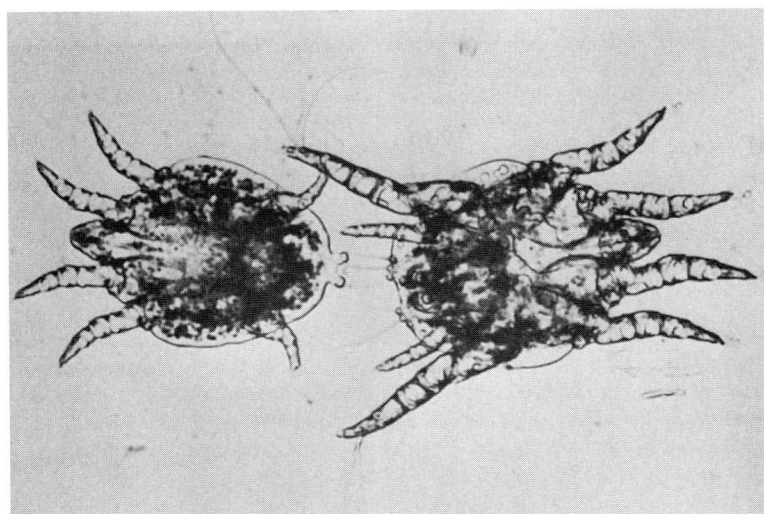

FIGURE 6–22. Larger male *O. cynotis* mite approaching a deutonymph.

The life cycle lasts 3 weeks. The egg is laid with a cement that sticks it to the substrate. After a 4-day incubation, it hatches to produce the six-legged larva. At this point, the larva feeds actively for 3 to 10 days, rests for 10 to 30 hours, and hatches to the protonymph, which has eight legs, although the last pair are small. After a simple active and resting stage, the protonymph molts into the deutonymph. The deutonymph is usually approached by the male adult (Fig. 6–22), and the two become attached (end to end) by the pair of dorsal posterior suckers on the body of the nymph and those on the rear legs of the adult male mite. If a male adult is produced from the deutonymph, the attachment has no physiologic significance; however, if a female mite emerges, copulation occurs at that moment, and the female mite becomes egg bearing. Female mites that are not attached, and thereby do not permit copulation at the moment of ecdysis, do not lay eggs. Sexual dimorphism occurs only in the adult form. The first four legs of all stages bear unjointed, short stalks and suckers, but only the adult male mites have suckers on the rear legs. Adults have approximately a 2-month life span.

The mites feed on epidermal debris and tissue fluid from the superficial epidermis. In this way, the host is exposed to, and immunized against, mite antigen.[107, 110] There is no delayed hypersensitivity, but a reaginic antibody develops early in the disease and precipitating antibodies later in its course.

As the mites feed, the epithelium of the ear canal is irritated and the canal fills with cerumen, blood, and mite debris. This discharge has the classic coffee grounds appearance (see Fig. 6–4G). Clinical symptoms are variable, especially in cats. Some cats with massive amounts of discharge show no clinical signs, whereas other cats have intense otic pruritus with minimal discharge (see Fig. 6–4H). Dogs tend to have otic pruritus with minimal discharge. Lesions may be restricted to the external ear canal, but mites are commonly found on other areas of the body, especially on the neck, rump, and tail.[7, 101] These ectopic mites often cause no disease, but some animals have a pruritic dermatitis, which can resemble flea bite hypersensitivity, atopy, or food hypersensitivity (see Figs. 6–23 and 6–19A). Dogs and cats that have *O. cynotis* infestations often have positive intradermal skin test reactions to other mites: *Dermatophagoides farinae*, *D. pteronyssinus*, and *Acarus siro*.[101a, 107a] These reactions become negative after the *O. cynotis* infestation is eliminated. Other conditions to be ruled out include pediculosis, *Pelodera* dermatitis, scabies, and chigger bites. Ear mites are highly contagious and especially prevalent in the young. The mites are not host specific,[9] so all contact animals should be presumed to be infected. Mites can cause a transient papular dermatitis in humans[104] or rarely become a true otic parasite.[105]

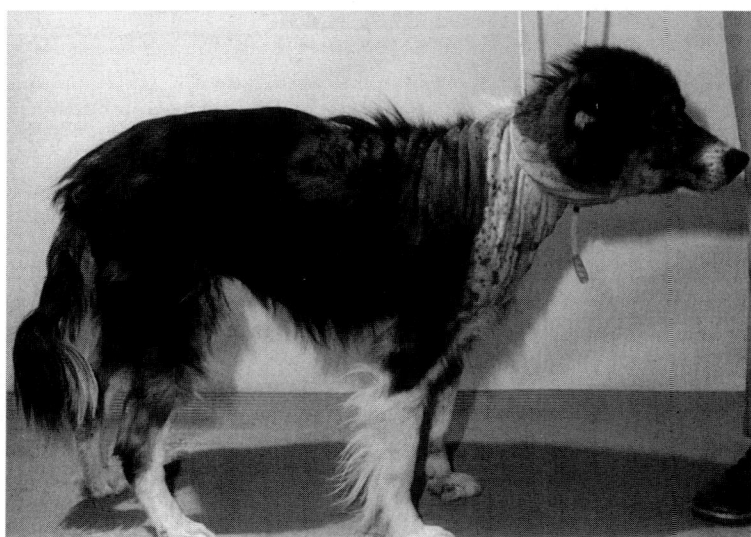

FIGURE 6–23. Otodectic mange. Dog with severe generalized disease.

Various treatment options exist, and selection depends on the number of animals involved and the severity of the clinical signs. With only one or two animals involved, the otic route of treatment is used. If the ear canals are filled with debris, they should be cleaned with an appropriate ceruminolytic agent. The mite infestation can be addressed with one of many otic parasiticides, baby oil, a neomycin sulfate–thiabendazole–dexamethasone solution (Tresaderm), or various steroid-antibiotic-antifungal ear products.[102, 106, 108] The thiabendazole in Tresaderm is thought to have both ovicidal and adulticidal activity. The products containing no parasiticide are thought to work by smothering the mite.[108] Animals with severe otic pruritus or secondary bacterial or yeast infections usually are treated with the polypharmaceutical agents. Specific instructions depend on the product used. Because all stages beyond the egg should be susceptible to the agent, treatment should only be needed for 7 to 10 days unless there is a secondary infection. With this short course of treatment, body treatment with an appropriate flea spray, foam, or dip is necessary to prevent reinfestation of the ear canal by the ectopic mites.[109]

In multiple animal situations, cases with skin disease, or when otic products cannot or will not be used, ivermectin can effectively eradicate the mites.[6, 101] Although aural administration is commonly used, relapses can be seen because of the irregularities in drug absorption.[103] Near 100% efficacy is seen with oral (weekly for three doses), subcutaneous (two doses at 14-day intervals), or topical (pour-on product—two doses at 14-day intervals) administration. Although no data are available, high-dose milbemycin should be effective in animals sensitive to high-dose ivermectin. Moxidectin (0.2 mg/kg) was given orally or subcutaneously, twice at a 10-day interval, with excellent tolerance and efficacy.[107a] The spot application form of fipronil also is effective.[109] Others indicate that the application of 2 to 4 drops of the fipronil spot-on product in both ears, repeated in 10 to 30 days, is effective.[96a, 101b, 101c] Selamectin (2 treatments at a 30-day interval) was very effective for the treatment of *Otodectes* infestations in cats and dogs.[43a]

Pneumonyssoides caninum

P. caninum is a mite of unknown incidence.[117] In one study, the mite was found in 7% of dogs undergoing necropsy for unrelated reasons.[112] It inhabits the nasal passages and sinuses of dogs, and most infested dogs are asymptomatic. When signs result, they include serous to catarrhal rhinitis-sinusitis, sneezing, reverse sneezing, excessive lacrimation, and other signs that could be confused with those of respiratory allergy.[115] The aerophagia associated with the respiratory signs predisposes the dog to gastric dilatation-volvulus.[113]

Some dogs have facial pruritus.[114, 118] Diagnosis is by mite identification grossly[114] at rhinoscopy or in nasal flushes. The mites may be impossible to demonstrate in some dogs, and response to acaricidal therapy allows a presumptive diagnosis to be made. The only effective treatments are ivermectin or milbemycin.[111, 116]

Environmental Mites

Many species of free-living mites can be found in grains, in hay and straw, and in the house. These mites can cause skin disease by accidental parasitism on mammals[119] or by the induction of allergic reactions when the exoskeletons, body parts, or excreta are ingested, absorbed percutaneously, or inhaled.[3, 120] The latter methods are most important, especially with *D. pteronyssinus* and *D. farinae*, the two most common species of house dust mites. Dogs with an atopy-like condition (see Chap. 8) often show positive reactions to these mites, but the absolute significance of those reactions is uncertain.

Environmental mites may be susceptible to parasiticides used in flea control programs, but the natural habitat of these mites makes their eradication difficult. Hay and straw mite problems can be resolved by removing the hay and straw or by using fresh straw, which should contain the natural foodstuffs of these mites.[117] Food storage mites can be eliminated only by destroying the food. House dust mite populations can be decreased by removal of carpets and frequent and thorough vacuuming of floors, furniture, and bedding. These cleaning procedures may help but do not completely resolve the pet's problem because the basis for the dermatitis is allergy and not direct parasitism.

Cheyletiellosis

Cheyletiella dermatitis (walking dandruff) is usually a mild, nonsuppurative mite-induced dermatitis produced by *Cheyletiella* spp. living on the surface of the skin.

Cause and Pathogenesis

Cheyletiella mites are large mites that affect cats, dogs, rabbits, and humans.[131] The incidence of the disease is unknown because signs are so variable, but it is probably less prevalent now because of the widespread use of flea control products, which also kill this mite. The three species of mites may travel freely among various host species.[9, 35, 122, 127] In general, *Cheyletiella yasguri* is considered the species found in dogs[123]; *C. blakei*, the species in cats[126]; and *C. parasitivorax*, the species in rabbits. Experimental transfer of *C. yasguri* between dogs and rabbits suggests that the various species do not have extreme host specificity.[123] All species can transiently affect contact humans.[124]

The large mites (385 µm) have four pairs of legs bearing combs instead of claws (Fig. 6–24). The most diagnostic feature of *Cheyletiella* spp. is the accessory mouthparts or palpi that terminate in prominent hooks (Fig. 6–25). The heart-shaped sensory organ on genu I is diagnostic of *C. yasguri*, the cone-shaped sensory organ is diagnostic of *C. blakei*, and the global sensory organ is diagnostic of *C. parasitivorax*.

Free-living cheyletids (e.g., *Cheyletus eruditis*) can also infest cats and dogs.[125] These mites are not reported to produce clinical signs. The free-living cheyletids must be differentiated from *Cheyletiella* mites, which they closely resemble. In the free-living cheyletids, the palptarus bears one or two combs.[125]

The mites do not usually burrow but live in the keratin layer of the epidermis and are not associated with hair follicles. They move about rapidly in pseudotunnels in epidermal debris but periodically attach themselves firmly to the epidermis, pierce the skin with their stylet chelicerae, and become engorged with a clear colorless fluid. The ova are smaller than louse nits and are attached to hairs by fine fibrillar strands. In contrast, louse eggs are cemented firmly to the host's hairs (see Fig. 2–28Z).

Cheyletiella mites are not predacious on other mites. The entire life cycle is completed on one host and goes through the typical egg, larval, nymphal, and adult stages. The life cycle is approximately 21 days. The mite is an obligate parasite, because larvae, nymphs, and adult male mites are thought to die soon after leaving the host. Adult female mites are more hardy and may live free of their host for up to 10 days or more.[6, 122, 127]

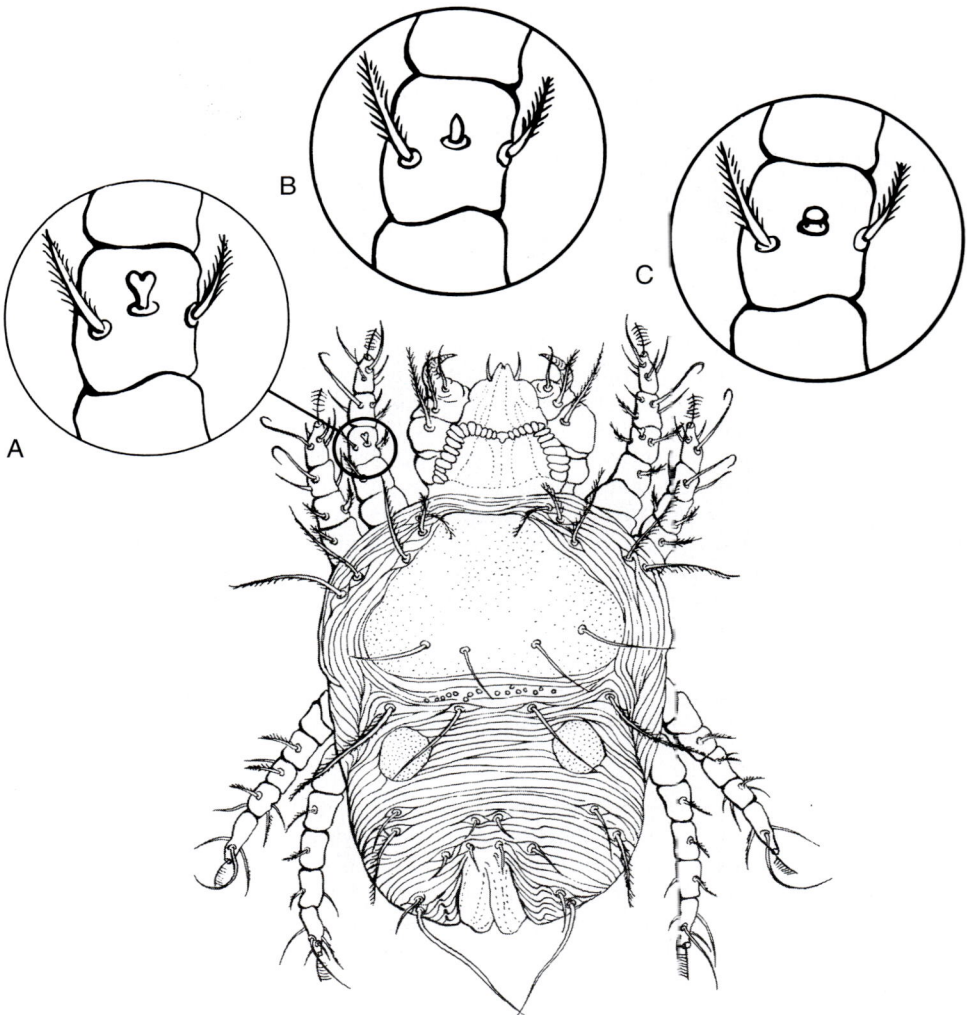

FIGURE 6–24. Artist's sketch of adult female *Cheyletiella yasguri* mite, showing characteristic saddle-shaped body and diagnostic hooks of the accessory mouthparts. Insert A shows the heart-shaped sense organ on genu I that typifies *Cheyletiella yasguri*. Insert B shows the conical sense organ on genu I that typifies *Cheyletiella blakei*. Insert C shows the global sense organ on genu I that typifies *Cheyletiella parasitivorax*.

Eggs that are shed into the environment with the pet's hair may be important sources of reinfestation.[35] Stein[132] reported seeing *Cheyletiella* mites crawling in and out of the nostrils of cats and thus added a new twist to the epidemiology and therapy of the disease.

The mites are highly contagious, especially between young host animals, and humans may be affected, too. Both dogs and cats may be a source of human infection.[124] In one survey, 27 of 41 catteries that had problems with a pruritic dermatitis had animals with cheyletiellosis.[128] In 20% of these situations, humans cases were also found. *C. blakei* was isolated in all cases. There is no doubt that the public health aspects of this parasite are important, because frequent contact with infected animals may produce an uncomfortable skin disease in humans. Human infestations vary in severity, but after direct contact with infested animals has occurred, grouped, erythematous macules form on the arms, the trunk, and the buttocks (see Fig. 6–19*F*). These rapidly develop a central papule that

Parasitic Skin Diseases • 455

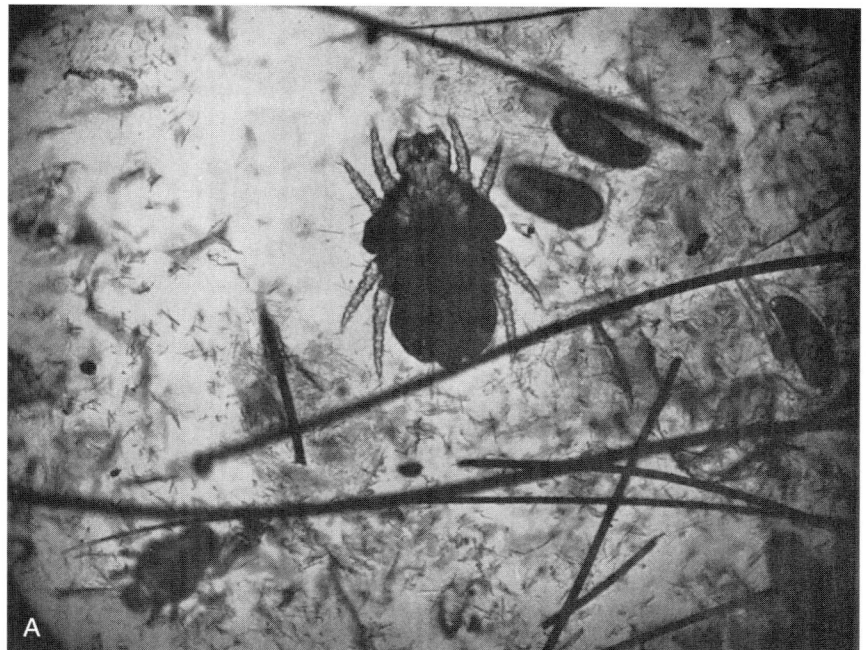

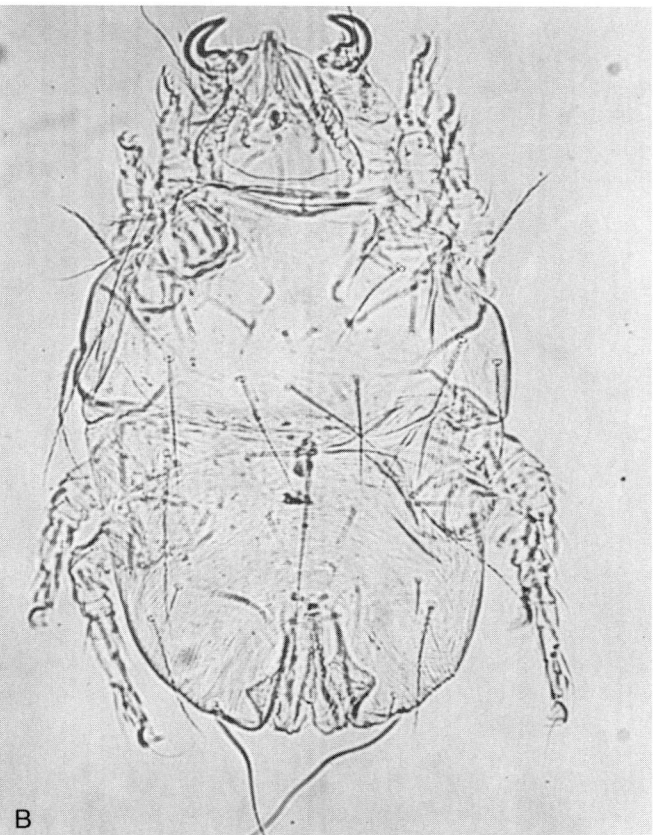

FIGURE 6–25. *A*, *C. yasguri* adult, larva, and eggs from skin scraping (low power). *B*, *C. yasguri* adult mite showing the diagnostic hooks of the accessory mouthparts.

becomes vesicular and then pustular, finally rupturing to produce a yellow crusted lesion that is frequently excoriated because of the intense pruritus. Although the lesions are severely inflamed, they are well demarcated from surrounding skin. Older lesions have an area of central necrosis, which is highly diagnostic. Constant animal contact is usually needed to maintain human infections. With no further infestation, lesions subside in 3 weeks.

Symptoms in dogs and cats are variable and range from virtually none to an intensely pruritic dermatitis. Any breed of animal can be affected, but there may be an increased frequency in Cocker spaniels.[127] Initially, most infested animals develop a dorsally oriented dry scaling with minimal or no pruritus (see Fig. 6–19D). These initial signs are probably due to inflammation caused by the mites' feeding. Because a cat's natural grooming removes both scale and mites and eggs (both can be found in feces), these initial signs tend to be less noticeable and disease progression is often slower than in the nongrooming dog. With time, the scaling becomes more severe and widespread (see Fig. 6–20E), hair loss can occur, and the level of pruritus tends to increase. In some animals, the intensity of the pruritus is well out of proportion to the number of mites present, suggesting the development of a hypersensitivity to the mite.[35] Animals in this latter group can have an exfoliative erythroderma or a scabies-like condition with the same distribution of lesions and intensity of pruritus. Some cats have a widespread papulocrustous eruption (miliary dermatitis).[9, 127] Other cats have self-induced dorsal hypotrichosis ("fur-mowing") with little or no skin lesions.

Diagnosis

The diagnosis is confirmed by identifying the mite or its eggs. This process can be difficult, especially in cats. Techniques used to identify the mite include direct examination of the animal with a powerful magnifying glass and examination of superficial skin scrapings obtained with a scalpel, acetate tape impressions, a large amount of hair and scale collected with a flea comb, or fecal flotations.[130] In the feces, *Cheyletiella* eggs resemble hookworm eggs but they are three to four times larger (230 by 100 μm) and are often embryonated. The success rate of each technique depends on the length of the animal's coat, the size of the area sampled, and most important, the number of mites present.

The most reliable method appears to be the flea combing technique, but this test can be negative in 15% of dogs[129] and 58% of cats.[130] Hair and scale collected in the comb can be evaluated in two ways. The first involves transferring the material to a Petri dish, covering it with mineral oil, and examining its contents with a dissecting microscope. In the second method, the hair and debris are dissolved by treating the sample with 10% potassium hydroxide in a warm water bath for approximately 30 minutes. After this treatment, fecal flotation solutions are added and the solution is centrifuged at 1500 rpm for 10 minutes. The surface layer is examined microscopically at low power for mites or eggs. Each method has advantages and disadvantages, and no studies have been done to compare the two methods. In the absence of positive mite identification, a therapeutic trial may be necessary to confirm or negate the diagnosis.

The differential diagnosis depends on the clinical presentation. If just scaling is present in dogs, the differential diagnosis includes primary seborrhea, intestinal parasitism, poor nutrition, demodicosis, otodectic mange, pediculosis, and flea infestation. If intense pruritus occurs, scabies, flea bite hypersensitivity, and food hypersensitivity must also be considered. For cats, diabetes mellitus and liver disease must be included if seborrhea is present, whereas feline scabies and the other differential diagnostic possibilities for miliary dermatitis must be considered with pruritus.

Histopathologic study reveals varying degrees of superficial perivascular dermatitis (hyperplastic or spongiotic). In some cases, an interface lichenoid lymphoplasmacytic dermatitis is seen. Mite segments are occasionally found within the hyperkeratotic stratum corneum (Fig. 6–26). Eosinophils vary in number, from few to many.

Treatment

In many instances, *Cheyletiella* infestation can be resolved by the weekly application of various pesticides to all dogs and cats in contact with the mites. Product selection and its

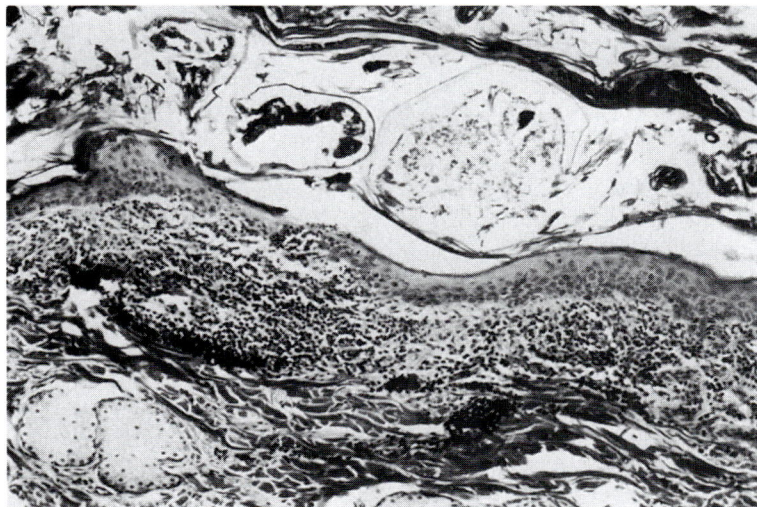

FIGURE 6–26. Cheyletiellosis in a dog. Note sections of mites within the stratum corneum.

route of administration depend on the species, the age of the animals, and the nature of the animals' coat and dermatitis. Lime sulfur dips or the various flea products are usually effective when applied weekly for 3 to 4 weeks. One treatment with fipronil spray or spot-on is effective.[96a, 101b, 121] Conventionally, environmental treatment was not recommended.

Many veterinarians have recognized cases in which these treatments did not work or relapses occurred. These problems can result from poor pesticide application, resistance to pesticide, nasal sequestration of mites, or reinfestation from the environment. One investigator reported the failure of some routine flea products, the need to treat some animals for long periods, and the isolation of live mites from furniture.[35] She recommended flea-type environmental treatments every second week and treatment of animals with lime sulfur, pyrethrins, or amitraz (dogs only) for 6 to 8 weeks.

If relapse occurs, nasal sequestration is known, the owners are physically disabled, or kennels or catteries are infested, satisfactory control usually necessitates the use of ivermectin at 200 to 300 μg/kg.[6, 129] Two injections at 14-day intervals or three oral doses given weekly should be sufficient. Milbemycin remains unproven but should be effective.

Canine Demodicosis

Demodicosis (demodectic mange, follicular mange, or red mange) is an inflammatory parasitic disease of dogs characterized by the presence of larger than normal numbers of demodectic mites. The initial proliferation of mites may be due to a genetic or immunologic disorder.

Cause and Pathogenesis

• **Parasite.** The mite *Demodex canis* is part of the normal fauna of canine skin and is present in small numbers in most healthy dogs.[187–189] Two other mites with different morphologic features have been recognized in some dogs with generalized demodicosis.[146, 165, 174] These mites could be mutants of *D. canis* or additional species of mite that have gone unrecognized. The skin of dogs with demodicosis is ecologically favorable to the reproduction and growth of demodectic mites. They seize this opportunity to colonize the hair follicles and to populate the skin by the thousands. The resulting alopecia and erythema are known as demodicosis. The entire life cycle of the mite is spent on the skin.[199] The parasite resides within the hair follicles and rarely in the sebaceous glands, where it subsists by feeding on cells, sebum, and epidermal debris. The variant mites appear to inhabit only the surface keratin and not the hair follicles.

Four stages of *D. canis* may be demonstrated in skin scrapings (Fig. 6–27). Fusiform eggs hatch into small, six-legged larvae, which molt into eight-legged nymphs and then

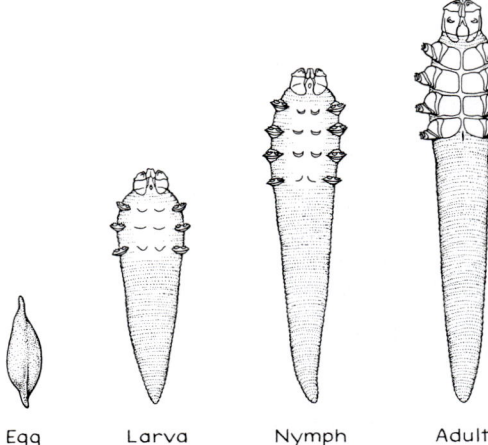

FIGURE 6–27. Adult and immature forms of *Demodex canis.*

Egg   Larva   Nymph   Adult

into eight-legged adults (Fig. 6–28).[189] The male adult measures 40 by 250 μm and the female adult is 40 by 300 μm. Mites (all stages) may be found in the lymph nodes, the intestinal wall, the spleen, the liver, the kidney, the urinary bladder, the lung, the thyroid gland, blood, urine, and feces. However, mites found in these extracutaneous sites are usually dead and degenerate, and represent simple drainage to these areas by blood or lymph.

In the late 1980s, a short-tailed demodicid mite was identified in the dog and is being recognized more frequently.[146, 147, 174, 199a] The mite ranges from 90 to 148 μm in length,[147] which is a third to one-half as long as the typical *D. canis* mite. Beyond its size, this mite seems to share the features of *D. canis* (e.g., acquired at birth, follicular residence). Some dogs show both types of mite on skin scraping.

In the 1990s, a long-bodied demodicid mite was identified in dogs.[165, 183a] This mite is 334 to 368 μm in length. Histologically, it is found in hair follicles.

• **Transmission.** *D. canis* is a normal resident of a dog's skin and ear canal. Transmission occurs from the bitch to nursing neonates by direct contact during the first 2 or 3 days of neonatal life.[156] Mites may be demonstrated in the hair follicles of puppies by the time they are 16 hours old. The mites are first observed on the muzzle of the puppies, which emphasizes the importance of direct contact and nursing. When puppies were taken by cesarean section and raised away from the infected bitch, they did not harbor mites, indicating that in utero transmission does not occur.[187, 201] Similarly, mites cannot be demonstrated in stillborn puppies.[198] Although mites can be transferred to normal adults by the application of mite-laden solutions to their skin or by close confinement with a dog with generalized demodicosis,[19, 153] progressive disease does not occur. Any lesions that occur resolve spontaneously.[198, 201]

Sako[199] found the thermotactic zone of *D. canis* to be between 16° and 41°C (60° to 106°F). Movement of the mites ceased at environmental temperatures below 15°C (59°F). Under various laboratory and artificial conditions, mites could live away from dogs for as long as 37 days.[199] However, these mites lost their ability to infect (invade the hair follicles of) dogs. On a more practical note, after they are on the surface of the skin, mites are rapidly killed by desiccation in 45 to 60 minutes at 20°C (68°F) and a relative humidity of 40%.[188]

Efforts to study the mite have been hampered by the inability to keep it alive in the laboratory. Recently, dog skin grafted to nude mice supported the growth and development of *Demodex canis*, which should allow detailed studies on the pathology and immunology of demodicosis.[143]

• *Types of Demodicosis.* Two types of demodicosis are generally recognized: localized and generalized. The course and the prognosis of the two types are vastly different. Localized demodicosis occurs as one to several small, circumscribed, erythematous, scaly nonpruritic to pruritic areas of alopecia, most commonly on the face and the forelegs. The

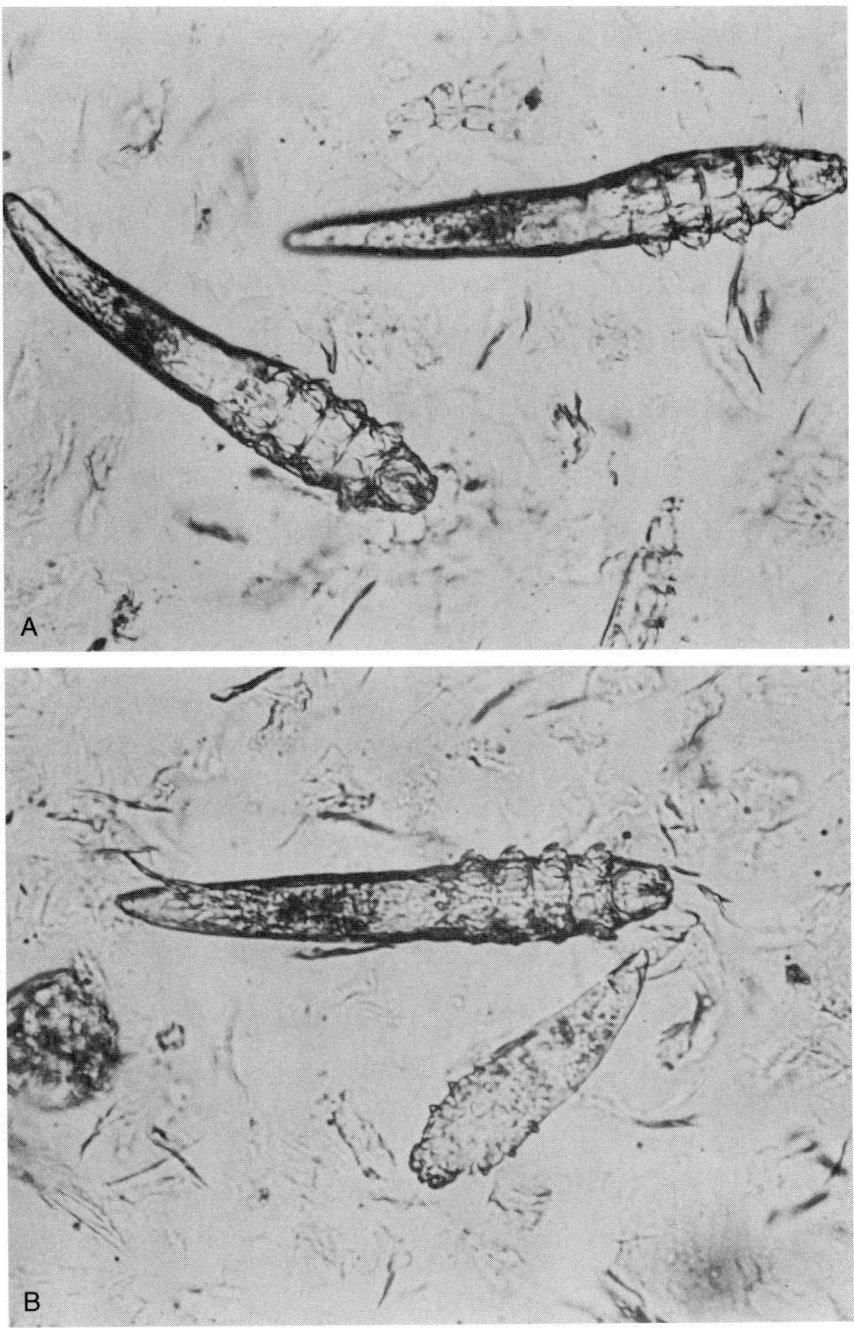

FIGURE 6–28. *Demodex canis* ($\times$ 500). *A,* Two adults (four pairs of legs). *B,* Adult and larva (three pairs of stubby legs).

Illustration continued on following page

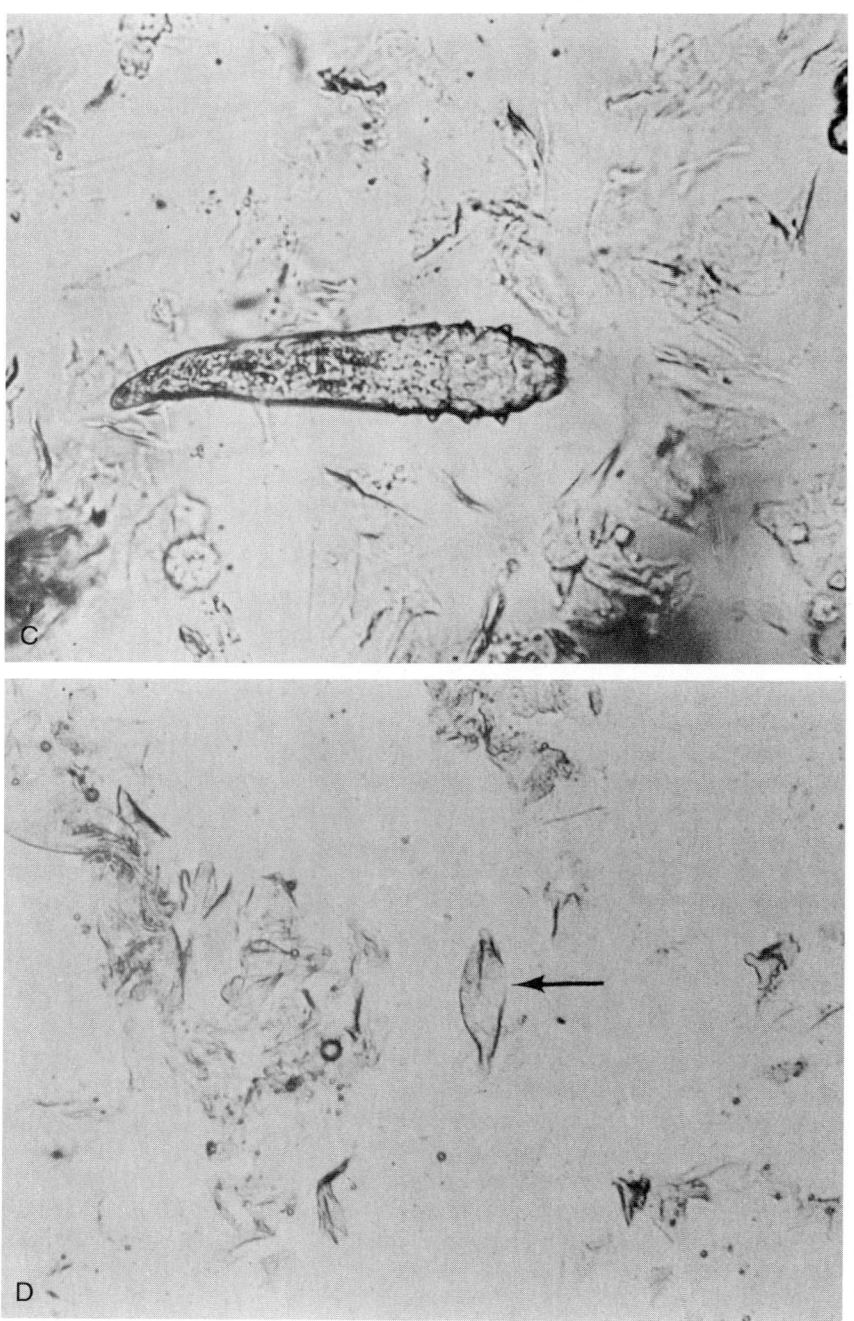

FIGURE 6–28. *Continued. C,* Nymph (four pairs of stubby legs). *D,* Egg *(arrow).*

course is benign and most cases resolve spontaneously. In a small number of cases, the localized proliferation of mites occurs only in the ear canals.[136] These dogs have a ceruminous otitis externa, which may be pruritic. Treatment usually is needed. Generalized demodicosis usually covers large areas of the body but can be more localized, especially when the disease first starts. A dog who has many localized lesions has involvement of an entire body region (e.g., facial area), or has complete involvement of two feet or more has generalized demodicosis. There is no uniformly accepted standard as to how many localized lesions are needed before generalized disease is diagnosed. Six or fewer usually indicates localized disease, whereas 12 or more is indicative of generalized disease. The intermediate group must be evaluated on an individualized basis. The disease may stay restricted in its scope or may become more generalized. Even with this relative localization of the lesions, the pathogenesis, prognosis, and treatment regimens remain the same as that for dogs with widespread demodicosis.

Generalized demodicosis usually starts during puppyhood (3 to 18 months). If the lesions do not resolve spontaneously or receive adequate treatment, the patient carries the disease into adulthood. It is not uncommon to make the diagnosis of generalized demodicosis in dogs older than 2 years of age. The majority of these cases occur in dogs between 2 and 5 years of age, and most of these dogs have had a chronic skin disease. These dogs typically have had the demodicosis from puppyhood but went undiagnosed. Dogs who first experience the disease at 4 years of age or older have true adult-onset demodicosis.

True adult-onset generalized demodicosis is rare, but when it occurs, it can be as serious as the juvenile form. In these cases, the dog has tolerated and controlled the demodectic mites as part of its normal cutaneous fauna for years. If the resistance of the host decreases, the mites suddenly multiply by the thousands. One can speculate that some internal diseases may cause immunosuppression or otherwise lower the dog's capacity to control the number of mites, and adult-onset demodicosis occurs. Each year the authors see multiple cases of adult-onset demodicosis, especially with a facial or pedal presentation, in which skin scrapings have not been performed. If one does not scrape the old dog with pyoderma or other skin disease, the diagnosis will be missed.

Disorders recognized in dogs with adult-onset demodicosis include hypothyroidism, naturally occurring or iatrogenic hyperadrenocorticism, leishmaniasis, and malignant neoplasia or treatment thereof.[133, 152, 171, 181a, 190] In more than 50% of cases, no underlying disease can be documented at the time the demodicosis is diagnosed.[172] In these cases, the dog should be monitored carefully because the malignancy or systemic illness may become obvious weeks to months into treatment. Although the condition may resolve spontaneously in some mildly affected dogs with the resolution of the underlying disease, most will require treatment. If no cause for the demodicosis can be found, the odds of successful treatment are reduced.[152]

In demodectic pododermatitis, the disease is confined to the paws, although some dogs have a higher than normal population of mites in their clinically normal skin. Demodectic pododermatitis can occur as a result of generalized demodicosis, in which the lesions heal everywhere except on the paws. The foot can be involved, especially in Old English sheepdogs, without generalized lesions. The digital, interdigital, and plantar involvements are almost always complicated by secondary bacterial infections (see Fig. 6–29G and H).

Demodicosis is more common in purebred dogs, and certain breeds have far more frequent disease than other breeds. In the Cornell population, the 10 breeds with the highest statistical risk of generalized demodicosis are the Shar pei, West Highland white terrier, Scottish terrier, English bulldog, Boston terrier, Great Dane, Weimaraner, Airedale terrier, Alaskan malamute, and Afghan hound.[177] Demodicosis is commonly diagnosed in other breeds (e.g., Doberman pinscher), but the frequency in those breeds is not out of proportion to the number of dogs within that breed. In other clinics, the Doberman pinscher is at risk so the local statistics must always be kept in mind.[185]

A hereditary predisposition has been observed regularly in breeding kennels. Certain breeders can predict which litters will have the disease. In an affected litter, all or some of the siblings experience generalized demodicosis. Elimination of affected or carrier dogs (both parents and siblings) from a breeding program greatly reduces or eliminates the incidence of demodicosis in that population of dogs. By following this strict culling program, some kennels have virtually eliminated the disease from their line. Analysis of the incidence data from one collie kennel (WHM) and one beagle kennel (DWS) conducted by the authors suggested an autosomal recessive mode of inheritance.

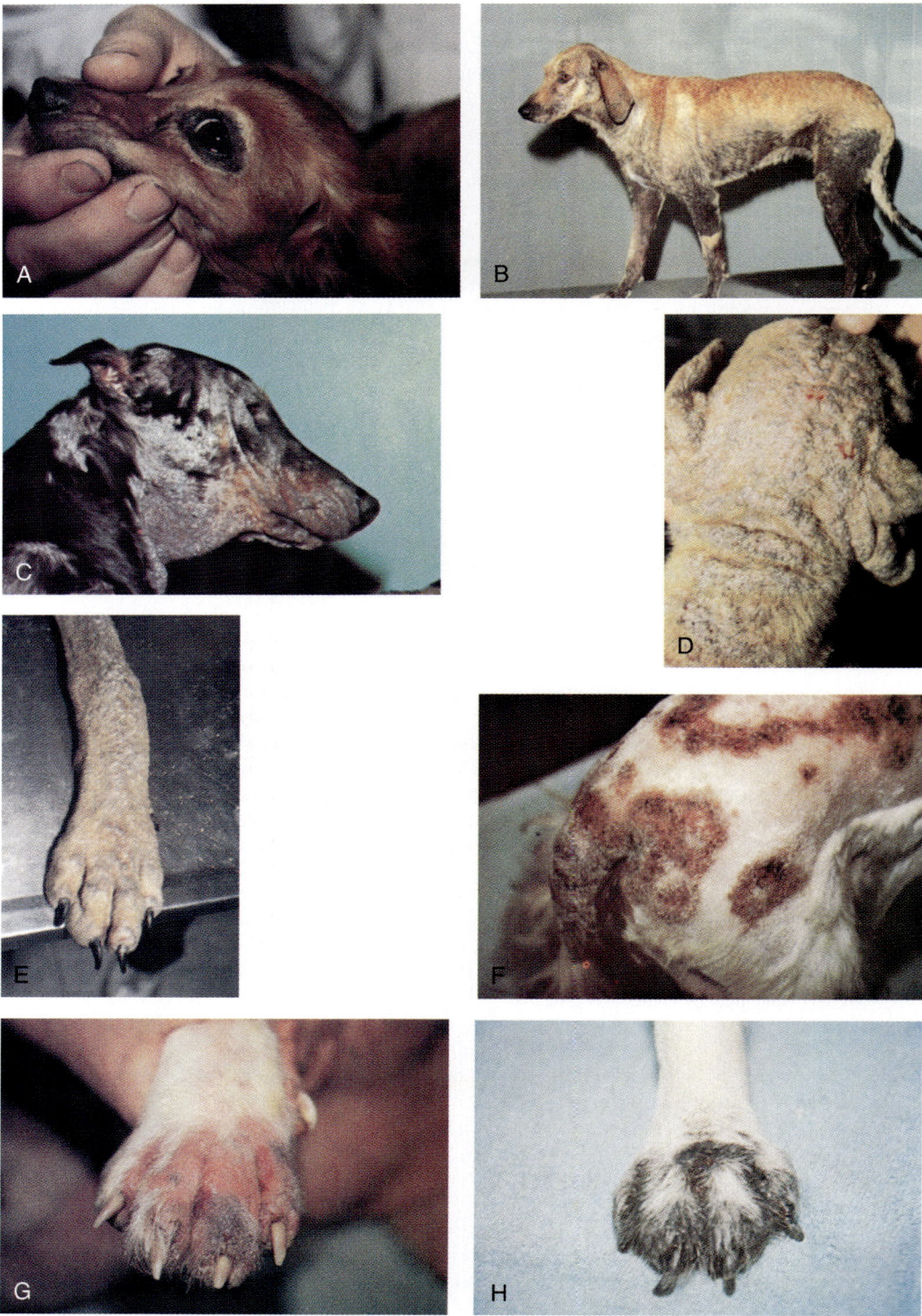

FIGURE 6–29. *A*, Periocular alopecia and hyperpigmentation in a dog with localized demodicosis. *B*, Hound-cross with chronic generalized demodicosis. *C*, A 9-month-old Doberman pinscher whose face is disfigured by the effects of the disease. The loose fold of skin at the throat containing numerous pustules is characteristic. *D*, Follicular papules, crusts, and alopecia over the dorsal neck and top of the head of a dog with generalized demodicosis. *E*, Follicular papules, crusts, and alopecia on the leg of a dog with generalized demodicosis. *F*, Well-demarcated, alopecic, crusted patches of generalized demodicosis with pyoderma on the rump of a West Highland White terrier. These lesions are not easily recognized unless the hair is clipped away. *G*, Canine demodectic pododermatitis. Erythema, alopecia, hyperpigmentation of a paw. *H*, Chronic pododermatitis in a dog with demodectic pododermatitis.

Other predisposing factors suggested for demodicosis include age, short hair, poor nutrition, estrus, parturition, stress, endoparasites, and debilitating diseases. In two studies, dogs relapsing after or not responding to treatment with ivermectin or milbemycin were intact females.[183, 183b] Most of these factors are difficult to evaluate and many are highly unlikely to be predisposing factors. Length of hair coat, size and activity of sebaceous glands, sex of the animal, and biotin deficiency have no effect on the development or progression of demodicosis.[201] In fact, the great majority of clinical cases are seen in purebred dogs that are receiving excellent diets and are otherwise in generally good condition.

If most dogs harbor the *Demodex* mite as part of their normal fauna, the question must be answered why some dogs develop demodicosis and other dogs do not. Differences in the virulence of some *Demodex* strains have been considered but seem unlikely. In litters with demodicosis, some puppies have serious disease whereas others remain normal. Because these normal puppies have been exposed to the same mite population as their affected littermates, demodicosis cannot be solely associated with the strain of mite. The induction of demodicosis in dogs treated with antilymphocyte serum[148] demonstrated the probable role of immunodeficiency in this disease. The development of demodicosis in adult dogs undergoing immunosuppressive treatments[190] or having cancer or serious metabolic disorders[152, 158] supported this theory. However, broad-based immunosuppression does not explain most cases of demodicosis. If puppies with generalized demodicosis were compromised immunologically, they should develop viral disorders, pneumonias, or other systemic infections and they do not.[201, 202] Likewise, most adult dogs having cancer, especially of the lymphoreticular system, or undergoing immunosuppressive treatment for autoimmune disorders or cancer should develop demodicosis and they do not. A mite-specific immunoincompetence of varying severity helps explain these disparities. Immunologic studies that support this theory are described in the following sections.

- **Nonspecific Immunity.** Nonspecific immunity in canine demodicosis has been studied in the neutrophil and complement systems. No absolute deficiencies of neutrophils or abnormalities in neutrophil morphologic features have been observed.[201, 202] Additionally, dogs with proven neutrophil dysfunction do not develop demodicosis. Limited complement studies have not shown any association of complement deficiency with demodicosis.[205, 207]

- **Humoral Immunity.** Dogs with generalized demodicosis typically have normal to elevated numbers of plasma cells in their skin, bone marrow, lymph nodes, and spleen.[201, 202] When these dogs are vaccinated with Aleutian mink disease virus or canine distemper-infectious canine hepatitis vaccine, they can mount a normal antibody response.[148] The number of IgE-bearing mast cells in the skin of dogs with demodicosis is identical to that found in specific pathogen-free dogs.[163] Most dogs with generalized demodicosis have a hyperglobulinemia and show a reactive serum protein electrophoretic pattern.[201] Dogs with IgM or IgA deficiency do not appear to be predisposed to demodicosis.[205] All of these studies demonstrate that humoral immunodeficiency is not the cause of demodicosis and that many of these dogs have hyperreactive B cell responses. This hyperreactivity may be the result of T cell hyporeactivity.

- **Cellular Immunity.** Dogs with chronic generalized demodicosis have depressed T cell function, as measured by the in vitro lymphocyte blastogenesis (IVLB) test[148, 149, 166, 201, 202] or skin testing with phytohemagglutinin, concanavalin A, or dinitrochlorobenzene.[149, 164, 206] Because these dogs are rarely lymphopenic and have no hypocellularity of the T cell areas of the lymph nodes and spleen, the deficiency appears to be one of function rather than numbers.

The IVLB test can be performed by various methods, is subject to a variety of technical problems, and does not give identical results in dogs of the same breed and age.[133] Accordingly, studies using this test should be performed in a large number of dogs and the results must be evaluated by appropriate statistical analysis. Much of the work on the IVLB in dogs with demodicosis was not subject to such careful scrutiny, and the conclusions drawn may not be valid.

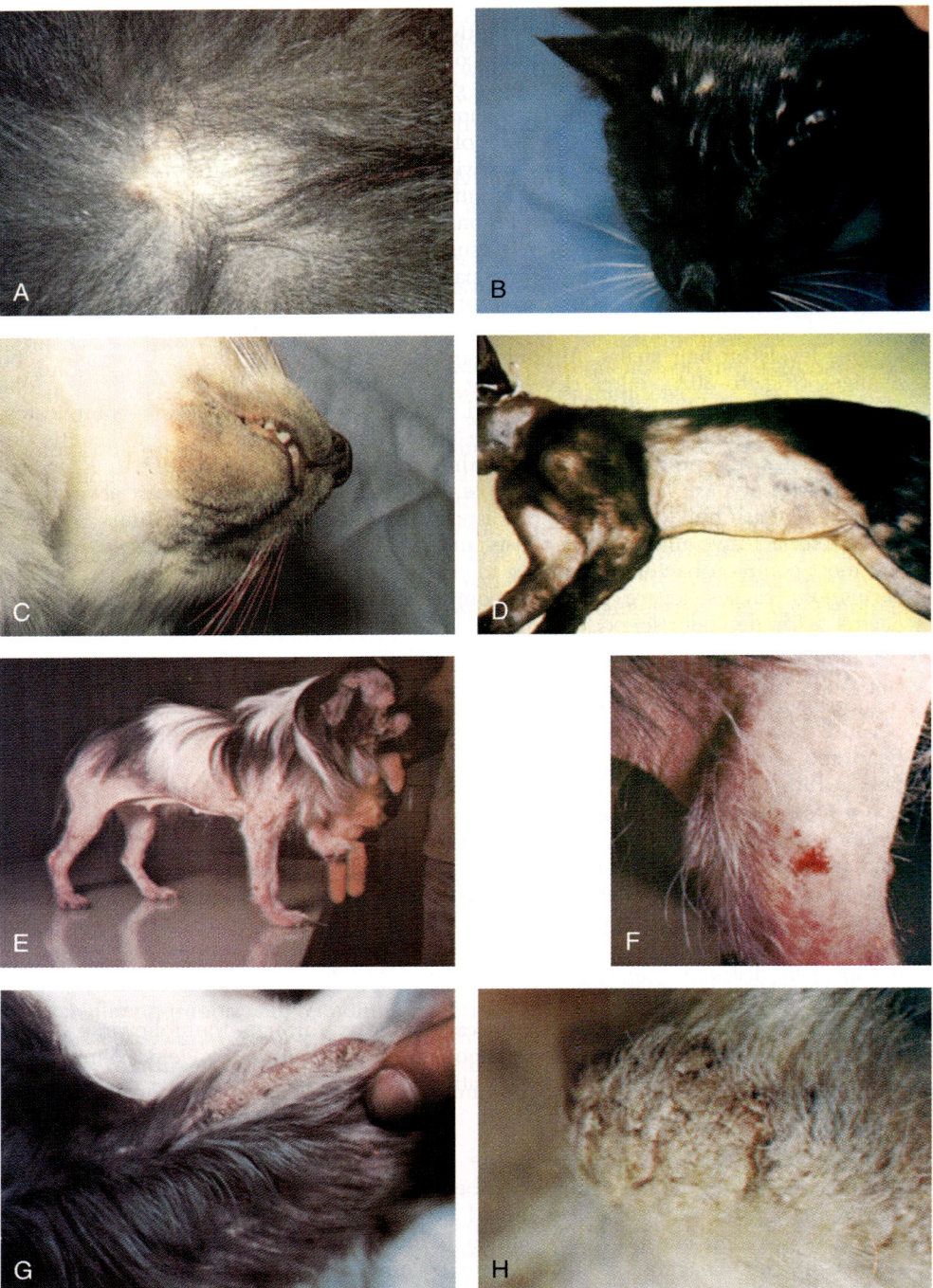

FIGURE 6–30. *A*, Diffuse scaling, follicular casts, and focal erythema and alopecia over the back of a dog with generalized demodicosis. *B*, Feline demodicosis. Alopecia and scaling of forehead and ears. *C*, Feline demodicosis. Alopecia and hyperpigmentation of chin and lip. *D*, Bilaterally symmetric alopecia in a cat with generalized demodicosis. (Courtesy B. Stein.) *E*, Canine scabies 4 weeks after onset in a Japanese spaniel. Fourteen dogs in a kennel were affected. This illustrates the typical distribution pattern. *F*, Closer view of same patient as in *E*, showing area on elbow where diagnostic skin scraping was made. The typical papular "rash" is well illustrated in this view. *G*, Ear margin showing characteristic grayish yellow crusts on affected skin. *H*, Crusted lesions on the elbow that are typical of a chronic case.

tosis (hair casts) is selected for sampling. In heavily infested dogs, a large number of mites will be trapped in the explanted follicular keratin. This testing can be negative in mildly diseased dogs and should never be used during therapeutic monitoring as a replacement for the skin scraping.

Skin scraping appears to be a straightforward, easy laboratory procedure; however, every year, the authors continue to receive cases on referral that somehow had negative findings on scraping and were misdiagnosed. Adequate skin scrapings are mandatory in all cases of canine pyoderma and seborrhea complex. When negative skin scraping findings are obtained from a Shar pei or from a dog with fibrotic lesions, especially in the interdigital region, a skin biopsy specimen should be examined before demodicosis is ruled out.

Clinical laboratory tests in young dogs with demodicosis usually show no consistent abnormalities. Anemia of chronic disease, elevations in white blood cell numbers, hyperglobulinemia, and depressed baseline thyroid hormone levels are found in many dogs. The depressed thyroid hormone values are usually the result of the demodicosis (euthyroid sick syndrome; see Chap. 10) and not its cause. In cases of adult-onset demodicosis, these routine tests become more significant in identifying the cause of the demodicosis. If baseline thyroid hormone levels are depressed, additional thyroid testing should be performed because hypothyroidism can trigger demodicosis in the adult dog.[152, 195] Unexplained elevations in liver enzyme activity should lead to the consideration of adrenal function tests (see Chap. 10) for hyperadrenocorticism, a common cause of adult-onset demodicosis.[152, 158]

Histopathology

Skin biopsy specimens from dogs with localized or generalized demodicosis show follicles containing mites and keratinous debris (Figs. 6–31 and 6–32). Dogs with demodicosis have an active local cutaneous response that increases with the severity of clinical disease.[142, 150] Three commonly recognized patterns of inflammation are interface mural folliculitis, nodular dermatitis, and suppurative folliculitis and furunculosis.[142] Interface mural folliculitis, in which plasma cells, lymphocytes, macrophages, mast cells, and eosinophils are found around the follicles and lymphocytes are found infiltrating the epithelium, is a consistent finding and the infiltrating lymphocytes are $CD3^+$ and $CD8^+$.[141] Perifollicular granulomas surrounding mite fragments can be seen in approximately 25% of cases, and 20% have a suppurative furunculosis as the main pattern. Perifollicular melanosis is

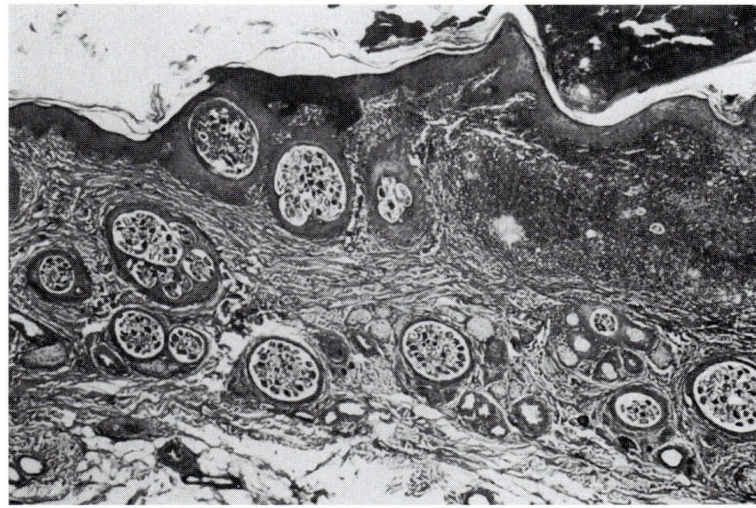

FIGURE 6–31. Demodicosis in a dog. Note hair follicles containing numerous mite segments and a pyogranuloma due to follicular rupture (upper right).

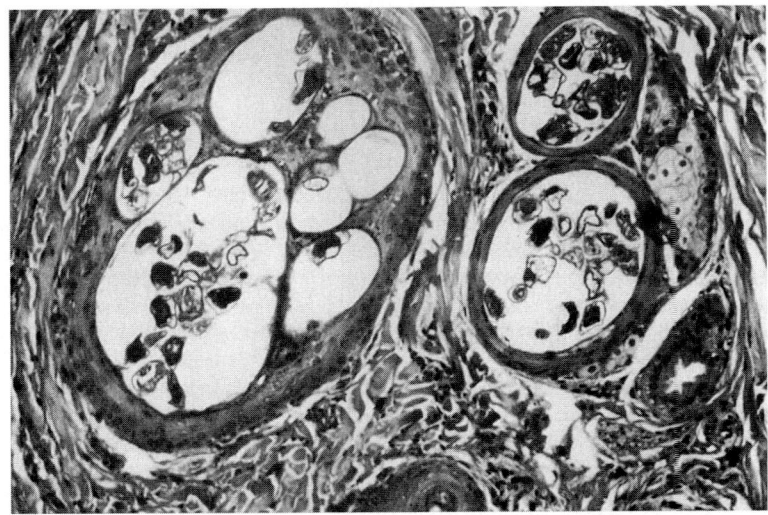

FIGURE 6–32. Demodicosis in a dog. Note numerous mite segments within hair follicles.

also a common finding in skin biopsy specimens from dogs with generalized demodicosis (Fig. 6–33).[142, 144]

To date, skin biopsy is not reliable in differentiating localized from generalized demodicosis or in indicating whether spotaneous resolution is likely. However, if mites are numerous and there is minimal to absent cellular response or eosinophils are

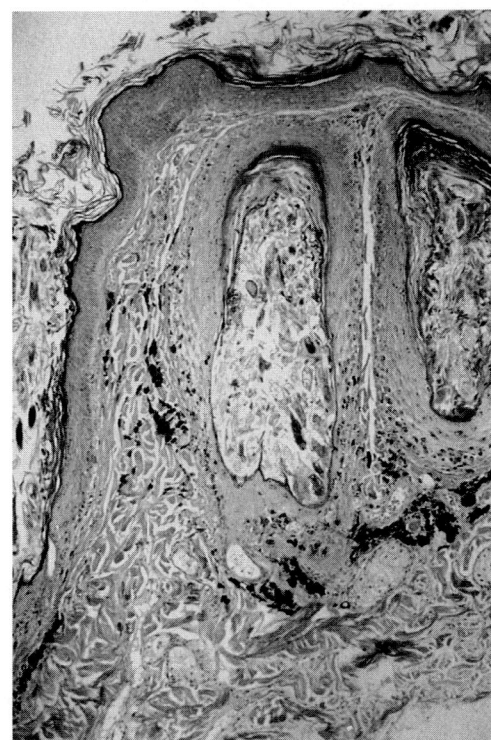

FIGURE 6–33. Demodicosis. Interface mural folliculitis and perifollicular melanosis. Mite fragments are visible in lumen of the follicle.

absent, especially when there is a furunculosis, the dog likely has severe immunosuppression.

Differential Diagnosis
Because skin scrapings easily reveal mites in the vast majority of cases of demodicosis, the disease should not be confused with other disorders. Generalized pyoderma may resemble demodicosis, and demodicosis should be suspected in every case of folliculitis. Dermatophytosis resembles patches of localized demodicosis. Superficial abrasions in young dogs sometimes resemble the erythematous patches of localized demodicosis. Conversely, demodicosis may be mistaken for abrasions. Muzzle folliculitis or furunculosis (acne) or early lesions of juvenile cellulitis on the face of young dogs sometimes resemble pustular demodicosis, and certain demodectic pustules on the abdomen and inside surface of the thighs resemble canine impetigo. Differentiation can be made by examination of exudative cytology and skin scrapings. Contact dermatitis exhibits erythematous papules that occasionally resemble squamous demodicosis. Pemphigus complex, lupus erythematosus, and dermatomyositis facial lesions can also mimic demodicosis.

Clinical Management
- **Localized Demodicosis.** This is a mild disease that usually heals spontaneously in 6 to 8 weeks but may wax and wane in a localized area for months. There is no difference in healing between treated and untreated cases. There is no evidence that treatment of localized demodicosis prevents generalization in cases so destined. If the clinician believes that some form of treatment is indicated, a mild topical parasitide used to treat ear mites or benzoyl peroxide gel (OxyDex gel, Pyoben gel) can be gently massaged into the alopecic area once a day. The medication should be rubbed in the direction of the hair growth so that as few hairs as possible are pulled out. The owner should be informed that the medications and the rubbing necessary to apply them worsen the lesions for 2 to 3 weeks. This does not affect the outcome of the disease, because the lesions only appear to be getting larger. It is important to check the general health status of the dog at this time, paying special attention to diet, endoparasite problems, and vaccination needs. Amitraz is not a rational nor approved treatment for localized demodicosis, and its use here may allow the mites to develop resistance to it.

At a return visit 4 weeks later, the veterinarian can determine whether there are any indications of generalized demodicosis. The skin scraping at the beginning of localized demodicosis often reveals numbers of live adult mites and immature forms. After 4 weeks of treatment, skin scrapings from healing cases should show fewer mites, fewer immature forms, and sometimes no live mites. If the lesions are spreading and the mite count (including the ratio of immature to adult) is high, the condition may be progressing to generalized demodicosis.

- **Generalized Demodicosis.** This can be the most serious non-neoplastic skin disease a veterinarian will treat. Although the prognosis for generalized demodicosis has improved dramatically since the mid-90s, it still is not an easily treated disease and the owner should be made aware of this from the onset. With intense treatment, most cases, probably near 90%, can be cured, but it may take nearly a year. Depending on the dog and the drug used, treatment can cost many hundreds of dollars and involve many hours of work on the owner's part. A common problem in the treatment of generalized demodicosis is premature cessation of therapy and, in many instances, occurs because the owner did not understand the entire course of treatment. These frustrations can be minimized by having an indepth discussion about the costs and requirements of treatment before any is undertaken.

Not all dogs need miticidal treatments. More than 30% to 50% of dogs younger than 1 year of age with generalized demodicosis recover spontaneously. In dogs with a familial history of demodicosis, the condition may resolve spontaneously, but the rate probably is much lower than that seen with no familial history. Intact females may experience exacerbation or relapse of disease when they come into estrus and may be more resistant to treatment.[183, 183b] Ovariohysterectomy is strongly recommended. No data are available to indicate whether treatment accelerates the dog's self-cure, and this significant rate of self-cure can confound therapeutic studies. Studies that do not specify the age of the dogs or the extent of disease cannot be evaluated critically. To euthanize 6- to 12-month-old dogs because they have severe generalized demodicosis is unwarranted, because some of them recover spontaneously if secondary pyodermas and seborrheas are controlled and the general health status is good. Dogs older than 1 to 2 years of age or dogs with adult-onset generalized demodicosis require treatment.

Before the institution of any treatment for the demodicosis, the dog's general health and management should be improved, if necessary. This is especially true for dogs with adult-onset disease. Their disease was triggered by some systemic disorder, and resolution of the underlying condition allows the demodicosis to resolve spontaneously or to respond better to treatment.

Dogs with demodicosis need to be examined and have skin scrapings performed at regular intervals, typically every 2 to 4 weeks. To determine the efficacy of treatment, the skin scrapings should always be done at the same sites and the results should be recorded in tabular fashion. A sheet of paper with the dog schematic for identification of the scraping sites and tabulation of results is most helpful.

The pyoderma and seborrhea seen in dogs with demodicosis is a result of the mite infestation and cannot be cured until the mites are eradicated. However, these problems should be addressed before topical acaricidal treatment to make the skin less irritable and to allow better penetration of the dip. Antibiotic selection varies with the case, but bactericidal agents should be selected because of the probable immunosuppressed state of the dog. Because of the high frequency of deep pyodermas in these dogs, courses of treatment of 6 to 8 weeks are commonplace. Because of the expense of this long-term treatment, the temptation is to use suboptimal dosages or a shortened course of treatment. Both measures can result in more serious infections and should be avoided.

How long does one wait for the condition to resolve spontaneously? If a dog still has clinical disease by the time it is 12 months of age, the odds of spontaneous resolution are remote. In most dogs, the need for treatment will be known much sooner. After the first 4 to 6 weeks of observation, when most dogs worsen because subclinical lesions become clinical, the dog who is destined to self-cure will show continual clinical improvement and reduction in its mite burden. If the mite count remains static or starts to increase, spontaneous resolution is unlikely.

Over the years, dozens of treatments have been used in demodicosis. Many were of no value, and some effective ones are no longer available.[201] New treatments are always being studied to increase our cure rate, which is approximately 90%.[186, 197, 200] Lufenuron failed to produce clinical improvement or decrease mite counts in dogs with generalized demodicosis, even though skin levels of the compound were about 10 times those in blood.[200]

Miticidal treatments can be given orally or applied topically. Treatments must continue until skin scrapings are negative and then for an additional 30 days or longer. Dogs always achieve clinical cure weeks before parasitologic cure. Parasitologic cure means that skin scrapings from the dog contain no live or dead mites at any stage of development. Demodex skeletons are translucent and can be overlooked if full illumination is used. The diaphragm on the condenser should be closed down to increase the contrast and visibility of the skeletons. A minimum of four to six sites should be negative at the same time to declare parasitologic cure. Site selection varies from case to case but always should include at least one from the face and front feet.

Amitraz is the only licensed product in the United States and Canada for the treatment of generalized demodicosis. The drug is diamide, N'-(2,4-dimethylphenyl)-N-[[(2,4-dimethylphenyl)imino]methyl]-N-methylmethanidamide.[19] It is marketed in the United States and Canada as Mitaban. Slightly different formulations of amitraz are marked worldwide as Ectodex Dog Wash or Taktic.[139] Amitraz is also available in a 9% antitick collar, and claims for its efficacy in the treatment of demodicosis have been made.[155] Unfortunately, this simple method of treatment is ineffective.[162]

In the United States and Canada, Mitaban is licensed for use at 250 ppm with an application frequency of 14 days. To achieve maximal results, it is imperative to follow this protocol:

1. Dogs with medium-length or long coats should be clipped closely to allow the aqueous solution to contact the skin and penetrate the hair follicle better.
2. All crusts are removed. In some cases, tranquilization or anesthesia is necessary, because some crusts adhere tightly and removal without anesthesia is painful. Remember to avoid sedating agents that are α-adrenergic agonists (e.g., benzodiazepines, xylazine), which can cause synergistic toxicity.
3. The entire dog is washed with a medicated shampoo designed to kill bacteria and remove scales and exudates. Soaking in a whirlpool bath or a gentle stream of water is beneficial. Even though the skin may appear raw and irritated after the above-mentioned procedures, the medication can have optimal contact with the affected skin. The dog is gently dried with a towel. Alternatively, the cleaning preparation can be done the day before treatment.
4. Amitraz solution is applied by wetting and sponging. The solution must be applied to the entire body—to normal as well as to affected areas of skin. Although the solution is not irritating, it is mandatory for persons applying amitraz to wear protective gloves and to work in a well-ventilated area. Amitraz causes a transitory sedative effect for 12 to 24 hours, especially after the first treatment, and some dogs become pruritic after the first few applications. Other side effects are rare and include allergic reactions (urticaria and edema), skin irritation, and a variety of systemic signs. Severe reactions or intoxications can be treated with yohimbine, atipamezole, and other appropriate supportive measures.[18, 28] The occurrence or severity of the side effects usually diminishes with subsequent applications. Rarely, dogs have increasingly severe reactions to amitraz dips: marked weakness, ataxia, and somnolence. If amitraz therapy is still desirable, dogs can be pretreated with yohimbine, which can prevent or markedly reduce the severity of these adverse effects. Exposure to amitraz can cause contact dermatitis, migraine-like headaches, or asthma-like attacks in some people. If there is demodectic pododermatitis, the paws can be immersed in a small pan containing amitraz solution and gently massaged to facilitate penetration. One should not rinse the feet or the body. The medication should remain on the skin for 2 weeks. Although about half the drug is retained in the skin for 2 weeks, some may be lost if the dog gets wet or swims. In this case, a new application may be given before the next treatment is due.
5. Although it is not necessary to repeat clipping and shampooing before each treatment, it makes sense to remove any new crusts before each treatment.

With this protocol, reported clinical cure rates vary from zero to nearly 90%.[153, 182, 203] More frequent applications at this or higher concentrations increases the recovery rate.[169, 170] When used weekly at a concentration of 500 or 1000 ppm, cure rates approaching 100% are reported.[139, 145, 161] These therapeutic modifications are an extralabel drug use, increase the labor intensity of treatment, and markedly increase the cost of treatment. The aqueous solution may not be effective in the ears or on the feet. In these cases, amitraz in mineral oil (1:9) can be effective.

Some percentage of dogs are not cured of their generalized demodicosis with the licensed amitraz protocol. When cure is not attainable, four options are available: euthanasia, control with regularly scheduled dips every 2 to 4 weeks, extralabel use of Mitaban or another EPA-registered parasiticide, or use of an avermectin or milbemycin. It is a violation of United States federal law to use an EPA-registered pesticide in a manner inconsistent with its labeling, even when treating generalized demodicosis. Accordingly, the extralabel use of an EPA-registered pesticide should be the last resort.

Some investigators retreat amitraz treatment failures with that chemical but at a higher frequency (every seventh day), either at the licensed strength (250 ppm) or at higher concentrations (500, 750, or 1000 ppm). As mentioned earlier, these therapeutic modifications can cure some initial treatment failures. The product information on Mitaban shows an increasing frequency of side effects as the topical concentration increases. Most side effects are transient and of low frequency at concentrations less than 1250 ppm. It is rare for a dog who tolerated dipping at 250 ppm every 14th day to experience clinical side effects when Mitaban is used at 500 ppm every seventh day. No published data are available on higher concentrations of Mitaban, but it can probably be used safely at 750 or 1000 ppm, as the European products are.[139] The cure rate is increased with the extralabel use of amitraz, but some dogs, perhaps as many as 20%, do not attain negative scraping results or experience relapse when treatment is stopped.[169]

In the early 90s, pilot studies on the efficacy of orally administered ivermectin or milbemycin were conducted with the hope of finding a therapeutic alternative for dogs who could not tolerate amitraz or be cured by it.[157, 178, 191] The results of those studies were so positive that it is now commonplace to treat generalized demodicosis with either product. The reader is reminded that this is an extralabel drug usage, and treatment should not be undertaken without satisfaction of the guidelines for extralabel usage. Because these drugs are simple to use and return the dog to clinical normalcy very quickly, it is imperative that the owner understand all aspects of the disease and its treatment. Because treatment is simple and straightforward, some owners do not understand why they should not use the dog for breeding. The authors will not treat any dog with any drug if it is to be used for breeding. An even more common problem is premature cessation of treatment because the dog looked normal. All dogs look normal well before skin scrapings are negative with parasitologic cure lagging behind clinical cure by 0.5 to 6 months.[135, 154, 159, 160] If the owner stops treatment too soon, a relapse will occur.

Data on the response of approximately 350 dogs treated with milbemycin are available for review.* Within the group, dogs of all breeds, including the breeds that are sensitive to high-dose ivermectin; either sex; and various ages at onset of disease and onset of treatment were treated with dosages varying from 0.5 to 2.0 mg/kg given daily. Treatment courses ranged from 60 to 300 days. Clinical cure rates varied from 15% to 92%, depending on the dosage used and the age at onset of disease. Dogs with adult-onset disease respond more poorly to treatment than dogs with juvenile-onset disease.[179] Cure rates were higher with the higher dosages. In all studies, a small percentage of dogs showed no real response to treatment. If a low dosage was being used, a dosage increase often resulted in clinical cure, but some dogs never achieved cure at 2 mg/kg. It is unknown what higher dosages might have done for those dogs.

Published data on the efficacy of ivermectin are more limited, with approximately 100 cases available for review.[154, 159, 176, 183b, 191, 196] Dosages used vary from 0.35 to 0.6 mg/kg/day and treatment courses ranged from 35 to 210 days. The rate of clinical cure varied from 83% to 100%. Preliminary data on an alternate-day protocol, in which the dog receives 0.45 to 0.6 mg/kg, suggest that daily treatment may not be necessary.[204]

As new avermectins and milbemycins become available or different formulations of the available ones are investigated, other potentially effective treatments will become available. The pour-on formulation of ivermectin is very effective in the treatment of nonfollicular mites of the dog and cat but performed very poorly when it was applied three times weekly at a dosage of 1.5 mg/kg to dogs with generalized demodicosis.[192] Only two of the 12 treated dogs achieved parasitologic cure. In other studies moxidectin, another milbemycin, was given orally to dogs at dosages between 0.2 and 0.4 mg/kg/day.[135, 135a] All dogs were cured, but details on long-term follow-up were unavailable. Transient side effects included lethargy, anorexia, ataxia, and stupor. In another study, nine dogs were given 0.3 mg/kg/day, with an 88% cure rate.[138]

In all the studies published, the rate of clinical cure exceeds the true cure rate, with relapses occurring in 10% to 45% of the cases. Although a relapse can occur at any time, most seem to occur within the first 3 months of the discontinuation of treatment. These relapses are probably due to insufficient treatment. The skin scraping, the only test

---

*See references 140, 157, 160, 167, 178, 179, 183.

available to determine parasitologic cure, is extremely crude and results can and will vary from veterinarian to veterinarian, from site to site, and with an even so slight variation of technique on the same dog. Even if the skin scrapings from a dog are without flaw, the scraping represents the parasitologic status of only 4 to 6 small areas of its skin and mites could be present a few inches away. In some cases, especially those with refractory pedal disease, skin biopsy is used to determine the end of treatment. Obviously, this type of testing is impractical in most cases.

For these and other reasons, treatment is not stopped when negative scrapings are obtained but is continued for some additional period of time, usually 2 to 4 weeks. The duration of the treatment after negative scraping should probably be based on the length of treatment, and the authors believe it always should be 4 or more weeks. Cure rates are higher when treatment is prolonged for 30 to 60 days beyond negative skin scrapings.[183b]

If a dog relapses within the first 3 months, more aggressive treatment with the same drug may cure it. If the second treatment results in relapse or if the first relapse occurred 9 or more months after treatment was stopped, further treatment with the drug is not likely to cure the dog. If the dog was initially treated with milbemycin, additional treatments with ivermectin can cure the dog and vice versa.

If all of the above-mentioned methods fail and the owner still wants to try to cure the dog, he has the option of using the farm animal formulation of amitraz (Taktic, Hoechst-Roussel).[175] A 1250-ppm aqueous solution of the amitraz is applied to one half of the animal's body on a rotating basis. If the feet are involved, they are treated daily. When this protocol was used on 71 dogs, 56 (79%) were cured, with a mean course of treatment of 3.7 months. No serious side effects were noted.

One of the authors (DWS) has consulted on cases of canine generalized demodicosis wherein daily avermectin or milbemycin therapy had been combined with weekly amitraz dips. The dogs developed severe neurotoxicity. In other cases, especially when the ivermectin is given once or twice weekly, no toxicity was noted with concurrent amitraz dips.[170] The use of concurrent intensive macrocyclic lactone and amitraz therapy should be used cautiously or be avoided.

Dogs who achieve negative skin scraping results cannot be declared cured of their disease until at least 12 months after treatment is stopped. During this waiting period, any skin lesions that develop should be scraped and the administration of immunosuppressive drugs should be avoided. Two dogs relapsed 13 and 18 months, respectively, following successful treatment.[183b]

With current treatments, not all dogs can be cured of their demodicosis. The addition of immunostimulants like levamisole, thiabendazole, *Propionibacterium acnes* (Immunoregulin, ImmunoVet), vitamin E, and muramyldipeptide-parapoxvirus combinations does nothing to increase the cure rate.[181, 203a] The failure rate will be influenced by the nature and vigor of the treatment, but probably 10% of dogs are incurable with any protocol. For these dogs, the owner must choose between euthanasia or chronic maintenance therapy. No data are available on the success and safety of long-term maintenance protocols with milbemycin or ivermectin, but the authors have had some patients under control for over 4 years with no adverse effects. In these cases, either the milbemycin or ivermectin is given every second to third day.

The concurrence of demodicosis and allergic skin disease (e.g., atopy) is an occasional therapeutic challenge for the clinician. Clearly, glucocorticoids need to be avoided, if at all possible. Symptomatic control of allergic pruritus should be attempted with antihistamines or omega-3/omega-6 fatty acids, or both. Remember, heterocyclic antidepressants are also monoamine oxidase inhibitors and may be contraindicated in conjunction with amitraz.

Generalized demodicosis is hereditary in young dogs. Until the mode of inheritance is established, preventive measures are impossible if affected dogs and their littermates are used for breeding. If the disease has a recessive mode of inheritance, some normal puppies in the litter will be truly normal, whereas other puppies will be carriers and will pass on the trait. Because no test is available to separate normal animals from carriers, all puppies from litters in which one or more pups is clinically affected should be culled from breeding programs. Dermatologists do not treat dogs for generalized demodicosis if they

Feline Demodicosis

Feline demodicosis is caused by (1) *Demodex cati*,[214, 216] (2) *Demodex gatoi*,[211, 215] and (3) an undescribed *Demodex* sp.[210a, 215]

D. cati is much like *D. canis*, with minor taxonomic differences (Fig. 6–34A). The ova are slim and oval (see Fig. 6–34B) rather than spindle shaped, and all immature life stages are narrower in *D. cati* than in *D. canis*. It is a rare disease that usually affects the eyelids, the periocular area, the head, and the neck (see Fig. 6–30B and C).[217] Lesions are variably pruritic and consist of patchy erythema, scaling, crusting, and alopecia. It is the localized type of demodicosis and is usually self-limited. Feline demodicosis may also occur as a ceruminous otitis externa.[219] Lime sulfur solution or mild parasiticides used for ear mites can be used to treat the lesions. Amitraz in mineral oil (1:9) is an effective otic miticide; it has not, however, been approved for use in cats.

Generalized feline demodicosis is rare and not usually as severe as the canine form.[213, 221, 225] Cases may be more common in purebred Siamese and Burmese cats.[225] Lesions are found primarily on the head but may be on the neck, the trunk, and the limbs. The lesions consist of circumscribed macules and patches with alopecia, scaling, erythema, hyperpigmentation, and crusting. Some cats develop generalized lesions. Pruritus is variable. In two cases, large numbers of mites were found in scrapings of the ear canal of healthy cats.[214] Generalized demodicosis due to *D. cati* is usually associated with

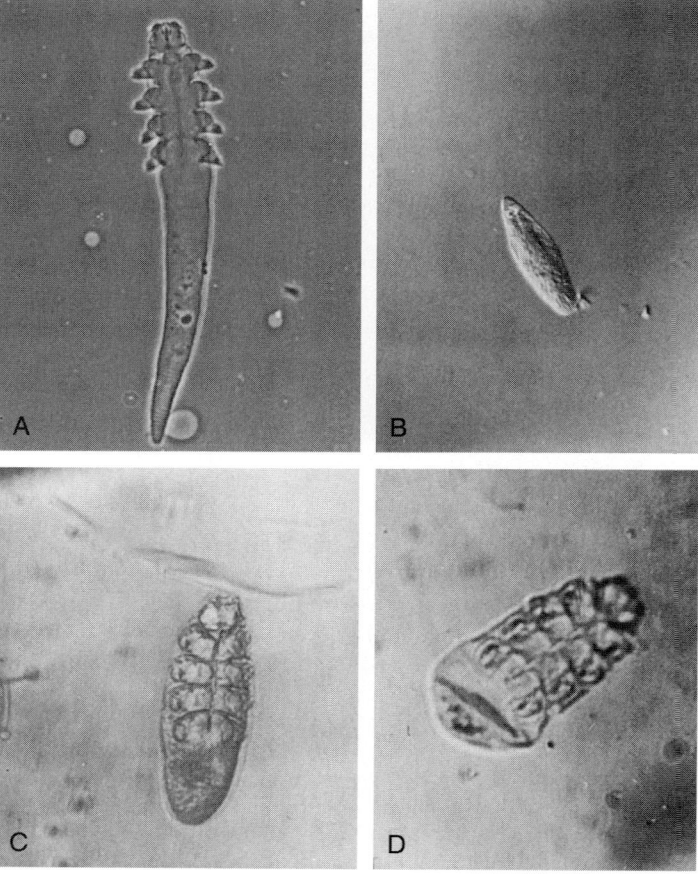

FIGURE 6–34. *A*, Adult *Demodex cati* in skin scraping. It is similar to *D. canis*, except for a somewhat slimmer abdomen. (Courtesy J. Georgi.) *B*, *D. cati* ovum in skin scraping. It is slim and oval rather than spindle shaped. (Courtesy J. Georgi.) *C* and *D*, *Demodex gatoi* in skin scraping from a cat. This mite is morphologically similar to *Demodex criceti*, which is found on hamsters. Note blunt, rounded abdomen.

underlying disease: diabetes mellitus,[213] feline leukemia virus infection, systemic lupus erythematosus, hyperadrenocorticism, feline immunodeficiency virus infection, or squamous cell carcinoma in situ.[188, 210, 213, 218, 223, 226] In some cases, no underlying cause can be found. One case had raised exudative lesions on the lips and chin.[208] Mites and a *Staphylococcus* organism were obtained, and the cat had a marked lymphopenia associated with long-term therapy for a respiratory tract infection. Clinicians should be aware of its possible association with serious systemic disease. Histologic examination reveals varying degrees of perifolliculitis and folliculitis, with mites in hair follicles (Fig. 6–35).

Some cats respond in a short time spontaneously with mild remedies such as topical lime sulfur dips, carbaryl shampoos, malathion dips, and rotenone.[213, 221] The apparent ease with which generalized demodicosis can be treated in some cats may be explained by the often superficial location of mites in the skin of cats as compared with that in the skin of dogs. Treatment with amitraz dips at 125 ppm or 250 ppm on a weekly basis also can be beneficial.[96a, 212]

The second species of mite causing feline demodicosis is *Demodex gatoi*, and it bears a close taxonomic resemblance to *Demodex criceti*, which is found in the epidermal pits in the stratum corneum of hamsters.[215, 220, 224] The mites affecting cats are shorter and have broad, blunted abdomens (see Fig. 6–34C and D), unlike the slim, elongated abdomens of *D. cati*.[211, 220] They are superficially located and inhabit only the stratum corneum. In nonpruritic cats, skin scrapings reveal numerous mites and ova, the latter being indicative of rapid reproduction.[215] Because of their small size and translucency, the mite can be overlooked if the slide is scanned rapidly with the four-power objective at full light intensity. The 10-power objective should be used, and the iris diaphragm should be closed down to increase the contrast. In pruritic cats, especially those that lick their skin, no mites may be seen.[209] In these cases, a contact cat at home should be examined because the mite is contagious[221, 222] or a therapeutic trial should be started.

The clinical signs of disease due to *D. gatoi* may be suggestive of feline scabies or allergic skin disease, with severe pruritus; alopecic, scaly, excoriated, and crusted lesions are seen, often concentrated on the head, the neck, and the elbows. Other cases have multifocal erythema and hyperpigmentation, with broken, stubby hairs located on the proximal rear legs, the flanks, and the ventral abdomen. Some are cases of symmetric alopecia with or without scaling (see Fig. 6–30D), which mimics feline symmetric alopecia, psychogenic alopecia, or hypersensitivity reactions.

Histologically, minimal inflammation is observed. The epidermis may be irregularly acanthotic and hyperkeratotic, with mites in the stratum corneum (Fig. 6–36). No mites are found in the hair follicles.

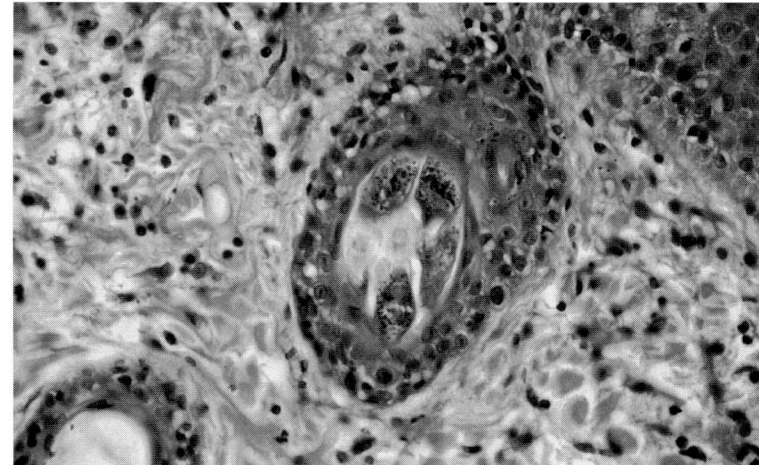

FIGURE 6–35. Feline demodicosis. Interface mural folliculitis and *Demodex cati* mites in the hair follicle.

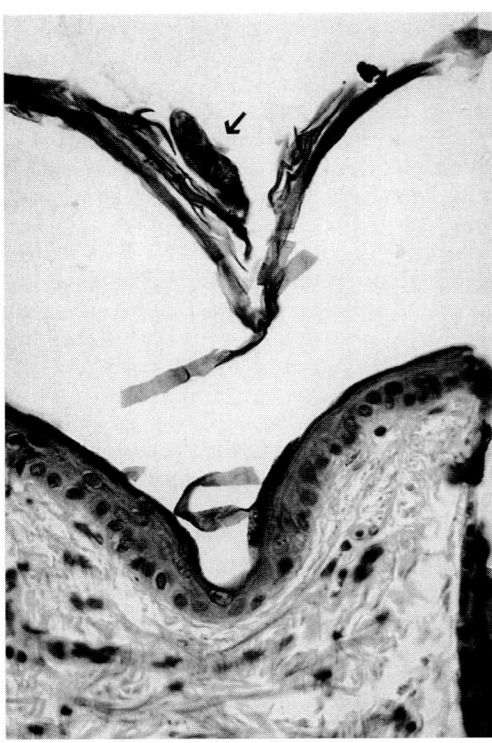

FIGURE 6-36. Feline demodicosis. *Demodex gatoi (arrow)* in the surface keratin layer.

Differential diagnosis of the second type of feline demodicosis must include all feline dermatoses that are associated with excessive grooming such as psychogenic alopecia, atopy, food hypersensitivity, feline scabies, contact dermatitis, flea bite hypersensitivity, and the demodicosis caused by *D. cati.* Careful skin scrapings are paramount in the work-up for each of these conditions to make a proper diagnosis. Because the mite can be difficult to find in cats that groom excessively, a short therapeutic trial with lime sulfur is indicated before complicated testing like dietary restriction is undertaken. If the cat has demodicosis, a positive response should be seen after three treatments.

Because *D. gatoi* is contagious, all cats in the household should be treated simultaneously. Although ivermectin has been suggested as an effective treatment,[216] most investigations use lime sulfur dips weekly for 4 to 6 weeks.[209, 222, 223] Amitraz dips, 125 to 250 ppm, are also effective.[96a]

The third, presently undescribed, *Demodex* mite from the cat superficially resembles *D. gatoi,* but is larger and possesses other anatomical differences.[210a, 215]

Canine Scabies

Canine scabies (sarcoptic mange) is a nonseasonal, intensely pruritic, transmissible infestation of the skin of dogs caused by the mite *Sarcoptes scabiei var. canis* (Fig. 6-37). The mite is transferable to other species.[228, 241] Recent molecular analyses support the conspecificity of *Sarcoptes* mites, and indicate that this genus consists of a single heterogeneous species.[250a]

Cause and Pathogenesis

The causative mite belongs to the family Sarcoptidae, as does *Notoedres cati,* the cause of feline scabies. Because these mites have much in common, their 17- to 21-day life cycles are presented together. Copulation of adults occurs in a molting pocket on the surface of the skin. The fertilized female mite excavates a burrow through the horny layer of the

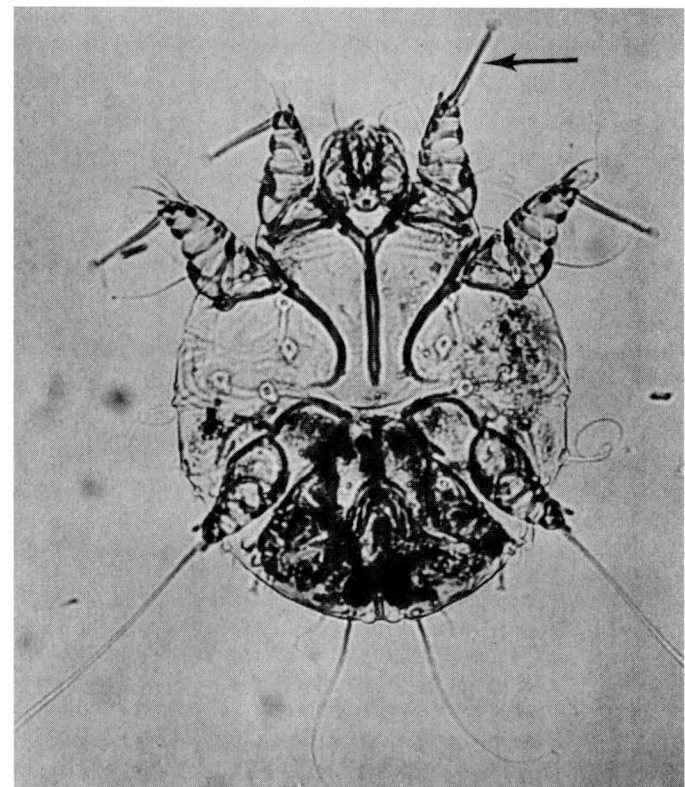

FIGURE 6–37. Adult *Sarcoptes scabiei* var. *canis*. Note the long unjointed stalks and suckers.

skin at a rate of 2 to 3 mm/d and lays eggs in the tunnel behind her. The eggs hatch as larvae and burrow to the surface of the skin, where they travel about feeding and eventually resting in a molting pocket. Nymphs also wander about the skin, but they may stay in the molting pocket until they are mature. Mites prefer skin with little hair, so they are most common on the ears, the elbows, the abdomen, and the hocks. As the disease spreads and hair is lost, they may eventually colonize large areas of the host's body. The entire life cycle may be complete in only 3 weeks.

Adult mites are small (200 to 400 μm), oval, and white with two pairs of short legs anteriorly that bear long unjoined stalks with suckers (see Figs. 6–37). The stalks are of medium length in *N. cati* (see Fig. 6–44). Two pairs of posterior legs are rudimentary and do not extend beyond the border of the body. The posterior legs carry long bristles, not suckers, although the fourth pair of legs of the male mite have suckers. The anus of *S. scabiei* var. *canis* is terminal, whereas that of *N. cati* has a dorsal location—an important point of differentiation.

Scabies mites have hosts of preference but can cause disease in other species. *S. scabiei* var. *canis* is known to cause disease in cats, foxes, and humans.[6, 237, 244] Likewise, dogs can be infected by mites from foxes and possibly even humans.[233] Reactions in humans occur within 24 hours after brief direct exposure and are characterized by pruritic papules on the trunk and arms (Fig. 6–38D). Pruritus is severe, especially when the skin is warm—as it is in bed at night or after a warm shower. Mites burrow but usually remain on the aberrant host for only a few days. The lesions regress spontaneously in 12 to 14 days, if only a few mites were transmitted and contact with affected dogs is terminated. However, with many mites and prolonged repeated contact, the human lesions persist for long periods. Canine *Sarcoptes* mites can live on human beings for at

478 • Parasitic Skin Diseases

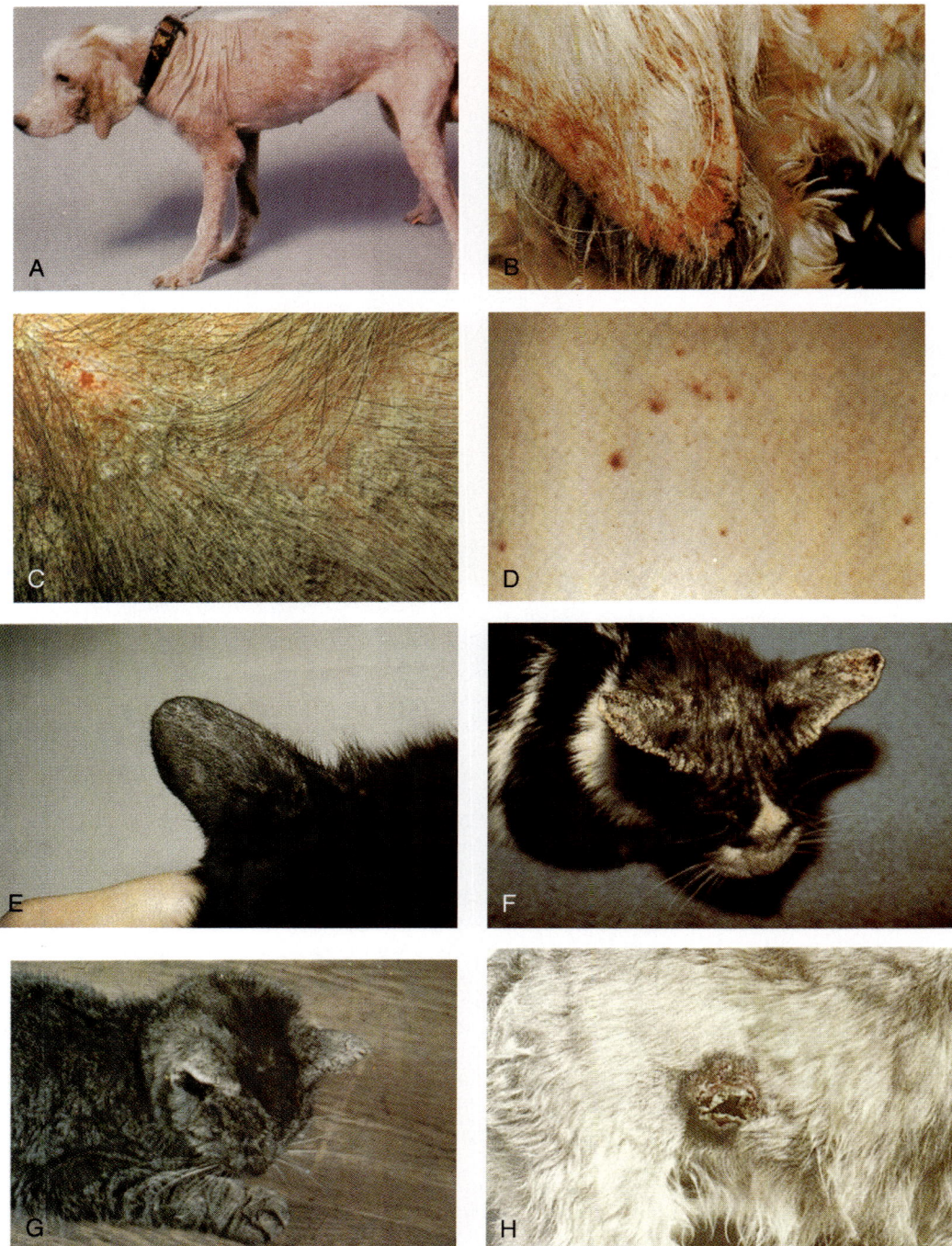

FIGURE 6–38. *A*, Generalized erythema and alopecia of dog with extensive scabies. *B*, Margin of the ear (pinna) is a characteristic site. *C*, Grayish crusts on the body mimic seborrheic dermatitis. Hemorrhagic area is from skin scraping (positive). *D*, Crusted papules on human skin (forearm), the typical lesion of canine scabies in humans. *E*, Pinnal alopecia, scale, and crust in an early case of feline scabies. *F*, Chronic feline scabies. Note marked crusting and excoriation on pinnae and head. *G*, Dry, crusted lesions on the edges of the ears and face are typical of feline scabies. *H*, Spider bite. Focal area of necrosis and slough in the flank of a dog.

least 6 days and produce ova during that time.[240] There is one report, however, of a child with Norwegian scabies caused by *S. scabiei* var. *canis*.[245] Similar mites were found on three dogs in the household and on all other members of the family.

The off-host survival time of scabies mites depends on the relative humidity and temperature. Female mites and nymphs generally survive longer than do male mites or larvae, and low temperature and high humidity prolong survival.[227] At 10° to 15°C (50 to 59°F), female mites and nymphs could survive for 4 to 21 days, depending on the humidity.[249] At room temperature (20° to 25°C, 68° to 77°F), all stages can survive for 2 to 6 days. These mites can be point sources of infection for other animals.[35, 127]

Clinical Features

The distribution pattern of canine scabies typically involves the ventral portions of the abdomen, the chest, and the legs.[236, 241] The ears and the elbows, favorite habitats of mites, are almost always affected and are premiere places for obtaining diagnostic scrapings (see Fig. 6–30E to H). However, some animals have no ear lesions. The disease spreads rapidly and can involve the entire body (see Fig. 6–38A), but the dorsum is usually spared. Alopecia is present, and early skin lesions are characteristic. These are pruritic, reddish papulocrustous eruptions (see Fig. 6–30F). Typically, they have thick yellowish crusts, and the intense and constant itching soon produces extensive excoriation (see Fig. 6–38B and C). These patients are miserable because they are constantly scratching themselves. Itching is thought to be more severe in warm environments (e.g., indoors or by the stove). In long-term cases, hyperpigmentation of the affected skin is common. Most patients also have a generalized lymphadenopathy.

The incubation period for scabies is unknown. When fox mites were transferred to dogs, there was a lag period of 6 to 11 days before signs developed, and those were mild.[233] In the natural situation, infested dogs should start to itch a few days after infection. The pruritus is at a low level and is proportional to the number of mites. As the number of mites increases, the pruritus becomes more severe, but there is some point at which the pruritus explodes in severity. Typically, the intense pruritus develops 21 to 30 days after exposure. In experimental studies, infected dogs seroconverted 2 to 5 weeks after infection and 1 to 3 weeks after clinical signs developed.[234] If these data are coupled with the more rapid seroconversion and self-cure of dogs at reinfection, it is clear that the intense pruritus of scabies is due to hypersensitivity to the mite.[230, 234, 235, 250]

Some dogs never have the classic lesions of scabies. They scratch incessantly and have few, if any, real lesions other than mild erythema and occasional excoriations. They are often treated for an allergy with systemic corticosteroids but without benefit. These dogs have had scabies ever since they came in contact with an infected dog or environment, but mites are not found in skin scrapings. Thorough grooming may have removed superficial mites and crusts, so only a few mites remain—enough to cause pruritus but too few to find. These dogs respond rapidly and dramatically to proper antiscabies therapy.

In cats, *S. scabiei* infestation is rare and variable in clinical presentation (Fig. 6–39).[219, 244] There are pruritic pinnal and facial papules; severe pododermatitis with or without claw abnormalities; generalized crusts, scale, and pruritus; and self-induced hair loss with no skin lesions. Temporary transmission from cats to humans has been reported. Affected cats are often immunosuppressed before infestation.

Diagnosis

Scabies mites can be difficult to demonstrate, especially when the patient is intensely pruritic, has had the disease for a long time, or has received multiple baths or dips. Scabies should be considered in any dog with nonseasonal, intense pruritus, especially when the pruritus does not stop with the administration of 1.1 mg/kg of prednisone. However, nearly 30% of dogs may respond to steroid treatments.[236] When scabies is a differential diagnostic possibility, it can be excluded only by the animal's failure to respond to adequate treatment.

A helpful, although nonspecific, test for scabies is the pinnal-pedal reflex. The edge of the dog's pinna is rubbed or scratched and the test is positive if the dog's hindleg attempts to scratch the ear region. Between 75% and 90% of dogs with scabies and ear

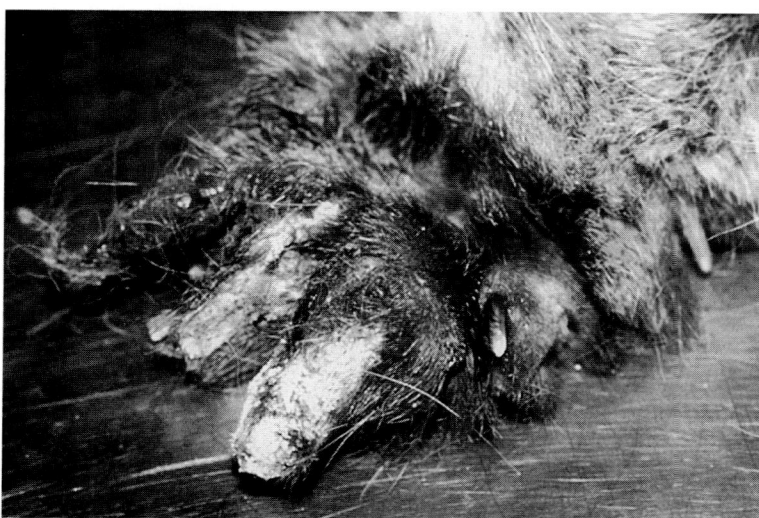

FIGURE 6–39. Scabies. Digital crusting, onychogryphosis, and onychorrhexis in a cat with *Sarcoptes scabiei* var. *canis* infection. (Courtesy H. P. Huang.)

lesions have a positive pinnal-pedal reflex.[243] The test may be negative if no ear lesions are present. Because hypersensitivity to the mite appears to be important in the pruritus of scabies and mites of various species may share some cuticular or fecal antigens, reports on the diagnostic accuracy of skin testing with house dust mite antigen have arisen. In one study of 20 dogs with scabies, 15 showed positive intradermal and serologic reactivity to house dust mites that was lost when the scabies was treated.[250] The authors have only been able to show dust mite reactivity in approximately 30% of their cases.[243] Testing with a *Sarcoptes suis* extract resulted in approximately 30% reactivity in infected dogs in one study.[231] The serodiagnostic rate in these dogs also was approximately 30%.

The absolute confirmation of the diagnosis necessitates that some stage of the mite or its feces be seen via skin scrapings. Multiple scrapings are necessary. For scraping, one should choose skin sites that have not been excoriated. In these areas, one should look for red, raised papules with yellowish crusts on top (see Fig. 6–38C). The ear margins, the elbows, or the hocks are primary scraping sites because the mites seem to prefer these areas. Large amounts of material are collected and spread on slides with mineral oil, and every field should be examined carefully. One mite, one egg (Fig. 6–40), or dark brown oval fecal pellets (Fig. 6–41) are diagnostic. Depending on the number of scrapings taken, mites may be seen in only 20% of cases.[243] A few patients have mites in the feces. An enzyme-linked immunosorbent assay (ELISA) test exists for the diagnosis of scabies and is reported to be 92% sensitive and 96% specific,[235] although some studies report a much lower rate.[231] Seroconversion can take up to 5 weeks after inoculation, so testing should not be performed too early.

Histologic examination may be useful but is rarely conclusive, unless actual mites are seen in the biopsy specimen. One should always select an active papule, undisturbed by excoriation, as the biopsy specimen. Mites may rarely be found in the superficial epidermis and the stratum corneum (Fig. 6–42). Early on, histopathologic changes are minimal. In developed cases, approximately 50% of biopsies have marked spongiosis and a perivascular-to-interstitial, heavily eosinophilic dermatitis.[247] A very suggestive histopathologic clue is the presence of focal areas of epidermal edema, exocytosis, degeneration, and necrosis (epidermal "nibbles") (Fig. 6–43). Eosinophils vary in number, from few to many, probably relative to recent glucocorticoid therapy. Focal parakeratotic hyperkeratosis is often pronounced.

Differential diagnosis should include contact dermatitis, atopy, food hypersensitivity, *Malassezia* dermatitis, *Pelodera* dermatitis, cheyletiellosis, otodectic dermatitis, and dirofilariasis. Any one of these dermatoses at a particular stage might resemble scabies. Failure

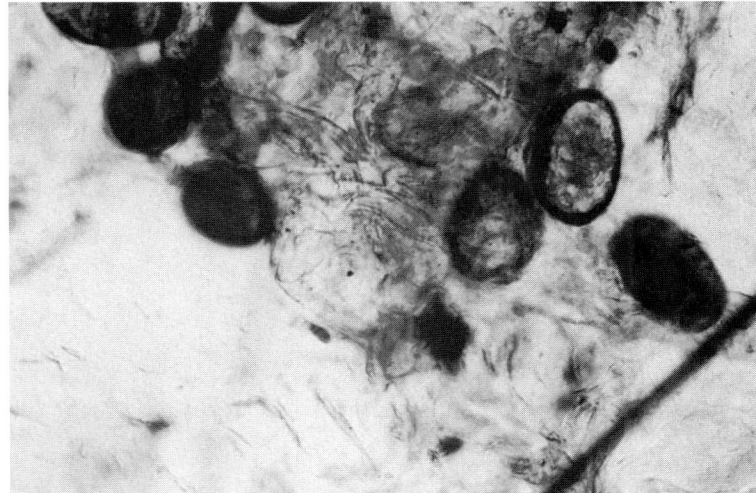

FIGURE 6–40. Multiple *S. scabiei* ova in skin scraping.

to find mites should not eliminate the diagnosis of scabies, and doing so is a common mistake. Many such cases are erroneously treated as an allergy. Careful history, physical examination, or appropriate cultures, biopsy, and examination of scrapings, and especially response to acaricidal medicaments, usually satisfactorily resolve the diagnostic problem.

Treatment

Although dogs develop an immunity to the scabies mite, which can lead to spontaneous resolution, the condition does not resolve spontaneously in all dogs, so eradication of the mites is indicated.[229] Treatment should be started as soon as the diagnosis is made or suspected. This disease is highly contagious in a kennel or a hospital. The only licensed method of treatment for canine scabies is the repeated application of a topical parasiticide. If the dog has a dense coat, the hair should be clipped. All patients should be bathed with an antiseborrheic shampoo to remove crusts and other debris, and then an acaricidal dip should be applied thoroughly and allowed to soak every inch of the skin surface. Spot treatment is ineffective. Particular care should be taken around the ears and the eyes; the

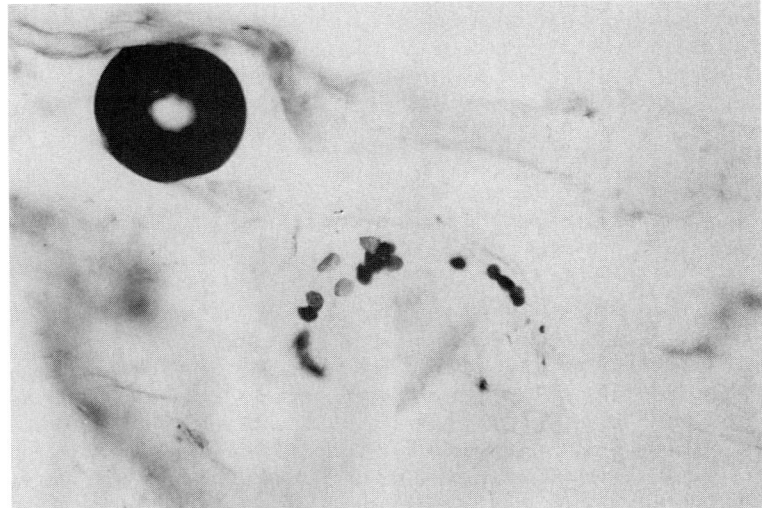

FIGURE 6–41. *S. scabiei* fecal pellets (scybala) in linear arrangement in skin scraping.

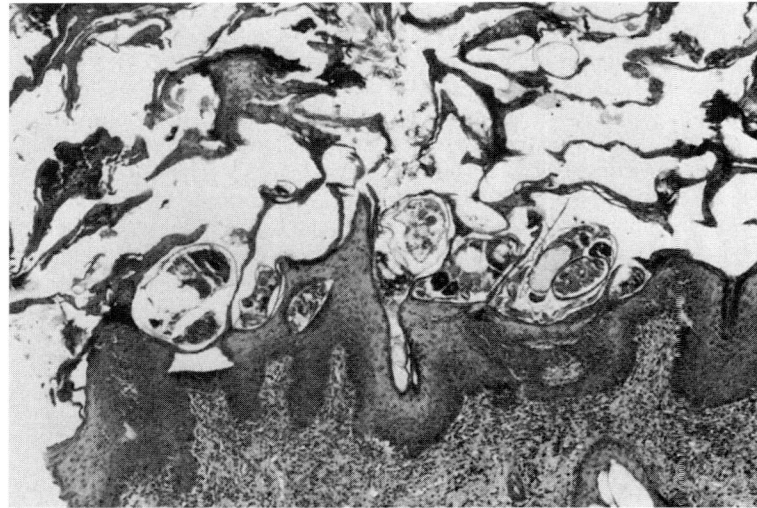

FIGURE 6–42. Canine scabies. Note mite segments within stratum corneum.

skin in those regions is often severely infected yet delicate and easily irritated by parasiticidal dips. Administration of systemic corticosteroids in full antiallergic dosages (1.1 mg/kg of prednisone or prednisolone daily) for 2 to 3 days is useful to provide relief from scratching and to stop self-mutilation until the mites are eliminated.

Many of the proven scabicides are no longer available for veterinary use, and mite resistance to some pesticides, especially the organophosphates, has been suggested. These problems limit the number of dips available, and no topical treatment can be considered 100% effective. Weekly administration of lime sulfur, organophosphate, or permethrin dips can be effective. Amitraz is reported to be an effective agent when used at 250 ppm once to three times at 2-week intervals.[242] Other reportedly effective topicals include fipronil spray and herbal treatments.[238, 239] Regardless of which treatment is selected, it should be used until the pruritus is vastly reduced or eliminated. Typically a 4- to 6-week course of treatment is satisfactory.

Topical treatments are very labor intense, especially when the dog has a dense coat. The owner's physical abilities or the dog's lifestyle, for example, swims daily, sometimes

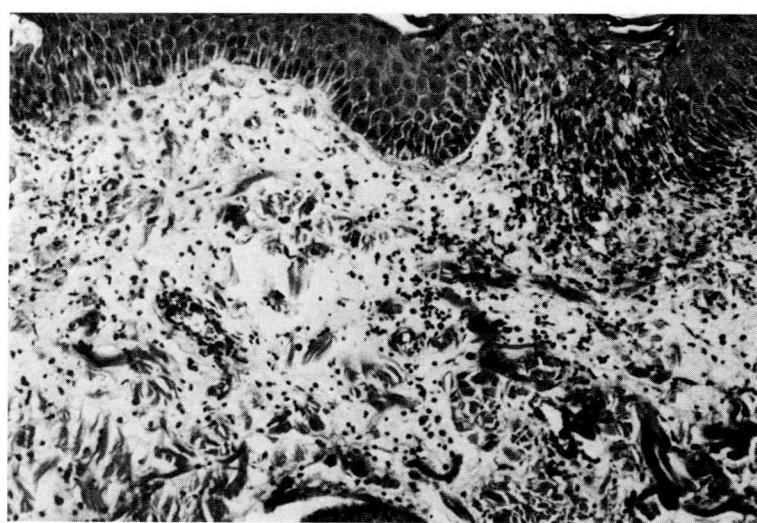

FIGURE 6–43. Canine scabies. Hyperplastic perivascular dermatitis with focal epidermal necrosis and exocytosis ("nibbles").

eliminates this route of treatment. High-dose ivermectin or milbemycin can be effective in these cases.[6, 35] Because of the expense of milbemycin, ivermectin receives widest use but cannot be used in ivermectin-sensitive breeds.[5] Ivermectin is given at dosages of 0.2 to 0.4 mg/kg subcutaneous twice at 14-day intervals or orally three times at 7-day intervals. The pour-on formulation applied twice at 14-day intervals at a dosage of 0.5 mg/kg is also effective.[248] One 0.2 mg/kg dose of doramectin given subcutaneously or intramuscularly reportedly is 100% effective.[244a]

Milbemycin oxime has been used as an alternate oral treatment for dogs sensitive to high-dose ivermectin. At dosages below 3 mg/kg, adverse reactions in any breed of dog are very rare.[116] In the initial clinical study, dogs were given 2 mg/kg either twice at 14-day intervals or three times at 7-day intervals, and all dogs were cured.[246] Another group of 56 dogs were treated with the three-dose protocol, and a 29% failure rate was reported.[232] Additional treatments were needed to cure the failures. If milbemycin is used, the owner should be asked to report after the third dosage. If the dog is still pruritic, additional treatments should be dispensed and these will result in cure.[263]

Recent studies indicated that two applications of selamectin at a 30-day interval cured 93% to 100% of the cases of canine scabies,[43a] and that fipronil spray was also curative.[238]

Most cases of scabies in a single-pet household can be resolved by treatment of the animal alone. In multiple-dog households, all contact dogs should be treated, even if they exhibit no signs, because asymptomatic carriers have been identified. Because the parasite can live in the environment for up to 21 days, cleaning and applying an environmental pesticide may be indicated.[35] This is most important when numerous mites are found on scraping, especially when multiple dogs are involved.

Humans who do not have lesions at the onset of treatment of the dog should not develop any. If lesions were present, they may persist for 7 to 14 days, but new lesions should not develop. Development of new lesions indicates inadequate treatment of the dogs, environmental infestation, or true human scabies, which could have been transferred to the dogs. The owners should be referred to a human dermatologist.

Feline Scabies

Feline scabies (notoedric mange) is a contagious parasitic disease of cats caused by *N. cati*.

Cause and Pathogenesis

N. cati (Fig. 6–44) primarily attacks cats but may also infect foxes, dogs, and rabbits.[2, 252] It causes transient lesions in humans. The mites are obligate parasites that probably survive off the host for only a few days. The disease is highly contagious by direct contact, and characteristically affects whole litters and both sexes of adult cats. Affected animals

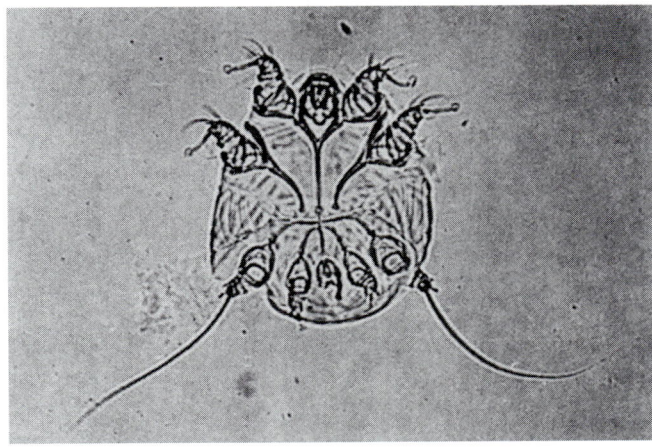

FIGURE 6–44. Adult *Notoedres cati*. Note the medium-length stalks, the striated integument, and the lack of a terminally located anus. The mite is smaller than *S. scabiei* var. *canis*.

have large numbers of mites, which are easily found on skin scrapings.[252] Notoedric mange appears in epizootics; it is rarely diagnosed in some parts of the country but is endemic and common in others.

The mite belongs to the family Sarcoptidae, and because its basic life cycle and structure are similar to those of canine scabies, the two are discussed together in the section entitled Cause and Pathogenesis of Canine Scabies. The main features of taxonomic differentiation for the clinician are that *N. cati* mites are smaller than *Sarcoptes canis* and have medium-length unjointed sucker-bearing stalks on their legs. They also have more body striations and, most important, have a dorsal anus as compared with the terminal anus of *Sarcoptes*.[1] The abundant mites are much easier to find on skin scrapings than they are in cases of *S. canis*.

Clinical Features

The distribution is typical. Lesions first appear at the medial proximal edge of the pinna of the ear (see Fig. 6–38*E*). They spread rapidly to the upper ear, the face, the eyelids, and the neck (see Fig. 6–38*F* and *G*). They also extend to the feet and the perineum. This probably results from the cat's habits of washing and of sleeping in a curled position.

Female mites burrow into the horny layer of the epidermis between hair follicles. These burrows appear on the skin surface in the center of minute papules. The skin soon becomes thickened, wrinkled, and folded and later is covered with dense, tightly adhering, yellow to gray crusts (see Fig. 6–38*G*). There is partial alopecia in affected areas. Intense pruritus develops, and the excoriations produced by scratching may become secondarily infected. As the disease progresses, the hair loss and skin lesions spread until large areas of the body are involved. Peripheral lymphadenopathy is usually present.

Diagnosis

The distribution of lesions and the intensity of the pruritus are highly suggestive. Identification of the mites is diagnostic. Scrapings should be examined with the 10-power objective with reduced light because the mites are small and become less visible with intense light. The differential diagnosis should rule out *Otodectes* infection, cheyletiellosis, atopy, food hypersensitivity, pemphigus foliaceus or erythematosus, and systemic lupus erythematosus.

Histopathologic study reveals varying degrees of superficial perivascular or superficial interstitial dermatitis (hyperplastic or spongiotic). Mite segments may be found within the superficial epidermis (Fig. 6–45). Eosinophils vary in number from few to many, probably reflecting recent glucocorticoid administration. Focal parakeratotic hyperkeratosis is usually pronounced.

Treatment

Many parasiticidal agents are contraindicated because of extreme toxic effects in cats. Sulfur in various forms is usually safe. With the cat under sedation, the hair is clipped, if necessary, and the cat is bathed in warm water and soap to loosen scales and debris. A 2% to 3% warm water solution of lime sulfur should be applied and allowed to dry on the skin. The dip is repeated every seventh day until the condition is resolved. Six to eight treatments may be necessary. All cats on the premises must be treated, because cats in preclinical stages of the disease might be carriers. The response to treatment is usually rapid and complete if all cats are thoroughly treated and re-exposure is prevented. Amitraz as used in demodicosis can be effective. Ivermectin given subcutaneously twice or thrice, or one subcutaneous dose of doramectin at 0.2 to 0.3 mg/kg is effective.[6, 250b, 251]

SPIDERS

Spiders are arachnids that inhabit woodpiles, old buildings, and refuse areas. The four species of spiders that are medically important in the United States are the black widow (*Latrodectus mactans*), the red-legged widow (*Latrodectus bishopi*), the brown recluse (*Loxosceles reclusa*), and the common brown spider (*Loxosceles unicolor*).[254, 258]

Spider bites occur most commonly on the forelegs and the face. Bites of spiders of

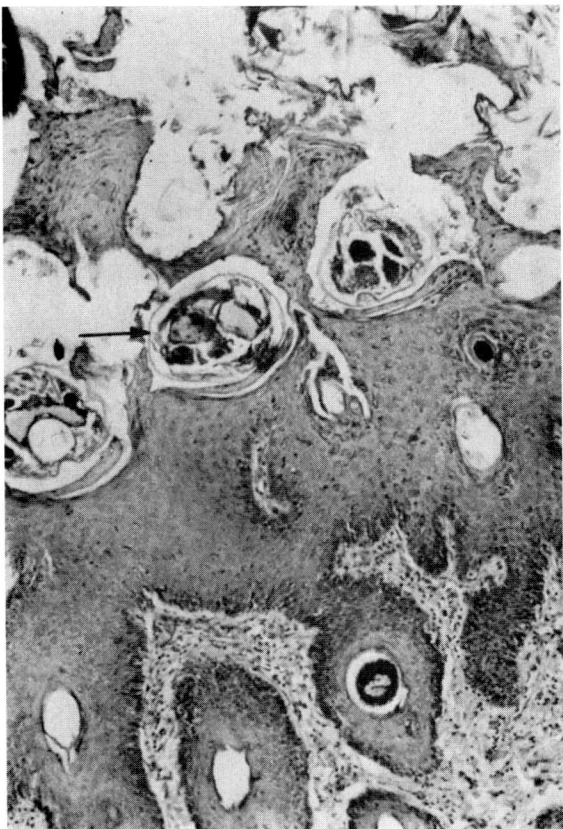

FIGURE 6–45. Histopathologic section of cat skin with three *N. cati* mites in the stratum corneum. The arrow points to the central mite. Note extensive acanthosis, hyperkeratosis, parakeratosis, prominent rete ridges, and infiltration of inflammatory cells in the superficial dermis. (Courtesy B. Bagnall.)

the genus *Latrodectus* (the widows) initially consist of two small puncture marks with local erythema. The local reaction may develop into granulomatous nodules within a few days. Bites of spiders of the genus *Loxosceles* (the brown spiders) initially appear as puncture marks surrounded by local erythema.[253] Within a few hours, they become vesicular and painful. The next day, the lesions turn black and become necrotic, and a large indolent ulcer develops (see Fig. 6–38*H*). Skin biopsy reveals a nodular to diffuse necrotizing dermatitis and panniculitis (Fig. 6–46).

Systemic reactions to spider bites may be severe. They may be manifested by salivation, nausea and diarrhea, ataxia and convulsions, or paralysis, any of which occur within 6 to 48 hours. Generalized urticaria can result from the ingestion or bites of less venomous spiders.

Although spider bites are rarely recognized and reported, they are probably underdiagnosed in veterinary medicine.[255] Diagnosis should be based on history and the physical examination findings. An extremely painful local swelling should increase the suspicion of spider bite.[256] Recommended early bite wound therapy includes local infusion with 2% lidocaine and triamcinolone acetonide.[257] Systemic support with the administration of analgesics, calcium gluconate, and epinephrine and glucocorticosteroids may be needed. In the case of bites of *Latrodectus* spp., the local infusion of 1 ml of antivenin is recommended.[257] Chronic ulcers may take months to heal and may be best treated by surgical excision.

The numbers of spiders can be controlled by cleaning up woodpiles and outdoor sites; by eliminating scattered debris; and by spraying insecticides under appliances, in cupboards, in cracks in basement and attic floors, and outdoors under eaves and in window wells and woodpiles.

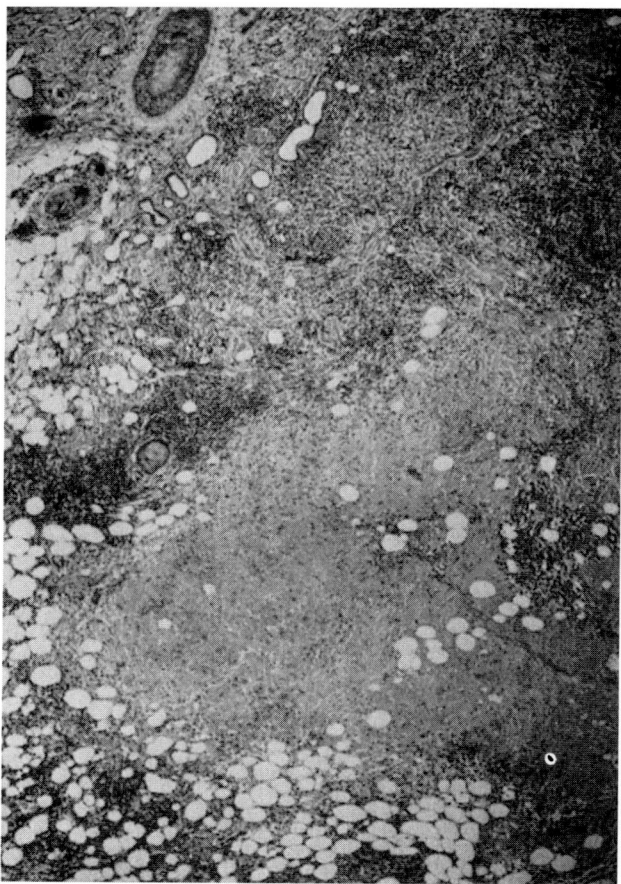

FIGURE 6–46. Spider bite, histologic view. Nodular area of necrotizing dermatitis and panniculitis.

Insects

The numerous species of insects play important roles in the health of animals as vectors of disease and as irritants to the skin.[2, 10] Insect's heads bear appendages and sensory organs, such as antennae and simple or compound eyes. The structure of the masticatory mouthparts varies, depending on the feeding habits. The thorax typically carries two pairs of wings and three pairs of legs. The abdomen is segmented and terminates in the male hypopygium or the female ovipositor. The body is encased in hard chitinous plates connected by flexible membranes.

The life cycles of insects are of three types: direct development, incomplete metamorphosis, and complete metamorphosis. In the first type, the newly hatched insect is a small replica of the adult. Incomplete metamorphosis occurs in primitive insects, and the larvae differ from adults in size, proportion, and lack of wings. Complete metamorphosis is found in more specialized species. The wormlike larva differ from the adult in regard to feeding habits. After several molts, the larva pupates and emerges as an adult. The larva and the pupa possess characteristic hairs, bristles, and appendages, which are of taxonomic importance. The duration of adult pupal and larval stages varies with the species and the environment.

Insects have medical importance because of the damage they can do to the skin and because their stings, bites, or body parts can be allergens. Insect hypersensitivity, aside from flea bite hypersensitivity, has received much attention and helps explain the severe skin reactions to seemingly trivial bites.[3] Equally as important, insects seem to be a source of inhaled allergen for some dogs or cats with atopy-like conditions. These animals have the classic signs of atopy but either show no intradermal or serologic reactions to common inhaled allergens or do not respond to immunotherapy. Ants, moths, houseflies, butterflies, and cockroaches are probably important as strictly inhaled allergens. Mosquitos, biting flies, and honeybees can cause disease through both their bites and the inhalation of their body parts. Hypersensitivity to these insects can be documented by intradermal tests.[3, 318] It remains to be seen how effective immunotherapy can be.

PEDICULOSIS

Pediculosis is infestation with lice (Fig. 6–47A).

Cause and Pathogenesis

Lice are small, degenerate, dorsoventrally flattened, wingless insects that do not undergo true metamorphosis. The eyes are reduced or absent, and each leg bears one or two claws. There is one pair of spiracles on the mesothorax and usually six pairs on the abdomen. Lice are host specific and spend their entire life on their host. They survive only a few days if separated from the host. Lice are spread by direct contact or by contaminated brushes, combs, and bedding. The operculated white eggs (nits) are cemented firmly to the hairs of the host. In contrast, *Cheyletiella* ova are smaller and loosely attached to the hair shafts (see Figs. 2–28Y and Z). The nymph hatches from the egg, undergoes three ecdyses (molting), and becomes the adult. The entire cycle lasts 14 to 21 days.

Lice are divided into two suborders: Anoplura, or sucking lice, and Mallophaga, or biting lice.

Anoplura

These have mouthparts adapted for sucking the blood of the host. With heavy infestations, they produce sufficient anemia to cause weakness, and some animals become distraught and ill-tempered because of the chronic irritation. The only species found commonly on dogs is *Linognathus setosus* (Figs. 6–48A and 6–49C).

Mallophaga

These so-called biting lice feed on epithelial debris and hair, but some species also have mouthparts adapted for drawing blood from their hosts. Because they are active, they may cause more irritation than do sucking lice, and rubbing by their host may cause alopecia. *Trichodectes canis* (see Fig. 6–49A) is the common biting louse of dogs. It may act as the intermediate host of the dog tapeworm, *D. caninum*. *Felicola subrostratuas* infests cats (Fig. 6–50; also see Fig. 6–48B) and may either be asymptomatic or cause severe pruritus with dermatitis and hair loss on the back. *Heterodoxus spiniger* may be found on dogs in warm climates only (see Fig. 6–49B). A single case of *Phthirus pubis* (human pubic louse) infesting a dog has been reported. The dog, which had no clinical signs, slept in the bed of its owner, who was infested with the louse.[260]

Clinical Features

Lice can be highly irritating to the host and can cause intense itching. They accumulate under mats of hair and around the ears and body openings. Sucking lice produce anemia and severe debilitation, especially in young animals. Sucking lice do not move rapidly and are easily seen and caught (see Fig. 6–47A). Biting lice, however, move rapidly and may be difficult to find and capture.

Lice produce a few direct lesions, but excoriations and secondary dermatitis from scratching may be severe. Pediculosis may look like miliary dermatitis in cats and like flea bite hypersensitivity in dogs. Papules and crusts may be found (see Fig. 6–47B). Debilitated, anemic, and frustrated patients are often ill-tempered and difficult to handle. The patient's coat is often dirty, matted, and ill-kept, as this is a disease of neglect often associated with overcrowding and poor sanitation. The animal has a mousy odor, especially when wet.

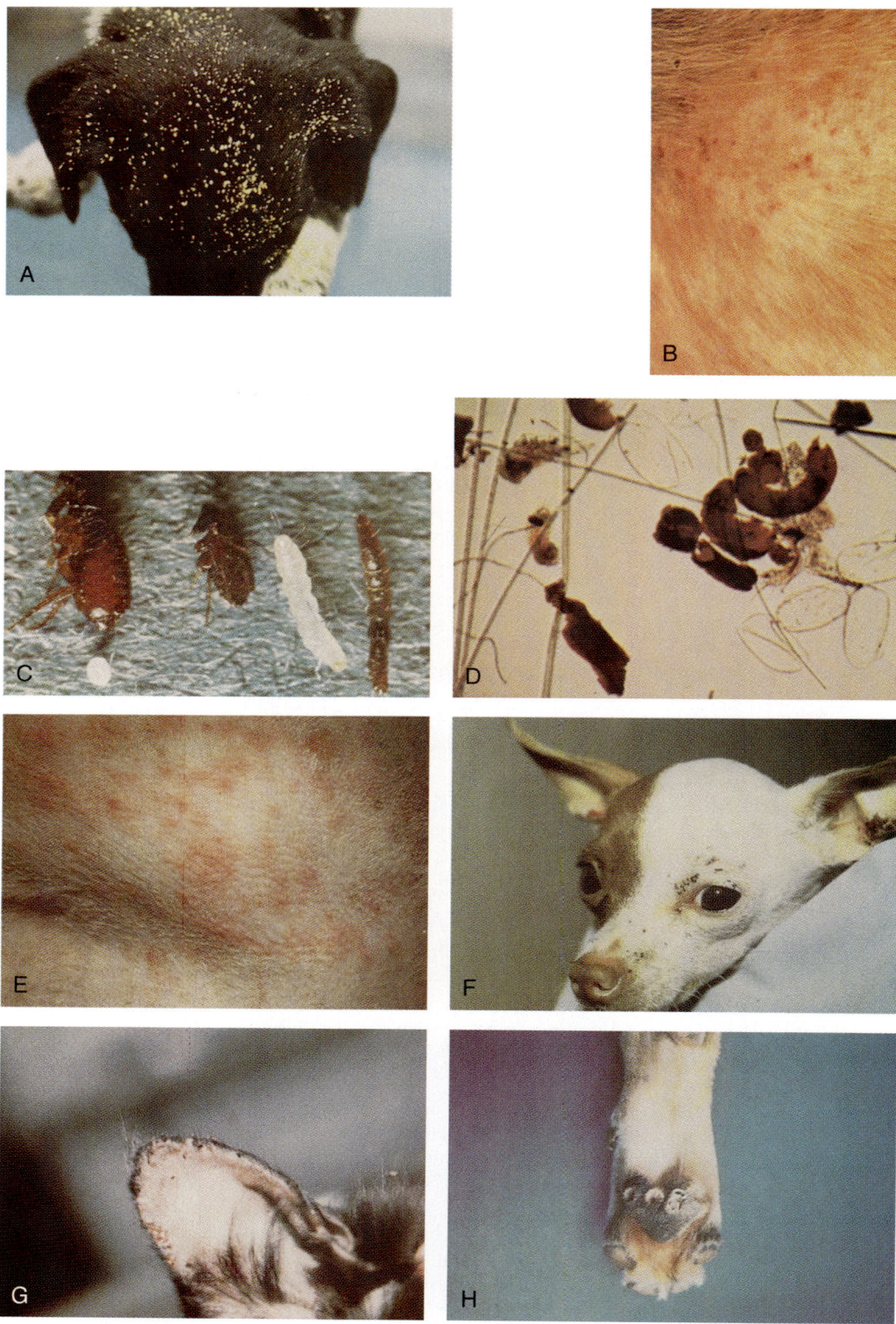

FIGURE 6–47. *A*, Multiple louse nits on the head of a dog. (Courtesy J. King.) *B*, Multiple erythematous, crusted papules on the back of a dog with pediculosis. *C*, Stages of life cycle of the flea *(from left to right):* Adult female with egg, adult male, mature larva ready to pupate (white), young larvae after first blood meal (red).

Legend continued on opposite page

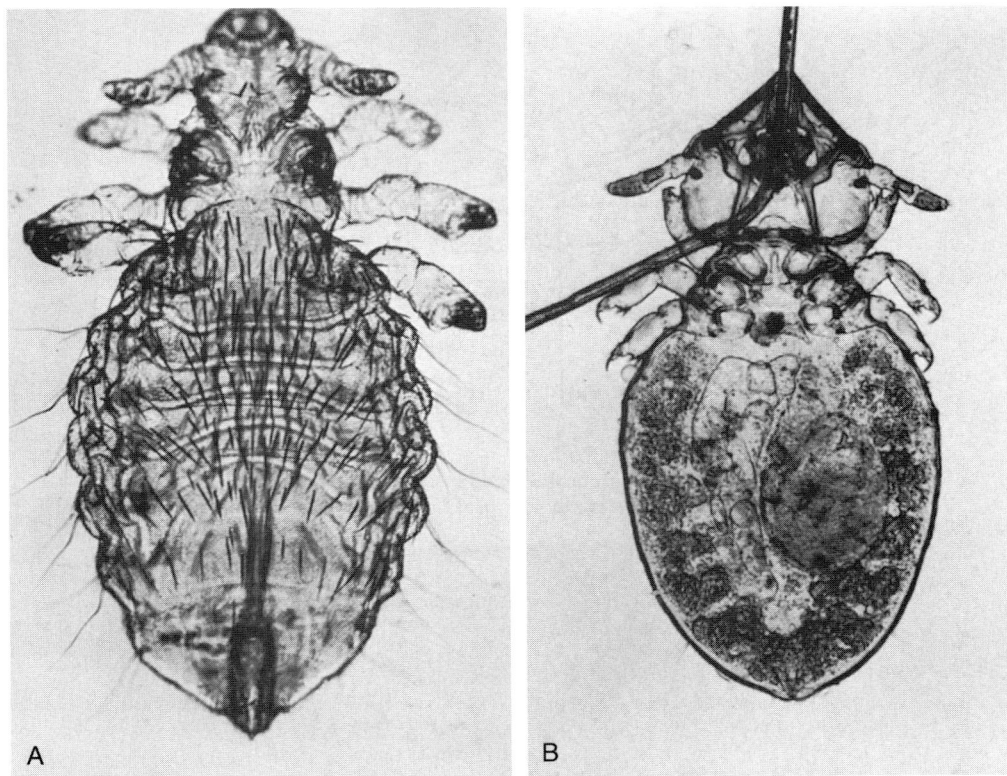

FIGURE 6–48. *A*, *L. setosus*, adult male. *B*, *F. subrostrata*, egg-bearing female.

In some cases, animals are asymptomatic carriers or have only seborrhea sicca with variable pruritus. Pediculosis is often more prevalent in the winter months, perhaps owing to the growth of longer, heavier haircoats and closer contact among animals. In addition, the high ambient and skin surface temperature during summer can be lethal to lice.

Pediculosis is a rare diagnosis in most veterinary practices. Lice are easily killed by common flea shampoos, sprays, or powders; consequently, owners usually eliminate these parasites with routine grooming care. More insecticidal shampoos are used today than were used many years ago, and louse infestation has decreased proportionately.

Diagnosis

Diagnosis is made by physical examination to find and identify the lice. The acetate tape impression method of immobilizing lice for identification is described in Chapter 2.

Differential diagnosis of pediculosis should include seborrhea, scabies, flea bite hypersensitivity, cheyletiellosis, and *Dermanyssus, Lynxacarus,* or *Trombicula* infestations. Skin scrapings and acetate tape examinations should resolve any diagnostic questions. Histopathologic examination reveals varying degrees of superficial perivascular dermatitis (hyperplastic or spongiotic). Eosinophils are usually prominent.

FIGURE 6–47. *Continued.* The pupa is not illustrated. *D*, Empty flea egg cases *(lower right)*, young yellow-white larvae *(upper left)*, and blood fecal crusts from adult fleas to be used as larval food. *E*, Erythematous papules on the abdomen of a dog with flea-bite hypersensitivity. *F*, Sticktight fleas *(Echidnophaga gallinacea)* on the face of a dog. (Courtesy G. Kunkle.) *G*, Multiple crusted papules on the margin of the pinna of a cat with European rabbit flea infestation. (Courtesy R. Harvey.) *H*, Multiple ulcers due to *Tunga penetrans* on the metacarpal pad of a dog. (Courtesy J. King.)

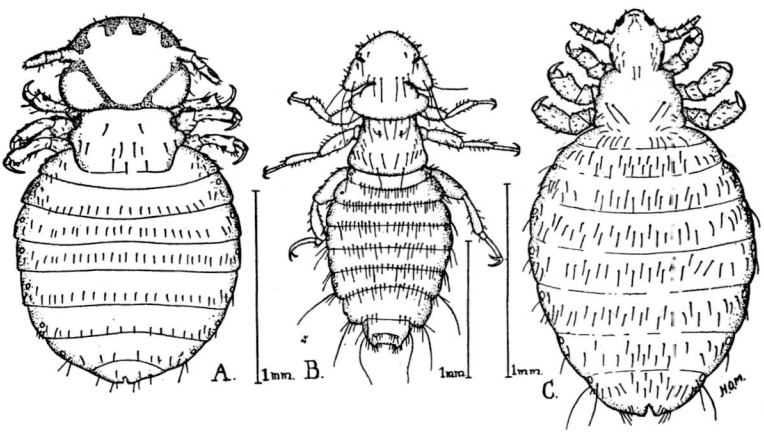

FIGURE 6–49. Dog lice. A, *Trichodectes canis*. B, *Heterodoxus spiniger*. C, *Linognathus setosus*. (From Lapage G: Monnig's Veterinary Helminthology and Entomology, 5th ed. Williams & Wilkins Co., Baltimore, 1962.)

Treatment

All affected animals and other animals in close association with them should be treated. Thick mats and hair tags should be clipped away. After a regular soap and water shampoo, the animal should be soaked or sprayed thoroughly with a good insecticide. Lice are susceptible to almost all parasiticidal agents. Ivermectin was reported to be effective when given at 0.2 mg/kg subcutaneously once.[262]

Cats

Cats can be treated with pyrethrin or carbamate shampoos. After being dried, cats can be sprayed or dusted with products containing pyrethrins. Treatment should be repeated within 10 to 14 days, because not all the nits may be killed and any that remain will have hatched by that time. Two percent lime sulfur dips are also effective. Fipronil spray should be effective.[96a, 258a]

Dogs

Stronger medications with residual action can be used on dogs, although lice are easily killed with the preparations noted above. Bathing the dog with a shampoo containing synergized pyrethrin or a pyrethroid is effective. Dogs can then be dipped or sprayed with any residual flea dip or fipronil.[101b, 259, 261] Imidacloprid was reported to be effective against *T. canis* (biting) and *L. setosus* (sucking) infestations on dogs.[261a]

It is advisable to clean bedding, the premises, and grooming implements thoroughly at least once, even though lice do not live long when they are off the host.

FLEAS

Fleas are small, brown, wingless insects with laterally compressed bodies (Fig. 6–51). Male fleas are smaller than female fleas, and the chitinous head bears antennae, eyes,

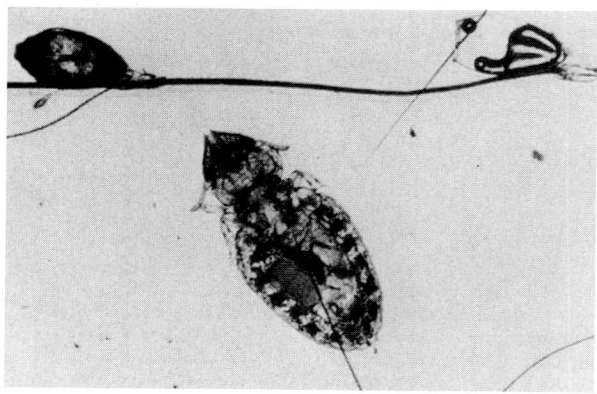

FIGURE 6–50. *Felicola subrostrata*, egg-bearing female. On the left is an intact egg; on the right, an empty case.

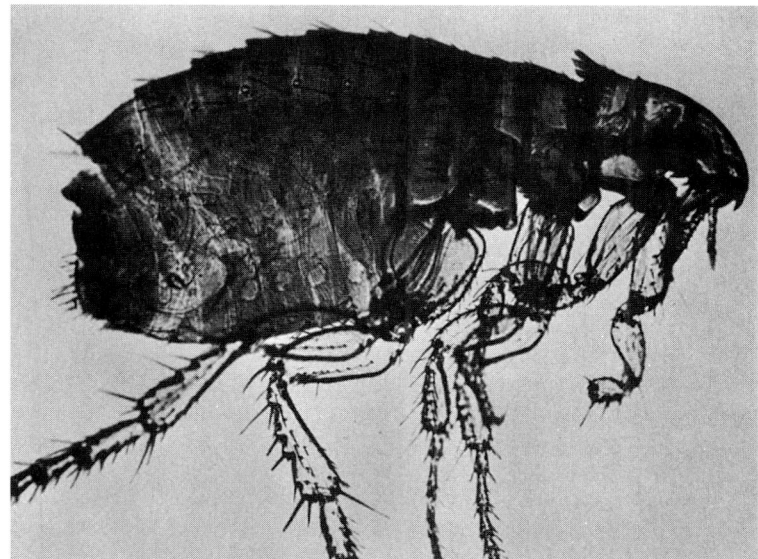

FIGURE 6-51. *Ctenocephalides felis felis* adult.

combs, and suctorial mouthparts. The prothoracic and genal combs are useful taxonomically. Each segment of the three-sectioned thorax bears a pair of powerful legs terminating in two curved claws. The structure adapts fleas for powerful jumping, which enables them to transfer from host to host. Because of their dependence on the host for protection and food, fleas spend their entire adult life on the host or other contact animals.[275]

There are more than 2000 species and subspecies of fleas worldwide. Although dogs and cats could be transient hosts for virtually any species of flea, only *Ctenocephalides felis, C. canis, Pulex* spp., and *Echidnophaga gallinacea* are of medical concern in most pets. The rabbit flea, *Spilopsyllus cuniculi,* is problematic in some parts of Europe and Australia.[283, 313]

Worldwide, *Ctenocephalides* spp. are of greatest medical concern. Surveys on flea-infested dogs and cats have shown that *C. felis felis* is the most common species, with prevalence figures of greater than 92% in dogs and 97% in cats.[30, 31, 273, 280, 292] *C. canis* is far less common but can be the predominant species.[297] *E. gallinacea*, the sticktight poultry flea, can occasionally infest pets, especially in warm climates.[296] For transfer to occur, the pet's environment must be or have been occupied by birds. *Pulex irritans*, the human flea, is an uncommon finding on most dogs. Given the choice between infesting humans or dogs, *P. irritans* appears to prefer the dog but transfers from the dog to contact humans. Because *P. irritans* may be important as a plague vector, the infestation of pets may have some public health significance.

Fleas develop by complete metamorphosis from the egg to the adult through three larval stages and one pupal stage. Details of the life cycle are illustrated in Figure 6–47C. The biology of only *C. felis felis* has been well described, and developmental data may not apply to other species. The female flea lays her eggs on the host and usually while the dog or cat rests or sleeps. These eggs are ovoid, white, and 0.5 mm in length. Because they are not sticky, the eggs fall from the host into the environment, where the life cycle is completed. Development is independent of the host's presence but is dependent on the macroenvironmental and microenvironmental conditions. Ambient temperature and relative humidity are critical for the flea's development and its timing. Because of their negative phototactism and positive geotropism, flea larvae move deep into carpets, down cracks in wood floors, and under the soil surface or organic debris outside.[308] In these protected environments, the local temperature and humidity can be different from those of the gross environment and the life cycle can be completed more rapidly than expected.

All stages of the flea are sensitive to environmental conditions.[310] In general, temperatures between 20° and 30°C with a relative humidity of less than 70% are ideal. Except at very high (greater than 35°C) or very low (less than 8°C) temperatures, relative humidity is more critical for survival. For example, 50% of flea eggs will hatch at 35°C with a humidity of 75%, but none hatch if the humidity is reduced to 33% or 50%. Provided that the temperature does not fall below or exceed the viable limits of the flea, variations of temperature slow or accelerate development. For example, at a humidity of 75%, 50% of larvae pupate within 34 days when the temperature is 13°C, whereas 80% pupate within 8 days at 32°C. In warm climates, such as north-central Florida, cat fleas survive outdoors all year round, even surviving light frosts in protected microhabitats such as inside a doghouse or under a mobile home.[296a]

Flea eggs usually hatch in 1.5 to 10 days.[275, 310] Low temperatures (less than 0°C) for 24 to 36 hours are lethal to most eggs. Newly hatched larvae move to dark protected areas, where they feed on organic debris, other larvae, and most important, adult flea feces (see Fig. 6–47D). Larvae are capable of moving over 40 cm in carpet. Two molts are completed before the third larval instar enters the pupal phase. The larval phase is completed in 5 to 10 days if sufficient food is available and the climate is ideal. Larvae are the Achilles heel of the flea, and outside of the laboratory, less than 25% usually survive.[310] Dryness (less than 33% relative humidity), high heat (greater than 35°C), and extreme cold (less than 8°C) are lethal to the larvae in a short period of time.

At the end of the larval phase, the third instar produces a silklike cocoon in which pupation occurs. If the larva is disturbed, it can develop as a naked pupa which decreased its chances of survival slightly. At 80% humidity and 27°C, adult cat fleas can start to emerge in 5 days. Peak emergence occurs at day 8 to 9. The pupal stage is more resistant to desiccation than other stages but will die at the temperature extremes (3°C or less; 35°C or higher). Emergence is not automatic but depends on the presence of appropriate stimuli, especially temperature and physical pressure. Without the proper stimulus, the adult flea can remain in the cocoon for as long as 140 days. These pre-emerged adults can emerge rapidly when the proper stimulus occurs, leading to a massive explosion in the number of fleas.

In most households, *C. felis felis* takes 3 to 4 weeks to complete its life cycle, with extremes of 12 to 174 days recorded.[30-32] The newly emerged adults require a host for long-term survival. Under standard household conditions, most nonhosted, nonfed adult fleas do not survive after 12 days. Elevations in temperature or reductions in humidity hasten the unfed fleas' death. If the fleas have fed for a few days before separation from the host, they die much more rapidly in the environment. If fleas are not removed from the host, they can survive for more than 100 days.

The female flea starts egg production 24 to 36 hours after her first blood meal. As long as the female is not removed from the host, reproduction will continue for over 100 days, although the fecundity decreases with increasing time. Production varies, with peaks of 40 to 50 eggs per day recorded. Under environmental conditions that allow a 21-day life cycle, one mating female flea who lays 20 eggs per day, 50% of which hatch to females, can be responsible for an infestation of more than 20,000 adults and more than 160,000 preadult forms in 60 days.

The biology of *E. gallinacea* is slightly different. After copulation, the female flea burrows into the skin, where the eggs are laid. The eggs hatch on the host, but the larvae fall into the environment, where the remainder of the life cycle is completed.[296]

Ctenocephalides canis is the most common flea isolated from dogs in Ireland and Greece.[267, 297] The ideal temperature and relative humidity for the development of *C. canis* are 25°C (77°F) and 75%, respectively. When reared on cats, *C. canis* did not develop beyond the first larval stages.

Most species of fleas move freely around their host's body and can be found virtually anywhere. *E. gallinacea* has a preference for the facial region (see Fig. 6–47F). During feeding, the flea releases material into the dermis to prevent blood clotting. *S. cuniculi*, the rabbit flea, has a preference for the pinna and periauricular areas (see Fig. 6–47G). *Tunga penetrans* burrows into the skin and produces significant damage at the site of attachment (see Fig. 6–47H).[285, 305]

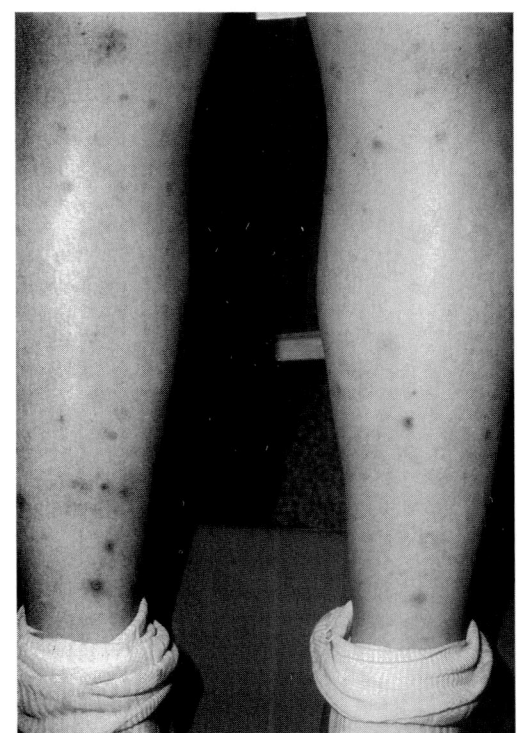

FIGURE 6–52. Flea bites on the legs of a girl. The back is another commonly affected area when the sofa is infested.

The flea's saliva contains a variety of substances that can be irritating or allergenic (see Fig. 6–47E). Signs associated with flea feeding are variable and depend on the number of fleas present, the tolerance of the host for skin irritation, and most important, the presence or absence of hypersensitivity to the flea saliva (see Chap. 8). Nonallergic individuals can harbor variable numbers of fleas with little or no clinical response to them. These animals are at risk for a blood loss anemia. Seventy-two female fleas can consume a total of 1 ml of blood per day. All animals, but especially those of small size, can lose a considerable amount of blood per day when they are heavily infested. However, the irritant nature of the flea's bite is usually somewhat protective for the animal. As the flea population increases, the animal's grooming behavior or scratching increases, which dislodges the flea and decreases the population feeding at any one time. Aside from the blood loss and skin damage they cause, fleas are intermediate hosts for the tapeworm *Dipylidium caninum* and can be vectors for *Rickettsia typhi*, *R. felis*, *Bartonella hinselar*, and various infectious agents.[277, 304] With heavy infestations, the owner will be bitten (Fig. 6–52).

FLEA CONTROL

Fleas are ubiquitous and, depending on the climate, can cause a seasonal or nonseasonal problem for pets and their owners. Any animal that contacts other dogs or cats, frequents grooming parlors or kennels, or is exercised in areas open to other pets or wildlife should be considered exposed. Preventive environmental and animal treatments can minimize or abort more serious problems. Measures discussed later can be both prophylactic and therapeutic, but need to be used much more vigorously when the pet and its local environment are heavily infested. Prevention is the key to good flea control.

Although fleas have a finite life span; often are groomed off and swallowed, especially by cats; and have a decreased reproductive efficiency when feeding on an allergic animal,[288, 300] they cannot be ignored and do not go away by themselves. Control necessitates routine regular treatment of all pets in the house, the house, and the yard. Effective on-animal treatments can eventually eliminate environmental fleas provided that untreated animals do not reinfest the area.[275d] Poor treatment in any one area, especially the house, can make the whole program unsatisfactory. Most programs employ the use of pesticides on the animals and in their environment.

Most pesticides have some residual activity, and levels can build up in the animal and its environment with repeated use. It is paramount that the veterinarian be aware of all pesticides used on the animal and its environment.[30-32] If the same type of insecticide (e.g., organophosphate) is used on both the pet and the environment, intoxication can result from absorption from both sites.

External Environment

Because flea eggs fall to the ground, the infested pet's yard can be seeded with fleas by the pet itself or by stray dogs, cats, or feral animals.[275, 310] Feral animals, especially opossums and raccoons, are a very common point source of infestation for a yard. Fleas can survive the winter in the animal's burrow.[302] During the spring and summer, the flea's rate of reproduction increases as the animal starts to roam through neighborhoods at night. As the animal stops at a garbage can or under a deck, it drops flea eggs into the environment and can pick up some adult fleas to worsen its own infestation. Eggs dropped into the yard may or may not develop. Flea larvae are sensitive to heat and desiccation. Relative humidities below 50% and temperatures above 35°C (95°F) are lethal to flea larvae. Accordingly, adults should not develop on paved areas, on deck surfaces, or in short-cut, sun-exposed lawn. Eggs that fall in protected areas (e.g., under decks, in crawl spaces, and in tall vegetation) can develop. All woodlands and uncultivated fields should be considered infested.

Obviously, the most effective outdoor treatment is prevention, but yards visited by untreated pets or feral animals will need treatment. The first and most environmentally sound step in outdoor flea control involves restriction of the pet from the trouble spots. Crawl spaces, areas under decks, and garden areas should be fenced off, and pets should not be allowed to roam in woods or fields. Exercise in short-cut, sun-exposed fields is allowed. Areas that cannot be avoided by the pet should be cleaned of organic debris frequently and treated with a pesticide registered for outside use. Powder, liquid, and granular formulations of carbamates or organophosphates are available.[30-32] Nonmicroencapsulated liquids have a shorter residual action than do the powder or granular formulations. Recently, a novel biopesticide system for outdoor flea control has been marketed (Interrupt, Veterinary Product Laboratories). This product contains harmless nematodes called *Steinernema carpocapsae*, which kill flea larvae and pupae in the grass and soil.[311] The efficacy of this system is not known.[286]

A commonly overlooked outdoor point source of infestation is the family vehicle. If the pet travels with the family, the vehicle can be seeded with eggs. It is ill-advised to apply a residual pesticide inside the vehicle. Fumes that could develop when the vehicle sits in the sun with the windows closed could make the passengers ill. The vehicle should be vacuumed thoroughly and frequently. If a pesticide is necessary, only short-acting, low-toxicity agents (e.g., pyrethrin) should be applied. The vehicle should be well ventilated before use.

Internal Environment

The house is usually most difficult in the flea control process, especially if the household has multiple pets. Although the infestation is heaviest in areas where the pets rest, any area that is traversed or casually visited must also be treated. If cats are present, virtually every square foot of the house can be infested.

Thorough cleaning is mandatory. Vacuuming with a powerful machine equipped with a beater bar can reduce the flea burden significantly by removing some eggs, larvae, and adults, and by stimulating pre-emerged adults to emerge. All areas should be vacuumed, but special attention should be paid to the furniture, the floor beneath the furniture, the baseboard areas, and all carpets, especially those with a long nap. The vacuum should be emptied after the cleaning. Carpet cleaning can be beneficial. Steam kills larval stages, but most nonprofessional steam cleaners do not produce true steam. Carpet temperatures from these machines may be too low to kill larvae. Even if the cleaning is not larvicidal, it removes organic debris and flea feces, the foodstuff of the larvae. One drawback to carpet cleaning is that the local humidity in the carpet can be increased to the ideal flea level for days to weeks. Any newly deposited eggs or missed pre-emerged stages may accelerate their development because of this environmental improvement. Accordingly, cleaned carpets should be treated with a pesticide. During the cleaning phase, the pet's bedding should be washed or replaced. Preliminary information suggests that flea traps may be of some benefit, but environmental ultrasonic devices are of no use.[270]

Unless the household is devoid of carpets and upholstered furniture, pesticides are necessary. Owners have the choice of applying the agents themselves or hiring a professional. Professional services probably costs more but, when owners put a dollar value on their time and realize that most professional services use products not available to the general public and usually include retreatment visits in the initial price quote, professional treatment becomes cost competitive. An added advantage is that professional treatment can last longer.[269] If professional services are employed, the owner should provide the clinician with the names of the products used to ensure that they are compatible with the animal products being administered.

Health and environmental concerns have led to the use of various nontraditional pesticides, especially sodium borate. The borate compounds have rapid ovicidal and larvicidal activity, probably through a dehydrating mechanism. Ingested crystals also kill larvae. Owner-applied and professionally applied products are available. The professionally applied product (Rx for Fleas, Inc.) is guaranteed for 1 year, provided that the carpets are not cleaned, and has a reported efficacy of greater than 99%.[30–32]

Most homeowners want to attack the flea problem themselves, and a wide variety of pesticides and methods of delivery are available. Whatever plan is developed, it must address the displaced adult flea, the pre-emerged adults, and all the immature forms. Insecticides with little residual action, so-called quick kill products, have no place in a flea control program as the sole agent, except for spot treatment of trouble areas such as the pet's sleeping area. Products selected should be either residual insecticides or quick kill products coupled with an insect growth regulator. Because of health and environmental concerns and local variations in pesticide regulations from state to state and nation to nation, the numbers and types of household pesticides change from year to year. Products available last year, especially those containing organophosphates, may not be available this year. In general, most environment products now contain pyrethrins or pyrethroids, which necessitate inclusion of a growth regulator.

Insect growth regulators prevent the pupation of flea larvae.[24, 30, 37, 41, 282, 294, 309] If these products are applied in the house before fleas are introduced, infestation should be aborted. Methoprene is degraded by sunlight and should be reapplied at least every 30 weeks. Fenoxycarb and pyriproxyfen are sunlight stable and last 6 to 12 months. When the household is already infested, growth regulators alone are not sufficient.

A wide variety of insecticide plus growth regulator products are available through veterinarians, pet stores, and other outlets. The insecticide kills displaced adult fleas and some pre-emerged adults provided that the cocoon is saturated, whereas the growth regulator prevents larval development. However, because neither component affects larvae that have just pupated and some pre-emerged adults probably do not emerge during the period of activity of the insecticide, fleas may be seen in the house shortly after the treatment. If the house was massively infested, fleas can be expected in 5 to 14 days[30–32] and retreatment with a quick kill insecticide is necessary. If the infestation was mild, this retreatment may not be necessary.

The most common complaint heard when owners treat their house is that the product did not work because they continue to see fleas. Although this apparent failure may be a result of insect resistance to the parasiticide,[40] the continued infestation most likely results from poor application and not an inferior product. Thorough treatment of a house takes a great deal of time and effort, and most uneducated owners apply the products incorrectly.

Perhaps the biggest setback in good flea control was the development of the fogger.

The advertisements for these products have stressed their ease of use but not their drawbacks. These room aerosols treat unnecessary areas (e.g., tabletops) and miss vital spots (e.g., under furniture, in room corners, and in closets). These problems are magnified when the owner uses only the number of foggers necessary to cover the number of square feet of the house with no regard to intervening walls and passageways, which interrupt aerosol dispersion.

The most effective methods of indoor flea control involve hand-directed spraying of the pesticide. Products are available in aerosol cans, hand-operated sprays, and concentrates for dilution and application via hand-pressurized spray tanks. If large areas are to be treated, hand-operated sprays are the poorest method of delivery because hand fatigue occurs. The spraying should start in the center of the room and work toward the walls. All trouble spots (e.g., under furniture) should be sprayed carefully. Foggers can be used to decrease the amount of spraying necessary in large rooms. After the corners of the rooms and trouble spots are hand sprayed, a well-designed fogger can be discharged to cover unobstructed areas.

Owners should be instructed to follow the manufacturer's directions carefully. Specific schedules for retreatment should be developed and followed. This is often the weak link in the program. Many clients postpone retreatment until new fleas are seen. At this point, the fleas are established, and retreatment is much more labor intensive and expensive.

Fleas orient and move toward a light source, even more so when the light source is suddenly and temporarily interrupted (which mimics the shadow cast by a passing host).[275a] Cat fleas are most sensitive to light with a wavelength between 510 to 550 nm (green light). Intermittent light traps collect over 86% of the fleas released into a 3 × 3 m carpeted room within 20 hours, whereas nonblinking commercial flea traps collect less than 14% of released fleas.[275a]

Animal

None of the available flea eradication products for animal use is 100% effective in killing fleas over the entire time till the next application. Hence, good environmental control to limit the number of fleas reaching the animal is needed. Another problem with these products is that their residual efficacy under field conditions can be far shorter than that found in the laboratory. In dogs who swim frequently, most topical products have no residual effect. Accordingly, the best pesticide to use in any particular situation is one that satisfies safety concerns and has limited restrictions on its use. Products that indicate some frequency of application but allow use as necessary give the veterinarian maximal flexibility.

Ideally, all dogs and cats in the household should be treated with the same vigor, even if only one animal has problems. Failure to treat the other animals, especially if they are allowed to roam outside, is a point source of infestation for the troubled pet via environmental seeding of eggs. In households with a large number of pets, most owners do not treat the apparently unaffected animals with the same vigor as they do the allergic ones. The owners should be encouraged to use the most effective method of control on the normal animals that their situation allows.

All animal flea control programs should be designed to prevent all flea bites. The number of fleas in the environment plus the owner's willingness and ability to do the treatments determine whether the goal is achievable. The key is regular use of the product. Haphazard use of an excellent product gives poor results. Before the specifics of a program are designed, the owner should be questioned about what he or she can do on a regular basis. Product selection is based on the owner's constraints. Despite the utmost care, some flea control programs do not perform as expected, especially in multiple animal households. At the onset of any control program, therapeutic monitoring with a flea comb is indicated to determine if the agents selected are effective and, if so, what the optimum frequency of application should be. The animal is combed once or twice weekly, and if fleas or flea dirt are seen before the next scheduled application of product, the timing of application is changed. If fleas are still found after the modification, there is some fatal flaw in the program and it should be reevaluated in its entirety. Regular use of a flea comb can decrease flea populations on shorthaired animals. A thorough, 10-minute combing can remove up to 81% of the fleas from shorthaired dogs.[275b]

Since the last edition of this text, flea control has been revolutionized with the marketing of long-acting residual products. The safety, ease of usage, and efficacy of these products is so high the use of conventional products almost seems like malpractice. However, in households with large numbers of dogs, cats, or both, the new products can be too expensive for some owners to use on all of their pets and a more conventional program must be designed. The discussion on conventional products follows that of the newer products.

Spot Application Products

Spot application products contain an insecticide in a proprietary vehicle. The product is applied to one or two spots over the animal's dorsum, and the vehicle with its admixed insecticide diffuses in a concentration-dependent manner over the animal's entire body. The various products' technical information indicates the rate of coverage varies from 12 to 72 hours. Available products include imidacloprid, fipronil, selamectin, or permethrin as their insecticide.

Imidacloprid (Advantage, Bayer) is marketed in various size tubes containing different volumes of a 9.1% w/w solution. It is licensed for both dogs and cats. The target dosage is 10 mg/kg, which is achieved by using a larger volume in animals with a greater body weight. Imidacloprid is strictly an insecticide with no activity against ticks or other arachnids. Company data show that efficacy is achieved within 12 hours of application and persists for 30 days. Efficacy figures vary from 95% to 100% depending on the species and week after application. The efficacy starts to decline as the time to reapplication approaches. According to the manufacturer, weekly immersion in water or a cleansing bath at day 4 after application has little effect on residual effectivity. Contact dermatitis has occasionally been seen at the site of application in both cats and dogs. Squames impregnated with imidacloprid drop off into the environment and are larvacidal.[288a] Because of this, environmental control can, at times, be achieved with the topical application of imidacloprid to pets.[275b, 281a]

Various studies in dogs[20, 264, 289, 290, 299a] and cats[290, 293, 295] corroborate the manufacturer's efficacy data. However, the authors and others have seen animals with a significant flea burden within 14 days of application. These fleas could have been destined to die but had not had sufficient time to do so or could indicate that the duration of action is significantly less than 30 days in a subset of the population. Imidacloprid is at its highest concentration directly after application and is bound to hairs and keratinocytes. If epidermal turnover is increased or hairs are lost, the surface concentration of imidacloprid will decrease. Likewise, daily swimming, excessive licking, or frequent bathing, especially with medicated shampoos, would be expected to reduce the surface concentration. Because the efficacy and duration of action are dose dependent,[264] it should not be surprising that some animals will need more frequent application. The authors have heard some investigators say that they tell all of their clients with pets with skin disease to apply imidacloprid every 14 days. Because this approach increases the cost of treatment, the authors suggest that the rate of application be determined on an individual basis. Owners are asked to flea comb their pets once to twice weekly and reapply product when needed. Recent studies indicate that (1) imidacloprid exhibits significantly and consistently greater flea kill at 6, 12, and 24 hours than selamectin,[275f] and (2) fleas stop feeding within 3 to 5 minutes on imidacloprid treated dogs, but continue to feed during the first hour on fipronil or selamectin treated dogs.[301a]

Fipronil (Frontline, Merial) is available in a 0.25% spray or a 10% spot application product (Top Spot). It is licensed for both dogs and cats. Fipronil is both an insecticide and acaricide, and is effective against fleas, ticks, and mites. Fipronil is stored in the sebaceous glands, and sebaceous secretion can replenish the skin surface supply.[11] Suggested frequency of application depends on the environmental flea burden, sensitivity of the animal to the bite of the flea, and the need to control ticks. Typically, fipronil is applied monthly for maximum efficacy. Manufacturer's data indicate a 24-hour lag phase to maximal efficacy with a 93% to 95% efficacy at the 30-day point. Because the sebaceous glands replenish the drug lost at the skin's surface, water immersion or bathing is reported to have minimal impact on efficacy for at least 30 days. Toxicity may be seen if animals (especially kittens, puppies, small breeds) are overdosed with fipronil spray.

Efficacy figures vary with the species examined, the formulation used, and whether the home environment was natural or simulated. In the simulated home environment, monthly application of the spot application product kept treated cats completely free of fleas.[284, 291] In the clinical situation, efficacy figures vary from approximately 70% to 88% for 30 day trials.[299, 307] If the evaluation point is extended to 60 days, the efficacy drops to near 60%.[306] With the spot application formulation, flea-free rates of 62%, 47%, and 28% were noted in one study at 30, 60, and 90 days, respectively, after application.[266] As with imidacloprid, the authors have examined animals with significant flea burdens despite the recent application of the fipronil spot application product.

It must be emphasized that neither imidacloprid nor fipronil (a) kill the majority of fleas before they are able to consume some quantity of blood, or (b) provide a noticeable repellent effect on fleas.[265a, 275c, 301a] Selamectin (Revolution, Pfizer) was reported to be highly effective in the control and prevention of flea infestations in dogs and cats.[43a]

Selamectin (Revolution, Pfizer) is a semisynthetic avermectin applied to the skin every 30 days for control of heartworms, fleas, ticks, select intestinal parasites, and some nonfollicular parasitic mites. Transdermally absorbed product circulates in the blood and concentrates in the sebaceous glands, where it is stored as a reservoir to replenish the skin. In flea control, peak efficacy is not seen for 36 to 42 hours after application. The product is reported to kill adult fleas, reduce egg production in fleas not killed, and have an environmental larvicidal activity. Manufacturer's data show high efficacy (>97%) for all of these claims.

Permethrin spot application products are available in veterinary (Defend Exspot Insecticide for Dogs, Schering-Plough) and over-the-counter formulations. The concentration of the permethrin varies from 45% to 60% and some products also contain methoprine or pyriproxyfen.[294] These products are toxic to cats, and no dog and cat contact should be allowed until the product is completely dry. Frequency of application depends on the product with figures ranging from 7 days to once monthly. Efficacy figures vary with product and range from 81% to 90% with weekly application.[39, 271]

Flea Collars

Flea collars are available to kill fleas (e.g., insecticidal collars), repel fleas (e.g., ultrasonic devices), or kill flea eggs laid on the animal (e.g., growth regulator collars). Ultrasonic collars are of no value.[274] Under ideal situations, insecticidal collars can reduce the flea burden by 50% to 90% but do not eliminate it.[278, 298] For the pet that is allergic to fleas, reduction probably is not sufficient and the insecticide in the collar can preclude the use of other similar products. Insecticidal collars should be reserved for contact animals, especially free-roaming cats, when the owner does not routinely use other methods of control. Collars containing methoprene or pyriproxyfen with or without an insecticide are available. These are environmental control agents applied to the animals' body. Pyriproxyfen can kill adult fleas, but both agents are aimed at sterilizing the eggs that the flea lays.[33] The methoprene collars inhibit 94% to 99.5% of egg development for over 130 days.[16, 301] Manufacturer's data suggest 100% efficacy for the pyriproxyfen collar for over 1 year.[34]

A noninsecticidal device was released on the European market: the Catan Dog's tag. It was marketed as a non-chemical and nontoxic method to control flea infestations. Product literature claimed efficacy approaching 90% during the first few months that the tag was worn. The tag was claimed to become activated and to produce some type of square-wave field that repelled or eliminated fleas and ticks. However, studies conducted in the United States demonstrated that the tag had no effect on adult fleas, egg production, or egg viability.[275e]

Flea Shampoos or Cream Rinses

Insecticidal shampoos are excellent grooming products but have a limited place in a serious flea control program. With correct use (e.g., 15-minute contact time), the shampoos will kill the fleas on the animal's body. In one study, a deltamethrin shampoo killed 100% and 95% of the fleas and ticks, respectively, and provided more than 95% residual activity for 2 to 3 weeks.[281] It remains to be seen if the residual activity would be similar in the clinical situation. Because the bathing must be followed by the application of some other insecticide, one must question the use of most flea shampoos. They often cost more than grooming products and have been known to cause reactions, so they cannot be considered an innocuous part of the program.

Insecticidal cream rinses are available and claim residual activity against fleas for up to 7 days but their true efficacy is unknown.

Flea Powders

Flea powders contain talc and various insecticides and repellents. Effective application puts the product on the skin, where it can have prolonged residual activity if it is not removed. Powders have limited applicability in animals with dense undercoats, short coats, or significant areas of hair loss. Because the talc absorbs sebum, repeated application of powder dulls the coat and dries the skin. Many powders have been reformulated with higher concentrations of active ingredients. Caution should be exercised when using these stronger products, because too-frequent application can lead to a high residual concentration of insecticides. Very little powder is used today.

Systemic Flea Products

The only systemic flea control product available worldwide is lufenuron (Program, Novartis). It is given by mouth to dogs and cats once monthly or by injection every 6 months to cats. The product concentrates in the animal's fat and is released from there so effective blood levels are maintained for at least 30 days with the oral product.[15, 26, 43] As the flea feeds, it absorbs the compound with the animal's blood and is passed in the flea's feces. In female fleas, lufenuron sterilizes the eggs. Prehatched larvae that feed on the medicated feces will develop endocuticular defects and will die.[15] The cytotoxicity of lufenuron affects cuticle, epidermal cells, chorion, and vitelline membrane of unhatched larvae.[301b] Although lufenuron causes mortality in adult fleas—weakened endocuticle, decreased resiliency of cuticle to expansion during blood feeding and egg production—this is only seen after 7 days of continuous blood feeding at blood concentrations of more than 2 ppm.[273a] These conditions are unlikely to occur in the clinical situation with recommended use of lufenuron. Reported efficacy on lufenuron varies from study to study but exceeds 95% in all.[21, 43, 268, 268a, 276, 279, 303, 312]

The primary place of lufenuron in a flea control program is the prevention of an indoor and outdoor environmental infestation. If the animal already has a few fleas and some eggs have been layed, the lufenuron alone may be sufficient to control the situation after 30 or more days, but most practitioners would add on adulticide to hasten the response time.

Because the various adulticides described in this section usually are not 100% effective, the concurrent use of lufenuron or another highly effective growth regulator is indicated to prevent the development of a strain of fleas resistant to the insecticide.

Until imidacloprid and fipronil were available, two systemic organophosphates received fairly wide usage. One product contained cythioate and was given by mouth twice weekly, whereas the other contained fenthion and was applied to the skin for transdermal absorption every 14 days. Although these products had some efficacy in flea control programs, they were nowhere near as effective as the newer products and were removed from the market in the United States.[7]

Over the years, various lay products containing garlic, thiamine, brewers' yeast, sulfur, and other natural ingredients have been touted as systemic flea repellents.[30–32] There is no clinical evidence that these products are effective.

Liquid Products

Various proprietary, nonproprietary, and homemade liquid flea control products are used. Although home remedies (e.g., Skin-So-Soft, Avon) can have some efficacy, data on other commonly used products (e.g., pennyroyal oil) are not available and some, like tea tree oil, can be toxic.[12] The proprietary products rarely contain a single active ingredient and usually are mixtures of insecticides, repellents, and potentiators. Each product is labeled for species and age range use and directions for its application. Intoxication can occur if the animal is sensitive to one ingredient or if the label directions are not followed.[17, 30] These products come in aerosol sprays, hand-pumped sprays, foams, and dips. As with any other product, its efficacy is influenced by its formulation and how well it is applied.

Aerosol sprays are of no real use; the other modes of application have use in different situations. Dips, or more appropriately rinses, are the most effective, in that a uniform concentration of the product can easily be applied to the skin, regardless of the nature of the haircoat. Drawbacks include the smell of the product, the tendency for dips to dry the coat and the skin, the long drying time, and the limited number of products licensed for cats. Because most cats hate repeated dippings, the limited number of products is of minimal concern.

Hand-pumped sprays are basically prediluted dips that are usually more cosmetically pleasing and expensive.[265] Most animals can be dipped just as effectively with these sprays as they can with traditional dips, but application time increases significantly. This method is ineffective in animals with dense undercoats, and many cats resent the use of sprays. If an owner likes the spray method but finds the prepackaged products too expensive to use regularly, the owner can be instructed to make his or her own spray from a dip concentrate, provided that the label instructions do not exclude this use. The owner purchases a misting spray bottle and marks it clearly with a permanent marker. The dip's dilution instructions are followed, but only that amount necessary to treat the animal or fill the reservoir bottle is made. Some dips allow reuse of diluted emulsions, whereas other dips make no reference to it or specifically prohibit it. In situations in which reuse of the dip is prohibited, only that volume necessary to treat the animals should be made. These homemade sprays have the odor and coat-drying problems of the dip, but their relatively low cost may offset the disadvantages.

As mentioned earlier, fipronil is in both a spot application and spray formulation. The spray formulation is just as hard to apply as a conventional product but its long duration of activity makes it very valuable.[287]

Flea foams (mousse) are special liquids that leave the can as a foam, which is applied to the hair. As the foam is massaged into the coat, the bubbles burst and the liquid reaches the skin. If the foam is applied correctly, the coat is left damp. This formulation is of most value in small animals, especially cats, who resent the application of traditional liquids. When it is used twice weekly, successful control can be expected in over 80% of cats.[272]

• DIPTERA (FLIES)

Medically, flies form a most important order of arthropods because they transmit or are intermediate hosts for many bacterial, viral, protozoal, and helminthic disease agents. However, their effects on skin are minor and are limited to bites (mosquitoes, stable flies, black flies, and deer flies) and myiasis.

The reaction to insect bites varies, because some animals are less attractive or less susceptible to certain flies. The local lesion is an irritant reaction that may become less severe with repeated exposures. The systemic reaction to injected antigen, however, often increases with repeated exposures (e.g., to bee and mosquito antigens), and severe local edema or anaphylaxis may develop.

The primary lesion is a wheal or papule around a bleeding point (Fig. 6–53D). The reaction may be transient or may persist for weeks. In the latter case, a pseudocarcinomatous hyperplasia develops, with scaling and alopecia. A superficial and deep perivascular or diffuse dermal infiltrate of eosinophils, plasma cells, and lymphocytes may be present.

Fly Dermatitis

Adult male and female stable flies *(Stomoxys calcitrans)* are peculiarly adapted for attacking the skin of the host and sucking blood.[2, 10] The rasping teeth and blades of the labella tear open the skin, and the labella and whole proboscis are plunged into the wound to

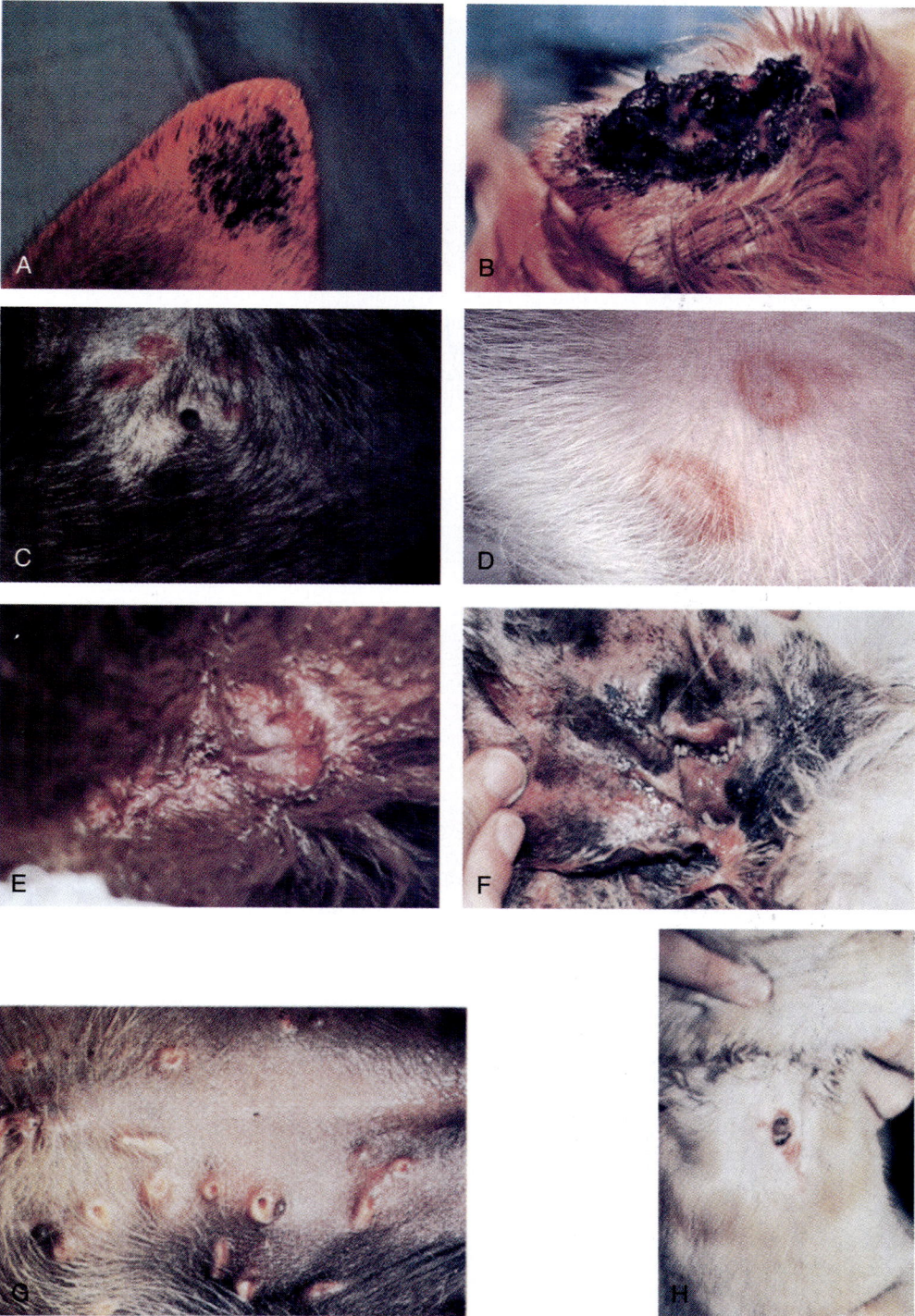

FIGURE 6-53. *A*, Fly dermatitis on a German shepherd's pinna. Hemorrhagic crusts form from the oozing blood and serum that result from the rasping mouthparts of stable flies *(Stomoxys calcitrans)*. *B*, Collie with folded ear shows extensive fly-bite lesions at the fold of the ear with secondary pyoderma. *C*, Multiple erythematous fly bites on a dog's abdomen. *D*, Multiple ecchymotic black fly bites on the glabrous skin of a canine abdomen. *E*, Myiasis. Moist exudative skin lesions attract flies. Note many white fly larvae on the surface of skin and hair. *F*, Myiasis *(Sarcophaga* sp.) complicating otitis externa in a dog. *G*, Multiple crateriform ulcers due to *Cordylobia anthropophaga* on the abdomen of a dog. (Courtesy J. Van Heerden.) *H*, *Cuterebra* sp. larva protruding from a fistula in the ventral neck region of a cat (area has been clipped).

suck blood. The entire action is highly irritating to the host and conducive to spreading disease.

The flies usually attack the face or the ears of dogs. The multiple bites are commonly found on the tips of the ears (see Fig. 6–53A) or at the folded edge of the skin in dogs whose ears are tipped over (such as Shetland sheepdogs and collies) (see Fig. 6–53B). Erythema and hemorrhagic crusts, caused by oozing serum and blood, are typical lesions. Pruritus varies from mild to severe, presumably reflecting the absence or presence of sensitization. Affected dogs are always housed outdoors and are often confined so that they cannot escape the fly attacks.

Ordinary fly repellents, flea products containing permethrin, or citronella in Vaseline applied to the affected skin help prevent repeated bites.[14, 39, 319] The patient should be housed indoors during the day, if possible, until the lesions heal. Topical medications such as antibiotic-corticosteroid ointment (Panalog) may be beneficial. The affected skin should be kept clean and dry. The source of the flies should be investigated, and straw piles, manure pits, and other likely areas can be sprayed with an insecticide.

Black flies (*Simuliidae* spp.) are tiny biting flies that reproduce in shaded areas with running water. They are seasonal in early spring and summer and, during that time, cause severe reactions in people and animals. Their bites are concentrated on hairless areas such as the abdomen (see Fig. 6–53C), the head, the ears, and the legs (see Fig. 6–53D). The lesions are intensely pruritic papules, crusts, and ulcers, with hemorrhage and severe excoriation that result in circumscribed areas of necrosis. Some animals have highly diagnostic annular, macular lesions characterized by a small, pinpoint puncture, surrounded by a larger blanched zone of edema, with a highly erythematous rim. Pruritus is variable. Black flies tend to swarm, and animals bitten by a swarm can die (Fig. 6–54). Histologically, black fly bites are characterized by a perivascular, predominantly eosinophilic, dermatitis with marked superficial dermal edema and purpura (Fig. 6–55). Horsefly (*Tabanus*), deer fly (*Chrysops*), and mosquito bites tend to be less reactive than are black fly bites, but they are all diagnosed, managed, and prevented in the same way as described for stable flies.

Mosquito Dermatitis

Most animals develop a pruritic papule only at the site of the mosquito's bite. Some cats apparently are hypersensitive to some mosquito salivary antigen (see Chap. 8) and develop a pruritic, erosive, crusting dermatitis of the bridge of the nose; papular to nodular lesions on the pinnae; crusted papular pinnal lesions; or hyperkeratosis and swelling of the

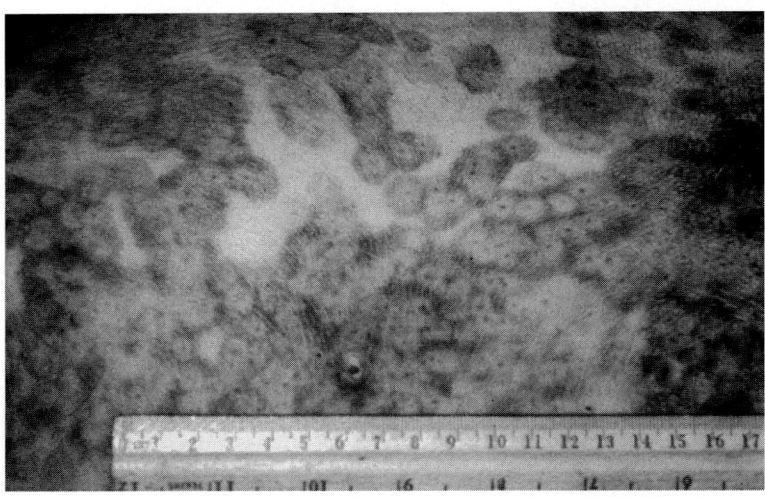

FIGURE 6–54. Black fly bites. Multiple lesions in a dog who was swarmed and died as a result of the bites. (Courtesy E. Clark.)

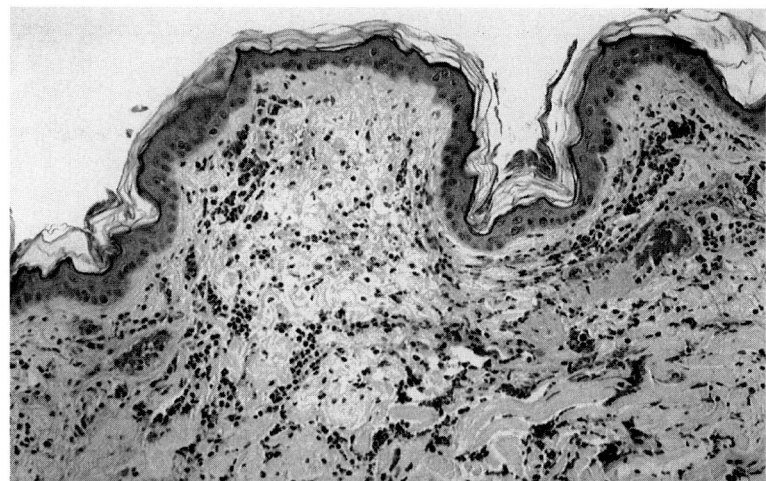

FIGURE 6–55. Black fly bite. Perivascular, predominantly eosinophilic, dermatitis with marked superficial dermal edema and purpura.

pads.[315, 316, 319] Lesions resolve with or without treatment when the cat is isolated from mosquitos and recur within 24 hours of new bites.

Histologically, the lesions are characterized by an eosinophilic interstitial to diffuse dermatitis with or without intraepidermal eosinophilic microabscesses or nodular eosinophilic granulomas with collagen flame figures. Infiltrative and necrotizing eosinophilic mural folliculitis is a common finding. Affected cats show positive intradermal test reactions to mosquito extracts.

Lesional resolution is hastened by the administration of glucocorticoids but may be incomplete with continued mosquito feeding. Unless the cat tolerates repeated applications of insect repellents, management changes are necessary. Because mosquitos feed primarily from dusk to dawn, the cat should be kept in a screened cage or room during those hours.

Myiasis

Although maggots can have medical use,[328] natural infection is detrimental to the patient's health. The adult forms of many dipterous flies place eggs on the wet, warm skin of debilitated, weakened animals with draining wounds or urine-soaked coats (see Figs. 6–53E and F).[325] Animals that are attractive are not equally so at all stages to all flies. As the skin breaks down and liquefies, it becomes a more ideal habitat to further attract a second or third species of fly. Calliphorids (blowflies) feed on only dead tissue, whereas sarcophagids (flesh flies) attack living tissue.[325] True screwworms, *Cochliomyia hominovorax*, have been eliminated from large areas of North America but exist in other areas. They are obligate parasites of living tissue and are never common in dogs and cats.[322] *Habronema* larvae can rarely cause disease in animals housed near horses.[83] Specific identification is not important in the treatment of most myiasis cases. If necessary, larvae can be kept until adult flies develop, or the posterior aspect of the larvae can be examined for posterior spiracles and stigmal plates that are taxonomically significant.

The larvae found in cutaneous myiasis are highly destructive and produce lesions over extensive areas with punched-out round holes (see Fig. 6–53G) in the skin.[7, 317, 325] These holes may coalesce to form broad defects with scalloped margins. The larvae may be found under the skin and in the tissues (Figs. 6–56 and 6–57). Favorite locations are around the nose, eyes, mouth, anus, and genitalia, or adjacent to neglected wounds (see Figs. 6–53E and F). Severely infested animals may die of shock, intoxication, or infection.[325] Myiasis is always a disease of neglect.

Treatment necessitates clipping hair away from the lesions and cleaning them with an antibacterial shampoo or wound flush. If the patient is stable, the diseased tissue should

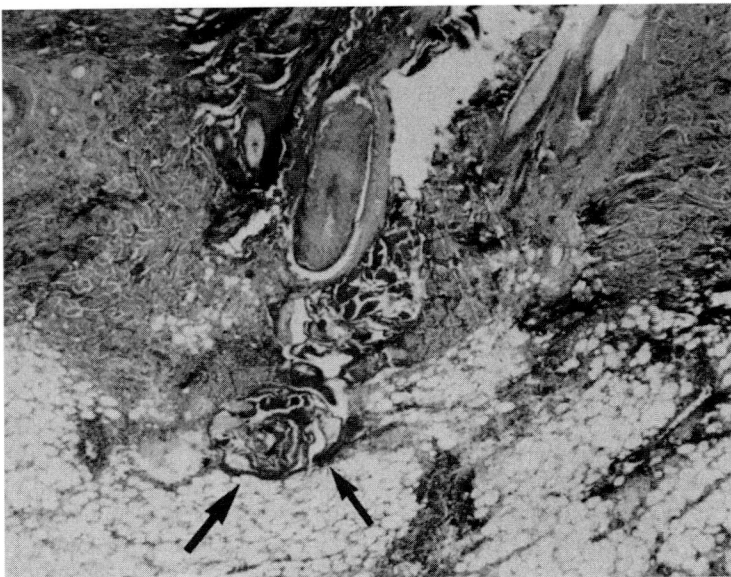

FIGURE 6-56. *Sarcophaga* sp. larva *(arrow)* surrounded by necrotizing dermatitis.

be surgically debrided. Larvae should be mechanically removed. Ivermectin (0.2 to 0.4 mg/kg)[327] or pyrethrin or pyrethroid sprays will kill any maggots that were missed.[325] Daily routine wound care is necessary, and the patient should be housed in screened, fly-free quarters. Usually, healing is rapid and complete, but one should also be concerned about the original cause. Fecal or urinary incontinence, a continually wet coat, fold dermatoses, or constant salivation or lacrimation, together with poor hygiene, can predispose the animal to myiasis. These underlying factors must be corrected as a primary part of therapy.

Some larvae, especially those of *Cordylobia anthropophaga* (see Fig. 6–53G), *Dermatobia hominis*, several species of *Cuterebra* (see later) and *Wohlfahrtia*, and possibly *Habronema* spp., can penetrate normal skin and produce single to multiple nodular to necrotic lesions.[77, 320, 321, 323, 324, 326, 330] Dogs and cats can act as transport for flies via their encysted larvae and introduce them to new countries. Treatment of individual lesions is

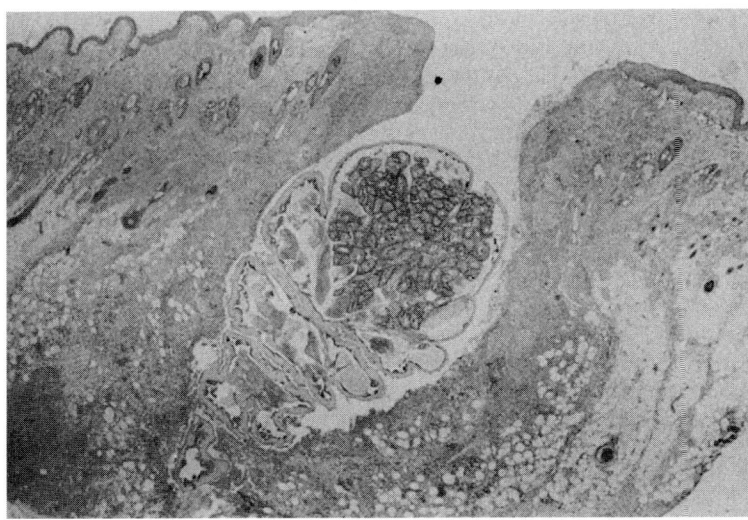

FIGURE 6-57. *C. anthropophaga* larva surrounded by necrotizing dermatitis and panniculitis. (Courtesy J. Van Heerden.)

the same as that mentioned earlier. In situations in which repeated infection with *Cordylobia* can be expected, administration of high-dose ivermectin (0.4 mg/kg) every third week can prevent infection.[329]

Cuterebra Species Infestation

Adult *Cuterebra* flies are large and beelike with vestigial mouthparts, but they neither bite nor feed. They are not directly attracted to a host species but deposit eggs on stones or vegetation near the entrance to the burrows or nests of animals to which they are probably attracted at night. Animals become infested as they pass through areas contaminated with the eggs of *Cuterebra* spp. Larvae enter the body via natural body openings, by skin penetration, or by ingestion as the animal grooms contaminated fur.[2, 10, 331] The natural hosts are usually rabbits and other rodents, and in these animals, the parasites exhibit host and site specificity.[333] Rabbit *Cuterebra* are less host specific and usually affect cats and dogs.

Because cats and dogs are abnormal hosts, the larvae undergo aberrant migrations and have been reported in the brain, the pharynx, the nostrils, and the eyelids.[332, 333] Typical cases involving the skin are usually localized to the regions of the head, the neck, or the trunk. Cases usually occur in late summer or fall, when the larvae enlarge and produce a swelling of 1 cm in diameter, which develops a fistula (see Fig. 6–53H).

Treatment involves incising or spreading the fistulous opening and extracting the grub with a mosquito forceps. Care should be taken to avoid crushing the larva because retained parts may produce allergic or irritant reactions. The infected wound should be treated, but healing is slow.

Identification is usually possible because the second instar larvae are 5 to 10 mm in length and cream to gray in color, with 10 to 12 visible body segments, the first 8 to 10 of which are encircled by 3 to 4 rows of scattered dark spines and spinules. They have well-developed cranial mouth hooks but no head capsule or legs. Molting occurs, and the third instar is the dark, thick, heavily spined larvae that the clinician sees in the subcutaneous or submucosal pocket.

HYMENOPTERA (BEES, WASPS, AND HORNETS)

These venomous insects are not parasitic. They possess membranous wings and mouthparts for chewing, sucking, and licking. The ovipositor of the female insect is adapted for stinging. The female insect has paired venom glands that express a toxin during the sting. When bees and certain wasps sting, the tip of the abdomen and the whole poison apparatus break off and remain in the wound. The gland may continue to express poison, so the stinger should be removed from the skin as soon as possible. Other wasps and hornets may sting repeatedly because they remain intact. Local redness, edema, and inflammation soon develop, and in some animals, angioedema, anaphylaxis, or secondary immune-mediated hemolytic anemia can occur. Intoxication is possible with a large number of stings.[303a, 334] If cardiac and respiratory impairment result, the patient may die.

Facial eosinophilic folliculitis and *furunculosis* has been described in dogs (see Chap. 8) and is thought to be due to the sting or bite of venomous insects, including bees, wasps, hornets, flies, and ants.[3, 319, 335] Dogs have an acute onset of a pruritic papular to nodular facial dermatitis.[336] Lesions may be single or multiple, are crusted, and may be ulcerated if the patient traumatizes them. Grossly, the lesions cannot be differentiated from those of other causes of folliculitis or furunculosis, but cytologic evaluation of the exudate shows numerous eosinophils and no signs of infection. Histologically, an eosinophilic folliculitis or furunculosis is seen, often accompanied by areas of collagen flame figures and mucinosis.[335] Lesions resolve slowly without treatment. If the patient is pruritic, the administration of topical or oral corticosteroids hastens the resolution of the lesions. The stinger should be removed, if it can be located. In severe cases with anaphylaxis, epinephrine should be given intramuscularly and glucocorticoids should be administered intravenously. If urticaria is present, epinephrine or large doses of prednisolone followed by a rapid-acting antihistamine should be administered systemically. The applica-

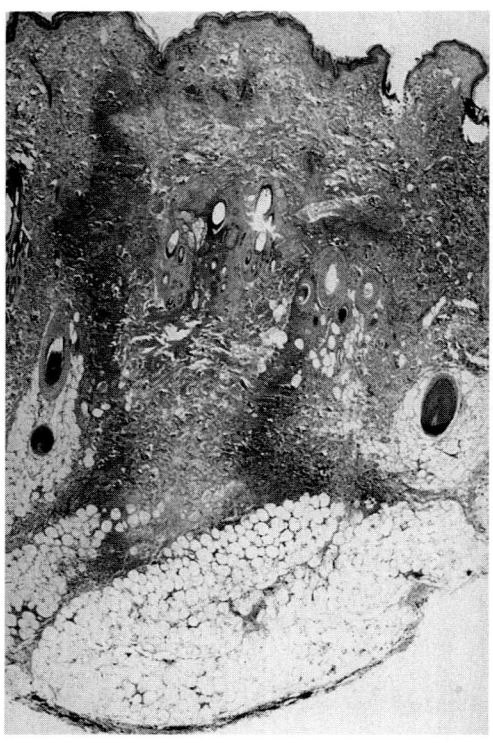

FIGURE 6–58. Fire ant sting. Vertically oriented linear bands of full-thickness dermal necrosis. (Courtesy P. Rakich.)

tion of cold compresses may relieve local pain. Subsequent bites or multiple bites make the reaction more severe.

ANTS

The fire ant *(Solenopsis invicta)* is found in South America and the southeastern United States.[337] These ants inhabit urban and rural settings. When their nest is disturbed, they swarm out, cover nearby objects, and deliver numerous stings. Fire ants attach themselves by pinching skin with their mandibles; they then arch their bodies and inject venom through an abdominal stinger. The venom is primarily composed of a unique alkaloid (solenopsin A) that is cytotoxic and hemolytic.

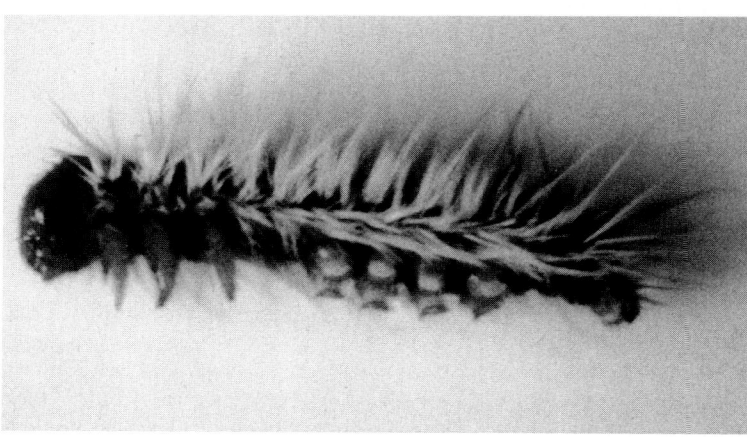

FIGURE 6–59. *Thaumetopoea* spp. caterpillar. (Courtesy J. P. Boutet.)

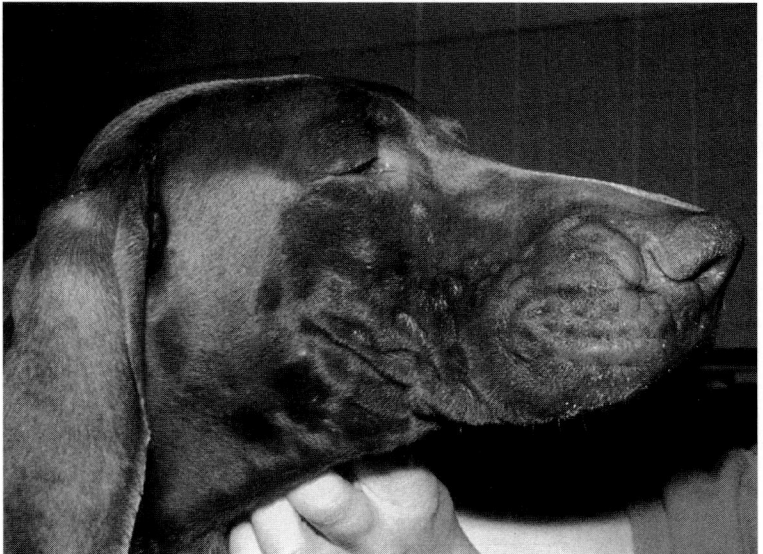

FIGURE 6–60. Urticarial and angioedematous lesions on the face of a dog with caterpillar dermatitis. (Courtesy L. Poisson.)

In dogs, the initial fire ant sting is painless, but it is followed within 15 minutes by erythematous, pruritic swellings less than 1 cm in diameter.[337] These swellings enlarge to be up to 2 cm in diameter in about 6 hours; they then regress and disappear within 48 hours.

Histopathologic findings include vertically oriented, linear bands of full-thickness dermal necrosis with surrounding edema and numerous eosinophils (Fig. 6–58).[337]

CATERPILLARS

The caterpillar larvae of certain Lepidoptera (butterflies and moths) can cause skin reactions.[338, 339] Such reactions are recognized commonly in dogs, rarely in cats, in the Mediterranean region of Europe. Pine and oak caterpillars (*Thaumetopoea* spp.) (Fig. 6–59) are most frequently involved. Bristles from these caterpillars contain thaumatopine, which causes mast cell degranulation and histamine release.

Animals (and humans) may be envenomated on direct contact with the caterpillars or their nests, or by contact with airborne bristles. Most cases of skin reactions are seen in the spring in young, curious dogs. Clinical signs include the sudden onset of facial pruritus, urticaria, or angioedema (Fig. 6–60). The lips and muzzle are most severely affected. In addition, the tongue is swollen and ptyalism is pronounced. In severe cases, necrotic areas may develop in the skin and on the lateral and distal portions of the tongue.

Therapy includes the use of glucocorticoids, antihistamines, and in severe cases, epinephrine.

• REFERENCES

General

1. Bowman DD: Georgis' Parasitology for Veterinarians, 7th ed. W.B. Saunders Co., Philadelphia, 1999.
2. Foley RH: Parasitic mites of dogs and cats. Comp Cont Educ 13:783, 1991.
3. Griffin CE: Insect and arachnid hypersensitivity. In: Kwochka KW, MacDonald JM (eds): Current Veterinary Dermatology. Mosby–Year Book, St. Louis, 1993, p 133.
4. Moriello KA: Common ectoparasites of the dog. Part I, Fleas and ticks. Canine Pract 14:7, 1987.
5. Paradis M: Ivermectin in small animal dermatology. Part I. Pharmacology and toxicology. Comp Cont Ed 20:193, 1998.
6. Paradis M: Ivermectin in small animal dermatology. Part II. Extralabel applications. Comp Cont Ed 20:459, 1998.
7. Scott DW, Miller WH Jr, Griffin CE: Muller and

Kirk's Small Animal Dermatology, 5th ed. W. B. Saunders, Co., Philadelphia, 1995.
8. Scott DW: Feline dermatology 1972–1982: Introspective retrospections. J Am Anim Hosp Assoc 20:537, 1984.
9. Sosna CB, Medleau L: Symposium on external parasites. Vet Med 87:537, 1992.
10. Soulsby EJL: Helminths, Arthropods, and Protozoa of Domesticated Animals, 7th ed. Lea & Febiger, Philadelphia, 1982.

Antiparasitic Treatments

10a. Beal MW, et al: Respiratory failure attributable to moxidectin intoxication in a dog. J Am Vet Med Assoc 215:1813, 1999.
11. Birckel P, et al: Skin and hair distribution of 14c-fipronil by microautoradiography following topical administration to the Beagle dog. J Vet Pharmacol Ther 20:155, 1997.
12. Bischoff K, Guale F: Australian tea tree (*Melaleuca alternifolia*) oil poisoning in three purebred cats. J Vet Diagn Invest 10:208, 1998.
13. Bossard RL, et al: Review of insecticide resistance in cat fleas. J Med Entomol 35:415, 1998.
14. Brown M, Hebert AA: Insect repellents: An overview. J Am Acad Dermatol 36:243, 1997.
14a. Cadiergues MC, et al: Efficacy of an adulticide used alone or in combination with an insect growth regulator in simulated home environments. Am J Vet Res 60:1122, 1999.
15. Dean SR, et al: Mode of action of lufenuron on larval cat fleas. J Med Entomol 35:720, 1998.
16. Donahue WA, Young R: Assessing the efficacy of (S)-methoprene collars against flea egg hatch on pets. Vet Med 91:1000, 1996.
17. Dorman DC, et al: Fenvalerate/N, N-diethyl-m-toluamide (Deet) toxicosis in two cats. J Am Vet Med Assoc 196:100, 1990.
18. Duncan KL: Treatment of amitraz toxicosis. J Am Vet Med Assoc 203:1115, 1993.
19. Folz SD, et al: Evaluation of a new treatment for canine scabies and demodicosis. J Vet Pharmacol Ther 1:199, 1978.
20. Franc M, Cadiergues MC: Antifeeding effect of several insecticidal formulations against *Ctenocephalides felis* on cats. Parasite 5:83, 1998.
21. Franc M, et al: Pharmacokinetics of a new long-acting formulation of lufenuron and dose-activity relationship using experimental infestation by *Ctenocephalides felis*. J Vet Pharmacol Ther 20:80, 1997.
22. Franc M, Cadiergues MC: Susceptibility of the cat flea, *Ctenocephalides felis*, to four pyrethroids. Parasite 4:91, 1997.
23. Frank LA, Kania SA: The effect of ivermectin on lymphocyte blastogenesis and T-cell subset ratios in healthy dogs. Vet Aller Clin Immunol 5:27, 1997.
24. Garg RC, et al: Pharmacologic profile of methoprene, an insect growth regulator, in cattle, dogs, and cats. J Am Vet Med Assoc 194:410, 1989.
25. Halliwell REW, Carlotti DN: Insect growth regulators: New products and new approaches for flea control on dogs. Prat Méd Chir Anim Comp 33:293, 1998.
26. Hink WF, et al: Evaluation of a single oral dose of lufenuron to control flea infestations in dogs. Am J Vet Res 55:822, 1994.
27. Hsu WH, Schaffer DD: Effects of topical application of amitraz on plasma glucose and insulin concentrations in dogs. Am J Vet Res 49:139, 1988.
28. Hugnet C, et al: Toxicity and kinetics of amitraz in dogs. Am J Vet Res 57:1506, 1996.
29. Kawada H, Hirano M: Insecticidal effects of insect growth regulators methoprene and pyriproxyfen on the cat flea. J Med Entomol 33:819, 1996.
30. MacDonald JM, Miller TA: Parasiticide therapy in small animal dermatology. In: Kirk RW (ed): Current Veterinary Therapy 9. W.B. Saunders Co., Philadelphia, 1986, p 571.
31. MacDonald JM: Flea allergy dermatitis and flea control In: Griffin CE, et al (eds): Current Veterinary Dermatology. Mosby–Year Book, St. Louis, 1993, p 57.
32. MacDonald JM: Flea control: An overview of treatment concepts for North America. Vet Dermatol 6:121, 1995.
33. Meola R, et al: Toxicity and histopathology of the growth regulator pyriproxyfen to adults and eggs of the cat flea. J Med Entomol 33:670, 1996.
34. Miller TA, Blagburn BL: Ovisterilant efficacy of pyriproxyfen collars on dogs and cats. Proc Annu Memb Meet Am Acad Vet Dermatol Am Coll Vet Dermatol 12:63, 1996.
35. Moriello KA: Treatment of *Sarcoptes* and *Cheyletiella* infestations. In: Kirk RW, Bonagura JD (eds): Kirk's Current Veterinary Therapy XI: Small Animal Practice. W.B. Saunders Co., Philadelphia, 1992, p 558.
36. Mueller RS, Bettenay SV: A proposed new therapeutic protocol for the treatment of canine mange with ivermectin. J Am Anim Hosp Assoc 35:77, 1999.
37. Palma KG, et al: Mode of action of pyriproxyfen and methoprene on eggs of *Ctenocephalides felis* (Siphonaptera: Pulicidae). J Med Entomol 30:421, 1993.
38. Rosenbaum MR, Kerlin RL: Erythema multiforme major and disseminated intravascular coagulation in a dog following application of a d-limonene-based insecticidal dip. J Am Vet Med Assoc 207:1315, 1995.
39. Ross DH, et al: Efficacy of a permethrin and pyriproxyfen product for control of fleas, ticks, and mosquitos on dogs. Canine Pract 22:53, 1997.
40. Schwinghammer KA, et al: Comparative toxicity of ten insecticides against the cat flea, *Ctenocephalides felis*. J Med Entomol 22:512, 1985.
41. Shaaya E: Interference of the insect growth regulator methoprene in the process of larval-pupal differentiation. Arch Insect Biochem Physiol 22:233, 1993.
42. Shipstone MA, Masson KV: The use of insect development inhibitors as an oral medication for control of the fleas *Ctenocephalides felis*, *Ct. canis* in the dog and cat. Vet Dermatol 6:131, 1995.
43. Stansfield DG: A review of the safety and efficacy of lufenuron in dogs and cats. Canine Pract 22:34, 1997.
43a. Thomas CA: Revolution: A unique endectocide providing comprehensive convenient protection. Compend Cont Edu Pract Vet 21(Suppl): 2, 1999.
43b. Thomas CA: Revolution safety profile. Compend Cont Edu Pract Vet 21(Suppl): 26, 1999.
44. Tranquilli JW, et al: Assessment of toxicosis induced by high-dose administration of milbemycin oxime in collies Am J Vet Res 52:1170, 1993.
45. Turnbull GJ: Animal studies in the treatment of poisoning by amitraz and xylene. Hum Toxicol 2:579, 1983.

Hookworm Dermatitis

46. Bowman DD: Hookworm parasites of dogs and cats. Comp Cont Educ 14:585, 1992.
47. Matthews BE: Mechanics of skin penetration by hookworm larvae. Vet Dermatol Newsl 6:75, 1981.

Pelodera Dermatitis

48. Bourdeau P: Cas de dermatite à rhabitides (*Pelodera strongyloides*) chez un chien. Point Vét 16:5, 1984.
49. Horton ML: Rhabditic dermatitis in dogs. Mod Vet Pract 61:158, 1980.
50. Pasyk K: Dermatitis rhabditidosa in an 11-year-old girl. Br J Dermatol 98:107, 1978.
51. Smith JD, et al: Larva currens; cutaneous strongyloides. Arch Dermatol 112:1161, 1976.

Strongyloides stercoralis—like Infection

52. Malone JB, et al: *Strongyloides stercoralis*—like infection in a dog. J Am Vet Med Assoc 176:130, 1980.
53. Mansfield LS, et al: Ivermectin treatment of naturally acquired and experimentally induced *Strongyloides stercoralis* infections in dogs. J Am Vet Med. Assoc 20:726, 1992.

Anatrichosomiasis

54. Hendrix CM, et al: *Anatrichosoma* sp. infection in a dog. J Am Vet Med Assoc 191:984, 1987.

Schistosomiasis

55. Harmon RRM: Parasites, worms, and protozoa. In: Rook A, et al (eds): Textbook of Dermatology. Blackwell Scientific Publications, Oxford, 1979.
56. Hoeffler DF: Swimmer's itch. Cutis 19:461, 1977.

Dracunculiasis

57. Beyer TA, et al: Massive *Dracunculus insignis* infection in a dog. J Am Vet Med Assoc 214:366, 1999.
58. Giovengo SL: Canine dracunculiasis. Comp Cont Educ 15:726, 1993.
59. Muhammad G: *Dracunculus medinensis* in a bull terrier (a case report). Indian Vet J 67:967, 1990.
60. Panciera DL, Stockham SL: *Dracunulus insignis* infection in a dog. J Am Vet Med Assoc 192:78, 1988.

Dirofilariasis

61. Bredal WP, et al: Adult *Dirofilaria repens* in a subcutaneous granuloma on the chest of a dog. J Small Anim Pract 39:595, 1998.
62. Coles LD, et al: Adult *Dirofilaria immitis* in hind leg abscesses of a dog. J Am Anim Hosp Assoc 24:363, 1988.
63. Elkins AD, et al: Interdigital cyst in the dog caused by an adult *Dirofilaria immitis*. J Am Anim Hosp Assoc 26:71, 1990.
64. Mozos E, et al: Cutaneous lesions associated with canine heartworm infection. Vet Dermatol 3:191, 1992.
65. Scott DW: Nodular skin disease associated with *Dirofilaria immitis* infection in the dog. Cornell Vet 59:233, 1979.
66. Scott DW, Vaughn TC: Papulonodular dermatitis in a dog with occult filariasis. Comp Anim Pract 1:31, 1987.
67. Seavers A: Cutaneous syndrome possibly caused by heartworm infestation in a dog. Aust Vet J 76:18, 1997.

Other Filarial Infections

68. Carmichael J, Bell FR: Filariasis in dogs in Uganda. J S Afr Vet Assoc 14:12, 1943.
69. Cazelles C, Montagner C: Deux cas de filariose cutanée associée à une leishmaniose. Point Vét 27:343, 1995.
70. Gardiner CH, et al: Onchocerciasis in two dogs. J Am Vet Med Assoc 203:828, 1993.
71. Hargis AM, et al: Dermatitis associated with microfilariae (*Filioidea*) in 10 dogs. Vet Dermatol 10:95, 1999.
72. Kamalu BP: Canine filariasis caused by *Dirofilaria repens* in southeastern Nigeria. Vet Parasitol 40:335, 1991.
72a. Tarello W: La dirofilariose sous-cutanée à Dirofilaria (Nochtiella) repens chez le chien. Revue bibliographique et cas clinique. Rec Méd Vét 150:691, 1999.

Miscellaneous Helminthic Infections

73. Amato JF, et al: Two cases of fistulated abscesses caused by *Lagochilascaris major* in the domestic cat. Mem Inst Oswaldo Cruz 85:471, 1990.
74. Bate M, et al: *Gnathostoma spinigerum* in a dog's leg. Aust Vet J 60:285, 1983.
75. Bauer C, et al: *Taenia crassiceps* metacestodes in the subcutis of a dog. Kleintierprax 43:37, 1998.
76. Chermette R, et al: Subcutaneous *Taenia crassiceps* cysticercosis in a dog. J Am Vet Med Assoc 203:263, 1993.
77. Chermette R, et al: Quelques parasitoses canines exceptionnelles en France: III—cysticercose proliférative du chien à *Taenia crassiceps*: À propos de trois cas. Prat Méd Chir Anim Comp 31:125, 1996.
78. Craig TM, et al: Parasitic nematode (*Lagochilascaris major*) associated with a purulent draining tract in a dog. J Am Vet Med Assoc 181:69, 1982.
79. Dell'Porto A, et al: Ocorrencia de *Lagochilascaris major* Leiper, 1910 em Gato (Felis catus domesticus L) no estado de Sao Paulo, Brasil. Rev Fac Med Vet Zootec 25:173, 1988.
80. Hovorka I, Dubinsky P: Helminths of domestic dogs and cats in the urban area of Kosice and the National Park in the year 1992. Folia Vena 25:195, 1995.
81. Mog S, et al: Subcutaneous migration of an adult *Paragonimus kellicoti* in a dog from Wisconsin. Vet Pathol 34:5, 1997.
82. Moisan PG, et al: Incidental subcutaneous gordiid parasitism in a cat. J Vet Diagn Invest 8:270, 1996.
83. Sanderson TP, et al: Cutaneous habronemiasis in a dog. Vet Pathol 27:208, 1991.

Parasitic Ticks

84. Atwell R, et al: The effect of fipronil on *Ixodes holocyclus* on dogs in Northern NSW. Aust Vet Practit 26:155, 1996.
84a. Barriga OO: Evidence and mechanisms of immunosuppression in tick infestation. Gen Anal Biomed Eng 14:139, 1999.
85. Barsanti JA: Botulism, tick paralysis and acute polyradiculoneuritis. In: Kirk RW (ed): Current Veterinary Therapy VII. W.B. Saunders Co., Philadelphia, 1980, p 773.
86. Blagburn BL, et al: Efficacy of the preventic (9 per cent amitraz) collar for control of *Rhipicephalus sanguineus* and *Dermacentor variabilis* infestations on dogs. In: Proceedings of the 1993 North American Veterinary Conference, Vol. 7, 1993, p 387.
86a. Estrada-Peña A, Ascher F: Comparision of amitraz-impregnated collar with topical administration of fipronil for prevention of experimental and natural infestations by the brown dog tick (*Rhipicephalus sanguineus*). J Am Vet Med Assoc 214:1799, 1999.
87. Rodriguez JM, Perez M: Use of ivermectin against a heavy *Ixodes ricinus* infestation in a cat. Vet Rec 135:140, 1994.
88. Searle A, et al: Results of a trial of fipronil as an adulticide on ticks (*Ixodes holocyclus*) naturally at-

tached to animals in the Brisbane area. Aust Vet Practit 25:157, 1995.
89. White SD, et al: *Otobius megnini* infestation in three dogs. Vet Dermatol 6:33, 1995.

Dermanyssus gallinae
90. DeClerg J, Nachtegaele L: *Dermanyssus gallinae* infestation in a dog. Canine Pract 18:34, 1993.
90a. Nordenfors H, et al: Effects of temperature and humidity on oviposition, molting, and longevity of *Dermanyssus gallinae* (Acari: Dermanyssidae). J Med Entomol 36:68, 1999.
91. Ramsay GW, Mason PC: Chicken mite (*D gallinae*) infesting a dog. N Z Vet J 23:155, 1975.
92. Tucci EC, Guimaraes JH: Biology of *Dermanyssus gallinae* (DeGeer, 1778). Rev Brasil Parasitol Vet 7:27, 1998.

Lynxacarus radovsky
93. Bowman WL: The cat fur mite (*Lynxacarus rhadovsky*) in Australia. Aust Vet J 54:403, 1978.
94. Craig TM, et al: *Lynxacarus rhadovsky* infestation in a cat. J Am Vet Med Assoc 202:613, 1993.
95. Foley RH: An epizootic of a rare fur mite in an island's cat population. Feline Pract 19:17, 1991.
96. Pereira M: The cat fur mite (*Lynxacarus radovskyi*) in Brazil. Feline Pract 24:24, 1996.

Trombiculiosis
96a. Beugnet F, Bourdeau P: Les ectoparasites du chat. Prat Méd Chir Anim Comp 34:427, 1999.
97. Fleming EJ, et al: Miliary dermatitis associated with *Eutrombicula* infestation in a cat. J Am Anim Hosp Assoc 27:529, 1991.
98. Greene RT, et al: Trombiculiasis in a cat. J Am Vet Med Assoc 188:1054, 1986.
99. Lowenstine LJ, et al: Trombiculosis in a cat. J Am Vet Med Assoc 175:289, 1979.
100. Nuttall TJ, et al: Treatment of *Trombicula autumnalis* infestation in dogs and cats with a 0.25 per cent fipronil spray. J Small Anim Pract 39:237, 1998.

Otodectes cynotis
101. Bensignor E: Dermatite feline à *Otodectes cynotis*. Point Vét 28:85, 1996.
101a. Bourdeau P, et al: The probable role of environmental conditions in the efficacy of treatment of *Otodectes cynotis* infestation in dogs? An example with moxidectin (Cydectin) in 50 dogs. Proc Annu Cong Eur Soc Vet Dermatol Eur Coll Vet Dermatol 15:149, 1998.
101b. Bourdeau P, Lecanu JM: Treatment of multiple infestations with *Otodectes cynotis*, *Cheyletiella yasguri*, and *Trichodectes canis* with fipronil (Frontline Spot-On; Merial). Proc Br Vet Dermatol Study Group, Autumn 1999, p 35.
101c. Coleman GT, Atwell RB: Use of fipronil to treat ear mites in cats. Aust Vet Practit 29:166, 1999.
102. Faulk RH, et al: Effect of Tresaderm against otoacariasis: A clinical trial. Vet Med (SAC) 73:307, 1978.
103. Gram DB, et al: Treating ear mites in cats: A comparison of subcutaneous and topical ivermectin. Vet Med 89:1122, 1994.
104. Harwick RP: Lesions caused by canine ear mites. Arch Dermatol 114:130, 1978.
105. Lopez RA: Of mites and man. J Am Vet Med Assoc 203:606, 1993.
106. Pappas C Jr, Katz TL: Evaluation of a treatment for the ear mite, *Otodectes cynotis*, in kittens. Feline Pract 23:21, 1995.
107. Powell MB, et al: Reaginic hypersensitivity in *Otodectes cynotis* infestation of cats and mode of mite feeding. Am J Vet Res 41:877, 1980.
107a. Saridomichelakis MN, et al: Sensitization to dust mites in cats with *Otodectes cynotis* infestation. Vet Dermatol 10:89, 1999.
108. Scherk-Nixon M, et al: Treatment of feline otoacariasis with 2 otic preparations not containing miticidal active ingredients. Can Vet J 38:229, 1997.
109. Vincenti P, Genchi C: Efficacité du fipronil (Frontline spot on) dans le traitement de la gale des oreilles (*Otodectes cynotis*) chez le chien et le chat. Proc GEDAC 13:5, 1998.
110. Weisbroth SH, et al: Immunopathology of naturally-occurring otodectic otoacariasis in the domestic cat. J Am Vet Med Assoc 165:1088, 1974.

Pneumonyssoides caninum
111. Bredal W, Vollset I: Use of milbemycin oxime in the treatment of dogs with nasal mites (*Pneumonyssoides caninum*) infection. J Small Anim Pract 39:126, 1998.
112. Bredal WP: The prevalence of nasal mite (*Pneumonyssoides caninum*) infection in Norwegian dogs. Vet Parasitol 76:233, 1998.
113. Bredal WP: *Pneumonyssoides caninum* infection: A risk factor for gastric dilatation-volvulus in dogs. Vet Res Commun 22:225, 1998.
114. Bussieras J, Chermette R: Quelques parasitoses canines exceptionnelles en France: I—infestation par *Pneumonyssoides caninum*. Prat Méd Chir Anim Comp 30:427, 1995.
115. Gunnarsson L, et al: Experimental infection of dogs with the nasal mite *Pneumonyssoides caninum*. Vet Parasitol 77:179, 1998.
116. Gunnarsson LK, et al: Clinical efficacy of milbemycin oxime in the treatment of nasal mite infection in dogs. J Am Anim Hosp Assoc 35:81, 1999.
117. Marks SI, et al: *Pneumonyssoides caninum*: The canine nasal mite. Compend Cont Educ 16:577, 1994.
118. Mundell AC, et al: Ivermectin in the treatment of *Pneumonyssoides caninum*. A case report. J Am Anim Hosp Assoc 26:393, 1990.

Environmental Mites
119. Kunkle GA, et al: Dermatitis in horses and man caused by the straw itch mite. J Am Vet Med Assoc 181:467, 1982.
120. Vollset I: Immediate type hypersensitivity in dogs induced by storage mites. Res Vet Sci 40:123, 1986.

Cheyletiellosis
121. Chadwick AJ: Use of 0.25 per cent fipronil pump spray formulation to treat canine cheyletiellosis. J Small Anim Pract 38:261, 1997.
122. Cohen SR: *Cheyletiella* dermatitis (in rabbit, cat, dog, man). Arch Dermatol 116:435, 1980.
123. Foxx TS, Ewing SA: Morphologic features, behavior, and life history of *Cheyletiella yasguri*. Am J Vet Res 30:269 1969.
124. Lee BW: *Cheyletiella* dermatitis: A report of 14 cases. Cutis 47:111, 1991.
125. McGarry JW: Recurrent infestation of a cat by *Cheyletus eruditus* (Shrank 1781). Vet Rec 125:18, 1989.
126. McKeever PJ, Allen SK: Dermatitis associated with *Cheyletiella* infestation in cats. J Am Vet Med Assoc 174:718, 1979.
127. Moriello KA: Cheyletiellosis. In: Griffin CE, et al (eds): Current Veterinary Dermatology. Mosby–Year Book, St. Louis, 1993, p 90.
128. Ottenslot TRF, Gil D: Cheyletiellosis in long-haired cats. Tidsch Diergeneeskd 103:1104, 1978.

129. Paradis M, Vileneuve A: Efficacy of ivermectin against *Cheyletiella yasguri* infestation in dogs. Can Vet J 29:633, 1988.
130. Paradis M, et al: Efficacy of ivermectin against *Cheyletiella blakei* infestation in cats. J Am Anim Hosp Assoc 26:125, 1990.
131. Smiley RL: A review of the family Cheyletiellidae (Acarina). Ann Entomol Soc Am 63:1056, 1970.
132. Stein B: Personal communication, 1982.

Canine Demodicosis

133. Barriga OO, et al: Evidence of immunosuppression by *Demodex canis*. Vet Immunol Immunopathol 32:37, 1992.
134. Barta O, et al: Lymphocyte transformation suppression caused by pyoderma—failure to demonstrate it in uncomplicated demodectic mange. Comp Immunol Microbiol Infect Dis 6:9, 1983.
135. Bensignor E, Carlotti DN: Moxidectine in the treatment of generalized demodicosis in dogs: A pilot study: 8 cases. In: Kwochka KW, et al (eds): Advances in Veterinary Dermatology III. Butterworth Heinemann, Oxford, 1998, p 554.
135a. Bensignor E, Carlotti DN: Conduite à tenir face à une démodecie chez le chien. Point Vét 30:667, 1999.
136. Brockis DC: Otitis externa due to *Demodex canis*. Vet Rec 135:464, 1994.
137. Burkett G, et al: Immunology of dogs with juvenile-onset generalized demodicosis as determined by lymphoblastogenesis and CD4:CD8 ratios. J Vet All Clin Immunol 4:46, 1996.
138. Burrows M: Evaluation of the clinical efficacy of moxidectin in the treatment of generalized demodicosis in the dog. Proc Aust Coll Vet Sci, 1997.
139. Bussieras J, Chermette R: Amitraz and canine demodicosis. J Am Anim Hosp Assoc 22:779, 1986.
140. Carlotti DN, et al: Therapy of generalized demodicosis with variable oral doses of milbemycine oxime in 88 dogs. In Kwochka KW, et al (eds): Advances in Veterinary Dermatology III. Butterworth Heinemann, Oxford, 1998, p 583.
141. Caswell JL, et al: A prospective study on the immunophenotype and temporal changes in the histologic lesions of canine demodicosis. Vet Pathol 34:279, 1997.
142. Caswell JL, et al: Canine demodicosis: A reexamination of the histopathologic lesions and description of the immunophenotype of infiltrating cells. Vet Dermatol 6:9, 1995.
143. Caswell JL, et al: Establishment of *Demodex canis* on canine skin engrafted onto scid-beige mice. J Parasitol 82:911, 1996.
144. Cayatte SM, et al: Perifollicular melanosis in the dog. Vet Dermatol 3:165, 1992.
145. Chen C: A review of canine demodicosis. Proc Annu Memb Meet Am Acad Vet Dermatol Am Coll Vet Dermatol 14:13, 1998.
146. Chen C: A short-tailed demodectic mite and *Demodex canis* infestation in a Chihuahua dog. Vet Dermatol 6:227, 1995.
147. Chesney CJ: Short form of *Demodex* species mite in the dog: Occurrence and measurements. J Small Anim Pract 40:58, 1999.
148. Corbett R, et al: Cellular immune responsiveness in dogs with demodectic mange. Transplant Proc 7:557, 1975.
149. Corbett RB, et al: The cell-mediated immune response: Its inhibition and *in vitro* reversal in dogs with demodectic mange. Fed Proc 35:589, 1976.
150. Day MJ: An immunohistochemical study of the lesions of demodicosis in the dog. J Comp Path 116:203, 1997.
151. Dodds J: Bleeding disorders: Their importance in everyday practice. Proc Am Anim Hosp Assoc 44:147, 1977.
152. Duclos DD, et al: Prognosis for treatment of adult-onset demodicosis in dogs: 34 cases (1979–1990). J Am Vet Med Assoc 204:616, 1994.
153. Folz SD: Demodicosis (*Demodex canis*). Comp Cont Educ 5:116, 1983.
154. Fondati A: The efficacy of daily oral ivermectin in the treatment of 10 cases of generalized demodicosis in adult dogs. Vet Dermatol 7:99, 1996.
155. Franc M, Soubeyroux H: Le traitement de la démodécie du chien par un collier à 9 pourcent amitraz. Rev Méd Vét 137:583, 1986.
156. Gaafer SM, Greeve J: Natural transmission of *Demodex canis* in dogs. J Am Vet Med Assoc 148:1043, 1966.
157. Garfield RA, Reedy LM: The use of oral milbemycin oxime (Interceptor) in the treatment of chronic generalized demodicosis. Vet Dermatol 3:231, 1992.
158. Guaguère E: La démodécie du chien adulte. A propos de 22 cas. Prat Méd Chir Anim Comp 26:411, 1991.
159. Guaguère E: Efficacy of daily oral ivermectin treatment in 38 dogs with generalized demodicosis: A study of relapse rates. In: Kwochka KW, et al (eds): Advances in Veterinary Dermatology III. Butterworth Heinemann, Oxford, 1998, p 453.
160. Guaguère E: La démodecie canine; stratégie thérapeutique. Prat Méd Chir Anim Comp 30:295, 1995.
161. Hamann F, et al: Canine demodicosis. Kleintierpraxis 42:745, 1997.
162. Havrileck B, et al: Suivi immunitaire individuel de chiens démodéciques par intradermoréactions à la phytohemagglutinin. Applications au prognostic. Rev Méd Vét 140:599, 1989.
163. Healy MC, Gaafar SM: Demonstration of reaginic antibody (IgE) in canine demodectic mange: An immunofluorescent study. Vet Parasitol 3:107, 1977.
164. Healy MC, Gaafar SM: Immunodeficiency in canine demodectic mange. II. Skin reactions to phytohemagglutinin and concanavalin A. Vet Parasitol 3:133, 1977.
165. Hiller A, Desch CE: A new species of *Demodex* mite in the dog: Case report. Proc Annu Memb Meet Am Acad Vet Dermatol Am Coll Vet Dermatol 13:118, 1997.
166. Hirsch DC, et al: Suppression of *in vitro* lymphocyte transformation by serum from dogs with generalized demodicosis. Am J Vet Res 36:195, 1975.
167. Holm B: Clinical efficacy of milbemycine oxime in the treatment of generalized demodicosis in the dog: A retrospective study of 40 cases (1993–1995). In Kwochka KW, et al (eds): Advances in Veterinary Dermatology III. Butterworth Heinemann, Oxford, 1998, p 582.
168. Krawiec DR, Gaafar SM: Studies on immunology of demodicosis. J Am Anim Hosp Assoc 16:669, 1980.
169. Kwochka KW, et al: The efficacy of amitraz for generalized demodicosis in dogs: A study of two concentrations and frequencies of application. Comp Cont Educ 2:234, 1980.
170. Kwochka KW: Demodicosis. In: Griffin CE, et al (eds): Current Veterinary Dermatology. Mosby–Year Book, St. Louis, 1993, p 72.

171. Lemarie SL: Canine demodicosis. Comp Cont Ed 18:354, 1996.
172. Lemarie SL, et al: A retrospective study of juvenile- and adult-onset generalized demodicosis in dogs (1986:91). Vet Dermatol 7:3, 1996.
173. Lemarie SL, Horohov DW: Evaluation of interleukin-2 production and interleukin-2 receptor expression in dogs with generalized demodicosis. Vet Dermatol 7:213, 1996.
174. Mason KV: A new species of *Demodex* mite with *D. canis* causing canine demodicosis: A case report. Proc Annu Memb Meet Am Acad Vet Dermatol Am Coll Vet Dermatol 9:92, 1993.
175. Medleau LM, et al: Efficacy of daily amitraz therapy for generalized demodicosis in dogs: Two independent studies. J Am Anim Hosp Assoc 31:246, 1995.
176. Medleau L, et al: Daily ivermectin for treatment of generalized demodicosis in dogs. Vet Dermatol 7:209, 1996.
177. Miller WH, Jr, et al: Dermatologic disorders of the Chinese Shar Peis: 58 cases (1981–1989). J Am Vet Med Assoc 200:986, 1992.
178. Miller WH Jr, et al: Efficacy of milbemycin oxime in the treatment of generalized demodicosis in adult dogs. J Am Vet Med Assoc 203:1426, 1993.
179. Miller WH Jr, et al: Clinical efficacy of increased dosages of milbemycin oxime for treatment of generalized demodicosis in adult dogs. J Am Vet Med Assoc 207:1581, 1995.
180. Mojzisova S, et al: Studies on the immunology of canine demodicosis. In: Kwochka, KW, et al (eds): Advances in Veterinary Dermatology III. Butterworth Heinemann, Oxford, 1998, p 498.
181. Mojzisova J, et al: The immunomodulatory effect of levamisole with the use of amitraz in dogs with uncomplicated generalized demodicosis. Vet Med (Praha) 42:307, 1997.
181a. Mozos E, et al: Leishmaniosis and generalized demodicosis in three dogs: A clinicopathological and immunohistochemical study. J Comp Pathol 120:257, 1999.
182. Muller GH: Demodicosis treatment with Mitaban liquid concentrate (amitraz). J Am Anim Hosp Assoc 19:435, 1983.
183. Mueller RS, Bettenay SV: Milbemycin oxime in the treatment of canine demodicosis. Aust Vet Practit 25:122, 1995.
183a. Mueller RS, Bettenay SV: An unusual presentation of canine demodicosis caused by a long-bodied *Demodex* mite in a Lakeland terrier. Aust Vet Practit 29:128, 1999.
183b. Mueller RS, et al: Daily oral ivermectin for treatment of generalised demodicosis in 23 dogs. Aust Vet Practit 29:132, 1999.
184. Muse R, Walder EJ: Nodular granulomatous dermatitis and generalized demodicosis in a dog. Proc Annu Memb Meet Am Acad Vet Dermatol Am Coll Vet Dermatol 14:75, 1998.
185. Nayak DC, et al: Prevalence of canine demodicosis in Orissa (India). Vet Parasitol 73:347, 1997.
186. Nayak DC, et al: Therapeutic efficacy of some homeopathic preparations against experimentally produced demodicosis in canines. Indian Vet J 75:342, 1998.
187. Nutting WB: Hair follicle mites (Acari: Demodicidae) of man. Int J Dermatol 15:79, 1976.
188. Nutting WB: Hair follicle mites (*Demodex* spp.) of medical and veterinary concern. Cornell Vet 66:214, 1976.
189. Nutting WB, Desch CE: *Demodex canis*: Redescription and reevaluation. Cornell Vet 68:139, 1978.
190. Owen LN: Transplantation of canine osteosarcoma. Eur J Cancer 5:615, 1969.
191. Paradis M, et al: Efficacy of daily ivermectin treatment in a dog with amitraz-resistant, generalized demodicosis. Vet Dermatol 3:85, 1992.
192. Paradis M, Page N: Topical (pour-on) ivermectin in the treatment of canine generalized demodicosis. Vet Dermatol 9:55, 1998.
193. Paulik S, et al: Evaluation of canine lymphocyte blastogenesis prior and after *in vitro* suppression by dog demodicosis serum using ethidium bromide fluorescence assay. Vet Med (Praha) 41:7, 1996.
194. Paulik S, et al: Lymphocyte blastogenesis to concanavalin A in dogs with localized demodicosis according to curation of disease. Vet Med (Praha) 41:245, 1996.
195. Reecy NR, et al: Serum thyroxine levels in canine demodicosis. Indian J Anim Sci 61:1300, 1991.
196. Ristie Z, et al: Ivermectin for treatment of generalized demodicosis in dogs. J Am Vet Med Assoc 207:1308, 1995.
197. Roy S, et al: Therapeutic evaluation of herbal ectoparasiticides against canine demodicosis. Indian Vet J 73:871, 1996.
198. Sako S, Yamane O: Studies on the canine demodicosis. III. Examination of the oral-internal infection, intrauterine infection, and infection through respiratory tract. Jpn J Parasitol 11:499, 1962.
199. Sako S: Studies on the canine demodicosis. IV. Experimental infection of *Demodex folliculorum var. canis* to dogs. Trans Tottori Soc Agri Sci 17:45, 1964.
199a. Saricomichelakis M, et al: Adult-onset demodicosis in two dogs due to *Demodex canis* and a short-bodied demodectic mite. J Small Anim Pract 40:529, 1999.
200. Schwassmann M, et al: Use of lufenuron for treatment of generalized demodicosis in dogs. Vet Dermatol 8:11, 1997.
201. Scott DW, et al: Studies on the therapeutic and immunologic aspects of generalized demodectic mange in the dog. J Am Anim Hosp Assoc 10:233, 1974.
202. Scott DW, et al: Further studies on the therapeutic and immunologic aspects of generalized demodectic mange in the dog. J Am Anim Hosp Assoc 12:203, 1976.
203. Scott DW, Walton DK: Experiences with the use of amitraz and ivermectin for the treatments of generalized demodicosis in dogs. J Am Anim Hosp Assoc 21:535, 1985.
203a. Scott DW: Treatment of canine demodicosis: Then and now. Proc Annu Memb Meet Am Acad Vet Dermatol Am Coll Vet Dermatol 15:111, 1999.
204. Tapp T, et al: Efficacy of alternate day oral ivermectin in the treatment of generalized demodicosis. Proc Annu Memb Meet Am Acad Vet Dermatol Am Coll Vet Dermatol 14:25, 1998.
205. Totman M, et al: Secondary immunodeficiency in dogs with enteric, dermatologic, infectious, or parasitic diseases. J Vet Med B 45:321, 1998.
206. Wilkie BN, et al: Deficient cutaneous response to PHA-P in healthy puppies from a kennel with a high prevalence of demodicosis. Can J Comp Med 43:415, 1979.
207. Wolfe JH, Halliwell REW: Total hemolytic comple-

ment values in normal and diseased dog populations. Vet Immunol Immunopathol 1:287, 1980.

Feline Demodicosis

208. Bailey RG, Thompson RC: Demodectic mange in a cat. Aust Vet J 57:49, 1981.
209. Beale KM: Contagion and occult demodicosis in a family of 2 cats. Proc Annu Memb Meet Am Acad Vet Dermatol Am Coll Vet Dermatol 14:99, 1998.
210. Chalmers S, et al: Demodicosis in two cats seropositive for feline immunodeficiency virus. J Am Vet Med Assoc 194:256, 1989.
210a. Chesney CJ: An unusual species of demodex mite in a cat. Vet Rec 123:671, 1988.
211. Conroy JD, et al: New *Demodex* sp. infesting a cat: A case report. J Am Anim Hosp Assoc 18:405, 1982.
212. Cowman LA, et al: Generalized demodicosis in a cat responsive to amitraz. J Am Vet Med Assoc 192:1442, 1988.
213. Chesney CJ: Demodicosis in the cat. J Small Anim Pract 30:689, 1989.
214. Desch C, Nutting WB: *Demodex cati*, Hirst, 1919: A redescription. Cornell Vet 69:280, 1989.
215. Desch CE Jr, Stewart TB: *Demodex gatoi*: new species of hair follicle mite (*Acari: Demodecidae*) from the domestic cat (*Carnivora: Felidae*). J Med Entomol 36:167, 1999.
216. Foley RH: Feline demodicosis. Comp Cont Ed 17: 481, 1995.
217. Gabbert N, Feldman BF: A case report—Feline *Demodex*. Feline Pract 6:32, 1976.
218. Guaguère E, et al: *Demodex cati* infestation in association with feline cutaneous squamous cell carcinoma *in situ*: A report of five cases. Vet Dermatol 10:61, 1999.
219. Kontos V, et al: Two rare disorders in the cat: Demodectic otitis externa and Sarcoptic mange. Feline Pract 26:18, 1998.
220. McDougal BJ, Novak CP: Feline demodicosis caused by an unnamed *Demodex* mite. Comp Cont Educ (SAC) 8:820, 1986.
221. Medleau L, et al: Demodicosis in cats. J Am Anim Hosp Assoc 24:85, 1988.
222. Morris DO: Contagious demodicosis in three cats residing in the same household. J Am Anim Hosp Assoc 32:350, 1996.
223. Morris DO, Beale KM: Feline demodicosis—a retrospective of 15 cases. Proc Annu Memb Meet Am Acad Vet Dermatol Am Coll Vet Dermatol 13:127, 1997.
224. Nutting WB: *Demodex crecti*, notes on its biology. J Parasitol 44:328, 1958.
225. Stogdale L, Moore DJ: Feline demodicosis. J Am Anim Hosp Assoc 18:427, 1982.
226. White SD, et al: Generalized demodicosis associated with diabetes mellitus in two cats. J Am Vet Med Assoc 191:448, 1987.

Canine Scabies

227. Arlian LG, et al: Survival of adults and developmental stages of *Sarcoptes scabiei var. canis* when off the host. Exp Appl Acarol 6:181, 1989.
228. Arlian LG, et al: Cross infestivity of *Sarcoptes scabiei*. J Am Acad Dermatol 10:979, 1984.
229. Arlian LG, et al: The development of protective immunity in canine scabies. Vet Parasitol 62:133, 1996.
230. Arlian LG, et al: Characterization of lymphocyte subtypes in scabietic skin lesions of naive and sensitized dogs. Vet Parasitol 68:347, 1997.
231. Beck W, Hiepe TH: Untersuchungen zu einem intrakutantest mit einer *Sarcoptes*-milbenextrakt-lösung (*Acari: Sarcoptidae*) als methode zum nachweis an *Sarcoptes*—räude erkrankter hunde. Tierärztl Wschr 111:174, 1998.
232. Bergvall K: Clinical efficacy of milbemycin oxime in the treatment of canine scabies: A study of 56 cases. Vet Dermatol 9:231, 1998.
233. Bornstein S: Experimental infection of dogs with *Sarcoptes scabiei* derived from naturally infected wild red foxes (*Vulpes vulpes*): Clinical observations. Vet Dermatol 2:151, 1991.
234. Bornstein S, Zakrisson G: Humoral antibody response to experimental *Sarcoptes scabiei var. vulpes* infection in the dog. Vet Dermatol 4:107, 1993.
235. Bornstein S, et al: Evaluation of an enzyme-linked immunosorbent assay (ELISA) for the serological diagnosis of canine sarcoptic mange. Vet Dermatol 7: 21, 1996.
236. Carlotti DN, Bensignor E: La gale sarcoptique du chien: étude retrospective de 38 cas. Prat Méd Chir Anim Comp 32:117, 1997.
237. Charlesworth EN, Johnson JL: An epidemic of canine scabies in man. Arch Dermatol 110:574, 1974.
238. Curtis CF: Use of 0.25 per cent fipronil spray to treat sarcoptic mange in a litter of five-week-old puppies. Vet Rec 139:43, 1996.
239. Das SS: Effect of a herbal compound for treatment of sarcoptic mange infestations on dogs. Vet Parasitol 63:303, 1996.
240. Estes SA, et al: Experimental canine scabies in humans. J Am Acad Dermatol 9:397, 1983.
241. Folz SD: Canine scabies (*Sarcoptes scabiei* infestation). Comp Cont Educ 6:176, 1984.
242. Folz SD, et al: Evaluation of a sponge-on therapy for canine scabies. J Vet Pharmacol Ther 7:29, 1984.
243. Griffin CE: Scabies. In Griffin CE, et al (eds): Current Veterinary Dermatology. Mosby–Year Book, St. Louis, 1993, p 85.
244. Huang HP, et al: *Sarcoptes scabiei* infestation in a cat. Feline Pract 26:10, 1998.
244a. Jagannath MS, Yathiraj S: Clinical evaluation of doramectin in the treatment of ectoparasites of canines. Indian Vet J 76:333, 1999.
245. Maldonado RR, et al: Norwegian scabies due to *Sarcoptes scabiei var. canis*. Arch Dermatol 113:1733, 1977.
246. Miller WH Jr, et al: Treatment of canine scabies with milbemycin oxime. Can Vet J 37:219, 1996.
247. Morris DO, Dunstan RW: A histomorphological study of sarcoptic acariasis in the dog: 19 cases. J Am Anim Hosp Assoc 32:119, 1996.
248. Paradis M, et al: Topical (pour-on) ivermectin in the treatment of canine scabies. Can Vet J 38:379, 1997.
249. Paradis M: Scabies and *Cheyletiella*. Proc Annu Memb Meet Am Acad Vet Dermatol Am Coll Vet Dermatol 13:48, 1997.
250. Prélaud P, Guaguère E: Sensitization to the house dust mite, *Dermatophagoides farinae*, in dogs with sarcoptic mange. Vet Dermatol 6:205, 1995.
250a. Zahler M, et al: Molecular analyses suggest monospecificity of the genus *Sarcoptes* (*Acari: Sarcophidae*). Int J Parasitol 29:759, 1999.

Feline Scabies

250b. Delucchi L, Castro E: Use of doramectin for treatment of notoedric mange in five cats. J Am Vet Med Assoc 216:215, 2000.
251. Ferrero O, et al: Doramectina en el tratamiento de la sarna notoedrica del gato. Rev Med Vet (Argent) 77:106, 1996.
252. Foley RH: A notoedric manage epizootic in an island's cat population. Feline Pract 19:8, 1991.

Spiders

253. Berger RS: The unremarkable brown recluse spider bite. J Am Med Assoc 225:1109, 1973.
254. King KE: Spider bites. Arch Dermatol 123:41, 1987.
255. Meerdink GL: Bites and stings of venomous animals. In Kirk RW (ed): Current Veterinary Therapy VIII. W.B. Saunders Co., Philadelphia, 1983.
256. Muir G: Red back spider bite in a cat. Cont Ther Ser 191:56, 1996
257. Northway RB: A therapeutic approach to venomous spider bites. Vet Med (SAC) 80:38, 1985.
258. Wong RC, et al: Spider bites (in depth review). Arch Dermatol 123:98, 1987.

Pediculosis

258a. Bordeau W: Traitement d'un cas de phtiriose à Trichodectes canis par le fipronyl chez un chat. Point Vét 30:655, 1999.
259. Cooper PR, Penaliggon J: Use of fipronil to eliminate recurrent infestation by *Tricodectes canis* in a pack of bloodhounds. Vet Rec 139:95, 1996.
260. Frye FL, Furman DP: Phthiriasis in a dog. J Am Vet Med Assoc 152:1113, 1968.
261. Majumder P, et al: Control of lice infestation in dog with Butox (Deltamethrin) in South Tripura. Indian J Anim Health 33:65, 1994.
261a. Mencke N: Efficacy of Advantage against natural infestations of dogs with lice: a field study from Norway. Compend Cont Edu Pract Vet 22(Suppl): 18, 2000.
262. Shastri UV: Efficacy of ivermectin against lice infestation in cattle, buffaloes, goats, and dogs. Indian Vet J 68:191, 1991.
263. Shipstone M, et al.: Milbemycin oxime as a treatment for canine scabies. Aust Vet Practit 27:170, 1997.

Fleas

264. Arther RG, et al: Efficacy of imidacloprid for removal and control of fleas (*Ctenocephalides felis*) on dogs. Am J Vet Res 58:848, 1997.
265. Ascher F, et al: Knock-down effect of a 2 per cent permethrin spray used for flea allergy dermatitis therapy. In Kwochka KW, et al (eds): Advances in Veterinary Dermatology III. Butterworth Heinemann, Oxford, 1998, p 566.
265a. Ascher F, et al: Antifeeding effect of modern insecticides. Proc Br Vet Dermatol Study Group, Spring 1998, p 20.
266. Atwell R, et al: The use of topical fipronil in field studies for flea control in domestic dogs. Aust Vet Practit 27:175, 1997.
267. Baker KP, Elharam S: The biology of *Ctenocephalides canis* in Ireland. Vet Parasitol 45:141, 1992.
268. Blagburn BL, et al: Efficacy of lufenuron against developmental stages of fleas (*Ctenocephalides felis felis*) in dogs housed in simulated home environments. Am J Vet Res 56:464, 1995.
268a. Blagburn BL, et al: Dose titration of an injectable formulation of lufenuron in cats experimentally infested with fleas. Am J Vet Res 60:1513, 1999.
269. Bourdeau P: Indoor control of *Ctenocephalides felis*: Comparison of three products (foggers, fumigation) in a replicated room. In: Kwochka KW, et al (eds): Advances in Veterinary Dermatology III. Butterworth Heinemann, Oxford, 1998, p 575.
270. Brown CR, et al: The efficacy of ultrasonic pest controllers for fleas and ticks. J S Afr Vet Assoc 62:110, 1991.
271. Carlotti DN, et al: Intéret d'une formulation de permethrine en spot-on dans le traitement de la dermatite par allergie aux piqûres de puce chez le chien: Une étude prospective de 24 cas. Prat Méd Chir Anim Comp 32:83, 1997.
272. Carlotti DN, et al: Therapy and prevention of flea allergy dermatitis with a new permethrin formulation (foam) in 12 cats. In Kwochka KW, et al (eds): Advances in Veterinary Dermatology III. Butterworth Heinemann, Oxford, 1998, p 574.
273. Chesney CJ: Species of flea found on cats and dogs in south west England: Further evidence of their polyxencus state and implications for flea control. Vet Rec 136:356, 1995.
273a. Dean SR, et al: Mode of action of lufenuron in adult *Ctenocephalides felis* (Siphonaptera: Pulicidae). J Med Entomol 36:486, 1999.
274. Dryden MW, et al: Effects of ultrasonic flea collars on *Ctenocephalides felis* on cats. J Am Vet Med Assoc 195:1717, 1989.
275. Dryden MW: Host association, on-host longevity and egg production of *Ctenocephalides felis felis*. Vet Parasitol 34:117, 1989.
275a. Dryden MW, Broce AB: Development of a flea trap for collecting newly emerged *Ctenocephalides felis* (Siphonaptera: Pulicidae) in homes. J Med Entomol 30:901, 1993.
275b. Dryden MW, et al: Techniques for estimating on-animal populations of *Ctenocephalides felis* (Siphonaptera: Pulicidae). J Med Entomol 31:631, 1994.
275c. Dryden MW: Laboratory evaluations of topical flea control products. Proc Br Vet Dermatol Study Group, Spring 1998, p 14.
275d. Dryden MW, et al: Control of fleas on pets and in homes by use of imidacloprid or lufenuron and a pyrethrin spray. J Am Vet Med Assoc 215:36, 1999.
275e. Dryden M: Investigations of alternative flea control methodologies. Proc Annu Kansas St Univ Conf Vet 61:37, 1999.
275f. Everett R, et al: Comparative evaluation of the speed of flea kill of Advantage (imidacloprid) and Revolution (selamectin) on dogs. Compend Cont Edu Pract Vet 22(Suppl): 9, 2000.
276. Fisher MA, et al: Evaluation of flea control programmes for cats using fenthion and lufenuron. Vet Rec 138:79, 1996.
277. Foley JE, et al: Seroprevalence of *Bartonella henselae* in cattery cats: Association with cattery hygiene and flea infestation. Vet Quart 20:1, 1998.
278. Franc M, Cadieurques MC: Comparative activity in dogs of deltamethrin- and diazinon-impregnated collars against *Ctenocephalides felis*. Am J Vet Res 59:59, 1998.
279. Franc M, Cadiergues M: Use of injectable lufenuron for treatment of infestations of *Ctenocephalides felis* in cats. Am J Vet Res 58:140, 1997.
280. Franc M, et al: Répartition des espèces de puces rencontrées chez le chien en France. Rev Méd Vét 149:135, 1998.

281. Franc M, Cadiergues MC: Activity of deltamethrin shampoo against *Ctenocephalides felis* and *Rhipicephalus sanguineus* in dogs. Vet Parasitol 81:341, 1999.
281a. Guaguère E, et al: Efficacité de l'imidaclopride dans le traitement de la dermatite par allergie aux piqûres de puces chez le chien. Prat Méd Chir Anim Comp 34:231, 1999.
282. Guerrini VH, Kriticos CM: Effects of azadirachtin on *Ctenocephalides felis* in the dog and cat. Vet Parasitol 74:289, 1998.
283. Harvey RG: Dermatitis in a cat associated with *Spilopsyllus cuniculi*. Vet Rec 126:89, 1990.
284. Harvey RG, et al: Prospective study comparing fipronil with dichlorvos/fenitrothin and methoprene/pyrethrins in control of flea bite hypersensitivity in cats. Vet Rec 141:628, 1997.
285. Hastriter MW: Establishment of the tungid flea, *Tunga monositus*, in the United States. Great Basin Naturalist 57:281, 1997.
286. Henderson G, et al: The effects of *Steinernema carpocapsea* (Weiser) application to different life stages on adult emergence of the cat flea *Ctenocephalides felis* (Bouche). Vet Dermatol 6:159, 1995.
287. Herrmann R, et al: Efficacy of a 0.25 per cent fipronil spray in the control of flea allergy dermatitis in the dog. Kleintierpraxis 43:199, 1998.
288. Hinkle NC, et al: Host grooming efficacy for regulation of cat flea populations. J Med Entomol 35:266, 1998.
288a. Hopkins T: Imidacloprid topical formulation: larvicidal effects against *Ctenocephalides felis* in the surroundings of treated dogs. Compend Cont Edu Pract Vet 19:410, 1997.
289. Hopkins T: Imidacloprid and resolution of signs of flea allergy dermatitis in dogs. Canine Pract 23:18, 1998.
290. Hopkins TJ, et al: Efficacy of imidacloprid to remove and prevent *Ctenocephalides felis* infestations on dogs and cats. Aust Vet Practit 26:150, 1996.
291. Hutchinson MJ, et al: Evaluation of flea control strategies using fipronil on cats in a controlled simulated home environment. Vet Rec 142:356, 1998.
292. Imai S, et al: Species distribution of flea infested to dogs and cats in Japan. J Jpn Vet Med Assoc 48:775, 1995.
293. Jacobs DE, et al: Comparison of flea control strategies using imidacloprid or lufenuron on cats in a controlled simulated home environment. Am J Vet Res 58:1260, 1997.
294. Jacobs DE, et al: A novel approach to flea control on cats, using pyriproxyfen. Vet Rec 139:559, 1996.
295. Jacobs DE, et al: Duration of activity of imidacloprid, a novel adulticide for flea control, against *Ctenocephalides felis* on cats. Vet Rec 140:259, 1997.
296. Kalkofen UP, Greenberg J: *Echidnophaga gallinacea* infestations in dogs. J Am Vet Med Assoc 165:447, 1974.
296a. Kern WH, et al: Outdoor survival and development of immature cat fleas (Siphonaptera: Pulicidae) in Florida. J Med Entomol 36:207, 1999.
297. Koutinas A, et al: Flea species from dogs and cats in northern Greece: Environmental and clinical implications. Vet Parasitol 58:109, 1995.
298. Lebreux B, et al: Evaluation of the efficacy of a diazinon + pyriproxyfen collar in the treatment and control of flea infestation in cats. J Vet Pharm Therap 20:157, 1997.
299. Le Nain S, et al: Efficacy of a 0.25 per cent fipronil formulation in the control of flea allergy dermatitis in the dog. In Kwochka KW, et al (eds): Advances in Veterinary Dermatology III. Butterworth Heinemann, Oxford, 1998, p 570.
299a. Liebisch A, Reimann U: The efficacy of imidacloprid against flea infestation on dogs compared with three other topical preparations. Canine Pract 25:8, 2000.
300. McDonald BJ, et al: An investigation on the influence of feline flea allergy on the fecundity of the cat flea. Vet Dermatol 9:75, 1998.
301. Maskiell G: Clinical impressions of s-methoprene-impregnated collars and lufenuron for flea control in dogs and cats. Aust Vet Practit 25:142, 1995.
301a. Mehlhorn H: Mode of action of imidacloprid and comparison with other insecticides (i.e., fipronil and selamectin) during in vivo and in vitro experiments. Compend Cont Edu Pract Vet 22(Suppl): 4, 2000.
301b. Meola RW, et al: Effect of lufenuron on chorionic and cuticular structure of unhatched larval *Ctenocephalides felis* (Siphonaptera: Pulicidae). J Med Entomol 36:92, 1999.
302. Metzger ME, Rust MK: Effect of temperature on cat flea development and overwintering. J Med Entomol 34:173, 1997.
303. Nishida Y et al: Disinfestation of experimentally infested cat fleas, *Ctenocephalides felis*, on cats and dogs by oral lufenuron. J Vet Med Sci 57:655, 1995.
303a. Noble SJ, Armstrong PJ: Bee sting envenomation resulting in secondary immune-mediated hemolytic anemia in two dogs. J Am Vet Med Assoc 214:1026, 1999.
304. Noden BH, et al: Molecular identification of *Rickettsia typhi* and *R. felis* in co-infected *Ctenocephalides felis*. J Med Entomol 35:410, 1998.
305. Pampiglione S, et al: *Tunga penetrans* (Insecta: Siphonaptera) in pigs in São Tomé (Equatorial Africa): Epidemiological, clinical, morphological, and histopathological aspects. Rev Elev Méd Vét Pays Trop 51:201, 1998.
306. Postal JM, et al: Field efficacy of a mechanical pump spray formulation containing 0.25 per cent fipronil in the treatment and control of flea infestation and associated dermatologic signs in dogs and cats. Vet Dermatol 6:153, 1995.
307. Postal JM, et al: Field efficacy of a 10 per cent fipronil spot-on formulation in the treatment and control of flea infestation. In Kwochka KW, et al (eds): Advances in Veterinary Dermatology III. Butterworth Heinemann, Oxford, 1998, p 568.
308. Robinson WH: Distribution of cat flea larvae in the carpeted household environment. Vet Dermatol 6:145, 1995.
309. Ross DH, et al: Topical pyriproxyfen for control of the cat flea and management of insecticide resistance. Feline Pract 26:18, 1998.
310. Rust MK, Dryden MW: The biology, ecology, and management of the cat flea. Ann Rev Entomol 42:451, 1997.
311. Silverman J, et al: Infection of cat flea, *Ctenocephalides felis* (Bouche) by *Neoaplectana carpocapsai* Weiser. J Nematol 14:394, 1982.
312. Smith RD, et al: Impact of an orally administered insect growth regulator (lufenuron) on flea infestations of dogs in a controlled simulated home environment. Am J Vet Res 57:502, 1996.
313. Studdert VP, et al: Dermatitis of the pinnae of cats in Australia associated with European rabbit flea. Vet Rec 123:624, 1988.
314. Sture GH, et al: Dose selection of VK-124-114, a

Mosquito Dermatitis

315. Mason KV, et al: Mosquito bite-caused eosinophilic dermatitis in cats. J Am Vet Med Assoc 198:2086, 1991.
316. Nagata M, Ishida T: Cutaneous reactivity to mosquito bites and its antigens in cats. Vet Dermatol 8:19, 1997.

Fly Dermatitis

317. Penny DS: Fly strike in a dog. Vet Rec 125:79, 1989.
318. Pucheu-Haston CM, et al: Allergic cross-reactivities in flea-reactive canine serum samples. Am J Vet Res 57:1000, 1996.
319. White SD, Bourdeau P: Hypersensibilités aux piqûres de diptères chez les carnivores. Point Vét 27:203, 1995.

Myiasis

320. Bourdeau, P, et al: Myiase à Dermatobia hominis. Rec Méd Vét 164:901, 1988.
321. Bragagna P, et al: Furuncular myiasis in a dog: Case report. Praxis Vet 18:20, 1997.
322. Chermette R: A case of canine otitis due to screw-worm, Cochliomyia hominivorax, in France. Vet Rec 124:641, 1989.
323. Dongus H, et al: Cordylobia anthropophaga als erreger einer Hautmyiasis bei einem Hund in Deutschland. Tierartztl Prax 24:493, 1996.
324. Fox MT, et al: Tumbu fly (Cordylobia anthropophaga) myiasis in a quarantined dog in England. Vet Rec 130:100, 1992.
325. Hendrix CM: Facultative myiasis in dogs and cats. Comp Cont Educ 13:86, 1991.
326. Hendrix CM, et al: Furunculoid myiasis in a dog caused by Cordylobia anthropophaga. J Am Vet Med Assoc 207:1187, 1995.
327. Jayagopala R, et al: Ivermectin in cutaneous myiasis of dogs. Indian Vet J 70:557, 1993.
328. Mulder JB: The medical marvels of maggots. J Am Vet Med Assoc 195:1497, 1989.
329. Nivoix R, Chermette R: Use of ivermectin for prevention of cutaneous tumbu fly (Cordylobia anthropophaga) myiasis in dogs. In: Kwochka KW, et al (eds): Advances in Veterinary Dermatology III. Butterworth Heinemann, Oxford, 1998, p 471.
330. Roosje PJ, et al: A case of Dermatobia hominis in a dog in the Netherlands. Vet Dermatol 3:183, 1992.

Cuterebra Species Infestation

331. Baird CR: Development of Cuterebra ruficrus (Dipterae Cuterebridae) in six species of rabbits and rodents with a morphological comparison of C. ruficrus and C. jellisoni third instars. J Med Entomol 9:81, 1972.
332. Fitzgerald SD, et al: A fatal case of intrathoracic cuterebriasis in a cat. J Am Anim Hosp Assoc 32:353, 1996.
333. Kazocos KR, et al: Cuterebra species as a cause of pharyngeal myiasis in cats. J Am Anim Hosp Assoc 16:773, 1980.

Hymenoptera (Bees, Wasps, and Hornets)

334. Cowell AK, et al: Severe systemic reactions to Hymenoptera stings in three dogs. J Am Vet Med Assoc 198:1014, 1991.

Canine Facial Eosinophilic Folliculitis and Furunculosis

335. Gross TL: Canine eosinophilic furunculosis of the face. In Ihrke PJ, Mason IS, White SD (eds): Advances in Veterinary Dermatology, Vol 2. Pergamon Press, Oxford, 1993, p 211.
336. Holtz CS: Eosinophilic dermatitis in a Siberian husky cross Calif Vet 44:11, 1990.

Ants

337. Rakich PM, et al: Clinical and histologic characterization of cutaneous reactions to stings of the imported fire ant (Solenopsis invicta) in dogs. Vet Pathol 30:555, 1993.

Caterpillars

338. Chermette R, Chareyre G: A propos des chenilles processionnaires. Point Vét 26:9:1993.
339. Poisson L, et al: Quatre cas d'envenimation par les chenilles processionnaires du pin chez le chien. Point Vét 25:992, 1994.

Chapter 7
Viral, Rickettsial, and Protozoal Skin Diseases

These dermatoses are apparently rare in dogs and cats. Additionally, many of those that have been reported are associative or circumstantial in nature. This chapter is a brief overview of proven and suspected skin diseases of viral, rickettsial, and protozoal origin in dogs and cats.

• VIRAL DISEASES

Feline Leukemia Virus Infection

The feline leukemia virus (FeLV) is an oncogenic immunosuppressive retrovirus.[1, 22] Although it can induce skin tumors (lymphoma, fibrosarcoma), FeLV most commonly affects the skin by its cytosuppressive actions. Clinical signs include chronic or recurrent gingivitis or pyoderma (folliculitis, abscess, paronychia), poor wound healing, seborrhea, exfoliative dermatitis, generalized pruritus, and cutaneous horns.[40] The viral origin of the cutaneous horns was proved by positive gp70 immunochemical staining.[12]

A pruritic crusting dermatitis has been described in six FeLV-positive cats.[19] The lesions are scaly, erosive, and crusted, and vary in distribution. All cases have some involvement of the face (Fig. 7–1A) or head, either around the lips or perioral skin, pinnae, or preauricular skin. Other commonly involved sites include the feet or footpads, mucocutaneous junctions of the anus or prepuce, legs, or trunk (see Fig. 7–1B). At presentation, the cats usually are otherwise healthy.

The differential diagnosis depends on the distribution and the extent of the lesions and the owner's ability to assess whether the skin lesions preceded the pruritus. If pruritus is apparently primary, allergic disorders, feline scabies, *Cheyletiella*, and demodicosis should be considered. With crusting first, drug reaction, superficial pemphigus, systemic lupus erythematosus, and exfoliative dermatitis of thymoma must be considered.

All cats are FeLV positive on serology,[49] but skin biopsies are necessary to prove that the skin lesions are viral in origin. Histologically, the epidermis is irregularly hyperplastic and usually heavily crusted (Fig. 7–2). A characteristic feature is syncytial-type giant cell formation in the epidermis and outer root sheath of the hair follicles to the level of the isthmus (Fig. 7–3). Keratinocytes within and around the giant cells often are apoptotic. Involved skin shows positive gp70 staining while nonlesional skin from these cats or other FeLV-positive cats with no skin disease is negative.

The skin lesions respond poorly to treatment with antibiotics, glucocorticoids, or other agents. With time, the cats often show signs of internal disease, e.g., anorexia, lethargy, but none is found at necropsy.

Feline Immunodeficiency Virus Infection

Feline immunodeficiency virus (FIV) is another retrovirus that causes a variety of cytosuppressive disorders in the cat.[1, 48, 49] The most common clinical sign is chronic or recurrent oral disease (gingivitis, periodontal disease, stomatitis).[39, 42] Reported dermatologic signs include chronic or recurrent abscesses, chronic bacterial infections of the skin and ears, an

The diagnosis of cowpox is based on the results of diagnostic tests. Serum samples and fresh biopsy or scab material in viral transport medium are submitted to an appropriate diagnostic laboratory for serologic examination and viral isolation, respectively. Serologic tests cannot differentiate cowpox from other orthopox viruses. Histopathologic examination of secondary lesions usually supports the diagnosis, and orthopoxvirus involvement can be demonstrated by immunohistochemical techniques[5] or electron microscopy. Virus isolation is the only method of making a precise diagnosis.

There is no specific therapy for cowpox infection. If secondary bacterial infections of the skin or other organs occur, appropriate antibacterial therapy should be instituted. Severely ill animals, which typically have an underlying immunosuppressive disorder, require intense supportive care and may have to be euthanized. Glucocorticoids are contraindicated.

Feline cowpox has zoonotic potential for contact cats, dogs, and humans.[4a, 14, 19a, 44, 45, 45a] In humans, these contact infections are uncommon; they can be serious, however, especially if the individual is immunologically compromised. Lesions are typically nodular and occur most commonly on the hands and arms. A fatality in a human receiving corticosteroids has been documented.[44] Accordingly, all infected cats should be isolated and handled carefully. The cowpox virus can remain viable under dry temperature conditions for several years, but it is susceptible to various disinfectants, especially to hypochlorite solutions.[5] Dogs develop solitary, asymptomatic, self-healing ulcerated nodules.[42a, 45]

No data are available to indicate whether infection confers long-lasting immunity. To prevent possible reinfection, hunting should be prohibited.

Feline Infectious Peritonitis

Feline infectious peritonitis is a systemic viral disease caused by strains of coronaviruses. Effusive and noneffusive forms are most common[1] Skin lesions other than those associated with debility have not been reported. Several cats that have been experimentally infected have developed ulcerative lesions around the head and neck (Fig. 7–7).[2] Histopathologic tests showed changes typical of a superficial vasculitis, and viral antigen was demonstrated in blood vessel walls by immunohistochemical techniques.

Canine Distemper

Canine distemper is caused by a paramyxovirus.[1] In addition to severe respiratory, gastrointestinal, and neurologic disorders, the virus may produce skin lesions in some animals.

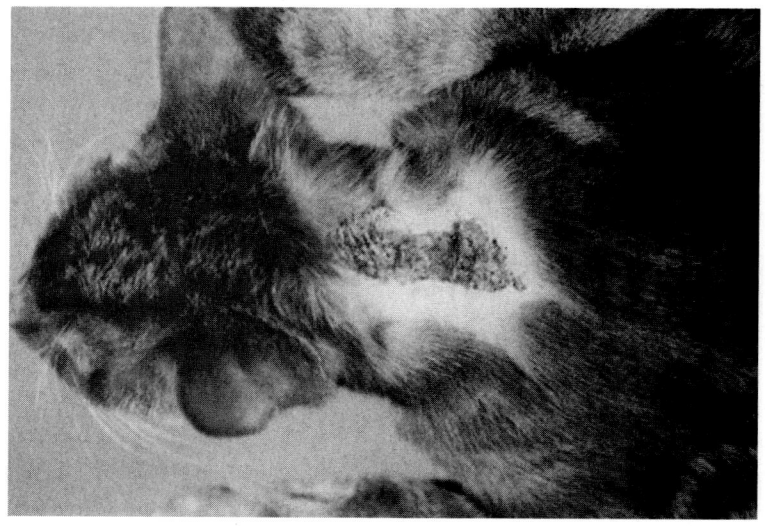

FIGURE 7–7. Well-demarcated necrosis and ulceration over the dorsal neck of a cat with feline infectious peritonitis.

Viral, Rickettsial, and Protozoal Skin Diseases • 523

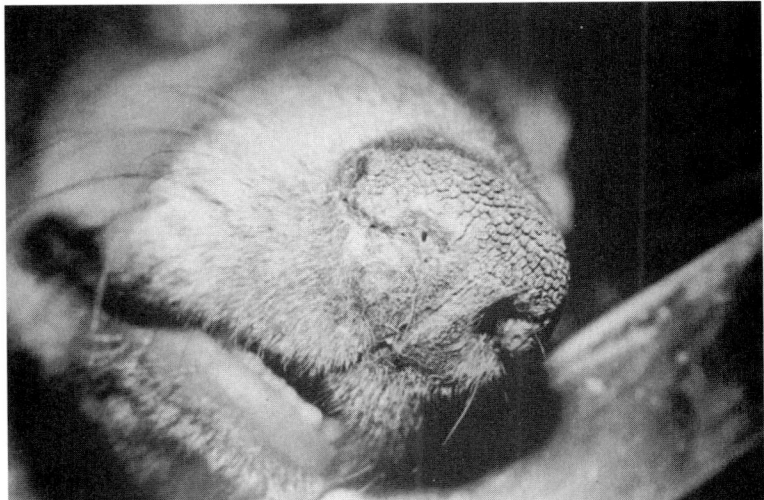

FIGURE 7–8. Nasal hyperkeratosis in a dog with canine distemper.

Because of their general debility, some dogs, and especially very young puppies, develop widespread impetigo (see Fig. 7–1F). The classic skin manifestation of distemper is the so-called hard pad disease, in which the dog develops nasal (Fig. 7–8) and footpad (Fig. 7–9) hyperkeratosis of varying severity. Although a variety of diseases (e.g., pemphigus foliaceus, lupus erythematosus, drug eruption) induce nasodigital hyperkeratosis, animals with those disorders are often not as systemically ill as dogs with distemper and have more widespread skin lesions. Distemper, leishmaniasis, necrolytic migratory erythema (see Chap. 10), and generic dog food skin disease (see Chap. 17) all can produce the nasodigital lesions and similar systemic signs of illness. The index of suspicion for distemper should be high when the pads are much harder to the touch than the degree of hyperkeratosis would suggest and the dog's vaccination history is poor.

Histologically, the skin or pad surface is covered with marked orthokeratotic and parakeratotic hyperkeratosis, and acidophilic cytoplasmic inclusion bodies are commonly seen in keratinocytes.[26] The inclusion bodies are variable in size and are round to irregular in outline. Nuclear inclusions are rare. Occasional multinucleated syncytial giant cells can

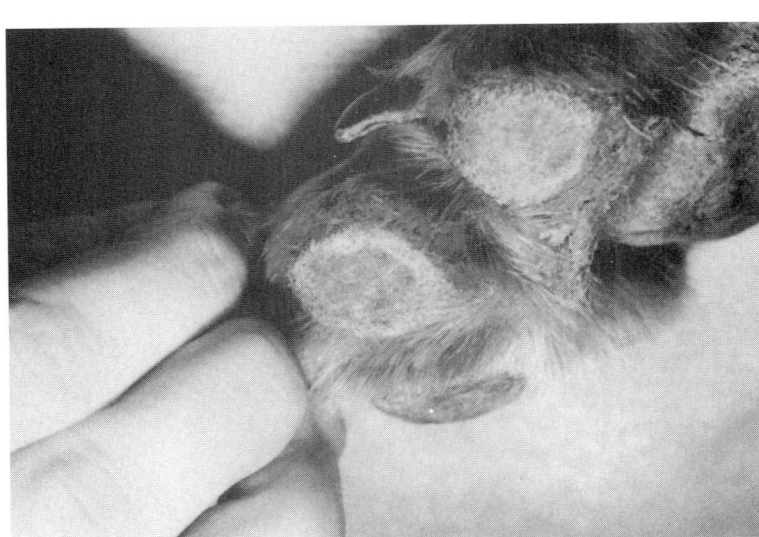

FIGURE 7–9. Digital hyperkeratosis in a dog with canine distemper.

be seen in the epidermis. Immunohistochemical detection of canine distemper virus in haired skin and footpad epithelium was reported to be very reliable for the antemortem diagnosis of distemper.[19b]

Contagious Viral Pustular Dermatitis

Contagious viral pustular dermatitis (orf, contagious ecthyma) is a disease that is found primarily in sheep and goats and is caused by a parapoxvirus.[41] Contagious viral pustular dermatitis was reported in a pack of hounds allowed to feed on sheep carcasses.[46] Lesions consisted of circular areas of acute moist dermatitis, ulceration, and crusts, typically around the head. Skin biopsy revealed epidermal hyperplasia, ballooning degeneration, acantholysis within the stratum spinosum, and marked infiltration of neutrophils. Saline suspensions of skin biopsies were applied to the scarified skin of a normal sheep. Crusts removed from the inoculation sites were processed for electron microscopy, and parapoxvirus virus particles were readily seen. One cat with parapoxvirus infection has been documented.[20] The cat had multiple large crusted lesions over the face and back. Further details were not provided.

Therapy for contagious viral pustular dermatitis is topical and varies according to the symptoms involved. The usual course of the disease in animals is 1 to 4 weeks. The disease may be transmitted to humans if broken skin is exposed to lesion material or contaminated objects. Generally, contagious viral pustular dermatitis is a benign disease in humans and results in the formation of a solitary lesion, especially on the hands. Lesions in humans are characterized by maculae that progress through a papular, nodular, and papillomatous stage. The lesions are usually centrally umbilicated and occasionally are bullous. Complications of contagious viral pustular dermatitis in humans include regional lymphadenopathy, lymphangitis, secondary bacterial infection, and rarely, generalized or systemic disease.

Pseudorabies

Pseudorabies is an acute, fatal viral disease caused by an α-herpesvirus.[1] Pigs are the main reservoir of infection. Dogs and cats can be infected by contact with an infected animal or, more typically, by eating raw pork products or offal. Incubation periods range from 2 to 10 days,[20a, 23] and death typically occurs within 48 hours of the onset of clinical signs.[32]

Early work suggested that intense, maniacal upper body pruritus was the cardinal feature of the disease in dogs.[23] More recent work, however, showed that this sign occurred in only 52% of affected dogs.[32] Ptyalism was a universal finding, followed by restlessness, anorexia, ataxia, and a variety of other neurologic abnormalities. When present, the pruritus is intense and leads to self-mutilation, typically of the head and ears. In cats, the neurologic signs seem to predominate and pruritus is rare.[1, 20a]

The diagnosis can be confirmed by virus isolation. Treatment is usually not attempted; when it is, the result is unrewarding. Prevention by means of strict hygienic procedures is of paramount importance.

Mumps

Mumps is a human viral disease caused by a paramyxovirus, and there are reports of clinical disease in dogs from households where humans had mumps.[1] One author (WHM) examined a dog with parotid salivary gland enlargement, a probably vesicular cheilitis, and positive antibody titer to the mumps antigen. Only epidermal collarettes were present on the lips, so biopsies were not performed. The skin lesions resolved spontaneously as the salivary gland returned to normal.

Feline Rhinotracheitis Infection

Feline rhinotracheitis is an infection with an α-herpesvirus resulting in upper respiratory disease.[29] Occasionally, a cat develops oral and cutaneous ulcers.[1, 16, 38] The cutaneous ulcers are usually superficial and multiple, and can occur anywhere on the body, including the footpads. Stress or trauma to the skin might precipitate the development of the ulcers. Skin biopsies reveal epidermal ulceration with subjacent dermal necrosis and a mixed inflammatory infiltrate. Basophilic intranuclear inclusion bodies may be visualized in the keratinocytes or dermal histiocytes. Herpesvirus can be cultured from the skin; more diagnostically, it can be seen in the keratinocytes via electron microscopy.[12]

An ulcerative and necrotizing facial dermatitis or stomatitis has been associated with herpesvirus 1 infection in cats.[21, 42c, 47] Affected cats may or may not have active or historical ocular or respiratory signs. The disorder is recognized most often in adult cats but kittens can be affected. Typically, crusted skin lesions involve the nasal planum, bridge of the nose, and periocular skin (see Fig. 7–1G). When the crusts are removed, the exposed skin is inflamed and ulcerated (see Fig. 7–1H). Similar lesions can be found elsewhere on the body.

Exfoliative erythema multiforme has occurred in cats following upper respiratory infections. Generalized exfoliation and erosions occur that histologically showed individual cell apoptosis and lymphocytic epitheliotropism. The lesions spontaneously resolve after the infection is cleared.[36]

With intercurrent respiratory signs, the diagnosis is straightforward. In the absence of respiratory signs, the differential diagnosis would include the FeLV dermatitis, drug reaction, erythema multiforme, pemphigus vulgaris, and systemic lupus erythematosus. Diagnosis is via skin biopsy. Serologic test results do not confirm active infection nor that the skin disease is due to the virus. In skin biopsies, an ulcerative, often necrotic, dermatitis and suppurative folliculitis and furunculosis is seen (Fig. 7–10). *Demodex cati* mites may be visible within the follicular lumen.[47] There is a perivascular-to-interstitial mixed inflammatory cell dermatitis with many eosinophils. In the surface and follicular epithelium, multinucleated keratinocytic giant cells can be seen (Fig. 7–11) and amphophilic intranuclear (Cowdry type A) inclusion bodies can be seen in the giant cells (Fig. 7–12) and other keratinocytes. A unique feature of this disease is necrosis of epitrichial sweat glands (Fig. 7–13). Ultrastructural studies demonstrate intranuclear virions consistent with herpesvirus. Polymerase chain reaction (PCR) testing in affected cats was strongly positive for herpesvirus 1.[21, 42c] However, the use of PCR as a diagnostic test for feline herpesvirus–associated disease is of limited value because of the occurrence of healthy carriers.[7a] An immunohistochemical test was reported to be accurate.[42c]

In adult cats, the disorder can be triggered by stress or corticosteroid usage. Correction of these problems with the use of antibiotics and other symptomatic treatments may allow for spontaneous healing. Other agents suggested include lysine (250 mg of the formulation without propylene glycol orally q24h), α-interferon, and acyclovir.[38, 47] These treatments may or may not be beneficial.

Feline Calicivirus Infection

Oral ulceration is reported to be more common with calicivirus infection than with rhinotracheitis.[1] Sporadic reports associate infection with skin lesions of the feet or perineum.[13, 25] The tissues are swollen, tender, and ulcerated. Although calicivirus was isolated from the skin in one case, no histopathologic tests were performed to demonstrate whether the virus was causal or a contaminant. Because some infected cats can develop a presumed immune-mediated arthropathy,[25] it is reasonable to assume that the virus can induce primary skin lesions.

Canine Papillomavirus Infection

Papillomaviruses belong to the papovavirus family and are either known to cause or suspected to cause oral papillomatosis, cutaneous papillomas, and cutaneous inverted papillomas in dogs (see Chap. 20).[34b] At least two strains of virus and probably more exist in the dog.[24a] In classic oral papillomavirus infection, self-cure is the rule, provided that the host is immunocompetent.[34a] Two additional syndromes have been recognized that are probably associated with papillomavirus infection in dogs.

The first syndrome involves the development of multiple warts on the footpads of

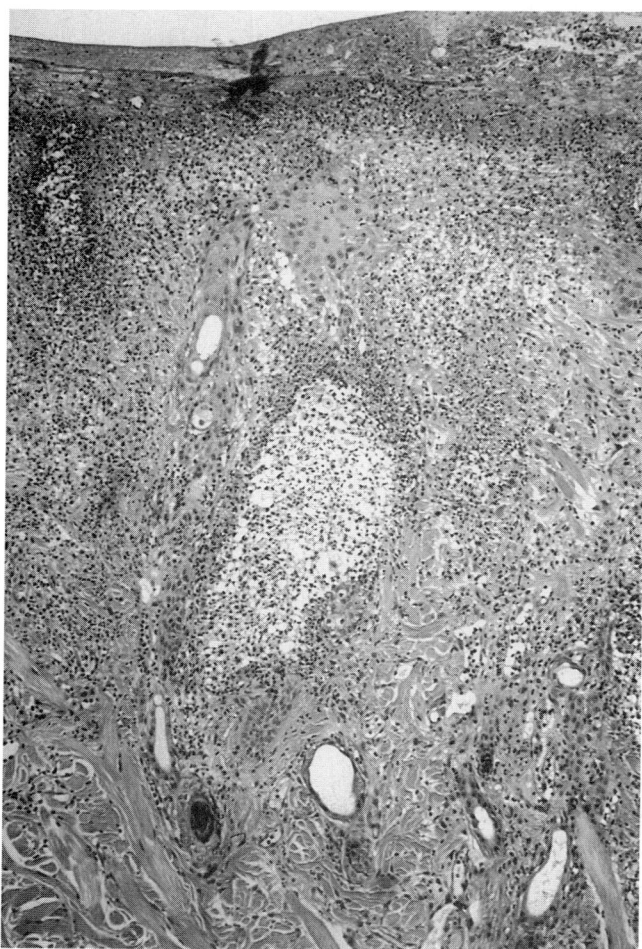

FIGURE 7–10. Suppurative, necrotizing folliculitis and furunculosis in a cat with herpes dermatitis.

young dogs.[2] Affected dogs are 1 to 2 years of age at the onset of symptoms. They develop discrete, firm, hyperkeratotic, often hornlike lesions on multiple pads of two or more paws (Fig. 7–14A). In the dogs studied, lesions were not detected elsewhere. If the lesions are large or involve the weight-bearing surface of the pad, lameness can occur. The lesions wax and wane in severity, and individual lesions may spontaneously resolve but new ones develop. Histologically, the lesions have the characteristics of viral papillomas; to date, however, efforts to demonstrate the virus have been unrewarding. Treatment with topical keratolytic or softening (e.g., water and petrolatum) agents removes the hyperkeratotic debris, softens the lesions, and decreases the dog's discomfort, but it does not appear to alter the course of infection. Topical dimethyl sulfoxide (DMSO) and oral etretinate have been of no benefit in the few dogs treated. Spontaneous resolution of all lesions has not been recognized and it is unknown whether immunotherapy would be of benefit.[3]

The second syndrome involves the development of multiple discrete and pigmented papules, plaques, or nodules (Fig. 7–15). The cases recognized have occurred in young adult dogs (3 to 5 years) with no prior history of skin disease.[2, 17, 24a, 33] In one dog, lesions developed while the dog was receiving a corticosteroid and spontaneously regressed within 3 weeks of drug withdrawal.[37] Lesions can be singular but typically are multiple from the onset, involved any skin surface, and became more numerous with time. Histologically, the lesions are sharply demarcated and characterized by surface and infundibular follicular

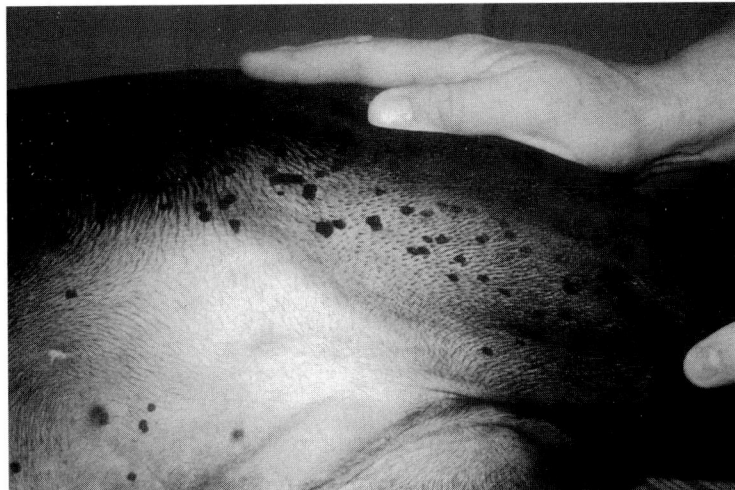

FIGURE 7–15. Multiple pigmented plaques due to papillomavirus infection in a Shar pei.

intensely pruritic papulocrustous dermatitis.[51] With its immunosuppressive nature, some German shepherd dogs develop recurrent German shepherd pyoderma until the ehrlichiosis is resolved (see Chap. 4). The facial dermatitis had histologic features seen in lupus erythematosus, but the dog was antinuclear antibody (ANA) negative and positive for *Ehrlichia canis*. Doxycycline, an antibiotic with very little direct effect on the skin, resulted in resolution of the skin lesions This highlights the need to consider infectious agents when the skin lesions clinically and histologically resemble those seen in lupus.

Feline Haemobartonellosis

Feline haemobartonellosis (feline infectious anemia) is an acute or chronic disease of domestic cats characterized by fever, depression, anorexia, and macrocytic hemolytic anemia.[1] It is caused by the rickettsial agent *Haemobartonella felis*. Cutaneous hyperesthesia and alopecia areata have been reported to occur in cats with acute and chronic haemobartonellosis[53]; however, no pictures, photomicrographs, or details of any kind were provided to substantiate these cutaneous diagnoses.

● PROTOZOAL DISEASES

Feline Toxoplasmosis

Toxoplasmosis is a multisystemic disease caused by the coccidian *Toxoplasma gondii*.[1, 99] Toxoplasmosis has been rarely reported to cause various cutaneous lesions in humans[61] and in cats.[2, 78] Histopathologic findings in cats were reported to be necrotizing dermatitis and vasculitis with *Toxoplasma* (Fig. 7–17). PCR-based techniques are available for the rapid and accurate diagnosis of toxoplasmosis.[90]

FIGURE 7–14. *A*, Discrete wartlike lesion on the edge of the pad of a puppy. *B*, A focal hyperpigmented and crusted lesion associated with papillomavirus infection in a cat. Note that the pigmentary change extends beyond the crusting. *C*, Oral ulceration in a dog with Rocky Mountain spotted fever. (Courtesy C. Foil.) *D*, Multifocal ulceration of the scrotum in a dog with Rocky Mountain spotted fever. *E*, Edema, purpura, and scaling on the scrotum of a dog with babesiosis. (Courtesy D. Carlotti.) *F*, Exfoliative dermatitis on the head and pinnae of a dog with leishmaniasis. (Courtesy Z. Alhaidari.) *G*, Mucocutaneous ulceration in a dog with visceral leishmaniasis. (Courtesy A. Koutinas.) *H*, Purpura, ulceration, and crusting on the paw of a dog with leishmaniasis. (Courtesy Z. Alhaidari.)

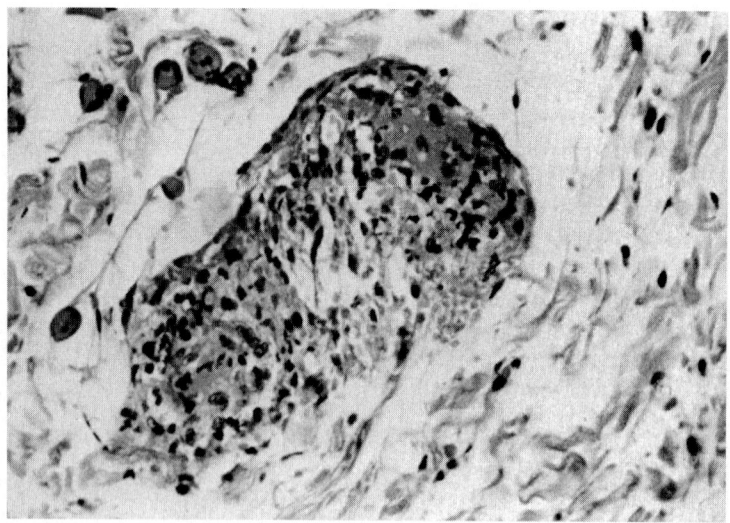

FIGURE 7–16. Leukocytoclastic vasculitis in a dog with Rocky Mountain spotted fever.

Canine Caryosporosis

Coccidia of the genus *Caryospora* have a complicated life cycle involving rodents, reptiles, and raptors.[1, 76] Infection occurs by ingestion of an infected host and results primarily in diarrhea. These organisms have been suspected[121, 123] or identified[76] in puppies that developed pustules, plaques, or nodules on the skin of the trunk. The tissue reaction was pyogranulomatous with eosinophils, and numerous organisms in various stages were identified in macrophages and connective tissue cells (Fig. 7–18).

Canine Neosporosis

Neosporosis is caused by *Neospora caninum*.[1, 58, 75, 80, 99a, 108, 120] Because its tachyzoites and tissue cysts resemble those of *Toxoplasma gondii*, the organism has doubtless existed unrecognized for years. Its complete life cycle is unknown. Infection occurs via vertical transmission or postnatal inoculation, the latter being most important.[58, 117] Exposure to cats may increase the risk of infection.[117] In one study, about 15% of normal dogs were

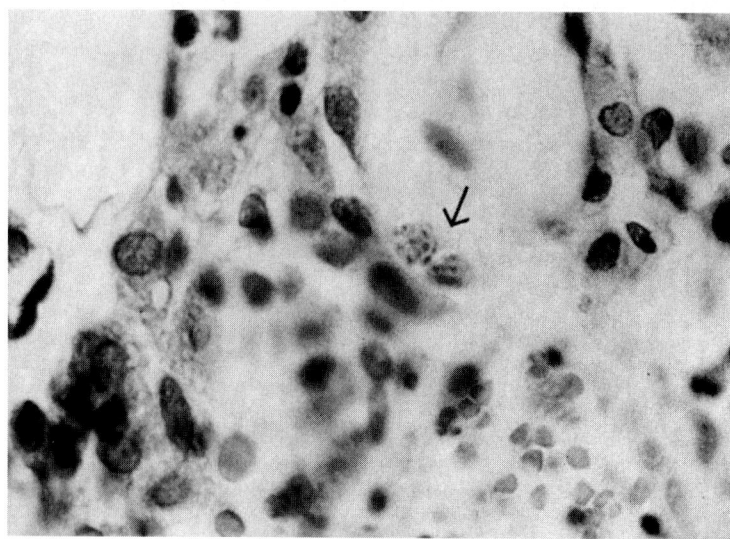

FIGURE 7–17. *Toxoplasma gondii* tachyzoites (*arrow*) in endothelial cells of a cat with cutaneous toxoplasmosis.

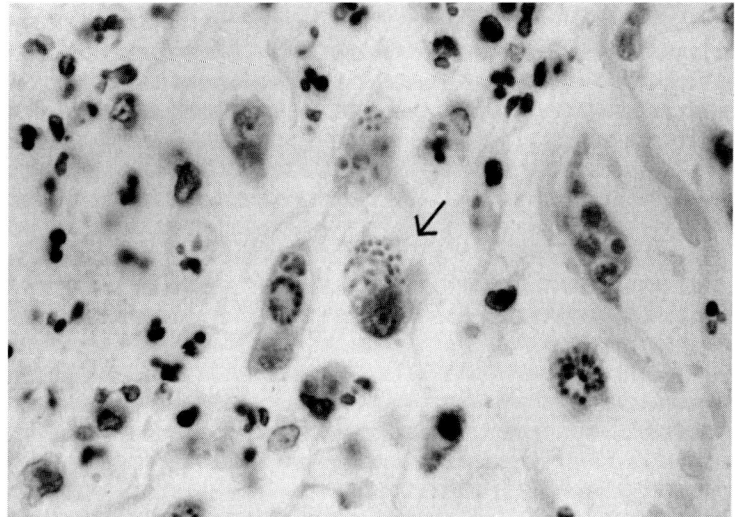

FIGURE 7–18. Tachyzoites *(arrow)* of *Caryospora* in pyogranulomatous dermatitis of a dog. (Courtesy J. Dubey.)

serologically positive. Sporozoites penetrate cells and change into tachyzoites, which divide rapidly and cause tissue damage. Tachyzoites then become bradyzoites within tissue cysts.

Dogs of any age can be infected, but clinical signs are more severe in young dogs. Neurologic and muscular signs predominate, but pneumonia, hepatitis, myocarditis, or dermatitis can also be seen.[89, 120] Skin disease has been described in a small number of dogs. Most had widespread draining nodules,[79, 87, 99a, 112, 113, 115] but one had a rapidly spreading, ulcerative dermatitis of the eyelids, neck, thorax, and perineum.[75] The lesions may be pruritic.

Histologically, nodular lesions are characterized by a pyogranulomatous dermatitis. Tachyzoites can be seen within keratinocytes, macrophages, neutrophils, and rarely, in endothelial cells. The dog with ulcerative lesions had an eosinophilic necrotizing dermatitis with severe congestion, thrombosis, and infarction.[75] To differentiate neosporosis from toxoplasmosis, immunohistochemical or ultrastructural studies are needed. Serologic tests are available to determine the rate of infection.[119] A titer of ≥1:800 by indirect fluorescent antibody testing is considered strongly suggestive of active infection.[99a]

Susceptibility testing of *N. caninum* to various antimicrobial agents has been performed but detailed studies on the *in vitro* versus *in vivo* correlation of these data are not available.[98] Susceptibility testing suggests that sulfamethoxazole, azithromycin, canthromycin, erythromycin, doxycycline, minocycline, and clindamycin hydrochloride can be of benefit. Several cases were treated with a 21-day[115] or 45-day[79] course of clindamycin (12.5 to 18.5 mg/kg, orally, q12h) with resolution of the lesions.[79, 99a] Combination therapy with pyrimethamine (0.25 to 0.5 mg/kg, orally, q12h) and sulfadiazine (30 mg/kg, orally, q12h) is also reported to be effective.[99a] When this combination is used, folinic acid (5 mg/day) or brewer's yeast (100 mg/kg/day) is given to prevent bone marrow suppression.[99a]

Canine Sarcocystosis

Sarcocystis organisms are widespread in nature, especially in cattle and sheep.[1] Dogs and cats become infected by ingesting tissue cysts (sarcocysts). *Sarcocystis* species are typically not pathogenic for dogs and cats, although there has been one report of a dog with chronic diarrhea who developed multiple cutaneous abscesses over the whole body and especially on the hind limbs.[77] Biopsy showed severe necrotizing, fibrinosuppurative dermatitis with numerous neutrophils and fewer eosinophils and macrophages. Vessels were

Canine Babesiosis

Canine babesiosis is a tickborne hematozoan disease caused by three species of *Babesia*[1, 101]: *Babesia canis*, which is worldwide in its distribution, and *Babesia gibsoni* and *Babesia vogeli*, which are more restricted. Infection induces a parasitemia that results in varying clinical signs. Asymptomatic carriers exist.

Aside from the oral or cutaneous petechial and ecchymotic hemorrhages associated with thrombocytopenia or disseminated intravascular coagulation, skin lesions are rare. Skin lesions are due to subjacent leukocytoclastic vasculitis with or without vascular necrosis.[67] Clinical signs include edema, ecchymosis, ulceration, and necrosis (see Fig. 7–14E), which can be seen on the pinnae, axillae, groin, limbs, or scrotum.[67, 69] As in ehrlichiosis, dogs with babesiosis can have some of the clinical features of systemic lupus erythematosus and may have a positive ANA titer. Accordingly, all dogs with suspect lupus erythematosus should have serologic tests for appropriate rickettsial or protozoal diseases before the diagnosis of systemic lupus is made.

Treatment with pentamidine isothionate resolved the skin lesions in the reported case.[67] Other babesiacides may also be effective.

Leishmaniasis

Leishmaniasis is a serious protozoal infection caused by a variety of *Leishmania* spp.[1, 82, 94, 122] Disease is most common in humans and dogs but can be seen in cats and other domestic animals. The disease is worldwide in distribution. In the Old World, most cases in dogs occur in the Mediterranean basin and Portugal, but reports have originated in France, Germany, Switzerland, the Netherlands, and other countries. In the New World, the disease is endemic in South and Central America; endemic foci have been reported in Texas, Oklahoma, Ohio, Michigan, and Alabama.[65] Dogs imported from endemic areas may develop the disease months or years later, so cases could be recognized anywhere. The disease is transmitted to humans and animals by bloodsucking sandflies of the genus *Lutzomyia* in the New World and *Phlebotomus* in the Old World. The frequency of infection increases during warm months when the vector load is high.[57] Domestic and wild dogs, rodents, and other wild mammals are the reservoir. Twenty percent of seropositive asymptomatic dogs have *Leishmania* organisms in clinically normal skin.[84a] Because of the occurrence of open lesions, some investigators have expressed concern regarding the possibility of direct or mechanical transmission from dog to dog or from dog to humans. Leishmaniasis in HIV-positive humans is an emerging disease.[118b] The possibility that humans act as a reservoir for other humans and animals has been put forth.[74]

In general, tissue damage in leishmaniasis is due to granulomatous inflammation and immune complex deposition. It has been hypothesized that dogs with subclinical or latent leishmaniasis may develop cutaneous lesions at the sites of external trauma and resultant inflammatory processes, because amastigotes in blood cells are transported to the inflamed areas.[115a] This mechanism could partly explain the distribution of inflammatory and ulcerative lesions at pressure points, which is common in canine leishmaniasis.

The incubation period varies from weeks to several years with a gradual onset of signs and continual progression. The disease primarily affects dogs less than 5 years old. Rural animals, especially those who spend the night outdoors, are at an increased risk.[133] From 10 to more than 50% of seropositive dogs have no clinical signs of disease and may remain healthy for prolonged periods of time, if not permanently.[84a, 94a, 123a] Skin lesions occur in over 80% of dogs with visceral involvement.[1, 72, 73, 94, 110, 116] The most common finding is an exfoliative dermatitis with silvery white, asbestos-like scaling. The exfoliation can be generalized but usually is most pronounced on the head, pinnae, and extremities (see Fig. 7–14F). Nasodigital hyperkeratosis may accompany the scaling, and the involved skin can be hypotrichotic to alopecic. Periocular alopecia (lunettes) is common. The next most common presentation is an ulcerative dermatitis (see Fig. 7–14G and H). Other findings include onychogryposis (Fig. 7–19), paronychia, sterile pustular dermatitis, nasal depigmentation with erosion and ulceration, and nodular dermatitis.[86, 94a] Secondary bacterial pyoderma occurs in about 25% of the dogs.[94a]

Systemic signs of illness are many and varied. Over 50% of involved dogs show decreased endurance, weight loss, and somnolence.[1, 71, 72, 94, 94a] Because of the parasitemia and the host's immunologic response to the organism, physical abnormalities are varied. Generalized lymphadenopathy and hepatosplenomegaly are common findings. Other abnormalities include muscle wasting, cachexia, intermittent fever, keratoconjunctivitis, and lameness. Because of the *Leishmania*-induced cell-mediated immunodeficiency, these dogs can be predisposed to generalized demodicosis in all of its forms.[106a]

Cats are resistant to experimental infection, and reports of spontaneous cases are rare.[59, 93, 96, 111] The majority of cases had a nodular or crusting dermatitis of the lips, nose, eyelids, and pinnae. A generalized exfoliative dermatitis can also be seen.

Because immunodeficiency is not a prerequisite for infection, dogs with leishmaniasis show an immunologic response to the organism. Resistance or susceptibility to clinical leishmaniasis appears to be associated with the stimulation of a T helper-1 or T helper-2 cell response, respectively.[94a] IL-2 and TNF-α seem to play a protective role.[94a] With infection, serum levels of anti-*Leishmania* IgG, IgM, IgA, and circulating immune complexes increase and, with high titer, predispose to renal disease.[102, 103, 105] With infection, the number of $CD21^+$, $CD5^+$, $CD4^+$, and $CD8^+$ cells decreases and the degree of incompetence seems to influence the severity of clinical signs.[62, 63, 66, 106] Early in experimental infection, the dog develops a cell-mediated immune response to the organism but this can disappear with the onset of clinical signs.[118] With a persistent cell-mediated response, the dog's clinical signs are absent or milder and the number of organisms found in the tissues is fewer.[62, 66, 85]

The differential diagnosis includes pemphigus foliaceus, systemic lupus erythematosus, zinc-responsive dermatosis, necrolytic migratory erythema, sebaceous adenitis, and lymphoma. Laboratory findings usually include nonregenerative anemia, hyperglobulinemia, hypoalbuminemia, and proteinuria.

Tests for immune-mediated diseases (Coomb's tests, ANA, lupus erythematosus preparation, rheumatoid factor) can be positive in dogs with leishmaniasis.[65, 94a] The frequency of a clinically insignificant positive ANA titer varies from 16% to over 80% of dogs tested.[72, 94, 104] Because many of the clinical signs of leishmaniasis overlap with those of systemic lupus erythematosus, immunodiagnostic test results must be interpreted carefully when a dog comes from an endemic area.

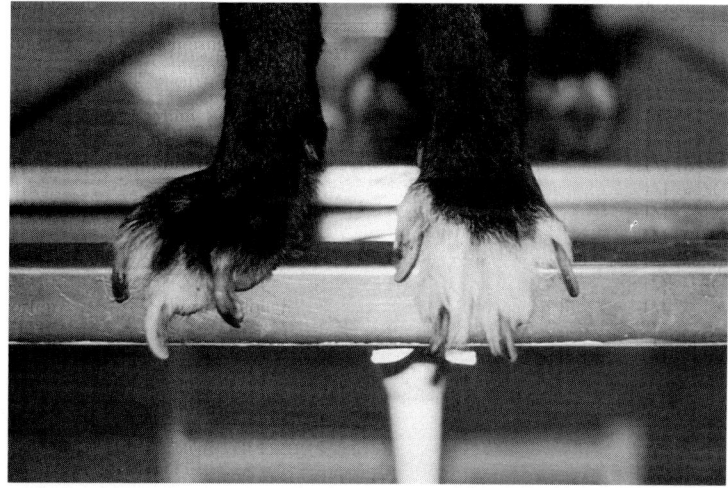

FIGURE 7–19. Onychogryposis in a dog with leishmaniasis. (Courtesy A. Koutinas.)

Demonstration of anti-*Leishmania* antibodies, positive skin test reaction,[68] or the organism itself confirms the diagnosis. Although dogs can have positive serologic test results in the absence of clinical disease, spontaneous elimination of the parasite is rare; therefore, positive test results indicate infection.[1] Various serologic tests are available (IFA, ELISA, Dot-ELISA) and the published sensitivity and specificity vary with the test, population being studied, and investigator.[60, 84, 94, 118a, 127, 128] No test is 100% accurate, with false-negative results reported in more than 10% of infected dogs tested. The test method also dictates whether the test can be used to monitor response to treatment. For that purpose, the indirect immunofluorescence test (IFA) is recommended.[83, 131] Amastigotes are most easily seen with Giemsa's stain and are found most often in smears from lymph nodes or bone marrow (Fig. 7–20). Identification in other tissues is more difficult and often unrewarding. Lymph node cytology is positive in about 85% of the clinically ill dogs, whereas IFA is positive in about 97%.[94a] In early clinical disease, cytology may be positive when serology is negative.[94a] There is no correlation of severity of clinical signs with serological titer.[94a]

Skin biopsy findings vary considerably. Orthokeratotic and parakeratotic hyperkeratosis are usually prominent; the inflammatory infiltrate typically consists of macrophages with fewer numbers of lymphocytes and plasma cells. Granulomatous perifolliculitis (Fig. 7–21), interstitial dermatitis, superficial and deep perivascular dermatitis, lichenoid interface dermatitis, nodular dermatitis, lobular panniculitis, suppurative folliculitis, and intraepidermal pustular dermatitis (Fig. 7–22) are the nine inflammatory patterns that have been recognized in leishmaniasis; this large number reflects the clinical variability of the disease.[94] The three most common patterns are granulomatous perifolliculitis, superficial and deep perivascular dermatitis, and interstitial dermatitis. It is common for a dog to have more than one pattern of inflammation present. In the perifollicular pattern, total obliteration of the sebaceous glands occurs in approximately 45% of the cases. This sebaceous destruction no doubt contributes to the high frequency of clinical exfoliation. The *Leishmania* organisms are found intracellularly and extracellularly in approximately 50% of cases. They are round to oval, 2 to 4 μm in size, and contain a round, basophilic nucleus and a small, rodlike kinetoplast. Although they are visible in routine stains, *Leishmania* organisms are best seen when Giemsa stain is used. Immunohistochemical techniques facilitate the identification of the organism.[64] PCR is at least as sensitive as immunohistochemical detection of *Leishmania* in biopsy specimens, and may be positive when the latter is negative.[119a]

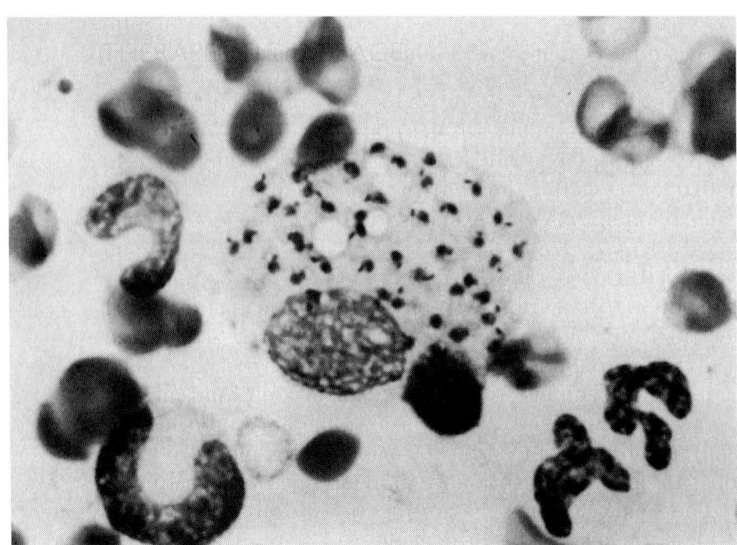

FIGURE 7–20. Macrophage containing numerous Leishman-Donovan bodies. (Courtesy T. French.)

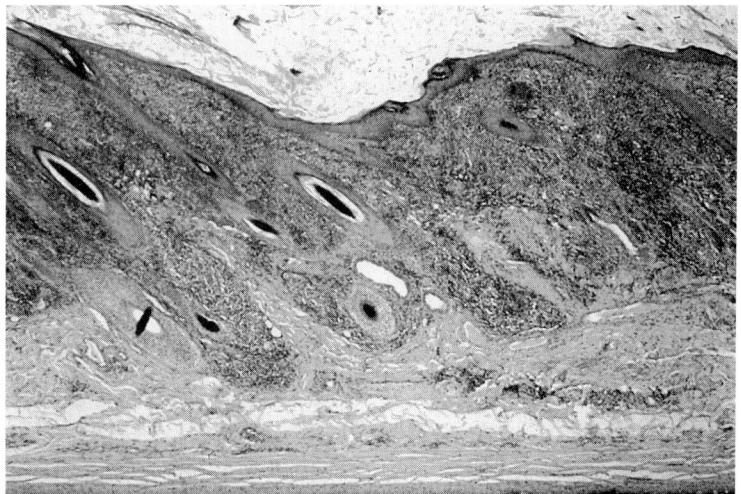

FIGURE 7–21. Perifollicular granulomatous dermatitis in a dog with visceral leishmaniasis.

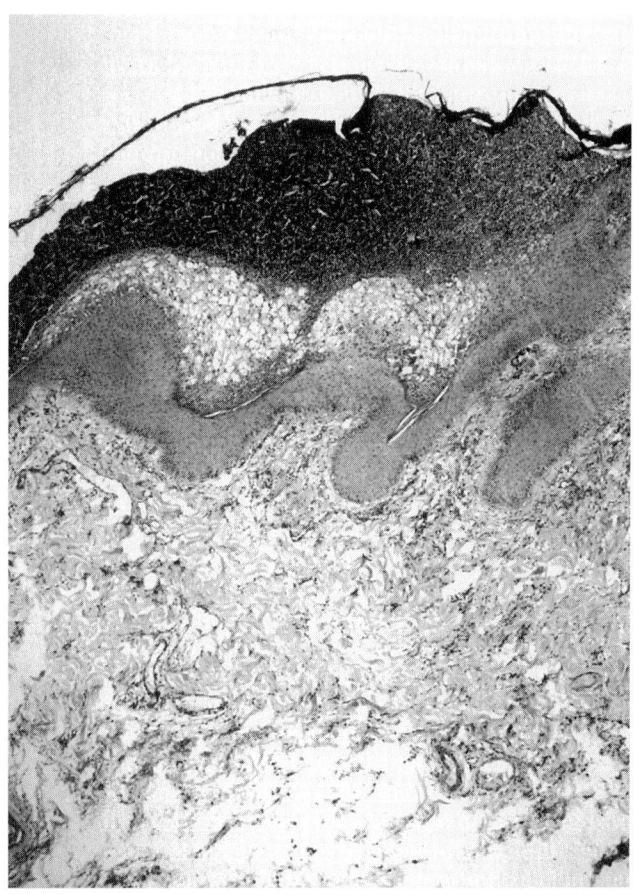

FIGURE 7–22. Intraepidermal pustular dermatitis in a dog with visceral leishmaniasis.

Dogs with visceral leishmaniasis show increased levels of IgG-2 specifically directed against O-acetylated sialic acids during active disease, and these antibodies have 96.6% sensitivity and 75% specificity.[71]

At present, canine leishmaniasis is considered an incurable disease in the vast majority of cases. Treatments can bring about a clinical cure, but relapses months to years after treatment are to be expected. These relapses are probably due to incomplete eradication of the parasite, but could also represent reinfection. Accordingly, with the poor prognosis for cure and the possible reservoir status of the dog for human infection, euthanasia may be indicated. In endemic areas, insect control measures can be beneficial in reducing the rate of insect feeding and, hopefully, infection.[92]

When treatment is indicated, the most widely used treatment is meglumine antimonate.[1, 82] Dosages vary with the study and range from 20 to 50 mg/kg given subcutaneously twice daily to 200 to 300 mg/kg given intravenously every other day.[73a, 118b, 124, 126] Remission rates approaching 85% can be achieved with a large number of injections,[73, 124] but parasitologic cure rates are much lower. Studies in humans and dogs have suggested that the antileishmanial activity of liposome-encapsulated meglumine antimonate is vastly superior to that of the unencapsulated drug.[70, 125] Other drugs that have been used in canine leishmaniasis include aminosidine,[114, 132] amphotericin B,[95] allopurinol,[67a, 97, 129, 130] metronidazole, and ketoconazole. Allopurinol has been receiving widest attention because of its low cost and safety.[100] With daily dosages of 11 to 15 mg/kg, clinical cure is achieved in most cases, but parasitologic cure is rare. Various drug combinations have been studied, with meglumine antimonate and allopurinol receiving widest usage.[73, 73a, 88, 109] In one study, the combination of meglumine and allopurinol was more effective than either product alone.[73a] The addition of allopurinol improves the clinical response rate, and its use on a daily basis for 1 week each month appears to prevent relapse. However, the rate of parasitologic cure is not impacted. The most helpful new treatment is an admixture of chemotherapy and immunotherapy with LiF2 antigen, an antigen derived from *L. infantum*.[107] Simultaneous use of this antigen and meglumine resulted in parasitologic cure in all cases tested.

There is no correlation between serologic titers and clinical signs in treated or untreated dogs.[94a] High titers often persist in clinically cured animals and cannot be used to monitor progress of therapy or to confirm complete cure.[94a] Antigen-specific lymphoproliferative responses do reappear in successfully treated dogs.[118a] *Leishmania* organisms can often be demonstrated cytologically, by culture, or by PCR in successfully treated dogs.[67a, 118b] Thus, these dogs remain important carriers and reservoirs.

Successful treatment of feline leishmaniasis has not been reported.

• REFERENCES

General Textbook Sources
1. Greene CE: Infectious Diseases of the Dog and Cat, 2nd ed. W. B. Saunders Co, Philadelphia, 1998.
2. Scott DW, et al: Muller and Kirk's Small Animal Dermatology, 5th ed. W. B. Saunders, Co, Philadelphia, 1995.

Viral Diseases
3. Agut M, et al: Autovaccination as a treatment in canine papillomavirus dermatological disease: A study of nine cases. Biomed Letters 54(213):23, 1996.
4. Baer KE, Helton K: Multicentric squamous cell carcinoma *in situ* resembling Bowen's disease in cats. Vet Pathol 30:535, 1993.
4a. Baxby D, Bennett M: Cowpox: A re-evaluation of the risks of human infection based on new epidemiological information. Arch Virol 13:1, 1997.
4b. Began M, et al: The population dynamics of cowpox virus infection in bank voles: Testing fundamental assumptions. Ecology Letters 1:82, 1998.
5. Bennett M, et al: Feline cowpox virus infection. J Small Anim Pract 31:167, 1990.
6. Bennett M, Baxby D: Feline and human cowpox. Vet Ann 35:229, 1995.
7. Bennett, M, et al: The laboratory diagnosis of orthopox virus infection in the domestic cat. J Small Anim Pract 26:653, 1985.
7a. Burgesser KM, et al: Comparison of PCR, virus isolation, and indirect fluorescent antibody staining in the detection of naturally occurring feline herpesvirus infections. J Vet Diagn Invest 11:122, 1999.
8. Canese MG, et al: Feline poxvirus infection. A case report. Schweizer Archiv fur Tierheilkunde 139:454, 1997.
9. Carney HC, et al: Papillomavirus infection of aged Persian cats. J Vet Diagn Invest 2:294, 1990.
10. Carpenter JL, et al: Cutaneous xanthogranuloma and viral papilloma on an eyelid of a cat. Vet Dermatol 3:187, 1992.

11. Chalmers S, et al: Demodicosis in two cats seropositive for feline immunodeficiency virus. J Am Vet Med Assoc 194:256, 1989.
11a. Chantrey J, et al: Cowpox-reservoir hosts and geographic distribution. Epidemiol Infect 122:455, 1999.
12. Clark EG, et al: Primary viral skin disease in three cats caused by three different viruses and confirmed by immunohistochemical and/or electron microscopic techniques on formalin-fixed tissue. Proc Annu Memb Meet Am Acad Vet Dermatol Am Coll Vet Dermatol 9:56, 1993.
13. Cooper LM, Sabine M: Paw and mouth disease in a cat. Aust Vet J 48:644, 1972.
14. Egberink HF, et al: Isolation and identification of a poxvirus from a domestic cat and a human contact case. J Vet Med [Br] 33:237, 1986.
15. Egberink HE, et al: Papillomavirus associated skin lesions in a cat seropositive for feline immunodeficiency virus. Vet Microbiol 31:117, 1992.
16. Flecknell PA, et al: Skin ulceration associated with herpesvirus infection in cats. Vet Rec 104:313, 1979.
17. Gross TL, et al: Multifocal intraepidermal carcinoma in a dog histologically resembling Bowen's disease. Am J Dermatopathol 8:509, 1986.
18. Gross, TL, et al: Veterinary Dermatopathology. Mosby–Year Book, Inc., St. Louis, 1992, p 340.
19. Gross TL, et al: Giant cell dermatosis in FeLV-positive cats. Vet Dermatol 4:117, 1993.
19a. Groux D, et al: La poxvirose féline: À propos de deux cas. Prat Méd Chir Anim Comp 34:215, 1999.
19b. Haines DM, et al: Immunohistochemical detection of canine distemper virus in haired skin, nasal mucosa, and footpad epithelium: A method for antemortem diagnosis of infection. J Vet Diagn Invest 11:396, 1999.
20. Hamblet CN: Parapoxvirus in a cat. Vet Rec 132:144, 1993.
20a. Hara M, et al: A natural case of Aujeszky's disease in the cat in Japan. J Vet Med Sci 53:947, 1991.
21. Hargis AM, et al: Ulcerative facial and nasal dermatitis and stomatitis in cats associated with feline herpes 1. Vet Dermatol 10:267, 1999.
21a. Hinrichs U, et al: Necrotizing pneumonia in a cat caused by an orthopox virus. J Comp Pathol 121:191, 1999.
22. Hoover EA, Mullins JI: Feline leukemia virus infection and diseases. J Am Vet Med Assoc 199:1287, 1991.
23. Howard DR: Pseudorabies in dogs and cats. In: Kirk RW (ed): Current Veterinary Therapy IX. W. B. Saunders Co, Philadelphia, 1986, p 1071.
24. LeClerc SM, et al: Papillomavirus infection in association with feline cutaneous squamous cell carcinoma in situ. Proc Annu Memb Meet Am Acad Vet Dermatol Am Coll Vet Dermatol 13:125, 1997.
24a. LeNet JL, et al: Multiple pigmented cutaneous papules associated with a novel canine papillomavirus in an immunosuppressed dog. Vet Pathol 34:8, 1997.
25. Love DN, et al: Feline calicivirus associated with pyrexia, profound anorexia, and oral and perineal ulceration in a cat. Aust Vet Pract 17:136, 1987.
26. Maeda, H, et al: Distemper skin lesions in a dog. J Vet Med A 42:247, 1994.
27. Maenhout T, et al: Drie Gevallen Van Koepokkeninfektie bij de Kat in Belgie. Vlaams. Diergenerskd Tijdschr 60:66, 1991.
28. Maggs DJ, et al: Evaluation of serologic and viral detection methods for diagnosing feline herpesvirus-1 infection in cats with acute respiratory tract or chronic ocular disease. J Am Vet Med Assoc 214:502, 1999.
29. Maggs DJ: Update of feline herpesvirus (FHV-1). Proc Am Coll Vet Int Med 16:613, 1998.
30. Mancianti F, et al: Mycological findings in feline immunodeficiency virus-infected cats. J Med Vet Mycol 30:257, 1992.
31. Miller WH Jr, et al: Multicentric squamous cell carcinomas in situ resembling Bowen's disease in five cats. Vet Dermatol 3:177, 1992.
32. Monroe WE: Clinical signs associated with pseudorabies in dogs. J Am Vet Med Assoc 195:599, 1989.
33. Nagata M, et al: Pigmented plaques associated with papillomavirus infections in dogs: is this epidermodysplasia verruciformis? Vet Dermatol 6:179, 1995.
34. Naidoo J, et al: Characterization of orthopoxviruses isolated from feline infections in Britain. Arch Virol 125:261, 1992.
34a. Nicholls PK, et al: Naturally occurring, nonregressing canine oral papillomavirus infection: Host immunity, virus characterization, and experimental infection. Virol 265:365, 1999.
34b. Nicholls PK, Stanley MA: Canine papillomavirus—a centenary review. J Comp Pathol 120:219, 1999.
35. Nowotny N, et al: Poxvirus infection in the domestic cat: Clinical, histopathological, virological, and epidemiological studies. Wien Tierärztl Mschr 81:362, 1994.
36. Olivry T: Newly recognized feline dermatoses: selected topics. Proc DVM Fall Seminar, Keywest, 1997, p 29.
37. Orth G, et al: Multiple pigmented cutaneous papules associated with a novel canine papillomavirus in an immunosuppressed dog. Vet Pathol 34:8, 1997.
38. Power HT: Newly recognized feline skin diseases. Proc Annu Memb Meet Am Acad Vet. Dermatol Am Coll Vet Dermatol 14:31, 1998.
39. Sato R, et al: Oral administration of bovine lactoferrin for treatment of intractable stomatitis in feline immunodeficiency virus (FIV)-positive and FIV-negative cats. Am J Vet Res. 57(10):1443, 1996.
40. Scott DW: Feline dermatology 1900–1978: A monograph. J Am Anim Hosp Assoc 6:331, 1980.
41. Scott DW: Large Animal Dermatology. W. B. Saunders Co, Philadelphia, 1988.
42. Setsuko TOI, et al: Histopathological features of stomatitis in cats spontaneously infected with feline immunodeficiency virus. J Jpn Vet Med Assoc 47:331, 1994.
42a. Smith KC, et al: Skin lesions caused by orthopoxvirus infection in a dog. J Small Anim Pract 40:495, 1999.
42b. Sundberg JP, et al: Feline papillomas and papillomaviruses. Vet Pathol 37:1, 2000.
42c. Suchy A, et al: Diagnosis of feline herpesvirus infection by immunohistochemistry, polymerase chain reaction, and in situ hybridization. J Vet Diagn Invest 12:186, 2000.
43. Thomsett LR: Feline poxvirus infection. In: Kirk RW (ed): Current Veterinary Therapy IX. W. B. Saunders Co, Philadelphia, 1986, p. 605.
44. Vestey JP, et al: What is human catpox/cowpox infection? Int J Dermatol 30:696, 1991.
45. von Bomhard D, et al: Zur Epidemiologie, Klink, Pathologie und Virologie der Katzen-Pocken-Infektion. Kleintierpraxis 37:219, 1992.

45a. Wienecke R, et al: Cowpox virus infection in an 11-year-old girl. J Am Acad Dermatol 42:892, 2000.
46. Wilkinson GT, et al: Possible "orf" (contagious pustular dermatitis, contagious ecthyma of sheep) infection in the dog. Vet Rec 87:766, 1970.
47. Wojciechowski J, et al: Herpesvirus dermatitis in a cat. Proc 14th Am Acad Vet Dermatol Am Coll Vet Dermatol, 1998, p 85.
48. Yamamoto JK, et al: Epidemiologic and clinical aspects of feline immunodeficiency virus infection in cats from the continental United States and Canada and possible mode of transmission. J Am Vet Med Assoc 194:213, 1989.
49. Zenger E: FIP, FELV, FIV: Making a diagnosis. Proc Am Coll Vet Int Med 16:407, 1998.

Rickettsial Diseases

50. Breitschwerdt EB, et al: Prednisolone at anti-inflammatory or immunosuppressive dosages in conjunction with doxycycline does not potentiate the severity of Rickettsia rickettsii infection in dogs. Antimicrob Agents Chemother 41:141, 1997.
51. Carlotti DN, Bensingnor, E: Manifestations dermatologiques de l'ehrlichiose canine. Prat Méd Chir Anim Comp 31:325, 1996.
52. Greene CE, et al: Rocky Mountain spotted fever in dogs and its differentiation from canine ehrlichiosis. J Am Vet Med Assoc 186:465, 1985.
53. Gretillati S: Feline haemobartonellosis. Feline Pract 14:22, 1984.
54. Frank LA: Cutaneous lesions associated with ehrlichiosis in a dog. Vet Allergy Clin Immunol 4:90, 1997.
55. Rutgers C, et al: Severe Rocky Mountain spotted fever in five dogs. J Am Anim Hosp Assoc 21:361, 1985.
56. Weiser ID, et al: Dermal necrosis associated with Rocky Mountain spotted fever in four dogs. J Am Vet Med Assoc 195:1756, 1989.

Protozoal Diseases

57. Acedo-Sanchez C, et al: Changes in antibody titres against Leishmania infantum in naturally infected dogs in southern Spain. Vet Parasitol 75:1, 1998.
58. Barber JS, Trees AJ: Naturally occurring vertical transmission of Neospora caninum in dogs. Intrnatl. J Parasitol 28:57, 1998.
59. Barnes JC, et al: Diffuse cutaneous leishmaniasis in a cat. J Am Vet Med Assoc 202:416, 1993.
60. Bernadina WE, et al: An immunodiffusion assay for the detection of canine leishmaniasis due to infection with Leishmania infantum. Vet Parasitol 73:207, 1997.
61. Binazzi M: Profile of cutaneous toxoplasmosis. Int J Dermatol 25:357, 1986.
62. Bourdoiseau G, et al: Specific IgG1 and IgG2 antibody and lymphocyte subset levels in naturally Leishmania infantum-infected treated and untreated dogs. Vet Immunol Immunopathol 59:21, 1997.
63. Bourdoisea G, et al: Lymphocyte subset abnormalities in canine leishmaniasis. Vet Immunol Immunopathol 56:345, 1997.
64. Bourdoiseau G, et al: Immunohistochemical detection of Leishmania infantum in formalin-fixed, paraffin-embedded sections of canine skin and lymph nodes. J Vet Diagn Invest 9:439, 1997.
65. Bravo L, et al: Canine leishmaniasis in the United States. Comp Cont Educ 15:699, 1993.
66. Cabral M, et al: The immunology of canine leishmaniasis: Strong evidence for a developing spectrum from asymptomatic dogs. Vet Parasitol 76:173, 1998.
67. Capelli, JL, et al: La babésiose canine, maladie à complexes immuns: À propos d'un cas de vascularite à manifestations cutanées. Prat Méd Chir Anim Comp 31:231, 1996.
67a. Cavaliero T, et al: Clinical, serologic, and parasitologic follow-up after long-term allopurinol therapy of dogs naturally infected with Leishmania infantum. J Vet Intern Med 13:330, 1999.
68. Cardoso L, et al: Use of a leishmanin skin test in the detection of canine Leishmania-specific cellular immunity. Vet Parasitol 79:213, 1998.
69. Carlotti DN, et al: Skin lesions in canine babesiosis. In: Ihrke PJ, et al (eds): Advances in Veterinary Dermatology, Vol 2. Pergamon Press, Oxford, 1993, p 229.
70. Chapman WL, et al: Antileishmanial activity of liposome-encapsulated meglumine antimonate in the dog. Am J Vet Res 45:1028, 1984.
71. Chatterjee M, et al: Diagnostic and prognostic potential of antibodies against O-acetylated sialic acids in canine visceral leishmaniasis. Vet Immunol Immunopathol 70:55, 1999.
72. Ciaramella P, et al: A retrospective clinical study of canine leishmaniasis in 150 dogs naturally infection by Leishmania infantum. Vet Rec 141:539, 1997.
73. Denerolle P: Leishmaniose canine: difficultés du diagnostic et du traitement (125 cas). Prat Méd Chir Anim Comp 31:137, 1996.
73a. Denerolle P, Bourdoiseau G: Combination allopurinol and antimony treatment versus antimony alone and allopurinol alone in the treatment of canine leishmaniasis (96 cases). J Vet Intern Med 13:413, 1999.
74. Dietze R, et al: Effect of eliminating seropositive canines on the transmission of visceral leishmaniasis in Brazil. Clin Infect Dis 25:1240, 1997.
75. Dubey JP, et al: Newly recognized fatal protozoan disease of dogs. J Am Vet Med Assoc 192:1296, 1989.
76. Dubey JP, et al: Caryospora-associated dermatitis in dogs. J Parasitol 76:552, 1990.
77. Dubey JP, et al: Fatal cutaneous and visceral infection in a rottweiler dog associated with a sarcocystis-like protozoan. J Vet Diagn Invest 3:72, 1991.
78. Dubey JP, Carpenter JL: Histologically confirmed clinical toxoplasmosis in cats: 100 cases (1952–1990). J Am Vet Med Assoc 203:1556, 1993.
79. Dubey JP, et al: Canine cutaneous neosporosis: clinical improvement with clindamycin. Vet Dermatol 6:37, 1995.
80. Dubey JP, Lindsay DS: A review of Neospora caninum and neosporosis. Vet Parasitol 67:1, 1996.
81. Edelhofer VR, et al: Importierte Leishmaniose-fälle bei Hunden in Österreich—eine rerospektive studie von 1985–1994. Wien Tierärztl Mschr 82:90, 1995.
82. Ferrer L: Leishmaniasis. In: Kirk RW, Bonagura JD (eds): Kirk's Current Veterinary Therapy XI. W. B. Saunders Co, Philadelphia, 1992, p 266.
83. Ferrer L, et al: Serological diagnosis and treatment of canine leishmaniasis. Vet Rec 136:514, 1995.
84. Fisa R, et al: Serological diagnosis of canine leishmaniasis by dot-ELISA. J Vet Diagn Invest 9:50, 1997.
84a. Fisa R, et al: Epidemiology of canine leishmaniasis in Catalonia (Spain). The example of the priorat focus. Vet Parasitol 83:87, 1999.
85. Fondevila D, et al: Epidermal immunocompetence in

canine leishmaniasis. Vet Immunol Immunopathol 56: 319, 1997.
86. Font A, et al: Canine mucosal leishmaniasis. J Am Anim Hosp Assoc 32:131, 1996.
87. Fritz D, et al: *Neospora caninum*: Associated nodular dermatitis in a middle-aged dog. Can Pract 22:21, 1997.
88. Ginel PJ, et al: Use of allopurinol for maintenance of remission in dogs with leishmaniasis. J Small Anim Pract 39:271, 1998.
89. Ginel PJ, et al: Use of allopurinol for maintenance of remission in dogs with leishmaniasis. J Small Anim Pract 39:271, 1998.
90. Greig B, et al: *Neospora caninum* pneumonia in an adult dog. J Am Vet Med Assoc 206:1000, 1995.
91. Hyman JA, et al: Specificity of polymerase chain reaction identification of *Toxoplasma gondii* infection in paraffin-embedded animal tissues. J Vet Diagn Invest 7–275, 1995.
92. Killick KR, et al: Protection of dogs from bites of phlebotomine sandflies by deltamethrin collars for control of canine leishmaniasis. Med Vet Entomol 22: 105, 1997.
93. Kirkpatrick CE, et al: *Leishmania chagasi* and *L. donovani*: Experimental infections in domestic cats. Exp Parasitol 58:125, 1984.
94. Koutinas AF, et al: Skin lesions in canine Leishmaniasis (Kala-Azar): A clinical and histopathologic study on 22 spontaneous cases in Greece. Vet Dermatol 3: 121, 1993.
94a. Koutinas AF, et al: Clinical considerations on canine visceral leishmaniasis in Greece: A retrospective study of 158 cases (1989–1996). J Am Anim Hosp Assoc 35:376, 1999.
95. Lamothe J: Essai de traitement de la leishmaniose canine par l'amphotéricine B (39 cas). Prat Méd Chir Anim Comp 32:133, 1997.
96. Laruelle-Magalon C, Toga I: Un cas de leishmaniose féline. Prat Méd Chir Anim Comp 31:255, 1996.
97. Lester SJ, Kenyon JE: Use of allopurinol to treat visceral leishmaniasis in a dog. J Am Vet Med Assoc 209:615, 1996.
98. Lindsay DS, et al: Examination of the activities of 43 chemotherapeutic agents against *Neospora caninum* tachyzoites in cultures cells. Am J Vet Res 55:976, 1994.
99. Lindsay DS, et al: Feline toxoplasmosis and the importance of the *Toxoplasma gondii* oocyst. Comp Cont Educ Pract Vet 19:488, 1997.
99a. Lindsay DS, et al: *Neospora caninum* and the potential for parasite transmission. Compend Contin Educ Pract Vet 21:317, 1999.
100. Liste F, Gascon M: Allopurinol in the treatment of canine visceral leishmaniasis. Vet Rec 137–23, 1995.
101. Lobetti RG: Canine babesiosis. Comp Cont Educ Pract Vet 20:418, 1998.
102. Lopez R, et al: Circulating immune complexes and renal function in canine leishmaniasis. J Vet Med B 43:469, 1996.
103. Lucena R, et al: Third component of complement serum levels in dogs with leishmaniasis. J Vet Med [Am] 41:48, 1994.
104. Lucena R, et al: Antinuclear antibodies in dogs with leishmaniasis. J Vet Med A 43:255, 1996.
105. Margarito JM, et al: Levels of IgM and IgA circulating immune complexes in dogs with leishmaniasis. J Vet Med B 45:263, 1998.
106. Martínez-Moreno A, et al: Humoral and cell-mediated immunity in natural and experimental canine leishmaniasis. Vet Immunol Immunopathol 48:209, 1995.
106a. Mozos E, et al: Leishmaniasis and generalized demodicosis in three dogs: A clinicopathological and immunohistochemical study. J Comp Pathol 120:257, 1999.
107. Neogy AB, et al: Exploitation of parasite-derived antigen in therapeutic success against canine visceral leishmaniasis. Vet Parasitol 54:367, 1994.
108. Odin M, Dubey JP: Sudden death associated with *Neospora caninum* myocarditis in a dog. J Am Vet Med Assoc 203:831, 1993.
109. Oliva G, et al: Comparative efficacy of meglumine antimoniate and aminosidine sulphate, alone or in combination, in canine leishmaniasis. Ann Trop Med Parasitol 92:165, 1998.
110. Opitz M: Hautmanifestationen bei der Leishmaniose des Hudes. Tierärztl Prax 24:284, 1996.
111. Ozon C, et al: Disseminated feline leishmaniasis due to *Leishmania infantum* in southern France. Vet Parasitol 75:273, 1998.
112. Perl S, et al: Pyogranulomatous dermatitis associated with *Neospora caninum* in a dog. World Small Anim Vet Assoc 21:417, 1996.
113. Perl S, et al: Cutaneous neosporosis in a dog in Israel. Vet Parasitol 79:257, 1998.
114. Poli A, et al: Comparison of aminosidine (paromomycin) and sodium stibogluconate for treatment of canine leishmaniasis. Vet Parasitol 71:263, 1997.
115. Poli A, et al: *Neospora caninum* infection in a Bernese cattle dog from Italy. Vet Parasitol 79:79, 1998.
115a. Prats N, Ferrer L: A possible mechanism in the pathogenesis of cutaneous lesions in canine leishmaniasis. Vet Rec 137:103, 1995.
116. Pumarola M, et al: Canine leishmaniasis associated with systemic vasculitis in two dogs. J Comp Pathol 105:279, 1991.
117. Rasmussen K, Jensen AL: Some epidemiologic features of canine neosporosis in Denmark. Vet Parasitol 6:345, 1996.
118. Rhalem A, et al: Immune response against *Leishmania* antigens in dogs naturally and experimentally infection with *Leishmania infantum*. Vet Parasitol 81: 173, 1999.
118a. Rhalem A, et al: Analysis of immune responses in dogs with canine visceral leishmaniasis before, and after, drug treatment. Vet Immunol Immunopathol 71:69, 1999.
118b. Riera C, et al: Serological and parasitological follow-up in dogs experimentally infected with *Leishmania infantum* and treated with meglumine antimoniate. Vet Parasitol 84:33, 1999.
119. Romand S, et al: Direct agglutination test for serologic diagnosis of *Neospora caninum* infection. Parasitol Res 84:50, 1998.
119a. Roura X, et al: Detection of *Leishmania* infection in paraffin-embedded skin biopsies of dogs using polymerase chain reaction. J Vet Diagn Invest 11:385, 1999.
120. Ruehlmann D, et al: Canine neosporosis: a case report and literature review. J Am Anim Hosp Assoc 31:174, 1995.
121. Sangster LT, et al: Coccidia associated with cutaneous nodules in a dog. Vet Pathol 22:186, 1985.
122. Sellon R: Leishmaniasis in the United States. In: Kirk GW, Bonagura JD (eds): Current Veterinary Therapy XI. W. B. Saunders Co, Philadelphia, 1992, p 271.

123. Shelton GC, et al: A coccidia-like organism associated with subcutaneous granulomata in a dog. J Am Vet Med Assoc 152:263, 1968.
123a. Sideris V, et al: Asymptomatic canine leishmaniasis in greater Athens area, Greece. Eur J Epidemiol 15:271, 1999.
124. Slappendel RJ, Teske E: The effect of intravenous or subcutaneous administration of meglumine antimonate (Glucantime) in dogs with leishmaniasis. A randomized clinical trial. Vet Quart 19:10, 1997.
125. Valladares JE, et al: Pharmacokinetics of liposome-encapsulated meglumine antimonate after intramuscular and subcutaneous administration in dogs. Am J Trop Med Hyg 57–403, 1997.
126. Valladares JE, et al: Pharmacokinetics of meglumine antimoniate after administration of a multiple dose in dogs experimentally infected with *Leishmania infantum*. Vet Parasitol 75:33, 1998.
127. Vercammen F, et al: Development of a slide ELISA for canine leishmaniasis and comparison with four serological tests. Vet Rec 141:328, 1997.
128. Vercammen F, et al: A sensitive and specific 30-min Dot-ELISA for the detection of anti-*Leishmania* antibodies in the dog. Vet Parasitol 79:221, 1998.
129. Vercammen F, et al: First evaluation of the use of allopurinol as a single drug for the treatment of canine leishmaniasis. Vlaams Diergeneeskd Tijdschr 64:208, 1995.
130. Vercammen F, De Deken R: Treatment of canine visceral leishmaniasis with allopurinol. Vet Rec 137:252, 1995.
131. Vercammen F, De Deken R: Antibody kinetics during allopurinol treatment in canine leishmaniasis. Vet Rec 138:264, 1996.
132. Vexenat JA, et al: Clinical recovery and limited cure in canine visceral leishmaniasis treated with aminosidine (paromomycin). Am J Trop Med Hyg 58:448, 1998.
133. Zaffaroni E, et al: Epidemiological patterns of canine leishmaniosis in Western Liguria (Italy). Vet Parasitol 81:11, 1999.

Chapter 8

Skin Immune System and Allergic Skin Diseases

The subject of immunodermatology has seen a tremendous emergence of new discoveries, findings, and laboratory techniques. An adequate review of this information is decidedly beyond the scope of this chapter. For the practitioner, student, and academician interested in details, numerous texts on immunology and immunodermatology are available, and a number of review articles can be recommended.* In this discussion, we confine ourselves to a brief overview of the concepts regarding immunology of the skin. To comprehend this discussion or to read the current scientific literature on many cutaneous diseases, the reader has to understand some newer terminology about cell surface antigens, cytokines, and adhesion molecules, which are basic components of all immunologic discussions.

• SURFACE ANTIGENS (DETERMINANTS) OR RECEPTOR TERMINOLOGY

The understanding of current literature involving immune responses requires an understanding of cell surface determinants, which are referred to by the cluster differentiation (CD) nomenclature. This nomenclature is applied to antigens that have been detected on the surface of cells with monoclonal antibodies, and these are usually assigned a number. Initially these antigens were studied and shown to be specific to or limited to a specific group of cell types. This allowed us to identify what types of cells are present in tissues or exudates. Further studies have allowed us to recognize the function and, in many cases, the structure of these antigens. It is now known that many of the surface molecules are various immunoglobulins, carbohydrates, enzymes, adhesion molecules to bind with other cells, and receptors for the various immunoglobulins and chemicals (cytokines) secreted by cells to communicate with surrounding cells. In humans, this list of cell surface determinants has grown to well over 100 and appears to grow faster each year. Work in dogs and cats is allowing us to recognize some of these determinants in small animals as well (Table 8–1).[10, 21, 52]

Cytokines

Cytokines are secreted from cells and function in communicating with surrounding cells (Table 8–2). They are soluble proteins or glycoproteins that affect the growth, differentiation, function, and activation functions of other cells. These soluble hormone-like molecules were initially discovered in association with lymphocytes and called *lymphokines* or with monocytes and called *monokines*. Because it was discovered that many other cells produced the same substances, these terms, and others such as *secretory regulins* and *peptide regulatory factors,* were no longer considered appropriate.

Cytokines are transiently produced and exert their biological activities via specific cell-surface receptors of target cells, which may be expressed only after activation of the

---

*See references 4, 5, 9, 14, 16, 20, 22, 23, 30, 36, 42, 49, 50, 54, 58, 60, 61, 69, 72, 75–77.

Table 8–1 GLOSSARY OF LEUKOCYTE ANTIGENS[52]

ANTIGEN FAMILY	ANTIGEN	COMMENT
CD1	CD1a CD1b CD1c	CD1 antigens are expressed in cortical thymocytes but not on mature T cells. CD1 molecules are the best markers of dendritic/APC, although subpopulations of B cells and monocytes express CD1c.
TCR/CD3	TCR$\alpha\beta$ TCR$\gamma\delta$ CD3	The T-cell receptor/CD3 complex is only expressed on the surface of mature T cells. There are two types of TCR: $\alpha\beta$ and $\gamma\delta$; each is associated with the CD3 complex, which is the signal transduction portion of both types of receptor.
CD4	CD4	Expressed by MHC class II–restricted T-helper cells. Macrophages and dendritic/APC can upregulate CD4 in some instances.
CD5	CD5	Expressed by almost all mature T cells; a minor subset of B cells can express CD5 (B1 cells). CD5 binds to CD72 which is expressed on B cells.
CD8	CD8α CD8β	Expressed by MHC class I–restricted T cytotoxic cells. T cells usually express CD8$\alpha\beta$ heterodimers.
β_2 Integrins	CD11a CD11b CD11c CD18	The β_2 integrins (CD11/CD18) are the major adhesion molecule family of leukocytes. Most leukocytes express one or more members of this family. CD18 is the β_2 subunit that pairs with one of four α-subunits to form a heterodimer. The α-subunits are: CD11a (all leukocytes), CD11b (granulocytes, monocytes, some macrophages), CD11c (granulocytes, monocytes, dendritic antigen-presenting cells). Macrophages and granulocytes express 10-fold more CD18 than do lymphocytes.
CD14	CD14	Receptor for LPS (endotoxin) and LPS binding protein complexes. CD14 is expressed on monocytes, subsets of macrophages, and subsets of B cells.
CD21	CD21	CD21 is a C3dg receptor (CR2) that complexes with components of the B-cell antigen receptor complex (sIg, CD79a, CD79b), CD19, and CD35 (CR1). CD21 is expressed on mature B cells and follicular dendritic cells of the germinal center.
Link	CD44	A broadly expressed adhesion receptor (for hyaluronate) on many cell types; involved in lymphocyte trafficking and activation.
CD45	CD45 CD45RA CD45R	CD45 is the leukocyte common antigen family. CD45RA is one of these isoforms. CD45RA is expressed by all B cells and by 100% of B-cell lymphomas involving lymph nodes. In skin disease, CD45RA is expressed by mast cell tumors, plasmacytomas, and rarely by T-cell lymphomas.
β_1 Integrins	CD49d-like	VLA family (CD49a-f) members (α-subunits) occur as heterodimers with the β_1-integrin subunit. VLA-4 (CD49d) is broadly expressed on leukocytes. VLA-4 is upregulated on memory T cells.
ICAM	CD50 CD54	Intracellular adhesion molecule (ICAM) family consists of at least four members. ICAM-1 (CD54) is broadly expressed (leukocytes, endothelium) and is a major ligand of CD11a. CD54 is upregulated on endothelium, leukocytes, and even on epithelium in inflammation (by inflammatory cytokines) and is important in leukocyte transmigration. Expression of CD54 on dendritic/APC enhances T-cell activation through CD11a. ICAM-3 (CD50) is expressed broadly by leukocytes but rarely occurs on endothelium.
NCAM	CD56	Neural cell adhesion molecule isoform; marker of NK cells in humans.
Thy-1	CD90	Thy-1 expression varies considerably among different species. Dogs express Thy-1 on thymocytes and T cells (similar to mice); expression of Thy-1 in human T cells is lost at the early stages of thymocyte maturation; peripheral T cells lack Thy-1 expression. Thy-1 is highly expressed by dermal dendritic/APC and fibroblasts. It is an important marker in proliferative-diseases of dendritic/APC in dogs (e.g., cutaneous and systemic histiocytosis). Thy-1 is expressed also by monocytes and eosinophils but not by neutrophils in the dog.
MHCII		Major histocompatibility complex (MHC) class II molecules present exogenously derived antigen CD4⁻ T cells. MHC class II molecules are highly expressed on dendritic/APC, B cells, resting (dog and cat!) and activated T cells (dog, cat, and human), and monocytes. Granulocytes do not express MHC class II. MHC class II can be upregulated on epithelial cells (e.g., keratinocytes) and endothelial cells by interferon-γ.

Table continued on following page

Skin Immune System and Allergic Skin Diseases • 545

● Table 8–1 **GLOSSARY OF LEUKOCYTE ANTIGENS** Continued

ANTIGEN FAMILY	ANTIGEN	COMMENT
BCR/CD79	CD79a	The B-cell receptor complex (BCR) consists of surface Ig (sIg) complexed with two invariant molecules that function as signal transduction molecules (CD79a, CB79b). CD79a (MB-1) is expressed throughout all stages of B-cell development and persists into the plasma cell stage (despite absent or diminished sIg on plasma cells). CD79a is a useful marker for establishing the diagnosis of B-cell lymphoma because it is present in the BCR of all B cells regardless of the isotype of the sIg receptor (background associated with Ig stains in tissues is also not an issue). CD79a is useful in the diagnosis of cutaneous plasmacytoma (about 80% have focal to diffuse expression).

cell.[7–9, 31, 50, 54, 80, 85] Each mediator usually has multiple overlapping activities. Numerous cytokines have been described, and typically they may perform several different functions, depending on the tissue they interact with and the other cytokines that may be present. In different environments, the same cytokine may even have opposite effects.[7–9, 50, 80]

Cytokines may affect the same cell in a permissive, inhibitor, additive, or suppressive manner. Cytokines are involved in virtually every facet of immunity and inflammation, including antigen presentation, bone marrow differentiation, cellular recruitment and activation, adhesion molecule expression, and acute-phase reactions (see Table 8–2).[7] The particular cytokines produced in response to an immunologic insult determine whether an immune response develops and whether the response is humoral, cell-mediated, or allergic. Certain cell types, particularly T lymphocytes, may secrete different patterns of cytokines, and this has been used to subclassify these cells and their associated different functions. A large group of cytokines have been identified that have as their sole or major purpose the direction of the movement of cells involved in inflammation and the immune response. These have been called *chemokines* (Table 8–3).[3, 50]

Adhesion Molecules

Glycoproteins critical for cell-to-cell and cell-to-matrix adhesion, contact, and communication, adhesion molecules play an integral role in cutaneous inflammation and immunology (see Chap. 1) (Table 8–4).[19, 31, 78, 82] The *integrin family* includes membrane glycoproteins with α and β subunits, such as vascular cell adhesion molecule-1 (VCAM-1) on endothelial cells, which binds T lymphocytes and monocytes via vascular leukocyte adherin-4 (VLA-4), and fibronectin and laminin, which bind keratinocytes and mast cells. The *immunoglobulin gene superfamily* contains intercellular adhesion molecule-1 (ICAM-1) found on keratinocytes, Langerhans' cells, and endothelial cells, which binds leukocytes via leukocyte function-associated antigen-1 (LFA-1) or CD11a/CD18. The *selectin family* includes lectin adhesion molecule-1 (LECAM-1 or L-selectin) on lymphocytes, which binds endothelial leukocyte adhesion molecule-1 (ELAM-1 or E-selectin) and Gmp-140 (P-selectin) as a "homing" mechanism. The *cadherin family* members are important in desmosome function (see Chap. 1).

Major Histocompatibility Complex

The major histocompatibility complex (MHC) is a cluster of genes that encodes a range of molecules of fundamental importance to the immune system.[15] MHC class I loci encode the classic histocompatibility antigens, which are expressed by all nucleated cells of the body and are target antigens in the rejection of incompatible tissue grafts. Products of the MHC class III loci include a number of factors of the complement pathways, two cytokines (TNF-α and TNF-β), and two heat-shock proteins. The MHC class II loci

Table 8–2. IMMUNOLOGIC PROPERTIES OF CYTOKINES

CYTOKINE	PROPERTIES
Interleukins	
IL-1	Immunoaugmentation (promotes IL-2, IFN-α, colony-stimulating factor (CSF) production by T cells); promotes B-cell activation (promotes IL-4, IL-5, IL-6, IL-7 production and immunoglobulin synthesis); stimulates macrophages and fibroblasts; induces arachidonate metabolism
IL-2	Activates T and natural killer (NK) cells; promotes cell growth and immunoglobulin production; activates macrophages
IL-3	Promotes growth of early myeloprogenitor cells, eosinophils, mast cells, and basophils
IL-4	Promotes B-cell activation and IgE switch; promotes T-cell growth; synergistic with IL-3 for mast cell growth
IL-5	Eosinophilic growth; B-cell growth and chemotaxis; T-cell growth
IL-6	Terminal differentiation factor for cells and polyclonal immunoglobulin production; enhances IL-4 induced IgE production; promotes T-cell proliferation and cytotoxicity; promotes NK-cell activity; activates neutrophils
IL-7	Lymphopoietin
IL-8	Chemoattractant for neutrophils, T lymphocytes, basophils; increases histamine release from basophils
IL-9	Maturation of erythroid progenitor cell tumor growth; synergistic with IL-3 for mast cell growth
IL-10	Downregulation (inhibits production of IL-1, IL-2, IL-4, IL-5, IL-6, IL-8, IL-12, TNF-α, IFN-γ, MHC class II expression)
IL-11	Megakaryocyte, lymphocyte, and plasma cell growth
IL-12	Cytotoxic lymphocyte maturation; NK-cell activation and proliferation
IL-13	Similar to IL-4; enhances production of MHC class II and integrins; reduced production of IL-1 and TNF; activation of eosinophils
IL-14	Expands clones of B cells and suppresses immunoglobulin secretion
IL-15	Proliferation; increased cytotoxicity of T cells, NK cells; expression of ICAM-3; B-cell growth and differentiation
IL-16	Chemoattractant, growth factor
IL-17	Autocrine proliferation and activation
IL-18	Similar to IL-12; inhibits IgE production by increasing IFN-γ
Colony-Stimulating Factors	
Granulocyte CSF	Neutrophil growth
Monocyte CSF	Monocyte growth
Granulocyte-monocyte CSF	Monomyelocytic growth
Basic fibroblast growth factor (bFGF)	Fibroblast growth and matrix production
Platelet-derived growth factor	Proliferation; chemoattractant for fibroblasts; active in wound healing
Stem cell factor	Chemoattractant; with IL-3 stimulates growth; also has histamine-releasing activity
Transforming growth factor	Inhibits IL-2-stimulated growth; switch factor for IgA but inhibits IgM and IgG production; counteracts IL-4 stimulation of IgE; inhibits cytotoxicity
Interferons	
IFN-α	Antiviral; antiproliferative; immunomodulating (activation of macrophages; proliferation of B cells; stimulation of NK cells); inhibit fibroblasts
IFN-β	Antiviral; antiproliferative; immunomodulating (activation of macrophages, proliferation of B cells, stimulation of NK cells); inhibit fibroblasts
IFN-γ	Immunomodulation (activation of macrophages; proliferation of B cells; stimulation of NK cells); antiproliferative; antiviral; inhibit fibroblasts; inhibits IL-4-mediated expression of IgE receptors and the IgE switch
Tumor Necrosis Factors	
TNF-α	Inflammatory, immunoenhancing, and tumoricidal
TNF-β	Inflammatory, immunoenhancing, and tumoricidal
TNF-$\beta_{1,2,3}$	Fibroplasia and immunosuppression

Table 8–3. CHEMOKINES AND THEIR ACTIONS

CHEMOKINE	TARGET CELLS	BIOLOGICAL EFFECTS
CXC (α) Family		
BCA-1 (B-cell–attracting chemokine-1)	B lymphocytes	Chemotaxis
β-TG (β-thromboglobulin)	Neutrophils	Chemotaxis; activation
	Fibroblasts	Chemotaxis; proliferation; activation
CTAP-III (connective tissue-activating peptide III)	Neutrophils	Chemotaxis; activation
	Fibroblasts	Chemotaxis; proliferation; activation
ENA-78 (epithelial cell-derived neutrophil-activating peptide 78)	Neutrophils	Chemotaxis
GCP-2 (granulocyte chemotactic protein 2)	Neutrophils	Chemotaxis; activation
GRO-α, β, ∂ (growth regulated oncogene)	Neutrophils	Chemotaxis; activation
	Basophils	Chemotaxis; activation
	T lymphocytes	Chemotaxis
IL-8 (interleukin-8)	Neutrophils	Chemotaxis; activation
	Basophils	Chemotaxis; inhibition of histamine release
	T lymphocytes	Chemotaxis; inhibition of IL-4 synthesis
	B lymphs/B-CELL	Chemotaxis; inhibition of growth and IgE production
	Keratinocytes	Chemotaxis; expression of HLA-DR
IP-10 (interferon-inducible protein 10)	Activated T lymphocytes	Chemotaxis
	Monocytes	Chemotaxis
	NK cells	Chemotaxis; activation
MIG (monokine induced by γ-interferon)	Activated T lymphocytes	Chemotaxis
	NK cells	Chemotaxis
NAP-2 (neutrophil-activating peptide 2)	Neutrophils	Chemotaxis; activation
PF-4 (platelet factor 4)	Neutrophils	Chemotaxis; activation
	Monocytes	Chemotaxis
	Fibroblasts	Chemotaxis
	Basophils	Modulation of histamine release
SDF-1 (stromal cell-derived factor 1)	T lymphocytes	Chemotaxis
C-C (β) Family		
Ckβ8 (chemokine β8)	Monocytes	Chemotaxis
	Resting T lymphocytes	Chemotaxis
Eotaxin	Eosinophils	Chemotaxis
	Basophils	Chemotaxis; activation
Eotaxin-2	Eosinophils	Chemotaxis
	Basophils	Chemotaxis; activation
	Resting T lymphocytes	Chemotaxis
HCC-2	Monocytes	Chemotaxis
	T lymphocytes	Chemotaxis
	Eosinophils	Chemotaxis
	Monocytes	Chemotaxis
MCP-1 (monocyte chemoattractant protein 1)	Monocytes	Chemotaxis
	Basophils	Activation
	T lymphocytes	Chemotaxis
	NK cells	Chemotaxis; activation
	Dendritic cells	Chemotaxis
MCP-2	Monocytes	Chemotaxis
	T lymphocytes	Chemotaxis
	Eosinophils	Chemotaxis; activation
	Basophils	Chemotaxis; activation
	NK cells	Chemotaxis; activation
	Dendritic cells	Chemotaxis
MCP-3	Monocytes	Chemotaxis
	T lymphocytes	Chemotaxis
	Eosinophils	Chemotaxis

Table continued on following page

Table 8–3 CHEMOKINES AND THEIR ACTIONS Continued		
CHEMOKINE	TARGET CELLS	BIOLOGICAL EFFECTS
MCP-3 Continued	Basophils	Chemotaxis; activation
	NK cells	Chemotaxis; activation
	Dendritic cells	Chemotaxis
MCP-4	Eosinophils	Chemotaxis; activation
	Monocytes	Chemotaxis
	T lymphocytes	Chemotaxis
	Basophils	Chemotaxis; activation
MIP-1α (macrophage inflammatory protein 1α or LD-78; also known as endogenous pyrogen)	T lymphocytes	Chemotaxis
	Monocytes/macrophages	Chemotaxis
	B lymphocytes	Increased IgE/IgG4 production
	NK cells	Chemotaxis; activation
	Basophils	Activation
	Dendritic cells	Chemotaxis
MIP-1β	NK cells	Chemotaxis; activation
	Dendritic cells	Chemotaxis
	B lymphocytes	Increased IgE/IgG4 production
NIP-3α (also known as Exodus of liver and activation-regulated chemokine [LARC])	T lymphocytes	Chemotaxis
	Dendritic cells	Chemotaxis
RANTES (regulated upon activation normal T cells expressed and presumably secreted)	Eosinophils	Chemotaxis
	T lymphocytes	Chemotaxis
	Monocytes	Chemotaxis
	Basophils	Chemotaxis
	NK cells	Chemotaxis; activation
	B lymphocytes	Increased IgE/IgG4 production
	Dendritic cells	Chemotaxis
SLC (secondary lymphoid tissue chemokine)	T lymphocytes	Chemotaxis
STCP-1 (stimulated T-cell chemotactic protein)	Activated T lymphocytes	Chemotaxis
C (γ) Family		
Lymphotactin	Lymphocytes	Chemotaxis
	Activated NK cells	Chemotaxis; activation
CX3C Family		
Fractalkine	Monocytes	Chemotaxis
	T lymphocytes	Chemotaxis

encode a series of transmembrane molecules with restricted expression by cells of the immune system, particularly the antigen-presenting cells: Langerhans' cells, dendrocytes, macrophages, and B lymphocytes.

In normal skin, low numbers (mean, 1.6 cells/HPF) of MHC class II and Langerhans' cells were demonstrated.[15] Increased numbers of MHC class II and Langerhans' cells were visible in the epidermis of dogs with discoid lupus erythematosus, allergic skin disease, and deep bacterial pyoderma, but not in pemphigus foliaceus.[15]

Skin-Associated Lymphoid Tissue

The immune system and its inflammatory component are complex models of biological activity and interaction. There is a tendency to dissect the immune response into its individual components and to discuss them as autonomous functional units. Immune responses are interwoven and interdependent, however, and manipulation of one component influences others. Newer studies have shown that the skin itself is a very integral and active component of the immune system. These observations led to the hypothesis that the skin, like the gastrointestinal tract, may be a functioning lymphoid organ; as such, it has been called skin-associated lymphoid tissue (SALT).[9, 53] Even prior to the development

Table 8-4 CELL ADHESION MOLECULES

ADHESION MOLECULES	CD	FAMILY	DISTRIBUTION	FUNCTION
VLA-1	CD49a	Integrin	ECs, monocytes, macrophages, activated T/B cells	Cell-matrix adhesion
VLA-2	CD49b	Integrin	ECs, EPs, activated T cells	Cell matrix adhesion
VLA-3	CD49c	Integrin	ECs, EPs	Cell-matrix adhesion
VLA-4	CD49d	Integrin	Leukocytes	Cell-cell and cell-matrix adhesion
VLA-5	CD49e	Integrin	ECs, EPs, lymphocyte, monocytes, macrophages	Cell-matrix adhesion
VLA-6	CD49f	Integrin	ECs, EPs, T lymphocytes, mast cells	Cell-matrix adhesion
LFA-1	CD11a/CD18	Integrin	Leukocytes	Adhesion of leukocytes of ECs
MAC-1	CD11b/CD18	Integrin	Monocytes, macrophages, granulocytes, Langerhans' cells	Adhesion of leukocytes to ECs
gp150,95	CD11c/CD18	Integrin	Monocytes, macrophages, granulocytes, Langerhans' cells	Adhesion of leukocytes to ECs
ICAM-1	CD54	IgG superfamily	Monocytes, EPs, fibroblasts	Cell-cell adhesion
ICAM-2	CD102	IgG superfamily	ECs, leukocytes	Adhesion of leukocytes to ECs
ICAM-3	CD50	IgG superfamily	EC, leukocytes, Langerhans' cells	Adhesion of leukocytes to ECs
VCAM-1	CD-106	IgG superfamily	Activated ECs	Adhesion of leukocytes to ECs
PECAM-1	CD31	IgG superfamily	ECs, leukocytes	Initiation of EC-EC adhesion, platelet-monocyte/neutrophil-EC adhesion
MAdCAM-1		IgG superfamily	ECs	Adhesion of leukocytes to ECs
E-selectin	CD62E	Selectin	ECs	Adhesion of leukocytes to ECs; rolling phenomenon
P-selectin	CD62P	Selectin	Platelets, ECs	Adhesion of platelets to monocytes and neutrophils; adhesion of leukocytes to ECs; rolling phenomenon
L-selectin	CD62L	Selectin	Leukocytes	Leukocyte-EC adhesion; lymphocyte homing
Cadherins		Cadherin	EPs	EP-EP adhesion

CD, cluster of differentiation; VLA, very late activation; ICAM, intercellular adhesion molecule, VCAM-1, vascular cell adhesion molecule 1; PECAM-1, platelet-endothelial cell adhesion molecule 1; MAdCAM-1, mucosal address in cell adhesion molecule 1; PSGL, P-selectin glycoprotein ligand 1; EC, endothelial cell; EP, epithelial cell.

of the SALT concept, it was suggested that the skin functions as a primary immunologic organ. The term *skin immune system* (SIS) has also been proposed to describe the components of the skin, excluding the regional lymph nodes, that constitute SALT.[9] In the following discussions, we attempt to briefly review the specifics of the skin immune system so that the reader is familiar with the tremendous gains in knowledge and future avenues for work that will lead to further discoveries.

SKIN IMMUNE SYSTEM

The SIS contains two major components, the cellular and the humoral. The cellular component comprises keratinocytes, epidermal dendritic cells (Langerhans' cells), dermal dendrocytes, lymphocytes, tissue macrophages, mast cells, endothelial cells, and granulocytes (see Chap. 1). The humoral components include immunoglobulins, complement components, fibrinolysins, cytokines, eicosanoids, neuropeptides, and antimicrobial peptides. Virtually all inflammatory and some noninflammatory skin diseases involve alterations of, or an interaction between, one or both parts of the SIS. As a result, it becomes inappropriate to consider immunologic disease as a category if one is to include all skin diseases that involve the immune system. Therefore, this chapter presents those diseases classically described as allergic (hypersensitive), and Chapter 9 deals with the immune-mediated skin diseases.

The epidermis is often considered the producer of the effective barrier between the outside world and the body's inside environment. In this role, the epidermis acts as a mechanical barrier because it is often the first component of the body exposed to environmental agents such as viruses, bacteria, toxins, insects, arachnids, and allergens. The epidermis also plays an active role in the body's immunologic response to these external factors.

Before the immune system can respond to these external factors, however, their presence has to be recognized. Recognition may occur at one of two levels: on the surface of the epidermis or in the dermis. If an intact epidermis is present, it would seem most likely that recognition of an environmental agent occurs in the epidermis. For many immunologic responses, including helper T-cell induction, antigens must first be processed for presentation to lymphocytes. Classically, this occurs by macrophages, which express MHC class II antigens, but other cells with MHC class II antigens may be involved. Because macrophages are present in the dermis and do not normally reside in the epidermis, this function is served by another cell, the Langerhans' cell. Even before Langerhans' cells are reached, external stimuli will likely encounter keratinocytes, which we now realize do more than act as a physical barrier.

Keratinocytes

Keratinocytes do much more than produce keratin, surface lipids, and intercellular substances (see Chap. 1). They are intimately associated with Langerhans' cells and play a major role in the SIS. It is now clear that keratinocytes produce a wide variety of cytokines that have important roles in mediating cutaneous immune responses, inflammation, wound healing, and the growth and development of certain neoplasms.[2,68] Keratinocytes also produce eicosanoids, prostaglandin (PG) E_2, and neuropeptides such as propiomelanocortin and α-MSH. Though some of these are proinflammatory, some—such as prostaglandin E_2 and the neuropeptides—also have anti-inflammatory effects.[68] Keratinocytes, especially when perturbed by exposure to interferon-γ (IFN-γ), express MHC II antigens.[9] This expression is required for cells to be antigen-presenting cells for T-cell responses.

Though keratinocytes are capable of phagocytosis, their role as antigen-processing cells is unlikely because they do not efficiently process and present surface MHC II–bound peptide antigens and have not been shown to be able to activate naive T cells. However, they can induce proliferation of allogenic CD4+ T cells. There is evidence that keratinocytes expressing MHC II surface molecules may induce tolerance. Keratinocytes may also be stimulated to produce the leukocyte adhesion molecule, ICAM-1.

Besides production of these immunologically important cell-surface markers, keratinocytes have been shown to be very capable producers of a variety of cytokines. They are the primary epidermal source for cytokines.[9] Probably the most immunologically important is interleukin-1 (IL-1). Keratinocytes store IL-1, which is readily released after damage to the cells. In fact, release of IL-1 from keratinocytes is essentially a primary event in skin disease.[47] Other cytokines derived from keratinocytes include IL-3, IL-6, IL-7, IL-8, IL-10, IL-12, IL-15, IL-16, IL-18, tumor necrosis factor α (TNF-α), and a variety of growth factors and granulocyte-monocyte-macrophage stimulating and activating factors.[9,44,47,50,68,80]

Depending on what cytokines are produced, keratinocytes may affect the type of immune response. Keratinocytes produce both IL-12 and IL-10, which may skew which type of T cells are activated or downregulate inflammation, depending on what stage T cells are exposed to them. Keratinocytes may also play a role in tissue repair by production of multiple growth factors. Therefore, it becomes apparent that keratinocytes are important in stimulating and controlling inflammation and repair of tissue. Considering the diverse functions, activities, and mediators produced by keratinocytes, it has become obvious that the epidermis plays a major role in the immune response and that keratinocytes do not function only as a mechanical barrier to environmental substances.[9, 68, 85]

Langerhans' Cells

Langerhans' cells are interdigitating dendritic cells, which appear as suprabasilar clear cells on skin sections stained routinely with hematoxylin and eosin (H&E) (see Chap. 1). They are members of a family of highly specialized antigen-presenting cells called *dendritic cells*.[37] They are localized at the interface between organism and environment, and they are important sentinels of the immune system. Langerhans' cells are the major antigen-presenting cells of the epidermis and the only epidermal cell capable of activating naive T cells. They are bone marrow–derived monocyte/macrophage-type cells.

The Langerhans' cell is characteristically identified in the epidermis by the electron-microscopic presence of Birbeck granules. These granules are often absent in the dog (see Chap. 1). In the dog, cutaneous dendritic antigen-presenting cells include both epidermal and dermal Langerhans' cells that express abundant CD1 molecules. Because CD1c may also be expressed on canine monocytes, CD1a is considered the best marker for canine Langerhans' cells. The function of the CD1 surface receptors has been elucidated.

CD1 receptors appear to be a third method of antigen presentation that is specialized and may play a more important role in cutaneous disease. A unique feature of CD1 antigen presentation is the ability to present nonpeptide antigens to T cells.[51] The epidermal Langerhans' cells do not express CD90 (Thy 1), whereas the dermal Langerhans' cells do.[52] Langerhans' cells express MHC class II antigens as well as receptors for C3b, Fc-IgG, and Fc-IgE. The main function of Langerhans' cells is antigen-specific T-cell activation. Antigenic peptides derived from endogenous protein synthesis (e.g., viral antigens, transplantation antigens, tumor-associated antigens) are generally presented in the context of MHC class I molecules, which are expressed on the surface of essentially all nucleated cells and recognized by CD8+ antigen-specific cytotoxic T cells. Exogenous antigens (not synthesized within antigen-presenting cells [e.g., extracellular bacteria, bacterial toxins, dermatophytes, vaccines, pollens, dust mites]) are presented via CD4+ helper cells that recognize antigenic peptides bound to MHC class II antigen selectively expressed by professional antigen-presenting cells (e.g., macrophages, dendritic cells, B cells).[9, 21, 37, 50, 54, 68]

Langerhans' cells bind epidermal antigens and then present the antigens along with co-stimulatory molecules, the so-called second signal to the lymphoid tissues (regional lymph node), where helper T-cell lymphocytes in particular are activated. MHC II molecules are produced in the endoplasmic reticulum, where they then migrate to the Golgi and endolysosomal compartments. The processed protein results in antigen peptides that are incorporated into the MHC II molecules at various points in this migration from endoplasmic reticulum to the cell surface. At the surface, the antigenic peptide/MHC II complex is presented to the T-cell receptor on the surface of the T cell, resulting in antigen-specific T-cell activation. Effective T-cell activation requires co-stimulators and cytokines that promote clonal expansion of the antigen-specific T cell. The co-stimulator or second signal is often supplied by the expression of the B7 family of cell surface molecules. These molecules may be expressed after Langerhans' cells are exposed to lipopolysaccharide, TNF-α, and IL-1B as well as other signals. Langerhans' cells produce cytokines such as IL-1 and some lipid mediators that direct the T-cell response.

Langerhans' cells express high levels of E-cadherin (other dendritic cells do not), which is important in selective adhesion to keratinocytes.[37] Epidermal Langerhans' cells are thus highly specialized cells expressing molecules that allow them to home to skin and localize in the epidermis. Tissue injury, microbial infection, and other perturbations of epidermal homeostasis provide a "danger" signal leading to local production of proinflammatory cytokines, which in turn induce mobilization and migration of Langerhans' cells to lymphoid tissue.

In humans, quantitative immunohistochemical studies demonstrated differences in Langerhans' cells in dermatitis due to internal versus external antigen sources.[59] Evaluation of skin biopsy specimens revealed significantly more Langerhans' cells and spongiosis in contact dermatitis (external antigen source) compared with drug reactions (internal antigen source).

Lymphocytes

Lymphocytes are all derived from a common stem cell in the bone marrow and may be divided into three main types: B (bursa- or bone marrow–derived) cells, T (thymus-dependent) cells, and natural killer (NK) cells.

B cells are characterized by possessing unique surface immunoglobulins, Fc receptors, CD79 or B-cell receptor complex, and C3b receptors. B cells mature into *plasma cells* after recognition of its specific antigen and activation, which produce the immunoglobulins IgG, IgM, IgA, and IgE, and they are responsible for antibody immunity.

The growth and development of B cells occurs in two phases. The first is antigen-independent and yields B cells that express IgM and IgD. These initial antibodies constitute the majority of the primary antibody response to antigens but are low affinity. The second phase, or memory response, is a response to a specific antigen that, with T cells, induces differentiation into IgA-, IgG-, and IgE-secreting or memory B cells.[13, 50, 51, 54] The second phase requires T-cell activation and is partly controlled by cytokines released by T cells, with IL-1, IL-2, IL-4, IL-5, and IL-10 all playing roles in growth or differentiation. IL-4 and IL-13 are particularly important for B cells to switch into IgE-producing plasma cells, and this effect is enhanced by IL-5, IL-6, and TNF-α.[13, 50] IL-4 also induces the switch to IgG4, and this precedes the switch to IgE.[13] In human beings, B lymphocytes are rarely found in normal skin and, even in dermatologic disease, are much less common than T cells.[9] Considering the relative increase in the frequency of plasma cells in canine compared with human cutaneous disease, however, the importance of B lymphocytes in the dog may be relatively greater. Humoral immunity is described as providing primary defense against invading bacteria and neutralization activity against circulating viruses.

NK cells are large granular lymphocytes that do not express antigen-specific receptors but do have receptors that recognize the self MHC I molecule. When they encounter nucleated cells with self MHC I molecules, these receptors inhibit killing (killer inhibitory receptors). Many viral or tumor cells fail to express self MHC I and are killed. NK cells also have receptors for Fc receptors and may mediate antibody-dependent cytotoxicity.[21, 51]

T cells are formed in the thymus, express CD3 or T-cell receptor when mature, and are divided into two major types: helper and suppressor or cytotoxic T lymphocytes. The two major types are differentiated by their activity and their T-cell receptors, which is the part of the T cell that recognizes an antigen. Classically, T cells are considered responsible for cell-mediated immunity, activation of memory B cells, and stimulation of NK cells.

T cells play a central role in directing and modifying the immune response. Functions of T cells include (1) helping B cells make antibody and directing what type of antibody is made (helper T cells), (2) suppressing B-cell antibody production (suppressor T cells), (3) directly damaging "target" cells, (4) mediating delayed hypersensitivity reactions, (5) suppressing delayed hypersensitivity reactions mediated by other T cells, (6) regulating macrophage function, (7) modulating the inflammatory response with chemokines and cytokines, (8) inducing graft rejection, and (9) producing graft-versus-host reactions. T-cell lymphokines may amplify or dampen phagocytic activity, collagen production, vascular permeability, and coagulation phenomena. T cells can kill microorganisms and other cells, or they can recruit effector cells to perform this function. T-cell function is known to be suppressed by numerous infections (staphylococcal pyoderma, demodicosis, blastomycosis, canine distemper, feline leukemia virus infection, feline immunodeficiency virus infection), cancers, and drugs.[30, 51, 53, 76]

As T cells mature in the thymus, they develop surface receptor molecules. The receptor molecules expressed on a T cell are critical in determining the future function of the cell. CD3 represents the T-cell receptor complex and marks all mature T cells. MHC II–expressing T helper cells express CD4, and MHC I–restricted cytotoxic T cells express CD8. CD28 is considered the major co-stimulator molecule required for the second signal from the antigen-presenting cells. CD28 is thought to react with the B7 receptor on the antigen-presenting cells. We also know that subpopulations of helper and cytotoxic T cells exist. These subpopulations have different cytokine production profiles. The initial separation and most studied are the Th1 and Th2 subpopulations of CD4+ T cells; Th2 cells produce IL-4, IL-5, and IL-10, whereas Th1 cells produce IL-2, IFN-γ, and TNF-α.[9, 50, 54] However, we now recognize that CD8 and γ-δ T cells also have type 1 and type 2 profiles.[80]

The type and diversity of T-cell receptors present on lymphocytes is an area of active research and one of the most relevant markers of T-cell populations. Terminology one sees regarding T-cell receptors refers to the structure of the T-cell receptor, which is usually a heterodimer consisting of two protein chains, most commonly in humans α and β and, less commonly, γ and δ. These protein chains are divided into variable, diversity, joining, and constant regions. With polymerase chain reaction technology, T cells in tissue are now being studied by their variable region of the T-cell receptor complex, which represents a small group of antigens. These antigens are most likely representing what is initiating, or the target of, the inflammation.[51]

Tissue Macrophages

The end stage of the mononuclear phagocyte system (MPS) is the tissue macrophage which, in the dermis, has also been considered the precursor cell to the dermal dendrocyte.[9, 54] In blood, lymph nodes, and other tissues, there are dendritic macrophage type cells that are also thought to be part of the MPS.[24] These cells are all bone marrow–derived and pass through the blood circulation as monocytes which, in general, are CD14+. These cells have a wide variety of activities and morphologic appearances, especially in inflammation. Tissue macrophages, epithelioid cells, and multinucleated histiocytic giant cells are all MPS cells found in a variety of inflammatory diseases. They serve the critical function of the afferent arm of the immune system in processing and presenting antigens, especially for T-cell activation, yet are also important in the efferent arm of the immune response.

The MPS also plays major roles in wound healing, granulopoiesis, erythropoiesis, and antimicrobial defense (especially against intracellular pathogens). Monocytes and macrophages may secrete numerous enzymes, cytokines, inflammatory mediators, histamine-releasing factors, and inhibitors when stimulated. Some mediators upgrade inflammation, whereas others inhibit inflammatory activity in order to prevent too much tissue destruction from inflammation.

Mast Cells

Mast cells are derived from hematopoietic stem cells in the bone marrow and migrate as immature unrecognizable cells in the blood and then localize in connective or mucosal tissues (see Chap. 1). Once present in tissue, they proliferate and differentiate into mature recognizable mast cells.[35] The regulation of mast cell proliferation and differentiation is the subject of much research. Cytokines from fibroblasts, stem cell growth factor, T cells, and IL-3 are particularly important.

Though mast cells were recognized many years ago, their role in preventing disease or homeostasis was unknown. Mast cells combine characteristics of both innate and acquired immune responses: They can (1) bind certain bacteria and phagocytose/kill them, (2) elaborate and secrete several biologically active products, and (3) serve as an antigen-presenting cell and promote clonal expansion of CD4+ helper T cells.[35, 48, 63] Their role in disease has been recognized for many years, and the importance of mast cells in immediate hypersensitivity diseases is well documented. Their role in other skin diseases, however, such as contact dermatitis and bullous pemphigoid, and in the process of fibrosis has only recently been recognized.[50] This relates to the diverse effects and interactions mast cells have with other cells and structures of the skin (Fig. 8–1).

Mast cells serve as repositories for or synthesizers of numerous inflammatory mediator

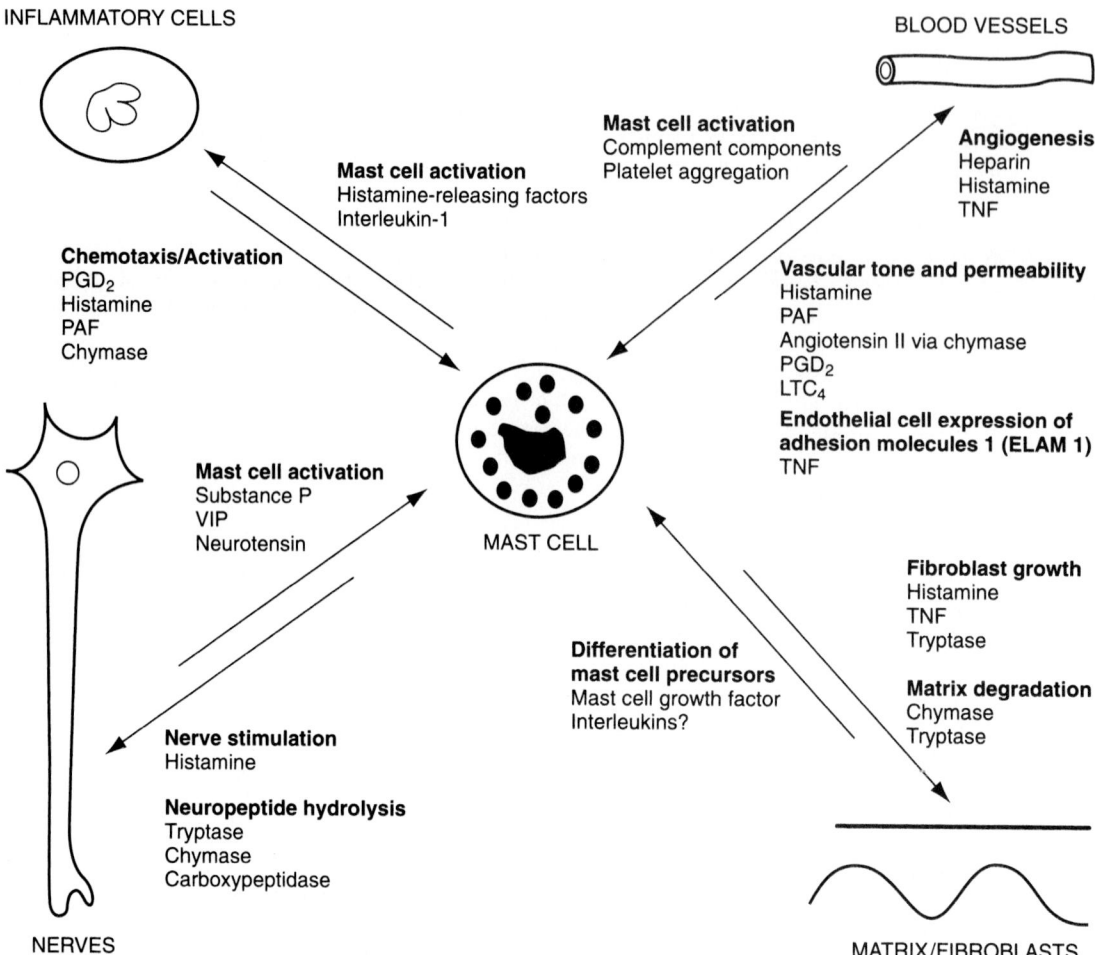

FIGURE 8–1. Schematic representation of the documented interactions of human mast cells with other cells and structures in skin. Factors identified in rodent species only are not shown. (From Goldstein SM, Wintroub BV: The cellular and molecular biology of the human mast cell. In: Fitzpatrick, TB, et al, ed: Dermatology in General Medicine V. McGraw-Hill, New York, 1993, p 365.)

substances. The mediators present vary by species studied and according to the type of the mast cells (see later).[50] Some mediators are universally present, such as histamine, leukotrienes, eosinophil chemotactic factor of anaphylaxis, and proteolytic enzymes. There are two main categories of mediators. Preformed mediators are produced and stored in mast cell granules, which are modified lysosomes that develop from the Golgi apparatus (Table 8–5).[50] Mast cells also produce mediators that are newly synthesized at the time of activation and degranulation (Table 8–6). More recently, it has been recognized that mast cells have the potential to synthesize many cytokines—IL-1, IL-2, IL-3, IL-4, IL-5, IL-6, IL-8, IL-10, IL-13, granulocyte macrophage colony-stimulating factor, TNF-α, IFN-γ— and many chemokines (e.g., macrophage inflammatory protein (MIP) 1-α).[12,48] Cytokine production may result in stored cytokines or secretion independent from mediators generated from degranulation.

There are differences in cytokine profiles for the different types of mast cells, further adding to the heterogeneity of mast cells.[12] Mast cells, therefore, may play many roles in the mediation of immune and inflammatory responses. Classically, they are known for the recruitment of eosinophils and neutrophils, immunoglobulins, and complement from the circulation and the regulation of the immunologic response (see Tables 8–5 and 8–6). In

● Table 8-5 **PREFORMED MEDIATORS OF HUMAN MAST CELLS**

MEDIATOR	FUNCTION
Histamine	H_1 and H_2 receptor–mediated effects on smooth muscle, endothelial cells, and nerve endings
Tryptase	Cleaves C3 and C3a; degrades VIP and CGRP kallikrein-like activity; activates fibroblasts
Chymases	Function unclear; cleave neuropeptides, including substance P
Carboxypeptidase	Acts in concert with other neutral proteases
Acid hydrolases	Break down complex carbohydrates
Arylsulfatase	Hydrolyses aromatic sulfate esters
ECF-A	Eosinophil chemotaxis and "activation"
Neutrophil chemotactic factor	Neutrophil chemotaxis and "activation"
Heparin	Anticoagulant, anticomplementary; modifies activities of other preformed mediators
Chondroitin sulfate	Function unknown
Cytokines (e.g., TNF-α, IL-4, IL-3, IL-5, and IL-6)	See Table 8–2

addition, mast cells can (1) produce IL-12 to drive Th1 responses, (2) produce IL-4, which is essential for the conversion of Th0 to Th2 cells, (2) produce IL-5 and IL-10 to drive Th2 responses, and (4) activate B cells without surface contact.

Mast cells may be divided in rodents morphologically and functionally into type I (atypical, mucosal) and type II (typical, connective tissue) cells.[9, 50, 54] *Mucosal* and *connective tissue* are misleading terms because both types of mast cells occur in mucosa and connective tissue. A more precise differentiation of mast cells has been based on the proteases, tryptase and chymase, present in the cells.[63] MC_T mast cells contain tryptase and are the predominant type found in the lung and small intestinal mucosa. MC_{TC} cells contain tryptase and chymase and are the predominant type in the skin, blood vessels, and gastrointestinal submucosa. However, because of differences in human and rodent mast cell proteases, this classification has been largely limited to human mast cells, though dog mast cells do have chymase and tryptase.[35]

Mast cell degranulation may be initiated by a variety of substances, including allergens

● Table 8-6 **PHARMACOLOGIC ACTIVITIES OF NEWLY GENERATED MAST CELL MEDIATORS**

MEDIATOR	ABBREVIATION	PHARMACOLOGIC ACTIONS
Prostaglandin D_2	PGD_2	Bronchoconstriction; peripheral vasodilation; coronary and pulmonary vasoconstriction; inhibition of platelet aggregation; neutrophil chemoattraction; augmentation of basophil histamine release
Prostaglandin F_2	9-α, 11-β-PGF_2	Bronchoconstriction; peripheral vasodilation; coronary vasoconstriction; inhibition of platelet aggregation
Thromboxane A_2	TXA_2	Vasoconstriction; platelet aggregaction; bronchoconstriction
Leukotriene B_4	LTB_4	Neutrophil chemotaxis, adherence and degranulation; augmentation of vascular permeability
Leukotriene C_4	LTC_4	Bronchoconstriction; increase in vascular permeability; arteriolar constriction
Leukotriene D_4	LTD_4	Bronchoconstriction; increase in vascular permeability
Leukotriene E_4	LTE_4	Weak bronchoconstriction; enhancement of bronchial responsiveness; increase in vascular permeability
Platelet-activating factor	PAF	Platelet aggregation; chemotaxis and degranulation of eosinophils and neutrophils; increase in vascular permeability; bronchoconstriction; engenders hypotension

cross-linking two surface IgE (or IgGd) molecules, complement components C3a and C5a, eosinophil major basic protein, some hormones (estrogen, gastrin, somatostatin), substance P, and a group of cytokines called *histamine-releasing factors*.[30, 50, 54] Other exogenous compounds known to cause mast cell degranulation include anti-IgE, compound 48/80, opiates, concanavalin A, and calcium ionophores. The different types of mast cells may be affected differently, depending on the compound that causes degranulation. Variability in degranulation, the mediators released, quantity, and time course may occur. Another secretory mechanism for histamine release has been described.[50] It has been called piecemeal secretion and transfer to the cell surface by microvesicles. There is also variability in the response of different mast cells to inhibition of mast cell degranulation with the drug cromolyn. Intestinal mast cells were most affected, whereas MC_T mast cells from the lung were mildly affected, and skin MC_{TC} mast cells were not affected.[63]

The heterogeneity of mast cells has been demonstrated in dog skin, though it has not been studied to the degree of human or rodent mast cells, and further work is warranted.[35, 50] This is an important distinction because many differences are species-specific. The skin of atopic dogs contains at least two subsets of mast cells that are distinguished in the following ways: (1) histologically, by metachromatic staining properties in different fixatives, and (2) functionally, by response to antigen in vivo (see discussion of canine atopy). Three mast cell subtypes are distinguished in normal canine skin based on their content of the mast cell–specific proteases, chymase and tryptase: tryptase mast cells, chymase mast cells, and tryptase/chymase mast cells.[41]

Interestingly, histamine has two types of effects on hypersensitivity reactions, proinflammatory and anti-inflammatory. The proinflammatory effects of histamine are mediated through histamine 1 (H_1) receptors and resultant decreases in intracellular cyclic adenosine monophosphate (cAMP). Also, H_1 receptors mediate pruritus, and the trauma associated with pruritus may lead to further tissue and keratinocyte damage. The anti-inflammatory effects of histamine (inhibition of the release of inflammatory mediator substances from mast cells, neutrophils, lymphocytes, and monocyte-macrophages) are mediated through H_2 receptors and resultant increases in cAMP. Canine and feline blood vessels possess both H_1 and H_2 receptors.[53]

Endothelial Cells

The vascular endothelium is now known to be a very active cell type that is important in inflammation, immune responses, and tissue repair (see Chap. 1).[18, 50, 54, 71] In response to various cytokines, endothelial cells express adhesion molecules (integrins, selectins, and immunoglobulin supergene family [intercellular adhesion molecules]) on their surfaces. The selectins (E-selectin and P-selectin) are expressed on endothelial cells after certain inflammatory stimuli and act to slow down and cause rolling of leukocytes along the vascular endothelium.

The leukocyte activation results in integrin expression and binding to immunoglobulin supergene family molecules such as ICAM-1 and VCAM-1 on endothelial cells, resulting in adhesion. Transendothelial migration occurs after adhesion.[6] Then, in response to chemokines, the migrating lymphocytes, monocytes, and granulocytes move toward the site of inflammation. Without this ability to home, the circulating effector cells could not respond to an immunologic or inflammatory event. In addition, activated endothelial cells can synthesize and secrete numerous substances such as cytokines (including IL-1, IL-6, and IL-8), fibronectin, collagen IV, proteoglycans, blood clotting factors, growth factors, and granulocyte-macrophage colony-stimulating factor. Defects in endothelial cell adhesion molecule expression may result in disorders that mimic immunodeficiencies owing to defective migration of lymphocytes, monocytes, or granulocytes (see Chap. 4).

Granulocytes

Neutrophils have, as their major roles, the function of phagocytosis and subsequent destruction and elimination of phagocytized material. In a sense, they are the scavengers

Table 8-7	CHEMOATTRACTANTS FOR NEUTROPHILS
Bacterial products	Lipid chemotactic factors (e.g., HETE) from mast cells
C5a (derived from complement activation; tissue, virus, and bacterial enzymes cleave C5)	Lysosomal proteases
C3a	Collagen breakdown products
C567	Fibrin breakdown products
Kallikrein	Plasminogen activator
Denatured protein	Prostaglandins
Lymphokines	Leukotrienes (especially LTB$_4$)
Monokines	Immune complexes
Neutrophil chemotactic factor (NCF) from mast cells	
ECF-A from mast cells	

of immunologically identified debris. They are considered most important in containing infection. Owing, however, to their numerous chemoattractants (Table 8-7) and intracellular products (Table 8-8) that may be released at sites of inflammation, neutrophils are omnipresent participants in most immune and virtually all inflammatory reactions.[30, 50, 54, 74]

Neutrophil dysfunctions have been described in dogs with pyoderma and generalized demodicosis (see Chap. 4) but are likely secondary to the skin disease. In addition, primary (hereditary) neutrophil dysfunctions are described (see Chap. 4).

Eosinophils, effector cells in hypersensitivity reactions, also participate in the downgrading of inflammation and defense of the host against extracellular parasites.[9, 50, 54] They are also phagocytic (immune complexes, mast cell granules, aggregated immunoglobulins, and certain bacteria and fungi). Eosinophils have a tremendous ability to communicate with surrounding cells by the expression of surface receptors and cytokine secretion. Over 60 receptors for a variety of adhesion molecules, immunoglobulin Fc receptors, cytokines, and lipid mediators have been found on the eosinophil membrane.[39] Eosinophil chemotaxis has been the subject of much research. Currently, a number of molecules are considered good candidates for eosinophil chemotaxis in vivo. These include platelet-activating factor (PAF), leukotriene (LT)B4, LTD4, hydroxyeicosatetraenoic acids (HETEs), and the C-C subfamily of chemokines.[39] The C-C chemokines considered most potent and selective for eosinophil chemotaxis are eotaxin, regulated upon activation of normal T cells expressed and presumably secreted (RANTES), monocyte chemoattractant protein (MCP)-3, and MCP-4.[39] Interestingly, the response of eosinophils from normal people is less to some chemotaxins than eosinophils from allergic people. This may reflect priming of eosinophils by some cytokines such as IL-3, IL-5, and granulocyte macrophage colony-stimulating factor.[39] Eosinophils are noteworthy for their preformed mediators stored within at least two types of eosinophilic granules but, like other inflammatory cells, they also newly synthesize leukotrienes and a variety of cytokines when activated (Table

Table 8-8	NEUTROPHIL PRODUCTS
Antimicrobial Enzymes	*Hydrolases*
Lysozyme	Cathepsin B
Myeloperoxidase	Cathepsin D
	N-acetyl-β-glucosaminidase
Proteases	β-glucuronidase
Collagenolytic proteinase	β-glycerophosphatase
Collagenase	
Elastase	*Others*
Cathepsin G	Lactoferrin
Leukotrienes	Eosinophil chemotactic factor
Gelatinase	Leukotrienes
	Pyrogen
	Prostaglandins
	Thromboxanes
	Platelet-activating factor

8–9). Degranulation can occur by three different mechanisms, though it appears that cytotoxic degranulation occurs commonly in vivo.[39]

Major basic protein (also found in basophils), eosinophil cationic protein, eosinophil-derived neurotoxin, and eosinophil peroxidase are potent toxic mediators and all have been shown to be effective at killing a variety of parasites. Eosinophil proteases may contribute to host tissue damage and wound healing because the collagenase degrades type I and III collagen and gelatinase degrades type XVII collagen. Additionally, eosinophil degranulation results in the production of membrane-derived mediators such as leukotrienes and PAF.

Basophils, major effector cells in some hypersensitivity reactions, may also play a role in downgrading delayed-type hypersensitivity reactions.[50] Basophils are somewhat similar to mast cells in that they have high-affinity receptors for IgE and contain high levels of histamine, but they also are the only leukocytes to share features once thought specific for eosinophils. Basophils contain major basic protein and the Charcot-Leyden crystals (lysophospholipase).[39] Basophils express over 30 surface receptors and have preformed granule-stored mediators and newly synthesized mediators after degranulation or activation. Basophils degranulate in four distinct morphologic patterns, none of which is cytotoxic.[25] Basophils are important in host defense. This has been most conclusively shown in the rejection of ticks. In skin diseases, basophils are particularly important in cutaneous basophil hypersensitivity, a T cell–controlled reaction important in host responses to various ectoparasites. The late-phase allergic reaction is thought to play a major, if not *the* major, role in chronic allergic skin or respiratory disease.[56] Basophils are a key cell involved in late-phase reactions.[11]

Humoral Components

The humoral components as described in the SIS include immunoglobulins (see Chap. 4), complement components, fibrinolysins, cytokines, eicosanoids, neuropeptides, and antimi-

Table 8–9 SECRETORY PRODUCTS OF EOSINOPHILS

Granule Proteins	Lipid Mediators
Major basic protein	Leukotriene B_4 (small amount)
Eosinophil peroxidase	Leukotriene C_4
Eosinophil cationic protein	Leukotriene C_5
Eosinophil-derived neurotoxic	5-HETE
β-glucuronidase	5,15- and 8,15--diHETE
Acid phosphatase	5-oxy- 15-hydroxy 6,8,11,13,-ETE
Arylsulfatase	Prostaglandins E_1 and E_2
Cytokines*	6-Keto-prostaglandin F_1
IL-1	Thromboxane B_2
IL-3	PAF
IL-4	*Enzymes*
IL-5	Elastase (questionable)
IL-6	Charcot-Leyden crystal protein
IL-8	Collagenase
IL-10	92-kD Gelatinase
IL-16	*Reactive Oxygen Intermediates*
GM-CSF	Superoxide radical anion
RANTES	H_2O_2
TNF-α	Hydroxy radicals
TGF-β	
TGF-β1	
MIP-1α	

*Physiologic significance of these cytokines needs to be confirmed.
HETE, hydrocyeicosatetraenoic acid; ETE, eicosatetraenoic acid; diHETE, dihydroxyeicosatetraenoic acid; TNF, tumor necrosis factor; TGF, transforming growth factor; MIP, macrophage inflammatory protein; PAF, platelet activating factor.
From Kita H, Gleich GJ: The eosinophil: Structure and function. In: Kaplan AP (ed): Allergy II. W.B. Saunders, Philadelphia, 1997, p. 153.

crobial peptides.[9, 50] The changes observed in inflammation, however, are mediated by numerous substances derived from the plasma, from cells of the damaged tissue, and from infiltrating monocytes, macrophages, lymphocytes, and granulocytes.

The interactions among cells, neurons, expression of cell receptors, cytokines, and other soluble mediators determine the inflammatory response. Some mediators augment inflammation, and others suppress it. Some mediators antagonize or destroy other mediators, and others amplify or generate other mediators. All mediators and cells normally act together harmoniously to maintain homeostasis and to protect the host against infectious agents and other noxious substances. Many mediators may be preformed and stored with the effector cells; other mediators are produced only in response to damage or appropriate receptor activation. A complete summary of all inflammatory mediator substances is beyond the scope of this chapter; the interested reader is referred to the various references.

Complement is a group of plasma and cell membrane proteins that induce and influence immunologic and inflammatory events.[30, 50, 54, 76] The critical step in the generation of biological activities from the complement proteins is the cleavage of C3. There are two pathways for the cleavage of C3. The classic pathway requires the presence of immunoglobulin and immune complexes. The alternative (properdin) pathway does not require immunoglobulin and may be directly activated by bacteria, viruses, and some abnormal cells. There is also a pathway to amplify C3 cleavage, and an effector sequence. The final effect of this sequence is the production of a membrane attack complex, which causes cell lysis.

As the effector sequence progresses, a variety of complement components are formed that have other effects. These other components play a role in neutralization of viruses, solubilization of immune complexes, and interaction with receptors on other cells. Many inflammatory cells have receptors for degradation products of C3 and C5. These activated receptors are important in phagocytosis, immune regulation, and mast cell and basophil degranulation. Hemolytic complement levels in dogs are reported to be decreased with enteropathies, hepatopathies, systemic lupus erythematosus, and systemic glucocorticoid therapy.[30, 53, 81] A genetically determined (autosomal recessive) deficiency of C3 has been reported in Brittany spaniels that experience recurrent bacterial skin and otic infections and sepsis (see Chap. 4).

Immune complexes are a heterogeneous group of immunoreactants formed by the noncovalent union of antigen and antibody.[9, 17, 30, 50, 53, 54] Many factors influence the formation, immunochemistry, biology, and clearance of these reactants. Circulating immune complexes influence both the afferent and efferent limbs of the immune response and can mediate tissue damage in certain pathologic states. Circulating immune complexes can be measured by a number of generally unavailable techniques, including C1q-binding, solid-phase C1q, conglutinin, and Raji cell assays. Circulating immune complexes have been detected in numerous human dermatoses and probably play an important role in the pathogenesis of systemic lupus erythematosus and vasculitis. Circulating immune complexes have been demonstrated in 6% of a normal dog population, in contrast with 25% of a population of sick dogs,[53] as well as in numerous conditions such as diabetes mellitus, hypothyroidism, arthropathies, nephropathies, neuropathies, mycotic and parasitic infections, systemic and discoid lupus erythematosus, cutaneous vasculitis, generalized demodicosis, and bacterial pyoderma.[17, 53]

Lipid mediators (PAF and eicosanoids) are newly synthesized unstored molecules derived from cell membranes. Cell membranes contain phospholipids, one of which is phosphatidylcholine, the parent molecule of PAF. Arachidonic acid is stored in cells as an ester in phospholipids and is the dominant fatty acid attached to the glycerol portion of PAF. Though arachidonic acid is also present in other phospholipids, this is a major source in inflammatory cells. After specific receptor stimulation and after cellular injury, phospholipases cause the degradation of phospholipids. Phospholipase A_2 enzymes break down phosphatidylcholine into a molecule of free arachidonic acid and one of PAF. Phospholipase C activity also results in free arachidonic acid, but it is the predominance of phospholipase A that contributes the most to the generation of inflammatory mediators.

Glucocorticoids inhibit the action of phospholipases, possibly by the induction of lipocortin, at pharmacologically achieved levels. This is thought to be a major anti-inflammatory mechanism of glucocorticoid therapy.[1, 9, 23, 50, 54]

PAF is not an eicosanoid but a phospholipid that also acts as an inflammatory mediator. It is produced from a variety of cells although, in humans, neutrophils and eosinophils produce the largest amounts.[9, 50, 54] PAF primes cells to have augmented responses to other stimuli and has its greatest effects on eosinophils and monocytes. It is an extremely potent eosinophil chemoattractant and stimulates their degranulation and release of leukotrienes. A chemoattractant for mononuclear cells, PAF stimulates their release of IL-1, IL-4, and TNF-α.

The metabolites of the oxidation of arachidonic acid are called eicosanoids and are potent biological mediators of a variety of physiologic or pathologic responses. Though arachidonic acid and the oxidative enzymes to degrade it are found in all human cells, only mast cells, leukocytes, endothelial cells, epithelial cells, and platelets have enough to play a major role in allergic diseases.[1, 9, 23, 50, 54] Free arachidonic acid is oxidized by one of three enzyme classes. The two most studied and important are cyclooxygenase and lipoxygenase. The third is monooxygenase, and this does result in *cis/trans*-dienols (HETE) formation which, in the human epidermis, leads to the formation of 12-HETE.[55]

The eicosanoids include two main types of molecules, the prostanoids and leukotrienes. Prostanoids (prostaglandins and thromboxanes) are derived by the metabolism of arachidonic acid by cyclooxygenase. Two forms of cyclooxygenase are known, cyclooxygenase-1 in the endoplasmic reticulum and cyclooxygenase-2 in the nuclear envelope, and they serve different functions and are preferentially important in different tissues. Aspirin and the nonsteroidal anti-inflammatory drugs primarily function by blocking cyclooxygenase. Cyclooxygenase metabolism results in PGH_2 formation, which is subsequently metabolized by specific terminal enzymes that result in the formation of PGE_2, PGF_2, PGD_2, PGI_2 or thromboxane A_2. Different cell types have variations in which an enzyme system is present and, therefore, which metabolites are produced. Each final metabolite has one or more specific receptors, and new therapeutic agents such as misoprostol are being developed as agonists or antagonists for these specific receptors.[1, 55]

Leukotrienes (LTA, LTB, LTC, LTD, and LTE) and their precursors—hydroperoxyeicosatetraenoic acids (HPETEs) and HETEs—are derived by the metabolism of arachidonic acid by the three enzymes of lipoxygenation, 5-, 12-, and 15-lipoxygenase. Different tissues express variable levels of the cytosolic lipoxygenases. The 5-lipoxygenase pathway predominates in neutrophils, monocytes, macrophages, and mast cells, whereas the 15-lipoxygenase pathway predominates in eosinophils and in endothelial and epithelial cells. The 12-lipoxygenase pathway predominates in platelets. The 5-lipoxygenase pathway results in the production of LTA_4 which, depending on the enzymes present in the cells, is converted to LTB_4 or LTC_4. LTD_4 and LTE_4 are produced from LTC_4.

Typically, eicosanoids have autocrine and paracrine functions that are important locally for host defense, and then they are inactivated or degraded. Abnormalities in production or control mechanisms may occur, however, leading to local or systemic tissue damage and disease. The actions of eicosanoids are diverse and variable according to the species, tissue, cellular source, the presence of stereospecific receptors, and the generation of secondary mediators.[1, 50, 55, 73] The understanding of how they function in disease is further complicated by the complex interactions that occur but that are not included in many laboratory studies, as well as by the fact that—because of their autocrine and paracrine functions—they must be measured in the involved tissue. The effects of arachidonic acid formation and some of the activities that eicosanoids may have in skin disease are summarized in Table 8–10.[9, 50, 54, 55]

Aging and the Skin Immune System

With advancing age, the immune system of animals and humans undergoes characteristic changes, usually resulting in decreased immunocompetence, which is called *immunosenescence*.[26, 30, 70] An age-associated decrease in immunoresponsiveness is commonly ac-

● Table 8-10 EFFECTS OF EICOSANOIDS IN SKIN DISEASE

EICOSANOID	EFFECT
$LTC_4/D_4/E_4$	Vascular dilation and increased permeability
LTB_4	Leukocyte chemotaxis and activation; increased endothelial adherence of leukocytes; stimulates keratinocyte proliferation; enhances NK-cell activity; hyperalgesia
12-HETE	Stimulates smooth muscle contraction
15-HETE	Hyperalgesia; inhibits cyclooxygenase; inhibits mixed lymphocyte reaction; stimulates suppressor T cells; inhibits NK-cell activity
15-HPETE	Suppresses T-lymphocyte function and Fc receptors
PGE_2	Plasma exudation; hyperalgesia; stimulates cell proliferation; suppresses lymphocyte and neutrophil function
PGF_2	Vasoconstriction; synergy with histamine and bradykinin on vascular permeability; stimulates cell proliferation
PGD_2	Smooth muscle relaxation
PGD_2/PGI_2	Suppression of leukocyte function; vasodilation and increased permeability

cepted for T lymphocytes but also claimed for B lymphocytes, Langerhans' cells, and other components of the immune system. Some studies have shown that aging humans and mice have increased susceptibility to infections or malignancies as well as elevated titers of autoantibodies, suggestive of higher susceptibility to autoimmune diseases.

● TYPES OF HYPERSENSITIVE REACTIONS

Clinical hypersensitivity disorders were divided on an immunopathologic basis, by Gell and Coombs, into four types[9, 30, 42, 76]:

Type I: immediate (anaphylactic)
Type II: cytotoxic
Type III: immune complex
Type IV: cell-mediated (delayed)

Subsequently, two other types of hypersensitivity reactions have been described: late-phase reactions and cutaneous basophil hypersensitivity. Clearly, these six reactions are oversimplified because of the complex interrelationships among the effector cells and the numerous components of the inflammatory response.

In most pathologic events, immunologically initiated responses almost certainly involve multiple components of the inflammatory process. In reality, many diseases may involve a combination of reactions, and their separation into distinct pathologic mechanisms rarely occurs. For example, IgE (classically involved in type I hypersensitivity reactions) and Langerhans' cells (classically involved in type IV hypersensitivity reactions) may interact in a previously unrecognized fashion in the development of human and canine atopic dermatitis. Even the classic type IV reaction is not as straightforward as we used to think because evidence suggests that mast cells, eosinophils, and basophils may play a role.

Realization that this scheme has become a simplistic approach to immunopathology has provoked other investigators to modify the original scheme of Gell and Coombs, often to a seemingly hopeless degree of hairsplitting.[53] In this section, we briefly examine the classic Gell and Coombs' classification of hypersensitivity disorders, because (1) it is still somewhat applicable to discussions of cutaneous hypersensitivity diseases and (2) it is still the immunopathologic scheme used by most authors and by major immunologic and dermatologic texts.

Type I (anaphylactic, immediate) hypersensitivity reactions are classically described as those involving genetic predilection, reaginic antibody (IgE) production, and mast cell degranulation. A genetically programmed person absorbing a complete antigen (e.g., ragweed pollen) responds by producing a unique antibody (reagin, IgE). IgE is homocytotropic and avidly binds membrane receptors on tissue mast cells and blood basophils.

Expense may also be an important factor. Total body bathing and/or rinses are required for regional or generalized pruritus and often reduce pruritus by removing surface debris, microbial byproducts, and allergens that may contribute to the pruritic load. Hydrocortisone (1%) shampoo is not significantly absorbed and may help treat allergic reactions.[156] Treatment with ointments, creams, lotions, and sprays may be possible for localized areas. Topical glucocorticoids are most effective, but are generally limited to localized hypersensitivity reactions. A 0.01% fluocinolone shampoo was applied to allergic dogs—twice weekly for 6 months—with no adverse effects.[87a] Topical therapy unfortunately is often overlooked and not presented as an option to clients. Appropriately administered topical therapy can greatly reduce the need for systemic treatment in many patients.

Fatty Acids

A large number of studies have shown that fatty acids are beneficial in the management of cases of pruritus in dogs and cats.[94, 95, 108, 117, 122, 124, 128, 136, 140, 143, 146] In most of these studies, the pruritus was due to hypersensitivity reactions, most commonly atopic disease. Fatty acids and their role in normal skin and coat is discussed in Chapter 3. Because these agents are relatively benign, diets or supplements containing appropriate amounts and ratios should be used in most allergic dogs and cats.

The proposed mechanism, besides the inhibition of arachidonic acid metabolism, relates to metabolic byproducts of fatty acid metabolism. Supplements used for pruritus usually contain one or both of γ-linolenic acid (GLA) and eicosapentaenoic acid (EPA). GLA is found in relatively high concentrations in evening primrose, borage, and black currant oils. It is elongated to dihomo(D)GLA, which directly competes with arachidonic acid as a substrate for cyclooxygenase and 15-lipoxygenase. The result of DGLA metabolism is the formation of prostaglandin E_1 and 15-hydroxy-8,11,13-eicosapentaenoic acid, both of which are thought to have anti-inflammatory effects.[162] An increase in various immune response parameters was reported in older dogs that were fed a diet rich in omega-6/omega-3 fatty acids at a ratio of 5:1.[38]

EPA, which is usually supplied by using cold water marine fish oils, also competes as a substrate for cyclooxygenase and 5- and 15-lipoxygenase. The metabolism of EPA by the lipoxygenase enzymes results in the formation of LTB_5 and 15-hydroxyeicosapentaenoic acid. These two products are thought to inhibit LTB_4, which is a potent proinflammatory mediator. This mechanism was reviewed by White,[162] and Figure 3–2 demonstrates the interactions of GLA, EPA, and arachidonic acid.

The use of fatty acids for atopic disease and chronic pruritus has been extensively studied. The beneficial effect has been documented in multiple double-blind or placebo-controlled studies.[93–95, 111, 115, 116, 140, 141, 146] In addition, multiple open uncontrolled studies have been published. In five separate clinical trials in North America, DVM Derm Caps were effective in 11% to 27% of the allergic dogs treated.[124, 126, 136, 143, 146] In cats, omega-6 and omega-3 fatty acid–containing products have been effective in more than 50% of allergic patients.[108–110, 128, 137, 147] How well fatty acids work depends on many variables (dose, omega-6:omega-3 ratio, animal's diet), with 10% to 80% of atopic animals realizing varying degrees of clinical improvement. The benefit is maximized if other contributing diseases such as food hypersensitivity, flea bite hypersensitivity, bacterial pyoderma, and *Malassezia* dermatitis are controlled. Overall, it is probably safe to inform clients that about 20% of the dogs, and about 50% of the cats, with allergic pruritus experience improvement. There is also evidence that higher doses of GLA and EPA enhance the results. These doses may be 4 to 10 times the manufacturer's recommendations.[93–95, 116, 137, 140, 141] Another factor that is important is the type of diet the animal is receiving. Dogs receiving lower-fat diets may respond better to the supplements.[137]

Although the benefits of these products are clear, which fatty acid, which combination of fatty acids, what ratio of omega-6 to omega-3, and what dose of these agents are most effective remain inconclusive. Several studies compared different types of supplements. In one study evaluating four different supplements, no one product was effective in all cases, and response could not be predicted.[146] Failure to respond to one product does not preclude a favorable response to another product. This study suggested that a single dose and type or blend of fatty acids that would be effective in all patients does not exist. Therefore, multiple trials may be best. In the dog, various doses (up to three times the manufacturer's recommendation) of only omega-6 fatty acids have not been effective in controlling pruritus.[117, 140] With recommended doses of omega-3 fatty acids, canine allergic pruritus was not controlled.[117] However, large doses (up to seven times those usually given) of omega-3 fatty acids effectively controlled pruritus in 30% to 60% of dogs.[116] Whereas twice the manufacturer's dose of an omega-6 and omega-3 fatty acid–containing product was no more effective than the recommended dose,[144] other studies reported that 2 to 10 times the recommended dose may be necessary to control allergic pruritus in dogs.[93–95]

Another area that still needs investigation is the importance or effect of combining the fatty acids with other elements, such as vitamins and minerals (so-called "cofactors"). Some manufacturers and authors[118] have claimed that the right combination of cofactors maximizes the beneficial effects of the fatty acids. No controlled studies to determine this, and what cofactors are most important, have been presented. In one double-blind study, a fatty acid product containing cofactors was no more effective than products that did not contain cofactors.[146] Three different fatty acid products were compared in atopic dogs in one study and no significant differences were noted, though the products differed somewhat in dose and whether omega-3 or omega-6 fatty acids predominated.[93–95] Other formulations claim to improve fatty acid absorption, such as by miscillization. Again, controlled studies are needed. How long one should try a product has also not been definitively determined. Although some dogs and cats show a favorable response within 1 to 2 weeks, an adequate therapeutic trial might necessitate 9 to 12 weeks.*

Although fatty acids may be solely effective for controlling pruritus and inflammation in some animals, their roles in synergistic therapy should be considered. Little has been done to study their synergistic role, but it has been suggested that they should frequently be tried in combination with other antipruritic agents for managing allergic pruritus.[27] A synergistic effect was documented between fatty acids and antihistamines.[136, 139, 144, 150] A synergistic effect with glucocorticoids was also described.[96, 122, 147, 148]

The risks and side effects of fatty acid supplementation are few. The most serious, although rarely reported, side effect is pancreatitis.[27] This has not been reported with the diets that have incorporated omega-6 and omega-3 fatty acids to appropriate ratios. With large doses, an increase in weight or diarrhea may occur. With supplements containing fish oil, some clients have reported an unpleasant odor or increased eructation ("fish breath").

A beneficial role of fatty acids has been documented, and they play an important role in managing pruritic dogs and cats. Because of their low potential for risk and their good potential for benefit, trial therapy with the optimized diets or supplements is often warranted. Their exact role, indications, and optimal use still need to be elucidated. In addition, the practitioner is presented with numerous different formulations and products from which to choose. Until more studies are performed, it is best to use diets with the proper ratio or products with proven efficacy and develop one's own clinical intuition about effectiveness and indications.

In addition to fatty acid supplementation, controlling the fatty acids in the diet may be beneficial. This has been confirmed in a study that used evening primrose oil at four times the recommended dose (150 mg/kg/day).[107] Ten atopic dogs were stabilized on a commercial canned diet and evening primrose oil supplementation. The dogs were then divided into two groups that had their diets switched to either Science Diet w/d (Hills) or a leading commercial dry dog food. The dogs consuming w/d continued to improve while the dogs consuming the dry dog foods worsened. Altering the fatty acid ratios and quantities in pet rations, and not using supplements, may be the most effective and least expensive method of assessing the efficacy of these agents. Studies showed that an omega-

---

*See references 94, 95, 108, 111, 122, 124, 128, 136, 140, 143, 146.

6:omega-3 ratio of 5–10:1 was the optimum ratio to result in less proinflammatory cytokines and greater levels of anti-inflammatory cytokines.[158, 161] This was then used to formulate a line of diets that have been evaluated and found to be beneficial in up to 44% of pruritic dogs.[142, 151]

In one study,[151] commercial dog foods were found to vary so greatly in both their quantity and ratio of omega-6 and omega-3 fatty acids, that achieving the proper anti-inflammatory quantity and ratio of these fatty acids with commercial supplements would be impossible (specific details of quantities and ratios *not* listed for the majority of diets) or impractical (such large doses required that it would be economically unfeasible). Thus, if one really wants to know whether a dog will respond to omega-6/omega-3 fatty acids, the only "sure" way is to feed a commercial diet that has known beneficial quantities and ratios (e.g., Eukanuba lamb and rice, Eukanuba f/p). Because fatty acids may have a synergistic or additive effect with other treatments, they are often recommended as part of a treatment plan.

Fatty acid supplements have also been reported to be effective in the management of feline atopy. Although fewer studies have been reported in cats than in dogs, current information would indicate that 50% to 75% of treated cats have a good response to products containing omega-3/omega-6 fatty acids.[109, 110, 128] It appears that this response may be due to the omega-3 fatty acids because a double-blinded, placebo-controlled study with evening primrose oil (omega-6, GLA) showed no beneficial effect after 12 weeks of therapy.[116] In addition, it has been reported that cats also benefit from the synergistic effects of combining fatty acids (DVM Derm Caps Liquid) with either chlorpheniramine or glucocorticoids.[147, 150] As a result of these good therapeutic results, the possible synergistic effects achievable, and the safety of these products, any cat that will readily ingest a liquid fatty acid supplement in its daily diet should initially be treated with it. If the supplement alone fails to control the pruritus adequately, antihistamines or glucocorticoids can be added.

Nonsteroidal Anti-Inflammatory Agents

Nonsteroidal anti-inflammatory agents are classically used to decrease pain and inflammation but have shown little benefit for pruritus or atopic disease. A number of nonsteroidal drugs have been used to treat canine atopy. Little or no work has been done to document the effect of some of these, including orgotein (metalloprotein, nonsteroidal anti-inflammatory), phenothiazine tranquilizers, barbiturates, and levamisole.[53, 58] Studies of nonsteroidal antipruritic agents in dogs with hypersensitivity skin disease indicated that aspirin (25 mg/kg orally q8h), vitamin E (400 IU orally q12h), zinc methionine (Zinpro, 1 tablet/9.1 kg orally q24h), vitamin C (25 mg/kg orally q12h), papaverine (150 to 300 mg/dog q12h), doxycycline (3 mg/kg q12h), and the combination of tetracycline and niacinamide are rarely effective.[53, 88, 146a, 148] So far, lipoxygenase inhibitors have not been shown efficacious in canine atopy, though they are in human asthma.[103] It was reported that oxatomide—a mast cell stabilizer—was effective at 15 to 30 mg every 12 hours for controlling pruritus in allergic cats.[150, 153]

Some recently evaluated nonsteroidal agents include pentoxifylline and misoprostol. *Pentoxifylline* (Trental) has a variety of effects, and the benefits may result from different mechanisms, depending on the disease being treated (see Chap. 3). It has been used for the treatment of contact hypersensitivity and atopic disease in dogs. For canine atopic disease, the response to pentoxifylline is not dramatic, but the drug does appear to have some benefit in a percentage of cases and may work best in combination with other treatments and as a steroid-sparing drug. A double-blind, placebo-controlled study in atopic dogs did show efficacy, though the condition of none of the dogs was completely controlled.[239] It was effective in dogs with contact hypersensitivity at 10 mg/kg q12h, but not q24h.[119] Because of cost, it was discontinued in these dogs. Attempts to lower the dose after a favorable response were not made. Ten mg/kg q8h should be an effective dose and may possibly be lowered to q12h.[97]

Misoprostol acts as a PGE_1 analog. PGE_1 inhibits production of IL-1 and TNF-α in some models of inflammation and inhibits production of LTB_4 by activated neutrophils. Of particular interest in allergic disease are its effects on decreasing histamine release, inhibiting eosinophil chemotaxis and survival, and inhibition of cutaneous late-phase allergic reactions.[87, 134] Because late-phase allergic reactions may be involved in the pathogenesis of canine atopic disease, misoprostol might be useful. Misoprostol (Cytotec, Searle) is available in 100-μg and 200-μg tablets. It has been used primarily to treat gastric ulcers and, in combination protocols, to induce abortions.[92] It was used in an open trial for the treatment of canine atopic disease.[132] In this study of 18 dogs treated with misoprostol at 6 μg/kg q8h, over 50% had greater than 50% reduction of pretreatment pruritus and lesion scores. However, in none of the dogs was pruritus reduced by more than 75%, and in only one dog was the lesion score reduced by more than 75%. The drug is sensitive to water and oxygen and should not be compounded with water or broken open in advance of use. The greatest risks with misoprostol are for inducing abortions (it should not be used in pregnant animals) and for causing diarrhea. In humans, life-threatening diarrhea was caused in patients with inflammatory bowel disease treated with misoprostol. In dogs, 33% experienced side effects, most commonly vomiting and diarrhea, but they were mild enough that the drug was not discontinued.

Antihistamines

Histamine is a potent chemical mediator that has variable actions, depending on what receptors and tissues are stimulated. The effects of histamine can be blocked in three ways: by physiologic antagonists, such as epinephrine; by agents that reduce histamine formation or release from mast cells and basophils; and by histamine receptor antagonists. We used to think that most antihistamines worked by this latter effect. Now we have learned that most of the older first-generation antihistamines also function by preventing mediator release from mast cells and basophils.[104] In veterinary dermatology, the primary indication for antihistamine therapy is the treatment of pruritus mediated by stimulation of histamine H_1 receptors, usually associated with hypersensitivity reactions.[130, 147, 148, 153]

First-generation (classic, or traditional) antihistamines are H_1 blockers. However, not all the effects of histamine are antagonized by H_1 blockers. Because antihistamines are metabolized by the liver, they should be used with caution in patients with hepatic disease. In addition, their anticholinergic properties contraindicate their use in patients with glaucoma, gastrointestinal atony, and urinary retentive states. Some antihistamines are teratogenic in various laboratory animals. No information on teratogenicity is available for dogs and cats; however, this issue should be considered before treating pregnant bitches and queens. Finally, the efficacy of antihistamines is notoriously unpredictable and individualized in a given patient. Part of this variation may be dose-related because antiallergic effects are concentration dependent and some dose ranges are antiallergic whereas others may enhance mediator release.[104] Thus, the clinician may try several antihistamines and doses before finding the one that is beneficial for a given patient.

Antihistamines block the physiologic effects of histamine. At least three different types of histamine receptors have been recognized. The role of H_3 receptors is just being uncovered, and they are primarily located in the central nervous system, where they affect a variety of nerve terminals and may affect neurotransmitter release.[104] Their role in dermatology has yet to be determined. The H_1-receptor antagonists are used in small animal dermatology. This is because H_1 receptors are primarily responsible for pruritus, increased vascular permeability, release of inflammatory mediators, and recruitment of inflammatory cells.[155]

In addition to their histamine-blocking action, some of these agents have sedative, antinausea, anticholinergic, antiserotoninergic, and local anesthetic effects. As mentioned previously, most block mediator release if present prior to allergen challenge and if at the appropriate concentration. Most of the second-generation, or nonsedating, antihistamines block mediator release to some degree.[155] However, the effects may differ with the variable or tissue being evaluated (i.e., different results may occur with various sources of mast cells, basophils, or eosinophils). Variable results may also depend on the method used to induce cellular responses, such as immunoglobulin E (IgE)-induced release or nonantibody inducers, though most also decrease the response to nonimmunologic stimuli.[104, 155] Cetirizine, a second-generation antihistamine, is particularly effective in blocking the allergen-induced late-phase cutaneous reaction and in decreasing the influx of eosinophils in response to allergens.[90]

A number of open uncontrolled or open controlled comparative studies have been reported.[123, 127, 129, 138, 143, 159] These indicated that the first-generation antihistamines, chlorpheniramine (0.4 mg/kg q8h), diphenhydramine (2 mg/kg q8h), and hydroxyzine (2 mg/kg q8h), may each be effective in up to 10% of the dogs with allergic pruritus. A double-blind, placebo-controlled study in 30 dogs revealed that the placebo was totally ineffective, whereas clemastine fumarate (Tavist) at 0.05 mg/kg q12h was effective in 30% of the cases.[135] Two other open clinical trials confirmed the effectiveness of clemastine in dogs.[129, 136] Trimeprazine tartrate (Temaril) at 0.12 mg/kg q12h was effective in only 3% of dogs with allergic pruritus.[135] Cyproheptadine hydrochloride (Periactin) at 0.1 mg/kg q12h and terfenadine (Seldane) at 5 mg/kg q12h were ineffective in double-blind, placebo-controlled studies.[145, 149] Terfenadine overdose in the dog was associated with vomiting, agitation, weakness, ataxia, and premature ventricular contractions but did respond to supportive care.[133]

Antihistamines may also be used to act synergistically with, or reduce required doses of, glucocorticoids.[135, 147, 148] In one study, the addition of trimeprazine to ongoing, alternate-day prednisone regimens in allergic dogs allowed an average 30% reduction in the prednisone dosage in 75% of patients.[135] Antihistamines can also be used synergistically with other nonsteroidal anti-inflammatory agents that work by different mechanisms.[136, 139, 144, 147, 148, 150] In one open clinical trial, dogs that responded to neither chlorpheniramine nor a fatty acid–containing supplement (DVM Derm Caps) when these were administered as individual drugs were given the same two drugs in combination.[144] Approximately 30% of the dogs responded well. This synergistic effect has also been documented with other nonsteroidal anti-inflammatory agents. A study compared the response of pruritic dogs to clemastine, a fatty acid supplement (DVM Derm Caps), or a combination of both.[136] Response to the combination was good in 10% of the dogs that did not respond to the individual agents.

Second-generation (nonsedating) antihistamines are also H_1 blockers but, because they are poorly lipid soluble and minimally cross the blood-brain barrier at recommended doses, they exert much less sedative action and anticholinergic effects than do first-generation antihistamines. For some reason, second-generation antihistamines have not been useful in dogs to date. Terfenadine (Seldane) at 5 mg/kg q12h,[135] astemizole (Hismanal) at 0.25 mg/kg q24h,[135] and loratadine (Claritin) at 10 mg/kg q24h[153] were all ineffective in placebo-controlled studies in dogs with allergic pruritus. Terfenadine and astemizole have been pulled from the United States market because of severe interactions with some other drugs. In addition to not having any greater efficacy in dogs and cats, second-generation antihistamines are also more expensive, and some authors do not think these agents are worth using.[113]

Adverse effects vary in incidence and severity with individual patients and individual drugs. Sedation and anticholinergic effects are the primary side effects from antihistamines. Trembling, increased pruritus, and panting have also been reported. Excitation may occur in rare cases. Doxepin and chlorpheniramine appear to cause a higher incidence of side effects. Drowsiness may lessen or resolve with continued therapy. For other side effects, and when drowsiness persists, the drug should be discontinued. Once the side effects have resolved, resuming therapy at a lower dose may still effectively control the pruritus without causing the side effects. Overdosage of hydroxyzine has been reported to cause ataxia, hyperesthesia, tremors, and hypersalivation.[91] Cardiovascular adverse effects (tachycardia, arrhythmias, hypertension) are very rare and usually seen only with overdosing. Although the adverse effects of antihistamines in dogs and cats are varied and numerous, they are rarely severe enough to necessitate stopping treatment.

H_2-receptor blockers appear to have little use in allergic diseases. In a study of 15 dogs with allergic skin disease, cimetidine alone was helpful in only one dog, and no dog responded better to the combination of H_2 (cimetidine) and H_1 (diphenhydramine) blockers than to the H_1 blocker alone.[123]

Antihistamines are also effective in cats.[61, 89, 121, 130, 147, 152, 153] In contrast with dogs, cats are relatively sensitive to these drugs, and antihistamines other than those described n this discussion should be used with caution. There seem to be more side effects in cats than dogs, and care in their use has been recommended. However, two reports have described using multiple types of antihistamines in cats. One author reported using multiple antihistamines in cats and indicated that problems were encountered with only cyproheptadine and hydroxyzine.[89] One study demonstrated an excellent response to chlorpheniramine at 2 mg/cat q12h in 73% of atopic cats.[125] Many other investigators have also reported favorable, though not as good, results with chlorpheniramine; therefore, it is considered the antihistamine of choice in the atopic cat. Cyproheptadine was evaluated in 20 allergic cats and was effective in controlling pruritus in 9 (45%) but produced side effects in 8 cats.[152]

Side effects with cyproheptadine included polyphagia, sedation, vomiting, and vocalization. Results of an open clinical trial indicated that clemastine (0.1 mg/kg q12h) was effective in 50% of cats with allergic pruritus.[129] Similar to dogs, synergistic effects may occur with other nonsteroidal treatments. Fifty percent of the cats that responded to neither chlorpheniramine nor DVM Derm Caps liquid, when these were administered individually, responded well when the two drugs were used in combination.[150] Because of the effects on eosinophils, cetirizine has been considered as a potential antihistamine to try in cats, but no published reports are available as to efficacy.

There is marked individual variation in different antihistamines when used to treat dogs or cats with chronic pruritus or allergic diseases. To maximize the percentage of dogs and cats that will respond to antihistamines, multiple different drugs should be evaluated. Antihistamine trials are often run consecutively, evaluating each drug for at least 2 weeks. Which antihistamines are evaluated in any given pet is a factor of efficacy, cost, and frequency of treatment administration. The most commonly recommended antihistamines are those with relatively high (A) and moderate (B) efficacy as indicated in Table 8–12.

Antidepressants

A variety of the psychotropic drugs have been used to treat some hypersensitivity disorders, especially if stress or a psychogenic component may be present. This category of drugs is discussed in detail in Chapter 15. The drugs that have been evaluated the most are the heterocyclic (tricyclic) antidepressants (amitriptyline, doxepin) and fluoxetine, another antidepressant that is structurally different from the heterocyclic antidepressants but that has a similar mechanism of action. Amitriptyline hydrochloride (generic or Elavil) at 1 mg/kg q12h was effective in 16% of the allergic dogs treated.[127] Another small pilot study with the serotonin uptake inhibitor fluoxetine hydrochloride (Prozac) at 1 mg/kg q24h showed it to be effective in 30% of dogs with allergic pruritus.[154] Doxepin was reported to be ineffective in one placebo-controlled study,[135] though in anecdotal reports it may be effective at 2 mg/kg q12h. Amitriptyline has also been used in the cat with a wide variation of success reported.[89, 121, 153] Some have indicated that amitriptyline is associated with many side effects in cats, particularly when given twice daily.[61] Amitripty-

● Table 8–12 **ANTIHISTAMINES FOR DOGS AND CATS**

ANTIHISTAMINE	DOG	CAT
Clemastine	A—0.05 to 0.1 mg/kg q12h	A—0.67 mg/cat q12h
Chlorpheniramine	A—0.4 mg/kg q8h	A—2 mg/cat q12h
Cyproheptadine	—	A—2 mg/cat q12h
Diphenhydramine	B—2.2 mg/kg q8h	—
Hydroxyzine	A—2.2 mg/kg q8h	B—10 mg/cat q12h

A, Generally effective; B, May be effective.

line was evaluated at 10 mg/cat q24h for recurrent idiopathic cystitis in 15 cats.[101] Two of the 15 cats experienced somnolence that resolved when the dose was decreased to 5 mg/cat q24h. Nine cats stayed on the drug 12 months: 7 of these had increased body weight and 8 had decreased coat quality due to decreased grooming, but serum biochemistry and hematologic abnormalities were not observed.

In general, the potentially more serious side effects of these drugs are induction of cardiac arrhythmias, such as promotion of heart block by slowing of cardiac conduction, and anticholinergic effects including dry mouth, urine retention, and reduced tear production. They also lower the seizure threshold and enhance monamine oxidase inhibitor (e.g., amitraz) toxicity, in addition to having the metabolic effects and side effects that are inherent with first-generation antihistamines. Up to 30% of animals treated with these agents may show vomiting, diarrhea, lethargy, hyperexcitability, polydipsia, aggression, personality changes, and anorexia. An exception is amitriptyline, which rarely produces side effects in dogs.[127] Electrocardiographic abnormalities were not detected in dogs treated with amitriptyline or clomipramine.[139a]

Systemic Glucocorticoids

Hypersensitivity diseases typically respond well to systemic glucocorticoids, and this is the treatment of choice for acute hypersensitivity diseases. It is also the treatment for many recurrent but short-duration (under 4 months/year) disorders. It is only indicated in the treatment of long-term, perennial hypersensitivity diseases when safer options are not effective or practical. If long-term therapy is required, short-acting oral glucocorticoids (prednisone, prednisolone, or methylprednisolone) are preferred (see Chap. 3). Some human patients with atopic dermatitis cases are resistant to glucocorticoids because of altered receptor binding.[102]

Glucocorticoids are the mainstay of therapy in cats with allergic diseases when avoidance is not possible.[147] The most common reason they are not used is that owners are concerned about the risks of glucocorticoids (inappropriately extrapolated from experiences in humans or dogs) and the occasional objectionable side effects. Other contraindications to their use in the cat are concurrent infections (viral, bacterial, fungal), diabetes mellitus, pancreatitis, renal failure and, perhaps, pregnancy.[147]

The simplest glucocorticoid treatment is with repositol methylprednisolone acetate (Depo-Medrol, Pharmacia & Upjohn) given subcutaneously or intramuscularly at 20 mg/cat or 5 mg/kg.[53, 121, 147] It may be given as needed, but not more frequently than every 8 weeks, and preferably every 12 weeks. Alternatively, or if methylprednisolone acetate is ineffective, triamcinolone acetonide (Vetalog), 5 mg/cat q8–12wk as needed, may be used. In cases that do not respond adequately or in which injectable glucocorticoids produce adverse side effects, or when clients prefer, oral glucocorticoids may be used (see Chap. 3). Most commonly, prednisone or prednisolone (2.2 mg/kg q24h) is given until the patient is in remission (5 to 10 days), followed by an alternate-day regimen. Some authors prefer oral prednisolone and use injectable glucocorticoids only as a last resort or in cats that will not take oral medications.[89] These authors have seen diabetes mellitus occur following one glucocorticoid injection. One of us (D.W.S.) uses injectable methylprednisolone acetate as his first choice glucocorticoid for the cat and has never seen diabetes mellitus after a single injection. Some cats will not take pills well, and liquid glucocorticoids such as dexamethasone, 0.25 mg/cat q12h then tapered to q72h, has been recommended.[121] We have used dexamethasone at 0.2 mg/kg q24h, then tapered, with good effect even in cats that do not respond to prednisone or prednisolone. In cats that are particularly difficult to pill, injectable dexamethasone or triamcinolone may be added to butter, cheese, or chicken/fish broth and given orally.

Cyclosporine

Cyclosporine (Sandimmune or Neoral, Novartis) is used for a wide variety of dermatologic diseases in humans, including atopic dermatitis.[106, 114] There have also been anecdotal reports of efficacy for atopic dermatitis in dogs. The drug is discussed in more detail in

Chapters 3 and 9. It has been suggested that a mechanism of action in the treatment of atopic dermatitis involves the inhibition of mast cell degranulation by affecting the interaction between mast cells and nerves.[105, 157]

Cyclosporine given orally has been shown effective in a number of humans with atopic dermatitis.[98, 160] It has been less effective when used topically, though a similar acting topical drug, FK506 in ointment form (Tacrolimus), appears to have some efficacy. The oral dosage being tried for atopic dogs is 5 to 10 mg/kg daily. After a response is seen, tapering to as low as 10 mg/kg q48h may be effective. Because this is an expensive drug, the reduction to the lowest effective levels is usually important. Additionally, the expense and marginal efficacy usually limit its use to cases of treatment failure with, or adverse reaction to, standard treatment protocols. Though the use of cyclosporine has not been described for cats with allergic disease, it should be considered. Side effects in cats may be serious (nephrotoxicity, gastrointestinal, upper respiratory infection)[121] but usually occur at higher doses (10–20 mg/kg/day). Lower doses for atopy (5 mg/kg/day) may be tolerated better and be less expensive.

Required doses of cyclosporine are greatly reduced by the simultaneous administration of ketoconazole in dogs and cats (see Chap. 3).[120a]

Other Specific Therapies

Chronic allergic diseases, even in acute phases, predispose to secondary infections with *Malassezia* or bacteria, most often *Staphylococcus intermedius* (see Chaps. 4 and 5). When present, whether as infection or just overgrowth, they may contribute significantly to the pruritus and inflammation. It is important to recognize and treat specifically for these problems; otherwise, therapies directed at the underlying hypersensitivity or pruritus will be much less effective. Parasitic diseases, besides causing a hypersensitivity reaction themselves, may aggravate other allergies by allergic or nonallergic mechanisms (see Chap. 6). These also must be identified and controlled for optimal success with antiallergy treatment protocols.

• HYPERSENSITIVITY DISORDERS

Urticaria and Angioedema

Urticaria (hives) and angioedema are variably pruritic, edematous skin disorders that are immunologic or nonimmunologic. They are uncommon in the dog and extremely rare in the cat. In fact, we have seen only one confirmed case of angioedema in the cat that was not associated with snake bites or vasculitis.

CAUSE AND PATHOGENESIS

Urticaria and angioedema result from mast cell or basophil degranulation, though the mast cell is considered the major effector cell. They may result from many stimuli, both immunologic and nonimmunologic.[23, 50, 53, 164, 167] Immunologic mechanisms include type I and III hypersensitivity reactions. Nonimmunologic factors that may precipitate or intensify urticaria and angioedema include physical forces (pressure, sunlight, heat, cold, exercise), psychological stresses, genetic abnormalities, and various drugs and chemicals (aspirin, narcotics, foods, food additives). A case of chronic urticaria and eosinophilic dermatitis was reported in a dog and attributed to diethylcarbamazine drug reaction.[168] Chronic idiopathic urticaria in humans may be associated with autoantibodies to the high-affinity IgE receptor (Fc epsilon RI α).[167] Humans with chronic urticaria were more likely to have exposure to dogs and cats and have positive titers to *Toxocara canis*.[169] The relationship is supported by a favorable response of many of these patients to parasiticidal therapy. Factors reported to have caused urticaria and angioedema in dogs and cats are listed in Table 8–13.[53, 61, 163–166]

● Table 8–13 **FACTORS REPORTED TO HAVE CAUSED URTICARIA AND ANGIOEDEMA IN DOGS AND CATS**

Foods
Drugs (penicillin, ampicillin, tetracycline, vitamin K, propylthiouracil, amitraz, ivermectin, moxidectin, radiocontrast agents, HyLyt°efa shampoo)
Antisera, bacterins, and vaccines (panleukopenia, leptospirosis, distemper-hepatitis, rabies, feline leukemia)
Stinging and biting insects (bee, hornet, mosquito, black fly, spider, ant)
Hairs from processionary caterpillar
Allergenic extracts°
Blood transfusions
Plants (nettle, buttercup)
Intestinal parasites (ascarids, hookworms, tapeworms)
Infections (staphylococcal pyoderma, canine distemper)°
Sunlight°
Excessive heat or cold°
Estrus°
Dermatographism°
Atopy°
Psychogenic factors°
Vasculitis, food allergy-induced°

°Reported in dogs only.

CLINICAL FEATURES

No age, breed, or sex predilections have been reported for urticaria and angioedema in dogs and cats. Clinical signs may be acute (most common) or chronic. In humans, acute urticaria and angioedema are empirically defined as episodes lasting less than 6 weeks, whereas chronic episodes last longer. Urticarial reactions are characterized by localized or generalized wheals, which may or may not be pruritic and usually do not exhibit serum leakage or hemorrhage (Figs. 8–2 and 8–3A). Characteristically, the wheals are evanescent lesions, with each lesion persisting less than 24 hours. Urticarial lesions occasionally are erythematous or assume bizarre patterns (serpiginous, linear, arciform, annular, papular) and coalesce to cover large areas as plaques (see Fig. 8–3B). Hair may appear raised in these areas. Angioedematous reactions are characterized by localized or generalized large, edematous swellings, which may or may not be pruritic and exhibit serum leakage or hemorrhage (Fig. 8–4).

DIAGNOSIS

The differential diagnosis for urticaria includes folliculitis, vasculitis, erythema multiforme, lymphoreticular neoplasia, and mast cell tumor. Staphylococcal folliculitis often manifests as slightly raised tufts of hair (tufted papules) and is the most common cause of misdiag-

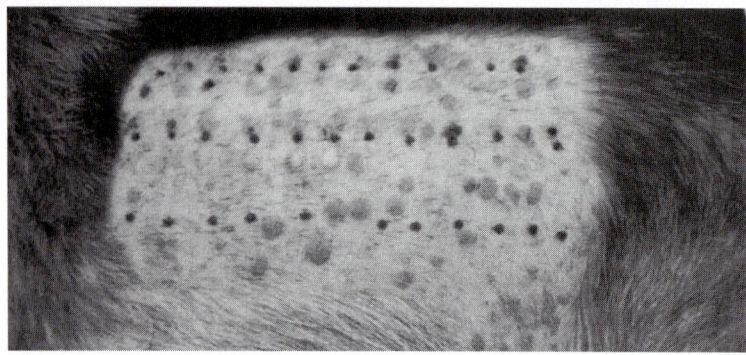

FIGURE 8–2. Numerous wheals in a dog with urticaria that occurred following clipping, marking with ink, and giving intradermal injections of allergens.

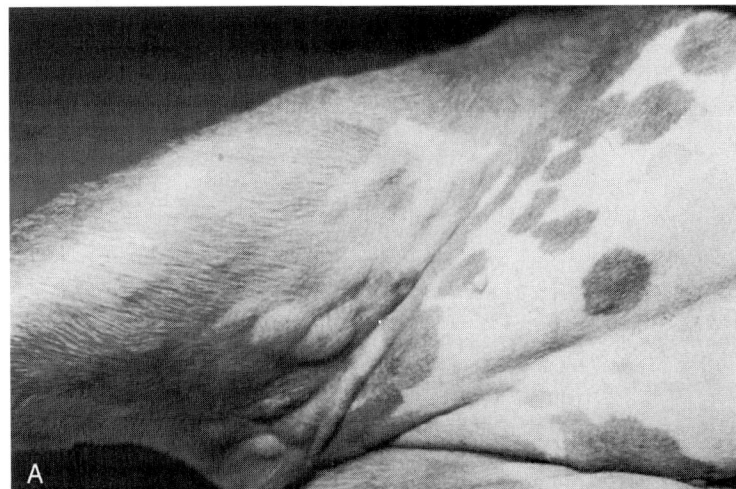
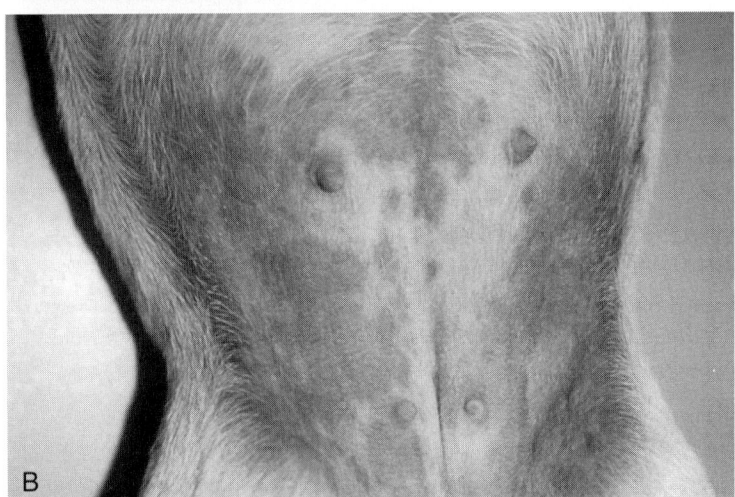

FIGURE 8–3. *A*, Urticaria in groin following amitraz dip. *B*, Urticaria with coalescing lesions forming plaques in a dog with atopy and food hypersensitivity. Urticarial "attacks" were associated with ingesting allergenic foods.

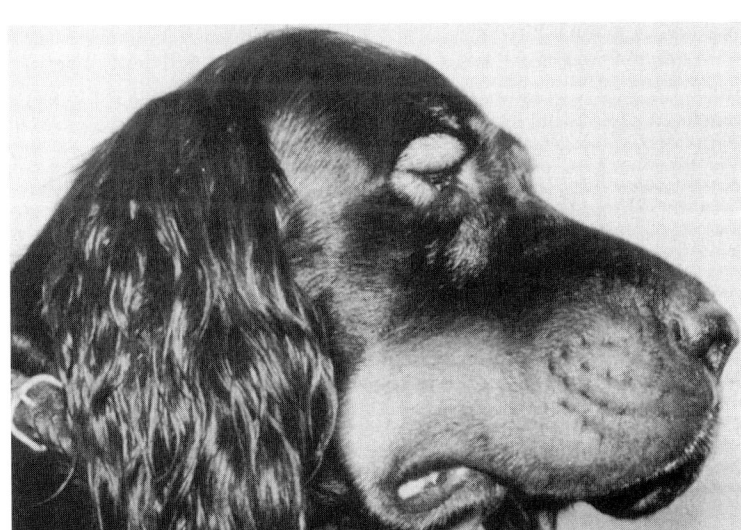

FIGURE 8–4. Angioedema due to phenamidine administration. Note swollen lips and eyelids. (Courtesy of D. N. Carlotti.)

nosed "urticaria" in dogs with short haircoats. Juvenile cellulitis, infectious cellulitis, mast cell tumor, and lymphoreticular neoplasia are the most common considerations in the differential diagnosis of angioedema. Definitive diagnosis is based on history, physical examination, and pursuit of the etiologic factors listed in Table 8–13. A specific or tentative etiologic diagnosis can usually be made in acute cases, but chronic urticaria and angioedema are extremely frustrating diagnostic challenges, with 75% to 80% of such cases in human patients defying specific etiologic diagnosis. A thorough hypoallergenic diet trial should be performed.

Histopathology

Skin biopsy shows a variable, nondiagnostic pattern, from simple vascular dilatation and edema in the superficial and middle dermis to pure superficial perivascular to interstitial dermatitis with varying numbers of mononuclear cells, neutrophils, mast cells, and eosinophils (uncommon).[28, 83, 84] Leukocytoclastic vasculitis is rare. Eosinophilic vasculitis has been observed in multiple cases that have involved food-induced urticaria.[163] Direct immunofluorescence testing of urticarial lesions in humans usually yields negative results but occasionally reveals immunoglobulin, complement, or both in blood vessel walls (especially when the histologic reaction is vasculitis).

CLINICAL MANAGEMENT

The prognosis for urticarial reactions is favorable because general health is not usually affected. The prognosis for angioedema varies with severity and location. Angioedematous reactions involving the nasal passages, pharynx, and larynx may be fatal.

Therapy consists of (1) elimination and avoidance of known etiologic factors and (2) treatment of symptoms with epinephrine (epinephrine 1:1000 at 0.1 to 0.5 ml subcutaneously or intramuscularly), glucocorticoids (prednisolone or prednisone at 2 mg/kg, given orally, intramuscularly, or intravenously), or both. Antihistamines have not been adequately evaluated for efficacy in treating chronic urticaria. They are ineffective for the treatment of acute reactions but may be useful for the prevention of future reactions or in the management of chronic cases. Some cases of chronic urticaria in dogs respond well to antihistamine therapy, although several agents may have to be tried to find the one that works best for a given patient. Pentoxifylline (10 mg/kg q8–12h) has been helpful if vasculitis is present.

Canine Atopic Disease

Atopic disease (atopy, allergic inhalant dermatitis) is a genetically programmed disease of dogs in which the patient becomes sensitized to environmental antigens that in nonatopic animals create no disease.[58, 61, 67a, 247] Additionally, atopy has been defined as a reaginic antibody-mediated disease.[29] Though allergen-specific IgE has been classically associated with the disease, more components of the immune system appear to be important. Some evidence supports the importance of allergen-specific IgG.[58, 208, 264, 310–312] The role of Langerhans' cells, T cells, and eosinophils, as well as changes in the inflammatory milieu with chronicity, are also being recognized as important components of the disease process.[176, 218, 234, 256–259, 267]

CAUSE AND PATHOGENESIS

Strong breed predilections, familial involvement, and limited breeding trials have demonstrated that canine atopy is genetically programmed.* A pilot study failed to demonstrate any clear-cut relationship between any single dog leukocyte-antigen type and canine atopy,

---

*See references 30, 61, 67a, 201–203, 277, 281, 306, 314.

but the combination of haplotypes DL-A3 and R15 was found significantly more often in atopic dogs.[304a] The heritability of the development of high-IgE response to antigen immunization has been documented in a colony of beagle dogs.[202, 203, 314] In Beagles, the high-IgE response appears to be a dominant trait, but the development of clinical dermatitis occurs in only approximately 40% of the offspring.[202, 203] A critical aspect of high-IgE induction is that immunization with the offending allergen had to occur shortly after birth and, if delayed until 3 to 4 months age, was ineffective.[314] In humans, the genetics of allergy appears to be complex, with multiple genetic traits likely being responsible.[50] This has been supported by work showing genetic differences in mast cell protein production in human patients with atopic dermatitis as compared with mast cells from patients with allergic asthma or rhinitis.[238]

In addition to genetics, other factors are important in the development of clinical atopy. One study has shown an association between the month of birth and the incidence of canine atopy.[303] Dogs studied that were born during the onset of pollen seasons more commonly experienced atopy than control dogs. This finding suggested that dogs may be particularly susceptible to primary sensitization during the first 4 months of life, which was supported by the work with the high-IgE beagle model.[314] Birth during nonpollen seasons would tend to disfavor the development of sensitization, whereas birth during pollen seasons would tend to increase the incidence of sensitization. These two features also suggest that what a dog becomes sensitized to may relate to what allergens are in high levels at this time.

Parasitic diseases may augment the production of IgE to other environmental allergens.[29] This observation has also been supported in studies in cats.[430] Viral infections, or at least vaccination with modified live viral vaccines, have been shown to augment production of IgE specific for environmental allergens.[27, 61, 67a, 210, 211] Interestingly, as in Beagle dogs, most of these dogs do not experience clinical signs while housed in a laboratory environment (O.L. Frick, personal communication, 1991). Thirty percent of the high-IgE responder Beagles spontaneously develop IgE to house dust mites, whereas all the colony dogs, both high- and low-IgE responders, develop house dust mite–specific IgG.[314] These findings document that natural exposure to house dust mites was present in all animals and, therefore, the development of house dust mite–specific IgE is related to other factors. Even when high-IgE responders with dermatitis were bred to each other, dermatitis only developed in some of the offspring.[314]

When Beagles are fed the offending allergen, IgE is not induced, but IgG is.[204] The presence of clinical signs is not always apparent in allergic humans, and disease may be present at the microscopic level in asymptomatic rhinitis patients.[194] We have seen many cases in which, when secondary infections are controlled, the owners considered their dogs asymptomatic until educated about signs of pruritus and asked to observe more closely. This may explain some of the dogs that have allergen-specific IgE but not significant clinical disease. At least in humans, the amount of allergen exposure and size of allergen may also contribute to the development of atopy as well as the type of symptoms manifested.[291]

The increase in environmental pollutants and indoor allergens has been postulated as another reason for the increase in incidence and development of atopic dermatitis in humans.[176, 212, 275] Considering all these studies, it is interesting to consider the potential impact of the following situations. Migrating ascarid larvae and intestinal worm infestations are more common in young dogs with developing immune systems, which is also when most dogs go through the most rigorous vaccination time in their life. Both factors occurring in puppies may help explain the high incidence of atopic disease in dogs.

Canine atopy has been classified as a type I hypersensitivity reaction. Genetically predisposed dogs absorb percutaneously, inhale, and possibly ingest various allergens that provoke allergen-specific IgE or IgG production. Canine IgE is (1) not precipitated in the presence of antigen, (2) inactivated at 56°C, (3) not complement fixing, (4) antigenically similar to human IgE, and (5) capable of passively transferring atopic sensitivities to normal dogs by Prausnitz-Küstner (P-K) testing.[30, 58, 61, 67a, 346] It has been traditional to espouse the primary importance of allergen-specific IgE, though total IgE level is not elevated.*

The lack of elevated serum total IgE levels in atopic dogs is because normal dogs have very high total IgE levels as compared with humans because of parasite-induced IgE, and the relatively minute levels of allergen-specific IgE—though enough to create disease—are not enough to change total IgE levels. Serum IgE levels are lower in laboratory dogs that live in confined environments with limited exposures and strict deworming programs.[214a, 270] IgE levels increase with age up to 4 years.[270] Allergen-specific IgE, as measured by commercial laboratories, may not be elevated in atopic dogs.[195] However, numerous studies show that allergen-specific IgE is associated with atopic disease.[204, 216, 236, 314, 322] Canine IgE also binds to epidermal Langerhans' cells in lesional atopic skin.[256, 257]

These findings are compelling evidence for the pathogenic role played by allergen-specific IgE in canine atopic disease. However, the absolute requirement for IgE is questioned because of several observations in human or canine atopics: (1) atopy has been recognized in patients with agammaglobulinemia[50]; (2) allergen-specific IgE cannot even be detected in many atopic dogs and normal dogs experimentally sensitized to allergens[61, 67a, 310, 311]; and (3) abnormally increased serum IgE levels generally do not fluctuate consistently during exacerbations, remissions, or treatment.[23, 50, 292] However, allergen-specific IgE may decrease in response to hyposensitization.

It has also been stated that allergen-specific IgG (IgGd subclass) is key.[58] Willemse and associates[310, 311] demonstrated a reaginic antibody, confirmed by passive cutaneous anaphylaxis (PCA) and P-K testing, in the IgGd subclass. Unfortunately, determining that the results became negative after IgG absorption, which would have proven that the reaginic antibody was an IgG, was not done. There also is controversy regarding the role and specificity of IgGd.[34, 268, 376] Another study showed that positive intradermal skin test reactions and detectable IgE and IgGd to *Dermatophagoides farinae*, *D. pteronyssinus*, and house dust antigen occurred with similar frequency in normal and atopic dogs.[236] However, allergen-specific IgGd was found in normal dogs in greater amounts than allergen-specific IgE. In addition, a high percentage of atopic dogs had detectable IgGd to various antigens despite negative intradermal skin test reactions. Allergen-specific IgG also increased in dogs undergoing hyposensitization.[225] Allergen-specific IgE had a higher specificity and predictive value than allergen-specific IgGd, and the authors concluded that allergen-specific IgE was a more useful test in canine atopic disease.[236]

The subclass profile of allergen-specific IgG antibodies was studied in atopic dogs.[199] The IgG response to house dust mites was dominated by IgG4 antibodies, and the response to timothy grass was predominantly IgG1 and IgG4. The data suggested a degree of IgG subclass restriction in the humoral response of atopic dogs, which may be dependent on the nature of the allergen.

The advent of in vitro tests that measure serum allergen-specific IgE levels has offered another tool to assess IgE production. In a number of studies, these tests have shown that normal dogs also produce allergen-specific IgE and that the titers do not correlate with clinical disease.[337] These observations in dogs, and other work in humans, have shown that heterogeneity of IgE exists, and perhaps only one or some select types are involved in atopic disease.[9, 29, 50, 182, 216, 236] It is hypothesized that two basic types of IgE would exist: IgE− and IgE+. Individuals with serum and tissue-bound IgE− would have minimal or no skin disease, whereas those with IgE+ would have atopic skin disease. A number of studies in dogs and cats have supported this concept of IgE heterogeneity, and this offers an explanation for the variation in serum IgE results in atopic and normal dogs and the frequent lack of correlation between serologic and skin test results.[215, 216, 236, 261, 431] Another possibility is that the sensitivity to IgE and the ability of target cells to degranulate may constitute the underlying abnormality in atopic disease.

The classic description of the pathogenesis of atopy is that IgE (or IgGd) fixes to

---

*See references 29, 30, 58, 61, 67a, 200, 222, 254, 376.

tissue mast cells, especially in the skin, the primary target organ of canine atopy. When mast cell–fixed IgE reacts with its specific allergen or allergens, mast cell degranulation and release or production of many pharmacologically active compounds ensues. This occurs after intradermal injection of allergen and is the basis of positive reactions. The role of mast cells is further supported by a study in atopic dogs correlating cutaneous mast cell density with the pattern of the typical clinical lesions. There are relatively more mast cells on the pinnae and ventral interdigital skin of the paws than any other regions.[170] However, the histology and the clinical appearance of the immediate lesion (wheal) induced by intradermal allergen presentation does not mimic the clinical disease.[67a] In contrast, the recognition that late-phase reactions to intradermal injections or patch test reactions produce lesions that clinically, histologically, and immmunophenotypically resemble the spontaneous disease in humans and dogs has led to newer theories regarding the pathogenesis of atopic dermatitis (see later).

In humans and dogs, it has been shown that IgE fixes to epidermal Langerhans' cells.[235, 256, 257, 267] In atopic humans, this is mediated by the expression of high-affinity IgE receptors on Langerhans' cells, and aeroallergen-specific IgE enhances the antigen-presenting capabilities of these cells.[231, 246] In dogs, epidermal eosinophil microaggregates and increased Langerhans' cells have been found in lesional atopic skin. Even clinically normal atopic skin has increased numbers of Langerhans' cells.[15, 256, 257, 267] Dermal increases in eosinophils also occur, though the mean percentage is 3.86% of all dermal inflammatory cells, which is similar to the findings in a previous study.[253, 257]

Similar to what is found in atopic humans, there is also an increase in the endothelial cell expression of ICAM-1, but not MHC II, in atopic dogs. There are increased numbers of T cells in lesional skin of atopic dogs, with an increase in the CD4/CD8 T cells ratio, and increased numbers of α, β T cells (type 2), as in atopic humans. Additionally, lesional skin from atopic dogs has relatively more CD8+ cells and γ, δ T cells (type 1) than human atopics.[257, 267, 286] These observations support the concept of percutaneous allergen activation of atopic disease and a similar pathogenesis in both dogs and humans. It is likely that atopic dermatitis is caused by a combination of immediate and late-phase contact reactions to aeroallergens.[256–259]

In humans, the genetic abnormality in atopic dermatitis appears to be an immunologic skin dysfunction that has been induced by bone marrow transplantation.[197] Abnormalities of the SIS in atopic humans include (1) endothelial cells that abnormally express adhesion molecules, (2) an increase in T cells that are predominantly T helper cells, (3) hyperstimulatory epidermal Langerhans' cells and increased dermal Langerhans' cells, (4) B-cell overproduction of IgE, (5) IgE on Langerhans' cells, and (6) Langerhans' cells with IgE that may be able to stimulate T cells locally.*

In the atopic patient, this ability could lead to an exaggerated T-lymphocyte response. Special stains of skin samples from humans with atopic dermatitis have revealed that lesional skin contains increased numbers of activated helper T cells of the subclass Th2.[245, 246] These helper T cells may preferentially induce IgE-producing B cells by themselves, thus resulting in the production of IL-4, IL-5, and IL-10.[9, 54, 245, 246] These interleukins stimulate mast cell and eosinophil activation and proliferation. Though eosinophils are often not detected in routine lesional skin from human atopic dermatitis patients, they do play a role in the inflammation. This assessment is based on the presence of eosinophil major basic and cationic proteins in human atopic lesional skin (confirming that eosinophils had been present) and the finding of eosinophils in early lesions at atopy patch test sites.[9, 50, 54, 229]

The T-cell subclass is not a constant finding, and recent work has shown that, in chronic lesions, there is more of a mixture. Thus, early lesions are dominated by Th2 cells, but a switch to both Th1 and Th2 occurs in chronic skin lesions. This has also been observed in the dog, in which a Th2 cytokine profile (IL-4 and IL-5 cytokine gene transcripts) are more prevalent in atopic dog skin, but a Th1 cytokine profile (IFN-γ) was

---

*See references 9, 50, 54, 178, 182, 197, 239, 245, 246.

found primarily in chronic skin lesions.[259] It is obvious that the pathogenesis is much more complex than genetically programmed alterations in IgE production.

Immediate intradermal test reactions do not mimic the clinical lesions in the atopic dog and, in many cases, they are not pruritic, suggesting that intradermally deposited antigen does not reproduce the natural disease.[67a] In humans, similar changes to naturally occurring lesions can be induced at allergen patch test (the so-called "atopy patch test") sites in patients with atopic dermatitis, but not in normal patients or patients with rhinitis or asthma.[23, 59, 228] Though these tests are quite specific, their sensitivity is variable. When results are positive, the changes induced by the patch tests mimic the clinical lesion, the microscopic findings, and the cellular phenotype that occurs in the natural disease. In addition, the time course of lesion development shows initial infiltration with IL-4–containing T cells, eosinophils, and later IFN-γ–containing T cells, similar to the natural disease in human atopics.[228, 232, 297]

These findings are in contrast with the late-phase reactions following intradermal injection of allergen, with resultant mast cell degranulation and subsequent neutrophilic infiltrates. These and other observations have led to the conclusion that the mast cell plays a minor role in atopic dermatitis and that the atopy patch test is a better model to study atopic disease.[245] Additionally, these observations strongly support the role of percutaneous absorption and the pathogenesis after helper T-cell and eosinophil activation. Only one patch test study has been published in dogs.[209] Six of 10 normal dogs experienced positive intradermal skin test reactions to house dust mites, and 1 of 6 "positive" dogs experienced a positive patch test reaction. Only 1 of 18 atopic dogs experienced a positive patch test reaction to antigens they were positive to with intradermal testing. These findings were not very supportive of the percutaneous penetration theory. The predominance of skin lesions in canine atopy occurring in contact areas would support the importance of percutaneous penetration of allergen.[27, 30, 67a] Therefore, the percutaneous absorption of antigen may better explain the clinical disease, and future studies in dogs may yield a new understanding of the pathogenesis of canine atopy.

In atopic humans, the water-retaining capacity of even clinically normal skin is significantly decreased, and transepidermal water loss is increased.[173, 205] It has been suggested that the skin of atopic humans is inherently functionally abnormal.[23] In dogs, preliminary studies have indicated that the baseline hydration of nonlesional atopic skin is the same as that in the skin of normal dogs.[193]

A summary of current thought as to the possible pathogenesis of atopic skin disease might go as follows:

Percutaneously absorbed allergens (allergen penetration probably enhanced by inherent defect of epidermal barrier function) encounter allergen-specific IgE on Langerhans' cells, whereupon the allergens are trapped, processed, and presented to allergen-specific T lymphocytes. There is a subsequent preferential expansion of allergen-specific Th2 cells, which produce IL-3, IL-4, IL-5, IL-6, IL-10, and IL-13. The imbalance in allergen-specific Th2 cells (with a resultant increase in IL-4–stimulated production of allergen-specific IgE) and allergen-specific Th1 cells (with a resultant decrease in INF-γ inhibition of allergen-specific IgE production) culminates in enhanced production of allergen-specific IgE by B lymphocytes.[32, 178, 182, 183, 274, 295] With chronicity, changes occur in cytokine expression with lower levels of IL-13 and increased IFN-γ.[176, 259, 297]

Though percutaneous absorption of allergen is the most likely route of allergen exposure, the ability of inhaled allergens to induce skin disease should not be overlooked. In both dogs and humans, inhalation of allergen has been shown to cause exacerbation of the cutaneous lesions as well as respiratory symptoms.[184, 242, 298]

An older theory focused on β-adrenergic blockade as the underlying abnormality of atopy.[61, 67a] Though it is not accepted as the major pathologic abnormality, it may play a role in the pathogenesis. Szentivanyi proposed the β-adrenergic theory of atopic disease in 1968.[53] He suggested that the heightened sensitivity of atopic human beings to various pharmacologic agents could be due to a blockage of β-adrenergic receptors in the tissues. Since that time, there has been an explosion of investigative effort in the field of the cyclic nucleotides.[9, 50, 54, 61, 67a] In brief, the cyclic nucleotides cyclic adenosine monophosphate (cAMP) and cyclic guanosine monophosphate (cGMP) appear to serve as the intracellular effectors of a variety of cellular events. They are viewed as exerting opposing influences in a number of systems.

A number of pharmacologic agents are known to act via various cell receptors to influence intracellular levels of cAMP and cGMP. In general, substances that elevate intracellular cAMP levels (β-adrenergic drugs, prostaglandin E, methylxanthines, histamine, and other mediator substances) or reduce intracellular cGMP levels (anticholinergic drugs) tend to stabilize the cells (lymphocytes, monocyte-macrophages, neutrophils, mast cells) and inhibit the release of various inflammatory mediators. On the other hand, substances that reduce cAMP levels (α-adrenergic drugs) or elevate cGMP levels (cholinergic drugs, ascorbic acid, estrogen, levamisole) tend to labilize the cells and promote the release of inflammatory mediators. Further studies in the area of cyclic nucleotides and biological regulation may produce significant advances in the areas of disease pathomechanism and control of immunologic inflammation.

Studies in a Basenji-Greyhound model of atopy have revealed the following findings: (1) airway hypersensitivity to methacholine, citric acid, and leukotrienes, (2) elevated blood histamine and leukotriene levels after antigen challenge, (3) blunted cAMP response to β-adrenergic agents, (4) adenylate cyclase activities and β-adrenergic receptor numbers and affinities similar to those in normal dogs, and (5) elevated levels of phosphodiesterase.[61, 67a, 184, 191] These studies suggest that the blunted cAMP responses in atopic dogs are due to increased phosphodiesterase activity rather than to defects in the β-adrenergic receptor-adenylate cyclase system.

Katz introduced the concept of allergic breakthrough.[30, 61, 67a] Normally, according to this concept, IgE antibody production is maintained at a low magnitude after sensitization because of the existence of a normal suppressive or "damping" mechanism that exists specifically to limit the quantity of IgE antibodies produced during any particular response. If any one of a number of possible perturbations (respiratory viral infections, endoparasites, hormonal fluctuations) disturbs this damping mechanism so as to diminish the overall damping capabilities to a sufficiently low level, and if, when the damping threshold is lowered, the individual becomes exposed to sufficient levels of allergen, sensitization resulting in allergic breakthrough occurs. This may explain why some atopic dogs experience a temporary worsening of their disease after their annual vaccinations.

It has been suggested that atopic dogs have a Δ-6 desaturase deficiency and metabolize fats differently than nonatopic dogs.[99, 162] In addition, atopic dogs have lower levels of plasma triglycerides than normal dogs after being fed corn oil, suggesting impaired fat absorption or increased plasma clearance.[302] The existence of two subsets of atopic dogs has been proposed.[151] Atopic dogs were fed an omega-3/omega-6 fatty acid–containing diet to control their pruritus. Nonresponders had a smaller increase in plasma fatty acids, suggesting an even more pronounced abnormality in fat absorption/metabolism/clearance. Both responders and nonresponders appeared to have a Δ-5 desaturase deficiency, whereas nonresponders also appeared to have a Δ-6 desaturase deficiency. The proposed Δ-5 desaturase deficiency was also recognized by others.[296] It was also reported that the metabolism of omega-3 fatty acids was differentially regulated among breeds of dogs.[38] All of these considerations could help explain the variable responses of atopic dogs to omega-3/omega-6 fatty acid supplementation.

Atopic dogs are known to be prone to secondary bacterial pyoderma and *Malassezia* infections. A variety of abnormalities present in atopic dogs may explain these infections. Atopic dog corneocytes have greater adherence for *S. intermedius*,[242] and the numbers of *S. intermedius* are increased on the skin of symptomatic atopic dogs.[241] However, the numbers of *S. intermedius* and corneocyte adhesion appear to be normal in atopic dogs whose condition is in remission with glucocorticoids.[220] Intradermal injection of histamine causes increased percutaneous penetration of staphylococcal antigens in normal dogs, suggesting that the inflamed skin of atopic dogs would also be more accessible to staphylococcal antigens and, perhaps, staphylococcal pyoderma.[240] Cell-mediated immunity is depressed.[251]

A similar situation occurs in human patients with atopic dermatitis. It has been shown that, in dogs, many of these abnormalities are the result of the allergic reaction and not a primary abnormality.[249–252] Atopic humans often have exaggerated responses to patch or intradermal testing with *Malassezia* antigens, and flares of their dermatitis may respond to antiyeast therapy.[274] A similar phenomenon is likely to occur in atopic dogs and the presence of an immunologic response has been demonstrated by intradermal testing and with in vitro tests for *Malassezia* specific IgE (see Chap. 5).[243, 254] Atopic dogs had higher serum levels of *Malassezia*-specific IgE than nonatopic dogs or dogs with *Malassezia* dermatitis without atopic disease, and the level was not related to numbers of organisms present.[254] *Malassezia* surface counts have been reported to be both higher than or equal to those in normal dogs (see Chap. 5).

Superantigens are a group of bacterial and viral proteins that are characterized by the capacity to stimulate large numbers of T cells.[287] They bind directly to MHC class II molecules on antigen-presenting cells and cross-link the antigen-presenting cell with T cells expressing certain receptors, leading to polyclonal T-cell activation. When staphylococcal superantigens are applied to intact human skin, dermatitis is produced. Furthermore, in the presence of superantigens, keratinocytes potently activate T-cells. Thus, superantigens play a role in the induction and exacerbation of inflammatory skin disease.

Bacterial exotoxins also amplify allergen-specific IgE production.[226] During exposure to allergens, IFN-γ production is decreased, leading to a predominance of Th2-like cytokines. Bacterial toxins bridge Th2 cells and B cells, inducing B-cell activation. Bacterial toxins also upregulate B7.2 expression on B cells and enhance IgE synthesis. IgE binds to CD23, allowing nonspecific B cells to become potent antigen-presenting cells via the co-stimulatory molecule, B7.2. As a result, Th2-like cells may expand and induce more B cells to switch to IgE production, with subsequent overproduction of IL-4 and allergen-specific IgE. Staphylococcal superantigen-induced inflammation may explain the antibiotic-induced reduction in inflammation and pruritus in atopic dogs that have no clinical signs of infection.

The average serum histamine concentration in atopic dogs was reported to be equal to that of normal dogs (15.3 ± 7.75 ng/ml)[253] or lower (1.46 ng/ml) than that of normal dogs (3.66 ng/ml).[273] The average response of the serum histamine concentration of atopic dogs to nasal aerosols of antigens that had given positive results on intradermal skin testing was 0.98 ng/ml (before antigenic exposure) to 2.70 ng/ml (10 to 20 minutes after exposure).[273] Nasal exposure to antigens that did not give positive reactions on intradermal skin testing resulted in average values of 0.76 ng/ml prior to exposure and 1.48 ng/ml post exposure.[273] Cutaneous histamine concentrations were always greater in atopic dogs than in normal dogs but did not correlate with plasma histamine concentrations.[253]

Some studies showed increased mast cell "releasibility" of histamine in atopic dogs,[201a, 224, 299] whereas another indicated that cutaneous mast cells from atopic dogs do not release any more histamine after incubation with atopic serum and anti-IgE than nonatopic dog mast cells.[181] Total histamine content of skin mast cells is higher in atopic than in normal dogs.[201a] Cutaneous mast cell density, as estimated by toluidine blue staining, was identical in atopic and normal dogs.[305] Cutaneous mast cell density, as estimated by subtypes (based on protease content: tryptase and chymase), was lower in atopic than normal dogs.[305]

Leukocyte (basophil) histamine release was found to be significantly greater in atopic and artificially hypersensitized dogs than in normal dogs, though the total histamine content of leukocytes was not statistically significantly different among the three groups.[227] It was concluded that leukocyte releasibility is a disorder of immunoregulation intrinsic to the atopic state and unrelated to the concentration of serum or tissue IgE.

Serum IgA levels may be low in atopic dogs.[185, 222] The significance of this is unknown, though the lowering of local immune responses or an increase in antigen absorption and presentation could potentially result. In one study, serum IgA levels were the same in atopic and normal dogs and skin IgA concentrations were significantly greater in atopics.[247a]

Canine atopy may be best described as a multifactorial disease in which genetically predisposed dogs exhibit a combination of cutaneous IgE-mediated immediate and late-phase reactions to environmental antigens. Immunologic abnormalities, antigenic stimuli, altered physiologic and pharmacologic reactions, and genetic predisposition all play a role in the pathogenesis.

CLINICAL FEATURES

Atopy is universally recognized and, in areas with fleas, is the second most common hypersensitivity skin disorder of dogs, probably affecting around 10% of the canine population.[29, 43, 58, 61, 67a, 187, 190, 192, 255, 277, 282, 283, 300, 359a, 402] The true incidence is unknown, and most estimates are likely low when one considers that many atopic dogs are never presented to the veterinarian because they have mild symptoms or because they present for only intermittent otitis externa, which is usually not attributed to atopic disease.[194, 248] Certain breeds are known to have a predilection for canine atopy, including Boxers, Chihuahuas, Gordon setters, Yorkshire terriers, Chinese Shar peis, Cairn terriers, West Highland white terriers, Scottish terriers, Lhasa apsos, Shih tzus, Wirehaired fox terriers, Dalmatians, Pugs, Irish setters, Boston terriers, Golden retrievers, English setters, Labrador retrievers, Cocker spaniels, Miniature schnauzers, Belgian Tervurens, Shiba inus, and Beaucerons.* Canine atopy is reportedly more common in females than in males, though some studies show no sex predilections.

The age of onset of clinical signs in atopic dogs varies from 4 months to 7 years, with about 70% of the dogs first manifesting clinical signs between 1 and 3 years of age. An exception to this general rule would be the Akita, Chow Chow, Golden retriever, and Shar Pei breeds, wherein the signs of atopy may begin as early as 2 months of age.[67a, 306] This may partly reflect the environment (allergen load) that the puppies are raised in and is more common when both parents are atopic.[27, 61, 67a] Older dogs may occasionally experience atopy, especially if they have changed environments.[306] Clinical signs may initially be seasonal or nonseasonal, depending on the allergens involved. About 80% of all atopic dogs eventually have nonseasonal clinical signs.[27, 58, 61, 67a, 282] About 80% of the atopic dogs initially manifest clinical signs in the period from spring to fall, and about 20% begin in winter.[61, 67a, 192, 282]

The initial lesion is pruritus in areas with either no visible lesion, slightly erythematous macules, or more diffuse erythema (Fig. 8–5A and B). An exception to the rule is the atopic English bulldog, which often presents with erythema, edema, and other secondary skin lesions but little or no history of pruritus. Though somewhat controversial, the presence of a primary papular rash should suggest another or coexistent disease. The exception is very small papules, best observed with a magnifying lens that may be present in areas of erythroderma or erythematous macules. The skin lesions in atopic dogs are usually those associated with self-trauma, secondary bacterial pyoderma, secondary *Malassezia* dermatitis, and secondary seborrheic skin disease.[27, 34, 61, 67a, 282]

The self-trauma, chronic inflammation, and secondary bacterial pyoderma or *Malassezia* dermatitis may result in complete or partial alopecia, salivary staining, papules, pustules, circular crusted papules, hyperpigmentation, and lichenification (see Figs. 8–5C and D). In general, the presence of lichenified, crusty, or greasy plaques is associated with secondary bacterial pyoderma or *Malassezia* dermatitis (see Fig. 8–5E). Pruritus usually involves the face (see Fig. 8–5A and C), paws (see Fig. 8–5B and D), distal extremities, anterior elbows (see Fig. 8–5F), and ventrum, or some combination thereof (see Figure 8–5G).

One study suggested that the pattern of disease in house dust mite–hypersensitive dogs was more a ventral contact pattern and that the pattern of all skin disease overall had no absolute association with the diagnosis of flea bite hypersensitivity or atopy from pollens or house dust mites.[180] This study also reported dorsal lumbar involvement in 39% of the atopic dogs. Generalized cutaneous involvement may eventually be present in about 40% of these dogs.[67a, 277, 402] Atopic otitis externa (see Fig. 8–5H) and conjunctivitis may

---

*See references 187, 192, 201, 255, 282, 283, 306, 359a.

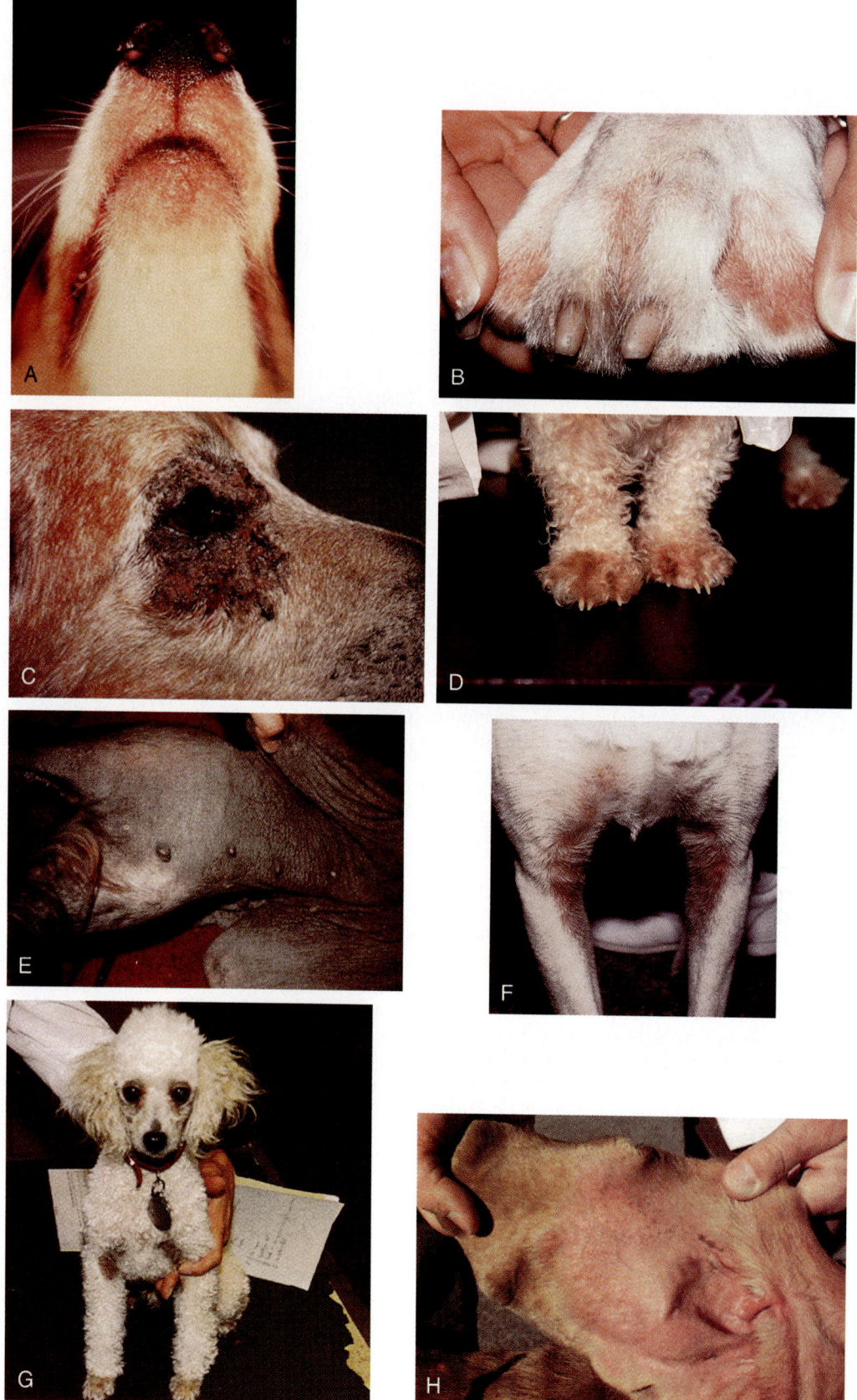

FIGURE 8–5. *See legend on opposite page*

be present in about 40% to 80% of these dogs.* Secondary bacterial pyoderma (folliculitis, furunculosis), pyotraumatic dermatitis, or acral lick dermatitis may be present in as many as 68% of atopic dogs.† Marked seborrhea occurs in 12% of atopic dogs.[27, 67a, 282] Close inspection, however, reveals that most atopic dogs have mild scaling in most pruritic areas. The haircoat is often dryer in these areas as well, though in some dog breeds (especially German shepherd, Chinese Shar Pei, Lhasa apso, Shih tzu) it may be greasy.[27] Hyperhidrosis may be present in 10% to 20% of atopic dogs.[61, 67a, 282]

Seborrheic skin disease, hyperhidrosis, secondary bacterial infections, and secondary *Malassezia* infections may complicate canine atopy, and there is a predisposition for atopic dogs to have an increased number of *Malassezia* organisms on their skin.[307] This is particularly apparent in skin scrapings from the interdigital area. The *Malassezia* contributes to the objectionable odor of atopic dogs and more commonly involves the ears, paws, claw folds, and ventral neck (Fig. 8–6). Brown staining of the claws at the claw fold is suggestive of *Malassezia* paronychia.[214] The yeast may also contribute as an allergen, exacerbating the atopic disease and pruritus directly, even without obvious yeast overgrowth.[243, 254] In one study, 27.7% of atopic dogs had anal sacculitis.[192]

Some atopic dogs experience a seasonally recurrent pruritic bacterial folliculitis or furunculosis. Antibiotic therapy resolves the skin lesions and the pruritus. Whether these atopic dogs are truly nonpruritic and asymptomatic without their infections, or whether their owners tolerate or ignore low levels of licking, chewing, and scratching (perhaps believing them to be normal for their dogs), is unclear. In any case, these dogs are skin test–positive, and successful hyposensitization or anti-inflammatory drug therapy prevents recurrence of the bacterial skin disease.

Noncutaneous clinical signs reported to occur occasionally in atopic dogs include rhinitis, asthma, cataracts, urinary and gastrointestinal disorders, and hormonal hypersensitivity.[27, 58, 67a, 282] We have also seen cases with reverse sneezing that resolves with a favorable response to hyposensitization. Atopic female dogs may exhibit irregular estrus cycles, low conception rates, and high incidence of pseudopregnancy.[61, 67a] It has not been determined what proportion of the secondary infections, seborrhea, and noncutaneous signs are induced or influenced by previous therapies used.

DIAGNOSIS

The differential diagnosis is lengthy, considering the wide variation of presenting signs and secondary complications that may occur—for example, pruritic facial dermatitis, pruritic pododermatitis, pruritic otitis externa, pruritic ventral dermatitis, pruritic generalized dermatitis, seborrhea, recurrent superficial bacterial pyoderma, and *Malassezia* dermatitis. The more common considerations in the differential diagnosis, however, are (1) flea bite hypersensitivity, (2) food hypersensitivity, (3) scabies, (4) insect hypersensitivity, (5) contact dermatitis (primary irritant or hypersensitivity), (6) intestinal parasite hypersensitivity, (7) bacterial folliculitis, and (8) *Malassezia* dermatitis. In dogs under 12 months of age, endoparasitic hypersensitivity, insect hypersensitivity, scabies, and food hypersensitivity are the major possibilities to pursue. In our experience, and that of most of the veterinary literature, flea bite hypersensitivity only rarely causes facial dermatitis, conjunctivitis, or

---

*See references 7, 61, 67a, 192, 248, 277, 282, 402.
†See references 27, 34, 61, 67a, 277, 282, 283.

FIGURE 8–5. Canine atopy. *A*, Mild erythroderma of the muzzle, an early lesion of atopic disease in a commonly affected site. *B*, Erythematous macules, and mild digital alopecia interdigitally. *C*, Periocular alopecia and hyperpigmentation from chronic rubbing of the eyes. *D*, Paw licking results in rust-colored digital hairs. *E*, Secondary bacterial pyoderma or *Malassezia* dermatitis is usually present in these ventral thoracic and abdominal lichenified lesions. *F*, Licking of the anterior elbows is a common site of pruritus in atopic dogs. *G*, Classic presentation of face, axillae, and paws. *H*, Pinnal erythema with secondary accumulations of excessive cerumen.

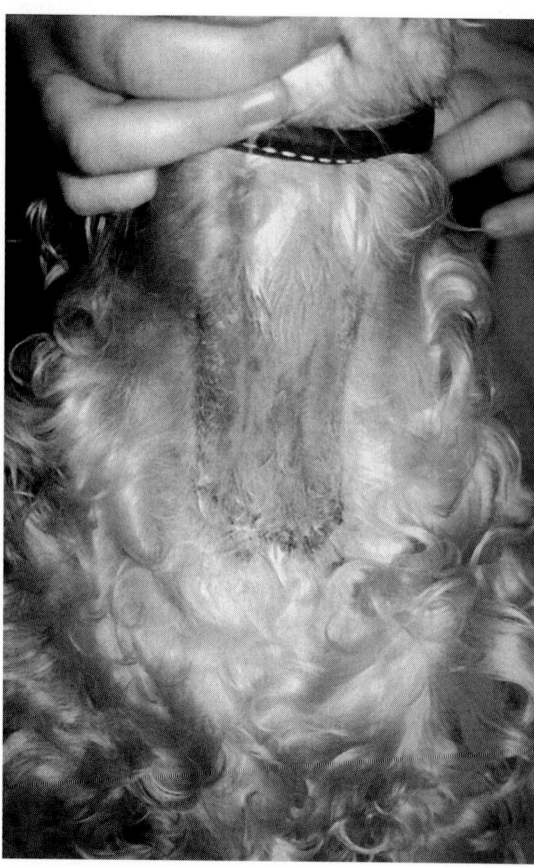

FIGURE 8-6. Ventral neck lesions with *Malassezia* dermatitis in an atopic dog.

otitis externa, but many atopic dogs (as many as 75%) have concurrent flea bite hypersensitivity.[30, 61, 67a, 186] Therefore, when these other cutaneous reaction patterns are present in a flea-hypersensitive dog, atopy may also be present and is most rapidly ruled out by intradermal skin testing. In addition, atopic dogs may have concurrent food hypersensitivity.[61, 67a, 186, 517, 518]

The diagnosis is based on history, physical examination, ruling out other possible diagnoses, and intradermal testing.[34, 61, 67a, 268, 376] It cannot be overemphasized that allergy tests are never a substitute for a meticulously gathered history, a thorough physical examination, and a careful and complete elimination of other diagnoses and concurrent problems. Owing to the generally low specificity of commercial in vitro tests, they should not be used for diagnosis of atopic disease.[26, 67a] Peripheral and tissue eosinophilias are rare in atopic dogs unless the dogs have concurrent ectoparasitisms, insect hypersensitivities, or endoparasitisms.[61, 67a]

A tentative diagnosis of canine atopy can be based on history, clinical signs, and laboratory tests to rule out other possibilities. A definitive diagnosis of atopy and revelation of the allergens involved may be made with intradermal (skin) testing and, to some extent, in vitro (serologic) allergy tests. The intradermal test is thought to be superior to the scratch, prick, and in vitro allergy tests.[58, 61, 67a] Because of the very common occurrence of "false-positive" (clinically insignificant) reactions obtained, in vitro allergy testing should not be used alone to diagnose atopy, but it may be helpful in determining which allergens to include in a hyposensitization formula.

Intradermal Allergy Testing

A limited number of studies have been conducted to document optimal intradermal testing procedures. Unfortunately, different commercial allergen sources were sometimes used, making comparisons impossible, and the studies have not directly compared different commercial sources of allergens. Whichever company is used should be consulted for information regarding their testing concentrations. Multiple studies have been conducted with a variety of different commercial allergens, and differences do occur.[61, 67a, 324, 376, 393] Even with the same allergen source, some results have differed.[30, 61, 216, 330, 332] It is likely that some differences among studies with the same allergens reflect the animals' exposure to significant allergen levels that may induce positive but clinically insignificant reactions.[30, 61, 216, 332] This is supported by the observation in humans of patients with known allergy having no symptoms but still having histologic evidence of disease.[194]

Preferably the allergen companies should have results of independent studies because differences may occur. Studies with aqueous allergens made by Greer Laboratories have shown that, for most allergens, 0.05 ml of 1000 protein nitrogen units (PNU) per ml is not reactive in most normal dogs and cats. Exceptions are mold mix 2, which probably should not be used, and house dust. When house dust antigen was used at a strength of greater than or equal to 250 PNU/ml, approximately 50% of atopic *and* normal dogs experienced positive intradermal reactions.[319, 330] If house dust is used, it should be used at 125 PNU/ml or less. House dust mite is currently preferred by many authors.[34, 58, 61, 67a] House dust is a heterogenous mixture of animal and human danders, molds, house dust mites, insect debris, bacteria, food particles, breakdown products of clothing, and inorganic substances, and each lot can vary in its antigenicity and irritability.[390, 391]

House dust mites are thought to be the major allergenic component. House dust has been used for years to test and hyposensitize dogs and cats.[61, 67a] One study showed that the reactivities of house dust and house dust mite allergens in atopic dogs were very comparable.[391] This same study indicated that there was a strong positive correlation between reactions to house dust mite and flea antigen but not between house dust and kapok or mixed feathers. Other allergens that have given controversial results are cattle hair, wool, feathers, tobacco, and cat dander as causes of false-positive (irritant) skin test reactions.[27, 58, 61, 67a] Cattle hair, wool, feathers, and mold mixes should be used at 250 to 500 PNU/ml. In general, the recommended aqueous test allergen concentration is 1000 PNU/ml or 1:1000 weight/volume (w/v).

- **Allergen Selection.** Skin test allergen selection is an important subject. Consultations with allergen firms and national pollen charts reviewing prevalence of pollens in the practice area help the clinician decide what to test for. A good veterinary reference is the book by Reedy and colleagues, *Allergic Skin Diseases of Dogs and Cats, 2nd edition*. It is important to select allergens from a reputable allergen supply house and then not to switch because experience with one source becomes important. Tremendous unresolved problems surround the standardization of allergenic extracts, including standards for raw material collection, methods of measuring the purity of raw materials, techniques for identifying many substances, a variety of methods of manufacturing, and determination of allergen stability and potency.[27, 30, 50, 58, 61, 67a] Bioactivity of commercial products varies from 10-fold to 1000-fold, and no relationship was found between bioactivity and concentrations declared in PNU or w/v.[58, 61, 67a]

Testing with allergen *mixes* is not recommended.[27, 58, 61, 67a, 376] Such mixes frequently result in false-negative reactions because individual allergens within the mix may be in a concentration too dilute for detection. More important, the patient may be allergic to only one of the allergens within the mix, making hyposensitization based on the mix result less specific. In fact, one most likely ends up hyposensitizing with allergens that the pet is not allergic to and, potentially, inducing new allergies. One report, however, has indicated that treating normal dogs with irrelevant antigens administered according to a common hyposensitization protocol induced neither skin test positivity nor clinical signs of allergy.[329] Skin testing with commercial "regional" allergen kits that use mixes is unsatisfactory. Instead, discussions with the supply house regarding the most important allergens for the practice area may be the most appropriate way to perform cost-effective and accurate tests for the client's budget.

Allergens commonly reported to be important in dogs are house dust mites, house dust, human dander, feathers, kapok, molds, weeds, grasses, and trees.° In the United States, most animals are multisensitive.[61, 67a, 279, 282] Polysensitization was originally reported to be rare in Europe.[58, 374] In fact, it was reported that European dogs were often sensitive only to house dust mites and, even when other allergens had given positive reactions, hyposensitization was frequently undertaken using only house dust mites and re-evaluated in 1 year.[58, 374] Recent publications, however, indicate that multisensitivity is the rule in some European countries.[192, 277, 386] The most important allergens in Europe are reported to be house dust, house dust mite, and human dander.† House dust mite is also the most important allergen in the United States and Japan.[61, 67a, 359a]

The two species of house dust mites commonly tested are *D. farinae* and *D. pteronyssinus*. Though both of these mites are members of the family *Pyroglyphidae*, they each have multiple allergenic epitopes for humans. In humans, there are two main groups of allergens that may have partial cross-reactivity between different species for allergens within the same group. In dogs, it has also been shown that *Dermatophagoides* mites cross-react with the mite *Blomia tropicalis*.[325] Studies have shown that dogs and humans recognize different major allergens from *Dermatophagoides* mites and that these antigens are not cross-reactive.[336, 337, 368, 369] However, the results of one in vitro study in atopic dogs in Japan indicated strong cross-reactivity between *D. farinae* and *D. pteronyssinus*.[359b]

In contrast, another study indicated that 69% of *D. farinae*–positive dogs had detectable serum IgE to a 30-kD protein thought to be Der F 1.[361] This is an important distinction because the trend in human medicine is to test for these specific allergenic epitopes. It would not be appropriate to extrapolate and use these specific tests in dogs unless the importance of that allergenic epitope is documented in the dog. Dogs react much more commonly to *D. farinae* than to *D. pteronyssinus* but not to the major allergens (Der F I and Der F II; Der P I and Der P II) recognized by humans.[368, 369] Of the house dust mite–hypersensitive dogs, 90% are found to react to a protein of 80 to 90 kD.[336, 337, 368, 369]

Another house dust mite major allergen has been detected in the dog.[361] It is a 109-kD protein chitinase. Another potential complicating factor when comparing studies on house dust mite studies is the variation in commercial extracts. This was shown in a study in dogs based on antigen-specific IgG tests.[385] Different commercial extracts varied in the number of protein bands detected. Comparing extracts from three companies also showed slightly different results in a group of normal laboratory reared dogs that would, theoretically, have very limited exposure to house dust mite allergen.[332]

Other mites are also important contributors to the arachnid levels in house dust. The mite *Euroglyphus maynei* has been found in numerous countries and, in England, has been reported to be the predominant species of mites in many homes. Though it is often found living with the *Dermatophagoides* spp. and it is a member of the same family, it does have multiple distinct allergens recognized by humans. No studies have been reported in the dog. The mite *Blomia tropicalis* is a glyciphagid house dust mite that is found in tropical and subtropical climates. It was found in 44% of examined houses in San Diego and, in Brazil, was found as the dominant house dust mite species. Several studies have shown some cross-reactivity with the *Dermatophagoides* spp. mites, but multiple species-specific allergens are also found. It is possible that these other house dust mites, which can be present in high numbers, may be important allergens in atopic dogs in certain regions. One study showed that dogs reacted to *B. tropicalis* in a country where this mite is not found and showed that at least some of this is due to cross-reactivity to *Dermatophagoides* spp.[325]

Storage mites may also play a role in atopy or act as a separate disease (see Storage Mite Dermatitis). In addition, other insect antigens (see Insect Hypersensitivity) have been reported to cause positive reactions in many atopic dogs as well as in atopic suspects that were skin test negative to all other commonly tested allergens.[27, 192, 392, 593, 594] Cock-

---

°See references 27, 34, 58, 61, 67a, 186, 192, 277, 279, 282, 337, 354, 370, 383.
†See references 58, 186, 192, 255, 277, 354, 386.

● Table 8–14 **REASONS FOR FALSE-NEGATIVE INTRADERMAL SKIN TEST REACTIONS**

Subcutaneous injections
Too little allergen:
    Testing with mixes
    Outdated allergens
    Allergens too dilute (1000 PNU/ml recommended)
    Too small volume of allergen injected
Drug interference:
    Glucocorticoids
    Antihistamines
    Tranquilizers
    Progestational compounds
    Any drugs that lower blood pressure significantly
Anergy (testing during peak of hypersensitivity reaction)
Inherent host factors
    Estrus, pseudopregnancy
    Severe stress (systemic diseases, fright, struggling)
Endoparasitism or ectoparasitism? ("blocking" of mast cells with antiparasitic IgE?)
Off-season testing (testing more than 1 to 2 months after clinical signs have disappeared)
Histamine "hyporeactivity"

roaches (*Blatella germanica, B. orientalis, Suppela suppellectillium, Periplaneta americana*) have been shown to be important allergens in humans and to cross-react with house dust, possibly because of cockroach particles present in house dust.[237] Twenty-five atopic dogs were skin tested with cockroach antigen, and results were positive in four, though these same four also yielded positive results to house dust mites.[237] One case of canine atopy was related to marijuana exposure.[338] Some dogs are reactive only to molds.[277, 408]

It is essential to remember that a positive skin test reaction means only that the patient has skin-sensitizing antibody, mast cells that degranulate on antigen exposure, and target tissue that responds to the released mediators. A positive reaction does not necessarily mean that the patient has clinical allergy to the allergen(s) injected. Thus, it is essential that positive skin test reactions be interpreted in light of the patient's history. By the same token, a negative skin test reaction does not necessarily mean that the patient is not atopic. Ten percent to 30% of the otherwise classically atopic dogs may have negative skin test reactions.[27, 58, 61, 67a] This group probably reflects either failure (by limiting the number of test allergens used) to challenge dogs with the appropriate allergens or the intervention of various factors known to produce false-negative reactions, as listed in Table 8–14.

Many factors may lead to false-positive or false-negative skin test reactions in dogs (see Table 8–14; Table 8–15).[34, 58, 61, 67a] These factors must be carefully considered when skin testing is performed. False-positive reactions to house dust mite have been reported in up to 60% of dogs with scabies.[67a, 374, 375] The most common cause of negative skin test

● Table 8–15 **REASONS FOR FALSE-POSITIVE INTRADERMAL SKIN TEST REACTIONS**

Irritant test allergens (especially those containing glycerin; also some house dust, feather, wool, mold, and all food preparations)
Contaminated test allergens (bacteria, fungi)
Skin-sensitizing antibody only (prior clinical or present subclinical sensitivity)*
Poor technique (traumatic placement of needle; dull or burred needle; too large a volume injected; air injected)
Substances that cause nonimmunologic histamine release (narcotics)
"Irritable" skin (large reactions seen to all injected substances, including saline control)
Dermatographism
Mitogenic allergen

*These reactions would be more appropriately called "clinically insignificant."

reactions is the recent administration of certain drugs: glucocorticoids, antihistamines, progestagens. Ketoconazole does not interfere with intradermal test results.[358] There are no reliable withdrawal times for these drugs. Guidelines have been arbitrarily determined by clinicians, with rare studies conducted to confirm them. One study that evaluated hydroxyzine inhibition of intradermal test results for flea allergen demonstrated suppression up to 10 days.[320] Even this study has to be interpreted carefully because some authorities think that different allergens may be more easily suppressed and that flea antigen in particular is less inhibited by drugs.[565]

General rules of thumb for drug withdrawal times prior to skin testing are: 3 weeks for oral and topical glucocorticoids, 8 weeks for injectable glucocorticoids, 10 days for antihistamines, and 10 days for products and diets containing omega-3/omega-6 fatty acids. Cutaneous reactivity to histamine was not significantly reduced in normal or pruritic dogs treated topically with a 1% hydrocortisone conditioner.[156] If the dog has any cutaneous signs of iatrogenic Cushing's syndrome, such as atrophy, striae, loss of elasticity, or peeling and scaling, it is preferable to wait until these signs are improved prior to testing. Allergens must also be stored properly in glass and not allowed to freeze repetitively.[30, 352] Although it has been reported that the biological activity of allergens stored in plastic syringes decreased faster than those stored in glass syringes,[326, 349, 379] no significant differences occurred in skin test reactivity.[379]

Studies of intradermal test reactions in normal dogs have generally yielded the following findings: (1) no breed differences, (2) either no age differences or decreased reactivity with increasing age, (3) either no sex differences or increased reactivity of females to some allergens, (4) decreased reactivity to some allergens with increasing haircoat pigmentation, (5) decreased reactivity to histamine in hospitalized dogs compared with normal household dogs (stress related?), (6) weekly intradermal injections of allergens resulting in multiple positive reactions to allergens that originally tested negative (usually after weekly injections for 8 weeks), and (7) previous treatment with allergens not inducing positive reactions.[61, 67a, 318, 319, 329, 382] Although many commercial skin test antigens contain measurable amounts of histamine, the quantity is not sufficient to cause false-positive skin test reactions.[372]

Clearly, intradermal testing is not a procedure to be taken lightly. It requires keen attention to details and possible pitfalls, together with experience and lots of practice. Intradermal testing, however, is the preferred method of diagnosing canine atopy.[*] Whereas clinically insignificant positive reactions in normal dogs are very common with serologic testing, they occur in only 10% to 15% of normal dogs with intradermal testing.[67a, 383, 384] Clinicians who cannot conduct skin tests on dogs on a weekly or biweekly basis will probably be unhappy with the results. In experienced hands, however, the intradermal test is a powerful tool in the diagnosis and management of canine atopy. When possible, cases should be referred to clinicians who specialize in this subject. When this is not possible, the use of serum in vitro tests is appropriate as long as atopic disease has been clinically diagnosed and the test results are carefully interpreted. These data are then used to select allergens for hyposensitization, with success rates being similar to those achieved with intradermal testing (see later).

- **Procedure for Intradermal Allergy Testing.** A commonly used procedure for intradermal testing is as follows:

    1. Make sure the patient at least reacts to histamine. One-twentieth (0.05) ml of 1:100,000 histamine phosphate is injected intradermally. A wheal 10 to 20 mm in diameter should be present at 15 to 30 minutes after injection. If the histamine wheal is small (less than 10 mm) to absent, postpone intradermal skin testing and test the animal with histamine weekly until the expected reaction is seen. *A positive reaction does not invariably indicate that testing will be unaffected by*

---

*See references 27, 61, 67a, 190, 195, 265, 331, 339, 363, 376.

previous drugs. Rarely, cutaneous reactivity to histamine returns prior to cutaneous reactivity to allergen.

2. Chemical restraint is helpful and may decrease the endogenous release of glucocorticoids. One study has indicated that intradermal skin testing performed in nonsedated dogs provoked hypercortisolemia, which was inhibited by prior sedation.[340] The hypercortisolemia produced in nonsedated dogs did not change intradermal skin test reactions, however. The combination of xylazine hydrochloride (Rompun, 0.25 to 0.5 mg/kg IV) and atropine sulfate is usually satisfactory for skin testing and is probably the most common form of chemical restraint employed.[61, 67a, 318, 321] Other acceptable chemical restraint protocols include thiamylal (17.5 mg/kg IV) with or without maintenance with halothane, isoflurane, or methoxyflurane; tiletamine-zolazepam (4 mg/kg IV); and medetomidine (Dormitor, 10 μg/kg IV).[321, 327, 328, 366, 387] Place the animal in lateral recumbency for testing.

3. The skin over the lateral thorax is the preferred test site. Because different areas of skin vary in responsiveness, the site used should be consistent from patient to patient. Gently clip the hair with a No. 40 blade, using *no* chemical preparation to clean the test site. Use a felt-tipped pen to mark each injection site. Place injection sites at least 2 cm apart, avoiding dermatitic areas.

4. Using a 26- to 27-gauge, 0.38-inch (0.9 cm) needle attached to a 1-ml disposable syringe, carefully inject, intradermally, 0.05 ml of saline or diluent control (negative control) and 0.05 ml of 1:100,000 histamine phosphate (positive control) and all the appropriately mixed test allergens. Skin testing–strength antigens should have been made fresh from concentrate within 12 weeks of use. Read the test sites at 15 and 30 minutes. Prevent the animal from traumatizing the test area.

5. By convention, a 2-plus (2+) or greater reaction is considered to be potentially significant and must be carefully correlated with the patient's history. With experience, positive reactions may be "guesstimated" by visual inspection. It is strongly recommended, however, that the novice measure the diameter of each wheal in millimeters. A positive skin test reaction may then be objectively defined as a wheal having a diameter that is equal to or larger than that halfway between the diameters of the wheals produced by the saline and histamine controls. In addition to the objective assessment of size, a subjective assessment of erythema and turgidity of the wheals is also used in determining a positive reaction. The size of positive skin test reactions does *not* necessarily correlate with their clinical importance. Late-phase immediate reactions (6 hours) and delayed skin test site reactions (24 to 48 hours after injection) occasionally occur and are of unknown significance. Pruritus at some positive reaction sites occasionally occurs and can be managed with cold compresses or topical steroids. Systemic reactions (anaphylaxis) to intradermal skin testing are extremely rare in dogs.

In Vitro Testing

- **Serologic Allergy Tests.** The radioallergosorbent test (RAST), enzyme-linked immunosorbent assay (ELISA), and liquid-phase immunoenzymatic assay are three tests that detect relative levels of allergen-specific IgE in the serum. The RAST and ELISA attach the allergens to be tested to a solid substrate such as a paper disk or polystyrene well. The liquid-phase immunoenzymatic assay (VARL) does not use a solid phase initially but mixes a labeled allergen with the patient's serum.[315] The combined labeled allergen-antibody complex is subsequently bound by the label to the plastic well. This method in humans has been shown to decrease the incidence of false-positive results due to background, nonspecific, "sticky" IgE.[27, 315] This liquid-phase assay also avoids the conformational distortions of antigens and resultant hiding of epitopes inherent to solid-phase techniques.

A small number of studies conducted with the early assays have shown problems with reproducibility of some commercial ELISA, RAST, and VARL assays.[316, 344, 373] These companies have made changes, but newer independent studies that show that these problems have been alleviated have not been presented. Although these tests are purported to be species specific, one study revealed that the canine RAST, but not the ELISA, indicated that all horses, goats, cats, and humans tested were also allergic![316] With all of the technologies involving the determination of allergen-specific IgE, virtually all normal dogs, all dogs with any kind of skin disease, and all atopic dogs, have at least one, and usually multiple, positive reactions.[316, 323, 331, 344, 353, 363, 376]

In a study evaluating a commercial ELISA test, results were positive in 7 of 12 normal dogs and negative in 10 of 36 atopic dogs, yielding an overall sensitivity of only 72.2% and a specificity of only 41.6%.[341, 342] Total serum IgE levels are very much higher in dogs than in human beings, with the mean level in normal dogs reported to be about 190 μg/ml, which is similar to that found in atopic dogs.[29, 30, 61, 67a, 253] The highest serum IgE levels are found in dogs with endoparasitism. Serial determinations of serum IgE concentrations in West Highland white terriers from 6 weeks to 3 years of age did not predict the development of atopy.[201] It has also been shown in the dog that the higher levels of total IgE contribute to an increased incidence of false-positive or irrelevant serologic reactions.[27, 345, 357] Total IgE levels in cats are also reported to be very high (175 to 850 μg/ml).[315]

According to some researchers, false-positive results are rarely obtained with the ELISA for allergen-specific IgGd in nonatopic dogs.[208, 318] This has become a controversial point in Europe because another researcher has shown that many normal dogs have allergen-specific IgGd.[236] Investigators in the United States, however, reported that allergen-specific IgG was detectable in the majority of nonatopic as well as all atopic dogs.[225] The results of serologic allergy testing correlate poorly or moderately with those of intradermal allergy testing.[316, 323, 331, 344, 348, 353, 363, 376] Some laboratories with monoclonal antibodies, mixed monoclonal antibodies, and FcεRIα-based systems for detecting the canine IgE have reported improved overall correlation with intradermal testing, from 75% to 90%, though there is still a variation depending on the allergen being tested.* The variation between individual allergens relates to their "stickiness" for background IgE.

In part, the discrepancies between serologic and intradermal testing may be explained by numerous difficulties in technique, sensitivity, and so forth. It is also important, however, to realize that they test for two different things, so complete correlations are not expected (Table 8–16). IgG anti-IgE immune complexes are present in atopic dogs, which may lead to inaccurate measurement of IgE.[350] In addition, considering that some dogs with negative intradermal skin test results or poor results with hyposensitization based on intradermal skin tests respond well to hyposensitization based on in vitro test results, it is valuable to have this alternative test available.[27] The differences may also indicate that two types of IgE are present, that tissue-bound IgE does not correlate with circulating levels, that tests have different sensitivities for different allergens, or that immediate skin test reactivity and the presence of allergen-specific antibodies are no more than secondary features (epiphenomena) of atopy.[27, 29, 30, 61, 67a] However, the results of breeding lines of high-IgE responder dogs and their natural development of skin disease after the development of their IgE response suggest that IgE is important in the pathogenesis of canine atopic disease.[394, 395]

The point, here, is that false- or irrelevant positive reactions are to be expected with serologic allergy testing. Hence, it is absolutely critical that (1) the candidates for testing undergo meticulous work-up so that atopy is the only possible remaining diagnosis and (2) the test results obtained be very carefully evaluated in light of the patient's dermatologic history. These tests are not used for the diagnosis of atopy but to detect what an animal produces allergen-specific IgE to as a way to select allergens for hyposensitization.[27, 67a, 190, 195, 363]

Results with newer techniques have improved, the results with some allergens having more positive results but most having fewer positive results.[360] The technologic variables being evaluated and applied to commercial tests include such things as[200, 315, 322, 335, 347, 351, 388, 389, 394, 395]

---

*See references 322, 325a, 351, 367, 389, 394, 395.

Table 8–16 COMPARISON OF INTRADERMAL AND IN VITRO ALLERGY TESTS IN DOGS

FEATURE	INTRADERMAL	IN VITRO
Detects reaginic antibody	Yes	Yes
Detects presence of reaginic antibody in serum	No	Yes
Detects presence of cutaneous mast cells with reaginic antibody present on them	Yes	No
Determines capability of inducing a cutaneous type I hypersensitivity reaction on exposure to antigen	Yes	No
Test results are inhibited by antihistamines and glucocorticoids	Yes	No*
Sensitivity (per cent)	70–90	70–100
Specificity (per cent)	>90	0–90
Risk to patient	Rare but possible anaphylaxis or sedative reaction	Only serum sample required
Availability	Limited to certain practices; often requires referral	Excellent
Cost per antigen tested	Inexpensive	Relatively expensive
Clinic overhead	Relatively high	Little to none

*Chronic administration of glucocorticoids can reduce test scores or cause negative results.

1. Using monoclonal anticanine IgE antibodies instead of polyclonal antibodies
2. Using mixtures of monoclonal antibodies to detect IgE
3. Using the Fc receptor to detect IgE
4. Processing the patient's serum through a column of ascarid antigen to remove parasitic IgE
5. Processing the patient's serum through a column with protein A to remove IgG

These techniques have been shown to improve the testing comparisons for the respective companies and compared with intradermal test results. Limited studies have compared two different commercial serologic tests and, in general, the comparisons were made to intradermal test results. No studies have been conducted between commercial companies with the different technologies based on the effectiveness of hyposensitization. However, multiple studies have shown that the results of hyposensitization based on serologic test results in atopic dogs are similar to that with intradermal testing results, including one double-blinded comparison.* These studies have used a wide variety of the commercial tests available, and all appear to have similar results. Interestingly, even the different technologic variables do not appear to significantly influence the results of hyposensitization because all the reports using the different companies appear similar in response rates. Some companies offer group testing, but there is no place for such testing because it leads to inappropriate treatment recommendations.

Another issue has been the effects of antipruritic therapies on in vitro test results. In general, antihistamines, fatty acids, and other nonsteroidal drugs may be given without affecting these tests. Short-term treatment with anti-inflammatory doses of glucocorticoids probably does not influence the results of serologic allergy testing,[364] but long-term treatment may cause false-negative reactions.[27, 290, 344, 360, 389] It is also likely that there are individual responses to clinically used glucocorticoid regimens. In one report, 50% of a group of dogs that tested negative with an in vitro test experienced positive test results when kept off of glucocorticoids for at least 1 month.[360]

In summary, serologic allergy tests have numerous advantages over intradermal testing, including (1) no patient risk (no need to sedate; no risk of anaphylactic reactions), (2) convenience (no need to clip patient's haircoat, chemically restrain patient, or keep patient at clinic while preparing for, performing, and evaluating test), (3) lower likelihood that results will be influenced by prior or current drug therapy, (4) the ability to be used

*See references 27, 265, 290, 317, 363, 378, 400, 408–410.

in patients with widespread dermatitis or dermatographism, and (5) similar results of hyposensitization therapy in carefully clinically diagnosed atopic dogs. Canine IgE was reported to be stable in serum samples subjected to 25 freeze/thaw cycles and when incubated at 25°C for up to 10 days.[223] The disadvantages of serologic tests are that they are more expensive per item tested and that false-positive (clinically insignificant) results are exceedingly common. Therefore, these tests are not appropriate to use for diagnosing atopic disease but only for management.

Attempts to create in-office allergy screening tests have varied in their success at correlating with in vitro or intradermal test results, or in discriminating between atopic and nonatopic dogs.[*] Even though these tests may have some value, they are limited because hyposensitization still requires complete testing with individual allergens and the diagnosis should not be made with tests but on clinical grounds.

Considering all the current available information, we and others suggest that intradermal testing is still the preferred method for diagnosis of canine atopy.[61, 67a, 195, 265, 323, 331] When intradermal testing is not available, when intradermal testing gives negative results in an otherwise classically atopic dog, or when hyposensitization based on intradermal testing is unsuccessful, serologic allergy testing may be useful. Because intradermal testing is not readily available, the response rate to hyposensitization based on in vitro testing is preferred over the option of lifelong therapy with glucocorticoids. When serologic testing is used, it is for the selection of allergens in dogs in which the clinical diagnosis of atopic disease is strong. If one is attempting to use a test to help confirm the diagnosis of atopic disease, an intradermal test should be performed.

- **Basophil Degranulation Test.** The in vitro basophil degranulation test has been reported to show promise in the diagnosis of canine atopy.[57, 58] The original test requires fresh blood, must be run within 24 hours, is time consuming and labor intensive, and is unlikely to become anything more than a research tool. The demonstration that canine sera also binds to human basophils has made the test potentially more practical because only serum will be needed.[377, 381] Preliminary results in dogs showed an 89% correlation with intradermal test results.[377] A technique utilizing flow cytometry for the detection of CD63 on human basophils activated by passive sensitization with canine serum is being evaluated and may lead to this test being faster and less expensive and more readily available.[380] However, further work is needed to determine whether it improves hyposensitization or diagnostic efficacy compared with other tests.

Major and Minor Diagnostic Criteria

Because of the difficulties associated with the in vivo and in vitro diagnosis of atopy, the concept of major and minor diagnostic features has been introduced in an attempt to provide consistency in the diagnosis of atopy in dogs and humans.[312] For dogs, the following criteria have been proposed:

At least three of the following *major* features should be present:

- Pruritus
- Facial and/or digital involvement
- Lichenification of the flexor surface of the tarsus or the extensor surface of the carpus
- Chronic or chronically relapsing dermatitis
- An individual or familial history of atopy
- A breed predilection

At least three of the following *minor* features should also be present:

- Onset of signs before 3 years of age
- Facial erythema and cheilitis
- Bacterial conjunctivitis
- A superficial staphylococcal pyoderma

---

*See references 341, 342, 351, 362, 367, 371, 394.

- Hyperhidrosis
- Immediate skin test reactivity to inhalant allergens
- Elevated allergen-specific IgGd
- Elevated allergen-specific IgE

To date, only one study has evaluated these criteria.[266, 268] Atopic dogs and nonatopic dogs were evaluated, and the sensitivity and specificity of each of the Willemse criteria were statistically analyzed. The authors concluded that pruritus, breed predilection, conjunctivitis, pyoderma, and skin and serologic test results were not useful criteria. These authors suggested that the diagnostic criteria be revised as follows:

- Major Criteria
    Bilateral lesions of the plantar surface of the interdigital spaces of the front paws
    Onset of signs between 6 months and 3 years of age
    Peribuccal erythema or erythema of the medial surface of the pinnae
    Anitis
    Recurrent dermatitis for greater than 2 years

- Minor Criteria
    Familial history
    Exacerbation when the dog contacts vegetation (e.g., grass, weed).
    Rhinitis
    History of urticaria/angioedema
    Acral lick dermatitis
    Hyperhidrosis
    Lichenification of the fold of the hock and/or the cranial surface of the carpus

In a study of 91 atopic dogs from Greece, lesions on the carpus and tarsus were negatively associated with skin test positivity.[277]

The reliability of using the Willemse major and minor criteria to diagnose canine atopy and not other diseases has still never been proven. Additionally, it has been suggested that a tentative diagnosis of atopic disease requires ruling out other major possibilities because the criteria just listed determine what patients may have atopy, but they do not exclude the possibility of some other diagnoses.[27, 67a] We do not use these criteria.

Histopathology

Skin biopsy of atopic dogs reveals variable degrees of superficial perivascular dermatitis (pure, spongiotic, hyperplastic) with lymphocytes and histiocytes usually predominating (see Fig. 8–7A and B.[28, 67a, 83, 84, 282] Mast cells may be increased in number. Though statistically there is a very mild tissue eosinophilia,[253, 257] it is not usually noted during routine histopathologic examination. The presence of a significant tissue eosinophilia suggests another or concurrent disease. Focal intraepidermal aggregates of eosinophils or Langerhans' cells may be visible.[256, 257] The presence of numerous neutrophils, plasma cells, or both indicates infection, usually secondary bacterial pyoderma. Therefore, histopathology is more helpful in suggesting that further diagnostics are indicated and does not confirm a diagnosis of atopy. Similar dermal changes of a milder degree may occur in clinically normal skin from atopic dogs. Histopathologic findings consistent with secondary bacterial pyoderma (suppurative folliculitis, perifolliculitis, intraepidermal pustular dermatitis) or *Malassezia* dermatitis are common in specimens of skin from atopic dogs.

CLINICAL MANAGEMENT

Prognostically, atopic dogs have about an 80% chance of experiencing nonseasonal disease. Natural desensitization is rare. One placebo-controlled study, however, revealed that about 20% of atopic dogs experience an improvement of greater than 50% after receiving an immunotherapy placebo for 9 months.[412] In general, over 90% of atopic dogs can be satisfactorily controlled. The client, however, must be made aware that treatment is

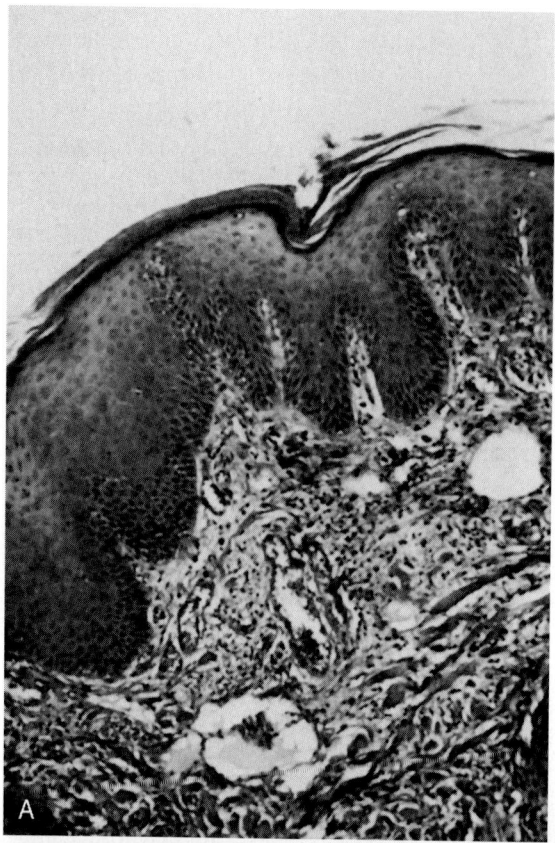

FIGURE 8–7. *A*, Canine atopy. Hyperplastic perivascular dermatitis. (From Scott DW: Observations on canine atopy. J Am Anim Hosp Assoc 17:91, 1981.) *B*, Canine atopy. Perivascular accumulation of mononuclear cells. (From Scott DW: Observations on canine atopy. J Am Anim Hosp Assoc 17:91, 1981.)

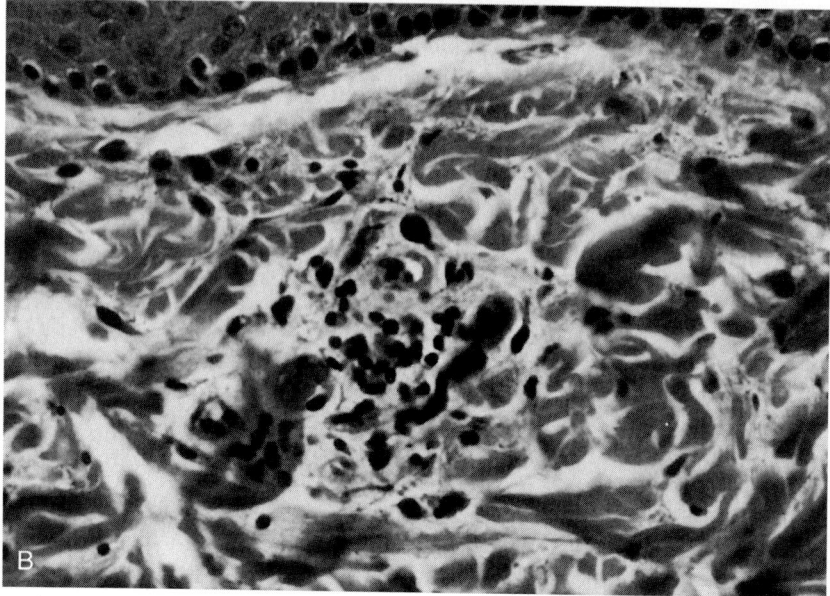

usually required for life and that therapeutic modifications over the life of the dog are to be expected.

Before the clinician discusses the details of therapy with the client, it is imperative to mention that some allergens may be tolerated by an individual without any disease manifestations, but a small increase in that load (one or more allergens) may push the individual over the pruritic threshold and initiate clinical signs.[61, 67a] Equally important when considering the cause of dermatologic disorders is the concept of summation of effect—for example, a subclinical hypersensitivity in combination with a flea infestation, a mild bacterial pyoderma, or a dry environment may produce marked discomfort that would be absent if any one of the disorders existed alone.[61, 67a] Thus, it is important to evaluate all possible contributions to the clinical signs in "allergic" dogs.

Education of the client is of key importance to the successful long-term control of the atopic dog. The following are the key points that should be discussed with clients that own atopic dogs.

Education Points to Consider

1. Atopic disease is a life-long problem.
2. It is controlled, not cured.
3. Many aggravating factors may cause flare-ups.
   a. Allergen load/exposure
   b. Stress
   c. Boredom
   d. Changes in heat, humidity
   e. Skin trauma
4. Concurrent diseases complicate the control and require different therapies.
   a. Fleas
   b. Food hypersensitivity
   c. Bacterial pyoderma
   d. *Malassezia*
      1. Dermatitis
      2. Otitis
      3. Paronychia
   e. Secondary bacterial otitis externa
   f. Fold dermatitis
   g. Pododermatitis
   h. Urine retention and skin irritation
   i. Anal sac disease
5. Different aspects of the disease and complicating factors are what cause client and owner dissatisfaction.
   a. This may have profound effects on how the case is handled.
   b. These need to be identified.
6. Clients must be agreeable and able to give or complete the treatment.
   a. This may have profound effects on how the case is handled.

Therapy for atopy includes various combinations of avoidance, topical therapies (see Chap. 3), hyposensitization, fatty acids and antihistamines (see Therapy for Hypersensitivity Diseases), systemic glucocorticoids (see Chap. 3), and occasionally immunosuppressive drugs (see Chap. 9).[27, 34, 61, 67a] In most cases, a single drug does not give the safest and most efficacious results, and the clinician should approach the management of the atopic dog with a complete treatment plan.[27, 213] Development of a treatment plan needs to consider multiple variables, including seasonality, distribution and amount of involved skin, cost, willingness and ability of the client to administer the treatment, acceptability to the patient, and risk to the patient. Optimally, the clinician incorporates avoidance, topical therapy (especially shampooing), and fatty acids into the treatment plan.

Avoidance

Avoidance of allergens is not always possible or practical. Such manipulations and their benefits are not generally possible without accurate identification of the offending allergen(s) by allergy testing. Because many patients have multiple reactivities and most allergens cannot be avoided, the effective use of this approach is rarely possible as a sole therapy. It is still an important aspect of the management, however, because it often decreases the allergen load. Additionally, some patients may greatly benefit from avoidance of confirmed allergens such as feathers (pillows, birds), cats (dander), newsprint (newspaper), and tobacco smoke.[27, 61, 67a, 175, 282] With other allergens, complete elimination may be impossible, but a decrease in exposure may be achievable (Table 8–17).[175]

Cat allergen can be common and persistent even in environments where cats no longer live.[177] Cat allergen is very stable and ubiquitous, and is found in dust samples and clothing from homes where cats have never been kept.[197a] Thus, avoidance may require more than is often considered. However, attempts at controlling sources may be helpful. For example, house dust mite exposure can be decreased by keeping the pet outdoors more or at least out of bedrooms and off fabric furniture; mold exposure can be decreased by removing or cleaning mildewed items, houseplants, and carpeting in bathrooms and by keeping bread refrigerated; cotton exposure can be decreased by avoiding laundry rooms and closets and by making sure that the dog's bedding is made from synthetic material. In atopic humans involved in a controlled trial wherein vacuuming and miticide were used in an attempt to eradicate house dust mites, the number of mites decreased but the patients derived no clinical benefit.[196]

Other studies, including a double-blinded, placebo-controlled study, have shown that if mites can be reduced by greater than 90%, benefit occurs, but the control measures require more than vacuuming, and just limiting mite numbers in one area of the house is not likely to be beneficial.[288, 294] If the same is true in dogs, the complete home environment must change, not just areas where the dog sleeps or stays within the house. For house dust mites, this is best accomplished by (1) minimizing carpets throughout the house and having polished floors, (2) having as little fabric-upholstered furniture as possible with wood, vinyl, or leather furniture preferred, especially sofas, (3) reducing humidity below 45%, and (4) covering pillow cases and mattresses with impermeable covers. This is often not possible or practical, and other techniques of treating carpets with a variety of acaricides, including benzyl benzoate and pirimiphos, have been described. Treating carpets and fabric furniture with acaricides may reduce mite levels by 70% to 90% for a

Table 8–17. PRACTICAL ENVIRONMENTAL MANAGEMENT FOR THE ATOPIC CANINE

ALLERGEN	AVOIDANCE SUGGESTIONS
House dust House dust mite	Keep dog out of room when cleaning/vacuuming for several hours Use plastic zippered cover over dog bed Wash bedding in hot water (>70°C) Avoid letting dog sleep on overstuffed furniture (if dog sleeps on human's bed, use plastic mattress/pillow covers) Avoid stuffed toys Keep dog overnight or during working hours in uncarpeted rooms Frequently damp-mop the dog's "holding" room Run air conditioner during hot and humid weather
Molds	Keep dog out of damp basements Keep dog away from barns Keep dog away while lawn is mowed Avoid dusty dog foods Clean and disinfect humidifiers Avoid having large numbers of house plants Avoid using as the dog's "holding" room any room with a high moisture level (bathroom, laundry room) Keep dog out of crawl spaces under house Use dehumidifiers Clean with chlorine bleach solutions
Pollens	Keep dog out of fields Keep grass cut short Rinse dog off after periods in high grasses/weeds Keep dog indoors at dusk and early morning during heavy pollen season Use air conditioners Keep dog away while mowing lawn

Modified from Bevier DE: Long-term management of atopic disease in the dog. Vet Clin North Am Small Anim Pract 20:1491, 1990.

month but do not eliminate house dust mite allergen.[288] Tannic acid in carpets has been used to denature house dust mite proteins.[313]

Topical Therapy

Topical therapy is used in two main ways. The first is through shampoos and rinses, which remove allergens from the skin and help to eliminate dry skin.[27, 67a] The second is through topical antipruritic agents, which are usually most effective for treating localized areas of pruritus. These therapies are covered in Chapter 3. In general, most atopic dogs should be bathed at least every 1 or 2 weeks. It should be remembered that atopic dogs often have sensitive, easily irritated skin. Hypoallergenic and colloidal oatmeal-containing shampoos are preferred. Shampoos and rinses containing the local anesthetic, pramoxine, are useful.[284]

- **Hyposensitization.** Hyposensitization (immunotherapy), which has been described as the mainstay of therapy in canine atopy, is indicated in animals in which avoidance of antigens is impossible, signs are present for more than 4 to 6 months of the year, and other antipruritic drugs are unsatisfactory.* This and avoidance are the only forms of therapy that stop the allergic reaction, in contrast with most medical therapies that counteract the effects of the allergic reaction. In humans, hyposensitization may even prevent the development of new allergies, though this has not been shown in the dog.[397] In fact, some dogs that respond well to hyposensitization stop responding because of new hypersensitivities that, in turn, do respond to a new immunotherapy formulation based on repeat allergy testing.

Virtually no attempts have been made to standardize hyposensitization regimens in the dog or to scientifically compare their merits. Thus, published regimens vary in the form of allergen used (aqueous, alum precipitated, propylene glycol suspended, glycerinated), the number and frequency of injections given in the induction phase, the dose of allergen administered, the potency of allergenic extract, and the route of administration (subcutaneous, intramuscular, intradermal). The vast majority of clinicians use only the subcutaneous route when hyposensitizing for atopy. Numerous authors have written about the benefits of hyposensitization, with most reporting a 50% to 80% rate of good to excellent responses, whether based on intradermal or serologic testing.† A double-blind study of hyposensitization in atopic dogs (alum-precipitated allergens vs. an alum-based placebo) reported that 59% of the dogs experienced a good response with the vaccine and 21% of the dogs experienced a good response with the placebo.[412] It is well accepted that hyposensitization is an effective, valuable, and relatively safe treatment for atopic dogs.

The mechanism of action of hyposensitization is complex, with a variety of end-organ, humoral, and cellular changes occurring in humans.[403] Various hypotheses were proposed in the past, such as (1) humoral desensitization (reduced levels of IgE), (2) cellular desensitization (reduced reactivity of mast cells and basophils), (3) immunization (induction of "blocking antibody"), (4) tolerization (generation of allergen-specific suppressor cells), and (5) some combination thereof.[50, 61, 67a] In humans hyposensitized for atopy, the organ changes that correlate best with the clinical response are skin, nasal, and conjunctival sensitivity to titrated doses of allergen. At the cellular level, an increase in allergen-induced CD25+CD8+ T lymphocytes correlates with a favorable response.[403] Atopic humans successfully treated with IFN-γ or cyclosporine usually have no decrease and, often, an increase in IgE levels.[292] This suggests the beneficial effect is not humoral but cellular (switch from Th2 to Th1 cytokine profile).

Three forms of allergens have been used for hyposensitization of atopic dogs.[34, 61, 67a] *Aqueous allergens*, which are rapidly absorbed, necessitate smaller doses, and require multiple, frequent injections, constitute by far the most commonly used type today. A variety of hyposensitization dose protocols are used, but most of the aqueous regimens are modifications of the schedule shown in Table 8–18. Some specialists, including ourselves, use just the two more potent concentrations and keep the intervals at no more than 14

---

*See references 27, 34, 61, 67a, 175, 188, 396, 398.
†See references 27, 34, 61, 67a, 188, 290, 306, 363, 370, 398, 399, 402, 404, 405, 407, 408, 409, 413.

● Table 8–18 HYPOSENSITIZATION SCHEDULE FOR AQUEOUS ALLERGENS*

INJECTION NO.	DAY NO.	VIAL 1 (100 to 200 PNU/ml)†	VIAL 2 (1000 to 2000 PNU/ml)	VIAL 3 (10,000 to 20,000 PNU/ml)
1	1	0.1 ml		
2	2	0.4 ml		
3	4	0.4 ml		
4	6	0.8 ml		
5	8	1.0 ml		
6	10		0.1 ml	
7	12		0.2 ml	
8	14		0.4 ml	
9	16		0.8 ml	
10	18		1.0 ml	
11	20			0.1 ml
12	22			0.2 ml
13	24			0.4 ml
14	26			0.8 ml
15	28			1.0 ml
16	38			1.0 ml
17	48‡			1.0 ml

*Injections are given subcutaneously.
†Protein nitrogen unit (PNU) value of each vial represents the total of *all* allergens used.
‡Thereafter, repeat injections (1.0 ml) every 20 to 40 days, as needed.

days for the first 4 months of therapy. In addition, we use different schedules depending on the size of the dog; Table 8–19 is one example of a small dog schedule. A preliminary study used a rush protocol that takes only 6 hours to reach the maximum concentration of 20,000 PNU/ml. This was reportedly done in 6 research and 14 clinical cases with no

● Table 8–19 HYPOSENSITIZATION SCHEDULE FOR DOGS UNDER 20 POUNDS

DAY	DATE	ITCH	VOLUME	DAY	DATE	ITCH	VOLUME
Vial 1				*Five-Day Interval*			
1			0.1	30			0.5
3			0.2	35			0.5
5			0.3	40			0.7
7			0.4	*Ten-Day Interval*			
9			0.6	50			0.7
11			0.8	60			0.7
13			1.0	70			0.7
Vial 2				80			0.7
15			0.1	*Fourteen-Day Interval*			
17			0.2	94			0.7
19			0.3	108			0.7
21			0.4	122			0.7
23			0.5	136			0.7
25			0.5	150			0.7

- Grade itch on scale of 0 (none) to 10 (most severe this pet has had in the past).
- *Note:* it is possible to go higher than 10 if the itching is getting worse than ever before.
- Call at 4 weeks and report grade of itching.
- Call if itch goes up by more than 2 levels.
- Call prior to giving any more shots if there are adverse reactions.
  - Vomiting, diarrhea, anxiousness, weakness are possible reactions.
  - Reactions will usually occur within 1 to 2 hours after shot is given.
- Recheck appointments should be made around day 60 and day 120.
- Watch for pattern of itching in relation to when shots are given.
- Itch increases before shot is due, or after shot is given.
- Itch decreases after shot is given.

increase in adverse reactions nor loss of efficacy noted.[401] This type of protocol may be indicated for cases requiring rapid hyposensitization because of particularly severe or life-threatening allergic reactions such as venomous insect bites.

Alum-precipitated allergens are intermediate in action between the aqueous allergens and emulsion allergens. They are more slowly absorbed than the aqueous allergens; as a result, larger doses, fewer and less frequent injections, and more rapid hyposensitization are possible. Concern has been expressed about the possible carcinogenicity of alum precipitates, which are increasingly less available today. In the United States, alum-precipitated formulations for immunotherapy are available for only a small number of allergens. In Europe, however, they are the allergens most commonly used and recommended.[58, 412, 413] It has been reported that successful hyposensitization with these allergens was improved with a low-dose protocol.[411]

Emulsion allergens (aqueous allergens in propylene glycol, glycerin, or mineral oil) are the most slowly absorbed, allowing the largest doses, the least number of injections, and the most rapid hyposensitization.

By convention, in the past no more than 10 allergens were used at once for hyposensitization.[61, 67a] This has changed over the years as more investigators have used more allergens, even up to 30.° Success has safely been achieved with the inclusion of up to 30 or more allergens in aqueous vaccines for atopic dogs.[67a] In fact, larger numbers may increase the success rate. In one report,[396] dogs were treated with up to 40 allergens, and the response rate was 72% in dogs treated with 1 to 10 allergens, 86% in dogs treated with 11 to 20 allergens, and 78% in dogs treated with 21 or more allergens. However, two other studies did not find any difference in success based on number of allergens in the vaccine.[404, 410] It has also been reported that, in animals with greater than 12 positive results, treatment failures to the first set of antigens may respond when a second set containing more allergens than the animal is allergic to are added as a new treatment set.[400] In animals with multiple sensitivities (e.g., 20 to 30 or more), the allergens should be selected on the basis of history, the probable presence of that allergen in the environment, the frequency at which the allergen is known to react in that region, and the duration of the allergen's presence.

Cross-reactivity may also be used in the decision. In general, cross-reactivity tends to stay within families or closer relationships so that genera of the same family have some cross-allergenicity, and species of the same genus have even greater cross-reactivity. Because grasses have fewer families, they tend to be the most cross-reactive, but the three main grass families tend to be different.[403] Bermuda grass is in the family Eragrostoideae and does not cross with the Festucoideae, the more common northern pasture grasses. Pancoideae, which includes Johnson and Bahia grass, cross-reacts somewhat with the other two families. Weeds are less cross-reactive than grasses, and trees are the least cross-reactive. All this information is based on allergens that commonly are found in humans, and this may not be the same in the dog, as has been discussed for house dust mites allergens.

Besides cross-reactivity, another issue is the effects allergens may have when combined. Studies have shown that molds, and to some degree insect allergens, contain proteases that may break down other allergens, especially pollens.[403, 406] In the one veterinary study, though protease degradation was documented, the author stated that success with hyposensitization had apparently not been affected, as compared with other published studies by the mixing of the mold allergens with other allergens (M. R. Rosenbaum, personal communication, 1996).

Depending on each individual dog's response, and which form of the allergen is being used, a beneficial response may occur as early as 2 weeks or as late as 18 months after hyposensitization is begun.† "Booster" injections of allergens are administered as needed (when clinical signs first begin to reappear) and, depending on the form of allergens

---

°See references 61, 67a, 396, 400, 405, 407, 409.
†See references 27, 34, 61, 67a, 188, 306, 370, 398, 400, 402, 405, 407–409, 412.

involved and the vaccine protocol being used, boosters may be needed every week to every 6 months. When aqueous allergens are used, animals that require injections more frequently than every 10 days are usually given smaller volumes of allergen.[27] In general, we use 0.1 ml/day for these short intervals. Experience with the patient allows the owner and the veterinarian to predict how long the patient will be asymptomatic after booster injections. Boosters are then administered shortly before clinical signs would be expected to flare up.

Intervals between boosters may vary at different times of the year. It is also important to not overtreat and cause adverse reactions. In one study, decreasing the dose, with or without decreasing the frequency, was done in all dogs that experienced any adverse reactions, and the response rate increased significantly in that group of dogs.[407] Adjusting the hyposensitization treatment for each individual case is the most appropriate way to maximize the response and, even when adverse reactions are absent and no exacerbations prior to injections are observed, trying different protocols may increase efficacy.[400]

In general, atopic dogs require lifetime administration of vaccine. There is no strong indication that sex, age, or duration of signs affects the success of hyposensitization, though evidence is growing that age or duration may be important. This is true for human patients with asthma and rhinitis who are hyposensitized.[403] There is some evidence that long-term disease (clinical signs for 5 years or more) and older age at the onset of clinical signs (over 5 years old) indicate a poorer response to hyposensitization.[306, 402, 404, 409] One of us (C.E.G.) thinks that severity is more important, also somewhat related to chronicity, and that dogs with excessive scarring do poorly.

Much of the inability to identify important variables may reflect the lack of studies with large-enough numbers to see differences in these groups. Boxers and West Highland white terriers have been reported to show a poorer response to hyposensitization.[413] One study evaluated 144 dogs on hyposensitization for over 1 year and divided the dogs by breed into four groups: retrievers, spaniels, terriers, or other.[410] The retrievers experienced significantly less response to hyposensitization (46% moderate or marked improvement) than did spaniels (69%), terriers (76%) and other (70%) groups.

Some authors report that the likelihood of successful hyposensitization is greater in animals with few positive reactions; others disagree.[396, 398, 404, 409, 413] One study indicated that low reactors (less than eight weak to moderate positives) responded better overall than high reactors (more than eight strong reactions) but had a lower percentage of dogs with an excellent response.[408] However, one of us (C.E.G.) thinks that animals with numerous reactions, but reactions primarily limited to pollens, do better. Regional variations may also occur. One of us (C.E.G.) with practices in Las Vegas and southern California has observed a better success rate in Las Vegas (80%) than in southern California (60%) with the same protocols.

Response to immunotherapy is allergen-specific.[363, 398, 413] Thus, response to hyposensitization was much better in atopic dogs when it was based on allergy testing (70% good to excellent responses) than when it was administered with standard regional allergens with no regard to allergy testing (18%, identical to placebo response).[317] The response to specific types of allergens has not been well studied. Though controversial, it has been reported that pollen-hypersensitive dogs do better than dogs with other types of hypersensitivity.[61, 402] One study reported that mold-hypersensitive dogs did very poorly.[402] However, another study reported similar success rates with hyposensitization in dogs that were only mold-hypersensitive and those that were hypersensitive to various other allergens.[408]

Follow-up and compliance is critical to achieve the maximum success rate. One report indicated that the compliance rate corresponds to the success rate.[405] Similar observations have been made by ourselves and other investigators.[407] Besides educating clients about compliance and follow-up, it is important that they are educated about what to watch for. Patterns of pruritus or signs related to when shots are given, overall level of pruritus, changes in pattern of pruritus, and adverse reactions must be watched for.[400]

Adverse reactions to hyposensitization are uncommon but may occur in up to 5% of patients.[61, 188, 334, 396] Minor reactions may occur in 25% of these dogs.[407] Adverse reactions include (1) intensification of clinical signs for a few hours to a few days, (2) local reactions (edema with or without pain or pruritus) at injection sites, and (3) anaphylaxis. Serious reactions have been reported to occur in less than 1% to 1.25% of these dogs.[29, 396] Adverse reactions are treated according to symptom. Intensification of clinical signs is the most common side effect. It may indicate that the animal's maximum tolerance dose of allergens has been exceeded and that the final hyposensitizing dose achieved needs to be lowered. In humans, most studies on the possible long-term adverse effects of hyposensitization have failed to demonstrate any clinical or immunologic abnormalities. One study of 20 consecutive human patients with polyarteritis nodosa, however, revealed that, in six patients, the onset of vasculitis symptoms coincided with hyposensitization for atopy.[67a] Multiple other studies have failed to demonstrate any immunologic abnormalities.[403]

In the severely affected, nonseasonally atopic dog, it may be necessary to control the symptoms with systemic glucocorticoids during hyposensitization. As long as oral prednisolone, prednisone, or methylprednisolone doses are kept as low as possible and administered on an alternate-day basis (see Chap. 3), hyposensitization can still be successful.[61, 67a] Avoiding glucocorticoids during at least the first few weeks of therapy allows one to identify mild reactions and make adjustments, which is a good reason to try and avoid those drugs early on.

Systemic Antipruritic Agents

Many atopic dogs require a systemic antipruritic agent, either as a sole agent or used in conjunction with other treatments for an additive effect.[61, 67a, 188] These agents were discussed earlier in this chapter, but some points are important to consider when treating atopic disease.

Systemic glucocorticoids are usually very effective for the management of atopy. They are, however, the most dangerous of the treatments commonly used to treat atopy. As such, their use should be limited to cases with active seasons lasting less than 4 to 6 months or for which safer options are not effective. Prednisolone or prednisone is administered orally (1 mg/kg q24h) in the morning until pruritus is controlled (3 to 10 days) and then on an alternate-day (morning) regimen as needed (see Chap. 3). This schedule is relatively safe compared with long-acting corticosteroids. Many atopic dogs have more than one disease, and these drugs are less effective if there is any bacterial pyoderma or *Malassezia* dermatitis present. Any animal not responding to rational treatments should be re-examined to determine whether secondary infections or other complicating factors are present. Efficacy of treatment may change as seasons and allergen loads change or as other complicating factors occur. Clients need to be aware of this, and encouraged to treat minor flare-ups early. Combinations with topical therapy, fatty acids, and antihistamines are often more effective than single therapies.

Other Experimental and Therapeutic Agents

In humans with atopic dermatitis, studies have demonstrated therapeutic benefits of cyclosporine,[212] leukotriene antagonists,[189] INF-γ,[212, 217, 271, 292] injectable allergen-antibody complexes,[233] thymopentin,[212, 293] extracorporeal photochemotherapy,[269] and Chinese herbal therapy.[212, 219] A double-blind trial in atopic dogs showed no benefit with homeopathic drops that apparently had pollens in them.[174] Other therapies being evaluated experimentally include peptide immunotherapy, anticytokine and cytokine receptor therapies, phosphodiesterase inhibitors, and anti-IgE therapy.[198, 200, 235]

In dogs, misoprostol (6 μg/kg q8h) produced at least 50% reduction in pruritus in over 50% of patients;[132] arofylline (phosphodiesterase-4 inhibitor, 1 mg/kg q12h) was as effective as prednisone but produced frequent gastrointestinal side effects[207]; pentoxifylline (10 mg/kg q8h) did not satisfactorily control pruritus[239]; the combination of tetracycline and niacinamide (250 to 500 mg of each q8h) was ineffective[88]; cyclosporine (5 to 10 mg/kg/day) may be useful in severe, medically refractory cases (see Chap. 3).

Feline Atopy

Feline atopy (feline atopic disease) was first described in 1982, and in recent years it has been shown that feline IgE exists.[389, 416, 423, 424, 426, 430, 431, 447] It is also likely that feline IgE is heterogeneous, which helps to explain some of the differences found when testing for feline atopy.[216, 433] Feline atopy is a pruritic skin and/or respiratory disease in cats that, in that aspect, is similar to human atopy.[422, 433, 434, 444] Many affected cats experience positive intradermal test reactions to environmental allergens.

The incidence of this disease is controversial, with some investigators stating it to be the most common cause of allergy in the cat (73% of all allergic cats) or second in incidence to flea bite hypersensitivity.[439, 444] An inherited predisposition has not been documented, though reports of cases with familial involvement suggest a genetic component.[453] This lack of well-documented genetic component is a major difference from other species with atopic disease.

CAUSE AND PATHOGENESIS

Feline atopy is caused by an exaggerated or inappropriate response of the affected cat to environmental allergens, presumably involving skin-sensitizing IgE.[433, 438] The most common environmental allergens are nonseasonal (positive reactions in over 90% of cats tested).[419, 442, 453] In a study of 28 atopic cats, 50% were mainly positive to nonseasonal allergens and 48% were reactive to both nonseasonal and seasonal allergens.[442] This study also reported immediate reactivity to flea allergen in 40% of the cats. In a study of 66 atopic cats, 50% were hypersensitive to fleas, 58% to only nonseasonal allergens, 39% to nonseasonal and seasonal allergens, and 5% to only pollens.[444] House dust mite reactions (predominantly *Dermatophagoides farinae*) are the most prevalent of the nonseasonal reactions, and generally 80% or greater of the atopic cats test positive.[419, 433, 444]

Other environmental allergens, even tobacco, may also cause reactions in some cats.[433, 443, 444] Normal cats rarely experience positive reactions to Greer Laboratories house dust mite antigens at 1000 PNU/ml and, in eight normal cats, the VARL result was totally negative.[343, 421] Using the basophil degranulation test, 17% of healthy cats experienced positive reactions to house dust mites and 33% of the cats with eosinophilic granuloma experienced positive results, but this was not statistically significant.[440] It has also been shown that cats with *Otodectes* infestation produce hypersensitivity reactions that may cross-react with house dust mites. This could possibly explain some positive reactions to house dust mites in normal cats.[278]

Initially, the results of intradermal testing led to the hypothesis that this disease was mediated by reaginic antibody.* The determination of feline IgE and its role in skin disease had been shown by a number of studies using P-K testing, PCA testing, and ultrastructural studies demonstrating cutaneous mast cell degranulation only at sites of positive intradermal allergen injections.[389, 416, 418, 430, 433, 447] A study with a monoclonal antibody against a putative feline IgE showed reactivity against feline IgA and IgM as well.[424] More recent studies have documented a specific polyclonal antifeline IgE as well as the ability of the Fcε RI-α assay to detect feline IgE.[216, 389, 428, 431]

IgE heterogeneity also exists in cats.[216] Skin lesions of atopic cats have an increased number of Langerhans' cells, MHC class II dermal dendritic cells, and a predominance of CD4+ T cells.[446, 448-450, 452] Th2 cells and IL-4 expression may also play a role in feline atopy, similar to the situation in humans and dogs.[448] These observations and some preliminary results of patch testing with aeroallergens in cats suggest that the pathogenesis is similar to that in humans and dogs.[446, 448-450] Studies in cats have shown that the highest number of dermal mast cells is found in skin from caudal pinnae, which may explain some of the head and neck lesions that may be visible when cats scratch at the pinnae.[427, 435]

CLINICAL FEATURES

No breed or sex predilections have been demonstrated. Young cats appear to be predisposed; 75% of the atopic cats with miliary dermatitis in one study experienced clinical signs between 6 and 24 months of age.[453] The most consistent feature of atopy is pruritus, which 100% of the cats with skin disease demonstrate.[61, 67, 414, 419, 438] The pruritus,

---

*See references 61, 67a, 416, 423, 424, 445, 453.

however, may not be obvious to the owner, particularly in cats presenting with noninflammatory alopecia, and some cats are presented for respiratory disease alone. In these cases, other indirect evidence of pruritus may be found, such as vomiting from hair balls, hair in feces, tufts of hair in the cat's hiding areas, hair in the cat's teeth, and trichograms revealing broken and chopped-off distal ends of hairs, suggesting licking and chewing as the cause of the hair loss.

The clinical lesions of feline atopy are quite variable. The four most commonly reported cutaneous reaction patterns are self-induced alopecia (fur mowing) (Fig. 8–8B), eosinophilic granuloma complex lesions (Fig. 8–8C), miliary dermatitis, and initially nonlesional pruritus of the face, neck, and pinnae (Fig. 8–8A).* Some cats manifest various combinations of these four patterns.[61, 67a] Erythematous macules, papules, and excoriations may also be visible, usually in association with one or more of the more common lesions. Recurrent swelling of the chin or lower lip (eosinophilic granuloma) may occur. The pruritus and lesions may be localized or generalized.

Localized involvement often includes the abdomen, groin, lateral thorax, and caudal thighs. The head, neck, and forelegs are also commonly involved. Although the pinnae are commonly affected, the ear canals are usually spared. Some cats manifest a recurrent, pruritic, ceruminous otitis externa that is typically misdiagnosed as ear mite infestation. Rarely, cats manifest an erythematous papulopustular eruption characterized clinicopathologically as a sterile eosinophilic folliculitis and furunculosis.[454] Noncutaneous signs may also be observed. Sneezing was reported in 50% of the cases in one study, and conjunctivitis may also be present.[419] Chronic coughing and feline asthma may occur in as many as 7.4% of the atopic cats, with or without concurrent skin disease.[30, 433, 434, 444] As more asthmatic cats are carefully tested for atopy, this percentage will likely increase. Lymphadenopathy is common in chronic cases that have miliary dermatitis, excoriations, or eosinophilic plaques.[433, 453] Though secondary bacterial pyoderma is rarely reported as a complication of feline atopy, one of us (C.E.G.) frequently encounters it in chronic cases with lymphadenopathy.

The incidence of concurrent diseases is quite controversial. A wide variation in the incidence of concurrent food hypersensitivity has been reported. One study showed that 25% of atopic cats may have concurrent food hypersensitivity, flea bite hypersensitivity, or both.[419] Another retrospective survey of multiple practitioners indicated that 48% of atopic cats had a component of food hypersensitivity.[434] In a prospective study of 66 atopic cats, 8% had concurrent food hypersensitivity and 50% had concurrent flea bite hypersensitivity.[444] Only one cat in this study had all three diseases. In another prospective study, 100% of the atopic cats had concurrent flea bite hypersensitivity and none was food hypersensitive.[439] A study of 29 allergic cats reported that only one (3%) had concurrent food hypersensitivity.[415] The concurrent presence of flea bite hypersensitivity and/or food hypersensitivity can greatly complicate the diagnostic work-up as well as the therapeutic regimen.

DIAGNOSIS

The wide variation of clinical lesions reported in atopic cats requires the consideration of a lengthy differential diagnosis for feline atopy. It is more practical to consider the presenting lesion and history and then to develop a differential diagnosis. The most common presentations are clinically noninflammatory alopecia, eosinophilic granuloma complex lesions (see Chap. 18), miliary dermatitis, and pruritus of the face or pinnae. The common differential diagnoses for these presentations include flea bite hypersensitivity, food hypersensitivity, cheyletiellosis, otodectic mange, dermatophytosis, and psychogenic alopecia.

The diagnosis of feline atopy is based on a compatible history and physical findings along with ruling out the two major alternatives, flea bite hypersensitivity and food hypersensitivity.[61, 67a, 433, 441] Currently, a definitive diagnosis requires a positive intradermal

---

*See references 61, 67a, 414, 419, 420, 433, 434, 438, 441, 453.

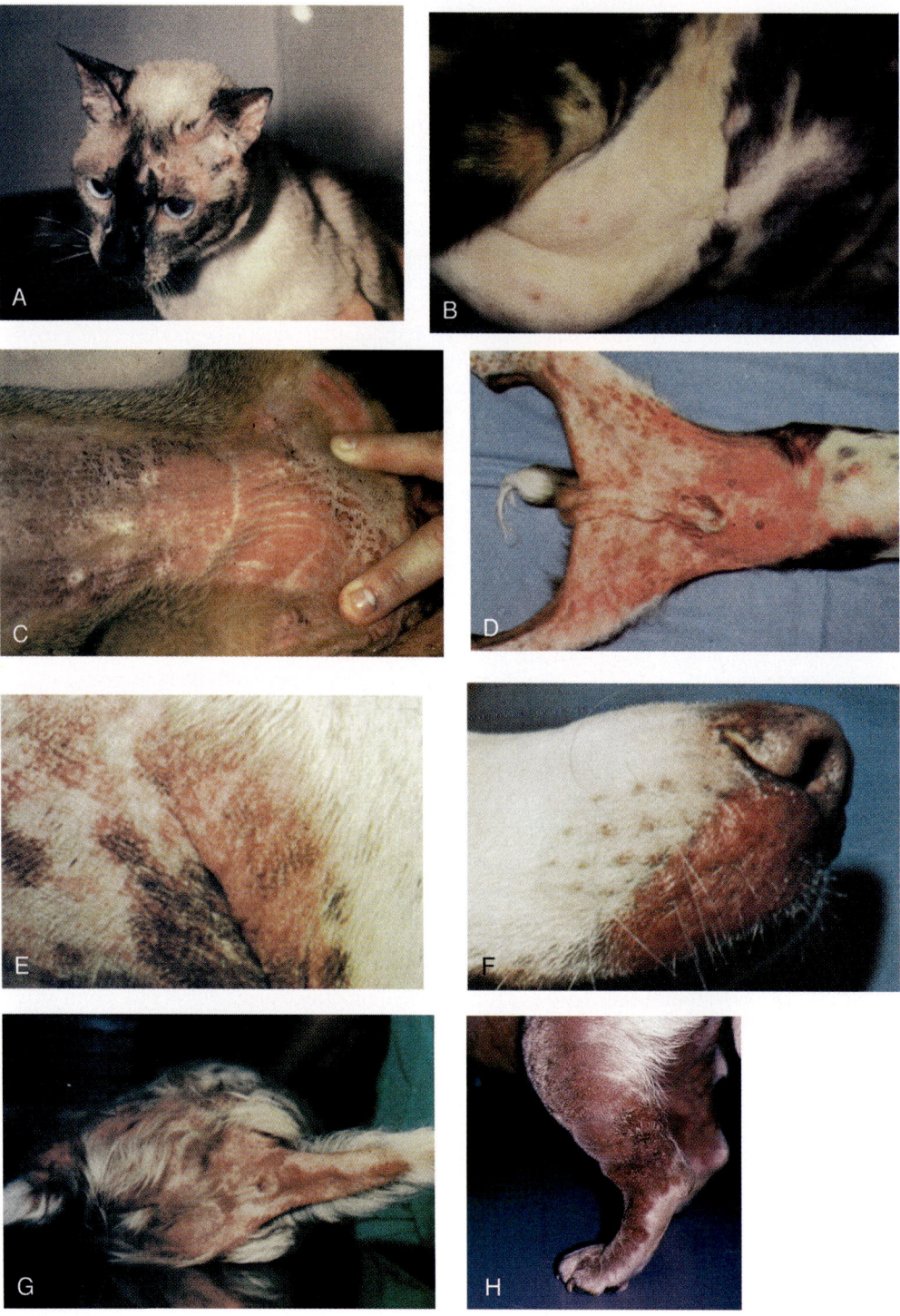

FIGURE 8-8. *A*, Feline atopy. Facial excoriations. *B*, Feline atopy. Self-induced symmetric alopecia. Note enlarged mammary glands, as this cat was receiving, but not responding to, megestrol acetate. *C*, Feline atopy. Eosinophilic plaques and alopecia. Note the linearity to the lesions that occur from licking and the spaces that correspond to skin folds that the tongue does not reach while the cat is curled to lick its abdomen. *D*, Contact hypersensitivity affecting the glabrous skin with papules and patches of erythema. *E*, Contact hypersensitivity. Axilla of affected dog shows erythema and papules—the primary lesions. *F*, Plastic dish dermatitis. The erythematous patch on the lip and alopecia are caused by contact with a plastic dish during eating. Note partial depigmentation of the tip of the nose. *G*, Erythema and alopecia over the perineum, ventral tail, and caudal thighs of a dog with food hypersensitivity. *H*, Severe edema, erythema and alopecia in a food hypersensitivity-induced eosinophilic vasculitis.

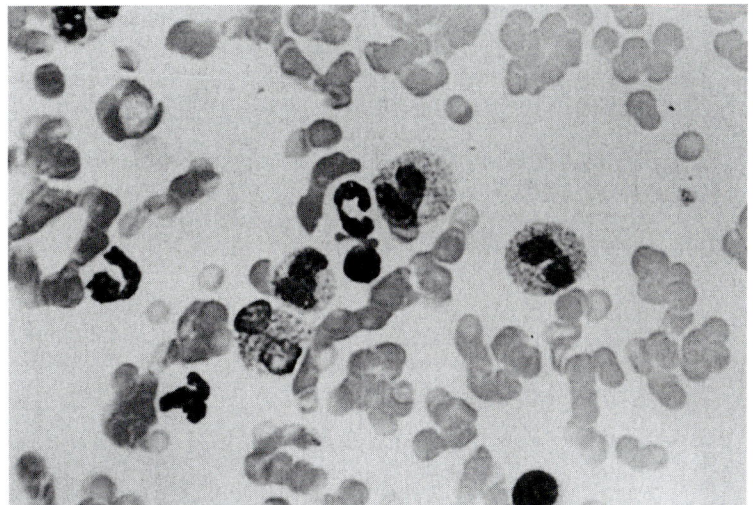

FIGURE 8–9. Feline atopy. Cytologic examination reveals numerous eosinophils and lesser numbers of nondegenerate neutrophils.

allergy test reaction, though it is likely that this requirement is not met in some atopic cats because the test is difficult to interpret in many cats.[61, 67a, 456] Good flea control and a poor response to a 9- to 13-week hypoallergenic diet, respectively, are required to rule out the two alternatives. In some cases, this approach may not be practical because it requires keeping the cat indoors. In vitro tests are not used to diagnose atopy but only to help select allergens when hyposensitization is being considered. Cytologic examination of skin lesions usually reveals eosinophils and occasionally basophils, though this picture is not specific for atopy but may also occur with food and flea bite hypersensitivity (Fig. 8–9). The presence of degenerate neutrophils with intracellular bacteria indicates secondary bacterial pyoderma. Peripheral eosinophilia is often present, unless the patient has recently received glucocorticoids.[67a]

Allergy Testing

Intradermal skin testing has been considered the optimal method for diagnosing atopic conditions in cats.* Experience with intradermal skin testing is limited in the cat compared with the dog. One study evaluated testing solutions in normal cats and, overall, the same protocol for aqueous allergens as that used in the dog was considered effective for the cat.† Age, allergen, coat color, and sex have a minor effect on skin test reactivity.[416] Some normal cats reacted to low concentrations of allergen, particularly house dust, firebush, and flea. However, it was shown that at least some of the reactions in normal cats are not irritant but most likely are mediated by reaginic antibodies, because they could be passively transferred.[416, 430]

- **Procedure.** The technique for feline intradermal allergy testing is similar to that described in the dog, with the following exceptions:

  1. Sedation with ketamine, ketamine and diazepam, tiletamine-zolazepam, or a general gas anesthetic is usually used for restraint.[61, 67a, 415, 437, 453]
  2. Extra care should be taken to make sure that all the injections are intradermal.
  3. The test site should be examined at 5 and 20 minutes post injection because feline reactions sometimes occur and fade rapidly, within 10 minutes.
  4. Reactions, including those to histamine, are often much subtler (less erythema and turgidity) than those in dogs.

---

*See references 61, 67a, 414, 415, 425, 438, 442.
†See references 61, 67a, 416, 419, 436, 445, 453.

A study has shown that intradermal skin testing in cats, with and without prior sedation, produced marked increases in the concentrations of plasma cortisol, corticotropin, and α-melanocyte-stimulating hormone.[456] This may explain the typically weak responses to skin testing in cats compared with dogs. It is also interesting that some atopic cats are as reactive as any dog. Whether this reflects a different group of atopic cats or has any prognostic significance has yet to be determined. Immediate skin test reactivity in cats was reported to return 2 weeks after stopping oral prednisone administration and 4 weeks after the injection of methylprednisolone acetate.[417]

Serum In Vitro Testing

Commercially available serologic allergy tests (RAST, ELISA) that claim to diagnose feline atopy by detecting allergen-specific IgE are available. Only recently has it been shown that cats have allergen-specific IgE.[423, 424, 426, 430–432] *D. farinae*–specific IgE was detected in all atopic, all normal, and all laboratory cats immunized with *D. farinae*, suggesting heterogeneity of IgE antibodies in cats.[430] The presence of *D. farinae*–specific IgE does not distinguish among healthy, atopic, and *D. farinae*–immunized cats and does not correlate with intradermal skin testing with *D. farinae*.[433] Serum IgE concentrations in cats are increased by *Toxocara cati* infestations and by modified live virus vaccines.[433, 441] In vitro tests have been compared with skin tests with variable results, generally poorer than those obtained with intradermal skin testing.

A study compared the results of intradermal skin tests and a commercially available serologic allergy test (ELISA) in atopic cats and concluded that the ELISA was not a useful diagnostic test.[425] In another report evaluating the VARL, only 1 of 8 normal cats reacted, whereas 6 of 12 suspected atopic cats reacted.[343] However, in experimentally induced hypersensitivity or flea bite hypersensitivity, respectively, in vitro results were similar to or more accurate than those obtained with intradermal testing.[360, 430] Overall, these commercial tests have not been evaluated in cats to the degree that they have in the dog and, at this time, should probably not be used to diagnose atopy but only for the selection of allergens for hyposensitization. Cats with confirmed allergic skin disease have significantly more IgGd directed against house dust, flea, and pollens than normal cats and cats with nondermatologic illnesses.[429]

Only one study has reported results of hyposensitization based on in vitro testing, wherein success rates were similar to those based on intradermal testing.[434] Though we have not reviewed the percentages, we have also seen cats respond well to hyposensitization based on in vitro tests. In cats, results of intradermal testing are often difficult to interpret, which appears to be a disadvantage compared with in vitro testing. This also makes the determination of in vitro sensitivity and specificity suspect if one uses the often difficult-to-analyze results of intradermal skin testing as the standard. In addition, a blinded study on the reproducibility of intradermal skin testing in cats has not been reported. We have seen cats with poor intradermal test results but positive in vitro VARL tests and good responses to hyposensitization. If only intradermal testing had been done, hyposensitization would not have been possible in these cats. Thus, in vitro tests do have a place in the approach to suspected atopic cats.

Basophil Degranulation Test

The in vitro basophil degranulation test has been reported to show promise in the diagnosis of feline atopy.[57, 58] The original test requires fresh blood, must be run within 24 hours, is very time consuming and labor intensive, and is unlikely to become anything more than a research tool. The demonstration that feline sera also binds to human basophils makes the test potentially more practical because only serum is needed.[377, 380] Preliminary results in cats showed a 76.5% correlation with intradermal skin test results.[377]

Histopathology

Skin biopsies of atopic cats are not diagnostic but are valuable for looking for evidence of some of the alternative diagnoses.[28, 67a, 84, 455] Additionally, the histopathologic findings may vary according to the clinical lesion sampled. Biopsy specimens from clinically noninflammatory alopecic areas typically have a normal to slightly hyperplastic epidermis with a mild superficial perivascular dermatitis wherein lymphocytes or mast cells are predominant (Fig. 8–10B). Inflammatory lesions (facial and pinnal pruritus, miliary dermatitis) reveal moderate to marked epidermal hyperplasia, spongiosis, serocellular crusts, erosions or ulcerations, and variable degrees of superficial or deep perivascular dermatitis, wherein eosinophils are usually the dominant inflammatory cell (Fig. 8–10A).[455]

Intraepidermal mast cells have also been seen in skin specimens from atopic cats, primarily those with eosinophilic plaques.[64] This finding is not specific for feline atopy. Specimens from atopic cats with eosinophilic granuloma complex lesions reveal changes typical of those lesions (see Chap. 18). In some cats, eosinophilic folliculitis and furunculosis are prominent.[455] To date, atopy, food hypersensitivity, and flea bite hypersensitivity cannot be differentiated histologically.

CLINICAL MANAGEMENT

The prognosis for feline atopy is good, although some cases are extremely difficult to manage. Concurrent flea bite hypersensitivity, food hypersensitivity, and bacterial pyoderma greatly interfere with achieving a favorable therapeutic response, and care should be taken to alleviate these complications. Treatment is usually required for life, during which multiple different therapies may be used. The treatment plan may involve the use of avoidance (see Canine Atopic Disease), glucocorticoids, antihistamines, fatty acids (see Therapy of Allergic Diseases), and hyposensitization.[61, 67a, 147, 433]

The treatment selected varies according to many client and patient factors. Generally, the differences in risks of therapy among the different treatments is not gravely important because cats appear relatively resistant to the acute and chronic side effects of glucocorticoids.[6a, 67a] In addition, glucocorticoid regimens tend to be less expensive and more convenient than the alternative forms of therapy. As a result, many atopic cats are managed with some form of glucocorticoid therapy.[6a, 67a] Topical therapy is uncommonly

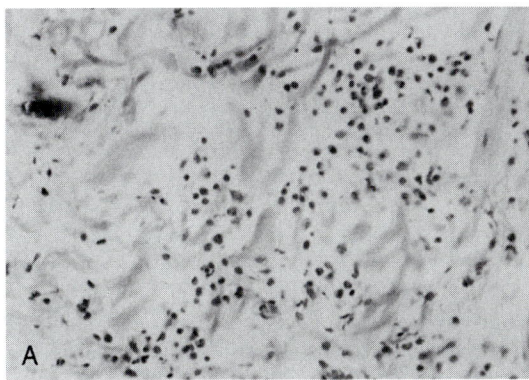
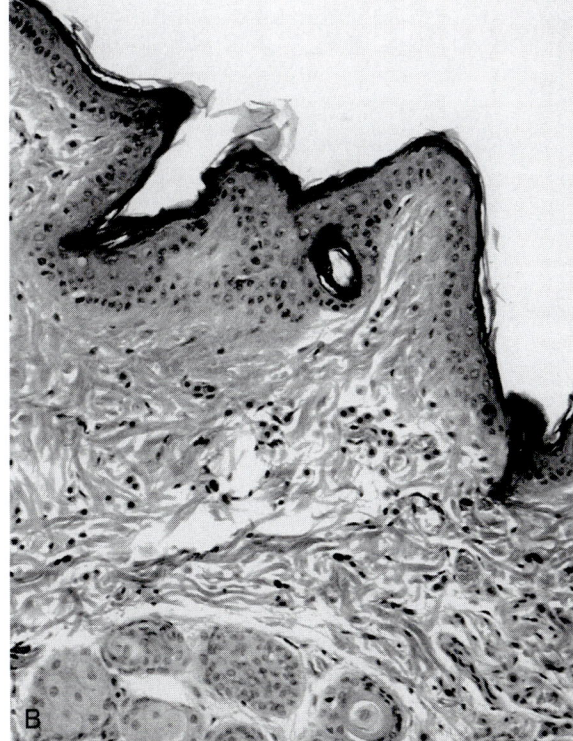

FIGURE 8–10. Feline atopy. A, Miliary dermatitis reaction pattern. Perivascular and interstitial infiltrations of predominantly eosinophils. B, Fur-mowing reaction pattern. Mild perivascular accumulations of mast cells and lymphocytes. Note the epidermis is normal.

used in the cat owing to the actual or perceived difficulty in bathing cats. In cats that tolerate bathing, however, and whose owners are willing, this practice can have a very beneficial effect. Cats may also present the problem of not tolerating long-term pilling or oral therapy. This is one indication for hyposensitization because we have seen numerous cats that tolerate injections q7-30d much better than oral medications. If glucocorticoids need to be avoided, antihistamines alone or in combination with fatty acids should be tried.

Hyposensitization is an option available in cases for which intradermal skin testing has determined what the cats are specifically allergic to. Hyposensitization utilizing either aqueous or alum-precipitated allergens is reported to give favorable responses in 70% of cases, though most studies concern small numbers of cats and do not involve long-term follow-up.* In one study of 29 cats with follow-up periods of greater than 1 year, 50% did not respond or were lost to follow-up prior to assessing response. Of those that stayed with hyposensitization, 47% responded with a moderate or better response.[415] It was also reported that the response at 12 months was similar to that in the literature but decreased with the longer follow-up periods.[415]

Hyposensitization based on serum in vitro testing has also been reported effective, with 75% of the cases improving over 50%.[434] This study also indicated that different response rates may occur, depending on the type of lesions present. In this report, though the numbers were small, 100% of linear eosinophilic granulomas and 95% of the indolent ulcers responded well; the poorest response was in cats with self-induced alopecia, with 53% responding. Most interesting was the 90% response in cats with asthma. Further work looking at the different presentations of atopy is needed to confirm these observations.

In some cats, hyposensitization is the best option other than repositol glucocorticoids because it is given by injection and relatively infrequently (once the maintenance dose is reached). Many cats tolerate the injections better than long-term oral medications. Some dermatologists use the same immunotherapy protocol that they use for the dog; others use a schedule similar to the one they use for small dogs (see Canine Atopy). One of us (C.E.G.) has found that many of the cases that respond to hyposensitization stay improved, even with a lower volume (0.5 ml) of maintenance injections, and uses a different protocol in cats from even the small dog protocol (Table 8–20).

Anecdotal reports indicate that chlorambucil or cyclosporine may be useful in severely atopic cats that do not respond to conventional therapies (see Chaps. 3 and 9).[433, 441]

Contact Hypersensitivity

Contact hypersensitivity (allergic contact dermatitis) is a rare, variably pruritic, maculopapular or lichenified dermatitis usually affecting sparsely haired skin in contact areas.

CAUSE AND PATHOGENESIS

Only a few reports of naturally occurring contact hypersensitivity in dogs and cats have been documented by patch testing, yet this is a common and well-studied problem in human dermatology.[67a, 458] Much of the veterinary literature and data on naturally occurring *allergic contact dermatitis* in dogs and cats are of dubious validity and value. In reality, there is often a huge overlap between what has been called contact hypersensitivity and primary irritant contact dermatitis in the veterinary literature.[29, 30, 61, 67a] Though experimentally induced irritant and allergic contact dermatitis can look histologically very different in dogs and humans at 24 hours, the chronic lesions in natural cases may be impossible to differentiate.[472, 483]

Classically, contact hypersensitivity represents a type IV hypersensitivity reaction wherein histologically lymphocytes are the dominant cell type.[9, 23, 30, 49, 53, 58, 61, 67a, 76, 457, 458, 472]

---

*See references 414, 419, 433, 434, 436, 438, 442, 445, 453.

Table 8–20 HYPOSENSITIZATION SCHEDULE FOR CATS

DAY	DATE	ITCH	VOLUME	DAY	DATE	ITCH	VOLUME
Vial 1				Five-Day Interval			
1			0.1	30			0.5
3			0.2	35			0.5
5			0.3	40			0.5
7			0.4	Seven-Day Interval			
9			0.6	47			0.5
11			0.8	54			0.5
13			1.0	61			0.5
Vial 2				68			0.5
15			0.1	Ten-Day Interval			
17			0.2	78			0.5
19			0.3	88			0.5
21			0.4	98			0.5
23			0.5	108			0.5
25			0.5	118			0.5

- Grade itch on scale of 0 (none) to 10 (most severe this pet has had in the past).
- *Note:* it is possible to go higher than 10 if the itching is getting worse than ever before.
- Call at 4 weeks and report grade of itching.
- Call if itch goes up by more than 2 levels.
- Call prior to giving any more shots if there are adverse reactions
  - Vomiting, diarrhea, anxiousness, weakness are possible reactions.
  - Reactions will usually occur within 1 to 2 hours after shot is given.
- Recheck appointments should be made around day 60 and day 120.
- Watch for pattern of itching in relation to when shots are given.
- Itch increases before shot is due, or after shot is given.
- Itch decreases after shot is given.

Most of the work on the pathogenesis of contact hypersensitivity has been performed in laboratory animals. In contrast with irritant reactions, allergic contact reactions are characterized by a immunologic reaction to a hapten, usually a small, chemically reactive, lipid-soluble molecule that binds to a protein to become a complete antigen.[472] The hapten protein complex binds to, and most likely is pinocytosed by, epidermal Langerhans' cells, which induces an increase in Langerhans' cell size, MHC II expression, and IL-1β synthesis.

The initial presentation and processing of the hapten is called the *afferent phase* of allergic contact reactions. This phase is thought to require transfer of stimulated hapten-containing Langerhans' cells from the skin to regional lymph nodes. This emigration from skin to lymph nodes may be initiated by TNF-α.[458] These T cells are stimulated to express skin-homing ligands that direct their movement to the skin. Langerhans' cell numbers are decreased in contact hypersensitivity because of their emigration to the lymph nodes but not in primary irritant contact dermatitis.[458]

The *efferent phase* or *elicitation phase* occurs in response to exposure to hapten in an already sensitized animal. Though some Langerhans' cell migration may occur, much of this reaction may occur locally. The activated memory T cells are recruited to the site of hapten exposure by expression of adhesion molecules, such as VCAM-1, E-selectin, and ICAM-1 on the vascular endothelium. ICAM-1 is also expressed on keratinocytes and may result in the diapedesis of lymphocytes. TNF-α is rapidly released from Langerhans' cells and keratinocytes after hapten exposure and stimulates the expression of E-selectin and VCAM-1 on the endothelial cells.[211, 458, 472] TNF-α is also released from cells in response to substance P, a neuropeptide that may be released as a result of the interaction between Langerhans' cells and nerve fibers.[458] Other epidermal cytokines involved include IL-6 and MIP. Which cytokines are associated with allergic contact and not irritant contact dermatitis is an area receiving extensive study. It appears that the differences in IL-1β, IL-6, IL-12, and IFN-γ may be key factors.[472] The production of IL-12 may be central to the development of a Th1 cell response.[458]

Newer information blurs the distinction between immunologic and nonimmunologic events and makes differentiation problematic.[477] The clinical and histopathologic features overlap greatly. Langerhans' cells are just as actively involved in irritant as allergic reactions (decreased numbers, apposition of lymphocytes). Virtually all cytokines identified in allergic reactions are also present in irritant reactions (ICAM-1, IL-2, TNF-α, LFA-1). The percentage of T-cell subtypes, Langerhans' cells, macrophages, and activated antigens are not significantly different. Even patch testing produces the same cytokine profile and so forth. Some authors conclude that the difference between irritant and allergic reactions is more conceptual than demonstrable.[477]

The last phase of naturally occurring contact hypersensitivity is the *resolution phase*. Less is known about this phase, though IL-10 may play an important role as it interferes with Th2 cell cytokine production. IL-10 is upregulated in keratinocytes in the late phase of allergic contact reactions. Basophils, which begin to migrate into late lesions, may also be involved in stimulating resolution.[472]

In dogs, histopathologic examination has given conflicting and confusing results.[67a] In a Danish study wherein positive patch test reactions underwent biopsy and histopathologic examination, the neutrophil was the dominant inflammatory cell.[482] In another histopathologic study of experimentally induced contact hypersensitivity to DNCB in dogs, the histopathology was similar to that seen in humans and laboratory animals, with lymphocytes and macrophages predominating.[483] Limited case studies in the dog have also implicated eosinophils as a cellular component of contact hypersensitivity in the dog.[461, 463, 465, 470, 475] These contrasting findings most likely reflect the problems of differentiating cases of contact-induced atopic disease and irritant dermatitis from true type IV hapten-induced contact hypersensitivity. Further work in this area is needed.

It has been noted that atopy is present in about 20% of the dogs with contact hypersensitivity.[474] This is in contrast with humans, wherein atopic dermatitis is associated with a lower incidence of contact hypersensitivity.[458] Whether this reflects similar breed predispositions, similarities in basic immunologic pathogenesis between contact hypersensitivity and atopic disease, misdiagnosis of contact atopic disease as contact hypersensitivity, or abnormalities in the epidermal barrier of atopic dogs that predispose to penetration of haptens that cause contact hypersensitivity remains to be determined. In fact, canine atopy itself may be a type of contact hypersensitivity, a type I (immediate) contact hypersensitivity (see Canine Atopy), and can cause positive patch test results, which could easily confuse the diagnosis.

Experimental attempts to induce contact hypersensitivity in dogs and cats have given inconsistent results. Nobreus and colleagues,[473] using a modified "maximization technique" of intradermal and topical sensitization, successfully sensitized dogs to dinitrochlorobenzene. They showed that the sensitization could be transferred to normal dogs with thoracic duct lymphocytes and that sensitization could be suppressed with antilymphocyte serum. Krawiec and Gaafar[466] as well as Conroy[483] successfully sensitized dogs to dinitrochlorobenzene with either intradermal and topical or topical challenge. Schultz and Adams[479] reported that helminth antigens, tissue antigens, viral antigens, bacterial antigens, fungal antigens, protein antigens, dinitrochlorobenzene, and mitogens had been used experimentally and clinically in dogs and cats to elicit delayed-type hypersensitivity responses in the skin, with limited reproducibility or irreproducible results. Schultz and Maguire[478] induced delayed-type hypersensitivity in normal cats with dinitrochlorobenzene.

Spontaneous, well-documented cases of contact hypersensitivity are rare in the veterinary literature. Though poison ivy and poison oak may be transferred to humans from dogs carrying the oleoresins in their haircoats, only rare cases occur in the dog, and documentation of these by patch testing has not been published. Other plants, however, have rarely been documented as a cause of contact hypersensitivity. Kunkle and Gross[467] reported a beautifully documented case of naturally occurring contact hypersensitivity to *Tradescantia fluminensis* (wandering Jew plant) in a dog. Sensitivity to *Hippeastrum* (Amaryllidaceae) leaves and bulbs was documented in a dog in the Netherlands.[486] Three cases were described with positive patch to plants belonging to the *Commelinceae* family (*Commelina diffusa* [spreading dayflower], *Murdannia nudiflora* [doveweed], and *Trades-*

cantia fluminensis [wandering Jew]).[469] One dog was also atopic, all three dogs tested had a favorable response to pentoxifylline, and one underwent a biopsy of the positive patch test site that was characterized by an eosinophilic infiltrate. Asian jasmine was also shown to be a cause in a case documented with patch testing and resolution upon avoidance.[470] Interestingly, in this last case, multiple intraepidermal eosinophilic microabscesses were revealed on histopathologic examination of the patch test site.

Dandelion leaves were well documented as a cause in one dog.[465] Cedar wood was also reported as a cause of contact hypersensitivity, although patch testing was not performed to document the case.[463] Indoor or synthetic products that contain allergens are a major cause of disease in humans but, again, are rarely documented to cause disease in dogs. In a Danish study, confirmed contact hypersensitivity to the following substances was documented: thiuram mix, cobalt chloride, nickel sulfate, quinoline mix, colophony, black rubber mix, wood alcohols, epoxy resin, balsam of Peru, carba mix, formaldehyde, fragrance mix, ethylenediamine, primin, wood tar, and naphthyl mix.[481, 482] Two other dogs were patch test positive to colophony, a pine oil resin, and this correlated with reaction to cleaning products.[462] Two different reports described reactions caused by exposure to cement.[462, 475]

Well-documented cases were also reported in three dogs that were allergic to synthetic textiles, though the allergenic component was not identified.[465] Carpet deodorizer and a plastic shopping bag were suspected, but not proven, to be contact allergens in a dog[464] and cat,[471] respectively. Bleach has also been reported to cause reactions in two dogs.[462] Neomycin is a commonly mentioned but rarely documented contact allergen in dogs and cats.[476, 485] Because it is often present in otic preparations, neomycin is most frequently incriminated as a cause of "allergic contact otitis externa." Contact dermatitis accounted for about 43% and 27%, respectively, of the idiosyncratic cutaneous adverse drug reactions recognized in dogs[166] and cats.[165]

It can be concluded from the preceding summary of investigations that contact hypersensitivity *can* be induced in dogs and cats, but only with difficulty and with inconsistent results compared with tests on humans and guinea pigs. The incidence of naturally occurring disease is much lower than in humans and rarely as well documented as in humans. Additionally, the pathogenesis of the lesions needs to be studied because there may be species differences or even multiple pathogenic mechanisms in the dog, as evidenced by the strikingly different histopathologic findings reported from clinical lesions or in positive patch tests. It is likely that some of the cases reported with positive patch tests may reflect contact atopic disease and not true hapten-induced contact hypersensitivity.[483]

CLINICAL FEATURES

Naturally occurring contact hypersensitivity is reported to account for about 1% to 10% of all canine dermatoses[61, 67a, 462, 468, 474, 485] and to be rare in cats. We consider it a very rare disease. A 1993 symposium on contact hypersensitivity in the dog presented very small numbers of cases, and most case reports were very old.[461, 463, 465, 470, 475] Walton[484] reported that over 20% of his cases of canine contact hypersensitivity occurred in yellow Labrador retrievers. In a study of 22 cases (confirmed by closed patch testing) of contact hypersensitivity in dogs in Denmark,[481] 50% of the dogs were German shepherds, whereas this breed accounted for only 16% of the purebred registered dogs. Other breeds described but not documented to be at increased risk are Wirehaired fox terriers, Scottish terriers, West Highland white terriers, and Golden retrievers.[474] These are breeds also at risk for atopy. French poodles are also reported to be at risk.[474, 482] No age or sex predilection has been documented.

Although contact hypersensitivity can be produced in dogs after a 3- to 5-week sensitization period, the sensitization period for dogs and cats with naturally occurring disease exceeds 2 years in over 70% of cases.[61, 67a, 474, 481, 484] Substances reported to cause naturally occurring "allergic contact dermatitis" in dogs and cats are listed in Table 8–21. Again, virtually none of these substances, other than those previously listed, has been well-

Table 8-21	SUBSTANCES REPORTED TO CAUSE NATURALLY OCCURRING "ALLERGIC CONTACT DERMATITIS" IN DOGS AND CATS
SUBSTANCE CATEGORY	EXAMPLES
Plants	Pollens and resins (grasses, trees, weeds), jasmine blooms, poison ivy, poison oak, wandering Jew, dandelion leaves, Asian jasmine, cedar wood, *Hippeastrum*
Medications	Numerous topicals (especially neomycin, bacitracin, thiabendazole, tretinoin, miconazole, polyhydroxidine, tetracaine and other "caines"); numerous otic preparations, soaps, shampoos (especially those containing tars, creosols, and benzoyl peroxide); petrolatum, lanolin, disinfectants, insecticides (shampoos, dips, sprays, flea and tick collars and medallions; especially d-limonene, rotenone)
Highly chlorinated water	
Home furnishings	Fibers (wool, nylon, synthetics), dyes, mordants, finishes, polishes, cleansers, rubber and plastic products, detergents, cat litter, collars (leather, metal), deodorants, cement, nickel, dichromate

documented with patch testing, and even less with typical histopathology of the positive patch test sites. None reported on results of intradermal testing with similar extracts or of testing with protein-free extracts. Such studies may help to determine whether these animals have type IV hypersensitivity or IgE-mediated diseases.

Clinical signs of contact hypersensitivity include varying degrees of dermatitis, which tend to be confined to hairless or sparsely haired areas of skin in contact regions: ventral aspect of paws (*not* pads) (Fig. 8-11B); ventral abdomen (see Fig. 8-8D), thorax (see Fig. 8-8E), tail, and neck; scrotum (see Fig. 8-11C and D); point of chin; perineum; and lateral aspect of pinnae. However, with chronicity, lesions may spread to involve larger areas that may seem less typical of a contact pattern and involve normally haired areas. Importantly, these cases have a history of slowly spreading into these adjacent areas as hair loss progresses at the margins of erythematous pruritic lesions. If the allergen is in a topical medicament in liquid, aerosol, or powder form, cutaneous reactions may also be visible in haired areas as well (see Fig. 8-11A). Reactions to rubber or plastic dishes and rawhide chew toys are usually confined to the lips and nose (see Fig. 8-8F). Lesions in ring patterns around the neck, though now less common with the newer collars, used to be a problem with flea collars, particularly in cats (see Fig. 8-11E).

Acute skin lesions consist of various combinations of erythema, macules, papules, and, rarely, vesicles. Although vesicles are the classic lesions in most species, they are rare in dogs and cats and often manifest themselves only at the microscopic level in acute lesions. Chronic lesions are often alopecic plaques that may be hyperpigmented or hypopigmented, excoriated, and lichenified. Secondary bacterial pyoderma, *Malassezia* dermatitis, seborrheic skin disease, or combinations of these may be present.[474, 481, 484, 485] Pruritus varies from mild to intense. Contact hypersensitivities may be seasonal or nonseasonal, depending on the allergens involved. In households with several dogs or cats, involvement of a single animal would suggest hypersensitivity, whereas clinical signs in several animals would point to irritant reactions or contagious disease.

DIAGNOSIS

The differential diagnosis includes primary irritant contact dermatitis, atopy, food hypersensitivity, canine scabies, insect hypersensitivity, *Pelodera* dermatitis, hookworm dermatitis, staphylococcal folliculitis, and *Malassezia* dermatitis. Definitive diagnosis is based on history, physical findings, and results of provocative exposure and patch testing with appropriate histopathology. Provocative exposure involves avoiding contact with suspected allergenic substances for up to 14 days.[61, 67a, 468, 474, 485]

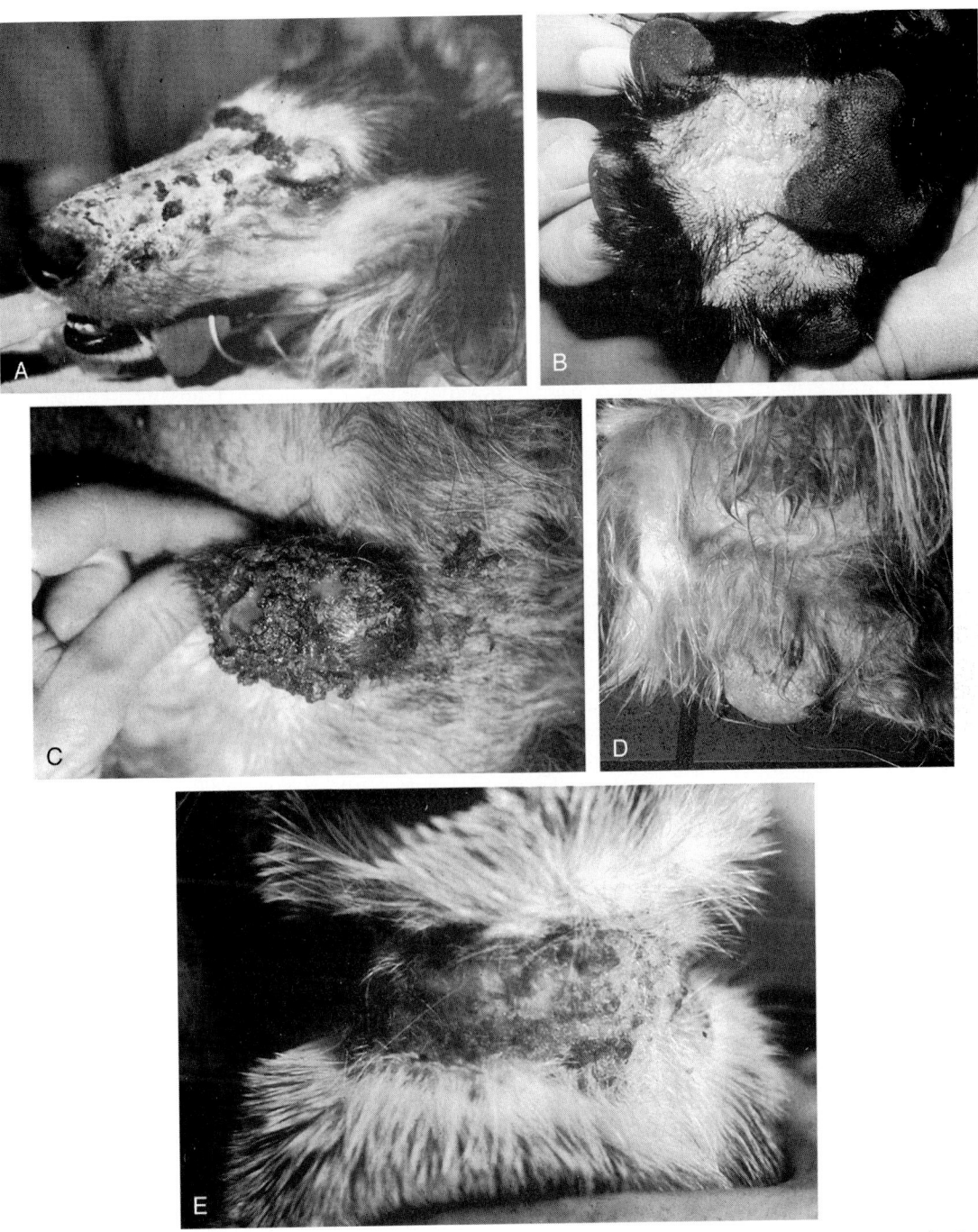

FIGURE 8–11. Contact dermatitis. *A*, Contact dermatitis due to neomycin (Panolog) on the bridge of the nose of a dog. *B*, Alopecia, erythema, and lichenification of the ventral paws, one of the common patterns of disease in contact dermatitis. *C*, Crusting, erythema, erosions of the scrotum form contact dermatitis, a commonly affected site in male dogs and it may be the only area of involvement. *D*, Canine brucellosis. Scrotal ulceration due to licking. *E*, Alopecia, erythema, erosions, and crusting in a cat with a flea collar reaction demonstrating the classic ring of lesions around the neck.

The animal is first bathed with a nonirritating, hypoallergenic shampoo to remove all possible allergenic substances from the skin and haircoat, then placed in a "nonallergenic" environment for up to 14 days. The animal is then re-exposed to its normal environment or to suspect substances, one at a time, and is observed for an exacerbation of the dermatosis over 7 to 10 days. Provocative exposure is time consuming, requires a patient and dedicated owner, and is frequently impossible to undertake. Additionally, without biopsy or patch testing, provocative exposure does *not* reliably distinguish among contact allergy, atopic disease, and irritant skin reactions. To better define the reactions, skin biopsy specimens taken from acute lesions induced by the exposure should be studied.

The patch test is the method for documenting contact hypersensitivity.[9, 50, 61, 67a, 474, 481, 482, 484, 485] In the classic closed patch test, the test substance is applied to a piece of cloth or soft paper that is then placed directly on intact skin, covered with an impermeable substance, and affixed to the skin with tape. After 48 hours, the patch is removed and the condition of the underlying skin examined. Owing to the logistical problems of applying and securing patch test substances to dogs and cats, patch testing is rarely done. The sliding of the material and irritation from tape leads to much misinterpretation of results. The use of ether to remove the tape and the adhesive (Scanpar) tends to minimize but not eliminate these problems.[474]

Walton[484] recommended open patch testing in the dog and listed suggested allergen concentrations and vehicles for canine patch testing. In open patch testing, the allergen is merely rubbed into a suitable marked test site of normal skin and the test site is then examined daily over 5 days. Walton[484] reported that positive patch test reactions in dogs are much less inflammatory than those in human beings and guinea pigs, usually consisting of mild erythema and edema and variable degrees of pruritus. In a Danish study, 63% of the affected dogs were monosensitive and 23% were sensitive to two allergens.[482]

For now, performing closed patch tests with suspected allergens in their natural state is probably the most sensible way to proceed. The dorsolateral thorax is gently clipped, and suspected allergens are applied to the skin (preferably with Scanpar), taped in place, and secured under a body bandage. The test materials are removed in 48 hours, and the test sites are observed for the following 3 to 5 days. Optimally, test sites should undergo biopsy, but more fulminant reactions can be considered positive. The nature of the reaction is not determined without biopsy of these acute lesions. Additionally, substances eliciting positive reactions should be tested on normal animals to make sure that they are not irritants.

A standardized patch test kit has been recommended for dogs.[474, 482] Limited testing with this kit in control dogs had been undertaken until a study indicated that 83.3% of normal dogs responded to one or more allergens, suggesting that this human kit is not appropriate for testing in dogs at the recommended strengths.[459] Further work at different strengths is warranted before this test can be used in the dog, and it has not been evaluated in cats. Additionally, many of the documented causes of contact hypersensitivity in dogs would have been missed by the test because the allergens were local plants or materials not included in this standard battery. Therefore, a complete work-up still requires that materials from the dog's local environment be tested in addition to the standardized battery. These natural materials can be chopped up, mixed with petrolatum, and applied with the Finn Chambers or placed in the center of a 2-inch gauze pad.

Histopathology

In experimentally induced contact hypersensitivity in dogs and cats, skin biopsy revealed varying degrees of superficial perivascular dermatitis, with mononuclear cells predominating.[466, 478, 483] In other attempts to induce type IV hypersensitivity reactions in dog and cat skin, however, biopsies revealed varying degrees of superficial perivascular dermatitis in which neutrophils prevailed.[479] Reports of natural cases also have revealed significant numbers of eosinophils.[465, 469, 470, 483]

In naturally occurring contact hypersensitivity of dogs, cats, and human beings, skin biopsy is nondiagnostic, showing varying degrees of superficial perivascular dermatitis (spongiotic, hyperplastic) wherein neutrophils, mononuclear cells, or eosinophils may predominate.[23, 28, 61, 67a, 458] Specimens taken from positive patch test reaction sites in dogs with spontaneous contact hypersensitivity revealed that neutrophils were the dominant dermal inflammatory cell and were commonly associated with neutrophilic exocytosis and even focal epidermal necrosis.[482] These changes are unexpected and suggestive of irritant contact dermatitis. No significant differences are found in the number of mononuclear inflammatory cells or in their subclasses in skin from humans with allergic or primary irritant contact dermatitis.[9, 50] Histopathologic findings consistent with secondary bacterial pyoderma, *Malassezia* dermatitis, seborrheic skin disease, or combinations of these may be present.

CLINICAL MANAGEMENT

The prognosis for contact hypersensitivity depends on the offending allergen. Therapy of contact hypersensitivity in dogs and cats may include avoidance of allergens or the use of glucocorticoids. Avoidance of allergens is preferable but may be impossible, either because of the nature of the substances or because they cannot be identified. In such instances, pentoxifylline or glucocorticoids are usually effective but are often needed for life. In some animals, management may consist of topical glucocorticoids alone (see Chap. 3). Other animals require systemic glucocorticoids. Prednisolone or prednisone may be administered orally at 1 mg/kg (dog) or 2 mg/kg (cat) daily for 5 to 7 days and then on an alternate-day regimen as needed (see Chap. 3). Pentoxifylline (a methylxanthine derivative) suppresses the production of TNF-α by leukocytes and keratinocytes. It also downregulates adhesion molecule expression, and the oral administration of the drug in humans with contact hypersensitivity gives variable results.[460, 480] Pentoxifylline (10 mg/kg q8h) was shown effective in preventing the development of contact hypersensitivity in the canine.[469] Topical application of pentoxifylline was ineffective in treating humans with contact hypersensitivity.[460]

Hyposensitization to certain contactants has been shown to be possible in humans.[22, 50] Such hyposensitization, however, is usually limited and temporary. In general, attempts to hyposensitize human beings, dogs, and cats to contactants have been totally unsuccessful.*

Canine Food Hypersensitivity

Food hypersensitivity (adverse food reaction, food allergy, food intolerance) is a nonseasonal, pruritic skin disorder of dogs that is associated with the ingestion of a substance found in the dog's diet.[496, 501, 529] Presumably it is a hypersensitivity reaction to an antigenic ingredient. This may not always be the case, however, and toxic food reactions and nontoxic, nonimmunologic reactions (intolerances) may also be occurring and be incorrectly called food hypersensitivity. Toxic reactions are usually dose related, occur in any individual, and are often associated with histamine or bacterial toxins in the food.

In one study of North American commercial pet foods, the histamine contact varied from 0.6 to 65.5 μg/g.[502] This amount is probably insufficient to cause histamine toxicosis but might be enough to enhance existing pruritus in some animals. Food intolerances are an individual sensitivity to a food that may occur by a variety of nonimmunologic mechanisms, including metabolic, pharmacologic, and idiosyncratic. Their clinical differentiation from allergy is rarely accomplished or necessary.[61, 67a, 504, 505, 523] The term *food hypersensitivity* is still accepted, however, because of its common usage and because of the difficulty differentiating between hypersensitivity and intolerance in practice.[67a, 505]

CAUSE AND PATHOGENESIS

Diet has long been recognized as a cause of hypersensitivity-like skin reactions in dogs, cats, and human beings. Although the pathomechanism of food hypersensitivity is unclear,

---

*See references 22, 50, 61, 67a, 481, 482, 484.

type I hypersensitivity reactions are well documented and the most common type of hypersensitivity reactions in humans, although type III and IV reactions have been suspected. Cutaneous type I reactions are associated with both immediate and late-phase reactions.[61, 67a, 505, 523] Immediated (within minutes to hours) and delayed (within several hours to days) reactions to foods have also occurred in the dog and cat.[61, 67a, 491, 517, 535]

Why the skin is a frequent target of food-induced hypersensitivity is not well known, though it has been recognized in humans that cutaneous lymphocyte antigen is induced on T cells when cutaneous disease is present but not on T cells in food-related respiratory disease.[523] Whether sensitization occurs in the intestinal mucosa or to absorbed allergen is unknown. Normally the gut possesses several mechanisms that make up the intestinal mucosal barrier, which blocks the absorption or the entering of foreign antigens into the body. Antigens are normally broken down by the effects of gastric acid enzymes, pancreatic and intestinal enzymes in the gut lumen, and intestinal cell lysosomal activity. Intestinal peristalsis also acts to decrease absorption of potential antigens by removing antigens trapped in the intestinal mucous.

The intestinal mucosal barrier is composed of a protective mucous coating overlying the epithelial cells, which are sealed together by tight junctions. Together the mucous and epithelial cells block the passage of most macromolecules. This is supported by an immunologic response of secretory IgA from the plasma cells in the lamina propria. Secretory IgA binds antigens and removes them in the intestinal mucus or, for those antigens that pass through the intestinal barrier, secretory IgA binds antigen and is removed from the circulation through the liver and bile.[489, 504, 505, 523] Antigens bypassing these protective mechanisms stimulate an immune response which, for many molecules, results in tolerance or anergy by activation of suppressor (CD8) T cells or suppressor cytokine profiles (such as IL-4, IL-10, and TGF-β) from Th2 and Th3 cells.[489] Abnormalities in the barrier or immune response may result in sensitization. Therefore, damage to the normal defense barriers along with ingestion of food molecules at the same time most likely contributes to which molecules become antigenic.

The type of molecule also plays a role because most food hypersensitivity reactions are directed against complex glycoproteins. The protection is delayed in human infants because, in the first month of life, there is predominantly an IgM response, which is not as effective as secretory IgA in trapping and removing antigens.[523] Children have immature intestinal mucosal barriers that are less efficient in handling and processing food proteins.[523]

Despite these defenses, an immunologic response to a variety of food antigens often occurs both in normal individuals and those with proven food hypersensitivity.[504, 505, 523] In rodents, it has been shown that antigen-presenting cells in the mononuclear phagocytic system stimulate gut CD8+ T cells that play a role in the development of immune tolerance; if overloaded with multiple antigens, this may prevent the induction of tolerance to subsequent exposed antigens. This observation has led to the suggestion that, if a similar mechanism occurred in human infants, the observation of increased incidence of food hypersensitivity in 4-month-old human infants fed a variety of solids foods could be explained.[523]

Another consideration in animals, in which gastrointestinal parasitism and viral enteritis are relatively common, is that a damaged intestinal tract allows the bypassing of the normal defense mechanisms and antigens would overload the gut mononuclear phagocytic system. The predisposition to develop IgE antibody may be enhanced by a concurrent parasitic infection.[29] This has been shown experimentally wherein endoparasites favor the development of IgE to orally administered allergens in atopy-prone dogs[495] and in cats.[531] Poor digestion results in larger protein molecules and, because food hypersensitivity to small proteins and amino acids is rare, these may be more capable of inducing a hypersensitivity reaction.[521]

Additionally, because endoparasitism and viral enteritis occur in young dogs and food hypersensitivity often develops in young dogs, it becomes a tempting hypothesis that needs to be studied. Attention has also been focused on a heterogeneous group of cytokines called histamine-releasing factors.[61, 504, 505] After being initially generated by chronic antigenic exposures, these cytokines can cause histamine release in the absence of the provoking antigen, and this release can continue for some time after the antigen is removed. Such a mechanism could explain the long delay (10 to 13 weeks) reported between the initiation of a hypoallergenic diet and clinical improvement in some food-hypersensitive dogs. This mechanism is also thought to play a role in cutaneous hyperirritability with chronic ingestion of the offending food allergens.[523]

Highly inbred, high IgE-producing atopic Spaniel-Basenji colony dogs were immunized subcutaneously with food antigen extracts in alum.[495] The dogs then experienced clinical manifestations of food hypersensitivity after oral challenge with the foods. However, these dogs experienced only gastrointestinal signs.

Compared with what is known in humans, little is known about the food allergens that are important in small animals. Most commonly, the allergen is a water-soluble glycoprotein present in the food, and this glycoprotein may become recognizable only after digestion or heating and preparation of the food. The size of the allergenic glycoproteins in humans is generally large, with a molecular weight greater than 12,000 daltons. This has not been confirmed in the dog. A company report of nine food-hypersensitive dogs described reactions to allergens most likely with molecular weights greater than 1400 daltons in casein, fish, and egg.[487] In the three casein-hypersensitive dogs, the offending allergen was determined to have a molecular weight between 1100 and 4500 daltons. This determination was based on patients reacting to a diet containing a hydrolysate with 98% of the proteins being less than 4500 daltons but not to a casein hydrolysate with 99.7% of the proteins being less than 1100 daltons.

In another study, a low-molecular-weight hydrolyzed diet was used to diagnose food hypersensitivity in 69% of 29 suspected food-hypersensitive dogs.[500] Rosser challenged 7 food-hypersensitive dogs with a hydrolyzed diet in which 98.8% of the proteins were smaller than 1400 daltons—with no exacerbations.[487]

The documentation of a hypersensitive mechanism is rarely confirmed in the dog. Food intolerance is also likely in the dog and may mimic food hypersensitivity reactions. In humans, food intolerance is thought to account for the majority of adverse food reactions, though their importance in cutaneous diseases has not been studied in depth.

We are beginning to acquire information on the dietary items responsible for food hypersensitivity in dogs, though studies are still limited in size or scope of items challenged. Good studies are difficult because few owners are willing to separate a diet into its components and to feed each item individually to identify the responsible allergen. In addition, challenges are open and, in humans, the placebo effect has been shown to be very high when attempting to determine dietary allergens. Therefore, documentation is based on three positive double-blinded, placebo-controlled food challenges.[523] In vitro (serologic) test results cannot be relied on to detect allergens that cause hypersensitivity because they are positive in most normal dogs and in most dogs with other skin diseases.[527] These test results are also positive in most dogs with proven hypersensitivity to food, but not to the important allergens as determined by test meal investigations.[527]

The largest prospective study to date evaluated 25 food-hypersensitive dogs with seven different diet ingredients.[509] The challenge was to a standard group of dietary ingredients (beef, chicken, chicken eggs, cow milk, wheat, soy, corn) and not necessarily to all the ingredients the dog had been eating prior to the diagnosis. Eighty percent of the dogs reacted to one or two, and 64% of the dogs reacted to two or more, of these seven foods, and the mean number of reactions in all dogs was 2.4. No dogs reacted to more than five proteins, but we have seen a few cases that reacted to numerous proteins, and one of us (C.E.G.) had a patient that, over a 2-year period, experienced hypersensitivity reactions to virtually every protein it was fed and ended up malnourished until treated with corticosteriods and fed the foods it was hypersensitive to.

In another study, one dog was hypersensitive to nine food items.[516] Beef was the most common reactant (60% of the dogs), but reactions were also detected with soy (32%), chicken (28%), milk (28%), corn (25%), wheat (24%), and eggs (20%).[509] This is similar to other reports that show that, in general, the most common offending foods are those most commonly found in the diets being fed: beef, dairy products, chicken, milk, wheat, chicken eggs, corn, and soy.[488, 491, 496, 506, 509, 516, 526, 529] Interestingly, 9% of the dogs in one study reacted to a rice product.[49]

Another study also found that 50% of eight food-allergic dogs reacted to fish (herring and catfish).[524] We have also seen a few cases with well-documented reactions to potato, a concern with the move toward potato-based hypoallergenic diets. It should also be realized that most cases do not get challenged with more than a few ingredients, and many foods are not routinely tested in provocative challenge. Table 8–22 lists dietary items reported to have caused food hypersensitivity in dogs. Though food additives (including preservatives) are often blamed by the public (particularly by naturalists), these substances are rarely documented to cause food hypersensitivity in dogs. One dog was documented to react to the additive gum carrageenan.[529]

CLINICAL FEATURES

It has been estimated that food hypersensitivity accounts for (1) as many as 1% of all canine and feline dermatoses in a general practice and (2) about 10% of all canine allergic skin diseases (excluding parasitic allergy).[61, 67a, 488, 492] Studies have indicated that food hypersensitivity in dogs and cats accounted for about 5% of all skin diseases and 15% of the allergic dermatoses.[491, 493] Food hypersensitivity is the third most common hypersensitivity skin disease in dogs after flea bite hypersensitivity and atopy.

The actual incidence is difficult to determine because food hypersensitivity often occurs concurrently with other allergic diseases and symptoms may ameliorate or become clinically acceptable when the concurrent allergy is controlled. In contrast, the other allergy may be clinically irrelevant when the food hypersensitivity is controlled—thus, the incidence reported may depend on the diagnostic approach selected by the clinician or investigator. Concurrent flea bite hypersensitivity or atopic disease occurs in up to 75% of cases.[491, 516, 517, 520, 529] Because many clients do not complete an adequate elimination diet, some cases go unrecognized.

No age or sex predilections have been documented for canine food hypersensitivity. Though there is no age predilection, it is important to note that many cases occur in young dogs. In four studies, between 33% and 52%, respectively, of the food hypersensitive dogs experienced clinical signs at 1 year of age or less.[493, 506, 517, 529] The index of suspicion for food hypersensitivity is above that of atopic disease when pruritus occurs in dogs under 6 months of age.[67a, 506, 517] Most investigators have not found a breed predilection.[69, 491, 528] Other investigators, however, found that American Cocker spaniels, English Springer spaniels, Labrador retrievers, Collies, Miniature schnauzers, Chinese Shar Peis, Poodles, West Highland white terriers, Wheaten terriers, Boxers, Dachshunds, Dalmatians, Lhasa apsos, German shepherds, and Golden retrievers were at increased risk.[493, 506, 517, 529]

Food hypersensitivity can cause a wide variety of lesions and can be considered in any nonseasonal pruritic dog.[67a, 491, 492, 513, 529] However, it is also important to recognize that

● Table 8–22 **DIETARY ITEMS THAT HAVE CAUSED FOOD HYPERSENSITIVITY IN THE DOG**

Artificial food additives (gum carrageenan)	Horse meat
Beef	Kidney beans
Canned foods	Lamb and mutton
Chicken	Oatmeal
Corn	Pasta
Cow's milk	Pork
Dairy products (whey)	Potatoes
Dog biscuits	Rabbit
Dog foods (including prescription canned and dry d/d)	Rice flour and rice
Eggs	Soy
Fish (variety)	Turkey
Food preservatives	Wheat

food hypersensitivity may be episodic or seasonal, such as when offending food items are given sporadically or when perennial food hypersensitivity symptoms are minimal but aggravated to a clinically significant level with concurrent seasonal atopic disease.[61, 67a, 496] Pruritus, with or without a primary eruption, is the only consistent finding. There is no classic set of cutaneous signs pathognomonic for food hypersensitivity in the dog. A variety of primary and secondary skin lesions are noted. These include papules, plaques, pustules, wheals, angioedema, erythema, ulcers, excoriation, lichenification, pigment changes, alopecia, scales, crusts, and moist erosions that appear as areas of pyotraumatic dermatitis (Fig. 8–12A; see Fig. 8–8G). Eosinophilic vasculitis presenting as urticaria, or any lesions of vasculitis, have been reported and seen by us in association with food hypersensitivity (see Fig. 8–8H).[163]

In general, the major complaint is pruritus, and the pruritus is nonseasonal and may be poorly responsive to glucocorticoids, though a favorable response should not decrease one's index of suspicion. If the offending food is a snack or table food, the signs can be episodic, depending on how often the dog eats it. Any distribution of skin involvement may occur, but the ears, rump, distal limbs, axillae, and groin appear commonly affected.[493, 506, 513, 517, 529] In some dogs, disease is limited to the ears or rump area.[496, 506, 517, 529]

Pruritic, bilateral otitis externa (frequently with secondary bacterial or *Malassezia* infections), along with secondary seborrheic skin disease, bacterial pyoderma, or both are common in conjunction with food hypersensitivity.[491, 493, 496, 506, 517, 529] Secondary bacterial pyodermas most commonly present as superficial folliculitis, though folliculitis and furunculosis as well as bacterial pododermatitis or acral lick dermatitis may occur. Some dogs present with only a recurrent bacterial pyoderma, with or without pruritus, wherein all clinical signs resolve with antibiotic therapy.[506, 529] Concurrent gastrointestinal disturbances (vomiting, diarrhea, colic) have been reported in 10% to 15% of these dogs.[61, 67a, 496, 529]

In experimentally induced food hypersensitivity, the most common abnormality was an increase in the number of bowel movements. When food-hypersensitive dogs were fed diets containing the offending allergen, they averaged about three bowel movements per day, versus 1.5 bowel movements per day when fed an allergen-free diet. One of us (C.E.G.) has observed that pruritic dogs with more than three bowel movements per day are more likely to have food hypersensitivities as part of the reason for their pruritus. In one study, 60% of the food-hypersensitive dogs with cutaneous and gastrointestinal signs defecated greater than or equal to six times a day.[516] In humans, the noncutaneous symptoms associated with food hypersensitivity are numerous ("tension-fatigue syndrome"), and malaise and dullness have been observed in dogs.[67a, 529]

Seizures have been rarely described as being responsive to hypoallergenic diets.[67a, 529] Rosser had two dogs with a seizure history in his 51 food-hypersensitive dogs, and we have seen seizures associated with food hypersensitivity.[517] It is interesting to note that well-documented upper and lower respiratory symptoms occur in humans with double-blinded, placebo-controlled food challenges, and this is not reported in veterinary texts.[61, 67a, 512, 523] This lack of recognition may reflect that the presence of respiratory symptoms has been a feature that strongly suggested atopic disease, and may have thus decreased an appropriate pursuit of food hypersensitivity in those dogs.

DIAGNOSIS

The differential diagnosis of canine food hypersensitivity consists of atopy, drug reaction, flea bite hypersensitivity, pediculosis, intestinal parasite hypersensitivity, scabies, *Malassezia* dermatitis, seborrheic skin disease, and bacterial folliculitis.

At present, the definitive diagnosis of food hypersensitivity in dogs is reliable only on the basis of elimination diets and provocative exposure testing. The necessary duration of a hypoallergenic diet is controversial.[496, 529] A 21-day protocol would have diagnosed only 26% of the food-hypersensitive dogs in Rosser's prospective study.[517] Studies have indicated that complete resolution or maximal improvement of clinical signs may require use of a hypoallergenic diet for 10 to 13 weeks.[493, 517] However, two of us (D.W.S. and W.H.M.) and others[496] believe that a significant degree of improvement should occur

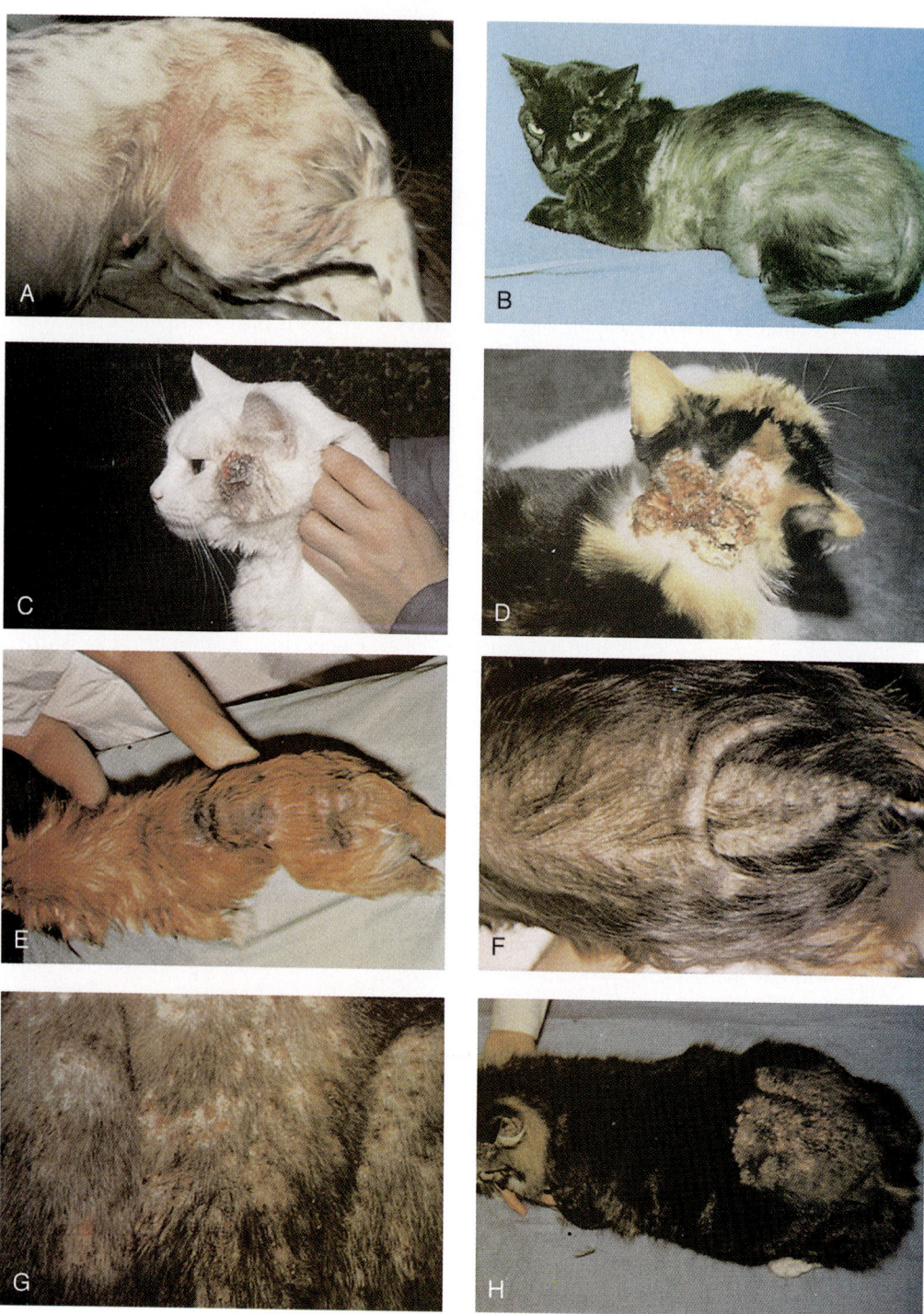

FIGURE 8-12. *A*, Erythema and alopecia over the lateral thighs of a dog with food hypersensitivity. *B*, Hypotrichosis of trunk and rump due to hair pulling in a cat with food hypersensitivity. *C*, Feline food hypersensitivity due to milk. Severe excoriation of the preauricular area. *D*, Feline food hypersensitivity due to fish. Severe excoriation of the neck. *E*, Chronic flea bite hypersensitivity in a Pekingese, showing alopecia, hyperpigmentation, and lichenification on the lower back and tail base. *F*, Canine flea bite hypersensitivity. After many seasons of affliction, areas of the lower back and tail become hairless, thickened, gray, and folded. *G*, Feline flea bite hypersensitivity. The individual miliary lesions are shallow excoriations covered with a small brown crust. Some crusts have been removed to show the lesion's base. *H*, Feline flea bite hypersensitivity. Numerous miliary lesions clustered on the back of a cat. Area has been clipped to expose lesions.

within 4 to 6 weeks, though maximum improvement may take 10 to 13 weeks. In another study of 20 dogs, 95% of dogs improved within 3 weeks or less.[500]

Hypoallergenic diets must be individualized for each patient on the basis of careful dietary history. However, hidden antigens must also be considered because some canned fish in water contain other proteins, such as vegetable and whey proteins present in canned tuna and hot dogs.[61] The objectives of the diet are (1) to feed the animals dietary substances that they are not commonly exposed to and (2) to feed the animals a diet that is free of additives (colorings, flavorings, preservatives). Switching from one commercial diet to another, or using commercially prepared "hypoallergenic" diets, is often not satisfactory. Frequently used components of a hypoallergenic diet include lamb, filleted whitefish, canned tuna fish in water, rabbit, venison, turkey, rice, potatoes, ostrich, yams, and pinto beans, depending on the dietary history.[67a, 488, 499, 528] These diets are usually not adequately balanced and, in young growing dogs, should not be fed without supplements.[522] Because the calcium content of such diets is particularly low, a nondairy calcium source as well as vitamins and essential fatty acids, at the minimum, should be added to the diet.

An alternative protocol, though not as accurate as feeding a carefully selected home-prepared diet, is to feed a commercially prepared, limited, and novel protein source diet. It has been suggested that one reason these commercial diets may not be as effective as home-prepared diets is contamination from processing in equipment used to make other foods.[490] Another concern is that the source of animal fats added to many of these diets could be contaminated with animal proteins other than those in the limited protein source. In young dogs, this may be preferred until they are older than 10 to 12 months, when the risks of a nonbalanced diet would be less.

A variety of limited and novel protein diets are now being manufactured by several companies, and they are very attractive because they are convenient and nutritionally complete.[492] Iams offers a fish and potato diet (Response f/p) as well as a kangaroo and oats diet (Response k/o). Innovative Veterinary Diets (IVD) offers a potato-based food with several novel proteins available, such as duck, lamb, venison, or rabbit; Waltham offers chicken and rice limited protein diets, and Master Foods offers a capelin (a type of fish in the salmon family) and tapioca dog food. Hills Pet Products Science Diets offer rice with egg, lamb, salmon, or duck dry dog foods.

New foods are constantly being produced, and the practitioner should intermittently check dog food companies at meetings, by telephone, or via their websites. It is critical, however, to understand that the reliability of these commercially prepared diets has either not been confirmed (the usual situation) or confirmed in limited trials in known food-hypersensitive dogs. Only a few studies have looked at the efficacy of some of these limited protein dog foods and, to date, none of the diets is 100% effective.

When known food-hypersensitive dogs were fed canned d/d (lamb and rice) or dry d/d (egg and rice) manufactured by Hill's Pet Products, 15% to 25% became pruritic again.[508, 520, 528] A study with a fish and potato diet (Response f/p, Iams) indicated that 50% of the previously confirmed food-hypersensitive dogs were more pruritic on this diet, and in 25% of the dogs the worsening of the clinical signs was confirmed to be due to the fish.[524] Capelin and tapioca (Pedigree canine selected protein 3, Master Food, Austria) was effective in 93.7% of food-hypersensitive dogs.[525] The differences in fish-based diets may reflect that, in humans, fish hypersensitivity may be limited to certain families or even species of fish.[523]

The commercial diets vary in the number of proteins as well as in their digestibility, and it has been recommended that diets with high digestibility be used.[521] Complete digestion results in the production of free amino acids and small peptides, which are probably poorer antigens.[521] Newer "hypoallergenic" diets have been formulated utilizing hydrolyzed proteins in an attempt to supply an adequate protein source that will not be capable of stimulating a food hypersensitivity. Exclude Veterinary Exclusion Diet (DVM Pharmaceuticals) utilizes hydrolyzed liver and casein and novel carbohydrate sources of pinto beans and oat groats; and CNM-HA (Purina) utilizes hydrolyzed soybean protein and corn starch so that the carbohydrate source will also have limited antigenicity. Though limited studies by the companies that have developed these diets suggest they may be beneficial, further independent work is needed. It has been suggested that the size of allergenic proteins in dogs may be smaller than it is in humans.

Feeding a strict diet is critical, and the dog's owner must be counseled to allow nothing but water and the limited diet to enter the dog's mouth. We see many referred dogs whose owners have become frustrated because they think that food hypersensitivity has been ruled out. However, on closer questioning, it is often determined that the dog is still eating the offending foods. The dogs may still be receiving treats such as rawhide chewies, flavored dietary supplements or medicines, or medication in food, such as cheese or a piece of hot dog. It must be remembered that medicines and supplements in gelatin (parts and pieces of cattle, swine, or horses) capsules must be withheld during the dietary trial. It is also important that the possibility of eating items while outside is eliminated and that all family members follow the diet guidelines.

Following a strict diet may be very difficult or impossible for some owners. In one study, 37% of owners that had been thoroughly counseled and thought they could provide an appropriate home-cooked diet dropped out prior to finishing the 8-week trial.[524] The major clinical sign being evaluated during the elimination diet is the pruritus. The level of pruritus should markedly decrease, but this may be gradual and may take 4 to 8 weeks to become evident. Because up to 75% of food-hypersensitive dogs have other concurrent hypersensitivities (especially atopy or flea bite hypersensitivity), the response to a hypoallergenic diet may be partial (for instance, 50% reduction in pruritus).[491, 493, 506, 513, 520] In other dogs, the pruritus may only decreased 25% to 50%, but the pattern of the pruritus may change.[499] The diagnosis is then highly suspected by feeding the animal its normal diet and seeing the dermatosis exacerbate in 10 to 14 days.[497, 506, 517]

In our experience, most well-documented cases of canine food hypersensitivity with multiple positive challenges have a recurrence of pruritus within 3 to 7 days. Rapid recurrences, though not given in days, were typical in another study.[509] Possibly, the cases requiring longer challenges represent food intolerance, which may be more dose related. As soon as an exacerbation is noted, the offending diet is discontinued. It is also important to then feed the hypoallergenic diet again, without any other therapeutic changes, and to see the lesions again resolve, confirming the diagnosis of food hypersensitivity. In general, dogs that experienced exacerbation within 2 days will only have to be back on the hypoallergenic diet a few days to again see the lesions or pruritus resolve. In humans, three positive challenges that are double-blinded and placebo-controlled are required to definitively document a food reaction because there is a significant placebo effect.[523]

When home-cooked diets are used, dogs may lose weight, be hungry, and experience a dull hair coat and scaly skin. Secondary infections must be controlled or response to the diet cannot be evaluated. Some dogs may experience new dietary sensitivities within 1 to 3 years.[496, 529]

Routine laboratory tests are not useful in diagnosing canine food hypersensitivity. Blood eosinophilia is rare in the dog.[61, 67a, 488] Prick, scratch, intradermal, and serologic (RAST, ELISA, VARL) tests with food allergens in dogs with food hypersensitivity are very inaccurate.[495, 497, 508, 511, 514, 527] In one study, about 75% of all normal dogs, dogs with various dermatoses, and dogs with food hypersensitivity experienced positive serologic (RAST, ELISA) test results for one or more foods.[527] Hence, serologic tests have a high sensitivity but a very low specificity. A monoclonal IgE ELISA (CMG Immunodot) was evaluated in proven food-hypersensitive dogs and yielded negative results in all instances, yielding a sensitivity of 0% and a positive predictive value of 0%.[514]

The lack of utility of these tests may reflect (1) different immunologic mechanisms at play (serologic tests only evaluate type I hypersensitivity) or (2) testing with inappropriate antigens (processing and digestion). One group of investigators was unable to demonstrate antigen-specific IgE antibodies in the serum of proven food-hypersensitive dogs using the P-K and oral P-K tests.[507] Numerous factors may influence the applicability of whole food extracts for skin testing and serologic testing, including the effects of cooking, processing, digestion, metabolism, additives, and contaminants on the original whole food substance. Gastroscopic food sensitivity testing has been described.[494, 503, 515] This modality would be inconvenient for routine clinical use, and further studies need to be conducted to determine its usefulness. The basophil degranulation test has also shown some promise for the diagnosis of food hypersensitivity, but larger, controlled studies are needed.[57, 58] This test is not currently available in the United States, requires rapid and special handling of blood, is very labor intensive, and is unlikely ever to be more than a research tool. New techniques may make this type of testing more available in the future.

Histopathology

Skin biopsy reflects the variability of the gross morphology of skin lesions. It is usually characterized by varying degrees of superficial perivascular dermatitis (pure, spongiotic, hyperplastic), with mononuclear cells or neutrophils usually predominating (Fig. 8–13A).[28, 67a, 83] Histopathologic changes consistent with secondary bacterial pyoderma, *Malassezia* dermatitis, or both of these are common. Occasionally, eosinophils are present, and an eosinophilic vasculitis may also occur in rare cases.[163] One dog with food hypersensitivity demonstrated an epitheliotropic lymphocytic infiltrate that mimicked epitheliotropic lymphoma (mycosis fungoides) immunophenotypically.[498] This confirms the variability that may occur histologically as well as clinically and emphasizes the need for a hypoallergenic trial prior to making a diagnosis of epitheliotropic lymphoma.

CLINICAL MANAGEMENT

The prognosis for food hypersensitivity is usually good. Therapy consists of avoiding offending foods or using systemic antipruritic agents. Once a hypoallergenic diet has been effective and challenge has confirmed the diagnosis, most clients will want to switch to a limited novel protein commercial diet. In general, we prefer provocative exposure testing to determine which ingredients are responsible. This allows the pet to eat a more varied diet in the future.

Hypoallergenic diets are formulated by adding single foodstuffs to the diet, one at a time, and evaluating each item for 10 to 14 days. In this way, a tolerable, varied diet can

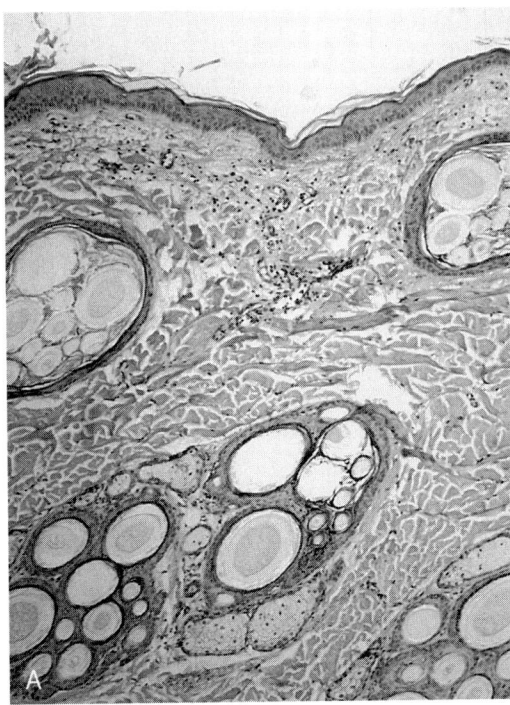
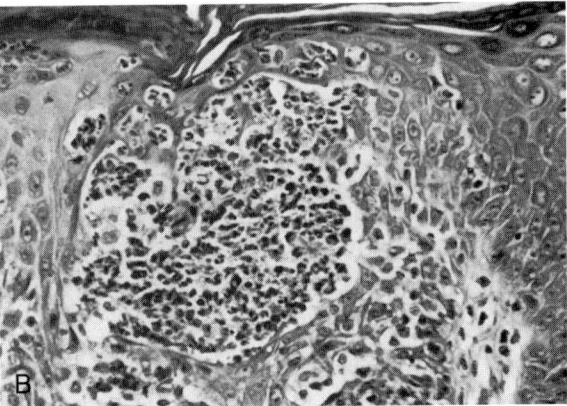

FIGURE 8–13. *A,* Canine food hypersensitivity (beef). Predominantly lymphocytic superficial perivascular dermatitis. *B,* Canine flea bite hypersensitivity. Epidermal eosinophilic microabscess.

usually be achieved over the course of 4 to 6 months. Such diets need to be balanced with vitamin, mineral, and fatty acid supplements prior to this prolonged challenge. Nonflavored, animal and vegetable protein-free vitamin supplements should be added, as well as calcium.[521] If the protein fraction is equal in quantity to the carbohydrate fraction, then calcium carbonate (2 g for 15 kg/day) may be used. As a compromise, animals can be "provoked" daily, for 10 to 14 days at a time, by being fed each of the major food items reported to cause food hypersensitivity in dogs (beef, dairy products, wheat, soy, corn, chicken, egg) to determine whether one or more of these items exacerbates the condition.[488, 506, 509] On the basis of information obtained from this provocation, a commercial food that does not contain the offending substance(s) can usually be selected. About 20% of food-hypersensitive dogs, however, cannot consume any commercial diet and must be maintained on a home-prepared diet.[493, 513, 517, 528] Occasionally, animals experience further dietary hypersensitivities and require re-evaluation by elimination diets and test meal investigations.

When hypoallergenic diets are not feasible, systemic glucocorticoids and/or antihistamines may be used to suppress clinical signs. Food hypersensitivity, however, may be difficult to control with these drugs. A complete response to systemic glucocorticoids occurs in only 50% of food-hypersensitive dogs.[491, 493, 506, 517]

Feline Food Hypersensitivity

Feline food hypersensitivity (food allergy, food intolerance) is a nonseasonal pruritic skin disorder of cats that has been described for many years.[61, 67a, 501] This condition is described as both uncommon and the third most common hypersensitivity in the cat. The reported incidence ranges from 1% to 6% of all feline dermatoses.[67a, 491, 493] It has also been described as being relatively more common in cats than in dogs.[512] A report of 34 cats with the cutaneous reaction patterns of miliary dermatitis, eosinophilic granuloma complex, and self-induced alopecia indicated that food hypersensitivity was the second most common cause, accounting for 17% of cases.[420] Flea bite hypersensitivity was diagnosed in 70% and atopy in 13% of the cats, respectively. In a prospective study of 25 cats recruited from referring veterinarians for suspicion of food hypersensitivity, 20 completed a diet trial and provocation and none was found to respond to a restricted protein (chicken and rice) commercial diet trial.[439] Additionally, 14 of these cats underwent intestinal permeability measurement and 13 were normal. Thirty five percent had flea bite hypersensitivity alone, and 35% had concurrent flea bite hypersensitivity and atopy. In another prospective evaluation of 61 pruritic cats and 12 cats with pruritus and vomiting or diarrhea, food hypersensitivity was pursued using diet trials with rice and chicken or venison and rice, as well as provocative exposure.[533] Food hypersensitivity was confirmed in 16% of the pruritic cats and in 42% of the pruritic cats with concurrent gastrointestinal signs. Such conflicting results suggest that further studies are warranted to determine the prevalence of these diseases.

CAUSE AND PATHOGENESIS

A type I hypersensitivity has been documented to occur in the cat.[526] The same report, however, also showed that IgG may also have been involved in the pathogenesis. It has also been shown that endoparasitism in cats with *Toxocara cati* at the time of oral antigen challenge increases the production of allergen-specific IgE.[531] There also is the induction of IgG and IgA. The presence of concurrent flea bite hypersensitivity, atopy, contact hypersensitivity, or a combination of them suggests that a predisposition to allergies of any type may be a factor.[491, 512, 517] It additionally suggests that the mechanism may involve more than a type I hypersensitivity because the associated diseases vary in their allergic mechanism.

In most clinical cases, the pathomechanism is not determined and, in fact, only the association between diet and pruritus or dermatitis is established. Food intolerance, as discussed in the dog, may also play a role in the pathogenesis. Very little controlled work

● Table 8–23	SUBSTANCES REPORTED TO HAVE CAUSED FOOD HYPERSENSITIVITY IN THE CAT
Dairy products (milk, cheese)	Lamb and mutton
Fish	Eggs
Beef	All commercial foods (various proteins, as well as preservatives and dyes)
Pork	Clam juice
Chicken	Cod liver oil
Rabbit	Benzoic acid
Horse meat	

has been done regarding the offending allergens or materials in the diets that result in the dermatitis. In two studies, provocative exposure testing showed fish, beef, and dairy products to be the most common allergens.[532, 538] In two studies, about 30% of the food-hypersensitive cats were unable to eat any commercially prepared diet without experiencing pruritus and dermatitis.[535, 538] Other studies have strongly implicated even such things as clam juice and lamb baby food.[491, 526, 534, 535] The frequent use and ready availability of commercial diets that contain lamb or other unusual protein sources is likely to induce some allergic reactions and make selecting a test diet more difficult. We and others[534] have seen cats present with or experience food hypersensitivity to lamb, both home-cooked and that found in commercial products. Table 8–23 lists all the foods currently reported to have caused food hypersensitivity in the cat.

CLINICAL FEATURES

The mean age of onset of feline food hypersensitivity is 4 to 5 years, with no age predilection documented. In one study, however, 46% of the cats experienced the disease by 2 years of age.[535] Siamese or Siamese cross cats may be at risk because they accounted for 30% of the cases in two studies,[491, 535] and in one study such cats had a relative risk factor of 5.0.[535] No sex predilection has been documented.

The most consistent clinical finding is pruritus, which is present in 100% of such cases. The pruritus is typically nonseasonal. Some cat owners like to rotate the commercial diets fed to their cats so as to provide variety, however. This practice can result in an irregularly recurrent pruritic dermatosis. Pruritus most commonly involves the face (see Fig. 8–12C), head, pinnae, and neck (see Fig. 8–12D), or combinations of these.* Generalized pruritus may also occur.[30, 61, 67a, 512] The other common cutaneous reaction patterns are self-induced alopecia (see Fig. 8–12B), miliary dermatitis, and eosinophilic granuloma complex lesions. Some cats develop an exfoliative dermatitis characterized histologically by a lymphocytic mural folliculitis (see Chap. 11). Rarely, cats manifest an erythematous papulopustular eruption characterized clinicopathologically as a sterile eosinophilic folliculitis and furunculosis.[454, 455] Other reported nonpruritic signs are angioedema, urticaria, and conjunctivitis.[30, 535] Gastrointestinal (usually diarrhea but also vomiting) disease is present in 10% to 15% of cases.[61, 67a, 532] In a prospective study of 73 pruritic cats, 33% of the food hypersensitive cats had concurrent gastrointestinal signs.[533]

Lymphocytic-plasmacytic colitis may be a manifestation of food hypersensitivity in cats.[530] In one cat with abdominal alopecia from excessive grooming and chronic diarrhea, alimentary lymphosarcoma was diagnosed on two occasions from biopsy taken by duodenoscopy, but the cat responded to an elimination diet.[537] Sneezing, malaise, and dullness have been reported.[61, 67a, 491] Peripheral lymphadenopathy, which can be quite marked, may be present.[453] Up to 25% of food-hypersensitive cats have other concurrent hypersensitivities, especially atopy or flea bite hypersensitivity.[491, 535] These multiple hypersensitivities can greatly complicate the diagnostic work-up. About 50% of food-hypersensitive cats do not completely respond to systemic glucocorticoids.[491, 493, 535]

---

*See references 492, 493, 513, 532, 535, 538, 539.

DIAGNOSIS

The differential diagnosis varies according to the clinical presentation. The most common alternatives are atopy, flea bite hypersensitivity, psychogenic alopecia and dermatitis, dermatophytosis, otodectic mange, cheyletiellosis, and notoedric mange. The diagnosis is suggested by using an elimination diet trial that results in a significant reduction in the clinical signs. The diagnosis is confirmed if clinical signs recur when the cat is fed its previous diet.

Hypoallergenic diets must be individualized for each cat according to previous dietary history. Some common favorites are lamb or ham baby food, ham, ostrich, ground rabbit, lobster, and venison. One of these may be fed alone or mixed in a blender with potato or rice. Studies have shown that these diets are not nutritionally balanced, and feeding them to young growing animals could lead to a deficiency disease.[522] Therefore, it may be prudent to recommend that the diet be at least supplemented with taurine tablets, calcium tablets (dicalcium phosphate), safflower oil, and a multiple vitamin that does not contain additives.

Commercially prepared "hypoallergenic" diets are not reliable. In some cases, however, such a diet is all the client will agree to try. In these cases, a canned diet may be more preferable to dry diets because there are less preservatives.[490] These diets also appear to be more palatable to cats. Examples of canned diets for cats include lamb with carbohydrates diets (Hills prescription d/d, rice; Innovative Veterinary Diet, potato; Iams response formula l/b, barley; Wysong, rice and quinoa). Innovative Veterinary Diets also make potato with venison or rabbit. Dry cat foods similar to most of the canned diets may be found. In these instances, the client should be told that negative results do not rule out the possibility of food hypersensitivity and that a diet with totally different ingredients from the cat's previous diet should be used.

The number of commercially prepared "hypoallergenic" diets is increasing daily, or so it seems.[492] It is essential to remember that, with very few exceptions, these diets have not been scientifically evaluated in confirmed food-hypersensitive cats. To our knowledge, only two commercial diets have been evaluated in cats—canned d/d for dogs and feline d/d, manufactured by Hill's Pet Products—and about 20% of the cats became pruritic and dermatitic while consuming these products.[536, 538] A capelin (fish) and tapioca dry cat food was also evaluated and was effective in three of three cats.[525] However, this diet is not very palatable to cats. A chicken and rice diet failed to document food hypersensitivity in any of 20 cats with compatible clinical signs.[439] Baby foods have often been used as hypoallergenic foods.[67a] However, baby foods with added onion powder are to be avoided because they can induce Heinz body anemia in cats.[510] In many cases, to adequately perform the dietary trial, the cat may have to remain completely indoors.[512] Studies have shown that the previously recommended 3-week dietary trial is not adequate.[491, 493, 535] Improvement may occur rapidly, gradually, or late, but the diet should be continued for 9 to 13 weeks so that maximum response is achieved. Cats that have concurrent atopy or flea bite hypersensitivity show a partial response. To confirm the diagnosis, the cat is then fed its former diet for 10 to 14 days to see whether the pruritus or dermatitis is reproduced.[493, 535]

Intradermal allergy testing and serologic tests are thought to suffer from the same problems as discussed for canine food hypersensitivity—that is to say, they are *worthless!*

Histopathology

Skin biopsy is not diagnostic but is especially useful for ruling out other diagnostic possibilities.[28, 67a, 83, 455] The histopathologic findings are quite variable, as are the clinical lesions (see Feline Atopy). The most common reaction pattern is a superficial or deep perivascular dermatitis wherein eosinophils are the dominant inflammatory cell.[455] Some cases lack eosinophils, whereas others are primarily composed of a dense infiltrate of mast cells that may be misinterpreted as mast cell neoplasia.[28] Eosinophilic folliculitis and furunculosis occasionally is a feature of feline food hypersensitivity.[28, 455] Biopsy specimens from eosinophilic granuloma complex lesions show the typical histopathologic findings for those lesions (see Chap. 18). Some cats have a lymphocytic mural folliculitis (see Chap. 11).

CLINICAL MANAGEMENT

The optimal treatment for feline food hypersensitivity is the avoidance of the offending allergen(s). This is best accomplished by feeding a limited protein source commercial diet, alleviating the problem of having to balance a home-prepared diet. Examples of limited-protein diets are Feline d/d (Hill's Pet Products); the Innovative potato-based diets with rabbit, lamb, duck, and venison; Waltham's limited protein diets with capelin and tapioca, or chicken and rice; chicken formula cat food (Iams). Fortunately, the pet food industry has been responding to this problem by developing new diets with atypical protein sources in them. About 30% of food-hypersensitive cats, however, cannot be successfully managed with any commercially prepared diet.[535] It is especially important that a home-prepared diet to be fed in the long term be balanced and, at the minimum, supplemented with calcium, taurine, essential fatty acids, vitamins, and minerals. The supplements required depend on the diet, and consultation with a nutrition text or nutritionist may be necessary.

A hypersensitivity to a component of the new diet may develop,[534] and it has been suggested that this development is more common in cats than dogs.[512] One of us (C.E.G.) has seen a cat that experienced new allergies to three consecutive diets over 2 years, at which point the client elected to treat with glucocorticoids for the long term. In other situations, avoidance is impossible because the cat is outdoors and finds other sources of allergenic substances to eat. In these cases, systemic glucocorticoids, antihistamines, or fatty acids may be used (see Chap. 3). The efficacy of antihistamines and fatty acids for the management of food-hypersensitive cats has not been reported. In cases that require high levels of systemic glucocorticoids or that do not respond to them, however, antihistamines and fatty acids may have a beneficial effect.

Parasitic Hypersensitivity

Parasites are known to be potent inducers of IgE and often elicit an eosinophilic response.[29, 30] Therefore, it is not surprising that they commonly induce hypersensitivity reactions in dogs and cats. Numerous ectoparasites of dogs and cats have types of hypersensitivity as very important and integral parts of their pathogenesis. Most are covered in this chapter, but one classic example of a parasite that creates most of its disease as a result of hypersensitivity is scabies, covered in Chapter 6.

CANINE FLEA BITE HYPERSENSITIVITY

Flea bite hypersensitivity (flea allergy dermatitis) is a pruritic, papular dermatitis in dogs that becomes sensitized to allergens produced by fleas. It is the most common hypersensitivity skin disorder of dogs in parts of the world where fleas are common. In one report looking at the prevalence of fleas and flea hypersensitivity in the United Kingdom in winter, fleas were found in 4.7% to 19.3% of the dogs, and the prevalence of flea bite hypersensitivity ranged from 1.8% to 11.4%.[570] This suggests that approximately half of dogs with fleas experience flea bite hypersensitivity.

Cause and Pathogenesis

Flea saliva and whole flea extracts contain several potentially antigenic substances, including polypeptides, amino acids, aromatic compounds, and fluorescent materials. However, very little flea salivary antigen is present in whole flea extract ($<0.5\%$).[542, 547] These substances are complete antigens and not haptens as was previously described for the guinea pig. Multiple studies have shown that at least 15 different antigens are present.* Gel filtration of flea saliva revealed that allergens were present in a high-molecular-weight fraction (about 4000 to 1,500,000 daltons) and in a highly fluorescent aromatic fraction (<1000 daltons). Individual dogs may react to completely different groups of allergens, though the most consistently reacting allergens appear in the range of 8 to 90 kD.† Only one salivary antigen—at 40 kD—was worthy of "major allergen" designation, binding IgE from about 60% of the dogs.[549] It was also demonstrated that *Ctenocephalides felis felis*, *Pulex irritans*, and *Pulex simulans* shared one or more antigens, and that guinea pigs and human beings sensitized to one type of flea reacted to all species.[67a]

The newest breakthrough has been the development of a new technique for collecting flea saliva and the subsequent studies with the saliva.[547, 548] This led to the purification, characterization, and cloning of a major flea salivary antigen as well as the use of this antigen in intradermal skin testing, serologic testing, and immunotherapy.[547, 548, 562, 566, 567] What still needs to be evaluated is whether any nonsalivary antigens are also important. If they are and they do not cross-react, they would be missed.

Most dogs that are hypersensitive to flea saliva have immediate skin test reactions to the intradermal injection of flea antigen, and these reactions correlate with clinical disease. In one study, allergen-specific IgE to flea saliva correlated with clinical disease, but allergen-specific IgG to flea saliva was very common in dogs and did not correlate with clinical disease.[566] However, another study indicated that antiflea IgE and IgG levels were similar in normal and flea-hypersensitive dogs.[568] One of the cat flea salivary antigens has been cloned and has been designated Ctef1.[567] The genes have been cloned into *Escherichia coli*, and a recombinant source for pure allergen rCtef1 is available (Heska Corporation). This allergen has been shown to be a major allergen in both experimentally induced and naturally occurring flea bite hypersensitivity, with greater than 90% of such dogs reacting. In addition, ELISA inhibition with the rCtef1 allergen removes 90% of the antiflea saliva IgE.

The orderly sequence of flea bite hypersensitivity that develops in guinea pigs does not occur in dogs and cats,[29, 30, 61, 67a] and dogs and cats rarely, if ever, achieve natural desensitization.[61, 67a] Many flea-hypersensitive dogs also experience delayed skin test reactions to flea antigen, and up to 30% experience only a delayed reaction.[30, 67a, 541] Whether or not this is to the same salivary allergen that produces immediate reactions has not been described. Biopsy specimens taken from skin lesions that are 4 to 18 hours old show changes compatible with cutaneous basophil hypersensitivity, and specimens from lesions that are 24 to 48 hours old show changes compatible with a delayed-type hypersensitivity reaction.[30, 551, 556] It has been suggested that late-phase IgE-mediated reactions are also involved in canine flea bite hypersensitivity.[29] It is likely that animals do not experience skin lesions as a result of flea infestation unless they are flea-hypersensitive. Skin samples from flea-hypersensitive dogs and normal dogs were tested for leukotriene C4 levels.[559] Sites tested were from normal-appearing skin that was a control site or injected with flea antigen or bacterial lipopolysaccharide. Surprisingly, all three sites had significantly less leukotriene C4 in the flea-hypersensitive dogs.

Studies of intradermal skin test reactions to flea antigen and of the serum levels of antiflea IgE and IgG in flea-naive dogs, experimentally maintained dogs, as well as dogs kept as pets or in animal shelters, with and without flea bite hypersensitivity, have indicated that dogs continually exposed to fleas and flea-naive dogs have low antibody levels and negative intradermal test reactions compared with flea-hypersensitive dogs.[29, 30, 555] These observations suggest that continually exposed dogs may become partially or completely immunologically tolerant. Experimentally, intermittent flea exposure was shown to induce both immediate and delayed intradermal reactions, and converting from intermittent to continuous exposure did not eliminate these reactions.[29, 30, 555] It has been sug-

---

*See references 29, 30, 67a, 517, 549, 550, 556, 563, 564, 568.
†See references 29, 547, 549, 550, 563, 564, 568.

gested that, if a dog has an abundance of fleas and no evidence of a hypersensitivity reaction, it might be prudent to refrain from introducing a diligent flea-control program.[30, 67a]

Whereas up to 40% of the normal dog population in flea-endemic areas may have positive intradermal skin test reactions to flea antigen, up to 80% of the atopic dogs in the same area may be positive.[29, 30] This finding suggests that the atopic state may predispose dogs to flea bite hypersensitivity. In other studies, however, only 14% to 36% of atopic dogs were also flea hypersensitive.[386, 541] This may partly relate to flea exposure because one of us (C.E.G.) has looked at flea-positive incidence in atopic dogs in southern California versus Las Vegas, a flea-free environment. Less than 10% of positive flea reactions were found in the Nevada dogs, with most having history of traveling to flea environments. In contrast, multiple surveys over years in the southern California dogs have shown that more than 50% react positively to fleas, though not all of these dogs prompted a clinical diagnosis of flea hypersensitivity.

Clinical Features

Most authors indicate that no breed or sex predilections are apparent.[61, 67a] In a French study, however, Setters, Fox terriers, Pekingese, spaniels, and Chow Chows were predisposed.[571] Although dogs may experience flea bite hypersensitivity at any age, it is rare for clinical signs to develop in animals less than 6 months of age. The most common age of onset is 3 to 5 years.

Canine flea bite hypersensitivity is characterized by a pruritic, papular dermatitis.[61, 67a, 541, 565] The flea bite induces a wheal or papule that persists for up to 72 hours. Crusts may develop on the surface of the papules. Chronic pruritus may lead to alopecia, lichenification, crusting, and hyperpigmentation. Lesions are typically confined to the dorsal lumbosacral area, caudomedial thighs, ventral abdomen, and flanks (see Fig. 8–12E and F). One study showed dorsal lumbar involvement in only 76% of flea-hypersensitive dogs, but this was not a distinguishing feature because 39% of atopic dogs also had dorsal lumbar involvement.[180] This study showed that facial involvement also occurred in 34% of the dogs with flea-bite hypersensitivity, but that paw disease was present in only 1.2% of the dogs. Crusted papules in the umbilical area may be particularly suggestive of flea bite hypersensitivity.

Generalized cutaneous signs may be present in severely hypersensitive animals. Pyotraumatic dermatitis ("hot spots"), secondary bacterial pyoderma, and secondary seborrhea are common in chronic cases. Owing to the constant, excessive chewing, some dogs wear down their incisors. Fibropruritic nodules occasionally occur in chronic cases and are usually present in the dorsal lumbar area (see Chap. 20).

The presence of otitis externa or pedal pruritus strongly suggests the presence of another concurrent hypersensitivity, such as atopy or food hypersensitivity.[67a] This has been supported by two studies.[180, 248] Flea bite hypersensitivity may be distinctly seasonal (summer and fall) in areas of the world with cold winters, though one study showed that disease may be present year round, even in these climates.[570] In warm climates, or where household infestation persists, flea bite hypersensitivity may be nonseasonal, although clinical signs are still usually more severe in summer and fall.

Diagnosis

The differential diagnosis includes food hypersensitivity, atopy, drug reaction, pediculosis, cheyletiellosis, intestinal parasite hypersensitivity, *Malassezia* dermatitis, and bacterial folliculitis.

Definitive diagnosis is based on history, physical examination, intradermal skin testing with flea antigen, and response to therapy. The morphology and distribution of the skin lesions are very suggestive. The presence of fleas or flea dirt is also a helpful, optimal finding. It has also been suggested that a diagnosis requires evidence of fleas.[20] A recent bath or dip or vigorous grooming, however, may eliminate the fleas and flea dirt. In fact, 15% of dogs with flea bite hypersensitivity do not have evidence of flea infestation (fleas, flea excrement) at the time of examination.[541] In our opinion, not finding evidence of fleas does not rule out the diagnosis, but it does cause one to question the diagnosis. More importantly, the mere presence of fleas on a pruritic dog does not mean the animal has flea bite hypersensitivity. In fact, the diagnosis of flea hypersensitivity does not preclude the presence of another disease. When fleas consistently are not seen on flea-hypersensitive dogs and the client has performed adequate flea control, the persistence of pruritus should prompt the clinician to look for a concurrent hypersensitivity such as atopy or food hypersensitivity. Eosinophilia is often present.[67a]

- **Allergy Testing.** Intradermal testing is an excellent method to help confirm the diagnosis of flea bite hypersensitivity. In the United States, one commercial aqueous flea antigen (Flea Antigen, Greer Laboratories) has emerged as a very reliable product.[30, 61, 67a] This product is injected intradermally (0.05 ml of 1:1000 w/v aqueous solution), along with positive (histamine) and negative (saline) controls, and skin reactions are read at 15 and 30 minutes and at 12, 24, and 48 hours. The majority of flea-hypersensitive dogs have both immediate and delayed reactions. About 30% have only delayed reactions. The delayed reactions are often very mild compared with the typical immediate reaction. The only change may be mild erythema or increased dermal thickness.

Other investigators have evaluated the Greer flea antigen in normal and flea-hypersensitive dogs.[573] Three grading systems were used to assess positive intradermal reactions: (1) an intradermal reaction at least 3 mm larger than the negative control, (2) an intradermal reaction at least 5 mm larger than the negative control, and (3) an intradermal reaction at least equal to the half-way point between size of the positive and negative control reactions. The grading system wherein a positive reaction was defined as being at least 5 mm larger than the negative control was the most accurate, being positive in 94% of the flea-hypersensitive dogs and none of the normal dogs. When the "half-way point" grading system was used, 100% of the hypersensitive and 67% of the normal dogs showed positive results.

Recently, another whole body flea antigen was tested and the skin threshold concentration was found to be 1000 NU (Noon units)/ml.[574] This antigen was then tested in 21 dogs with skin disease other than flea bite hypersensitivity and 24 flea-hypersensitive dogs with the diagnosis based on clinical findings. Intradermal testing had an sensitivity of 88%, a specificity of 90%, and an overall accuracy of 89% in diagnosing flea hypersensitivity.

It is essential to remember that a positive test reaction only means that the patient has skin-sensitizing antibody or a cellular response to flea antigen. It does not necessarily mean that the patient has clinical hypersensitivity. Thus, although virtually all flea-hypersensitive dogs and cats have positive skin test reactions to flea antigen, so does a portion of the normal dog population, and so do some dogs with other dermatoses. In one study, 24% of normal dogs had positive intradermal reactions to flea antigen.[576a] Two years later, most of these dogs were still normal, suggesting that positive intradermal reactions were not predictive of future flea bite hypersensitivity. Current or recent administration of drugs, especially glucocorticoids and progestogens, can cause false-negative intradermal test reactions. In some cases, a positive reaction in a dog on glucocorticoid therapy is still produced.[558, 565] With negative reactions, however, testing should be repeated after a longer period of steroid withdrawal. It is also recommended to test for house dust or house dust mites at the same time.[43, 67a] This limited intradermal test with saline, histamine, flea, and house dust mite antigens allows for the recognition of many dogs that have concurrent atopy. A positive house dust mite reaction occurs in about 50% of atopic dogs.

In vitro (serologic) tests are offered for diagnosis of flea bite hypersensitivity. Results appear to vary greatly from company to company, and this at least partly reflects the allergen utilized. Most normal and flea-hypersensitive dogs have high levels of IgG reactive with flea salivary proteins, which presents huge technical problems in assays that attempt to measure antiflea IgE.[389] In an experimental laboratory evaluation, the in vitro tests were valuable if the flea antigen was optimized by partial purification.[29] First, they detect only IgE-mediated disease, and up to 30% of flea-hypersensitive dogs primarily have delayed intradermal reactions. Second, in contrast with results with other allergen tests, one of us (C.E.G.) has seen many negative results in flea-hypersensitive dogs that had positive immediate intradermal skin test reactions. Lastly, some normal dogs had positive serologic test results, suggesting that both sensitivity and specificity need to be further evaluated. A recently developed assay utilizes two proprietary technologic breakthroughs in the development of an in vitro flea allergy test for IgE-mediated disease.[566] This study compared 18 flea-hypersensitive dogs with positive intradermal skin test reactions to 49 experimental dogs with no history of flea exposure. The serologic tests had a sensitivity of 78%, specificity of 91%, and overall accuracy of 88% when compared with intradermal skin test results with the same flea salivary antigen.

It appears that a good intradermal test will give better sensitivity with similar accuracy and be faster and less expensive than the in vitro test. Whether these differences reflect that intradermal testing detects more than IgE-mediated disease, or the obvious differences in whole body flea extract versus flea salivary extracts, remains to be determined.

• **Histopathology.** Skin biopsy is nondiagnostic, revealing varying degrees of superficial perivascular (pure, spongiotic, hyperplastic) to interstitial dermatitis, with eosinophils often being a predominant cell type.[28, 67a, 83, 551] In addition, eosinophilic intraepidermal microabscesses in association with epidermal edema and necrosis (epidermal nibbles) may be visible (see Fig. 8–13B). Histopathologic findings consistent with secondary bacterial pyoderma (suppurative folliculitis, intraepidermal pustular dermatitis) are common.

Clinical Management

In general, it has been classically thought that flea bite hypersensitivity in dogs tends to worsen as the animals age. Clinical signs begin a little earlier in the season, persist a little longer, and tend to become progressively more severe. Naturally occurring desensitization is apparently rare. This concept has come into question, however, with some evidence that occasional dogs improve as they age.[29] Additionally, dogs with other concurrent allergies, atopic disease, or food hypersensitivity may tolerate flea exposure much better if those diseases are adequately controlled.

Therapy of flea bite hypersensitivity may include flea control (see Chap. 6), systemic glucocorticoids, and hyposensitization.[565] Of course, the single most effective therapy would be separating the fleas from the pet or eliminating the fleas. This involves concentrating extermination efforts on the indoor and outdoor premises. Aggressive flea control programs are necessary, and newer therapies have made the treatment of flea bite hypersensitivity without glucocorticoids a reality (see Chap. 6).[552, 561] Ultrasonic collars and a recent noninsecticidal metal tag (Catan Dog's tag) on the European market are of no benefit.[546] Light traps assist in monitoring and controlling flea populations.[545, 546] Regular use of a flea comb can dramatically reduce flea populations, especially in shorthaired dogs.[545a] A thorough 10-minute combing can remove 81.5% of fleas.

Some topical therapies have been shown efficacious for flea-hypersensitive dogs. Permethrin spot applications or spray, fipronil (Frontline, Merial), and imidacloprid (Advantage, Bayer) have all been shown effective for flea bite hypersensitivity. However, some outdoor dogs require very aggressive use of these products, and only those that are approved for frequent application (permethrin sprays and imidacloprid) may be used legally in some of these cases. Repellents need to be applied frequently to dogs that visit outdoor areas that cannot be adequately treated for fleas. In one study, neither imidacloprid, fipronil spray, nor fipronil spot-on provided noticeable repellent effect on fleas.[540]

Signs of developing insecticide resistance include (1) clients presenting pruritic flea-hypersensitive dogs that the clinician has not seen since prescribing one of the new insecticides, and (2) clinicians noticing that products that used to control fleas and flea bite hypersensitivity for 1 month now only work for 2 weeks.[569] As resistance develops, it takes longer for fleas to die and they are able to feed and inject antigen. Anecdotal reports from the southern United States indicate that this is occurring, with clinicians indicating that imidacloprid or fipronil now must be applied every 1 to 2 weeks to be totally effective.

Prednisolone or prednisone is given orally at 1 mg/kg daily for 5 to 7 days and then in an alternate-day regimen (see Chap. 3), as needed. Dogs with severe flea bite hypersensitivity and heavy flea exposure may require 2.2 mg/kg daily to achieve remission and then need much higher alternate-day dosages. If glucocorticoids are undesirable or unsatisfactory, some flea-hypersensitive dogs may respond to antihistamines (chlorpheniramine, 0.4 mg/kg q8h orally; diphenhydramine, 2.2 mg/kg q8h orally; or hydroxyzine, 2.2 mg/kg q8h orally) or omega-3/omega-6 fatty acid-containing products (see Chap. 3).

The efficacy of hyposensitization in canine flea bite hypersensitivity is still controversial. Enthusiastic proponents and outspoken critics abound.[61, 67a] Initial double-blind controlled studies in dogs showed that hyposensitization with aqueous[554] and alum-precipitated[557, 572] whole flea antigens is rarely effective as well as being expensive and time-consuming. Hyposensitization was used for only 3 to 4 months in these studies, however, a much shorter time than that used for atopy (see Canine Atopy). A double-blind, placebo-controlled study utilizing C. felis salivary antigens in a rush immunotherapy protocol did show efficacy compared with a placebo-treated group.[562] This study certainly indicated the potential for flea hyposensitization. On the basis of current information, treatment of canine flea bite hypersensitivity with commercially available whole flea extracts should be viewed as a last-ditch therapeutic effort. It would seem most appropriate that, if hyposensitization were to be tried, the flea salivary antigens (Heska Corp.) should be used.

FELINE FLEA BITE HYPERSENSITIVITY

It has long been thought that feline flea bite hypersensitivity (flea allergy dermatitis) is the most common feline hypersensitivity disease in areas where fleas are present, causing a variety of clinical syndromes, all characterized by pruritus.[67a] In one study, 70% of cats referred for suspicion of food hypersensitivity actually had flea bite hypersensitivity alone or with other diseases based on response to flea control.[439] However, in a study of 88 cats with allergic skin disease, 9% had only flea bite hypersensitivity, but 47% had flea bite hypersensitivity as one component of their skin disease, and atopic disease was the most prevalent problem.[444] In the United Kingdom, fleas were found on 18% to 26% of the cats, even in winter.[570] The prevalence of flea bite hypersensitivity in the same study varied from 6% to 14%.

Cause and Pathogenesis

Though much research has been conducted on flea bite hypersensitivity in the dog and guinea pig, very little has been done in the cat.[29, 61, 67a] This is particularly interesting because cats are used to maintain both research and commercial populations of the cat flea, Ctenocephalides felis felis. The guinea pig and dog have very different immunopathogenic responses to flea antigen; therefore, it may be inappropriate to assume that cats will react as the other species would. Most flea-hypersensitive cats have immediate positive intradermal test reactions to flea antigen. Experimental sensitization of cats to flea bites resulted in lesions in all the continuously exposed cats and no lesions in the intermittently exposed cats, which is in contrast with what has been described in dogs.[578] Interestingly, all the intermittently exposed cats experienced positive intradermal skin test reactions, but only 60% had positive in vitro test results with the same flea salivary allergen. Overall, when tested with flea salivary allergen, 88% were positive on intradermal skin testing, and 88% were positive on the serum in vitro assay. Based on intradermal skin test results, the serum test had an overall accuracy of 82%. This study also evaluated one flea-hypersensitive cat serum for heat lability of the positive serum. Heat inactivation at 56°C greatly diminished and heat inactivation at 57°C abolished the reaction, indicating this was a IgE-mediated reaction. In one study, delayed skin test reactions were reported in three of seven flea-hypersensitive cats at both 24 and 48 hours.[577] Even some normal cats with negative intradermal test results have mild histopathologic changes at the site of intradermal flea extract injections or flea bites, suggesting that subclinical reactions occur.[577]

Clinical Features

No age, breed, or sex predilections have been reported. Papulocrustous eruptions are usually considered the most typical lesions of flea bite hypersensitivity in the cat (see Fig.

8–12G).[67a] This cutaneous reaction pattern, called *miliary dermatitis*, is particularly common in cats and may be caused by a number of specific diseases (Table 8–24). However, in one prospective study of perennially pruritic cats, the most prevalent reaction pattern was symmetric alopecia in flea-hypersensitive cats, but papulocrustous lesions were statistically more prevalent in the cats with flea bite hypersensitivity and atopic disease.[439] Alopecia, excoriations, crusts, and scales may also be found. Alopecia may also occur as a result of cats excessively grooming to remove fleas. It has been shown that flea-hypersensitive cats are more effective at removing fleas than flea-naive cats. Additionally, the hypersensitive cats produce an unknown factor that results in the production of fewer flea eggs.[579] Pigment changes may occur, and multifocal small melanotic macules are evidence of previous inflammatory sites. Lesions are typically confined to the dorsal lumbosacral area (see Fig. 8–12H), caudomedial thighs, ventral abdomen, flanks, and neck. Generalized cutaneous signs may be present in severely hypersensitive animals.

Flea-hypersensitive cats may also present with (1) self-induced symmetric alopecia (little or no dermatitis) or (2) eosinophilic granuloma complex lesions (indolent ulcer, eosinophilic plaque, eosinophilic granuloma, or some combination of these three lesions) (see Chap. 18).[61, 67a, 581] In addition, any given cat may manifest various combinations of these reaction patterns. Secondary bacterial pyoderma occurs occasionally. Cats with flea bite hypersensitivity may experience moderate to marked peripheral lymphadenopathy.[453] Rarely, cats manifest an erythematous papulopustular eruption characterized clinicopathologically as a sterile eosinophilic folliculitis and furunculosis.[454] Because infiltrative eosinophilic mural folliculitis occurs at the site of flea bite sites and intradermal injections of flea antigen within 24 hours, this appears to be a reaction to flea antigen.[577] Disease often becomes more severe as the cats age. Cats with flea bite hypersensitivity may have concurrent atopy and/or food hypersensitivity, which can greatly complicate the diagnostic work-up as well as the therapeutic regimen.

Diagnosis

The differential diagnosis depends on which clinical syndrome is being examined. Most commonly, the differential diagnosis for miliary dermatitis (see Table 8–24) must be considered, with atopy, food hypersensitivity, cheyletiellosis, and dermatophytosis being the primary alternatives in most cases. The diagnosis is based on the history and physical findings. The presence of fleas, flea dirt, flea eggs, or infestation with the tapeworm *Dipylidium caninum* all provide circumstantial evidence. Recent bathing or grooming, however, may remove all evidence of fleas. Neither does the mere presence of fleas on a cat with one of the typical cutaneous reaction patterns confirm that the fleas are causing

● Table 8–24 **DIFFERENTIAL DIAGNOSIS OF WIDESPREAD PAPULOCRUSTOUS DERMATITIS ("MILIARY DERMATITIS") IN THE CAT**

Hypersensitivity reactions	Flea bite hypersensitivity
	Atopy
	Food hypersensitivity
	Drug reaction
	Intestinal parasite hypersensitivity
	Pemphigus foliaceus
	Feline hypereosinophilic syndrome
Ectoparasitisms	Cheyletiellosis
	Otodectic mange
	Trombiculosis
	Cat fur mite
	Pediculosis
Infections	Dermatophytosis
	Staphylococcal folliculitis
Dietary imbalances	Biotin deficiency
	Fatty acid deficiency

the dermatosis. Cytologic examination of papulocrustous lesions and eosinophilic granuloma complex lesions usually demonstrates numerous eosinophils and occasional basophils (Fig. 8–14). Eosinophilia, occasionally with basophilia, is often present.

Intradermal allergy testing with flea antigen, as described for the dog, produces a positive immediate reaction.[61, 67a, 578, 580, 581] One should remember that a positive intradermal reaction to flea antigen only means that the cat is sensitized to the antigens; it does not prove that the cat has clinical flea bite hypersensitivity. In one study, 36% of the clinically normal cats that had been exposed to fleas had a positive immediate skin test reaction to flea antigen.[580] In another study, 17% of specific pathogen-free cats also had positive intradermal skin test reactions and serologic test results for flea salivary antigen.[578] It is also useful to test at the same time with house dust mite to investigate the possibility of concurrent atopy.[43, 67a] Limited evaluation of serum in vitro testing for feline flea bite hypersensitivity has shown poor predictive value. However, preliminary studies with the canine $Fc\epsilon\ RI\text{-}\alpha$ receptor-based serologic tests have shown an overall predictive value of 82% and a better correlation with the clinical presentation than did intradermal testing with the same antigen.[578]

- **Histopathology.** Skin biopsy is not diagnostic but typically shows varying degrees of superficial or deep perivascular to interstitial dermatitis with numerous eosinophils and mast cells.[28, 67a, 83, 455, 477] Infiltrative mural eosinophilic folliculitis may be visible at the sites of flea bites and delayed skin test reactions.[577] Cats presenting with clinical lesions of indolent ulcer, eosinophilic plaque, and eosinophilic granuloma have dermatohistopathologic findings consistent with these entities (see Chap. 18).

Clinical Management

Therapy of flea bite hypersensitivity includes vigorous flea control and is most successful in cats kept predominantly indoors or in a controlled environment (see Chap. 6).[67a, 565] Flea control has been revolutionized with the advent of more effective topical and systemic formulations for killing fleas, eggs, and larvae, but still more aggressive therapy may be required for the flea-hypersensitive outdoor cat.[575] For roaming outdoor cats, imidacloprid (Advantage, Bayer) applied every 1 to 2 weeks has been effective for many cases in our experience. Anecdotally, fipronil (Frontline, Merial) is also very effective at more frequent intervals, but this goes against EPA-labeled use and is illegal. Fipronil spray and imidacloprid spot-on are excellent adulticides but did not kill the majority of fleas before they were able to consume at least some quantity of blood.[543] Flea repellents are helpful, but they must be applied daily and are not tolerated by many cats. Regular use of a flea comb can dramatically reduce flea populations, especially in shorthaired cats.[545a] A thorough 10-minute combing can remove up to 81.5% of the fleas.

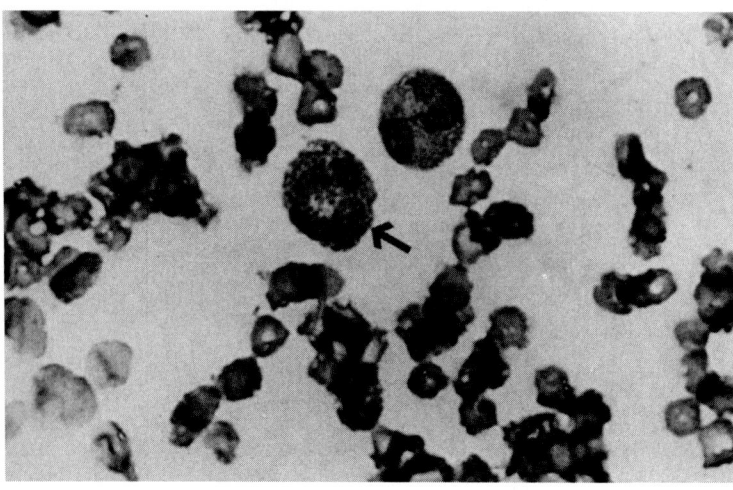

FIGURE 8–14. Feline flea bite hypersensitivity. Cytologic examination reveals numerous eosinophils and smaller numbers of basophils (*arrow*).

Repositol methylprednisolone acetate (5 mg/kg or 20 mg/cat subcutaneously every 12 weeks) or oral prednisone or prednisolone (2.2 mg/kg q24h orally for 5 to 7 days then on an alternate-day basis) is most commonly used for short-term relief of the hypersensitivity or when flea control is ineffective (see Chap. 3). With severe flea infestations, the dosages of these glucocorticoids may have to be doubled or a different glucocorticoid may be needed (see Chap. 3) to achieve an adequate response. Chlorpheniramine (2 to 4 mg/cat q12h orally), clemastine (0.68 mg/cat q12h orally), or hydroxyzine (2 mg/kg q12h orally) may also be effective.[125, 137, 147, 153, 181] Omega-6/omega-3 fatty acid–containing products may also be useful.[108, 128] Hyposensitization in cats has been shown to be ineffective for most cases, though an occasional cat may have a dramatic response.[576]

TICK BITE HYPERSENSITIVITY

Cutaneous hypersensitivity reactions to tick bites have been recognized in dogs and humans.[22, 61, 67a, 592, 598] The proposed pathomechanism of these reactions involves cutaneous basophil hypersensitivity and type III and type IV hypersensitivity responses. No age, breed, or sex predilections have been reported.

Cutaneous hypersensitivity reactions to tick bites in dogs and cats may be characterized by (1) focal areas of necrosis and ulceration, (2) nodules that may or may not be erythematous, pruritic, and ulcerated, and (3) pruritic pododermatitis. Diagnosis is based on history and physical examination.

Skin biopsy may reveal leukocytoclastic vasculitis with hemorrhage, necrosis, and ulceration (type III reaction) or nodular to diffuse dermatitis due to granulomatous or pyogranulomatous inflammation (type IV reaction), often with numerous eosinophils and lymphoid hyperplasia. Tick mouth parts are seldom found in biopsy specimens.

Therapy includes tick removal and control. Surgical excision or glucocorticoids are effective for severe or persistent reactions.

FELINE MOSQUITO BITE HYPERSENSITIVITY

Feline mosquito bite hypersensitivity has been described as a clinical entity in cats.[582–585] The original descriptions of this syndrome came from Australia,[586] but not until 1988 was the etiology confirmed.[583] This is an uncommon, seasonal, predominantly pinnal and facial dermatitis of cats.

Cause and Pathogenesis

Two excellent studies have documented the mosquito as the cause of this syndrome.[583, 585] Lesions were shown to resolve without treatment when affected cats were confined to a mosquito-free environment. After challenge with mosquito bites, lesions developed at the sites of the bites. In addition, previously normal haired skin was shaved and challenged with mosquito bites. Again, these sites developed the typical lesions. Wheals were seen within 20 minutes, papules occurred at 12, 24, and 48 hours, and papulocrustous lesions developed at 48 hours.[585] Intradermal allergy testing with mosquito antigen indicates that one component of the pathogenesis may involve a type I hypersensitivity.[583, 585] In one study, P-K testing results were positive in three of three cats tested and negative with control cat serum.[585] Histopathologic findings, however, include an initially perivascular, then diffuse to nodular dermatitis with an intense eosinophilic infiltrate and foci of collagen flame figures. These latter findings do not occur in typical type I reactions, suggesting that more is involved in the pathogenesis of this disorder.

Clinical Features

To date, no age, breed, or sex predilections have been recognized. The largest reported series of 26 cases had a median age of 3.3 years with a range of 9 months to 8 years.[585] It is interesting to note that all 26 cats in this study had dark hair on their pinnae. The disease is seasonal, coinciding with the mosquito season. Affected cats usually are kept outdoors or allowed access to the outdoors, though the disease has been reported in an indoor cat.[585] Pruritus is usually present, but the severity is variable. The earlier lesions consist of erythematous papules to plaques that often have an erosive or ulcerated, necrotic, or crusted appearance (Fig. 8–15E). Chronic lesions include nodules, pigment changes (melanoderma or, most commonly, leukoderma), alopecia, and scaling (Fig. 8–15F). The development of multiple lesions often results in a polycyclic plaque or patch of alopecia interspersed with areas of acute lesions, scales, or crust. These lesions are usually found on the pinnae (primarily the convex surface, but the concave surface may be affected), bridge of the nose and, rarely, the eyelids and footpads.[583–585] The nasal planum and nasal philtrum may be involved and have small punctate crusted depressions. Footpads may also be affected with swelling, hyperkeratosis, fissures, and pigment changes. Less commonly, the chin and lips may be affected.[582] Lymphadenopathy and, in acute cases, pyrexia may occur.

Diagnosis

The major components of the differential diagnosis are pemphigus foliaceus or erythematosus, atopy, food hypersensitivity, and dermatophytosis. In endemic areas, feline poxvirus infection is also an alternative. The clinical presentation is fairly distinctive, and the tentative diagnosis is relatively well confirmed by keeping the cat indoors or hospitalized for 5 days, at which point the lesions are much improved. If confinement is not possible, the use of repellents on the affected areas may help establish the diagnosis. In other cases, this may be impossible or ineffective, and ruling out other possible diagnoses by biopsy and other laboratory tests helps establish a diagnosis. Peripheral eosinophilia occurred in 16 of 18 cats.[585] Hypergammaglobulinemia was present in all cats tested.[585]

- **Histopathology.** Skin biopsy reveals severe superficial and deep eosinophilic inflammation that is initially perivascular, then interstitial, and finally diffuse.[28, 67a, 583–585] Infiltrative eosinophilic mural folliculitis and furunculosis, dermal mucinosis, and flame figures are often present (Fig. 8–16). The finding of eosinophilic folliculitis and furunculosis is uncommon in eosinophilic granulomas of other causes and, when found in cats and dogs, is more often associated with arthropods bites or insect stings.[584] Similar histopathologic changes can occasionally occur in cats with atopy, food hypersensitivity, and flea bite hypersensitivity.[454, 455]

Clinical Management

Confinement indoors during the mosquito season, or at least during the peak mosquito feeding time, is beneficial. If this is not possible, repositol methylprednisolone acetate (20 mg/cat or 5 mg/kg subcutaneously) is usually effective and relatively safe because this entity is a seasonal problem. Alternatively, oral glucocorticoids may be used (see Chap. 3). In all cases, but especially those in which glucocorticoids cannot be used, mosquito repellents in the form of pyrethrins with MGK 264, dimethyl metatolulimide (DEET), or butoxypolypropylene are helpful. Repellents do not need to be applied to the whole body, only to the shorthaired and sparsely haired areas.

INSECT AND ARACHNID HYPERSENSITIVITY

Numerous insects and arachnids that may stimulate an immune response exist in the normal dog and cat environment.[592, 594, 598] These hypersensitivity reactions induce a pruritic disease that involves short or sparsely haired areas.

Cause and Pathogenesis

Insects and arachnids are known to produce a number of potentially allergenic substances that may be present in their saliva, feces, or exoskeletons (body/wing parts, hairs).[587, 593, 594, 597] Dogs have been shown to develop IgE antibodies to a variety of these allergens.[593, 594] In humans, the insect allergens may be injected (by bite or sting), inhaled, or absorbed percutaneously and induce the allergic reaction.[50] How allergen access occurs in dogs and cats has not been documented but is thought to be similar to what occurs in

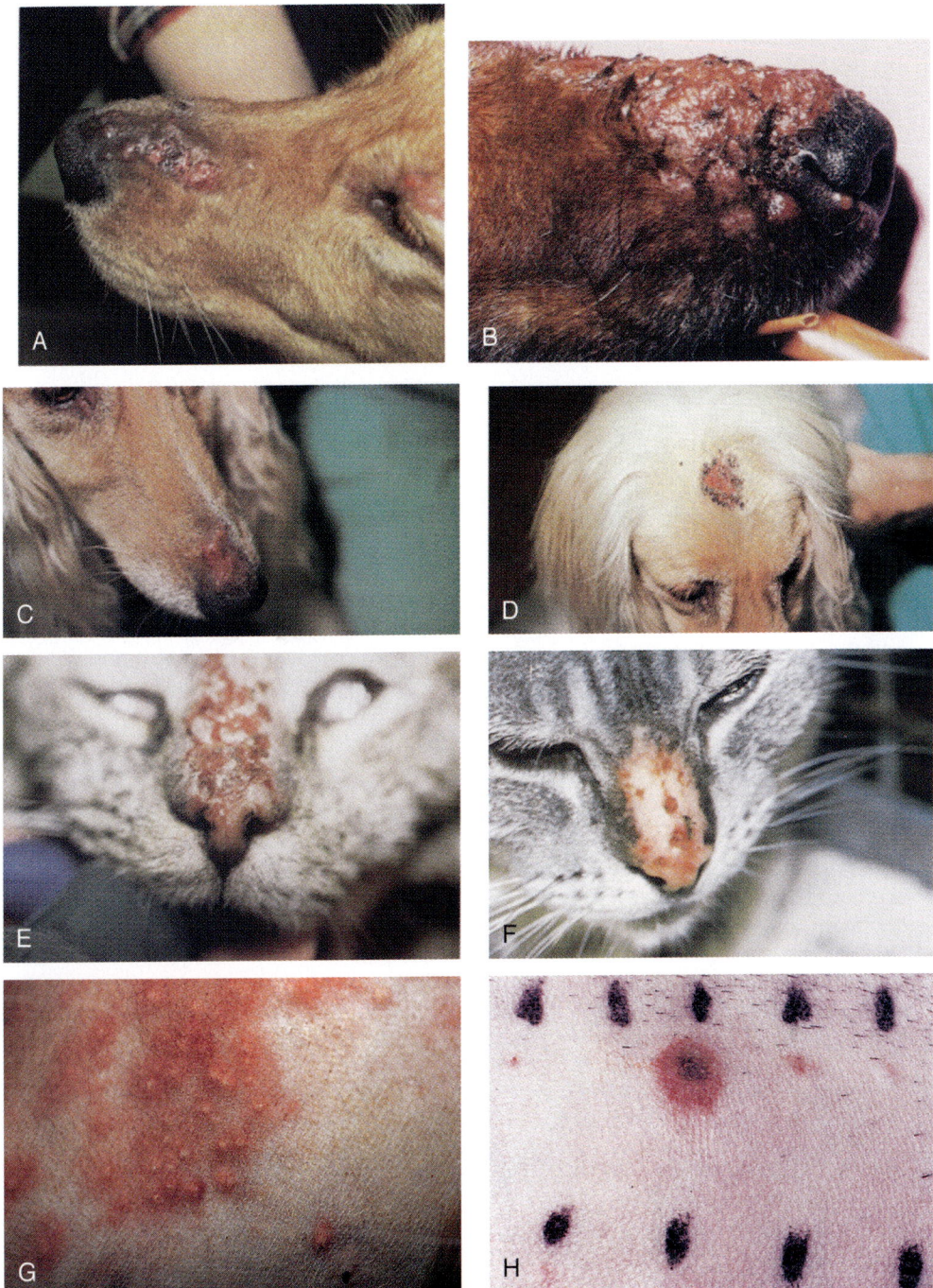

FIGURE 8–15. *A*, Canine eosinophilic furunculosis of the face. Multiple papules and ulcers on the bridge of the nose and upper eyelid associated with exposure to wasps. *B*, Canine eosinophilic furunculosis of the face. Erythematous papules and ulcerated, oozing nasal plaque. (Courtesy of K. V. Mason.) *C*, Erythematous papules on bridge of nose of a dog with cutaneous dirofilariasis. *D*, Ulcerated, crusted nodule on head of a dog with cutaneous dirofilariasis. *E*, Feline mosquito bite hypersensitivity. Plaquelike swelling, ulceration, and depigmentation of bridge of nose and nasal planum. *F*, Feline mosquito bite hypersensitivity. Note presence of mosquito on depigmented, alopecic bridge of nose and nasal planum. (Courtesy of K. V. Mason.) *G*, Multiple erythematous pustules on the abdomen of a dog with bacterial hypersensitivity. (From Scott DW, et al: Staphylococcal hypersensitivity in the dog. J Am Anim Hosp Assoc 14:766, 1978.) *H*, Hemorrhagic bulla skin test reaction 48 hours after the intradermal injection of *Staphylococcus aureus* bacterin-toxoid (Staphoid A-B) in a dog with bacterial hypersensitivity. (From Scott DW, et al: Staphylococcal hypersensitivity in the dog. J Am Anim Hosp Assoc 14:766, 1978.)

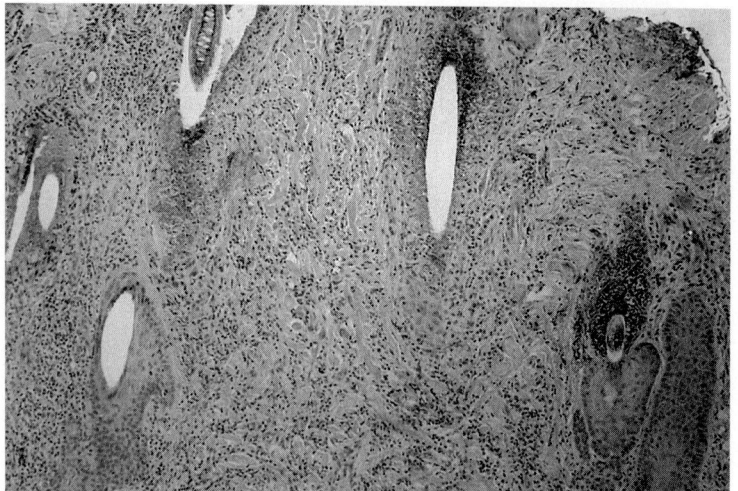

FIGURE 8–16. Feline mosquito bite hypersensitivity. Infiltrative, necrotizing eosinophilic mural folliculitis and furunculosis.

humans. These hypersensitivities are common in atopic animals and may even be considered a subcategory of atopy.

In about 50% of suspected atopic dogs in the southwestern United States that have negative intradermal test reactions to routine allergens (pollens, molds, epithelia, flea, and house dust mites), positive intradermal reactions to one or more insects or arachnids are present.[594] Another report from the eastern United States indicated that results in 15.6% of atopic dogs were negative or only weakly positive to traditionally tested allergens, including flea and house dust mite.[590] Fourteen percent of these dogs with negative or weakly positive results had positive reactions to at least one of the insects tested. In contrast, a study conducted in the northeastern United States determined that results in 63% of the atopic dogs tested with regional aeroallergens and insects were positive to one or more insects, but none of the dogs had a positive reaction for insects alone.[602]

Another study evaluated intradermal injections of insect allergens to flea, fire ant, blackfly, deerfly, horsefly, mosquito, *Culicoides* spp., house dust mite, black ant, caddis fly, cockroach, housefly, and moth.[392] It showed that normal pet dogs had the same incidence of reactions as atopic dogs, except to fleas. This study also tested with a *Dermataphagoides farinae* antigen at 1:50,000 w/v/ml and found no difference in incidence of positive reactions between normal and atopic dogs. This is in contrast with one other study that showed significantly more reactions to *D. farinae* antigen in atopic dogs.[330] In experimental studies on house dust mite reactions in laboratory and normal pet dogs, normal laboratory Beagles were negative to house dust mite antigen, whereas normal house pets were more likely to be positive.[216] This may reflect real IgE reactions that are due to either a clinically insignificant type of IgE or a sensitivity not associated with clinical disease for other reasons.[194, 216] Another study in 15 normal laboratory Beagles recorded no positive reactions to insects with the same allergens that caused numerous positive reactions in 10 atopic dogs.[345, 593]

Cross-reactivity among a variety of insects (house fly, horsefly, deerfly, caddis fly, black fly, black ant, fire ant, moth, mosquito, cockroach, and flea) was evaluated.[601] Black fly, black ant, cockroach, and flea were found to have significant cross-reactivity. Mites such as *Otodectes* and *Sarcoptes* are known to produce hypersensitivity reactions that may cross-react with house dust mites.[278, 375, 595] Though cross-reactivity could explain some cases seen clinically, it still would be expected that, if the animal were hypersensitive to house dust mite, those intradermal test results would be positive as well. More studies are awaited to further evaluate cross-reactivity. Allergens for cockroach are being identified in humans and hopefully will be evaluated in dogs to determine whether they are different.[591]

Further evidence that insect/arachnid hypersensitivity is a real clinical entity would be the response to therapy. One of us (C.E.G.) and others have seen cases with positive insect avoidance/repellent reactions that respond to insect therapy.[590, 592] Even better evidence that this is IgE-mediated hypersensitivity would be beneficial response to hyposensitization. Evidence against this is found in one study that indicated no difference in immunotherapy success rates in two groups of insect-positive dogs when insects were left out or included in the hyposensitization formula.[602] One of us (C.E.G.) has several cases that were only or mainly insect-hypersensitive that have responded to hyposensitization, but further studies are needed to adequately answer this question.

Clinical Features

No age, breed, or sex predilections have been described. The onset may be sudden and occasionally is historically correlated with an increase in insect or arachnid numbers in the animal's environment. The primary symptom is pruritus, though erythematous maculopapular dermatitis may be present. Depending on the offending allergen, these cases may be seasonal, with clinical signs being worst in warm weather. Chronic pruritus can lead to secondary alopecia, crusting, lichenification, and secondary bacterial pyoderma. Occasionally in chronic cases, nodules or firm plaques are present. Glabrous skin or short-haired areas are more commonly affected. As a result, the abdomen, groin, axillae, face, distal extremities, and pinnae are most commonly affected.

Diagnosis

The differential diagnosis consists of atopy, scabies, food hypersensitivity, bacterial folliculitis and furunculosis, and contact hypersensitivity. A helpful feature differentiating this type of hypersensitivity from atopy that may occur in some cases is the presence of a papular dermatitis not associated with bacterial folliculitis.

The diagnosis is suggested by a compatible history and physical findings and is confirmed by positive intradermal test reactions to insect or arachnid antigens. Intradermal allergy testing, as described for atopy, is performed with the antigens listed in Table 8–25. Cytologic examination of a specimen taken from a papule may reveal a mixture of neutrophils and eosinophils.

- **Histopathology.** Histopathology has not been reported for a large group of cases but, in limited numbers of animals, a hyperplastic superficial perivascular dermatitis with mononuclear cells, mast cells, and some eosinophils was found. Nodular and plaque-like lesions show a multinodular lymphocytic to granulomatous dermatitis with numerous eosinophils.

Clinical Management

Avoidance, if possible, is the treatment of choice, but some insect and arachnid allergens are significantly aerosolized during peak seasons, making their avoidance impossible.[597]

- Table 8–25 **RESULTS OF INTRADERMAL TESTS TO INSECTS AND ARACHNIDS IN 193 SUSPECT ATOPIC DOGS***

ANTIGEN	NO. OF DOGS WITH 3 OR 4+ REACTIONS	PNU
Black fly	11.4	1000
Mosquito	7.8	1000
Deer fly	9.3	1000
Horsefly	17.1	1000
Red ant	5.7	1000
Black ant	4.2	1000
Housefly	Not done	1000
Cockroach	Not done	1000

*Southern California.

Avoidance is best accomplished by keeping the animals indoors as much as possible and utilizing an aggressive insect control regimen such as described for flea control (see Chap. 6). Medical management with glucocorticoids is usually effective. Prednisone, 1 mg/kg q24h until the condition is controlled (3 to 7 days), then on an alternate-day regimen, is most commonly used. Antihistamines and fatty acids (see Chap. 3) may also be tried, though their efficacy is not as good.

Storage Mite–Related Hypersensitivity

Storage mites are mites known to infest foodstuffs. Classically, the storage mites belong to the family *Tyroglyphidae*, though other families of mites are also important invaders of foodstuffs. Multiple genera and species exist. These mites infest flour, grains, cereal foods, cheese, dried fruits, dried meats, jams, and jellies. Several of these mites occur in large enough numbers and frequency to be important sources of environmental allergens. The species studied the most in dogs are *Acarus siro, Glycyphagus domesticus*, and *Tyrophagus putrescentiae*.[61, 304, 354, 604] *Acarus siro*, also called the grain or flour mite, is one of the most frequently encountered and feeds on many foodstuffs as well as fungi and molds. *Tyrophagus putrescentiae*, also known as the mold mite or copra mite, is another common food-infesting mite found worldwide that likes foods with high fat or protein content. This mite has been found in most foodstuffs that the other mites are reported to infest, as well as well as brewer's yeast and herring meal, which are frequently added to dog foods. *Glycyphagus domesticus* is also called the grocer's itch mite and furniture mite. It has a food preference for rolled oats, brewer's yeast, and vegetable fibers, including some commonly used as furniture stuffing. It establishes larger infestations with higher moisture levels and is found in association with damp structures and mildew.

With the advent of dog foods containing newer ingredients such as rice, other mites may be important to consider. The scaly grain mite, *Suideasia nesbetti*, is found in rice and bran. The predatory mite, *Cheyletus eruditus*, is the most common predator of the food-infesting mites. This mite may become more prevalent than the grain or mold mite, especially as food is stored at lower moisture contents. In certain situations, there are many other mites that may be more numerous than these common ones. Similar to the situation with house dust mites, regional differences are likely to exist and, if cross-reactivity is poor, other important allergens may be waiting to be identified.

The source of allergen for testing may be as important as which mites one is testing for. One of us (C.E.G.) tested 20 atopic dogs with *Tyrophagus putrescentiae* from HAL in June–July 1995, with only 2 (10%) having a 3+ reaction and no dogs having 2+ or 4+ reactions. During the same two months in 1996, 25 atopic dogs were tested with ALK allergens, and 7 (28%) had 3+ or greater reactions to *T. putrescentiae* and an additional 5 dogs had 2+ reactions. In one study, 36.9% and 55.4% of atopic dogs reacted to intradermal injections of *A. siro* and *T. putrescentiae*, respectively.[192] In Greece, 48.4% of atopic dogs reacted to *A. siro* but, because the prevalence of this mite is very low in Greek homes, it was suggested that this may represent cross-reactivity with *D. farinae* or other mites.[277]

- **Clinical Features.** Clinical presentation appears similar to atopic dermatitis. One report included several dogs presenting primarily for diarrhea.[304] This report also suggested that lip and muzzle pyoderma may be a manifestation of storage mite dermatitis.
- **Diagnosis.** Appropriate clinical signs and intradermal testing are currently the preferred method of making a tentative diagnosis. However, because one major source for these mites is dry dog food, a diet trial to home-prepared or canned dog food may also be conducted.
- **Therapy.** Therapy includes avoidance as well as the routine drugs used for the management of the atopic dog. Specific studies on hyposensitization have not been reported. One pruritic dog with a positive intradermal test reaction to storage mites responded to changing the diet from dry food to canned food only.[588] This dog experienced relapse when challenged with commercial dry dog foods containing lamb and rice but improved when fed home-cooked lamb and rice or canned lamb and rice.

Otodectic Acariasis

Hypersensitivity appears to play a role in some cases of otodectic acariasis (otodectic mange, ear mites) in cats (see Chaps. 6 and 19).[67a, 598] Clinically, cats occasionally experience a widespread, pruritic, papulocrustous dermatitis associated with *Otodectes cynotis* infestation.[67a] Immunologically, passive cutaneous anaphylaxis reactions to *O. cynotis* antigen were reported in cats with experimentally induced ear mite infestations, demonstrating the existence of reaginic antibody.[600] In addition, cats may have facial or generalized pruritic dermatitis that responds to ivermectin. *Otodectes* mites may be difficult to find in some cases.

Canine Eosinophilic Furunculosis of the Face

Canine eosinophilic furunculosis of the face is an acute, predominantly nasal and muzzle disease that appears severe but is generally self-limiting or exquisitely responsive to glucocorticoids.

- **Cause and Pathogenesis.** This syndrome was initially described in nine dogs in which the common potential inciting feature was exposure to bees or wasps.[607] Since then, other reports or observations have been made.[67a, 605, 606, 608] Cases have been seen in winter (no flying insects present), wherein the dogs had been seen playing with or following spiders.[67a, 606] A similar-looking but chronic case was seen in which intradermal allergy test reactions to blackfly and horsefly were positive.[67a] Eosinophils were numerous on cytologic evaluation of this dog. Because of the chronic history of the case and the lack of histopathologic evaluation, however, it may represent a different syndrome. However, another report did include a dog with a 3-month duration of nodules.[606] Eosinophilic furunculosis of the face has been proposed to be some type of hypersensitivity reaction to an attack by some insect or arthropod.[607, 609] However, some dogs apparently have no known or possible exposure to insects and arthropods.[605, 608] The condition is generally of short duration and not recurrent. Hence, if it is a hypersensitivity reaction, these cases either resolve with no persistent sensitivity or the animals learn to avoid the offending arthropod/insect. The exact pathomechanism is unknown, and further studies are needed regarding both pathomechanism and etiology.

- **Clinical Features.** Age of onset was under 2 years in about 50% of the affected dogs. Specific breed predilections are not yet determined but, typically, large or midsize breeds are affected. Toy and miniature breeds have not been described with this syndrome. No sex predilection has been determined. Onset is very acute; often the dog is normal when it goes outside but returns home within hours with fully developed lesions. The severity of the reaction often peaks within 24 hours, and the course with just antibiotics or without treatment is 14 to 21 days. The dogs present with papules, nodules, plaques, and varying degrees of ulceration, serum exudation, hemorrhage, and crusts (see Fig. 8–15A and B). Pruritus may be absent or intense, and the lesions may be painful.[605–608] Early lesions were described as erythematous or hemorrhagic blisters or papules. Lesions are present on the bridge of the nose, on the muzzle, and often periocularly (see Fig. 8–16A and B). Occasionally, lesions may be on the trunk (especially the relatively glabrous ventral abdomen and thorax [Fig. 8–17B]), extremities (Fig. 8–17A and C), pinnae, and lips.[605, 608] Most dogs are otherwise healthy, but some may be febrile, anorexic, and lethargic.[605, 608] Recurrences have not been reported, though one dog with more generalized lesions and compatible histopathology seen by one of us (C.E.G.) did have two episodes.

- **Diagnosis.** The differential diagnosis is staphylococcal nasal folliculitis and furunculosis. If lesions persist, dermatophytosis may also be considered. Eosinophilic furunculosis of the face has a striking history and appearance, however, making a clinical diagnosis rather simple. Cytologic examination reveals numerous eosinophils. Occasionally, degenerate neutrophils with intracellular bacteria are present, but they probably reflect a secondary bacterial pyoderma. Blood eosinophilia was present in seven of nine dogs examined.[605, 608]

Histopathology. Skin biopsy and examination reveals infiltrative eosinophilic mural

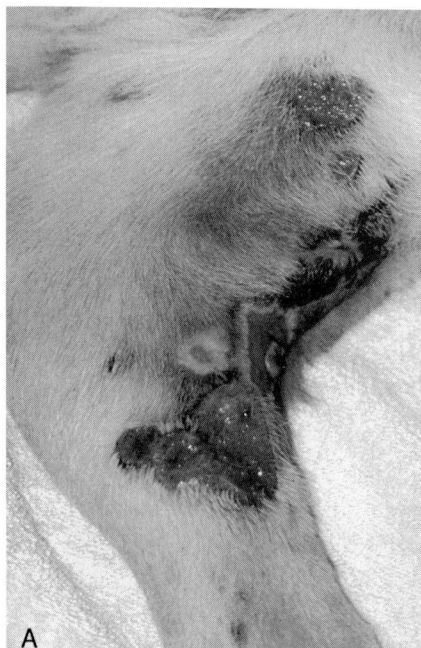
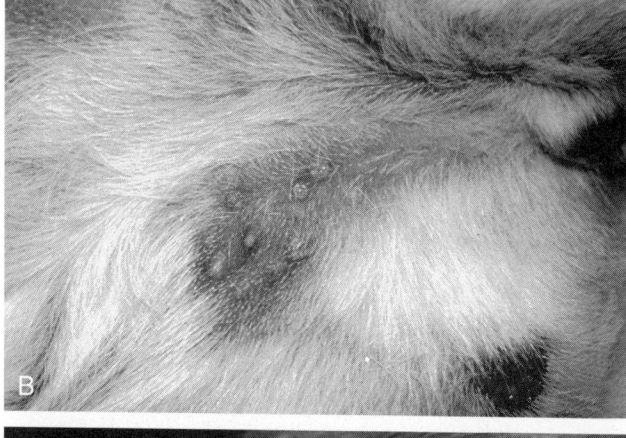
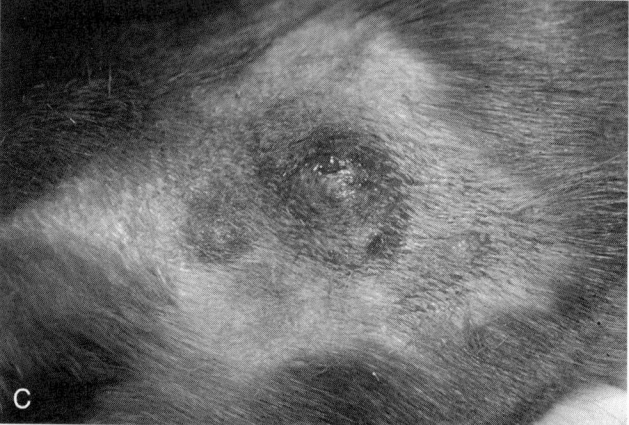

FIGURE 8–17. Case of eosinophilic furunculosis and eosinophilic vasculitis. Lesions developed acutely while dog was boarded in a kennel. Suspected spider or insect bite on the rear leg, where lesions were initially most severe (*A*) but also developed lesions on the pinnae, abdomen (*B*), face and shoulder (*C*).

folliculitis, luminal eosinophilic folliculitis, and eosinophilic furunculosis (Fig. 8–18).[28, 607] Neutrophils, lymphocytes, and macrophages are also present in smaller numbers. Marked dermal and subcutaneous mucinosis and ulceration are common. Focal or multifocal areas of dermal hemorrhage and flame figures are also often found.

• **Clinical Management.** The prognosis is excellent. Systemic glucocorticoid therapy is very effective, with the majority of dogs responding rapidly within 24 to 48 hours, and lesions being completely resolved with 10 to 14 days. Oral prednisone, 1 to 2 mg/kg q24h until lesions have greatly resolved, then on an alternate-day basis for 10 more days, is usually effective, although repositol glucocorticoids could potentially be used because long-term therapy is not required.

INTESTINAL PARASITE HYPERSENSITIVITY

Various intestinal parasites (ascarids, *Coccidia*, hookworms, tapeworms, whipworms) of dogs, cats, and humans may rarely be associated with pruritic dermatoses.[22, 61, 67a, 598] The pathomechanism of these dermatoses is unknown, but a type I hypersensitivity reaction is likely. Although the pathomechanism is unknown, a clear relationship between the parasite and the dermatosis is established, because (1) eliminating the parasites cures the dermatosis and (2) re-infestation with the parasite reproduces it.

Clinical signs may consist of (1) generalized or multifocal pruritic, papulocrustous dermatitis, (2) pruritic seborrheic skin disease, (3) pruritic urticaria, or (4) pruritus without skin lesions. Other signs referable to intestinal parasitism may or may not be present. No age, breed, or sex predilections have been reported.

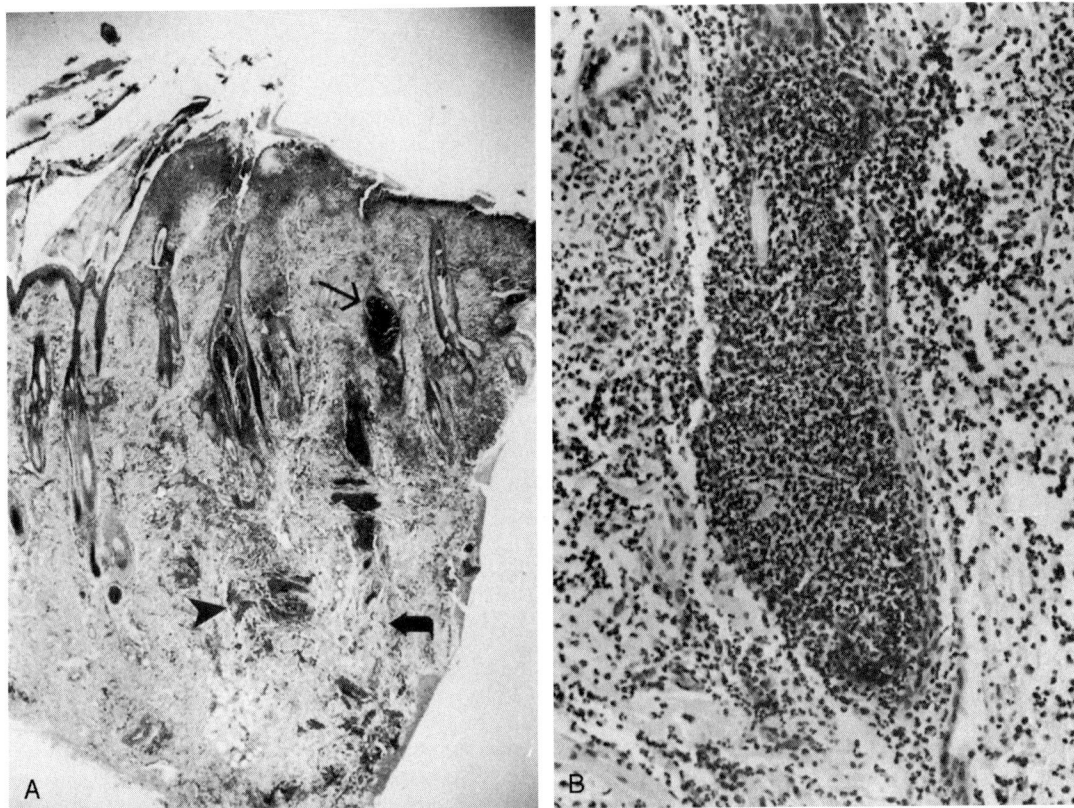

FIGURE 8–18. Canine eosinophilic furunculosis of the face. A, Note marked accumulation of eosinophils in follicles (*upper thin arrow*), numerous collagen flame figures (*notched arrow*), and prominent mucinosis of the middle and deep dermis (*curved arrow*). B, Canine eosinophilic furunculosis of the face. Hair follicle has been literally replaced by eosinophils.

Diagnosis is based on history, physical examination, fecal examinations, and response to therapy. Skin biopsy is nondiagnostic, revealing varying degrees of superficial perivascular dermatitis (pure, spongiotic, hyperplastic), often with small to large numbers of eosinophils.

Therapy includes elimination of the parasites and treatment of symptoms with topical (shampoos, soaks) and systemic medicaments (glucocorticoids), as indicated.

FILARIASIS

Dirofilariasis

Numerous rare skin disorders associated with *Dirofilaria immitis* infection (heartworm disease) have been described in dogs (see Chap. 6).[61, 67a, 598, 599] The pathomechanism of these skin disorders is unknown, although a hypersensitivity to *D. immitis* microfilaria has been suggested. No age, breed, or sex predilections have been reported.

Cutaneous syndromes reported in association with dirofilariasis in dogs include (1) a pruritic, ulcerative, nodular dermatitis of the head, trunk, and limbs (see Fig. 8–15C and D), (2) a pruritic papulocrustous dermatitis resembling canine scabies, (3) a pruritic ulcerative dermatitis of the head and limbs, (4) an erythematous, alopecic dermatitis of the chest and limbs, (5) interdigital cyst, and (6) seborrheic skin disease.

Diagnosis is based on history, physical examination, demonstration of *D. immitis* microfilaria in peripheral blood and in skin specimens, ruling out of other possible causes of the dermatosis, and response to therapy for dirofilariasis. Most dogs with dirofilariasis

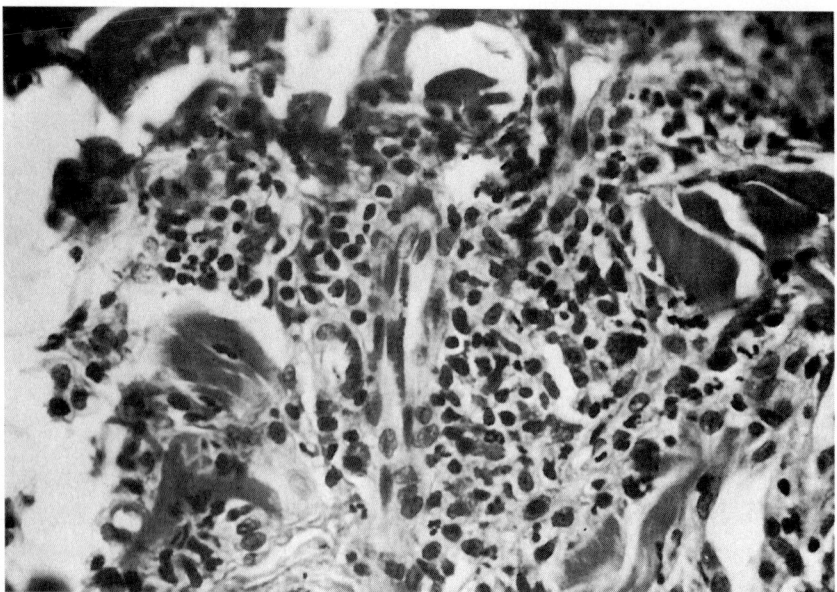

FIGURE 8–19. Canine cutaneous dirofilariasis. Perivascular pyogranuloma with microfilarial segment within blood vessel.

have peripheral eosinophilia and serum hypergammaglobulinemia.[20] About 50% of affected dogs also have peripheral basophilia. In about 20% of the dogs with dirofilariasis, microfilaria cannot be demonstrated in peripheral blood (occult dirofilariasis) owing to an immune-mediated reaction against microfilarial antigen. Various ELISA methods for the detection of adult *D. immitis*–associated antigens (Filarochek, Mallinckrodt; Dirochek, Synbiotics; ClinEase-CH, Norden; CITE, Agri Tech Systems) are very useful for the detection of occult dirofilariasis.[20]

Histologic examination of the nodular form of cutaneous dirofilariasis reveals superficial and deep perivascular to nodular dermatitis.[28, 67a, 83] Eosinophils are numerous. Pyogranulomas may be situated perivascularly, with microfilaria present intravascularly (Fig. 8–19) or interstitially surrounding extravascular microfilaria (Fig. 8–20).

Therapy consists of the administration of adulticidal and microfilaricidal drugs. Cutaneous lesions heal within 5 to 8 weeks after the completion of microfilaricidal therapy.

Filarioidea Dermatitis

A report in 10 dogs with a filarial nematode in the skin other than *Dirofilaria* or *Dipetalonema* was published (see Chap. 6).[596] All the dogs came from the southwestern United States. The dogs presented with single or multiple, alopecic papules or plaques and varying degrees of erythema, crusts, scarring, and ulceration. Eighty percent were pruritic. All dogs had dorsal lesions. These dogs were heartworm antigen–negative and yielded positive histopathologic results, with filarial segments in microgranulomas or free in the dermis or subcutaneous tissue. In one case, an adult nematode was found in the tissue that was identified as an *Acanthocheilonema* spp. Of the dogs treated and followed, all responded to ivermectin therapy or surgical excision with steroids and antibiotics.

Hormonal Hypersensitivity

Hormonal hypersensitivity is a very rare, pruritic, papulocrustous dermatitis of dogs and humans associated with hypersensitivity reactions to sex hormones.[22, 61, 67a, 610]

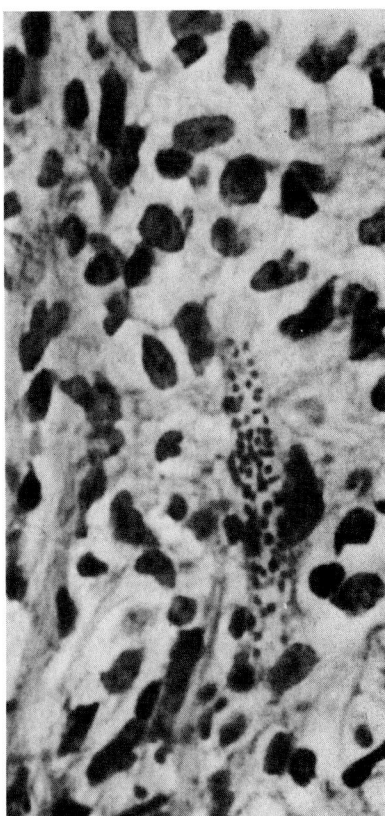

FIGURE 8–20. Canine cutaneous dirofilariasis. Extravascular microfilaria within a granuloma.

CAUSE AND PATHOGENESIS

Although the pathomechanism of the dermatitis in dogs is unknown, results of intradermal allergy testing and basophil degranulation testing to progesterone suggest that type I and type IV hypersensitivity reactions to endogenous progesterone, estrogen, or testosterone are involved.[67a, 610, 615, 616] In humans, a variety of skin disorders have been described, including urticaria, erythema multiforme, stomatitis, pruritic erythematous dermatitis, and vesicles.[611–614] Reactions have been predominantly to progesterone, but estrogens may also be involved. Cases are associated with antiprogesterone antibodies (usually IgG), positive patch and prick test results, positive basophil degranulation to progesterone, and passive cutaneous transfer of skin test reactivity (positive P-K test result) to normal humans.[57, 58, 67a, 616]

CLINICAL FEATURES

No age or breed predilections have been reported, but over 90% of the reported cases have occurred in intact females. Affected females often have a history of repeated pseudopregnancy, irregular estral cycles, or both. Dermatologic signs include a pruritic, erythematous, often papulocrustous eruption that usually begins in the dorsal rump, perineal, genital, and caudomedial thigh regions, is bilaterally symmetric, and progresses cranially (Figs. 8–21 and 8–22). The feet, face, and ears are commonly affected in chronic cases. Enlargement of the vulva and nipples is common (Fig. 8–23). In female dogs, the dermatologic signs usually coincide initially with estrus, pseudopregnancy, or both but tend to become more severe and protracted with each episode until the dog may have

646 • Skin Immune System and Allergic Skin Diseases

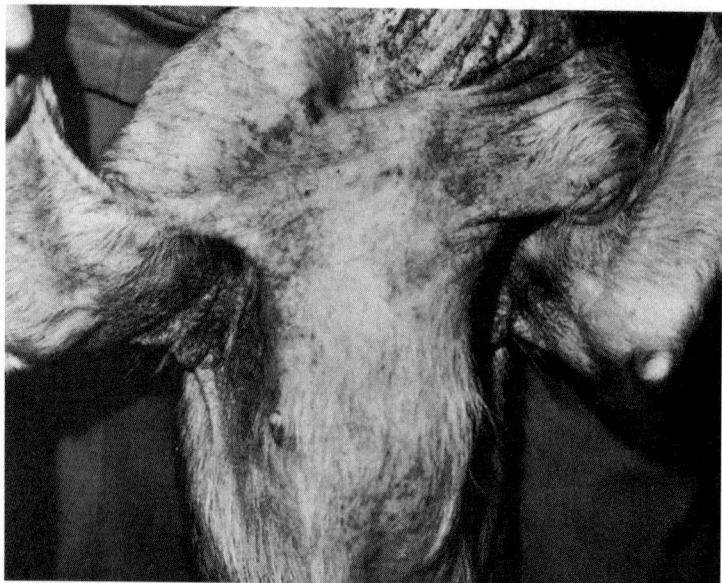

FIGURE 8–21. Canine hormonal hypersensitivity. Traumatic and inflammatory alopecia, hyperpigmentation, and lichenification of ventral neck and chest, axillae, and medial forelimbs.

some degree of pruritic dermatitis at all times. In male dogs, dermatologic signs are nonseasonal.[616]

DIAGNOSIS

The differential diagnosis includes flea bite hypersensitivity, food hypersensitivity, atopy, drug eruption, and staphylococcal folliculitis. Definitive diagnosis is based on history, physical findings, intradermal allergy test results, and response to therapy. Intradermal allergy testing has been performed with aqueous progesterone (0.025 mg), estrogen

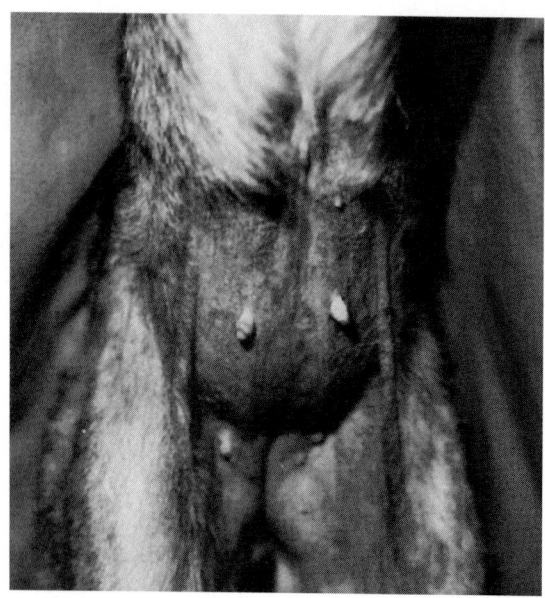

FIGURE 8–22. Canine hormonal hypersensitivity. Traumatic and inflammatory alopecia with enlarged nipples.

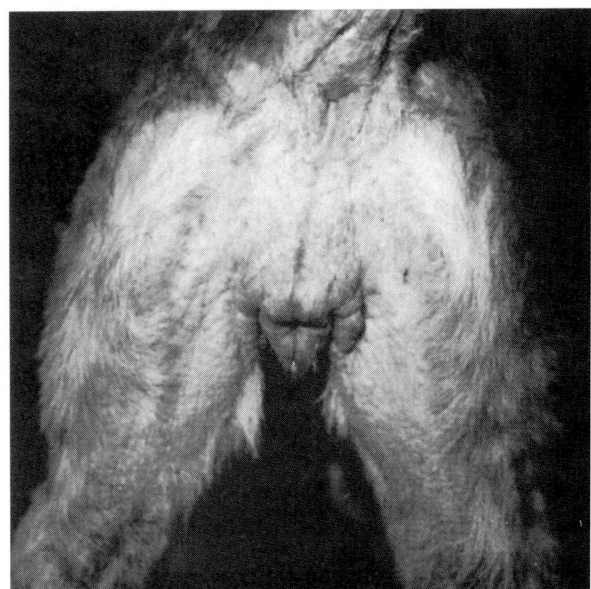

FIGURE 8–23. Canine hormonal hypersensitivity. Inflammatory and traumatic alopecia with lichenification and vulvar enlargement.

(0.0125 mg), and testosterone (0.05 mg), and the skin is observed for immediate and delayed hypersensitivity reactions.[67a, 616] These hormones, however, are currently unavailable in aqueous form. The basophil degranulation test was useful in establishing the diagnosis in five bitches[67a, 615]; however, this test is currently only a research tool (see discussion of canine atopy).

Histopathology

Histopathology is nondiagnostic, revealing varying degrees of superficial perivascular dermatitis (pure, spongiotic, hyperplastic), with neutrophils or mononuclear cells predominating.

CLINICAL MANAGEMENT

The prognosis of hormonal hypersensitivity is favorable if neutering can be performed.[67a, 610, 615, 616] Therapy consists of ovariohysterectomy or castration and treatment of symptoms with topical and systemic medicaments, as indicated. Response to neutering is dramatic; marked improvement occurs within 5 to 10 days. Response to systemic glucocorticoids is often unsatisfactory. In females, response to repositol testosterone (1.0 mg/kg intramuscularly) is a useful presurgical diagnostic aid, with dramatic relief of pruritus occurring within 7 days. A similar response can be produced in males with the oral administration of estrogen.[616]

Bacterial Hypersensitivity

Bacterial hypersensitivity (staphylococcal hypersensitivity) is a rare, severely pruritic, pustular dermatitis in dogs associated with a presumed hypersensitivity reaction to staphylococcal antigen.

CAUSE AND PATHOGENESIS

In humans, bacterial antigens are thought to elicit type I, II, III, and IV hypersensitivity reactions in the skin.[23, 67a] The pathomechanism of bacterial hypersensitivity in dogs is unclear, although evidence supporting the existence of a type III, and perhaps a type I, hypersensitivity reaction has been reported.[30, 620] Dogs with recurrent bacterial pyoderma may have elevated levels of circulating immune complexes,[17] and these immune complexes may contain staphylococcal (*S. intermedius*) antigens that stimulate canine neutrophils.[617a] Such staphylococcal immune complexes could precipitate vasculitis. Two studies of normal dogs, dogs with nonrecurrent staphylococcal pyoderma, dogs with bacterial hypersensitivity, and dogs with recurrent staphylococcal pyoderma associated with atopy measured the levels of circulating antistaphylococcal IgE and IgG.[617b, 618a] The levels of IgG were elevated in all dogs that had experienced a staphylococcal infection, but IgE levels were only elevated in dogs with bacterial hypersensitivity or recurrent pyoderma associated with atopy.

Staphylococci are one group of bacteria known to produce a number of toxins that function as superantigens. The role of bacterial superantigens needs to be investigated because they can induce T-cell activation in an antigen-nonspecific way. Superantigens applied to human skin, either normal or atopic, induce dermatitis but, in atopic patients, dermatitis also occurs in other allergic sites where the superantigens were not applied.[621] Exotoxins A, C, and toxic shock syndrome toxin-1 have been detected in some canine *S. intermedius* isolates from normal dogs or dogs with atopy or bacterial pyoderma.[617] There was no relationship with pruritus or type of lesion. Mason and Lloyd demonstrated that the degranulation of canine cutaneous mast cells caused an increased epidermal permeability to staphylococcal antigens.[241]

Obviously, *S. intermedius* behaves as an antigen for some dogs. Theoretically, antistaphylococcal IgE, fixed to the surfaces of cutaneous mast cells and in the presence of staphylococcal antigens, could cause the degranulation of mast cells, the liberation of inflammatory mediators, the depression of local bacteriocidal mechanisms, and the augmentation of the absorption of staphylococcal antigens. These circumstances could encourage the persistence of infection and a vicious cycle of inflammation and pruritus.

CLINICAL FEATURES

Clinical signs associated with canine bacterial hypersensitivity are intense pruritus in conjunction with a superficial or deep pustular and seborrheic dermatitis.[619, 620] Erythematous pustules and hemorrhagic bullae are present with bacterial hypersensitivity (see Fig. 8–15G and H). Annular or arciform areas of central erythema or hyperpigmentation, alopecia, and scaling that spread peripherally and often coalesce are very common but nondiagnostic. Some lesions may exhibit associated palpable purpura. Rarely, a dog manifests only an antibiotic-responsive, generalized, nonlesional pruritus.[618] Helpful historical clues are prior pyogenic infection, poor or incomplete response to systemic glucocorticoids, and rapid response to appropriate systemic antibiotics. Relapse after cessation of short-term antibiotic therapy is common.

Approximately 50% to 80% of these dogs have concurrent diseases that appear to predispose them to, or to intensify, the bacterial hypersensitivity.[619, 620] Examples of such diseases include seborrheic skin disease, hypothyroidism, other hypersensitivities (atopy, food hypersensitivity, flea bite hypersensitivity), and foci of chronic infection (anal sacculitis, gingivitis, tonsillitis, lip folds, otitis externa).

DIAGNOSIS

The differential diagnosis consists of bacterial folliculitis, demodicosis, dermatophytosis, seborrheic skin disease, subcorneal pustular dermatosis, sterile eosinophilic pustulosis, pemphigus foliaceus, atopy, food hypersensitivity, scabies, and flea bite hypersensitivity. Definitive diagnosis is based on history, physical examination, and results of bacterial culture, skin biopsy, and intradermal allergy testing. All reported cases of canine bacterial hypersensitivity have grown pure cultures of either coagulase-positive *Staphylococcus* spp. (most cases) or coagulase-negative *Staphylococcus* spp. (rare cases).

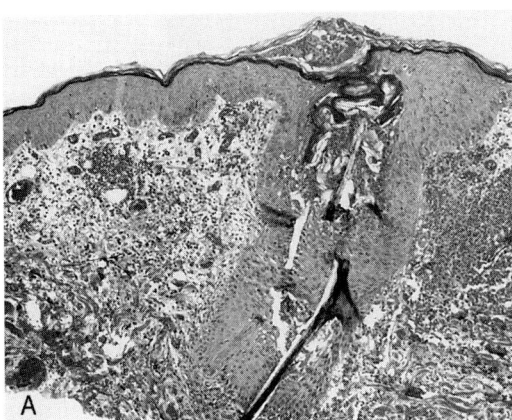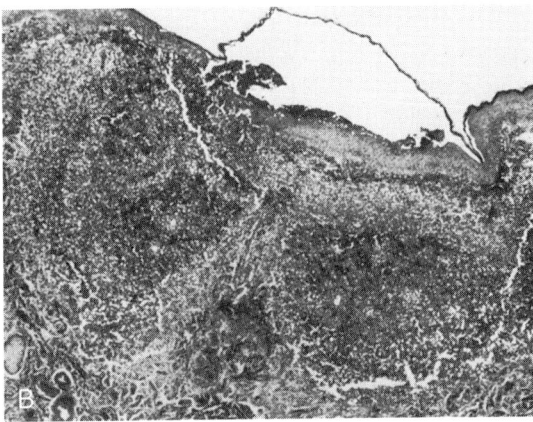

FIGURE 8–24. Bacterial hypersensitivity in a dog. *A*, Suppurative luminal folliculitis with neutrophilic vasculitis and purpura. *B*, Subepidermal hemorrhagic bulla. (*B*, from Scott DW, et al: Staphylococcal hypersensitivity in the dog. J Am Anim Hosp Assoc 14:766, 1978.)

Histopathology

Skin biopsy reveals varying degrees of vasculitis and intraepidermal pustular dermatitis or folliculitis and furunculosis (Fig. 8–24).[620] The vasculitis is usually mixed (neutrophils and mononuclear cells), significant leukocytoclasis is common, and fibrinoid degeneration is rare (Fig. 8–25).

Intradermal Allergy Testing

Intradermal allergy testing with a staphylococcal cell wall toxoid product (Staphoid A–B) had been useful for diagnosing canine bacterial hypersensitivity.[619–620] However, this prod-

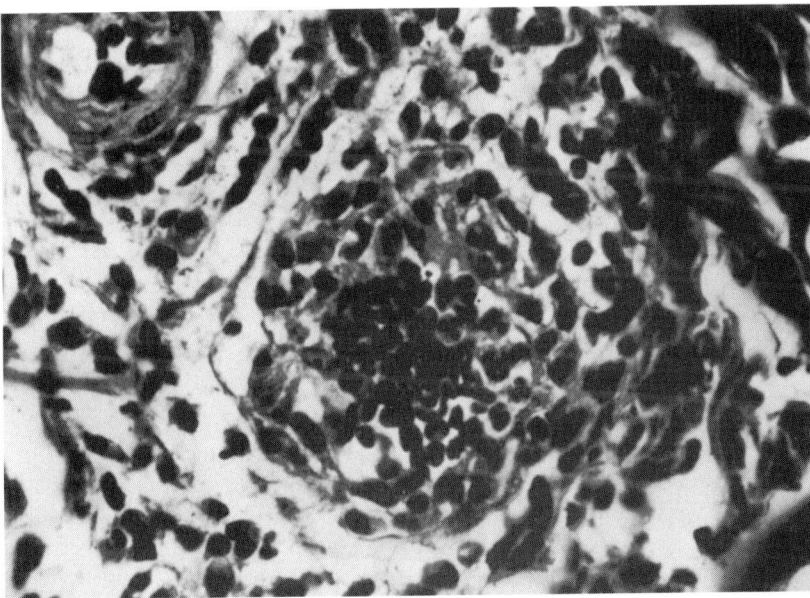

FIGURE 8–25. Canine bacterial hypersensitivity. Mixed-cell (neutrophils, mononuclear cells) vasculitis with endothelial swelling and degeneration and vacuolization of vessel wall. (From Scott DW, et al: Staphylococcal hypersensitivity in the dog. J Am Anim Hosp Assoc 14:766, 1978.)

uct is no longer available. The product was diluted with an equal volume of sterile saline, and 0.1 ml of the mixture was injected intradermally. In virtually all dogs, normal or dermatitic from *any* cause, an immediate wheal and flare reaction developed that persisted for 12 to 18 hours and appeared to be an irritant in nature. At 24 to 72 hours after injection, however, dogs with bacterial hypersensitivity experienced erythematous, indurated, oozing, pruritic reactions that often turned red-purple, became necrotic, and ulcerated (Arthus reaction) (see Fig. 8–15H). Diagnostic skin testing with bacterial antigens presents problems resulting from a lack of uniformity of staphylococcal antigens, the complex antigenic structure of staphylococci and their metabolites, and various nonimmunologic cutaneous reactions.[30, 67a]

CLINICAL MANAGEMENT

Treatment of canine bacterial hypersensitivity may vary, depending on the existence of concurrent diseases and the age of the dog. In those cases in which an underlying disease can be detected and successfully managed, a 3- to 8-week course of appropriate systemic antibiotics is often curative. In cases in which no underlying disease can be detected but the dog is less than 1 year of age, such a course of antibiotic therapy may still be curative.

When no underlying disease can be detected, however, and the dog is over 1 year of age, the idiopathic bacterial hypersensitivity will probably have to be managed for life with repeated antibiotic or biological therapy. Biological therapy is preferred, because repeated antibiotic therapy can lead to increasing bacterial drug resistance, rising drug expense, and euthanasia. In the past, biological therapy with Staphoid A–B had been reported to be successful in 67% to 88% of mature dogs with idiopathic bacterial hypersensitivity.[67a, 619–620] This product is no longer available. An alternative treatment approved for the dog is Staphage Lysate (Delmont Labs) (see Chap. 4). When biological therapy is unsuccessful, the therapy of choice for recurrent bacterial hypersensitivity is chronic antibiotic administration (see Chap. 4).

Fungal Hypersensitivity

Cutaneous hypersensitivity reactions to fungi are thought to be important in humans, but the importance of such reactions in dogs and cats is unknown.[23, 67a] Hypersensitivity to *Candida albicans* infections has been suspected in some cases of paronychia and gingivitis in dogs and cats, in which the tissue response was out of proportion to the degree of infection found.[67a] Fungal kerions are thought to represent hypersensitivity reactions to dermatophytes. Hypersensitivity reactions have been suspected in the pruritic widespread papulocrustous eruptions (miliary dermatitis) in cats associated with *Microsporum canis* infections.[67a] *Malassezia* dermatitis may also be, in part, a hypersensitivity reaction (see Atopic Disease and Chap. 5).

• REFERENCES

General

1. An S, Goetzl EJ: Lipid mediators of hypersensitivity and inflammation. In: Middleton E, et al (eds): Allergy Principles and Practice V. C.V. Mosby, St. Louis, 1998, p. 168.
2. Ansel J, et al: Cytokine modulation of keratinocyte cytokines. J Invest Dermatol 94:101S, 1990.
3. Bacon KB, Schall TJ: Chemokines as mediators of allergic inflammation. Int Arch Allergy Immunol 109: 97, 1996.
4. Benjamin E, et al: Immunology, A Short Course III. Wiley-Liss, New York, 1996.
5. Beutner EH, et al: Immunopathology of the Skin III. Churchill Livingstone, New York, 1987.
6. Bochner BS: Cellular adhesion in inflammation in allergic inflammation. In: Middleton E, et al (eds): Allergy Principles and Practice V. C. V. Mosby, St Louis, 1998, p. 94.
7. Borish L, Rosenwasser LJ: Update on cytokines. J Allergy Clin Immunol 97:719, 1996.
8. Borish L, Rosenwasser LJ: Cytokines in allergic inflammation. In: Middleton E, et al (eds): Allergy Principles and Practice V. C.V. Mosby, St. Louis, 1998, p. 108.
9. Bos JD: Skin Immune System. CRC Press, Boca Raton, 1989.
10. Cannon AG, Affolter VK: What does "CD" mean?

Proc Annu Memb Meet Am Acad Vet Dermatol Am Coll Vet Dermatol 14:133, 1998.
11. Charlesworth EN, et al: Cutaneous late-phase response to allergen: Mediator release and inflammatory cell infiltration. J Clin Invest 83:1519, 1989.
12. Church MK, et al: Mast cell-derived mediators in allergic inflammation. In: Middleton E, et al (eds): Allergy Principles and Practice V. C.V. Mosby, St. Louis, 1998, p. 146.
13. Corrigan CJ: Biology of lymphocytes. In: Middleton E, et al (eds): Allergy Principles and Practice V. C.V. Mosby, St. Louis, 1998, p. 228.
14. Dahl MV: Immunodermatology II. Year Book Medical Publishers, Chicago, 1988.
15. Day MJ: Expression of major histocompatibility complex class II molecules by dermal inflammatory cells, epidermal Langerhans' cells and keratinocytes in canine dermatological disease. J Comp Pathol 115:317, 1996.
16. Day MJ: A Color Atlas of Clinical Immunology of the Dog and Cat. Iowa State University Press, Ames, 1999.
17. DeBoer DJ, et al: Circulating immune complex concentrations in selected cases of skin disease in dogs. Am J Vet Res 49:143, 1988.
18. Dore M, et al: Production of a monoclonal antibody against canine GMP-140 (P-selectin) and studies of its vascular distribution in canine tissues. Vet Pathol 30:213, 1993.
19. Elangbam CS, et al: Cell adhesion molecules—update. Vet Pathol 34:61, 1997.
20. Ettinger SJ, Feldlman EC: Textbook of Veterinary Internal Medicine IV. W.B. Saunders, Philadelphia, 1995.
21. Fadok VA: Immunology can be fun! The star wars approach to immune function. Proc Annu Memb Meet Am Acad Vet Dermatol Am Coll Vet Dermatol 15:81, 1999.
22. Fitzpatrick TB, et al: Dermatology in General Medicine III. McGraw-Hill, New York, 1993.
23. Freedberg IM, et al: Fitzpatrick's Dermatology in General Medicine V. McGraw-Hill, New York, 1999.
24. Gant VA, et al: Biology of monocytes and macrophages. In: Middleton E, et al (eds): Allergy Principles and Practice V. C.V. Mosby, St. Louis, 1998, p. 295.
25. Grant JA, Huamin L: Biology of basophils. In: Middleton E, et al (eds): Allergy Principles and Practice V. C.V. Mosby, St. Louis, 1998, p. 277.
26. Greeley EH, et al: The influence of age on the canine immune system. Vet Immunol Immunopathol 55:1, 1996.
27. Griffin CE, et al: Current Veterinary Dermatology. Mosby Year Book, Inc., St. Louis, 1993.
28. Gross TL, et al: Veterinary Dermatopathology: A Macroscopic and Microscopic Evaluation of Canine and Feline Skin Disease. Mosby Year Book, Inc., St. Louis, 1992.
29. Halliwell REW: Clinical and immunological aspects of allergic skin diseases in domestic animals: In: von Tscharner C, Halliwell REW (eds): Advances in Veterinary Dermatology I. Ballière-Tindall, Philadelphia, 1990, p. 91.
30. Halliwell REW, Gorman NT: Veterinary Clinical Immunology. W.B. Saunders, Philadelphia, 1989.
31. Hargis AM, Liggit HD: Cytokines and their role in cutaneous injury. In: Ihrke PJ, et al (eds): Advances in Veterinary Dermatology II. Pergamon Press, New York, 1993, p. 325.
32. Hauser C, et al: T helper cells grown with hapten-modified cultured Langerhans' cells produce interleukin 4 and stimulate IgE production by B cells. Eur J Immunol 19:245, 1989.
33. Hauser C, Orbea HA: Superantigens and their role in immune-mediated diseases. J Invest Dermatol 101:503, 1993.
34. Prélaud P: Allergologie Canine. Masson, Paris, 1999.
35. Hill PB, Martin RJ: A review of mast cell biology. Vet Dermatol 9:145, 1998.
36. Ihrke PJ, et al: Advances in Veterinary Dermatology II. Pergamon Press, New York, 1993.
37. Jakob T, Udey MC: Epidermal Langerhans' cells: From neurons to nature's adjuvants. Adv Dermatol 14:209, 1999.
38. Kearns RJ, et al: Effect of age, breed, and dietary omega-6 (n-6): Omega-3 (n-3) fatty acid ratio on immune function, eicosanoid production and lipid peroxidation in young and aged dogs. Vet Immunopathol 69:165, 1999.
39. Kita H, et al: Biology of eosinophils. In: Middleton E, et al (eds): Allergy Principles and Practice V. C.V. Mosby, St. Louis, 1998, p. 242.
40. Kondo S, Sauder DH: Epidermal cytokines in allergic contact dermatitis. J Am Acad Dermatol 33:786, 1995.
41. Kube P, et al: Distribution, density, and heterogeneity of canine mast cell depending on fixation techniques. Histochem Cell Biol 110:129, 1998.
42. Lewis RM, Picut CA: Veterinary Clinical Immunology. Lea & Febiger, Philadelphia, 1989.
43. Locke PH, et al: Manual of Small Animal Dermatology. British Small Animal Veterinary Association, Shurdington, 1993.
44. Luger TA, Schwartz T: Evidence for an epidermal cytokine network. J Invest Dermatol 95:100S, 1990.
45. Martin LB, et al: Eosinophils in allergy: Role in disease, degranulation, and cytokines. Int Arch Allergy Immunol 109:207, 1996.
46. McEwan BJ, et al: The response of the eosinophil in acute inflammation in the horse. In: von Tscharner C, Halliwell REW (eds): Advances in Veterinary Dermatology I. Baillière-Tindall, Philadelphia, 1990, p. 176.
47. McKenzie RC, Sauder DN: The role of keratinocyte cytokines in inflammation and immunity. J Invest Dermatol 95:105S, 1990.
48. Mécheris DB: Unravelling the mast cell dilemma: Culprit or victim of its generosity? Immunol Today 18:212, 1997.
49. Middleton E, et al: Allergy Principles and Practice IV. Mosby Year Book, Inc., St. Louis, 1993.
50. Middleton E, et al: Allergy Principles and Practice V. C.V. Mosby, St Louis, 1998.
51. Modlin RL: Lymphocytes. In: Freedberg IM, et al (eds): Fitzpatrick's Dermatology in General Medicine V. McGraw-Hill, New York, 1999, p. 400.
52. Moore PF, et al: The use of immunological reagents in defining the pathogenesis of canine skin diseases involving proliferation of leukocytes. In: Kwochka KW, et al (eds): Advances in Veterinary Dermatology III. Butterworth Heinemann, Boston, 1998, p. 77.
53. Muller GH, et al: Small Animal Dermatology IV. W.B. Saunders, Philadelphia, 1989.
54. Nickoloff BJ: Dermal Immune System. CRC Press, Boca Raton, 1993.
55. Pentland AP: Arachidonic acid metabolism. In:

Freedberg IM, et al (eds): Fitzpatrick's Dermatology in General Medicine V. McGraw-Hill, New York, 1999, p. 432.
56. Peters SP, et al: Late-phase allergic reactions. In: Middleton E, et al (eds): Allergy Principles and Practice V. C.V. Mosby, St. Louis, 1998, p. 342.
57. Prélaud P: The basophil degranulation test in the diagnosis of canine allergic skin disease. In: von Tscharner C, Halliwell REW (eds): Advances in Veterinary Dermatology I. Baillière-Tindall, Philadelphia, 1990, p. 117.
58. Prélaud P: Les Dermites Allergiques du Chien et du Chat. Masson, Paris, 1991.
59. Prieto VG, et al: Quantitative immunohistochemical differences in Langerhans' cells in dermatitis due to internal versus external antigen sources. J Cutan Pathol 25:301, 1998.
60. Reedy LM, Miller WH Jr: Allergic Skin Diseases of Dogs and Cats. W.B. Saunders, Philadelphia, 1989.
61. Reedy LM, et al: Allergic Skin Diseases of Dogs and Cats, 2nd ed. W.B. Saunders, Philadelphia, 1997.
62. Saint-Andre Marchal I, et al: Feline Langerhans' cells migrate from skin and vaginal mucosa to regional lymph nodes during experimental contact sensitization with fluorescein isothiocyanate. Vet Dermatol 9:9, 1998.
63. Schwartz LB, et al: Biology of mast cells in allergic inflammation. In: Middleton E, et al (eds): Allergy Principles and Practice V. C.V. Mosby, St. Louis, 1998, p. 261.
64. Scott DW: Epidermal mast cells in the cat. Vet Dermatol 1:65, 1990.
65. Scott DW: Feline dermatology 1979–1982: Introspective retrospections. J Am Anim Hosp Assoc 20:537, 1984.
66. Scott DW: Feline dermatology 1983–1985: "The secret sits." J Am Anim Hosp Assoc 23:255, 1987.
67. Scott DW, et al: La dermatite miliaire féline: Une modalité de réaction cutanée. Point Vét 19:284, 1987.
67a. Scott DW, et al: Muller and Kirk's Small Animal Dermatology V. W.B. Saunders, Philadelphia, 1995.
68. Stingl G, et al: The epidermis: An immunologic microenvironment. In: Freedberg IM, et al (eds): Fitzpatrick's Dermatology in General Medicine V. McGraw-Hill, New York, 1999, p. 343.
69. Stone J: Dermatology, Immunology and Allergy. Mosby Year Book, Inc., St. Louis, 1985.
70. Sunderkötter C, et al: Aging and the skin immune system. Arch Dermatol 133:1256, 1997.
71. Swerlick RA, Lawley TJ: Role of microvascular endothelial cells in inflammation. J Invest Dermatol 100:111S, 1993.
72. Thiers BH, Dobson RL: Pathogenesis of Skin Disease. Churchill Livingstone, New York, 1986.
73. Thomsen MK: Species specificity in the generation of eicosanoids: Emphasis on leukocyte-activating factors in the skin of allergic dogs and humans. In: Ihrke PJ, et al (eds): Advances in Veterinary Dermatology II. Pergamon Press, New York, 1993, p. 63.
74. Thomsen MK: The Role of Neutrophil-Activating Mediators in Canine Health and Disease. Ballerup, Copenhagen, 1991.
75. Thompson JP: Basic immunologic principles of allergic disease. Semin Vet Med Surg 6:247, 1991.
76. Tizard IR: Veterinary Immunology: An Introduction V. W.B. Saunders, Philadelphia, 1997.
77. von Tscharner C, Halliwell REW: Advances in Veterinary Dermatology I. Baillière-Tindall, Philadelphia, 1990.
78. Walsh LJ, Murphy GF: Role of adhesion molecules in cutaneous inflammation and neoplasia. J Cutan Pathol 19:161, 1992.
79. Wassom DL, Grieve RB: *In vitro* measurement of canine and feline IgE: Review of Fcϵ RIα-based assays for detection of allergen-reactive IgE. Vet Dermatol 9:173, 1998.
80. Williams IR, et al: Cytokines and chemokines. In: Freedberg IM, et al (eds): Fitzpatrick's Dermatology in General Medicine V. McGraw-Hill, New York, 1999, p. 384.
81. Wolfe JH, Halliwell REW: Total hemolytic complement values in normal and diseased dog populations. Vet Immunol Immunopathol 1:287, 1980.
82. Yager JA: The skin as an immune organ. In: Ihrke PJ, et al (eds): Advances in Veterinary Dermatology II. Pergamon Press, New York, 1993, p. 3.
83. Yager JA, Scott DW: The skin and appendages. In: Jubb KVF, et al (eds): Pathology of Domestic Animals IV. Academic Press, New York, 1993, p. 531.
84. Yager JA, Wilcock BP: Color Atlas and Text of Surgical Pathology of the Dog and Cat. Wolfe, Spain, 1994.
85. Yager JA: The skin as an immune organ. In: Kwochka KW, et al (eds): Pergamon Press, Oxford, 1996, p. 3.
86. Zunic M, et al: Immune responses in the lymphoid organs of dogs with experimentally induced IgE-mediated allergy. Proc Annu Memb Meet Am Acad Vet Dermatol Am Coll Vet Dermatol 13:78, 1997.

Allergic Therapy

87. Alam R, et al: Selective inhibition of the cutaneous late but not immediate allergic response to antigens by misoprostol, a PGE analog—results of a double-blind placebo-controlled study. Am Rev Respir Dis 148:1066–1070, 1993.
87a. Beale KM, et al: Safety of long-term administration of a 0.01% fluocinolone shampoo in allergic dogs. Vet Dermatol 11:3, 2000.
88. Beningo KE, et al: Observations on the use of tetracycline and niacinamide as antipruritic agents in atopic dogs. Can Vet J 40:268, 1999.
89. Betttenay SV: Feline atopy. In: Bonagura JD (ed): Kirk's Current Veterinary Therapy XIII. W.B. Saunders, Philadelphia, 2000, p. 564.
90. Bierman CW, et al: Effect of H_1 receptor blockade on late cutaneous reactions to antigen: A double-blind controlled study. J Allergy Clin Immunol 87:151, 1991.
91. Bloom PB: Hydroxyzine poisoning in 3 dogs. Proc Annu Memb Meet Am Acad Vet Dermatol Am Coll Vet Dermatol 15:29, 1999.
92. Boeckh A: Misoprostol. Comp Cont Educ Small Anim Pract 21:66, 1999.
93. Bond R, Lloyd DH: Double-blind comparison of three concentrated essential fatty acid supplements in the management of canine atopy. Vet Dermatol 4:185, 1994.
94. Bond R, Lloyd DH: A double-blind comparison of olive oil and a combination of evening primrose oil and fish oil in the management of chronic atopy. Vet Rec 131:558, 1992.
95. Bond R, Lloyd DH: Randomized single-blind comparison of an evening primrose oil and fish oil combination and concentrates of these oils in the management of canine atopy. Vet Dermatol 3:215, 1992.
96. Bond R, Lloyd DH: Combined treatment with con-

centrated essential fatty acids and prednisone in the management of canine atopy. Vet Rec 134:30, 1994.
97. Rees CA, et al: Disposition and hematologic effects of a single intravenous or oral dose pentoxifylline administration in normal dogs. Proc Annu Memb Meet Am Acad Vet Dermatol Am Coll Vet Dermatol 15:89, 1999.
98. Boguniewicz M, Leung DYM: Atopic dermatitis. In: Middleton E, et al (eds): Allergy Principles and Practice V. C.V. Mosby, St. Louis, 1998, p. 1123.
99. Campbell KL, et al: Effects of oral sunflower oil on serum and cutaneous fatty acid concentration profiles in seborrheic dogs. Vet Dermatol 3:29, 1992.
100. Chalmers SA, Medleau L: Feline atopic dermatitis: Its diagnosis and treatment. Vet Med 89:342, 1994.
101. Chew DJ, et al: Amitriptyline treatment for severe recurrent idiopathic cystitis in cats. J Am Vet Med Assoc 213:1282, 1998.
102. Clayton MH, et al: Altered glucocorticoid receptor binding in atopic dermatitis. J Allergy Clin Immunol 96:421, 1995.
103. DeBoer DJ, et al: Inability of short-duration treatment with a 5-lipoxygenase inhibitor to reduce clinical signs of canine atopy. Vet Dermatol 5:13, 1994.
104. Estelle F, Simons R: Anithistamines. In: Middleton E, et al (eds): Allergy Principles and Practice V. C.V. Mosby, St. Louis, 1998, p. 612.
105. Garcia G, et al: Inhibition of histamine release from dispersed canine skin mast cells by cyclosporine A, rolipran and salbutamol, but not by dexamethasone or sodium cromoglycate. Vet Dermatol 9:81, 1998.
106. Granlund H, et al: Long-term follow-up of eczema patients treated with cyclosporine. Acta Dermatol Venerol 78:40–43, 1998.
107. Harvey RG: personal communication, 1990.
108. Harvey RG: Management of feline miliary dermatitis by supplementing the diet with essential fatty acids. Vet Rec 128:326, 1991.
109. Harvey RG: Effect of varying proportions of evening primrose oil and fish oil on cats with crusting dermatosis ("miliary dermatitis"). Vet Rec 133:208, 1993.
110. Harvey RG: A comparison of evening primrose oil and sunflower oil for the management of papulocrustous dermatitis in cats. Vet Rec 133:571, 1993.
111. Harvey RG: A blinded, placebo-controlled study of the efficacy of borage seed oil and fish oil in the management of canine atopy. Vet Rec 144:405, 1999.
112. Héripret D: Les antiprurigineux non steroïdiens. Prat Méd Chir Anim Comp 28:73, 1993.
113. Héripret D, Vroom M: Antipruritic therapy. In: Kwochka KW, et al (eds): Advances in Veterinary Dermatology III. Butterworth Heinemann, Boston, 1998, p. 417.
114. Lim KK, et al: Cyclosporine in the treatment of dermatologic disease: An update. Mayo Clin Proc 71:1183–1191, 1996.
115. Logas DB, Kunkle GA: Double-blinded study examining the effects of evening primrose oil on feline pruritic dermatitis. Vet Dermatol 4:181, 1993.
116. Logas DB, Kunkle GA: Double-blinded crossover study with marine oil supplement containing high-dose eicosapentaenoic acid for the treatment of canine pruritic skin disease. Vet Dermatol 5:99, 1994.
117. Lloyd DH, Thomsett LR: Essential fatty acid supplementation in the treatment of canine atopy: A preliminary study. Vet Dermatol 1:41, 1989.
118. Lloyd DH: Essential fatty acids and skin disease. J Small Anim Pract 30:207, 1989.
119. Marsella R, et al: Use of pentoxifylline in the treatment of allergic contact reactions to plants of the Commelinceae family in dogs. Vet Dermatol 8:121, 1997.
120. Marsella R: Effects of ketoconazole on intradermal skin test and leukotriene C4 concentration in the skin of atopic dogs. In: Kwochka KW, et al (eds): Advances in Veterinary Dermatology III. Butterworth Heinemann, Boston, 1998, p. 549.
120a. McAnulty JF, Lensmeyer GL: The effects of ketoconazole on the pharmacokinetics of cyclosporine A in cats. Vet Surg 28:448, 1999.
121. Messinger LM: Therapy for feline dermatoses. Vet Clin North Am Small Anim Pract 25:981, 1995.
122. Miller WH Jr: Fatty acid supplements as anti-inflammatory agents. In: Kirk RW (ed): Current Veterinary Therapy X. W.B. Saunders, Philadelphia, 1989, p. 563.
123. Miller WH Jr: Nonsteroidal anti-inflammatory agents in the management of canine and feline pruritus. In: Kirk RW (ed): Current Veterinary Therapy X. W.B. Saunders, Philadelphia, 1989, p. 566.
124. Miller WH Jr, et al: Clinical trial of DVM Derm Caps in the treatment of allergic disease in dogs: A nonblinded study. J Am Anim Hosp Assoc 25:163, 1989.
125. Miller WH Jr, Scott DW: Efficacy of chlorpheniramine maleate for the management of pruritus in cats. J Am Vet Med Assoc 197:67, 1990.
126. Miller WH Jr, et al: Investigation on the antipruritic effects of ascorbic acid given alone and in combination with a fatty acid supplement to dogs with allergic skin disease. Canine Pract 17:11, 1992.
127. Miller WH Jr, et al: Nonsteroidal management of canine pruritus with amitriptyline. Cornell Vet 82:53, 1992.
128. Miller WH Jr, et al: Efficacy of DVM Derm Caps Liquid in the management of allergic and inflammatory dermatoses of the cat. J Am Anim Hosp Assoc 29:37, 1993.
129. Miller WH Jr, et al: A clinical trial on the efficacy of clemastine in the management of allergic pruritus in dogs. Can Vet J 34:25, 1993.
130. Miller WH Jr, Scott DW: Medical management of chronic pruritus. Comp Cont Educ 16:449, 1994.
131. Miller WH Jr, Scott DW: Clemastine fumarate as an antipruritic agent in pruritic cats: Results of an open clinical trial. Can Vet J 35:502, 1994.
132. Olivry T, et al: Treatment of canine atopic dermatitis with misoprostol, a prostaglandin E_1 analogue: An open study. J Dermatol Treat 8:243–247, 1997.
133. Otto CM, Greentree WF: Terfenadine toxicosis in dogs. J Am Vet Med Assoc 205:1004, 1994.
134. Pan PY, et al: The effects of short term treatment with the prostaglandin E1 (PGE1) analog misoprostol on inflammatory mediator production in murine lupus nephritis. Clin Immunol Immunopathol 75:125–130, 1995.
135. Paradis M, et al: Further investigations on the use of nonsteroidal and steroidal anti-inflammatory agents in the management of canine pruritus. J Am Anim Hosp Assoc 27:44, 1991.
136. Paradis M, et al: The efficacy of clemastine (Tavist), a fatty acid-containing product (DVM Derm Caps), and the combination of both products in the management of canine pruritus. Vet Dermatol 2:17, 1991.
137. Paradis M, Bettenay S: Nonsteroidal antipruritic drugs in small animals. In: Ihrke PJ, et al (eds): Ad-

vances in Veterinary Dermatology II. Pergamon Press, New York, 1993, p. 429.
138. Paterson S: Use of antihistamines to control pruritus in atopic dogs. J Small Anim Pract 35:415, 1994.
139. Patterson S: Additive benefits of EFAs in dogs with atopic dermatitis after partial response to antihistamine therapy. J Small Anim Pract 36:389, 1995.
139a. Reich MR, et al: Electrocardiographic assessment of antianxiety medication in dogs and correlation with serum drug concentration. J Am Vet Med Assoc 216:1571, 2000.
140. Scarff DH, Lloyd DH: Double blind, placebo controlled, crossover study of evening primrose oil in the treatment of canine atopy. Vet Rec 131:97, 1992.
141. Scarff DH, et al: A multicenter placebo-controlled practitioner study to investigate the effect of evening primrose oil in canine atopic dermatosis. In: Von Tscharner C, Halliwell REW (eds): Advances in Veterinary Dermatology I. Baillière-Tindall, Philadelphia, 1990, p. 481.
142. Schick RO, et al: Efficacy of an omega-3 fatty acid adjusted diet in pruritic dogs. Proc Annu Memb Meet Eur Soc Vet Dermatol Eur Coll Vet Dermatol 12:245, 1995.
143. Scott DW, Buerger RG: Nonsteroidal anti-inflammatory agents in the management of canine pruritus. J Am Anim Hosp Assoc 24:425, 1988.
144. Scott DW, Miller WH Jr: Nonsteroidal management of canine pruritus: Chlorpheniramine and a fatty acid supplement (DVM Derm Caps) in combination, and the fatty acid supplement at twice the manufacturer's recommended dosage. Cornell Vet 80:381, 1990.
145. Scott DW, et al: Failure of cyproheptadine hydrochloride as an antipruritic agent in allergic dog: Results of a double-blinded, placebo-controlled study. Cornell Vet 82:247, 1992.
146. Scott DW, et al: Comparison of the clinical efficacy of two commercial fatty acid supplements (Efa Vet and DVM Derm Caps), evening primrose oil, and cold water marine fish oil in the management of allergic pruritus in dogs: A double-blinded study. Cornell Vet 82:319, 1992.
146a. Scott DW, Cayatte SM: Failure of papaverine hydrochloride and doxycycline hyclate as antipruritic agents in pruritic dogs: Results of an open clinical trial. Can Vet J 34:164, 1993.
147. Scott DW, Miller WH Jr: Medical management of allergic pruritus in the cat, with emphasis on feline atopy. J S Afr Vet Assoc 64:103, 1993.
148. Scott DW, Miller WH Jr: Nonsteroidal anti-inflammatory agents in the management of canine allergic pruritus. J S Afr Vet Assoc 64:52, 1993.
149. Scott DW, et al: Failure of terfenadine as antipruritic agent in atopic dogs: Results of a double-blinded, placebo-controlled study. Can Vet J 35:286, 1994.
150. Scott DW, Miller WH Jr: The combination of an antihistamine (chlorpheniramine) and an omega-3/omega-6 fatty acid-containing product (DVM Derm Caps Liquid) for the management of pruritic cats. Results of an open clinical trial. N Z Vet J 43:29, 1995.
151. Scott DW, et al: Effect of an omega-3/omega-6 fatty acid-containing commercial lamb and rice diet on pruritus in atopic dogs: Results of a single-blinded study. Can J Vet Res 61:145, 1997.
152. Scott DW, et al: Observations on the use of cyproheptadine hydrochloride as an antipruritic agent in allergic cats. Can Vet J 39:634, 1998.
153. Scott DW, Miller WH Jr: Antihistamines in the management of allergic pruritus in dogs and cats. J Small Anim Pract 40:359, 1999.
154. Shoulberg N: The efficacy of fluoxetine (Prozac) in the treatment of acral lick and allergic inhalant dermatitis in canines. Proc Annu Memb Meet Am Acad Vet Dermatol Am Coll Vet Dermatol 6:31, 1990.
155. Simon FE, Simon KJ: Antihistamines. In: Middleton E, et al (eds): Allergy Principles and Practice IV. Mosby Year Book, St. Louis, 1993.
156. Thomas RC, Logas D: Effects of a 1% hydrocortisone conditioner in hematological and biochemical parameters, adrenil function testing, and cutaneous reaction to histamine in normal and pruritic dogs. Vet Dermatol 10:109, 1999.
157. Toyoda M, Morohashi M: Morphological assessment of the effects of cyclosporine A on mast cell–nerve relationship in atopic dermatitis. Acta Dermatol Venerol 78:321–325, 1998.
158. Turek JJ, Hayek MG: Effect of omega-6:omega 3 fatty acid ratios on cytokine production in adult and geriatric dogs. In: Reinhart GA, Carey DP (eds): Recent Advances in Canine and Feline Nutrition II. Orange Frazer Press, Wilmington, OH, 1998, p. 305.
159. Umesh KG, et al: Evaluation of terfendaine and hydroxyzine as antipruritic agents in dogs. Indian Vet J 75:345, 1998.
160. van Joost T, et al: Cyclosporine in atopic dermatitis. J Am Acad Dermatol 27:922, 1992.
161. Vaughn DM, et al: Evaluation of effects of dietary n-6 to n-3 fatty acids ratios on leukotriene B synthesis in dog skin and neutrophils. Vet Dermatol 5:163, 1994.
162. White P: Essential fatty acids: Use in management of canine atopy. Comp Cont Educ 15:451, 1993.

Urticaria and Angioedema

163. Nichols PR, et al: A retrospective study of canine and feline cutaneous vasculitis. Proc Annu Memb Meet Am Acad Vet Dermatol Am Coll Vet Dermatol 14:27, 1998.
164. Noxon JO: Anaphylaxis, urticaria, and angioedema. Semin Vet Med Surg 6:265, 1991.
165. Scott DW, Miller WH Jr: Idiosyncratic cutaneous adverse drug reactions in the cat: Literature review and report of 14 cases (1990–1996). Feline Pract 26:10, 1998.
166. Scott DW, Miller WH Jr: Idiosyncratic cutaneous adverse drug reactions in the dog: Literature review and report of 101 cases (1990–1996). Canine Pract 24:16, 1999.
167. Soter NA: Urticaria and angioedema. In: Freedberg IM, et al (eds): Fitzpatrick's Dermatology in General Medicine V. McGraw-Hill, New York, 1999, p. 1409.
168. Vitale CB, et al: Putative diethylcarbamazine-induced urticaria with eosinophilic dermatitis in a dog. Vet Dermatol 5:197, 1994.
169. Wolfrom E, et al: Chronic urticaria and *Toxocara canis* infection: A case-study. Ann Dermatol Venereol 123:240, 1996.

Canine Atopy
General

170. Auxilia ST, Hill PB: Mast cell distribution in normal dog skin: A possible explanation for the predilection sites of atopic dermatitis. Proceedings of the British Small Animal Veterinary Association, Birmingham, 1999, p. 236.
171. Ballauf B: Vergleich von Intrakutan—und Pricktest in der Allergiediagnostik beim Hund. Tierarztl Prax 19:428, 1991.

172. Becker AB, et al: Cutaneous mast cell heterogeneity: Response to antigen in atopic dogs. J Allergy Clin Immunol 78:937, 1986.
173. Berardesca E, Borroni G: Instrumental evaluation of cutaneous hydration. Clin Dermatol 13:323, 1995.
174. Bettenay S: A double-blinded trial evaluating homeopathic drops in the treatment of atopy in 20 dogs. In: Kwochka KW, et al (eds): Advances in Veterinary Dermatology III. Butterworth Heinemann, Boston, 1998, p. 508.
175. Bevier DE: Long-term management of atopic disease in the dog. Vet Clin North Am Small Anim Pract 20:1487, 1990.
176. Boguniewicz, M., Leung DYM: Atopic dermatitis: A question of balance. Arch Dermatol 134:870, 1998.
177. Bollinger RE, et al: Cat antigen in homes with and without cats may induce allergic symptoms. J Allergy Clin Immunol 97:907, 1996.
178. Bos JD, et al: Immune dysregulation in atopic eczema. Arch Dermatol 128:1509, 1992.
179. Bourdeau P, Paragon BM: Alternatives aux corticoïdes en dermatologie des carnivores. Rev Méd Vét 168:645, 1992.
180. Bourdeau P, et al: Relationships between the distribution of lesions and positive intradermal reactions in 307 dogs suspected of atopy and/or flea bite hypersensitivity. Proc Annu Memb Meet Eur Soc Vet Dermatol Eur Coll Vet Dermatol 15:157, 1998.
181. Brazis P, et al: Comparative study of histamine release from skin mast cells dispersed from atopic, ascaris-sensitive, and healthy dogs. Vet Immmunol Immunopathol 66:43, 1998.
182. Bruijnzeel-Koumen CAFM, et al: New aspects in the pathogenesis of atopic dermatitis. Acta Dermatol Venereol (Stockh) Suppl 144:58, 1989.
183. Bruijnzeel PLB, et al: The involvement of eosinophils in the patch test reaction to aeroallergens in atopic dermatitis: Its relevance for the pathogenesis of atopic dermatitis. Clin Exp Allergy 23:97, 1993.
184. Butler JM, et al: Pruritic dermatitis in asthmatic basenji-greyhound dogs: A model for human atopic dermatitis. J Am Acad Dermatol 8:33, 1983.
185. Campbell KL, et al: Immunoglobulin A deficiency in the dog. Canine Pract 16:7, 1991.
186. Carlotti DN, Castargent F: Analyse statistique de tests cutanés positifs chez 449 chiens atteints de dermatite allergique. Prat Méd Chir Anim Comp 27:53, 1992.
187. Carlotti D: La dermatite atopique du chien. Point Vét 17:5, 1985.
188. Carlotti DN: Traitement et suivi au long cours du chien à dermatite atopique. Prat Méd Chir Anim Comp 33(Suppl):359, 1998.
189. Carucci JA, et al: The leukotriene antagonist zafirlukast as a therapeutic agent for atopic dermatitis. Arch Dermatol 134:785, 1998.
190. Chalmers SA, Medleau L: An update on atopic dermatitis in dogs. Vet Med 89:326, 1994.
191. Chan SC, et al: Elevated leukocyte phosphodiesterase as a basis for depressed cyclic adenosine monophosphate responses in the basenji-greyhound dog model of asthma. J Allergy Clin Immunol 76:148, 1985.
192. Chandoga P, et al: The incidence of atopic diseases in dogs in the Košice region (Slovakia): Anamnestic and clinical aspects. Folia Vet 42:159, 1998.
193. Chesney CJ: Measurement of skin hydration in normal dogs and in dogs with atopy or a scaling dermatosis. J Small Anim Pract 36:305, 1995.
194. Ciprandi G, et al: Minimal persistent inflammation is present at mucosal level in patients with asymptomatic rhinitis and mite allergy. J Allergy Clin Immunol 96:6, 1995.
195. Codner EC, Lessard P: Comparison of intradermal allergy test and enzyme-linked immunosorbent assay in dogs with allergic skin disease. J Am Vet Med Assoc 202:739, 1993.
196. Collo MJ, et al: A controlled trial of house dust mite eradication using natamycin in homes of patients with atopic dermatitis: Effect on clinical status and mite populations. Br J Dermatol 121:199, 1989.
197. Cooper KD: Atopic dermatitis: Recent trends in pathogenesis and therapy. Dermatol Foundation 102:128, 1994.
197a. D'Amato G, et al: Clothing is a carrier of cat allergens. J Allergy Clin Immunol 98:577, 1997.
198. Davis FM: Anti-IgE treatment for allergic diseases. Proc Annu Memb Meet Am Acad Vet Dermatol Am Coll Vet Dermatol 14:57, 1998.
199. Day MJ, et al: Subclass profile of allergen-specific IgG antibodies in atopic dogs. Res Vet Sci 61:146, 1996.
200. DeBoer DJ: Advances in allergic skin disease. In: Kwochka KW, et al (eds): Advances in Veterinary Dermatology III. Butterworth Heinemann, Boston, 1998, p. 147.
201. DeBoer DJ, Hill PB: Serum immunoglobulin E concentrations in West Highland white terrier puppies do not predict development of atopic dermatitis. Vet Dermatol 10:275, 1999.
201a. DeMora F, et al: Skin mast cell releasibility in dogs with atopic dermatitis. Inflam Res 45:424, 1996.
202. De Weck AL, et al: Genetics and regulation of the IgE response leading to experimentally induced atopic-like dermatitis in beagle dogs. Proc Annu Memb Meet Am Acad Vet Dermatol Am Coll Vet Dermatol 13:76, 1997.
203. De Weck AL, et al: Dog allergy, a model for allergy genetics. Int Arch Allergy Immunol 113:55, 1997.
204. De Weck AL, et al: Genetic and environmental aspects of IgE regulation in dogs. Proc Annu Memb Meet Eur Soc Vet Dermatol Eur Coll Vet Dermatol 15:111, 1998.
205. Elsner P, et al: Bioengineering of the Skin: Water and the Stratum Corneum. CRC Press, Boca Raton, 1994.
206. Esch RE: Canine allergy to house dust mites. Vet Allergy Clin Immunol 5:110, 1997.
207. Ferrer L, et al: Clinical anti-inflammatory efficacy of arofylline, a new selective phosphodiesterase-4 inhibitor, in dogs with atopic dermatitis. Vet Rec 145:191, 1999.
208. Fontaine J, Henroteaux M: Utilisation du dosage des anticorps anaphylactiques (IgG) pour le diagnostic d'atopie chez le chien. Ann Méd Vét 135:57, 1991.
209. Frank LA, McEntee MF: Demonstration of aeroallergen contact sensitivity in dogs. Vet Allergy Clin Immunol 3:75–80, 1995.
210. Frick OL, et al: Immunoglobulin E antibodies to pollens augmented in dogs by virus vaccines. Am J Vet Res 44:440, 1983.
211. Frick OL: Pathogenesis of chronic allergic reactions using the atopic dog as a model. Proc Am Acad Vet Allergy, 1991.
212. Graham-Brown RAC: Therapeutics in atopic dermatitis. Adv Dermatol 13:3, 1998.
213. Griffin CE: Atopic disease. Semin Vet Med Surg 6:290, 1991.
214. Griffin CE: *Malassezia paronychia* in atopic dogs.

Proc Annu Memb Meet Am Acad Vet Dermatol Am Coll Vet Dermatol 12:51, 1996.
214a. Griot-Wenk ME, et al: Total serum IgE and IgA antibody levels in healthy dogs of different breeds and exposed to different environments. Res Vet Sci 67:239, 1999.
215. Groeben H, et al: Dermal and airway responses to monoclonal antibodies specific for canine IgE. Vet Immunol Immunopathol 58:209, 1997.
216. Halliwell REW, et al: Induced and spontaneous IgE antibodies to *Dermatophagoides farinae* in dogs and cats: Evidence of functional heterogeneity of IgE. Vet Dermatol 9:179, 1998.
217. Hanifin JM, et al: Recombinant interferon therapy for atopic dermatitis. J Am Acad Dermatol 28:189, 1993.
218. Hanifin JM: Biochemical and immunologic mechanisms in atopic dermatitis: New targets for emerging therapies. J Am Acad Dermatol 41:72, 1999.
219. Harper, J: Traditional Chinese medicine for eczema. Br Med J 308:489, 1994.
220. Harvey RG, Noble WC: A temporal study comparing the carriage of *Staphylococcus intermedius* on normal dogs with atopic dogs in clinical remission. Vet Dermatol 5:21, 1994.
221. Héripret D: Les antiprurigineux non stéroïdiens. Prat Méd Chir Anim Comp 28:73, 1993.
222. Hill PB, et al: Concentrations of total serum IgE, IgA, and IgG in atopic and parasitized dogs. Vet Immunol Immunopathol 44:105, 1995.
223. Hill PB, DeBoer DJ: Quantification of serum total IgE concentration in dogs by use of an enzyme-linked immunsorbent assay containing monoclonal murine-anticanine IgE. Am J Vet Res 55:944, 1994.
224. Hirshman CA, et al: Enhanced bronchoalveolar lavage mast cells histamine releasibility in allergic dogs with and without airway hyperresponsiveness. J Allergy Clin Immunol 81:829, 1988.
225. Hites MJ, et al: Effect of immunotherapy on the serum concentrations of allergen-specific IgG antibodies in dog sera. Vet Immunol Immunopathol 22:39, 1989.
226. Hofer MF, et al: Staphylococcal toxins augment specific IgE responses by atopic patients exposed to allergen. J Invest Dermatol 112:171, 1999.
227. Jackson HA, et al: Canine leukocyte histamine release: Response to antigen and to anti-IgE. Vet Immunol Immunopathol 53:195, 1996.
228. Junghans V, et al: Epidermal cytokines Il-1β, TNF-α, and IL-12 in patients with atopic dermatitis: Response to application of house dust mite antigens. J Invest Dermatol 111:1184, 1998.
229. Kapp A, et al: Eosinophil cationic protein in sera of patients with atopic dermatitis. J Am Acad Dermatol 24:555, 1991.
230. Kapp A, et al: Altered production of immunomodulating cytokines in patients with atopic dermatitis. Acta Dermatol Venereol (Stockh) 144:97, 1989.
231. Klubal, R, et al: The high-affinity receptor for IgE is the predominant IgE-binding structure in lesional skin of atopic dermatitis patients. J Invest Dermatol 108:3, 1997.
232. Langeveld-Wildschut EG, et al: Evaluation of the atopy patch test and the cutaneous late-phase reaction as relevant models for the study of allergic inflammation in patients with atopic eczema. J Allergy Clin Immunol 98:1019, 1996.
233. Leroy BP, et al: A novel therapy for atopic dermatitis with allergen-antibody complexes: A double-blind, placebo-controlled study. J Am Acad Dermatol 28:232, 1993.
234. Leung DYM: Atopic dermatitis: The skin as a window into the pathogenesis of chronic allergic diseases. J Allergy Clin Immunol 96:302, 1995.
235. Leung DYM, et al: Atopic dermatitis (atopic eczema). In: Freedberg IM, et al (eds): Fitzpatrick's Dermatology in General Medicine V. McGraw-Hill, New York, 1999, p. 1464.
236. Lyon TM, Halliwell REW: Allergen-specific IgE and IgGd antibodies in atopic and normal dogs. Vet Immunol Immunopathol 66:203, 1998.
237. Magalono-Laruelle C: Sensibilisation à la blatte chez le chien atopique. Prat Méd Chir Anim Comp 30:331, 1995.
238. Mao XQ, et al: Association between genetic variants of mast cell chymase and eczema. Lancet 348:581, 1996.
239. Marsella R, et al: Double-blinded placebo-controlled cross-over study on the effects of pentoxifylline in canine atopy. Proc Annu Memb Meet Am Acad Vet Dermatol Am Coll Vet Dermatol 15:91, 1999.
240. Mason IS, Lloyd DH: Factors influencing the penetration of bacterial antigens through canine skin. In: von Tscharner C, Halliwell REW (eds): Advances in Veterinary Dermatology I. Baillière-Tindall, Philadelphia, 1990, p. 370.
241. Mason IS, Lloyd DH: The role of allergy in the development of canine pyoderma. J Small Anim Pract 30:216, 1992.
242. McEwan NA: Bacterial adherence to canine corneocytes. In: von Tscharner C, Halliwell REW (eds): Advances in Veterinary Dermatology I. Baillière-Tindall, Philadelphia, 1990, p. 454.
243. Morris DO, et al: Type-1 hypersensitivity responses to *Malassezia pachydermatis* extracts in atopic dogs. Proc Annu Memb Meet Am Acad Vet Dermatol Am Coll Vet Dermatol 13:74, 1997.
244. Mudde GC, et al: IgE positive Langerhans' cells and Th2 allergen specific T cells in atopic dermatitis. J Invest Dermatol 99:103, 1992.
245. Mudde GC, et al: Advances in the pathogenesis and therapy of atopic dermatitis in humans and dogs. Proc Annu Memb Meet Am Acad Vet Dermatol Am Coll Vet Dermatol 14:41, 1998.
246. Mudde GC, et al: Allergen presentation by epidermal Langerhans' cells from patients with atopic dermatitis is mediated by IgE. Immunology 69:335, 1990.
247. Mueller RS: Diagnosis and management of canine atopic disease. Aust Vet Practit 23:20, 1993.
247a. Mueller RS, et al: Serum and skin IgA concentrations in normal and atopic dogs. Aust Vet J 75:906, 1997.
248. Muse R, et al: The prevalence of otic manifestations and otitis externa in allergic dogs. Proc Annu Memb Meet Am Acad Vet Dermatol Am Coll Vet Dermatol 12:33, 1996.
249. Nimmo-Wilkie JS, et al: *In vitro* lymphocyte stimulation by concanavalin A and with histamine as a co-mitogen in dogs with atopic dermatitis. Vet Immunol Immunopathol 28:67, 1991.
250. Nimmo-Wilkie JS, et al: Abnormal cutaneous response to mitogens and a contact allergen in dogs with atopic dermatitis. Vet Immunol Immunopathol 28:97, 1991.
251. Nimmo-Wilkie JS, et al: Altered spontaneous and histamine-induced *in vitro* suppressor-cell function in

dogs with atopic dermatitis. Vet Immunol Immunopathol 30:129, 1992.
252. Nimmo-Wilkie JS, et al: Changes in cell-mediated immune responses after experimentally-induced anaphylaxis in dogs. Vet Immunol Immunopathol 32:325, 1992.
253. Nimmo-Wilkie JS, et al: Morphometric analyses of the skin of dogs with atopic dermatitis and correlations with cutaneous and plasma histamine and total serum IgE. Vet Pathol 27:179, 1990.
254. Nuttal TJ: *Malassezia* specific IgE levels in normal and atopic dogs. Proc Annu Memb Meet Eur Soc Vet Dermatol Eur Coll Vet Dermatol 15:155, 1998.
255. Ohlén BM: Diagnostiering och behandling vid atopi hos hund i Sverige. Svensk Veterinär 44:299, 1992.
256. Olivry T, et al: Langerhans' cell hyperplasia and IgE expression in canine atopic dermatitis. Arch Dermatol. Res. 288:579–585, 1996.
257. Olivry T, et al: Characterization of the cutaneous inflammatory infiltrate in canine atopic dermatitis. Am J Dermatopathol 19:477–486, 1997.
258. Olivry T, et al: Characterization of the cutaneous inflammatory infiltrate during IgE-mediated late-phase reactions in dogs with atopic dermatitis. Proc Annu Memb Meet Am Acad Vet Dermatol Am Coll Vet Dermatol 14:71, 1998.
259. Olivry T, et al: Toward a canine model of atopic dermatitis: amplification of cytokine-gene transcripts in the skin of atopic dogs. Exper Dermatol 8:204, 1999.
260. Peng Z, et al: Measurement of ragweed-specific IgE in canine serum by use of enzyme-linked immunosorbent assays containing polyclonal and monoclonal antibodies. Am J Vet Res 54:239, 1993.
261. Peng Z, et al: Heterogeneity of polyclonal IgE characterized by differential charge, affinity to protein A, and antigenicity. J Allergy Clin Immunol 100:87, 1997.
262. Reference deleted.
263. Prélaud P, Sainte-Laudy J: Dermatite atopique du chien: Méthodes de diagnostic *in vitro*. Prat Méd Chir Anim Comp 23:441, 1988.
264. Prélaud P, Sainte-Laudy J: IgG spécifiques de l'acarien de la poussière de maison, *Dermatophagoides farinae*, chez les chiens atopiques et nonatopiques. Rev Méd Vét 140:1117, 1989.
265. Prélaud P: Traitement de l'atopie canine. Prat Méd Chir Anim Comp 28:461, 1993.
266. Prélaud P, et al: Reevaluation of diagnostic criteria of canine atopic dermatitis. Proc Annu Memb Meet Eur Soc Vet Dermatol Eur Coll Vet Dermatol 14:169, 1997.
267. Prélaud P, Olivry T: Etiopathogénie de la dermatite atopique canine. Prat Méd Chir Anim Comp 33(Suppl):315, 1998.
268. Prélaud P: Diagnostic de la dermatite atopique canine: Un diagnostic clinique. Prat Méd Chir Anim Comp 33(Suppl):331, 1998.
269. Prinz B, et al: Long-term application of extracorporeal photochemotherapy in severe atopic dermatitis. J Am Acad Dermatol 40:577, 1999.
270. Racine BP, et al: Influence of sex and age on serum total immunoglobulin E concentration in beagles. Am J Vet Res 60:93, 1999.
271. Reinhold U, et al: Systemic interferon treatment in severe atopic dermatitis. J Am Acad Dermatol 29:58, 1993.
272. Rhodes KH, et al: Comparative aspects of canine and human atopic dermatitis. Semin Vet Med Surg 2:166, 1987.
273. Rhodes KH, et al: Investigation into the immunopathogenesis of canine atopy. Semin Vet Med Surg 2:199, 1987.
274. Rokugo M, et al: Contact sensitivity to *Pityrosporum ovale* in patients with atopic dermatitis. Arch Dermatol 126:627, 1990.
275. Ruzicka T: Atopic eczema between rationality and irrationality. Arch Dermatol 134:1462, 1998.
276. Sager N, et al: House dust mite specific reactivity in the skin of subjects with atopic dermatitis: Frequency and lymphokine profile in the allergen patch test. J Allergy Clin Immunol 89:801, 1992.
277. Saridomichelakis MN, et al: Canine atopic dermatitis in Greece: Clinical observations and the prevalence of positive intradermal test reactions in 91 spontaneous cases. Vet Immunol Immunopathol 69:61, 1999.
278. Saridomichelakis MN, et al: Sensitization to dust mites in cats with *Otodectes cynotis* infestation. Vet Dermatol 10:89, 1999.
279. Schick RO, Fadok VA: Responses of atopic dogs to regional allergens: 268 cases (1981–1984). J Am Vet Med Assoc 189:1493, 1986.
280. Schwartzman RM: Immunologic studies of progeny of atopic dogs. Am J Vet Res 45:375, 1984.
281. Schwartzman RM, et al: The atopic dog model: Report of an attempt to establish a colony. Int Arch Allergy Appl Immunol 72:97, 1983.
282. Scott DW: Observations on canine atopy. J Am Anim Hosp Assoc 17:91, 1981.
283. Scott DW, Paradis M: A survey of canine and feline skin disorders seen in a university practice: Small Animal Clinic, University of Montreal, Saint-Hyacinthe, Quebec, (1987–1988). Can Vet J 31:830, 1990.
284. Scott DW, et al: A clinical study of the efficacy of two commercial veterinary pramoxine cream rinses in the management of pruritus in atopic dogs. Canine Pract 25:15, 2000.
285. Shaw SC: The role of house dust mite allergens in canine allergic disease. In: Kwochka KW, et al (eds): Advances in Veterinary Dermatology III. Butterworth Heinemann, Boston, 1998, p. 505.
286. Sinke JD, et al: Immunophenotyping of skin-infiltrating T-cell subsets in dogs with atopic dermatitis. Vet Immunol Immunopathol 57:13, 1997.
287. Skov L, Baadsgaard O: Superantigens: Do they have a role in skin diseases? Arch Dermatol 131:829, 1995.
288. Solomon, W. R, Platts-Mills TAE: Aerobiology and inhalant allergens. In: Freedberg IM, et al (eds): Fitzpatrick's Dermatology in General Medicine V. McGraw-Hill, New York, 1999, p. 367.
289. Sousa CA: Atopic dermatitis. Vet Clin North Am Small Anim Pract 18:1049, 1988.
290. Sousa CA, Norton AL: Advances in methodology for diagnosis of allergic skin disease. Vet Clin North Am Small Anim Pract 20:1419, 1990.
291. Sporik R, et al: Exposure to house-dust mite allergen (der p I) and the development of asthma in childhood: A prospective study. N Engl J Med 323:502, 1990.
292. Stevens SR, et al: Long-term effectiveness and safety of recombinant human interferon gamma therapy for atopic dermatitis despite unchanged serum IgE levels. Arch Dermatol 134:799, 1998.

293. Stiller MJ, et al: A double-blind, placebo-controlled clinical trial to evaluate the safety and efficacy of thymopentin as an adjunctive treatment in atopic dermatitis. J Am Acad Dermatol 30:597, 1994.
294. Tan BB, et al: Double-blind controlled trial of effect of house dust-mite allergen avoidance on atopic dermatitis. Lancet 347:15, 1996.
295. Tanaka Y, et al: Immunohistochemical studies on dust mite antigen in positive reaction site of patch test. Acta Dermatol Venereol (Stockh) Suppl 144:93, 1989.
296. Tangbøl O, et al: The fatty acid profile of subcutaneous fat and blood plasma in pruritic dogs and dogs without skin problems. Can J Vet Res 62:275, 1998.
297. Thepen T, et al: Biphasic response against aeroallergen in atopic dermatitis showing a switch from initial Th2 response to a Th1 response in situ: An immunocytochemical study. J Allergy Clin Immunol 97:828, 1996.
298. Tupker RA, et al: Induction of atopic dermatitis by inhalation of house dust mite. J Allergy Clin Immunol 97:1064, 1996.
299. Turner CR, et al: Dermal mast cell releasibility and end organ responsiveness in atopic and nonatopic dogs. J Allergy Clin Immunol 83:643, 1989.
300. Umesh KG, et al: Epidemiological and therapeutic aspects of canine atopy. Indian Vet J 72:56, 1995.
301. van der Heijden FL, et al: High frequency of IL-4 producing CD4+ allergen-specific T lymphocytes in atopic dermatitis lesional skin. J Invest Dermatol 97:389, 1991.
302. van den Broek AHM, Simpson JW: Fat absorption in dogs with atopic dermatitis. In: von Tscharner C, Halliwell REW (eds): Advances in Veterinary Dermatology I. Ballière-Tindall, Philadelphia, 1990, p. 155.
303. Van Stee EW: Risk factors in canine atopy. Calif Vet 37:8, 1983.
304. Vollset I, et al: Immediate type hypersensitivity in dogs induced by storage mites. Res Vet Sci 40:123, 1986.
304a. Vriesendorp HM, et al: Serological DLA typing of normal and atopic dogs. Transplant Proc 7:375, 1975.
305. Welle MM, et al: Mast cell density and subtypes in the skin of dogs with atopic dermatitis. J Comp Pathol 120:187, 1999.
306. White SD, Bourdeau P: L'atopic chez le chien: Données actualisées. Point Vét 27:191, 1995.
307. White SD, et al: Comparison via cytology and culture of carriage of Malassezia pachydermatis in atopic and healthy dogs. In: Kwochka KW, et al (eds): Advances in Veterinary Dermatology III. Butterworth Heinemann, 1998, p. 291.
308. Willemse A: Canine atopic disease: Investigations of eosinophils and the nasal mucosa. Am J Vet Res 45:1867, 1984.
309. Willemse A, van den Brom WE: Investigations of the symptomatology and the significance of immediate skin test reactivity in canine atopic dermatitis. Res Vet Sci 34:261, 1983.
310. Willemse A, et al: Allergen specific IgGd antibodies in dogs with atopic dermatitis as determined by the enzyme linked immunosorbent assay (ELISA). Clin Exp Immunol 59:359, 1985.
311. Willemse A, et al: Induction of non-IgE anaphylactic antibodies in dogs. Clin Exp Immunol 59:351, 1985.
312. Willemse A: Atopic skin disease: A review and a reconsideration of diagnostic criteria. J Small Anim Pract 27:771, 1986.
313. Woodfolk JA, et al: Chemical treatment of carpets to reduce allergen: Comparison of the effects of tannic acid and other treatments on proteins derived from dust mites and cats. J Allergy Clin Immunol 96:3, 1995.
314. Zunic M, et al: Studies of atopy in genetically high IgE responder dogs. Proc Annu Memb Meet Am Acad Vet Dermatol Am Coll Vet Dermatol 14:53, 1998.

Testing

315. Alaba O: Allergies in dogs and cats: Allergen-specific IgE determination by VARL Liquid Gold compared with ELISA/RAST. Vet Allergy Clin Immunol 5:93, 1997.
316. Ackerman L: Diagnosing inhalant allergies: Intradermal or in vitro testing. Vet Med 83:779, 1988.
317. Anderson RK, Sousa CA: In vitro versus in vivo testing for canine atopy. In: Ihrke PJ, et al (eds): Advances in Veterinary Dermatology II. Pergamon Press, New York, 1993, p. 425.
318. August JR: The intradermal test as a diagnostic aid for canine atopic disease. J Am Anim Hosp Assoc 18:164, 1982.
319. August JR: The reaction of canine skin to the intradermal injection of allergenic extracts. J Am Anim Hosp Assoc 18:157, 1982.
320. Barbet JL, Halliwell REW: Duration of inhibition of the immediate skin test reactivity by hydroxyzine hydrochloride in dogs. J Am Vet Med Assoc 194:1565, 1989.
321. Beale KM, et al: Effects of sedation on intradermal skin testing in flea-allergic dogs. J Am Vet Med Assoc 197:861, 1990.
322. Bevier DE, et al: Fcϵ RIα-based ELISA technology for in vitro determination of allergen-specific IgE in a population of intradermal skin-tested normal and atopic dogs. Comp Cont Educ Pract Vet 19(Suppl):10, 1997.
323. Bond R, et al: Evaluation of two enzyme-linked immunosorbent assays for the diagnosis of canine atopy. Vet Rec 135:130, 1994.
324. Bourdeau P, et al: Positive skin reactions to allergenic challenge in healthy dogs: Part I—Intradermal skin testing. In: Kwochka KW, et al (eds): Advances in Veterinary Dermatology III. Butterworth Heinemann, Boston, 1998, p. 444.
325. Bourdeau P, Blumstein P: Nonspecific sensitization to house dust mites in dogs: A study of 170 intradermal skin testing to Blomia tropicalis in France. Proc Annu Memb Meet Am Acad Vet Dermatol Am Coll Vet Dermatol 15:19, 1999.
325a. Bunde CJW, et al: Comparison of intradermal skin testing and a new ELISA for specific IgE. Vet Allergy Clin Immunol 5:1, 1997.
326. Campbell KL, Hall IA: Effect of storage of allergens in plastic and glass syringes on the results of intradermal skin testing in dogs. Proc Annu Memb Meet Am Acad Vet Dermatol Am Coll Vet Dermatol 9:48, 1993.
327. Codner EC, et al: Effect of tiletamine-zolazepam sedation on intradermal allergy testing in atopic dogs. J Am Vet Med Assoc 201:1857, 1992.
328. Codner EC, McGrath CJ: The effect of tiletamine-zolazepam anesthesia on the response to intradermally injected histamine. J Am Anim Hosp Assoc 27:189, 1991.
329. Codner EC, Lessard P: Effect of hyposensitization with irrelevant antigens on subsequent allergy skin

329. test results in normal dogs. Vet Dermatol 3:209, 1992.
330. Codner EC, Tinker MK: Reactivity to intradermal injections of extracts of house dust and house dust mite in healthy dogs and dogs suspected of being atopic. J Am Vet Med Assoc 206:812, 1995.
331. Codner EC, Griffin CE: Serologic allergy testing for dogs. Comp Cont Educ Pract Vet 18:237, 1996.
332. Curtis CF, et al: Evaluation of the response to intradermally injected environmental mite allergen solutions in healthy kenneled dogs. In: Kwochka KW, et al (eds): Advances in Veterinary Dermatology III. Butterworth Heinemann, Boston, 1998, p. 510.
333. Darsow U, et al: Evaluating the relevance of aeroallergen sensitization in atopic eczema with the atopy patch test: A randomized, double-blind multicenter study. J Am Acad Dermatol 40:187, 1999.
334. DeBoer DJ: Survey of intradermal skin testing practices in North America. J Am Vet Med Assoc 195:1357, 1989.
335. Dérer M, et al: Monoclonal anti-IgE antibodies in the diagnosis of dog allergy. Vet Dermatol 9:185, 1998.
336. Esch RE, et al: Isolation and characterization of a major dust mite (*Dermatophagoides farinae*) allergenic fraction in dogs. Proc Annu Memb Meet Am Acad Vet Dermatol Am Coll Vet Dermatol 13:87, 1997.
337. Esch RE, Grier TJ: Clinical utility of *in vitro* canine IgE assays. Vet Allergy Clin Immunol 5:31, 1997.
338. Evans AG: Allergic inhalant dermatitis attributable to marijuana exposure in a dog. J Am Vet Med Assoc 195:1588, 1989.
339. Ferguson EA: A review of intradermal skin testing in the UK. Vet Dermatol Newsl 14:13, 1992.
340. Frank LA, et al: Comparison of serum cortisol concentration before and after intradermal testing in sedated and nonsedated dogs. J Am Vet Med Assoc 200:507, 1992.
341. Ginel PJ, et al: Correlation between intradermal and in-hospital serological testing in atopic dogs. In: Kwochka KW, et al (eds): Advances in Veterinary Dermatology III. Butterworth Heinemann, Boston, 1998, p. 441.
342. Ginel PJ, et al: Evaluation of a commercial ELISA test for the detection of allergen-specific IgE antibodies in atopic dogs. J Vet Med B 45:421, 1998.
343. Griffin CE: *In vitro* versus *in vivo* testing for atopy. Proc Annu Memb Meet Am Acad Vet Dermatol Am Coll Vet Dermatol 12:50, 1996.
344. Griffin CE: RAST and ELISA testing in canine atopy. In: Kirk RW (ed): Current Veterinary Therapy X. W.B. Saunders, Philadelphia, 1989, p. 592.
345. Griffin CE, et al: The effect of serum IgE on an *in vitro* ELISA test in the normal canine. In: von Tscharner C, Halliwell REW (eds): Advances in Veterinary Dermatology I. Baillière-Tindall, Philadelphia, 1990, p. 137.
346. Griot-Wenk ME, et al: Characterization of two dog IgE-specific antibodies elicited by different recombinant fragments of the epsilon chain in hens. Vet Immunol Immunopathol 64:15, 1998.
347. Guaguère E, et al: Canine atopy: *In vitro* testing using a monoclonal anti-IgE. In: Kwochka KW, et al (eds): Advances in Veterinary Dermatology III. Butterworth Heinemann, Boston, 1998, p. 454.
348. Halliwell REW, Kunkle GA: The radioallergosorbent test in the diagnosis of canine atopic disease. J Allergy Clin Immunol 62:236, 1978.
349. Halliwell REW: Canine allergic skin diseases. Proc Kal Kan Symp Treat Small Anim Dis 11:33, 1987.
350. Hammerberg B, et al: Auto-IgG anti-IgE and Ig X IgE immune complex presence and effects on ELISA-based quantitation of IgE in canine atopic dermatitis, demodectic acariasis and helminthiasis. Vet Immunol Immunopathol 60:33, 1997.
351. Hämmerling, R., de Weck AL: Comparison of two diagnostic tests for canine atopy using monoclonal anti-IgE antibodies. Vet Dermatol 9:191, 1998.
352. Johnson CA: The effects of constant and variable temperature on the biological activity of allergens stored in plastic and glass syringes. Proc Annu Memb Meet Am Acad Vet Dermatol Am Coll Vet Dermatol 11:18, 1995.
353. Kleinbeck ML, et al: Enzyme-linked immunosorbent assay for measurement of allergen-specific IgE antibodies in canine serum. Am J Vet Res 50:1831, 1989.
354. Koch HJ, Peters S: 207 Intrakutnatests bei Hunden mit Verdacht auf atopische dermatitis. Kleinterpraxis 39:25, 1994.
355. Kunkle G, et al: Steroid effects on intradermal skin testing in sensitized dogs. Proc Annu Memb Meet Am Acad Vet Dermatol Am Coll Vet Dermatol 10:41, 1994.
356. Lyon TM, Halliwell REW: Allergen-specific IgE and IgGd antibodies in atopic and normal dogs. Vet Immunol Immunopathol 66:203, 1998.
357. MacDonald JM, Angarano DW: Comparison of intradermal testing with commercial *in vitro* allergy testing (ELISA) in parasitized nonallergic beagle dogs. Proc Annu Memb Meet Am Acad Vet Dermatol Am Coll Vet Dermatol 6:46, 1990.
358. Marsella R, et al: Double-blinded pilot study on the effects of ketoconazole on intradermal skin test and leukotriene C4 concentration in the skin of atopic dogs. Vet Dermatol 8:3, 1997.
359. Mason IS, Lloyd DH: Evaluation of compound 48/80 as a model of immediate hypersensitivity in the skin of dogs. Vet Dermatol 7:81, 1996.
359a. Masuda K, et al: Positive reactions to common allergens in 42 atopic dogs in Japan. Vet Immunol Immunopathol 73:193, 2000.
359b. Masuda K, et al: IgE sensitivity and cross-reactivity to crude and purified mite allergens (Derf1, Derf2, Derp1, Derp2) in atopic dogs sensitive to *Dermatophagoides* mite allergens. Vet Immunol Immunopathol 72:303, 2000.
360. McCall C: One years experience with IgE Fc RI testing. Proc Annu Memb Meet Am Acad Vet Dermatol Am Coll Vet Dermatol 14:51, 1998.
361. McCall C, et al: Characterization and cloning of the major house dust mite (*Dermatophagoides farinae*) allergen for dogs. Proc Annu Memb Meet Am Acad Vet Dermatol Am Coll Vet Dermatol 15:111, 1999.
362. Miller WH Jr, et al: Evaluation of an allergy screening test for use in atopic dogs. J Am Vet Med Assoc 200:931, 1992.
363. Miller WH Jr, et al: Evaluation of the performance of a serologic allergy system in atopic dogs. J Am Anim Hosp Assoc 29:545, 1993.
364. Miller WH Jr, et al: The influence of oral corticosteroids or declining allergen exposure on serologic allergy test results. Vet Dermatol 3:327, 1992.
365. Mills AC, McKeever PJ: Comparison of intradermal skin testing in non-sedated and sedated dogs. Proc Annu Memb Meet Am Acad Vet Dermatol Am Coll Vet Dermatol 10:46, 1994.

366. Moriello KA, Eicker SW: Influence of sedative and anesthetic agents on intradermal skin test reactions in dogs. Am J Vet Res 52:1484, 1991.
367. Mueller RS, et al: Comparison of intradermal testing and serum testing for allergen-specific IgE using monoclonal IgE antibodies in 84 atopic dogs. Aust Vet J 77:90, 1999.
368. Noli, C. et al.: The significance of reactions to purified fractions of Dermatophagoides pteronyssinus and Dermatophagoides farinae in canine atopic dermatitis. Vet Immunol Immunopathol 52:147, 1996.
369. Noli C: Spécificité de l'allergie aux acariens de la poussière de maison chez le chien. Prat Méd Chir Anim Comp 33(Suppl):305, 1998.
370. Ohlén BM: Projekt allergitester i Sverige. Svensk Veterinär 44:365, 1992.
371. Paradis M, Lécuyer M: Evaluation of an in-office allergy screening test in nonatopic dogs having various intestinal parasites. Can Vet J 34:293, 1993.
372. Phillips MK, et al: Cutaneous histamine reactivity, histamine content of commercial allergens, and potential for false-positive skin test reactions in dogs. J Am Vet Med Assoc 203:1288, 1993.
373. Plant JD: The reproducibility of three in vitro canine allergy tests: A pilot study. Proc Annu Memb Am Acad Vet Dermatol Am Coll Vet Dermatol 10:16, 1994.
374. Prélaud P: Tests cutanés d'allergie immédiate chez le chien: Minimiser erreurs et deceptions. Prat Méd Chir Anim Comp 27:529, 1992.
375. Prélaud P, Guaguère E: Sensitization to the house dust mite Dermatophagoides farinae in dogs with sarcoptic mange. Vet Dermatol 6:205, 1995.
376. Prélaud P: Méthodes de diagnostic biologique en allergologie canine. Prat Méd Chir Anim Comp 33(Suppl):281, 1998.
377. Prost C: Allergy diagnosis in companion animals: Clinical experience with the basophil activation model. Vet Dermatol 9:213, 1998.
378. Rachofsky MA: Comments on in vitro allergy testing. Dermatol Dialogue, Winter 1993/1994, p. 4.
379. Rees CA, et al: The effects of temperature and type of syringe on the biologic activity of stored allergens. Vet Allergy Clin Immunol 5:12, 1997.
380. Saint-Laudy J: Passive antibody transfer on human leukocytes: Application to small animal allergy diagnosis by flow cytometry. Vet Dermatol 9:213, 1998.
381. Sainte-Laudy J, Prost C: Binding of canine anaphylactic antibodies on human basophils: Application to canine allergy diagnosis. Vet Dermatol 7:185, 1996.
382. Schmeitzel LP: The effects of multiple intradermal skin tests on skin reactivity. Vet Allergy, Summer 1986, p. 1.
383. Schwartzman RM, Lillard S: Polyclonal anti-IgE antibody results in an allergen-specific ELISA. Canine Pract 20:17, 1995.
384. Schwartzman RM: The ELISA as an aid to the diagnosis of canine atopic disease. Vet Allergy Clin Immunol 3:81–90, 1995.
385. Shaw SC: The role of house dust mite allergens in canine allergic disease. In: Kwochka KW, et al (eds): Advances in Veterinary Dermatology III. Butterworth Heinemann, Boston, 1998, p. 505.
386. Sture GH, et al: Canine atopic disease: the prevalence of positive intradermal skin tests at two sites in the north and south of Great Britain. Vet Immunol Immunopathol 44:293, 1995.
387. Vogelnest LJ, et al: The suitability of Domitor (medetomidine) sedation for facilitating intradermal skin testing in dogs. Proc Annu Memb Meet Am Acad Vet Dermatol Am Coll Vet Dermatol 14:37, 1998.
388. Wassom DL: Principles and history of the Fc epsilon Receptor (FceRI) for IgE detection. Comp Cont Educ Pract Vet 19(Suppl):6, 1997.
389. Wassom DL, Grieve RB: In vitro measurement of canine and feline IgE: Review of Fcε RIα-based assays for detection of allergen-reactive IgE. Vet Dermatol 9:173, 1998.
390. Wellington J, et al: Determination of skin threshold concentration of an aqueous house dust mite allergen in normal dogs. Cornell Vet 81:37, 1991.
391. Wellington JR, et al: Dermatophagoides mites in house dust as an allergen source in atopic dogs. Cornell Vet 81:429, 1991.
392. Willis EL, Kunkle GA: Intradermal reactivity to various insect and arachnid allergens in dogs from the southeastern United States. J Am Vet Med Assoc 209:1431, 1996.
393. Willemse A, van den Brom WE: Evaluation of the intradermal allergy test in normal dogs. Res Vet Sci 32:57, 1982.
394. Zunic M: Comparison between IMMUNODOT tests and the intradermal skin test in atopic dogs. Vet Dermatol 9:201, 1998.
395. Zunic M, Honel A: Diagnosis of canine atopy: In vitro testing using CMG IMMUNODOT. Proc Annu Memb Meet Am Acad Vet Dermatol Am Coll Vet Dermatol 13:39, 1997.

Hyposensitization

396. Angarano DW, MacDonald JM: Immunotherapy in canine atopy. In: Kirk RW, Bonagura JD (eds): Current Veterinary Therapy XI. W.B. Saunders, Philadelphia, 1991, p. 505.
397. DesRoches A: Specific immunotherapy prevents the onset of new sensitization in monosensitized children. J Allergy Clin Immunol 95(1):309, 1995.
398. Ferguson EA: A retrospective comparison of the success of two different hyposensitization protocols in the management of canine atopy. Proc Br Vet Dermatol Study Grp 16:26, 1994.
399. Garfield RA: Injection immunotherapy in the treatment of canine atopic dermatitis: Comparison of 3 hyposensitization protocols. Proc Annu Memb Meet Am Acad Vet Dermatol Am Coll Vet Dermatol 8:7, 1992.
400. Griffin CE: Hyposensitization. Calif Vet 52:1, 1998.
401. McDonald JM: Rush hyposensitization in the treatment of canine atopy. Proc Annu Memb Meet Am Acad Vet Dermatol Am Coll Vet Dermatol 15:95, 1999.
402. Mueller RS, Bettenay SV: Long-term immunotherapy in 146 dogs with atopic dermatitis—a retrospective study. Aust Vet Practit 26:128, 1996.
403. Nelson HS: Immunotherapy for inhalant allergens. In: Middleton E, et al (eds): Allergy Principles and Practice V. C.V. Mosby, St. Louis, 1998, p. 1050.
404. Nuttal TJ: A retrospective survey of hyposensitization therapy. In: Kwochka KW, et al (eds): Advances in Veterinary Dermatology III. Butterworth Heinemann, Boston, 1998, p. 507.
405. Reedy LM: Personal experiences with injection immunotherapy. Proc Annu Memb Meet Am Acad Vet Dermatol Am Coll Vet Dermatol 15:99, 1999.
406. Rosenbaum MR, et al: Effects of mold proteases on the biological activity of allergenic pollen extracts. Am J Vet Res 57:1447, 1996.

407. Rosser EJ: Aqueous hyposensitization in the treatment of canine atopic dermatitis: A retrospective and prospective study of 100 cases. In: Kwochka KW, et al (eds): Advances in Veterinary Dermatology III. Butterworth Heinemann, Boston, 1998, p. 169.
408. Schwartzman RM, Mathis L: Immunotherapy for canine atopic dermatitis: Efficacy in 125 atopic dogs with vaccine formulations based on ELISA allergy testing. Vet Allergy Clin Immunol 5:123, 1997.
409. Scott KV, et al: A retrospective study of hyposensitization in atopic dogs in a flea-scarce environment. In: Ihrke PJ, et al (eds): Advances in Veterinary Dermatology II. Pergamon Press, New York, 1993, p. 79.
410. Scott KA, Rosychuk RAW, et al: Hyposensitization: The Colorado State University experience with emphasis on efficacy by breed. Proc Annu Memb Meet Am Acad Vet Dermatol Am Coll Vet Dermatol 15:107, 1999.
411. Wagner R: A retrospective survey of hyposensitization therapy using low concentrations of alum-precipitated allergens. Proc Annu Memb Meet Am Acad Vet Dermatol Am Coll Vet Dermatol 15:89, 1998.
412. Willemse A, et al: Effect of hyposensitization on atopic dermatitis in dogs. J Am Vet Med Assoc 184:277, 1984.
413. Willemse T: Hyposensitization of dogs with atopic dermatitis based on the results of in vivo and in vitro (IgGd ELISA) diagnostic tests. Proc Annu Memb Meet Am Acad Vet Dermatol Am Coll Vet Dermatol 10:61, 1994.

Feline Atopy/Allergic Diseases

414. Bettenay S: Diagnosing and treatment feline atopic dermatitis. Vet Med 86:488, 1991.
415. Bettenay S: Response to hyposensitization in 29 atopic cats. In: Kwochka KW, et al (eds): Advances in Veterinary Dermatology III. Butterworth Heinemann, Boston, 1998, p. 517.
416. Bevier DE: The reaction of feline skin to the intradermal injection of allergenic extracts and passive cutaneous anaphylaxis using the serum from skin test positive cats. In: von Tscharner C, Halliwell REW (eds): Advances in Veterinary Dermatology I. Ballière-Tindall, Philadelphia, 1990, p. 126.
417. Bevier DE: Effect of methylprednisolone acetate and oral prednisone on immediate skin test reactivity in cats. Proc Annu Memb Meet Am Acad Vet Dermatol Am Coll Vet Dermatol 10:45, 1994.
418. Bevier DE, Dunstan S: Ultrastructural changes in feline dermal mast cells during antigen-induced degranulation in vivo. In: Kwochka KW, et al (eds): Advances in Veterinary Dermatology III. Butterworth Heinemann, Boston, 1998, p. 213.
419. Carlotti D, Prost C: L'atopie feline. Point Vét 20:777, 1988.
420. Chalmers S, Medleau L: Recognizing the signs of feline allergic dermatoses. Vet Med 84:388, 1989.
421. Codner EC: Reactivity to intradermal injections of extracts of house dust mite and flea antigen in normal cats and cats suspected of being allergic. Proc Annu Memb Meet Am Acad Vet Dermatol Am Coll Vet Dermatol 12:26, 1996.
422. Corcoran BM, et al: Feline asthma syndrome: A retrospective study of the clinical presentation in 19 cats. J Small Anim Pract 36:481, 1995.
423. DeBoer DJ, et al: Feline IgE: Preliminary evidence of its existence and cross-reactivity with canine IgE. In: Ihrke PJ, et al (eds): Advances in Veterinary Dermatology II. Pergamon Press, New York, 1993, p. 51.
424. DeBoer DJ, et al: Monoclonal antibodies against feline immunoglobulin E. Proc Annu Memb Meet Am Acad Dermatol Am Coll Vet Dermatol 10:11, 1994.
425. Foster AP, O'Dair H: Allergy testing for skin disease in the cat: In vivo versus in vitro tests. Vet Dermatol 4:111, 1993.
426. Foster AP, et al: Studies on the isolation and characterization of a reaginic antibody in a cat. Res Vet Sci 58:70, 1995.
427. Foster AP: A study of the number and distribution of cutaneous mast cells in cats with disease not affecting the skin. Vet Dermatol 5:17, 1994.
428. Bevier D, et al: Fcε RIα-based ELISA technology for in vitro determination of allergen-specific IgE in normal cats and correlation to intradermal skin test results: Preliminary findings. Comp Cont Educ Pract Vet 19(Suppl):17, 1997.
429. Foster AP, et al: Allergen-specific IgG antibodies in cats with allergic skin disease. Res Vet Sci 63:239, 1997.
430. Gilbert S, Halliwell REW: Assessment of an ELISA for the detection of allergen-specific IgE in cats experimentally sensitized against house dust mites. In: Kwochka KW, et al (eds): Advances in Veterinary Dermatology III. Butterworth Heinemann, Boston, 1998, p. 520.
431. Gilbert S, Halliwell REW: Production and characterization of polyclonal antisera against feline IgE. Vet Immunol Immunopathol 63:223, 1998.
432. Gilbert S, Halliwell REW: Feline immunoglobulin E: Induction of antigen-specific antibody in normal cats and levels in spontaneously allergic cats. Vet Immunol Immunopathol 63:235, 1998.
433. Gilbert S, et al: L'atopie féline. Prat Méd Chir Anim Comp 34:15, 1999.
434. Halliwell REW: Efficacy of hyposensitization in feline allergic diseases based upon results of in vitro testing for allergen-specific immunoglobulin E. J Am Anim Hosp Assoc 33:3, 1997.
435. Koeman JP, et al: Quantity and distribution of mast cells and eosinophils in feline allergic miliary dermatitis. In: Kwochka KW, et al (eds): Advances in Veterinary Dermatology III. Butterworth Heinemann, Boston, 1998, p. 480.
436. McDougal BJ: Allergy testing and hyposensitization for three common feline dermatoses. Mod Vet Pract 67:629, 1986.
437. Mueller RS, et al: Effect of tiletamine-zolazepam anesthesia on the response to intradermally injected histamine in cats. Vet Dermatol 2:119, 1991.
438. Mueller RS: Diagnosis and management of feline atopy. Aust Vet Practit 27:138, 1997.
439. O'Dair H, et al: An open prospective investigation into aetiology in a group of cats with suspected allergic skin disease. Vet Dermatol 7:193, 1996.
440. Prélaud P: In vitro allergy testing to Dermatophagoides farinae and flea in 99 cases of feline eosinophilic granuloma complex. Proc Annu Memb Meet Eur Soc Vet Dermatol Eur Coll Vet Dermatol 14:170, 1997.
441. Prélaud P, et al: Le chat allergique. Prat Méd Chir Anim Comp 34:437, 1999.
442. Prost C: Les dermatoses allergiques du chat. Prat Méd Chir Anim Comp 28:151, 1993.
443. Prost C: Hypersensitivity to tobacco in six dogs and two cats: A social disease. Proc Annu Memb Meet Eur Soc Vet Dermatol Eur Coll Vet Dermatol 10:70, 1993.
444. Prost C: Diagnosis of feline allergic diseases: A study

of 90 cats. In: Kwochka KW, et al (eds): Advances in Veterinary Dermatology III. Butterworth Heinemann, Boston, 1998, p. 516.
445. Reedy LM: Results of allergy testing and hyposensitization in selected feline skin diseases. J Am Anim Hosp Assoc 18:618, 1982.
446. Roosje PJ, et al: Feline atopic dermatitis: A model for Langerhans' cell participation in disease pathogenesis. Am J Pathol 151:927, 1997.
447. Roosje PJ, Willemse T: Cytophilic antibodies in cats with miliary dermatitis and eosinophilic plaques: Passive transfer of immediate-type hypersensitivity. Vet Q 17:66, 1995.
448. Roosje PJ, et al: A role of Th2 cells in the pathogenesis of allergic dermatitis in cats? Cong Br Netherlands Soc Immunol 86(1):98, 1995.
449. Roosje PJ, et al: MHC Class II+ and CD1A+ cells in lesional skin of cats with allergic dermatitis. World Cong Vet Dermatol 3:59, 1996.
450. Roosje PJ, et al: Immunopathogenesis of feline atopic dermatitis current concepts. Proc Annu Memb Meet Eur Soc Vet Dermatol Eur Coll Vet Dermatol 15, Speaker's Notes, 1998.
451. Roosje PJ, et al: Increased numbers of CD4+ and CD8+ T cells in lesional skin of cats with allergic dermatitis. Vet Pathol 35:268, 1998.
452. Saint-Andre I, et al: Quantitative assessment of CD18 positive major histocompatibility complex class II positive and CD1a positive epidermal dendritic cells in the cat. In: Kwochka KW, et al (eds): Advances in Veterinary Dermatology III. Butterworth Heinemann, Boston, 1998, p. 524.
453. Scott DW, et al: Miliary dermatitis: A feline cutaneous reaction pattern. Proc Annu Kal Kan Semin 2:11, 1986.
454. Scott DW, et al: Sterile eosinophilic folliculitis in the cat: An unusual manifestation of feline allergic skin disease? Comp Anim Pract 19:6, 1989.
455. Scott DW: Analyse du type de réaction histopathologique dans le diagnostic des dermatoses inflammatoires chez le chat: Étude sur 394 cas. Point Vét 26:57, 1994.
456. Willemse T, et al: Changes in plasma cortisol, corticotropin, and α-melanocyte-stimulating hormone concentrations in cats before and after physical restraint and intradermal testing. Am J Vet Res 54:69, 1993.

Contact Hypersensitivity

457. Baadsgaard O, Wang T: Immune regulation in allergic and irritant skin reactions. Int J Dermatol 30:161, 1991.
458. Belisto DV: Allergic contact dermatitis In: Freedberg IM, et al (eds): Fitzpatrick's Dermatology in General Medicine V. McGraw-Hill, New York, 1999, p. 1447.
459. Bourdeau P, et al: Positive reactions to allergenic challenge in healthy dogs. Part 2—Patch test. In: Kwochka KW, et al, (eds): Advances in Veterinary Dermatology III. Butterworth Heinemann, Boston, 1998, p. 445.
460. Brehler R, et al: Topically applied pentoxifylline has no effect on allergic patch responses. J Am Acad Dermatol 39:1017, 1998.
461. Calderwood-Mays MB, et al: Carpet deodorant contact dermatitis in a cat. Proc Annu Memb Meet Am Acad Vet Dermatol Am Coll Vet Dermatol 9:67, 1993.
462. Carlotti DN, et al: Scrotal contact dermatitis in the dog: A report of 6 cases. Proc Annu Memb Meet Am Acad Vet Dermatol Am Coll Vet Dermatol 15:51, 1999.
463. Clark EG, et al: Cedar wood-induced allergic contact dermatitis in a dog. Proc Annu Memb Meet Am Acad Vet Dermatol Am Coll Vet Dermatol 9:68, 1993.
464. Comer KM: Carpet deodorizer as a contact allergen in a dog. J Am Vet Med Assoc 193:1553, 1988.
465. Dunstan RW, et al: Histologic features of allergic contact dermatitis in four dogs. Proc Annu Memb Meet Am Acad Vet Dermatol Am Coll Vet Dermatol 9:69, 1993.
466. Krawiec DR, Gaafar SM: A comparative study of allergic and primary irritant contact dermatitis with dinitrochlorobenzene (DNCB) in dogs. J Invest Dermatol 65:248, 1975.
467. Kunkle GA, Gross TL: Allergic contact dermatitis to Tradescantia fluminensis (wandering Jew) in a dog. Comp Cont Educ 5:925, 1983.
468. Kunkle GA: Contact allergic dermatitis. Vet Clin North Am Small Anim Pract 18:1061, 1988.
469. Marsella R, et al: Use of pentoxifylline in the treatment of allergic contact reactions to plants of the Commelinceae family in dogs. Vet Dermatol 8:121, 1997.
470. Merchant SR, et al: Eosinophilic pustules and eosinophilic dermatitis secondary to patch testing a dog with Asian jasmine. Proc Annu Memb Meet Am Acad Vet Dermatol Am Coll Vet Dermatol 9:64, 1993.
471. Michaud AJ: Plastic shopping bag as a possible contact allergen in a cat. Feline Pract 19:6, 1991.
472. Mydlarski PR, et al: Contact dermatitis. In: Middleton E, et al (eds): Allergy Principles and Practice V. C.V. Mosby, St Louis, 1998, p. 1135.
473. Nobreus N, et al: Induction of dinitrochlorobenzene contact sensitivity in dogs. Monogr Allergy 8:100, 1974.
474. Olivry T, et al: Allergic contact dermatitis in the dog. Vet Clin North Am Small Anim Pract 20:1443, 1990.
475. Olivry T: Allergic contact dermatitis to cement: A delayed hypersensitivity to dichromates and nickel. Proc Annu Memb Meet Am Acad Vet Dermatol Am Coll Vet Dermatol 9:63, 1993.
476. Prélaud P: Dermatite de contact à la néomycine chez un chat. Action Vét 21:1169, 1991.
477. Rietschel RL: Irritant contact dermatitis. Mechanisms in irritant contact dermatitis. Clin Dermatol 15:557, 1997.
478. Schultz KT, Maguire HC: Chemically-induced delayed hypersensitivity in the cat. Vet Immunol Immunopathol 3:585, 1982.
479. Schultz RD, Adams LS: Immunologic methods for the detection of humoral and cellular immunity. Vet Clin North Am Small Anim Clin 8:721, 1978.
480. Schwartz A, et al: Pentoxifylline suppresses irritant and contact hypersensitivity reactions. J Invest Dermatol 101:549, 1993.
481. Thomsen MK, Kristensen F: Contact dermatitis in the dog: A review and clinical study. Nord Vet Med 38:129, 1986.
482. Thomsen MK, Thomsen HK: Histopathological changes in canine allergic contact dermatitis patch test reactions: A study on spontaneously hypersensitive dogs. Acta Vet Scand 30:379, 1989.
483. Walder EJ, Conroy JD: Contact dermatitis in dogs and cats: Pathogenesis, histopathology, experimental induction and case reports. Vet Dermatol 5:149, 1994.
484. Walton GS: Allergic contact dermatitis. In: Kirk RW

(ed): Current Veterinary Therapy VI. W.B. Saunders, Philadelphia, 1977, p. 571.
485. White PD: Contact dermatitis in the dog and cat. Semin Vet Med Surg 6:303, 1991.
486. Willemse T, Vroom MA: Allergic dermatitis in a Great Dane due to contact with hippeastrum. Vet Rec 122:490, 1988.

Canine Food Hypersensitivity

487. Rosser EJ: Protein hydrolysates in canine diets to diagnose and prevent food allergy. Monograph, Allergy Concepts, Inc., 1999.
488. August JR: Dietary hypersensitivity in dogs: Cutaneous manifestations, diagnosis, and treatment. Comp Cont Educ 7:469, 1985.
489. Batt R, et al: Food allergy and intolerance—the gut perspective. Waltham Focus, Focus on Skin and Coat, April, 1999, p. 31.
490. Brown CM, et al: Nutritional management of food allergy in dogs and cats. Comp Cont Educ 17:637, 1995.
491. Carlotti DN, et al: Food allergy in dogs and cats: A review and report of 43 cases. Vet Dermatol 1:55, 1990.
492. Denis S, Paradis M: L'allergie alimentaire chez le chien et le chat. I: Revue de la literature. Méd Vét Québec 24:11, 1994.
493. Denis S, Paradis M: L'allergie alimentaire chez le chien et le chat. II: Étude rétrospective. Méd Vét Québec 24:15, 1994.
494. Elmwood CM, et al: Gastroscopic food sensitivity testing in 17 dogs. J Small Anim Pract 35:199, 1994.
495. Ermel RW, et al: The atopic dog: A model for food allergy. Lab Anim Sci 47:40, 1997.
496. Fadok VA: Diagnosing and managing the food-allergic dog. Comp Cont Educ Pract Vet 16:1541, 1994.
497. Ferguson E, Scheidt VJ: Hypoallergenic diets and skin disease. In: Ihrke PJ, et al (eds): Advances in Veterinary Dermatology II. Pergamon Press, New York, 1993, p. 459.
498. Ghernati I, et al: A case of food allergy immunohistopathologically mimicking mycosis fungoides. In: Kwochka KW, et al (eds): Advances in Veterinary Dermatology III. Butterworth Heinemann, Boston, 1998, p. 432.
499. Griffin CE: Diagnosis and management of food allergy. Proceedings of the European School of Advanced Veterinary Studies, 1999.
500. Groh M, Moser E: Diagnosis of food allergy in the nonseasonally symptomatic dog using a novel antigen, low molecular weight diet: A prospective study of 29 cases. Vet Allergy Clin Immunol 6:5, 1998.
501. Guaguère E, Prélaud P: Les intolérances alimentaires. Prat Méd Chir Anim Comp 33(Suppl):389, 1998.
502. Guilford WG, et al: The histamine content of commercial pet foods. N Z Vet J 42:201, 1994.
503. Guilford WB, et al: Development of gastroscopic food sensitivity testing in dogs. J Vet Intern Med 8:414, 1994.
504. Halliwell REW: Comparative aspects of food intolerance. Vet Med 87:893, 1992.
505. Halliwell REW: Management of dietary hypersensitivity in the dog. J Small Anim Pract 33:156, 1993.
506. Harvey RG: Food allergy and dietary intolerance in dogs: A report of 25 cases. J Small Anim Pract 33:22, 1993.
507. Hillier A, Kunkle GA: Inability to demonstrate food antigen-specific IgE antibodies in the serum of food allergic dogs using the PK and oral PK tests. Proc Annu Memb Meet Am Acad Vet Dermatol Am Coll Vet Dermatol 10:28, 1994.
508. Jeffers JG, et al: Diagnostic testing of dogs for food hypersensitivity. J Am Vet Med Assoc 198:245, 1991.
509. Jeffers JG, et al: Responses of dogs with food allergies to single-ingredient dietary provocation. J Am Vet Med Assoc 209:608, 1996.
510. Kaplan AJ: Onion powder in baby food may induce anemia in cats. J Am Vet Med Assoc 207:1405, 1995.
511. Kunkle G, et al: Validity of skin testing for diagnosis of food allergy in dogs. J Am Vet Med Assoc 200:677, 1992.
512. MacDonald JM: Food allergy. In: Griffin CE, et al (eds): Current Veterinary Dermatology. Mosby Year Book, St. Louis, 1993, p. 121.
513. Merchant SR, Taboada J: Food allergy and immunologic diseases of the gastrointestinal tract. Semin Vet Med Surg 6:316, 1991.
514. Mueller R, Tsohalis J: Evaluation of serum allergen-specific IgE for the diagnosis of food adverse reactions in the dog. Vet Dermatol 9:167, 1998.
515. Olsen JW: Clinical use of gastroscopic food sensitivity testing in the dog. Proc Am Acad Vet Allergy, 1991.
516. Paterson S: Food hypersensitivity in 20 dogs with skin and gastrointestinal signs. J Small Anim Pract 36:529, 1995.
517. Rosser EJ Jr: Diagnosis of food allergy in dogs. J Am Vet Med Assoc 203:259, 1993.
518. Rosser E: Food allergy in dogs and cats: A review. Vet Allergy Clin Immunol 6:21, 1998.
519. Rosser EJ Jr: Foreword in Allergy Concepts, Inc.: Protein hydrolysates in canine diets to diagnose and prevent food allergy. Monograph, Allergy Concepts, Inc., 1999.
520. Roudebush P, Schick R: Evaluation of a commercial canned lamb and rice diet for the management of adverse reactions to food in dogs. Vet Dermatol 5:63, 1994.
521. Roudebush P, et al: Protein characteristics of commercial canine and feline hypoallergenic diets. Vet Dermatol 5:69, 1994.
522. Roudebush P, et al: Results of a hypoallergenic diet survey of veterinarians in North America with a nutritional evaluation of homemade diet prescriptions. Vet Dermatol 3:23, 1992.
523. Sampson HA: Adverse reactions to foods. In: Middleton E, et al (eds): Allergy Principles and Practice V. C.V. Mosby, St Louis, 1998, p. 1162.
524. Tapp T, et al: Comparisons of a commercial limited antigen diet versus a home prepared diet in the diagnosis of canine food hypersensitivity. Vet Allergy Clin Immunol (accepted 1999).
525. Wagner R, Horvath C: Capelin and tapioca 1 dry food in dogs and cats with food allergy. Proc Annu Memb Meet Am Acad Vet Dermatol Am Coll Vet Dermatol 15:32, 1999.
526. Walton GS: Skin responses in the dog and cat to ingested allergens: Observations of 100 confirmed cases. Vet Rec 81:709, 1967.
527. White SD, Mason IS: Dietary allergy: In: von Tscharner C, Halliwell REW (eds): Advances in Veterinary Dermatology I. Ballière-Tindall, Philadelphia, 1990, p. 404.
528. White SD: Food hypersensitivity in 30 dogs. J Am Vet Med Assoc 188:695, 1986.
529. White SD: Food allergy in dogs. Comp Cont Educ Pract Vet 20:261, 1998.

furunculosis in three cases. J Small Anim Pract 36: 119, 1995.
606. Fondati A, Mechelli L: Cutaneous arthropod reactions in the dog: 6 cases. In: Kwochka KW, et al (eds): Advances in Veterinary Dermatology III. Butterworth Heinemann, Boston, 1998, p. 576.
607. Gross TL: Canine eosinophilic furunculosis of the face. In: Ihrke PJ, et al (eds): Advances in Veterinary Dermatology II. Pergamon Press, New York, 1993, p. 239.
608. Guaguère E, et al: Furonculose éosinophilique chez le chien: Étude rétrospective de 12 cas. Prat Méd Chir Anim Comp 31:413, 1996.
609. Hotz CS: Eosinophilic dermatitis in a Siberian husky. Calif Vet 44:11, 1990.

Hormonal Hypersensitivity

610. Chamberlain KW: Hormonal hypersensitivity in canines. Canine Pract 1:18, 1974.
611. Coustou D, et al: Dermatitis caused by estrogens. Ann Dermatol Venerol 125:505, 1998.
612. Lee CW, et al: Autoimmune progesterone dermatitis. J Dermatol 19:629, 1992.
613. Miura MT, et al: Two cases of autoimmune progesterone dermatitis: Immunohistochemical and serological studies. Acta Dermatol Venerol 69:308, 1989.
614. Moghadam BK, et al: Autoimmune progesterone dermatitis and stomatitis. Oral Surg Oral Med Oral Pathol Oral Radiol Endocrinol 85:537, 1998.
615. Prost C, et al: Hypersensibilité hormonale et allergie alimentaire chez une chienne Labrador. Prat Méd Chir Anim Comp 30:411, 1995.
616. Scott DW, Miller WH Jr: Probable hormonal hypersensitivity in two male dogs. Canine Pract 17:14, 1992.

Bacterial Hypersensitivity

617. Burkett G, Frank LA: Comparison for production of *Staphylococcus intermedius* exotoxin among clinically normal dogs, atopic dogs with recurrent pyoderma, and dogs with a single episode of pyoderma. J Am Vet Med Assoc 213:232, 1998.
617a. DeBoer DJ, et al: Immunomodulatory effects of staphylococcal antigens and antigen-antibody complexes on canine mononuclear and polymorphonuclear leukocytes. Am J Vet Res 55:1690, 1994.
617b. Halliwell REW: Levels of IgE and IgG antibodies to staphylococcal antigens in normal dogs and dogs with recurrent pyoderma. Proc Annu Memb Meet Am Acad Vet Dermatol Am Coll Vet Dermatol 3:5, 1987.
618. Miller WH Jr: Antibiotic-responsive generalized nonlesional pruritus in a dog. Cornell Vet 81:389, 1991.
618a. Morales CA, et al: Antistaphylococcal antibodies in dogs with recurrent staphylococcal pyoderma. Vet Immunol Immunopathol 41:137, 1994.
619. Pukay BP: Treatment of bacterial hypersensitivity by hyposensitization with *Staphylococcus aureus* bacterin-toxoid. J Am Anim Hosp Assoc 21:479, 1985.
620. Scott DW, et al: Staphylococcal hypersensitivity in the dog. J Am Anim Hosp Assoc 14:666, 1978.
621. Strange P, et al: Staphylococcal enterotoxin B applied on intact normal and intact atopic skin induces dermatitis. Arch Dermatol 132:27, 1996.

Chapter 9

Immune-Mediated Disorders

Immune-mediated dermatoses are well recognized* but uncommon skin diseases in dogs and cats. These dermatoses have been reported to account for 1.4% and 1.3%, respectively, of all canine and feline dermatoses examined by the dermatology service at a university small animal practice.[56] They have been subdivided into primary or autoimmune, and secondary or immune-mediated, the latter believed to be primarily diseases wherein tissue destruction results from an immunologic event that is not directed against normal self-antigens.[25, 65]

In autoimmune disease, antibodies or activated lymphocytes develop against normal body constituents and induce the lesions of the disease by passive transfer.[18, 59] This may result from failure to eliminate high-affinity self-reactive lymphocytes in primary lymphoid organs or failure to regulate the activity of low-affinity self-reactive lymphocytes.[9] A major level of control of the autoreactive clones of lymphocytes is suppression by suppressor T cells that are specific for those clones.[25, 65]

The development of autoimmune diseases is a reflection of a lack of control or a bypass of the normal control mechanisms. Over the years, a variety of possible defects have been described, but the exact abnormal mechanism and what induces these diseases still remain unknown. Some of the possibilities include (1) suppressor T cell bypass, (2) suppressor T cell dysfunction, (3) abnormal major histocompatibility complex (MHC) II expression or interaction, (4) cytokine and receptor ligand abnormalities, (5) autoantigen modification, (6) cross-reacting antigens, (7) inappropriate interleukin (IL)-2 production, (8) idiotype/anti-idiotype imbalance, (9) mutations in receptor affinity, and (10) failure of clonal deletion of low-affinity autoreactive thymocytes.† In addition, there is sexual dimorphism in the immune response, with female sex hormones tending to accelerate immune responses and male sex hormones tending to suppress responses.[3]

In secondary immune-mediated diseases, the antigen is foreign to the body. Most commonly, the inciting antigens are drugs, bacteria, and viruses that stimulate an immunologic reaction that results in host tissue damage.[6, 25, 47, 65] Superantigens are gene products that are recognized by a large fraction of T cells and have the potential to interfere with the recognition and elimination of conventional antigens.[28] These gene products may play a role in the genesis of immune-mediated diseases. So-called "epitope spreading" may also be important in autoimmune diseases.[118] In this situation, patients' bodies make antibodies against one protein early in their disease. Then, as the disease evolves, patients' bodies make additional antibodies against molecules that are similar in structure or even unlike in structure but physically closely associated within the tissue.

• DIAGNOSIS OF IMMUNE-MEDIATED SKIN DISEASE

The diagnosis of the these dermatoses requires demonstration of characteristic dermatopathologic changes and, optimally, the autoantibodies, immune complexes, or mediators

---

*See references 21, 22, 24, 25, 29, 30, 32, 34, 38, 47, 55–57, 59, 66, 67.
†See references 1, 4, 6, 8, 9, 12, 15, 17, 25, 26, 27, 35, 37, 39, 41–43, 48, 58, 59, 61, 65, 68, 70

(e.g., cytotoxic T cells) of the immunologic injury. Establishing the presence of characteristic dermatopathology requires cutaneous biopsy (see Chap. 2). In general, the following guidelines should be observed[20]:

1. Multiple biopsies should always be taken.
2. Samples should be selected from the most representative lesions of the suspected immune-mediated diseases.
3. Punch biopsy samples should be taken as gently as possible; wedge biopsy by scalpel excision may be necessary.
4. Whenever possible, biopsy specimens should be taken when the animal is not under the effects of any glucocorticoid or immunosuppressive therapy.[20, 47, 56]
5. Dermatopathologic examination should be performed by a veterinary pathologist who has a special interest in dermatopathology or by a veterinary dermatologist trained in dermatopathology.

Establishing the mediator of the immunologic damage may require biopsy and/or analysis of the patient's serum for auto or abnormal antibodies. The biopsies for immunopathologic examination often must be processed in special ways that may require fresh tissue, frozen tissue, or specially fixed samples, depending on the test to be performed. The veterinary immunopathology laboratory will be able to tell you what is required. Tests used to detect the presence of autoantibodies or various immunoreactants (e.g., immunoglobulins, complement components, microbial antigens) in skin lesions include immunofluorescence and immunohistochemical (immunoperoxidase) testing (Fig. 9–1).[7, 45, 73] In general, the following guidelines are used for collecting these biopsy specimens:

1. Biopsy specimens for direct antibody testing should be selected from areas not secondarily infected and generally representing the earliest lesion typical for that disease; a possible exception is discoid lupus erythematosus, wherein older lesions may be preferred. Vasculitis lesions less than 24 hours old are best. For bullous diseases, the blister itself is not sampled; instead, the adjacent normal skin or erythematous skin is used.
2. Sites wherein immunoglobulins are often present in normal tissue (e.g., nasal planum of dogs and cats, footpads of dogs) should not be sampled or should be interpreted appropriately (see Chap. 1).[33, 47]
3. Samples for direct immunofluorescence testing need to be fixed and mailed in Michel's fixative. Samples for direct immunoperoxidase testing may be formalin-fixed. The results of studies of tissues processed by quick-freezing and of those kept in Michel's fixative for up to 2 weeks are comparable.[10, 47] Studies in dogs and cats suggest that specimens may reliably be preserved in Michel's fixative for at least 7 to 14 days. In some instances, specimens have successfully been preserved for 4 to 8 years.[31, 47] The pH of Michel's fixative must be carefully maintained at 7.0 to 7.2 to ensure accurate results.[55, 56]
4. Samples for direct antibody detection should be sent to a veterinary immunopathology laboratory.

Testing for abnormal antibody or immune complex deposition is considered highly valuable in human medicine for many of the immune-mediated dermatoses. For the similar canine and feline diseases, however, their value has been considerably less. Reports from veterinary immunopathology research laboratories show that techniques and results appear to be improving.[51, 59, 140] However, these tests are fraught with numerous procedural and interpretational pitfalls, including method of specimen handling, choice of substrates used, method of substrate handling, specificity of conjugates, fluorescein-protein-antibody concentrations, and unitage of conjugates. An in-depth discussion of these factors is beyond the scope of this chapter; the reader is referred to Beutner and colleagues for details.[5]

The incidence of positive results in the canine disorders typically varies from about 25% to 90% for direct immunofluorescence testing.[19, 47, 55, 56] Positive results are

Immune-Mediated Disorders • **669**

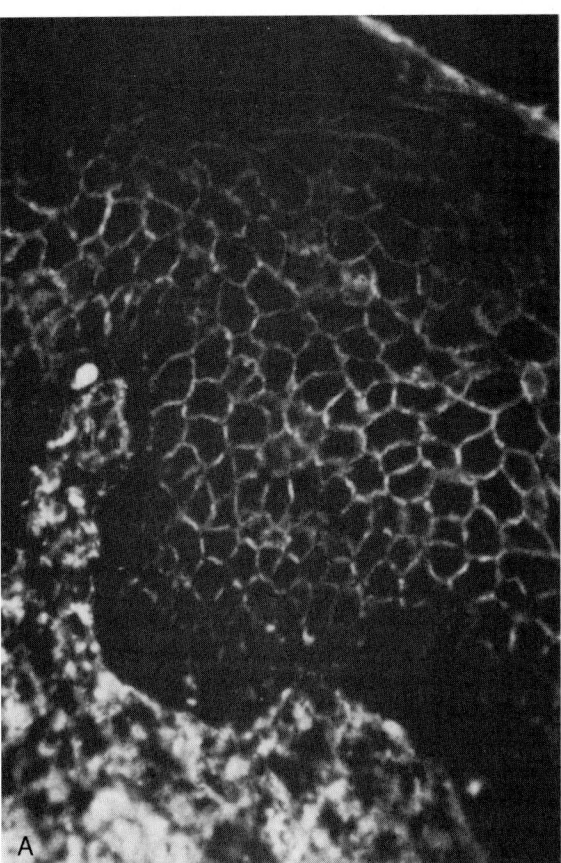

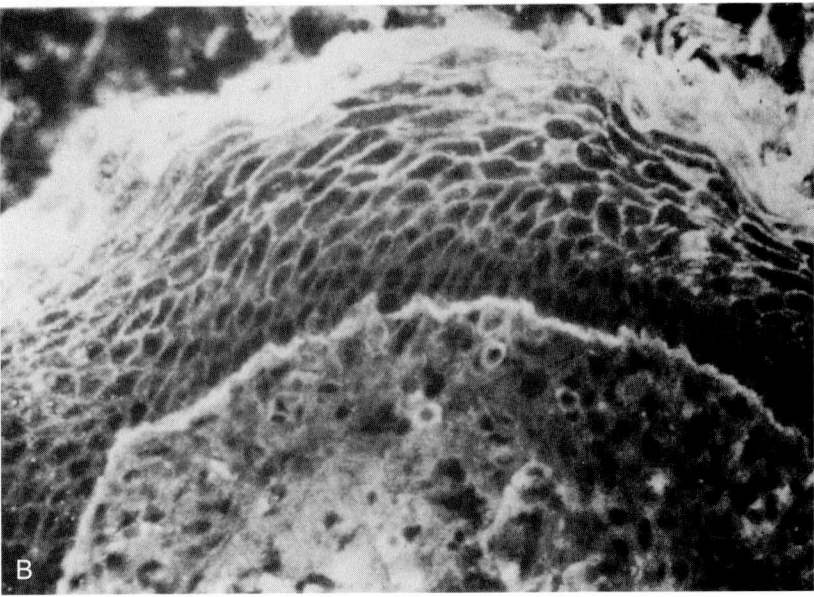

FIGURE 9–1. *A,* Canine pemphigus vulgaris. Direct immunofluorescence testing reveals host IgG within the intercellular spaces of epidermis. *B,* Canine pemphigus erythematosus. Direct immunofluorescence testing reveals host IgG within the intercellular spaces of epidermis and along the basement membrane zone. (*A* and *B,* from Scott DW, Lewis RM: Phemphigus and pemphigoid in a dog and man: Comparative aspects. J Am Acad Dermatol 5:148, 1981.) *Figure continues on following page*

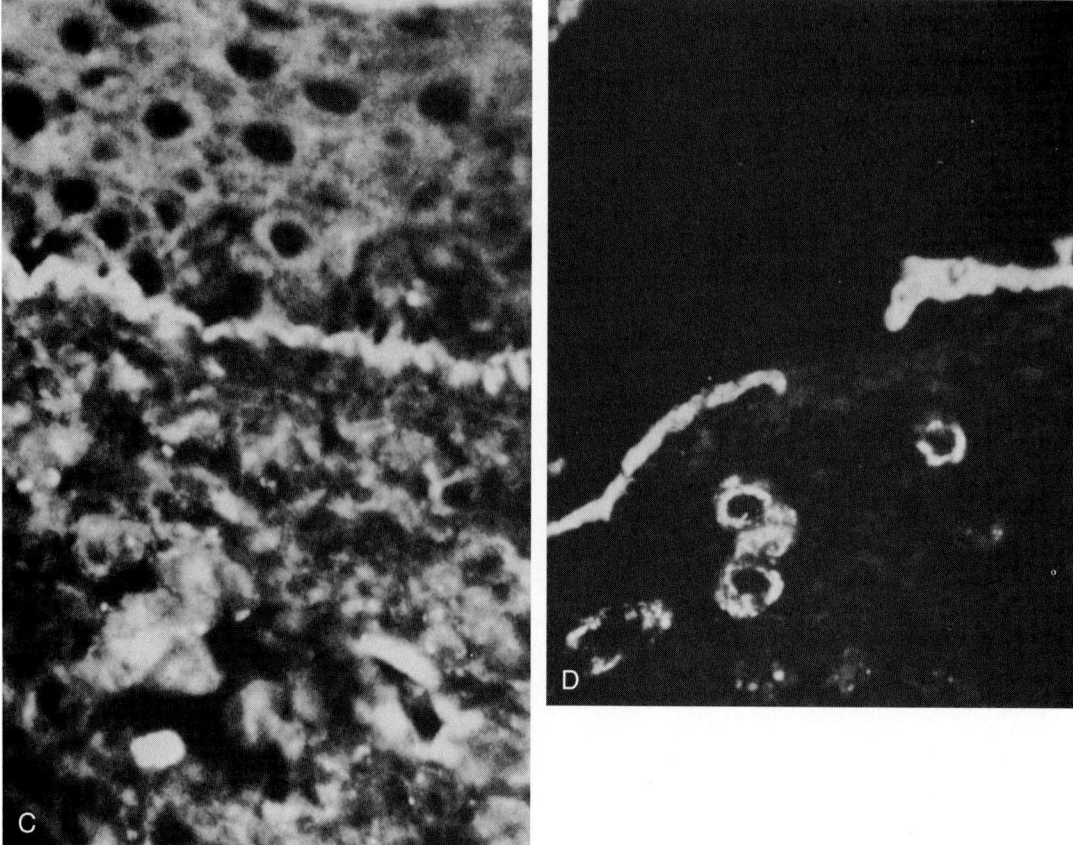

FIGURE 9–1. *Continued. C,* Canine bullous pemphigoid. Direct immunofluorescence testing reveals host IgG deposited at the basement membrane zone. (From Scott DW, et al: Observations on the end therapy of canine pemphigus and pemphigoid. J Am Vet Med Assoc 180:48, 1982.) *D,* Canine cutaneous vasculitis. Direct immunofluorescence testing reveals host IgG within blood vessel walls.

much more commonly achieved with the immunoperoxidase technique. With this technique, however, the incidence of false-positive results is also much higher.[23, 44] In fact, the intercellular and basement membrane zone deposition of immunoglobulins or complement can be detected from time to time in a wide variety of inflammatory dermatoses.[44, 47, 55, 56, 73]

In order to appropriately interpret these tests, one needs a good biopsy specimen for histopathologic examination. However, if one has an appropriate specimen for histopathologic examination, further testing and expense is usually not necessary. Thus, we, as well as others,[46] do not think that these tests need to be routinely done in the work-up of a suspected case of immune-mediated skin disease in a dog or cat.

Autoimmune dermatoses are classified on the basis of the specific autoallergens being targeted.[59, 117, 155, 191] This cannot be determined on the basis of routine immunofluorescence or immunohistochemical testing. Specific identification requires techniques such as immunoprecipitation and immunoblotting. This is rarely done in routine veterinary diagnostic laboratories and is limited to certain veterinary immunologic research laboratories. As a result, we may still be lumping together different diseases or variants that share clinical, histopathologic, and routine immunopathologic features.

Indirect immunofluorescence testing (testing serum for the presence of circulating autoantibody) in the past rarely yielded positive results in dogs and cats, and results were conflicting. Therefore, it was not recommended as a cost-effective test.[19, 47, 55, 56] More recently, results have been positive in a variety of diseases, including pemphigus foliaceus,[138, 139] pemphigus vulgaris,[59, 167, 168] paraneoplastic pemphigus,[125] bullous pemphigoid,[180, 185] epidermolysis bullosa acquisita,[191] and alopecia areata.[380, 382] The only disease in which more than a few cases have been studied is canine pemphigus foliaceus, wherein the most recent study reported 63% of the cases to yield positive results.[138, 140]

Now that the technology is available, we should consider obtaining tissue and serum samples for researchers who are performing these tests correctly and frequently. Only then will we be able to determine whether the variants described in humans also exist in dogs and cats and whether their differentiation leads to prognostic or therapeutic value. Results of immunopathologic testing can never be appropriately interpreted in the absence of histopathologic findings.[46, 47] On the other hand, histopathologic findings are sufficiently characteristic to be diagnostic in the majority of cases.[22, 47, 71]

The clinician's time and the owner's money are better spent in the careful selection and procuring of representative skin specimens and their forwarding to a knowledgeable dermatopathologist. As techniques that are more sensitive become readily available, this type of testing will undoubtedly become more common. For now, we recommend collecting serum from dogs and cats with active suspected autoimmune disease and saving it in the freezer. After other test results are reviewed, and with the recommendation of the pathologist, the indirect immunofluorescence test may still be performed by an appropriate laboratory or the serum may be submitted to appropriate research centers to support future progress. This sample may also be used at a later date as a pretreatment sample for some serum biochemical parameters.

• THERAPY OF IMMUNE-MEDIATED SKIN DISEASES

As a group, all of these immune-mediated dermatoses are characterized by an inappropriate immune response that, to be adequately controlled, may require the use of potent immunosuppressive and immunomodulating drugs.[16, 76] In the past, this primarily meant high levels of glucocorticoids and, occasionally, cyclophosphamide or azathioprine. These initial attempts at treatment, although often successful, led to many side effects (see Chap. 3). In recent years, however, a variety of different treatment approaches have been evaluated, and now more therapeutic options are available to the clinician for the management of some of these diseases. The diseases are not all optimally treated in the same way, however, nor do they carry the same prognosis. Therefore, it is important that the clinician make as specific a diagnosis as possible. Although much work on new approaches to the management of these diseases is underway in human medicine, very little of this information is being applied in veterinary medicine.

The drugs used to treat immune-mediated skin diseases are generally called *immunosuppressive agents*. However, the exact mechanism of some of these drugs is unknown. They may act in methods different from those of the more classic immunosuppressive agents. They are considered together because, whatever their mechanism of action, they share the feature of being beneficial in managing the immune-mediated skin diseases.

Glucocorticoids are the most common class of drugs used as immunosuppressive agents. They are discussed in Chapter 3. However, many other drugs are used in practice, and some are effective only in specific diseases (Table 9–1). A special use of glucocorticoids for the initial treatment of some severe immune-mediated dermatoses is pulse therapy. Glucocorticoid pulse therapy (11 mg/kg methylprednisolone sodium succinate given intravenously over 1 hour for 3 consecutive days) was used to induce remissions in cases of canine pemphigus that had not responded to oral glucocorticoids.[79] This therapy is expensive and not without complications (see Chap. 3).

Cyclophosphamide

Cyclophosphamide (Cytoxan, Bristol-Meyers Squibb) is metabolized to alkylating agents that inhibit mitosis by interfering with DNA replication and ribonucleic acid (RNA)

Table 9-1 IMMUNOSUPPRESSIVE DRUGS AND INDICATIONS

DRUG	INDUCTION DOSE	INDICATIONS
Glucocorticoids		Short-term use in severe cases of autoimmune disease
Prednisone	2.2–6.6 mg/kg q24h	
Prednisolone	2.2–6.6 mg/kg q24h	
Triamcinolone	0.2–0.6 mg/kg q24h	
Dexamethasone	0.2–0.6 mg/kg q24h	
Cyclophosphamide	1.5–2.5 mg/kg q48h	Undesirable for long-term use, short-term use only in severe cases
Azathioprine	1.5–2.5 mg/kg q24h (low dose in dogs >30 kg; high dose in dogs <15 kg)	All immune-mediated disorders; not for use in cats
Chlorambucil	0.1–0.2 mg/kg q24–48h (in cats usually 0.2 mg/kg q48h)	All, but especially feline diseases
Cyclosporine	5–10 mg/kg q24h	All
Chrysotherapy		
Aurothioglucose	1 mg/kg IM	Feline pemphigus foliaceus and erythematosus; plasma cell stomatitis; plasma cell pododermatitis; canine pemphigus complex (second choice)
Auranofin	3–6 mg q24h	
Dapsone	1 mg/kg q8h (in dogs); 1 mg/kg q24h (with caution, in cats)	Subcorneal pustular dermatosis; leukocytoclastic vasculitis; pemphigus complex
Sulfasalazine	22–44 mg/kg q8h (in dogs)	Subcorneal pustular dermatosis; vasculitis
Vitamin E	100–400 mg q12h	Discoid lupus erythematosus; pemphigus erythematosus; epidermolysis bullosa
Tetracycline and niacinamide	In dogs >10 kg: 500 mg q8h each In dogs <10 kg: 250 mg q8h each	Discoid lupus erythematosus; pemphigus erythematosus; sterile pyogranuloma syndrome; sterile panniculitis; uveodermatologic syndrome; lupoid onychodystrophy; German shepherd metatarsal fistulae; vasculitis
Sun avoidance		Discoid lupus erythematosus; pemphigus erythematosus; systemic lupus erythematosus

transcription and replication.[74–76] It is used alone or in combination with other chemotherapeutic agents for the treatment of various neoplasms, as well as for its immunosuppressive activity in nonmalignant diseases and organ transplantation.[77, 82] Able to kill cells in all phases of the cell cycle, this type of cytotoxic drug is more effective in slow-growing tumors than phase-specific drugs that act during only a specific time of the cell cycle. It is most effective against rapidly dividing cells. Lymphocytes are especially sensitive to cyclophosphamide. The drug is immunosuppressive to both the humoral and cell-mediated immune systems, but it is more effective against B cells than against T cells. Cyclophosphamide suppresses antibody production. Maximal effect occurs if the drug is given shortly after the antigenic stimulus, when it suppresses primary and secondary humoral responses.

Major toxic sequelae include sterile hemorrhagic cystitis, bladder fibrosis, teratogenesis, infertility, alopecia and poor hair growth, nausea, inflammation of the gastrointestinal tract, increased susceptibility to infections, and depression of the bone marrow and hematopoietic systems. Cats may lose their whiskers. Hemorrhagic cystitis occurs in up to 30% of dogs on chronic therapy of more than 2 months' duration.[75] Its effects should be monitored with periodic hemograms and urinalyses.

Clinical indications include lymphoreticular neoplasms, for which the drug is best combined with glucocorticoids or vincristine. It can be given with high doses of glucocorticoids to achieve remission of severe cases of immune-mediated diseases such as systemic lupus erythematosus, vasculitis, pemphigus complex, bullous pemphigoid, idiopathic thrombocytopenia, hemolytic anemia, gammopathies, and rheumatoid arthritis.[77, 82] The potential for hemorrhagic cystitis and bladder fibrosis makes this drug less desirable for long-term (>3 to 4 months) use than azathioprine or chlorambucil.[76] Because dogs with immune-mediated skin disease will be on lifelong or months of therapy, we rarely use this drug. The protocol for neoplasms is 50 mg/m^2 of body surface area given orally q24h for 4 days, then no treatment for 3 days; this sequence is repeated weekly. For immunosuppression, the oral dosage is 1.5 to 2.5 mg/kg. Dosage frequency varies from every other day to 4 days on and 3 days off.[47, 75, 76]

Chlorambucil

Chlorambucil (Leukeran, Glaxo Wellcome) is an orally administered alkylating agent.[77] Its cytotoxic effect is due to cross-linking of DNA.[74–76] Compared with other alkylating agents, it is slow acting and less toxic. Although serious toxicity is rare at usual doses, myelosuppression is possible. Consequently, patients should initially be monitored with hemograms every 2 to 4 weeks. Anorexia, vomiting, and diarrhea have been reported at daily dosing but often resolve with alternate-day dosing.[80] Alopecia and delayed hair growth after clipping have been reported, and Poodles and Kerry blue terriers are reported to be at greater risk.[75] Chlorambucil is available only in a 2-mg tablet, making it most useful in small dogs and cats.

Chlorambucil may be useful in the pemphigus complex, bullous pemphigoid, discoid and systemic lupus erythematosus, immune-mediated vasculitis, and cold agglutinin disease, as well as in lymphocyte and plasma cell malignancies.[77] It is especially helpful in cats because they do not tolerate azathioprine as well as dogs. The size of the tablet is very good for use in most cats. It is most commonly combined with a glucocorticoid and, occasionally, with azathioprine (dogs only!). Chlorambucil may be used to replace cyclophosphamide if hemorrhagic cystitis develops during the use of that drug. The oral dosage in dogs and cats is 0.1 to 0.2 mg/kg q24h to q48h.[76–78, 81]

Azathioprine

Azathioprine (Imuran, Glaxo Wellcome) is a synthetic modification of 6-mercaptopurine that can be given orally or by injection.[76, 77, 84] However, for skin diseases, the oral route is usually used. It is metabolized in the liver to 6-mercaptopurine and other active metabolites. 6-Mercaptopurine is then metabolized by three enzyme systems. Xanthine oxidase and thiopurine methyltransferase (TPMT) produce inactive metabolites. Humans and possibly dogs that have absent (homozygous) or low (heterozygous) TPMT activity are more likely to experience myelosuppression.[87] Ten percent of the normal dogs sampled in one study had low (heterozygous) TPMT activity (9 to 1.3 U/ml RBC; normal, 15.1 to 26.6).[87] The drug antagonizes purine metabolism, thereby interfering with DNA and RNA synthesis.[75]

Azathioprine primarily affects rapidly proliferating cells, with its greatest effects on cell-mediated immunity and T lymphocyte–dependent antibody synthesis. Primary antibody synthesis is affected more than secondary antibody synthesis. Azathioprine is preferred over 6-mercaptopurine because it has a more favorable therapeutic index, and 6-mercaptopurine is less effective when given orally in humans.

Even so, azathioprine is a potent drug with potential toxicities, which include anemia, leukopenia, thrombocytopenia, vomiting, hypersensitivity reactions (especially of the liver), pancreatitis, elevated serum alkaline phosphatase concentrations, skin rashes, and alopecia. The most common significant side effect is diarrhea, which may be hemorrhagic. This often responds to dose reductions or temporary discontinuation of the drug.[85] More than 90% of patients experience anemia and lymphopenia, but usually not to the degree that treatment needs to be discontinued. It has also been suggested that patients that are not responding to therapy, that are not lymphopenic, and that are otherwise tolerating the drug very well should have their dose of azathioprine increased.[85] Long-term therapy is associated with the development of demodicosis, recurrent bacterial pyoderma, or dermatophytosis in at least 10% of cases.[85] Pancreatitis may occur, though this has been reported in dogs that were also receiving glucocorticoids.[86] We have also noted pancreatitis in a few dogs and, in some cases, azathioprine could be continued when the glucocorticoid was discontinued without further episodes of pancreatitis.

Patients should be monitored initially every 2 weeks with complete blood counts and platelet counts.[77, 85] After the patient's condition is stable, monitoring can be tapered to once every 4 months. If other symptoms occur, or at least yearly, a chemistry panel should also be run. Hepatitis and pancreatitis are the major conditions to monitor with chemistry panels.

In small animals, azathioprine may be beneficial for pemphigus complex, bullous pemphigoid, and both types of lupus erythematosus, as well as other autoimmune and immune-mediated disorders.[77] It is most commonly used in cases of canine pemphigus foliaceus that do not respond to glucocorticoids. Azathioprine is usually not used alone but is combined with systemic glucocorticoids. There is often a lag phase, with clinical improvement occurring in 3 to 6 weeks.

After remission is achieved, the dosages of both drugs are tapered, but initially, unless side effects are a problem, the glucocorticoid dosage is tapered to levels approaching 1 mg/kg q48h. The oral dosage of azathioprine for dogs is 2.5 mg/kg q24h until clinical response is achieved, and then it is continued every other day for a month or longer. Slow tapering down to as little as 1 mg/kg q72h may be achieved. Slow tapering to the lowest dose possible decreases side effects and the expense of therapy. Glucocorticoids can be given on the alternate days when azathioprine is not given. A switch to chrysotherapy has been recommended if high-dose prednisone in combination with azathioprine at 1 mg/kg q24h for 3 months, then at 2 mg/kg q24h for 3 months, is ineffective.[36] Another option is to continue to increase the azathioprine dose if the complete blood counts are relatively normal, especially if the patient is not lymphopenic.[85]

Cats are susceptible to azathioprine toxicity (including fatal leukopenia and thrombocytopenia), and this drug should be used very cautiously, if at all, in this species.[83, 84]

Cyclosporine

Cyclosporine (Sandimmune, Novartis) is effective in preventing human organ transplantation rejection (see Chap. 3).[76, 88, 91] In animal models, it has been used with similar excellent results.[90] It has also been evaluated for the treatment of immune-mediated skin diseases, and its systemic use is discussed in Chapter 3. Initial studies in dogs and cats with immunologic dermatoses such as pemphigus foliaceus, pemphigus erythematosus, and discoid lupus erythematosus have shown cyclosporine by itself to be rarely effective.[77, 90] It is usually used concurrently with glucocorticoids.

Topical cyclosporine, available as a veterinary product in a 0.2% ointment (Optimmune, Schering-Plough), has been used to treat keratoconjunctivitis sicca. Some of the benefit may reflect the vehicle used.[92] A study treating canine nictitans plasmacytic conjunctivitis showed a significant response in clinical symptoms as well as a reduction in post-treatment plasma cell infiltrates.[89] No controlled studies with topical cyclosporine for immune-mediated skin diseases have been published. However, we and others have seen cases of localized disease in lupus erythematosus and pemphigus erythematosus that improved when topical cyclosporine was added to the treatment regimen.

Leflunomide

Leflunomide is active in a wide range of immune disorders in murine and human models.[76] It has antiproliferative effects on T cell–dependent and T cell–independent antibody synthesis, inhibits pyrimidine synthesis, and antagonizes the action of IL-3, IL-4, and tumor necrosis factor (TNF)-α. When used with prednisone and cyclosporine, leflunomide virtually eliminates allograft rejection responses. One of the metabolites of leflunomide is highly gastroenterotoxic for dogs; thus the dose and dosage regimen must be closely followed. The dosage for dogs is about 2 to 6 mg/kg/day orally until a serum trough level of 30 μg/ml is achieved.

Chrysotherapy

Chrysotherapy is the use of gold as a therapeutic agent. Gold compounds are capable of modulating many phases of immune and inflammatory responses, but the exact mechanisms of this effect are unknown.[76, 96, 97] Gold is available in two dosage forms, which have dissimilar pharmacokinetics: The oral compound auranofin (Ridaura, SmithKline Beecham) contains 29% gold, and the parenteral compound aurothioglucose (Solganal, Schering) contains 50% gold. Neither form is approved for use in dogs and cats, but their distribution, metabolism, and actions have been established in humans and laboratory animals. Studies in humans show that the oral forms are 25% absorbed and attain blood levels with a 21-day half-life, but only small amounts can be detected in tissues and skin.[100] In a few clinical trials in dogs with immune-mediated dermatoses, the results with oral gold were equivocal, but no adverse side effects were observed.[101] The parenteral form is 100% absorbed but has only a 6-day half-life in blood. It is 95% protein-bound and is well distributed to cells of the mononuclear phagocytic system, liver, spleen, bone marrow, kidneys, and adrenal glands. Much lower levels are detected in skin.

In humans, gold may act at several levels of the inflammatory and immune response. Auranofin appears to have an additional immunomodulating action, whereas gold sodium thiomalate inhibits IL-5–mediated eosinophil survival, but both oral and parenteral golds inhibit bacteria, the first component of complement, and the epidermal enzymes that may be responsible for blister formation in pemphigus.[96, 99] Gold inhibits phagocytosis by macrophages.[75] Gold also reduces the release of inflammatory mediators, such as lysosomal enzymes, histamine, and prostaglandin; inactivates complement components; interferes with immunoglobulin-synthesizing cells; inhibits antigen- and mitogen-induced T-cell proliferation; and suppresses IL-2 and IL-2 receptor synthesis.[76, 96–98]

Toxic effects are worrisome in humans, because 33% of patients have some adverse reaction, although 80% of these reactions are minor. Most common are skin eruptions, oral reactions, proteinuria, and bone marrow depression. During the induction phase, a hemogram and urinalysis should be checked weekly and monthly thereafter.[93, 97] In over 100 dogs treated with injectable gold salts, the most common side effect was pain at the injection site.[36] In addition, two dogs experienced reversible thrombocytopenia, and four dogs experienced fatal toxic epidermal necrolysis when switched immediately from azathioprine to aurothioglucose therapy for pemphigus foliaceus.[36, 94] This may be enhanced by previous or concurrent administration of azathioprine.[77, 96] We have seen aurothioglucose-related erythema multiforme in both dogs and cats and, in one dog and one cat, it manifested primarily as oral ulceration and erythema.

Parenteral gold (aurothioglucose) has been reported to be effective for the treatment of cases of canine and feline pemphigus that were unresponsive to glucocorticoids or azathioprine and prednisone combination therapy.[36, 78, 97, 101] It has been useful for the treatment of canine bullous pemphigoid and feline plasma cell pododermatitis.[77, 95, 96] Although most adverse reactions develop late in therapy, it is suggested that a small test dose of 1 mg be given intramuscularly to patients with less than 10 kg of body weight and that 5 mg be given to larger patients in the first week. Dosage is increased to 1 mg/kg intramuscularly weekly until remission occurs. If no response occurs after 12 weeks of therapy, the dosage can be increased to 1.5 to 2 mg/kg.[77] After remission, one dose is given every 2 weeks and then once monthly for several months.

It is advisable to halt medication administration eventually for observation because some patients go into complete remission, whereas other animals can be maintained on a reduced dosage. Two points of caution: (1) The treatment takes 6 to 12 weeks for full effect to occur, so that other medication—typically glucocorticoids—should be maintained, if needed, at full dosage until this lag period is passed; and (2) gold compounds should not be administered simultaneously with other cytotoxic drugs (such as azathioprine and cyclophosphamide) because toxicity is thereby enhanced.

The oral form of gold (auranofin) has been used in only a few dogs with pemphigus (at 3 to 6 mg/day) with little success. It has been recommended at 0.12 to 0.2 mg/kg q12h but is only available as a nonbreakable 3-mg capsule.[101] In addition, this oral form is expensive.

Gold is seldom the first-choice drug for pemphigus. Patients are usually started on a glucocorticoid regimen, with azathioprine added to reduce the steroid dosage. In cases with excessive side effects, or when azathioprine and prednisone are ineffective, gold is a logical choice. It may be especially useful in cats.[77, 95] Gold injections should be delayed for 4 weeks after the discontinuation of azathioprine.[36]

Sulfones and Sulfonamides

DAPSONE

Dapsone (Dapsone tablets, Jacobus) is an anti-inflammatory, antibacterial chemical (4,4'-diaminodiphenyl sulfone). It inhibits the action of lysosomal enzymes; neutrophil chemotaxis; degranulation of mast cells; synthesis of IgG, IgA, and prostaglandin; activation of the alternative complement pathway; and T cell responses.[109] It is an antioxidant scavenger and also inhibits proteases. It inhibits the incorporation of choline into cell membranes, resulting in disrupted phospholipid synthesis.[105] It has been suggested that dapsone interferes with myeloperoxidase-halide–mediated toxicity, inhibits neutrophil chemotaxis, inhibits IL-1–stimulated adhesion of neutrophils to endothelial cells, inhibits adherence of neutrophils to antibodies deposited in the skin, and inhibits integrin-mediated neutrophil adherence.[47, 107]

Dapsone is useful in various diseases characterized by accumulations of neutrophils and, in some cases, eosinophils.[96, 105] In humans, it is most efficacious for dermatitis herpetiformis and erythema elevatum diutinum. It is erratically effective for a wide variety of other human skin diseases, including leukocytoclastic vasculitis, bullous lupus erythematosus, bullous pemphigoid, discoid lupus erythematosus, subcorneal pustular dermatosis, linear IgA bullous dermatosis, and relapsing polychondritis.[105] In these cases, the human dosage regimen starts low and rapidly builds to 150 mg/day. This dosage is held until response occurs and then is gradually decreased and stopped after 4 to 10 months. In many cases, there is no relapse. Treatment with dapsone is also effective in human leprosy and some cases of rheumatoid arthritis.

In dogs, dapsone has been used with benefit in cases of subcorneal pustular dermatosis, leukocytoclastic vasculitis, linear IgA pustular dermatosis, and pemphigus foliaceus and erythematosus.[103, 108] Dapsone is most useful in the first two diseases, although not all cases were controlled. In the last three diseases, only about half the cases showed benefit. However, in some cases of pemphigus that were successfully treated with immunosuppressive combinations (such as azathioprine with corticosteroids), the addition of dapsone permitted lowering the dose of the corticosteroid.

Dapsone is not approved for use in dogs and cats in the United States, but reports suggest a dosage of 1 mg/kg q8h (dogs only!) orally for 2 to 4 weeks until lesions clear, and then a reduction of the frequency of administration to q12h or q24h. Others have used the drug once daily or every 48 hours in combination with prednisone. The less frequent administration may be warranted because a study in normal dogs showed a half-life of 13 hours after intravenous administration.[104] In one dog given approximately 5 mg/kg, bioavailability was 99.5% and half-life was 11.5 hours.[104] The maintenance dosage should be further reduced to q48h, then once or twice weekly, or even stopped, because toxicity is somewhat dose-related.

Potential toxicity can be serious. During induction, mild anemia, leukopenia, and moderate elevations of serum alanine aminotransferase levels may be expected, but this does not necessitate stopping treatment if the animal remains clinically normal. Blood dyscrasias, thrombocytopenias, skin reactions, and hepatic toxicity can be serious but appear to be rare.[106, 108] Patients should be monitored every 2 weeks during induction therapy with hemograms and platelet counts, blood urea nitrogen determination, urinalysis, and serum alanine aminotransferase determination. Cats are especially susceptible to dapsone toxicity, with hemolytic anemia and various neurotoxicities reported. A dosage of 1 mg/kg q24h orally is recommended.

SULFASALAZINE

Sulfasalazine (Azulfidine, Pharmacia) is converted in the colon to sulfapyridine 5-aminosalicylate, which has anti-inflammatory action.[108] The dosage is 10 to 20 mg/kg q8h orally.[47, 108] The dosage may be reduced or even changed to every other day while maintaining clinical remission. A serious side effect with long-term administration is the production of keratitis sicca. Thus, tear production should be checked regularly. In one report, two cases with subcorneal pustular dermatosis were managed satisfactorily with sulfasalazine after becoming refractory to dapsone.[108] Sulfasalazine has also been used successfully in the management of neutrophilic vasculitis.[102, 108]

TETRACYCLINE AND NIACINAMIDE

The combination of tetracycline and niacinamide has been recommended for the treatment of discoid lupus erythematosus and pemphigus erythematosus in dogs. Reported results are variable, but 25% to 65% of cases have an excellent response.[110–112] It has also been effective in some cases of pemphigus foliaceus when added to azathioprine and prednisone regimens. Some cases of vesicular cutaneous lupus erythematosus ("idiopathic ulcerative dermatosis") in collies and Shetland sheepdogs respond well to tetracycline and niacinamide.

This combination has also been used with success in some dogs with lupoid onychodystrophy, German shepherd dog metatarsal fistulae, sterile panniculitis, sterile granulomatous/pyogranulomatous dermatitis, vasculitis, and cutaneous histiocytosis (see Chap. 3). The precise mechanism of action is unknown. However, tetracyclines possess various anti-inflammatory and immunomodulatory properties, including suppression of in vitro lymphocyte blastogenic transformation and antibody production, suppression of in vivo leukocyte chemotactic responses, inhibition of the activation of complement component 3, inhibition of lipases and collagenases, and inhibition of prostaglandin synthesis.[110] Niacinamide has been shown to block antigen-IgE–induced histamine release in vivo and in vitro, prevent degranulation of mast cells, inhibit phosphodiesterases, and decrease protease releases.[112]

The initial dosage for dogs weighing more than 10 kg is 500 mg of tetracycline and 500 mg of niacinamide given q8h. If response is favorable, the dosage may be decreased to q12h and then to q24h. Although no studies have been reported, one of us (C.E.G.) noted that this combination may have shown benefit when used concurrently with vitamin E or glucocorticoids. It was also reported that tetracycline alone may be beneficial in treating discoid lupus erythematosus.[111] Side effects are uncommon, although vomiting, anorexia, lethargy, and diarrhea have been reported and are primarily due to the niacinamide.[80, 111, 112] One of us (C.E.G.) also saw two cases of anorexia with increased liver enzyme activity that resolved with discontinuation of therapy. In one case, tetracycline administration was continued, suggesting that the niacinamide was responsible for the adverse reactions.

Antimalarials

Several antimalarials have been useful for the treatment of humans with discoid lupus erythematosus, dermatomyositis, polymorphous light eruption, solar urticaria, and scleroderma.[113] There are also anecdotal reports of response with cutaneous leishmaniasis, cutaneous cryptococcosis, epidermolysis bullosa, and lymphocytic skin infiltrations.[114] Antimalarials may have future use in problem cases involving animals with such diseases.

Their specific mode of action is unknown, but the drugs stabilize lysosomal membranes and thus are anti-inflammatory. They inhibit protein synthesis, viral replication, and cell-mediated immunity. They do not affect the development of primary or secondary antibody response but do inhibit complement. Consequently, they may inhibit the formation of immune complexes, which explains their effectiveness in systemic lupus erythematosus and related autoimmune disorders. The drugs are seldom used alone for first-line therapy and, in humans, are usually given with salicylates or small doses of corticosteroids. Side effects are numerous, the most serious affecting the eyes.

The drugs most commonly used in humans are quinacrine hydrochloride (Atabrine hydrochloride, Winthrop), chloroquine (Aralen, Winthrop), and hydroxychloroquine sulfate (Plaquenil sulfate, Winthrop). Their place in veterinary dermatology has yet to be determined, although anecdotal reports suggest that the antimalarials may be beneficial in canine lupus erythematosus.[96] No case reports or studies supporting their efficacy have been reported.

Colchicine

Colchicine has been useful for the treatment of humans with leukocytoclastic vasculitis, epidermolysis bullosa acquisita, linear IgA bullous dermatosis, dermatitis herpetiformis, and relapsing polychondritis.[116] It may have future use in problem cases involving animals with such diseases.

Colchicine is an alkaloid that suppresses neutrophil chemotactic and phagocytic functions via disruption of microtubule assembly and elongation, increasing cellular cyclic AMP levels and inhibiting lysosomal degranulation. It also inhibits immunoglobulin secretion, IL-1 production, histamine release, and human leukocyte antigen (HLA)-DR expression. The main side effects are gastrointestinal.

Early clinical reports in dogs involved the use of a colchicine analog in cases of "eczema."[115] These reports are not interpretable.

• AUTOIMMUNE DISEASES

Pemphigus Complex

The pemphigus complex is a group of uncommon autoimmune diseases described in dogs and cats that is comparable to the human disease. Although there are similarities, many significant differences exist. These disorders are vesiculobullous to pustular disorders of the skin or mucous membranes characterized by acantholysis (loss of cohesion between keratinocytes). In humans, there are at least eight varieties of pemphigus, whereas dogs and cats have at least five varieties.[59, 155, 169]

CAUSE AND PATHOGENESIS

In humans, the pemphigus complex is characterized histologically by intraepithelial acantholysis leading to vesicle formation and immunologically by the presence of autoantibodies to components of the keratinocyte desmosome, both bound in the skin and circulating in the serum.[117, 118, 155] The clinical lesions, both in severity and in body location, appear to relate to which components of the desmosome the autoantibodies are targeting.[117, 146, 155, 165] For instance, humans with mucosal dominant pemphigus vulgaris have antibodies against desmoglein III, those with pemphigus foliaceus produce antibodies against desmoglein I, and patients with mucocutaneous pemphigus vulgaris produce both.[117] Using a neonatal mouse model, the injection of antidesmoglein III IgG alone is not efficient at inducing gross skin lesions, whereas combining both antidesmoglein III and antidesmoglein I does produce lesions.[117] As pemphigus vulgaris progresses to cutaneous involvement, antidesmoglein I antibodies are produced, possibly because of epitope spreading.

In dogs and cats, only pemphigus vulgaris causes an intraepidermal vesicle or bulla. The other forms of pemphigus are typically associated with intraepidermal pustules, a major distinction between the human and the canine and feline diseases.[22, 127, 130] In the past, pemphigus antibody was not readily demonstrated in the skin or serum of many dogs and cats.[96] In humans, negative immunologic findings raise serious doubts about the diagnosis for some variants of pemphigus. However, as the techniques to find serum autoantibodies improve, the frequency of detection increases.[137, 138, 140] These two differences raise questions about the pathologic similarities and the accuracy of the diagnosis based on just clinical and histopathologic findings between the human and animal diseases. Part of the discrepancy also relates to sensitivity and technique because we appear to be finding more cases with detectable serum autoantibodies, and these autoantibodies do target similar or identical structures as in the human diseases.[59, 125, 138, 167, 168] Further studies comparing cases with and without appropriate immunologic findings are needed to determine whether we have multiple similar diseases or the identification primarily relates to the sensitivity of the techniques being used.

Pemphigus antigens are heterogeneous (85 to 260 kd) and present in all mammalian and avian skin, and those identified specifically are associated with desmosomal components.[59, 125, 126, 155] In humans, regional variation exists in the expression of both pemphigus foliaceus and pemphigus vulgaris antigens, which also differ from each other.[136] This regional difference and the specific profile of the patient's autoantibodies correlate with, and help to explain, the distribution of lesions in clinical disease.[117, 146] Canine skin has been shown to have similar antigens.[59, 167, 168] The pemphigus vulgaris and pemphigus foliaceus antibodies from human patients reproduce their respective clinical, histopathologic, and immunopathologic syndromes when injected into neonatal mice. Antibodies to some of these antigens are not associated with pathology, however.

The pathomechanism of blister formation in pemphigus is unknown, though it has been proposed to be as follows: (1) the binding of pemphigus antibody on the antigen, (2) internalization of the pemphigus antibody and fusion of the antibody with intracellular lysosomes, and (3) resultant activation and release of a keratinocyte proteolytic enzyme (plasminogen activator or another factor), which diffuses into the extracellular space and converts plasminogen into plasmin, which hydrolyzes the adhesion molecules.[18, 124, 167, 168] The resultant loss of intercellular cohesion leads to acantholysis and blister formation within the epidermis. The pemphigus antibody-induced acantholysis is not dependent on complement or inflammatory cells. Experimentally, however, complement potentiates the acantholysis. Urokinase-type plasminogen activator receptors were shown to have increased expression in the skin lesions of humans with pemphigus vulgaris and pemphigus foliaceus.[174] Other studies have shown that plasminogen activator activity does not correlate with lesion development, and studies conducted in genetically engineered mouse models also have suggested that direct interference with the antibody targets creates similar lesions.[18]

In desmoglein III^{null} mice, treatment with human pemphigus vulgaris serum induces extensive acantholysis and blistering, suggesting that autoantibodies against cell-surface molecules other than desmoglein I and desmoglein III can induce pemphigus vulgaris.[148] Patients with pemphigus vulgaris and pemphigus foliaceus have IgG antibodies that precipitate cholinergic receptors.[148] Because cholinergic receptors control keratinocyte adhesion and motility, their inactivation by autoantibodies may elicit cell signals that cause desmosomal disassembly. Although keratinocyte desmosomal cadherins (desmoglein I and III) hold the cells together, desmoglein III^{null} mice do *not* experience spontaneous acantholysis and blisters. In addition, activation of cholinergic receptors can prevent, stop, and reverse the acantholysis elicited by pemphigus antibodies in vitro. Thus, the acantholysis in pemphigus may be mediated by at least two complementary pathogenic pathways: (1) anticholinergic receptor autoantibodies that weaken intercellular adhesion between keratinocytes via inactivation of the cholinergic receptor–mediated physiologic control of cadherin (desmoglein) expression and/or function, which causes dyshesion, cell detachment, and rounding up (acantholysis), and (2) autoantibodies to other adherence molecules (e.g., desmoglein) that prevent the formation of new desmosomes.

Ultraviolet light irradiation exacerbates the acantholysis induced by anti-desmoglein I and anti-desmoglein III autoantibodies in patients with pemphigus erythematosus, pemphigus foliaceus, and pemphigus vulgaris.[139, 153a]

What initiates the autoantibody formation is still unknown, though a virus spread by an insect vector is suspected in an endemic form of pemphigus foliaceus (fogo selvagem) in South America.[18, 145] It has been suggested that the black fly may play the role of vector. This hypothesis has been supported by an epidemiologic study correlating exposure to black flies as a risk factor for endemic pemphigus foliaceus.[145]

Genetic factors in humans and dogs also appear to be important. In humans, both pemphigus foliaceus and pemphigus vulgaris have HLA associations, and some populations may be susceptible to pemphigus vulgaris due to differences in their immune response genes.[18] Although this has not been demonstrated in dogs, breed predispositions and familial cases have been shown.[47, 150] Other factors thought to be involved in the pathogenesis of some cases of pemphigus are drug provocation (especially penicillamine and phenylbutazone), ultraviolet light, and emotional upset.[5, 18, 47, 139, 157, 163, 164] Drugs and chronic skin disease both seem to be important in the pathogenesis of some cases of canine and feline pemphigus.[130, 131] Interestingly, drug-induced disease in humans is less commonly associated with classic immunopathologic findings.[172] Possibly, the human drug-induced form is more similar to animal pemphigus. The most commonly incriminated drugs are those with highly reactive sulfhydryl moieties (e.g., penicillamine) and those with an amide component (e.g., captopril, penicillins, cephalosporins).

Diet has been implicated as a cause of pemphigus in humans.[158, 170] The molecular structure of many food ingredients is similar to that of known pemphigus-inducing drugs. For instance: *thiols* contained in garlic, onion, leek, and chive; *isothiocyanates* in mustard, horseradish, turnip, radish, cabbage, cauliflower, and Brussels sprouts; *phenols* in mango, cashews, and many food additives; and *tannins* in tea, coffee, ginseng, certain berries, banana, pear, apple, and avocado. Interestingly, most humans with fogo selvagem live close to rivers, many of which contain high levels of tannins because of decomposing leaves and other vegetable matter.[170] Heat and humidity cause tannin decomposition. Perhaps consumption of such substances is more important than black flies!

Owing to the thinness, or other characteristics, of canine and feline epidermis, intraepidermal vesicles, bullae, and pustules are fragile and transient. Thus, clinical lesions usually include erosions and ulcers bordered by epidermal collarettes.

DIAGNOSIS

The pemphigus complex is uncommon in dogs and cats, accounting for about 0.6% to 1% of all canine and feline skin disorders seen at university small animal clinics.[56, 59] In general, the various forms of pemphigus have relatively distinct clinical differences. Certain diagnostic features, however, can be applied to the whole group. The most important diagnostic aspects are the history, physical examination, and histopathologic findings. Detection of pemphigus antibody by direct immunofluorescence or immunohistochemical testing may also be helpful but, owing to costs, technical problems, and relatively poor diagnostic sensitivity and specificity at routine laboratories, these tests are not routinely recommended. If they are performed, however, all the pemphigus variants should show an intercellular deposition of IgG or complement components (see Fig. 9–1A).[47, 163, 164] In three of seven dogs with pemphigus foliaceus, the IgG was of the IgG2 or IgG4 subtypes.[13]

Occasionally, immunoglobulins of other classes are found. Indirect immunofluorescence testing infrequently yields positive results unless a research laboratory is used; even then, results are still not routinely positive.[59] Pemphigus erythematosus may show deposition of immunoreactants along the basement membrane zone in addition to the intercellular findings (see Fig. 9–1B). Microscopic examination of direct smears from intact vesicles or pustules or from recent erosions often reveals numerous nondegenerate neutrophils, occasionally numerous eosinophils, and numerous acantholytic keratinocytes.[55, 164] One or two acantholytic keratinocytes may be visible in an occasional high-power microscopic field during microscopic examination in any suppurative condition, but when these cells are present in clusters or large numbers in several microscopic fields, they are strongly suggestive of pemphigus.

Skin biopsy may be diagnostic or strongly supportive in pemphigus.[22, 47, 55, 164] Intact vesicles, bullae, or pustules are essential. Because these lesions are so fragile and transient, it may be necessary to hospitalize the animal so that it can be carefully scrutinized for 2 to 4 hours for the presence of primary lesions. When a bullous lesion is observed, biopsy must be performed immediately. Multiple biopsies and serial sections greatly increase the chances of demonstrating diagnostic histologic changes.

Electron-microscopic examination of pemphigus lesions has suggested that dissolution of the intercellular cement substance is the initial pathologic change, followed by the retraction of tonofilaments, disappearance of desmosomes, and acantholysis.[163, 164]

Results of routine laboratory determinations (hemogram, serum chemistries, urinalysis, serum protein electrophoresis) are nondiagnostic, often revealing mild to moderate leukocytosis and neutrophilia, mild nonregenerative anemia, mild hypoalbuminemia, and mild to moderate elevations of α_2, β, and γ globulins.[163, 164]

CLINICAL MANAGEMENT OF PEMPHIGUS: GENERAL COMMENTS

The prognosis for canine pemphigus appears to vary with the form and severity of the disease.[55, 163, 164] The natural course of untreated cases is unclear. Veterinarians have long recognized refractory mucocutaneous erosive or ulcerative disorders and severe exfoliative dermatoses that have resulted in the death or euthanasia of affected dogs and cats. Retrospectively, many of those dogs and cats may have had pemphigus vulgaris or pemphigus foliaceus. On the basis of the small numbers of cases documented in the veterinary literature, (1) pemphigus vulgaris appears to be a severe disease that is often fatal and, even with treatment, many animals fail to respond and are euthanized, (2) pemphigus foliaceus is less severe but, without therapy, may be fatal, and (3) pemphigus erythematosus and panepidermal pustular or pemphigus vegetans are usually benign disorders that rarely produce systemic signs and readily respond to treatment.[36, 47, 59]

Because the prognosis and treatment for the different forms varies, it is important to make a specific diagnosis. Suspect drug-induced cases of pemphigus may not require prolonged therapy and seem more likely to allow treatment to be permanently discontinued after remission has been maintained for 6 months. Too few cases of paraneoplastic pemphigus have been described to allow comment, though this condition carries a very poor prognosis in humans.

Therapy of canine and feline pemphigus is often difficult, requiring large doses of systemic glucocorticoids with or without other potent immunomodulating drugs.[47, 55, 163, 164] Side effects of these drugs are common, varying from mild to severe, and close physical and hematologic monitoring of the patient is critical. Additionally, therapy must usually be maintained for prolonged periods, if not for life. Thus, the therapeutic regimen must be individualized for each patient, and owner education is essential.

Large doses of glucocorticoids (2 to 6 mg/kg prednisone orally q24h in dogs; 4 to 8 mg/kg prednisone q24h in cats) induce remission in most patients. However, severe glucocorticoid side effects and the inability to achieve safe alternate-day maintenance regimens render these drugs unacceptable in at least 50% of cases. In our referral dermatology practices, only 30% to 40% of cases are adequately controlled with glucocorticoids alone.

When glucocorticoids are ineffective or undesirable, other immunomodulating drugs can be used in an attempt to reduce the dosage or eliminate the need for glucocorticoids. Azathioprine is often the drug of choice in this situation in dogs. Azathioprine should be used either not at all or very cautiously in cats, because even small doses (1 mg/kg orally q48h) may produce fatal leukopenia or thrombocytopenia.[121] Chlorambucil is effective in dogs and cats and is the preferred treatment in the cat.[154] Chrysotherapy (use of gold salts) is also useful, especially in cats and cases that cannot be controlled with azathioprine and prednisone.[34, 36, 47, 132, 156]

In animals in which significant nasal depigmentation has occurred and photodermatitis has become an aggravating factor, photoprotection is an important therapeutic adjunct.[55, 153a, 163, 164] Avoidance of sunlight between 8 AM and 5 PM is helpful. The use

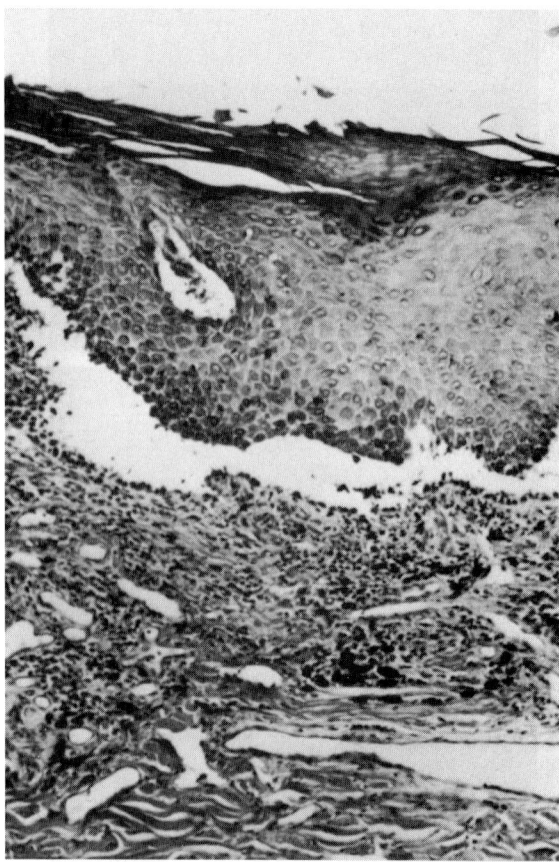

FIGURE 9–3. Canine pemphigus vulgaris. Suprabasilar acantholysis and cleft formation. (From Scott DW, et al: Pemphigus vulgaris without mucosal or mucocutaneous involvement in two dogs. J Am Anim Hosp Assoc 18:401, 1982.)

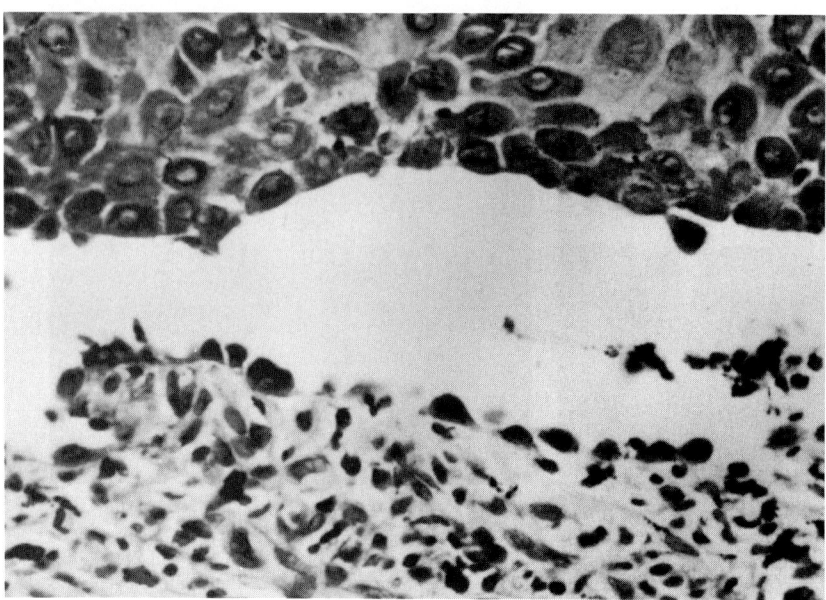

FIGURE 9–4. Canine pemphigus vulgaris. Suprabasilar cleft with basilar epidermal cells remaining attached to the dermis like a row of "tombstones." (From Scott DW, et al: Pemphigus vulgaris without mucosal or mucocutaneous involvement in two dogs. J Am Anim Hosp Assoc 18:401, 1982.)

most difficult form to put into and keep in remission. Systemic glucocorticoids alone or in combination with azathioprine are the initial treatments of choice in dogs, whereas systemic glucocorticoids alone or in combination with chlorambucil are preferred in cats. Combination therapy is usually required. Heparin (100 IU/kg q12h subcutaneously) was shown to have at least a temporary beneficial effect in one medically resistant case of pemphigus vulgaris.[151]

PEMPHIGUS VEGETANS

Pemphigus vegetans has been reported in the dog but is considered to be extremely rare.[160, 164] In 1998, it was suggested that these cases represent the newly proposed variant, panepidermal pustular pemphigus, though some clinical features were different.[59] No age, breed, or sex predilections are apparent. Pemphigus vegetans is a vesiculopustular disorder that evolves into verrucous vegetations and papillomatous proliferations, which ooze and are studded with pustules (see Fig. 9–2E and F). The Nikolsky sign may be present. Pruritus and pain are variable, and the dogs are usually otherwise healthy. Pemphigus vegetans is thought to represent a more benign or abortive form of pemphigus vulgaris in an animal that has more resistance to the disease.

Diagnosis

The differential diagnosis of pemphigus vegetans includes bacterial and fungal granulomas, benign familial chronic pemphigus, and cutaneous neoplasia (especially lymphoreticular neoplasia and mast cell tumor).

The definitive diagnosis of pemphigus vegetans is based on history, physical examination, direct smears, biopsy, and immunofluorescence or immunohistochemical testing.

Pemphigus vegetans is characterized histopathologically by papillated epidermal hyperplasia, papillomatosis, and intraepidermal microabscesses that predominantly contain eosinophils and acantholytic keratinocytes (Figs. 9–5 and 9–6).[71, 160, 163]

Management

Too few cases of pemphigus vegetans have been described for specific recommendations to be made, but initially, systemic glucocorticoids would be indicated. In one report, three

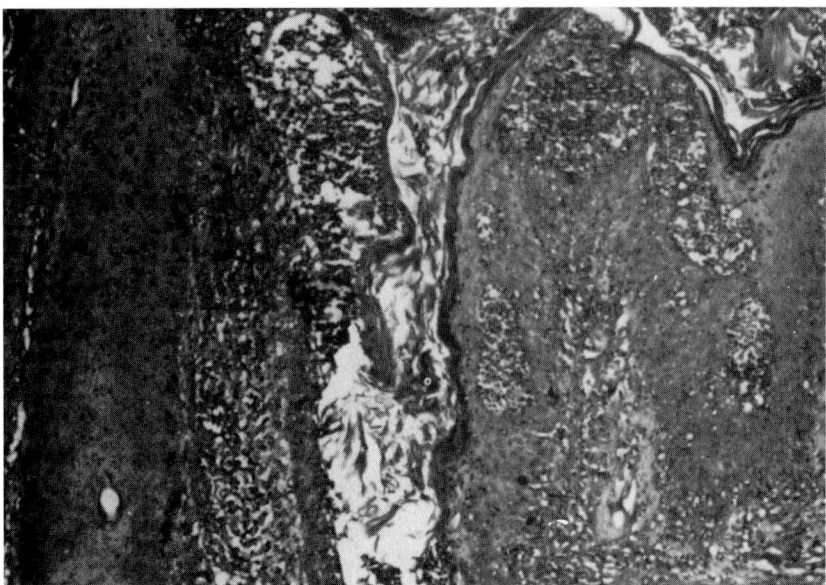

FIGURE 9–5. Canine pemphigus vegetans. Seven intraepidermal eosinophilic microabscesses. (From Scott DW, Lewis RM: Pemphigus and pemphigoid in dog and man: Comparative aspects. J Am Acad Dermatol 5:148, 1981.)

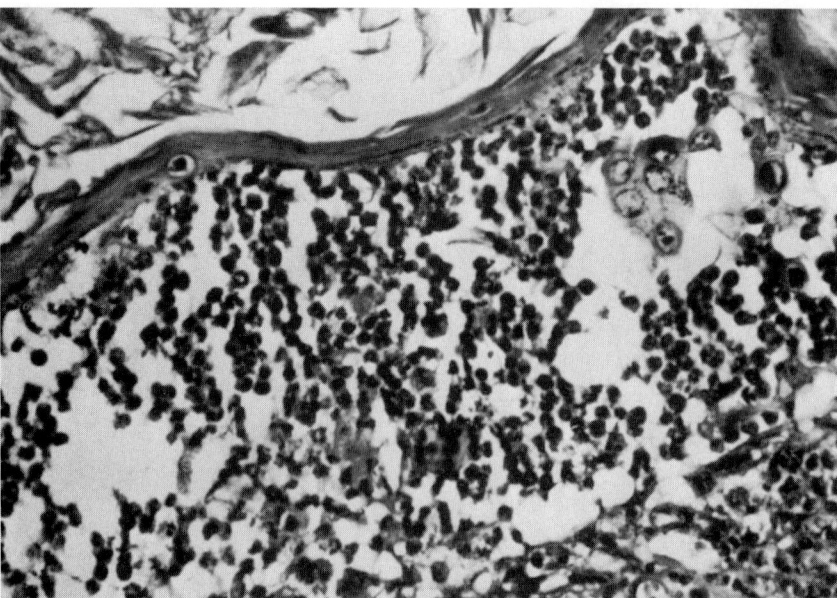

FIGURE 9–6. Canine pemphigus vegetans. Intraepidermal microabscess containing predominantly eosinophils and a few acantholytic keratinocytes. (From Scott DW: Pemphigus vegetans in a dog. Cornell Vet 67:374, 1977.)

cases were mentioned and all responded readily to tapering dosages of glucocorticoids.[36] If glucocorticoids are not effective, azathioprine would be added.

PANEPIDERMAL PUSTULAR PEMPHIGUS

In a 1991 report, 16 cases of putative pemphigus vegetans were described.[149] To us, however, many of the dogs in these cases appeared to have "deep" pemphigus erythematosus or pemphigus foliaceus. The diagnosis of pemphigus vegetans was based on histopathology because of the presence of pustules in the epidermis and follicular infundibula. Dunstan[127] has referred to this group as having pemphigus vegetans/erythematosus and considers this entity more similar to human pemphigus vegetans, Hallopeau type. He and others[173] have proposed the name *panepidermal pustular pemphigus*. One case evaluated immunopathologically had autoantibodies against desmoglein I, similar to pemphigus foliaceus.[169] Based on the clinical findings and limited immunopathologic studies, this entity cannot be distinctly characterized. We still believe that these dogs simply have pemphigus foliaceus or pemphigus erythematosus.

PEMPHIGUS FOLIACEUS

Pemphigus foliaceus is the most common form of pemphigus and is perhaps the most common immune-mediated dermatosis in dogs and cats.[55, 120, 121, 129, 133, 135, 147, 156] It has been reported to account for as high as 1% to 1.5% of all cases at a dermatology referral practice or as low as 0.04% of the hospital canine population.* The major pemphigus foliaceus antigen is desmoglein I, a 150-kd glycoprotein from the cadherin group of adhesion molecules.[59, 141] The same antigen is the target of the autoantibodies in the dog.[138, 168] No age or sex predilections have been reported. In *dogs,* Akitas, Chow Chows, Dachshunds, Bearded collies, Newfoundlands, Doberman pinschers, the Finnish spitz, and

---

*See references 55, 120, 121, 129, 133, 135, 147, 156.

Schipperkes may be predisposed.[55, 135] The mean age of onset is about 4 years, with 65% of the affected dogs experiencing disease at 5 years or less.[135]

Pemphigus foliaceus is characterized by pustular dermatitis (see Fig. 9-2G). This is an important differentiation from human pemphigus foliaceus, which starts with erythema and vesicles and may progress to pustules. Canine and feline pemphigus foliaceus does not have a vesicular phase—it is a pustular, crusting disease.

Three forms of pemphigus foliaceus appear to exist in the canine.[131] The first is spontaneous canine pemphigus foliaceus. Akitas and Chow Chows may be prone to this form. The disease develops in dogs with no previous history of skin disease or drug exposure. The second form, drug-induced pemphigus foliaceus, may be more common in Labrador retrievers and Doberman pinschers. Drug-induced pemphigus is becoming more frequently recognized, with several cases associated with the administration of trimethoprim/sulfonamides.° The third form occurs in dogs with a history of chronic skin disease. These dogs often have had one or more years of usually pruritic or allergic skin disease. They suddenly experience "more severe disease with new features" that ends up being diagnosed as pemphigus foliaceus. These dogs with chronic, disease-associated pemphigus foliaceus often have been exposed to multiple drugs, so their disease may occasionally be drug-induced, though a cause-and-effect relationship is not obvious, nor does the eruption go away when the drugs are stopped. No seasonality or environmental risk factors were found in a study of pemphigus foliaceus in dogs and cats.[152]

Pemphigus foliaceus usually begins on the face and ears (Fig. 9-7B); it commonly involves the feet, clawbeds, footpads (villous hyperkeratosis or "hard pad") (see Fig. 9-7C to E), and groin and becomes multifocal or generalized (see Fig. 9-7A) within 6 months in many animals. Very early lesions consist of erythematous macules that rapidly progress through a pustular phase (see Fig. 9-2G) and end up as dry, yellow or honey-colored to brown crusts (see Fig. 9-2H). There are usually scales, alopecia, and erosions bordered by epidermal collarettes. The Nikolsky sign may be present. Mucocutaneous orientation is uncommon, and oral cavity involvement is very rare. Some dogs and cats with pemphigus foliaceus present with only footpad lesions and may be lame.[119, 134] Paronychia and involvement of the nipples are common in cats.[132] Various claw abnormalities (onychodystrophy, onychorrhexis, onychogryposis) occasionally occur in dogs. Nasal depigmentation is common and may result in photodermatitis (see the following discussion of pemphigus erythematosus). Pruritus and pain are variable, and secondary bacterial pyoderma and peripheral lymphadenopathy may be present. Severely affected animals may be anorectic, depressed, or febrile. The disease commonly has a waxing/waning course. There may be hours to days when numerous new pustules form, followed by days to weeks of crusting during which few new lesions are found.

Diagnosis

The differential diagnosis of pemphigus foliaceus includes bacterial folliculitis, dermatophytosis, demodicosis, dermatophilosis, seborrheic skin disease, benign familial chronic pemphigus, pemphigus erythematosus, discoid and systemic lupus erythematosus, dermatomyositis, and cutaneous adverse drug reaction. Dermatophytosis can mimic the histopathology as well as the clinical findings (see Chap. 5).[153] In addition, pemphigus foliaceus could be confused with subcorneal pustular dermatosis, sterile eosinophilic pustulosis, linear IgA pustular dermatosis, necrolytic migratory erythema, leishmaniasis, and zinc-responsive dermatitis.

The definitive diagnosis of pemphigus foliaceus is based on history, physical examination, direct smears, skin biopsy, immunofluorescence or immunohistochemical testing, and demonstration of the antigen being targeted (desmoglein I). Pemphigus foliaceus is characterized histologically by intragranular or subcorneal acantholysis with resultant cleft and vesicle or pustule formation (Figs. 9-8 and 9-9).[22, 71, 164] Within the vesicle or pustule, cells from the stratum granulosum may be attached to the overlying stratum corneum

---

°See references 11, 49, 52, 252, 269, 286, 287.

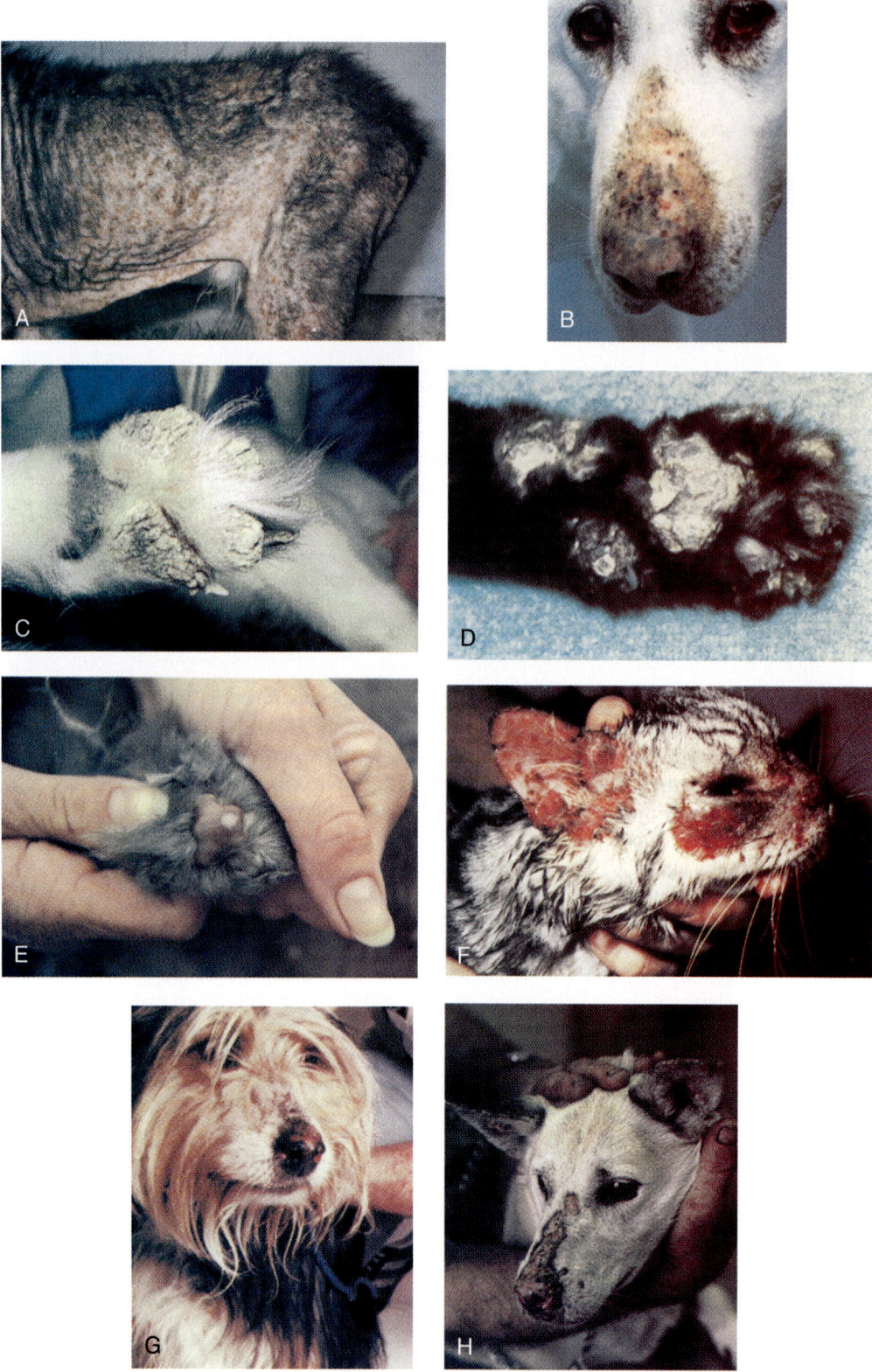

FIGURE 9–7. Legend on opposite page

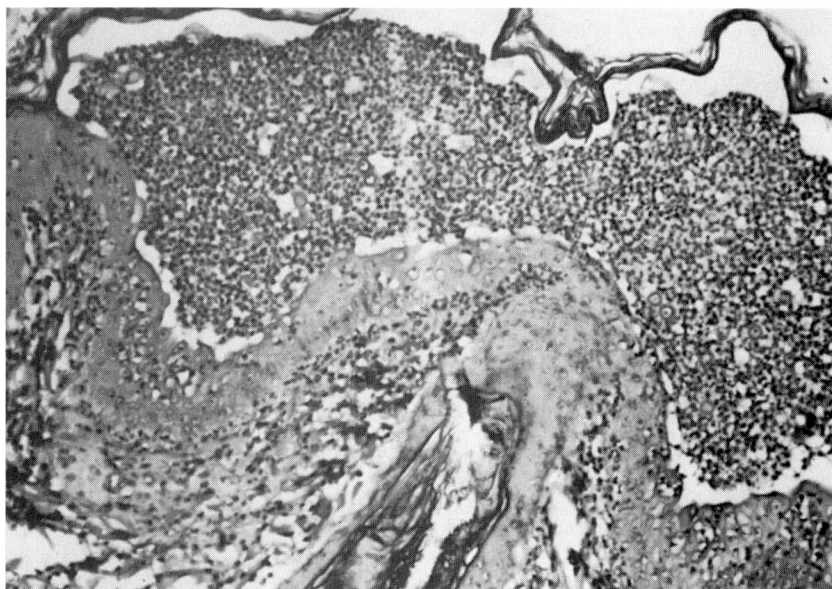

FIGURE 9–8. Canine pemphigus foliaceus. Numerous neutrophils and acantholytic keratinocytes within a subcorneal pustule. (From Scott DW, Lewis RM: Pemphigus and pemphigoid in dog and man: Comparative aspects. J Am Acad Dermatol 5:148, 1981.)

(granular cell "cling-ons") (Fig. 9–10A and B). Either neutrophils or eosinophils may predominate within the vesicle or pustule. Other helpful histopathologic findings in canine and feline pemphigus foliaceus are (1) eosinophilic exocytosis and microabscess formation within the epidermis or follicular outer root sheath or both, (2) frequent involvement of the follicular outer root sheath in the acantholytic and pustular process, and (3) acantholytic, dyskeratotic granular epidermal cells ("grains") at the surface of erosions (Fig. 9–11).

Management

The initial treatment of choice for pemphigus foliaceus depends on the clinical presentation. Milder localized cases may be treated with topical steroids, whereas more extensive disease is usually treated with oral prednisone.[156, 164] The induction dose should be maintained until the disease is inactive, though alopecia and residual crusts may be present. After induction, the dosage is tapered to an alternate-day regimen. In cats, patients failing to respond to prednisone may respond to dexamethasone (0.2 to 0.4 mg/kg q24h) or triamcinolone (0.4 to 0.8 mg/kg q24h) and can be safely maintained by administration of either product every second or third day. It has been suggested that oral triamcinolone may be superior to prednisone and prednisolone; however, this needs to be evaluated.[131] Oral glucocorticoids are ineffective or unsatisfactory in at least 50% of cases. In the dog, the next most common treatment is the addition of azathioprine for combination immunosuppressive therapy. In the cat, chlorambucil or chrysotherapy is used. If dogs do not

---

FIGURE 9–7. A, Pemphigus foliaceus. Generalized papules, pustules, erosions, and crusts. B, Pemphigus foliaceus. Note symmetric dermatitis involving bridge of the nose and periocular regions. C, Hyperkeratosis of the footpads in a dog with pemphigus foliaceus. D, Hyperkeratosis of the footpads in a cat with pemphigus foliaceus. E, Pustule on footpad of a cat with pemphigus foliaceus. F, Erythema, alopecia, erosion, and crusting of the face and ear of a cat with pemphigus erythematosus. (From Scott DW, et al: Pemphigus erythematosus in the dog and cat. J Am Anim Hosp Assoc 16:815, 1980.) G, Nasal erythema, ulceration, crusting, and depigmentation in a dog with pemphigus erythematosus. H, Pemphigus erythematosus demonstrating nasal depigmentation without crusting—typical of discoid lupus erythematosus—and crusted areas on nasal planum and pinna—suggestive of pemphigus foliaceus.

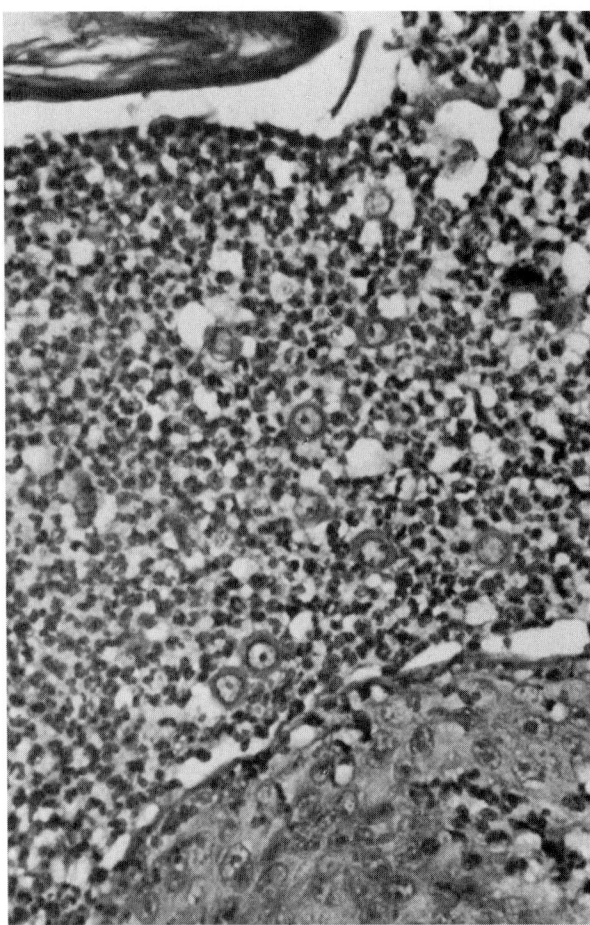

FIGURE 9–9. Canine pemphigus foliaceus. Numerous acantholytic keratinocytes within subcorneal pustule.

respond to azathioprine and glucocorticoids, gold salt injections may be warranted, but only after waiting for 4 weeks after discontinuing the azathioprine.[36] It has been stated that about 10% of patients with canine and feline pemphigus foliaceus fail to respond to any treatment and are euthanized.[120]

PEMPHIGUS ERYTHEMATOSUS

Pemphigus erythematosus is thought to represent a more benign form of pemphigus foliaceus.[18, 128, 164] Some workers have also suggested it may represent a crossover syndrome between pemphigus and lupus erythematosus because of histopathologic and immunopathologic findings. It has also been suggested to be a mild form of pemphigus foliaceus. The antigen target has not been definitely identified in humans or dogs though, in humans, it is believed to be similar to pemphigus foliaceus.[18, 59] Pemphigus erythematosus has been reported in dogs and cats.[55, 161, 164] No age or sex predilections are known. In dogs, collies and German shepherds may be predisposed.[55] This disease has been considered to be photoaggravated in some cases, similar to canine discoid lupus erythematosus. This was confirmed in a study demonstrating in vivo and in vitro sensitivity to UVB.[139]

Pemphigus erythematosus is characterized by erythematous, pustular dermatitis of the face and ears (see Fig. 9–7F). Because the primary lesions are transient, dogs and cats typically present with oozing crusts, scales, alopecia, and erosions bordered by epidermal collarettes. The Nikolsky sign is infrequently present. Pruritus and pain are variable. The disease involves, and is often limited to, the facial/nasal region. The nose frequently becomes depigmented, whereupon photodermatitis becomes an aggravating factor (see

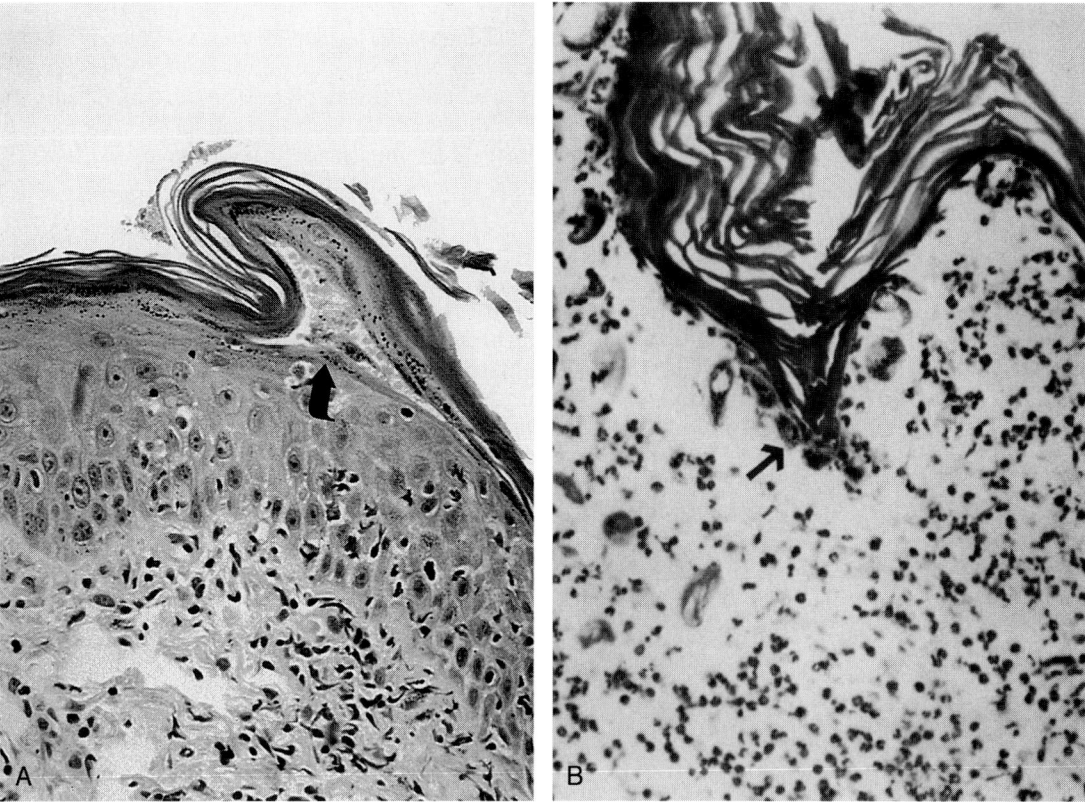

FIGURE 9–10. Canine pemphigus foliaceus. *A*, Early pallor and intragranular cleft formation (*arrow*). *B*, Intragranular acantholysis produces a "subcorneal" pustule with numerous keratinocytes from the stratum granulosum still adherent (granular "cling-ons") to the overlying stratum corneum (*arrow*).

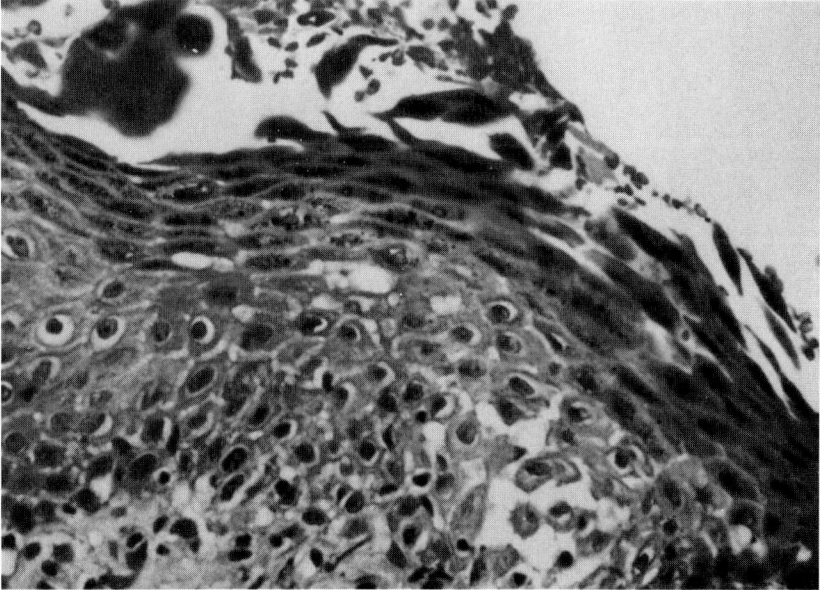

FIGURE 9–11. Canine pemphigus erythematosus. Acantholytic keratinocytes ("grains") within stratum granulosum at the surface of an erosion. (From Scott DW, Lewis RM: Pemphigus and pemphigoid in dog and man: Comparative aspects. J Am Acad Dermatol 5: 148, 1981.)

Fig. 9–7G and H). If the nasal region is primarily involved, the condition is often worse in sunny weather and the dog may be misdiagnosed as having nasal solar dermatitis ("collie nose"). Often the depigmentation is an early sign in pemphigus erythematosus. This is in contrast with pemphigus foliaceus, wherein the depigmentation comes later. In addition, the crusting is often milder than what occurs in pemphigus foliaceus. Oral cavity involvement has not been reported, and affected animals are usually otherwise healthy. Occasional animals have isolated skin lesions distant from the face and ears, such as on the paws or genitalia.

Diagnosis

The differential diagnosis of pemphigus erythematosus includes bacterial folliculitis, dermatophytosis, demodicosis, benign familial chronic pemphigus, facial pemphigus foliaceus, discoid and systemic lupus erythematosus, dermatomyositis, drug reaction, leishmaniasis, and zinc-responsive dermatitis.

The definitive diagnosis of pemphigus erythematosus is based on history, physical examination, direct smears, skin biopsy, and immunofluorescence or immunohistochemical testing. Pemphigus erythematosus is histologically identical to pemphigus foliaceus, except that it often has a lichenoid cellular infiltrate of mononuclear cells, plasma cells, and neutrophils or eosinophils or both (Fig. 9–12). Immunopathologically these cases may have a low positive antinuclear antibody titer and basement membrane immunoglobulin deposition.[55]

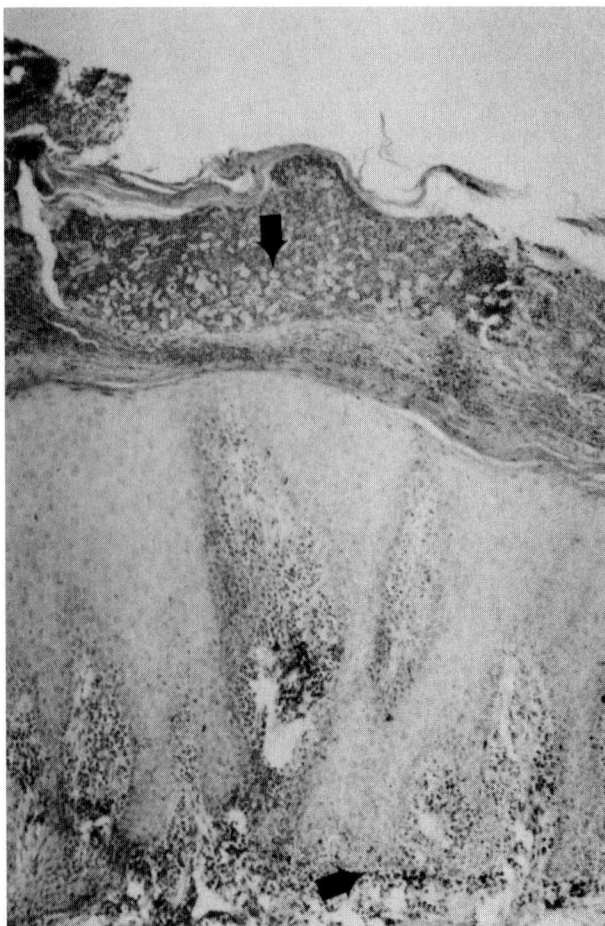

FIGURE 9–12. Canine pemphigus erythematosus. Note the combination of histopathologic patterns: intraepidermal pustular dermatitis with numerous acantholytic keratinocytes (*upper arrow*), and interface dermatitis (*lower arrow*).

Management

The initial therapeutic options for pemphigus erythematosus are different than for most immune-mediated diseases. This is an important reason to try to establish a definitive diagnosis rather than just a diagnosis of "pemphigus."

Pemphigus erythematosus may initially be treated with sun avoidance and topical glucocorticoids. In dogs, the combination of tetracycline and niacinamide is effective in up to 25% of cases. If this combination is not effective, vitamin E, then a short course of systemic glucocorticoids, may be added to the regimen. Once in remission, the initial therapeutic protocols may be effective in keeping the disease in remission. Topical cyclosporine has also been helpful in some cases.

PARANEOPLASTIC PEMPHIGUS

This form of pemphigus was first characterized in humans in 1990 and recently described in dogs.[123, 125, 143, 171] The diagnostic criteria established in humans include severe oral ulceration with polymorphous skin eruptions; histology that includes intraepithelial acantholysis, keratinocyte apoptosis, and vacuolar interface changes; direct immunofluorescence testing findings that include the intercellular deposition of IgG within the epithelium and C3 in a granular pattern along the basement membrane zone; and indirect immunofluorescence findings that include IgG deposition in the intercellular spaces on monkey esophagus and rodent urinary bladder.[155] The immunofluorescence findings on rodent urinary bladder have a specificity of 83% and a sensitivity of 75%; thus, false-positive and false-negative results occur.[155] Immunoprecipitation studies are needed to confirm the diagnosis by identifying the characteristic antigen complex: desmoplakins I (250 kd) and II (210 kd), bullous pemphigoid antigen I (230 kd), envoplakin (210 kd), periplakin (190 kd), desmoglein III (130 kd), and an unidentified (170 kd) transmembrane antigen.[155] Antibodies from human patients reproduce the cutaneous lesions when injected into newborn mice.[159]

The pathogenesis of paraneoplastic pemphigus is unknown. It has been hypothesized that antitumor immune responses cross-react with normal epithelial proteins, perhaps associated with anomalous expression of desmosomes and/or desmoplakins by the neoplasms and/or dysregulated cytokine production (e.g., IL-6) by neoplastic cells.[155] Autoantibodies against desmoglein III and the 170-kd protein probably initiate acantholysis and cell membrane damage, resulting in autoantibody formation against desmoplakins. The antidesmoplakin antibodies then enter keratinocytes and bind target autoantigens by an epitope-spreading phenomenon.

A canine case was shown to have three serum autoantibodies important in human paraneoplastic pemphigus: antibodies that recognize the 210-kd, 190-kd, and 170-kd proteins.[125] The best documented canine case had a concurrent lymphoma.[143] Two cases of pemphigus foliaceus were suspected to be paraneoplastic pemphigus. One was associated with a Sertoli cell tumor,[171] the other was associated with a mammary carcinoma.[123] In humans, paraneoplastic pemphigus is usually associated with malignancies, especially lymphomas (Table 9–2).[155] Unless the associated neoplasm can be cured, immunosuppressive therapy is not very effective.[155, 159]

● Table 9–2 **NEOPLASIA ASSOCIATED WITH HUMAN PARANEOPLASTIC PEMPHIGUS**

LYMPHOCYTIC NEOPLASIA	NONLYMPHOCYTIC NEOPLASIA
Non-Hodgkin's lymphoma	Poorly differentiated sarcoma
Chronic lymphocytic leukemia	Waldenström's macroglobulinemia
Castleman's tumor	Inflammatory fibrosarcoma
Thymoma	Bronchogenic squamous cell carcinoma
Hodgkin's disease	Round cell liposarcoma
T cell lymphoma	

Autoimmune Subepidermal Bullous Dermatoses

The classification of autoimmune blistering diseases is based on the antigen(s) targeted by pathogenic autoantibodies. The autoimmune subepidermal bullous diseases represent different nosologic entities.[18, 51, 185, 191] Studies conducted by Olivry and colleagues have demonstrated that canine subepidermal bullous diseases include bullous pemphigoid (autoantibodies against bullous pemphigoid antigen 2 [Type XVII collagen]), epidermolysis bullosa acquisita (autoantibodies against Type VII collagen), bullous systemic lupus erythematosus (IgG autoantibodies against the noncollagenous aminoterminus of Type VII collagen), linear IgA bullous dermatosis (IgA and IgG autoantibodies against the extracellular portion of bullous pemphigoid antigen 2, from which the intracellular, transmembrane, and NC16A domains have been removed by proteolysis), and mucous membrane pemphigoid (autoantibodies against a 97-kd antigen—possibly the C-terminus of bullous pemphigoid antigen 2—in the lower lamina lucida).[51, 183, 191] These entities are similar clinically, histopathologically, and on routine immunofluorescence or immunohistochemical testing. However, they are different diseases, and studies of larger numbers of cases may reveal important prognostic and therapeutic differences.

The use of salt-split skin as a substrate for indirect immunofluorescence testing is a practical contribution to the study of autoimmune subepidermal bullous diseases.[175, 191] A 1-molar solution of NaCl splits skin through the lamina lucida, allowing the recognition of autoantibodies that bind to the roof (epidermal), floor (dermal), or combined both sides of the split.

BULLOUS PEMPHIGOID

Bullous pemphigoid is a very rare autoimmune, vesiculobullous, ulcerative disorder of skin or oral mucosa or both that has been reported in dogs, cats, and humans.[18, 47, 180, 184, 185] It has been reported to account for 0.01% to 0.1% of all canine dermatology cases.[56, 59] However, it should be noted that the majority of reported cases were diagnosed on the basis of clinical, histopathologic, and immunopathologic findings, not on the basis of the specific antigen being targeted. It is likely that some of these cases were not true bullous pemphigoid as determined by the presence of autoantibodies to specific bullous pemphigoid antigens. Olivry has studied the immunopathology and antigen targeting of 20 dogs with subepidermal blistering diseases: Only 15% had true bullous pemphigoid, suggesting that this disease is even rarer than previously thought.[183]

Cause and Pathogenesis

Bullous pemphigoid is characterized histologically by subepidermal vesicle formation and immunologically by the presence of one or two autoantibodies against antigens at the basal cell hemidesmosomes of skin and mucosa.[5, 18] The bullous pemphigoid antigens are present in all mammalian and avian skin and are associated with hemidesmosomes and the lamina lucida of the basement membrane.[5, 179]

The first antigen is bullous pemphigoid antigen 1 (BPAg 1, BP230), which is a 230-kd intracellular antigen that is a homolog to desmoplakin I.[18, 188] Serum antibodies to this antigen have not yet been described in animals. The second bullous pemphigoid antigen (BPAg 2, BP180), also called collagen XVII, is a 180-kd hemidesmosomal transmembranous molecule.[188] In humans, circulating IgE and IgG4 autoantibodies are the major immunoglobulins preferentially targeting two distinct epitopes on BP180, and the levels of these autoantibodies parallel disease activity.[178a] Canine and feline cases of bullous pemphigoid exhibit antibodies to this latter molecule.[169, 177, 184, 185] The cause of antibody production is still unknown, but genetic factors have been determined in humans and dogs.

The proposed pathomechanism of blister formation in bullous pemphigoid is as follows: (1) the binding of complement-fixing pemphigoid antibody to the antigen of the hemidesmosomes, (2) complement fixation and activation, (3) activation of mast cells and release of chemotactic cytokines, (4) chemoattraction of neutrophils and eosinophils, and

(5) release of proteolytic enzymes from the infiltrating leukocytes, which disrupt dermo-epidermal cohesion, resulting in dermo-epidermal separation and vesicle formation.[5, 18, 47, 176] In humans, elevated concentrations of eosinophil cationic protein, major basic protein, and neutrophil-derived myeloperoxidase and elastase were detected in blister fluid and serum of patients with bullous pemphigoid, suggesting that the release of these substances from activated granulocytes may be important in the pathogenesis of blister formation.[178] An eosinophil-derived enzyme, gelatinase, may be involved in cleaving the Type XVII collagen.[177, 187] Human pemphigoid antibodies, when injected into rabbit cornea or guinea pig skin, locally produce the clinical, histologic, and immunopathologic features of bullous pemphigoid.[5, 18]

Other factors thought to be involved in the pathogenesis of some cases of bullous pemphigoid are drug provocation (especially sulfonamides, penicillins, and furosemide) and ultraviolet light.[5, 18, 157, 186] Bullous pemphigoid–like drug eruptions have been reported in dogs, though the exact antigenic target was not determined and these cases may not have been true bullous pemphigoid.[268, 269, 282]

Clinical variants occur in humans, and their differentiation is proceeding based on the more advanced methods of detecting target antigens. The past confusion and overlap between some of these "variants"—such as cicatricial pemphigoid and herpes gestationis, which do share, at least partially, the target antigens noted in bullous pemphigoid—are beginning to be worked out.[181, 188, 190] This also is the case in the canine, wherein Olivry's group has recognized mucous membrane pemphigoid. This disease has been known as cicatricial pemphigoid in humans and is still the name preferred by some investigators.[190] Mucous membrane pemphigoid is one of the most common forms of autoimmune basement membrane zone disease in dogs.[183] It is phenotypically distinct, yet immunologically heterogeneous, as in humans. Six cases of mucous membrane pemphigoid have been recognized in dogs: four of them exhibited antibodies against the NC16A domain of BP180 and one of them had antibodies against the C-terminus of BP180.[183]

Clinical Features

Bullous pemphigoid is very rare in the dog, accounting for about 0.1% of all canine skin disorders at one university small animal clinic[56] and 0.01% of all canine dermatology cases at another.[59] Canine bullous pemphigoid has no reported age or sex predilections, although collies and, perhaps, Doberman pinschers appear to be predisposed to it.[47, 182, 186] The disease in collies and shelties must be separated from so-called ulcerative dermatosis of collies and Shetland sheepdogs (probably vesicular cutaneous lupus erythematosus).[203]

Bullous pemphigoid is a vesiculobullous, ulcerative disorder that may affect the oral cavity, mucocutaneous junctions, skin, or any combination thereof (Fig. 9–13A and B). About 80% of affected dogs have oral cavity lesions at the time of diagnosis. In Olivry's confirmed cases of canine bullous pemphigoid, only one third exhibited oral involvement, which is in contrast with cases of canine mucous membrane pemphigoid that exhibit consistent mucosal involvement with no or minimal skin lesions.[183] Oral cavity involvement has been recognized either after or at the same time as the cutaneous signs and rarely as the initial event. Cutaneous lesions occur most commonly in the axillae and groin, also the common sites for vesicular cutaneous lupus erythematosus of collies and Shetland sheepdogs. Ulcerative paronychia, onychomadesis, or footpad ulceration may occur.

An insidious, chronic, clinically benign form of cutaneous bullous pemphigoid has been recognized in dogs, with lesions confined to the axillae, groin, or isolated mucocutaneous areas such as the anus and prepuce.[47, 186] Cases of bullous pemphigoid may be severe and clinically indistinguishable from pemphigus vulgaris and other subepidermal blistering diseases. In true bullous pemphigoid, the vesicles and bullae are less fragile and transient than those occurring in vesicular cutaneous lupus erythematosus of collies and sheepdogs.[183] In contrast with the flaccid blisters of pemphigus vulgaris, the blisters of bullous pemphigoid are tense.[183] The presence of intact vesicles or bullae is more suggestive of subepidermal bullous diseases and, with further study, we will hopefully be able to better clinically differentiate these diseases. When vesicles and bullae have ruptured, the

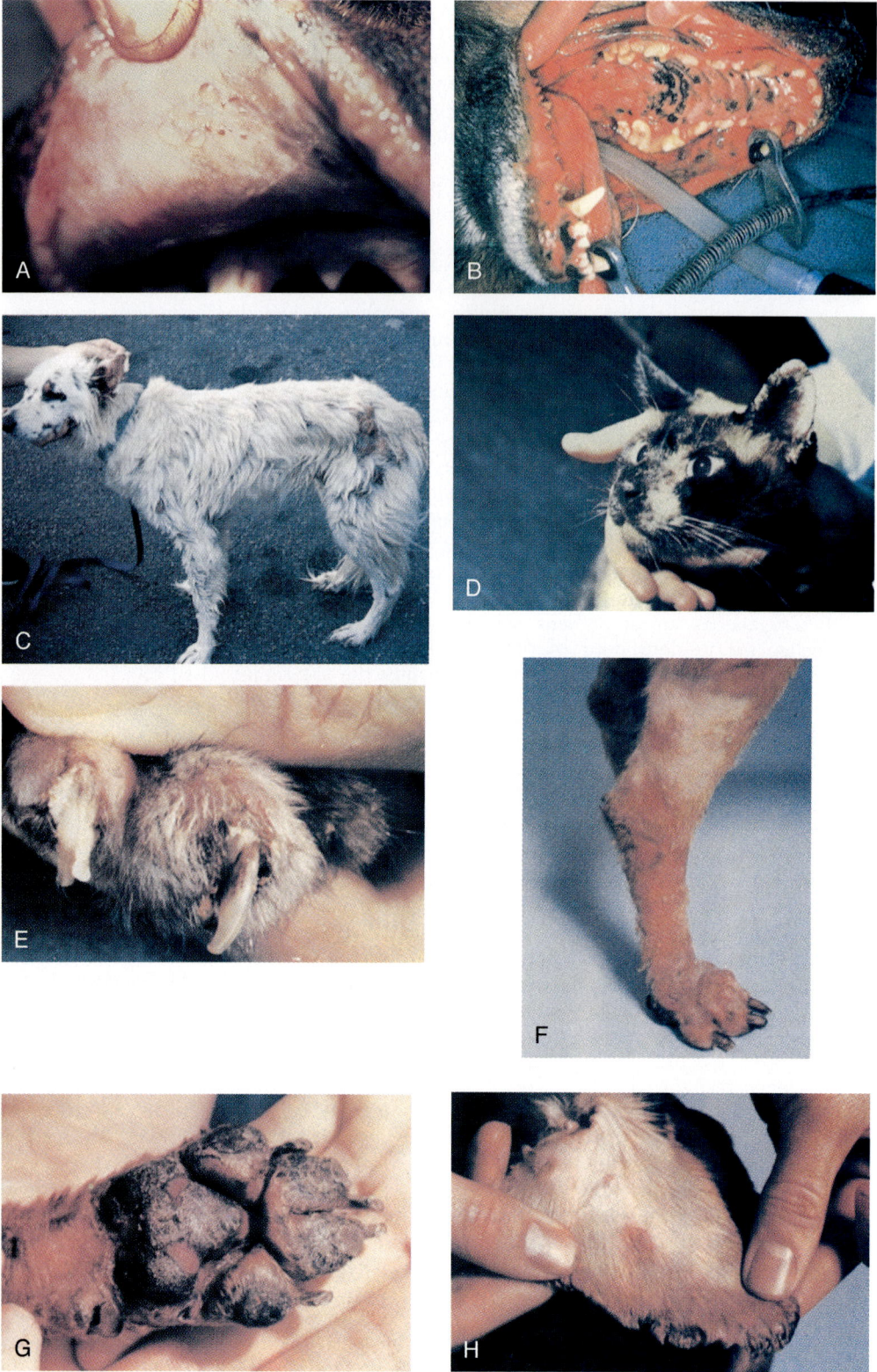

FIGURE 9-13. *Legend on opposite page*

clinician sees ulcers bordered by epithelial collarettes. The pseudo-Nikolsky sign may be present.

Pruritus and pain are variable, and secondary bacterial pyoderma is common. Severely affected dogs may be anorectic, depressed, or febrile and may die because of fluid, electrolyte, and protein imbalances and septicemia.

Results of routine laboratory determinations (hemogram, serum chemistries, urinalysis, serum protein electrophoresis) are nonspecific, often revealing mild to moderate leukocytosis and neutrophilia, mild nonregenerative anemia, mild hypoalbuminemia, and mild to moderate elevations of α_2, β, and γ globulins.[55, 186] Peripheral eosinophilia is rare.[55, 186]

Diagnosis

The differential diagnosis includes pemphigus vulgaris, systemic lupus erythematosus, epidermolysis bullosa acquisita, linear IgA bullous dermatosis, erythema multiforme, toxic epidermal necrolysis, idiopathic ulcerative dermatosis (vesicular cutaneous lupus erythematosus) of collies and Shetland sheepdogs, drug reaction, epitheliotropic lymphoma, candidiasis, and the numerous causes of canine ulcerative stomatitis. Definitive diagnosis of bullous pemphigoid is based on history, physical examination, skin (or mucosal) biopsy, demonstration of basement membrane fixed autoantibodies, and circulating antibodies that target the bullous pemphigoid antigens. Microscopic examination of direct smears from intact vesicles, bullae, or recent ulcers does not reveal acantholytic keratinocytes.

Bullous pemphigoid is characterized histologically by subepidermal cleft and vesicle formation (Figs. 9–14 and 9–15).[18, 22, 47, 186] Acantholysis does not occur. Inflammatory infiltrates vary from mild and perivascular to marked and lichenoid (Fig. 9–16). Tissue eosinophilia is common in canine bullous pemphigoid. In contrast, cases of mucous membrane pemphigoid have noninflammatory blisters, and epidermolysis bullosa acquisita cases have neutrophil-rich vesicles.[183, 191] Feline bullous pemphigoid has only a few eosinophils.[184] Subepidermal vacuolar alteration (subepidermal "bubblies") has been suggested as the earliest prevesicle histopathologic finding.[47] Olivry thinks that the first lesion of canine bullous pemphigoid might be eosinophil degranulation at the basement membrane zone (Fig. 9–17).[183]

Electron-microscopic examination of pemphigoid lesions has revealed the following features: smudging, thickening, and interruption of the basement membrane zone; fragmentation and disappearance of anchoring fibrils, anchoring filaments, and hemidesmosomes; basal cell degeneration; and separation occurring within the lamina lucida.[47, 186]

Direct immunofluorescence or immunohistochemical testing reveals a linear deposition of immunoglobulin, and usually complement, at the basement membrane zone of skin or mucosa in 50% to 90% of patients (see Fig. 9–1C).[5, 18, 55, 186] However, this is not specific for bullous pemphigoid. Complement component C3 is the most commonly demonstrated immunoreactant. The presence of IgG is expected.[180, 184, 185] It would appear to be important to test with all classes of immunoglobulins, because in some dogs, results are positive for only IgM or IgA (though in light of the more recent studies, these cases may not have truly been bullous pemphigoid). It is also important to sample intact vesicles and bullae as well as perilesional tissue. Indirect immunofluorescence testing frequently yielded negative results in the past, though a definitive diagnosis should include the demonstration of circulating IgG autoantibodies to the bullous pemphigoid antigen(s).[180, 185] In one study, the IgG subtypes were predominantly IgG2 or IgG4.[13]

FIGURE 9–13. *A*, Bullae on the labial mucosa of a dog with bullous pemphigoid. (From Scott DW, Lewis RM: Pemphigus and pemphigoid in dog and man. Comparative aspects. Am Acad Dermatol 5:148, 1981.) *B*, Canine bullous pemphigoid. Severe ulcerative stomatitis and cheilitis. *C*, Systemic lupus erythematosus in a dog with arthritis and generalized erythematous, alopecic, and focally ulcerative skin lesions. *D*, Alopecia, erythema, crusting, and depigmentation of the face and ear of a cat with systemic lupus erythematosus. *E*, Bacterial paronychia in a cat with systemic lupus erythematosus. (*D* and *E*, from Scott DW, et al: A glucocorticoid-responsive dermatitis in cats, resembling systemic lupus erythematosus in man. J Am Anim Hosp Assoc 15:157, 1979.) *F*, Erythema, alopeica, and ulceration of the hind leg of a dog with systemic lupus erythematosus. *G*, Ulcerated footpads of a dog with systemic lupus erythematosus. *H*, Necrosis of the margin of the pinna in a dog with systemic lupus erythematosus.

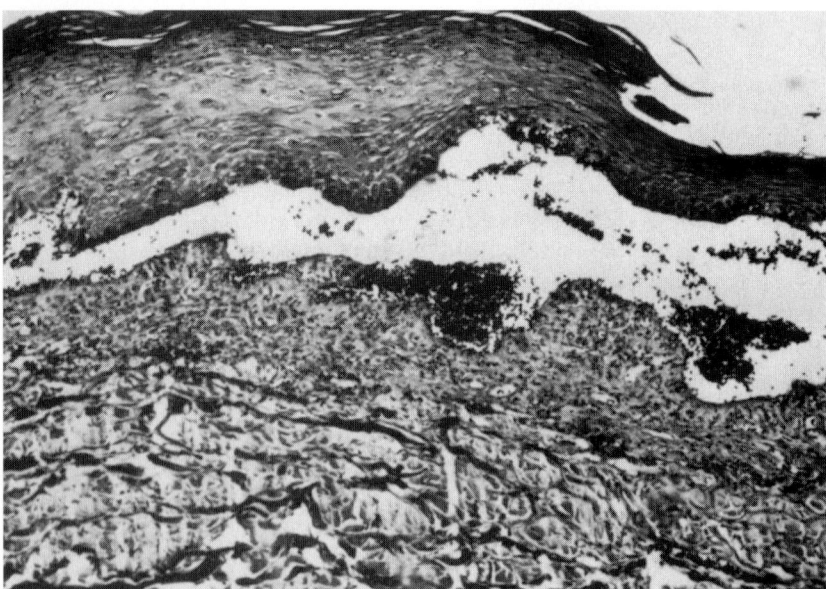

FIGURE 9–14. Canine bullous pemphigoid. Subepidermal vesicle and lichenoid band of inflammatory cells. (From Scott DW, Lewis RM: Pemphigus and pemphigoid in dog and man: Comparative aspects. J Am Acad Dermatol 5:148, 1981.)

Clinical Management

The natural course of untreated cases is unclear. Veterinarians have long recognized refractory mucocutaneous ulcerative disorders that resulted in the death or euthanasia of affected dogs. Retrospectively, some of these dogs may have had bullous pemphigoid. On the basis of the small number of cases documented in the veterinary literature, canine bullous pemphigoid is usually a severe disease. The prognosis for true bullous pemphigoid is not yet established, but it appears to be a more localized and more benign disease than epidermolysis bullosa acquisita.[183] Extensive cases may be fatal unless treated. Therapy of canine bullous pemphigoid may be difficult, requiring large doses of systemic glucocorticoids with or without other potent immunomodulating drugs. In one study of nine dogs

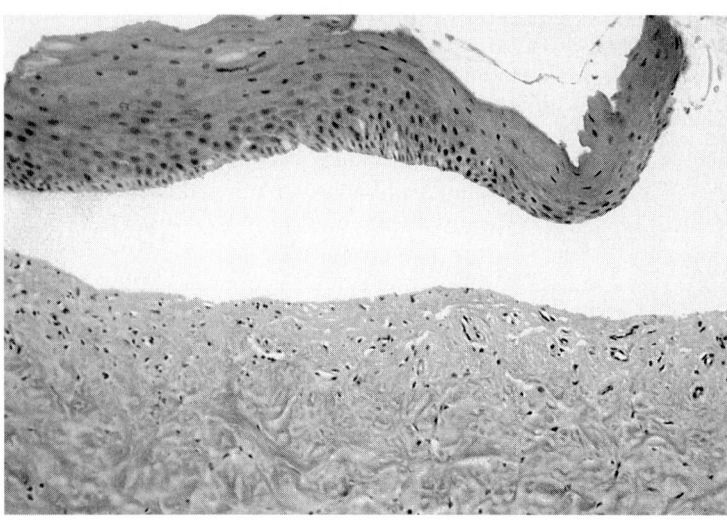

FIGURE 9–15. Feline bullous pemphigoid. Subepidermal vesicle, cell-poor. (Courtesy Dr. T. Olivry.)

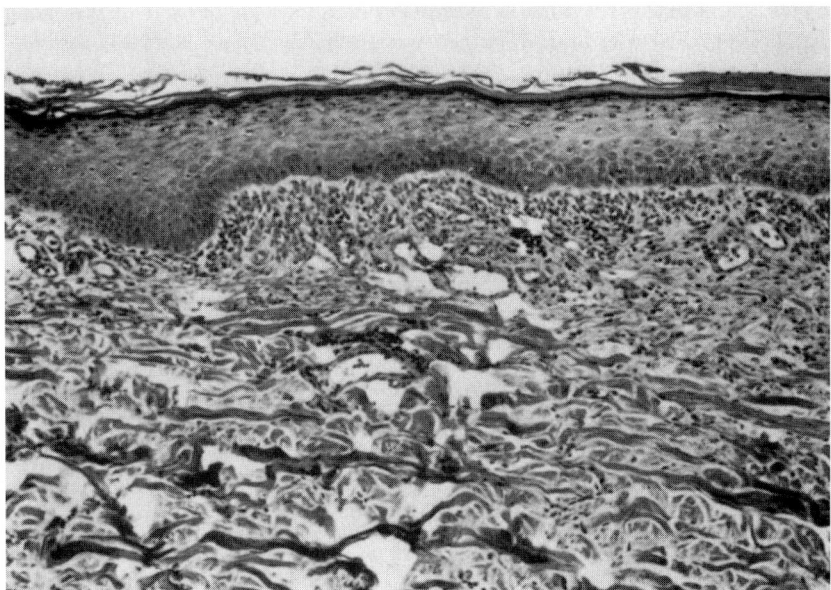

FIGURE 9-16. Canine bullous pemphigoid. Subepidermal vacuolar alteration (subepidermal "bubblies") and lichenoid band of inflammatory cells.

with subepidermal blistering disease believed to be bullous pemphigoid,[186] the following observations were made: 1 mg/kg prednisolone, given orally q12h, was ineffective for controlling the disease, and 3 mg/kg prednisolone, given orally q12h, was effective for controlling the disease. Two of the nine dogs requiring the larger dose were euthanized, however, because of unacceptable side effects, and another two died after 7 to 10 days of therapy (from acute pancreatitis). Thus, systemic glucocorticoids were unsatisfactory for treatment in four of nine dogs (44%).

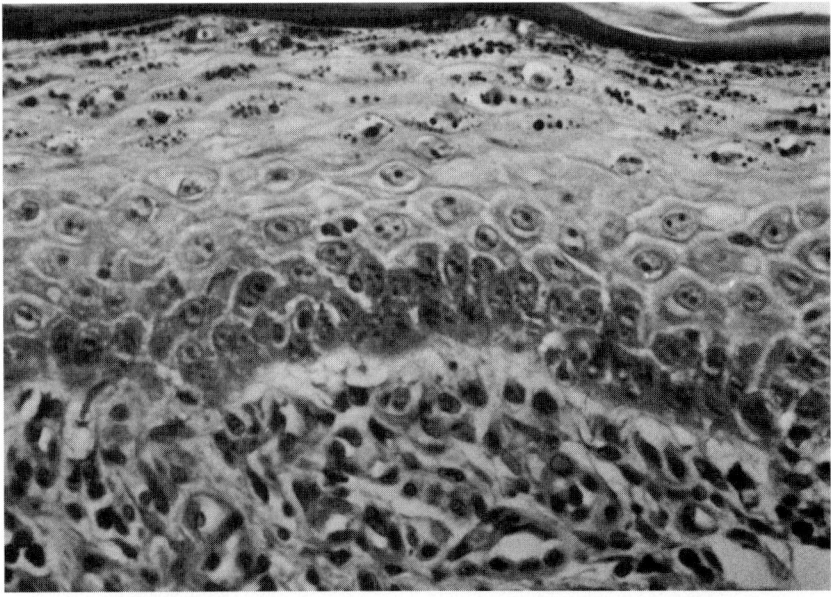

FIGURE 9-17. Canine bullous pemphigoid. Subepidermal vacuolar alteration.

Suspected bullous pemphigoid cases have, in our experience, usually required combinations of immunosuppressive agents. One case (seen by C.E.G.) even required glucocorticoids, azathioprine, and chlorambucil to be kept in remission. Therapy usually must be maintained for prolonged periods if not for life. Thus, the therapeutic regimen must be individualized for each patient, and owner education is essential. Mild cases of canine bullous pemphigoid may be successfully managed with topical glucocorticoids or relatively low doses of systemic glucocorticoids (2.2 mg/kg/day of prednisolone or prednisone orally for induction), and therapy may occasionally even be terminated.[55, 186]

Tetracycline and erythromycin have been reported to be beneficial in the treatment of bullous pemphigoid in humans.[18, 189] It is thought that the benefit derived from these drugs is related to their ability to inhibit neutrophil chemotaxis and random migration and to increase dermo-epidermal cohesion and inhibit proteases that might be involved in blister formation.

Because (1) cutaneous lesions of bullous pemphigoid in humans can be induced by exposure to ultraviolet light and (2) canine bullous pemphigoid may worsen with exposure to ultraviolet light, it may be prudent to avoid direct exposure to sunlight between 8 AM and 5 PM.[18, 47, 186] The limited number of identified cases of true canine bullous pemphigoid have not been photosensitive.[183] Until a definitive diagnosis is made, sun avoidance still should be recommended.

EPIDERMOLYSIS BULLOSA ACQUISITA

Epidermolysis bullosa acquisita is a subepidermal blistering disease. It is thought to be one of the most common causes of autoimmune subepidermal blistering in dogs (25% of the cases).[183] In humans, it is an acquired autoimmune disease that was clinically similar to the childhood form of epidermolysis bullosa—hence the name—even though it is not hereditary or a disease typically found in children.[192] It is characterized by the chronic development of subepidermal blisters that may be induced by trauma and by fragile skin. In humans, the epidermal separation was similar to that of bullous pemphigoid, and even direct immunofluorescence test findings were similar.[192] Immunoelectron microscopy revealed the antibody deposits to be located at the anchoring fibrils, separating this disease from bullous pemphigoid. Subsequent studies have shown that the autoantibodies target type VII collagen within the anchoring fibrils of the basement membrane zone.[192]

A case of epidermolysis bullosa acquisita was described in a 1-year-old, intact male Great Dane that experienced an acute onset and rapid progression of skin lesions.[191] There was generalized urticaria, vesiculation, and cutaneous sloughing, resulting in ulcers. Ulcerations were most pronounced in the oral cavity (Fig. 9–18) and on the footpads.

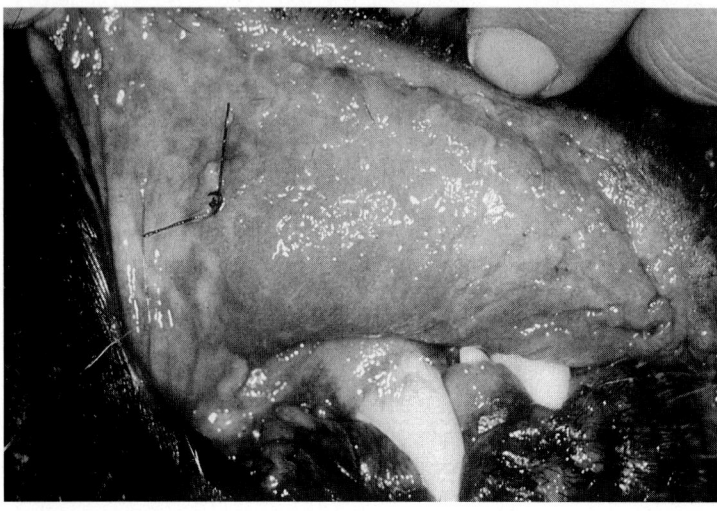

FIGURE 9–18. Canine epidermolysis bullosa acquisita. Severe ulceration of oral cavity. (Courtesy Dr. T. Olivry.)

The dog was also febrile and lethargic. Treatment with prednisone (5 mg/kg/day), antibiotics, and dapsone was not satisfactory, so euthanasia was performed at the owner's request. Histopathology and collagen IV staining revealed that the subepidermal vesicles were occurring in the sublamina densa (Fig. 9–19). A mild, bandlike infiltrate of neutrophils and lymphocytes was visible at the base of subepidermal vesicles. In more severe lesions, neutrophil microabscesses were visible in the superficial dermis. Direct immunofluorescence testing revealed IgG, IgM, IgA, and C3 at the basement membrane zone. Indirect immunofluorescence testing (IgG and IgA at the basement membrane zone of dog lip and tongue, but *not* with monkey esophagus), indirect protein A immunogold electron microscopy, Western immunoblotting, and recombinant collagen VII-NC1 enzyme-linked immunosorbent assay (ELISA) were all used to confirm that the autoantibodies targeted collagen VII in the anchoring fibrils.[191, 192a] Olivry has recognized four more cases, and four of the five dogs exhibited a generalized phenotype that did not respond to treatment.[183] One dog had a localized variant (predominantly head region) that responded completely to prednisone (2 mg/kg/day), thus resembling the Brunsting-Perry epidermolysis bullosa acquisita in humans.[183a]

LINEAR IgA BULLOUS DERMATOSIS

A 3-year-old, spayed female mongrel dog was presented for vesicles, erosions, ulcers, and crusts on the lips, pinnae, axillae, sternum, groin, extremities, footpads, and tongue.[51] Histologic examination revealed mixed inflammatory, hemorrhagic, subepidermal vesicles. Circulating IgA and IgG autoantibodies targeted the 120-kd linear IgA bullous dermatosis antigen (LAD-1) in the upper lamina lucida.

MUCOUS MEMBRANE PEMPHIGOID

A 1-year-old, intact male Australian shepherd was presented for vesicles, erosions, and crusts on the periorbital, perinasal, and pinnal skin as well as the oral mucosa.[51] Histologic examination revealed large subepidermal vesicles and focal neutrophilic subepidermal microabscesses. Circulating IgG autoantibodies targeted a 97-kd antigen in the lower lamina lucida.

Lupus Erythematosus

Lupus erythematosus is a term that encompasses a group of diseases that have different clinical syndromes that share a similar underlying autoimmune process.[218] The appropriate terminology and classification of the syndromes and cases with these disorders have led to,

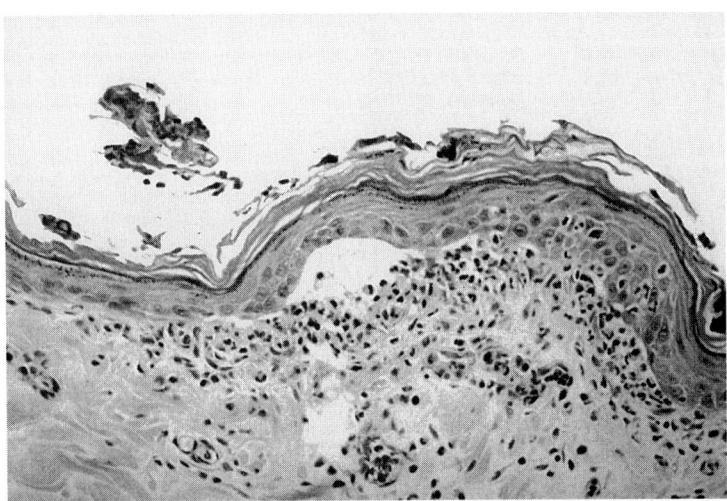

FIGURE 9–19. Canine epidermolysis bullosa acquisita. Subepidermal clefting and neutrophil infiltrate. (Courtesy Dr. T. Olivry.)

and still create, differing views and controversy. The terminology and a classification system used in humans, described by Sontheimer, is beginning to be used in veterinary medicine.[203, 218, 219]

In Sontheimer's system, the basis is that there is lupus erythematosus, which may be systemic or cutaneous (Table 9–3). The systemic form of lupus erythematosus may be associated with any of the lupus-related skin diseases or many nonspecific cutaneous lesions. The lupus erythematosus–related skin disease might be nonspecific or be one of the forms of cutaneous lupus erythematosus that are specific skin syndromes, characterized by certain clinical and histopathologic findings. The different forms of cutaneous lupus erythematosus vary as concerns the probability of associated systemic disease. In the dog, we have classically recognized two main forms of cutaneous lupus erythematosus, though newer forms are being recognized but are not as well studied.[203, 212, 213]

Lupus erythematosus is an uncommon autoimmune disorder of dogs, cats, and humans that has polyclonal lymphocytic involvement. The exact etiology is unknown but, in humans, all forms are characterized by a variety of autoantibodies to nuclear antigens and/or immune complex deposition. Genetic associations have been described in humans and dogs. In humans, the different forms of cutaneous lupus erythematosus have different genetic markers. Other precipitating factors include viral infections, drugs, hormones, chemical exposure, and cigarette smoking.[18, 219]

The pathogenesis of skin lesions in lupus erythematosus is unclear. All three forms of cutaneous lupus erythematosus in humans, as well as canine cutaneous lupus erythematosus, are often exacerbated by exposure to ultraviolet radiation.[47, 195, 219] In humans, it has been demonstrated that the lymphocytes infiltrating skin lesions of discoid and systemic lupus erythematosus are predominantly T cells and that helper T cells predominate in discoid lupus, whereas suppressor T cells predominate in the systemic variety.[5, 18] In the dog, plasma cells are prominent, a feature not shared with humans, suggesting that B lymphocytes may be important and that a different pathogenesis may be occurring.

Five characteristics of cutaneous lupus erythematosus are (1) photosensitivity (lesions may be produced by sunlight in both the UVB and UVA spectrums), (2) keratinocyte damage (associated with contiguous T lymphocytes and macrophages), (3) lymphohistiocytic infiltration, (4) autoantibody production, and (5) immune complex deposition.[18, 206, 211, 216, 224] Skin lesions may be induced or exacerbated with ultraviolet light exposure. Infusion of antinuclear antibodies (ANAs) does not produce skin lesions, however, and immune complexes appear at the basement membrane zone after dermatohistopathologic changes appear (up to 6 weeks *after* inflammatory changes appear).

A current hypothesis for the pathogenesis of skin lesions in genetically susceptible individuals is as follows:

1. Ultraviolet light (both UVB and UVA) penetrating to the level of epidermal basal cells induces, on the keratinocyte surface, the enhanced expression of intercellular adhesion molecule-1 (ICAM-1) and of autoantigens (e.g., Ro) previously found only in the nucleus or cytoplasm (e.g., native and denatured DNA).
2. Specific autoantibodies to these antigens that are present in plasma and in tissue fluid, bathing the epidermis, attach to keratinocytes and induce antibody-dependent cytotoxicity of keratinocytes.
3. Injured keratinocytes release IL-2 and other lymphocyte attractants, accounting for the resultant lymphohistiocytic infiltrate.
4. Injured keratinocytes release increased amounts of TNF-α, IL-1, and IL-6, which are associated with elevations of ANA, increased B cell activity, and higher production of IgM.[18, 211, 216] Inappropriate activation of apoptosis occurs.

Immunopathologic studies of cutaneous and oral mucosal lupus erythematosus lesions in humans have revealed a predominance of helper T cells and macrophages and a near absence of B cells and Langerhans' cells.[18] In humans, retroviral antigen has been demonstrated at the basement membrane zone of skin lesions and evidence has been presented suggesting that the immune deposits are complement-activating and may be functional

● Table 9-3 **THE GILLIAM CLASSIFICATION OF SKIN LESIONS ASSOCIATED WITH LUPUS ERYTHEMATOSUS (LE)**

LE-Specific Skin Disease (Cutaneous LE [CLE])

Acute cutaneous LE (ACLE)
    Localized ACLE (malar rash; butterfly rash)
    Generalized ACLE (lupus rash; maculopapular lupus rash; photosensitive lupus dermatitis)
Subacute cutaneous LE (SCLE)
    Annular SCLE (lupus marginatus; symmetric erythema centrifugum; autoimmune annular erythema; lupus erythematosus gyratus repens)
    Papulosquamous SCLE (disseminated LE; psoriasiform LE; pityriasiform LE; and maculopapular photosensitive LE)
Chronic cutaneous LE (CCLE)
    Classic discoid LE (DLE)
        Localized DLE
        Generalized DLE
    Hypertrophic DLE/verrucosus DLE
    Lupus panniculitis/lupus profundus
    Mucosal DLE
        Oral DLE
        Conjunctival DLE
    Lupus tumidus (urticarial plaque of LE)
    Chilblains LE (chilblains lupus)
    Lichenoid DLE (LE/lichen planus overlap, lupus planus)

LE-Nonspecific Skin Disease

Cutaneous vascular disease
    Vasculitis
        Leukocytoclastic
            Palpable purpura
            Urticarial vasculitis
        Periarteritis nodosa–like cutaneous lesions
    Vasculopathy
        Degos' disease-like lesions
        Secondary atrophy blanche (livedoid vasculitis, livedo vasculitis)
    Periungual telangiectasia
    Livedo reticularis
    Thrombophlebitis
    Raynaud's phenomenon
    Erythromelalgia
Nonscarring alopecia
    "Lupus hair"
    Telogen effluvium
    Alopecia areata
Sclerodactyly
Rheumatoid nodules
Calcinosis cutis
LE-nonspecific bullous lesions
Urticaria
Papulonodular mucinosis
Cutis laxa/anetoderma
Acanthosis nigricans (secondary to type B insulin resistance)
Erythema multiforme (Rowell's syndrome)
Leg ulcers
Lichen planus

Alternative or synonymous terms are listed inside parenthesis.
From Sontheimer RD: The lexicon of cutaneous lupus erythematosus: A review and personal perspective on the nomenclature and classification of the cutaneous manifestations of lupus erythematosus. Lupus 6:84, 1997.

and involved in the inflammatory response.[5, 18] Fibronectin, type IV collagen, and type VII collagen are all altered at the basement membrane zone of lesional skin.[210]

In one study of cutaneous lupus erythematosus in humans,[197] there was a marked increase in Ki-67 (a protein essential for cell proliferation) and p53 (a protein that can regulate cell proliferation and downregulate bcl-2) and a marked decrease in bcl-2 (a protein that promotes cell survival and inhibits apoptosis). It was hypothesized that basal keratinocytes, damaged by antibody-dependent cellular cytotoxicity, become hyperproliferative (thus expressing Ki-67), which induces the expression of p53 which, in turn, downregulates bcl-2 and activates an apoptotic pathway in the epidermis.

SYSTEMIC LUPUS ERYTHEMATOSUS

Systemic lupus erythematosus is the most severe form of the lupus diseases because it involves more than cutaneous lesions and may present with a wide array of clinical symptoms that reflect multiple organ or tissue damage.

Cause and Pathogenesis

The etiology of systemic lupus erythematosus appears to be multifactorial, with genetic predilection, immunologic disorder (T cell deficiency, B cell hyperactivity, deficiencies of complement components), viral infection, and hormonal and ultraviolet light modulation all playing a role.[5, 18, 47, 193, 195, 199, 208] B lymphocyte hyperactivity results in a plethora of autoantibodies formed against numerous body constituents. The most well-studied are the ANA, which are found in up to 100% of the cases reported. The study of these antibodies utilizing newer techniques, such as immunoblotting and immunoprecipitation, has revealed that a number of nuclear components are targeted, including double-stranded DNA, histones, and extractable nuclear antigens.[195, 209, 220, 226] These latter may be more important in the dog and include a group of ribonuclear proteins (RNPs), the small nuclear RNP complexes (snRNPs), and heterogeneous nuclear RNPs (hnRNPs).[195, 226]

Studies in dogs with systemic lupus have showed that, in the active phase of disease, there is a marked lymphopenia that, though it affects both CD4+ and CD8+ T cells, more severely involves CD8+ cells.[194] This results in an altered (increased) CD4/CD8 ratio (mean of 6 with disease; mean of 2.3 in normals). The decrease in CD8+ T lymphocytes is directly related to disease severity, and an increase in these cells is associated with a good response to therapy. Additionally, the percentage of active phase T cells increases with successful treatment.[194] This T cell imbalance persisted in cases of spontaneous inactivity or treated dogs that responded poorly but normalized in dogs that responded well to treatment.[194]

In humans, a number of drugs (especially procainamide, hydralazine, isoniazid, penicillamine, several anticonvulsants, and contraceptives) are known to precipitate or exacerbate systemic lupus erythematosus.[5, 18] Vaccination with a modified live virus product containing distemper, hepatitis, parainfluenza, and parvovirus antigens was suspected to have precipitated systemic lupus erythematosus in a dog.[47] Tissue damage in systemic lupus erythematosus appears to be due to a Type III hypersensitivity reaction. The New Zealand black mouse, the F1 hybrid of the New Zealand black mouse, and the New Zealand white mouse experience a lupus-like disease that has many similarities to systemic lupus erythematosus in humans.[5, 18, 47, 216]

In the dog, the serologic abnormalities associated with spontaneous canine systemic lupus erythematosus can be transmitted both to normal dogs and to mice by means of cell-free extracts, thus suggesting an infective agent.[25, 47] As yet, however, none of these dogs has developed overt systemic lupus erythematosus, indicating that other factors are involved in the pathogenesis of the clinical entity. It has been reported that dogs with systemic lupus erythematosus have lower levels of circulating thymic factors than do normal dogs, analogous to the situation in humans.[18, 47, 195]

In a colony of dogs obtained by the mating of a male and female, each having systemic lupus erythematosus, the F1 generation had no clinical signs; with subsequent breeding, a few dogs in the F2 generation were affected; and clinical signs were common and marked in the F3 generation.[202] Affected dogs had depressed suppressor T cell activity, decreased levels of serum thymulin, and a decreased percentage of circulating T cells.[202]

In the colony of dogs at Lyon, France, greater than 50% of the dogs are ANA carriers, and 25% to 30% of the dogs experience disease.[196] In the same colony, there is a strong association between dog leukocyte antigen (DLA) phenotypes and the occurrence of systemic lupus erythematosus (DLA-A7 positively associated, DLA-A1 and DLA-B5 negatively associated).[196, 222] A high incidence (47.6%) of ANA positivity was also found in an English Cocker spaniel breeding colony.[199]

Clinical Features

The clinical signs associated with systemic lupus erythematosus are varied and changeable. Because of this phenomenal clinical variability and ability to mimic numerous diseases, systemic lupus erythematosus has been called the "great imitator."

- **Dog.** Systemic lupus erythematosus is an uncommon disease in dogs.[25, 47, 56, 217] The incidence has been estimated at 0.03% of the canine population.[195, 217] There is no age predilection (average, 5 years) and, at least in some studies, males have been overrepresented at a ratio of 7:3.[195] Breed predilections have also been described for collies, Shetland sheepdogs, Poodles, and German shepherd dogs.[47, 195, 217] The most common manifestations are fever (constant or irregularly cyclic), polyarthritis (nonerosive, nondeforming), proteinuria (>0.5 g/L), and skin disease, being present in greater than 50% of cases.[47, 195, 217] Consequent muscle wasting can make the dogs look much older than they are. Other relatively common manifestations include anemia, leukopenia, peripheral lymphadenopathy, splenomegaly, and oral ulcers.[47, 195, 217] Other syndromes reported in association with canine systemic lupus erythematosus are pericarditis, thrombocytopenia, polymyositis, myocarditis, pneumonitis, pleuritis, neurologic disorders (seizures, meningitis, myelitis, psychoses, polyneuropathy), and lymphedema.

The cutaneous manifestations of canine systemic lupus erythematosus are extremely diverse. They include seborrheic skin disease, alopecia, diffuse or regional erythema, cutaneous or mucocutaneous vesiculobullous or ulcerative disorders, footpad ulcers and hyperkeratosis, discoid lupus erythematosus, refractory secondary bacterial pyodermas, panniculitis (lupus profundus), and nasal dermatitis (see Fig. 9–13C, F to H).[47, 195, 217] Skin lesions may be multifocal or generalized and commonly involve areas of skin poorly protected by hair: face (especially nose, lips, pinnae if erect), limbs (especially cranial aspect of thoracic limbs), axillae, groin, and ventral abdomen. They may be exacerbated or induced by exposure to sunlight. Pruritus is variable, and scarring is common. Occasionally, dogs experience acute facial or hemifacial edema.

A 4-year-old, castrated male Bichon Frisé with systemic lupus erythematosus had erosions and ulcers of lips, external auditory meati, lateral thorax, axillae, prepuce, metatarsi, and footpads.[51, 213] Histopathologic findings were early noninflammatory subepidermal blisters and late subepidermal vesicles with subjacent neutrophils. IgG autoantibodies against the noncollagenous aminoterminus of type VII collagen (bullous systemic lupus erythematosus antigen) were detected. It was suggested that this was analogous to so-called *type I–bullous systemic lupus erythematosus* in humans.

- **Cat.** Systemic lupus erythematosus is rarely reported in cats.[56, 214, 225] The incidence has been estimated to be 0.06% of all feline hospital visits.[214] There is no apparent sex predilection, and affected cats range from 1 to 12 years old. Siamese, Persian, and Himalayan cats may be predisposed. Syndromes reported include hematologic abnormalities, neurologic or behavioral abnormalities, fever, lymphadenopathy, polyarthritis, myopathy, oral ulceration, conjunctivitis, renal failure, and subclinical pulmonary disease.

About 20% of affected cats have cutaneous lesions.[56, 214, 225] Dermatologic abnormalities include seborrheic skin disease, exfoliative erythroderma, and erythematous, scaling, crusting, alopecic, scarring dermatitis most commonly involving the face (see Fig. 9–13D), pinnae, and paws (see Fig. 9–13E).

Diagnosis

The differential diagnosis of cutaneous systemic lupus erythematosus is lengthy, owing to the varied and changeable cutaneous manifestations of the disorder. Typical alternative diagnoses are seborrheic skin disease, dermatophytosis, bacterial folliculitis, demodicosis, food hypersensitivity, scabies, pemphigus vulgaris, bullous pemphigoid, epidermolysis bullosa acquisita, discoid lupus erythematosus, erythema multiforme, necrolytic migratory erythema, leishmaniasis, toxic epidermal necrolysis, candidiasis, and epitheliotropic lymphoma.

The definitive diagnosis of systemic lupus erythematosus is often one of the most challenging tasks in medicine. The disease is so variable in its clinicopathologic presentations that any dogmatic diagnostic categorization is impossible. The clinicopathologic abnormalities that are demonstrated depend on the organ systems involved and may include anemia (nonregenerative or hemolytic) with or without a positive direct Coombs' test result, thrombocytopenia with or without a positive platelet factor-3 test result or antiplatelet antibody, leukopenia or leukocytosis, proteinuria, hypergammaglobulinemia (polyclonal), and sterile synovial exudate obtained by arthrocentesis.[47, 205] A positive lupus-type anticoagulant test result was reported in a dog with hemolysis, pulmonary thromboembolism, nephrotic syndrome, polyarthropathy, and thrombocytopenia.[221] The lupus erythematosus (LE) cell test may yield a positive result in up to 60% of patients, but it is variable from day to day, is steroid-labile, and lacks sensitivity and specificity. The assay has been discontinued in many of the leading laboratories in human medicine.[47]

The ANA test is currently considered the most sensitive serologic test for systemic lupus erythematosus.[25, 47, 195, 207] It yields a positive result in up to 100% of cases of active systemic lupus erythematosus. It is *not* the most specific of tests,[47, 207] yielding positive results in up to 20% of dogs with infectious diseases (particularly leishmaniasis) and up to 16% of control dogs.[195] In general, results from different laboratories cannot be compared. It is important to record the titer (and compare it with normals for the same laboratory; some normal dogs may have high titers) and the pattern of nuclear fluorescence. The homogeneous, then reticulonodular patterns are the most common in canine systemic lupus erythematosus, but titers and patterns appear to have little or no specificity in dogs and cats.[47, 195] Other authors indicate that the speckled and homogeneous ANA patterns are the most common in dogs with autoimmune connective tissue diseases.[207]

There is no clear, constant correlation between clinical disease activity and positive ANA titer, though there is usually a progressive decrease in titer with successful therapy.[47, 195, 204, 207, 223] Any decrease in ANA titer always occurs after clinical remission. It must be remembered that ANA can be detected from time to time with probably any disease as well as in healthy animals.[47, 195, 214] Thus, a positive ANA titer must always be interpreted in light of other critical historical, physical, and laboratory data.

Preparations of the protozoan *Crithidia luciliae* have become commercially available for assaying patient sera for antibodies against native DNA. Large surveys employing this substrate in dogs and cats have not been reported, although preliminary reports indicate that the assay is rarely positive in dogs with systemic lupus erythematosus and in those with positive ANA titers,[47] suggesting that dogs rarely form antibodies against native DNA. Positive results with this test occurred in a 6-year-old female Beauceron with systemic lupus erythematosus as well as in two of her female puppies.[198] The standard Farr test (radioimmunoassay) for the measurement of antinative DNA antibodies in humans is unsatisfactory in dogs, resulting in numerous false-positive results.[47] Newer techniques employing specific reagents in an ELISA format did not reveal anti–double-stranded DNA antibodies but did detect IgG antibodies to the individual histones H_1, H_{2A}, H_3, and H_4.[209]

About 10% of human patients with systemic lupus erythematosus are ANA-negative.[18, 47] These patients have unique anticytoplasmic antibodies (anti-Ro), which are not detected when traditional ANA test substrates (mouse or rat liver) are employed; as a result, special substrates (calf thymus, normal human lymphocytes, human epithelial tissue culture line) are needed for such patients. The importance of this autoantibody system in dogs and cats is unknown. It could, however, explain the negative ANA results occasionally obtained in dogs with systemic lupus erythematosus.[56, 217]

In one study, sera from 131 dogs were evaluated for ANA and extractable nuclear antigens (ENAs), including the Ro ribonuclear protein antigen.[227] The ENA was only positive in 46% of the dogs with systemic lupus erythematosus, and none were Ro-positive. ENAs were not specific for systemic lupus erythematosus, however, because results were positive in 5% of healthy dogs and 11% of dogs with other diseases. However, the newer techniques have shown that, in the dog, antihistone antibodies are positive in 65% and anti-ENA antibodies are detected in greater than 40% of cases.[195, 209, 227]

In humans, antihistone autoantibodies have an association with drug-induced systemic lupus erythematosus.[219] Two anti-ENA antibodies are highly specific for canine systemic lupus erythematosus: The anti-Sm antibodies are found in 16% of cases and anti-hnRNP G is found in 20% of cases (this autoantibody is not usually tested for in commercially available anti-ENA tests in human medicine).[195, 209] Another novel canine autoantibody, anti-hnRNP I, was found in a Schnauzer with polyarthritis.[220] These studies demonstrate that dogs may manifest different autoantibodies than humans and that testing techniques may have to be adapted for the canine (and, presumably, the cat).

Investigators have attempted to better understand lupus erythematosus in humans by studying subsets of patients on the basis of one clinical characteristic (or set of them), histopathologic or immunopathologic findings, or serologic studies.[5, 18] The use of this subset approach may allow the clinician to gain insight into prognosis, improved therapy, or presumed pathogenesis. Currently, three subsets of cutaneous lupus erythematosus are recognized in humans: chronic cutaneous (discoid) lupus erythematosus, subacute cutaneous lupus erythematosus, and acute cutaneous lupus erythematosus. Their recognition is important because the different probability of systemic disease does correlate with which autoantibodies are detected.[219]

The suggestion that the disease previously described as idiopathic ulcerative dermatosis of collies and Shetland sheepdogs should be renamed *canine vesicular cutaneous lupus erythematosus*, and that it may be similar to subacute lupus erythematosus in humans, was based on clinical and histopathologic findings (see Chap. 12).[203] Serologic studies were not performed in the canine study but, in humans, this type of cutaneous lupus erythematosus is highly associated with anti-Ro antibodies (70% to 90% of cases), and approximately 50% of the patients will experience systemic lupus erythematosus, though usually not severe and lacking renal disease.[219] A study reviewing the histopathology of dogs with so-called hereditary lupoid dermatosis of German shorthaired pointers suggested that this disease be renamed *exfoliative cutaneous lupus erythematosus* (see Chap. 12).[212] The applicability of such subsets to the canine and feline diseases awaits further study.

The dermatohistopathologic changes in systemic lupus erythematosus vary with the type of gross morphologic lesions and may be nondiagnostic.[18, 22, 72, 217] The most characteristic finding is interface dermatitis (hydropic, lichenoid, or both), which may involve hair follicle outer root sheaths (Figs. 9–20 to 9–22). Apoptosis of basal and suprabasal cells may occur, and occasionally these apoptotic cells are associated with lymphocytic satellitosis.[50] Other common findings are subepidermal vacuolar alteration (subepidermal bubbles), focal thickening of the basement membrane zone (Fig. 9–23), and dermal mucinosis. Uncommon findings are intrabasal to subepidermal vesicles, leukocytoclastic vasculitis, and lupus erythematosus panniculitis (see Chap. 18). In humans, these changes are often not present until the skin lesions are at least 6 weeks old.

Direct immunofluorescence or immunohistochemical testing reveals the deposition of immunoglobulin, complement, or both at the basement membrane zone, often known as a positive lupus band, in 50% to 90% of patients.[5, 18, 47, 55, 217] The variability in positive results reflects differences in laboratory techniques, lesion selection (age and activity of lesion), previous or current glucocorticoid therapy, and possibly other factors. In addition, immunoreactants may be found at the basement membrane zone of skin in many other conditions, including sun-damaged skin.

We saw a case of canine solar dermatitis that was positive for basement membrane fluorescence. Though there is some controversy, positive lupus band tests from lesional skin are not considered very diagnostic. However, in humans, positive results from nonlesional sun-protected sites correlate well with the diagnosis of systemic lupus erythematosus.[219] In dogs, C3 is the most commonly detected immunoreactant, with IgA and IgM being the most commonly detected immunoglobulins.[56, 217]

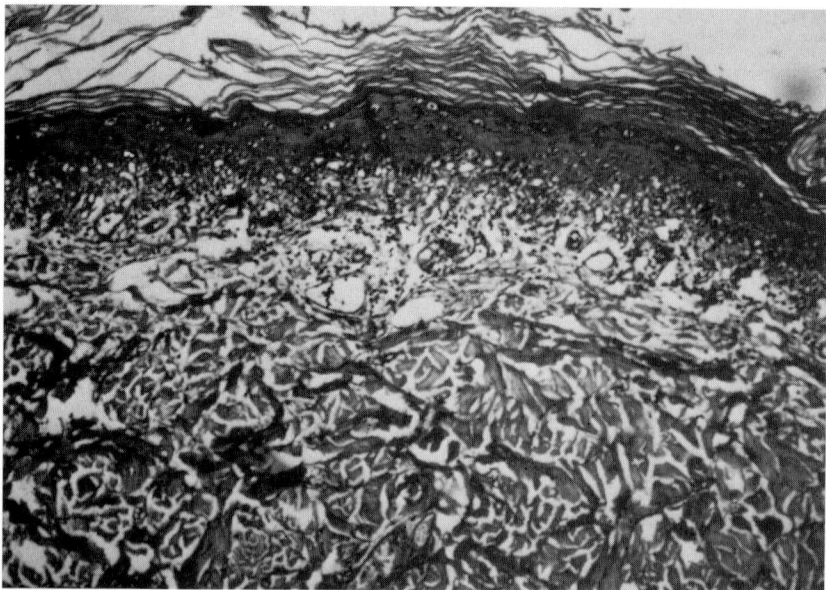

FIGURE 9–20. Canine systemic lupus erythematosus. Hydropic interface dermatitis.

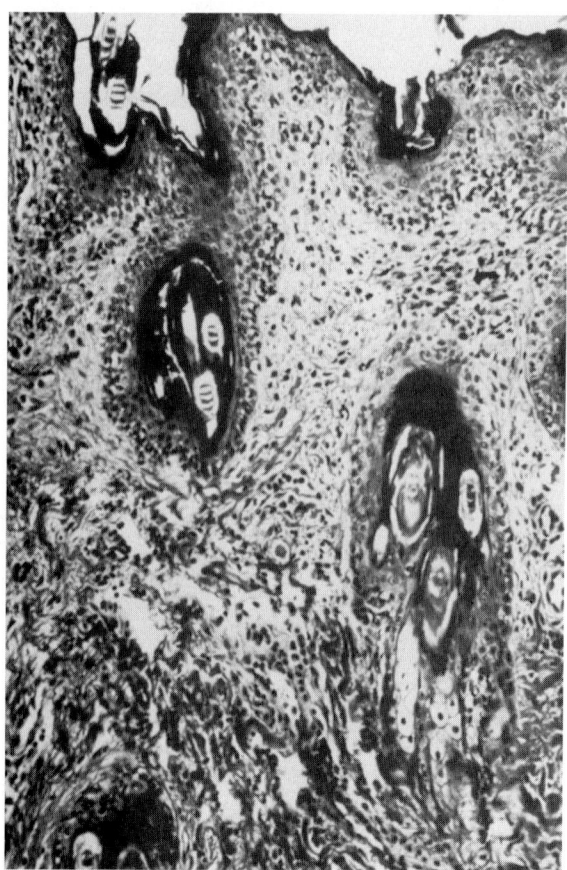

FIGURE 9–21. Feline systemic lupus erythematosus. Hydropic interface dermatitis. (From Scott DW, et al: A glucocorticoid-repsonsive dermatitis in cats, resembling systemic lupus erythematosus in man. J Am Anim Hosp Assoc 15:157, 1979.)

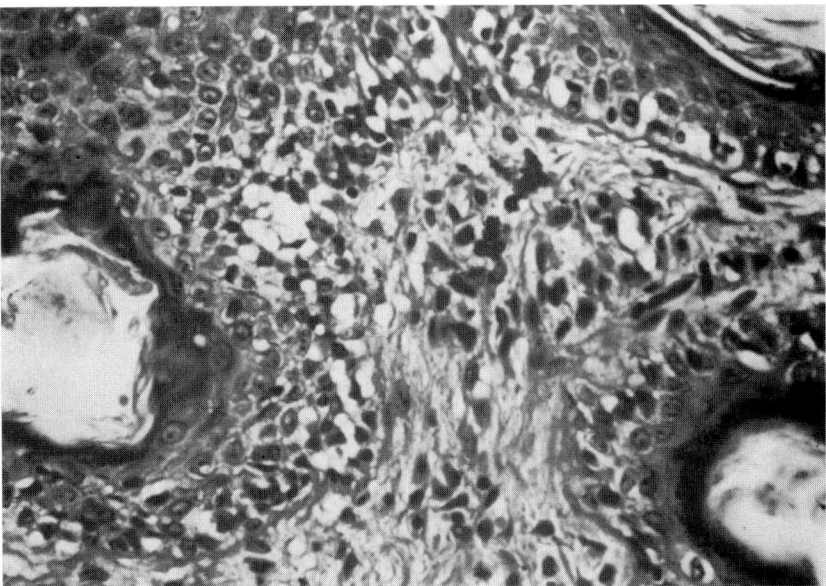

FIGURE 9–22. Feline systemic lupus erythematosus. Hydropic degeneration of epidermal basal cells. (From Scott DW, et al: A glucocorticoid-responsive dermatitis in cats, resembling systemic lupus erythematosus in man. J Am Anim Hosp Assoc 15:157, 1979.)

In humans, it is often possible to distinguish between systemic lupus erythematosus and discoid lupus erythematosus on the basis of direct immunofluorescence testing of lesional and sun-exposed normal skin. In human patients with systemic lupus erythematosus, sun-exposed normal skin may have positive lupus bands in up to 60% of cases,

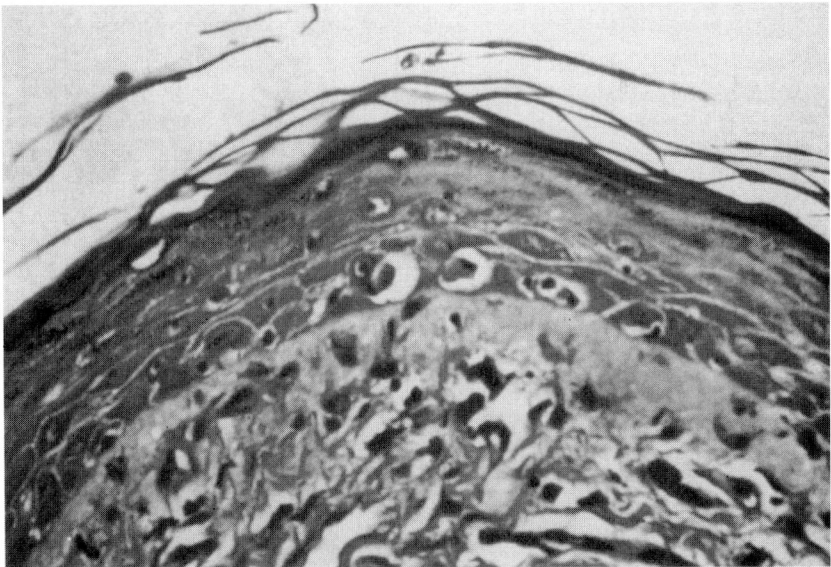

FIGURE 9–23. Canine systemic lupus erythematosus. Two large, apoptotic keratinocytes in stratum basale of epidermis can be seen in the center of the photograph. In addition, the basement membrane zone is thickened.

whereas this rarely occurs in discoid lupus erythematosus.[5, 18] This criterion is of no value in the hairy dog and cat, wherein normal skin is usually negative.[56, 217]

In humans, it is recommended that (1) biopsies not be taken from edematous lesions (only about 47% of such lesions are positive), (2) biopsies be taken from lesions over 1 month old (only about 30% are positive if less than 1 month old), (3) skin with telangiectases not be sampled (17% of such lesions are positive, regardless of their etiology), and (4) all glucocorticoid and immunomodulating therapy be terminated, if possible, 3 weeks prior to biopsy.[5, 18, 47]

Because no single laboratory test is diagnostic for systemic lupus erythematosus, a number of groups have produced sets of classification criteria for making the diagnosis.[25, 47] Although such criteria have acknowledged validity in humans, there is no such validation of criteria for dogs and cats. The veterinarian must rely on the recognition of multisystemic disease (especially joint, skin, kidney, oral mucosa, and hematopoietic system), positive ANA results, and confirmatory histopathologic and immunopathologic findings in involved skin and oral mucosa or both.[56, 217] Indirect immunofluorescence testing is negative in lupus erythematosus.

The American Rheumatism Association developed criteria for the diagnosis of systemic lupus erythematosus in humans, and these were modified in 1982. These have also been applied to dogs with minor modifications, primarily those reflecting the humoral immunologic responses of the canine (Table 9–4).[196] Dogs that experience four or more of the modified criteria during any given observation period have systemic lupus erythematosus. It has also been suggested that a probable diagnosis of systemic lupus erythematosus is appropriate if three criteria are present or polyarthritis with ANA is present. Though these criteria are helpful guidelines, they must be used cautiously. In humans, numerous situations that may lead to a false diagnosis based on the American Rheumatism

● Table 9–4 **CRITERIA FOR THE DIAGNOSIS OF CANINE SYSTEMIC LUPUS ERYTHEMATOSUS***

CRITERION	DEFINITION
Erythema	Redness in areas of skin that are thin or poorly protected by the haircoat (particularly the face)
Discoid rash	Depigmentation, erythema, erosions, ulcerations, crusts, and keratotic scaling that selectively affect the face (e.g., nasal planum, forehead, lips, and periocular region)
Photosensitivity	Skin rash resulting from an unusual reaction to sunlight
Oral ulcers	Oral or nasopharyngeal ulceration, usually painless
Arthritis	Nonerosive arthritis involving two or more peripheral joints characterized mainly by pain during movement (progressive forced flexion-extension); swelling or effusion are often not very marked
Serositis	Presence of a nonseptic inflammatory cavity effusion (pleuritis or pericarditis)
Renal disorders	Persistent proteinuria (>0.5 g/L or $>3+$ if quantification is not performed) or cellular casts (red blood cell, hemoglobin, or mixed)
Neurologic disorders	Seizures or psychosis in the absence of offending drugs or known metabolic disorders (e.g., uremia, ketoacidosis, or electrolyte imbalances)
Hematologic disorders	Hemolytic anemia (with reticulocytosis) or leukopenia ($<3000/mm^3$ total on two or more occasions) or lymphopenia ($<1000/mm^3$ total on two or more occasions) or thrombocytopenia ($<100,000/mm^3$ in the absence of offending drugs)
Immunologic disorders	Antihistone (antibody to histone at an abnormal titer) or anti-Sm (antibody to the Sm nuclear antigen) or anti-type 1 (antibody to a 43-kd nuclear antigen) or T cell subsets (a striking decrease in the CD8+ population [$<200/mm^3$] or a CD4+ : CD8+ ratio higher than 4.0)
Antinuclear antibodies (ANAs)	An abnormal titer of ANAs as shown by immunofluorescence or an equivalent assay in the absence of drugs known to be associated with their formation

*Adapted from the 1982 revised American Rheumatism Association Criteria.
From Chabanne L, et al: Canine systemic lupus erythematosus. Part II: Diagnosis and treatment. Compend Cont Educ Pract Vet 21:402, 1999.

Association criteria have been described. The presence of skin disease and subsequent diagnosis of systemic lupus erythematosus is particularly problematic, and other multipart classification schemes have been proposed.[218]

Clinical Management

The prognosis in systemic lupus erythematosus is generally unpredictable and depends on the organs involved.[47, 55, 196, 200, 217] In general, the earlier the diagnosis is made, the better the prognosis. In the dog, it appears that patients with joint, skin, or muscle disease respond more reliably to medication and are maintained in relatively long periods of clinical remission. On the other hand, dogs with severe hemolytic anemia, thrombocytopenia, or both often do not respond satisfactorily to systemic glucocorticoids and require other immunomodulating drugs, splenectomy, or both. Animals with glomerulonephritis regularly experience progressive renal failure in spite of therapy, and this finding indicates a poor prognosis.

Therapy of systemic lupus erythematosus must be individualized. The initial agent of choice is probably large doses of systemic glucocorticoids (e.g., 2 to 6 mg/kg prednisone q24h).[47, 55, 196, 217] When systemic glucocorticoids are unsatisfactory, other immunomodulating drugs may be useful: azathioprine (Imuran) given orally at 2.2 mg/kg q24h, then q48h (dog only), or chlorambucil (Leukeran) given orally at 0.2 mg/kg q24h, then q48h.[47, 55, 217] Splenectomy may be needed for patients with severe hemolytic anemia, thrombocytopenia, or both. Cyclophosphamide, 2 mg/kg q24h orally, 4 days a week, may be given for acute episodes of hemolytic anemia.[196] Vincristine, 0.01 to 0.025 mg/kg intravenously, once weekly, may be useful when thrombocytopenia is severe.[196]

Levamisole (Levasole), given orally at 2.5 mg/kg q48h, has occasionally been beneficial in dogs and humans with systemic lupus erythematosus.[47] The combination of levamisole, 2 to 5 mg/kg (maximum dose, 150 mg) q48h, with prednisone, has been reported to give good results in 75% of canine cases, with remissions lasting for months to years.[196, 200] The prednisone is initially dosed at 0.5 to 1.0 mg/kg twice daily, then tapered off over 1 to 2 months with long-term therapy consisting of just levamisole. Only 2 of 33 dogs treated experienced unacceptable side effects (neutropenia, excited behavior, and aggressiveness) from levamisole.[196, 200]

Chrysotherapy (injectable aurothioglucose, oral auranofin) has occasionally been used to reduce glucocorticoid requirements in dogs but would be contraindicated in patients with renal disease.[18, 34, 47] Aspirin has occasionally been effective in the management of cases in dogs and humans.[18, 47] Other drugs used in human patients—dapsone, antiandrogens, antimalarials, colchicine, and omega-3/omega-6 fatty acids—are of undetermined benefit in dogs and cats.[18, 47] Plasmapheresis has been used to enhance initial response to chemotherapy in dogs and humans with severe systemic lupus erythematosus.[18, 40] This technique, currently used as a research tool, is hazardous and expensive.

In murine lupus erythematosus, functional elimination of the helper T cell subset (CD4+) suppresses autoantibody formation and prevents or retards disease.[215] In humans, treatment with an anti-CD4 antibody induced a long-lasting decrease in disease activity in patients with severe cutaneous lupus erythematosus.[215]

Patients with systemic lupus erythematosus are prone to infections.[196, 217] Thus, infections must be identified quickly and treated aggressively.

The following statements can be made about prognosis. Over 40% of the dogs with systemic lupus erythematosus are dead within 1 year after the diagnosis is made, either as a result of natural (renal disease, septicemia) or drug-induced causes or owing to euthanasia.[47, 217] Dogs that respond well to therapy often do so with glucocorticoids alone and often experience long-term remission on alternate-day therapy.[47, 217] Some dogs, in whom disease was controlled well with therapy for several months, remain in prolonged drug-free remission.[47, 196, 217]

Several reports have indicated that people in close contact with dogs having systemic lupus erythematosus or high-titer ANA do not have greater clinical or serologic evidence of systemic lupus erythematosus compared with nonexposed human beings.[25, 47]

DISCOID LUPUS ERYTHEMATOSUS

Discoid lupus erythematosus (cutaneous lupus erythematosus) is the second most common immune-mediated dermatitis of the dog, although it remains uncommon. It has been described in the cat but appears to be very rare.

Cause and Pathogenesis

Canine discoid lupus erythematosus is a relatively benign cutaneous disease with no systemic involvement.[55, 233, 234] A relationship or progression to canine systemic lupus erythematosus has not been reported, nor has the disease been shown to be a good model for the human disorder. Sun exposure aggravates the disease in about 50% of cases, suggesting that photosensitivity plays a role in the pathogenesis. In humans, it has been demonstrated that the lymphocytes infiltrating skin lesions of discoid and systemic lupus erythematosus are predominantly T cells and that helper T cells predominate in discoid lupus, whereas suppressor T cells predominate in the systemic variety.[5, 18] In the dog, plasma cells are prominent, a feature not shared with humans, suggesting that B lymphocytes may be important and that a different pathogenesis may be occurring.

A 9-year-old Shetland sheepdog with discoid lupus erythematosus had, on indirect immunofluorescence testing, antibody deposition at the basement membrane zone. Western immunoblotting revealed that the 120-kd and the 85-kd proteins targeted by the autoantibody did not correspond with the known basement membrane zone components.[230] A current hypothesis concerning the pathogenesis of lesion formation is presented in the discussion of systemic lupus erythematosus.

Clinical Features

• **Dog.** There is probably no strong sex predilection, because both females[234] and males[231] have been reported to be predisposed. No age predilection has been reported. Collies, German shepherds, Shetland sheepdogs, Siberian huskies, Brittany spaniels, and German shorthaired pointers demonstrate predilection.[55, 231, 234] Discoid lupus erythematosus has been reported to account for 0.3% of the canine dermatoses examined at one university small animal practice.[56]

Clinical signs of canine discoid lupus erythematosus initially include depigmentation, erythema, and scaling of the nose (Fig. 9–24A). Early depigmentation manifests as a slate blue or gray color change (see Fig. 9–24B). A helpful early change is the conversion of the normally rough, cobblestone-like architecture of the nasal planum into a smooth surface (see Fig. 9–24C and D). Later lesions commonly include erosion, ulceration, and crusting. Initially, lesions tend to occur dorsally at the junction between the nasal planum and haired skin or along the ventral or medial aspects of the alar folds. Typically, with time, nasal involvement becomes more extensive and the lesions may spread up the bridge of the nose. Less commonly, lesions may be visible periocularly, on the pinnae (see Fig. 9–24F), on the distal limbs, and on the genitals. The lips may also be involved (see Fig. 9–24E), and small punctate ulcers may be detected in the oral cavity (see Fig. 9–24G), most commonly involving the tongue or palate (see Fig. 9–24E). Occasional dogs present only with lesions of both pinnae or with nasodigital hyperkeratosis.[228, 234, 235] Pruritus and pain are variable. Scarring and variable degrees of permanent leukoderma are common. Rarely, deeply ulcerated nasal lesions damage arterioles, resulting in episodic, pulsatile hemorrhage. Affected dogs are otherwise healthy.

Discoid lupus erythematosus in dogs is commonly exacerbated or precipitated by exposure to ultraviolet light. Thus, the disease often is more severe in the summer and in parts of the world with sunny climates. It is very likely that many dogs previously referred to as having nasal solar dermatitis, or "collie nose," actually had discoid lupus erythematosus, pemphigus foliaceus, and pemphigus erythematosus. Squamous cell carcinomas are reported to rarely develop in chronic discoid lupus erythematosus skin lesions (see Fig. 20–19B).[236] The cause of the rare development of squamous cell carcinoma is likely multifactorial.[232] In the reported cases, the discoid lupus had been active for years and no photoprotection had been used on the chronically inflamed, depigmented skin.[236] We have

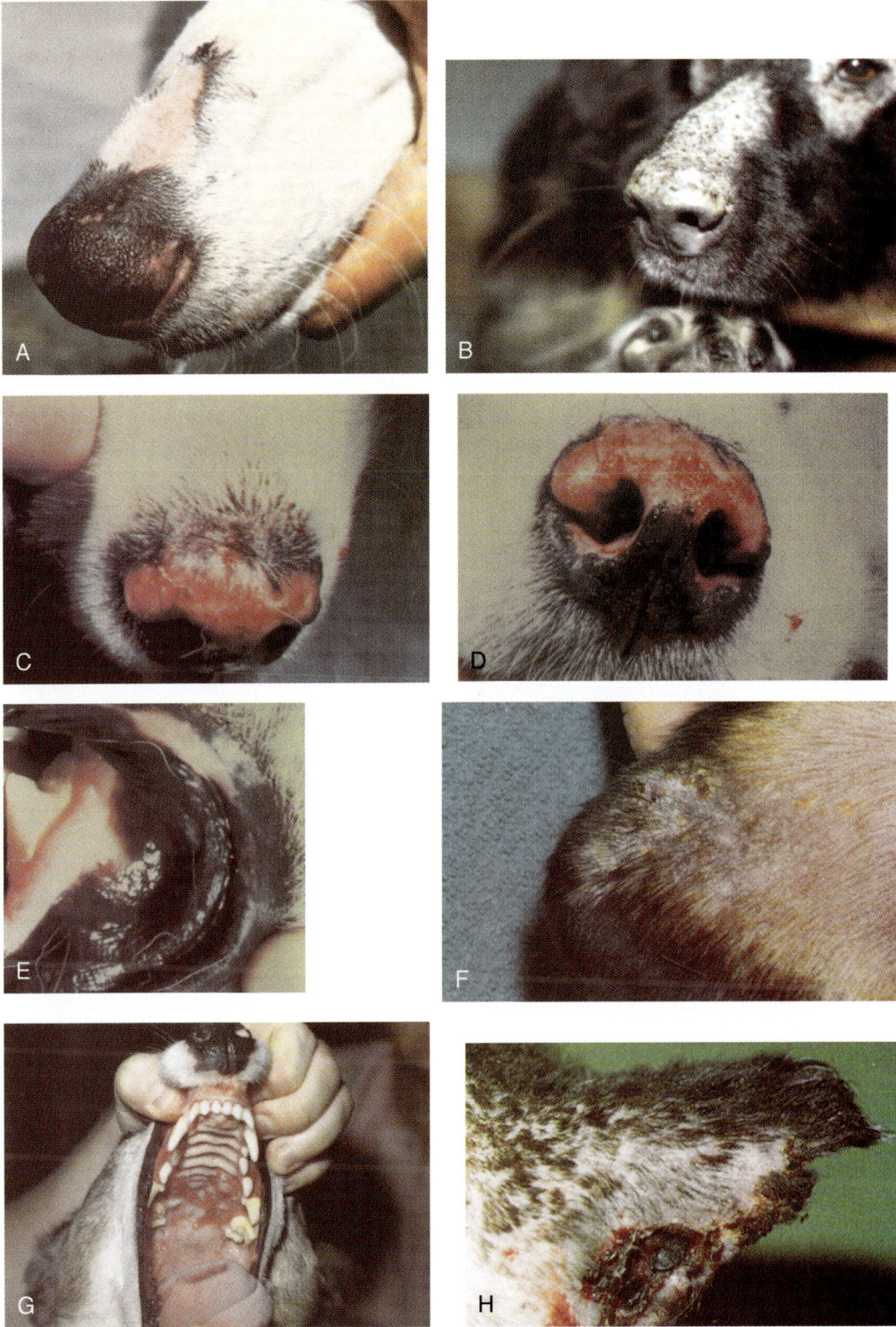

FIGURE 9–24. *A,* Early erythema, alopecia, scaling, and depigmentation in a borzoi with discoid lupus erythematosus. (From Griffin CE, et al: Canine discoid lupus erythematosus. Vet Immunol Immunopathol 1:79, 1979.) *B,* Discoid lupus erythematosus. Note gray-blue discoloration of skin around nostrils. *C,* Nasal erythema, ulceration, and depigmentation in a dog with discoid lupus erythematosus. *D,* Frontal view of nose of dog in *C. E,* Depigmentation of the lip in a dog with discoid lupus erythematosus. (*C* and *D,* From Walton DK, et al: Canine discoid lupus erythematosus. J Am Anim Hosp Assoc 17:851, 1981.) *F,* Discoid lupus erythematosus. Patchy alopecia, erythema, scale, and crust of pinna. *G,* Palatine ulcers in a dog with discoid lupus erythematosus. *H,* Cryoglobulinemia in a cat. Necrosis of pinnal margin.

also seen squamous cell carcinoma occur in the nasal lesions of chronic dermatomyositis. Thus, the depigmentation, ultraviolet light exposure, and chronic irritation may be more important than the disease affecting the nasal region.

• **Cat.** Discoid lupus erythematosus appears to be very rare in cats.[229, 239] No age, breed, or sex predilections are reported. Lesions are most common on the pinnae and face. They are erythema, scaling, crusting, and alopecia. Pruritus is variable. Nasal dermatitis and depigmentation are less common (Fig. 9–25). Lesions may be more severe when exposure to sunlight is increased. Affected cats are otherwise healthy.

Diagnosis

The most common differential diagnosis includes nasal solar dermatitis, nasal depigmentation, vitiligo-like disease, pemphigus erythematosus or pemphigus foliaceus, trauma, dermatomyositis, epitheliotropic lymphoma, drug reaction, uveodermatologic syndrome, contact dermatitis, and systemic lupus erythematosus.

Definitive diagnosis of discoid lupus erythematosus is based on history, physical examination, and skin biopsy. Immunopathology may be an aid to diagnosis but, in the dog, it is not thought to be required for a definitive diagnosis because both false-positive and false-negative results occur.[20, 233] Results of routine laboratory determinations (hemogram, serum chemistries, urinalysis, serum protein electrophoresis) are usually unremarkable. The ANA and LE cell tests almost always yield negative results; if positive, the ANA titer is low. One report indicated that 9% and 4% of the dogs with discoid lupus erythematosus were positive for anti-ENA and anti-Ro, respectively.[227]

Histopathology

Skin biopsy reveals interface dermatitis (hydropic, lichenoid, or both) (Figs. 9–26 and 9–27).[22, 71, 234] Focal hydropic degeneration of basal epidermal cells, pigmentary incontinence, focal thickening of the basement membrane zone, apoptotic keratinocytes, and marked accumulations of mononuclear cells and plasma cells around dermal vessels and appendages are important histopathologic features of discoid lupus erythematosus. Dermal mucinosis of variable degrees is also a common feature of discoid lupus erythematosus.

Immunopathologic testing reveals deposition of immunoglobulin, complement, or both at the basement membrane zone.[56, 231, 234] It would appear to be important to test for individual immunoglobulin classes because IgG, IgM, or IgA may be the only demonstrable immunoglobulin. In humans, it is recommended that (1) edematous lesions not be biopsied (only about 47% of such lesions are positive), (2) telangiectatic areas not be biopsied (about 17% of the telangiectatic skin lesions of any dermatosis are positive), and

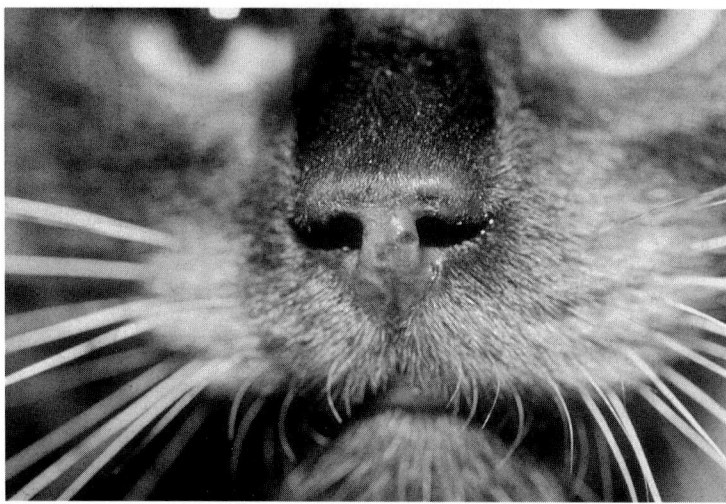

FIGURE 9–25. Feline discoid lupus erythematosus. Depigmentation, erythema, and mild erosion of nasal planum.

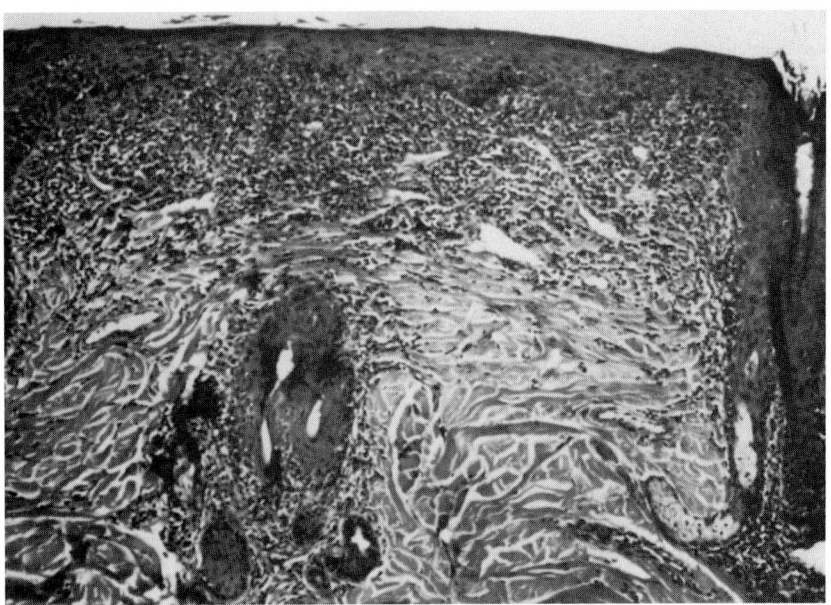

FIGURE 9–26. Canine discoid lupus erythematosus. Lichenoid interface dermatitis. (From Scott DW, et al: Linear IgA dermatoses in the dog. Cornell Vet 72:394, 1982.)

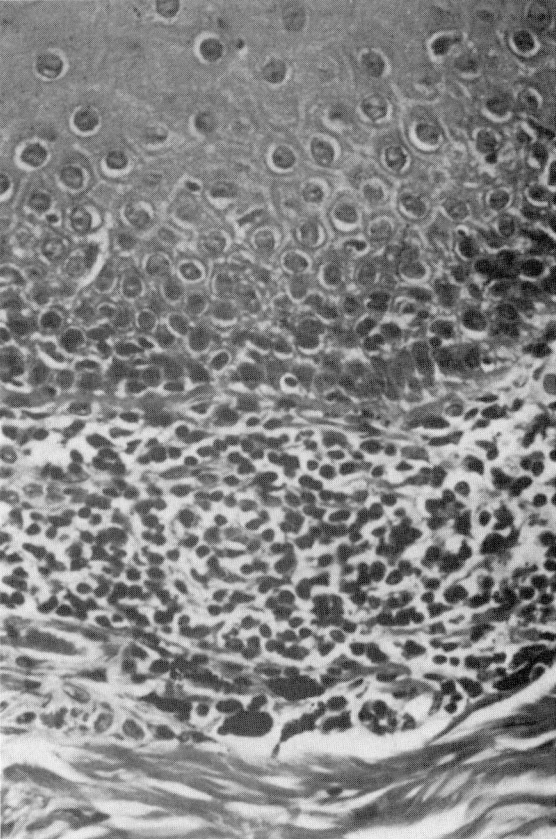

FIGURE 9–27. Canine discoid lupus erythematosus. Lichenoid interface dermatitis with thickening of the basement membrane zone. (From Walton DK, et al: Canine discoid lupus erythematosus. J Am Anim Hosp Assoc 17:851, 1981.)

(3) lesions less than 1 month old not be biopsied (only about 30% of such lesions are positive). In addition, topical or systemic glucocorticoid therapy may lead to false-negative immunopathologic findings.[20, 47, 56]

We do not think that immunopathologic testing is required for the diagnosis of discoid lupus erythematosus in most instances. Immunopathologic tests are also considered to be inferior to, and only supportive of, a diagnosis based on histopathologic criteria.[238, 240] Indirect immunofluorescence testing has generally been negative in discoid lupus erythematosus, though one dog having autoantibodies to the basement membrane zone has been reported.[230]

Clinical Management

The prognosis for discoid lupus erythematosus is usually good.[56, 231, 234] Therapy will probably need to be continued for life, and marked depigmentation predisposes to sunburn.

Therapy of discoid lupus erythematosus must be appropriate to the individual.[47, 56, 231, 233, 234] Mild cases may be controlled by, and all cases benefit from, avoidance of exposure to intense sunlight (from 8 AM to 5 PM), the use of topical sunscreens, and the use of topical glucocorticoids (see Chap. 3). Initially, topical glucocorticoid therapy is most successful when potent agents, such as betamethasone or fluocinolone in DMSO (Synotic), are applied every 12 hours.

After the dermatosis is in remission, topical glucocorticoids are applied as needed (once daily, q48h, and so forth), and less potent agents (e.g., 1% to 2% hydrocortisone) may be sufficient for maintenance. Anecdotal reports indicate that the topical application of 1% cyclosporine is effective.[232a] In some cases, a 1-month course of systemic prednisone (2.2 mg/kg orally q24h until remission is achieved, then q48h) is helpful. The topical agents may then be sufficient to maintain the remission. Though not frequently effective as the sole therapy, systemic vitamin E (400 to 800 IU daily) is recommended because it may have a beneficial effect.[234] Vitamin E appears to have a 1- to 2-month lag phase before its benefit is recognized clinically, and systemic glucocorticoids may be used concurrently during this period. Vitamin E should be administered 2 hours before or after feeding. Two of us (D.W.S., W.H.M.) have had good success in some cases with the oral administration of products containing omega-3/omega-6 fatty acids (DVM Derm Caps) and now use these products instead of vitamin E. Various combinations of fatty acids, vitamin E, and other treatments have been used successfully. In some cases, more potent drugs may be given initially, then remission maintained with fatty acids and vitamin E.

If these benign treatments are not effective in dogs, tetracycline and niacinamide in combination may be effective in up to 70% of the cases (see Chap. 3).[233] In dogs under 10 kg, the dosage is 250 mg of each drug q8h, and in dogs over 10 kg, the dosage is 500 mg of each q8h. The tetracycline-niacinamide combination produces its effects within 8 weeks.

In refractory cases in dogs and cats in which the owners think that better control is absolutely required, systemic glucocorticoids (2.2 to 4.4 mg/kg prednisolone or prednisone, given orally q24h) are often effective. For more severe or refractory cases, other systemic drugs may be added to the treatment regimen: azathioprine (2.2 mg/kg orally q24h, then q48h in dogs only) or chlorambucil (0.2 mg/kg orally q24h, then q48h). Owners should understand that discoid lupus erythematosus is rarely a life-threatening disease but that some of the potent immunomodulating drugs could cause severe side effects.

In humans, discoid lupus erythematosus is often responsive to antimalarial drugs—chloroquine (Aralen), hydroxychloroquine (Plaquenil), and quinacrine (Atabrine).[18] These drugs may be useful in the dog as well, but dosage, efficacy, and toxicity need to be carefully evaluated. Other drugs occasionally found to be beneficial in humans are retinoids, dapsone, and gold (oral or injectable).[18] The usefulness of these latter compounds in dogs is currently unknown.

Bilateral rotation flaps have been successfully used for the treatment of chronic, medically refractory cases of canine nasal dermatitis.[237]

VESICULAR CUTANEOUS LUPUS ERYTHEMATOSUS

Results of a clinicopathologic study of five Shetland sheepdogs and two collies with so-called "idiopathic ulcerative dermatosis" led the investigators to conclude that the syndrome should be renamed *vesicular cutaneous lupus erythematosus* (see Chap. 12).[203]

EXFOLIATIVE CUTANEOUS LUPUS ERYTHEMATOSUS

Results of recent pathologic and immunopathologic studies of German shorthaired pointers with so-called "hereditary lupoid dermatosis" led the investigators to conclude that the syndrome should be renamed *exfoliative cutaneous lupus erythematosus* (see Chap. 12).[212]

Cryoglobulinemia and Cryofibrinogenemia

CAUSE AND PATHOGENESIS

Cryoglobulins and *cryofibrinogens* are proteins that precipitate from serum and plasma, respectively, by cooling and redissolve on rewarming.[18, 47, 242, 245] Cryoglobulins have been classified into three types according to their characteristics. Type I cryoglobulins are composed solely of monoclonal immunoglobulins or free light chains (Bence Jones proteins) and are most commonly associated with lymphoproliferative disorders. Type II cryoglobulins are composed of monoclonal and polyclonal immunoglobulins and are most commonly associated with autoimmune and connective tissue disease. Type III cryoglobulins are composed of polyclonal immunoglobulins and occur with infections, autoimmune disorders, and connective tissue diseases. Essential forms also may occur where no underlying cause is identifiable. Cutaneous signs associated with cryoglobulins and cryofibrinogens are due to vascular insufficiency (obstruction, stasis, spasm, thrombosis) that occur from microthrombi and vasculitis.

CLINICAL FEATURES

Cryoglobulinemia and cryofibrinogenemia have been rarely reported to cause skin disease in dogs and cats.[47, 243–246] When associated with autoantibodies directed against erythrocytes (cold agglutinin disease, cold hemagglutinin disease, cryopathic hemolytic anemia), it is an autoimmune disorder associated with cold-reacting (usually IgM) erythrocyte autoantibodies. The cryopathic autoantibody is most active at colder temperatures (0° to 4°C) but has a wide range of thermal activity (0° to 37°C). Two forms are recognized in dogs.[25] The first is associated with cold agglutinins that are IgM antibodies. The second form is a nonagglutinating type, usually associated with IgG. The latter form is rarer and is not known to cause skin disease. A dog with combined cryoglobulinemia (IgG, IgM) and cryofibrinogenemia has been reported.[245] Cold agglutinin disease represents a Type II hypersensitivity reaction and has been associated with idiopathy and lead poisoning in dogs and with upper respiratory infection, lead poisoning, and idiopathy in cats.

Clinical signs of cryoglobulinemia and cryofibrinogenemia are variable and relate to anemia, intracapillary cold hemagglutination, or both. Skin lesions include pain, erythema, purpura, acrocyanosis, necrosis, and ulceration. Skin lesions generally involve the extremities (paws, pinnae, nose, tip of tail) (see Figs. 9–24H and 9–28A) and are precipitated or exacerbated by exposure to cold. Hemoglobinemia may also be present.

Tail-tip necrosis was reported in two litters of Birman kittens from the same queen.[241] Based on blood group testing of the queen and one of the toms, a presumptive diagnosis of neonatal isoerythrolysis involving cold agglutinins was made. The tip of the tail became necrotic within the first week of life. It was thought that the pinnae, paws, and nose of the neonates were protected from cold by close contact with the queen. The kittens survived pending the severity of any intravascular hemolysis.

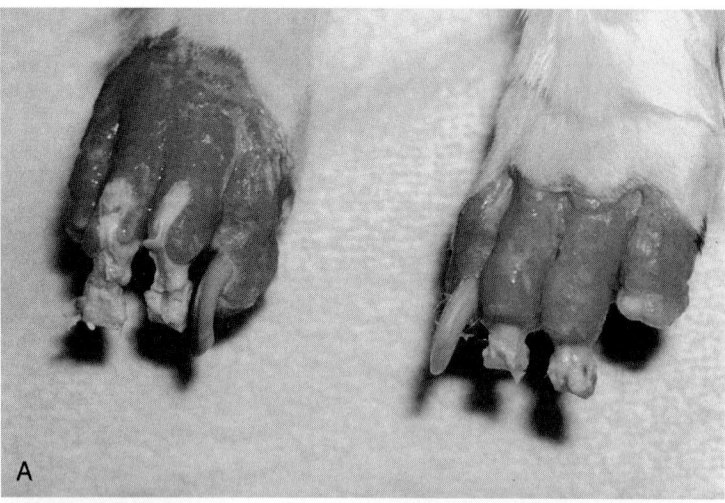
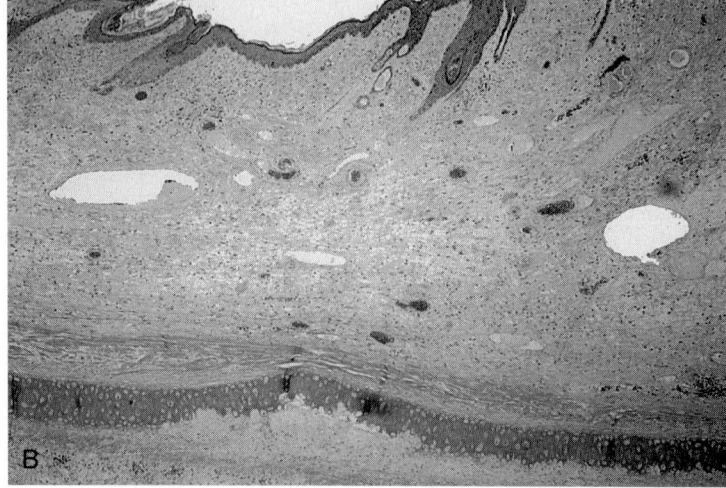

FIGURE 9–28. Cryoglobulinemia in a dog. *A,* Marked sloughing of skin and claws, with exposure of phalanges on front paws. *B,* Biopsy of pinna. Diffuse edema, extravasation of erythrocytes, thrombosed vessels, and homogenization of dermal collagen.

DIAGNOSIS

The differential diagnosis includes vasculitis, systemic lupus erythematosus, dermatomyositis, disseminated intravascular coagulation, and frostbite.

Definitive diagnosis of cold agglutinin disease is made by history, physical examination, and demonstration of significant titers of cold agglutinins. In vitro autohemagglutination of blood at room temperature can be diagnostic for cold-reacting autoantibodies. Blood in heparin or ethylenediaminetetra-acetic acid (EDTA) is allowed to cool on a slide, thus permitting the autoagglutination to be readily visible macroscopically. The reaction can be accentuated by cooling the blood to 0°C or reversed by warming the blood to 37°C. Doubtful cases can be confirmed via Coombs' test if the complete test is performed at 4°C and the Coombs reagent has activity against IgM. Caution in interpretation of the cold Coombs' test is warranted, because normal dogs and cats may have titers up to 1:100.[47, 247]

Cryoprecipitate levels may be crudely determined by allowing venous blood collected in a warm syringe to clot at 37°C for 30 minutes, then the serum and citrated plasma are cooled to 4°C and a gel-like precipitate is formed that will redissolve upon rewarming to 37°C.[245] The precipitate is removed, and the serum and plasma globulin and fibrinogen levels with and without the precipitate may be compared to give a level of cryoglobulin and cryofibrinogen. In 10 normal dogs, the mean levels were 0.106 gL^{-1} for cryoglobulin and 0.16 gL^{-1} for cryofibrinogen, whereas an affected dog had levels of 0.669 gL^{-1} and 0.3 gL^{-1}, respectively.[245]

HISTOPATHOLOGY

Skin biopsy usually reveals necrosis, ulceration, and often secondary suppurative changes. Fortuitously sampled sections may show vasculitis, thrombotic to necrotic blood vessels, or blood vessels containing an amorphous eosinophilic substance consisting largely of precipitated cryoglobulin.[18, 242, 245] Diffuse edema, extravasation of erythrocytes, and homogenization of dermal collagen also occur (see Fig. 9–28B).

CLINICAL MANAGEMENT

The prognosis for cryoglobulinemia and cryofibrinogenemia varies with the underlying cause. Therapy includes (1) correction of the underlying cause, if possible, (2) avoidance of cold, and (3) immunosuppressive drug regimens (e.g., glucocorticoids, azathioprine) (see Chap. 3).

Graft-Versus-Host Disease

Graft-versus-host disease is a well-recognized result of bone marrow transplantation in dogs and humans.[2, 18, 47, 249, 251] The disease occurs whenever lymphoid cells from an immunocompetent donor are introduced into a histoincompatible recipient that is incapable of rejecting them. The disease results from donor T cell responses to recipient transplantation antigens.

In dogs and humans, a bone marrow graft from a donor genetically identical for major histocompatibility (MHC) antigens is followed by significant graft-versus-host disease in about 50% of recipients, despite post-graft immunosuppressive therapy. Hence, minor histocompatibility antigens are important in the development of disease. The principal target organs are the skin, liver, and intestinal tract. In dogs, acute graft-versus-host disease develops about 2 weeks after grafting and is characterized by erythroderma, jaundice, diarrhea, and gram-negative infections. Chronic graft-versus-host disease develops about 3 to 4 months after grafting and is characterized by exfoliative erythroderma, ulcerative dermatitis, ascites, and gram-positive infections.

Diagnosis is based on history, physical examination, and skin biopsy. Histopathologic findings in acute graft-versus-host disease include varying degrees of dermal lymphoid infiltrates, interface dermatitis (hydropic or lichenoid) with apoptosis and satellitosis. The lymphocytic exocytosis and apoptosis also target the follicular epithelium.[18, 47, 248, 250] These changes have been compared to and are similar to those occurring in erythema multiforme.[2] In chronic graft-versus-host disease, one finds variable sclerodermoid or poikilodermatous changes.

The immunohistochemistry of acute canine graft-versus-host disease has been studied in six dogs and is similar to that described in humans.[2, 249] Epidermal and follicular keratinocytes of affected skin upregulate ICAM-1, CD44, and MHC II, similar to what is found in erythema multiforme.[2] However, the overall lymphocytic infiltrate in these two diseases is different. Although both diseases have CD3+, CD8$\alpha\beta$+ and TCR-$\alpha\beta$+ T cells, graft-versus-host disease had fewer dermal CD4+ T cells, CD1+ and CD11+ dendritic cells, and no CD21+ B cells (which occurred in erythema multiforme). These findings suggested that the mechanism of disease is similar in the two diseases, though erythema multiforme has additional pathologic pathways.[2] Whether this relates to the stage of disease is unknown because the dogs with erythema multiforme may have had more chronic disease than the dogs with experimentally induced graft-versus-host disease.

Epidermal and follicular ICAM-1 expression may play a key role in tethering CD8+ T cells, enabling subsequent interactions between T cells and keratinocytes.[2, 249] Activated T cells produce a storm of cytokines, including IL-2, IL-3, IL-4, interferon (IFN)-α, and TNF-α. These mediators recruit and activate effector cells, including additional lymphocytes, macrophages, and natural killer cells that attack both host and donor tissue through contact-dependent mechanisms (such as perforin) or soluble mediators (such as TNF-α).

Therapy of graft-versus-host disease with various combinations of systemic glucocorticoids, azathioprine, cyclosporine, methotrexate, and antithymocyte serum have been only partially and unpredictably effective.[249, 251] A combination of mycophenolate mofetil and cyclosporine demonstrated synergism, but beneficial effects were still limited.[251] Leflunomide, when combined with prednisone and cyclosporine, has been reported to virtually eliminate allograft rejection responses.[76]

Cutaneous Adverse Drug Reaction

Cutaneous adverse drug reactions (drug eruption, drug allergy, dermatitis medicamentosa) in dogs and cats are uncommon, variably pruritic, and pleomorphic cutaneous or mucocutaneous reactions to a drug.[253, 257, 269, 270, 286, 287]

CAUSE AND PATHOGENESIS

Adverse reactions to drugs are common and, in humans, cutaneous reactions are one of the most common.[18] Drugs responsible for skin eruptions may be administered orally, topically, or by injection or inhalation. The incidence of cutaneous adverse drug reactions in dogs and cats was reported to be 2% and 1.6%, respectively, of all the canine and feline dermatology cases examined at one university practice.[286, 287] In humans, the incidence is reported to be 2.2% of all hospitalized patients and 3 per 1000 courses of drug therapy.[18] Even these numbers are suspect because few mechanisms can accurately record the incidence of drug reactions.[290]

Adverse drug reactions may be divided into two major groups: (1) *predictable*, which are usually dose-dependent and are related to the pharmacologic actions of the drugs, and (2) *unpredictable* or *idiosyncratic*, which are often dose-independent and are related to the individual's immunologic response or to genetic differences in the susceptibility of patients (idiosyncracy or intolerance), which are often related to metabolic or enzymatic deficiencies. Drug metabolites are generated by cytochrome P-450–mixed function oxidases (phase I enzymes) but also by other oxidative metabolizing enzymes, some of which are present in skin.[295] Reactive drug metabolites then need to be detoxified by phase II enzymes, such as epoxide hydrolase or glutathione-S-transferase, to prevent toxicity.

Thus, two places allow for inappropriate generation and/or accumulation of toxic reactants more toxic than the parent compounds. In humans, slow acetylation contributes to sulfonamide drug reactions and familial anticonvulsant drug reactions are linked to inherited detoxification defects.[295] A hypothesis for the drug reactions associated with sulfonamides and anticonvulsants includes (1) oxidation by cytochrome P-450 into chemically reactive metabolites (either in liver by hepatic cytochrome P-450 with secondary transfer to skin or in keratinocytes by epidermal cytochrome P-450), and (2) decreased detoxification of these reactive metabolites, which bind to proteins and induce an immunologic response.

Many cutaneous effects of certain drugs are predictable. For instance, many of the anticancer or immunosuppressive drugs can cause alopecia, purpura, poor wound healing, and increased susceptibility to infection through their effects on cellular biology.[18, 47, 254, 256, 277] Doxorubicin typically causes alopecia that begins on the head and extends to the ventral neck, thorax, and abdomen.[263, 274, 276] Hyperpigmentation and pruritus may also occur. Immunologic reactions involved in cutaneous drug reactions include Types I, II, III, and IV hypersensitivity reactions. Newer techniques may help to determine the underlying immune response in some types of drug reactions.[255] Additionally, other immunologic reactions may occur as evidenced by the drug-induced development of erythema multiforme, toxic epidermal necrolysis, and superficial suppurative necrolytic dermatitis of miniature Schnauzers. Though the mechanism for these reactions is unknown, it is thought that immunologic mechanisms may play a role. Human patients with systemic lupus erythematosus and atopy are thought to be predisposed to cutaneous drug reactions,[18] but no such observations have been made for the dog and cat.

Any drug may cause an eruption (Tables 9–5 and 9–6), though certain drugs are more frequently associated with cutaneous adverse drug reactions. The most common drugs recognized to produce idiosyncratic cutaneous adverse drug reactions in dogs are topical agents, sulfonamides (especially those that are trimethoprim-potentiated, such as Tribrissen), penicillins, cephalosporins, levamisole, and diethylcarbamazine.[287] In cats, the most common causes are topical agents, penicillins, cephalosporins, and sulfonamides.[286]

CLINICAL FEATURES

Cutaneous adverse drug reactions can mimic virtually any dermatosis (see Tables 9–5 and 9–6; Fig. 9–29A to H).* In humans, the most common morphologic patterns are exanthematous, urticaria or angioedema, and fixed drug eruption.[290] In dogs, the most common reactions were contact dermatitis, exfoliative dermatitis, pruritus with self-induced lesions, maculopapular eruptions, and erythema multiforme.[287] In cats, the most common reactions were contact dermatitis and pruritus with self-induced lesions.[286] No age or sex predilections have been reported for canine and feline cutaneous drug reactions.[286, 287] In general, no breed predilections are evident, though Poodles, Bichon Frisés, Yorkshire terriers, silky terriers, Pekingese, and Maltese terriers ("fuzzy" hair coats) are predisposed to local injection reactions (especially with rabies vaccine),[270, 287] Doberman pinschers to sulfonamide reactions,[260, 287] and miniature Schnauzers to sulfonamide, gold, and shampoo (superficial suppurative necrolytic dermatitis) reactions.[287, 294]

In one study of cutaneous adverse drug reactions in dogs,[287] the following breeds were found to be at increased risk: Shetland sheepdog, Dalmatian, Yorkshire terrier, miniature Poodle, miniature Schnauzer, Australian shepherd, Old English sheepdog, Scottish terrier, wirehaired Fox terrier, and Greyhound. Although humans with HIV infections are at increased risk for drug reactions, cats with cutaneous adverse drug reactions were not FIV-positive or FeLV-positive.[286]

Although no specific type of reaction is related to only one drug, certain reactions are more common with certain drugs. The syndrome of *superficial suppurative necrolytic dermatitis of miniature Schnauzers* has been associated only with shampoos (see Fig. 9–29H).[287, 294] Adult miniature Schnauzers of either sex show cutaneous and systemic signs within 48 to 72 hours after shampooing (usually insecticidal). Lesions, which may be widespread or primarily ventral, include erythematous papules and plaques that develop pustulosis, becoming painful, necrotic, and ulcerative. Lesions regress spontaneously within 1 to 2 weeks with symptomatic therapy. Systemic signs include pyrexia, depression, and neutrophilia.

Drug eruptions associated with systemic signs and a fatal outcome were reported in two dogs after carprofen (Rimadyl) therapy.[293] Skin lesions included small pustules, erythematous macules, crusts, and erosions that histologically had dermal neutrophilic infiltrates. Both dogs died in spite of immunosuppressive therapy. Both had neutrophilic infiltrates of the respiratory tract. It was proposed that these two cases had a carprofen-induced condition similar to Sweet's syndrome in humans.

Erythema multiforme and toxic epidermal necrolysis have been most common with administration of sulfonamides, cephalosporins, and levamisole (see Fig. 9–29E to G).† Three dogs, two treated with trimethoprim/sulfonamide, experienced superficial pemphigus that had features of erythema multiforme, including keratinocyte apoptosis and neutrophilic satellitosis.[11] A drug eruption in a dog with coccidioidomycosis treated with itraconazole had clinical and histologic changes compatible with erythema multiforme.[279]

Diethylcarbamazine and 5-fluorocytosine have been associated with fixed drug eruptions, especially on the scrotum of male dogs (Fig. 9–30A).[47, 271, 281] A hypersensitivity

---

*See references 47, 52, 265, 269, 273, 279, 282, 284–287.
†See references 49, 52, 56, 253, 269, 273, 287, 291, 323

Table 9-5   CUTANEOUS ADVERSE DRUG REACTIONS IN DOGS[40, 271, 307]

REACTION PATTERN	FREQUENCY*	DRUGS
Urticaria-angioedema	R	Penicillin, ampicillin, cephalosporins, sulfonamides, tetracycline, ivermectin, moxidectin, levamisole, barbiturates, etoposide, neostigmine, xylazine, phenamidine, cyclosporine, amitraz, polyhydroxidine, vaccines, bacterins, antisera, blood transfusions, radiographic contrast media, allergen extracts, vitamin K, hypoallergenic shampoo
Maculopapular (morbilliform)	U	Penicillins, sulfonamides, amoxicillin clavulanate, griseofulvin, 5-fluorocytosine, diethylcarbamazine, hydroxyzine, procainamide, cimetidine, various shampoos, amitraz
Erythroderma/exfoliative dermatitis	C	Various topical agents, sulfonamides, quinidine, levamisole, lincomycin, itraconazole, hydroxyzine, chlorpheniramine, acepromazine
Autoimmune-like	R	
Pemphigus foliaceus		Sulfonamides, ampicillin, penicillin, cephalosporins, diethylcarbamazine
Pemphigus vulgaris		Procainamide, thiabendazole, phenytoin
Bullous pemphigoid		Triamcinolone
Systemic lupus erythematosus		Sulfonamides, hydralazine, primidone, vaccine
Erythema multiforme	U	Sulfonamides, amoxicillin, amoxicillin clavulanate, cephalexin, chloramphenicol, enrofloxacin, erythromycin, gentamicin, lincomycin, tetracycline, aurothioglucose, diethylcarbamazine, ivermectin, levamisole, L-thyroxine, phenobarbital, chlorpyrifos, D-limonene, otic drops, itraconazole
Toxic epidermal necrolysis	R	Sulfonamides, ampicillin, penicillin, cephalexin, griseofulvin, levamisole, 5-fluorocytosine, D-limonene, aurothioglucose
Pruritus and self-induced lesions (allergy-like)	U	Sulfonamides, chloramphenicol, griseofulvin, acepromazine, primidone, levamisole, diethylcarbamazine, gentamicin, thyroid extracts, lincomycin, astemizole, phenobarbital, cephalexin, various topicals
Injection site reactions	U	
Panniculitis		Rabies vaccine, others
Vasculitis		Rabies vaccine, others
Atrophy		Glucocorticoids
Contact dermatitis/otitis externa	C	Numerous topicals (dermatologic and otic)
Vasculitis	U	
Local		Injectables (especially rabies vaccine)
Multifocal		Sulfonamides, ampicillin, erythromycin, penicillin, chloramphenicol, amoxicillin, enrofloxacin, gentamicin, ivermectin, metronidazole, phenobarbital, furosemide, itraconazole, loperamide (Imodium), metoclopramide, vaccines, enalapril, phenylbutazone
Fixed eruption	R	Diethylcarbamazine, ampicillin, amoxicillin clavulanate, cephalexin, 5-fluorocytosine, aurothioglucose, thiacetarsamide, L-thyroxine
Granulomatous mural folliculitis	R	Cefadroxyl, amitraz, shampoos, L-thyroxine
Lichenoid	VR	Drug combination
Miscellaneous		
Mucocutaneous dermatitis		Retinoids
Pressure point ulceration and onychomadesis		Bleomycin
Alopecia and increased susceptibility to infection		Glucocorticoids, numerous immunosuppressive agents
Flushing and pruritus		Doxorubicin

Table continued on opposite page

● Table 9-5 CUTANEOUS ADVERSE DRUG REACTIONS IN DOGS[40, 271, 307] Continued

REACTION PATTERN	FREQUENCY*	DRUGS
Hirsutism, papillomatosis, lymphoplasmacytoid dermatitis		Cyclosporine
Superficial suppurative necrolytic dermatitis		Shampoos
Epitheliotropic lymphoma–like		Ketoconazole, drug combination
Eosinophilic pustulosis		Ampicillin
Subcorneal to follicular neutrophilic pustulosis		Sulfonamides, carprofen
Urticarial eosinophilic dermatitis		Diethylcarbamazine
Sterile abscess		Sulfonamides
Scabies-like		Amoxicillin-clavulanate
Follicular necrosis and atrophy		Sulfonamides, levamisole

*C = common; R = rare; U = uncommon; VR = very rare.

reaction (probably Type III) associated with trimethoprim-sulfadiazine (Tribrissen) administration (probably sulfadiazine-related) has been recognized in Doberman pinschers (genetically programmed?).[260] Though idiosyncratic reactions to sulfonamides are considered relatively common, cutaneous manifestations occurred in only 9% of affected dogs in one study.[259] Interestingly, neither of these two dogs was a Doberman pinscher.

Cyclosporine has been reported to cause lymphoplasmacytoid dermatitis with malignant features (usually a solitary plaque or nodule) in dogs and humans.[262, 283] Methimazole may produce severe pruritus and excoriations of the face and neck of cats that are

● Table 9-6 CUTANEOUS ADVERSE DRUG REACTIONS IN CATS[40, 270]

REACTION PATTERN	FREQUENCY*	DRUGS
Urticaria-angioedema	VR	Tetracycline, penicillin, ampicillin, vaccines
Maculopapular (morbilliform)	R	Cephalexin, sulfonamides, penicillin, ampicillin, griseofulvin
Erythroderma/exfoliative dermatitis	U	Various topicals, penicillin
Autoimmune-like Pemphigus foliaceus	R	Ampicillin, cimetidine, doxycycline, cephalexin, sulfonamides
Erythema multiforme	R	Cephalexin, penicillin, aurothioglucose, amoxicillin, sulfonamides, griseofulvin, propylthiouracil
Toxic epidermal necrolysis	R	Cephaloridine, hetacillin, ampicillin, griseofulvin, penicillin, aurothioglucose, cephalexin, FeLV antiserum
Pruritus and self-induced lesions (allergy-like)	U	Methimazole, amoxicillin clavulanate, propylthiouracil, ampicillin, hetacillin, gentamicin
Injection site reactions	U	
Panniculitis		Vaccines, glucocorticoids
Vasculitis		Vaccines, ivermectin, antibiotics
Atrophy		Glucocorticoids, progestationals
Contact dermatitis/otitis externa	C	Numerous topicals (dermatologic and otic)
Vasculitis	R	
Local		Injectables
Multifocal		Penicillin, fenbendazole
Fixed eruption	VR	Clemastine, enrofloxacin
Lichenoid	VR	Drug combination
Miscellaneous		
Pinnal erythema		Ciprofloxacin, enrofloxacin
Generalized atrophy and fragility		Glucocorticoids, progestationals, phenytoin

*C = common; R = rare; U = uncommon; VR = very rare.

724 • Immune-Mediated Disorders

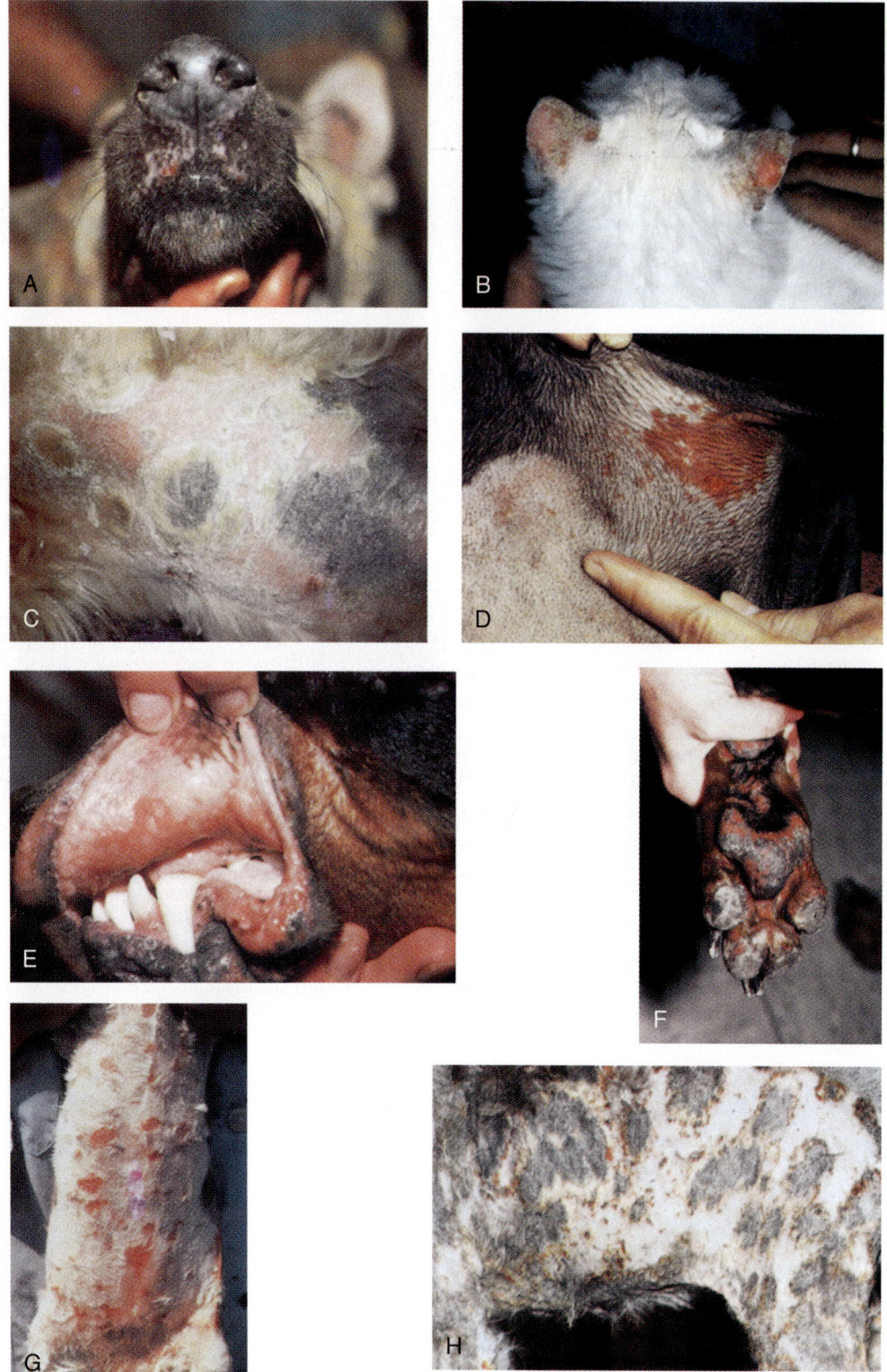

FIGURE 9-29. *Legend on opposite page*

only partially responsive to glucocorticoid treatment and mimic food hypersensitivity.[266] Drugs have also been reported to produce reactions that clinically, pathologically, and immunologically resemble pemphigus (see Figs. 9–29C and 9–30B) and pemphigoid.[252, 268, 272, 273, 275] Drug reactions (associated with ketoconazole in one case, multiple drugs in others) have occurred in dogs that were clinically and histologically indistinguishable from epitheliotropic lymphoma, as has been reported with various drugs in humans.[261, 280, 287] Lesions resolved spontaneously when the drugs were stopped. Chronic eosinophilic urticaria was associated with diethylcarbamazine.[292]

Unusual reactions to local injections are also well recognized (Fig. 9–31). One such reaction is the focal vasculitis and alopecia that follows the subcutaneous administration of rabies vaccine, especially in Poodles and Yorkshire and silky terriers (see discussion of vasculitis).[270] Another local reaction is the panniculitis associated with the subcutaneous administration of rabies vaccine in cats and dogs,[264] combined rhinotracheitis-calicivirus vaccine in cats,[289] and other products (see discussion of panniculitis in Chap. 18).[286, 287]

Plaquelike lesions with a distinctive interstitial granulomatous dermatitis histopathologic appearance have been associated with drug therapy in humans.[267] One of us (D.W.S.) has seen one such reaction in a dog being treated with amoxicillin clavulanate (Fig. 9–32).

Granulomatous mural folliculitis is a rare cutaneous reaction pattern apparently associated with drug administration (amitraz, cefadroxyl, topicals, L-thyroxine).[288] Lesions consist of large areas of well-circumscribed, coalescent alopecia; scaling; and hyperkeratosis (Fig. 9–33A and B). Foci of papules, plaques, erosions, and crusts may occur. Chronic lesions often have a smooth, shiny, cicatricial appearance.

Because drug reaction can mimic so many different dermatoses, an accurate knowledge of the medications given to any patient with an obscure form of dermatosis is imperative. Drug eruption may occur after a drug has been given for days or years or a few days after drug therapy is stopped. Eruptions most commonly occur within 1 to 3 weeks after initiating therapy.[286, 287] Some reactions (vasculitis, atrophic dermatosis, nodules, rabies vaccine reactions) may occur weeks to months after the drug is administered.[269, 270] At present, the only reliable test for the diagnosis of drug eruption is to withdraw the drug and watch for disappearance of the eruption (usually in 1 to 2 weeks). Occasionally, however, drug eruptions persist for weeks to months after the offending drug is stopped (e.g., reactions to vaccines and other injectables; lichenoid reactions).[269, 270, 286, 287] Purposeful readministration of the offending drug to determine whether the eruption will be reproduced is undesirable and may be dangerous.

DIAGNOSIS

The differential diagnosis is complex because cutaneous adverse drug reaction may mimic virtually any dermatosis. In general, no specific or characteristic laboratory findings indicate drug eruption. Results of in vivo and in vitro immunologic tests have usually been disappointing. The basophil degranulation test has been reported to be a valuable test for detecting some hypersensitivity-induced cutaneous adverse drug reactions[47] but is technically demanding and generally unavailable.

Helpful criteria for determining whether a drug eruption is likely are as follows[286, 287]:

1. Hypersensitivity or reactions occur in a minority of patients receiving the drug.

FIGURE 9–29. Drug reaction. A, Mucocutaneous depigmentation and ulcers due to triple sulfa. B, Pinnal erythema, crusting, and alopecia due to Tresaderm. C, Exfoliative erythroderma due to Tribrissen. D, Vasculitic purpura due to chloramphenicol. E, Ulcerative stomatitis and cheilitis associated with erythema multiforme major in a dog with *Klebsiella* otitis externa who had received numerous topical and systemic medications. F, Same dog as in E. Note ulcers on footpads. G, Multifocal ulcers on the ventral thorax and abdomen of a cat with erythema multiforme major due to cephalexin. (Courtesy E. Guaguère.) H, Superficial suppurative necrolytic dermatitis in a miniature Schnauzer following administration of an antiseborrheic shampoo.

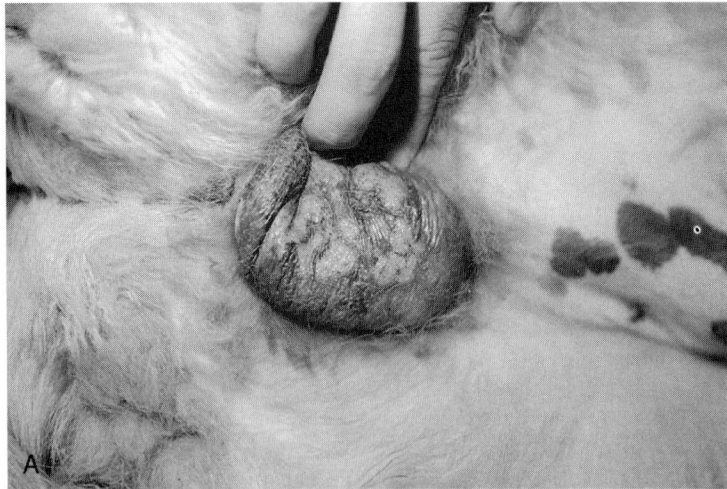
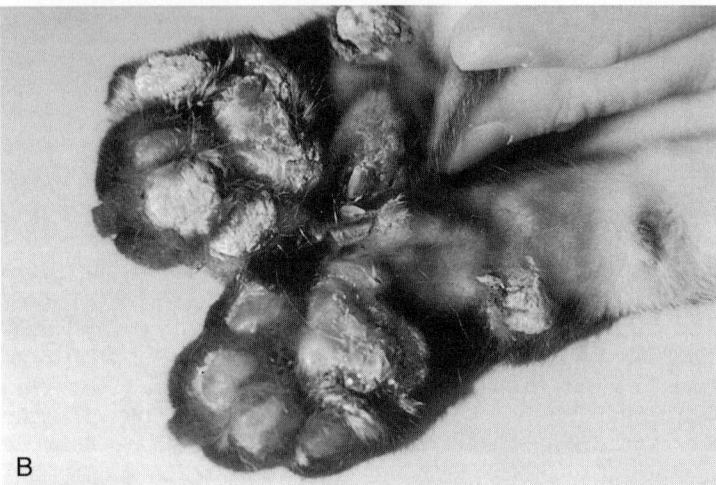

FIGURE 9–30. Cutaneous adverse drug reactions. *A*, Fixed drug eruption on scrotum of a dog associated with diethylcarbamazine. Well-circumscribed ulceration and depigmentation. *B*, Pemphigus foliaceus on the footpads of a cat in association with trimethoprim-sulfadiazine.

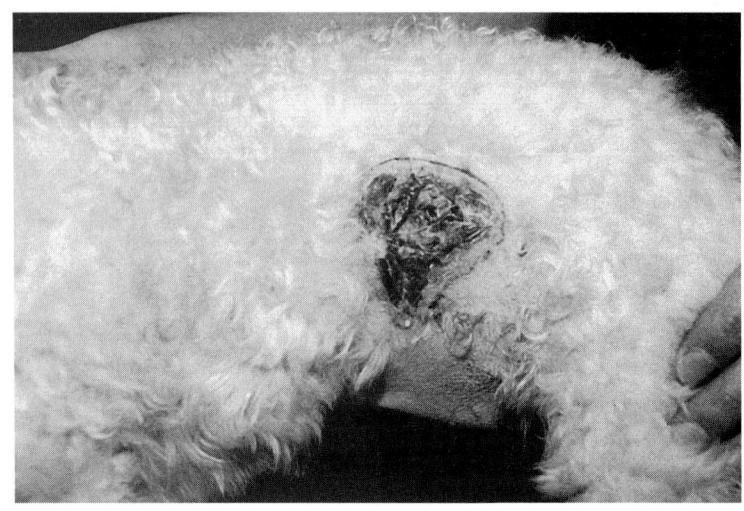

FIGURE 9–31. Local area of necrosis in the flank of a dog following administration of leptospirosis bacterin.

Immune-Mediated Disorders • 727

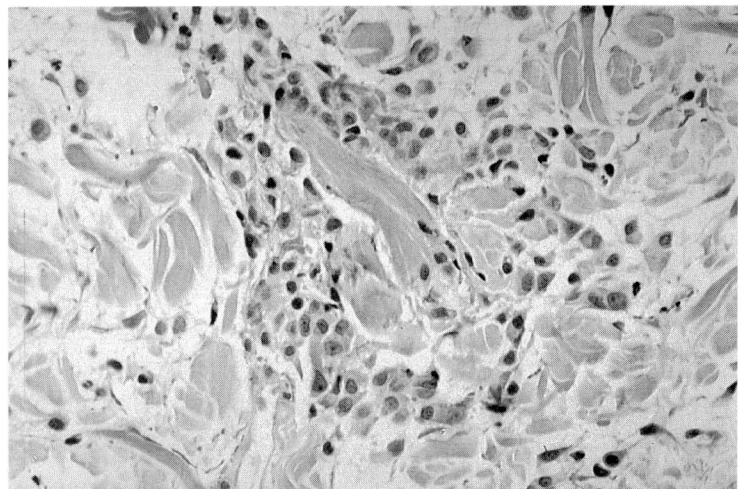

FIGURE 9–32. Granulomatous interstitial dermatitis in a dog associated with amoxicillin-clavulanate. Infiltrate of macrophages and lymphocytes around degenerate collagen fibers.

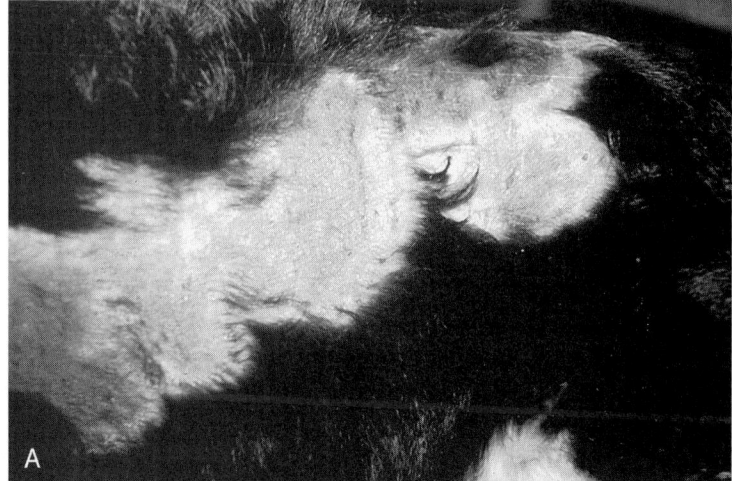

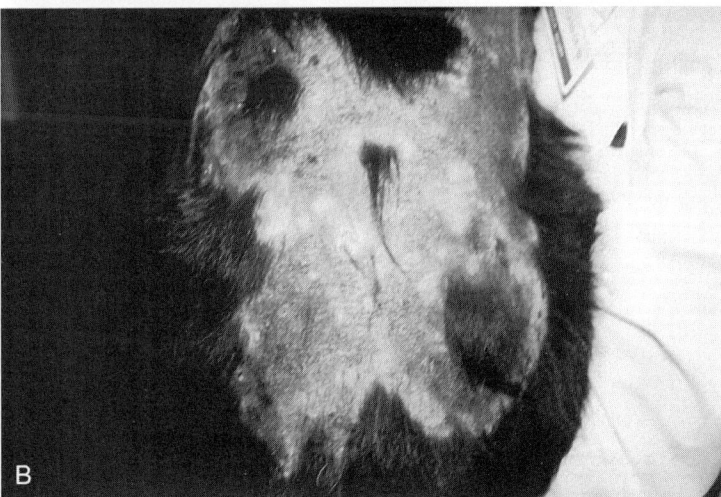

FIGURE 9–33. Granulomatous mural folliculitis in a dog associated with L-thyroxine. A, Well-circumscribed alopecia, scaling, and mild hyperpigmentation over the dorsolateral thorax. B, Similar lesions, including hyperkeratotic plaques, over the dorsal lumbosacral area.

2. Observed manifestations do not resemble known pharmacologic actions for the drugs.
3. Previous experience that the suspected drug is known for causing this type of cutaneous reaction.
4. Lack of alternative causes that could explain the cutaneous reaction that occurred with the suspect drug.
5. Appropriate timing—generally, cutaneous adverse drug reactions occur within the first 1 to 3 weeks of the initiation of therapy with the offending drug and while the drug is still being taken or is still present in the body. Prior exposure to the drug may have been tolerated without adverse effects and, if the reaction is a hypersensitivity reaction, prior exposure should have occurred so that sensitization could occur. If an animal has been previously sensitized, cutaneous reactions may be seen within hours to days of drug readministration.
6. Dechallenge. Resolution begins to occur within 1 to 2 weeks after the drug is discontinued. For some reactions—such as fixed drug, lichenoid, and local injection reaction—resolution may require several weeks.
7. Rechallenge. Reaction is reproduced by administration of small doses of the drugs or of cross-reacting drugs. Though this is the most definitive way to document the drug reaction, it is generally not recommended because more serious reactions may occur. In one study, 29% of cases of cutaneous adverse drug reaction in dogs were confirmed, often accidentally, by rechallenge.[287]

Identifying the specific cause of a cutaneous drug eruption can be difficult because many patients are receiving several drugs at the same time.[18, 252, 286, 287] In some cases, the reactions only occur with drug combinations and one drug will be tolerated.

Recently, possible causal drug exposure has been assessed by adaptation of drug implication criteria adopted by the French committee for pharmacologic surveillance in humans (Table 9–7).[278, 308]

Just as the clinical morphology of drug reactions varies greatly, so do the histologic findings. Histologic patterns recognized with cutaneous adverse drug reactions include

● Table 9–7 **PROPOSED CRITERIA FOR THE IMPLICATION OF DRUGS AS CAUSES OF CUTANEOUS ERUPTIONS**[262, 292]

Delay in Appearance of Lesions as Related to Drug Administration

Drug attributed a score of:
a. +1 (suggestive) if lesions began over 7 days after the first administration of the drug *or* less than 1 day after reexposure to a culprit medication.
b. 0 (inconclusive) if a specific assessment could not be made.
c. −1 (not suggestive) where criteria for "suggestive" (+1) not met.

Effect of Drug Interruption on Cutaneous Lesions

Drug attributed a score of:
a. +1 (suggestive) if lesions resolve solely with removal of suspect drug.
b. 0 (inconclusive).
c. −1 (incompatible) if patient does *not* improve upon drug elimination or if improvement occurs *without* removal of suspect drug.

Drug Rechallenge

Drug attributed a score of:
a. +1 (suggestive) if lesions recur with readministration of the suspect drug.
b. 0 (inconclusive) if no rechallenge performed.
c. −1 (incompatible) if rechallenge does not reproduce the lesions.

A positive total drug score (e.g., +1, +2, +3) is considered suggestive of drug causation.
A zero score is considered inconclusive.
A negative score (e.g., −1, −2, −3) is considered doubtful.

Drugs are given a numerical score of −3 to +3 based on the added values obtained from the three criteria.

perivascular dermatitis (pure, spongiotic, hyperplastic), interface dermatitis (hydropic, lichenoid), vasculitis/vasculopathy (Fig. 9–34), intraepidermal vesiculopustular dermatitis (Fig. 9–35), subepidermal vesicular dermatitis, interstitial dermatitis, and panniculitis. Eosinophils may be absent or numerous.[269, 270] In humans, eosinophils may be more prominent with drug-induced than with non–drug-induced pemphigus foliaceus.[157] Some syndromes—such as erythema multiforme, toxic epidermal necrolysis, and superficial suppurative necrolytic dermatitis—have their own characteristic histopathology. Superficial suppurative necrolytic dermatitis of miniature Schnauzers is characterized by parakeratosis, superficial epidermal suppuration and necrosis, epidermal edema, and suppurative perivascular and perifollicular dermatitis (Fig. 9–36).[294] Similar changes may occur in the follicular epithelium. Granulomatous mural folliculitis is characterized by infiltration and eventual replacement of follicular epithelium, and occasionally sebaceous glands, by granulomatous inflammation (Fig. 9–37).[288]

Direct immunofluorescence and immunohistochemical testing in drug reactions may reveal immunoreactants deposited in a variety of nondiagnostic patterns, especially in the walls of blood vessels and at the basement membrane zone.[269, 270, 286, 287]

CLINICAL MANAGEMENT

The prognosis for drug reaction is usually good unless other organ systems are involved or there is extensive epidermal necrosis. Therapy of drug reaction consists of (1) discontinuing the offending drug, (2) treating symptoms with topical and systemic medications as indicated, and (3) avoiding chemically related drugs.[286, 287] Drug reactions may be poorly responsive to glucocorticoids, though some immunologically mediated reactions respond to glucocorticoids, pentoxifylline, or immunosuppressive regimens (see Chap. 3).[252, 270]

Erythema Multiforme

Erythema multiforme is an uncommon, acute, usually self-limited eruption of the skin, mucous membranes, or both characterized by distinctive gross lesions and a diagnostic sequence of pathologic changes.

CAUSE AND PATHOGENESIS

Despite recognition of multiple etiologic and triggering causes, the pathogenesis of erythema multiforme is not fully understood. It is currently thought to represent a host-specific cell-mediated hypersensitivity reaction directed toward various antigens, including

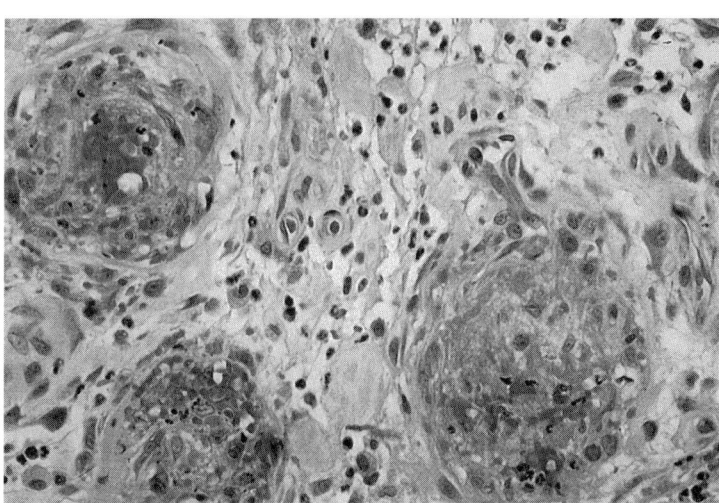

FIGURE 9–34. Vasculitis associated with trimethoprim-sulfamethoxazole in a dog. Note necrosis of vessel walls, thrombosis, and karyorrhectic neutrophils.

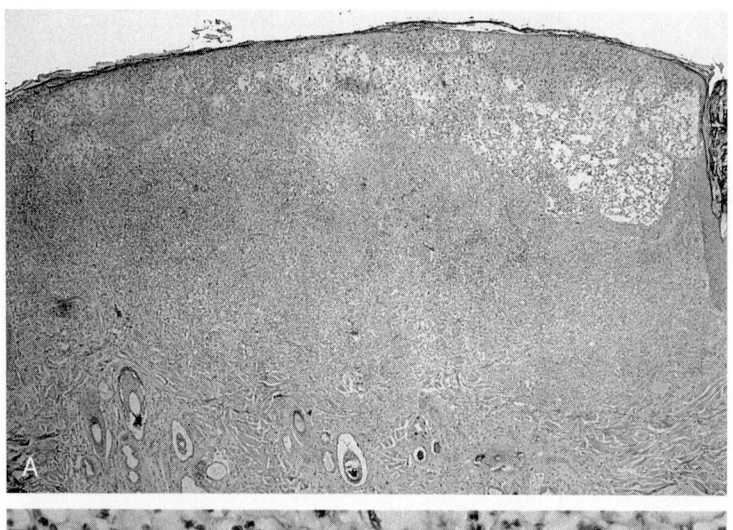

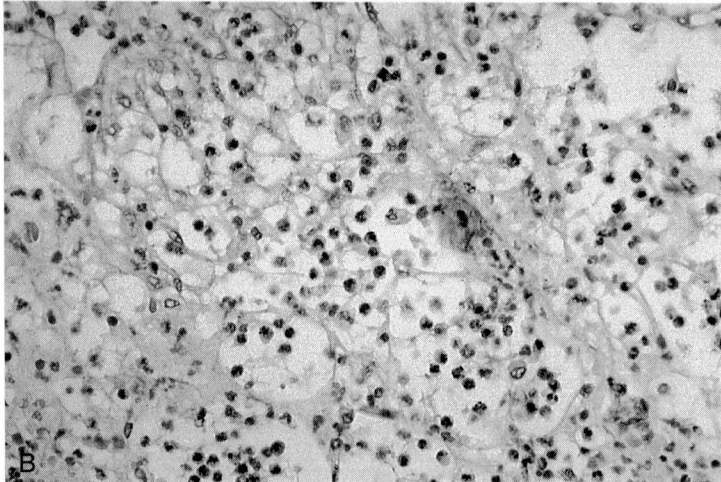

FIGURE 9–35. Sterile neutrophilic/eosinophilic pustulosis in a dog associated with trimethoprim-sulfadiazine. A, Intraepidermal pustules and dense interstitial dermatitis. B, Close-up of A. Pustules contain neutrophils and eosinophils.

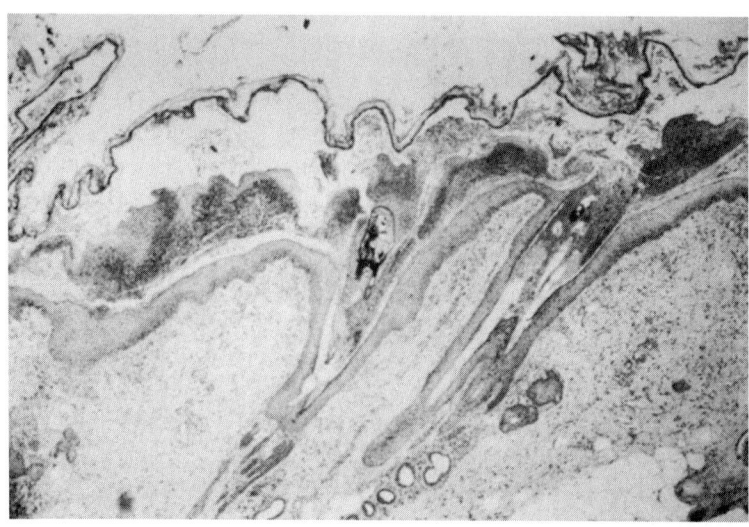

FIGURE 9–36. Superficial suppurative necrolytic dermatitis of miniature Schnauzers. Superficial suppuration and necrosis affecting the epidermis and hair follicle infundibulum.

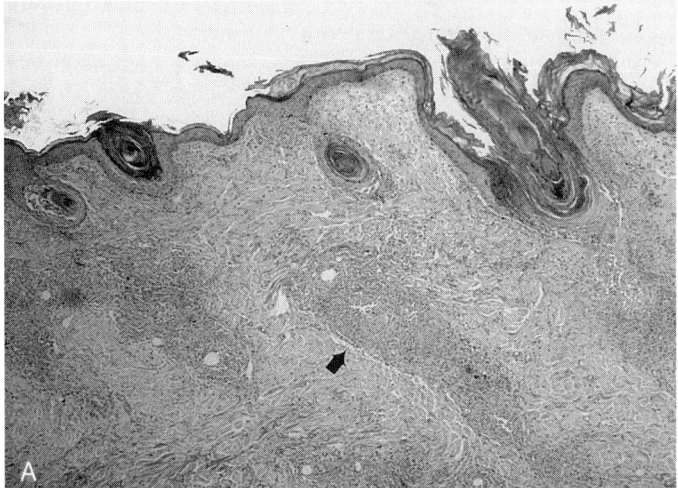
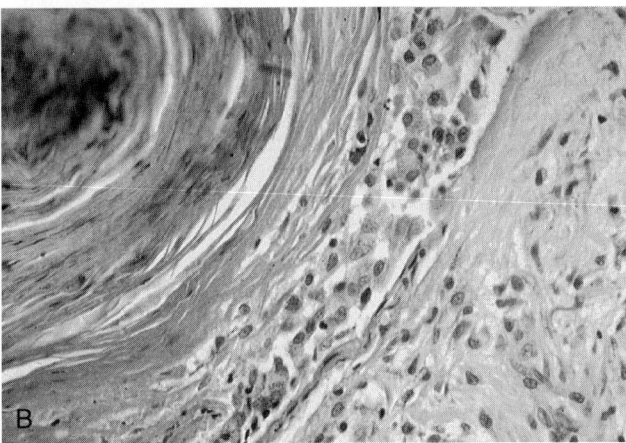
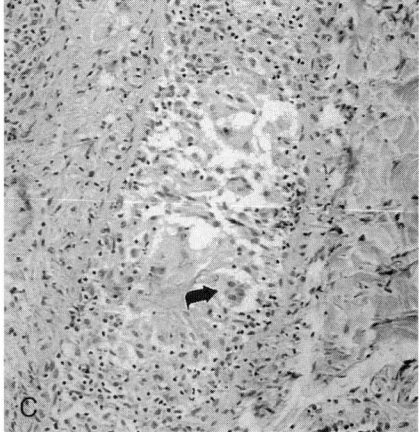

FIGURE 9–37. Granulomatous mural folliculitis in a dog associated with L-thyroxine. *A,* Hair follicles have been replaced by granulomatous infiltrate *(arrow). B,* Macrophages, often containing melanin, within follicular epithelium. Follicular keratin is excessive and ortho-to-parakeratotic (left). *C,* Hair follicle replaced by granulomatous infiltrate, including multinucleated histiocytic giant cells *(arrow).*

infections, drugs, foods, neoplasia, and connective tissue diseases.[2, 18, 56, 291, 323] Recent studies indicated that the immunohistochemical findings in skin lesions from dogs with erythema multiforme and acute graft-versus-host disease were similar.[2] Epidermal and follicular keratinocytes markedly expressed ICAM-1, MHC II and, to a lesser extent, CD1a. The expression of these molecules is likely to tether leukocytes and keep them in the epithelium. The simultaneous expression of MHC II and CD1a provides altered keratinocytes with the capability of antigen presentation. Keratinocytes in adjacent, noninflamed epidermis also expressed ICAM-1 and MHC II, suggesting that the upregulation of both adhesion molecules may represent an early phase in the development of erythema multiforme. CD44 was markedly upregulated in keratinocytes and infiltrating cells, and it is involved in T lymphocyte activation and site-specific extravasation of lymphocytes into tissues. Intraepithelial infiltrating cells were mainly CD3+, CD8-$\alpha\beta$+, TCR-$\alpha\beta$+ T lymphocytes, with smaller numbers of CD4+ T lymphocytes. CD1+, CD11c+ Langerhans' cells were increased in number. The majority of dermal infiltrating cells were also CD3+, CD8-$\alpha\beta$+, TCR-$\alpha\beta$+ T lymphocytes. CD1+, CD11c+ dermal dendrocytes were increased in number.

The phenotypic changes in keratinocytes in canine erythema multiforme indicate that alteration of the keratinocyte (e.g., by drugs, infectious agents) might be a primary factor in disease pathogenesis.[2] The upregulation of ICAM-1 and MHC II, perhaps through the production of IFN-α and TNF-β by CD8+ (cytotoxic) and CD4+ (helper) T lymphocytes, allows the tethering and keeping of lymphocytes in epithelium. Keratinocyte apoptosis is probably produced by signals from intraepithelial CD8+ T lymphocytes.

Studies in humans with erythema multiforme have shown that various basement membrane zone molecules—integrins α6 and β4, laminins 1 and 5, collagens IV and VII—are disrupted and fragmented.[312] A subset of humans with erythema multiforme have autoantibodies against desmoplakin I and II as well as suprabasilar acantholysis in skin biopsy specimens.[304]

The confusion with the pathogenesis and classification of erythema multiforme has been frustrating for human and veterinary medicine for years.[298, 306–308] In humans, erythema multiforme is usually divided into two subsets.[298, 306] An important distinction, in humans, is that the more common, mild, relapsing cutaneous disease of erythema multiforme (erythema multiforme "minor") is most often associated with viral infections, whereas the more severe forms involving mucosa and having more widespread cutaneous disease (erythema multiforme "major") are most often associated with drug eruptions.[306]

In addition, much confusion has existed over the relationship of erythema multiforme to the Stevens-Johnson syndrome (also called *erythema multiforme major* by some authors), toxic epidermal necrolysis (Lyell's syndrome), and "overlaps" of the latter two entities. Relying on some etiologic, clinical, and histopathologic similarities, it had been suggested that these conditions simply represent different aspects of a single spectrum of diseases.[297, 306, 315, 319, 320] However, this unitary concept has been disputed on clinical and histologic grounds.[297, 306, 315, 319, 320] Using standard histopathologic and immunohistochemical techniques, it was shown that the inflammatory infiltrates in the skin of humans with erythema multiforme and toxic epidermal necrolysis differed both in density and nature.[315, 321] In erythema multiforme, the cellular infiltrate was of high density (cell-rich) and rich in T lymphocytes, whereas in toxic epidermal necrolysis, the infiltrate was of low density (cell-poor) and dominated by macrophages and dermal dendrocytes.[315]

Support for a different pathomechanism has been shown in dogs as well.[50, 308] In a study of apoptosis in canine skin disease, investigators found that keratinocyte apoptosis was a feature of erythema multiforme but not of toxic epidermal necrolysis.[50] This at least suggests that these two diseases are not the same. However, before conclusions can be reached, more cases and some that share the histopathology of both disorders need to be studied.

Much of the confusion in classification has stemmed from the terminology that is applied to the various syndromes in humans and the lack of agreement on a clinical definition.[47, 306, 308] Hence, various authors consider the Stevens-Johnson syndrome and erythema multiforme major to be different or the same, and they divide erythema multiforme into "minor" and "major" variants or not.[297, 298] For this reason, some authors have proposed that the term *erythema multiforme* be used to describe all forms of the entity and that the Stevens-Johnson syndrome and toxic epidermal necrolysis be called Stevens-Johnson syndrome–toxic epidermal necrolysis, eliminating the terms *major* and *minor*.[306, 319] In veterinary medicine, this confusion has been compounded by the common acceptance of a diagnosis based primarily on histopathologic findings.[22, 72, 308]

The clinical separation of these different diseases is becoming more realistic in human medicine. The first point of separation is on presentation because most cases of erythema multiforme are relatively mild; have an acute onset of lesions, including classic target lesions; have no fever or prodromal symptoms; and, if there is mucosal involvement, it is usually mild and limited to the oral cavity.[306] These cases are self-limited, and lesions clear within 1 to 3 weeks.

The confusion has occurred in cases that are more widespread and may involve fever or prodromal symptoms. Recently, after the publication of a study in human patients requiring hospitalization for severe disease with lesions compatible with erythema multiforme or Stevens-Johnson syndrome–toxic epidermal necrolysis, a clinical classification was proposed and reviewed and a consensus on a clinical separation was reached.[298] However, these authors wrote of their classification that its "validity is unproven." Four types of lesions were found in these cases: typical target lesions, raised atypical target lesions, flat atypical target lesions, and macules with or without blisters. Two main features were used to separate these cases: the presence of typical target lesions and extent or body surface area of epidermal detachment.[298] Cases were classified into one of five categories, and the salient differentiating feature between what is erythema multiforme and the rest of Stevens-Johnson syndrome–toxic epidermal necrolysis cases was the presence of the typical target lesion in all cases of erythema multiforme. Additionally, all erythema multiforme cases involved less than 10% body surface area epidermal detachment.

When this classification scheme was used, a significant correlation between clinical findings, cause, and histology was found between erythema multiforme and Stevens-Johnson syndrome–toxic epidermal necrolysis. Erythema multiforme was primarily associated with infections, particularly herpesvirus, and Stevens-Johnson syndrome–toxic epidermal necrolysis was primarily associated with drug administration.[297, 298] Erythema multiforme lesions may also occur with lupus erythematosus in Rowell's syndrome.[300] Histopathologic findings in the erythema multiforme cases revealed a predominantly inflammatory mononuclear lichenoid infiltrate, and Stevens-Johnson syndrome–toxic epidermal necrolysis revealed predominantly epidermal necrosis with minimal inflammation.[297, 301, 321]

The human international consensus clinical classification has been adapted for use in dogs by a multicenter group (Canada, Europe, United States) (Table 9–8).[308] Possible causal drug exposure was addressed by adopting the drug implication criteria used in humans (see Table 9–7).[278] In this scheme, erythema multiforme cases have flat or raised target or polycyclic lesions, less than 50% of the body surface affected with an erythematous or purpuric macular or patchy eruption, and less than 10% of the body surface showing epidermal detachment. The erythema multiforme cases were subclassified into "minor" if one or no mucosal surface was involved and "major" if more than one mucosal surface was affected. All three forms of Stevens-Johnson syndrome–toxic epidermal necrolysis had greater than 50% of the body surface affected with macular or purpuric eruption, greater than one mucosal surface involved, and no target or polycyclic lesions.

With this classification scheme, it was shown that only 19% of erythema multiforme was associated with drug exposure, whereas 92% of Stevens-Johnson syndrome–toxic epidermal necrolysis cases were associated with drug exposure. Histopathologic findings showed an overlap between the groups, suggesting that, at least in this canine classification system, biopsy and histopathologic examination was not able to separate the two entities, though the erythema multiforme cases did have less epidermal necrosis and greater dermal inflammation than the Stevens-Johnson syndrome–toxic epidermal necrolysis cases. Further studies are indicated to document the validity and usefulness of this classification system in dogs. We and others[273] think that the histopathologic findings of erythema multiforme and toxic epidermal necrolysis in dogs, as in humans, are quite different.

A major distinction still to address is the typical target lesion. This appears to be a major feature for the diagnosis of erythema multiforme in humans but has not been addressed in the dog. The typical target lesion is defined as a highly regular, well-defined, round, wheal-like erythematous papule or plaque of less than 3 cm in diameter that has at

● Table 9–8 **PROPOSED CRITERIA FOR THE CLINICAL CLASSIFICATION OF ERYTHEMA MULTIFORME AND STEVENS-JOHNSON SYNDROME–TOXIC EPIDERMAL NECROLYSIS**[292]

CLINICAL LESIONS	EM min	EM maj	SJS	OVERLAP	TEN
Flat or raised, focal or multifocal, target or polycyclic lesions	Yes	Yes	No	No	No
Number of mucosal surfaces involved	None or 1	>1	>1	>1	>1
Erythematous or purpuric, macular or patchy eruption (percent of body surface)	<50	<50	>50	>50	>50
Epidermal detachment (percent of body surface)	<10	<10	<10	10–30	>30

EM min = erythema multiforme minor; EM maj = erythema multiforme major; SJS = Stevens-Johnson syndrome; OVERLAP = SJS-TEN overlap syndrome; TEN = toxic epidermal necrolysis.

least three different zones, which are composed of two concentric rings around a central disk (Fig. 9–38A). The central disk varies from erythematous to violaceous, dusky, purpuric, or necrotic and may vesiculate. The inner ring is edematous and pale, the outer ring ("halo") is erythematous.[298, 307] This "typical target lesion" has been detected in 15.9% of dogs with erythema multiforme.[323] This aspect needs to be more carefully reevaluated in veterinary medicine.

Erythema multiforme is uncommon in dogs and cats, accounting for only 0.4% and 0.11%, respectively, of all the canine and feline dermatology cases examined at a university practice.[323] Erythema multiforme has been recognized in dogs in association with infections, drug therapy (especially trimethoprim-potentiated sulfonamides, penicillins, and cephalosporins), and idiopathy (Table 9–9).[47, 56, 269, 291, 302, 308, 318, 322, 323] Two cases of drug-induced erythema multiforme have been associated with disseminated intravascular coagulation.[311, 318] Erythema multiforme has also been reported to be a manifestation of adverse reactions to dietary substances.[323] In one study, 22.8% of the cases of canine erythema multiforme were idiopathic.[323] A subgroup of idiopathic erythema multiforme has been described in old dogs, occasionally associated with an underlying disease, suggesting immune dysfunction.[22] In cats, erythema multiforme has been reported in association with drug therapy (cephalexin, penicillin, aurothioglucose, trimethoprim-sulfonamide, amoxicillin, griseofulvin, propylthiouracil) and herpesvirus infection wherein lesions may accompany upper respiratory signs and resolve when the respiratory disease resolves.[47, 323, 385]

CLINICAL SIGNS

Prodromal or concurrent clinical signs may reflect the underlying cause. As the term *multiforme* implies, the skin lesions are variable, but they are usually characterized by an acute, rather symmetric onset of (1) erythematous macules (see Fig. 9–38B) or slightly

● Table 9–9 **REPORTED ETIOLOGIC FACTORS FOR CANINE ERYTHEMA MULTIFORME**[40, 307]

Antibiotics
Amoxicillin
Amoxicillin clavulanate
Cephalexin
Chloramphenicol
Enrofloxacin
Erythromycin
Gentamicin
Lincomycin
Ormetoprim-sulfadimethoxine
Tetracycline
Trimethoprim-sulfadiazine
Trimethoprim-sulfamethoxazole

Infections
Pseudomonal otitis externa
Staphylococcal dermatitis
Anal sacculitis

Miscellaneous
Aurothioglucose
Chlorpyrifos
Beef and/or soy (in diet and chewable heartworm preventive)
Diethylcarbamazine
D-limonene
Idiopathic
Ivermectin
Levamisole
L-Thyroxine
Otic drops
Phenobarbital

Immune-Mediated Disorders • 735

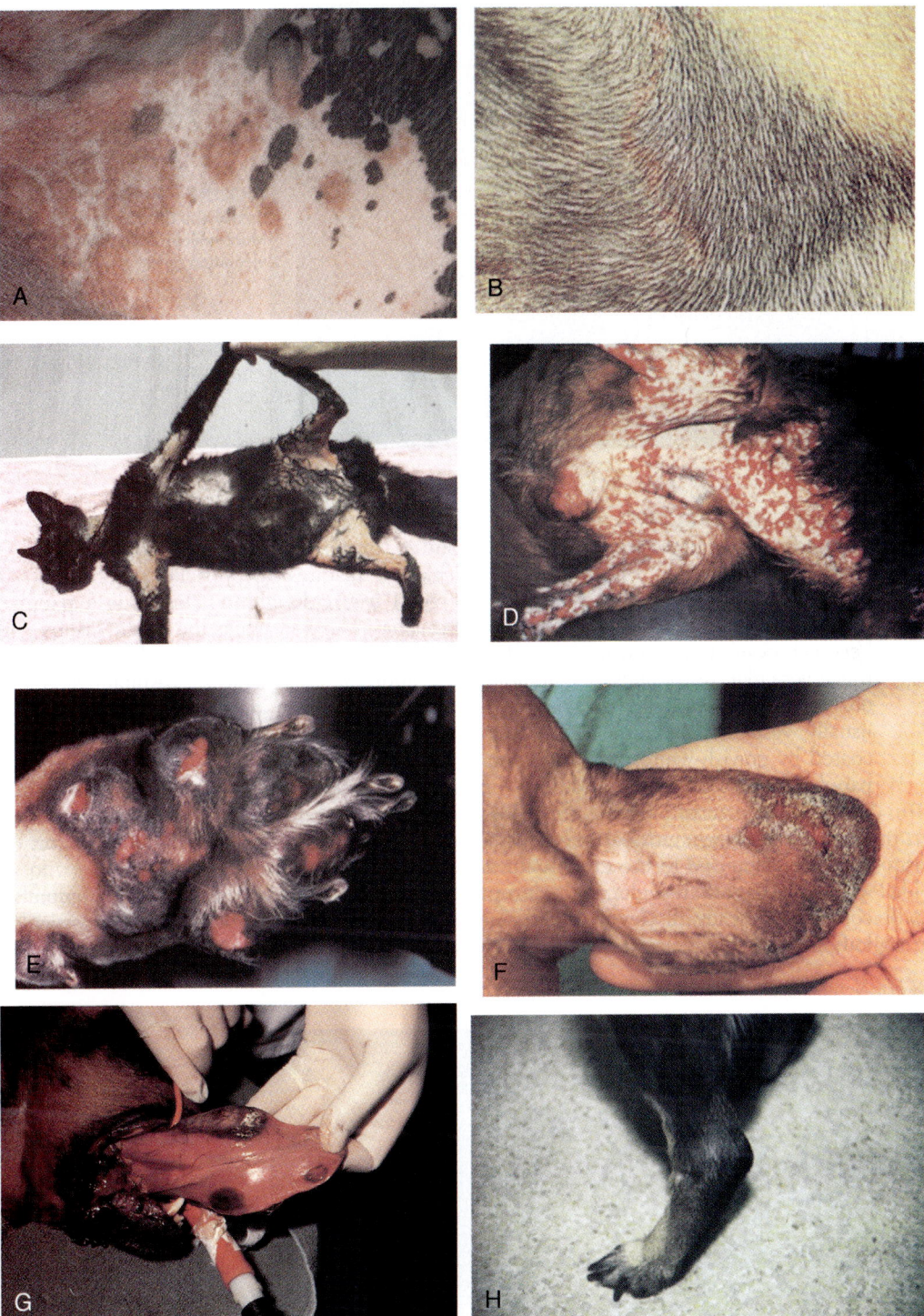

FIGURE 9–38. *A*, Erythema multiforme minor in a dog caused by Tribrissen, Annular, erythematous, target lesions in flank. *B*, Canine erythema multiforme due to cephalexin. Serpiginous erythema. *C*, Toxic epidermal necrolysis in a cat. (From Rosenkrantz WS: Cutaneous drug reactions. In: Griffin CE, et al [eds]: Current Veterinary Dermatology. Mosby–Year Book, St. Louis, 1993.) *D*, Severe ulceration of the ventrum, medial thighs, and scrotum of a dog with toxic epidermal necrolysis due to levamisole. (Courtesy G. T. Wilkinson.) *E*, Ulcerated footpads in a dog with idiopathic leukocytoclastic vasculitis. *F*, Cutaneous idiopathic vasculitis in a dog. Necrosis and ulceration tracing pinnal vasculature. *G*, Punctate ulcers on the tongue of a dog with idiopathic leukocytoclastic vasculitis. *H*, Pitting edema of the hock in a dog with vasculitis.

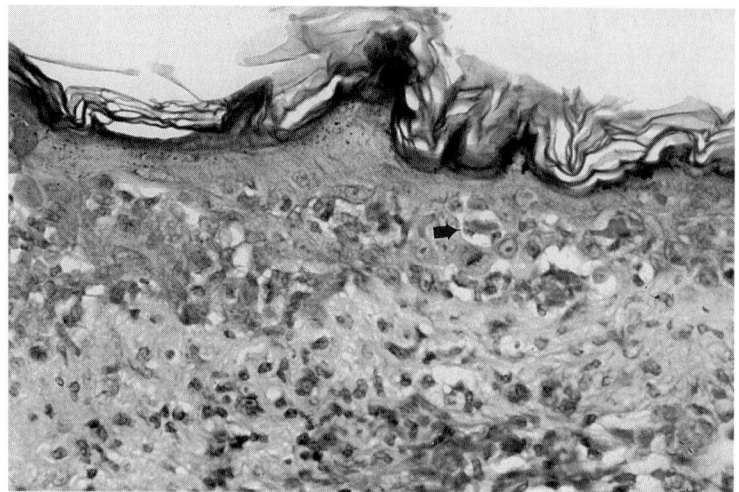

FIGURE 9–43. Erythema multiforme in a dog due to trimethoprim-sulfamethoxazole. Note hydropic degeneration, marked apoptosis (*arrow*) at all levels of epidermis, and lymphocytic exocytosis. Also note mild epidermal hyperplasia and normal stratum corneum.

and those without (i.e., idiopathic).[323] Maculopapular lesions are characterized histologically by hydropic interface dermatitis with prominent single-cell apoptosis of keratinocytes at all levels of the epidermis and satellitosis of lymphocytes and macrophages (Figs. 9–43 and 9–44). The infundibular region of hair follicle outer root sheath epithelium is often similarly affected. In the absence of necrosis, ulceration, and bacterial infection, the stratum corneum is orthokeratotic and normal, and the epidermis shows mild to moderate, regular hyperplasia. A superficial interstitial or, rarely, a dense lichenoid inflammatory infiltrate is visible.

Urticarial lesions are characterized by hydropic interface dermatitis and striking dermal edema (Fig. 9–45). Dermal collagen fibers become vertically oriented and attenuated, presenting a weblike appearance ("gossamer" collagen). *Vesiculobullous* lesions are characterized by segmental full-thickness coagulation necrosis of epithelium (Fig. 9–46). A superficial perivascular to interstitial accumulation of predominantly lymphohistiocytic cells is typical, and subepidermal cleft and vesicle formation may occur owing to separation of the necrotic epithelium from the underlying connective tissue at the basement membrane zone. Pigmentary incontinence is common.

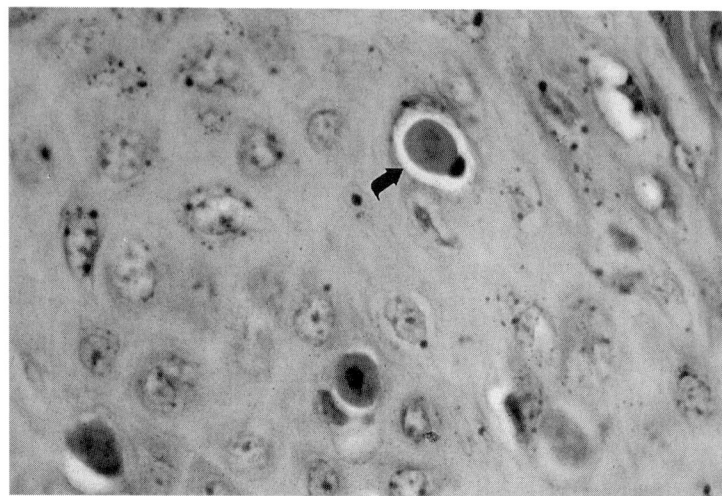

FIGURE 9–44. Erythema multiforme in a dog due to trimethoprim-sulfamethoxazole. Note apoptotic keratinocytes and one adherent lymphocyte ("satellitosis") (*arrow*).

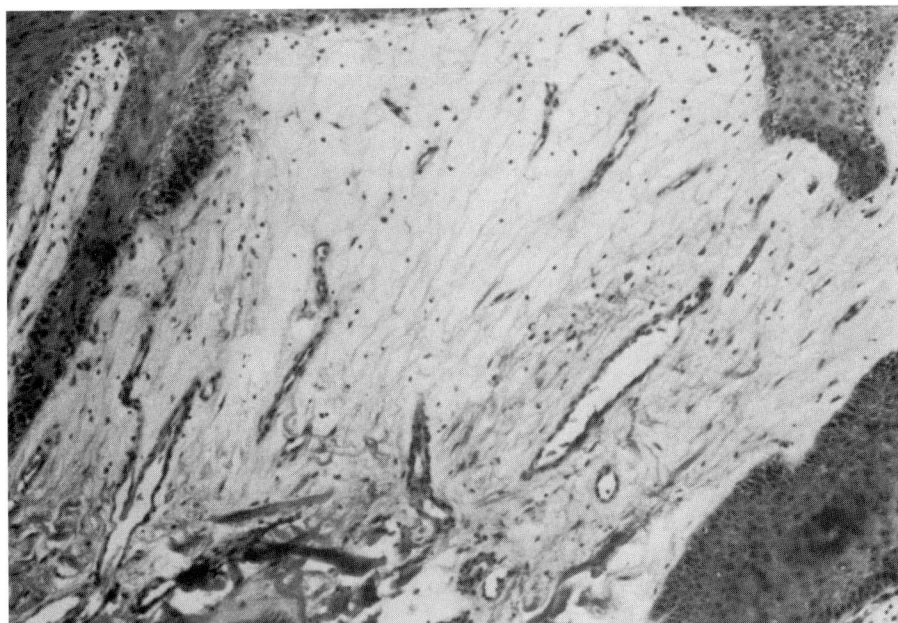

FIGURE 9–45. Canine erythema multiforme. Marked dermal edema with vertical stretching of collagen fibers ("gossamer collagen").

Direct immunofluorescence testing usually yields negative results but may demonstrate IgG, IgM, or C3 between epidermal keratinocytes, around globoid bodies in the superficial dermis, or in association with dermal blood vessel walls.[47, 273, 323]

CLINICAL MANAGEMENT

Erythema multiforme may run a mild course, spontaneously regressing within a few weeks. An underlying cause should be sought and corrected, whenever possible, a procedure that also results in spontaneous resolution of the erythema multiforme.[18, 47, 323]

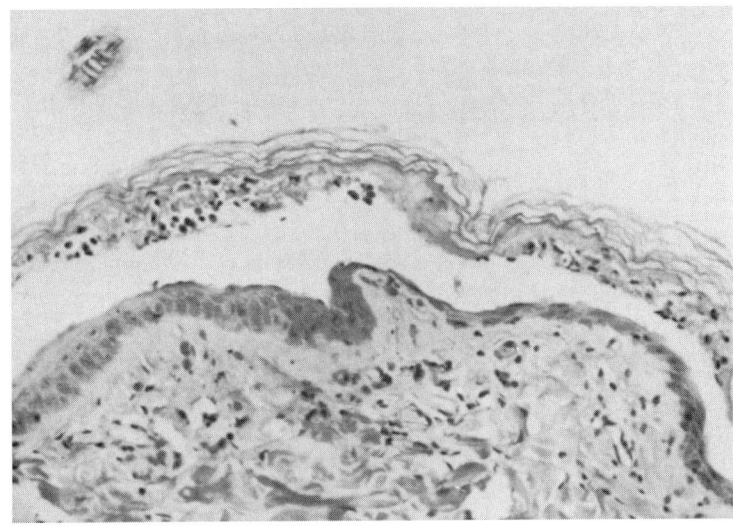

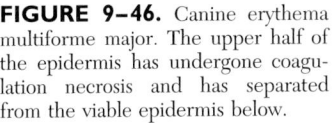

FIGURE 9–46. Canine erythema multiforme major. The upper half of the epidermis has undergone coagulation necrosis and has separated from the viable epidermis below.

Severe vesiculobullous cases of erythema multiforme require supportive care and an exhaustive search for underlying causes. When trigger factors can be identified and eliminated, the erythema multiforme usually resolves within 3 weeks.[323]

In human medicine, the use of immunosuppressive drugs, especially glucocorticoids, in the treatment of erythema multiforme continues to be controversial.[307, 323] Given the presumed immune-mediated pathogenesis of erythema multiforme, treatment with immunomodulating drugs would seem to make sense in cases in which elimination of potential trigger factors has been achieved yet the disease persists.[323] In fact, dogs with severe idiopathic erythema multiforme have been successfully treated with large doses of glucocorticoids and/or azathioprine.[323]

Anecdotal reports suggest that cyclosporine[253] or etretinate[316] may be useful in idiopathic erythema multiforme in dogs. We have used pentoxifylline successfully in a few cases, and this drug may warrant a trial prior to immunosuppressive drugs. All idiopathic cases should receive a novel antigen ("hypoallergenic") diet to rule out diet-related disease.[323] Even "idiopathic" cases have been known to spontaneously resolve after 4 to 12 months, suggesting that undocumented antigenic triggers had been eliminated.[323]

Toxic Epidermal Necrolysis

Toxic epidermal necrolysis is a rare, variably painful, extensive vesiculobullous and ulcerative disorder of skin and oral mucosa in dogs, cats, and human beings. Less extensive cutaneous with mucosal involvement is often called Stevens-Johnson syndrome, though confusion in the veterinary and human literature has equated this with more severe erythema multiforme.[319]

CAUSE AND PATHOGENESIS

In humans, toxic epidermal necrolysis has been temporally associated with drugs in 80% to 95% of cases.[307] Fifty percent of the cases of Stevens-Johnson syndrome are also drug-related.[307] A variety of drugs and causes have been associated with toxic epidermal necrolysis in dogs (see Table 9–9).[56, 282, 291, 317, 324] Flea dips were implicated in both a dog and cat that experienced toxic epidermal necrolysis.[305] Some cases are idiopathic.

Although the pathomechanism of toxic epidermal necrolysis is unknown, immunopathologic mechanisms have been suggested.[18] It has also been suggested that drug-induced erythema multiforme major and toxic epidermal necrolysis may relate to defective epidermal detoxification of drug byproducts.[307] Fadok proposed that apoptosis may be induced and that it is massive and sudden in toxic epidermal necrolysis, but localized and more gradual in erythema multiforme.[253] In humans, apoptosis seems to be the key mechanism leading to keratinocyte death, and TNF-α is a major cytokine involved in apoptosis.[309, 313, 314, 325]

Perforin (a cytoplasmic peptide contained in cytotoxic T lymphocytes and natural killer cells) has been suggested to play a role in keratinocyte apoptosis.[309] In addition, the role of calcium in the regulation of apoptosis is crucial, and the expression of calprotectin (a calcium-binding protein) is increased in the epidermis of patients with toxic epidermal necrolysis.[314] This information has led to the hypothesis that toxic drug metabolites stimulate keratinocytes to produce TNF-α and perturb calcium homeostasis, which leads to keratinocyte apoptosis in the absence of inflammatory cells. Other studies have suggested that the upregulation of keratinocyte Fas ("cell-surface death receptor," CD95) is the critical trigger of keratinocyte destruction.[325]

In dogs, one study could not demonstrate apoptosis in any of seven cases of toxic epidermal necrolysis, and it was thought that the epidermis in these cases was undergoing necrosis by a pathologic mechanism different from apoptosis.[50]

CLINICAL FEATURES

There are no apparent age, breed, or sex predilections. Clinically, toxic epidermal necrolysis is usually characterized by an acute onset of constitutional signs (pyrexia, anorexia, lethargy, depression) and a multifocal or generalized vesiculobullous disease (see Fig. 9–38C and D). This may be a major differentiating feature from erythema multiforme because, in humans, all cases of toxic epidermal necrolysis are preceded by pyrexia.[301] Vesicles and bullae, necrosis, and resultant ulcers with epidermal collarettes may be found anywhere in the skin and often involve the oral mucosa, mucocutaneous junctions, and footpads. Nikolsky's sign is usually present. Cutaneous pain is usually moderate to marked.

DIAGNOSIS

The differential diagnosis is relatively limited in severe cases with constitutional signs and acute history, and it includes burns, systemic lupus erythematosus, severe erythema multiforme, superficial suppurative necrolytic dermatitis, and epitheliotropic lymphoma.

Definitive diagnosis is based on history, physical examination, and skin biopsy. A hemogram usually reveals neutropenia or neutrophilia.[56] In humans, persistent neutropenia portends a fatal outcome.[18]

HISTOPATHOLOGY

Histopathologic findings in toxic epidermal necrolysis are identical, regardless of underlying cause. They consist of hydropic degeneration of basal epidermal cells, full-thickness coagulation necrosis of the epidermis, and minimal dermal inflammation (silent dermis or cell-poor inflammation) (Fig. 9–47).[22, 47, 71] Dermo-epidermal separation results in subepidermal vesicles (Fig. 9–48). This is in contrast with the cell-rich inflammation that occurs in erythema multiforme.[315, 323] The periodic acid–Schiff (PAS)-positive basement membrane zone, when present, is usually located at the floor of the vesicles. The infundibular region of hair follicle outer root sheath epithelium may be similarly affected. In humans, the atrichous sweat gland duct is often affected, but this has not been studied in animals.[296] It must be emphasized that toxic epidermal necrolysis is not usually the definitive diagnosis. It is imperative to remember that toxic epidermal necrolysis is only a cutaneous reaction pattern, and every attempt must be made to find the underlying cause.

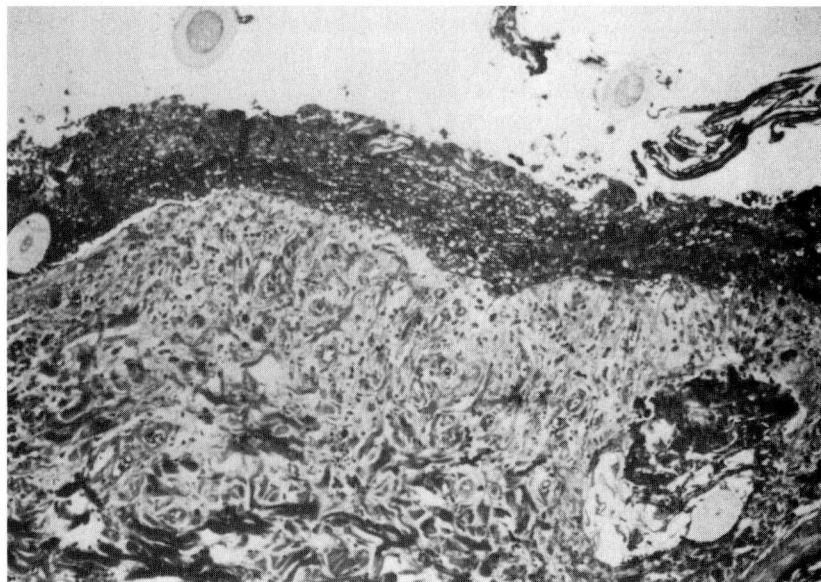

FIGURE 9–47. Canine toxic epidermal necrolysis (associated with staphylococcal endocarditis). Full-thickness epidermal coagulation necrosis with minimal inflammation. (From Scott DW, et al: Toxic epidermal necrolysis in two dogs and a cat. J Am Anim Hosp Assoc 15:271, 1979.)

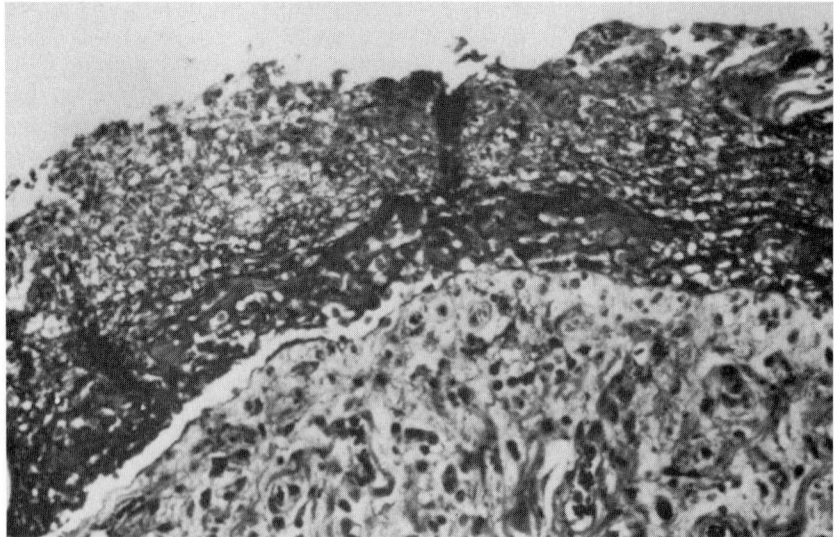

FIGURE 9–48. Canine toxic epidermal necrolysis (staphylococcal endocarditis). Full-thickness epidermal coagulation necrosis with subepidermal cleft formation. (From Scott DW, et al: Toxic epidermal necrolysis in two dogs and a cat. J Am Anim Hosp Assoc 15:271, 1979.)

Results of direct and indirect immunofluorescence testing are usually negative.[18, 56, 269] In humans, immunohistochemical studies have shown that the cell-poor infiltrate in toxic epidermal necrolysis contains predominantly macrophages and dermal dendrocytes, unlike the cell-rich infiltrate rich in T lymphocytes found in erythema multiforme.[315]

CLINICAL MANAGEMENT

The prognosis for toxic epidermal necrolysis is guarded to poor, pending identification of the underlying cause, with a mortality rate as high as 50% in humans.[307] The mortality is greatest in idiopathic cases, wherein a precipitating factor cannot be recognized and specifically corrected. The sequelae and prognosis are similar to those of a massive second-degree burn, owing to fluid, electrolyte, and colloid losses and to secondary infections and sepsis that compound the loss of epidermal barrier function. Mortality rates are lower when therapy in humans is conducted in specialty treatment centers for burn patients.[301, 303]

Treatment consists of (1) correction of the underlying cause and (2) symptomatic and supportive measures (e.g., fluids, antibiotics, topicals). The use of systemic glucocorticoids is controversial, some investigators thinking that these drugs are at best not helpful and, at worst, detrimental.[18] The incidence of sepsis resulting in a higher fatality rate is the greatest concern, so the severity and extent of involvement may relate to the decision as to whether to use glucocorticoids. The administration of systemic glucocorticoids may be indicated, however, in drug-induced cases.[18] Plasmapheresis has been beneficial in humans.[303] Intravenous immunoglobulin therapy has been reported to be effective in humans, presumably via Fas (CD95) blockade.[325] Recovery (depending on the identification and correction of the underlying cause) usually occurs in 2 to 3 weeks.

Vasculitis

Cutaneous vasculitis is an uncommon disorder in dogs that is characterized by purpura (often palpable), wheals, edema, papules, plaques, nodules, alopecia, scarring, necrosis, and ulceration, often involving the extremities. In some cases, the lesions are slightly purpuric, appearing erythematous but not blanching with diascopy. Cutaneous vasculitis is rare in cats.

CAUSE AND PATHOGENESIS

Vasculitides are classified histologically into neutrophilic, eosinophilic, lymphocytic, granulomatous, mixed forms, and cell-poor forms.[47, 72] The neutrophilic forms may be leukocytoclastic (neutrophil nuclei undergo karyorrhexis, resulting in "nuclear dust") or nonleukocytoclastic.[12, 18] In dogs, the nonleukocytoclastic form is more common, and two other forms of neutrophilic vasculitis occur.[72] In one there are associated skin lesions such as intraepidermal pustules, folliculitis, or neutrophilic spongiosis, and this pattern may be associated with bacterial skin infections or drug reactions. In the third neutrophilic form, the major lesion is thrombosis and resultant tissue ischemia. This pattern is more often associated with gram-negative septicemia and infections that target the endothelial cells.[72]

Eosinophilic vasculitis is associated with arthropod reactions, food hypersensitivity, eosinophilic granuloma, and mast cell tumors.[22, 72, 342] However, the "vasculitic" nature of these eosinophil-associated lesions has been challenged.[346] Interstitial granulomatous dermatitis with vasculitis associated with cyclosporine administration was observed in a dog with periocular edema and alopecia and a swelling at the base of one ear.[349] In humans, vasculitis is also categorized by the size of the affected vessel (large or small), though this has been considered of little value in the dog and cat.[72, 339] In most cases, cutaneous vasculitis involves small dermal blood vessels (postcapillary venules). Vasculitis can occur via immune and nonimmune mechanisms.[25, 330, 341] As a cause of cutaneous disease, vasculitis most commonly is thought to be immunologically mediated and the result of a drug reaction or infection.[25, 347]

The pathomechanism of most cutaneous vasculitides is assumed to involve Type III hypersensitivity reactions.[14, 60–64, 69] Type I hypersensitivity reactions may be important in the initiation of immune complex deposition in blood vessel walls. However, it appears to be more complex, and multiple mechanisms likely play a role. It has been postulated that differences in membrane receptors (probably adhesion molecules and cytokines) for immunoglobulin and complement on leukocytes may account for the different histologic appearances of neutrophilic and lymphocytic vasculitides.[5] Additionally, initial neutrophil-induced damage to endothelial cells could result in the expression of "not self" antigens, whereupon dendritic cells and T cells could initiate a secondary cell-mediated immune response, thus perpetuating the vascular disease and producing a lymphocyte-dominated infiltrate.[337] In cutaneous necrotizing vasculitis, endothelial cells show increased expression of ICAM-1 and E-selectin.[347] E-selectin is an adhesion molecule for neutrophils. In some cases and forms of vasculitis there has been an association with the presence of autoantibodies that react with neutrophil cytoplasmic structures (e.g., proteinase-3, myeloperoxidase) or endothelial cells.[337, 347]

Cutaneous vasculitis may be associated with coexisting disease (infections, food hypersensitivity, insect bites, malignancies, connective tissue disorders [such as lupus erythematosus]), precipitating factors (infections, drugs, vaccines), or it may be idiopathic (about 50% of all cases).* Infections may induce immune complex or septic vasculitis.[22, 72, 282] About 7.5% of the dogs treated with itraconazole at 10 mg/kg/day experience cutaneous vasculitis (lymphedema and/or necrotizing lesions on one or more limbs), whereas dogs treated with 5 mg/kg/day do not experience this reaction.[336] Focal cutaneous vasculitis reactions at the site of rabies vaccination have been described in dogs, and rabies viral antigen was detected in blood vessel walls.[351] In a retrospective study of cutaneous vasculitis in 18 dogs and 1 cat, food hypersensitivity was diagnosed in 2 dogs, adverse drug reaction in 2 dogs, rabies vaccine reaction in 4 dogs, and the condition was idiopathic in 10 dogs. The 1 cat had vaccine-related vasculitis.[342]

---

*See references 12, 18, 56, 72, 282, 330, 337, 340–342.

Certain breeds may be predisposed, such as Jack Russell terriers, Scottish terriers, German shepherd dogs, Greyhounds, Dachshunds, and Rottweilers.[56, 328, 343, 344, 350] Vaccine reactions are more commonly recognized in Poodles, silky terriers, Yorkshire terriers, Pekingese, and Maltese, which may reflect breed predilection, small body size, or the long period of anagen hair growth and "fuzzy" haircoat phenotype in these breeds.[287] In one survey, two of four cases were the Bichon breed, one Maltese and one Poodle.[342] The breed associations may suggest some genetic component to the etiology of some forms of vasculitis, as has been suggested in humans because of HLA associations.[347]

CLINICAL FEATURES

Skin is often the only organ system involved. However, other organ systems may be affected, wherein the skin lesions may represent the initial sign of a systemic disease. Skin lesions typically occur in dependent areas of the body, in skin over areas of pressure and normal "wear and tear," and in skin covering extremities (pinnae, tip of tail, and so forth) that are more susceptible to cold environmental influences. Cutaneous signs of vasculitis usually include palpable purpura, plaques, hemorrhagic bullae, papules or pustules, necrosis, punched-out (crateriform) ulcers, and occasionally acrocyanosis, especially involving the extremities (paws, pinnae, lips, tail, scrotum, and oral mucosa), and they may clearly be associated with vascular pathways (see Fig. 9–38E to G; Figs. 9–49 to 9–54).

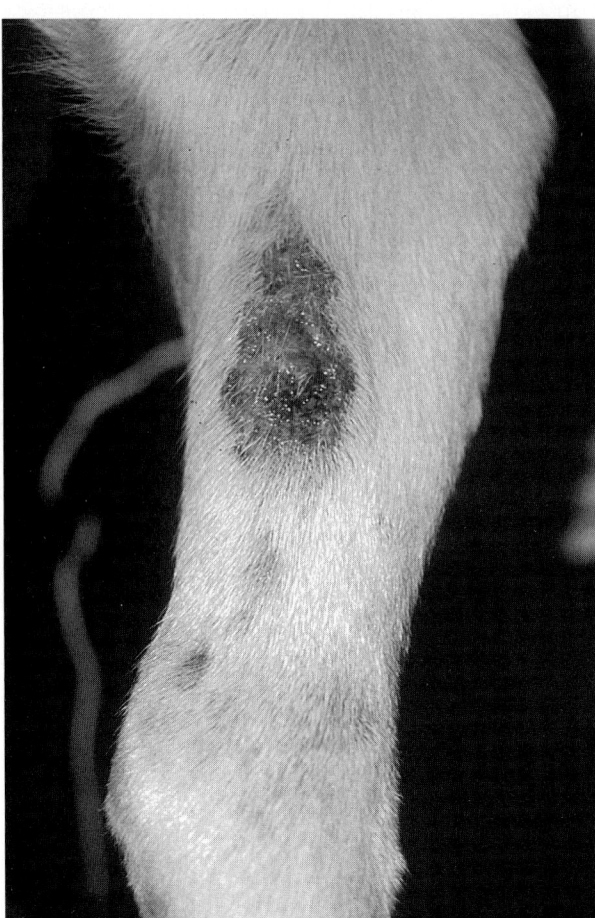

FIGURE 9–49. Ulcerated nodule on the leg of a dog with eosinophilic vasculitis.

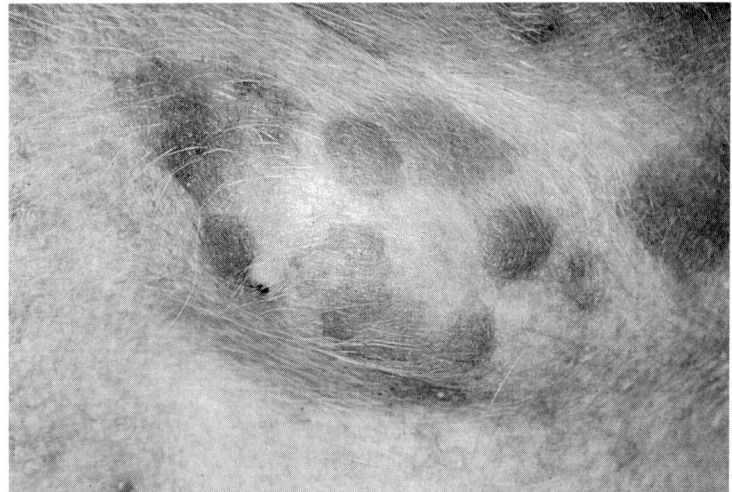

FIGURE 9–50. Purpuric hives in a dog with food hypersensitivity vasculitis.

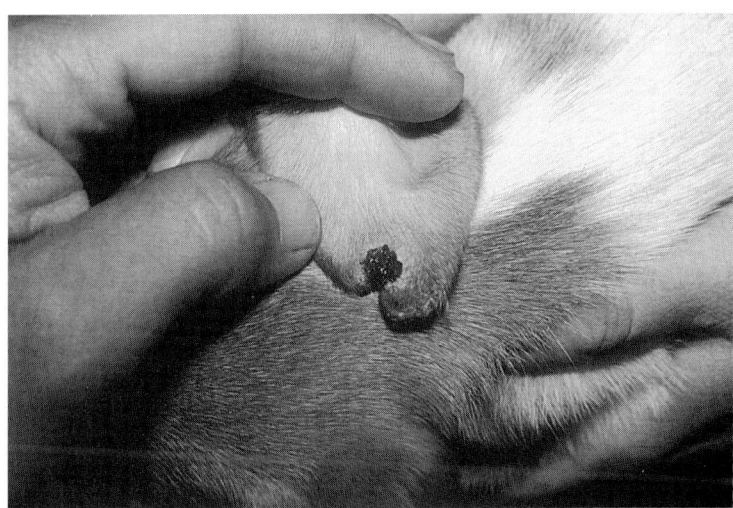

FIGURE 9–51. Pinnal lesions in a dog with vasculitis. The pinnal apex shows acrocyanosis and an infarct.

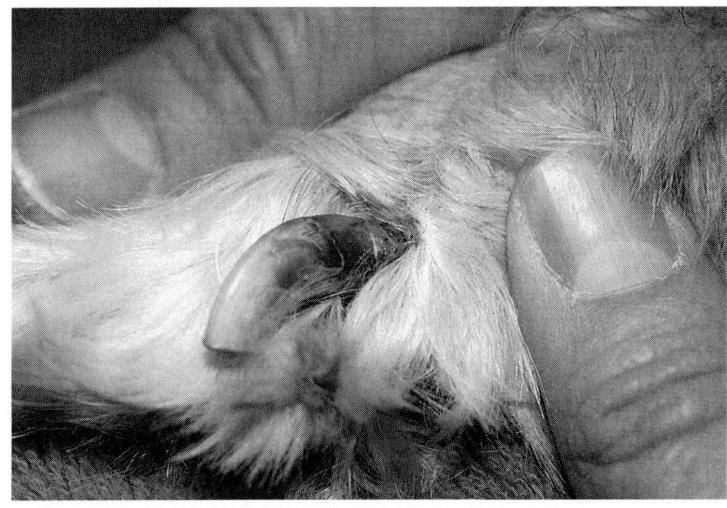

FIGURE 9–52. Subungual hemorrhage in a claw of a dog with symmetric lupoid onychodystrophy. This clinical appearance suggests vascular damage.

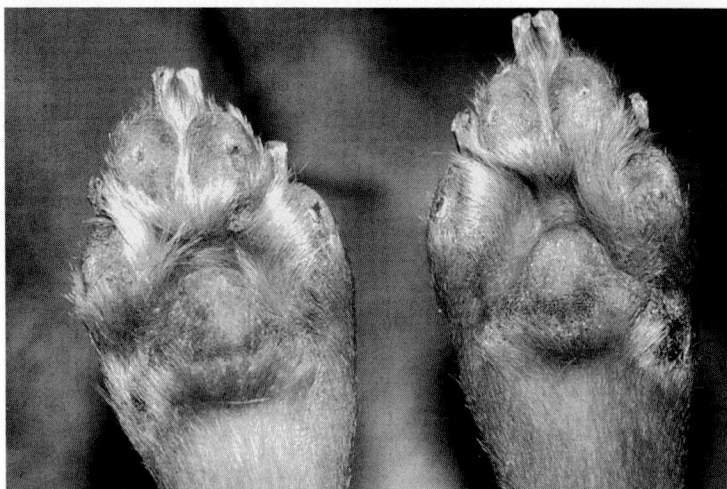

FIGURE 9–53. Footpads of a dog with vasculitis. Note multiple crusted depressions (pits) representing healed and healing infarcts.

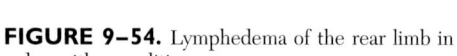

FIGURE 9–54. Lymphedema of the rear limb in a dog with vasculitis.

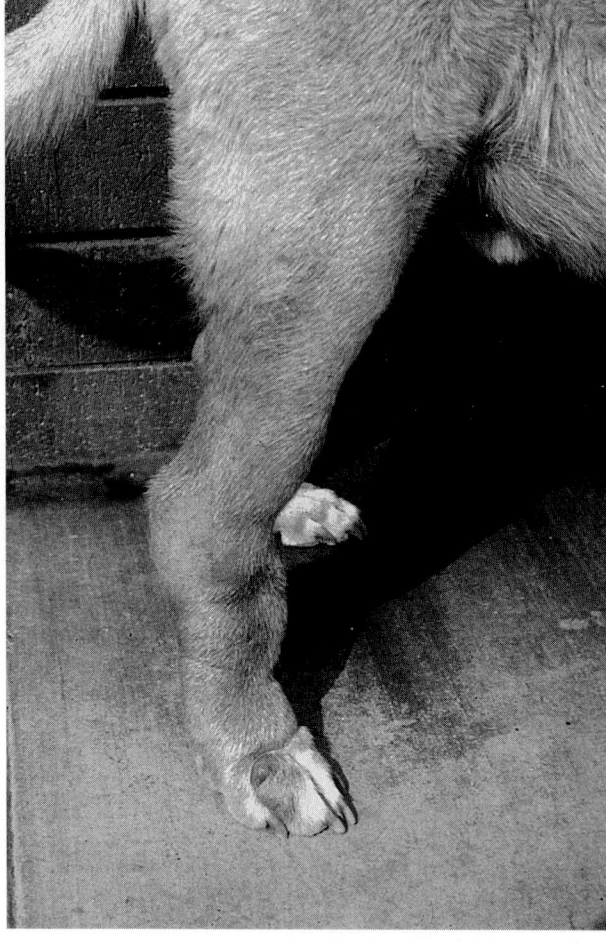

Pinnal lesions are often more prevalent on the apex and concave surface (see Fig. 9–51). Hemorrhages may occur within the claw (see Fig. 9–52). Pads may develop central punched-out ulcers (see Fig. 9–38E) or depressed scarred or crusted plaques (see Fig. 9–53). Generalized urticaria may occur and, in our experience as well as in the results of one study, this is more common with food hypersensitivity as the underlying etiology (see Fig. 9–50).[342] Edematous plaques and lymphedema may be present on the extremities or in the groin (see Figs. 9–38H and 9–54). The lesions may or may not be painful. In some animals, widespread erythema that may be purplish or cyanotic occurs. The erythematous skin does not blanch with diascopy, confirming its purpuric nature (Fig. 9–55).[330] Rarely, subcutaneous nodules are noted, which represent panniculitis caused by septal vasculitis.[330, 345] Constitutional signs may be present, including anorexia, depression, and pyrexia. Although extracutaneous signs are uncommon, polyarthropathy, myopathy, neuropathy, hepatopathy, thrombocytopenia, and anemia have been reported in some dogs and cats.[330, 338, 341] Any age, breed, or sex may be affected.

A *proliferative thrombovascular necrosis of the pinnae* has been recognized in dogs.[333, 334] The etiology is unknown, and there are no apparent age, breed, or sex predilections. Lesions begin on the apical margins of the pinnae and spread along the concave surface. An elongated necrotic ulcer is at the center of the lesions. There is often a thickened, scaly, hyperpigmented zone surrounding the ulcers (Fig. 9–56A and B). The

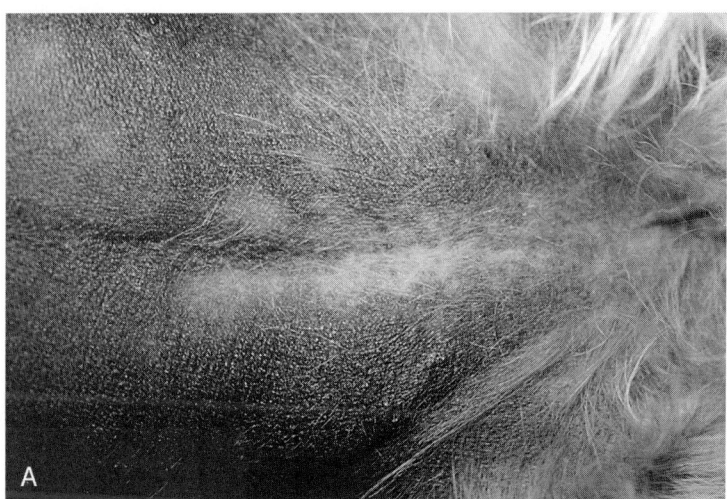
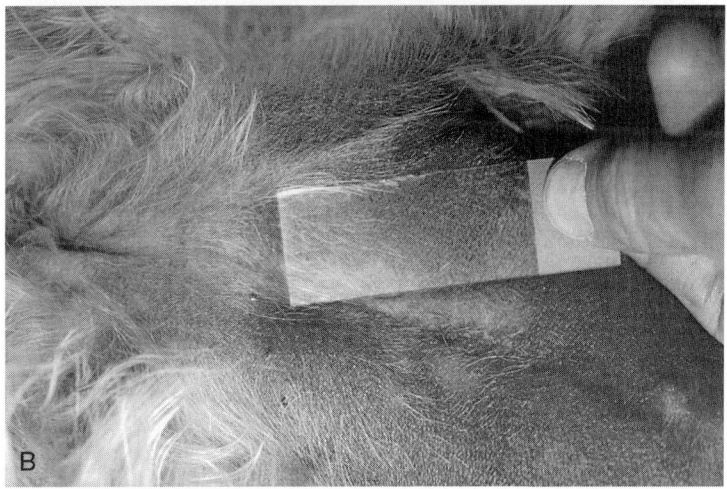

FIGURE 9–55. *A*, Abdomen of dog with drug–induced vasculitis and purpura. *B*, Erythema fails to blanch with diascopy, confirming dermal hemorrhage.

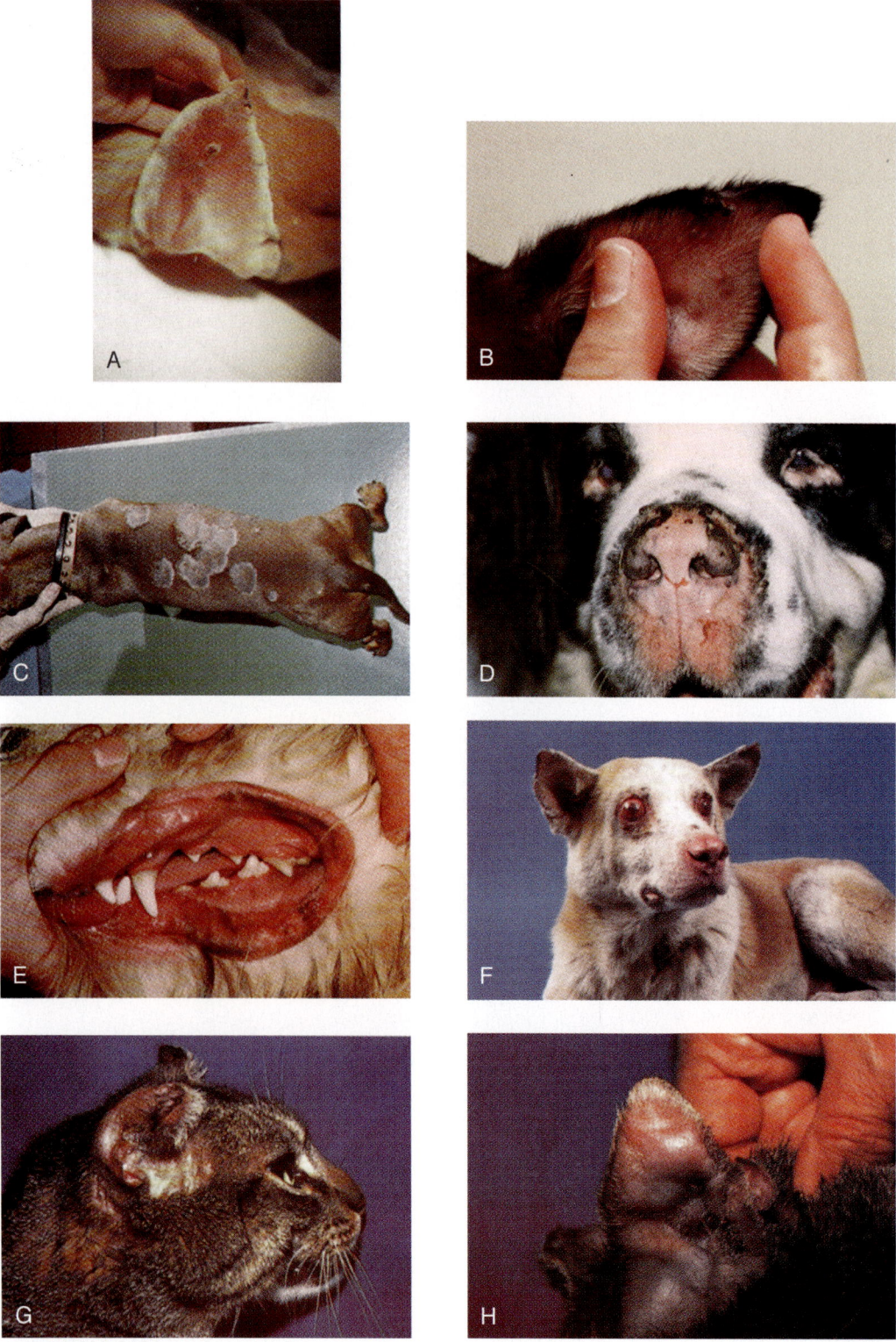

FIGURE 9–56. *A*, Pinnal thrombovascular necrosis with erythema of pinnal apex and linear crust on lateral surface and margin of pinna. *B*, Wedge-shaped hyperpigmented to erythematous plaque with ulceration of pinnal margin in a dog with pinnal thrombovascular necrosis. *C*, Canine linear IgA pustular dermatosis. Annular, coalescing areas of alopecia, scaling, crusting, and hyperpigmentation.

Legend continued on opposite page

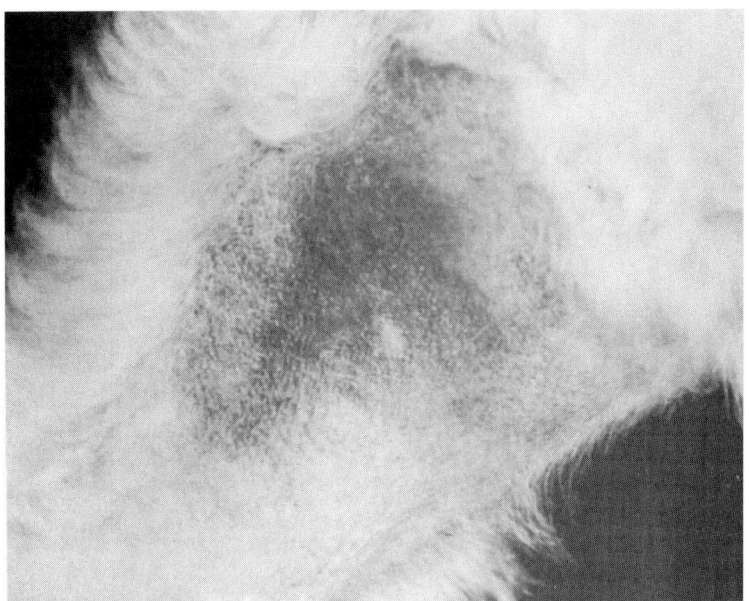

FIGURE 9–57. Alopecic, hyperpigmented plaque on caudomedial thigh of a Poodle due to postvaccinal vasculitis.

lesions are wedge-shaped, with the wide base at the pinnal apex. As the ulcer enlarges, the older areas undergo complete necrosis, resulting in a deformed pinnal margin.

A *focal cutaneous vasculitis and alopecia at the sites of rabies vaccination* has been described in dogs.[22, 253, 270, 327, 351] Poodles and Yorkshire and silky terriers appeared to be predisposed. Reactions were characterized by roughly annular areas of variable alopecia, hyperpigmentation, and, less commonly, scaling or erythema overlying a variably indurated dermis and subcutis. The caudal or lateral thigh, or the withers, are typically affected (Fig. 9–57). The lesions generally appear 3 to 6 months after the subcutaneous administration of vaccine and persist for months to years.

A *cutaneous and renal glomerular vasculopathy* ("Alabama rot," "Greenetrack disease") has been described in kenneled and racing, related and unrelated, Greyhounds (see Chap. 12).[328, 329] No age (6 months to 6 years) or sex predilections exist. Palpable purpura, with lesions pinpoint to 10 cm in diameter, is characterized by reddened areas that rapidly become dark red to purple to black and then slough. Lesions are multiple and most commonly occur on the limbs and, less commonly, the groin and trunk (Figs. 9–58 and 9–59). Within 1 to 2 days, the lesions ulcerate and discharge a serosanguineous fluid. The ulcers are well-demarcated and usually extend into the subcutis. Healing is slow, resulting in scar formation within 1 to 2 months. Many dogs experience pitting edema, especially distal to the stifle or elbow, on limbs that have ulcers. In most dogs, new lesions do not develop after the initial lesions resolve. Some dogs experience pyrexia, lethargy, polydipsia, polyuria, vomiting, dark or tarry stools, and acute renal failure. This syndrome is thought to be produced by verotoxin (shiga-like toxin) elaborated by *E. coli* in contaminated raw beef products (similar to the *hemolytic-uremic syndrome* in people).[329] A genetic predisposition may help explain the susceptibility of Greyhounds.[329]

Familial (autosomal recessive trait) cutaneous vasculopathy of German shepherd dogs

---

FIGURE 9–56. *Continued* D, Canine uveodermatologic syndrome. Depigmentation of nose, muzzle, and periocular skin. E, Canine uveodermatologic syndrome. Depigmentation of lips. F, Uveodermatologic syndrome in an Akita. (From MacDonald JM: Uveodermatologic syndrome in the dog. In: Griffin CE, et al [eds]: Current Veterinary Dermatology. Mosby–Year Book, St. Louis, 1993.) G, Feline auricular chondritis. Swollen, curled, misshapen pinnae. (Courtesy E. Guaguère.) H, Feline auricular chondritis. Swollen, violaceous pinna. (Courtesy E. Guaguère.)

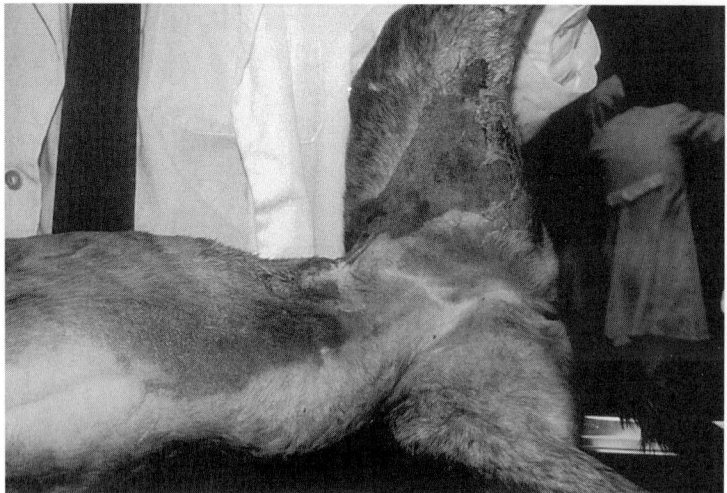

FIGURE 9–58. Cutaneous vasculopathy in a Greyhound. Large area of purpura on ventral abdomen, and well-circumscribed necrosis and ulceration of left medial thigh. (Courtesy B. Fenwick.)

FIGURE 9–59. Cutaneous vasculopathy in a Greyhound. Marked lymphedema of left hind leg, and multifocal necrosis and ulceration of right hind leg. (Courtesy B. Fenwick.)

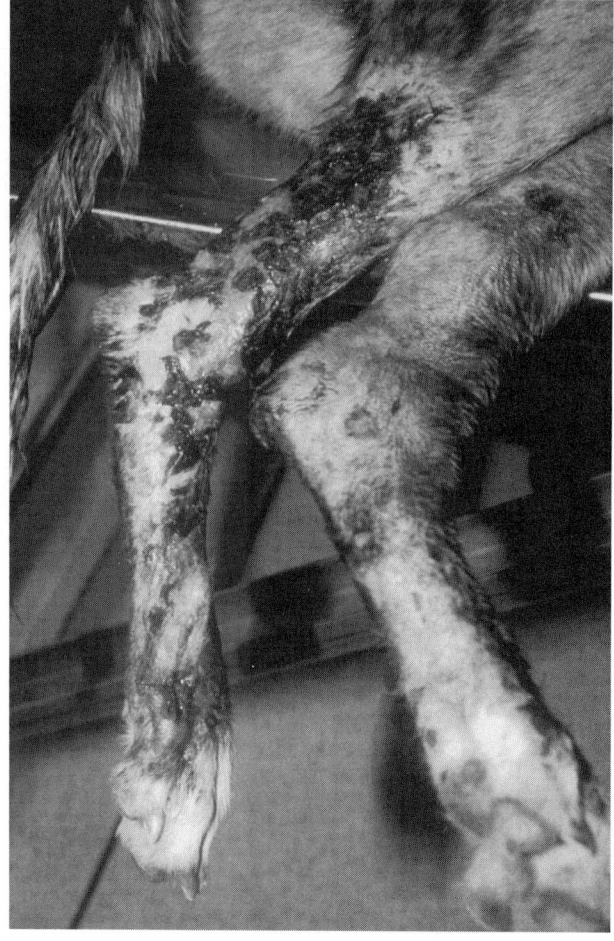

has been reported in young puppies.[350] These dogs experience pyrexia and lethargy, most commonly associated with swollen, depigmented foot pads. Alopecia, crusts, and ulceration may also occur, involving the pinnae, tail, and nasal planum. Footpad biopsies demonstrate varying degrees and combinations of nodular dermatitis, collagenolysis, vascular degeneration, vasculitis, and cell-poor interface dermatitis with basal cell apoptosis. The changes may partly reflect the stage of disease at the time of biopsy. The cause is not determined, though a variety of immunologic test results have been normal.

Ischemic dermatopathy is a syndrome that results from loss of blood supply from either vasculitis or vasculopathy. In some cases, a relationship between vasculitis and vasculopathy is present because both histopathologic lesions may occur in the same case and may reflect stage of lesion development at time of sampling.[72] This syndrome is exemplified by what has been called the prototypical form of ischemic dermatopathy, post-rabies vaccination alopecia.[348] In addition, lesions of canine dermatomyositis are thought to represent ischemic dermatopathy.[72, 332, 348] This has also been proposed for the vascular diseases that are considered cell-poor, such as familial German shepherd vasculopathy, some "lupoid" dermatoses, and the disease in Greyhounds.[72] To date, the reports primarily have been associated with vaccine reactions, with lesions occurring in a wider distribution than just at the site of vaccination.[332, 348] A typical postvaccinal lesion is visible at the site of injection about 2 to 8 months after vaccination, and multiple multifocal lesions develop within 1 to 5 months after the appearance of the injection site lesion. The lesions are various combinations of plaques, nodules, alopecia, scale, erosions, ulcers, crusts, hyperpigmentation, and scarring (see Fig. 9–57). Lesions may occur at the site of vaccination, pinnae (usually the apex and often the concave surface, especially at the pinnal margins), face, paw pads, tip of the tail, periocular region, and over bony prominences. Erosions and ulcers may be seen on the tongue. An associated ischemic, atrophic myopathy may be present.

DIAGNOSIS

The differential diagnosis includes coagulopathy, systemic lupus erythematosus, cold agglutinin disease, frostbite, disseminated intravascular coagulation, and lymphoreticular neoplasia. When urticarial lesions predominate, hypersensitivity disorders not associated with vasculitis are also differential diagnoses. Definitive diagnosis is based on history, physical examination, and skin biopsy. Histopathology reveals varying degrees of neutrophilic, eosinophilic, or lymphocytic vasculitis (Fig. 9–60), possibly reflecting the age of the lesions and the types of immunoreactants.[22, 71] Fibrinoid necrosis is not usually present.[47, 348] Involvement of deep dermal vessels may suggest systemic disease.

When the deep vasculature is affected, necrosis of appendages and subcutaneous fat may occur. The lesions most likely to show diagnostic changes are those from 8 to 24 hours old. In some biopsies, the diagnosis of vasculitis or vasculopathy is suspected on the basis of a cell-poor hydropic interface dermatitis, mural folliculitis, and the loss of definition and staining intensity and ultimate atrophy or necrosis of hair follicles ("fading follicles") (Fig. 9–61). Sebaceous and sweat glands may be similarly, but less frequently, affected. Hyalinization of dermal collagen and hypovascularity as demonstrated by decreased factor VIII staining of blood vessels may be present.[348] Once the diagnosis of cutaneous vasculitis has been established, it is imperative that underlying etiologic factors be sought and eliminated (Table 9–10).

Cutaneous vasculitis has been reported in dogs with bacteremia, systemic lupus erythematosus, rheumatoid arthritis, polyarteritis nodosa, Rocky Mountain spotted fever, ehrlichiosis, babesiosis, leishmaniasis, sarcocystosis, parvovirus and coronavirus infections, drug reactions, vaccine reactions, staphylococcal hypersensitivity, and as an idiopathic occurrence.[47, 56, 330, 335, 341] In addition, lymphocytic or eosinophilic vasculitis has been recognized in dogs with drug reaction, severe scabies and flea bite hypersensitivity, food hypersensitivity, and arthropod bites/stings.[47, 72, 342] In cats, cutaneous vasculitis has been associated with drug administration, vaccination (rabies, herpes virus-calicivirus-panleukopenia), infections (FeLV, FIV, FIP), and idiopathy.[335, 338, 341]

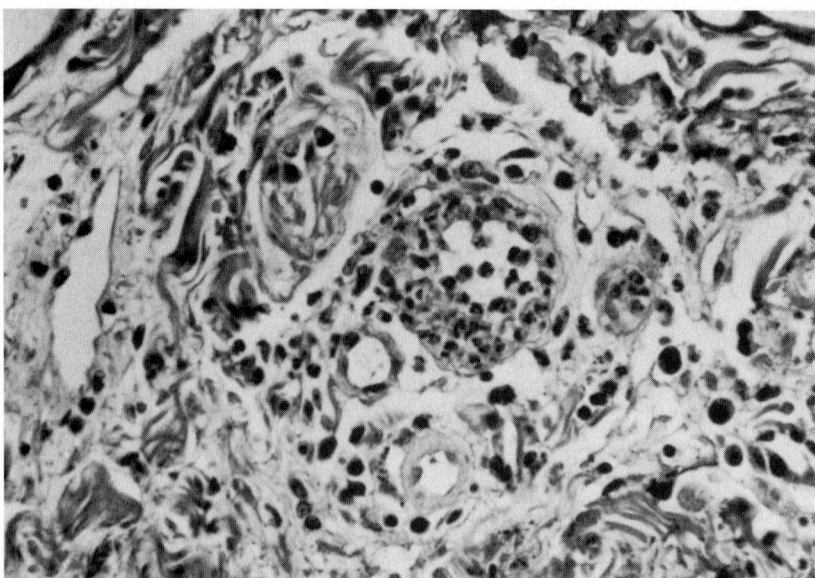

FIGURE 9–60. Canine cutaneous idiopathic leukocytoclastic vasculitis. Degeneration of blood vessel wall with leukocyclasis and "nuclear dust" formation. (From Manning TO, Scott DW: Cutaneous vasculitis in a dog. J Am Anim Hosp Assoc 16:61, 1980.)

Proliferative thrombovascular necrosis of the pinnae is characterized by arteriolar proliferation, sclerosis, hyaline degeneration, and eventually thrombosis.[333] No inflammatory vasculitis is present. *Focal vasculitis and alopecia subsequent to rabies vaccination* is characterized by vasculitis affecting the arterioles of the deep dermis and subcutis, septal panniculitis, fat necrosis, focal lymphoid nodules, and marked atrophy or necrosis of the overlying adnexa (see Fig. 9–61; Figs. 9–62 and 9–63).[341]

Cutaneous and renal glomerular vasculopathy is characterized by mild to severe changes in the arterioles and arteries of the deep dermis and subcutis.[328] These changes range from increased eosinophilia of the tunica media to pyknosis and karyorrhexis and, occasionally, fibrinoid necrosis. Vascular thrombosis and ischemia result in purpura and cutaneous infarcts. Many affected Greyhounds, especially those with azotemia, have thrombocytopenia, normocytic normochromic anemia, hypoalbuminemia, and increased serum creatine kinase activity.[329]

Direct immunofluorescence or immunohistochemical testing may demonstrate immunoglobulin, complement, or both in vessel walls and occasionally at the basement membrane zone in both the neutrophilic and lymphocytic forms of cutaneous vasculitis (see Fig. 9–1D).[5, 18, 56] In humans, the most common immunoreactants are C3, IgM, and fibrin in a granular pattern within the vessel wall.[341] These tests are usually not needed, however, and are not particularly useful for diagnosis. If they are performed, they are best done within the first 4 hours after lesion formation and no later than 24 hours.[47, 341] Studies in humans have shown that the intradermal injection of 0.02 ml of a histamine phosphate solution into the skin of patients with active cutaneous vasculitis was a reliable method for demonstrating the deposition of immunoreactants, with direct immunofluorescence testing of the injection site performed 4 hours after injection.[5]

Dogs with active vasculitis may have increased levels of circulating immune complexes, decreased levels of serum complement, and hypergammaglobulinemia.[47]

CLINICAL MANAGEMENT

It is difficult to predict the course of the disease in any individual case. A single episode lasting a few weeks may occur, or the disorder may be chronic or recurrent. The outcome

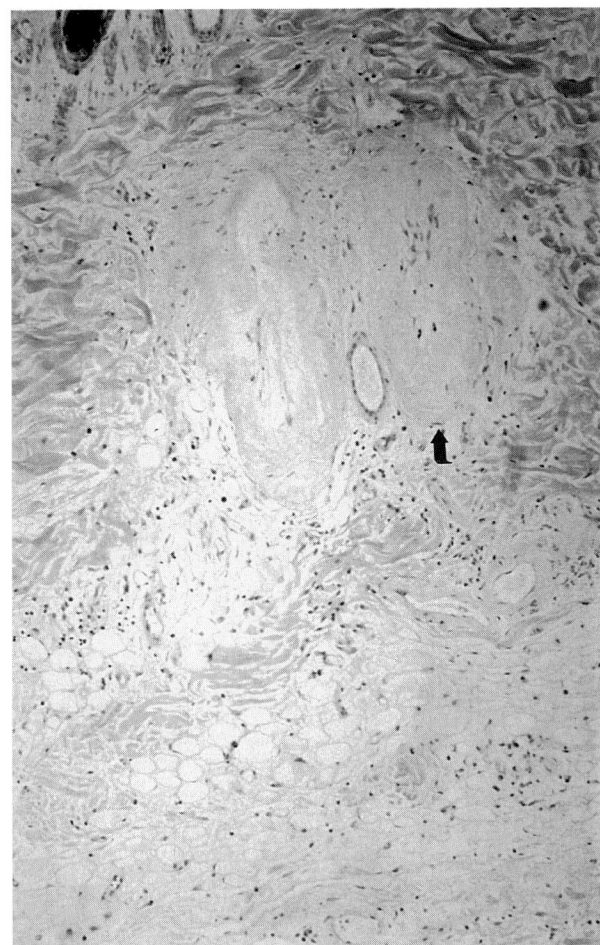

FIGURE 9–61. Rabies vaccine–induced vasculitis in a dog. Ischemic necrosis of hair follicles ("fading follicles") (*arrow*) with subjacent panniculitis.

depends on the extent of internal organ involvement (especially renal and neurologic) and the underlying or precipitating factor(s).

Treatment of vasculitis consists of correction of the underling cause and immunomodulatory drug treatment.[18, 56] In less severe cases, initial therapy with pentoxifylline is indicated because of its relative lack of side effects and some reports of success (see Chap. 3).[342, 348] Pentoxifylline was apparently effective in four of seven rabies vaccine–associated vasculitides (which required 2 to 5 months of therapy) but was of no benefit in leukocytoclastic vasculitides.[342, 348] In more severe cases of vasculitis, especially neutrophilic types, systemic prednisone or prednisolone (2 to 4 mg/kg orally q24h) is initially used, with or without pentoxifylline.[47, 330, 338] For cases that are refractory to glucocorticoids, sulfones such as dapsone (1 mg/kg orally q8h in dogs; 1 mg/kg orally q24h with caution in cats) or sulfasalazine (20 to 40 mg/kg orally q8h in dogs) may be effective.[47, 340, 341, 343] The combination of glucocorticoid and dapsone may be synergistic.[343] Large doses of vitamin E may be a useful adjunctive therapy.[341, 343] Cyclophosphamide has been useful in some patients,[47] and colchicine is often beneficial in humans.[18] Azathioprine has been effective in some dogs, as has the combination of tetracycline and niacinamide.[341] In some cases, therapy can be stopped after 4 to 6 months of treatment. Other patients require long-term maintenance therapy with lower drug doses and reduced frequency of administration (see Chap. 3). The vasculitis occurring with itraconazole therapy can often be eliminated by reducing the dose from 10 mg/kg/day to 5 mg/kg/day (see Chap. 5).

Table 9–10 ETIOLOGIC FACTORS FOR CUTANEOUS VASCULITIS

Infections
Bacterial
Mycobacterial
Fungal
Viral
Protozoal
Rickettsial

Injections of Foreign Proteins
Sera
Vaccines
Hyposensitization

Drugs
Antibiotics
Ivermectin
Vaccines
Metronidazole
Phenobarbital
Furosemide
Itraconazole
Phenylbutazone
Enalapril
Imodium
Metoclopramide
Fenbendazole

Allergy
Food
Insect/arthropod

Genetic
Hereditary pyogranuloma and vasculitis of Scottish terriers
Cutaneous and renal vasculopathy of Greyhounds
Familial vasculopathy of German shepherd dogs and Jack Russell terriers
Dermatomyositis

Immune-Mediated Diseases
Systemic lupus erythematosus
Discoid lupus erythematosus
Rheumatoid arthritis

Other Diseases
Plasma cell pododermatitis
Malignancies
Ulcerative colitis
Juvenile polyarteritis in beagle dogs

Proliferative thrombovascular necrosis of the pinnae is slowly progressive and usually unresponsive to all medical therapies that have been tried.[333] Anecdotal reports suggest that pentoxifylline or the combination of tetracycline and niacinamide are occasionally effective.[341] In our experience, pentoxifylline has been helpful to totally successful in thrombotic pinnal diseases, possibly through its effect of increasing peripheral perfusion and/or its anti-inflammatory effects.

If pentoxifylline is ineffective, the treatment of choice is partial surgical removal of the pinna. Relapses have occurred only when attempts were made to save as much tissue as possible. *Focal cutaneous vasculitis and alopecia subsequent to injections* may also respond (up to 75% reduction in lesion size) to pentoxifylline or may be treated by complete surgical excision, or it occasionally spontaneously resolves.[327, 348] It would be logical to *not* repeat the incriminated vaccine, unless required by law.[327, 341] One could

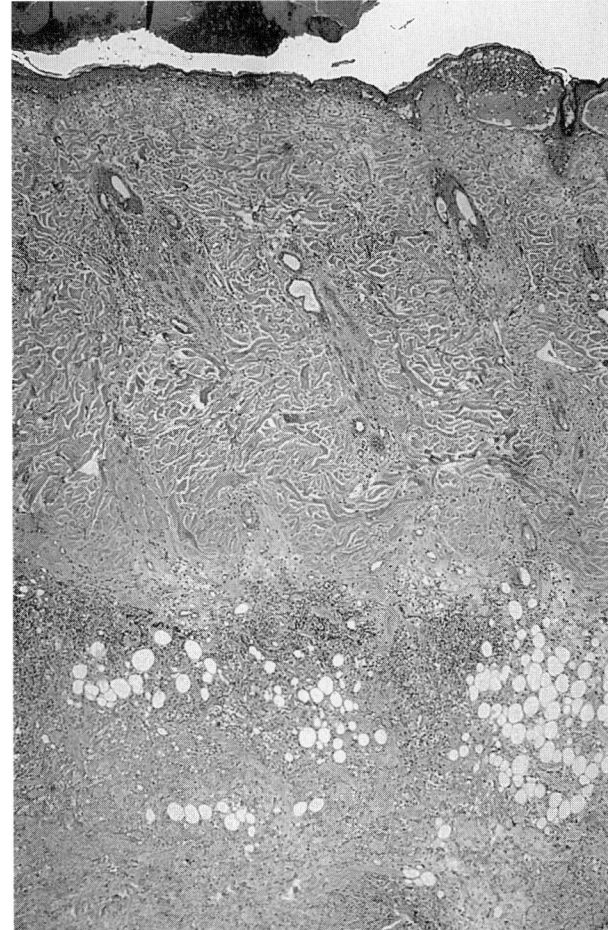

FIGURE 9-62. Rabies vaccine–induced vasculitis in a dog. Panniculitis with atrophied hair follicles and hydropic interface dermatitis.

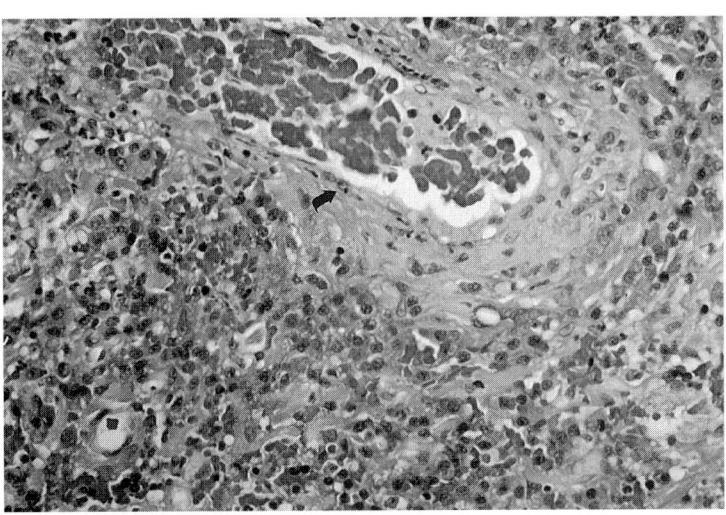

FIGURE 9-63. Rabies vaccine–induced vasculitis in a dog. Note karyorrhectic leukocytes within vessel wall (*arrow*).

avoid the local vaccine reaction by giving the product intramuscularly, but generalized reactions would still be possible.[327]

Canine Linear IgA Pustular Dermatosis

Linear IgA pustular dermatosis is a very rare idiopathic, sterile superficial pustular dermatosis of Dachshunds, characterized histologically by subcorneal pustules and immunologically by the deposition of IgA at the basement membrane zone of affected skin.[56, 352] It is not analogous to a similarly named dermatosis of humans.[5, 18]

Clinically, linear IgA pustular dermatosis is characterized by multifocal to generalized pustular dermatitis. The trunk is typically involved. Secondary skin lesions include annular areas of alopecia, erosion, epidermal collarettes, hyperpigmentation, scaling, and crusting (see Fig. 9–56C). Pruritus is minimal to absent, and the dogs are otherwise healthy. All cases to date have been recognized in adult Dachshunds of either sex.

The differential diagnosis includes bacterial folliculitis, dermatophytosis, demodicosis, pemphigus foliaceus, and subcorneal pustular dermatosis. Cytologic examination of pus reveals nondegenerate neutrophils, no microorganisms, and an occasional or no acantholytic keratinocytes. Diagnosis is based on culture (negative) and skin biopsy (intraepidermal pustular dermatitis, with numerous nondegenerate neutrophils and minimal acantholysis) (Fig. 9–64), and direct immunofluorescence or immunohistochemical testing (IgA deposited at the basement membrane zone).

Therapy consists of large doses of prednisolone or prednisone (2.2 to 4.4 mg/kg orally q24h, then an alternate-day regimen) or dapsone (1 mg/kg orally q8h, then as needed) (see Chap. 3). Interestingly, glucocorticoids may work in one case and not another. The same is true of dapsone.

Canine Uveodermatologic Syndrome

The uveodermatologic syndrome (Vogt-Koyanagi-Harada–like syndrome) is a rare, idiopathic syndrome of concurrent granulomatous uveitis and depigmenting dermatitis in dogs.[361, 364]

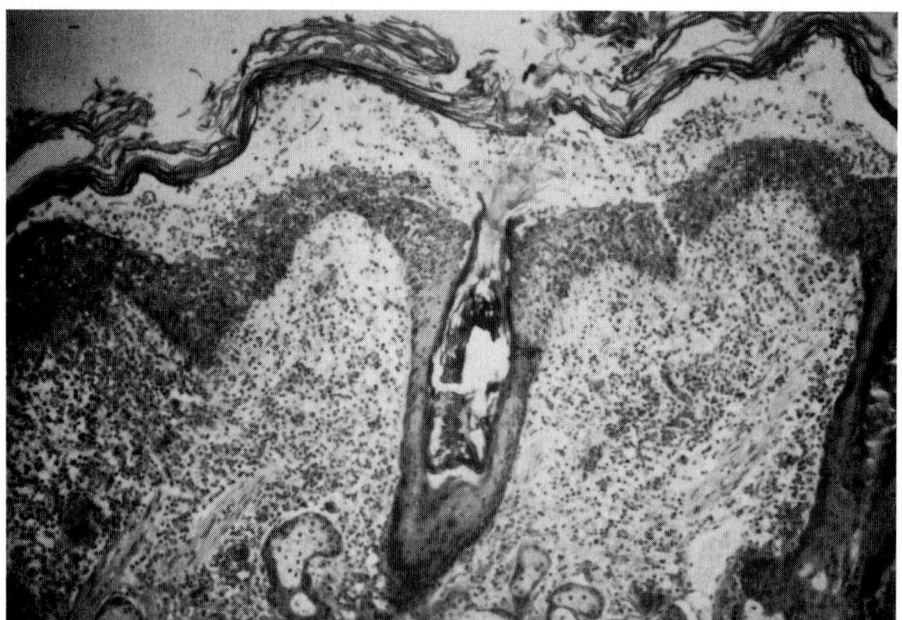

FIGURE 9–64. Canine linear IgA pustular dermatosis. Subcorneal pustular dermatitis.

CAUSE AND PATHOGENESIS

The cause of this syndrome is unknown. The syndrome has similarities to the Vogt-Koyanagi-Harada syndrome in humans, which is currently thought to represent an autoimmune disorder.[18, 353, 356, 358, 359, 364] In humans, cell-mediated hypersensitivity to melanin and melanocytes has been demonstrated, as have antibodies against melanin, gangliosides, and photoreceptors.[364] Antiretinal antibodies were demonstrated in a dog.[360]

CLINICAL FEATURES

In humans, the Vogt-Koyanagi-Harada syndrome has three phases: (1) a *meningoencephalitic* phase with prodromata of fever, malaise, headache, tinnitus, nausea, and vomiting, (2) an *ophthalmic* phase with photophobia, uveitis, decreased visual acuity, and potential blindness, and (3) a *dermatologic* phase with poliosis (90% of cases), alopecia (73%), and vitiligo (63%).[18, 364] The dermatologic signs are usually symmetric, especially involving the head, neck, and eyelids, and they usually mark the convalescent stage when the uveitis begins to abate. The pigmentary changes tend to be permanent.

In dogs, there are no apparent age (6 months to 13 years) or sex predilections, but Akitas, Chows, Samoyeds, and Siberian huskies appear to be predisposed.[352, 356, 358, 359, 361, 364] The syndrome is usually characterized by the acute onset of uveitis and concurrent or subsequent depigmentation of the nose, lips, eyelids, and occasionally the footpads, scrotum, prepuce, anus, and hard palate (see Fig. 9–56D to F). The cutaneous lesions usually appear within 10 days of the recognition of the ocular lesions, but they occasionally occur several months later.[364]

In one dog, a concurrent onychomadesis was present.[362] Oral ulcerations rarely occur.[358, 363] In most cases, skin lesions are mild, consisting of well-demarcated depigmentation with or without mild erythema and scale. Some cases, however, progress or even rapidly develop more marked dermatitis, with depigmented areas developing varying degrees of erosion, ulceration, and crusting. Perhaps some of the dermatitis may be associated with exposure to sunlight (photodermatitis).[47] Patchy leukotrichia may be present in the areas surrounding the cutaneous depigmentation. Rarely, leukoderma and leukotrichia are widespread.[354, 355, 361] Clinicopathologic evidence of a meningoencephalitic phase is rare in dogs, though one case with second cranial nerve deficits was reported.[357, 364] Clinical signs referable to the uveitis (anterior and posterior) may include photophobia, blepharospasm, lacrimation, conjunctival congestion, corneal edema, retinal detachment, glaucoma, cataract, and blindness.[364]

DIAGNOSIS

The definitive diagnosis is based on history, physical examination, and skin biopsy. Histopathologic findings in specimens taken from early skin lesions are characterized by lichenoid interface dermatitis, wherein large histiocytes are a major cellular component (Figs. 9–65 and 9–66).[22, 56, 71, 364] Pigmentary incontinence is pronounced, but hydropic degeneration of epidermal basal cells is rare. Cytology of aqueous humor in one case revealed an infiltrate of predominantly macrophages.[357] Histopathologic findings in the eye include granulomatous panuveitis and retinitis, and degenerative changes of the optic nerve and tract may occur.[364] Results of direct and indirect immunofluorescence testing are usually negative.[56]

CLINICAL MANAGEMENT

Patients with poorly controlled uveitis often experience posterior synechiae with secondary glaucoma, cataracts, and vision loss. Thus, aggressive early treatment is essential. Topical or subconjunctival glucocorticoids and topical cycloplegics (e.g., atropine) are beneficial in patients with anterior uveitis. Systemic glucocorticoids and azathioprine are needed to combat posterior uveitis and dermatologic signs.[359, 363] Topical cyclosporine was useful in

758 • Immune-Mediated Disorders

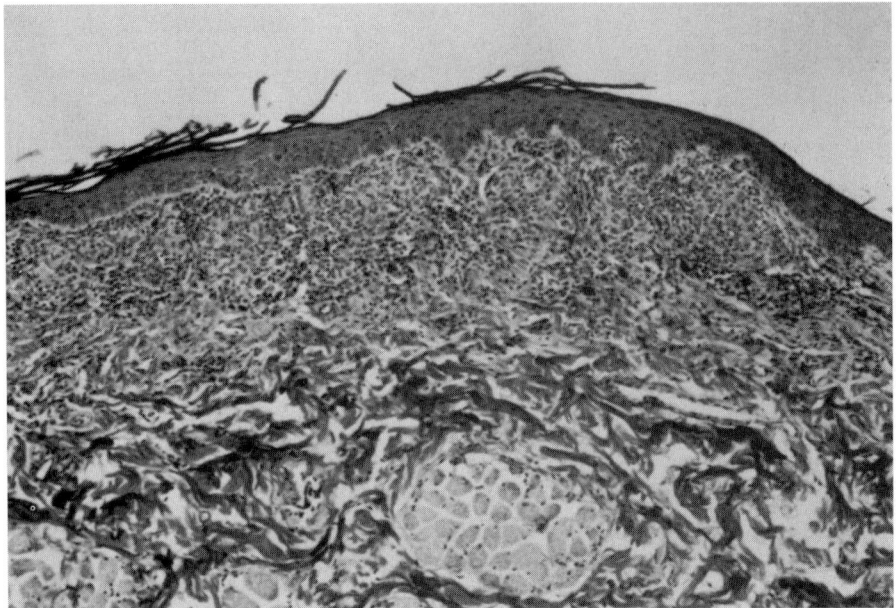

FIGURE 9–65. Canine uveodermatologic syndrome. Lichenoid interface dermatitis.

one dog.[361] If the disease is treated early, variable degrees of cutaneous repigmentation (sometimes complete) usually occur.[355, 361] Occasionally, these cases may respond to systemic glucocorticoids alone, but because blindness may result from delaying an effective therapy and because more aggressive therapy is often required, we recommend combination immunosuppressive therapy.[361]

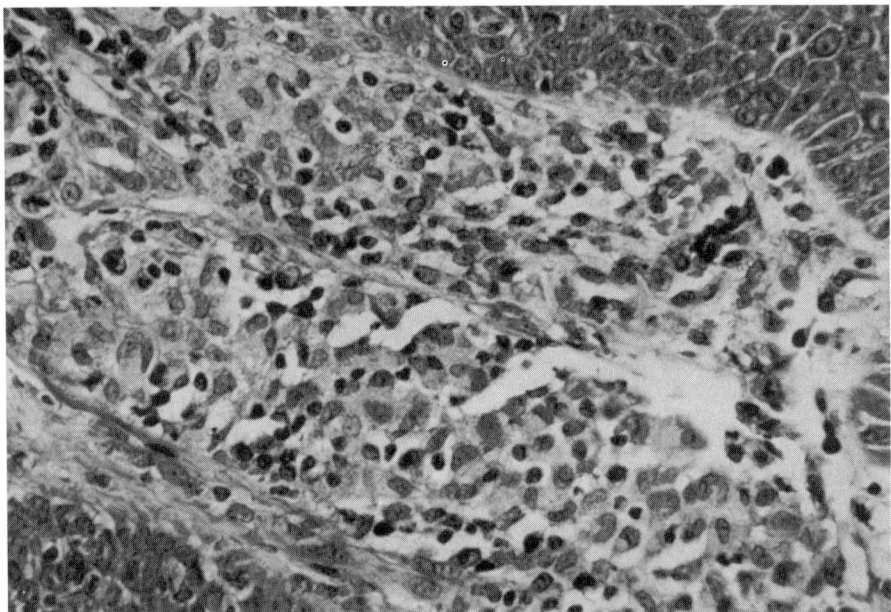

FIGURE 9–66. Close-up of Figure 9–65. Numerous histiocytes in lichenoid band.

Dogs usually require long-term alternate-morning oral glucocorticoid therapy (e.g., 0.25 to 1.1 mg/kg prednisone or prednisolone) to prevent recurrence.[56] We have seen some very good responses with the combination of tetracycline and niacinamide (see Chap. 3). This drug combination has allowed marked reduction in or discontinuation of systemic glucocorticoid therapy. The response of the skin lesions should not be used to assess response to therapy because uveitis may be active while the skin is improving.[356] Ophthalmic examinations should be periodically performed even when the cutaneous changes are in remission.

Auricular Chondritis

Auricular chondritis ("relapsing polychondritis") is a rare disease of cats and dogs characterized by inflammation and destruction of auricular cartilage.[18, 53, 368, 369] In humans, a somewhat similar condition is called *relapsing polychondritis*.[18] However, in cats, only the auricular cartilage is affected, and the condition has not been reported to have a relapsing nature. Hence, in cats, the term *relapsing polychondritis* is presently inappropriate.[371]

CAUSE AND PATHOGENESIS

Relapsing polychondritis is often classified among the immune-mediated diseases because of similarities to rheumatoid arthritis and lupus erythematosus as well as its favorable response to immunomodulatory therapy. In humans, antibodies against Type II collagen may be demonstrated in some cases.[18] In one dog, a definitive cause was not determined, though chronic otitis preceded the development of the auricular chondritis.[366]

CLINICAL FEATURES

Affected cats and the one dog presented with a history of swollen, erythematous, painful ears.[54, 366-368] When examined, the pinnae are swollen and meaty, erythematous to violaceous, and curled and deformed (see Fig. 9–56G and H; Fig. 9–67). Typically, both pinnae are affected, although one may be more severely affected than the other, or the condition may be initially unilateral, then bilateral.[365] Cats may be otherwise healthy or may show signs of pyrexia, lethargy, and anorexia. In cats, no age (1 to 14 years), sex, or breed predilections are evident.[365] The dog had a history of nonerosive polyarthritis and laxity of digital and carpal joints as well as otitis prior to the development of auricular chondritis.

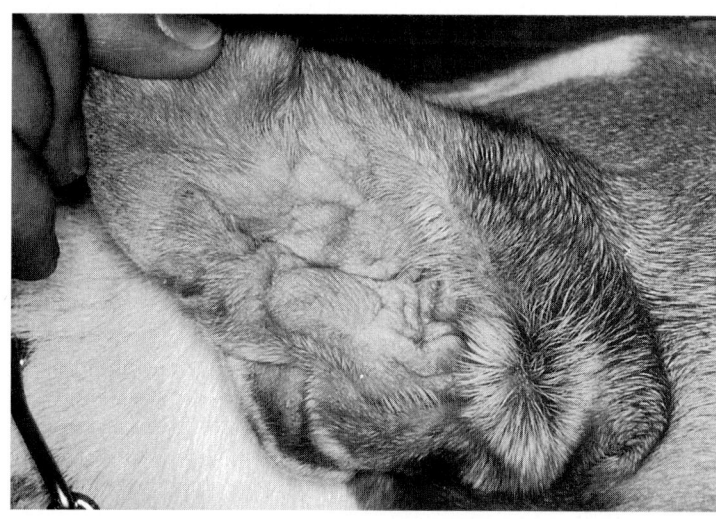

FIGURE 9–67. Auricular chondritis in a dog with suspect polychondritis.

DIAGNOSIS

Biopsies reveal lymphoplasmacytic inflammation, loss of cartilage basophilia, and cartilage necrosis (Fig. 9–68).[47, 365] Hematologic examinations may demonstrate variable degrees of neutrophilia, lymphocytosis, and hyperglobulinemia.[365] One cat was positive for ANA but also had concurrent FIV infection.[368] Direct immunofluorescence testing was negative in two cats.[371]

CLINICAL MANAGEMENT

Cats that are in no pain and show no systemic signs may do fine without therapy. Systemic glucocorticoids were ineffective in eight cats.[371, 375] Dapsone (1 mg/kg q24h) induced a remission in four cats, and no relapse occurred when therapy was stopped.[365, 368] Permanent deformity of the pinnae is to be expected, whether or not the cat is treated. Surgical excision was effective in eliminating the discomfort and gross lesions in the one dog.[365]

Immunoproliferative Enteropathy of Basenji Dogs

Immunoproliferative enteropathy of Basenjis is characterized by chronic intractable diarrhea, progressive emaciation, and gastropathy.[47, 370] An autosomal recessive inheritance of the condition has been hypothesized. A similar disease exists in humans.

Basenjis of either sex and a wide age range are affected. Skin lesions are variable and may consist of alopecia, hyperpigmentation, hyperkeratosis, and marginal necrosis and ulceration of the pinnae or a symmetric alopecia of the ventrum. The haircoat is often dry and dull.

Diagnosis is based on history, physical examination, and laboratory testing. Most affected dogs have hypergammaglobulinemia. Some dogs are hypothyroid. Intestinal biopsy reveals lymphoplasmacytic enteritis.

Dermatohistopathologic findings are nondiagnostic. Alopecic skin is characterized by endocrinopathic changes, probably reflecting hypothyroidism. Dermatitic pinnae are characterized by ulcerative perivascular dermatitis, necrosis, and changes consistent with secondary bacterial infection. Although the clinical appearance of the pinnae is suggestive of a vasculopathy, histologic evidence of vessel disease has not been reported.

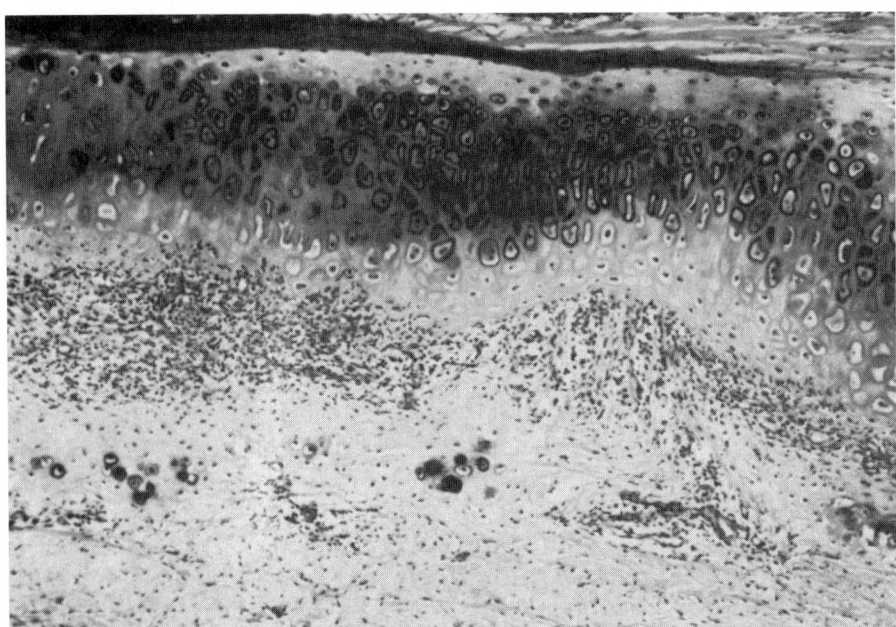

FIGURE 9–68. Feline auricular chondritis. Inflammation and necrosis of ear cartilage.

Therapy is provided according to symptoms and is often disappointing. Genetic counseling, avoidance of stress, and high-quality commercial diets are indicated. Systemic glucocorticoids may be beneficial.

Alopecia Areata

Alopecia areata is an uncommon disorder of dogs and cats characterized by patches of nonscarring hair loss that grossly is noninflammatory.

CAUSE AND PATHOGENESIS

Alopecia areata is of complex pathogenesis with immunologic targeting of anagen hair follicles and the relatively consistent finding of antifollicular autoantibodies (IgG class) as well as CD4+ and CD8+ cells in the affected follicles in humans.[373] T lymphocytes and antifollicular antibodies have also been documented in the dog.[374] In dogs, autoantibodies are directed against trichohyalin, inner root sheath, and hair matrix antigens.[373, 375, 376] This is different from the findings in humans and mice, wherein the outer root sheath and hair matrix are most often targeted.[373] CD4+ and CD8+ perifollicular lymphocytes and $\alpha\beta$, CD8+ intrabulbar T cells have been described in dogs.[373, 374] In addition, many CD1+ dendritic antigen-presenting cells are present in the perifollicular dermis.[373]

Other observations in humans supporting the immunologic basis are (1) accumulations of lymphoid cells (helper T cells) around hair bulbs during the active phase of the disease, (2) occasional association of alopecia areata with other immune-mediated diseases, (3) increased incidence of various autoantibodies in alopecia areata, (4) decreased numbers of circulating T cells, (5) abnormal presence of Langerhans' cells in the follicular bulb, (6) increased expression of class I and II MHC antigens (7) the deposition of C3 or IgG and IgM or both at the basement membrane zone of the hair follicles in lesional and normal scalp as revealed by direct immunofluorescence testing, and (8) the therapeutic benefit of inducing delayed-type hypersensitivity and immunosuppressive therapies. In addition, genetic, endocrine, and psychological factors have been thought to play a role in humans with alopecia areata.[18, 373] Morphologic abnormalities of melanocytes in follicular bulbs have been described in humans with alopecia areata. Cytokines IL-1α, IL-1β, and TNF-α are potent inhibitors of hair follicle growth and in vitro produce changes in hair follicle morphology similar to those in alopecia areata.[372a]

CLINICAL FEATURES

In dogs and cats, alopecia areata is characterized by focal or multifocal patches of asymptomatic, noninflammatory alopecia.[22, 47, 373] There are no apparent age or sex predilections. Though few cases have been reported, the Dachshund may be over-represented.[373] The alopecic areas are well circumscribed, and the exposed skin appears normal (Fig. 9–69). Chronically alopecic areas may become variably hyperpigmented.

Lesions may occur anywhere, especially the head, neck, and trunk. Lesions may be solitary or numerous and may be asymmetric or symmetric. Rarely, alopecia progresses to involve the majority of the body (Fig. 9–70). Hair growth may occur spontaneously, with the initially regrown hair being white, only to later be replaced by pigmented hair (Fig. 9–71).[373] Microscopic examination of hairs plucked from the margin of enlarging lesions reveals a mixture of normal telogen, dysplastic, and "exclamation point" hairs—short, stubby hairs with frayed, fractured, pigmented distal ends whose shafts undulate or taper toward the proximal end (Fig. 9–72). Occasionally, alopecia areata may be confined to the dark-haired areas of multicolored haircoats (Fig. 9–73). Claw changes compatible with trachyonychia (roughening, ridging, vertical striations) were seen in one dog and were compared to those occasionally occurring in humans with alopecia areata.[371]

DIAGNOSIS

The differential diagnosis includes traction alopecia, injection reactions, acquired pattern alopecia, topical steroid reaction, follicular dysplasia, dermatophytosis, demodicosis, staphy-

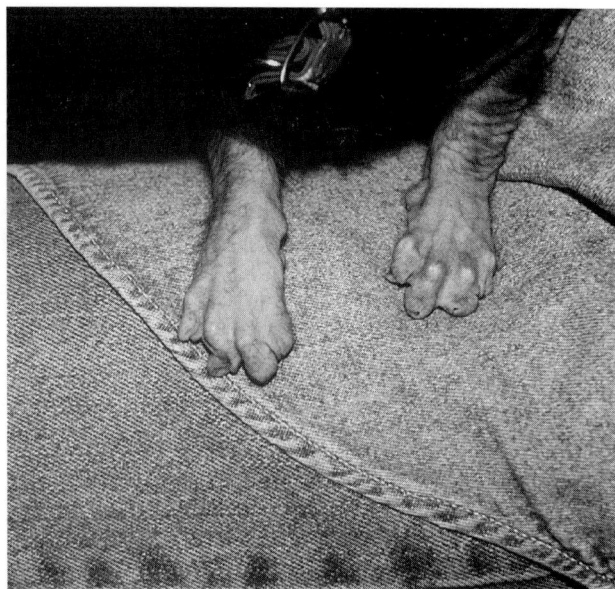

FIGURE 9–76. Same cat as in Figure 9–75. Alopecia of front legs. Note all claws have sloughed.

HISTOPATHOLOGY

The characteristic early histopathologic findings include a variably severe accumulation of lymphocytes, histiocytes, and fewer plasma cells that is most intense at the follicular isthmus (Fig. 9–77).[377, 378] In cats, small numbers of neutrophils and eosinophils may also be present. In early lesions, inflammation is marked, atrophic changes are mild to absent, and sebaceous glands are present. In late lesions, atrophic changes are severe, inflammation is mild, and sebaceous glands are often absent.

CLINICAL MANAGEMENT

This condition has failed to respond to topical and systemic glucocorticoids as well as chlorambucil.[377, 379] In cats, anecdotal reports indicate that cyclosporine may be effective.[379] Spontaneous remission has not been reported.

Amyloidosis

Amyloidosis is a generic term that signifies the abnormal extracellular deposition of one of a family of unrelated proteins that share certain characteristic staining properties and ultrastructural features.[12, 18, 381, 389] Amyloidosis is not a single disease entity, and amyloid may accumulate as a result of a variety of different pathogenetic mechanisms. In the dog and cat, most cases of amyloidosis are related to deposition of immunoglobulin light chains.[22, 25, 386]

CAUSE AND PATHOGENESIS

Different amino acid compositions of amyloid may occur.[385, 389] Amyloid deposits contain a nonfibrillar protein called amyloid-P, which is identical to a normal circulating plasma globulin known as serum amyloid-P (an elastase inhibitor that may help protect amyloid deposits from degradation and phagocytosis). Primary and myeloma-associated systemic amyloidosis have immunoglobulin light chains (mostly the lambda type) as precursors to the amyloid fibril protein, which is called *amyloid-L*. In secondary systemic amyloidosis

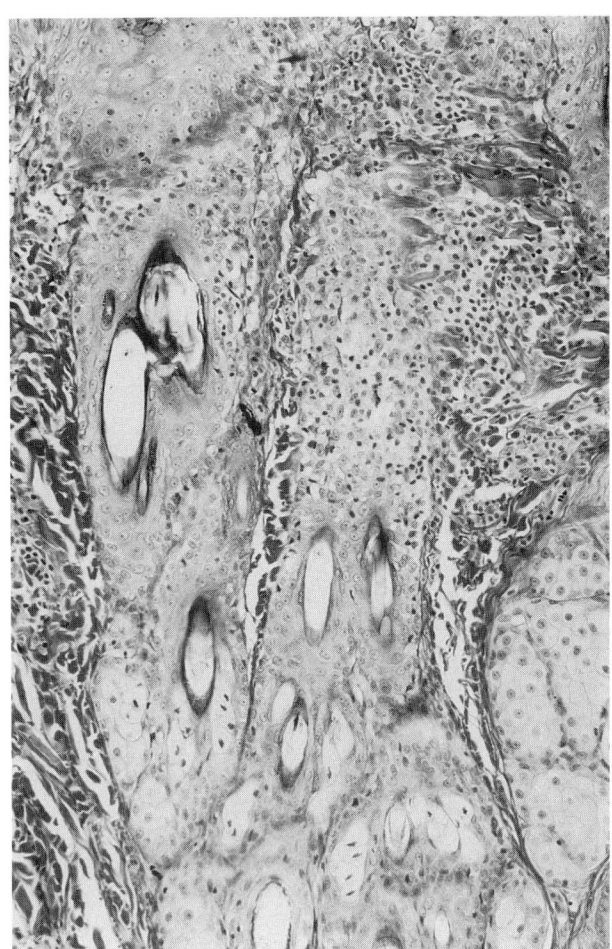

FIGURE 9–77. Same cat as in Figures 9–75 and 9–76. Note mural lymphocytic folliculitis.

(associated with chronic inflammation), a serum precursor protein, serum amyloid-A (a high-density lipoprotein and acute-phase reactant), forms the fibrils in the amyloid deposits. Serum amyloid-A is thought to be cleaved proteolytically by macrophages to amyloid-A and excreted extracellularly.

Although the pathogenesis of amyloidosis is unclear, it is morphologically related to cells of the mononuclear phagocytic system, plasma cells, and keratinocytes. Functional studies suggest that such cells play at least a partial role in the genesis of amyloidosis. Ultimately, amyloid deposits lead to changes in tissue architecture and function. In dogs and cats, amyloidosis is usually associated with chronic inflammatory disease, neoplasia, and accumulations of plasma cells.[22, 25, 381, 386] It has also been associated with a vasculitic syndrome.[387] It has also been suggested that vaccination reactions caused polyarthritis in 12 Akitas, 33% of which progressed to renal amyloidosis.[389] A familial tendency has been detected in Chinese Shar pei and beagle dogs and in Abyssinian and Siamese cats.[381, 382, 385, 387]

CLINICAL FEATURES

Most commonly, amyloidosis is an internal disease, usually affecting the kidneys, spleen, and liver, with death often resulting from the renal involvement.[25, 381] Cutaneous lesions are described in dogs with systemic amyloidosis and primary cutaneous disease.[22] Cutane-

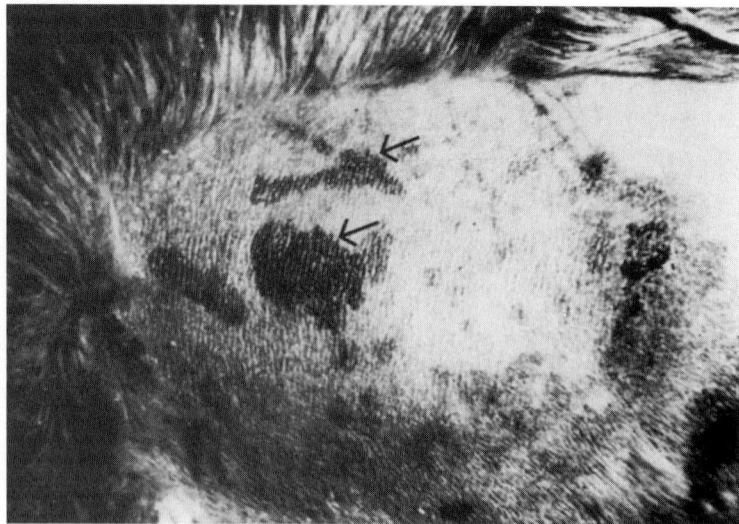

FIGURE 9–78. Canine cutaneous amyloidosis. Ecchymoses produced by traumatizing the skin (pinch purpura) (*arrows*). (Courtesy R. M. Schwartzman.)

ous lesions with systemic amyloidosis associated with a monoclonal gammopathy was reported in an adult female Cocker spaniel.[388] Cutaneous hemorrhage could be induced by flicking the abdominal skin briskly with a finger or by removing hair (Fig. 9–78). If the skin was traumatized severely, blood oozed through the skin within seconds and clotted immediately. Skin biopsy revealed an amorphous, homogeneous, eosinophilic superficial dermis. The walls of the blood vessels in the involved area were thickened by deposition of the homogeneous eosinophilic material (Fig. 9–79). The material was Congo red–positive (congophilia), and a green birefringence of the material was visible in Congo red–stained sections examined with polarized light (dichroism). A monoclonal serum IgG paraprotein was found. No treatment was given, and the dog remained unchanged for 14 months.

Mucocutaneous amyloidosis unassociated with monoclonal gammopathy was reported in a 3-year-old Brittany spaniel.[380] The dog had multiple, whitish to ulcerated papular and plaquelike lesions on the tongue and gingiva as well as oozing ulcers on the footpads, ventral surface of the interdigital spaces, and multiple pressure points (elbows, stifles).

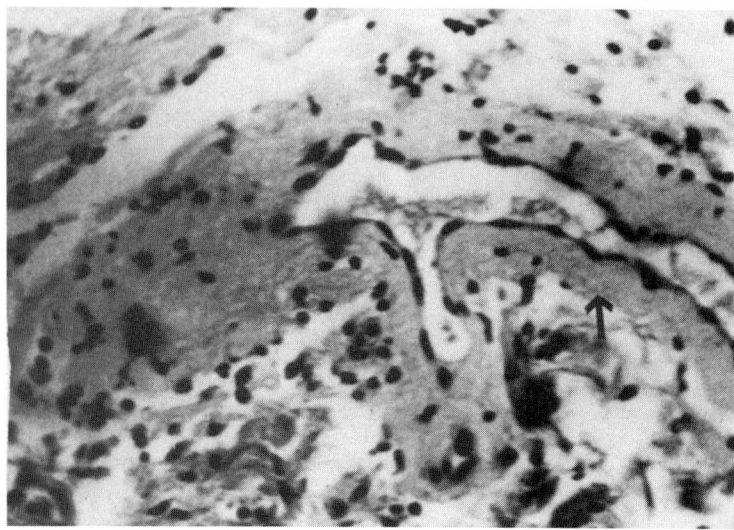

FIGURE 9–79. Canine cutaneous amyloidosis. Dermal blood vessel wall is markedly thickened by amyloid deposition (*arrow*). (Courtesy R. M. Schwartzman.)

A case of generalized amyloidosis was described in a 10-week-old German shepherd puppy.[384] It presented with swollen erythematous pads and reluctance to walk. Though amyloidosis was found at necropsy, the pads only showed chronic exudative inflammation.

Primary nodular cutaneous amyloidosis has been described as the most common type of cutaneous amyloidosis in dogs and cats.[22] Solitary or grouped dermal or subcutaneous nodules may occur anywhere but more commonly involve the ear. Some nodules may ulcerate secondary to necrosis. In humans, nodular amyloidosis is considered to be a plasmacytoma that locally produces immunoglobulin light chains as precursors to amyloid fibrils.[386, 389] This may be the case in dogs as well. The differential diagnosis for these lesions would be neoplasia, cysts, and infectious or sterile nodular granulomas. Diagnosis is made by histopathologic examination, which shows multiple dermal accumulations of amorphous eosinophilic material. Small numbers of plasma cells are found, as well as macrophages and small numbers of lymphocytes.

DIAGNOSIS

The diagnosis of amyloidosis is confirmed by biopsy.[22] Light-microscopic examination reveals the deposition of an eosinophilic amorphous substance that is congophilic and birefringent when polarized (Fig. 9–80).[389] Secondary—but not primary and myeloma-associated—amyloid loses its congophilia after pretreatment with potassium permanganate. Electron-microscopic examination reveals the characteristic presence of 7.5- to 10-nm-wide linear, nonbranching tubular fibrils, each fibril being composed of several filaments arranged in a β-pleated sheet configuration.[389]

CLINICAL MANAGEMENT

Solitary nodules unassociated with systemic disease can be successfully excised. Successful treatment of multiple lesions is not reported. In humans, skin lesions of both primary and myeloma-associated amyloidosis have responded to DMSO, which may inhibit amyloid synthesis or act to promote amyloid degradation.[389]

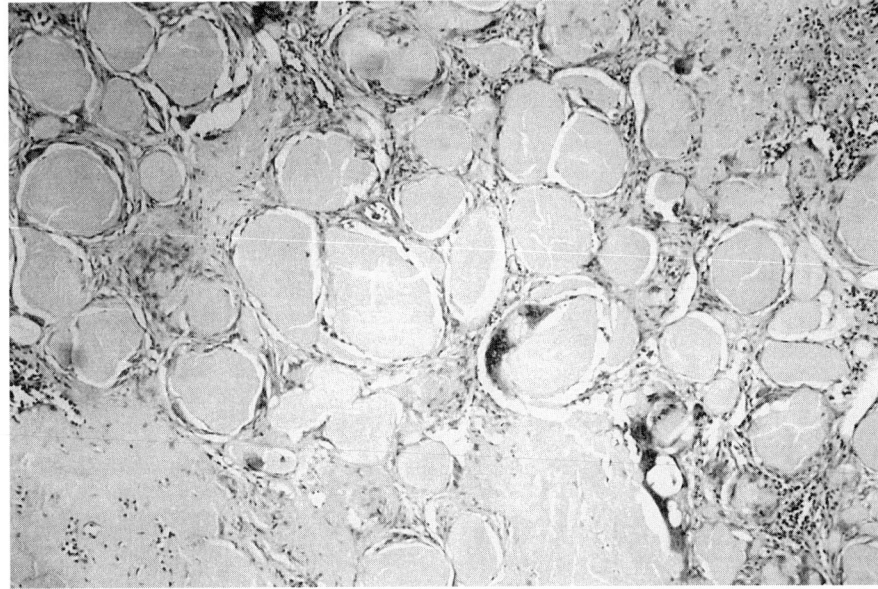

FIGURE 9–80. Canine cutaneous amyloidosis. Multiple "lakes" of homogeneous, fractured amyloid.

REFERENCES

General

1. Abdou NI: The idiotype-anti-idiotype network in human autoimmunity. J Clin Immunol 5:365, 1985.
2. Affolter VK, et al: Immunohistochemical characterization of canine acute graft-versus-host disease and erythema multiforme. In: Kwochka KW, et al (eds): Advances in Veterinary Dermatology III. Butterworth-Heinemann, Boston, 1998, p 103.
3. Ahmed SA, et al: Sex hormones, immune responses, and autoimmune diseases. Am J Pathol 121:531, 1985.
4. Ansel J, et al: Cytokine modulation of keratinocyte cytokines. J Invest Dermatol 94:101S, 1990.
5. Beutner EH, et al: Immunopathology of the Skin III. Churchill Livingstone, New York, 1987.
6. Bos JD: Skin Immune System. CRC Press, Boca Raton, FL, 1989.
7. Bradley GA, Calderwood Mays MB: Immunoperoxidase staining for the detection of autoantibodies in canine autoimmune skin disease: Comparison to immunofluorescence results. Vet Immunol Immunopathol 26:105, 1990.
8. Braquet P, et al: Perspectives in platelet-activating factor research. Pharmacol Rev 39:97, 1987.
9. Brunner CJ: Autoimmunity. In: Bonagura JD (ed): Kirk's Current Veterinary Therapy XII. W.B. Saunders Co., Philadelphia, 1995, p 554.
10. Caciolo PL, et al: Michel's medium as a preservative for immunofluorescent staining of cutaneous biopsy specimens in dogs and cats. Am J Vet Res 45:128, 1984.
11. Carlotti DN, et al: Drug-related superficial pemphigus in the dog: A report of 3 cases. Proc Annu Memb Meet Am Acad Vet Dermatol Am Coll Vet Dermatol 15:23, 1999.
12. Dahl MV: Immunodermatology II. Year Book Medical Publishers, Chicago, 1988.
13. Day MJ, Mazza G: Tissue immunoglobulin G subclasses observed in immune-mediated dermatopathy, deep pyoderma, and hypersensitivity dermatitis in dogs. Res Vet Sci 58:82, 1995.
14. DeBoer DJ, et al: Circulating immune complex concentrations in selected cases of skin disease in dogs. Am J Vet Res 49:143, 1988.
15. Dore M, et al: Production of a monoclonal antibody against canine GMP-140 (P-selectin) and studies of its vascular distribution in canine tissues. Vet Pathol 30:213, 1993.
16. Ettinger SJ, Feldman EC: Textbook of Veterinary Internal Medicine IV. W.B. Saunders Co., Philadelphia, 1995.
17. Fadok VA: TGFβ: The janus of cytokines. J Vet Allergy Clin Immunol 5:129, 1997.
18. Freedberg IM: Fitzpatrick's Dermatology in General Medicine V. McGraw-Hill, New York, 1999.
19. Griffin CE, Rosenkrantz WS: Direct immunofluorescence testing: A comparison of two laboratories in the diagnosis of canine immune-mediated skin disease. Semin Vet Med Surg 2:202, 1987.
20. Griffin CE: Diagnosis and management of primary autoimmune skin disease: A review. Semin Vet Med Surg 2:173, 1987.
21. Griffin CE, et al: Current Veterinary Dermatology. Mosby–Year Book, St. Louis, 1993.
22. Gross TL, et al: Veterinary Dermatopathology: A Macroscopic and Microscopic Evaluation of Canine and Feline Skin Disease. Mosby–Year Book, St. Louis, 1992.
23. Haines DM, et al: Avidin-biotin peroxidase complex immunohistochemistry to detect immunoglobulin in formalin fixed skin biopsies in canine autoimmune skin disease. Can J Vet Res 51:104, 1987.
24. Kwochka KW, et al (eds): Advances in Veterinary Dermatology III. Butterworth-Heinemann, Boston, 1998.
25. Halliwell REW, Gorman NT: Veterinary Clinical Immunology. W.B. Saunders Co., Philadelphia, 1989.
26. Hargis AM, Liggit HD: Cytokines and their role in cutaneous injury. In: Ihrke PJ, et al (eds): Advances in Veterinary Dermatology II. Pergamon Press, New York, 1993, p 325.
27. Hauser C, et al: T helper cells grown with hapten-modified cultured Langerhans' cells produce interleukin 4 and stimulate IgE production by B cells. Eur J Immunol 19:245, 1989.
28. Hauser C, Orbea HA: Superantigens and their role in immune-mediated diseases. J Invest Dermatol 101:503, 1993.
29. Henfry JI: Autoimmune skin disease in dogs. In Pract 13:131, 1991.
30. Hewicker-Trautwein M, et al: Zur diagnostic bullöser und nicht-bullöser autoimmuner Hautkrankheiten bei Hund und Katze. Kleintierpraxis 37:135, 1992.
31. Ihrke PJ, et al: The longevity of immunoglobulin preservation in canine skin utilizing Michel's fixative. Vet Immunol Immunopathol 9:161, 1985.
32. Ihrke PJ, et al (eds): Advances in Veterinary Dermatology II. Pergamon Press, New York, 1993.
33. Kalaher KM: The value of immunofluorescence testing. In: Kirk RW (ed): Current Veterinary Therapy XI. W.B. Saunders Co., Philadelphia, 1992, p 503.
34. Kristensen F, Mehl NB: Autoimmune lidelser hos hund og kat: Behandling med guldsalte. Dansk Vet Tidsskr 72:883, 1989.
35. Kromer G, et al: Is autoimmunity a side effect of interleukin 2 production? Immunol Today 7:199, 1986.
36. Kummel BA: Medical treatment of canine pemphigus-pemphigoid. In: Bonagura JD (ed): Kirk's Current Veterinary Therapy XII. W.B. Saunders Co., Philadelphia, 1995, p 636.
37. Lewis RM, Picut CA: Veterinary Clinical Immunology. Lea & Febiger, Philadelphia, 1989.
38. Locke PH, et al: Manual of Small Animal Dermatology. British Small Animal Veterinary Association, Shurdington, 1993.
39. Luger TA, Schwartz T: Evidence for an epidermal cytokine network. J Invest Dermatol 95:100S, 1990.
40. Matus RW, et al: Plasmapheresis in 5 dogs with systemic immune-mediated disease. J Am Vet Med Assoc 187:595, 1985.
41. McEwan BJ, et al: The response of the eosinophil in acute inflammation in the horse. In: von Tscharner C, Halliwell REW (eds): Advances in Veterinary Dermatology I. Baillière-Tindall, London, 1990, p 176.
42. McKenzie RC, Saunder DN: The role of keratinocyte cytokines in inflammation and immunity. J Invest Dermatol 95:105S, 1990.
43. Middleton E, et al: Allergy Principles and Practice IV. Mosby–Year Book, St. Louis, 1993.

44. Moore FM, et al: Localization of immunoglobulins and complement by the peroxidase antiperoxidase method in autoimmune and nonautoimmune canine dermatopathies. Vet Immunol Immunopathol 14:1, 1987.
45. Morrison LH: When to request immunofluorescence: Practical hints. Semin Cutan Med Surg 18:36, 1999.
46. Mottier S, von Tscharner C: Immunohistochemistry in skin disease: diagnostic value? In: von Tscharner C, Halliwell REW (eds): Advances in Veterinary Dermatology I. Baillière-Tindall, London, 1990, p 479.
47. Scott DW, et al: Muller and Kirk's Small Animal Dermatology V. W.B. Saunders Co., Philadelphia, 1995.
48. Nickoloff BJ: Dermal Immune System. CRC Press, Boca Raton, FL, 1993.
49. Noli C, et al: A retrospective evaluation of adverse reaction of trimethoprim-sulfonamide combinations in dogs and cats. Vet Q 17:123, 1995.
50. Noli C, et al: Apoptosis in selected skin diseases. Vet Dermatol 9:221, 1998.
51. Olivry T, et al: Heterogeneity of canine autoimmune subepidermal bullous diseases: Identification of targeted antigens defines novel clinicopathologic entities. Proc Annu Memb Meet Am Acad Vet Dermatol Am Coll Vet Dermatol 13:80, 1997.
52. Medleau L, et al: Trimethoprim-sulfonamide–associated drug eruptions in dogs. J Am Anim Hosp Assoc 26:305, 1990.
53. Scott DW: Feline dermatology 1979–1982: Introspective retrospections. J Am Anim Hosp Assoc 20:537, 1984.
54. Scott DW: Feline dermatology 1983–1985: "The secret sits." J Am Anim Hosp Assoc 23:255, 1987.
55. Scott DW, et al: Immune-mediated dermatoses in domestic animals: Ten years after. Part I. Compend Cont Educ Small Anim Pract 9:423, 1987.
56. Scott DW, et al: Immune-mediated dermatoses in domestic animals: Ten years after. Part II. Compend Cont Educ Small Anim Pract 9:539, 1987.
57. von Tscharner C, Halliwell REW (eds): Advances in Veterinary Dermatology I. Baillière-Tindall, Philadelphia, 1990.
58. Stone J: Dermatology, Immunology, and Allergy. Mosby–Year Book, St. Louis, 1985.
59. Suter MM, et al: Autoimmune diseases of domestic animals: An update. In: Kwochka KK, et al (eds): Advances in Veterinary Dermatology III. Butterworth-Heinemann, Boston, 1998, p 321.
60. Swerlick RA, Lawley TJ: Role of microvascular endothelial cells in inflammation. J Invest Dermatol 100:111S, 1993.
61. Thiers BH, Dobson RL: Pathogenesis of Skin Disease. Churchill Livingstone, New York, 1986.
62. Thomsen MK: Species specificity in the generation of eicosanoids: Emphasis on leukocyte-activating factors in the skin of allergic dogs and humans. In: Ihrke PJ, et al (eds): Advances in Veterinary Dermatology II. Pergamon Press, New York, 1993, p 63.
63. Thomsen MK: The Role of Neutrophil-Activating Mediators in Canine Health and Disease. Ballerup, Copenhagen, 1991.
64. Thompson JP: Basic immunologic principles of allergic disease. Semin Vet Med Surg 6:247, 1991.
65. Tizard IR: Veterinary Immunology: An Introduction V. W.B. Saunders Co., Philadelphia, 1996.
66. van den Broek, A: Autoimmune skin diseases in cats. In Pract 13:175, 1991.
67. Day MJ: A Color Atlas of Clinical Immunology of the Dog and Cat. Iowa State University Press, Ames, IA, 1999.
68. Walsh LJ, Murphy GF: Role of adhesion molecules in cutaneous inflammation and neoplasia. J Cutan Pathol 19:161, 1992.
69. Wolfe JH, Halliwell REW: Total hemolytic complement values in normal and diseased dog populations. Vet Immunol Immunopathol 1:287, 1980.
70. Yager JA: The skin as an immune organ. In: Ihrke PJ, et al (eds): Advances in Veterinary Dermatology II. Pergamon Press, New York, 1993, p 3.
71. Yager JA, Scott DW: The skin and appendages. In: Jubb KVF, et al (eds): Pathology of Domestic Animals IV. Academic Press, New York, 1993, p 531.
72. Yager JA, Wilcock BP: Color Atlas and Text of Surgical Pathology of the Dog and Cat: Dermatopathology and Skin Tumors. Wolfe Publishing, London, 1994.
73. Zipfel W, et al: Demonstration of immunoglobulins and complement in canine and feline autoimmune and nonautoimmune skin diseases with the direct immunofluorescence and indirect immunoperoxidase method. J Vet Med A 32:494, 1992.

Therapy

74. Miller E: The use of cytotoxic agents in the treatment of immune-mediated diseases of dogs and cats. Semin Vet Med Surg 12:157, 1997.
75. Plumb DC: Veterinary Drug Handbook III. Iowa State University Press, Ames, 1999.
76. Pedersen NC: A review of immunologic diseases of the dog. Vet Immunol Immunopathol 69:251, 1999.
77. Rosenkrantz W: Immunomodulating drugs in dermatology. In: Current Veterinary Therapy X. W.B. Saunders Co., Philadelphia, 1989, p 570.
78. Rosenkrantz WS: Pemphigus foliaceus. In: Griffin CE, et al (eds): Current Veterinary Dermatology. Mosby–Year Book, St. Louis, 1993, p 141.
79. White SD, et al: Corticosteroid (methylprednisolone sodium succinate) pulse therapy in 5 dogs with autoimmune skin disease. J Am Vet Med Assoc 191:1121, 1987.
80. White SD: Nonsteroidal immunosuppressive therapy. In: Bonagura JD (ed): Kirk's Current Veterinary Therapy XIV. W.B. Saunders Co., Philadelphia, 1999, p 536.

Alkylating Agents (Cyclophosphamide, Chlorambucil)

81. Rhodes KH, Shoulberg N: Chlorambucil: Effective therapeutic option for the treatment of feline immune-mediated dermatoses. Feline Pract 20:5, 1992.
82. Stanton ME, Legendre AM: Effects of cyclophosphamide in dogs and cats. J Am Vet Med Assoc 188:1319, 1986.

Azathioprine

83. Beale KM: Azathioprine toxicity in the domestic cat. In: von Tscharner C, Halliwell REW (eds): Advances in Veterinary Dermatology I. Baillière, London, 1990, p 457.
84. Beale KM: Azathioprine for treatment of immune-mediated diseases of dogs and cats. J Am Vet Med Assoc 53:1236, 1992.
85. Griffin CE: Pemphigus foliaceus: Recent findings on the pathophysiology and results of treatment. Proceedings of the University of Edinburgh, Edinburgh, 1993, p 85.
86. Moriello KA, et al: Acute pancreatitis in two dogs given azathioprine and prednisone. J Am Vet Med Assoc 191:695, 1987.

87. White SD, et al: Investigation into the role of thiopurine methyltransferase in the use of azathioprine in dogs: Phase one. Proc Annu Memb Meet Am Acad Vet Dermatol Am Coll Vet Dermatol 14:111, 1998.

Cyclosporine

88. Page EH, et al: Cyclosporine A. J Am Acad Dermatol 14:785, 1986.
89. Read RA: Treatment of canine nictitans plasmacytic conjunctivitis with 0.2% cyclosporine ointment. J Small Anim Pract 36:50, 1995.
90. Rosenkrantz WS, et al: Clinical evaluation of cyclosporine in animal models with cutaneous immune-mediated disease and epitheliotropic lymphoma. J Am Anim Hosp Assoc 25:377, 1989.
91. White JV: Cyclosporine: Prototype of a T-cell selective immunosuppressant. J Am Vet Med Assoc 189:566, 1986.
92. Williams DL: A comparative approach to topical cyclosporine therapy. Eye 11:453, 1997.

Gold Therapy

93. Fadok VA: Thrombocytopenia and hemorrhage associated with gold salt therapy for bullous pemphigoid in a dog. J Am Vet Med Assoc 181:261, 1982.
94. Kummel B: Treatment of autoimmune disease. Derm Dialogue 4:2, 1985.
95. Medleau L, et al: Ulcerative pododermatitis in a cat: Immunofluorescent findings and response to chrysotherapy. J Am Anim Hosp Assoc 18:449, 1982.
96. Muller GH, et al (eds): Small Animal Dermatology IV. W.B. Saunders Co., Philadelphia, 1989.
97. Scott DW: Chrysotherapy (gold therapy). In: Kirk RW (ed): Current Veterinary Therapy VIII. W.B. Saunders Co., Philadelphia, 1983, p 448.
98. Sfikakis PP, et al: Suppression of IL-2 and IL-2 receptor biosynthesis by gold compounds in in vitro activated human peripheral blood mononuclear cells. Arth Rheumatol 35:208, 1993.
99. Suzuki S, et al: Gold sodium thiomalate selectively inhibits IL-5 mediated eosinophil survival. J Allergy Clin Immunol 96:251, 1995.
100. Thomas I: Gold therapy and its indications in dermatology. J Am Acad Dermatol 16:845, 1987.
101. White S: Oral gold therapy. Derm Dialogue 5:2, 1986.

Sulfones/Sulfonamides

102. Fadok VA, Barrie J: Sulfasalazine-responsive vasculitis in the dog: A case report. J Am Anim Hosp Assoc 20:161, 1984.
103. Halliwell REW, et al: Dapsone for the treatment of pruritic dermatitis (dermatitis herpetiformis and subcorneal pustular dermatosis) in dogs. J Am Vet Med Assoc 170:698, 1977.
104. Hekman P, et al: Pharmacokinetics and bioavailability of dapsone in the beagle dog. J Small Anim Pract 30:92, 1989.
105. Katz SI: Sulfones. In: Freedberg IM, et al (eds): Fitzpatrick's Dermatology in General Medicine V. McGraw-Hill, New York, 1999, p 2790.
106. Lees GE, et al: Fatal thrombocytopenic hemorrhagic diathesis associated with dapsone administration to a dog. J Am Vet Med Assoc 174:49, 1979.
107. Thuong-Nguyen V, et al: Inhibition of neutrophil adherence to antibody by dapsone: A possible therapeutic mechanism of dapsone in the treatment of IgA dermatoses. J Invest Dermatol 100:349, 1993.
108. Scott DW: Sulfones and sulfonamides in canine dermatology. In: Kirk RW (ed): Current Veterinary Therapy IX. W.B. Saunders Co., Philadelphia, 1986, p 606.
109. Wozel G, Barth J: Current aspects of modes of action of dapsone. Int J Dermatol 27:547, 1988.

Tetracycline/Niacinamide

110. Humbert P, et al: The tetracyclines in dermatology. J Am Acad Dermatol 25:691, 1991.
111. Rosenkrantz WS: Discoid lupus erythematosus. In: Griffin CE, et al (eds): Current Veterinary Dermatology. Mosby–Year Book, St. Louis, 1993, p 149.
112. White SD, et al: Use of tetracycline and niacinamide for treatment of autoimmune skin disease in 31 dogs. J Am Vet Med Assoc 200:1497, 1992.

Antimalarials

113. Isaacson D, et al: Antimalarials in dermatology. Int J Dermatol 21:379, 1982.
114. Tannenbaum L, Tuffanelli DL: Antimalarial agents. Arch Dermatol 116:587, 1980.

Colchicine

115. Guilhan J, Orr J: Essais de traitement de l'eczéma des carnivores domestiques par le colchicoside. Bull Acad Vét France 30:29, 1957.
116. Sullivan TP, et al: Colchicine in dermatology. J Am Acad Dermatol 39:993, 1998.

Pemphigus Complex

117. Amagai M, et al: The clinical phenotype of pemphigus is defined by the antidesmoglein autoantibody profile. J Am Acad Dermatol 40:167, 1999.
118. Anhalt GJ: Making sense of antigens and antibodies in pemphigus. J Am Acad Dermatol 40:763, 1999.
119. August JR, Chickering WR: Pemphigus foliaceus causing lameness in 4 dogs. Compend Cont Educ Small Anim Pract 7:894, 1985.
120. Bensignor E, et al: Le pemphigus foliacé des carnivores domestiques. Ann Méd Vét 142:5, 1998.
121. Caciolo PL, et al: Pemphigus foliaceus in 8 cats and results of induction therapy using azathioprine. J Am Anim Hosp Assoc 20:571, 1984.
122. Carlotti DN, et al: Pemphigus vulgaris in the dog: A report of 8 cases. Proc Annu Memb Meet Am Acad Vet Dermatol Am Coll Vet Dermatol 15:21, 1999.
123. Carlotti DN, et al: Concurrent superficial pemphigus and multifocal cutaneous metastatic mammary carcinoma in a dog: A paraneoplastic disease? Proc Annu Memb Meet Am Acad Vet Dermatol Am Coll Vet Dermatol 15:75, 1999.
124. Crameri FM, Suter MM: Induction of acantholysis in a serum-free culture system. Proc Annu Memb Meet Am Acad Vet Dermatol Am Coll Vet Dermatol 10:63, 1994.
125. deBruin A, et al: Periplakin and envoplakin are target antigens in canine and human paraneoplastic pemphigus. J Am Acad Dermatol 40:682, 1999.
125a. Ding X, et al: The anti-desmoglein 1 autoantibodies in pemphigus vulgaris sera are pathogenic. J Invest Dermatol 112:739, 1999.
126. Dmochowski M, et al: Desmocollins I and II are recognized by certain sera from patients with various types of pemphigus, particularly Brazilian pemphigus foliaceus. J Invest Dermatol 100:380, 1993.
127. Dunstan RW: Controversies in immunologic diseases from a pathologist's perspective. Controversies in Veterinary Dermatology. Bad Kreuznach, 1992.
128. Fukuda E, et al: Pemphigus erythematosus in a Shetland sheepdog. J Vet Med (Tokyo) 51:24, 1998.
129. Greek JS: Feline pemphigus foliaceus: A retrospective

of 23 cases. Proc Annu Memb Meet Am Acad Vet Dermatol Am Coll Vet Dermatol 9:27, 1993.
130. Griffin CE: Controversies in immunologic diseases from a clinician's standpoint. Controversies in Veterinary Dermatology. Bad Kreuznach, 1992.
131. Griffin CE: Pemphigus foliaceus: Recent findings on the pathophysiology and results of treatment. Presentation, William Dick Bicentenary, Edinburgh, 1993.
132. Griffin CE: Recognizing and treating pemphigus foliaceus in cats. Vet Med 86:513, 1991.
133. Halliwell REW, Goldschmidt M: Pemphigus foliaceus in the canine: A case report and discussion. J Am Anim Hosp Assoc 13:431, 1977.
134. Ihrke PJ, et al: Pemphigus foliaceus of the footpads in 3 dogs. J Am Vet Med Assoc 186:67, 1985.
135. Ihrke PJ, et al: Pemphigus foliaceus in dogs: A review of 37 cases. J Am Vet Med Assoc 186:59, 1985.
136. Ioannides D, et al: Regional variation in the expression of pemphigus foliaceus, pemphigus erythematosus, and pemphigus vulgaris antigens in human skin. J Invest Dermatol 96:15, 1991.
137. Ischii K, et al: Characterization of autoantibodies in pemphigus using antigen-specific enzyme-linked immunosorbent assays with baculovirus-expressed recombinant desmogleins. J Immunol 159:2010, 1997
138. Iwasaki T, et al: The detection of the autoantigen targeted by patient sera from dogs with pemphigus foliaceus. Proc Annu Memb Meet Am Acad Vet Dermatol Am Coll Vet Dermatol 12:44, 1996.
139. Iwasaki T, Maeda Y: The effect of ultraviolet (UV) on the severity of canine pemphigus erythematosus. Proc Annu Memb Meet Am Acad Vet Dermatol Am Coll Vet Dermatol 13:86, 1997.
140. Iwasaki T, et al: Effect of substrate on indirect immunofluorescence test for canine pemphigus foliaceus. Vet Pathol 33:332, 1996.
141. Iwatsuki K, et al: Ultrastructural binding site of pemphigus foliaceus antibodies: Comparison with pemphigus vulgaris. J Cutan Pathol 18:160, 1991.
142. Koch PJ, et al: Targeted disruption of the pemphigus vulgaris antigen (desmoglein 3) gene in mice causes loss of keratinocyte cell adhesion with a phenotype similar to pemphigus vulgaris. J Cell Biol 137:1091, 1997.
143. Lemmens P, et al: Paraneoplastic pemphigus in a dog. Vet Dermatol 9:127, 1998.
144. Liang L, et al: The phosphodiesterase inhibitors pentoxifylline and rolipram prevent diabetes in NOD mice. Diabetes 47:570, 1998.
145. Lombardi C, et al: Environmental risk factors in endemic pemphigus foliaceus (fogo selvagem). J Invest Dermatol 18:847, 1992.
146. Mahoney MG, et al: Explanation for the clinical and microscopic localization of lesions in pemphigus foliaceus and vulgaris. J Clin Invest 103:461, 1999.
147. Manning TO, et al: Pemphigus diseases in the feline: Seven case reports and discussion. J Am Anim Hosp Assoc 18:433, 1982.
148. Nguyen T, et al: The pathophysiological significance of nondesmoglein targets of pemphigus autoimmunity. Arch Dermatol 134:971, 1998.
149. Mattise AW: Canine pemphigus vegetans: A report of 16 cases. Proc Annu Memb Meet Am Acad Vet Dermatol Am Coll Vet Dermatol 7:28, 1991.
150. Noxon JO, Myers RK: Pemphigus foliaceus in two Shetland sheepdog littermates. J Am Vet Med Assoc 194:545, 1989.
151. Olivry T, et al: Pemphigus vulgaris lacking mucosal involvement in a German shepherd dog: Possible response to heparin. Vet Dermatol 3:79, 1992.
152. Pascal A, et al: Seasonality and environmental risk factors for pemphigus foliaceus in animals: A retrospective study of 83 cases presented to the veterinary medical teaching hospital, University of California, Davis from 1976 to 1994. Proc Annu Memb Meet Am Acad Vet Dermatol Am Coll Vet Dermatol 11:24, 1995.
153. Poisson L, et al: Subcorneal neutrophilic acantholytic pustular dermatitis: An unusual manifestation of dermatophytosis resembling canine pemphigus foliaceus. In: Kwochka KW, et al (eds): Advances in Veterinary Dermatology III. Butterworth-Heinemann, Boston, 1998, p 456.
153a. Reis VMS, et al: UVB-induced acantholysis in endemic pemphigus foliaceus (fogo selvagem) and pemphigus vulgaris. J Am Acad Dermatol 42:571, 2000.
154. Rhodes KH, Shoulberg N: Chlorambucil: Effective therapeutic options for the treatment of feline immune-mediated dermatoses. Feline Pract 20:5, 1992.
155. Robinson ND, et al: The new pemphigus variants. J Am Acad Dermatol 40:649, 1999.
156. Rosenkrantz WS: Pemphigus foliaceus. In: Griffin CE, et al (eds): Current Veterinary Dermatology. Mosby-Year Book, St. Louis, 1993, p 141.
157. Ruocco V, Sacerdoti G: Pemphigus and bullous pemphigoid due to drugs. Int J Dermatol 30:307, 1991.
158. Ruocco V, et al: A case of diet-related pemphigus. Dermatology 192:373, 1996.
159. Schoen H, et al: Immunophoresis in paraneoplastic pemphigus. Arch Dermatol 134:706, 1998.
160. Scott DW: Pemphigus vegetans in a dog. Cornell Vet 67:374, 1977.
161. Scott DW, et al: Pemphigus erythematosus in the dog and cat. J Am Anim Hosp Assoc 16:815, 1980.
162. Scott DW, et al: Pemphigus vulgaris without mucosal or mucocutaneous involvement in two dogs. J Am Anim Hosp Assoc 18:401, 1982.
163. Scott DW, Lewis RM: Pemphigus and pemphigoid in dog and man: Comparative aspects. J Am Acad Dermatol 5:148, 1981.
164. Scott DW: Pemphigus in domestic animals. Clin Dermatol 1:141, 1983.
165. Shirakata Y, et al: Lack of mucosal involvement in pemphigus foliaceus may be due to low expression of desmoglein 1. J Invest Dermatol 110:76, 1998.
166. Stannard AA, et al: A mucocutaneous disease in the dog, resembling pemphigus vulgaris in man. J Am Vet Med Assoc 166:575, 1975.
167. Suter MM, et al: Ultrastructural localization of pemphigus antigens on keratinocytes *in vivo* and *in vitro*. Am J Vet Res 41:507, 1990.
168. Suter MM, et al: Identification of canine pemphigus antigens. In: Ihrke PJ, et al (eds): Advances in Veterinary Dermatology II. Pergamon Press, New York, 1993, p 367.
169. Suter MM, et al: Bullous autoimmune skin diseases in animals. Proc Annu Memb Meet Am Acad Vet Dermatol Am Coll Vet Dermatol 13:100, 1997.
170. Tur E, Brenner S: Diet and pemphigus. Arch Dermatol 134:1406, 1998.
171. Walder EJ, Werner A: A possible case of paraneoplastic skin disease with features of erythema multiforme and pemphigus folicaceus in a dog. Proc Annu Memb Meet Am Acad Vet Dermatol Am Coll Vet Dermatol 12:70, 1996.

172. Wolf R, et al: Drug-induced versus drug-triggered pemphigus. Dermatologica 182:207, 1991.
173. Wurm S, et al: Comparative pathology of pemphigus in dogs and humans. Clin Dermatol 12:515, 1994.
174. Xue W, et al: Functional involvement of urokinase-type plasminogen activator receptor in pemphigus acantholysis. J Cutan Pathol 25:469, 1998.

Autoimmune Subepidermal Bullous Dermatoses

175. Ghohestani RF, et al: Diagnostic value of indirect immunofluorescence on sodium chloride-split skin in differential diagnosis of subepidermal autoimmune bullous dermatoses. Arch Dermatol 133:1102, 1997.

Bullous Pemphigoid

176. Borreyo L, et al: Deposition of eosinophil granule proteins preceding blister formation in bullous pemphigoid: Comparison with neutrophil and mast cell granule proteins. Am J Pathol 148:897, 1996.
177. Chan LS, et al: Cloning of the cDNA encoding canine skin basement membrane bullous pemphigoid antigen 2 reveals molecular and immunologic identity in the human and canine NC16A domain. J Invest Dermatol 110:509A, 1998.
178. Czech W, et al: Granulocyte activation in bullous diseases: Release of granular proteins in bullous pemphigoid and pemphigus vulgaris. J Am Acad Dermatol 29:210, 1993.
178a. Dopp R, et al: IgG4 and IgE are the major immunoglobulins targeting the NC16A domain of BP180 in bullous pemphigoid: serum levels of these immunoglobulins reflect disease activity. J Am Acad Dermatol 42:577, 2000.
179. Hashimoto T, et al: Comparative study of bullous pemphigoid antigens among Japanese, British, and U.S. patients indicates similar antigen profiles with the 170-kd antigen present both in the basement membrane and on the keratinocyte cell membrane. J Invest Dermatol 100:38S, 1993.
180. Iwasaki T, et al: Canine bullous pemphigoid (BP)-identification of the 180 kd canine BP antigen by circulating autoantibodies. Vet Pathol 32:387, 1995.
181. Katz SI: Herpes gestationis (pemphigoid gestationis). In: Freedberg IM, et al (eds): Fitzpatrick's Dermatology in General Medicine V. McGraw-Hill, New York, 1999, p 686.
182. Kunkle G, et al: Bullous pemphigoid in a dog: A case report with immunofluorescent findings. J Am Anim Hosp Assoc 14:52, 1978.
183. Olivry T: personal communication 1999.
183a. Olivry T, et al: Novel localized variant of canine epidermolysis bullosa acquisita. Vet Rec 146:193, 2000.
184. Olivry T, et al: Novel feline autoimmune blistering skin disease resembling bullous pemphigoid in humans: IgG autoantibodies target the NC16A ectodomain of type XVII collagen (BP180/BPAG2). Vet Pathol 36:328, 1999.
185. Olivry T, et al: Canine bullous pemphigoid IgG autobodies target antigenic epitopes in the NC16A ectodomain of type XVII collagen (BP180/BPAg2). Proc Annu Memb Meet Am Acad Vet Dermatol Am Coll Vet Dermatol 14:115, 1998.
186. Scott DW: Pemphigoid in domestic animals. Clin Dermatol 5:155, 1987.
187. Stahle-Backdahl M, et al: 92-kd gelatinase is produced by eosinophils at the site of blister formation in bullous pemphigoid and cleaves the extracellular domain of recombinant 180-kd bullous pemphigoid autoantigen. J Clin Invest 93:2022, 1994.
188. Stanely JR: Bullous pemphigoid. In: Freedberg IM, et al (eds): Fitzpatrick's Dermatology in General Medicine V. McGraw-Hill, New York, 1999, p 666.
189. Thomas I, et al: Treatment of generalized bullous pemphigoid with oral tetracycline. J Am Acad Dermatol 28:74, 1993.
190. Yancy KB: Cicatricial pemphigoid. In: Freedberg IM, et al (eds): Fitzpatrick's Dermatology in General Medicine V. McGraw-Hill, New York, 1999, p 674.

Epidermolysis Bullosa Acquisita

191. Olivry T, et al: Canine epidermolysis bullosa acquisita: Circulating autoantibodies target the aminoterminal noncollagenous (NC1) domain of collagen VII in anchoring fibrils. Vet Dermatol 9:19, 1998.
192. Woodley DT, et al: Epidermolysis bullosa acquisita. In: Freedberg IM, et al (eds): Fitzpatrick's Dermatology in General Medicine V. McGraw-Hill, New York, 1999, p 702.
192a. Xu LT, et al: Molecular cloning and characterization of a cDNA encoding canine type VII collagen noncollagenous (NC1) domain, the target antigen of autoimmune disease epidermolysis bullosa acquisita (EBA). Biochim Biophys Acta 1408:25, 1998.

Systemic Lupus Erythematosus

193. Cohen PL: T- and B-cell abnormalities in systemic lupus. J Invest Dermatol 100:69S, 1993.
194. Chabanne L, et al: Abnormalities of lymphocyte subsets in canine systemic lupus erythematosus. Autoimmunity 22:1, 1995.
195. Chabanne L, et al: Canine systemic lupus erythematosus. Part I: Clinical and biologic aspects. Compend Cont Educ Pract Vet 21:135, 1999.
196. Chabanne L, et al: Canine systemic lupus erythematosus. Part II: Diagnosis and treatment. Compend Cont Educ Pract Vet 21:402, 1999.
197. Chung JH, et al: Apoptosis in the pathogenesis of cutaneous lupus erythematosus. Am J Dermatopathol 20:233, 1998.
198. Clercx C, et al: Nonresponsive generalized bacterial infection associated with systemic lupus erythematosus in a Beauceron. J Am Anim Hosp Assoc 35:220, 1999.
199. Day MJ: Inheritance of serum autoantibody, reduced serum IgA and autoimmune disease in a canine breeding colony. Vet Immunol Immunopathol 53:207, 1996.
200. Fournel C, et al: Canine systemic lupus erythematosus. Part I: A study of 75 cases. Lupus 1:133, 1992.
201. Hansson H: Antinuclear antibodies: Presence and specificity in autoimmune connective tissue disease in the dog. Vet Immunol Immunopathol 69:225, 1999.
202. Hubert B, et al: Spontaneous familial systemic lupus erythematosus in a canine breeding colony. J Comp Pathol 98:85, 1988.
203. Jackson HA, Olivry T: Cutaneous lupus erythematosus (ulcerative dermatitis) in the Shetland sheepdog and collie: A review and re-evaluation of the clinical and histological features. Proc Annu Memb Meet Am Acad Vet Dermatol Am Coll Vet Dermatol 15:31, 1999.
204. Jones DRE: Canine systemic lupus erythematosus: New insights and their implications. J Comp Pathol 108:215, 1993.
205. Kristensen AT, et al: Detection of antiplatelet anti-

206. Lehmann P, et al: Experimental reproduction of skin lesions in lupus erythematosus by UVA and UVB radiation. J Am Acad Dermatol 22:181, 1990.
207. McVey DS, Shuman W: Use of multiple antigen substrates to detect antinuclear antibody in canine sera. Vet Immunol Immunopathol 28:37, 1991.
208. Monier JC, et al: Systemic lupus erythematosus in a colony of dogs. Am J Vet Res 49:46, 1988.
209. Monestier M, et al: Autoantibodies to histone, DNA and nucleosome antigens in canine systemic lupus erythematosus. Clin Exp Immunol 99:37, 1995.
210. Mooney E, et al: Characterization of the changes in matrix molecules at the dermoepidermal junction in lupus erythematosus. J Cutan Pathol 18:417, 1991.
211. Norris DA: Pathomechanisms of photosensitive lupus erythematosus. J Invest Dermatol 100:58S, 1993.
212. Olivry T, et al: Interface dermatitis and sebaceous adenitis in exfoliative cutaneous lupus erythematosus (lupoid dermatosis) of German shorthaired pointers. Proc Annu Memb Meet Am Acad Vet Dermatol Am Coll Vet Dermatol 15:41, 1999.
213. Olivry T, et al: Bullous systemic lupus erythematosus (type-1) in a dog. Vet Rec 145:165, 1999.
214. Pedersen NC, Barlough JE: Systemic lupus erythematosus in the cat. Feline Pract 19:5, 1991.
215. Prinz JC, et al: Treatment of severe cutaneous lupus erythematosus with a chimeric CD4 monoclonal antibody, cM-T412. J Am Acad Dermatol 34:244, 1996.
216. Sauder DN, et al: Epidermal cytokines in murine lupus. J Invest Dermatol 100:42S, 1993.
217. Scott DW, et al: Canine lupus erythematosus. I: Systemic lupus erythematosus. J Am Anim Hosp Assoc 19:461, 1983.
218. Sontheimer RD: The lexicon of cutaneous lupus erythematosus: A review and personal perspective on the nomenclature and classification of the cutaneous manifestations of lupus erythematosus. Lupus 6:84, 1997.
219. Sontheimer RD: Lupus erythematosus. In: Freedberg IM, et al (eds): Fitzpatrick's Dermatology in General Medicine V. McGraw-Hill, New York, 1999, p 1993.
220. Soulard M, et al: The I protein of the heterogeneous nuclear ribonucleoprotein complex is a novel dog nuclear autoantigen. J Autoimmun 9:599, 1996.
221. Stone MS, et al: Lupus-type anticoagulant in a dog with hemolysis and thrombosis. J Vet Intern Med 8:57, 1994.
222. Teichner M, et al: Systemic lupus erythematosus in dogs: Association to the major histocompatibility complex class I antigen DLA-A7. Clin Immunol Immunopathol 55:255, 1990.
223. Thoren-Tolling K, Ryden L: Serum auto-antibodies and clinical/pathologic features in German shepherd dogs with a lupus-like syndrome. Acta Vet Scand 32:15, 1991.
224. Velthuis PJ, et al: Immunohistopathology of light-induced skin lesions in lupus erythematosus. Acta Dermatol Venereol (Stockh) 70:93, 1990.
225. Vitale CB, et al: Systemic lupus erythematosus in a cat: Fulfillment of the American Rheumatism Association criteria with supportive skin histopathology. Vet Dermatol 8:133, 1997.
226. Welin Henricksson E, et al: Autoantibody profiles in canine ANA-positive sera investigated by immunoblot and ELISA. Vet Immunol Immunopathol 61:157, 1998.
227. White SD, et al: Investigation of antibodies to extractable nuclear antigens in dogs. Am J Vet Res 53:1019, 1992.

Discoid Lupus Erythematosus

228. Guaguère E, Magnol JP: Lupus érythémateux discoïde à localisation auriculaire chez le chien. Prat Méd Chir Anim Comp 24:101, 1989.
229. Kalaher KM, Scott DW: Discoid lupus erythematosus in a cat. Feline Pract 19:7, 1991.
230. Iwasaki T, et al: A canine case of discoid lupus erythematosus with circulating autoantibody. J Vet Med Sci 57:1097, 1995.
231. Olivry T, et al: Le lupus érythémateux discoïde du chien: A propos de 22 observations. Prat Med Chir Anim Comp 22:205, 1987.
232. Rogers KS, et al: Squamous cell carcinoma of the canine nasal planum: Eight cases (1988–1994). J Am Anim Hosp Assoc 31:373, 1995.
232a. Rosenbaum M: Cyclosporine. Derm Dialogue, Summer 1999, p 5.
233. Rosenkrantz WS: Discoid lupus erythematosus. In: Griffin CE, et al (eds): Current Veterinary Dermatology. Mosby–Year Book, St. Louis, 1993, p 149.
234. Scott DW, et al: Canine lupus erythematosus. II: Discoid lupus erythematosus. J Am Anim Hosp Assoc 19:481, 1983.
235. Scott DW, et al: Unusual findings in canine pemphigus erythematosus and discoid lupus erythematosus. J Am Anim Hosp Assoc 20:579, 1984.
236. Scott DW, Miller WH Jr: Squamous cell carcinoma arising in chronic discoid lupus erythematosus nasal lesions in two German shepherd dogs. Vet Dermatol 6:99, 1995.
237. Stanley BJ, et al: Bilateral rotation flaps for the treatment of chronic nasal dermatitis in four dogs. J Am Anim Hosp Assoc 27:295, 1991.
238. Sugai SA, et al: Cutaneous lupus erythematosus: Direct immunofluorescence and epidermal basement membrane study. Int J Dermatol 31:260, 1992.
239. Willemse T, et al: Discoid lupus erythematosus in cats. Vet Dermatol 1:19, 1989.
240. Williams REA, et al: The contribution of direct immunofluorescence to the diagnosis of lupus erythematosus. J Cutan Pathol 16:122, 1989.

Cryoglobulinemia and Cryofibrinogenemia

241. Bridle KH, Littlewood JD: Tail tip necrosis in two litters of Birman kittens. J Small Anim Pract 39:88, 1998.
242. Cohen SJ, et al: Cutaneous manifestations of cryoglobulinemia: Clinical and histopathologic study of seventy-two patients. J Am Acad Dermatol 25:21, 1991.
243. Dickson NJ: Cold agglutinin disease in a puppy associated with lead intoxication. J Small Anim Pract 31:105, 1990.
244. Godfrey DR, Anderson RM: Cold agglutinin disease in a cat. J Small Anim Pract 35:267, 1994.
245. Nagata M, et al: Cryoglobulinaemia and cryofibrinogenaemia: A comparison of canine and human cases. Vet Dermatol 9:277, 1998.
246. Niemand S, et al: Kalteagglutinin-Krankheit bei einer Katz. Kleintierpraxis 30:259, 1985.
247. Zulty JC, Kociba GJ: Cold agglutinins in cats with haemobartonellosis. J Am Vet Med Assoc 196:907, 1990.

Graft-Versus-Host Disease

248. Horn TD, et al: Reappraisal of histologic features of the acute cutaneous graft-versus-host reaction based on an allogenic rodent model. J Invest Dermatol 103:206, 1994.
249. Johnson ML, Farmer ER: Graft-versus-host reactions in dermatology. J Am Acad Dermatol 38:369, 1998.
250. Langley RGB, et al: Apoptosis is the mode of keratinocyte death in cutaneous graft-versus-host disease. J Am Acad Dermatol 35:187, 1996.
251. Yu C, et al: Synergism between mycophenolate mofetil and cyclosporine in preventing graft-versus-host disease among lethally irradiated dogs given DLA-nonidentical unrelated marrow grafts. Blood 91:2581, 1998.

Cutaneous Adverse Drug Reaction

252. Affolter VK, von Tscharner C: Cutaneous drug reactions: A retrospective study of histopathologic changes and their correlation with the clinical disease. Vet Dermatol 4:79, 1993.
253. Affolter VK, Shaw SE: Cutaneous drug eruptions. In: Ihrke PJ, et al (eds): Advances in Veterinary Dermatology II. Pergamon Press, New York, 1993, p 447.
254. Baker JR, et al: Pathologic effects of bleomycin on the skin of dogs and monkeys. Toxicol Appl Pharmacol 25:190, 1973.
255. Barbaud AM, et al: Role of delayed cellular hypersensitivity and adhesion molecules in amoxicillin-induced morbilliform rashes. Arch Dermatol 133:481, 1997.
256. Barthold SW, et al: Reversible dermal atrophy in a cat with phenytoin. Vet Pathol 17:469, 1980.
257. Bureau of Veterinary Drugs: Suspected drug adverse reactions reported to the Bureau of Veterinary Drugs. Can Vet J 33:237, 1992.
258. Carlotti DN, Bensignor E: La gale sarcoptique du chien: Étude rétrospective de 38 cas. Prat Méd Chir Anim Comp 32:117, 1997.
259. Cribb AE: Idiosyncratic reactions to sulfonamides in dogs. J Am Vet Med Assoc 195:1612, 1989.
260. Giger U, et al: Sulfadiazine-induced allergy in six Doberman pinschers. J Am Vet Med Assoc 186:479, 1985.
261. Gordon KG, et al: Pseudomycosis fungoides in a patient taking clonazepam and fluoxetine. J Am Acad Vet Dermatol 34:304, 1996.
262. Gupta AK, et al: Lymphocytic infiltrates of the skin in association with cyclosporine therapy. J Am Acad Dermatol 23:1137, 1990.
263. Hammer AS, Cuoto CG: Diagnosing and treating canine hemangiosarcoma. Vet Med 87:188, 1992.
264. Hendrick MJ, Dunagan CA: Focal necrotizing granulomatous panniculitis associated with subcutaneous injection of rabies vaccine in cats and dogs: 10 cases (1988–1989). J Am Vet Med Assoc 198:304, 1991.
265. Henricks PM: Dermatitis associated with the use of primidone in a dog. J Am Vet Med Assoc 191:237, 1987.
266. Kunkle G: Adverse cutaneous reactions in cats given methimazole. Derm Dialogue Spring/Summer, 1993, p 4.
267. Magro CM, et al: The interstitial granulomatous drug reaction: A distinctive clinical and pathologic entity. J Cutan Pathol 25:72, 1998.
268. Mason KV: Subepidermal bullous drug eruption resembling bullous pemphigoid in a dog. J Am Vet Med Assoc 190:881, 1987.
269. Mason KV: Cutaneous drug eruptions. Vet Clin North Am Small Anim Pract 20:1633, 1990.
270. Mason KV, Rosser EJ: Cutaneous drug eruptions. In: von Tscharner C, Halliwell REW (eds): Advances in Veterinary Dermatology I. Ballière-Tindall, Philadelphia, 1990, p 426.
271. Mason KV: Fixed drug eruption in two dogs caused by diethylcarbamazine. J Am Anim Hosp Assoc 24:301, 1988.
272. Mason KV, Day MJ: A pemphigus foliaceus–like eruption associated with the use of ampicillin in a cat. Aust Vet J 64:223, 1987.
273. Mason KV: Blistering drug eruptions in animals. Clin Dermatol 11:567, 1993.
274. Mauldin GN, et al: Efficacy and toxicity of doxorubicin and cyclophosphamide used in the treatment of selected malignant tumors in 23 cats. J Vet Intern Med 2:60, 1988.
275. McEwan NA, et al: Drug eruption in a cat resembling pemphigus foliaceus. J Small Anim Pract 28:713, 1987.
276. Ogilvie GK, et al: Acute and short-term toxicoses associated with the administration of doxorubicin to dogs with malignant tumors. J Am Vet Med Assoc 195:1584, 1989.
277. Ogilvie GK, et al: Hypotension and cutaneous reactions associated with intravenous administration of etoposide in the dog. Am J Vet Res 49:1367, 1988.
278. Perez T, et al: Hypersensitivity reactions to drugs: Correlation between clinical probability score and laboratory diagnostic procedure. J Invest Clin Immunol 5:276, 1995.
279. Plotnick AN, et al: Primary cutaneous coccidioidomycosis and subsequent drug eruption to itraconazole in a dog. J Am Anim Hosp Assoc 33:139, 1997.
280. Rijlaarsdam U, et al: Mycosis fungoides–like lesions associated with phenytoin and carbamazepine therapy. J Am Acad Dermatol 24:216, 1991.
281. Roche E, Mason KV: Periocular alopecia caused by a fixed drug eruption. Aust Vet Pract 21:80, 1991.
282. Rosenkrantz WS: Cutaneous drug reactions. In: Griffin CE, et al (eds): Current Veterinary Dermatology. Mosby–Year Book, St. Louis, 1993, p 154.
283. Rosenkrantz WS, et al: Cyclosporine and cutaneous immune-mediated disease. J Am Acad Dermatol 14:1088, 1986.
284. Scott DW, et al: Drug eruption associated with sulfonamide treatment of vertebral osteomyelitis in a dog. J Am Vet Med Assoc 168:1111, 1976.
285. Scott DW: Drug eruption in a cat due to a miticide. Feline Pract 7:47, 1977.
286. Scott DW, Miller WH Jr: Idiosyncratic cutaneous adverse drug reactions in the cat: Literature review and report of 14 cases (1990–1996). Feline Pract 26:10, 1998.
287. Scott DW, Miller WH Jr: Idiosyncratic cutaneous adverse drug reactions in the dog: Literature review and report of 101 cases (1990–1996). Canine Pract 24:16, 1999.
288. Scott DW: Folliculite murale granulomateuse chez le chien: Manifestation d'un accident médicamenteux cutané? Méd Vét Québec 29:154, 1999.
289. Stanley RG, Jabara AG: Chronic skin reaction to a combined feline rhinotracheitis virus (herpesvirus) and calicivirus vaccine. Aust Vet J 65:128, 1988.
290. Stern RS, Wintroub BU: Cutaneous reactions to drugs. In: Freedberg IM, et al (eds): Fitzpatrick's

291. Van Hees J, et al: Levamisole-induced drug eruptions in the dog. J Am Anim Hosp Assoc 21:255, 1985.
292. Vitale CB, et al: Putative diethylcarbamazine-induced urticaria with eosinophilic dermatitis in a dog. Vet Dermatol 5:197, 1994.
293. Vitale CB, et al: Putative Rimadyl-induced neutrophilic dermatosis resembling Sweet's syndrome in 2 dogs. Proc Annu Memb Meet Am Acad Vet Dermatol Am Coll Vet Dermatol 15:69, 1999.
294. Walder E: Superficial suppurative necrolytic dermatitis in miniature schnauzers. In: Ihrke PJ, et al (eds): Advances in Veterinary Dermatology II. Pergamon Press, New York, 1993, p 419.
295. Wolkenstien P, et al: Metabolic predisposition to cutaneous adverse drug reactions. Arch Dermatol 131:544, 1995.

Erythema Multiforme and Toxic Epidermal Necrolysis

296. Akosa AB, Elhag AM: Toxic epidermal necrolysis: A study of the sweat glands. J Cutan Pathol 22:359, 1995.
297. Assier H, et al: Erythema multiforme with mucous membrane involvement and Stevens-Johnson syndrome are clinically different disorders with distinct causes. Arch Dermatol 131:539, 1995.
298. Bastuji-Garin S, et al: Clinical classification of cases of toxic epidermal necrolysis, Stevens-Johnson's syndrome and erythema multiforme. Arch Dermatol 129:92, 1993.
299. Becker DS: Toxic epidermal necrolysis. Lancet 351:1417, 1998.
300. Child FJ, et al: Rowell's syndrome. Clin Exp Dermatol 24:74, 1999.
301. Cote B, et al: Clinicopathologic correlation in erythema multiforme and Stevens-Johnson syndrome. Arch Dermatol 131:1268, 1995.
302. Delmage DA, Payne-Johnson CE: Erythema multiforme in a Doberman on trimethoprim-sulphamethoxazole therapy. J Small Anim Pract 32:635, 1991.
303. Egan CA, et al: Plasmapheresis as an adjunct treatment in toxic epidermal necrolysis. J Am Acad Dermatol 40:458, 1999.
304. Foedinger D, et al: Autoantibodies against desmoplakin I and II define a subset of patients with erythema multiforme major. J Invest Dermatol 106:1012, 1996.
305. Frank AA, et al: Toxic epidermal necrolysis associated with flea dips. Vet Hum Toxicol 34:57, 1992.
306. Fritsch PO, Ruiz-Maldonado R: Erythema multiforme. In: Freedberg IM, et al (eds): Fitzpatrick's Dermatology in General Medicine V. McGraw-Hill, New York, 1999, p 636.
307. Fritsch PO, Ruiz-Maldonado R: Stevens-Johnson syndrome and toxic epidermal necrolysis. In: Freedberg IM, et al (eds): Fitzpatrick's Dermatology in General Medicine V. McGraw-Hill, New York, 1999, p 644.
308. Hinn AC, et al: Erythema multiforme, Stevens-Johnson syndrome, and toxic epidermal necrolysis in the dog: Clinical classification, drug exposure, and histopathologic correlations. J Vet Allergy Clin Immunol 6:13, 1998.
309. Inachi S, et al: Epidermal apoptotic cell death in erythema multiforme and Stevens-Johnson syndrome. Arch Dermatol 133:845, 1997.
310. McMurdy MA: A case resembling erythema multiforme major (Stevens-Johnson syndrome) in a dog. J Am Anim Hosp Assoc 26:297, 1990.
311. Medleau L, et al: Erythema multiforme and disseminated intravascular coagulation in a dog. J Am Anim Hosp Assoc 26:643, 1990.
312. Mirowsk GW, et al: Altered expression of epithelial integrins and extracellular matrix receptors in oral erythema multiforme. J Cutan Pathol 23:473, 1996.
313. Paquet P, Piéraud GE: Soluble fractions of tumor necrosis factor-α, interleukin-6 and their receptors in toxic epidermal necrolysis: A comparison with second-degree burns. Int J Mol Med 1:459, 1998.
314. Paquet P, Piéraud GE: Epidermal calprotectin in drug-induced toxic epidermal necrolysis. J Cutan Pathol 26:301, 1999.
315. Paquet P, Piéraud GE: Erythema multiforme and toxic epidermal necrolysis: A comparative study. Am J Dermatopathol 19:127, 1997.
316. Power H: Practice tip. Derm Dialogue Winter 1993/1994, p 7.
317. Rachofsky MA, et al: Toxic epidermal necrolysis. Compend Cont Educ 11:840, 1989.
318. Rosenbaum MR, Kerlin RL: Erythema multiforme major and disseminated intravascular coagulation in a dog following application of a d-limonene-based insecticidal dip. J Am Vet Med Assoc 207:1315, 1995.
319. Roujeau J: The spectrum of Stevens-Johnson syndrome and toxic epidermal necrolysis: A clinical classification. J Invest Dermatol 102:28S, 1994.
320. Roujeau J: Stevens-Johnson syndrome and toxic epidermal necrolysis are severity variants of the same disease which differs from erythema multiforme. J Dermatol 24:726, 1997.
321. Rzony B, et al: Histopathologic and epidemiological characteristics of patients with erythema exudativum multiforme major, Stevens-Johnson syndrome and toxic epidermal necrolysis. Br J Dermatol 135:6, 1996.
322. Scott DW, et al: Erythema multiforme in the dog. J Am Anim Hosp Assoc 19:453, 1983.
323. Scott DW, Miller WH Jr: Erythema multiforme in dogs and cats: Literature review and case material from the Cornell University College of Veterinary Medicine (1988–96). Vet Dermatol 10:297, 1999.
324. Scott DW, et al: Toxic epidermal necrolysis in two dogs and a cat. J Am Anim Hosp Assoc 15:271, 1979.
325. Viard I, et al: Inhibition of toxic epidermal necrolysis by blockage of CD95 with human intravenous immunoglobulin. Science 282:490, 1998.

Vasculitis

326. Beale KM: Vasculopathy in two dogs associated with ivermectin administration. Proc Annu Memb Meet Am Acad Vet Dermatol Am Coll Vet Dermatol 15:39, 1999.
327. Bensignor E: What is your diagnosis? J Small Anim Pract 40:151, 1999.
328. Carpenter JL, et al: Idiopathic cutaneous and renal glomerular vasculopathy of greyhounds. Vet Pathol 25:401, 1988.
329. Cowan LA, et al: Clinical and clinicopathologic abnormalities in greyhounds with cutaneous and renal glomerular vasculopathy: 18 cases (1992–1994). J Am Vet Med Assoc 210:789, 1997.
330. Crawford MA, Foil CS: Vasculitis: Clinical syndromes in small animals. Compend Cont Educ 11:400, 1989.
331. Fondati A, et al: Familial cutaneous vasculopathy and demodicosis in a German shepherd dog. J Small Anim Pract 39:137, 1998.

332. Frank LA: Rabies vaccine-induced ischemic dermatitis in a dog. Vet Allergy Clin Immunol 6:9, 1998.
333. Griffin CE: Pinnal Diseases: The Complete Manual of Ear Care. Solvay Veterinary, Inc., Princeton, 1985, p 21.
334. Griffin CE: Pinnal diseases. Vet Clin North Am Small Anim Pract 24:897, 1994.
335. Guaguère E, et al: Lésions cutanées associées à des maladies internes chez le chien. Prat Méd Chir Anim Comp 32:275, 1997.
336. Legendre AM, et al: Treatment of blastomycosis with intraconazole in 112 dogs. J Vet Intern Med 10:365, 1996.
337. Lotti T, et al: Cutaneous small-vessel vasculitis. J Am Acad Dermatol 39:667, 1998.
338. Mathet JL, et al: Vascularite leucocytoclasique primaire à localisation cutanéo-muqueuse chez le chat: Á propos de deux cas. Prat Méd Chir Anim Comp 32:293, 1997.
339. Mandell BF, Hoffman GS: Systemic necrotizing arteritis. In: Freedberg IM, et al (eds): Fitzpatrick's Dermatology in General Medicine V. McGraw-Hill, New York, 1999, p 2034.
340. Manning TO, Scott DW: Cutaneous vasculitis in a dog. J Am Anim Hosp Assoc 16:61, 1980.
341. Morris DO: Cutaneous vasculitides. Proc Am Coll Vet Intern Med Forum 16:452, 1998.
342. Nichols PR, et al: A retrospective study of canine and feline cutaneous vasculitis. Proc Annu Memb Meet Am Acad Vet Dermatol Am Coll Vet Dermatol 14:27, 1998.
343. Parker WM, Foster RA: Cutaneous vasculitis in five Jack Russell terriers. Vet Dermatol 7:109, 1996.
344. Pedersen K, Scott DW: Idiopathic pyogranulomatous inflammation and leukocytoclastic vasculitis of the nasal planum, nostrils and nasal mucosa in Scottish terriers in Denmark. Vet Dermatol 2:85, 1991.
345. Rachofsky MA, et al: Probable hypersensitivity vasculitis in a dog. J Am Vet Med Assoc 194:1592, 1989.
346. Scott DW: Eosinophils in the walls of large dermal and subcutaneous blood vessels in biopsy specimens from cats with eosinophilic granuloma or eosinophilic plaque. Vet Dermatol 10:77, 1999.
347. Soter NA: Cutaneous necrotizing venulitis. In: Freedberg IM, et al (eds): Fitzpatrick's Dermatology in General Medicine V. McGraw-Hill, New York, 1999, p 2044.
348. Vitale CB, et al: Vaccine-induced ischemic dermatopathy in the dog. Vet Dermatol 10:131, 1999.
349. von Tscharner C, Haemmerling R: Granulomatous vasculitis in a West Highland white terrier. Proc Annu Memb Meet Am Acad Vet Dermatol Am Coll Vet Dermatol 14:85, 1998.
350. Weir JA, et al: Familial cutaneous vasculopathy of German shepherds: Clinical, genetic and preliminary pathologic and immunological studies. Can Vet J 35:763, 1994.
351. Wilcock BP, Yager JA: Focal cutaneous vasculitis and alopecia at sites of rabies vaccination in dogs. J Am Vet Med Assoc 188:1174, 1986.

Linear IgA Pustular Dermatosis

352. Scott DW, et al: Linear IgA dermatoses in the dog: Bullous pemphigoid, discoid lupus erythematosus and a subcorneal pustular dermatitis. Cornell Vet 72:394, 1982

Uveodermatologic Syndrome

353. Boldy KL, et al: Uveodermatologic syndrome in the dog: Clinical characteristics and treatment of a disorder similar to human Vogt-Koyanagi-Harada syndrome. Vet Focus 1:112, 1989.
354. Campbell KL, et al: Generalized leukoderma and poliosis following uveitis in a dog. J Am Anim Hosp Assoc 22:121, 1986.
355. Herrera DH, Duchene AG: Uveodermatological syndrome (Vogt-Koyanagi-Harada–like syndrome) with generalized depigmentation in a Dachshund. Vet Ophthalmol 1:47, 1998.
356. Kern TJ, et al: Uveitis associated with poliosis and vitiligo in six dogs. J Am Vet Med Assoc 187:408, 1985.
357. Lindley DM, et al: Ocular histology of Vogt-Koyanagi-Harada–like syndrome in an akita dog. Vet Pathol 27:294, 1990.
358. MacDonald JM: Uveodermatologic syndrome in the dog. In: Griffin CE, et al (eds): Current Veterinary Dermatology. Mosby–Year Book, St. Louis, 1993, p 217.
359. Morgan RV: Vogt-Koyanagi-Harada syndrome in humans and dogs. Compend Cont Educ 11:1211, 1989.
360. Murphy CJ, et al: Antiretinal antibodies associated with Vogt-Koyanagi-Harada-like syndrome in a dog. J Am Anim Hosp Assoc 27:399, 1991.
361. Slinckx J, Fontaine J: Un cas de syndrome uvéodermatologique ressemblant au syndrome Vogt-Koyanagi-Harada chez un fox terrier. Point Vét 30:243, 1999.
362. Tachikawa S, et al: Uveodermatologic (Vogt-Koyanagi-Harada-like) syndrome with sloughing of the nails in a Siberian husky. J Vet Med (Tokyo) 48:559, 1995.
363. Vercelli A, et al: Canine Vogt-Koyanagi-Harada–like syndrome in two Siberian husky dogs. Vet Dermatol 1:151, 1990.
364. Warmoes T: Modèle canine d'un syndrome de Vogt-Koyanagi-Harada. Point Vét 30:249, 1999.

Auricular Chondritis

365. Badoil F: Etude comparative chez l'homme et le chat de la polychondrite atrophiante chronique. Thèse, Ecole Nationale Vétérinaire de Lyon, 1996.
366. Boord MJ, Griffin CE: Aural chondritis or polychondritis dessicans in a dog. Proc Annu Memb Meet Am Acad Vet Dermatol Am Coll Vet Dermatol 14:65, 1998.
367. Bunge MM, et al: Relapsing polychondritis in a cat. J Am Anim Hosp Assoc 28:203, 1992.
368. Guaguère E, et al: Polychondrite auriculaire atrophiante: Á propos d'un cas chez un chat. Prat Méd Chir Anim Comp 27:557, 1992.
369. Lemmens P, Schrauwen E: Feline relapsing polychondritis: A case report. Vlaams Diergeneeskd Tijdschr 62:183, 1993.

Immunoproliferative Enteropathy of Basenji Dogs

370. Breitschwerdt EB, et al: Clinical and laboratory characterization of basenjis with immunoproliferative small intestinal disease. Am J Vet Res 45:267, 1984.

Alopecia Areata

371. DeJonghe SR, et al: Trachyonychia associated with alopecia areata in a Rhodesian ridgeback. Vet Dermatol 10:123, 1999.
372. Elston DM, et al: Eosinophils in fibrous tracts and near hair bulbs: A helpful diagnostic feature of alopecia areata. J Am Acad Dermatol 37:101, 1997.
372a. Madani S, Shapiro J: Alopecia areata update. J Am Acad Dermatol 42:549, 2000.
373. McElwee KJ, et al: Comparison of alopecia areata in

human and nonhuman mammalian species. Pathobiology 66:90, 1998.
374. Olivry T, et al: Antifollicular cell-mediated and humoral immunity in canine alopecia areata. Vet Dermatol 7:67, 1996.
375. Tobin DJ, et al: Hair follicle–specific antibodies in mammalian species with alopecia areata. J Invest Dermatol 108:654, 1997.
376. Tobin DJ, et al: Anti-trichohyalin antibodies in canine alopecia areata. In: Kwochka KW, et al (eds): Advances in Veterinary Dermatology III. Butterworth-Heinemann, Boston, 1998, p 353.

Pseudopelade

377. Gross TL, et al: Morphologic and immunologic characterization of a canine isthmus mural folliculitis resembling pseudopelade of humans. Vet Dermatol 11:17, 2000.
378. Power HT, et al: Novel feline alopecia areata–like dermatosis: Cytotoxic T lymphocytes target the follicular isthmus. In: Kwochka KW, et al (eds): Advances in Veterinary Dermatology III. Butterworth-Heinemann, Boston, 1998, p 538.
379. Power HT: Newly recognized feline skin diseases. Proc Annu Memb Meet Am Acad Vet Dermatol Am Coll Vet Dermatol 14:27, 1998.

Amyloidosis

380. Alhaidari Z, et al: Amylose cutanéomuqueuse chez un chien. Prat Méd Chir Anim Comp 26:341, 1991.
381. DiBartola SP, Benson MD: The pathogenesis of reactive systemic amyloidosis. J Vet Intern Med 3:31, 1989.
382. DiBartola SP, et al: Familial renal amyloidosis in Chinese Shar Pei dogs. J Am Vet Med Assoc 197:483, 1990.
383. Dodds JW: Amyloidosis. J Am Anim Hosp Assoc 31:100, 1995.
384. Gelens HC, et al: Reactive amyloidosis in a puppy, associated with a chronic inflammatory syndrome. J Am Anim Hosp Assoc 30:529, 1994.
385. Van der Linde-Sipman JS, et al: Generalized AA-amyloidosis in Siamese and Oriental cats. Vet Immunol Immunopathol 56:1, 1997.
386. Platz SJ, et al: Identification of lambda light chain amyloid in eight canine and two feline extramedullary plasmacytomas. J Comp Pathol 116:45, 1997.
387. Snyder PW, et al: Pathologic features of naturally occurring juvenile polyarteritis in beagle dogs. Vet Pathol 32:337, 1995.
388. Schwartzman RM: Cutaneous amyloidosis associated with a monoclonal gammapathy in a dog. J Am Vet Med Assoc 185:102, 1984.
389. Touart DM, Sau P: Cutaneous deposition diseases: Part I. J Am Acad Dermatol 39:149, 1998.

Chapter 10
Endocrine and Metabolic Diseases

Many hormones affect the skin and adnexa.[3] Although this chapter is limited to a discussion of endocrine influences on the skin, hormones also affect the rest of the body. The specific actions of many proven and alleged hormonal imbalances on the skin are often poorly understood. Additionally, confusion is intensified by (1) species differences, (2) lack of adequate, standardized, or readily available diagnostic tests, (3) conflicting data in the literature, and (4) the complex physiologic and pathophysiologic interrelationships between the endocrine glands and their hormonal products. The skin must also be regarded as having endocrine functions because it is a major site for the metabolism and interconversion of many of the steroids.

With the exception of some of the sex hormone dermatoses, animals with an endocrine or metabolic disorder have both dermatologic and constitutional signs of illness. Depending on the disease under consideration and the astuteness of the owner, the skin changes may be noticed months before the constitutional signs. Classically, endocrine disorders are associated with a symmetric, nonpruritic hair loss. Early on, however, the animal may have no hair loss but be presented for a localized (e.g., ceruminous otitis externa) or generalized seborrheic condition, recurrent bacterial infection, or some other cutaneous abnormality (e.g., cutaneous mucinosis). If there is an endocrine basis for the disorder under consideration, hair loss eventually accompanies the abnormality. Because most dogs and cats go through two hair cycles per year, hair loss should appear within 6 months of the presenting complaint. If the chronically affected animal has a perfectly normal coat, an endocrine causality is very unlikely and any abnormal laboratory data should be interpreted cautiously.

With a coat change, the hair in the involved areas is dull and dry and usually epilates easily. Epilated hairs may not regrow (e.g., hypothyroidism), may regrow very slowly (e.g., hyperadrenocorticism), or may regrow very abnormally (e.g., the woolly coat of adrenal hyperplasia-like syndrome). In hypothyroidism or hyperadrenocorticism, all hair follicles on the trunk are affected and advanced cases have a bilaterally symmetric truncal alopecia. Early in the course of the disease, the hair loss may be localized to regions of the body (e.g., flank and saddle areas) and necessitate the consideration of nonendocrine causes of hair loss. Eventually, the hair loss becomes more widespread. Because there is a topographic variation in the number and/or affinity of sex hormone receptors in dog skin, the sex hormone dermatoses have a more regionalized pattern of alopecia that persists in those areas for extended periods of time.

• FUNCTIONAL ANATOMY OF THE ENDOCRINE HYPOTHALAMUS AND HYPOPHYSIS

Anatomically and functionally, the hypothalamus and the hypophysis (pituitary gland) are most usefully thought of together as the "master gland" or the "endocrine brain."[1, 2] The important portion of the hypophysis as it relates to dermatology is the adenohypophysis (anterior pituitary, or pars distalis).

The hypothalamus contains a number of specialized cells that combine neural and secretory activity: the endocrine neurons. The endocrine hypothalamus produces hormones (adenohypophysiotropic releasing and inhibiting factors) that are transported as unstainable neurosecretions to the pituitary portal system and then to the adenohypophysis. Important hypothalamic releasing and inhibiting factors that control the adenohypophysis include the following:

- Corticotropin-releasing factor (CRF) (or adrenocorticotropic hormone–releasing factor [ACTH-RF], corticotropin-releasing hormone [CRH])
- Thyrotropin-releasing hormone (TRH) (or thyroid-stimulating hormone–releasing factor [TSH-RF], thyrotropin-releasing factor [TRF])
- Growth hormone–releasing factor (GHRF) (or somatotropin-releasing factor [SRF])
- Growth hormone–inhibiting factor (GHIF) (or somatotropin-inhibiting factor [SIF], somatostatin)
- Gonadotropin-releasing hormone (GnRH) (or follicle-stimulating hormone–releasing hormone [FSH-RH], luteinizing hormone–releasing hormone [LH-RH])
- Prolactin-releasing factor (PRF)
- Prolactin-inhibiting factor (PIF)

These hypophysiotropic factors are presently thought to be regulated by higher brain centers, adenohypophyseal hormones ("short-loop" feedback system), and target endocrine gland hormones ("long-loop" system).

By means of light microscopy and acidic or basic dye-staining characteristics, the adenohypophysis is seen to consist of three cell types: acidophils (producing growth hormone [GH] and prolactin), basophils (producing follicle-stimulating hormone [FSH], luteinizing hormone [LH], thyrotropin [TSH], ß-lipotropin, and corticotropin [ACTH]), and chromophobes (producing ACTH and ß-lipotropin).[2] When electron microscopy and immunohistochemical examination are used, the adenohypophysis is observed to consist of five cell types: thyrotrophs (producing TSH), corticotrophs (producing ACTH and ß-lipotropin), gonadotrophs (producing FSH and LH), somatotrophs (producing GH), and mammotrophs (producing prolactin).[1, 2] The release of adenohypophyseal hormones is thought to be regulated by hypophysiotropic factors from the hypothalamus and negative feedback by target endocrine gland hormones.

In general, three factors determine the secretory rates of the endocrine glands: (1) humoral feedback loops, (2) neurologic stimulation or suppression, and (3) genetic influence. The effects of hormones depend on many factors, including the chemical structure, the concentration in the blood, the method of transport in the blood, the quantity of unbound target cell receptors, the integrity of target cell postreceptor mechanism, and the rate of hormonal degradation and elimination.

Most peptide hormones (e.g., ACTH, TSH, FSH, LH, and TRH) initiate their actions by activating the cell membrane enzyme adenyl cyclase and the cyclic adenosine monophosphate system. Steroid hormones (e.g., glucocorticoids and sex hormones) pass through target cell membranes and bind to cytoplasmic receptors[395]; the resultant steroid-receptor complex binds to nuclear chromatin to initiate activity. Thyroid hormones pass into target cell cytoplasm to the nucleus, where they bind chromatin receptors and initiate activity.

The basic causes of endocrine disease include the following: (1) primary hyperfunction (e.g., hyperadrenocorticism due to functional pituitary and adrenal neoplasms and hyperestrogenism due to functional ovarian or testicular neoplasms), (2) secondary hyperfunction (e.g., hyperadrenocorticism due to bilateral adrenocortical hyperplasia), (3) primary hypofunction (e.g., congenital or acquired hypothyroidism and hypopituitarism due to cystic Rathke's cleft), (4) secondary hypofunction (e.g., secondary hypothyroidism due to hypopituitarism), (5) ectopic hypersecretion (e.g., ectopic ACTH syndrome), (6) failure of target cell response, (7) abnormal degradation of hormone (e.g., feminization due to chronic liver disease), (8) hormone interactions (e.g., antiandrogenic actions of progestogens), and (9) iatrogenic hormone excess (excessive glucocorticoids, progestogens, or estrogens).[1, 2]

• DIAGNOSIS OF ENDOCRINOPATHIES

The diagnosis of clinical endocrinopathies is usually based on finding an abnormal concentration of a hormone in the blood. The ideal endocrine assay does not exist. Although radioimmunoassay (RIA) and enzyme-linked immunosorbent assay (ELISA) are the most sensitive, specific, accurate, and precise available methods of measuring hormones, these techniques are usually species specific and must be specially validated for dogs and cats. Any laboratory not willing to provide validation information on request is best avoided.

Basal (resting) levels of serum and plasma hormones frequently do not distinguish normal individuals from those with an endocrinopathy. At any one moment in time, a dog with an endocrine disorder can have hormone levels within the normal range. Conversely, a normal dog may have a subnormal level. Basal blood hormone levels fluctuate in response to environmental, psychic, circadian, and drug-induced influences, and they vary with age, breed, sex, and so forth.° Thus, various stimulation and suppression tests are routinely employed to overcome this unreliability of basal blood hormone levels.

The endocrine system is very dynamic, and hormonal interactions are complex. It is not at all uncommon for one hormone, in deficiency or excess, to affect the levels of another hormone. Common examples include pseudohypothyroidism in the dog with hyperadrenocorticism[333] or decreased growth hormone levels in dogs with hypothyroidism,[87] sex hormone imbalances,[11] or adrenal disease.[383] The laboratory abnormalities usually disappear once the primary endocrine disorder is resolved. If the abnormalities persist or are associated with clinical signs, the dog may suffer from panhypopituitarism[356, 363] or have a polyglandular syndrome.[5, 7] In these syndromes, multiple glands become dysfunctional simultaneously and require individual treatment. When widespread clinicopathologic and endocrine abnormalities exist in the same patient, multiple laboratory evaluations are needed for the patient's complete evaluation.

• THYROID HORMONES

A deficiency of thyroid hormone action is the most common endocrine dermatosis of dogs, but it is rare as a naturally occurring disorder in cats.[1, 2, 106] The etiology of canine hypothyroidism is complex, with the most important cause being lymphocytic (autoimmune) thyroiditis.

Thyroid Physiology

Canine thyroid physiology is a complex subject and has been exhaustively reviewed.[101] It has been shown that dogs produce 3,5,3′,5′-tetraiodothyronine (thyroxine [T_4]), 3,5,3′-triiodothyronine (T_3), 3,3′,5′-triiodothyronine ("reverse" T_3 [rT_3]), 3,3′-diiodothyronine (3,3′-T_2), and 3′,5′-diiodothyronine (3′,5′-T_2).[1, 79, 83, 96]

The thyroid gland secretes all the T_4, but up to 60% of the daily T_3 requirement is formed via monodeiodination (thyroxine 5′-deiodinase) from T_4 in peripheral tissues. The preference of canine thyroid to secrete T_3 rather than T_4 is enhanced by TSH. T_3 is more potent and penetrates much faster into interstitial and intracellular spaces than does T_4. Iodine-deficient dogs show an 80% reduction in their serum T_4 levels, but their serum T_3 levels remain normal and the dogs remain eumetabolic. In addition, hypothyroid dogs being adequately maintained on only oral liothyronine (T_3) have *no* detectable serum T_4, whereas those maintained on only oral levothyroxine (T_4) show normal levels of both serum T_3 and T_4. Thus, T_3 is the major metabolically active thyroid hormone in dogs, with T_4 serving mainly as a prohormone.

In dogs, rT_3, which is metabolically inactive, is formed via monodeiodination (thyrox-

---

°See references 1, 2, 12, 14, 68, 91, 131, 133, 137, 183, 212.

ine 5-deiodinase) from T_4. In human beings and rodents, a number of conditions (chronic and acute illnesses, surgical trauma, fasting, starvation, fever, and glucocorticoid therapy) produce moderate to marked reduction of serum T_3 levels, mild to marked reduction of serum T_4 levels, and marked elevation of serum rT_3 levels.[28, 47, 48, 101, 162] In these circumstances, the patients are euthyroid and in no need of thyroid medication. This situation is called the euthyroid sick syndrome and is a common source of misdiagnosis when basal T_3 and T_4 serum levels are used to diagnose hypothyroidism. The euthyroid sick syndrome also occurs in dogs and cats.* It is thought that this metabolic switch in the sick patient is protective by counteracting the excessive calorigenic effects of T_3 in catabolic states and is caused by an inhibition of one or more iodothyronine ß-ring deiodinases, leading to both decreased production of T_3 from T_4 and decreased rT_3 degradation.

Studies in dogs have shown that T_2 is the major product of peripheral tissue deiodination of T_3 and rT_3. T_2 is metabolically inactive.

Information on thyroid physiology in cats is minimal, and naturally occurring feline hypothyroidism has been documented rarely. It is known that cats produce both T_3 and T_4.[11, 15, 17]

Thyroid Hormones and the Skin

Thyroid hormone plays a dominant role in controlling metabolism and is essential for normal growth and development.[1, 2] The primary mechanisms of action of thyroid hormone are stimulation of cytoplasmic protein synthesis and increase of tissue oxygen consumption. These effects are thought to be initiated by the binding of thyroid hormone to nuclear chromatin and by augmentation of the transcription of genetic information. Available data suggest that thyroid hormone plays a pivotal role in the differentiation and maturation of mammalian skin, as well as in the maintenance of normal cutaneous function.

Hypothyroidism results in epidermal atrophy and abnormal keratinization because of decreased protein synthesis, mitotic activity, and oxygen consumption in dogs and humans.[1, 2] The thyroid hormone–deficient epidermis is characterized by both abnormal lipogenesis and decreased sterol synthesis by keratinocytes.[136] Epidermal melanosis may occur in hypothyroid dogs and humans, but the pathogenic mechanism is unclear.[11] Sebaceous gland atrophy occurs in hypothyroid dogs and humans, and sebum excretion rates are reduced in hypothyroid humans and rats.[11, 32] Hypothyroid dogs have increased triglyceride levels because of impaired plasma clearance.[145] Alterations in plasma fatty acid levels also occur, with increases in oleic and linoleic acids and decreases in dihomo-γ-linolenic, arachidonic, and other elongation acids.[32] Similar changes occur in the cutaneous fatty acid concentrations. Thyroid hormones may regulate Δ-6-desaturase activity.

Thyroid hormone is necessary for the initiation of the anagen phase of the hair follicle cycle.[11] Anagen is not initiated in hypothyroid dogs, resulting in retention of the hair follicles in telogen and leading to failure of hair growth and alopecia. The oral or topical administration of T_4 to normal dogs increases both the growth rate of hair and the numbers of anagen hair follicles, especially in the flanks.[61]

In hypothyroid dogs, humans, and rats, glycosaminoglycans accumulate in the dermis, leading to an increase in the interstitial ground substance and a thick, myxedematous dermis.[1, 2] The exact cause of this tissue mucinosis is unknown, but because thyroid hormones are thought to restrain the synthesis and to increase the catabolism of glycosaminoglycans, decreased thyroid function should cause an accumulation in the dermis.

Thyroid hormone has been reported to heal the ulcers and to reduce the scarring associated with chronic radiodermatitis in humans and to improve the healing of deep dermal burns in rats.[11] These effects were thought to be due to actions of thyroid hormone on the proliferation and metabolism of fibroblasts and collagen synthesis. In

---

*See references 1, 2, 48, 65, 95, 101, 103, 132, 158.

humans, hypothyroidism is associated with a 50% reduction in plasma fibronectin levels.[11] Not surprisingly, the skin of hypothyroid dogs and human beings exhibits poor wound healing and easy bruising.

Bacterial pyoderma is a common complication of canine hypothyroidism.[11, 20, 101, 137] In various animal models, it has been reported that (1) the development of lymphoid tissue depends on the integrity of the thyroid gland, (2) thyroidectomy results in hypoplasia of lymphoid organs and thymus, and (3) depletion of thyroid hormones results in impaired neutrophil functions and B- and T-lymphocyte functions.

Uncomplicated canine hypothyroidism is characterized by the absence of pruritus. Tissue levels of histamine are decreased in experimental canine hypothyroidism.[11] Clinically, canine hypothyroidism is characterized by (1) bilaterally symmetric alopecia, (2) a dull, dry, easily epilated haircoat that fails to grow after clipping, (3) variable hyperpigmentation, (4) skin that is often dry, cool to the touch, thick, and puffy, (5) poor wound healing, (6) easy bruising, (7) frequent seborrheic skin disease, bacterial pyoderma, or both, and (8) variable changes of coat color. Histologically, the condition is characterized by various combinations of orthokeratotic hyperkeratosis, follicular keratosis, follicular dilatation, follicular atrophy, telogenization of hair follicles, excessive trichilemmal keratinization (flame follicles), epidermal melanosis, sebaceous gland atrophy, thick dermis, and increased dermal mucin (myxedema).[4, 16]

Thyroid Function Tests

Despite the routine and regular use of thyroid function tests in veterinary medicine since the early 1970s, the practitioner is still plagued with the problem of making an accurate but inexpensive diagnosis of hypothyroidism. After years of discussion on the inaccuracy of single sample measurements of any of the various thyroid hormones, the use of stimulation tests, either the TSH-response test or the TRH-response test, became routine. Although these tests were not foolproof, they had a high sensitivity and specificity for thyroid disease. In most parts of the world today, TSH is not available at any price and TRH, when available, is very expensive. Some preliminary work has been done with the new recombinant human TSH (rhTSH), and this hormone probably will be useful in testing dogs and cats.[141] Recombinant TRH (rhTRH) is also available but has not been tested. As one might imagine, these new hormones are very expensive and will not find their way into veterinary medicine until their costs decrease significantly.

Until a new function test becomes available, the practitioner has returned to the dark ages of thyroid testing where only single sample measurements are available for interpretation. However, great strides have been made since the 1970s. If samples are sent to qualified laboratories and seriously ill animals or those under the influence of drugs known to influence thyroid hormones are not tested, hypothyroidism or euthyroidism can be accurately diagnosed in over 95% of animals tested.

SERUM THYROID HORMONE DETERMINATIONS

RIA or ELISA methods are used to determine serum levels of total T_4 (TT_4), free T_4 (fT_4), total T_3 (TT_3), free T_3 (fT_3), and reverse T_3 (rT_3). Serum samples may be held at room temperature for at least 1 week with no significant deterioration.[25] Reported basal serum levels of thyroid hormones in dogs are as follows: TT_4, 1.5 to 4 $\mu g/dl$; fT_4, 0.3 to 1.7 ng/dl; TT_3, 75 to 160 ng/dl: and fT_3: 0.3 to 0.6 ng/dl. However, because not all laboratories may use the same assay kit or technique to determine their results, normal ranges can vary from laboratory to laboratory. Because normal levels of TT_3 and fT_3 are common in hypothyroid dogs,[23, 78, 102] these hormones appear to have little diagnostic specificity for hypothyroidism and will not be discussed further.

The sensitivity and the specificity of TT_4 measurements in the diagnosis of hypothyroidism have been studied extensively. These measurements can lead to erroneous diagnoses, especially if the patient's state of health and drug history are ignored. Low levels can occur with a variety of acute and chronic illnesses (euthyroid sick syndrome), including hyperadrenocorticism, diabetes mellitus, hypoadrenocorticism, liver disease, renal failure, various cutaneous and noncutaneous infectious diseases, and a variety of other conditions.

Drugs can decrease or falsely increase TT_4 levels by changing its production, binding, or metabolism. Anticonvulsants (phenobarbital, phenytoin, and diazepam) and glucocorticoids are the most common offenders, but salicylates, phenylbutazone, sulfonamide antimicrobials, radiocontrast agents, mitotane (o,p'-DDD), furosemide, various cardiac drugs, androgens, and estrogens, to name a few, have also been implicated.[48, 54, 75, 101, 102, 157] Of special concern in dogs with dermatologic disease are corticosteroids[95, 158] and the potentiated sulfonamides.[54, 70, 103, 157] Because dogs receive these or other medications because of illness, thyroid levels could be suppressed by both the disease and the drug.

Variations in TT_4 levels can occur with season,[1, 2, 11] time of day,[91, 99] breed,[1, 2, 12, 48, 101, 140] body size,[11, 133] age,[12, 133] and the reproductive status of bitches.[131, 160] With all these variables, it is not surprising that TT_4 measurements can be unreliable. Compounding the problems in measurement are those of interpreting test results. Most laboratories report their normal values in a range; some report the mean value and its standard deviation. If one interprets a test result that is just below the lower limit of the normal or below the mean as abnormal, the margin of error in that interpretation is high.

To reduce the frequency of the misdiagnosis of hypothyroidism, many laboratories suggest a gray zone of interpretation wherein the test results may not be accurate in the diagnosis of hypothyroidism. Typically used zones are 1.0 to 1.5 $\mu g/dl$ when the normal range is greater than 1.5 or values that fall between 1 and 2 standard deviations of the mean. By making the definition of hypothyroidism more stringent (e.g., a value below 1.0 $\mu g/dl$ or less than 2 standard deviations from the mean), the specificity of TT_4 increases. However, some normal dogs have TT_4 values within these stricter guidelines and some hypothyroid dogs are within the gray zone or normal range. Without strict guidelines, basal TT_4 measurements can be low in approximately 20% of euthyroid dogs[11] and be normal in 30% to 50% of hypothyroid dogs.[118] With stricter criteria, TT_4 is in the normal range in only approximately 10% of hypothyroid dogs.[43, 124] Unfortunately, the misdiagnosis rate of approximately 20% in the euthyroid dogs can still be expected.

In humans, serum thyroid hormone–binding protein levels are known to markedly influence serum thyroid hormone levels.[1, 101] Thyroid hormone–binding proteins in the dog have been identified by electrophoresis as thyroxine-binding globulin, thyroxine-binding prealbumin, albumin, inter-α-globulin, and two ß-globulin regions.[1, 2, 11, 101] Alteration in thyroid hormone–binding protein levels or the availability of binding sites on those proteins influences TT_4 measurements. If there is an insufficient amount of protein or the receptors are occupied by other hormones or drugs, the T_4 will not bind and will be rapidly metabolized by the liver. Because fT_4 is not immediately influenced by most of the disorders that alter protein levels or receptor availability, its levels should be normal in the euthyroid dog. It has been suggested that the fT_4 may be the better test to document true hypothyroidism in a dog with a drug history or other disorders.[165] It has been reported that glucocorticoids, phenylbutazone, salicylates, diazepam, primidone, phenytoin, androgens, and phenobarbital may decrease basal serum TT_4 levels by interfering with protein binding and that basal serum TT_4 levels may be elevated in pregnancy, in pseudopregnancy, in male dogs with functional Sertoli's cell testicular tumors, and in response to estrogen therapy, owing to increased protein-binding capacity.[1, 2, 11, 48, 131, 160]

In summary, basal serum levels of TT_4 are significantly influenced by numerous conditions that have nothing to do with thyroid disease and hypothyroidism. In the absence of classic historical, clinical, and clinicopathologic evidence of thyroid hormone deficiency, low basal serum TT_4 levels must be interpreted cautiously because approximately 20% of euthyroid dogs have low levels at any one measurement. To support the diagnosis, additional tests should be performed. To repeat, serum TT_3 levels are a particularly poor measure of thyroid dysfunction.[23, 118] Because TT_3 is predominantly an intracellular hormone and is preferentially produced in states of thyroid deficiency, TT_4 levels drop before TT_3 levels. In addition, TT_3 levels are more severely affected by nonthyroid illnesses and drugs and are inconsistently responsive to TSH and TRH stimulation.

Because the concentration of fT_4 appears to determine hormone availability to cells, and because total hormone concentrations may change with drugs, illness, and so forth without a change in fT_4, a direct or an indirect measurement of fT_4 provides a more consistent laboratory assessment of thyroid status than does the measurement of TT_4. The standard techniques for measurement of fT_4 are RIA, chemiluminescence, and equilibrium dialysis. Equilibrium dialysis is superior to RIA methods, but one report indicates that the chemiluminescence test is equivalent in accuracy to equilibrium dialysis.[117] In the early evaluations of fT_4 measured by RIA, between 11% and 20% of hypothyroid dogs with no confounding illnesses had normal fT_4 levels, whereas 0% to 8% of euthyroid dogs had low levels.[23, 43, 100, 118] Free-T4 measurements by dialysis or chemiluminescence are more accurate.

In two independent studies using large numbers of dogs, the sensitivity of fT_4 in the diagnosis of hypothyroidism was 98% whereas the specificity was either 92% or 93%.[89, 124] Those investigators and others[80, 117, 165] suggest that measurement of fT_4 may be the single most accurate test of thyroid function in the dog. Because some normal dogs and dogs with other endocrine diseases or nonthyroidal illness[107] have low fT_4 levels, low levels are not absolutely diagnostic for hypothyroidism.

In normal cats, basal serum TT_3 and TT_4 levels by RIA are reported to range from 15 to 60 ng/dl and 1.5 to 5 $\mu g/dl$, respectively.[1, 2, 11] T_4-binding serum globulins could not be found in the cat.[1, 2, 11]

In dogs, basal serum rT_3 levels by RIA are reported to be approximately 100 ng/dl.[1, 2] Serum rT_3 levels are expected to be elevated in the euthyroid sick syndrome.

SERUM THYROTROPIN DETERMINATION

In humans, the determination of serum TSH levels by RIA is the most sensitive and reliable indicator of hypothyroidism, often being abnormal for months before basal serum TT_4 levels and TSH stimulation test results are abnormal.[1, 2, 11] Serum TSH levels should be elevated in primary hypothyroidism and low to normal in secondary hypothyroidism. TSH is a species-specific protein that can cross-react with FSH and LH.[164] Assays using human reagents in dogs are inaccurate,[1, 2] and tests designed for the dog (cTSH) can vary depending on the specificity of the antibody used. Normal levels vary with the laboratory, but values of less than 0.5 ng/ml are typical. TSH levels are not influenced by time of day, but random fluctuations do occur, so a single measurement may not be indicative of the thyroid status of the dog.[29] In one study, it was estimated that a dog would have to be sampled approximately 40 times to get meaningful results.[72a] Early evaluations of the cTSH assay were disappointing and were no more predictive of hypothyroidism than measurement of TT_4.[126, 134] Although some studies showed 100% correlation of cTSH results with the final diagnosis,[72, 73] most showed inconsistent elevation in hypothyroid dogs and elevations in 10% to 30% of normal dogs.[127]

In primary hypothyroidism, TSH levels should increase to stimulate the glands to produce more hormone.[44] In secondary or tertiary disease, levels are low. Because the majority of hypothyroid dogs have primary disease, elevated cTSH levels are to be expected in most dogs. In a number of recent studies evaluating cTSH, fT_4, and/or TT_4, the sensitivity of cTSH in the diagnosis of hypothyroidism varied from 63% to 87%[42, 43, 89, 124, 144] whereas the specificity varied from 75% to 93%. In most instances, the TT_4 or fT_4 performed better, indicating that single measurements of cTSH are of questionable value.

To increase the discriminating value of cTSH, it has been suggested that the assay be run in conjunction with a TT_4 or fT_4.[42, 43, 89] The TT_4 or fT_4 would have to be low whereas the cTSH level would have to be elevated before the diagnosis of hypothyroidism would be acceptable. Because it would be harder for hypothyroid dogs to satisfy these more stringent requirements, the sensitivity of the testing would decrease but the specificity would increase. Similar increases in specificity have been reported when TT_4 and fT_4 are evaluated together.[23]

PROVOCATIVE THYROID FUNCTION TESTS

To overcome the unreliability of basal hormone measurement levels, various provocative tests of thyroid function have been developed.[165] There is controversy about the relative efficiency and accuracy of the various tests. Results are often difficult to compare because of variation in methods (different products used at different doses, different time intervals of sampling, and different laboratories performing and interpreting the tests). As mentioned earlier, the availability and/or expense of the hormones used in these tests has severely curtailed their use.

Thyrotropin Stimulation Test

TSH is a species-specific glycoprotein with a molecular weight of about 28,000 that is produced by the adenohypophysis.[118] The secretion of TSH is stimulated by hypothalamic TRH and is inhibited by hypothalamic somatostatin, thyroid hormones, glucocorticoids, dopamine, and stress. Bovine TSH is biologically active in dogs and cats.

The TSH stimulation test has been widely evaluated in dogs and is vastly superior to the determination of basal blood TT_4 and fT_4 levels in the diagnosis of hypothyroidism.* A commonly used procedure for conducting the TSH stimulation test in dogs is as follows: Serum samples for TT_4 determination are collected immediately before and 6 hours after the intravenous (IV) injection of 0.1 IU/kg or 1 to 2 units/dog[116] of bovine TSH. Because TSH can be frozen in conventional freezers for over 200 days without loss of biological potency, multiple dogs can be tested from one vial when these low doses are used. Single or repeated IV injections can rarely produce anaphylaxis,[67] so some investigators use the subcutaneous route.

Euthyroid dogs usually have pre-TSH serum TT_4 levels within or below the normal pre-TSH range for the laboratory performing the assay, and post-TSH serum TT_4 levels within the normal post-TSH range. Some investigators categorize the response to TSH as normal when the post-TSH TT_4 level increases by some specific amount, even if the post-TSH TT_4 value does not enter the normal post-TSH TT_4 range. The specific increase expected varies from laboratory to laboratory and cannot be used reliably elsewhere.[118] The commonly espoused criterion—that euthyroid dogs double their basal serum TT_4 levels after TSH stimulation—is unreliable. In general, measuring serum TT_3 levels before and after TSH administration is unreliable and not recommended. Little work has been done with fT_4.[117]

The TSH stimulation test usually achieves normal poststimulation serum TT_4 levels in dogs with the euthyroid sick syndrome and drug-related low basal serum TT_4 level.[1, 2, 11, 99, 165] In some cases, especially in dogs with hyperadrenocorticism or dogs being treated with glucocorticoids, both the pre-TSH and post-TSH serum TT_4 levels are below the expected normal ranges.[95, 120, 158, 207] However, the slope of the response parallels that of normal dogs. Glucocorticoids have been reported to suppress TRH secretion, suppress pituitary responsiveness to TRH, suppress TSH secretion, depress serum thyroid hormone–binding protein levels, suppress basal serum TT_4 and TT_3 levels, inhibit the conversion of TT_4 to TT_3, and increase serum rT_3 levels.

If a clinician wishes to perform a TSH stimulation test on dogs receiving thyroid hormone treatment, administration of the thyroid supplement should be stopped for at least 30 days. Cessation for 60 days may give more reliable results.[1, 2, 104] The TSH stimulation test can be conducted simultaneously with an ACTH stimulation test or a dexamethasone suppression test with no compromise in the accuracy of either procedure.[10, 13]

In cats, the following two protocols have been reported to be accurate measurements of thyroid function: (1) serum TT_4 determinations before and 6 hours after IV injection of either 1 IU or 1 IU/kg of bovine TSH[70, 146] and (2) serum TT_4 determinations before and 10 hours after intramuscular (IM) injection of 2.5 IU of bovine TSH.[6]

---

*See references 1, 2, 23, 24, 78, 102, 118.

Thyrotropin-Releasing Hormone Stimulation Test

TRH is a tripeptide produced by the hypothalamus.[1, 2] TRH stimulates the release of TSH and prolactin.[76] TRH secretion is enhanced by norepinephrine, histamine, serotonin, and dopamine, and it is probably inhibited by thyroid hormones.

In humans, serum TT_4 and TSH responses to exogenous TRH have been used to differentiate among primary, secondary, and tertiary hypothyroidism.[1, 2] Patients with primary hypothyroidism have low basal serum TT_4 levels and high basal serum TSH levels, neither of which responds to TRH stimulation. Patients with secondary hypothyroidism have low basal serum TT_4 and TSH levels, neither of which responds to TRH stimulation. Patients with tertiary hypothyroidism have low basal serum TT_4 and TSH levels, both of which respond to TRH stimulation.

A variety of different studies on the accuracy of the TRH stimulation test in separating euthyroid and hypothyroid dogs have been published.* This testing can be done in conjunction with other stimulation tests (e.g., ACTH stimulation test for hyperadrenocorticism) without impact on any test.[88] The TRH is given intravenously and samples are collected before and 4 or 6 hours after injection. Most authors suggest doses of 0.2 or 0.25 mg, but a dose of 0.05 mg/kg has also been suggested.[51, 165] Doses greater than 0.9 mg or greater than 0.1 mg/kg often cause various cholinergic side effects, including hypersalivation, coughing, miosis, vomiting, diarrhea, urination, tachycardia, and tachypnea.

In the early evaluations of this test, TT_4 levels only were determined. Basal TT_4 levels are expected to at least double in normal dogs, whereas this should not occur in hypothyroid dogs. When results of the TRH stimulation test were compared with the results of TSH stimulation tests performed in the same dogs, the TRH results were less predictable of hypothyroidism; the current sentiment is that the standard TRH stimulation test is not reliable for the diagnosis of hypothyroidism.[51, 147] Recent studies have focused on measurement of cTSH in response to TRH administration. In normal dogs, cTSH levels should increase over 150% after TRH administration, whereas very little change should occur in hypothyroid dogs.[69, 143] This small rate of change indicates that pituitary output of TSH is already at its maximum. Although this testing can be helpful in some cases, baseline measurement of cTSH is probably just as accurate.[143] Unless further modifications improve the accuracy of the TRH stimulation test, it has little or no use.

In normal cats, serum TT_4 levels were reported to show a reproducible doubling 4 hours after the IV injection of 0.1 mg/kg of TRH.[122, 146] TRH doses of 0.1 mg/kg or greater often produced the cholinergic side effects mentioned earlier for dogs.

THYROID BIOPSY

Primary and secondary canine hypothyroidism can be easily distinguished by histologic examination of a biopsy specimen of the thyroid.[1, 2, 11] In primary hypothyroidism, there is massive loss of follicular epithelium, usually associated with lymphocytic thyroiditis.[86] In secondary hypothyroidism, the follicles are distended with colloid, the follicular epithelium is flattened, and there is no vacuolation of the colloid. Normal dogs treated with systemic glucocorticoid have increased numbers of colloid droplets per thyroid follicular cell, suggesting inhibition of thyroid lysosomal hydrolysis of colloid.[11] In these dogs, basal serum TT_3 and TT_4 levels were decreased, but TSH and TRH stimulation test results were normal.

TESTS USED IN LYMPHOCYTIC THYROIDITIS

In dogs and human patients with lymphocytic thyroiditis, a number of immunologic evaluations have been conducted, including determination of serum levels of antithyroglobulin antibodies, serum levels of antimicrosomal and anticolloidal antibodies, in vitro

---

*See references 51, 69, 76, 78, 84, 102, 143, 147, 149.

lymphocyte blastogenesis to thyroid extract, delayed-type hypersensitivity skin test reactions to thyroid extract, and circulating immune complex levels.[1, 2, 30, 34, 55, 79, 161] In dogs, antithyroglobulin antibodies are demonstrable in more than 50% of cases of naturally occurring hypothyroidism by means of ELISA, hemagglutination, and indirect immunofluorescence techniques.[22, 36, 62–64]

Antibodies to T_4 or T_3 also may be detected.[34, 52, 79, 130] When present, these autoantibodies cause spurious elevations of the TT_4 or TT_3 values as measured by RIA.[80, 96] The patient looks either normal or hypothyroid but has TT_4 or TT_3 levels consistent with hyperthyroidism. Great Danes, Irish setters, Borzois, Doberman pinschers, and Old English sheepdogs may be predisposed. Interestingly, antithyroglobulin antibodies are also demonstrable in more than 40% of dogs with nonthyroidal endocrine disorders and healthy relatives of antibody-positive patients, as well as in 13% of hospitalized patients without endocrine disease. Screening for antithyroid antibodies may be useful in detecting family members that might experience hypothyroidism and helping to differentiate primary immune-mediated hypothyroidism (antibody-positive) from secondary and tertiary hypothyroidism (antibody-negative).

• GLUCOCORTICOIDS

Glucocorticoids are produced by the zona fasciculata of the adrenal cortex and are probably the most commonly used therapeutic agents in veterinary medicine.[1, 2, 306] Glucocorticoids are bound primarily to a high-affinity corticosteroid-binding globulin (80%) and serum albumin (10%).[213] The remaining 10% is free and metabolically active. Because most of the receptor sites on the corticosteroid-binding protein are open, cortisol production can increase fivefold before the free fraction increases. Hyperglucocorticoidism may be produced by hypersecretion of ACTH or ACTH-like substances (ectopic, idiopathic, functional pituitary neoplasm), hypersecretion of endogenous glucocorticoids (functional adrenocortical neoplasm), and exogenous glucocorticoid administration (iatrogenic).

Glucocorticoids and the Skin

The skin is a sensitive and specific indicator of hyperglucocorticoidism, reflecting both internal disease and inappropriate therapy.[1, 2, 11] The protein catabolic, antienzymatic, and antimitotic effects of glucocorticoids are manifested in numerous ways in dog and cat skin: (1) the epidermis becomes thinned and hyperkeratotic (because of suppressed deoxyribonucleic acid [DNA] synthesis, decreased mitoses, and keratinization abnormalities), (2) the basement membrane zone becomes thinned and disrupted, (3) pilosebaceous atrophy becomes pronounced, (4) the dermis becomes thinned and dermal vasculature becomes fragile (owing to inhibition of fibroblast proliferation, collagen, and ground substance production), and (5) wound healing is delayed. Unique to the dog, presumably through changes in protein structure, collagen and elastin fibers become attractive sites for mineralization, resulting in dystrophic calcinosis cutis.[71] In chronic cases, cutaneous ossification can occur.[211] Additionally, owing to the broad-spectrum anti-inflammatory and immunosuppressive effects of excessive glucocorticoids, patients have increased susceptibility to bacterial and fungal cutaneous infections.[1, 2, 11]

Clinically, hyperglucocorticoidism in dogs and cats is characterized by (1) thin, hypotonic skin, (2) easy bruising (petechiae and ecchymoses), (3) poor wound healing, (4) seborrhea sicca, (5) phlebectasias, and (6) increased susceptibility to bacterial infection, demodicosis, and perhaps dermatophytosis and *Malassezia* infection. In dogs, calcinosis cutis, bilaterally symmetric alopecia, easy epilation, comedones, and variable hyperpigmentation are features of hyperglucocorticoidism. In human patients, but not in dogs and cats, hypertrichosis and cutaneous striae are common features of hyperglucocorticoidism.

Histologically, hyperglucocorticoidism in dogs and cats is characterized by variable combinations of orthokeratotic hyperkeratosis, follicular keratosis, telogenization of hair follicles, excessive trichilemmal keratinization (flame follicles), thin dermis, and telangiectasia.[4, 16] The follicular dilatation, follicular atrophy, epidermal atrophy, epidermal melanosis, sebaceous gland atrophy, and dystrophic mineralization that occur in dogs are rare in cats.

Adrenal Function Tests

Adrenal function tests are basically of two types: those that are single measurements of basal glucocorticoid levels in blood or urine and those that are provocative, dynamic-response tests. Single measurements of basal glucocorticoid levels, although cheaper and easier to perform, are unreliable.[1, 2, 280, 343b] Many dogs with hyperadrenocorticism have elevated basal glucocorticoid levels, but some dogs have normal levels,[243] and dogs with nonadrenal disorders can have elevated levels.[186]

URINARY GLUCOCORTICOID DETERMINATION

In dogs, the major cortisol metabolites found in urine are cortol, 3-epiallocortol, cortolone, 3-epiallotetrahydrocortisol, and tetrahydrocortisol.[1, 2, 11] These metabolites are excreted mainly as glucuronides, and a major portion of this fraction is represented by steroids reduced at C-20. Thus, the use of steroid assay procedures that measure only those steroids having a dihydroxyketotic side chain, such as the Porter-Silber reaction, do not measure these cortisol metabolites in dogs. In cats, virtually all glucocorticoid metabolites are excreted in bile (99%), with only a small amount of Porter-Silber chromogens present as the free compounds in urine (1%).[1, 2, 15]

Assays of urinary steroids (17-ketosteroids and 17-hydroxycorticosteroids) necessitate 24-hour urine samples, metabolic cages, and collecting equipment; are easily contaminated; and must be performed before and after the administration of a provocative test agent. They are rarely used today.

The urinary cortisol to creatinine ratio was developed to avoid the need for 24-hour urine collection and to screen the patient for hyperadrenocorticism.[203, 237, 256] Normal dogs have low values (5.7 ± 0.9), whereas dogs with hyperadrenocorticism have high values (337.6 ± 72). However, values in dogs under stress,[320] with renal disease, or with other disorders can overlap those in dogs with Cushing's disease, so the test is not specific (positive predictive value, 87%).[236] Because values are not normal in dogs with hyperadrenocorticism, this ratio can be a useful screening test to exclude that diagnosis (negative predictive value, 100%).

BLOOD CORTISOL DETERMINATION

Blood cortisol levels in dogs and cats have been measured by three methods: fluorometry, competitive protein binding, and RIA.[1, 2] RIA is the method of choice and the one in general use. Basal blood cortisol levels by RIA in normal dogs and cats are approximately 0 to 8 μg/dl,[1, 2] but the normal values established for the laboratory performing the testing should always be used. Serum or plasma can be used in the testing, and freezing is unnecessary provided samples reach the laboratory within 8 days and are kept cold ($<20°C$).[11, 25] Most investigators separate the serum or plasma as quickly as possible and freeze it until the assay is performed.

Important considerations when interpreting blood cortisol levels include the following: (1) different laboratories may vary in their normal and abnormal values, (2) stress and nonadrenal illness can markedly elevate blood cortisol levels, (3) cortisol levels can vary with the patient's age, (4) episodic cortisol secretion occurs in normal dogs and dogs with hyperadrenocorticism, and (5) single measurements of blood cortisol are of limited value in the diagnosis of hyperadrenocorticism.* Although early data suggested rhythmic variation in cortisol secretion in dogs and cats,[1, 2, 11] it is now generally thought that these

---

*See references 1, 2, 11, 12, 183, 186, 212, 298.

species show little or no circadian variation in plasma concentrations of ACTH or cortisol.[246] These hormones appear to be secreted in an episodic baseline with 8 to 16 peaks per day.

CORTISOL RESPONSE TESTS

To overcome the unreliability of basal blood cortisol levels, various provocative tests have been developed.[1, 2, 280, 343b] Because some dogs with hyperadrenocorticism have an altered clearance of ACTH and dexamethasone[219] or may have low circulating cortisol levels,[275] no one test is absolutely diagnostic and all results must be evaluated in light of the patient's signs. Cortisol response tests are traditionally begun at 8 to 10 AM.

Corticotropin (ACTH) Stimulation Test

ACTH is a polypeptide with a molecular weight of about 4500 secreted by the adenohypophysis as part of a large prohormone, pro-opiomelanocortin, which also contains in its sequence ß-lipotropin, ß-endorphin, enkephalins, and α-MSH.[1, 2, 246]

The ACTH stimulation test (ACTH response test) reliably documents a diagnosis of hypoadrenocorticism or iatrogenic hyperadrenocorticism in dogs and cats. Basal blood cortisol levels are normal or low and show little or no response to ACTH. In addition, the ACTH stimulation test is useful for monitoring therapeutic response to adrenosuppressive treatments.[249, 273] Two commonly used protocols for ACTH stimulation are as follows: (1) plasma or serum cortisol samples collected before and 2 hours after the IM injection of 2.2 IU/kg of ACTH gel or (2) plasma or serum cortisol samples collected before and 1 hour after the IV or IM injection of synthetic ACTH (Cortrosyn).[224] The ACTH gel is currently difficult to obtain. The synthetic product is packaged in single-dose vials of 0.25 mg. Conventionally, the whole vial was administered. In many animals, this 0.25-mg dose was well above the 5 µg/kg needed to maximally stimulate the dog's adrenal glands.[248, 330] Because the product's bioavailability is maintained for 4 months in the refrigerator or for 6 months in the conventional freezer ($-20°C$), many investigators subdivide the vial and give only what is needed.[171, 248] The ACTH stimulation test can be performed concurrently with the TSH stimulation test while maintaining the accuracy of both tests.[10, 13]

In many of the older texts and papers, the ACTH stimulation test was considered inferior to the low-dose dexamethasone suppression test for the diagnosis of spontaneous hyperadrenocorticism in the dog.* This assessment was based on the fact that about 15% of cases with pituitary-dependent hyperadrenocorticism do not have an exaggerated response to ACTH administration; about 50% of cases with an adrenocortical tumor hyperresponded; and chronically ill or stressed animals can have elevated basal cortisol levels and may hyperrespond to ACTH. As was discussed in the thyroid testing section, more current methods of evaluation give the raw data and the sensitivity, specificity, and possibly the positive predictive value of the test. The positive predictive value is the probability that the positive test result was correct.

In one study comparing the accuracy of the ACTH stimulation test versus the low-dose dexamethasone suppression test in 40 dogs with hyperadrenocorticism (30 with pituitary-dependent disease, 10 with adrenal tumor) and 41 normal dogs, the sensitivities of both tests were nearly identical, 95% and 96%, respectively, but the specificity of the low-dose dexamethasone test was 76%, resulting in a positive predictive value of 76%. The ACTH stimulation test was more specific (91%), with a positive predictive value of 91%.[318] In another study on 20 dogs with pituitary-dependent disease, 59 dogs with nonadrenal disease, and 21 normal dogs, the positive predictive values for the ACTH stimulation test and low-dose dexamethasone suppression test were lower, 67% and 38%, respectively, but the ACTH stimulation test was superior.[239] Sensitivity and specificity data also was poorer. The poorer performance of both of these tests was due to the inclusion of the 59 dogs

---

*See references 183, 212, 235, 256, 272, 273, 280, 333, 343b.

with nonadrenal disease. About 35% had significantly elevated baseline cortisol levels, and 38% and 56% failed to show adequate suppression to dexamethasone at 4 or 8 hours, respectively. Eight dogs (14%) had abnormal ACTH response test results. Both of these and other studies validate the use of the ACTH stimulation test but highlight the need for careful evaluation of the results.

The ACTH stimulation test has been studied in normal cats and in a small number of cats with spontaneous hyperadrenocorticism.* Two protocols recommended for cats are as follows: (1) plasma or serum cortisol determinations before and 90 minutes after the IM injection of 2.2 IU/kg of ACTH gel and (2) plasma or serum cortisol determinations before and 90 minutes after the IV injection of 0.125 mg of synthetic ACTH. Other investigators reported no difference in the response of the healthy cats to 0.125 mg or 0.250 mg of synthetic ACTH IM (peak cortisol responses at 30 minutes after injection).[310] It was reported that cats with diabetes mellitus may hyperrespond to ACTH,[281] but another study failed to document this finding in diabetic and nondiabetic sick cats.[343]

Low-Dose Dexamethasone Suppression Test

The low-dose dexamethasone suppression test is used to confirm the diagnosis of spontaneous canine hyperadrenocorticism.[1, 2, 235, 256, 272, 280, 343b] In normal dogs, the low dose of dexamethasone consistently suppresses blood cortisol levels to less than 1 μg/dl for the 8-hour test period. The definition of suppression varies, but most investigators think that a reduction in the blood cortisol level to below 1.5 μg/dl or to less than 50% of the resting level indicates suppression. A commonly used protocol for the low-dose dexamethasone suppression test is to take plasma or serum cortisol samples before and 4 and 8 hours after the IV administration of 0.01 mg/kg of dexamethasone. The dexamethasone suppression test has been performed concurrently with the TSH stimulation test while preserving the accuracy of both tests.[10, 13]

As mentioned in the discussion of the ACTH stimulation test, the low-dose dexamethasone suppression test can be equally or more specific than the ACTH stimulation test but has a much lower specificity and positive predictive value in both normal dogs and dogs with nonadrenal disease.[183, 206, 218, 239, 242, 318] The test performs much more poorly in dogs with nonadrenal disease because (1) they have an accelerated clearance of dexamethasone, (2) they have a receptor insensitivity, or (3) their chronic illness has resulted in significant adrenocortical hyperplasia. As with all other tests, the results of the low-dose dexamethasone suppression test must be interpreted in light of the patient's clinical signs and not just accepted at face value.[1, 2]

The dexamethasone suppression test has been studied in a few normal cats and cats with spontaneous hyperadrenocorticism.[269, 270, 281, 310, 343b] One group of investigators reported that plasma cortisol responses of healthy cats to IV injections of dexamethasone at doses of 0.01 mg/kg, 0.1 mg/kg, and 1 mg/kg were similar (with peak suppression at 6 to 10 hours after injection).[310] It was reported that the results of dexamethasone suppression testing were not different in normal, diabetic, and nondiabetic sick cats.[343]

High-Dose Dexamethasone Suppression Test

The high-dose dexamethasone suppression test is used to differentiate between pituitary-dependent hyperadrenocorticism and that caused by the adrenocortical neoplasia in dogs.[1, 2, 235, 256, 272, 280, 343c] Because high-dose dexamethasone should cause suppression in both normal dogs and most dogs with pituitary-dependent disease, this test cannot be used to confirm the diagnosis of hyperadrenocorticism. The definition of suppression varies, but most investigators think that a reduction in the blood cortisol level to below 1.5 μg/dl or to less than 50% of the resting level indicates suppression. A commonly used protocol for the high-dose dexamethasone suppression test is to take plasma or serum cortisol samples before and 4 and 8 hours after the IV injection of 0.1 mg/kg of dexamethasone. Some investigators recommended a much higher dose, 1 mg/kg.[280] Although

---

*See references 1, 2, 11, 279, 281, 283, 284, 310, 342, 343b.

this larger dose increases the expense of the test, it does not clearly enhance the diagnostic accuracy of the test.[1, 2, 240] In fact, it has been suggested that the 1 mg/kg dose was less reliable than the 0.1 mg/kg dose.[11, 240]

Not all dogs with pituitary-dependent disease experience suppression in the expected fashion.[240, 280, 325] In a large study of 181 dogs with pituitary-dependent disease and 35 dogs with an adrenal tumor, suppression did not occur in 46 (25%) of the dogs with pituitary-dependent disease. Suppression did occur in 2 (6%) of the dogs with adrenal tumors.[125] The dogs with pituitary-dependent disease in which suppression did not occur might have had a tumor in the intermediate lobe, an area typically unresponsive to blood-borne ACTH and dexamethasone.[340]

PLASMA CORTICOTROPIN (ACTH) DETERMINATION

Plasma ACTH levels have been measured by RIA in normal dogs and in dogs with spontaneous hyperadrenocorticism.[1, 2, 11, 241, 256, 272, 280, 291, 333, 343c] Endogenous plasma ACTH levels are extremely useful in determining the cause of spontaneous canine hyperadrenocorticism, especially when interpreted together with the results of dexamethasone suppression testing. Plasma ACTH levels range from normal to elevated (greater than 40 pg/ml) in dogs with pituitary-dependent hyperadrenocorticism and range from low to undetectable (less than 20 pg/ml) in dogs with functional adrenocortical neoplasms. As is the case with plasma cortisol levels, plasma ACTH levels fluctuate episodically throughout the day, which results in some overlap of values between normal dogs and dogs with spontaneous hyperadrenocorticism. Plasma ACTH levels have been measured by RIA in normal cats and are reported to be approximately 20 to 100 pg/ml.[1, 2, 269–281, 342, 343c] Plasma ACTH levels were markedly elevated in one cat with pituitary-dependent hyperadrenocorticism.

Accurate determination of plasma ACTH necessitates proper collection and handling of the specimen and a carefully performed, difficult RIA technique. Conventionally, blood for ACTH assay was collected in heparin-containing or ethylenediaminetetra-acetic–containing plastic tubes and spun within 90 minutes at 4°C (39.2°F). The plasma must be promptly separated into plastic or polypropylene tubes and kept frozen until assayed. If aprotinin, a proteinase inhibitor, is added to the collection tubes, the separated and refrigerated (but unfrozen) plasma will not undergo any decrease in ACTH concentration provided that it reaches the laboratory within 4 days.[247] At −20°C (−4°F), the ACTH concentration of samples is maintained for only 30 days, so the assay must be performed quickly.[225]

CORTICOTROPIN-RELEASING FACTOR STIMULATION TEST

CRF is a peptide secreted in pulsatile fashion by the hypothalamus.[1, 2, 185] CRF secretion is stimulated by epinephrine and serotonin, and it is inhibited by glucocorticoids and serotonin antagonists (e.g., cyproheptadine).

The isolation and synthesis of CRF makes possible an additional diagnostic test to differentiate the two causes of spontaneous hyperadrenocorticism.[1, 2, 241, 280, 285, 343c] Synthetic ovine CRF was injected intravenously (0.1, 1, or 10 μg/kg) into normal dogs and produced peak plasma ACTH and cortisol levels within 30 to 60 minutes.[241] Preliminary information indicates that the CRF stimulation test is useful for distinguishing between canine pituitary-dependent hyperadrenocorticism (increased levels of ACTH and cortisol) and adrenocortical neoplasia (no response).[280] However, until a relatively inexpensive, single-dose, sterilized CRF preparation becomes available, the CRF stimulation test is of limited usefulness to most veterinarians.

OTHER ADRENAL FUNCTION TESTS

Attempts have been made to devise more foolproof, inexpensive, and time-efficient adrenal function tests for the dog and the cat. Tests evaluated include (1) the metyrapone response test, (2) the lysine-vasopressin test, (3) the insulin response test, (4) the glucagon response test, and (5) a combination of the ACTH response and dexamethasone suppression tests.[1, 2, 11, 197, 200, 201] However, these tests are inferior to the standard ACTH stimulation and dexamethasone suppression tests and cannot be recommended.

• GROWTH HORMONE

GH (somatotropin) is a polypeptide (molecular weight about 22,000) produced by the adenohypophysis.[1, 2] It has diametrically opposed intrinsic anabolic and catabolic activities. Its catabolic activity (enhanced lipolysis and restricted glucose transport caused by insulin resistance) is caused directly by the GH polypeptide, whereas its anabolic activity is mediated by somatomedins (insulin-like growth factors), which are primarily generated by the liver and controlled by GH.[346, 354, 355] The major function of GH is hormonal control of growth (in concert with thyroid hormones, insulin, cortisol, and sex steroids). GH is also important for the development of the thymus and T-cell function.[370, 371]

The secretion of GH is episodic and labile; it is affected by the sleep-wake cycle, physical activity, the animal's nutritional state, physical and emotional stress, and pregnancy.[1, 2] In a study of 500 normal dogs, pulsatile GH secretion was found during a 24-hour period.[347] About 30% of the dogs did not respond to clonidine and xylazine provocation, probably because the agents were administered in the postsecretory refractory period when the pituitary would not respond to further stimulation. Various neurotransmitters—norepinephrine, dopamine, and serotonin—as well as hypoglycemia, various amino acids, and progestogens stimulate GH secretion.

No significant changes occurred in the concentrations of GH in whole blood held at room temperature (20° to 22°C) or in refrigeration (4°C) for 24 hours; in plasma held at room temperature or in refrigeration for 8 days; or in plasma that went through four freeze/thaw cycles.[381]

Excessive GH secretion produces acromegaly.[354, 365, 375, 377] The skin becomes thickened, is myxedematous, and is thrown into exaggerated folds. These changes are most obvious on the face and the extremities. Hypertrichosis is common. Hyperpigmentation occurs in about 40% of human patients with acromegaly but has not been reported in dogs.[11] Histologically, acromegalic skin is characterized by increased dermal collagen and mucin and by hyperplasia of the epidermis and the appendages.[4, 16, 375]

In dogs, juvenile GH deficiency results in retention of the puppy coat, followed by bilaterally symmetric alopecia and hyperpigmentation, and by thin, hypotonic skin.[11, 355] Hyposomatotropism in the mature dog yields similar cutaneous findings, but the dog has a normal adult coat before the hair loss starts.[355, 359, 373, 376] Histologically, both entities are characterized by variable combinations of orthokeratotic hyperkeratosis, follicular keratosis, follicular dilatation, follicular atrophy, telogenization of hair follicles, excessive trichilemmal keratinization (flame follicles), epidermal melanosis, sebaceous gland atrophy, thin dermis, and decreased to absent elastin fibers in chronically affected dogs.[4, 16]

Specific RIA techniques for measuring canine GH have been developed.[11, 355, 376] Basal GH levels in normal dogs and cats are approximately 1 to 4.5 ng/ml.[1, 2, 11, 347, 355, 376] Neither breed nor sex causes variation in normal levels, but age has a profound effect. Dogs younger than 1 year have approximately double the levels in dogs older than 1 year.[347] Young dogs also have a twofold to fourfold greater increase in poststimulation GH levels as compared with mature dogs. Basal GH levels in pituitary dwarfs and hypophysectomized dogs may approximate these values as well. Thus, basal GH levels are inadequate for the documentation of GH deficiency.

To document GH deficiency, stimulation tests must be performed.[1, 2, 11, 361, 372] Clonidine hydrochloride (Catapres), an α-adrenergic and antihypertensive drug, has been used to stimulate GH release in dogs. Normal dogs showed a marked increase in plasma GH and insulin-like growth factor (IGF-1) levels within 15 to 30 minutes after IV injection of 20 to 30 μg/kg of clonidine, whereas no response occurred in pituitary dwarfs and hypophysectomized dogs. Because some normal dogs show no response to clonidine or xylazine provocation,[347] this test cannot be considered diagnostic for GH deficiency. Clonidine may cause severe hypotension and shock.[11] Xylazine (Rompun), a sedative hypnotic drug, gives similar results when injected intravenously at 100 to 300 $\mu g/kg$. The 300 $\mu g/kg$ xylazine dose may cause severe hypotension and shock in toy and miniature breeds of dogs.[11] More recently, testing with synthetic human or bovine GH-RF has been suggested.[344, 359] Either product is injected intravenously at 1 $\mu g/kg$, with sampling at 0, 15, and 30 minutes. Side effects have not been reported. Proper interpretation of GH levels also necessitates the assessment of thyroid and adrenal gland function.[1, 2, 355, 376] Both hyperglucocorticoidism and hypothyroidism impair GH secretion. In addition, pseudopregnancy, progestogen therapy, and sex hormone imbalances can cause elevation of basal plasma GH levels and poor response to xylazine.

In acromegaly, basal plasma GH levels have been markedly elevated, ranging from 11 to 1476 ng/ml.[354, 365, 375, 377] A hallmark of acromegaly is the nonsuppressibility of plasma GH levels during the administration of an IV glucose load. In canine acromegaly, plasma GH levels were not suppressed by the IV administration of 1 g of glucose per kilogram.[1, 2, 354]

Somatomedins are polypeptides (molecular weight, 5000 to 10,000) that can also be quantitated by RIA to assess GH status indirectly.[1, 2, 354–359] Insulin-like growth factor I (IGF-1) is most commonly assayed. IGF-1 plasma levels parallel body size in dogs; normal values for Cocker spaniels are 5 to 90 ng/ml as opposed to 230 to 330 ng/ml for normal German shepherds. IGF-1 production is impaired by glucocorticoids and estrogens, and levels are expected to be low or undetectable in GH-deficient states and elevated in acromegaly. Values have been normal in some dogs with presumed adult-onset hyposomatotropism.[359, 368]

• SEX HORMONES

Estrogens

Estrogens are present in both male and female animals and are produced by the ovarian follicles, the zona reticularis of the adrenal cortex, and Sertoli's and interstitial cells of the testicles.[1, 2, 418] They may also be made by peripheral aromatization of androgens. Pituitary FSH stimulates ovarian follicular growth and estrogen production in females and spermatogenesis in males.[1, 2] Hypothalamic GnRH stimulates the pituitary to release FSH. In turn, estrogen inhibits GnRH release, and inhibin (produced by ovarian follicles and testicular Sertoli's cells) inhibits FSH release.

Estrogens are reported to stimulate epidermal mitosis, to increase epidermal thickness in mice and humans, and to reduce epidermal thickness in rats and humans.[11, 418] Epidermal atrophy was produced in dogs by daily IM injections of 1 mg of diethylstilbestrol for 400 days.

Estrogens increase skin pigmentation in the guinea pig by increasing both free melanin and melanin within melanocytes, whereas ovariectomy has the opposite effect.[11] Cutaneous hyperpigmentation is a feature of clinical dermatoses associated with hyperestrogenism in dogs.

Estrogens reduce both sebaceous gland size and sebum production in rats and humans.[11] These effects appear to result from a local action on sebaceous glands rather than from a feedback suppression of endogenous androgens. The daily IM injection of 1 mg of diethylstilbestrol into dogs for 400 days produced marked sebaceous gland atrophy.

Estrogens suppress the initiation of anagen in rats, whereas ovariectomy has the opposite effect.[11, 418] In addition, the rate of hair growth is greater in spayed female rats than in intact normal female rats, and estradiol implanted into spayed female or castrated male rats reduces the growth rate. In dogs, estrogens administered orally, subcutaneously, intramuscularly, and topically produce alopecia. Bilaterally symmetric alopecia and easily epilated hair are striking features of clinical dermatoses associated with hyperestrogenism in dogs. There appears to be regional sensitivity of hair follicles to estrogenic abnormalities because these dermatoses follow a predictable pattern (see later). Evidence also suggests that these estrogen-sensitive areas of skin may have increased numbers of estrogen receptors.[390]

Estrogens are reported to increase the amount of dermal ground substance in mice and humans.[11] The daily IM injection of 1 mg of diethylstilbestrol in dogs for 400 days reduced the thickness of the subcutis.[386, 421] Estrogens are also known to affect thymic function, to enhance antibody production, and to inhibit suppressor T-cell function.[399]

Hyperestrogenism is thought to be the cause of two distinctive dermatoses in dogs: feminization of the male dog with a functional tumor of the testicle and hyperestrogenism of the intact female dog. Cutaneous changes in these syndromes include (1) bilaterally symmetric alopecia that begins in the perineal, genital, and ventral abdominal regions and spreads cranially and ventrally, (2) variable hyperpigmentation, (3) a dull, easily epilated haircoat that fails to regrow after clipping, (4) nipple hypertrophy, (5) pendulous prepuce, (6) vulvar enlargement, and (7) variable seborrheic skin disease. In male dogs, linear preputial dermatosis appears to correlate with the presence of hyperestrogenism and testicular neoplasia. Histologically, both syndromes are characterized by variable combinations of orthokeratotic hyperkeratosis, follicular keratosis, follicular dilatation, follicular atrophy, telogenization of hair follicles, excessive trichilemmal keratinization (flame follicles), epidermal melanosis, and sebaceous gland atrophy.[4, 16]

The vast majority of adrenalectomized and ovariectomized dogs maintained on only mineralocorticoids have normal skin and haircoats, indicating that estrogens or any other sex steroids are not necessary for normal skin and haircoats in dogs. However, hypoestrogenism has been hypothesized as an etiologic consideration in the estrogen-responsive dermatosis of spayed female dogs. Clinically, the dermatosis is characterized by (1) bilaterally symmetric alopecia that begins in the perineal, genital, and ventral abdominal areas and spreads cranially and ventrally, and (2) an easily epilated haircoat that fails to regrow after clipping. Histologically, the dermatosis is characterized by follicular keratosis and follicular dilatation with telogenization of hair follicles.[4, 16] In addition, spayed female cats with feline acquired symmetric alopecia may respond to estrogen replacement therapy.

Assays (RIA) for plasma or serum estrogens are commercially available.[1, 2] Most available assays measure only one type of estrogen (e.g., estradiol or estrone). Because numerous estrogenic substances are produced in the body, such assays may be unsatisfactory. Thus, one can readily understand why only 50% of the dogs with feminization due to functional Sertoli's cell neoplasm of the testicle could be shown to have hyperestrogenism (only estradiol was measured). Additionally, blood estrogen levels, along with the blood levels of the other sex steroids, fluctuate markedly during the day, necessitating multiple samples and unrealistic financial considerations.[400] Evidence has been presented that suggests that dogs can have so-called cutaneous hyperestrogenism (increased cutaneous estrogen receptors) in the absence of hyperestrogenism.[390] Reported values for blood estradiol in the dog and cat vary with the sex of the animal, whether it is neutered or intact, the stage of the estrous cycle, and the laboratory used.[418]

Androgens

Androgens are present in both male and female animals and they are produced by the interstitial cells of the testicle, by the zona reticularis of the adrenal cortex, and through peripheral conversion of other sex steroids.[1, 2, 418] Pituitary LH stimulates androgen secretion by testicular interstitial cells and ovulation and corpus luteum formation and maintenance.[1, 2] Hypothalamic GnRH stimulates the pituitary release of LH. In turn, androgens and progesterone inhibit LH release, and estrogens and androgens (via hypothalamic aromatization to estrogens) inhibit GnRH release.

Androgens are reported to stimulate epidermal mitosis in mice and rats.[11, 418] In humans, androgens are reported to increase epidermal mitotic activity and cell turnover time and thickness.

Androgens have no effect on pigmentation in the guinea pig, but are reported to stimulate pigmentation in specialized areas of the skin, such as the subcostal region of the male golden hamster and the scrotum of the ground squirrel.[11] In humans, androgens increase cutaneous pigmentation, especially in sexual skin, apparently owing to increased melanin synthesis and alteration of the packaging of melanosomes. Men with an androgen deficiency experience hypopigmentation.

Androgens enlarge the sebaceous glands in rats, rabbits, hamsters, mice, and humans and increase sebum production in humans and rats.[11] In humans, excessive androgens produce excessively oily skin, whereas androgen deficiency produces dry skin and hair. The action of androgens involves both an increase in the rate of formation of new sebaceous cells and an increase in the size of mature cells.

In rats, androgen administration retards the initiation of anagen, whereas gonadectomy enhances it.[11] However, neither castration nor treatment with testosterone has any effect on the rate of hair growth in rats. In humans, an excess of androgens results in accelerated hair growth, whereas androgen deficiency in men causes the hair to become sparse.[395]

Androgens are reported to increase the relative and total amounts of hyaluronic acid and dermal ground substance in mice.[11] In humans, androgens cause thickening of the dermis with demonstrable increase in skin collagen content. Androgens also inhibit various T-cell functions.[399]

In the testosterone-responsive dermatosis of male dogs, hypoandrogenism is an etiologic hypothesis. The dermatosis is characterized by (1) bilaterally symmetric alopecia that begins in the perineal, genital, and ventral abdominal areas and spreads cranially and ventrally, (2) a dull, dry, easily epilated haircoat that fails to grow after clipping, (3) thin hypotonic skin, and (4) seborrhea sicca. Alteration in coat color occurs in some dogs. Histologically, the dermatosis is characterized by orthokeratotic hyperkeratosis, epidermal atrophy, follicular atrophy, telogenization of hair follicles, sebaceous gland atrophy, and thin dermis.[4, 16] In addition, castrated male cats with feline acquired symmetric alopecia may respond to testosterone replacement therapy. Conversely, hyperandrogenism is presumed to be the cause of seborrhea oleosa in oversexed intact male dogs, and the condition resolves with castration.[11] Hyperandrogenism has also been demonstrated in intact male animals with hyperplasia of the circumanal glands and the tail gland.[419] Normal cats treated with mibolerone became virilized, showing thickening of the skin of the neck and clitoral hypertrophy.[1, 2]

Assays (RIA) for plasma or serum androgens are commercially available and are accompanied by the same interpretational, financial, and practical considerations as previously mentioned for estrogen assays. Values for blood testosterone in normal male dogs and cats are approximately 0.5 to 6 ng/ml, whereas those in normal female dogs and cats are usually less than 0.5 ng/ml.[1, 2, 11, 17, 409, 418]

Progesterone

Progesterone is present in both male and female animals, and it is produced by the corpus luteum of the ovary and by the zona reticularis of the adrenal cortex.[1, 2, 409, 418] The effects of progestational compounds on the skin have not been well studied. However, with the use of these compounds (e.g., megestrol acetate and medroxyprogesterone acetate) for the management of feline and canine skin disorders, the clinician must be alerted to some possible cutaneous side effects.

Progesterone is known to have immunosuppressive action, and various progesterone analogs are known to have glucocorticoid activity.[1, 2, 11, 323, 399] Progestational compounds have also been shown to bind to the intracellular cytosol receptor for dihydrotestosterone and to inhibit the enzyme 5-α-reductase, which converts testosterone to dihydrotestosterone. By binding androgen receptors in multiple tissues, progestational compounds may be androgenic, synandrogenic, or antiandrogenic, depending on the compound and the dose.

In the skin, topically applied progesterone was shown to suppress the sebum excretion rate significantly in women.[11] Medroxyprogesterone was reported to delay wound healing in rabbits. In the cat, subcutaneous injections of medroxyprogesterone acetate may produce local alopecia, atrophy, and pigmentary disturbances, and oral megestrol acetate administration can produce generalized cutaneous atrophy, alopecia, xanthomas, and poor wound healing. Bilateral flank alopecia was reported in a dog with hyperprogesteronemia and a testicular Sertoli's cell neoplasm.[393]

Assays (RIA) for plasma or serum progesterone are commercially available and are burdened by the same interpretational, financial, and practical considerations as previously mentioned for estrogen assays. Values for blood progesterone in female dogs and cats are approximately less than 5 ng/ml (in anestrus, estrus, and proestrus) and 10 to 50 ng/ml (in metestrus and pregnancy), and they are approximately less than 1 ng/ml in male dogs and cats.[1, 2, 418]

Sex Hormone Function Tests

As is the case with other endocrine tests, basal measurements of serum sex hormone levels can give misleading results, especially in intact dogs. Although stimulation tests with hCG[391] or GnRH[400] to evaluate reproductive performance are available, their value in dogs with gonadal or adrenal sex hormone dermatoses is largely unknown. To date, the testing that has received widest attention in these conditions is the sex hormone ACTH response as offered by the Endocrinology Laboratory at the University of Tennessee, College of Veterinary Medicine, Knoxville, TN 37901-1071.[374] Dogs are given either synthetic ACTH (0.5 IU/kg IV) or repository ACTH (2.2 mg/kg IM), and serum samples are collected before injection and again at 1 hour (synthetic ACTH) or 2 hours (gel ACTH) after injection. Samples are separated immediately, frozen, and mailed frozen to the laboratory by overnight mail. In addition to cortisol determinations, the laboratory measures prestimulation and poststimulation levels of progesterone, 17-hydroxyprogesterone, dehydroepiandrosterone sulfate, androstenedione, testosterone, and estradiol-17ß. Normal values are available for all hormones for intact or neutered male or female animals. The laboratory should be contacted before testing to make sure the protocol has not changed.

Gonadotropins and Prolactin

The gonadotropins, FSH (follitropin, molecular weight about 32,000) and LH (lutropin, molecular weight about 30,000), are produced by the adenohypophysis.[1, 2] Gonadotropin secretion is stimulated by hypothalamic GnRH and inhibited by estrogens, glucocorticoids, and androgens (via aromatization to estrogens in the hypothalamus). FSH secretion is also inhibited by inhibin from the ovarian follicle and testicular Sertoli's cells. LH secretion is inhibited by progestogens and androgens. In normal dogs and cats, serum FSH levels by RIA are reported to be approximately 40 to 70 ng/ml (higher in females in proestrus). Serum LH levels by RIA in normal dogs and cats are reported as follows: 0 to 3 ng/ml in intact male animals, 6 to 10 ng/ml in female animals in estrus, and less than 2 ng/ml in female animals in metestrus or anestrus.[1, 2] Gonadotropin deficiencies were detected with hypothalamic or pituitary disorders.

Prolactin is a polypeptide (molecular weight, ~22,500) produced by the adenohypophysis. Prolactin secretion is episodic and labile; it is stimulated by one or more hypothalamic releasing factors (including TRH) and inhibited by hypothalamic dopamine. In normal dogs and cats, serum prolactin levels by RIA are reported to be approximately 1 to 10 ng/ml.[1, 2] Hyperprolactinemia was found with hypothyroidism, pituitary neoplasms, and certain drug administrations (phenothiazines, cimetidine), resulting in galactorrhea, gynecomastia, and inhibition of FSH or LH secretion.

• CLINICAL ASPECTS OF ENDOCRINE SKIN DISEASES

Canine Hyperadrenocorticism

Hyperadrenocorticism (Cushing's disease, Cushing's syndrome) is a common disorder of the dog associated with excessive endogenous or exogenous glucocorticoids and is classically characterized by polyuria and polydipsia, bilaterally symmetric alopecia, thin hypotonic skin, and skeletal muscle wasting. More than 50% of cases have nontraditional clinical findings.[3, 14, 333, 334]

CAUSE AND PATHOGENESIS

Canine hyperadrenocorticism may occur naturally or may be iatrogenic.[1, 2, 235, 280, 343a] The naturally occurring type typically is associated with bilateral adrenocortical hyperplasia. In a small number of dogs, the hyperadrenocorticism is due to both adrenal and pituitary neoplasia.[220] Iatrogenic canine hyperadrenocorticism results from the misuse of exogenous glucocorticoids.[232]

In about 80% to 85% of dogs with spontaneous hyperadrenocorticism, the disorder results from excessive pituitary ACTH secretion, which produces bilateral adrenocortical hyperplasia (pituitary-dependent hyperadrenocorticism). This excessive ACTH secretion arises from either microadenomas or macroadenomas of the anterior pituitary gland.[180, 182, 199, 235, 246, 278, 280] Despite the high frequency of disease in certain breeds, the pituitary tumors appear to arise spontaneously with no genetically coded predisposition.[321] Approximately 90% of the pituitary tumors are functional, and large tumors cause neurologic signs in over 50% of patients.[314] The tumor can be found in either the pars distalis or the pars intermedia.[172, 180, 181, 246] ACTH secretion from the pars distalis is regulated by CRH and cortisol, whereas intermediate lobe secretion is regulated by tonic inhibition by primarily dopamine. It is estimated that upward of 30% of the pituitary tumors are located in the pars intermedia.[172, 180, 300, 312] Large pituitary tumors tend to secrete more ACTH than smaller ones, and the large ones, especially those of the intermediate lobe, are most resistant to stimulation by CRH or to dexamethasone suppression.[252, 253, 314, 322]

Canine pituitary-dependent hyperadrenocorticism has also been associated with pituitary adenocarcinomas. Except with large tumors, there appears to be no direct correlation among the size of the pituitary neoplasm, the degree of bilateral adrenocortical hyperplasia, and the severity of the clinical signs. The hypersecretion of ACTH results in bilateral adrenocortical hyperplasia that may be diffuse, nodular, or both. The zona glomerulosa is usually normal in width and histologic appearance, and enlargement is due to hyperplasia of the zona fasciculata and zona reticularis. In some cases, gross enlargement of the adrenals is absent. The adrenal cortex may be grossly and histologically normal but functionally abnormal.

Functional (cortisol-producing) adrenocortical neoplasms account for about 15% to 20% of the cases of naturally occurring canine hyperadrenocorticism. A threefold higher incidence of adrenal neoplasia in females has been demonstrated in one study.[194] They may be adenocarcinomas or adenomas and can occur in either gland. Older data suggested a higher frequency of occurrence in the right adrenal, but newer studies show no clear-cut predilection for one gland over the other.[277, 288, 291, 326] These neoplasms are thought to function autonomously, producing excessive amounts of cortisol, which results in negative feedback suppression of CRF (hypothalamus) and ACTH (pituitary) and in atrophy of the contralateral adrenal gland. Adrenocortical adenocarcinomas tend to be large, often extending into the adrenal vein and caudal vena cava, and they usually metastasize to the liver, lung, kidney, and lymph nodes. Dogs with bilateral adrenocortical adenomas or carcinomas have been reported rarely.[208] Intercurrent pheochromocytomas can also be found, and these dogs respond poorly to treatment.[173, 324]

By far, the most alarming cause of canine hyperadrenocorticism is the injudicious use of glucocorticoids for therapeutic purposes.[232, 306] Although iatrogenic hyperadrenocorticism appears to be less common than the 50% incidence rate cited in the past, it still is a problem for clinicians and pet owners. Long-term steroid use, whether by mouth,[266, 306] via injection,[244, 259, 306] or topically (eyes,[196, 214, 264, 268, 295] ears,[264] or skin[341]) can produce adrenocortical suppression, elevated levels of hepatic enzymes, and iatrogenic hyperadrenocorticism in dogs.

CLINICAL FEATURES

Naturally occurring canine hyperadrenocorticism is a disease of middle-aged and older dogs, but cases occur in young dogs. No definitive sex predilection has been documented, but many studies show a slightly higher frequency in female dogs.[272, 280, 333] Traditionally, Boxers, Boston terriers, Poodles, and Dachshunds are predisposed, but all breeds, even dogs of mixed breeding, can be affected. The occurrence of spontaneous hyperadrenocorticism in related Dachshunds,[333] Dandie Dinmont terriers,[303] and Yorkshire terriers[304] reinforces the concept of breed predisposition. Iatrogenic canine hyperadrenocorticism knows no age, sex, or breed predilection. It occurs most commonly in dogs with chronic pruritus because they are more likely to receive long-term systemic corticosteroids.

The clinical signs of hyperadrenocorticism are many and varied. Although some findings may be caused by the compressive or invasive effects of a pituitary or adrenal tumor, most signs are a direct result of excessive levels of cortisol and possibly other adrenal steroids. The signs at presentation depend on the dog's age and body size, the owner's power of observation, and the cause of the hyperadrenocorticism. Smaller breeds tend to have more classic and greater numbers of clinical signs than large breeds.[195] Old dogs are more sensitive to the catabolic effects of glucocorticoids and tend to experience signs more rapidly and markedly compared with younger dogs. Breeders and others with a keen interest in their dog's skin may detect subtle changes in the coat and present the dog for those changes before other signs have developed. At the other end of the spectrum is the dog owner who pays little attention to the animal and presents the animal only when the disease, and therefore the signs, are well advanced. In dogs with pituitary-dependent hyperadrenocorticism resulting from pituitary adenomas or loss of feedback control, signs tend to develop gradually, whereas the rate of occurrence can be more rapid and unpredictable with pituitary adenocarcinomas or adrenal tumors.

Polyuria and polydipsia (>100 ml/kg/day of water intake) are commonly the initial signs of hyperadrenocorticism and can precede easily recognized cutaneous changes by 6 to 12 months. Incidence figures vary from 32% to 82%.[241, 280] Concomitant with the polyuria and polydipsia, varying degrees of polyphagia develop in approximately 50% of affected dogs. In some chronic cases we have seen, the earliest sign of hyperadrenocorticism is apparently spontaneous improvement in the dog's allergies.

Cutaneous changes occur in most cases of hyperadrenocorticism, but not all are recognized by casual inspection of the skin. The most common change occurs in the coat. Early on, the coat loses its luster and healthy appearance and is more difficult to groom (Fig. 10–1A). Some Poodle owners comment that grooming appointments could be skipped because the hair was not growing as fast as normally. With time, hairs are lost, resulting in hypotrichosis to alopecia (see Fig. 10–1B and C). In most cases, the hair loss is symmetric and involves the trunk, sparing the head and distal extremities, but patchy hair loss or involvement of only the flank region[14] (see Fig. 10–30) or the face[332] can also occur. In one study of 60 dogs, 8 (13.3%) had nontruncal alopecia of the legs (see Fig. 10–1D) or face.[333] Short-coated dogs, in particular, tend to have a thinned or moth-eaten coat (see Fig. 10–1E).

Coat color change can occur as the initial cutaneous sign in some dogs. Black hairs turn auburn or rust colored and brown hairs lighten to tan or blonde (see Fig. 10–1F). This change in pigmentation can involve the entire length of the hair shaft or only the distal portions. In the latter case, the color change appears to be due to solar bleaching because the hairs are not shed as rapidly as normally. Uniform color change appears to be mediated by sex hormones. In our experience, coat color change with few other signs of hyperadrenocorticism is indicative of a gonadal sex hormone imbalance or adrenal neoplasia, especially adenocarcinomas. Clitoral hypertrophy (see Fig. 10–1G) is another strong indicator of an adrenal tumor.

Other cutaneous signs include thin, hypotonic skin (mimics dehydration, tends to wrinkle) (see Fig. 10–1E), hyperpigmentation, easy bruising (petechiae and ecchymoses), phlebectasias (see Fig. 10–1H), seborrhea (dry or greasy), comedones (Fig. 10–2A), poor wound healing, bacterial pyoderma (see Fig. 10–2B), calcinosis cutis (see Fig. 10–2C and

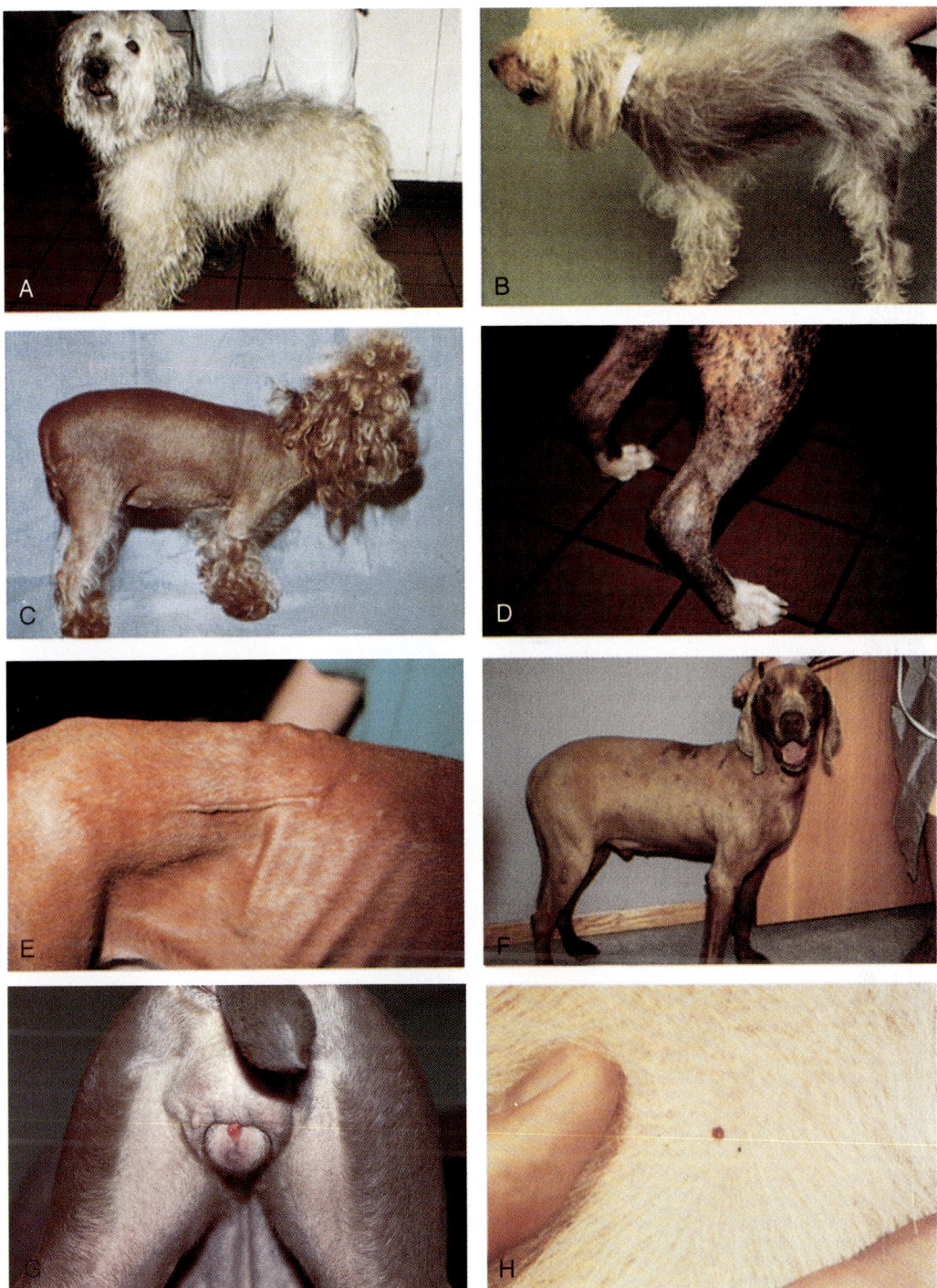

FIGURE 10–1. Hyperadrenocorticism. *A,* Soft-coated Wheaten terrier with an unmanageable coat. *B,* Marked truncal hypotrichosis and hyperpigmentation. *C,* Toy Poodle showing typical advanced alopecic pattern and hyperpigmented skin. This dog regrew a good haircoat with o,p'-DDD treatment. *D,* Distal extremity hair loss. *E,* Hypotrichotic and hypotonic skin. *F,* Generalized coat color change in a German shorthaired pointer. (Courtesy of R. Long.) *G,* Clitoral hypertrophy associated with an adrenal tumor. *H,* Phlebectasia.

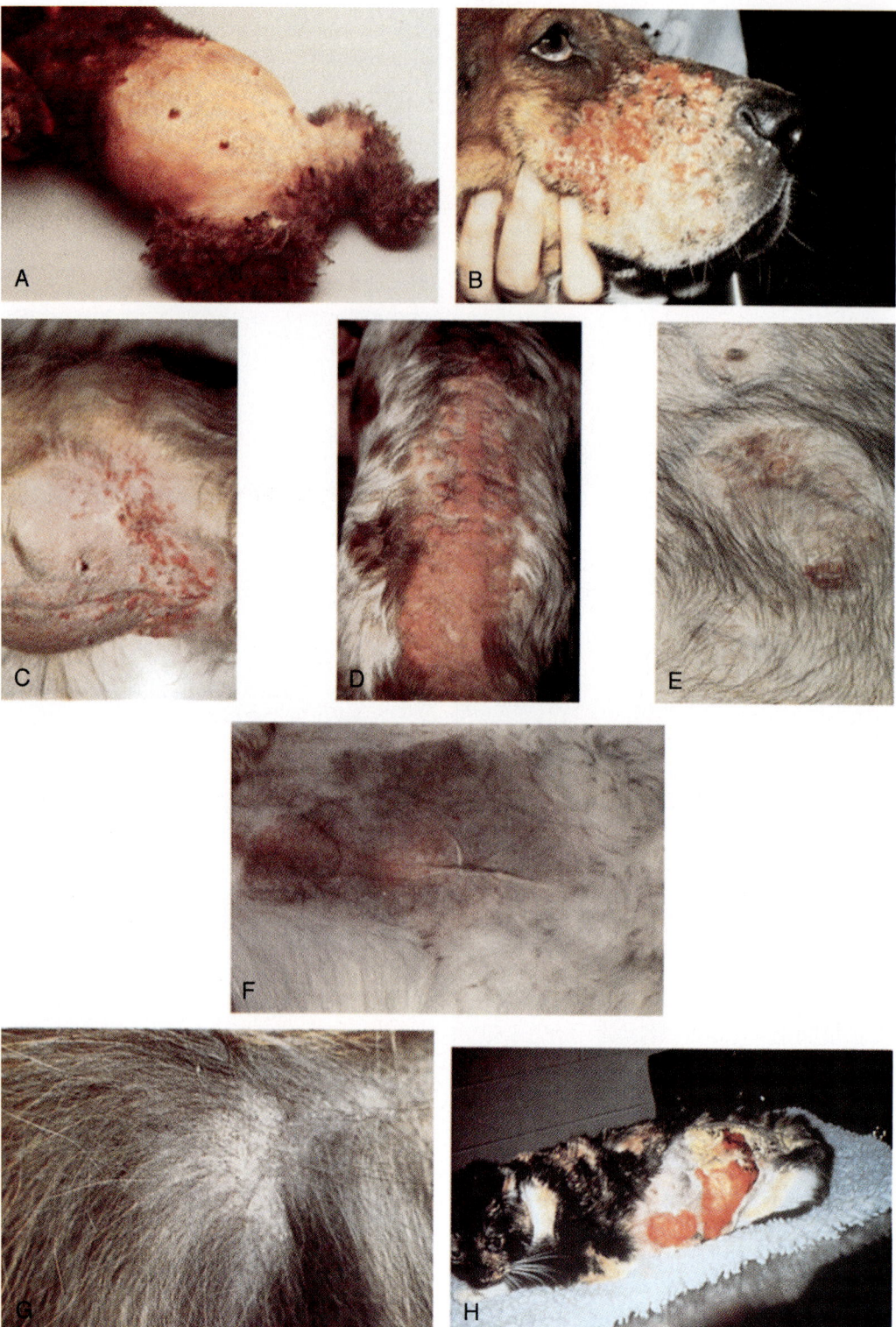

FIGURE 10–2. Hyperadrenocorticism. *A*, Comedones, alopecia, and potbelly. *B*, Severe facial furunculosis in a dog with Cushing's disease. *C*, Calcinosis cutis on the ventral abdomen. *D*, Calcinosis cutis along the caudal dorsum. *E*, Stria with focal ulceration. *F*, Thin, hypotonic skin with a central wrinkle, prominent vasculature, and a few petechiae in a cat with iatrogenic hyperglucocorticoidism. *G*, Hypotrichosis with scaling in a cat. *H*, Large traumatic wound in a cat with hyperadrenocorticism. (Courtesy of R. Rosychuk.)

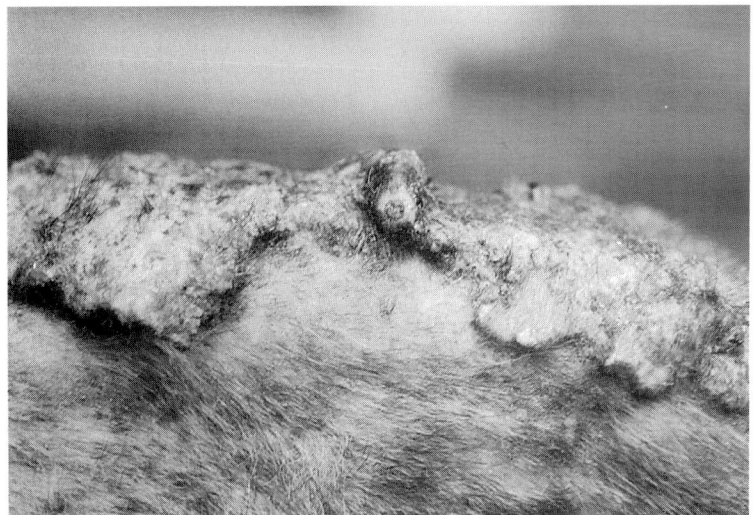

FIGURE 10-3. Cutaneous ossification over the dorsum of a dog with chronic iatrogenic hyperadrenocorticism. A bone saw was needed to take the biopsy samples.

D), and striae (see Fig. 10–2E). The striae may occur spontaneously or be the result of remodeling of a previous scar. In chronic cases, the calcinosis cutis persists and cutaneous ossification (Fig. 10–3) can occur.[211] Demodicosis (Fig. 10–4) may be a secondary confounding problem in more than 5% of cases.[11, 333] The older veterinary literature gives incidence figures for most of these conditions, figures that can be different from those generated today. For example, a study done in the 1980s on 300 dogs[280] reported comedones in 34% of the dogs, whereas a more recent study on 60 dogs showed a 5% incidence rate.[333] These disparate results do not mean that the signs of hyperadrenocorticism are changing but rather that most cases are diagnosed and treated earlier before the classic cluster of changes occurs.[256]

The skin infections in hyperadrenocorticism typically occur in the hypotrichotic to

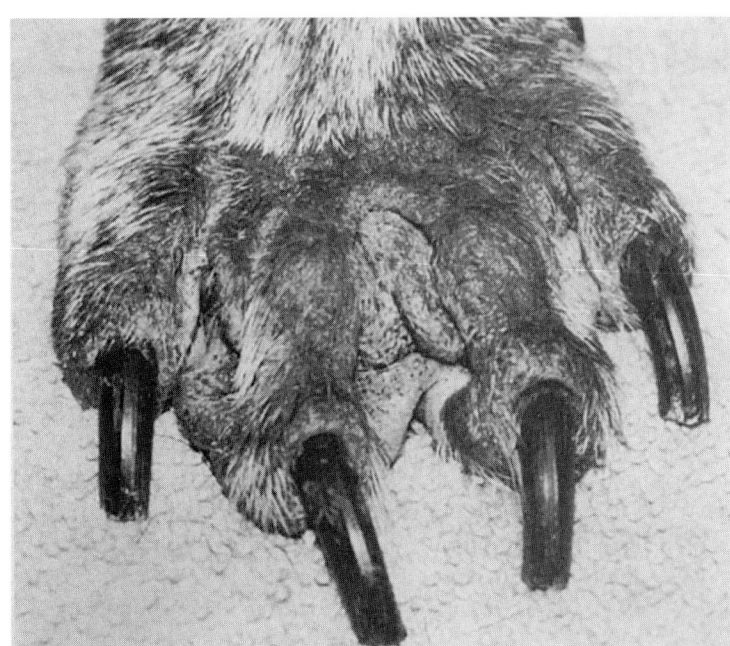

FIGURE 10-4. Adult-onset pedal demodicosis in a cushingoid dog.

alopecic areas, but some dogs do not have other skin lesions. Typically, the infection is follicular, but large, nonfollicular superficial pustules (bullous impetigo) with minimal inflammation may occur. The infections in these dogs respond poorly to treatment or recur shortly after treatment is discontinued. In cases in which the response to antibiotics is poor, multiple deep skin scrapings should be performed to check for demodicosis. Calcinosis cutis occurs in up to 40% of cases, but the incidence in cases presented early is much lower (1.7% to 8%).[333] It occurs most commonly over the dorsal neck, on the rump, and in the axillary and inguinal regions (see Fig. 10–2C and D). Early lesions are firm, whitish dermal papules to plaques. With time, the overlying skin reddens, ulcerates, and crusts. Old lesions can resemble pyoderma or pyotraumatic dermatitis and are often pruritic. Other causes of pruritus in hyperadrenocorticism are bacterial pyoderma, *Malassezia* dermatitis, seborrhea, and demodicosis.

Cutaneous phlebectasias occur in up to 40% of the dogs with hyperadrenocorticism, especially over the ventrum and medial thighs.[308] These vascular lesions are macular to papular, are erythematous, range up to 6 mm in diameter, are asymptomatic, and generally do not blanch with diascopy (see Fig. 10–1H). These lesions do not regress after effective treatment. Pressure sores (decubital ulcers) are common in large dogs with hyperadrenocorticism.[2]

Musculoskeletal abnormalities are common in canine hyperadrenocorticism.[1, 2, 272, 273] Lethargy and decreased exercise tolerance are common. Skeletal muscle atrophy and weakness occur, with atrophy being most pronounced over the head, shoulders, thighs, and pelvis. Abdominal enlargement (potbelly) is frequent (see Fig. 10–2A), with the abdomen being flaccid and the dog not being able to tense the abdomen normally. In addition, a cushingoid myotonia or pseudomyotonia may occur, which is characterized by muscle stiffness and proximal appendicular muscle enlargement. Lameness associated with osteoporosis and osteomalacia, with or without pathologic fractures, is rare. Chronic hyperadrenocorticism can exaggerate common problems such as anterior cruciate ligament rupture and patellar luxation.[2]

Persistent anestrus is frequent in intact bitches with hyperadrenocorticism.[2, 235, 280, 409] In addition, clitoral enlargement is not uncommon and presumably results from hypersecretion of adrenal androgens.[189] Clitoral enlargement does not occur with iatrogenic hyperadrenocorticism. Testicular atrophy is common in intact males.

Respiratory complications reported to occur with canine hyperadrenocorticism include excessive panting, bronchopneumonia, dystrophic mineralization and fibrosis, and pulmonary thrombosis.[3, 254, 274]

Behavioral changes may also occur (aggressiveness, depression, psychoses, and self-mutilation). Neurologic signs, including ataxia, blindness, head pressing, somnolence, Horner's syndrome, anisocoria, circling, hyperesthesias, and seizures, occasionally are apparent in naturally occurring canine hyperadrenocorticism and are caused by pituitary neoplasia or metastatic adrenocortical neoplasia.[190, 258, 271, 300] Old dogs with cognitive dysfunction have a higher frequency of hypothalamic-pituitary-adrenal (HPA) dysregulation, and some may have abnormal adrenal function tests.[299] Exophthalmos, indolent corneal ulcers, and keratopathy have also been reported in association with canine hyperadrenocorticism.[1, 2, 328]

Palpable hepatomegaly is a common feature of canine hyperadrenocorticism. Fasting hyperglycemia occurs in 40% to 60% of cases, with overt diabetes mellitus being noted in approximately 15% of dogs.[177, 265, 286] Other complications associated with hyperadrenocorticism include hypertension,[276] recurrent urinary tract infections, urolithiasis, and acute pancreatitis.[2, 3] Acute abdomen with or without hemoperitoneum is a rare manifestation of hemorrhage from an adrenocortical neoplasm.[316]

DIAGNOSIS

Before the onset of the cutaneous signs, the differential diagnosis of hyperadrenocorticism is basically that of polyuria and polydipsia: chronic renal disease, chronic liver disease, diabetes mellitus, diabetes insipidus (pituitary or renal), psychogenic polydipsia, hyperthyroidism, hypercalcemia, hypernatremia, hypokalemia, hypoadrenocorticism, polycythemia vera, and pyrexia.[1, 2, 11] With truncal alopecia and no polyuria and polydipsia, the differential diagnosis includes hypothyroidism, hyposomatotropism, and adrenal or gonadal sex hormone imbalance. Definitive diagnosis is based on history, physical examination findings, hemogram, urinalysis, serum chemistry studies, radiography, skin biopsy, and adrenal function tests. If the dog has some other condition (e.g., diabetes mellitus), that condition should be controlled before adrenal function tests are performed.[228] Many chronic diseases make it difficult to interpret test results.

Hemograms classically reveal leukocytosis (17,000 to 68,000/µl), neutrophilia (11,500 to 65,000/µl), lymphopenia (0 to 1000/µl), and eosinopenia (0 to 1000/µl).[1, 2, 11, 235, 272, 280, 333] Erythrocytosis (polycythemia), nucleated red blood cells, thrombocytosis, and hypersegmentation of neutrophil nuclei may also occur. Urinalysis usually reveals a low specific gravity (typically, 1.012). In addition, 50% of these dogs have urinary tract infection, usually manifested only by bacteriuria. Proteinuria is common. The urinary protein/creatinine ratio is increased in dogs with hyperadrenocorticism, but the elevation is not specific for that disorder.[233] Calcium crystals may be observed because these dogs are 10 times more likely to have uroliths.[229] About 15% of these dogs have glucosuria in association with concurrent diabetes mellitus. The urinary cortisol/creatinine ratio is typically elevated in hyperadrenocorticism. However, elevations are not specific for hyperadrenocorticism.[203, 237] Because the seemingly trivial stress of an office visit can falsely elevate the cortisol/creatinine ratio, owners should collect screening urine samples at home.[320]

Serum chemistry panel abnormalities may include mild to marked elevations in levels of cholesterol and triglycerides,[309] serum alanine transaminase, serum aspartate transaminase, and glucose, and a decreased blood urea nitrogen (BUN) level. Hypophosphatemia occurs in about 33% of dogs with spontaneous hyperadrenocorticism. Abnormal glucose tolerance test results and elevated serum insulin levels are common.

The serum alkaline phosphatase level is usually elevated in canine hyperadrenocorticism (80% to 95%) and is mainly due to a steroid-induced isoenzyme.[256, 311, 338] Because serum alkaline phosphatases can be increased by anticonvulsants or in diabetes mellitus, hepatic disease, and other nonadrenal illnesses, results of this testing cannot be considered diagnostic.[184, 267, 297] If the alkaline phosphatase isoenzymes are determined and the dog has elevations in both the liver and cortisol fractions, it has severe liver disease and may be more at risk for adverse reactions with o,p'-DDD treatment.[313]

Basal thyroid hormone levels (TT_4, fT_4, and TT_3) are usually low in canine hyperadrenocorticism.[1, 2, 207] These spuriously low thyroid hormone levels are caused by glucocorticoids and do not usually indicate concurrent hypothyroidism. The results of TSH stimulation tests are usually normal, but pre-TSH and post-TSH levels may be below the normal ranges. When the hyperadrenocorticism is corrected, thyroid hormone levels return to normal. Occasionally, a dog truly has concurrent hypothyroidism and requires thyroid hormone maintenance therapy.

Dogs with hyperadrenocorticism often have elevated systolic (180 to 280 mm Hg; normal, 170 or less) and diastolic (110 to 180 mm Hg; normal, 100 or less) blood pressures, which may predispose to thromboembolism, glomerulosclerosis, left ventricular hypertrophy, congestive heart failure, and retinal detachment.[235, 272, 280] The blood pressure may or may not normalize with treatment.[276] In dogs with cushingoid myopathies, electromyographic studies have revealed bizarre high-frequency discharges in association with histopathologic findings in skeletal muscle (atrophy, degeneration, and necrosis) and peripheral nerves (segmental demyelination).

Dogs with hyperglucocorticoidism have decreased blood GH levels, which respond poorly or not at all to xylazine or clonidine.[1, 2, 11, 260, 290, 368] The pituitary dysfunction in these dogs extends to other hormones and can influence serum gonadotropin (LH and FSH) levels, prolactin levels, and testosterone, estrogen, and progesterone levels.[2, 409] Serum testosterone responses to exogenous LH or human chorionic gonadotropin injections are normal in this situation.

Radiography may reveal (1) hepatomegaly; (2) osteoporosis and osteomalacia (especially of vertebrae, ribs, and flat bones), with or without pathologic fractures; (3) dystrophic mineralization of soft tissues (especially of the lung, the kidney, and the skin); and

(4) adrenocortical neoplasms. The success rate of demonstrating adrenal tumors with routine radiographic techniques varies from 27% to 57%.[256, 277, 326, 327] Mineralization in the area of an adrenal gland indicates tumor, but does not differentiate adenomas from adenocarcinomas, because the incidence of mineralization is similar for both. Special radiographic techniques (nephrotomography and x-ray computed tomography) are reported to be near perfect in detecting adrenal tumors.[256, 258, 288, 325–327] This testing does not differentiate adenomas from adenocarcinomas and is impractical for routine use.

Easy access to sensitive imaging techniques (ultrasonography, x-ray computed tomography, nuclear magnetic resonance) has greatly increased the clinician's ability to demonstrate and localize adrenocortical tumors and to evaluate the pituitary region.[334] Although brain imaging could be a routine part of the initial diagnostic work-up of an animal with hyperadrenocorticism, risk and cost efficacy must be evaluated carefully in the patients with no neurologic signs.[314] In two studies on 34 dogs with pituitary-dependent disease and no neurologic signs, pituitary masses were detected in 19 (56%) dogs.[174, 175] This compared with the 100% rate when central neurologic signs are present.[193] Thirteen dogs, 8 of which showed positive results initially, were re-evaluated in 1 year.[175] A mass was detected in 2 of the 5 dogs initially considered negative, and the previously documented mass had enlarged in only 4 of the 8 dogs. These data suggest that initial pituitary imaging is of little prognostic value in dogs not undergoing hypophysectomy. The primary place of pituitary imaging studies is in patients with neurologic signs, especially when those signs only occur after medical treatment has been instituted.[193] If the neurologic signs are due to drug toxicity, no mass will be detected.

Routine use of an abdominal ultrasonogram can also be questioned in dogs with classic clinical and laboratory signs of pituitary-dependent disease. It is of great diagnostic significance in patients when adrenocortical neoplasia, pituitary-dependent disease with an intercurrent pheochromocytoma, or nonadrenal illness with overlapping symptoms (e.g., hepatic encephalopathy, steroid-producing luteoma[339]) are suspected.[288, 326] In these latter conditions, both glands should be evaluated and compared with each other and the normal values established for dogs.[169, 222, 231] Because bilateral adrenal neoplasia[230] and intercurrent adrenal neoplasia and pituitary-dependent disease[173, 220, 324] has been documented, the evaluation should not stop when a mass is detected in one gland.

Dogs with hyperadrenocorticism may have significant elevations of coagulation factors I (fibrinogen), V, VII, IX, and X, as well as elevated levels of antithrombin III and plasminogen. These abnormalities may predispose the patient to hypercoagulability and thromboembolism.

Histopathology

Skin biopsy in canine hyperadrenocorticism may reveal many nondiagnostic changes consistent with endocrinopathy (orthokeratotic hyperkeratosis, epidermal atrophy, epidermal melanosis, follicular keratosis, follicular dilatation, follicular atrophy, telogenization of hair follicles, excessive trichilemmal keratinization, and sebaceous gland atrophy).[4, 16] Histopathologic findings highly suggestive of hyperadrenocorticism include dystrophic mineralization (of collagen fibers, basement membrane zone of epidermis and hair follicles), thin dermis, and absence of arrector pili muscles (Figs. 10–5 to 10–7). Histopathologic findings consistent with secondary pyoderma and foreign-body granuloma (associated with dystrophic mineralization) may be detected. Histopathologic characteristics of cutaneous phlebectasias range from marked dilatation and congestion of superficial dermal blood capillaries (macular stage) (Fig. 10–8) to a lobular proliferation of normal-appearing superficial dermal blood vessels, which may be encased by an epidermal collarette (papular stage).[308]

In many cases, especially with chronic disease, the tentative diagnosis of hyperadrenocorticism is straightforward and easily supported by the results of routine laboratory tests. At the other end of the spectrum is the dog with truncal alopecia, recurrent pyoderma, or seborrhea with no nondermatologic signs. Results of routine tests in these dogs often suggest a diagnosis of hyperadrenocorticism, but more than 30% of these dogs have no convincing hematologic or biochemical evidence of that disease.[333] In these dogs, the diagnosis must be confirmed or refuted by adrenal function tests.

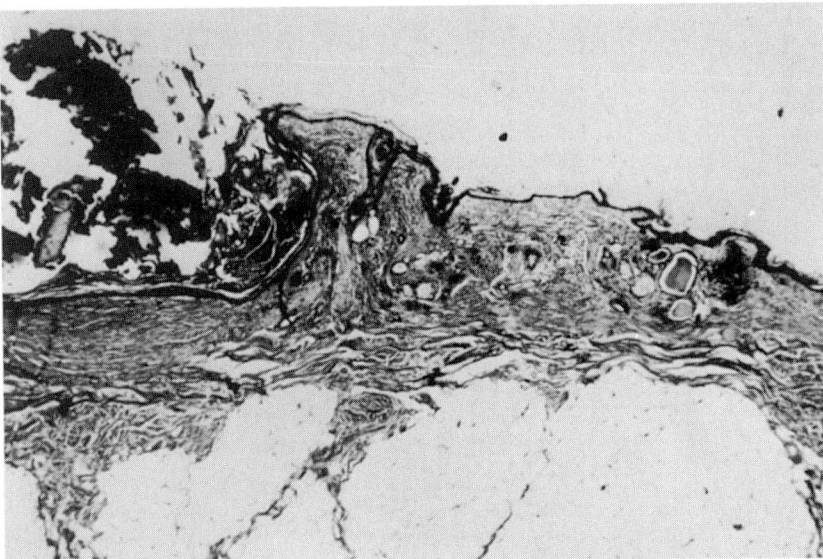

FIGURE 10-5. Canine hyperadrenocorticism. Note follicular keratosis and atrophy, absence of hair shafts, sebaceous gland atrophy, thin dermis, and dystrophic mineralization of dermis (*right*) and surface (*left*).

Adrenal Function Tests

Once spontaneous hyperadrenocorticism is suspected, the diagnosis is substantiated and further defined by a two-stage protocol. The objective of the first, or screening, stage is to confirm or rule out the diagnosis of hyperadrenocorticism.[343b] After the diagnosis is confirmed, the purpose of the second stage is to differentiate pituitary-dependent hyperadrenocorticism from that caused by adrenal neoplasia.[343c]

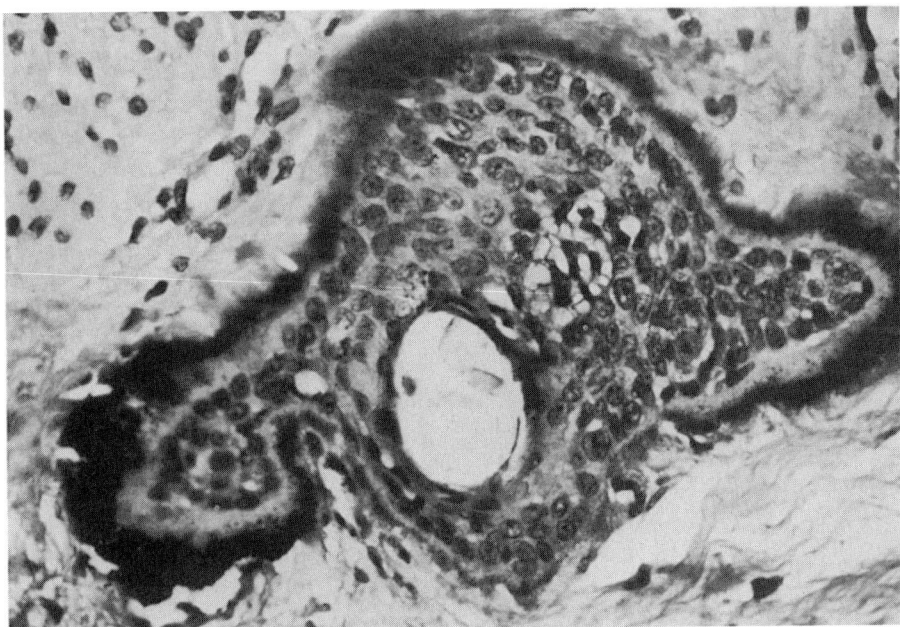

FIGURE 10-6. Canine hyperadrenocorticism. Dystrophic mineralization of the glassy membrane of a hair follicle.

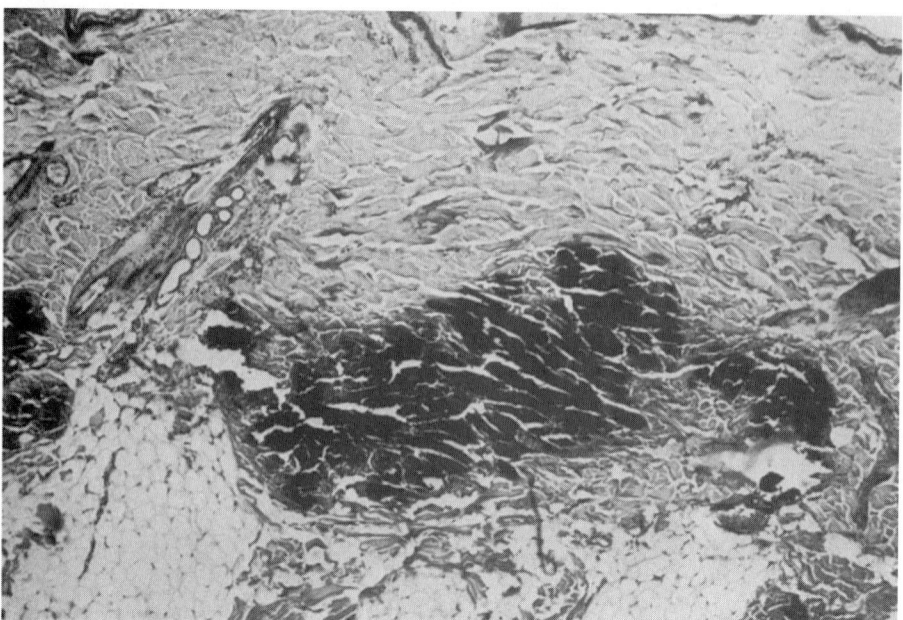

FIGURE 10–7. Dystrophic mineralization of dermal collagen.

Adrenal function tests are basically of two types: those that are single measurements of basal glucocorticoid levels in urine or blood and those that are provocative, dynamic-response tests of the glucocorticoid levels in blood. Aside from the urinary cortisol/creatinine ratio test, all cortisol evaluations are currently conducted on serum or plasma. Single measurements of plasma cortisol are completely unreliable. Normal dogs, dogs with nonadrenal disease, dogs recently hospitalized, and stressed dogs can have cortisol levels above normal levels, whereas up to 50% of dogs with hyperadrenocorticism can have levels within the normal range.[183, 212, 239, 280] Currently, the only single cortisol assessment that can be of diagnostic significance is the urinary cortisol to creatinine ratio. Normal dogs have low values (5.7 ± 0.9), whereas dogs with hyperadrenocorticism have high values (337.6 ± 72).[203, 237] However, because dogs under the stress of an examination,

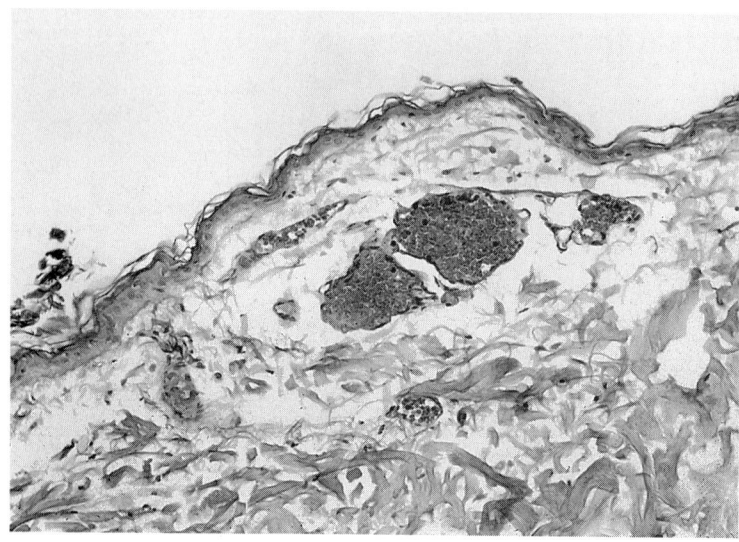

FIGURE 10–8. Cutaneous phlebectasia. Marked dilatation and congestion of superficial vessels.

with renal disease, and with other disorders can have values that overlap those found in hyperadrenocorticism, the test is not specific for hyperadrenocorticism and performs best in excluding that diagnosis.[320]

Single measurements of endogenous plasma ACTH levels can aid in the diagnosis of hyperadrenocorticism and the definition of its cause.[343c] Plasma concentrations deteriorate when the sample is unfrozen. The addition of aprotinin, a proteinase inhibitor, to the sample prevents concentration changes in unfrozen samples provided the sample remains cold and arrives at the laboratory within 4 days.[247] Plasma ACTH levels should be normal to elevated (>40 pg/ml) in dogs with pituitary-dependent hyperadrenocorticism and low to undetectable (<20 pg/ml) with adrenal neoplasia.[225, 280, 282] Unfortunately, not all dogs with hyperadrenocorticism have abnormal levels, and one study of 41 dogs with adrenal tumors showed that 30% of dogs had levels within the normal range.[333] Repetition sampling probably would increase the sensitivity of this testing but is cost prohibitive. Plasma ACTH levels should only be evaluated in conjunction with other tests.

- **Tests to Diagnose Hyperadrenocorticism.** The ACTH stimulation test reliably documents a diagnosis of iatrogenic hyperadrenocorticism or hypoadrenocorticism in dogs. Basal blood cortisol levels are low or normal and show little or no response to ACTH. Two commonly used ACTH stimulation test protocols for dogs are as follows: (1) plasma or serum cortisol determinations are collected before and 2 hours after the IM injection of 2.2 IU/kg of ACTH gel and (2) plasma or serum cortisol determinations are collected before and 1 hour after the IV injection of either 0.25 mg/dog or 5 µg/kg of synthetic ACTH.

In hyperadrenocorticism, dogs with pituitary-dependent bilateral adrenal hyperplasia should show an exaggerated response to the administration of ACTH.[280, 343b] Because adrenal tumors should secrete independently of ACTH, poststimulation values should show little change from the initial sample. Unfortunately, these theories do not absolutely hold in the clinical situation.

The low-dose dexamethasone suppression test is used to diagnose spontaneous hyperadrenocorticism in dogs.* Plasma or serum cortisol levels are determined before and 8 hours after an IV injection of 0.01 mg/kg of dexamethasone. Most investigators also draw a sample at 4 hours. In normal dogs, the low dose of dexamethasone consistently suppresses cortisol levels to less than 50% of baseline or less than 1 µg/dl for the test period. Because of differences in dexamethasone metabolism in dogs with hyperadrenocorticism and possibly other nonadrenal illnesses, the low-dose dexamethasone suppression test does not identify all dogs with hyperadrenocorticism.[218, 242] This testing can give false-positive results in uncontrolled diabetics and other chronically stressed dogs and is uninterpretable in the dog with iatrogenic hyperadrenocorticism.

One study on 216 dogs with hyperadrenocorticism used the low-dose dexamethasone suppression test to document hyperadrenocorticism and to discriminate between pituitary-dependent disease and adrenocortical neoplasia.[206] Thirty-five dogs had adrenal tumors, and 181 had pituitary-dependent disease. By definition, hyperadrenocorticism was documented if the cortisol level at 8 hours was greater than 1.4 µg/dl. Under these criteria, diagnosis was correct in 213 of the 216 (99%). To discriminate between pituitary-dependent disease and adrenal neoplasia, pituitary-dependent disease was diagnosed if the 4- or 8-hour sample was less than 50% of baseline or less than 1.4 µg/dl at 4 hours. None of the dogs with adrenal tumors satisfied the criteria for pituitary-dependent disease, but in many dogs with pituitary-dependent disease, adrenal tumor could have erroneously been diagnosed depending on which definition was being followed. This and many other studies show that the low-dose dexamethasone suppression test is not specific for hyperadrenocorticism, especially when dogs with chronic nonadrenal disorders are in the study population.[206, 239, 318]

In most cases, the low-dose test does not reliably discriminate between pituitary-dependent disease and adrenal neoplasia. One pattern, complete suppression at 4 hours

---

*See references 1, 2, 235, 255, 256, 280, 333, 343b.

with loss of suppression at 8 hours, has a high predictive value for pituitary-dependent disease.[280] Unless the dog shows this pattern, a high-dose dexamethasone suppression test, measurement of plasma ACTH levels, or some other testing must be performed to separate pituitary-dependent disease from adrenal neoplasia.

- **Tests to Differentiate the Cause of Hyperadrenocorticism.** Because the treatment of choice is different for pituitary-dependent hyperadrenocorticism and adrenal neoplasia, every effort should be made to define the cause of the hyperadrenocorticism. Unless the low-dose dexamethasone suppression test shows the diagnostic pituitary-dependent pattern or the imaging techniques (radiographs, ultrasonography, and so on) clearly demonstrate adrenal neoplasia or bilateral hyperplasia, further suppression testing is necessary.

Although various stimulation or suppression tests have been studied over the years,[11, 197, 200, 201, 256] the only test currently used is the high-dose dexamethasone suppression test.[343c] High-dose dexamethasone suppression testing is performed with the IV injection of 0.1 mg/kg of dexamethasone with sampling points at 0, 4, and 8 hours.[235, 272, 333] Some investigators recommend a dose of 1 mg/kg,[280] but there is no clear and convincing evidence that this dose increases the accuracy of the test in most dogs. Some investigators define suppression as a decrease in cortisol to less than 50% of the level at time zero, whereas other researchers use levels of less than 1.5 μg/dl. In theory, dogs with pituitary-dependent disease should demonstrate suppression completely at 4 hours and maintain or escape suppression at 8 hours. With adrenal neoplasia, partial or no suppression should occur. However, suppression is inadequate in 15% to 30% of dogs with pituitary-dependent disease.[179, 181, 240, 280, 285] In these cases, measurement of endogenous plasma ACTH levels can be helpful. However, one study showed that ACTH levels and high-dose dexamethasone testing gave contradictory results in 15% of dogs tested, so some dogs cannot be categorized by this testing.[333]

CRF stimulation testing can be useful in differentiating naturally occurring hypoadrenocorticism from the iatrogenic form[185, 241, 285] and pituitary-dependent hyperadrenocorticism from adrenal neoplasia. Intravenous injection of 1 μg/kg of CRF to normal dogs causes rapid elevations in both plasma ACTH and cortisol levels. Dogs with pituitary-dependent disease show prompt elevation in both ACTH and cortisol levels, whereas dogs with adrenal tumors should not respond. Clinically useful protocols will be developed when CRF becomes available for routine diagnostic use.

CLINICAL MANAGEMENT

The prognosis for untreated naturally occurring canine hyperadrenocorticism is poor, with death often occurring within 2 years (from such conditions as septicemia, diabetes mellitus, heart failure, pancreatitis, pyelonephritis, and thromboembolism).[249, 273] There is no clear and convincing evidence that treatment of the uncomplicated case prolongs survival time. However, successful treatment improves the quality of life for the dog and its owner. Death may be associated with adrenalectomy, hypophysectomy, o,p'-DDD administration, or concurrent diseases. In addition, death may occur at any time during or after therapy related to growth of a pituitary neoplasm or metastasis of an adrenocortical adenocarcinoma. Because hyperadrenocorticism is a disease of older dogs, many dogs die or are euthanized within 2 years of diagnosis as a result of any of the aforementioned conditions. Several independent studies on large numbers of dogs gave mean survival times of approximately 2 years, with ranges from 10 days to 8.2 years.[249, 280]

The cause of hyperadrenocorticism determines the treatment. Adrenocortical tumors should be surgically removed.[291, 301] When the tumor is undiagnosed, has metastasized, or cannot be removed because of the patient's health, medical treatment can be instituted, but the vigor of therapy and results are different from those obtained in treating pituitary-dependent disease.[202, 250] Before any specific treatment is undertaken, all intercurrent disorders (e.g., urinary tract infection and diabetes mellitus) should be identified and treatment of these conditions should be instituted.[3, 274] Although the problems identified may not respond completely to treatment until the hyperadrenocorticism is resolved, they can become life threatening to the patient if their control is not attempted.

Pituitary-Dependent Hyperadrenocorticism

Surgical treatment can be accomplished with either bilateral adrenalectomy or hypophysectomy.[1, 2, 198, 261-263] Both procedures necessitate a skilled surgeon, intensive intraoperative and postoperative monitoring and supportive care, lifelong hormone replacement therapy, and considerable expense. Because some residual cells can be left, clinical signs can persist or recur at a later date.

Radiation therapy offers a nonmedical alternative for dogs with pituitary-dependent disease.[190, 193, 216, 258, 314] Because of the specialized equipment needed, treatment centers are limited and the process is very expensive. Although irradiation can be used in any dog, it finds greatest use in dogs with neurologic signs secondary to macroadenomas. Protocols vary with the study, but doses between 44 and 48 Gy, fractionated in 11 or 12 doses, are typical. Side effects are minimal but, because response time is slow, some dogs deteriorate before the treatments can be completed. Small tumors appear to respond better than large ones.[314] Although improvement can occur in most treated dogs, the improvement may not be sufficient to return the dog to a normal life, and relapses occur in up to 50% of the cases.[193]

Pituitary-dependent hyperadrenocorticism has been treated with drugs that act on the central nervous system, adenohypophysis, and adrenal gland.[1, 2, 11, 280] Cyproheptadine hydrochloride (Periactin) is an antiserotonin agent that blocks serotonin-mediated CRF and ACTH release. The drug has been used to treat spontaneous canine hyperadrenocorticism (0.3 to 3 mg/kg/day orally), but most dogs were not helped.[312] Bromocriptine mesylate (Parlodel) is a potent dopamine receptor agonist that inhibits ACTH secretion. This drug has also been used to treat dogs with spontaneous hyperadrenocorticism (up to 0.1 mg/kg/day) with rare benefit.[1, 2, 11] Side effects with these drugs include vomiting, depression, behavioral changes, and changes in appetite. Because of their frequent side effects and infrequent benefit, these drugs appear to have limited usefulness in the management of hyperadrenocorticism.[2]

Trilostane, an inhibitor of 3β-hydroxysteroid dehydrogenase, is used in Europe for the treatment of hyperadrenocorticism in humans. In a preliminary study of five dogs with hyperadrenocorticism, all responded, even the one dog with a nonresectable adrenal tumor, to treatment with no side effects noted.[234] The dosage used varied from 2.6 to 4.8 mg/kg. In three dogs, the dosage was given twice daily until a response occurred, then the administration was reduced to once daily. The other two dogs received the drug once daily from the onset. With its apparent high degree of safety and efficacy, further studies are indicated.

The drug L-deprenyl (Anipryl, Pfizer Animal Health) is a selective irreversible monoamine oxidase-B (MAO-B) inhibitor. Because MAO-B is used in dopamine metabolism, its inhibition increases central dopamine concentration. L-deprenyl is used in the treatment of cognitive dysfunction in geriatric dogs and in dogs with hyperadrenocorticism.[180-182] Most old dogs with cognitive dysfunction have an inter-related to intercurrent HPA dysregulation.[299] Its use is contraindicated in patients taking other MAO inhibitors, which include amitraz and tricyclic antidepressants. These drugs should be withdrawn for at least 14 days before treatment is begun.[181]

As discussed previously, the release of ACTH from the pars intermedia is tonically inhibited by various neurotransmitters, especially dopamine.[178, 182] Dopamine inhibits ACTH secretion. It is estimated that 30% of dogs with pituitary-dependent hyperadrenocorticism have pars intermedia involvement with primary dopamine depletion, secondary excessive ACTH secretion, and tertiary bilateral adrenal hyperplasia. L-deprenyl restores the dopamine concentration, thus reducing ACTH secretion. If the hyperadrenocorticism is secondary to CRH-mediated ACTH secretion, L-deprenyl will have little or no effect.

Because there is no readily available test to determine if the patient in question has pars intermedia involvement, the only way to determine efficacy is by therapeutic trial.

Because approximately 70% of dogs with pituitary-dependent disease do not respond to this drug, and those that do do so slowly, it is suggested that L-deprenyl be used as a first-line agent in dogs with mild-to-moderate disease. With severe disease, other treatments should be used to put the disease into remission with consideration of L-deprenyl for long-term maintenance.[182] The drug is given daily at 1 mg/kg for an initial 30 to 60 days. If no response occurs, the dosage should be increased to 2 mg/kg for an additional trial period. In a report on 90 dogs, 38 needed the higher dosage.[180] Response is gradual and cumulative. Because the drug is very safe and not adrenolytic, response is determined by change in clinical signs and laboratory monitoring is not needed. Adverse reactions occur in approximately 5% of patients and include diarrhea, vomiting, listlessness, disorientation, decreased hearing, and restlessness.[181] In the 90 dog study, the owners and veterinarians of about 80% of those dogs thought the dog was better with treatment. In a different study of 10 dogs, only 2 improved.[292]

Ketoconazole is an antifungal imidazole drug that also inhibits adrenocortical steroidogenesis in dogs and humans.[2, 335] Normal dogs treated with 10 to 30 mg/kg/day of ketoconazole show significant decreases in basal cortisol levels and response to exogenous ACTH.[335] Similar response occurs when dogs with pituitary-dependent hyperadrenocorticism or adrenal neoplasia are treated.[204, 205] When 9 dogs with adrenocortical neoplasia and 11 dogs with pituitary-dependent hyperadrenocorticism were treated with 15 mg/kg every 12 hours for 15 days to 12 months, 18 dogs returned to clinical normalcy.[205] Two dogs with pituitary-dependent disease did not respond. In another study of 11 dogs, the 9 with pituitary-dependent disease all responded but experienced relapse within 1 year.[287] Two dogs with adrenal tumors did not respond. The protocol for the use of ketoconazole recommends that the drug be given at 5 mg/kg every 12 hours for 7 days to determine whether the dog shows any idiosyncratic reactions to its administration. If none occurs, the dose is increased to 10 mg/kg every 12 hours for 14 days. Response is determined by ACTH stimulation testing. Urinary cortisol/creatinine ratios cannot be used for monitoring.[168, 223] Because ketoconazole is an enzyme inhibitor and not an adrenolytic agent, it is imperative that the drug be given 1 to 3 hours before testing. If this testing shows poststimulation cortisol levels above the reference range, the dosage should be increased to 15 mg/kg every 12 hours for 14 days. If this dosage produces the desired suppression, it must be maintained on a daily basis. Although ketoconazole is safe and effective in the treatment of hyperadrenocorticism, its expense precludes its long-term use in many dogs. Its primary indications are cases of adrenal neoplasia in which surgery cannot be performed or in which metastasis has occurred and dogs who cannot tolerate other medical treatments.

The drug of choice for pituitary-dependent hyperadrenocorticism in dogs is o,p′-DDD (mitotane, Lysodren).[194, 249, 273, 280] This drug is a chlorinated hydrocarbon derivative that causes selective necrosis and atrophy of the zona fasciculata and zona reticularis of the adrenal cortex, whereas the zona glomerulosa (mineralocorticoid-producing zone) is relatively resistant. In a small number of dogs, this zone is destroyed with treatment and the dog is a permanent Addisonian.[174] The initial dosage of o,p′-DDD is 25 to 50 mg/kg/day for 7 to 10 days. The daily dose should be divided in half and administered every 12 hours with food.[329] Small doses of glucocorticoid (oral prednisone or prednisolone at 0.2 mg/kg/day, or oral hydrocortisone at 1 mg/kg/day) are often given during the initial 7 to 10 days of o,p′-DDD therapy to minimize the side effects associated with acute glucocorticoid withdrawal. Some authors advise against glucocorticoid use because it makes evaluation of early responses difficult and is necessary in only about 5% of cases.[2] In dogs with concurrent diabetes mellitus, treatment with o,p′-DDD reduces the daily insulin requirement and can predispose to insulin overdosage and hypoglycemia.[177] A low initial dosage of o,p′-DDD (25 mg/kg/day) and a higher daily maintenance dose of prednisone or prednisolone (0.4 mg/kg) or hydrocortisone (2 mg/kg) prevent the rapid reduction in circulating glucocorticoid levels and daily insulin requirements and allow for easier regulation of the diabetes.

The most common side effects observed during initial o,p′-DDD therapy include lethargy, vomiting, diarrhea, anorexia, and weakness.[249] Less common side effects include disorientation, ataxia, and head pressing. About 25% of dogs have one or more side effects during initial therapy, but the effects are relatively mild in most dogs. Side effects develop when plasma cortisol levels either fall below normal basal range (less than 1 μg/dl) or drop too rapidly into normal range (glucocorticoid withdrawal syndrome) and resolve promptly with glucocorticoid supplementation. If adverse signs occur during initial o,p'-DDD therapy, the drug administration should be stopped and the glucocorticoid dose doubled until the dog can be evaluated. If clinical signs persist longer than 3 days after increasing the glucocorticoid dose, other medical problems should be considered.

There are many ways to assess the effectiveness of initial o,p'-DDD therapy. Measurement of daily water consumption and eosinophil counts can be used but may be misleading because they only indirectly reflect circulating cortisol levels and not all cushingoid dogs manifest eosinopenia or polydipsia, especially while hospitalized. Urinary cortisol/creatinine ratios cannot be used for monitoring.[289] Most investigators perform an ACTH stimulation test to monitor the level of adrenal suppression. Because prednisone, prednisolone, and hydrocortisone all cross-react in most cortisol assays, glucocorticoid supplementation should not be given on the morning of ACTH stimulation testing. To ensure adequate control of hyperadrenocorticism with o,p'-DDD, both basal and post-ACTH cortisol levels should remain within the normal resting (basal) range.[172] After o,p'-DDD induction therapy and ACTH stimulation testing, o,p'-DDD administration should be discontinued and glucocorticoid supplementation should be continued until cortisol results are available.

About 15% of dogs still have exaggerated cortisol production after initial o,p'-DDD therapy.[249] In these dogs, daily o,p'-DDD therapy should be continued and ACTH stimulation tests repeated at 5- to 10-day intervals until basal and post-ACTH cortisol levels are in the normal range. This may necessitate as long as 30 to 50 days in some dogs.[249] In contrast, approximately 40% of dogs have basal and post-ACTH cortisol levels below normal range after initial o,p'-DDD therapy. In these dogs, o,p'-DDD administration should be stopped and glucocorticoid supplementation continued as needed until basal cortisol levels normalize. This usually takes about 2 to 6 weeks.

After normal cortisol levels are documented, o,p'-DDD is continued at a weekly maintenance dosage. The weekly maintenance dosage is that used for loading and should be divided in half and given twice weekly. During maintenance therapy with o,p'-DDD, glucocorticoid supplementation is rarely required. In the rare dog that manifests poor appetite, depression, weakness, and mild weight loss in spite of normal cortisol levels, alternate-morning doses of prednisone or prednisolone (0.4 mg/kg) are beneficial.

About 5% of the dogs treated with maintenance o,p'-DDD therapy experience iatrogenic hypoadrenocorticism characterized by low basal and post-ACTH cortisol levels and hyperkalemia or hyponatremia. These changes can occur after weeks or years of treatment but typically occur at about 5 months.[249] Adverse clinical signs resolve after stopping o,p'-DDD therapy and supplementation with appropriate doses of glucocorticoids and mineralocorticoids. Iatrogenic hypoadrenocorticism may be temporary or permanent, and further o,p'-DDD therapy is not indicated unless the hypoadrenocorticism resolves and basal and post-ACTH cortisol levels increase above normal range.

About 60% of dogs treated with initial loading and maintenance doses of o,p'-DDD experience relapse within 12 months of treatment as evidenced by recurrence of clinical signs and elevated basal and post-ACTH cortisol levels.[249, 293] Control is regained by daily treatment for 5 to 14 days, and then maintenance is reinstituted with larger dosages, typically 25% to 50% higher than that used previously. Approximately 40% of the dogs who experience relapse once do so one or more additional times.[249] Dosage adjustments allow control to be regained. In a study on 200 dogs treated with o,p'-DDD, 184 were well controlled with maintenance doses ranging from 26.8 to 330 mg/kg/week.[249] To ensure continued control and prevent serious relapse during o,p'-DDD therapy, ACTH stimulation testing should be repeated every 6 months during maintenance therapy. With careful monitoring, survival times exceeding 3 years can be expected.[194]

An alternative protocol for the use of o,p'-DDD has been developed to minimize the occurrence of relapses and the unexpected development of hypoadrenocorticism. High doses are given for extended periods to destroy the adrenal cortex intentionally, resolving the hyperadrenocorticism but causing permanent hypoadrenocorticism.[188, 293, 294] The o,p'-DDD is administered at 50 to 75 mg/kg/day for medium-sized to large dogs for 25 days. Dosages up to 100 mg/kg/day are recommended for toy breeds. The daily dosage is divided into three or four equal parts and is given with food. Glucocorticoid and mineralocorticoid replacement therapy is started on day 3 of treatment. Cortisone acetate is administered at 1 mg/kg every 12 hours until 1 week after the o,p'-DDD regimen is completed, and the dosage is then reduced to 0.5 mg/kg every 12 hours. Fludrocortisone (0.0125 mg/kg) and sodium chloride (0.1 mg/kg/day divided over two or three meals) is suggested therapy for the hypoadrenocorticism. Adjustments in treatment are made according to the animal's needs. Although this protocol is designed to destroy the adrenal cortex, the treatment is not uniformly successful because relapse rates near 30% within 1 year have been reported.[188, 293] Retreatment with the original dosage for 25 days and then once-weekly administration for 5 to 6 weeks should result in another remission. Because some dogs treated by the standard o,p'-DDD protocol need nearly 70 days of loading, some of the relapses with this new protocol may be due to an insufficient course of treatment. An ACTH stimulation test should be performed after the 25 days of treatment to ensure that adrenal suppression has occurred. Additional loading time is indicated if the adrenals hyperrespond to ACTH.

Aside from pituitary irradiation, none of the treatments described affects pituitary tumors, and their continued growth can be expected. Growth is slow but progressive. Large tumors can result in neurologic dysfunction with stupor, anorexia, and head pressing most commonly observed.[271] Other signs include pacing, circling, behavioral changes, weakness, seizures, ataxia, and adipsia. If these signs develop, pituitary irradiation is necessary for continued management.

Adrenocortical Neoplasia

The therapy of choice for adrenocortical neoplasia is adrenalectomy.[291, 301] The majority of dogs with clinical evidence of hyperadrenocorticism and nonsuppressible adrenal function tests have a unilateral adrenocortical tumor. Because bilateral adrenocortical tumors have been documented,[230] both adrenal glands should be evaluated carefully by ultrasound or other imaging studies before surgery is undertaken. During the evaluation, both adrenal glands should be compared in size and consistency with each other and with normal values for dogs. Despite the common conception that the gland contralateral to the tumor will be atrophied, that gland often is normal in size.[230] Dogs with symmetric and normal-sized glands should be evaluated for a steroid-producing tumor of another organ system (e.g., luteoma, a serious hepatic disorder with shunting, or an ectopic ACTH-producing tumor). A more problematic situation is when there is an obvious mass in one gland while the contralateral gland is normal sized or somewhat enlarged. Is this a dog with pituitary-dependent disease and an intercurrent pheochromocytoma[173, 324] or a dog with a unilateral adrenocortical tumor? Because dogs with pheochromocytomas are at increased risk during anesthesia, the clinical and laboratory data should be reviewed carefully. If any inconsistencies are found, additional testing for pheochromocytoma should be conducted before the dog is taken to surgery.

In one report, tumor cells were found in blood vessels in 22 of 37 adrenal tumors and 8 of the 26 dogs that survived the surgery experienced relapses in clinical signs.[319] Accordingly, all surgical candidates should be evaluated thoroughly before and during surgery for evidence of metastatic disease. During surgery, the viscera, especially the pancreas, should be handled carefully because these dogs are prone to potentially fatal pancreatitis. If the contralateral adrenal gland is atrophied, the dog will have to be supported as a glucocorticoid-deficient patient with maintenance and stress doses of glucocorticoids for 2 or more months. ACTH stimulation testing can be performed every 2 to 4 weeks to determine when the remaining adrenal gland has returned to normal function.

If the adrenal neoplasm is malignant, if the owner refuses surgery for the dog, or if the dog is considered an unsuitable surgical candidate, medical treatment may be beneficial. Although published data are limited, ketoconazole appears to be effective for both adenomas and adenocarcinomas.[205, 287] Because ketoconazole is an enzyme blocker and not an adrenolytic agent, tumor growth continues and metastasis, with all its sequelae, may occur. Because o,p'-DDD is an adrenolytic agent, it can be beneficial in some dogs with adrenal tumors. Reports of success with both the standard and new protocol have been reported.[202, 293] With the standard protocol, loading often takes longer and can necessitate dosages as high as 150 mg/kg/day. Relapses are common and, in general, maintenance dosages are much higher than those needed in pituitary-dependent disease. In a study of 32 dogs, 66% were considered to have a good to excellent response to o,p'-DDD, with a mean survival time of 16.4 months, and a final mean maintenance dosage of 35.3 to 1273 mg/kg/week.[250]

When severe calcinosis cutis is present, treatment with DMSO gel hastens resolution of the lesions.[170] A thin film of the gel is applied to the lesions once or twice daily until resolved.

Iatrogenic Hyperadrenocorticism

Therapy for canine iatrogenic hyperadrenocorticism necessitates ceasing excessive exogenous glucocorticoid administration. When glucocorticoid therapy is withdrawn, patients may be susceptible to hypothalamic-pituitary-adrenal insufficiency for 3 to 12 months and the dog may show signs of glucocorticoid insufficiency under normal living conditions or with stress. Some investigators anticipate these problems and institute replacement therapy with hydrocortisone (0.2 to 0.5 mg/kg/day) or prednisolone (0.1 to 0.2 mg/kg/day). The glucocorticoid administration is slowly withdrawn during 7 to 14 days. Other investigators, including ourselves, do not routinely use the steroid supplements unless surgery or some other known stressful situation is to occur. The glucocorticoid is dispensed and the owners are instructed to use the drug if the dog needs it, but most dogs do not.[232] Recovery usually occurs within 3 to 4 months. Exogenous ACTH should not be used in iatrogenic hyperadrenocorticism. The block after prolonged glucocorticoid therapy is not at the level of the adrenocortical response to ACTH but at the level of the ability of the hypothalamic-pituitary unit to resume release of CRF and ACTH. Therefore, ACTH supplementation may actually aggravate the problem.[1, 2, 11]

After the hyperadrenocorticism is controlled, the skin may initially show increasing scaling and pigmentation and new hair regrowth may be different from the normal color (for example, gray hair grows in black, black grows in red) and texture. With successful therapy, the cutaneous signs of hyperadrenocorticism, including calcinosis cutis, usually regress within 3 to 4 months. In the rare case that has progressed to cutaneous ossification, the skin lesions persist unless removed surgically. Some dogs with bacterial pyoderma have recurring episodes of infection for up to 1 year after the hyperadrenocorticism has been controlled. Noncutaneous signs should resolve slowly, but some signs may remain owing to the physiologic alterations.[176, 273]

Feline Hyperadrenocorticism

Both naturally occurring and iatrogenic hyperadrenocorticism are rare in the cat.

CAUSES AND PATHOGENESIS

Naturally occurring hyperadrenocorticism is a rare disease in the cat, with fewer than 100 cases reported.[187, 192, 226, 238, 251, 254a, 269, 270, 281, 331] With such a limited data base, it is difficult to make precise statements on the value of the various diagnostic tests and the best method of treatment. Approximately 80% of cats have pituitary-dependent hyperadrenocorticism resulting from a pituitary adenoma or adenocarcinoma, whereas the remainder have functioning adrenocortical tumors.[192, 343a] Both adrenocortical adenomas and adenocarcinomas have been reported, and in one case, progesterone secretion appeared to be responsible for the clinical signs.[178] One cat had a functioning adrenocortical adenoma in its remaining adrenal gland approximately 1 year after the other gland was removed for a similar tumor. Iatrogenic hyperadrenocorticism can be produced with only great difficulty in the cat,[221, 302, 307] possibly because of the lower number of low-capacity, high-affinity dexamethasone-binding receptors in this species.[317]

CLINICAL FEATURES

Naturally occurring hyperadrenocorticism typically occurs in middle-aged to old cats.[182a] No breed predisposition has been noted. Females appear to be at higher risk.[192, 226] The clinical syndrome is not as predictable as it is in the dog. The most common owner complaint is marked polyuria and polydipsia. Weight loss, anorexia, polyphagia, and depression also may be reported. On physical examination, muscle wasting and a potbelly are common findings. Skin changes occur in about half the cases and include alopecia (see Fig. 10–2F and G), thin skin (see Fig. 10–2F), fragile skin (Fig. 10–9A; see Fig. 10–2H), easy bruising (see Fig. 10–9B), recurrent abscessation, comedones, seborrhea, and hyperpigmentation.[226, 269, 270] The hair loss can be partial or complete and involve the entire trunk, the flank region, or the ventrum.[226] The increased fragility of the skin occurs in over 50% of the cases and is manifested by tearing during grooming or routine handling. Although data are limited, this extreme fragility may be more common in cats with adrenal tumors than in those with pituitary-dependent hyperadrenocorticism.[226]

Reports on cats with iatrogenic hyperadrenocorticism are rare.[221, 302, 307] These cases can have all of the clinical signs of the naturally-occurring disease (e.g., muscle wasting, polyuria and polydipsia, steroid-induced diabetes mellitus). Cutaneous signs seen include hair loss, thin hypotonic skin, medial curling of the ear tips, easy bruising, mild seborrhea sicca, and spontaneous tearing of the skin. Because medial curling of the pinna has not been reported in the naturally occurring cases, this may be of diagnostic significance.

DIAGNOSIS

In the absence of cutaneous signs, the primary differential diagnostic consideration is diabetes mellitus. Because approximately 90% of cats with naturally occurring hyperadrenocorticism are prediabetic or overtly diabetic because of the insulin antagonistic action of corticosteroids, the responsiveness of the cat to insulin is of key importance.[251] The diabetes mellitus in cats with hyperadrenocorticism is difficult to impossible to regulate without treatment of the hyperadrenocorticism. With successful treatment of the hyperadrenocorticism, the diabetes responds to insulin as expected or may spontaneously resolve.

With just hair loss, the differential diagnosis includes all causes of traumatic alopecia, telogen defluxion, diabetes mellitus, and advanced hyperthyroidism. Cutaneous asthenia, pancreatic neoplasia, hepatic lipidosis, progestogen administration,[323] and acquired skin fragility syndrome (see Chap. 18) must be considered when extreme fragility is noted.

In the cat, hemograms, serum chemistry panels, and urinalysis are of little diagnostic specificity.[226, 269, 270, 342] The liver enzyme elevations due to a steroid hepatopathy are inconsistent in the cat and can be masked by biochemical alterations caused by the frequently encountered diabetes mellitus.[184, 239, 302]

Histopathology

Skin biopsy results can vary. In some cases, the hair follicles are in anagen with no atrophic changes of the epidermis or pilosebaceous units. Other cats show profound atrophic changes. The most consistent abnormality is a decreased quantity of dermal collagen. The bundles in the superficial and deep dermis are thinner than normal, widely separated, and without normal organization.[4, 16, 226] On electron microscopy, collagen fibril diameters vary in size.

Adrenal Function Tests

All the various diagnostic tests used in the dog have all been used in cats, but the limited data available make determining the reliability of each test difficult.[182a, 198, 343b, 343c]

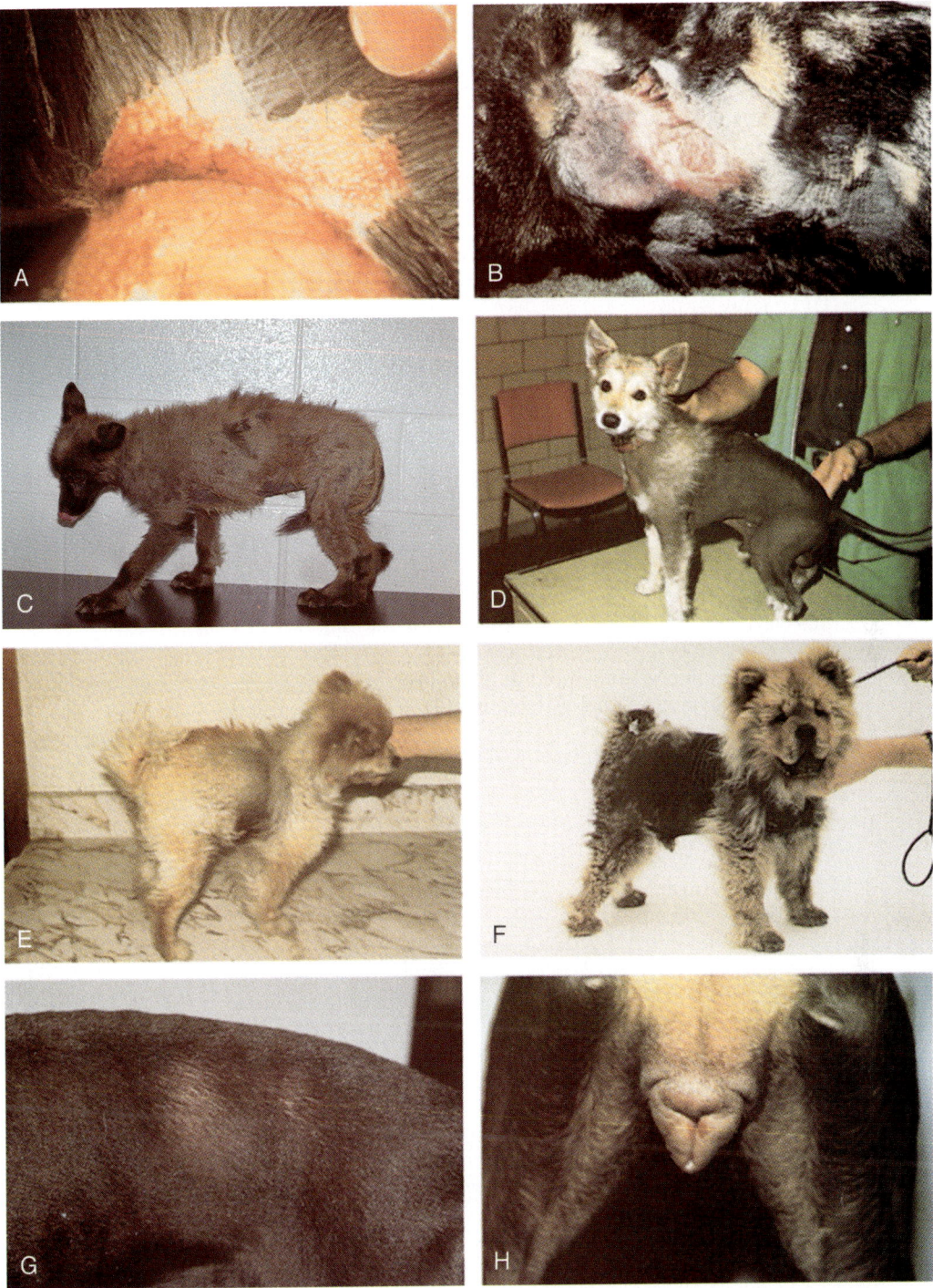

FIGURE 10–9. *A*, Close-up of the cat in Figure 10–2*H* showing the thin, fragile skin. (Courtesy of R. Rosychuk.) *B*, Bruising and ulceration (torn skin) on the back of a cat with iatrogenic hyperglucocorticoidism. The area has been clipped. (From Scott, DW: Feline dermatology 1900–1978: A monograph. J Am Anim Hosp Assoc 16:331, 1980.) *C*, Hair loss, hyperpigmentation, and absence of primary hairs in a dwarf. *D*, Profound hair loss and hyperpigmentation in an adult dwarf. *E*, Early hyposomatotropism. Note the loss of primary hairs and early hyperpigmentation. *F*, Chronic hyposomatotropism with profound hair loss and hyperpigmentation. *G*, Hyperestrogenism. Flank hypotrichosis. *H*, Same patient as in *G* with perineal hair loss and vulvar enlargement.

Cats excrete small amounts of cortisol in their urine.[217] With hyperadrenocorticism, the urinary cortisol/creatinine ratio is elevated above normal. However, the cortisol/creatinine ratio can also be elevated in nonadrenal disease (e.g., renal failure[227]), so this testing probably has the same place in the diagnosis of feline hyperadrenocorticism as it does in the dog. Hyperadrenocorticism can be dismissed when the urinary cortisol/creatinine ratio is normal, but elevations do not confirm that diagnosis. In the ACTH stimulation test, both the gel (2.2 IU/kg IM) and synthetic (125 μg IV) forms of ACTH have been used. Most protocols suggest that cortisol levels be determined before and 90 minutes after ACTH administration.[279, 283, 284, 310, 343b] Most cats with hyperadrenocorticism show an exaggerated response to ACTH, but a borderline or normal response can occur.[184, 238, 269] The cat with the progesterone-secreting adrenal tumor did not respond to ACTH.[178]

Three doses of dexamethasone have been used for suppression testing.[182a, 189, 251, 269, 296, 310] Cortisol samples are collected before, 3 to 6 hours, and 8 hours after IV administration. Suggested dosages vary from 0.01 to 0.1 mg/kg. Because upward of 20% of normal cats do not show adrenal suppression when 0.01 mg/kg of dexamethasone is given,[178, 296] some authors suggest 0.1 mg/kg for low-dose testing. Normal cats should have their cortisol levels suppressed to less than 1 μg/dl during the test period. Where studied, all cats with hyperadrenocorticism have failed to have their cortisol levels suppressed to normal levels. High-dose testing is conducted with either 0.1 or 1 mg/kg. Suppression to 50% or less of the baseline value suggests pituitary-dependent hyperadrenocorticism, but failure to suppress is not absolutely indicative of adrenal neoplasia.[296] Because so few cases have been studied, the accuracy of this cut-off point is open to question. Endogenous plasma ACTH levels were elevated in the 23 cats tested with pituitary-dependent disease and low in 3 with adrenal neoplasia.[184, 187, 281, 310] Normal or low values can occur in cats with adrenal tumors.[221]

Ultrasonographic examination of the adrenal glands in the cat can be difficult.[182a] Unilateral or bilateral adrenal enlargement, the latter being indicative of pituitary-dependent hyperadrenocorticism, may occur. Special radiographic techniques may be of additional diagnostic value, but this is unproved in cats.[258]

CLINICAL MANAGEMENT

Cats with hyperadrenocorticism often are presented late in the course of disease. At this point, the prognosis becomes much poorer because most cats have insulin-resistant diabetes mellitus, hyperfragility of the skin, or other degenerative changes. No medical treatment has been described that has had a high degree of success in the long-term management of cats with pituitary-dependent hyperadrenocorticism. When o,p'-DDD was administered orally (25 to 50 mg/kg/day) to four normal cats, two showed progressive adrenal suppression and two cats showed no response.[342] One cat experienced vomiting, diarrhea, and anorexia. The response in diseased cats is generally poor,[269] although anecdotal reports indicate success in some cases.[182a] Details of successful long-term management are available only for one cat.[305] After about 2 months of daily treatment with 37.5 mg/kg/day, the cat was maintained on a weekly dose of 50 mg/kg/week. With this treatment, all clinical signs resolved, but recurred when the drug was discontinued.

Ketoconazole is also of uncertain value.[182a] Even though normal cats show no cortisol suppression with a month's worth of treatment,[336] some diseased cats improve with treatment. When seven cats were given 20 to 30 mg/kg/day, four cats responded, two showed no response, and one experienced thrombocytopenia.[254a, 270, 315] Metyrapone, a blocker of adrenal conversion of 11-deoxycortisol to cortisol, has been used in five cats, with clinical response in three.[187, 257, 270] At dosages of 65 mg/kg every 12 hours, adrenal suppression can be documented in 5 days. Treatment for longer than 30 days has not been reported. Although L-deprenyl is reported to be safe in cats,[181] no reports on its use are available. Because intermediate lobe hormones in the cat are under dopaminergic control,[245, 337] L-deprenyl may be of some use.

Because of the limited success of medical treatments, most investigators recommend adrenalectomy as the treatment of choice. In cats with adrenal neoplasia, surgery should be curative with no need for maintenance therapy. In cats with pituitary-dependent disease, bilateral adrenalectomy must be performed and lifelong treatments for hypoadrenocorticism must be administered. Because the majority of cats with hyperadrenocorticism present poor surgical risks because of their diabetes mellitus and fragile skin, medical treatment with either ketoconazole or metyrapone should be considered. If either agent is effective, its administration should be continued until the skin is healed and the diabetes mellitus is controlled. After the cat's health is better, surgery should be performed. In the largest study reported, postoperative complications developed in all 10 cats.[191] Electrolytic irregularities were most common, but skin lacerations, pancreatitis, hypoglycemia, pneumonia, and venous thrombosis were also reported. If the cat survives the postoperative period, all clinical signs resolve in 2 to 4 months. In most cats, the diabetes mellitus becomes subclinical and no longer requires insulin.

There are no reports of cats with iatrogenic hyperadrenocorticism with signs of glucocorticoid or mineralocorticoid insufficiency on sudden cessation of treatment. Unless the cat is to undergo surgery near the time of glucocorticoid withdrawal, replacement therapy should not be needed.

Hypopituitarism

Hypopituitarism can be caused by failure or loss of one or more of the pituitary hormones.[1, 2, 352] The endocrine manifestations of hypopituitarism are related to the type and degree of hormonal deficiency and the stage in life at which the deficiency occurs.

Hypopituitarism may be caused by pituitary or hypothalamic deficiencies. Pituitary deficiencies may be caused by congenital hypoplasia, destructive lesions (infections, lymphocytic hypophysitis, infiltrative diseases, trauma, and neoplasms), vascular lesions, and the inherited disorder of German shepherds and Carnelian bear dogs. Hypothalamic deficiencies may be caused by trauma, encephalitis, aberrant parasite migration, hamartoma, neoplasia, and neurosecretory dysfunction.

Diagnosis of hypopituitarism is based on various clinical signs, responses of various target organs and pituitary hormones to challenges with pituitary and hypothalamic hormones and releasing factors, and various sophisticated radiographic techniques.[1, 2]

Pituitary Dwarfism

Canine pituitary dwarfism is a hereditary hypopituitarism associated with proportionate dwarfism, bilaterally symmetric alopecia and hyperpigmentation, and variable thyroidal, adrenocortical, and gonadal abnormalities.

CAUSE AND PATHOGENESIS

In the German shepherd and Carnelian bear dog, pituitary dwarfism is thought to be inherited as a simple autosomal recessive condition.[1, 2, 11, 14, 355] Most affected dogs appear to have a variably sized cyst (Rathke's cleft cyst) in the pituitary gland, resulting in varying degrees of anterior pituitary insufficiency. Because normal dogs can have Rathke's cysts and some dwarfs have either a hypoplastic or normal pituitary gland, the defect in some dwarfs may be due to dysfunctional cells.[11, 356, 360, 363] The clinical signs are related to GH deficiency, with or without concurrent thyroidal, adrenocortical, and gonadal abnormalities.

Immunodeficient dwarfism has been reported in an inbred colony of Weimaraners with GH deficiency and congenital absence of the thymic cortex.[370, 371]

CLINICAL FEATURES

Canine pituitary dwarfism has been reported in many breeds, but predominantly in the German shepherd and Carnelian bear dog.[1, 2, 11, 349] No sex predilection is evident.

For the first 2 to 3 months of life, the dog may appear normal and indistinguishable from normal litter mates. After this time, the dog fails to grow, the haircoat is notably shorter, and no primary hairs develop (Fig. 10–10). The puppy coat of secondary hairs is retained. This hair is soft, woolly, and easily epilated (see Fig. 10–9C). Primary hairs are often present on only the face and the distal extremities. Bilaterally symmetric alopecia then develops, especially in the wear areas of the neck and caudolateral aspects of the thighs. The alopecic skin is at first normally pigmented, then progresses through increasing degrees of hyperpigmentation (see Fig. 10–9D). The skin becomes thin, hypotonic, and scaly. Comedones may be numerous. These dogs may have behavioral abnormalities such as fear biting and aggressiveness. Gonadal status may vary from atrophic testicles or absence of estrus to normal findings. If there are concurrent deficiencies of TSH or ACTH, the dogs may manifest signs of hypothyroidism and adrenocortical insufficiency. As dwarfs grow older, they often become progressively more listless, dull, and inactive, and most dwarfs die between 3 and 8 years of age because of infections, degenerative diseases, or neurologic dysfunction.[2]

Immunodeficient dwarfism in Weimaraners is characterized by puppies that appear normal at birth, exhibiting a wasting syndrome at a few weeks of age.[370, 371] Clinical signs include unthriftiness, emaciation, lethargy, and persistent infections, usually resulting in death.

Delayed growth has been described in sibling German shepherd dogs.[364] Two dogs had histologic evidence of hypopituitarism, and two dogs had normal serum concentrations of growth hormone, T_4, and cortisol. In contrast with German shepherd dogs with pituitary dwarfism, these dogs had no dermatologic abnormalities and eventually reached normal stature.

DIAGNOSIS

The differential diagnosis includes congenital hypothyroidism with dwarfism, juvenile diabetes mellitus, gonadal dysgenesis, malnutrition, severe metabolic diseases (portacaval shunts, congenital renal disease, and congenital heart defects), and skeletal dysplasias (chondrodysplasia in Alaskan malamutes, pseudoachondroplastic dysplasia in Miniature poodles, and mucopolysaccharidosis).[1, 2] Definitive diagnosis is based on history, physical examination findings, laboratory test results, skin biopsy, radiography, the presence of insulin-induced hypoglycemia, and the results of GH stimulation tests. Depending on the degree of anterior pituitary insufficiency, affected dogs may have laboratory findings consistent with hypothyroidism and secondary adrenocortical insufficiency. Immunodeficient dwarf Weimaraners have deficient lymphocyte blastogenic responses to phytomitogens, as well as thymic cortical hypoplasia.[370, 371]

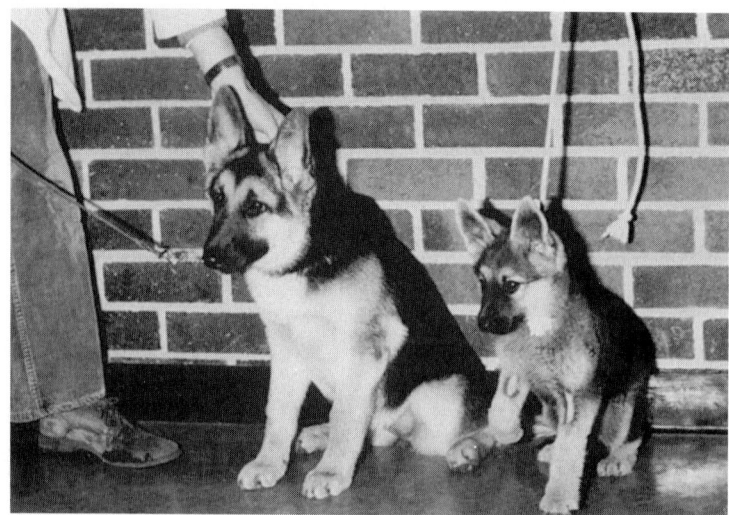

FIGURE 10–10. Pituitary dwarf with a normal littermate.

Histopathologic examination of the skin reveals changes consistent with endocrinopathy (orthokeratotic hyperkeratosis, follicular keratosis, follicular dilatation, follicular atrophy, telogenization of hair follicles, excessive trichilemmal keratinization, sebaceous gland atrophy, epidermal melanosis, and thin dermis).[16] A highly suggestive finding is the decreased amount and size of dermal elastin fibers (see Figs. 10–12 and 10–13). In cases with concurrent hypothyroidism, histopathologic findings may include vacuolated or hypertrophied arrector pili muscles.

Radiography may reveal delayed closure of growth plates of long bones, delayed eruption of permanent teeth, failure of the os penis to mineralize completely by 1 year of age, open fontanelles of the skull, and smaller-than-normal heart, liver, and kidney.[1, 2, 11, 349]

A characteristic metabolic abnormality of GH-deficient dogs is hypersensitivity to the hypoglycemic effect of insulin.[1, 2, 11, 355] The IV injection of regular insulin at 0.025 units/kg into GH-deficient dogs produces severe, prolonged hypoglycemia.

Basal plasma GH levels (by RIA) in normal dogs vary from 1 to 4.5 ng/ml in most reports.[1, 2, 11] However, basal GH levels in pituitary dwarfs and hypophysectomized dogs may come close to these values. Thus, basal GH levels are inadequate for the documentation of GH deficiency. Clonidine (an α-adrenergic antihypertensive drug) and xylazine have been used to stimulate GH release in the dog and to document the existence of GH deficiency.[1, 2, 11, 347, 355] Normal dogs show a marked increase in plasma GH and insulin-like growth factor (IGF-1) levels within 15 to 30 minutes after the IV injection of 10 to 30 μg/kg of clonidine or 100 to 300 μg/kg of xylazine, whereas pituitary dwarfs and hypophysectomized dogs do not respond.[368] Hypothyroidism, hyperadrenocorticism, and sex hormone abnormalities must always be ruled out because they can impair GH secretion. These hormones can be evaluated singularly or by the rapid sequential injection of the various stimulating or releasing hormones.[8, 9, 356]

The measurement of plasma IGF-1 levels could also be diagnostic (<5 ng/ml) for growth hormone deficiency, but test results must be evaluated in light of the size of the dog.[1, 2, 355] Heterozygous carriers of the pituitary dwarfism trait have intermediate levels of plasma IGF-1 compared with dwarfs and normal dogs. In some instances, it may be of value to assess both GH and IGF-1 levels.[1, 2, 368]

Human or bovine GHRF has been used to evaluate GH responses in the dog.[1, 2, 344, 359] When administered to normal dogs at a dose of 1 μg/kg, GHRF produced a twofold to fourfold increase in GH levels, whereas there was no response in dogs with hyposomatotropism.

CLINICAL MANAGEMENT

The owner should be made aware of the chronic nature of the disease, the general unavailability of GH for treatment, and the animal's shortened life expectancy. If the owner is willing to accept these possibilities, the dwarf dog can be kept as a pet. Concurrent hypothyroidism[348] or secondary adrenocortical insufficiency necessitate additional specific therapy with levothyroxine or glucocorticoids, respectively. If secondary adrenocortical insufficiency is present, this should always be treated first.

Bovine GH (10 IU subcutaneously, every other day for 30 days) and porcine GH (2 IU subcutaneously, every other day, or 0.1 IU/kg subcutaneously, three times weekly, for 4 to 6 weeks) have been used experimentally to treat canine pituitary dwarfism.[1, 2, 11, 349, 355] A beneficial response to GH in the skin and haircoat occurs within 6 to 8 weeks. However, growth plates close rapidly, and no appreciable increase in stature is achieved. Although not reported during the treatment of canine pituitary dwarfism, repeated injections of bovine and porcine GH could result in hypersensitivity reactions,[345] diabetes mellitus, or acromegalic-like bone changes.[351] Antibody production to bovine GH can occur and block its activity.[366]

Progestin administration to normal dogs increases growth hormone and IGF-1 concentrations in the blood (see Acromegaly).[348, 378, 379] These hormones arise from the mammary ductile epithelium. When four intact dwarf German shepherds, two male and two female, were given medroxyprogesterone acetate (5 or 10 mg/kg subcutaneously every third week), all dogs grew a normal coat.[358, 401] As expected, the progestin administration increased the plasma growth hormone and IGF-1 levels. The latter probably was responsible for the coat regrowth.[362] Long-term follow-up data was reported for two dogs. In these animals, a maintenance dosage of 5 mg/kg every sixth week was used. Both dogs maintained their haircoat and were healthy 3 to 4 years after the initiation of treatment. They both had repeated episodes of pyoderma, the male had some acromegalic features, and the bitch had to be neutered for a progestin-induced pyometra.[358] Refinement of the treatment protocol might eliminate some of the side effects.

Hyposomatotropism in the Mature Dog

Hyposomatotropism (pseudo-Cushing's syndrome, or GH-responsive dermatosis) is a rare condition resulting in a bilaterally symmetric alopecia in the mature dog.

CAUSE AND PATHOGENESIS

The cause and the pathogenesis of this disorder are unknown.* Clonidine or xylazine stimulation tests have documented inadequate or absent GH secretion in some but not all dogs.[368] When 95 dogs with clinical signs compatible with hyposomatotropism were studied, 32 (34%) had a normal GH response test result.[359] In addition, serum IGF-1 levels were normal in dogs with an abnormal GH response. IGF-1 should be decreased with true GH deficiency. When 12 normally coated Pomeranians and 7 with hyposomatotropism were studied, all dogs showed no significant increase in GH levels after xylazine or human GHRF administration.[372] All dogs also had abnormal adrenal sex hormone synthesis, suggestive of a partial deficiency of the 21-hydroxylase enzyme. These factors, coupled with normal pituitary morphologic findings in one of two dogs at necropsy,[11] shed doubts on the primary role of GH in this condition. The GH deficiency could be induced by the abnormal adrenal steroid synthesis[368, 383] or could be a coincidental endocrinopathy, which may or may not contribute to the hair loss in these dogs.[11, 412]

Two adult Poodles with typical clinical signs of adult-onset hyposomatotropism had fluctuating but low GH levels that showed no response to clonidine or GHRH, but the dogs had normal levels of IGF-1.[368] The authors suggested that both dogs had a mild and fluctuating hyperadrenocorticism with resultant glucocorticoid-caused suppression of somatostatin release.

CLINICAL FEATURES

Hyposomatotropism has been reported predominantly in male dogs of many different breeds, but especially in Chow Chow, Keeshond, Pomeranian, Miniature Poodle, Samoyed, and American water spaniel breeds.[345, 359] Because four of these breeds, namely the Chow Chow, Keeshond, Pomeranian, and Samoyed, are over-represented in adrenal hyperplasia-like syndrome, it is very likely that any growth hormone irregularity in these dogs is a coincidental or secondary problem. Age at onset is between 9 months and 11 years, with about 50% of the affected dogs being younger than 2 years of age. The first noticeable change in the coat is a gradual loss of primary hairs with retention of secondary hairs, giving the coat a puppy-like appearance. With time, all hairs are lost around the neck, pinnae, tail, and caudomedial thighs (see Fig. 10–9E). As those areas become alopecic, the truncal primary hairs are lost gradually and then the secondary hairs become more sparse. Complete truncal alopecia is uncommon, even in chronic cases. In many dogs, the exposed skin hyperpigments rapidly (see Fig. 10–9F). A small number of these dogs have hair loss, with or without hyperpigmentation, restricted symmetrically to the flank region (Fig. 10–11).[386, 412] Hairs in affected areas are often easily epilated. In chronic cases, the skin may be thin and hypotonic. In cases in which skin biopsies had

---

*See references 14, 345, 359, 368, 372, 373, 376.

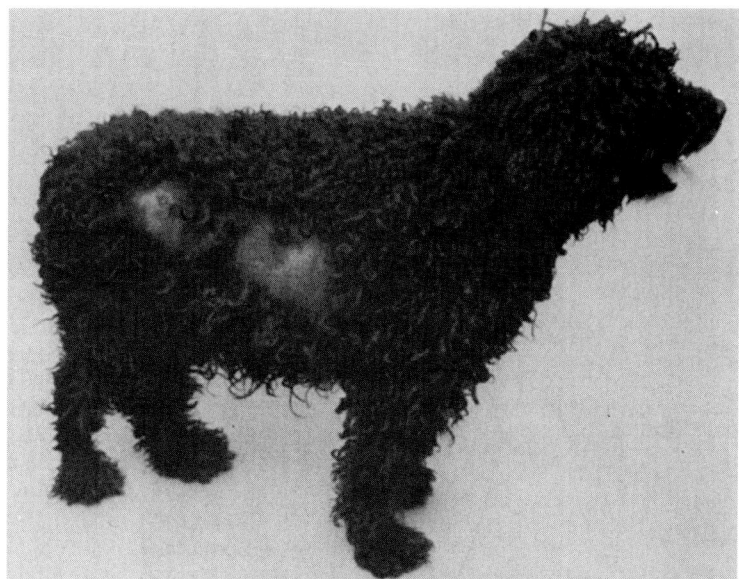

FIGURE 10–11. Hyposomatotropism. Symmetric flank alopecia.

been performed, the hair grew back over the biopsy sites. The dogs are normal except for the dermatologic signs.

Airedales, Boxers, and English bulldogs experience a seasonal disease in which flank alopecia and hyperpigmentation develop in winter or spring. The low GH levels in these dogs may be spurious because a seasonal follicular dysplasia is also described in these same breeds (see Chaps. 11 and 12). Alternatively, the low GH levels may be caused by the hormones responsible for the hair loss or may be real.[389] In the last case, the GH deficiency would be a co-contributor to the hair loss. By itself, it causes no hair loss but makes the hair follicles more sensitive to the effects of other hormones.

DIAGNOSIS

The differential diagnosis includes hypothyroidism, hyperadrenocorticism, and gonadal or adrenal hyperplasia-like syndrome. Definitive diagnosis is based on history, physical examination findings, laboratory results that rule out other conditions, skin biopsy, and response to therapy. Skin biopsy reveals changes consistent with endocrinopathy (orthokeratotic hyperkeratosis, follicular keratosis, follicular dilatation, telogenization of hair follicles, excessive trichilemmal keratinization, epidermal melanosis, sebaceous gland atrophy, and thin dermis).[16] A highly suggestive histopathologic finding is decreased amounts and small size of dermal elastin fibers (Figs. 10–12 and 10–13), but this finding may be present only in dogs that have been clinically affected for 2 years or longer.[376] Measurements of plasma GH and IGF-1 levels before and after the IV injection of clonidine or xylazine documents GH deficiency, but this testing is not routinely available in most laboratories. In dogs with seasonal GH deficiency (Airedales, Boxers, and English bulldogs), xylazine responses are suppressed during the period of hair loss but become normal with hair regrowth.[11] Hypothyroidism, hyperadrenocorticism, and sex hormone abnormalities must always be ruled out before GH test results are interpreted because these conditions impair GH secretion.[1, 2, 355, 376]

CLINICAL MANAGEMENT

Until the pathogenic mechanism of this disorder is completely defined, treatment recommendations are difficult. Some dogs with documented GH deficiency respond to GH supplementation, whereas others do not. Additionally, some dogs regrow the coat with

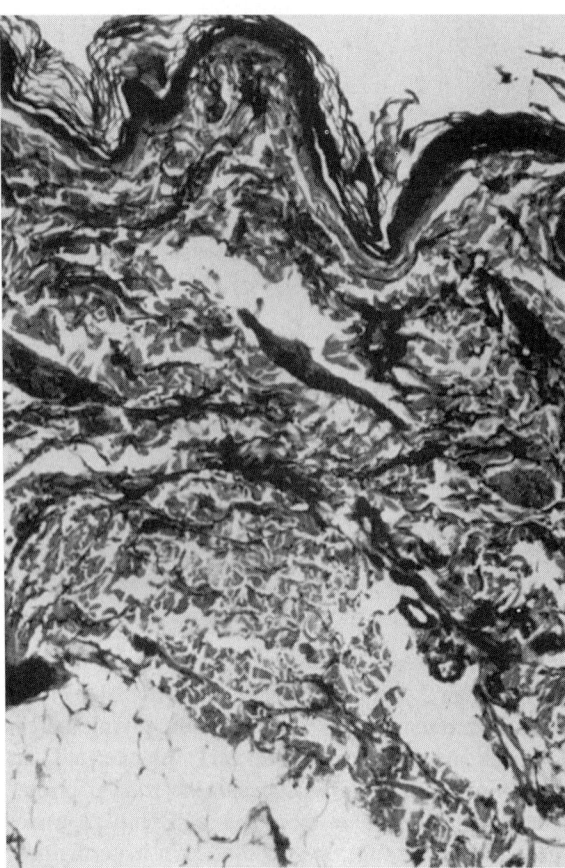

FIGURE 10–12. Normal canine skin. Numerous thick, long elastin bundles and fibers are present in the dermis (Verhoeff's stain). (From Parker WM, Scott DW: Growth hormone–responsive alopecia in the mature dog: A discussion of 13 cases. J Am Anim Hosp Assoc 16:824, 1980.)

neutering, testosterone supplementation, or treatment with o,p′-DDD.[373] In light of those facts and the fact that GH, beyond that marketed for milk production in cows, is not available to veterinarians on a routine and regular basis, most investigators suggest that these animals be treated initially as if they had a gonadal or adrenal sex hormone imbalance. If there is no response to those treatments, GH supplementation is indicated.

Response to bovine, porcine, and human GH has been reported,[345, 355, 372] although ovine GH was ineffective.[376] Original treatment protocols suggested that dogs weighing less than 14 kg be given 2.5 IU, whereas larger dogs receive 5 IU. These doses are given subcutaneously every other day for 10 treatments. Newer reports suggest dosages of 0.1 IU/kg three times weekly for 6 weeks[355] or 0.015 IU/kg twice weekly for the same period.[374] The recombinant bovine growth hormone available for dairy cattle cannot be diluted down to these doses. Because GH is a diabetogenic agent, a fasting blood sugar level should be obtained before treatment and weekly thereafter. If hyperglycemia occurs, the injections should be discontinued immediately; otherwise, an irreversible diabetic condition may develop. Other side effects include acromegaly and hypersensitivity to the protein of origin of the GH.[345, 368] The latter has occurred with both recombinant human and bovine growth hormone. Autoantibody production with loss of efficacy is another problem recognized with those agents.[262] If response is to occur, it should be seen within 3 months. Most dogs start to lose hair again within 3 to 36 months. Retreatment should produce another remission.

Although the pathogenic mechanism of this disorder is unknown, the high number of cases within certain breeds suggest some genetic influence.[359, 380] Affected dogs should not be used for breeding.

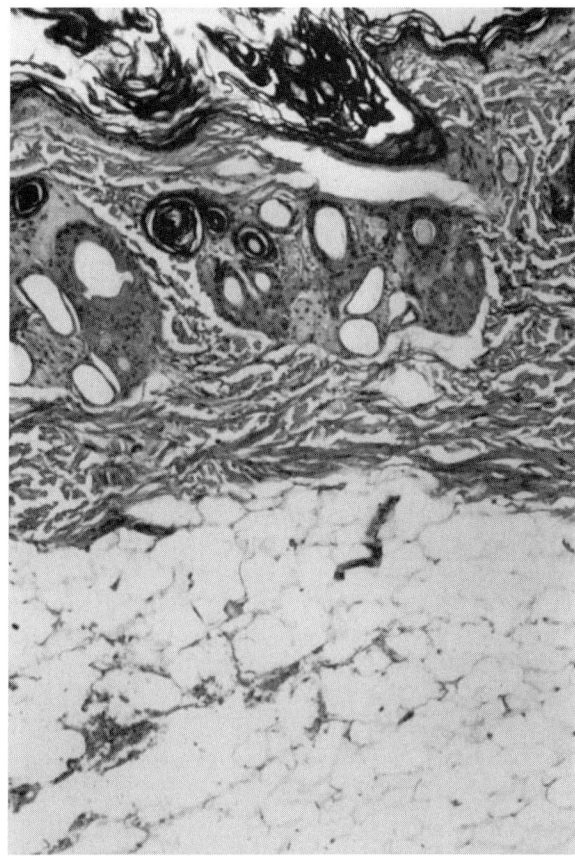

FIGURE 10-13. Hyposomatotropism (growth hormone–responsive dermatosis) in a dog. Marked absence of dermal elastin (Verhoeff's stain). (From Parker WM, Scott DW: Growth hormone–responsive alopecia in the mature dog: A discussion of 13 cases. J Am Anim Hosp Assoc 16:824, 1980.)

Acromegaly

Acromegaly is due to hypersecretion of GH in the mature animal. It is a rare disease in dogs and cats.

CAUSE AND PATHOGENESIS

Acromegaly is caused by hypersecretion of GH in the mature animal (after epiphyseal closure). Hypersecretion of GH results in an overgrowth of connective tissue, bone, and viscera. In the dog, acromegaly has been reported in association with injections of anterior pituitary gland extracts, acidophilic hyperplasia or adenoma of the anterior pituitary gland, diestrus in the intact cycling bitch, and administration of progestational compounds.* Some acromegalic changes were induced in two pituitary dwarfs treated with methylprogesterone acetate.[358] In these dogs, the growth hormone was produced by mammary tissue.[382] In the cat, acromegaly has been associated with pituitary tumors.[1, 2, 353, 365]

CLINICAL FEATURES

Canine Acromegaly

No breed or age predilections are evident, but most cases occur in middle-aged to old dogs. Because progestational stimulation is the most common cause of acromegaly in dogs,

---

*See references 1, 2, 351, 354, 357, 365, 375, 377, 378.

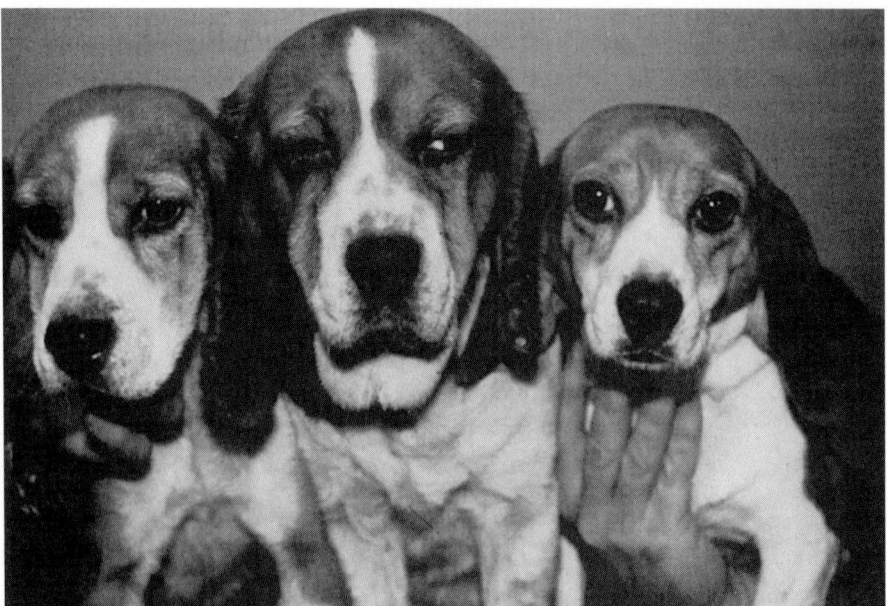

FIGURE 10–14. Acromegaly. Acromegalic beagle (*center*) and two normal littermates.

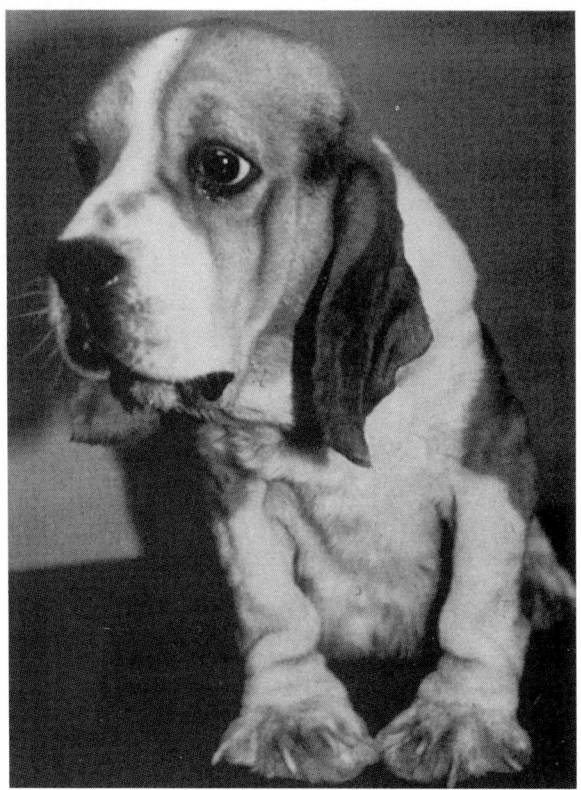

FIGURE 10–15. Acromegaly. Note large head and paws.

most cases occur in intact females. Male or female dogs being treated with progestational compounds are at risk. The most common signs noted include inspiratory stridor (due to soft tissue increases in the orolingual-oropharyngeal regions), increased body size (especially paws and skull) (Figs. 10–14 and 10–15), abdominal enlargement, polyuria, polydipsia, polyphagia, fatigue, frequent panting, prognathism, widening of the interdental spaces, and galactorrhea.[365] Cutaneous changes include thickened, myxedematous skin thrown into excessive folds, hypertrichosis, and thick hard claws.

Feline Acromegaly

No breed or age predilections are reported, but more than 90% of cases occur in male cats. Clinical signs include increased body size (especially paws and skull), prognathism, widened interdental spaces, organomegaly, dyspnea due to cardiac failure, cardiomegaly, neurologic signs with large tumors, and polyuria and polydipsia with or without renal failure.[365] Skin changes are the same as those described for the dog but are usually not marked.

Both dogs and cats with acromegaly can have insulin-resistant diabetes mellitus.[424] Although the diabetes occurs later than the other signs, it may be the only complaint at presentation. The changes in the skin or body may be subtle or pronounced but go unnoticed because they occur gradually.

DIAGNOSIS

The definitive diagnosis of acromegaly is based on history, physical examination findings, serum chemistry studies, skin biopsy, persistent elevation of plasma GH levels, altered response of GH levels to stimulation with clonidine, GHRH, or IV glucose administration.[1, 2, 354, 365, 375] Many acromegalic dogs have mild to moderate hyperglycemia and mild to severe elevations of serum alkaline phosphatase levels. Nonsuppressibility of plasma GH levels after an IV glucose load is considered a hallmark of acromegaly. The levels of plasma GH do not always correlate with the degree of acromegaly. GH levels may also be elevated in response to stress, acute illness, chronic renal and liver disease, diabetes mellitus, and starvation.[1, 2] The measurement of plasma IGF-1 levels (mean, 679 ± 116 ng/ml in acromegalic dogs; mean, 280 ± 23 ng/ml in normal German shepherds) could also be diagnostic but must be evaluated in light of the size of the dog.[1, 2, 354]

In dogs and human beings, histologic examination of acromegalic skin reveals collagenous hyperplasia, myxedema, and hyperplasia of the epidermis and appendages (Figs. 10–16 and 10–17).[375]

CLINICAL MANAGEMENT

Dogs with acromegaly associated with diestrus or with progestational compound treatment have responded well to ovariohysterectomy and to cessation of progestogen therapy, respectively.[357, 365] Soft tissue changes resolve slowly, but skeletal changes are likely to be permanent. Aside from pituitary irradiation, no successful form of treatment has been described for the cat.[215]

Sex Hormone Dermatoses

Dermatoses associated with sex hormones are uncommon and may be of gonadal or adrenal origin.[1, 2, 11, 14] Clinical signs typically include the absence of systemic signs and the presence of truncal alopecia, which may be generalized or regionalized. Regionalized, or patterned, hair loss is more common. The discussion lends itself to categorization by sex and gonadal status, but there is great overlap in each category.

828 • Endocrine and Metabolic Diseases

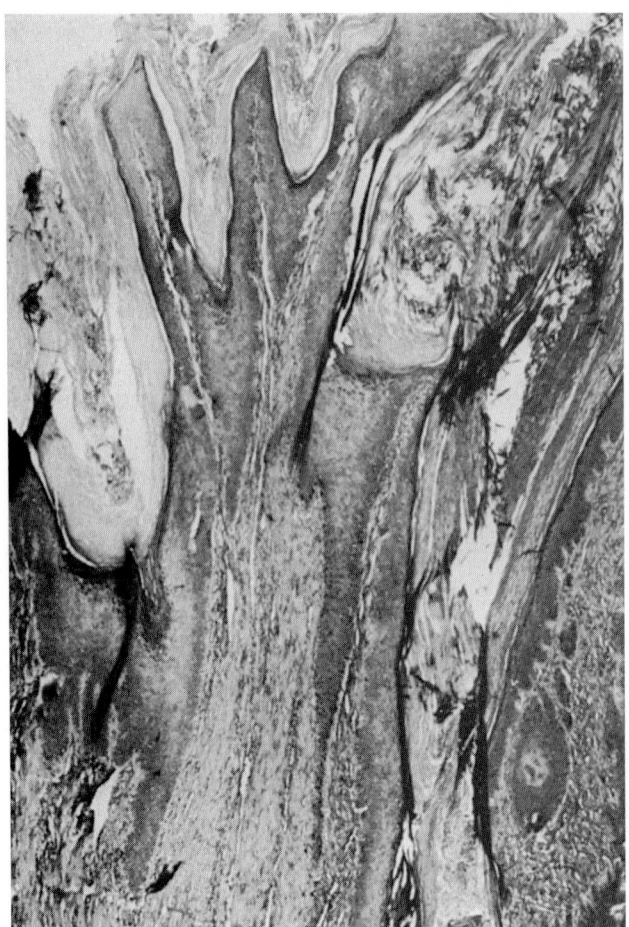

FIGURE 10-16. Acromegaly. Papillated hyperplasia and orthokeratotic hyperkeratosis.

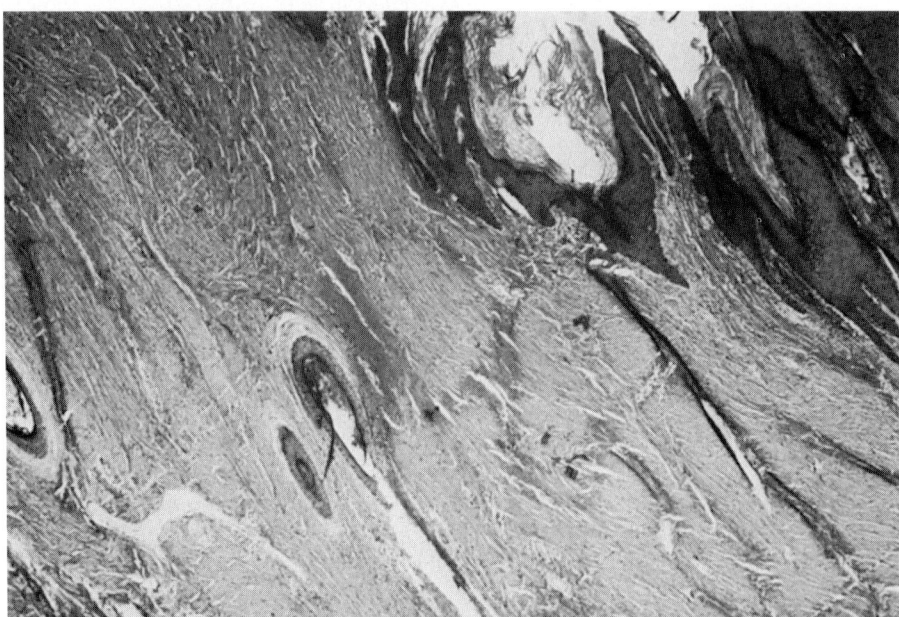

FIGURE 10-17. Acromegaly. Collagenous hyperplasia.

HYPERESTROGENISM IN FEMALE ANIMALS

Hyperestrogenism in the female dog is a rare disorder characterized by bilaterally symmetric alopecia, enlargement of the vulva and nipples, and estrous cycle abnormalities.[394, 396, 408, 414] Hyperestrogenism in the cat has been been reported only once.[403]

Cause and Pathogenesis

This disorder is usually associated with cystic ovaries and rarely with functional ovarian tumors.[396, 417] Most estrogen-producing ovarian neoplasms are granulosa-theca cell in origin, and 10% to 20% are malignant.[1, 2] These tumors may also produce progesterone, which causes mammary hypertrophy. Cases have been recognized in neutered females with normal adrenal function.[373] The cause of the hyperestrogenism is unknown, but it may be due to abnormalities in peripheral conversion of sex hormones or an ectopic source of production.

Estrogenic substances have been administered to dogs by a number of investigators, resulting in cutaneous syndromes identical to the naturally occurring disease. An identical syndrome may also occur with overdoses of estrogens used to treat mismating and urinary incontinence after ovariohysterectomy.[386, 421] Some dogs have cutaneous hyperestrogenism (normal blood estrogen levels) owing to increased numbers of cutaneous estrogen receptors.[390]

Clinical Features

Hyperestrogenism associated with polycystic ovaries usually occurs in the middle-aged, intact female dog. English bulldogs may be predisposed to the disorder.[1, 2] Hyperestrogenism associated with functional ovarian neoplasia usually occurs in older intact females, and no breed predilections are reported. The disorder is characterized by bilaterally symmetric alopecia beginning in the perineal, inguinal, and flank regions (see Fig. 10–9G and H). The hair loss remains confined to these areas for long periods but can progress to involve the entire trunk in chronic cases. Hairs in affected areas are easily epilated. In some dogs, the hair loss is confined to the flank area and the degree of hair loss can vary with the estrous cycle.

The nipples and vulva are enlarged (Fig. 10–18A), and comedones are usually numerous on the ventrum and vulvar skin. With additional progestational stimulation, the mammary glands enlarge. Secondary seborrheic changes can occur, but skin infections are uncommon. Estrous cycle abnormalities (irregular cycles, prolonged estrus, and nymphomania) often occur, and endometritis or pyometra may be seen. In the cat, truncal alopecia was associated with persistent estrus.[403]

Diagnosis

In the intact female, the diagnosis is straightforward if the dog has both estral and cutaneous changes. With a history of poor estrus, tumor or incompletely excised ovarian tissue, or estrogen administration without the history of same, the diagnosis is more difficult and the primary differential diagnostic considerations include hypothyroidism, hyperadrenocorticism, and follicular dysplasia. Definitive diagnosis is based on history, physical examination findings, laboratory test results that rule out other conditions, and response to therapy. Skin biopsy differentiates hyperestrogenism from follicular dysplasia and other nonendocrine follicular disorders but does not differentiate this condition from other endocrine disorders. Changes include orthokeratotic hyperkeratosis, follicular keratosis, follicular dilatation, follicular atrophy, telogenization of hair follicles, excessive trichilemmal keratinization, epidermal melanosis, and sebaceous gland atrophy (Fig. 10–19).[16] Elevated blood estrogen levels may support the diagnosis. An hCG response test can be useful in detecting hormonal changes in tumors that are not too large. Ultrasonography and laparoscopy are useful for delineating ovarian neoplasms.[1, 2, 396]

Clinical Management

Therapy for hyperestrogenism in the intact female dog consists of ovariohysterectomy. A good response is usually evident within 3 months but occasionally does not occur for 6

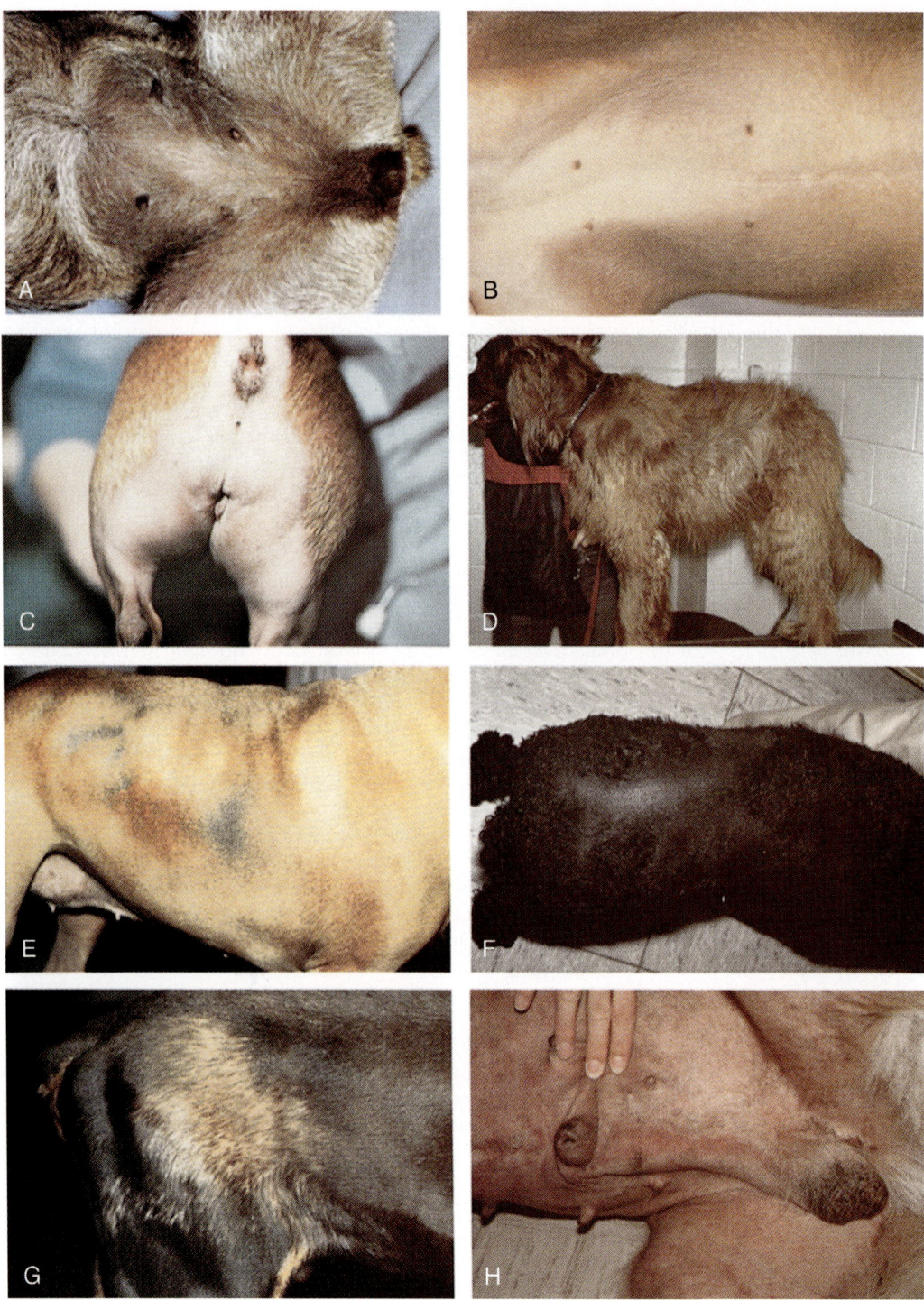

FIGURE 10–18. *A*, Hyperestrogenism. Note the hypertrophied, hyperpigmented vulva. *B*, Estrogen-responsive dermatosis. Ventral alopecia and juvenile nipples. *C*, Estrogen-responsive dermatosis. Perineal hair loss with small recessed vulva. *D*, Hypertrichosis in an estrogen-responsive Irish setter. *E*, Flank alopecia in an intact female with hypogonadism. *F*, Alopecia and hyperpigmentation in a bitch in overt pseudopregnancy. *G*, Testosterone-responsive dermatosis. Dull dry coat with coat color change. *H*, Linear preputial dermatosis in a dog with a Sertoli's cell tumor.

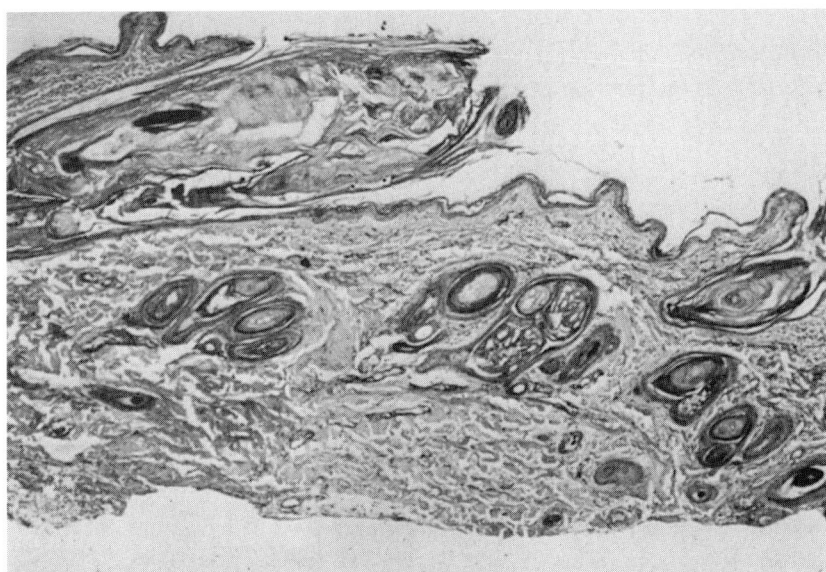

FIGURE 10-19. Hyperestrogenism in a dog. Note follicular keratosis and plugging, absence of hair shafts, and sebaceous gland atrophy.

months. Symptomatic therapy with topical antiseborrheic agents may be indicated. If an ovarian neoplasm is suspected, chest radiographs should be taken before surgery. No successful treatment of neutered females with nonovarian hyperestrogenism has been described.[373]

ESTROGEN-RESPONSIVE DERMATOSIS OF FEMALE ANIMALS

Estrogen-responsive dermatosis is a rare, bilaterally symmetric alopecia of unknown etiology seen in spayed female dogs.[412] The condition is extremely rare in cats.

Cause and Pathogenesis

The cause and the pathogenesis of estrogen-responsive dermatosis in female dogs are unknown.[375] Hypoestrogenism has been suggested as the cause of this endocrine-like dermatosis. In most cases, low estrogen levels cannot be documented. Investigators have seen positive responses to estrogen supplementation in some intact female animals that experience dermatoses before their first estrus, during pseudopregnancy, or in association with an abnormal estrous cycle. The role of estrogens in the response of those dogs is uncertain, and it is best to reserve the term estrogen-responsive dermatosis for neutered females.

Clinical Features

Estrogen-responsive dermatosis is usually first noticed when the dog is a young adult (2 to 4 years). No age or breed predilections are documented, but most reported cases involve Dachshunds and Boxers. In shorthaired dogs, the dermatosis is characterized by hypotrichosis that begins in the perineal and genital regions. Diffuse alopecia results and can affect the caudomedial thighs, the ventral abdomen, the thorax, the neck, and the postauricular region of the head (see Fig. 10-18B and C). Hairs in affected areas are easily epilated. The nipples and the vulva are often infantile. Some dogs have only bilateral flank alopecia. In longhaired dogs, the first noticeable change is loss of primary hairs, giving the coat a puppy-like quality. Hair loss starts in the flank region and progresses slowly (Fig. 10-20). Some Irish setters with this condition present for hypertrichosis with blending of the retained hairs (see Fig. 10-18D). Any dog with this condition can have secondary

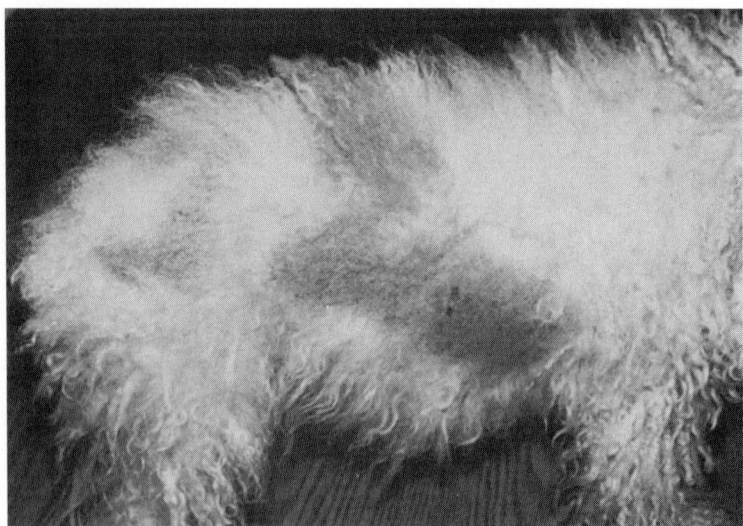

FIGURE 10–20. Estrogen-responsive dermatosis. Loss of primary hairs and flank alopecia.

seborrheic skin disease, but this is uncommon. Dogs with estrogen-responsive dermatosis are usually normal otherwise, but concurrent estrogen-responsive urinary incontinence occurs occasionally. In cats, symmetric truncal alopecia, especially of the ventrum, may occur.

Diagnosis

The differential diagnosis varies with the presentation. With persistent ventral hair loss, the primary differential diagnostic possibility is patterned baldness. Careful review of the history can help differentiate the conditions. In both cases, the dogs have normal puppy coats and shed them at the appropriate time. With patterned baldness, the coat that regrows is sparser and finer than normal and continues to worsen. In dogs with estrogen-responsive dermatosis, a normal adult coat develops that is maintained for variable periods of time before the hair loss begins. With other presentations, hypothyroidism, hyperadrenocorticism, hyposomatotropism, adrenal sex hormone imbalance, and follicular dysplasia must be considered. Definitive diagnosis is based on history, physical examination findings, laboratory test results that rule out other conditions, and response to therapy. Skin biopsy eliminates nonendocrine causes of the hair loss but otherwise is nondiagnostic, revealing orthokeratotic hyperkeratosis, follicular keratosis, follicular atrophy, follicular dilatation, and telogenization of hair follicles (Fig. 10–21).[4, 16]

Clinical Management

Traditionally, this condition has been treated with diethylstilbestrol, given orally at doses of 0.1 to 1 mg. Some investigators give the drug every other day, whereas other clinicians give it daily for 3 weeks, stop treatment for 1 week, and then repeat the cycle.[11] The latter scheme was developed to spare the bone marrow[413] because dogs are susceptible to sometimes irreversible bone marrow depression (thrombocytopenia, leukopenia, and anemia) with long-term administration. No data are available to indicate that either approach is safer or more effective. The drug is given as described until hair regrows, and then the frequency of administration is slowly reduced to a maintenance dose of once to twice weekly.

Diethylstilbestrol tablets are difficult if not impossible to obtain, and the small tablet size makes division into smaller doses difficult, often thus precluding the treatment of small dogs. Estradiol and various conjugated or esterified estrogens are available through pharmaceutical houses and may be beneficial in dogs. We have used estradiol in a few

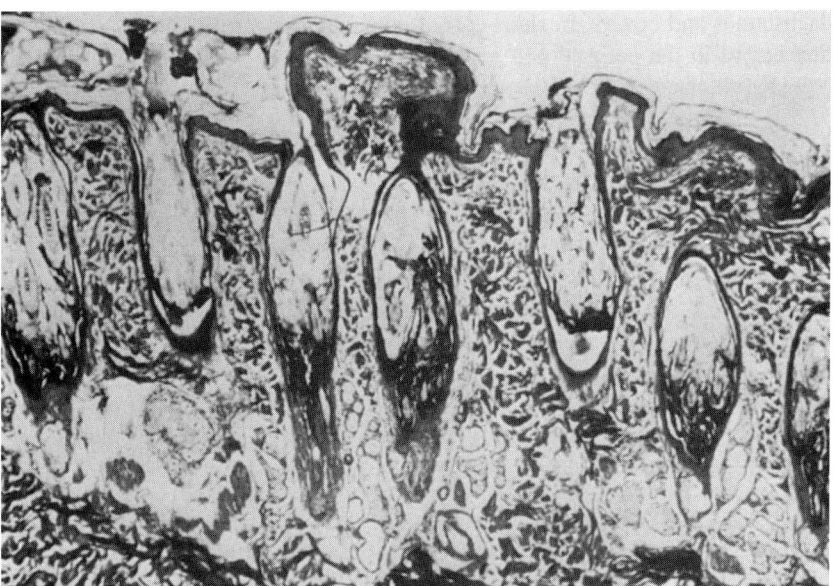

FIGURE 10–21. Estrogen-responsive dermatosis. Note follicular keratosis and plugging and absence of hair shafts.

dogs and noted a positive response with no apparent side effects. Before a substitute for diethylstilbestrol is dispensed, its potency relative to diethylstilbestrol should be determined. When estrogens cannot be used, response may occur with the daily administration of methyltestosterone or mibolerone (Cheque Drops, Upjohn). Methyltestosterone is given at 1 mg/kg with a maximal dose of 30 mg, whereas the mibolerone is given at 30 μg for dogs weighing less than 11 kg and at 50 μg for dogs weighing between 11 and 23 kg. The drug is given until hair regrows and then tapered to a maintenance level. These agents are controlled substances because of their anabolic nature and should be dispensed carefully.

HYPOGONADISM IN INTACT FEMALE ANIMALS

The term *hypogonadism* indicates a decrease or abnormality in the functional activity of the gonads. The condition can result from primary gonadal abnormalities or irregularities in the hormonal control mechanisms. Bitches with hypogonadism can present for infertility, coat changes, or both.

Cause and Pathogenesis

A variety of disorders of sexual development (primary hypogonadism) have been described.[1,2] Many conditions have been discovered at neutering or when the bitch's cycle failed to occur. Because the gonadal problem is identified early, coat changes are uncommon in these dogs. If the reproductive irregularity is overlooked, hair loss can occur. miniature Poodles, Terriers, and Dachshunds may be predisposed.[403]

Secondary hypogonadism is much more common. The dog's history includes an irregular estrous pattern, an increasing interestrous interval, or complete anestrus. If these estral irregularities develop after the dog has had a normal cycle for years, the hypogonadism is due to some systemic illness, typically of the endocrine system. Hypothyroidism and hyperadrenocorticism are the most common causes.[1,2]

All nonpregnant bitches go through a phase of pseudopregnancy in diestrus. In some dogs, the pseudopregnancy becomes clinical, with the development of preparturient behaviors and mammary activity. Dogs with clinical pseudopregnancy appear to have normal diestrus hormonal changes but, for some unknown reason, are sensitive to them.[1,2]

Clinical Features

The nature of the hair loss that can occur in these dogs varies with the cause of the cyclic abnormality. With primary hypogonadism, there are no clinical or cytologic signs of estrus. Hair loss starts early in life (younger than 3 years), first in the perineal and inguinal regions, with slow progression along the ventrum and trunk.[403] With irregular cycles or increasing interestrous intervals, the hair loss starts around the heat period, gradually worsens through the cycle, and then spontaneously resolves months after the cycle is completed.[403] As the interestrous interval increases, the length of the hair loss phase increases. With complete anestrus, the hair loss is persistent.

In dogs with short to medium-length coats, the hair loss associated with cyclic abnormalities occurs in the flank region and occasionally in the perineum (see Fig. 10–18E). In some dogs, the hair loss remains restricted to these areas, even with the development of complete anestrus, whereas it progresses to truncal alopecia in other dogs. The truncal alopecia is a late event and follows multiple cycles of hair loss and regrowth. In longhaired dogs, especially those with dense undercoats, the cutaneous manifestation of the cyclic abnormality is usually a change in the quality of the coat long before any hair loss is seen. The dog gradually loses its primary hairs on the trunk and has a puppy-like coat. When hair loss starts, it is usually first noted in the collar area, the flanks, and the posterior thighs. Progression to generalized truncal alopecia is slow.

In dogs with clinical pseudopregnancy, the hair loss usually is first noticed 4 to 6 weeks after estrus and involves the collar area, the rump, and the mammary region (see Fig. 10–18F).[412] An occasional dog has flank alopecia. The hair loss can become more widespread at subsequent estrous cycles. Behavioral and physical signs (mammary development and lactation) of clinical pseudopregnancy are present.

Diagnosis

When the hair loss is cyclic and has a temporal relationship to an estrous cycle or occurs in an intact but anestrous bitch, the diagnosis of an ovarian-induced hair loss is straightforward. Other differential diagnostic possibilities include excessive shedding and seasonal flank alopecia. When the hair loss is noncyclic, hypothyroidism, hyperadrenocorticism, hyposomatotropism, adrenal sex hormone imbalance, and follicular dysplasia must be considered. Skin biopsy eliminates nonendocrine causes of the hair loss but does not indicate an ovarian cause.

Because hypogonadism in the adult dog is typically secondary to an underlying endocrine disorder, all dogs with an increasing interestrous interval should be tested for hypothyroidism and hyperadrenocorticism. If results of these tests are normal, an ovarian dysfunction is likely. The tentative diagnosis can often be supported by measurement of sex hormone levels; with abnormalities in estrogen, progesterone, or testosterone levels[402, 403]; or by response to neutering.

Clinical Management

Dogs with hypogonadism experience coat regrowth with neutering or, if the hair loss is cyclic, do not lose their coat again. If the owner does not wish to neuter the dog and there is no other intercurrent endocrine disorder, the case should be referred to a theriogenologist for evaluation and treatment. Although there are reports of hair regrowth and return to estrous function with administration of GnRH (2 µg/kg IM twice at 10-day intervals), FSH (0.75 to 2 IU/kg IM daily until signs of proestrus occur), FSH (20 IU/kg IM for 10 days) followed by weekly injections of human chorionic gonadotropin (35 IU/kg), long-term efficacy of these treatments is unknown.[388, 403] If hypothyroidism or hyperadrenocorticism is documented, correction of that condition can return the dog to normal reproductive function with subsequent hair regrowth. In some dogs, the ovarian dysfunction persists and the animal must be neutered.

HYPERANDROGENISM IN MALE DOGS

Documented hyperandrogenism in the male dog is rare and has not been reported in the cat. It can cause circumanal gland and tail gland hyperplasia, with or without seborrhea oleosa, in dogs with testicular neoplasia.[412, 419] Hyperandrogenism is a suspected cause of seborrhea oleosa or truncal endocrine alopecia in oversexed intact male dogs.[11]

Cause and Pathogenesis

The circumanal glands and the tail gland of the dog are composed of the same glandular ("hepatoid") tissue. This tissue as well as the sebaceous glands is androgen responsive. Hypertestosteronemia, usually in association with testicular neoplasia (especially interstitial cell tumors),[418] results in glandular hyper-reactivity with hyperplasia and increased secretion.

Clinical Features

Dogs with idiopathic hyperandrogenism have severe seborrheic disease or, rarely, symmetric truncal hair loss.[384] The seborrhea is greasy and is most pronounced on the face, on the ears, and in the intertriginous areas (feet, axillae, and groin). Infection and pruritus are common, which worsens the condition. The hair loss in some dogs mimics that of other endocrine conditions. All dogs with idiopathic hyperandrogenism show hypersexual behavior, aggression to other dogs or humans, or both.

Hyperandrogenism due to testicular neoplasia causes circumanal gland hyperplasia. The glands around the anus enlarge uniformly, resulting in a donut-like appearance (Fig. 10–22). Tail gland hyperplasia appears as an oval enlargement of the dorsal surface of the proximal tail (Fig. 10–23). In advanced cases, the area becomes alopecic and greasy, and

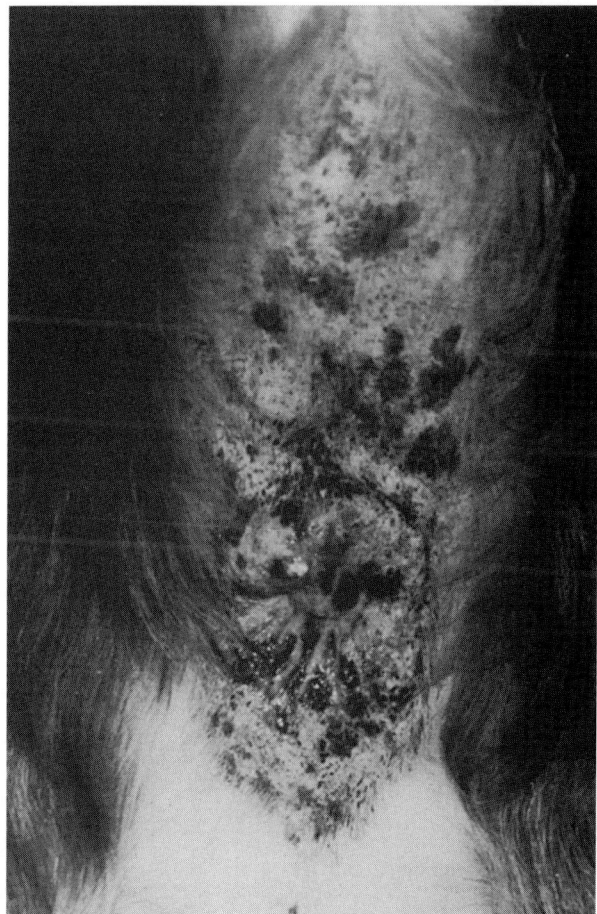

FIGURE 10–22. Dog with interstitial cell tumor of testicle and hypertestosteronemia. Circumanal gland hyperplasia and macular melanosis.

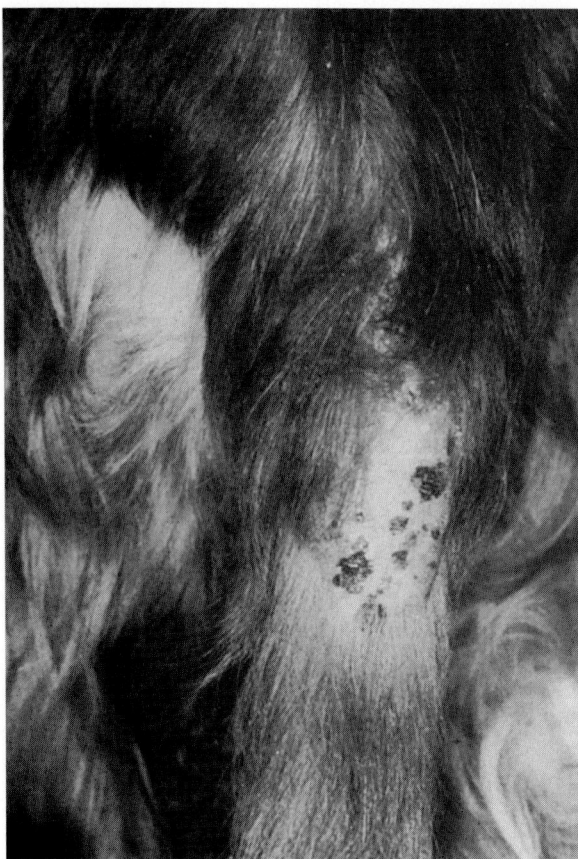

FIGURE 10-23. Same dog as in Figure 10-22. Alopecia, macular melanosis, and hypertrophy of tail gland.

the glandular hyperplasia can become so severe that multiple nodules or cysts or both occur in the area. Because circumanal glands can also be found in the perineum and the inguinal area, nodular lesions can be present elsewhere. Some dogs have macular melanosis of the tail gland, the perianal area, the scrotum, the ventral tail, and the ventral abdomen (Fig. 10-24) before, simultaneously with, or after the glandular hyperplasia occurs. A testicular mass can usually be palpated in these dogs but may not be appreciable when the skin lesions are first noted.

Diagnosis

Diagnosis is based on history, physical examination findings, determination of blood testosterone levels, and response to castration. Testicular ultrasonography may be helpful in detecting small nonpalpable tumors.[392] Histopathologic examination of the testicular tumor usually reveals an interstitial cell neoplasm. No cause of idiopathic hyperandrogenism has been found.

Clinical Management

Castration is indicated for these dogs. In idiopathic hyperandrogenism, the skin gradually returns to normal condition in 2 to 4 months, but the behavioral changes can last longer and may necessitate behavior modification. In seborrheic dogs, frequent bathing with an appropriate antiseborrheic shampoo hastens the dog's response. Castration of the dog with glandular hyperplasia prevents any worsening of the condition but may not return the dog to normal status. Some of the glandular hyperplasia is irreversible, as is the overlying hair loss. The macular melanosis fades slowly during 6 months.

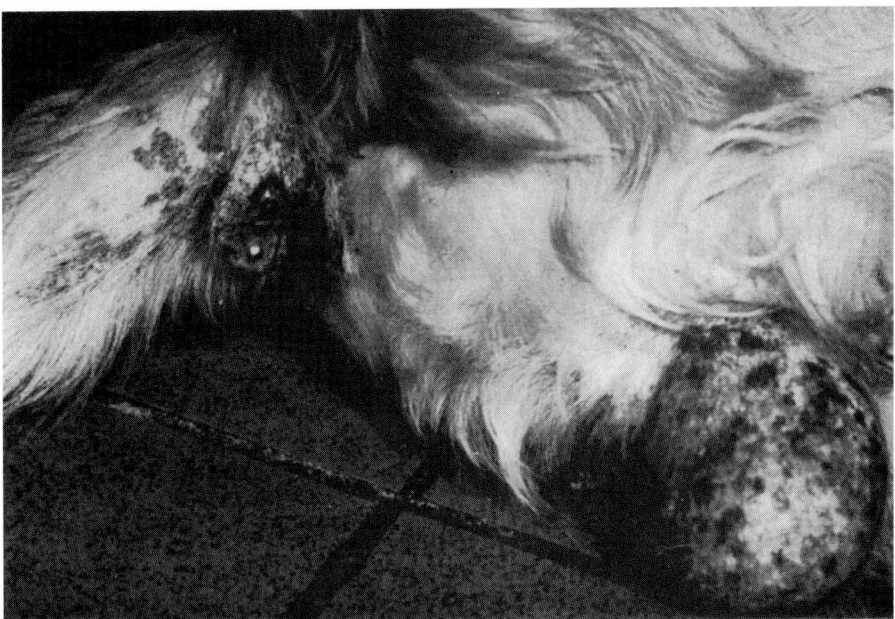

FIGURE 10-24. Same dog as in Figures 10-22 and 10-23. Note enlarged scrotum and macular melanosis of scrotum and perianal area.

TESTOSTERONE-RESPONSIVE DERMATOSIS OF MALE ANIMALS

Testosterone-responsive dermatosis (hypoandrogenism) is a rare, bilaterally symmetric alopecia of unknown cause in castrated male dogs.[402, 412] The condition is even rarer in the cat.

Cause and Pathogenesis

The cause and the pathogenesis of testosterone-responsive dermatosis in male dogs are unknown. Hypoandrogenism has been suggested but not documented as the cause of this endocrine-like dermatosis.

Clinical Findings

This condition is rare and occurs in old castrated males. Afghan hounds may be predisposed.[403] Some authors include intact dogs with testicular abnormalities or tumors in this category because some affected animals show transient response to testosterone, but we think that those cases should be described elsewhere (hypogonadism, testicular tumor) because they are not idiopathic. Castrated males with this condition first have a dull, dry coat with or without other seborrheic changes (Fig. 10-25). Dogs with dark brown or black haircoats often show coat color change to light brown or auburn, respectively, before hair loss is noted (see Fig. 10-18G). The hair loss in these dogs is truncal, is slowly progressive, and mimics that of other endocrine disorders. The skin may be thin and hypotonic. Rarely, the dog has hypertrichosis.

Diagnosis

The differential diagnosis includes hypothyroidism, hyperadrenocorticism, hyposomatotropism, and adrenal sex hormone imbalance. Definitive diagnosis is made by history, physical examination findings, laboratory test results that rule out other conditions, and response to therapy. Skin biopsy is nondiagnostic, revealing orthokeratotic hyperkeratosis, epidermal atrophy, follicular keratosis, follicular atrophy, follicular dilatation, telogenization of hair follicles, thin dermis, and sebaceous gland atrophy.[16]

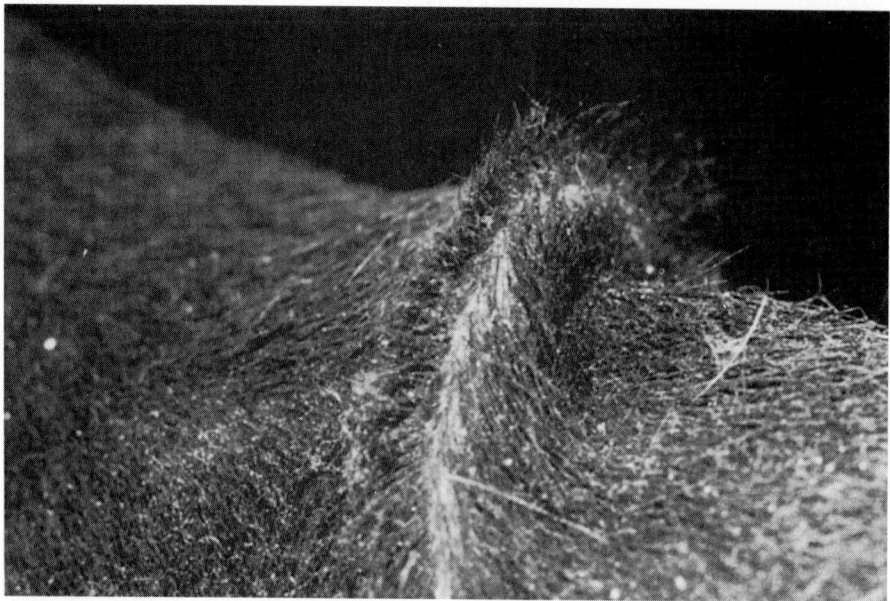

FIGURE 10–25. Testosterone-responsive dermatosis. Note thinning, hypotonicity, and scaling.

Clinical Management

Therapy consists of methyltestosterone given orally at 1 mg/kg, up to a maximal total dose of 30 mg, every other day.[11] Mibolerone (Cheque Drops, Upjohn) per the manufacturer's recommendations also is effective. A good response should be evident within 3 months. At this point, a maintenance dose may be established (once or twice weekly). Large doses of anabolic steroids may result in seborrhea oleosa, cholestatic liver disease, and behavioral changes (aggression). Because anabolic steroids are abused substances in humans, drug use should be monitored carefully.

TESTICULAR NEOPLASIA AND THE SKIN

Testicular neoplasia is common in the dog. Data suggest an approximately equal frequency of occurrence of interstitial cell tumors, seminomas, and Sertoli's cell tumors.[11, 405] A 10-year survey of all canine testicular tumors examined at the College of Veterinary Medicine at Cornell identified 1971 tumors with the following breakdown: interstitial cell tumor, 750 (38.1%); seminoma, 690 (35%); and Sertoli's cell tumor, 531 (26.9%).[11] Combinations of tumor types in the same or contralateral testicle occur in approximately 25% of cases.[405] Cryptorchid testes are more than 10 times more likely to develop tumor, especially Sertoli's cell tumor or seminoma. Canine testicular tumors, except for interstitial cell tumors, occur more frequently in the right testis in either the normal or cryptorchid location.[1, 2, 405]

Testicular tumors can reduce fertility[392] by direct destruction of the testis or by the abnormal secretion of hormones, can be malignant with metastatic potential, and can cause many cutaneous abnormalities, especially endocrine alopecia. Sertoli's cell tumors and seminomas are more likely to cause hair loss than are interstitial cell tumors. When the clinician examines an old male dog with a palpable scrotal testicular tumor or a marked testicular asymmetry suggesting an unidentified tumor, the basic quandary is whether the tumor is the cause of the hair loss or a coincidental finding with no dermatologic significance. When the dog has one or more of the following abnormalities, the tumor is likely to be functionally significant and the dog should be castrated: (1) puppy-like coat, (2) patterned alopecia, (3) coat color change, (4) linear preputial dermatosis, (5) macular melanosis, (6) uniform circumanal gland hyperplasia, (7) tail gland hyperplasia, and (8) numerous comedones.

Sex steroids appear to have preferential affinity for primary hair follicles. Disorders caused by sex steroids tend to cause the dog to lose its primary hairs first while retaining the secondary hairs, giving the puppy-like coat.

Because of the presumed sex and site variation in the numbers or affinity of sex hormone receptors in the skin of dogs, sex steroid imbalances induce hair loss in certain regions of the body and the alopecia tends to be confined to these areas for long periods.[11, 418] Coat color change can be explained by environmental bleaching or a direct effect of the sex hormones on pigment production and transfer. The latter is probably most important.

Linear preputial dermatosis is a term used to describe a linear narrow pigmentary change running from the preputial orifice along the ventral aspect of the prepuce to the scrotum (see Fig. 10–18H).[398] The exact mechanism of the development of the lesion is unknown (Fig. 10–26), but it is not associated with trauma and appears to be a specific cutaneous marker for testicular neoplasia, especially tumors that produce estrogens. If a dog has linear preputial dermatosis but its testes palpate normally or are intra-abdominal, a complete ultrasonographic evaluation of the patient is indicated to locate the neoplasm.[392]

Dogs with macular melanosis have multiple black macules around the anus, perineum, ventral proximal tail, inguinal area, and scrotum (see Fig. 10–24). Typically, these are sudden in onset and numerous. These lesions must be differentiated from lentigines. The latter have an identical clinical appearance but are distributed more widely and can occur in females. In addition, lentigines tend to have a gradual onset. The cause of macular

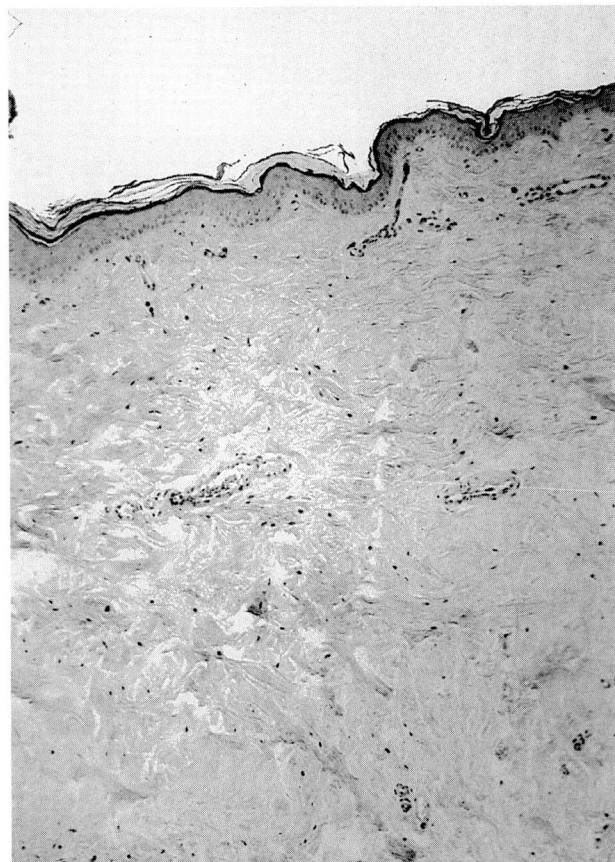

FIGURE 10–26. Linear prepucial erythema. Beyond some mild vascular dilatation and congestion, no histologic abnormalities are present.

melanosis is unknown. Circumanal and tail gland hyperplasia results from androgenic stimulation of the circumanal glands (see Figs. 10–22 and 10–23). This is most common with interstitial cell tumors.[419] Comedones are not specific for a sex hormone imbalance but are common in these disorders.

The change in coat quality and color, the patterned alopecia, and comedones are not specific to testicular tumor but also can occur in hypogonadism and adrenal sex hormone imbalance.[359, 374, 412] Testicular tumors can be functional but not yet palpable; thus, most investigators suggest castration of the intact male dog with sex hormone signs because it is diagnostic for neoplasia and therapeutic for both neoplasia and hypogonadism. If the patient is a poor surgical candidate or the owner refuses to neuter the dog, the condition may not be resolvable.

Sertoli's Cell Tumor

Sertoli's cell tumors were the least frequent in the Cornell review[11] but were the most common type of tumor to cause symmetric alopecia. Some dogs with these tumors have no hair loss.[392]

- **Cause and Pathogenesis.** A syndrome of endocrine alopecia and feminization occurs in about one third of dogs with a testicular Sertoli's cell tumor.[1, 2, 11] An identical clinical syndrome has been reported rarely in association with testicular interstitial cell tumors and seminomas. However, more than one type of tumor may be present in the testis simultaneously and bilateral testicular neoplasia is not uncommon. In addition, a hereditary syndrome of male pseudohermaphroditism, cryptorchidism, Sertoli's cell neoplasia, and feminization has been reported in Miniature schnauzers.[1, 2, 387]

Many investigators demonstrated increased levels of estrogens in the peripheral blood and the neoplastic tissue of dogs with Sertoli's cell testicular neoplasia and feminization. Hyperestrogenism results in the cutaneous, prostatic, behavioral, and hematologic abnormalities. Bilateral flank alopecia has been reported in a male dog with hyperprogesteronemia and a testicular Sertoli cell tumor.[393] Hair loss, feminization, and bone marrow suppression have been reported with hyperestrogenemia and a testicular interstitial cell tumor.[420]

- **Clinical Features.** Functional Sertoli's cell tumors are most common in cryptorchid testicles. The incidence of feminization increases from about 15% with scrotally located tumors to 50% in cases of inguinal and 70% in cases of abdominal location. Feminization is more likely with larger tumors and tends to be increasingly severe as tumor size increases. Although any breed of dog may be affected, Boxers, Shetland sheepdogs, Weimaraners, Cairn terriers, Pekingese, and Collies are predisposed.[1, 2, 11, 405, 422] The disease usually affects middle-aged to older dogs.

About 10% of dogs with Sertoli's cell tumors have one in both testicles, and about 20% have another tumor type. In the Cornell review,[11] approximately 20% of tumors had histologic features of malignancy, but metastasis occurred in only 8% of those cases. Blood estrogen levels are not always elevated. In addition, the hyperestrogenism could be a local (tissue level) effect with the peripheral aromatization of androgens to estrogens.

The functional Sertoli's cell tumor feminization syndrome is characterized by varying combinations of bilaterally symmetric alopecia, nipple enlargement, pendulous prepuce, and attraction of other male dogs (Fig. 10–27). It is important to emphasize that affected dogs may have alopecia, feminization, or both. The alopecia begins on the collar region, the rump, the perineum, and the genital area and progresses slowly (Fig. 10–28A). In some dogs, the hair loss is restricted to the flanks (see Fig. 10–28B). Generalized truncal hair loss is rare. Hairs in affected areas are easily epilated. The skin may be thin or of normal thickness. Pruritus, dermatitis, and hyperpigmentation are uncommon. Linear preputial dermatosis (see Fig. 10–18H) is a common but not consistent finding.

In addition to nipple enlargement and attraction of other male dogs, signs of feminization may include decreased libido and spermatogenesis. The tumor may be palpated in a retained or scrotal testicle. The non-neoplastic testicle is usually atrophied. Caution is warranted here because functional Sertoli's cell tumors may occur in palpably normal

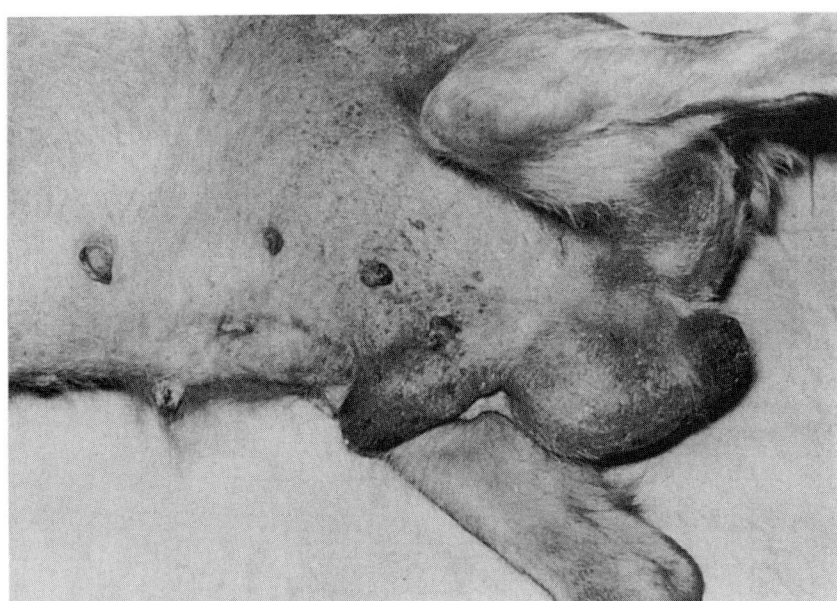

FIGURE 10–27. Intrascrotal testis with Sertoli's cell tumor constituting most of the scrotal mass. The small nodule at the posterior edge of the scrotum is the uninvolved but atrophied testis. Note the enlarged nipples.

scrotal testicles. The prostate is often enlarged (estrogen-induced squamous metaplasia) and infected, and there may be clinical signs referable to prostatomegaly, prostatitis, or both. Rarely, spermatic cord torsion with an intra-abdominal testicular Sertoli's cell tumor occurs, resulting in an acute abdomen.[406] Estrogen-induced bone marrow depression (thrombocytopenia, neutropenia, and anemia) is uncommon to rare, but is a life-threatening complication.[413] Pseudohermaphroditism in Miniature schnauzers consists of unilateral or bilateral cryptorchidism, small penis and prepuce, feminization, and endocrine alopecia.[1, 2, 387] These dogs may also have anorexia, depression, and pyrexia with concurrent pyometra.

- **Diagnosis.** A dog with a palpable testicular mass and one or more of the skin changes associated with a functional testicular tumor (e.g., patterned alopecia, linear preputial erythema) is no diagnostic challenge. When no tumor can be palpated, the diagnosis is more problematic and the differential diagnosis includes hypogonadism and adrenal sex hormone imbalance. Advanced cases can mimic cases of hypothyroidism or hyperadrenocorticism, but these are rare. Definitive diagnosis is based on history, physical examination findings, laboratory tests to rule out other disorders, and response to therapy. Ultrasonographic examination may delineate scrotal tumors that cannot be palpated.[392, 404] Skin biopsy is nondiagnostic, revealing orthokeratotic hyperkeratosis, follicular keratosis, follicular dilatation, follicular atrophy, telogenization of hair follicles, excessive trichilemmal keratinization, and sebaceous gland atrophy (Fig. 10–29).[16] Elevated blood estrogen levels may support the diagnosis. Diagnosis is confirmed by histopathologic examination of the neoplastic testicles.

- **Clinical Management.** Therapy consists of bilateral castration. Although the metastatic rate of these tumors is low, all dogs should be examined carefully before surgery. If the spermatic cord is thickened or the sublumbar lymph nodes are enlarged, spread may have already occurred. A good clinical response usually occurs within 3 months. Remission followed by relapse indicates functional metastases.[407] Concurrent prostatic or bone marrow disease must also be treated. Aplastic anemia or thrombocytopenia resulting from hyperestrogenism warrants a guarded prognosis because these often persist after surgery.[367]

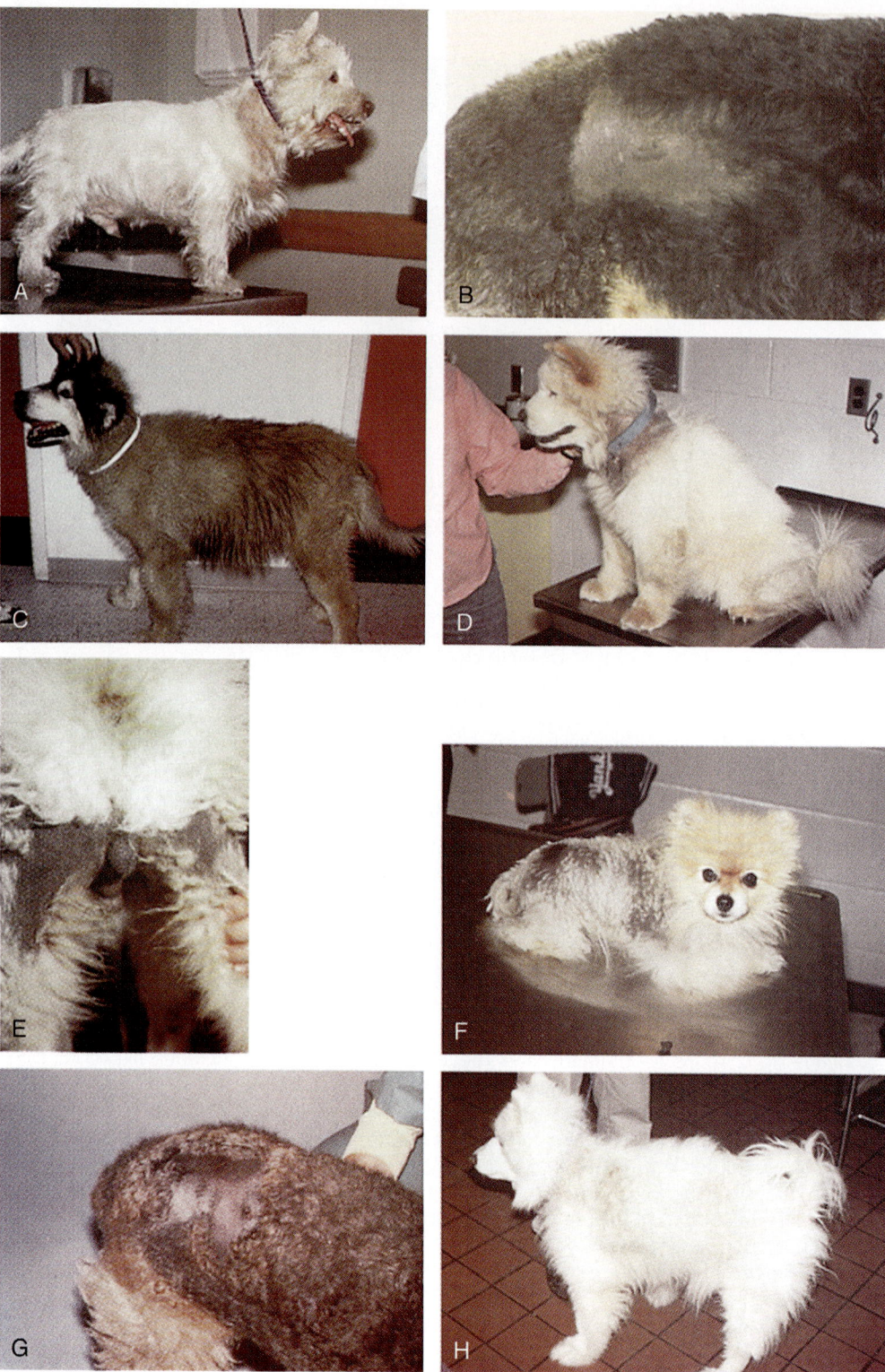

FIGURE 10-28. *A*, Sertoli's cell tumor. Hair loss in the collar area and along the ventrum. Pendulous prepuce. *B*, Flank alopecia in an Airedale terrier with a Sertoli's cell tumor. *C*, Male hypogonadism in a wooly malamute. *D*, Male hypogonadism. Coat color change, loss of primary hairs, and collar region alopecia. *E*, Male hypogonadism. Pronounced hair loss and hyperpigmentation on the posterior thighs. *F*, Male hypogonadism. Incomplete hair loss after 3 years of disease. *G*, Male hypogonadism. Hair loss over the rump. *H*, Adrenal sex hormone imbalance. Loss of primary hairs and mild hypotrichosis.

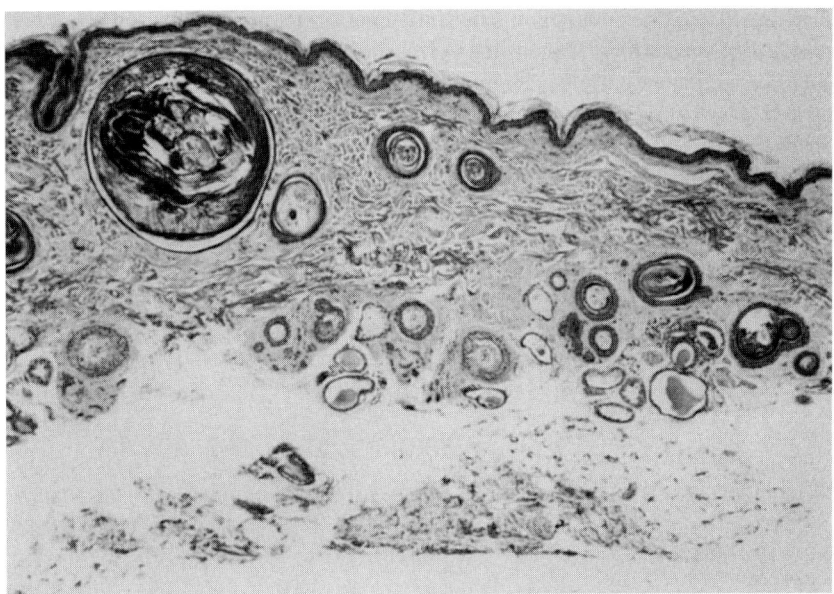

FIGURE 10-29. Skin from dog with functional Sertoli's cell testicular neoplasm syndrome. Note follicular keratosis and dilatation, absence of hair shafts, and sebaceous gland atrophy.

Therapy of pseudohermaphroditism in Miniature schnauzers may entail simultaneous castration and hysterectomy.

Seminomas

Seminomas are as common as interstitial cell tumors in dogs. They are more common in cryptorchid testes.[405] Boxers and German shepherds are predisposed. Reports indicate a low rate of malignancy but a tendency to be locally invasive.[405] In the Cornell study, 12.2% of the seminomas had histologic features of malignancy, and evidence of metastasis was recognized in 11% of those cases.[11]

Secretory activity in seminomas is rare. Most cases have no dermatologic signs. If there is secretion of estrogens, the clinical signs mimic those of Sertoli's cell tumors.

Interstitial Cell Tumors

Interstitial cell tumors are common.[405] Boxers are predisposed. Interstitial cell tumors have no tendency to develop in cryptorchid testes, and these tumors occur with equal frequency in the right or the left testicle. They are often multiple in the same testicle or can be found in both testes. Texts report rare evidence of malignancy, but 12.9% of the tumors in the Cornell study had histologic features of malignancy.[11] No metastatic lesions were reported.

In most cases, interstitial cell tumors cause no dermatologic abnormalities. When present, the signs include circumanal gland hyperplasia, tail gland hyperplasia, macular melanosis, or combinations of these (see Fig. 10-24). Additional findings can include prostate disease, circumanal adenoma, and perineal hernia. The association of perineal hernia with altered sex hormone levels has largely been disproved.[410] If estrogens or progesterone are produced in the testicle or by peripheral conversion, cutaneous signs of hyperestrogenemia or hyperprogesteronemia (hypoandrogenemia) may occur.[420]

HYPOGONADISM IN INTACT MALE ANIMALS

Of all the sex hormone–related dermatoses, hypogonadism (castration-responsive dermatosis, "woolly" syndrome, alopecia X) in the male dog is the most poorly understood.[373, 411, 412] Dogs with this condition can either have symmetrically small and atrophic testes or palpably normal testes.

Cause and Pathogenesis

Primary, noninflammatory testicular degeneration is rare in the adult dog.[1, 2] Dogs with symmetric atrophy have some systemic illness, especially hypothyroidism or hyperadrenocorticism, or nonpalpable bilateral secretory testicular tumors.

A syndrome of delayed gonadal maturation has been described, especially in Afghan hounds, Yorkshire terriers, and Miniature poodles.[403] The dogs never exhibit leg-lifting behavior, show no interest in a bitch in estrus, and experience hair loss early in life (younger than 3 years). The external genitalia are hypoplastic.

Most dogs with hypogonadal hair loss have palpably normal testes and can be successful stud dogs. Testicular pathologic changes are rare after castration. Measurement of serum estradiol, progesterone, and testosterone levels may show abnormalities in the levels of one or more hormones,[403, 411, 412] but normal values are possible.[373, 400] The hair loss in the dogs with normal levels may be due to abnormalities in the levels of some unmeasured sex steroid, abnormalities in peripheral conversion of the sex steroids, or some specific follicular receptor defect in which the follicle changes its sensitivity to sex hormones. In the breeds predisposed to this condition, the follicular sensitivity no doubt has some genetic influence. Because some of these dogs respond to melatonin supplementation, their pineal axis may also be at fault.

Clinical Features

There is no apparent breed predilection in dogs with atrophic hypogonadism. These dogs have truncal alopecia that mimics the type occurring in testosterone-responsive dermatosis, hypothyroidism, or hyperadrenocorticism.

Dogs with delayed gonadal maturation experience symmetric hair loss first in the perineal and inguinal regions.[403] The hair loss spreads slowly to involve the ventrum and then the trunk.

Hypogonadism with normal testes can occur in any breed, but Malamutes, Siberian huskies, Chow Chows, Samoyeds, Pomeranians, and Keeshonds appear to be over-represented. The age of onset is a very important piece of information, but many owners place it many months later then it actually was. Dogs seem to fall into two categories. In the first and possibly most common, onset of coat change is between 2 and 4 years of age. The coat changes in the second group start in late middle age or early old age. The initial clinical sign is usually change in coat quality and color. The primary hairs on the trunk are lost slowly while the secondary hairs are retained, giving the dog an overall puppy-like appearance (see Fig. 10–28C). The retained secondary hairs lose their luster, become crimped and fluffy, and take on a woolly appearance. Dark hairs lighten down to their roots, indicating a change in pigment deposition rather than environmental bleaching (see Fig. 10–28D).

Because these coat changes occur slowly over many months, some owners do not recognize them as abnormalities. They present the dog for hair loss and, when asked when the problem began, base their answer on hair loss only. Inspection of pictures taken of the dog months earlier might give a more accurate age at onset. Hair loss is noted on the collar area, the rump, the perineum, and the caudomedial thighs (see Fig. 10–28E). Progression of hair loss in these areas and elsewhere is slow. Rarely, dogs that have this condition for years experience complete truncal alopecia (see Fig. 10–28F). In some dogs, hair loss is restricted to the flank region (see Fig. 10–28G). Hyperpigmentation of the skin is variable and, when present, is diffuse. The testes are normal on palpation, and no other physical abnormalities are found.

Diagnosis

With atrophic hypogonadism, hypothyroidism and hyperadrenocorticism must be considered and ruled out by appropriate testing. If the dog has palpably normal testes, testicular neoplasia, adult-onset hyposomatotropism, adrenal sex hormone imbalances, and follicular dysplasia are the primary differential diagnostic possibilities. Skin biopsy is diagnostic for follicular dysplasia but of no help in the differential diagnosis of other conditions. Castration with histopathologic evaluation of the testes is both diagnostic and therapeutic for hypogonadism and testicular neoplasia. If no response occurs within 4 months of castration, the other differential diagnostic conditions should be investigated.

If the owner is unwilling to use castration as a diagnostic test, thyroid testing and measurement of serum estradiol, progesterone, and testosterone levels should be performed. These dogs are typically euthyroid, but some dogs have low or high resting TT_4 levels. Sex hormones, especially androgens, can interfere with the true measurement of TT_4 levels by changing the amount or affinity of binding proteins. With hyperandrogenemia or hypoestrogenemia, the baseline TT_4 level can be at or above normal limits. These changes do not occur in all dogs with hypogonadism and can be caused by other nongonadal disorders that alter thyroid hormone binding.

Although the hair loss in these dogs is due to a sex hormone abnormality, baseline serum levels of estrogen, testosterone, or progesterone may be normal. In some cases, hyperestrogenemia, or hyperprogesteronemia can be documented.[373, 411] In our experience, the likelihood of detecting a baseline sex hormone abnormality is influenced by the dog's breeding, the age at onset of coat changes, and the duration of disease. Because sex hormones levels vary during the day and the range of normal values is wide, it is difficult to document a baseline abnormality when the dog has only been affected for a short period of time. However, chronicity does not guarantee a detectable abnormality, especially when the dog is a Chow Chow, Samoyed, Pomeranian, or Keeshond and its coat change started within the first 4 years of life. These dogs are likely to have an intercurrent adrenal sex hormone abnormality (see Adrenal Hyperplasia–Like Syndrome). Too few cases have been recognized in the Malamute and Siberian husky to know whether to include them with the other breeds. Dogs of other breeds, especially when their coat change started in later life, are likely to have only a gonadal problem that can be documented by baseline sex hormone measurements. If baseline sex hormone levels are normal, results of GnRH stimulation tests[400] or ACTH stimulation testing can be useful.

Clinical Management

Correction of the underlying cause of the atrophic hypogonadism usually resolves the hair loss. If response is incomplete, testosterone supplementation may be necessary. Castration is curative for most dogs with normal testes, with hair regrowth in 2 to 4 months. If castration is not allowed, supplementation with testosterone[359] or treatment with human chorionic gonadotropin (50 IU/kg IM twice weekly for 6 weeks)[403] may be of some benefit. No reports are available on the long-term successful medical management of these cases.

As mentioned earlier, castration is curative for most dogs with palpably normal testes. Failures typically occur in the Chow Chow, Samoyed, Pomeranian, and Keeshond breeds. Some dogs respond completely to castration only to experience relapse within a few years.[373] Again, the four breeds mentioned seem to be over-represented. All dogs who do not respond to castration or experience relapse within a few years should be evaluated for adrenal hyperplasia–like syndrome. There are anecdotal reports that dogs with this condition respond to melatonin supplementation.[416] Because hair follicles have no melatonin receptors, but do have receptors for IGF-1 and sex hormones,[11, 350] the response probably is due to local or serum changes of the sex hormones. The latter has been demonstrated (see Chap. 3).[385] Because dogs with seasonal flank alopecia[412] (see Chap. 11) have normal serum sex hormone levels[389] but can respond to melatonin,[385, 416] a local alteration at the hair follicle level is probable. Oral treatment with 3 to 6 mg q8–12h should initiate hair growth within 6 weeks. If no response occurs, testosterone supplementation might be beneficial.

ADRENAL SEX HORMONE DISORDERS

These dogs have symmetric truncal alopecia, which mimics that seen in hyposomatotropism or the gonadal sex hormone dermatoses, but these patients do not respond to GH supplementation or neutering.[359, 373, 374]

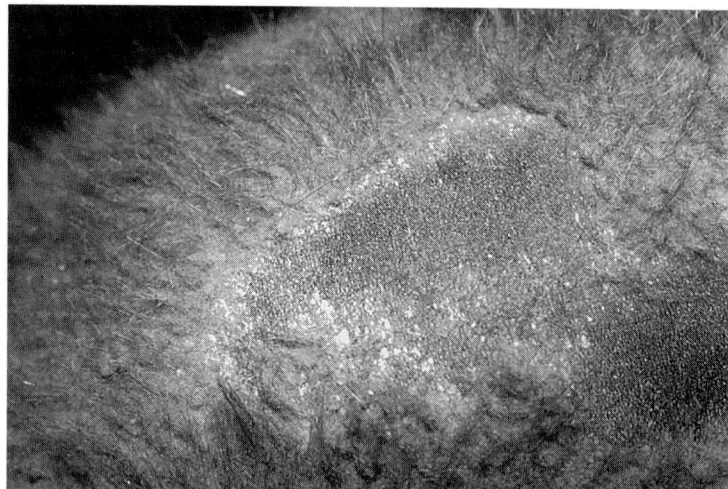

FIGURE 10-32. Adrenal hyperplasia-like syndrome. A puppy-like hair coat with hair loss in an adult dog. The hairless areas hyperpigmented very quickly.

loss in the frictional areas progresses, more primary hairs are lost on the trunk, giving the remaining coat a puppy-like appearance (Fig. 10–32). The retained secondary hairs are lost slowly, and all exposed skin tends to become hyperpigmented quickly. Complete truncal alopecia is rare and occurs only after years of disease. These dogs tend to regrow tufts of hair at sites damaged by skin biopsy or cutting trauma.

At the onset of the coat changes, these dogs are otherwise healthy. With long-standing disease, most dogs experience noticeable polyuria and polydipsia, but it is nowhere near as marked as that occurring in hyperadrenocorticism or diabetes mellitus. Some dogs, especially the Samoyeds (a breed with a tendency toward hyperprogesteronemia) in our case material, experience profound polyuria and polydipsia associated with insulin-resistant diabetes mellitus.

Diagnosis

The primary differential diagnostic possibilities if there is a persistent patterned alopecia with retention of the secondary hairs on the trunk include hyposomatotropism, gonadal sex hormone imbalance, adrenal sex hormone imbalance, and follicular dysplasia. The last disorder is excluded by skin biopsy.[4, 16]

Skin biopsies from these dogs show the classic changes of endocrinopathy (orthokeratotic surface and follicular hyperkeratosis, follicular dilatation, excessive trichilemmal keratinization, epidermal melanosis, and telogenization of hair follicles) and can also show some features of follicular dysplasia (dysplastic follicles with a tentacular or octopus-like appearance and abnormalities in melanization of the hairs, follicular epithelium, and sebaceous glands) (Fig. 10–33). The dysplastic-type changes can occur in any endocrine skin disease but tend to be more florid in adrenal hyperplasia–like syndrome.

Results of routine laboratory tests are typically normal, as are those of thyroid tests and the results of low-dose dexamethasone suppression testing. Dogs with diabetes mellitus undergo the biochemical changes of that disorder, and dogs in which estrogen levels are irregular might show the hematologic changes of estrogen toxicity. In chronic cases, the baseline and post-ACTH levels of cortisol can be elevated with changes mimicking a chronic stress pattern. This hypercortisolemia causes the low-level polyuria and polydipsia these dogs experience and can result in small elevations in serum alkaline phosphatase. The diagnosis is confirmed by the detection of abnormal concentrations of sex hormones, especially progesterone and estradiol, as determined by baseline testing[373] or in response to ACTH administration.[374] Baseline testing is least desirable because abnormalities do not show in all dogs and the testing cannot differentiate the gonadal or adrenal origin if the dog is intact.

Currently, the only laboratory with well-established normal values for sex steroids

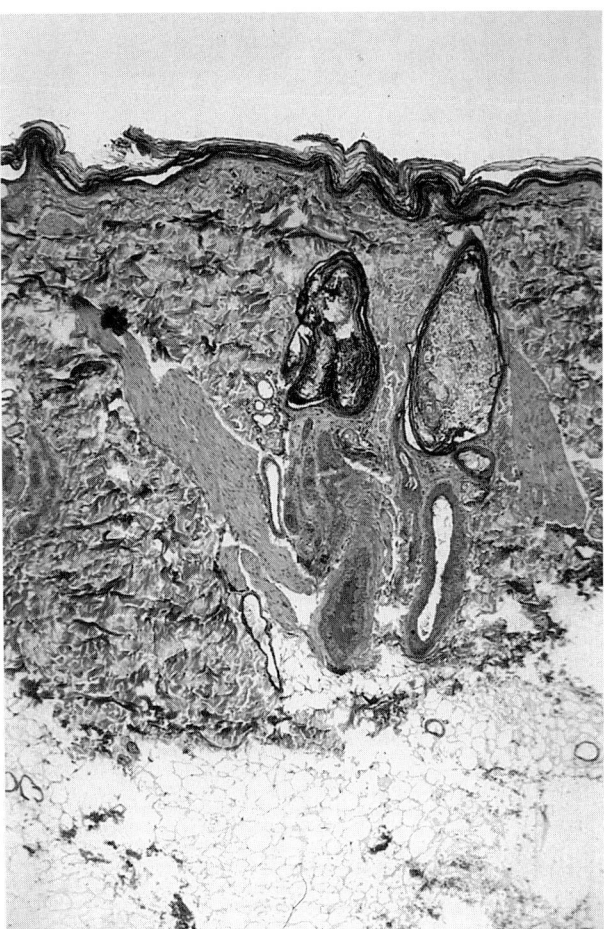

FIGURE 10–33. Adrenal hyperplasia-like syndrome. An admixture of endocrine (surface and follicular hyperkeratosis, follicular dilatation, and telogenization of hair follicles) and dysplastic (dysplastic follicles) changes. Abnormalities in melanization are also present.

before and after ACTH administration (Table 10–1) is the Endocrinology Laboratory at the University of Tennessee, College of Veterinary Medicine, Knoxville, TN 37901-1071. We have submitted pre- and post-ACTH samples to our regular endocrinology laboratories for sex hormone evaluation. Because these laboratories do not use the same assay techniques as the Tennessee laboratory, evaluate the same hormones, or have post-ACTH values that are as well established, the results developed therein are not directly comparable with those from Tennessee. However, the pattern of change in the Tennessee data (e.g., elevated progesterone baseline value that more than triples after ACTH administration) can be duplicated.

Clinical Management

In intact dogs, especially male dogs, neutering is the initial treatment of choice because many dogs experience hair regrowth for some period of time after surgery. If the hair loss initially occurred after neutering, recurred after regrowth following surgery, or did not improve after surgery, treatment options include methyltestosterone, GH, melatonin, o,p'-DDD, or observation. Bilateral adrenalectomy should be effective, but is unproven. Because GH is not readily available, the options are reduced. Treatments with melatonin or methyltestosterone may be beneficial in regrowing hair[359, 416] but do not alter the abnormal adrenal steroid production. These animals, like those who remain untreated, should be monitored for signs of bone marrow suppression or diabetes mellitus. Current recommendations for o,p'-DDD use indicate that the drug be given at daily doses of 15 to 25 mg/kg.[374] Response is determined by ACTH response testing for plasma cortisol at weekly intervals.

Table 10-1. MEAN (±SD) SEX HORMONE LEVELS* IN NORMAL DOGS BEFORE AND AFTER ACTH STIMULATION

MALES	INTACT (n = 10)		NEUTERED (n = 9)	
	Baseline	Post-ACTH	Baseline	Post-ACTH
Progesterone	0.4 (±0.5)	1.1 (±1.2)	0.1 (±0.0)	0.4 (±0.4)
17-hydroxyprogesterone	0.3 (±0.4)	1.4 (±0.9)	0.1 (±0.0)	0.6 (±0.3)
DHEAS	18.5 (±11.5)	20.8 (±11.0)	2.1 (±3.3)	2.9 (±4.3)
Androstenedione	13.3 (±10.1)	12.2 (±6.7)	4.8 (±1.5)	5.4 (±2.0)
Testosterone	3.1 (±4.2)	2.6 (±4.1)	0.0 (±0.0)	0.0 (±0.0)
Estradiol 17 β	18.7 (±14.6)	15.6 (±8.6)	43.1 (±10.0)	41.3 (±13.5)

FEMALES	INTACT (n = 5)		NEUTERED (n = 8)	
	Baseline	Post-ACTH	Baseline	Post-ACTH
Progesterone	0.3 (±0.1)	0.8 (±0.3)	0.1 (±0.1)	0.7 (±0.7)
17-hydroxyprogesterone	0.2 (±0.1)	1.5 (±0.4)	0.1 (±0.1)	0.9 (±0.3)
DHEAS	5.7 (±1.7)	7.8 (±1.68)	3.8 (±4.5)	5.0 (±4.7)
Androstenedione	6.5 (±8.0)	2.0 (±0.9)	6.5 (±3.7)	4.9 (±0.4)
Testosterone	0.1 (±0.0)	0.1 (±0.0)	0.0 (±0.0)	0.0 (±0.0)
Estradiol 17 β	24.8 (±9.4)	22.0 (±8.1)	40.3 (±8.2)	40.6 (±8.1)

*All levels are in ng/ml except estradiol 17 β levels, which are in pg/ml.

Modified with permission from Schmeitzel LP, et al: Congenital adrenal hyperplasia-like syndrome. In: Bonagura JD (ed): Kirk's Current Veterinary Therapy XII. W.B. Saunders, Philadelphia, 1995, p 600.

The goal of therapy is to reduce the baseline cortisol concentration to a low-normal range with some response to ACTH. One investigator suggested poststimulation values of 3 to 5 µg/dl,[374] whereas another investigator recommended 5 to 7 µg/dl.[368, 373] After the desired adrenal suppression has been achieved, drug administration is changed to weekly and then adjusted as needed to maintain the suppression. This treatment resulted in complete hair regrowth in 10 of 12 cases.[369]

Because these dogs are healthy and the o,p'-DDD treatment is expensive and not without risk, some owners elect not to treat their dog. If the dog's progesterone or estrogen metabolism is irregular, periodic laboratory evaluations for progesterone-induced diabetes mellitus or estrogen-induced bone marrow suppression is indicated. At the first sign of an abnormality, treatment must be instituted to prevent serious metabolic consequences. The untreated dog's hair loss progresses very slowly and eventually involves the majority of the trunk (Fig. 10–34). These dogs are at increased risk for frostbite, sunburn,

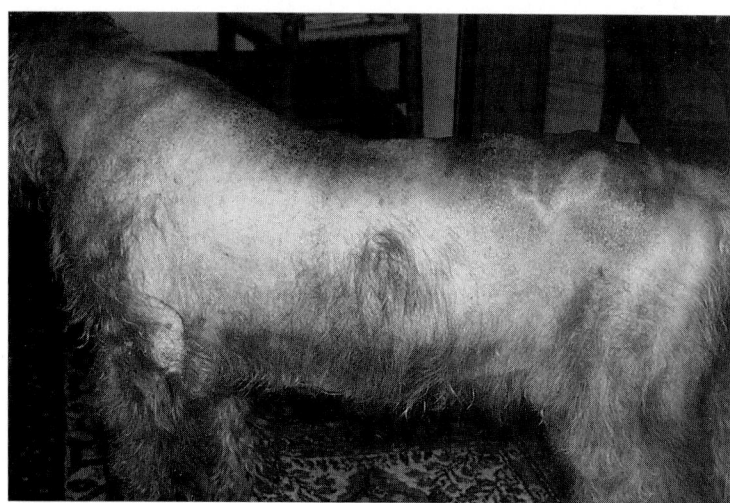

FIGURE 10–34. Adrenal hyperplasia-like syndrome. A 13-year-old Bouvier de Flanders with untreated disease for over 7 years. Note the islands of hair on the almost hairless trunk.

or other environmental insults, and their management must be adjusted accordingly. As mentioned earlier, they will experience polyuria and polydipsia that worsens slowly. At some point, the polyuria and polydipsia can become so severe that the dog loses its house training. Because the hair follicles in these dogs are still viable despite years of inactivity, late treatment results in coat regrowth and the elimination of the cortisol-induced polyuria and polydipsia.

RARE SEX HORMONE DERMATOSES

Early editions of this and other dermatology texts associated feline endocrine alopecia and idiopathic male feminizing syndrome with sex hormones.[11] The feline condition is discussed in Chapter 11 because it has no endocrine basis in the vast majority of cases. Occasionally, cats respond to estrogen or testosterone supplementation, but because of the hepatic sensitivity of cats to sex hormones and the rarity of the condition, all other causes of hair loss should be investigated first.

Dogs with idiopathic male feminizing syndrome experience hair loss of the rump, the perineum, and the ventral abdomen, which can progress to involve the entire ventrum, the neck, and the face.[11] The exposed skin is hyperpigmented and seborrheic. Moderate to severe pruritus, ceruminous otitis, and nipple enlargement are consistent findings. The testes and sex hormone levels in these dogs are normal. Skin biopsy reveals no evidence of endocrinopathy; instead, it reveals changes most consistent with hypersensitivity.[16]

Careful review of cases of presumed idiopathic male feminizing syndrome shows that pruritus precedes the skin lesions. In early cases, only the inguinal nipples are involved, which refutes an endocrine cause. Trauma during itching is the likely cause of the nipple hypertrophy. Most dogs with idiopathic male feminizing syndrome have hypersensitivity, with food hypersensitivity and hormonal hypersensitivity most likely. Resolution of signs with castration supports the latter diagnosis.

If the hair loss, hyperpigmentation, and seborrhea precede any pruritus and the nipple enlargement is uniform throughout all glands, endocrine disease must be considered. Hypothyroidism and estrogen-producing testicular neoplasia are the primary differential diagnostic considerations.

Canine Hypothyroidism

Hypothyroidism is the most common endocrine disorder of the dog and is characterized by a plethora of cutaneous and noncutaneous clinical signs associated with a deficiency of thyroid hormone activity.* It is also the most commonly overdiagnosed endocrine disease.

CAUSE AND PATHOGENESIS

Canine hypothyroidism may be naturally occurring or iatrogenic.[1, 2, 101] Naturally occurring, acquired primary hypothyroidism accounts for more than 90% of all cases of canine hypothyroidism. The two main causes of acquired primary hypothyroidism are lymphocytic thyroiditis and idiopathic thyroid necrosis and atrophy.

Lymphocytic (Hashimoto's) thyroiditis is a common cause of hypothyroidism in dogs.† Lymphocytic thyroiditis has long been recognized as a familial disorder of colony-raised Beagles with polygenic inheritance.[56] In one closed colony, approximately 10% of dogs were affected.[159] Dogs with thyroiditis are at increased risk for thyroid tumors, but it is unclear whether the neoplasia is triggered by the thyroiditis or some other genetic influence.[26] Lymphocytic thyroiditis is thought to be an autoimmune disorder in which humoral and cell-mediated autoimmunity are involved in the pathogenesis.

Antibodies to thyroglobulin, T_3, T_4, or combinations thereof can be detected.[130] Anti-

---

*See references 1, 2, 14, 20, 48, 68, 101, 111, 137.
†See references 22, 34, 52, 55, 62–64, 79.

thyroglobulin antibodies are demonstrable in the sera of more than 50% of dogs with naturally occurring hypothyroidism, and Great Danes, Irish setters, Borzois, Old English sheepdogs, and Doberman pinschers appear to be predisposed.[22, 36, 55] However, antithyroglobulin antibodies can be found in normal dogs or those with nonthyroidal endocrine diseases.[40, 71, 98] Antibodies have been detected in approximately 50% of clinically normal dogs related to dogs with hypothyroidism and in approximately 15% of randomly studied normal dogs. The prevalence of antithyroglobulin antibodies also was increased in dogs with various dermatoses.[22] Anti-T_3 antibodies and, rarely, anti-T_4 antibodies can also be detected in the serum of dogs with thyroiditis.[34, 52, 79, 130] Invariably, dogs with anti-T_3 antibodies have antithyroglobulin antibodies, but the reverse is not true.[52] These autoantibodies interfere with thyroid assays and lead to spurious results that suggest hyperthyroidism.[61] Twenty percent of the dogs with naturally occurring hypothyroidism also have circulating immune complexes.

Lymphocytic thyroiditis has been produced in normal dogs by injections of thyroglobulin or thyroid antigens with adjuvants, intrathyroid injections of antithyroglobulin antibodies, and intrathyroid injections of allogenic lymphocytes.[55, 64] Thyroid lesions in dogs with naturally occurring lymphocytic thyroiditis are characterized by multifocal to diffuse interstitial infiltration of lymphocytes, plasma cells, and macrophages associated with destruction of thyroid follicles, as well as by the presence of electron-dense deposits in the follicular basement membrane that resemble antigen-antibody complexes. The frequency and severity of laboratory abnormalities vary with the extent of involvement. Dogs with mild pathologic changes in the thyroid glands often have normal thyroid profiles.[56] Because lymphocytic thyroiditis is a focal disease and because inflammation is minimal in the late stages, it has been suggested that so-called idiopathic thyroid necrosis and atrophy may be an end stage of lymphocytic thyroiditis.

Naturally occurring secondary hypothyroidism accounts for less than 10% of all canine hypothyroidism and has been reported in association with pituitary dwarfism and pituitary neoplasia.[1, 2, 11] Other causes of canine hypothyroidism are rare.

CLINICAL FEATURES

Goitrous and nongoitrous congenital hypothyroidism has been reported in the Boxer, Bull mastiff, German shepherd, Scottish deerhound, and Giant schnauzer breeds.[33, 35, 60, 87, 92, 135] Mongrels can also be affected.[35]

Acquired hypothyroidism may affect any breed of dog. At Cornell University, breeds at risk for hypothyroidism, in decreasing order of relative risk, are the Chinese Shar pei, Chow Chow, Great Dane, Irish wolfhound, Boxer, English bulldog, Dachshund, Afghan hound, Newfoundland, Malamute, Doberman pinscher, Brittany spaniel, Poodle, Golden retriever, and Miniature schnauzer.[11] Other studies include the Airedale terrier, Cocker spaniel, Irish setter, Shetland sheepdog, Old English sheepdog, and Pomeranian.[48, 101] Antithyroglobulin antibodies are found more often in Great Danes, Borzois, Irish setters, Old English sheepdogs, and Doberman pinschers.[22, 48] German shepherd dogs and mongrels are thought to be at lower risk.[11] Familial hypothyroidism has been suspected in Great Danes, Doberman pinschers, and German shorthaired pointers.

There is no sex predilection for canine hypothyroidism, but neutered male and female dogs may be at higher risk than intact dogs.[48, 106] Although a dog of any age may be affected, the risk is greater for dogs between the ages of 6 and 10 years. The onset of hypothyroidism tends to be earlier (2 to 3 years old) in large and giant breeds and those breeds predisposed to the disorder.

The clinical signs associated with hypothyroidism are many and varied and involve multiple organ systems.* At presentation, the dog can have systemic illness with normal skin, dermatologic disease plus systemic signs of illness, or dermatologic disease only. In the latter case, the systemic signs may be unrecognized, may be attributed to the dog's

---

*See references 14, 20, 48, 68, 99, 101, 111, 113, 137.

aging, or may not exist. If there are no systemic signs, the cutaneous lesions may be due to hair follicle receptor insensitivity or local deiodination problems.[138] With this variability, hypothyroidism has rightfully been labeled "the great impersonator."

Although lethargy, mental depression, obesity, hypothermia, and thermophilia are classic manifestations of hypothyroidism,[45a] many hypothyroid dogs appear active and alert, are well fleshed or thin, and do not exhibit heat-seeking behavior.[106] In general, if a dog is obviously obese, it is probably not hypothyroid. The rectal temperature of most hypothyroid dogs is in the normal range.

The classic cutaneous signs of canine hypothyroidism include (1) bilaterally symmetric truncal alopecia, which tends to spare the extremities (Fig. 10-35B); (2) a dull, dry, brittle, easily epilated haircoat that fails to regrow after clipping (see Fig. 10-35C); (3) thick, puffy, nonpitting skin (myxedema) that is cool to the touch (see Figs. 10-35D and 10-36); (4) variable hyperpigmentation (see Fig. 10-35B); (5) seborrhea (see Fig. 10-35C); (6) susceptibility to skin infections (Fig. 10-37); and (7) lack of pruritus. However, the clinical variations from this classic picture are enormous and frequent.

Because receptors for thyroid hormones are found on sebocytes and cells of the outer root sheath and dermal papilla,[18] coat abnormalities can be expected in most, if not all, hypothyroid dogs. Growing hairs are decreased in diameter, and telogen hairs are maintained because initiation of anagen is prevented.[38] Although some laboratory dogs don't lose hair, hair loss is common in household dogs. Initially, the coat loses its normal sheen and luster and becomes dull, dry, and brittle. Shedding becomes more pronounced during nonshed periods, and the lost hairs either regrow more slowly than normally or are not replaced.

Noticeable hypotrichosis or alopecia occurs first in frictional areas, especially over pressure points, the ventrum, the perineum, and the tail (see Fig. 10-35E). Large and giant breeds often lose hair first on the lateral surface of the extremities (see Fig. 10-35F). With time, the hair loss becomes more widespread (see Fig. 10-35G) and involves the entire trunk in a symmetric distribution (see Fig. 10-35B). In advanced cases, all hairs except those on the head and distal extremities are lost. Most cases are presented earlier in the course of the disease and may have hypotrichosis or alopecia, which may be focal, multifocal, symmetric, or asymmetric (Figs. 10-38 to 10-40; see Fig. 10-35H). In some dogs, hair loss is restricted to the flank region (Fig. 10-41). An unusual finding is hypertrichosis in which, because of the retarded turnover of the hairs, the coat becomes thick and resembles a carpet (Fig. 10-42). Hypertrichosis occurs most commonly in Boxers and Irish setters. The coat can become lighter in color, especially at the tips of the hairs, because the retained hairs are more susceptible to environmental bleaching. This coat color change can occur in nonhypertrichotic hypothyroid dogs but is more common in dogs with sex hormone imbalances.

Because thyroid hormones influence serum and cutaneous fatty acid concentrations[32, 136, 145] and influence sebaceous gland function,[18] seborrheic changes are common in hypothyroid dogs. The altered lipid profile can result in dryness, greasiness, or seborrheic dermatitis. These changes usually occur in the ears (ceruminous otitis) (Fig. 10-43A), on the body (see Fig. 10-35C), or in both locations. On the body, the seborrheic changes can be focal, multifocal, or generalized. The seborrheic changes predispose the animal to secondary staphylococcal or *Malassezia* infections, which intensify the seborrheic signs.

Bacterial pyoderma occurs frequently in hypothyroid dogs.[11, 20] The bacterial pyoderma may be localized (e.g., pododermatitis or otitis externa), multifocal, or generalized and may be superficial (folliculitis) (see Fig. 10-37) or deep (furunculosis) (see Fig. 10-43B and C). The pathogenic mechanism of this increased susceptibility to bacterial pyoderma probably relates to an altered cutaneous barrier, immunologic hyporeactivity, or a combination of both. In various laboratory animals, it has been reported that depletion of thyroid hormone results in impaired B-lymphocyte and T-lymphocyte functions.[11] Because hypothyroid dogs do not appear to be at risk for noncutaneous infections, the skin infections in most dogs are probably due to a skin defect or alteration in local cutaneous immunity.[113] Rarely, a dog with bacterial pyoderma due to hypothyroidism has depressed neutrophil or T-lymphocyte function as assessed by bactericidal assay or in vitro lympho-

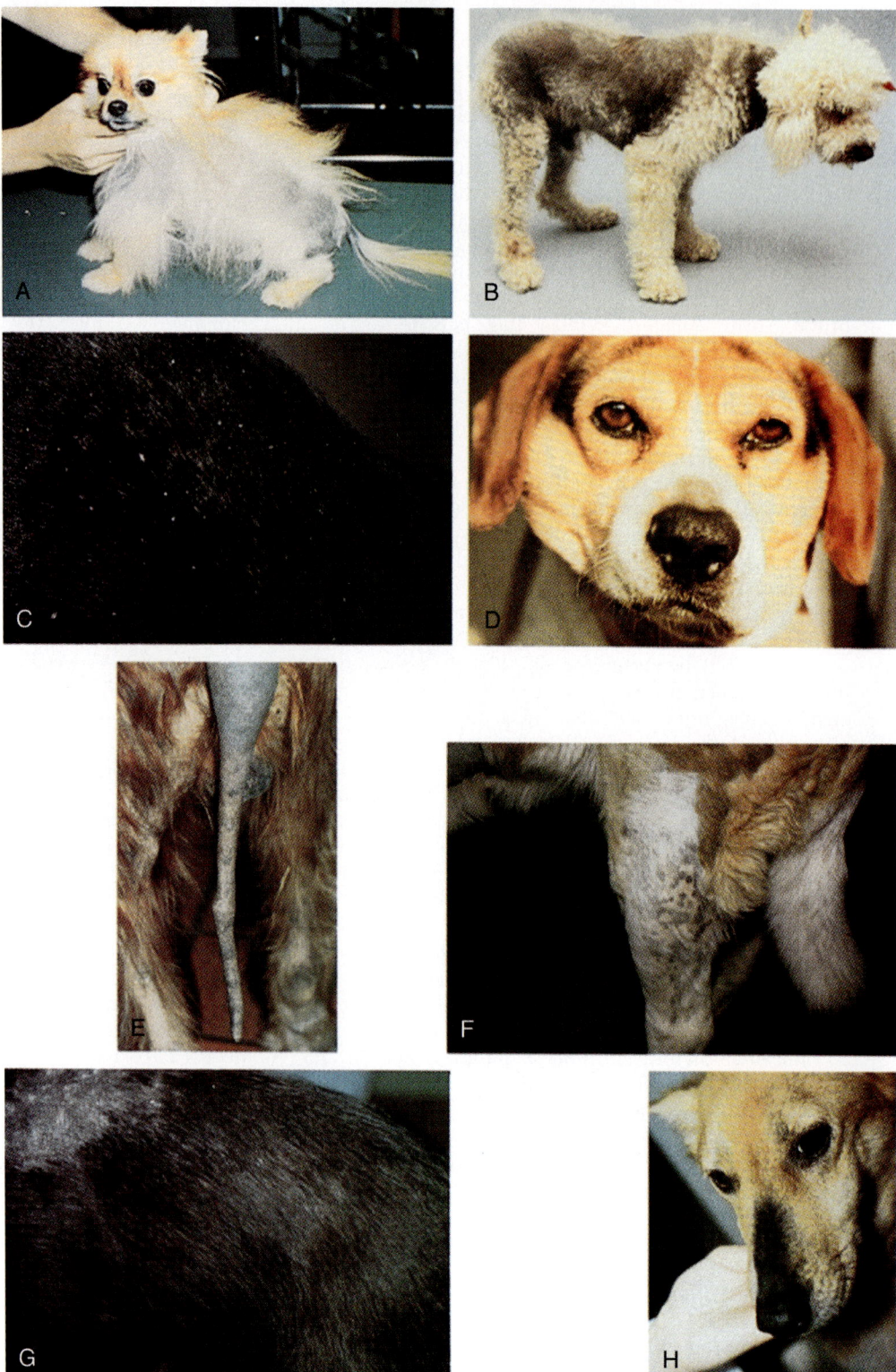

FIGURE 10-35. *A*, Adrenal sex hormone imbalance. Note similarities to Figures 10-9*E* and 10-28*F*. *B*, Hypothyroidism. Note symmetric truncal alopecia and hyperpigmentation. *C*, Hypothyroidism. Dull, dry, seborrheic coat. *D*, Hypothyroidism. Facial myxedema leading to a "tragic" expression. *E*, Hypothyroidism. "Rat tail." *F*, Hypothyroidism. Frictional hair loss of the distal limbs of a St. Bernard. *G*, Hypothyroidism. Truncal hypotrichosis and alopecia with secondary superficial folliculitis. *H*, Hypothyroidism. Nasal alopecia and hyperpigmentation. The area is cool to the touch.

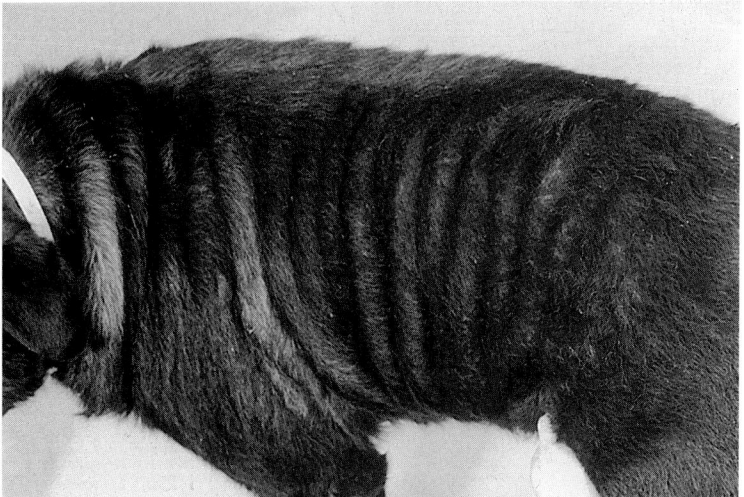

FIGURE 10–36. Hypothyroidism. Generalized myxedema in a mongrel dog.

cyte blastogenesis to phytomitogens, respectively.[11] The immunologic abnormalities return to normal with T_4 therapy. However, antibiotics are necessary to resolve the current infection, whereas T_4 therapy prevents further relapses. Some hypothyroid dogs experience a secondary *Malassezia* dermatitis in intertriginous areas or, less commonly, in a generalized distribution, or they have *Malassezia* otitis externa.[20] Some cases of adult-onset generalized demodicosis have been associated with hypothyroidism.[20]

When seborrhea, bacterial pyoderma, or *Malassezia* dermatitis are attributable to canine hypothyroidism, pruritus may be considerable. Poor wound healing is probably referable to defects in fibroblast function and collagen metabolism. Altered healing can be manifested by delayed healing of traumatic or surgical wounds or by the development of excessive fibrous tissue at points of minimal trauma. In the latter case, excessive scarring can occur in areas of deep follicular infection, or the dog can have excessive calluses at common pressure points and other less commonly affected areas such as the tuber ischium.[11, 111] Easy bruising may be associated with the collagen metabolism defects mentioned previously or with thrombasthenia and clotting factor defects that respond to thyroid hormone therapy.[35, 48, 101]

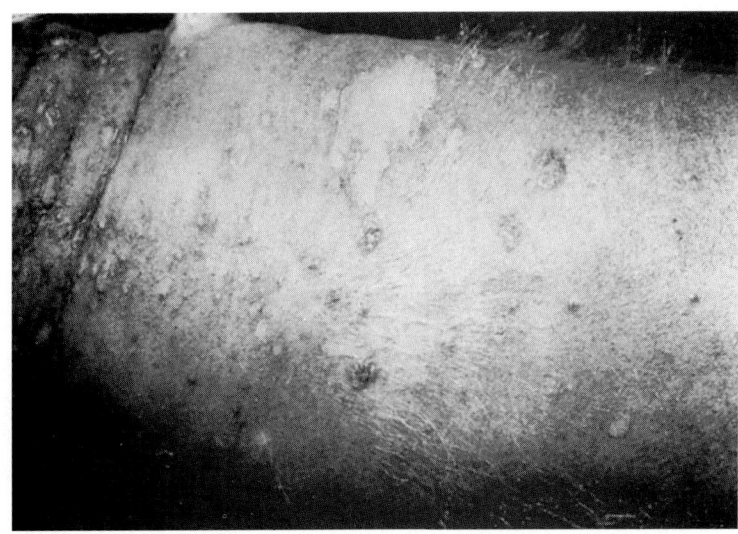

FIGURE 10–37. Hypothyroidism. Truncal alopecia with a secondary superficial folliculitis.

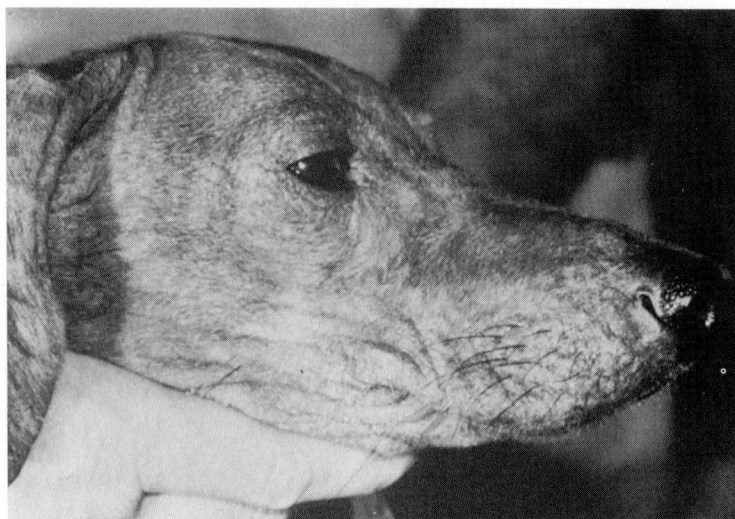

FIGURE 10–38. Hypothyroidism. Facial hair loss and scaling.

Other cutaneous signs commonly associated with hypothyroidism include hyperpigmentation, lichenification, comedones, and mucin accumulation.[14, 20, 137] The hyperpigmentation and lichenification are not specific for hypothyroidism, but reflect its chronicity. Although comedones can be numerous on the ventral abdomen of hypothyroid dogs, they usually accompany seborrheic changes on the trunk. In the absence of other seborrheic changes, numerous comedones are more frequently associated with hyperadrenocorticism or sex hormone dermatoses. Because thyroid hormones help to regulate the production of dermal glycosaminoglycans, hypothyroid dogs can accumulate hyaluronic acid in the dermis.[41, 46] This accumulation of mucin can lead to myxedema, in which the skin is thick, puffy (Fig. 10–36), and cool to the touch, or rarely mucinous vesication (see Fig. 10–43D).[20] The myxedematous changes are usually most pronounced on the face, where the skin of the forehead, eyelids, and lips droops, producing a tragic facial expression (see Fig. 10–35D).

The veterinary literature includes large lists of noncutaneous abnormalities associated with hypothyroidism. Aside from mental dullness, central nervous system signs are rare

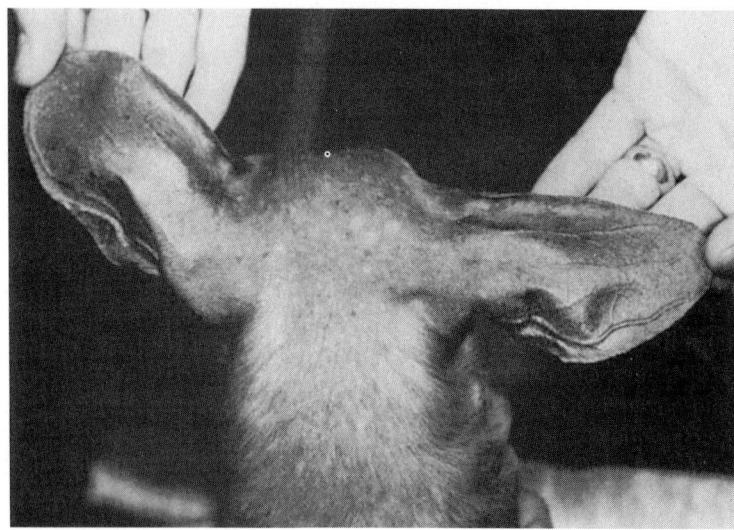

FIGURE 10–39. Hypothyroidism. Hair loss on the head and ears.

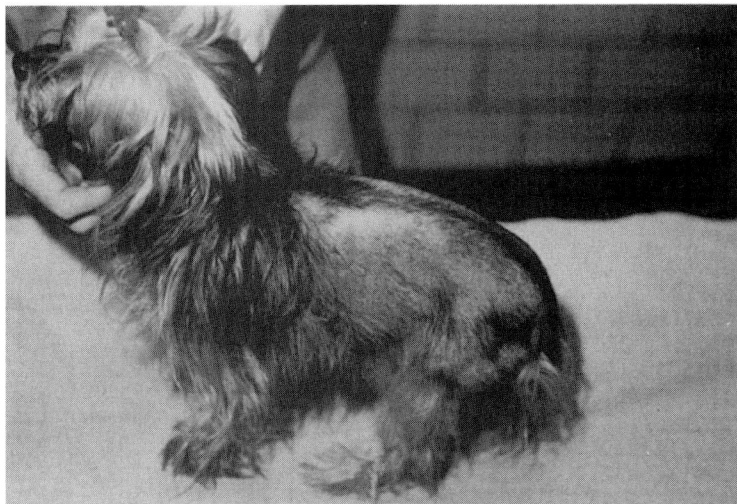

FIGURE 10–40. Hypothyroidism. Hair loss over the caudal dorsum.

in primary hypothyroidism and can be caused by atherosclerotic or myxedematous changes.[77, 85, 111, 113, 119, 163] The atherosclerotic changes are secondary to hyperlipidemia and can also affect the vessels in the heart, kidney, and gastrointestinal tract.[113, 166] Signs can include seizures, disorientation, circling, and coma. Myxedematous coma is of most concern because death can occur rapidly.[3, 35, 67a] Most cases have been reported in Doberman pinschers, and precoma signs include severe mental depression, hypoventilation, bradycardia, and hypothermia. Progression to coma can occur spontaneously or be precipitated by various drugs, disease, or anesthesia.

Neuromuscular disorders can occur with or without cutaneous signs. Cranial nerve abnormalities (head tilt, ataxia, facial palsy, and laryngeal paralysis), megaesophagus, unilateral lameness, paraparesis, tetraparesis, and myopathy with weakness and atrophy have all been associated with hypothyroidism.[27, 31, 48, 101] Depending on the cause and chronicity of the problem, these changes may or may not be reversible with treatment.

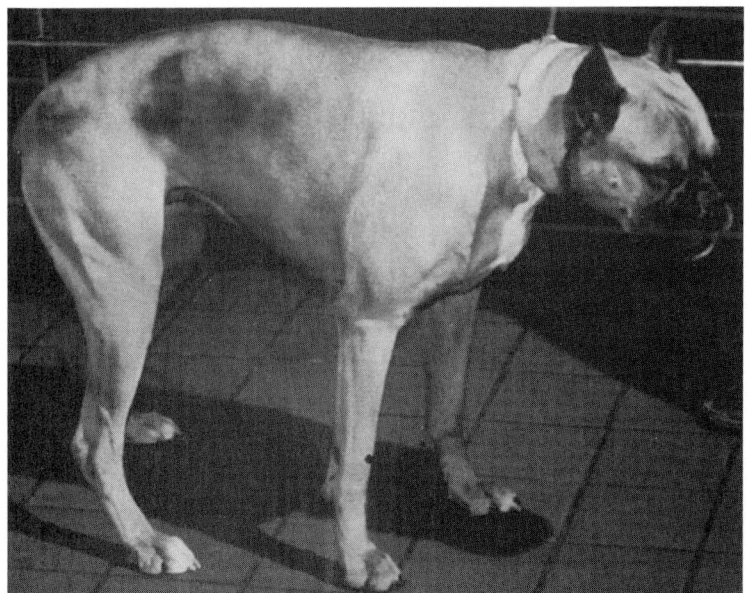

FIGURE 10–41. Hypothyroidism. Symmetric flank alopecia and hyperpigmentation.

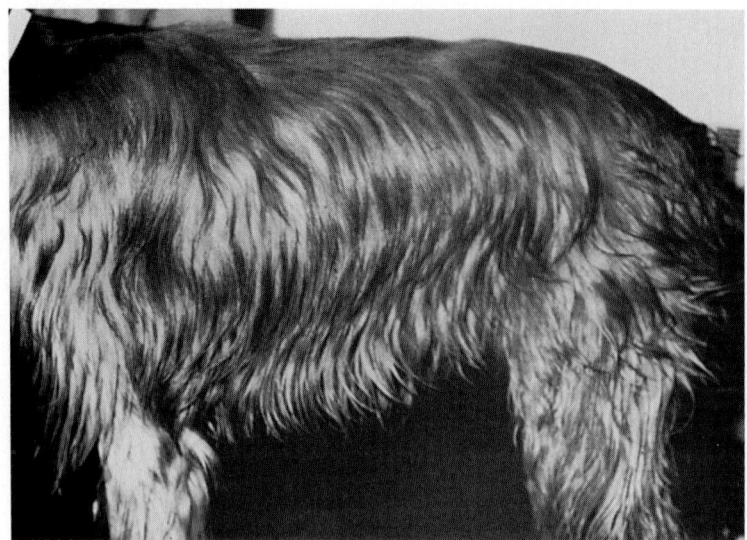

FIGURE 10–42. Hypertrichosis in an Irish setter with hypothyroidism.

The most common gastrointestinal sign of hypothyroidism in humans, but not in dogs, is constipation. In dogs, the most common gastrointestinal signs of hypothyroidism are diarrhea, vomiting, or both.[11, 48] These are occasional. Cardiovascular complications of hypothyroidism in dogs include bradycardia, weak apex beat, atherosclerosis, thrombosis, and cardiac arrhythmias associated with cardiomyopathy.[1, 2, 99, 101]

Ocular abnormalities that may be associated with canine hypothyroidism include corneal lipidosis, corneal ulceration, lipid aqueous flair, keratoconjunctivitis sicca, uveitis, and retinopathy.[1, 2, 48, 101, 113]

Hypothyroid dogs can have mild nonregenerative anemia or an increased bleeding tendency due to platelet dysfunction[150] or clotting factor defects (see Fig. 10–43E). Because T_4 amplifies production of factor VIII and factor VIII–related antigen, hypothyroidism could worsen the coagulation profile in a dog with von Willebrand's disease.[35, 48, 101] The theory that hypothyroidism induces acquired von Willebrand's syndrome has largely been discounted.[108, 109]

Classic reproductive changes associated with hypothyroidism include infertility, altered or absent estrous cycles, abortion, high puppy mortality, decreased spermatogenesis, and testicular atrophy.[2, 21] Gynecomastia and inappropriate galactorrhea can occur in up to 25% of intact, anestrous bitches and rarely in neutered female and male animals (Fig. 10–44).[1, 2, 11, 76] In these cases, the mammary changes are thought to be due to hyperprolactinemia induced by elevated levels of TRH.[37]

Renal lesions have been recognized in humans and laboratory animals with hypothyroidism.[11] Renal lesions and renal failure have also been recognized in association with canine hypothyroidism, especially in dogs with lymphocytic thyroiditis.

Hypothyroidism can exist singularly, occur intercurrently with another endocrine disease (e.g., diabetes mellitus),[50] be secondary to another endocrine disease (e.g., hyperadrenocorticism),[150] or be part of a polyglandular problem.[48, 113] In the latter case, diabetes mellitus, hypoadrenocorticism, and thyroiditis occur simultaneously and are thought to result from an autoimmune process. Typically, the signs of the hypoadrenocorticism predominate. Because hypoadrenocorticism and diabetes mellitus are causes of thyroid profile irregularities in euthyroid dogs, thyroid testing should be postponed in these dogs until the other conditions are regulated. Satisfactory control of one problem (e.g., diabetes mellitus) often necessitates correction of the other intercurrent conditions.[50]

Congenital hypothyroidism has been reported in both purebred and mongrel dogs.[33, 35, 60, 67, 92, 135] It may be goitrous or nongoitrous. During the first month of life, the puppies are fairly normal, but abnormalities are recognized quickly thereafter. The dogs

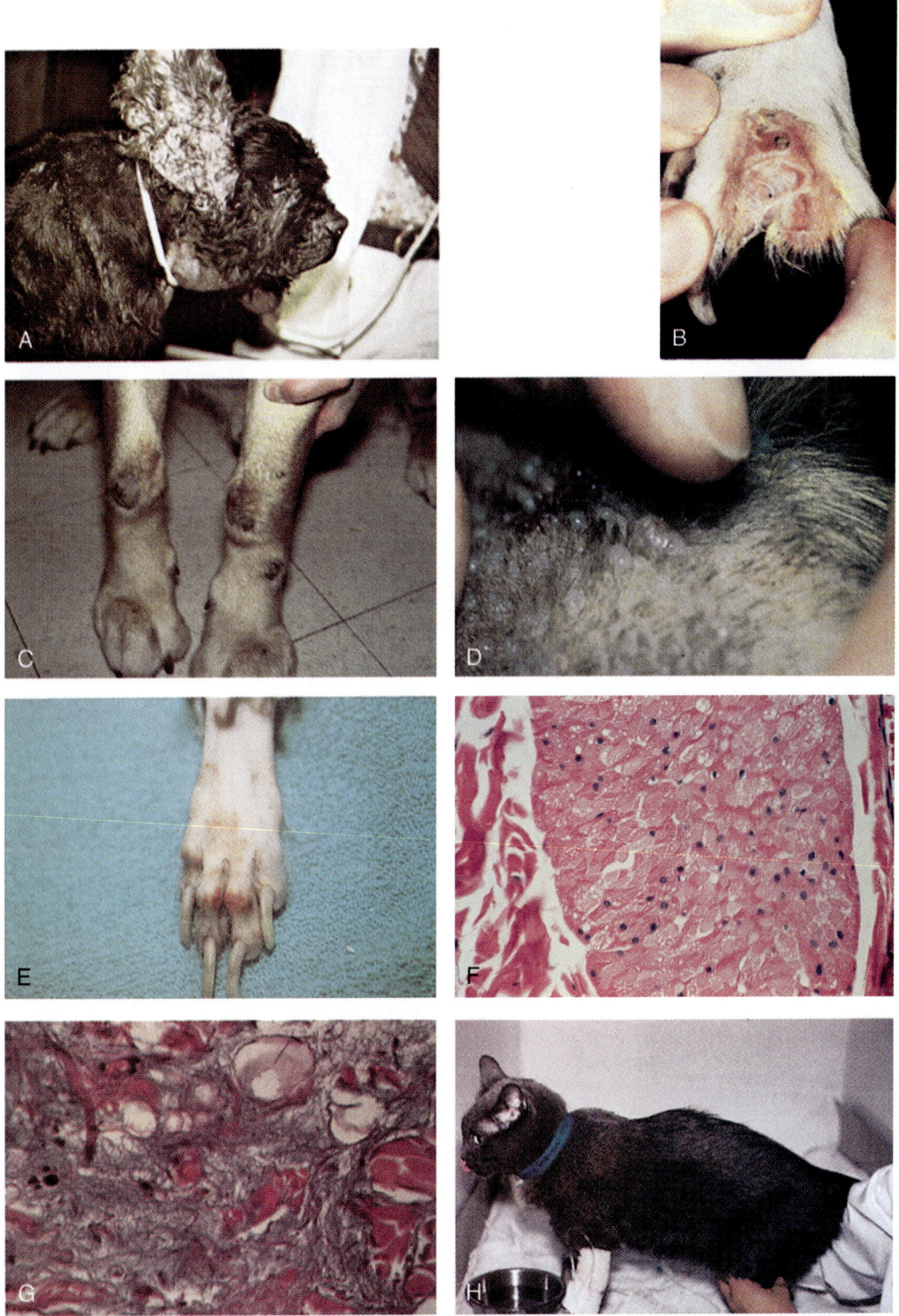

FIGURE 10–43. *A*, Severely hypothyroid black cocker spaniel, showing severe chronic otitis. *B*, Hypothyroidism. Interdigital furunculosis is the only sign of disease. *C*, Hypothyroidism. Symmetric areas of furunculosis mimicking acral lick dermatitis. *D*, Hypothyroidism. Mucinous vesiculation. *E*, Hypothyroidism. Bruising secondary to trauma. *F*, Hypothyroidism. Photomicrograph showing vacuolated arrector pili muscle. *G*, Hypothyroidism. Photomicrograph showing myxedema. *H*, Traumatic dorsal hair loss and scaling in a hyperthyroid cat.

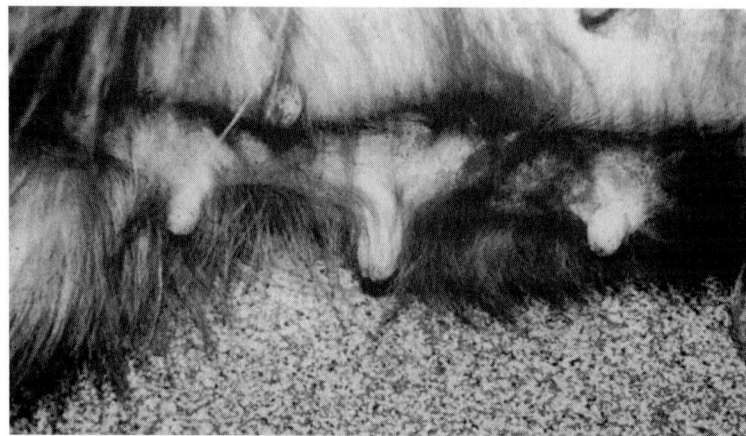

FIGURE 10-44. Hypothyroidism. Gynecomastia in a neutered female.

are somnolent, mentally retarded, disproportionately dwarfed, and lame. Other signs also are possible. Hair loss is not evident, but the coat is often different from that of the normal littermates. Early treatment is needed to prevent irreversible changes.

DIAGNOSIS

Because of the plethora of clinical signs in canine hypothyroidism, the differential diagnosis is exhaustive, as would be expected from a disease with such variable signs.[114] Definitive diagnosis necessitates thyroid biopsy but, because such testing is impractical, most clinicians rely on the history, physical examination findings, hematology, serum chemistry determinations, urinalysis, skin biopsy, and thyroid function tests. None of these tests is specific for primary hypothyroidism, and all have some margin of error. Because no one test is diagnostic, it is important to evaluate all test results in light of the patient's history and physical examination results.

The hemogram classically reveals a normocytic, normochromic, nonregenerative anemia (packed cell volume, 25% to 36%).[1, 2, 101] However, this is found in only approximately 30% of cases.[106] In addition, macrocytic and microcytic-hypochromic anemias may occur in canine hypothyroidism, possibly reflecting defects in vitamin B_{12} and folic acid metabolism or iron metabolism, respectively. Leptocytosis may be prominent in the anemic hypothyroid dog.

Another classic laboratory finding in hypothyroidism is hypercholesterolemia (260 to 1000 mg/dl).[1, 2, 45a, 101] However, serum cholesterol levels are greatly influenced by diet, can be elevated in other nonthyroid disorders, and are significantly elevated after a 24-hour fast in only about 50% to 75% of cases. Serum cholesterol levels tend to be elevated with severe degrees of thyroid failure. Analysis of serum lipids in lipemic hypothyroid dogs may reveal hypercholesterolemia, hypertriglyceridemia, and intense electrophoretic bands at the origin, β_1-lipoprotein, and α_2-lipoprotein positions.[32, 136, 145]

Serum creatine kinase activity is mildly to markedly elevated in less than 50% of dogs with hypothyroidism with or without concurrent clinical myopathy.[101, 106] Other serum enzyme levels that may be mildly to markedly elevated in hypothyroidism include lactate dehydrogenase, aspartate transaminase, alanine transaminase, and alkaline phosphatase levels. These elevations presumably result from the aforementioned hypothyroid myopathy and from the degenerative hepatopathies (fatty infiltration and cirrhosis) that may accompany canine hypothyroidism.

Urinalysis results usually are normal in canine hypothyroidism. A few dogs with lymphocytic thyroiditis have had proteinuria and immune complex glomerulonephritis.

Electrocardiographic examination of hypothyroid dogs may reveal bradycardia, low voltage in all leads, flat T waves, and arrhythmias.[1, 2, 101] Radiographic examination of animals with congenital hypothyroidism reveals epiphyseal dysgenesis.[1, 2]

Skin biopsy in canine hypothyroidism may reveal many nondiagnostic changes consistent with endocrinopathy (orthokeratotic hyperkeratosis, epidermal atrophy, epidermal melanosis, follicular keratosis, follicular dilatation, follicular atrophy, telogenization of hair follicles, excessive trichilemmal keratinization, and sebaceous gland atrophy).[4, 16, 137] Histopathologic findings highly suggestive of hypothyroidism include vacuolated, hypertrophied arrector pili muscles (see Fig. 10-43F), increased dermal mucin (mucinosis or myxedema) (see Fig. 10-43G), and a thick dermis. About 50% of the biopsy specimens from hypothyroid dog skin reveal variable degrees of inflammation, reflecting the common occurrence of secondary seborrhea, bacterial pyoderma, or both.

Thyroid Testing

Except for thyroid biopsy, no one thyroid test is diagnostic for primary hypothyroidism.[11, 68] Because peripheral hormone levels depend on thyroid production, protein binding, and rate of metabolism, basal measurements can be subject to a wide margin of error. Function studies (TSH or TRH stimulation tests) test the thyroid's secretory capacity and are most diagnostic but are not commonly used because of the expense and difficulty in obtaining TSH or TRH. All test results, including stimulation tests, must be evaluated critically, and if the results do not correlate well with the history and physical examination findings, the test should be repeated.[78]

Because stimulation tests are not available, basal measurements of TT_4, fT_4, TT_3, fT_3, and cTSH are the mainstay of testing. Because measurement of TT_3 and fT_3 has limited value in the diagnosis of hypothyroidism, these hormones will be eliminated from the discussion.[23, 78, 102] In the literature prior to 1995, most studies defined a normal range of values for TT_4 or fT_4 and evaluated their results based on this range.[23, 78, 100, 102, 118] Dogs with values in or above the normal range were considered euthyroid, whereas those with values below the lower limit of normal were not. These studies also reported their data as raw numbers of dogs that were or were not considered euthyroid or hypothyroid under the conditions of study. Both of these shortcomings caused some inaccuracy in the data.

Thyroid testing started to become popular in the late 1970s. In that era, statistical methods rarely were used in clinical studies, so the range of normal presented for the various thyroid tests was exactly that. The lower limit of normal was the lowest value recorded in the population of normal dogs tested. In most cases, the number of dogs used to develop the normal range was not available or was small. Today, we know that large numbers of observations are needed to statistically discriminate between two very similar conditions and that means values ± 1 or 2 standard deviations are a more accurate way of presenting the normal range of the data. Additionally, we know that raw data presentation does not account for random fluctuations in the population and that calculation of the test's sensitivity, specificity, positive predictive value, and negative predictive value is more informative and accurate.

If one accepts the range of normal values for TT_4, fT_4, or cTSH at their face value and defines a hypothyroid dog as one with a TT_4 or fT_4 below normal or a cTSH above normal, significant error is introduced. For example, when 51 euthyroid dogs were evaluated and the diagnosis of hypothyroidism was based on a subnormal TT_4 or fT_4 level, 20% of the dogs would have been called hypothyroid.[118] In that same study, 8% of the 24 hypothyroid dogs were called normal. In another study of 49 euthyroid dogs with skin disease and 9 hypothyroid dogs, low TT_4 or fT_4 levels were defined as a value less than the mean minus 2 standard deviations.[23] With these stricter criteria, none of the euthyroid dogs was considered hypothyroid. Three of the 9 hypothyroid dogs had a low TT_4 and 9 had a low fT_4 level. In all 9 of the hypothyroid dogs, diagnosis was correct if the definition of hypothyroidism was based on a low TT_4 or fT_4 level.

These and other studies indicate that we should request two or more thyroid tests for each patient and that we must be critical in our evaluation of these tests. Values just below normal are of unknown significance, and the accuracy of diagnosis increases as the definition of hypothyroidism becomes more stringent. Data in the gray zone (e.g., mean value minus 1 standard deviation) are not interpretable by themselves, and tests must be performed again at a later date or be evaluated with another thyroid hormone. If stimulation tests become available again, data in the gray zone should be evaluated by that testing.

To overcome shortcomings in sample size and account for random fluctuations in the population, most current papers present the sensitivity and specificity data of the test in question. Tests with a high sensitivity (e.g., 98%) but a low specificity (e.g., 75%) are of questionable value in discriminating between normal and disease states because abnormal values can be found in a significant percentage, in this case 25%, of normal individuals. Published sensitivity figures for TT_4 levels vary from 89% to 100%; the specificity varies from 75% to 82%.[43, 124] Figures for the sensitivity and specificity of fT_4 range from 80% to 98% and 92% to 94%, respectively.[43, 89, 124] Lastly, the sensitivity and specificity data for cTSH range from 63% to 87% and 75% to 93%, respectively.[42, 43, 89, 124, 144] Obviously, no one test is perfect, but a fT_4 level by dialysis has the highest degree of accuracy for any single test. Simultaneous evaluation of two or more tests (e.g., a thyroid panel) can markedly increase the specificity of the testing.[89, 144] This panel approach is necessary in epileptic dogs or those taking other medications that can influence hormone levels.[39, 53]

Because immune-mediated thyroiditis is a common cause of hypothyroidism, measurement of serum antithyroglobulin, anti-T_3, or anti-T_4 antibodies can be useful in documenting thyroiditis. In an evaluation of over 100,000 serum samples submitted for thyroid profiles, approximately 6% had autoantibodies.[130] Approximately 5% had antibodies to T_3, 0.3% had antibodies to T_4, and 0.9% had both T_3 and T_4 autoantibodies. Approximately 25% to 35% of euthyroid dogs have elevated levels, and approximately 50% of hypothyroid dogs have normal levels; thus, this testing cannot be used to document hypothyroidism.[45] Additionally, these autoantibodies can interfere with the accurate measurement of TT_3 or TT_4.[80] Although the dog has the clinical signs of hypothyroidism, its TT_3 or TT_4 is spuriously elevated into the hyperthyroid range. The fT_4 level in these dogs may be valid.

Function Studies

The TSH stimulation test is vastly superior to the determination of basal serum TT_4, fT_4, or cTSH levels for the diagnosis of hypothyroidism. Unfortunately, the TSH of bovine origin that was used in this testing is not available in many parts of the world. Recombinant human TSH stimulates the dog's thyroid gland when given intravenously at doses of 50 μg or greater.[141] However, this product is extremely expensive, which precludes its regular use. If bovine TSH is available, samples are collected before and 4 or 6 hours after the subcutaneous or intravenous administration of 0.1 IU/kg or 1 IU/dog.[27, 78, 102, 116, 118] Because reconstituted TSH maintains its potency when frozen in the standard freezer ($-20°C$ [$-4°C$]) for over 6 months,[30, 81, 116] large vials should be subdivided and frozen so the largest number of animals can be tested.

Traditionally, euthyroidism was diagnosed when the post-TSH TT_4 value was at least double the basal level. With this system, approximately 30% of euthyroid dogs can be called hypothyroid and approximately 50% of hypothyroid dogs are called normal.[118] It is more appropriate to base normalcy on either a rise in the post-TSH TT_4 to some predetermined value or an increase of at least some predetermined amount. Specific values for the end point of normalcy or the rise expected in normal dogs vary with the laboratory and the amount of TSH used. When one investigator used the 1.4 μg/dl rise suggested in another study[82] rather than the 1.9 μg/dl figure suggested by the testing laboratory, diagnosis was incorrect in 4 of 75 dogs.[118] Accordingly, test results must always be interpreted in light of the normal values developed by the testing laboratory.

A TSH (or TRH) stimulation test performed on a dog that is receiving thyroid hormone therapy will give spurious results. Because exogenous T_4 suppresses thyroid function,[105] the drug must be withdrawn for accurate testing. Most dogs can be accurately tested after a 30-day withdrawal period, but approximately 20% of dogs are still under the influence of the drug.[104] An 8-week withdrawal is satisfactory in all dogs.

The TRH stimulation test was developed as a less expensive and consistently available alternative to the TSH stimulation test.[84] Unfortunately, the test has not lived up to its expectation and is of little diagnostic value.[51] Serum TT_4 levels are determined before and

6 hours after the IV injection of 0.2 or 0.05 mg/kg (maximum, 1 mg)[51, 165] of TRH. The post-TRH TT_4 level in normal dogs should increase by 0.4 µg/dl or more or be at least 1½ times greater than the basal value.[1, 2, 84, 102] Although TRH testing in normal dogs gives good results, its accuracy in hypothyroid dogs often is not satisfactory.[51]

The diagnosis of hypothyroidism, as well as the distinction between primary and secondary hypothyroidism, can be based on thyroid biopsy.[86] Radioiodine uptake studies and other special radiographic techniques are also valuable but are not routinely available.

Although the response to thyroid hormone therapy is often listed as a diagnostic test of hypothyroidism, it can be unreliable. The metabolic effects of thyroid hormones may produce varying degrees of improvement in symptoms such as lethargy, depression, and obesity, regardless of their cause. In addition, thyroid hormone administration may produce varying degrees of hair growth in normal dogs and hair regrowth in dogs with numerous dermatoses that are unrelated to hypothyroidism.[61] However, the institution of treatment with prompt therapeutic monitoring of TT_4 levels might be of some diagnostic significance. When a hypothyroid dog is given 0.02 mg/kg of oral levothyroxine, its serum concentration of TT_4 should peak in 4 to 6 hours and be at or slightly above the upper limit of normal. In our experience, the post-pill TT_4 level of a euthyroid dog given the therapeutic dose of levothyroxine for a month will be significantly above normal. This markedly elevated post-pill TT_4 level does not guarantee the euthyroid state but should prompt the clinician to carefully evaluate the case before continuing the treatment.

CLINICAL MANAGEMENT

After treatment of primary hypothyroidism has been started, it is continued for the remainder of the patient's life.

In most cases, oral levothyroxine (T_4) is the drug of choice for hypothyroidism. Various treatment regimens can be found in the veterinary literature, but most suggest either once- or twice-daily administration of 0.02 mg/kg to a maximum daily dosage of 0.8 mg q12h.[49, 58, 59, 102, 112] Because supplementation is lifelong and owner compliance decreases when multiple treatments are needed each day, it is ideal to administer the T_4 once daily. When 12 thyroidectomized dogs were treated with 0.04, 0.02, or 0.01 mg/kg of levothyroxine either once or divided twice daily, variability in drug absorption and elimination was noted among the dogs.[97] Twice-daily administration resulted in drug concentrations closer to the physiologic range. However, most dogs respond favorably to the more convenient once-daily administration,[49, 58, 59, 112] and some dogs treated twice daily show signs of toxicity. Because of the rapid metabolic turnover rate of T_4 (10 to 16 hours in dogs, 7 days in humans), incomplete absorption from the gut, and marked fecal excretion, signs of overdosing are very uncommon at the typical therapeutic dosages and include anxiety, panting, polydipsia, polyuria, polyphagia, diarrhea, tachycardia, heat intolerance, pruritus, and pyrexia. These signs of hyperthyroidism disappear quickly when the dosage is modified appropriately.

Ultimately, the accuracy of any clinical diagnosis is proven by a positive response to a specific treatment. Although some euthyroid dogs experience temporary improvement in their coats and skin with T_4 supplementation, permanent resolution of all metabolic and dermatologic signs of hypothyroidism confirms the accuracy of the diagnosis. If the diagnosis of hypothyroidism is based on an evaluation with near 100% sensitivity and specificity, treatment can be started on a once-daily basis and clinical response can be expected. The question remains as to the best treatment protocol for the cases where thyroid testing cannot be performed, is inconclusive, or may be confounded by intercurrent disease or drug therapy. If once-daily treatment is instituted and the dog needs twice-daily administration, response to treatment will be incomplete and the accuracy of the diagnosis comes under question. To avoid this problem, it is best to start treatment on a twice-daily basis. If the diagnosis was correct, the dog will return to normal with the T_4 supplementation. Once the expected response occurs, the frequency or administration can be reduced to once daily to see if the response can be sustained. If the clinical signs start to recur with this modification, twice-daily treatments are needed.

Although no studies have used levothyroxine from different manufacturers in the same dogs, data suggest that bioavailability does vary with the product used.[96] Accordingly, the veterinary clinician should select an effective product and use it to the exclusion of all others. Because the clinician has little control over what product a pharmacy catering to humans dispenses, prescriptions for levothyroxine should not be written.

Most of the dermatologic and metabolic abnormalities in hypothyroid dogs are correctable with treatment. Some lesions (e.g., scars over pressure points) do not disappear entirely, but new ones should not develop. Dogs with attitudinal abnormalities (e.g., lethargy, depression) respond rapidly (within 2 to 4 weeks) to levothyroxine therapy. Response in the skin is slower, and the owner must be told to administer the drug for at least 3 months. Initial skin changes usually do not become apparent for approximately 4 weeks. Unless warned of this slow response time, many owners stop treatment after a month of no change because all other conditions they have treated in their pets have responded within this period. Most dogs are normal or nearly so by 3 to 4 months of treatment, but it can take longer to regrow the long-flowing coat of some breeds such as the Afghan hound.

Dogs with cardiac disease experience a change in cardiac function with treatment and should be started on *lower* doses of levothyroxine; otherwise, heart failure may be precipitated.[110] The following protocol for levothyroxine is recommended: 0.005 mg/kg every 12 hours for 2 weeks, then 0.01 mg/kg every 12 hours for 2 weeks, then 0.015 mg/kg every 12 hours for 2 weeks, then up to routine maintenance dosage. In addition, patients with concurrent hypoadrenocorticism should not be treated for hypothyroidism until their adrenal insufficiency is corrected and stabilized with medication. Thyroid hormone therapy can also necessitate altered doses of insulin[112] and certain anticonvulsants (phenytoin and phenobarbital) in cases being managed with those agents.[48]

Liothyronine (T_3) may also be used to treat canine hypothyroidism but is rarely indicated.[1, 2, 102] It should be given orally at 4 to 6 μg/kg every 8 hours, thus necessitating more frequent administration and greater expense.

Treatment of myxedema coma is a medical emergency.[1, 2, 35, 67a, 77, 113] Therapy consists of IV administration of levothyroxine or oral liothyronine by gastric tube, mechanical respiratory support, IV administration of glucocorticoids and broad-spectrum antibiotics, and passive rewarming.[67a]

The reasons for therapeutic failure with thyroid hormones are multiple. The most common reasons are incorrect diagnosis, failure to recognize other intercurrent endocrinopathies (e.g., hypothyroidism in a dog with a sex hormone imbalance), and insufficient therapy (e.g., insufficient course of treatment, wrong dosage, wrong frequency of administration, use of a product with poor bioavailability, and poor owner compliance). After the clinician has determined that the correct dosage of an appropriate medication was dispensed and that the clients are administering the medication appropriately, post-pill testing is the next step in determining why the dog's response was poor.

In dogs, TT_4 levels peak 4 to 6 hours after oral administration of levothyroxine and decline thereafter.[96] With the administration of a satisfactory dose of an absorbable product, the TT_4 level should be within the normal range at 4 to 6 hours. Values at or slightly above the upper limit of normal are expected.[59] Dogs given the medication once daily have higher peak values than dogs that receive that dosage divided into two equal doses.[96] If the peak TT_4 value is too high or low, dosage adjustments are necessary. The adequacy of a new dosage must be determined by additional post-pill testing in 2 to 4 weeks. Because the half-life of T_4 can vary from dog to dog, an adequate peak value in a dog receiving once-daily treatment does not necessarily guarantee that normal levels are maintained during the entire 24-hour period. If this dog's response is poor or incomplete, a 24-hour post-pill TT_4 value should be evaluated. If that TT_4 is well below normal, the single dose must be increased or the dog should be treated twice daily.

Dogs with autoantibodies to T_4 cannot be monitored by conventional post-pill testing because the autoantibodies interfere with the TT_4 assay. In these cases, free T_4 can be used for monitoring.[47] The post-pill fT_4 level should be at or slightly above the upper limit of normal at 4 to 6 hours. TSH levels can also be used for monitoring and should be within the normal range with appropriate T_4 replacement therapy. Because some hypothyroid dogs do not have elevated TSH levels and TT_4 levels may be too high despite normal TSH levels, monitoring via TSH levels is least desirable.

Post-pill testing is unnecessary in dogs that show a satisfactory response to treatment with no clinical signs of overdosage. If clinical signs return later in the dog's life, testing at that point is indicated. Hypothyroid dogs rarely show clinical signs of overdosage when they are given 0.02 mg/kg of levothyroxine twice daily. If signs occur, post-pill testing should be performed immediately. If the TT_4 value is greatly elevated above normal levels, the diagnosis of hypothyroidism must be questioned. Moderate elevations above normal levels indicate overdosage and suggest that the half-life of levothyroxine may be longer in this dog. Some investigators decrease the dosage but maintain the twice-daily administration, whereas other researchers reduce treatment to once daily. Too few dogs are recognized with this problem to allow for specific recommendations.

When normal dogs are given levothyroxine, their responsiveness to TSH decreases after 4 weeks of treatment and continued treatment results in increased unresponsiveness and histologic evidence of thyroid inactivity.[104, 105] Although unproved, clinical evidence suggests that unnecessary administration of levothyroxine for long periods eventually induces a secondary hypothyroidism, necessitating lifelong replacement therapy.

Treatment of secondary hypothyroidism is essentially the same as that described for primary hypothyroidism. Dietary iodine deficiency is corrected by supplementing dogs with dietary iodine at 34 µg/kg/day and cats with 100 µg/day.[11]

Feline Hypothyroidism

Other than congenital hypothyroidism, naturally occurring spontaneous hypothyroidism has been documented in only one cat.[128]

CLINICAL FEATURES

Signs of congenital hypothyroidism in cats are similar to signs in the dog.[19, 74, 122, 142, 148] The kittens are born normal, but are obviously different from their littermates by 4 to 6 weeks of age. Affected cats have a decreased rate of growth, with stunting, and become disproportionate dwarfs. They are lethargic, mentally dull, and have depressed appetites. Although they have full haircoats, the coat is dull and dry and has fewer primary hairs than normal. Unless treatment is instituted soon after signs begin, death can occur within 2 weeks. In one cat colony, autoimmune thyroiditis with an autosomal recessive mode of inheritance was documented.[142]

When experimental adult cats underwent thyroidectomy by radiation and were followed for 96 weeks, the systemic and cutaneous signs were far different from those in hypothyroid dogs.[153] Clinically, the cats were initially lethargic but returned to normal status spontaneously. No change in appetite or body weight was recognized. The cats groomed less than normal, which resulted in dorsal matting and seborrhea, and experienced alopecia of the pinnae, pressure points, and dorsal and lateral tail base region. With the sensitivity of the cat's thyroid axis to iodine levels,[151] iodine depletion can cause clinical signs. Experimentally deprived cats exhibited cutaneous changes more typical of the dog.[15] The coats became dry with easily epilated hairs, and symmetric alopecia developed on the lateral neck, the thorax, and the abdomen. The skin was dry, scaly, and thickened.

The cat with spontaneous adult-onset hypothyroidism resembled dogs with that disease.[128] The cat was lethargic, thermophilic, inappetent, and obese. The cat's face was puffy and the coat was dull, dry, seborrheic, and lighter in color than normal (Fig. 10–45). Hair regrowth at clipped sites was poor. The diagnosis was confirmed by TSH response test and thyroid biopsy.

DIAGNOSIS

Because naturally occurring acquired hypothyroidism is so rare in cats, no data exist on the diagnostic value of hemograms, chemistry profiles, and other tests used in the dog.

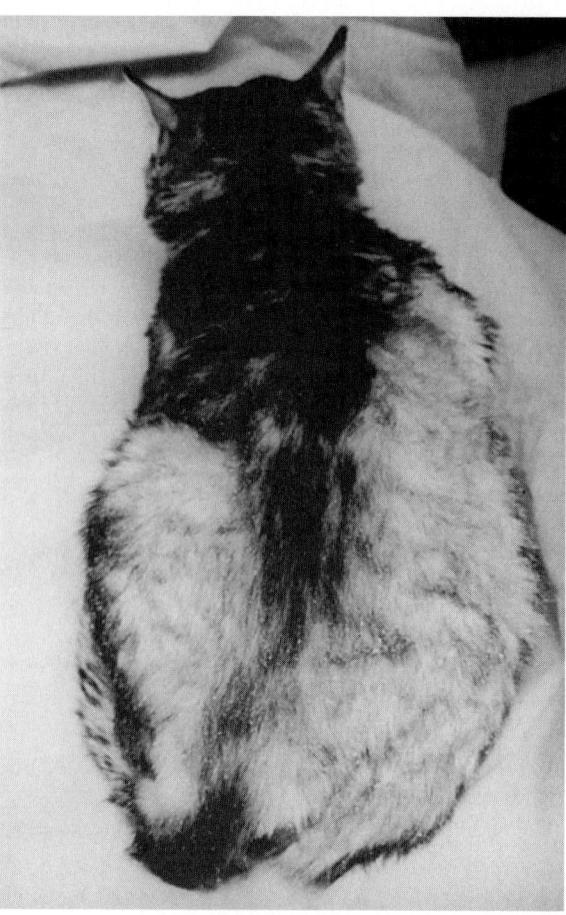

FIGURE 10-45. Hair loss and scaling in a cat with spontaneous hypothyroidism. (From Rand JS, et al: Spontaneous adult-onset hypothyroidism in a cat. J Vet Intern Med 7:272, 1993.)

Unlike puppies, kittens have adult cat levels of TT_4 and fT_4 from birth. TT_3 and fT_3 levels are low until 5 weeks of age.[167] As in the dog, isolated measurement of TT_4 has very poor discriminating value in the diagnosis of feline hypothyroidism. Cats with common nonthyroidal illnesses such as diabetes mellitus, liver disease, or renal disease have TT_4 values well below normal or normal.[93, 121, 152, 156] Measurement of fT_4 may be more reliable in the detection of hypothyroidism. In one study, fT_4 values were not decreased in cats with nonthyroidal illness.[93]

When either 1 IU/cat or 1 IU/kg of TSH is given intravenously, TT_4 levels peak at 6 hours. TT_3 and fT_4 levels peak at 7 hours. Total T_4 levels should double and fT_4 values should triple in euthyroid cats.[70, 146] When 0.1 mg/cat of TRH is given intravenously, TT_4 and fT_4 levels peak at 4 hours and increase onefold and twofold, respectively. Vomiting at the injection of TRH occurred in 4 of 13 cats.[146]

CLINICAL MANAGEMENT

Appropriate doses of thyroid hormones for cats have not been studied in detail. Cats bilaterally thyroidectomized for hyperthyroidism typically receive between 0.05 to 0.2 mg of levothyroxine every 24 hours or 30 µg of liothyronine every 8 hours.[148, 155] These doses should be adequate for cats with congenital or acquired hypothyroidism. The cat with spontaneous adult-onset disease was given 0.1 mg every 24 hours and returned to normal status after 3 months of treatment.[128] Typical of dogs, constitutional changes were noted after 1 week of treatment, whereas skin changes started about week 6 of treatment.

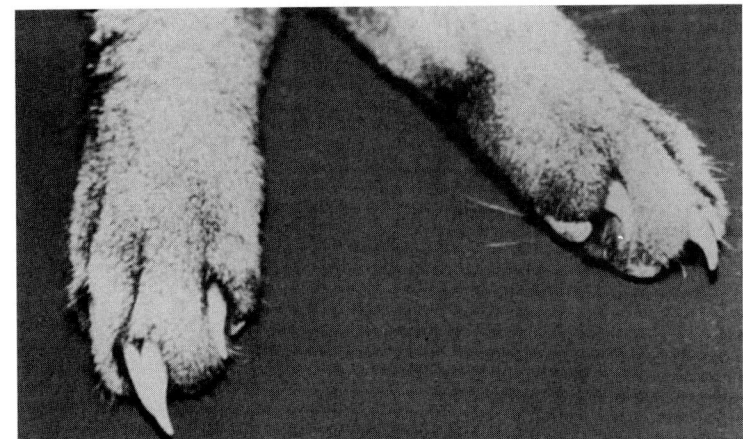

FIGURE 10-46. Overgrown claws in a hyperthyroid cat.

Feline Hyperthyroidism

Hyperthyroidism and diabetes mellitus are the most common endocrine disorders of the cat.[1, 2, 154] The cause of feline hyperthyroidism is usually a solitary thyroid adenoma or multinodular adenomatous hyperplasia of the thyroid. Thyroid carcinomas are rare. Clinical signs are due to an accelerated basal metabolic rate and increased sensitivity to catecholamines.

Feline hyperthyroidism occurs in older cats, 6 to 20 years of age, with no apparent breed or sex predilections. Common clinical signs include polyphagia, polydipsia, polyuria, weight loss, hyperactivity, tachycardia, vomiting, and diarrhea.[154] Cutaneous abnormalities occur in approximately 30% of cases and include excessive shedding and matting of the haircoat, focal or symmetric alopecia associated with excessive grooming (see Fig. 10-43H), increased rate of claw growth (Fig. 10-46), dry or greasy seborrhea, thin skin, and peripheral arteriovenous fistula.[1, 2, 154] In chronic cases, there is complete truncal alopecia with thin, hypotonic skin, mimicking hyperadrenocorticism (Fig. 10-47).[11]

Diagnosis is based on history, physical examination findings, and elevated basal TT_4, fT_4, or TT_3 levels. Common biochemical abnormalities in hyperthyroid cats include elevated levels of serum alkaline phosphatase, serum lactate dehydrogenase, and serum

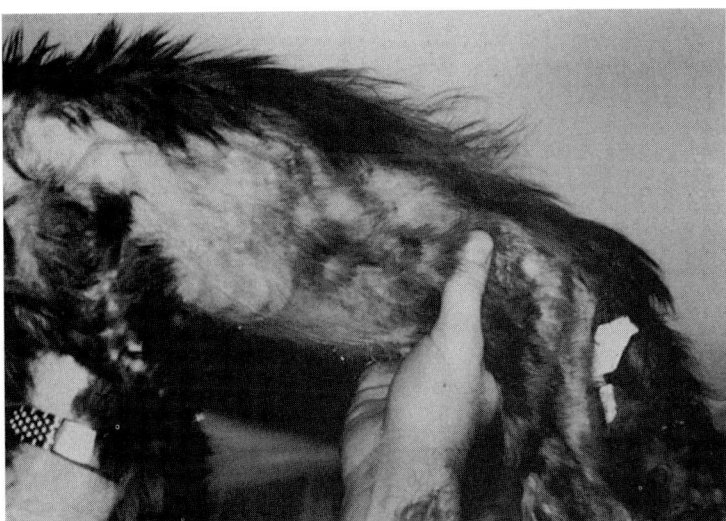

FIGURE 10-47. Truncal hair loss with thin hypotonic skin in a chronically hyperthyroid cat.

aspartate transaminase. More than 50% of hyperthyroid cats have TT_4 levels that overlap those of normal cats.[57] In these cases, hyperthyroidism can be diagnosed by fT_4 measurement, the T_3 suppression test, or the TRH stimulation test.[57] Because fT_4 levels can be increased in nonthyroidal disease, fT_4 should always be evaluated with the TT_4.[115, 123] The T_3 suppression test involves the oral administration of 15 to 25 µg of liothyronine every 8 hours for seven doses.[57, 129] A sample for TT_4 and fT_4 determinations is taken before the medication administration is started and then 2 to 4 hours after the seventh dose. Hyperthyroid cats show little or no change in their TT_4 or fT_4 levels, whereas euthyroid cats show a 50% reduction in TT_4 and fT_4 values. Hyperthyroid cats show no change in TT_4 levels after TRH administration.[57]

Therapy includes surgical excision, radioactive iodine treatment,[90] and the administration of antithyroid drugs (methimazole, carbimazole, stable iodine, and calcium ipodate).[94, 155]

Diabetes Mellitus

In human beings, diabetes mellitus is associated with a number of dermatologic disorders, including vascular complications (microangiopathy and atherosclerosis), necrobiosis lipoidica, granuloma annulare, scleredema, fibrovascular papillomas, yellow nails, rubeosis, bacterial and fungal infections, diabetic neuropathy, pruritus, idiopathic bullae, alopecia, xanthomatosis, and poor wound healing.[436] Up to 30% of humans with diabetes mellitus experience a skin disorder that is either an early indicator of undiagnosed diabetes or a complication of known diabetes. In dogs and cats, skin lesions have been reported to occur rarely or in as many as one third of cases.*

The most common dermatologic manifestations of diabetes mellitus in dogs and cats appear to be bacterial pyoderma (Fig. 10–48A), seborrheic skin disease (see Fig. 10–48B), thin and hypotonic skin, and varying degrees of alopecia (Fig. 10–49). The thin, hypotonic skin, with or without alopecia, probably results from protein catabolism. The seborrheic skin disease (usually generalized seborrhea sicca) is probably due to protein catabolism and abnormal lipid metabolism.

Diabetics are predisposed to infections, particularly those caused by coagulase-positive staphylococci and *Candida* spp.[11, 436, 441] This susceptibility appears to be due to abnormalities in neutrophil chemotaxis, phagocytosis, intracellular killing, and cell-mediated (T-cell) immune responses. These abnormalities may or may not be totally corrected through restoration of normoglycemia with insulin therapy.

Rarely, pruritus vulvae, xanthomatosis, and necrobiosis lipoidica have been reported in association with diabetes mellitus in dogs.[1, 2, 446, 455] Xanthomatosis has been reported in cats with naturally occurring and megestrol acetate–induced diabetes mellitus.

Necrolytic Migratory Erythema

Necrolytic migratory erythema is a term coined to describe the skin rash in humans with a glucagon-secreting pancreatic tumor (glucagonoma) or, rarely, hepatic cirrhosis and other miscellaneous gastrointestinal disorders. The rash has been recognized in dogs and the cat, but a standard nomenclature has not been accepted.[445] The terms *hepatocutaneous syndrome*,[11, 430, 442, 443] *superficial necrolytic dermatitis*,[4, 433] and *metabolic epidermal necrosis*[434, 447] are commonly used to describe the same condition. However, epidermal necrosis and necrolysis are *not* features of this disorder.

CAUSE AND PATHOGENESIS

The skin lesions in necrolytic migratory erythema are due to degeneration of the keratinocytes, which results in laminar high-level epidermal edema and degeneration. The specific

---

*See references 1, 2, 11, 17, 424, 446, 455.

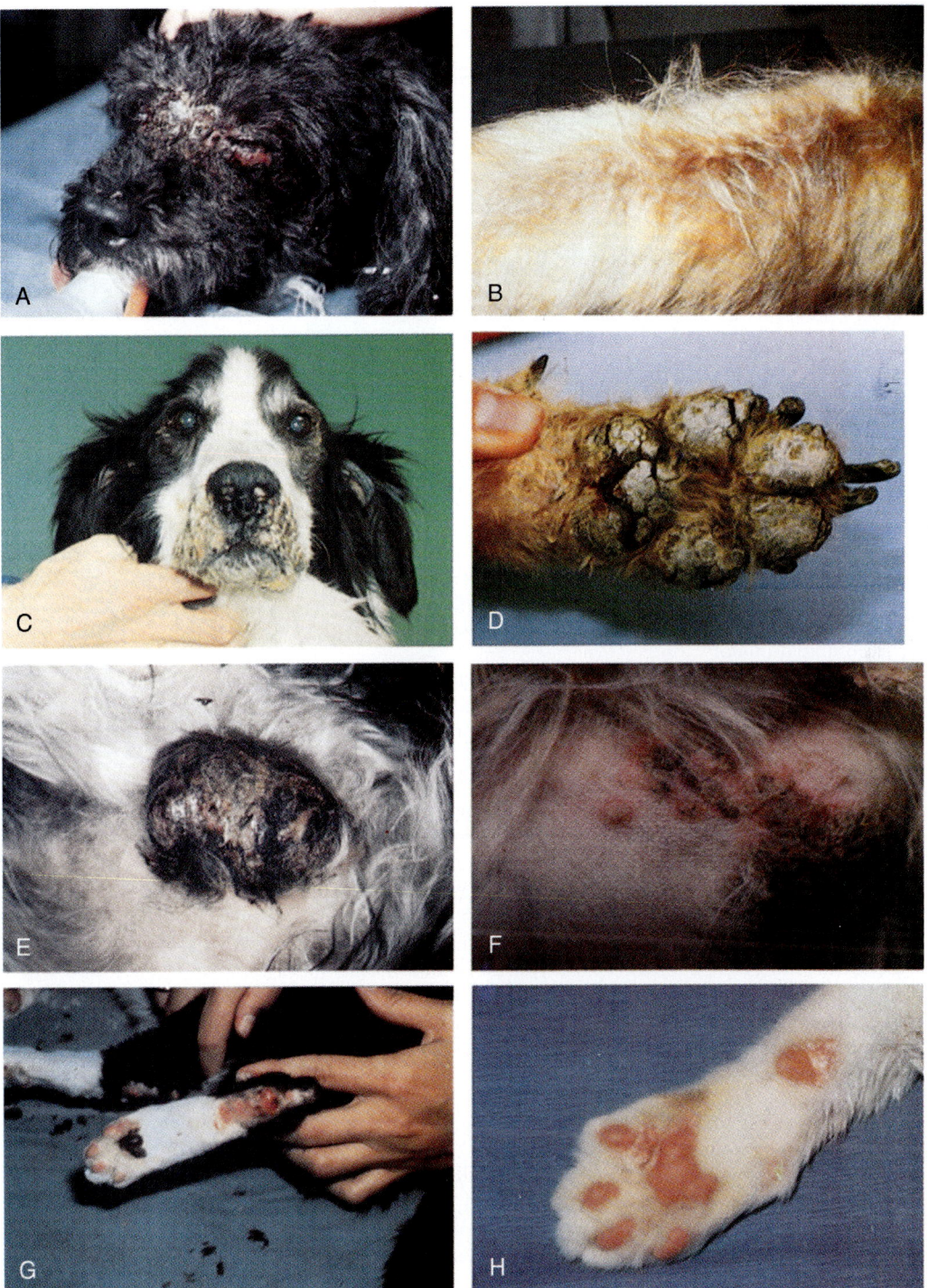

FIGURE 10–48. *A*, Diabetes mellitus. Severe facial bacterial pyoderma. *B*, Diabetes mellitus. Hypotrichosis with a greasy seborrhea. *C*, Necrolytic migratory erythema. Temporal muscle atrophy with crusting dermatitis of the periocular areas and muzzle. *D*, Necrolytic migratory erythema. Hyperkeratosis and fissuring of footpads. *E*, Necrolytic migratory erythema. Scrotal ulceration and crusting. *F*, Necrolytic migratory erythema. Intact and crusted vesicular lesions. *G*, Xanthomas of the hock region in a cat. (Courtesy of K. Helton.) *H*, Xanthomas of the pads of a cat. (Courtesy of D. Chester.)

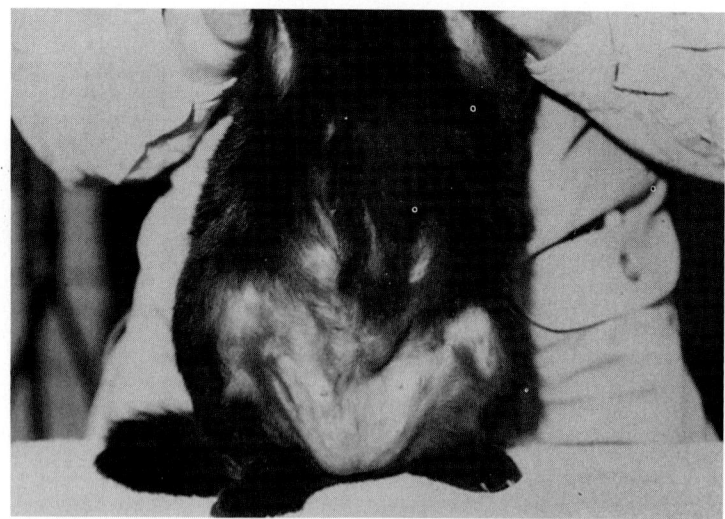

FIGURE 10–49. Diabetes mellitus in a cat. Abdominal hair loss.

cause of the degeneration is unknown but probably results from cellular starvation or some other nutritional imbalance. Cutaneous hypoaminoacidemia or deficiencies in biotin, essential fatty acids, or zinc have been proposed.[433, 442, 443] These nutritional deficiencies result from metabolic abnormalities caused by hyperglucagonemia, liver dysfunction, or combinations of these.

In humans, necrolytic migratory erythema is a cutaneous marker for an α_2-glucagon–producing islet cell tumor of the pancreas. Successful resection of the tumor corrects the metabolic irregularities associated with the hyperglucagonemia, and the eruption heals spontaneously. In a small percentage of patients, necrolytic migratory erythema occurs in association with hepatic cirrhosis and its associated hyperglucagonemia, pancreatitis, celiac sprue, or zinc deficiency.[450] A reverse in the incidence data appears to be true in dogs. Approximately 75 cases of necrolytic migratory erythema in dogs are reported in the veterinary literature, and only five (6.7%) have had a documented pancreatic tumor. The remainder of patients have hepatic disease that is well characterized ultrasonographically and histologically. Although the hepatopathy occasionally has been associated with the ingestion of mycotoxins or anticonvulsant medications, its cause in most dogs is unknown.[450] Dogs with glucagonomas typically have elevated plasma glucagon levels,[423, 444, 451, 452] whereas those with hepatic disease most often do not. The inability to consistently document hyperglucagonemia in the liver group probably relates to the highly efficient extraction of glucagon from the plasma by the liver.[450] The one case reported in the cat was associated with a pancreatic tumor.[447]

CLINICAL FEATURES

Necrolytic migratory erythema is typically seen in old dogs.[433, 442, 443, 454] No consistent breed predisposition has been identified. Skin disease is the presenting complaint in most dogs, although the eruption occasionally develops after the recognition of systemic illness, especially the polyuria and polydipsia associated with diabetes mellitus.[443] Skin lesions occur in areas of trauma, especially the muzzle, mucocutaneous areas of the face (see Fig. 10–48C), distal limbs, and footpads (see Fig. 10–48D). Lesions can also be in the mouth, on the pinnae, on the external genitalia (see Fig. 10–48E), on the elbows and hocks, and along the ventrum. Most lesions are crusted with subjacent erosion or ulceration, but intact vesicular lesions (see Fig. 10–48F) occur occasionally.

Routine laboratory evaluation of most dogs usually shows normocytic, normochromic, nonregenerative anemia; borderline or frank hyperglycemia; elevations in activity of liver enzymes, especially serum alkaline phosphatase and alanine aminotransferase; and hypoalbuminemia.[443] Dogs with liver disease have increased sulfobromophthalein retention or postprandial bile acid levels, abnormal liver anatomy on palpation, and a unique, pathognomonic "honeycomb" pattern on ultrasound evaluation of the liver.[450] Antinuclear antibody titers can be postive.[443, 444] In contrast, dogs with pancreatic tumors typically show no biochemical abnormalities other than hypoalbuminemia. The liver is normal by palpation and ultrasonography. Ultrasonographic identification of the pancreatic mass is extremely rare. Special laboratory tests show hypoaminoacidemia, variable plasma glucagon concentrations, and elevated insulin concentrations.[433]

The one case reported in the cat occurred in an 11-year-old with a short history of anorexia, depression, and skin disease.[447] The initial skin lesions involved the axillae, proximal front limbs, and dorsum. With time, the ventrum, lateral thorax, and groin became involved. The dorsal skin was thickened and covered with adherent white scales, whereas the lesions elsewhere were exudative, alopecic, and reddened. Clinical biochemical abnormalities were nonspecific, and none of the alterations typical in the dog was present. At necropsy, the liver was enlarged and a large pancreatic carcinoma was present at the junction of the left and right lobes.

DIAGNOSIS

The differential diagnostic considerations in the dog include pemphigus foliaceus, systemic lupus erythematosus, zinc deficiency, and generic dog food dermatosis. If the laboratory evaluation is performed before skin biopsy, all differential diagnostic considerations except systemic lupus erythematosus can be excluded because dogs with pemphigus foliaceus, zinc deficiency, and generic dog food dermatosis rarely have the abnormalities described. If all cases in the cat resemble the one reported, the differential diagnosis should include the exfoliative dermatitis associated with thymoma, FeLV- or FIV-associated dermatitis, pemphigus foliaceus, or acquired skin fragility syndrome with secondary bacterial folliculitis.

Cytologic examination of the vesicular fluid reveals complete acellularity in this disorder, whereas inflammatory cells occur in the other differential diagnostic conditions. Skin biopsy of early lesions shows diffuse parakeratotic hyperkeratosis, with high-level confluent vacuolation of keratinocytes resulting in a band of upper-level epidermal edema (Figs. 10–50 and 10–51).[4, 433] Dermal changes are usually minimal and include superficial edema and a perivascular accumulation of lymphocytes and plasma cells. Chronic lesions rarely show the epidermal edema and have marked parakeratotic hyperkeratosis, epidermal hyperplasia, and surface crusting. Chronic lesions may have a superficial interstitial to lichenoid inflammatory infiltrate. Bacteria, dermatophytes, or yeast may be visible in the superficial keratin layer.

CLINICAL MANAGEMENT

Necrolytic migratory erythema is a cutaneous marker for a serious internal disease with a short survival time. One study showed that most dogs died or were euthanized within 5 months of the development of skin lesions.[443] Cases due to an identifiable glucagonoma should be treated surgically. Because dogs with necrolytic migratory erythema often have subclinical pancreatitis, surgery can be difficult with a significant risk of postoperative complications.[432] Although too few cases have been reported, glucagonomas in dogs appear to metastasize quickly.[423, 444, 451, 452] In these cases, removal of the primary tumor can return the dog to normal for an extended but not indefinite period of time. One of us (W.H.M.) administered somatostatin (6 μg/kg subcutaneously q8h) to a dog with a metastatic tumor, and the skin lesions vastly improved within 14 days. Because of renal dysfunction and the high cost of the somatostatin ($100 per day), the treatments were not continued and the dog was euthanized.

Dogs with liver disease are more problematic. Treatment with corticosteroids usually improves the skin lesions but eventually precipitates a diabetic crisis.[454] Unless the hepatopathy is associated with mycotoxin ingestion, anticonvulsant medications, or some other

872 • Endocrine and Metabolic Diseases

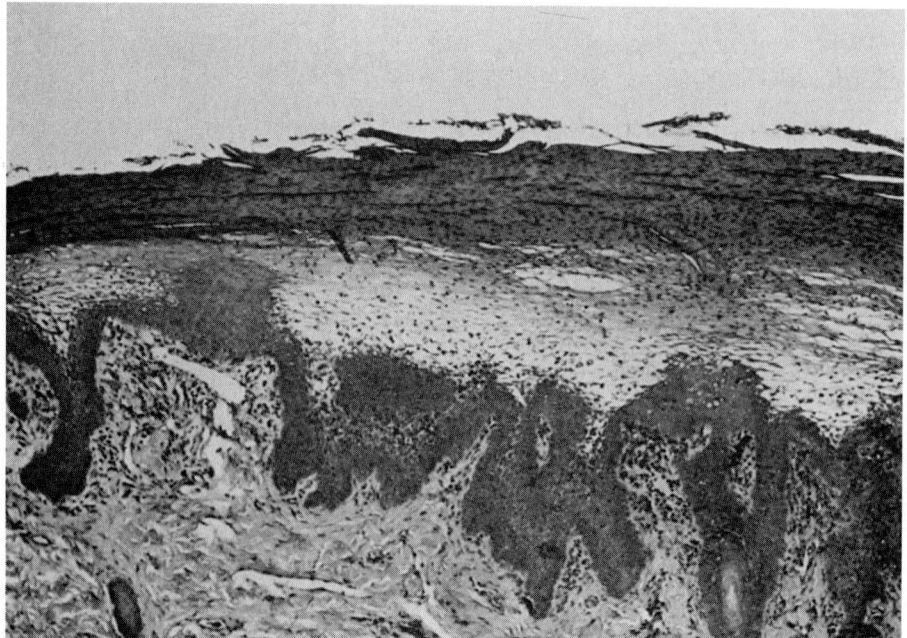

FIGURE 10–50. Canine necrolytic migratory erythema. Marked edema of the upper one half of epidermis with diffuse parakeratotic hyperkeratosis.

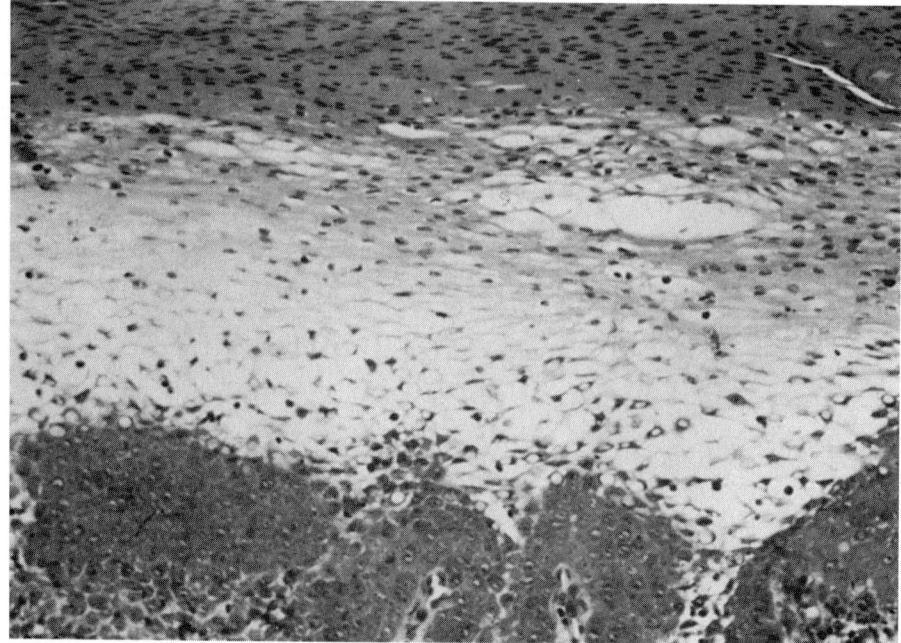

FIGURE 10–51. Close-up of Figure 10–50. Marked intercellular and intracellular edema with parakeratotic hyperkeratosis.

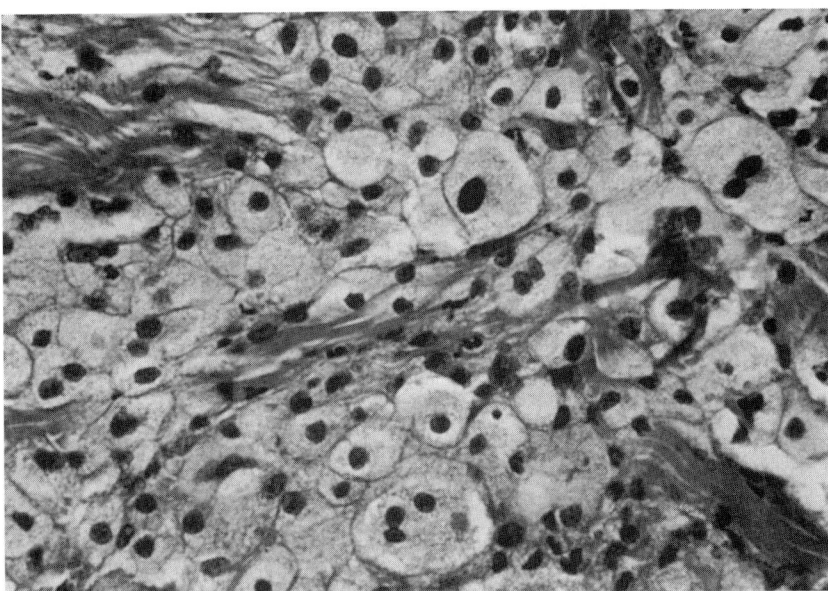

FIGURE 10–52. Feline xanthoma. Typical xanthoma cells.

resolvable condition, the animal cannot be cured. Because the skin lesions have a nutritional basis, supplementation can be of some benefit. The formula used most widely was developed at the University of California[433] and consists of high-quality protein (1 egg yolk/4.5 kg), a zinc supplement (e.g., zinc sulfate: 10 mg/kg/day), and a fatty acid supplement. If there is any clinical or biochemical evidence of pancreatitis, pancreatic enzymes can be added. Although amino acid hyperalimentation should be beneficial, it is very expensive and may not be of significant benefit.[450] If an amino acid profile is available, a supplement specifically formulated for the patient can be used. Some investigators use the commercially available large animal product (Aminosyn, Abbott) and administer 500 ml/dog over 6 to 8 hours.[449] Because the supplementation does not address the underlying hepatopathy, the disease progresses and eventually results in the animal's death.

Xanthomas

Xanthomas are benign granulomatous lesions associated with an abnormality in lipid metabolism. Xanthomatosis has been reported in cats with presumed hereditary hyperlipoproteinemia.[429, 431, 438] No reports of xanthomatosis in Miniature schnauzers with hyperlipidemia have been presented. Cases of apparently idiopathic xanthomas have been reported in the cat.[427, 429] Most cases of xanthomatosis in dogs[428] and cats[17, 437, 440] have been associated with the feeding of high-fat foods or treats[453] or with naturally occurring or drug-induced (megestrol acetate) diabetes mellitus.[145]

Lesions consist of multiple whitish or yellow papules, nodules, or plaques, which may be ulcerated (see Fig. 10–48G and H). The surrounding skin is erythematous, and the lesions can be painful or pruritic. The head, distal extremities, feet, and bony prominences are typically involved.

Histopathologically, there is a nodular to diffuse infiltration of foamy macrophages and variable numbers of multinucleate histiocytic giant cells (Fig. 10–52). Lipid lakes are often prominent throughout the affected dermis. Granulomatous inflammation and fibroplasia may also occur.

Lesions associated with diabetes mellitus or hyperlipoproteinemia resolve spontaneously with resolution of the underlying problem. Surgical removal without correction of the triggering cause usually results in relapse.[427] In cats with idiopathic hypertriglyceridemia and xanthomatosis,[431] feeding a low-fat commercial diet (Prescription Diet canine r/d [Hill's]) resulted in complete clinical remission within 30 days. New lesions developed each time a regular commercial cat food was given for even a short period of time.

Minoxidil in Canine Alopecia

Minoxidil is a vasodilator that has been used topically or orally to treat people with pattern baldness and alopecia areata.[448] Minoxidil is known to increase cutaneous blood flow, have direct effects on keratinocytes (prolong life in culture, stimulate differentiation, and increase mitotic activity of matrix cells), and suppress lymphocyte-mediated immunologic phenomena.

When neonatal descendants of Mexican hairless dogs were treated topically with 3% minoxidil daily for 1 month, all dogs grew hair.[439] Application to adult dogs of this breeding resulted in no hair growth. Other dogs with alopecia of undetermined cause have been treated with minoxidil.[425, 435] In the most detailed study,[435] all dogs had bilaterally symmetric alopecia isolated to the flank or dorsal lumbar regions, and all dogs were breeds (Boxer, Doberman pinscher, Staffordshire bull terrier, and Airedale terrier) prone to follicular dysplasia, some cases of which are seasonally recurrent (see Chaps. 10 and 11). Dogs were treated with 0.1 to 0.5 mg/kg of minoxidil given orally every 24 hours. Of 12 dogs studied, 4 had a good response, 2 had a partial response, 4 had no response, and 2 dogs spontaneously regrew their hair before treatment could be given. These data are difficult to interpret and could all be explained by a spontaneously waxing and waning follicular dysplasia. In addition, 50% of the treated dogs experienced moderate to severe side effects, including weakness, lethargy, and collapse. We do not recommend the use of oral minoxidil in dogs at this time.

• References

General References

1. Chastain CB, Ganjam VK: Clinical Endocrinology of Companion Animals. Lea & Febiger, Philadelphia, 1986.
2. Feldman EC, Nelson RW: Canine and Feline Endocrinology and Reproduction, 2nd ed. W.B. Saunders Co., Philadelphia, 1996.
3. Greco DS: Endocrine emergencies. Part II: Adrenal, thyroid, and parathyroid disorders. Comp Cont Educ 19:27, 1997.
4. Gross TL, et al: Veterinary Dermatopathology. Mosby Year Book, St. Louis, 1992.
5. Hess RS, Ward CR: Diabetes mellitus, hyperadrenocorticism, and hypothyroidism in a dog. J Am Anim Hosp Assoc 34:204, 1998.
6. Kemppainen RJ, et al: Endocrine responses of normal cats to TSH and synthetic ACTH administration. J Am Anim Hosp Assoc 20:737, 1984.
7. Kooistra HS, et al: Polyglandular deficiency syndrome in a boxer dog: Thyroid hormone and glucocorticoid deficiency. Vet Q 17:59, 1995.
8. Meij BP, et al: Assessment of a combined anterior pituitary function test in beagle dogs: Rapid sequential intravenous administration of four hypothalamic releasing hormones. Dom Anim Endocrinol 13:161, 1996.
9. Meij BP, et al: Thyroid-stimulating hormone responses after single administration of thyrotropin-releasing hormone and combined administration of four hypothalamic releasing hormones in beagle dogs. Dom Anim Endocrinol 13:465, 1996.
10. Moriello KA, et al: Determination of thyroxine, triiodothyronine, and cortisol changes during simultaneous adrenal and thyroid function tests in healthy dogs. Am J Vet Res 48:458, 1987.
11. Muller and Kirk's Small Animal Dermatology, 5th ed. W.B. Saunders Co., Philadelphia, 1995.
12. Quadri SK, Palazzolo DL: How aging affects the canine endocrine system. Vet Med 86:692, 1991.
13. Reimers TJ, et al: Changes in serum thyroxine and cortisol in dogs after simultaneous injection of TSH and ACTH. J Am Anim Hosp Assoc 18:923, 1982.
14. Rosychuk RAW: Cutaneous manifestations of endocrine disease in dogs. Compend Cont Educ Pract Vet 20:287, 1998.
15. Scott DW: Feline dermatology 1900–1978: A monograph. J Am Anim Hosp Assoc 16:331, 1980.
16. Scott DW: Histopathologic findings in the endocrine skin disorders of the dog. J Am Anim Hosp Assoc 18: 73, 1982.
17. Scott DW: Feline dermatology 1979–1982: Introspective retrospections. J Am Anim Hosp Assoc 20:537, 1984.

Thyroid Physiology and Disease

18. Ahsan MK, et al: Immunohistochemical localization of thyroid hormone nuclear receptors in human hair follicles and in vitro effect of l-triiodothyronine on cultured cell of hair follicles and skin. J Med Invest 44: 179, 1998.
19. Arnold U, et al: Goitrous hypothyroidism and dwarfism in a kitten. J Am Anim Hosp Assoc 20:735, 1984.
20. Beale KM: Dermatologic manifestations of hypothyroidism. In: Hypothyroidism: Diagnosis and Clinical Manifestations. Daniels Pharmaceuticals, St. Petersburg, 1993, p 16.

21. Beale KM, et al: Correlation of racing and reproductive performance in Greyhounds with response to thyroid function testing. J Am Anim Hosp Assoc 28:263, 1992.
22. Beale KM, et al: Prevalence of antithyroglobulin antibodies detected by enzyme-linked immunosorbent assay of canine serum. J Am Vet Med Assoc 196:745, 1990.
23. Beale KM, et al: Serum thyroid hormone concentrations and thyrotropin responsiveness in dogs with generalized dermatologic disease. J Am Vet Med Assoc 201:1715, 1992.
24. Beale KM, et al: Comparison of two doses of aqueous bovine thyrotropin for thyroid function testing in dogs. J Am Vet Med Assoc 197:865, 1990.
25. Behrend EN, et al: Effect of storage conditions on cortisol, total thyroxine, and free thyroxine concentrations in serum and plasma of dogs. J Am Vet Med Assoc 212:1564, 1998.
26. Benjamin SA, et al: Association between lymphocytic thyroiditis, hypothyroidism, and thyroid neoplasia in beagles. Vet Pathol 33:486, 1996.
27. Bichsel P, et al: Neurologic manifestations associated with hypothyroidism in four dogs. J Am Vet Med Assoc 192:1745, 1989.
28. Brent BA, Hershman JM: Thyroxine therapy in patients with severe nonthyroidal illnesses and low thyroxine concentration. J Clin Endocrinol Metab 63:1, 1986.
29. Bruner JM, et al: Effect of time of sample collection in serum thyroid-stimulating hormone concentrations in euthyroid and hypothyroid dogs. J Am Vet Med Assoc 212:1572, 1998.
30. Bruyette DS, et al: Effect of thyrotropin storage on thyroid-stimulating hormone response testing in normal dogs. J Vet Intern Med 1:91, 1987.
31. Budsberg SC, et al: Thyroxin-responsive unilateral forelimb lameness and generalized neuromuscular disease in four hypothyroid dogs. J Am Vet Med Assoc 202:1859, 1993.
32. Campbell KL, Davis CA: Effects of thyroid hormones on serum and cutaneous fatty acid concentrations in dogs. Am J Vet Res 51:752, 1990.
33. Chastain CB, et al: Congenital hypothyroidism in a dog due to an iodide organification defect. Am J Vet Res 44:1257, 1983.
34. Chastain CB, et al: Anti-triiodothyronine antibodies associated with hypothyroidism and lymphocytic thyroiditis in a dog. J Am Vet Med Assoc 194:531, 1989.
35. Chastain CB: Unusual manifestations of hypothyroidism in dogs. In: Kirk RW, Bonagura JD (eds): Kirk's Current Veterinary Therapy XI. W.B. Saunders Co., Philadelphia, 1992, p 327.
36. Conaway DH, et al: Clinical and histological features of primary progressive, familial thyroiditis in a colony of borzoi dogs. Vet Pathol 22:439, 1985.
37. Cortese L, et al: Hyperprolactinemia and galactorrhea associated with primary hypothyroidism in a bitch. J Small Anim Pract 38:572, 1997.
38. Credille KM, et al: Clinical, morphologic, morphometric, and cell proliferation assessment of hair follicles in canine hypothyroidism. J Invest Dermatol 110:581, 1998.
39. Daminet S, et al: Short-term influence of prednisone and phenobarbital on thyroid function in euthyroid dogs. Can Vet J 40:411, 1999.
40. Deeg C, et al: Canine Hypothyreose: Nachweis von Autoantikörpern gegen Thyreoglobulin. Tierarztl Prax 25:170, 1997.
41. Delverdier M, et al: Les mucinoses cutanées du chien et du chat: Étude histologique et histochimique à partir de 106 cas. Rev Méd Vét 146:33, 1995.
42. Dixon RM, et al: Comparison of endogenous serum thyrotropin (cTSH) concentrations with bovine TSH response test results in euthyroid and hypothyroid dogs. Proc Annu Meet Am Coll Vet Intern Med 15:668, 1997.
43. Dixon RM, Mooney CT: Evaluation of serum free thyroxine and thyrotropin concentrations in the diagnosis of canine hypothyroidism. J Small Anim Pract 40:72, 1999.
44. Dixon RM, et al: Serum thyrotropin concentrations: A new diagnostic test for canine hypothyroidism. Vet Rec 138:594, 1996.
45. Dixon RM, Mooney CT: Canine serum thyroglobulin autoantibodies in health, hypothyroidism, and nonthyroidal illness. Res Vet Sci 66:243, 1999.
45a. Dixon RM, et al: Epidemiological, clinical, haematological and biochemical characteristics of canine hypothyroidism. Vet Rec 145:481, 1999.
46. Doliger S, et al: Histochemical study of cutaneous mucins in hypothyroid dogs. Vet Pathol 32:628, 1995.
47. Engler D, Burger AG: The deiodination of the iodothyronines and of their derivatives in man. Endocrinol Rev 5:151, 1984.
48. Ferguson DC: An internal medical perspective of hypothyroidism. In: Hypothyroidism: Diagnosis and Clinical Manifestations. Daniels Pharmaceuticals, St. Petersburg, 1993, p 2.
49. Ferguson DC, Hoenig M: Reexamination of dosage regimens for l-thyroxine (T_4) in the dog: Bioavailability and persistence of TSH suppression. Proc Annu Meet Am Coll Vet Intern Med 15:668, 1997.
50. Ford SL, et al: Insulin resistance in three dogs with hypothyroidism and diabetes mellitus. J Am Vet Med Assoc 202:1478, 1993.
51. Frank LA: Comparison of thyrotropin-releasing hormone (TRH) to thyrotropin (TSH) simulation for evaluating thyroid function in dogs. J Am Anim Hosp Assoc 32:481, 1996.
52. Gaschen F, et al: Recognition of triiodothyronine-containing epitopes in canine thyroglobulin by circulating thyroglobulin autoantibodies. Am J Vet Res 54:244, 1993.
53. Gaskill CL, et al: Effects of phenobarbital treatment on serum thyroxine and thyroid-stimulating hormone concentrations in epileptic dogs. J Am Vet Med Assoc 215:489, 1999.
54. Gookin JL, et al: Clinical hypothyroidism associated with trimethoprim-sulfadiazine administration in a dog. J Am Vet Med Assoc 214:1028, 1999.
55. Gosselin SJ, et al: Autoimmune lymphocytic thyroiditis in dogs. Vet Immunol Immunopathol 3:185, 1982.
56. Graham PA, et al: Heterogeneity of thyroid function in beagles with lymphocytic thyroiditis. Proc Annu Meet Am Coll Vet Intern Med 15:667, 1997.
57. Graves TK, Peterson ME: Occult hyperthyroidism in cats. In: Kirk RW, Bonagura JD (eds): Kirk's Current Veterinary Therapy XI. W.B. Saunders Co., Philadelphia, 1992, p 334.
58. Greco DS, et al: The effect of levothyroxine treatment on resting energy expenditure of hypothyroid dogs. J Vet Intern Med 12:7, 1998.
59. Greco D: Use of endogenous thyrotropin and free thyroxine determinations for monitoring thyroid re-

59. placement treatment in dogs with hypothyroidism. In: Bonagura JD (ed): Kirk's Current Veterinary Therapy XIII. W.B. Saunders Co., Philadelphia, 1999, p 330.
60. Greco DS, et al: Congenital hypothyroid dwarfism in a family of Giant Schnauzers. J Vet Intern Med 5:57, 1991.
61. Gunaratnam P: The effect of thyroxine on hair growth on the dog. J Small Anim Pract 27:17, 1986.
62. Haines DM, et al: Survey of thyroglobulin autoantibodies in dogs. Am J Vet Res 45:1493, 1984.
63. Haines DM, et al: The detection of canine autoantibodies to thyroid antigens by enzyme-linked immunosorbent assay, hemagglutination, and indirect immunofluorescence. Can J Comp Med 48:262, 1984.
64. Haines DM, Penhale WJ: Experimental thyroid autoimmunity in the dog. Vet Immunol Immunopathol 9:221, 1985.
65. Hall IA, et al: Effect of trimethoprim/sulfamethoxazole on thyroid function in dogs with pyoderma. J Am Vet Med Assoc 202:1159, 1993.
66. Hansen SR, et al: Acute overdose of levothyroxine in a dog. J Am Vet Med Assoc 200:1512, 1992.
67. Hasler A, Rohner K: Schwerwiegende Reaktionen nach TSH-Stimulationstest beim Hund. Schweiz Arch Tierheilkd 134:423, 1992.
67a. Henik RA, Dixon RM: Intravenous administration of levothyroxine for treatment of suspected myxedema coma complicated by severe hypothermia in a dog. J Am Vet Med Assoc 216:713, 2000.
68. Héripret D: Diagnostic biologique de l'hypothyroïdie canine. Prat Méd Chir Anim Comp 32:31, 1997.
69. Hoenig M, Ferguson DC: Comparison of TRH-stimulated thyrotropin (cTSH) to TRH- and TSH-stimulated T_4 in euthyroid, hypothyroid, and sick dogs. Proc Annu Meet Am Coll Vet Intern Med 15:668, 1997.
70. Hoenig M, Ferguson DC: Assessment of thyroid functional reserve in the cat by the thyrotropin-stimulation test. Am J Vet Res 44:1229, 1983.
71. Iversen L, et al: Development and validation of an improved enzyme-linked immunosorbent assay for the detection of thyroglobulin autoantibodies in canine serum samples. Domest Anim Endocrinol 15:525, 1998.
72. Iversen L, et al: Evaluation of the analytical performance of an enzyme immunometric assay (EIA) designed to measure endogenous thyroid-stimulating hormone (TSH) in canine serum samples. J Vet Med Assoc 45:93, 1998.
72a. Iversen L, et al: Biological variation of canine serum thyrotropin (TSH) concentration. Vet Clin Pathol 28:16, 1999.
73. Jensen AL, et al: Evaluation of an immunoradiometric assay for thyrotropin in serum and plasma samples of dogs with primary hypothyroidism. J Comp Pathol 114:339, 1996.
74. Jones BR, et al: Preliminary studies on congenital hypothyroidism in a family of Abyssinian cats. Vet Rec 131:145, 1992.
75. Kantrowitz LB, et al: Serum total thyroxine, total triiodothyronine, free thyroxine, and thyrotropin concentrations in epileptic dogs treated with anticonvulsants. J Am Vet Med Assoc 214:1804, 1999.
76. Kaufman J, et al: Serum concentrations of thyroxine, 3,5,3'-triiodothyronine, thyrotropin, and prolactin in dogs before and after thyrotropin-releasing hormone administration. Am J Vet Res 46:486, 1985.
77. Kelly MJ, Hill JR: Canine myxedema stupor and coma. Comp Cont Educ 6:1049, 1984.
78. Kemppainen RJ: Laboratory diagnosis of hypothyroidism. In: Hypothyroidism: Diagnosis and Clinical Manifestations. Daniels Pharmaceuticals, St. Petersburg, 1993, p 10.
79. Kemppainen RJ, Young DW: Canine triiodothyronine autoantibodies. In: Kirk RW, Bonagura JD (eds): Kirk's Current Veterinary Therapy XI. W.B. Saunders Co., Philadelphia, 1992, p 327.
80. Kemppainen RJ, et al: Autoantibodies to triiodothyronine and thyroxine in a golden retriever. J Am Anim Hosp Assoc 32:195, 1996.
81. Kobayashi DL, et al: Serum thyroid hormone concentrations in clinically normal dogs after administration of freshly reconstituted versus previously frozen and stored thyrotropin. J Am Vet Med Assoc 197:597, 1990.
82. Larsson MG: Determination of free thyroxine and cholesterol as a new screening test for canine hypothyroidism. J Am Anim Hosp Assoc 24:209, 1988.
83. Laurberg P: Iodothyronine deiodination in the canine thyroid. Domest Anim Endocrinol 1:1, 1984.
84. Li WI, et al: Effects of thyrotropin-releasing hormone on serum concentrations of thyroxine and triiodothyronine in healthy, thyroidectomized, thyroxine-treated, and propylthiouracil-treated dogs. Am J Vet Res 47:163, 1986.
85. Liu SK, et al: Clinical and pathologic findings in dogs with atherosclerosis: 21 cases (1970–1983). J Am Vet Med Assoc 189:227, 1986.
86. Lucke VM, et al: Thyroid pathology in canine hypothyroidism. J Comp Pathol 93:415, 1983.
87. Medleau L, et al: Congenital hypothyroidism in a dog. J Am Anim Hosp Assoc 21:341, 1985.
88. Meij BP, et al: Thyroid-stimulating hormone responses after single administration of thyroid-releasing hormone and combined administration of four hypothalamic releasing hormones in beagle dogs. Domest Anim Endocrinol 13:465, 1996.
89. Melian C, et al: Evaluation of free T_4 and endogenous TSH as diagnostic tests for hypothyroidism in dogs. Proc Annu Meet Am Coll Vet Intern Med 15:667, 1997.
90. Meric SM, Rubin SI: Serum thyroxine concentrations following fixed-dose radioactive iodine treatment in hyperthyroid cats: 62 cases (1986–1989). J Am Vet Med Assoc 197:621, 1990.
91. Miller AB, et al: Serial thyroid hormone concentrations in healthy euthyroid dogs, dogs with hypothyroidism, and euthyroid dogs with atopic dermatitis. Br Vet J 148:451, 1992.
92. Mooney CT, Anderson TJ: Congenital hypothyroidism in a boxer dog. J Small Anim Pract 34:31, 1993.
93. Mooney CT, et al: Effect of illness not associated with the thyroid gland on serum total and free thyroxine concentrations in cats. J Am Vet Med Assoc 208:2004, 1996.
94. Mooney CT, Thoday KL: CVT update: Medical treatment of hyperthyroidism in cats. In: Bonagura JD (ed): Kirk's Current Veterinary Therapy XIII. W.B. Saunders Co., Philadelphia, 1999, p 333.
95. Moore GE, et al: Effects of oral administration of anti-inflammatory doses of prednisolone on thyroid hormone response to thyrotropin-releasing hormone and thyrotropin in clinically normal dogs. Am J Vet Res 54:1993.
96. Nachreiner RF, Refsal KR: Radioimmunoassay moni-

96. toring with thyroid hormone concentrations in dogs on thyroid replacement therapy: 2674 cases (1985–1987). J Am Vet Med Assoc 201:623, 1992.
97. Nachreiner RF, et al: Pharmacokinetics of L-thyroxine after its oral administration in dogs. Am J Vet Res 54:2091, 1993.
98. Nachreiner RF, et al: Prevalence of autoantibodies to thyroglobulin in dogs with nonthyroidal illness. Am J Vet Res 59:951, 1998.
99. Nelson RW, Ihle SL: Hypothyroidism in dogs and cats: A difficult deficiency to diagnose. Vet Med 82:60, 1987.
100. Nelson RW, et al: Serum free thyroxine concentration in healthy dogs, dogs with hypothyroidism, and euthyroid dogs with concurrent illness. J Am Vet Med Assoc 198:1401, 1991.
101. Panciera DL: Canine hypothyroidism. Part I. Clinical findings and control of thyroid hormone secretion and metabolism. Comp Cont Educ 12:689, 1990.
102. Panciera DL: Canine hypothyroidism. Part II: Thyroid function tests and treatment. Comp Cont Educ 12:943, 1990.
103. Panciera DL, Post K: Effect of oral administration of sulfadiazine and trimethoprim in combination on thyroid function in dogs. Can J Vet Res 56:349, 1992.
104. Panciera DL, et al: Thyroid function tests in euthyroid dogs treated with L-thyroxine. Am J Vet Res 51:22, 1989.
105. Panciera DL, et al: Quantitative morphologic study on the pituitary and thyroid glands of dogs administered L-thyroxine. Am J Vet Res 51:27, 1990.
106. Panciera DL: Hypothyroidism in dogs: 66 cases (1987–1992). J Am Vet Med Assoc 204:761, 1994.
107. Panciera DL: Thyroid-function testing: Is the future here? Vet Med 92:50, 1997.
108. Panciera DL, Johnson GS: Plasma von Willebrand factor antigen concentration in dogs with hypothyroidism. J Am Vet Med Assoc 205:1550, 1994.
109. Panciera DL, Johnson GS: Plasma von Willebrand factor antigen concentration and buccal mucosal bleeding time in dogs with experimental hypothyroidism. J Vet Intern Med 10:60, 1996.
110. Panciera DL: An echocardiographic and electrocardiographic study of cardiovascular function in hypothyroid dogs. J Am Vet Med Assoc 205:996, 1994.
111. Panciera DL: Clinical manifestations of canine hypothyroidism. Vet Med 92:44, 1997.
112. Panciera DL: Treating hypothyroidism. Vet Med 92:58, 1997.
113. Panciera DL: Complications and concurrent conditions associated with hypothyroidism in dogs. In: Bonagura JD (ed): Kirk's Current Veterinary Therapy XIII. W.B. Saunders Co., Philadelphia, 1999, p 327.
114. Panciera DL: Is it possible to diagnose canine hypothyroidism? J Small Anim Pract 40:152, 1999.
115. Paradis M, Page N: Serum free thyroxine concentrations measured by chemiluminescence in hyperthyroid and euthyroid cats. J Am Anim Hosp Assoc 32:489, 1996.
116. Paradis M, et al: Effects of administration of low dose of frozen thyrotropin on serum total thyroxine concentrations in clinically normal dogs. Can Vet J 35:367, 1994.
117. Paradis M, et al: Serum-free thyroxine concentrations, measured by chemiluminescence assay before and after thyrotropin administration in healthy dogs, hypothyroid dogs, and euthyroid dogs with dermatopathies. Can Vet J 37:289, 1996.
118. Paradis M, et al: Studies of various diagnostic methods for canine hypothyroidism. Vet Dermatol 2:125, 1991.
119. Patterson JS, et al: Neurologic manifestations of cerebrovascular atherosclerosis associated with primary hypothyroidism in a dog. J Am Vet Med Assoc 186:499, 1985.
120. Peterson ME, et al: Effects of spontaneous hyperadrenocorticism on serum thyroid hormone concentrations in the dog. Am J Vet Res 45:2034, 1984.
121. Peterson ME, Camble DA: Effect of nonthyroidal illness on serum thyroxine concentrations in cats: 494 cases (1988). J Am Vet Med Assoc 197:1203, 1990.
122. Peterson ME: Feline hypothyroidism. In: Kirk RW (ed): Current Veterinary Therapy X. W.B. Saunders Co., Philadelphia, 1989, p 1000.
123. Peterson ME, et al: Measurement of serum concentrations of total and free T_4 in hyperthyroid cats and cats with nonthyroidal disease. Proc Am Coll Vet Intern Med 16:701, 1998.
124. Peterson ME, et al: Measurement of serum total thyroxine, triiodothyronine, free thyroxine, and thyrotropin concentrations for diagnosis of hypothyroidism in dogs. J Am Vet Med Assoc 211:1396, 1997.
125. Quinlan WJ, Michaelson S: Homologous radioimmunoassay for canine thyrotropin: Response of normal and x-irradiated dogs to propylthiouracil. Endocrinology 108:937, 1981.
126. Rachofsky MA: Clinical relevance of results from the new canine specific endogenous TSH assay: A review of 79 cases. Proc Annu Memb Meet Am Acad Vet Dermatol Am Coll Vet Dermatol 4:1988.
127. Ramsey IK, et al: Thyroid-stimulating hormone and total thyroxine concentrations in euthyroid, sick euthyroid and hypothyroid dogs. J Small Anim Pract 38:540, 1997.
128. Rand JS, et al: Spontaneous adult-onset hypothyroidism in a cat. J Vet Intern Med 7:272, 1993.
129. Refsal KR, et al: Use of triiodothyronine suppression test for diagnosis of hyperthyroidism in ill cats that have serum concentrations of iodothyronines within normal range. J Am Vet Med Assoc 199:1594, 1991.
130. Refsal KR, et al: Thyroid hormone autoantibodies in the dog: Distribution with serum concentrations of thyroxine and thyrotropin in a laboratory survey. Proc Annu Meet Am Coll Vet Intern Med 16:700, 1998.
131. Reimers TJ, et al: Effects of reproductive state on concentrations of thyroxine, 3,5,3'-triiodothyronine and cortisol in serum of dogs. Biol Reprod 31:148, 1984.
132. Reimers TJ, et al: Effect of fasting on thyroxine, 3,5,3'-triiodothyronine, and cortisol concentrations in serum of dogs. Am J Vet Res 47:2485, 1986.
133. Reimers TJ, et al: Effects of age, sex, and body size on serum concentrations of thyroid and adrenocortical hormones in dogs. Am J Vet Res 51:454, 1990.
134. Richardson HW: Evaluation of endogenous cTSH assay RIA test kit in clinically normal and suspect hypothyroid dogs. Proc Annu Memb Meet Am Acad Vet Dermatol Am Coll Vet Dermatol 4:1988.
135. Robinson WF, et al: Congenital hypothyroidism in Scottish deerhound puppies. Aust Vet J 65:386, 1988.
136. Rosenberg RM, et al: Abnormal lipogenesis in thyroid hormone-deficient epidermis. J Invest Dermatol 86:244, 1986.
137. Rosychuk RAW: Dermatologic manifestations of canine hypothyroidism and the usefulness of dermato-

138. Rudas P, et al: Impaired local deiodination of thyroxine to triiodothyronine in dogs with symmetrical truncal alopecia. Vet Res Commun 18:175, 1994.
139. Ruschig S, Kraft W: Bestimmung von caninem Thyreoideastimulierendem Hormon (cTSH) im Blutserum des Hundes und seine Reaktion in TRH-Stimulationstest. Tierarztl Prax 24:479, 1996.
140. Sauvé F, et al: Evaluation de la function thyroidienne chez les chiens de race Terre-Neuve. Méd Vét Québec 27:77, 1997.
141. Sauvé F, Paradis M: Use of recombinant human thyroid-stimulating hormone for thyrotropin stimulation test in euthyroid dogs. Can Vet J 41:215, 2000.
142. Schumm-Draeger PM, Fortmeyer HP: Autoimmune thyroiditis—spontaneous disease models—cats. Exp Clin Endocrinol Diabetes 104:12, 1996.
143. Scott-Moncrieff JCR, Nelson RW: Change in serum thyroid-stimulating hormone concentration in response to administration of thyrotropin-releasing hormone to healthy dogs, hypothyroid dogs, and euthyroid dogs with concurrent diseases. J Am Vet Med Assoc 213:1435, 1998.
144. Scott-Moncrieff JCR, et al.: Comparison of serum concentrations of thyroid-stimulating hormone in healthy dogs, hypothyroid dogs, and euthyroid dogs with concurrent disease. J Am Vet Med Assoc 212:387, 1998.
145. Simpson JW, van den Broek AHM: Fat absorption in dogs with diabetes mellitus or hypothyroidism. Res Vet Sci 50:346, 1991.
146. Sparks AH, et al: Thyroid function in the cat: Assessment by the TRH response test and thyrotropin stimulation test. J Small Anim Pract 32:59, 1991.
147. Sparkes AH, et al: Assessment of dose and time responses to TRH and thyrotropin in healthy dogs. J Small Anim Pract 36:245, 1995.
148. Stephan I, Schutt-Mast I: Kongenitale Hypothyreose mit disproportioniertem Zwergwuchs bei einer Katze. Kleintierpraxis 40:701, 1995.
149. Stolp R, et al: Plasma cortisol response to thyrotropin releasing hormone and luteinizing hormone releasing hormone in healthy kennel dogs and in dogs with pituitary-dependent hyperadrenocorticism. J Endocrinol 93:365, 1982.
150. Sullivan P, et al: Altered platelet indices in dogs with hypothyroidism and cats with hyperthyroidism. Am J Vet Res 54:2004, 1993.
151. Tarttelin MF, et al: Serum free thyroxine levels respond inversely to changes in levels of dietary iodine in the domestic cat. N Z Vet J 40:66, 1992.
152. Thoday KL, et al: Radioimmunoassay of serum total thyroxine and triiodothyronine in cats: Assay methodology and effects of age, sex, breed, heredity, and environment. J Small Anim Pract 25:457, 1984.
153. Thoday KL: Feline hypothyroidism: An experimental study. Vet Dermatol Newsl 12(1), 1989.
154. Thoday KL, Mooney CT: Historical, clinical and laboratory features of 126 hyperthyroid cats. Vet Rec 131:257, 1992.
155. Thoday KL, Mooney CT: Medical management of feline hyperthyroidism. In: Kirk RW, Bonagura JD (eds): Kirk's Current Veterinary Therapy XI. W.B. Saunders Co., Philadelphia, 1992, p 338.
156. Thorneloe C, et al: Evaluation de la thyroxine totale par ELISA chez des chats normanx, hyperthyroïdiens et euthyroïdiens souffrant de maladies systemiques. Méd Vét Québec 27:119, 1997.
157. Torres SMF, et al: Hypothyroidism in a dog associated with trimethoprim-sulfadiazine therapy. Vet Dermatol 7:105, 1996.
158. Torres SMF, et al: Effect of oral administration of prednisolone on thyroid function in dogs. Am J Vet Res 52:416, 1991.
159. Vajner L: Lymphocytic thyroiditis in beagle dogs in a breeding colony: Findings of serum autoantibodies. Vet Med Czech 11:333, 1997.
160. Van Der Walt JA, et al: Functional endocrine modification of the thyroid following ovariectomy in the canine. J S Afr Vet Assoc 54:225, 1983.
161. Wall JR, Kuroki T: Immunologic factors in thyroid disease. Med Clin North Am 69:913, 1985.
162. Wartofsky L, Burman KD: Alterations in thyroid function in patients with systemic illness: The "euthyroid sick syndrome." Endocrinol Rev 3:164, 1982.
163. Wheatley T, Edwards OM: Mild hypothyroidism and oedema: Evidence for increased capillary permeability to protein. Clin Endocrinol 18:627, 1983.
164. Williams DA, et al: Validation of an immunoassay for canine thyroid stimulating hormone and changes in serum concentration following induction of hypothyroidism in dogs. J Am Vet Med Assoc 209:1730, 1996.
165. Yu AA, et al: Effect of endotoxin on hormonal responses to thyrotropin and thyrotropin-releasing hormone in dogs. Am J Vet Res 59:186, 1998.
166. Zeiss CJ, Waddle G: Hypothyroidism and atherosclerosis in dogs. Comp Cont Educ 17:1117, 1995.
167. Zerbe CA, et al: Thyroid profiles in healthy kittens from birth to 12 weeks of age. Proc Annu Meet Am Coll Vet Intern Med 16:702, 1998.

Adrenal Physiology and Disease

168. Angles JM, et al: Use of urine cortisol:creatinine ratio versus adrenocorticotropic hormone stimulation testing for monitoring mitotane treatment of pituitary-dependent hyperadrenocorticism in dogs. J Am Vet Med Assoc 211:1002, 1997.
169. Barthez PY, et al: Ultrasonographic evaluation of the adrenal glands in dogs. J Am Vet Med Assoc 207:1180, 1995.
170. Beale KM, Morris DO: Treatment of canine calcinosis cutis with dimethylsulfoxide gel. Proc Annu Memb Meet Am Acad Vet Dermatol Am Coll Vet Dermatol 14:97, 1998.
171. Behrend EN, et al: Effect of storage conditions on cortisol, total thyroxine, and free thyroxine concentrations in serum and plasma of dogs. J Am Vet Med Assoc 212:1564, 1998.
172. Behrend EN, Kemppainen RJ: Medical therapy of canine Cushing's syndrome. Comp Cont Educ 20:679, 1998.
173. Bennett PF, Norman EJ: Mitotane (o,p'DDD) resistance in a dog with pituitary-dependent hyperadrenocorticism and pheochromocytoma. Aust Vet J 76:101, 1998.
174. Bertoy EH, et al: Magnetic resonance imaging of the brain in dogs with recently diagnosed but untreated pituitary-dependent hyperadrenocorticism. J Am Vet Med Assoc 206:651, 1995.
175. Bertoy EH, et al: One-year follow-up evaluation of magnetic resonance imaging of the brain in dogs with pituitary-dependent hyperadrenocorticism. J Am Vet Med Assoc 208:1268, 1996.

176. Biewenga WJ, et al: Persistent polyuria in two dogs following adrenocorticolysis for pituitary-dependent hyperadrenocorticism. Vet Q 11:193, 1989.
177. Blaxter AC, Gruffydd-Jones TJ: Concurrent diabetes mellitus and hyperadrenocorticism in the dog: Diagnosis and management of eight cases. J Small Anim Pract 31:117, 1990.
178. Boord M, Griffin C: Progesterone secreting adrenal mass in a cat with clinical signs of hyperadrenocorticism. J Am Vet Med Assoc 214:666, 1999.
179. Bruyette DS, et al: L-deprenyl therapy of canine pituitary dependent hyperadrenocorticism. Poster, Am Coll Vet Intern Med Forum, Washington DC, 1993.
180. Bruyette DS, et al: Management of canine pituitary-dependent hyperadrenocorticism with l-deprenyl (Anipryl). Vet Clin North Am 27:273, 1997.
181. Bruyette DS, et al: Treating canine pituitary-dependent hyperadrenocorticism with l-deprenyl. Vet Med 92:711, 1997.
182. Bruyette DS: Anipryl versus lysodren. Proc Am Coll Vet Intern Med 16:525, 1998.
182a. Bruyette DS: An approach to diagnosing and treating feline hyperadrenocorticism. Vet Med 95:142, 2000.
183. Chastain CB, et al: Evaluation of the hypothalamic-pituitary-adrenal axis in clinically stressed dogs. J Am Anim Hosp Assoc 22:435, 1986.
184. Chauvet AE, et al: Effects of phenobarbital administration on results of serum biochemical analyses and adrenocortical function tests in epileptic dogs. J Am Vet Med Assoc 207:1305, 1995.
185. Chrousos GP, et al: Clinical applications of corticotropin-releasing factor. Ann Intern Med 102:344, 1985.
186. Church DB, et al: Effect of nonadrenal illness, anaesthesia and surgery on plasma cortisol concentrations in dogs. Res Vet Sci 56:129, 1994.
187. Daley CA, et al: Use of metyrapone to treat pituitary-dependent hyperadrenocorticism in a cat with large cutaneous wounds. J Am Vet Med Assoc 202:956, 1993.
188. den Hertog E, et al: Results of nonselective adrenocorticolysis by o,p′-DDD in 129 dogs with pituitary-dependent hyperadrenocorticism. Vet Rec 144:12, 1999.
189. Dow SW, et al: Perianal adenomas and hypertestosteronemia in a spayed bitch with pituitary-dependent hyperadrenocorticism. J Am Vet Med Assoc 192:1439, 1988.
190. Dow SW, et al: Response of dogs with functional pituitary macroadenomas and macrocarcinomas to irradiation. J Small Anim Pract 31:287, 1990.
191. Duesberg CA, et al: Adrenalectomy for treatment of hyperadrenocorticism in cats: 10 cases (1900–1992). J Am Vet Med Assoc 207:1066, 1995.
192. Duesberg C, Peterson ME: Adrenal disorders of the cat. Vet Clin North Am 27:321, 1997.
193. Duesberg CA, et al: Magnetic resonance imaging for diagnosis of pituitary macrotumors in dogs. J Am Vet Med Assoc 206:657, 1995.
194. Dunn KJ, et al: Use of ACTH stimulation tests to monitor the treatment of canine hyperadrenocorticism. Vet Rec 137:161, 1995.
195. Dunn KJ: Complications associated with the diagnosis and management of canine hyperadrenocorticism. In Practice 24:246, 1997.
196. Eichenbaum JD, et al: Effect in large dogs of ophthalmic prednisolone acetate on adrenal gland and hepatic function. J Am Anim Hosp Assoc 24:705, 1988.
197. Eiler H, et al: Stages of hyperadrenocorticism: response of hyperadrenocorticoid dogs to the combined dexamethasone suppression/ACTH stimulation test. J Am Vet Med Assoc 185:289, 1984.
198. Emms SG, et al: Adrenalectomy in the management of canine hyperadrenocorticism. J Am Vet Med Assoc 23:557, 1987.
199. Etreby MFE, et al: Functional morphology of spontaneous hyperplastic and neoplastic lesions in the canine pituitary gland. Vet Pathol 17:109, 1980.
200. Feldman EC: Evaluation of a combined dexamethasone suppression/ACTH stimulation test in dogs with hyperadrenocorticism. J Am Vet Med Assoc 187:49, 1985.
201. Feldman EC: Evaluation of a six-hour combined dexamethasone suppression/ACTH stimulation test in dogs with hyperadrenocorticism. J Am Vet Med Assoc 189:1562, 1986.
202. Feldman EC, et al: Comparison of mitotane treatment for adrenal tumor versus pituitary-dependent hyperadrenocorticism in dogs. J Am Vet Med Assoc 200:1642, 1992.
203. Feldman EC, Mack RE: Urine cortisol:creatinine ratio as a screening test for hyperadrenocorticism in dogs. J Am Vet Med Assoc 200:1637, 1992.
204. Feldman EC, Nelson RW: Use of ketoconazole for control of canine hyperadrenocorticism. In: Kirk RW, Bonagura JD (eds): Kirk's Current Veterinary Therapy XI. W.B. Saunders Co., Philadelphia, 1992, p 349.
205. Feldman EC, et al: Plasma cortisol response to ketoconazole administration in dogs with hyperadrenocorticism. J Am Vet Med Assoc 197:71, 1990.
206. Feldman EC, et al: Use of low- and high-dose dexamethasone tests for distinguishing pituitary-dependent from adrenal tumor hyperadrenocorticism in dogs. J Am Vet Med Assoc 209:772, 1996.
207. Ferguson DC, Peterson ME: Serum free and total iodothyronine concentrations in dogs with hyperadrenocorticism. Am J Vet Res 53:1636, 1992.
208. Ford SL, et al: Hyperadrenocorticism caused by bilateral adrenocortical neoplasia in dogs. Four cases (1983–1988). J Am Vet Med Assoc 202:789, 1993.
209. Frank LA, et al: Comparison of cortisol concentrations after administration of cosyntropin at low and high doses. Proc Annu Memb Meet Am Acad Vet Dermatol Am Coll Vet Dermatol 15:99, 1999.
210. Frank LA, Oliver JW: Comparison of serum cortisol concentrations in clinically normal dogs after administration of freshly reconstituted versus reconstituted and stored frozen cosyntropin. J Am Vet Med Assoc 212:1569, 1998.
211. Frazier KS, et al: Multiple cutaneous metaplastic ossification associated with iatrogenic hyperglucocorticoidism. J Vet Diagn Invest 10:303, 1998.
212. Garnier F, et al: Adrenal cortical response in clinically normal dogs before and after adaptation to a housing environment. Lab Anim 24:40, 1990.
213. Gayrard V, et al: Interspecies variations of corticosteroid-binding globulin parameters. Domest Anim Endocrinol 13:35, 1996.
214. Glaze MR, et al: Ophthalmic corticosteroid therapy: Systemic effects in the dog. J Am Vet Med Assoc 192:73, 1988.
215. Goossens MMC, et al: Cobalt 60 irradiation of pituitary gland tumors in three cats with acromegaly. J Am Vet Med Assoc 231:374, 1998.
216. Goossens MMC, et al: Efficacy of cobalt 60 radiotherapy in dogs with pituitary-dependent hyperadrenocorticism. J Am Vet Med Assoc 212:374, 1998.

217. Goossens MMC, et al: Urinary excretion of glucocorticoids in the diagnosis of hyperadrenocorticism in cats. Domest Anim Endocrinol 12:355, 1995.
218. Greco DS, et al: Dexamethasone pharmacokinetics in clinically normal dogs during low- and high-dose dexamethasone suppression testing. Am J Vet Res 54:580, 1992.
219. Greco DS, et al: Pharmacokinetics of exogenous corticotropin in normal dogs, hospitalized dogs with nonadrenal illness and adrenopathic dogs. J Vet Pharmacol Ther 21:369, 1998.
220. Greco DS, et al: Concurrent pituitary and adrenal tumors in dogs with hyperadrenocorticism: 17 cases (1978–1995). J Am Vet Med Assoc 214:1349, 1999.
221. Greene CE: Iatrogenic hyperadrenocorticism in a cat. Feline Pract 23:7, 1995.
222. Grooters AM, et al: Ultrasonographic characteristics of the adrenal glands in dogs with pituitary-dependent hyperadrenocorticism: Comparison with normal dogs. J Vet Intern Med 10:110, 1996.
223. Guptill L, et al: Use of urine cortisol:creatinine ratio to monitor treatment response in dogs with pituitary-dependent hyperadrenocorticism. J Am Vet Med Assoc 210:1158, 1997.
224. Hansen BL, et al: Synthetic ACTH (cosyntropin) stimulation tests in normal dogs: Comparison of intravenous and intramuscular administration. J Am Anim Hosp Assoc 30:38, 1994.
225. Hegstad RL, et al: Effect of sample handling on adrenocorticotropin concentration measured in canine plasma, using a commercially available radioimmunoassay kit. Am J Vet Res 51:1941, 1990.
226. Helton-Rhodes K, et al: Cutaneous manifestations of feline hyperadrenocorticism. In: Ihrke PJ, et al (eds): Advances in Veterinary Dermatology, Vol 2. Pergamon Press, New York, 1993, p 391.
227. Henry CJ, et al: Urine cortisol:creatinine ratio in healthy and sick cats. J Vet Intern Med 10:123, 1996.
228. Hess RS, Ward CR: Concurrent canine hyperadrenocorticism and diabetes mellitus: Diagnosis and treatment. Comp Cont Educ 20:701, 1998.
229. Hess RS, et al: Association between hyperadrenocorticism and development of calcium-containing uroliths in dogs with urolithiasis. J Am Vet Med Assoc 212:1889, 1998.
230. Hoerauf A, Reusch C: Ultrasonographic characteristics of both adrenal glands in 15 dogs with functional adrenocortical tumors. J Am Anim Hosp Assoc 35:193, 1999.
231. Hörauf A, Reusch C: Darstellung der nebennieren mittels Ultraschall: Untersuchungen bei gesunden Hunden, Hunden mit nicht-endokrinen Erkrankungen sowie mit Cushing-syndrom. Kleintier Praxis 40:351, 1995.
232. Huang H, et al: Iatrogenic hyperadrenocorticism in 28 dogs. J Am Anim Hosp Assoc 35:200, 1999.
233. Hurley KJ, Vaden SL: Evaluation of urine protein content in dogs with pituitary-dependent hyperadrenocorticism. J Am Vet Med Assoc 212:369, 1998.
234. Hurley K, et al: The use of Trilostane for the treatment of hyperadrenocorticism in dogs. Proc Annu Meet Am Coll Vet Intern Med 16:700, 1998.
235. Jensen RB, DuFort RM: Hyperadrenocorticism in dogs. Comp Cont Educ 13:615, 1991.
236. Jensen AL, et al: Evaluation of the urinary cortisol:creatinine ratio in the diagnosis of hyperadrenocorticism in dogs. J Small Anim Pract 38:99, 1997.
237. Jones CA, et al: Changes in adrenal cortisol secretion as reflected in the urinary cortisol/creatinine ratio in dogs. Dom Anim Endocrinol 7:559, 1990.
238. Jones CA, et al: Adrenocortical adenocarcinoma in a cat. J Am Anim Hosp Assoc 28:59, 1992.
239. Kaplan AJ, et al: Effects of disease on the results of diagnostic tests for use in detecting hyperadrenocorticism in dogs. J Am Vet Med Assoc 207:445, 1995.
240. Kemppainen RJ, Zenoble RD: Nondexamethasone-suppressible, pituitary-dependent hyperadrenocorticism in a dog. J Am Vet Med Assoc 187:276, 1985.
241. Kemppainen RJ, et al: Ovine corticotrophin-releasing factor in dogs: Dose-response relationships and effects of dexamethasone. Acta Endocrinol 112:12, 1986.
242. Kemppainen RJ, Peterson ME: Circulating concentration of dexamethasone in healthy dogs, dogs with hyperadrenocorticism and dogs with nonadrenal illness during dexamethasone suppression testing. Am J Vet Res 54:1765, 1993.
243. Kemppainen RJ, et al: Plasma free cortisol concentrations in dogs with hyperadrenocorticism. Am J Vet Res 52:682, 1991.
244. Kemppainen RJ, et al: Effects of single intravenously administered doses of dexamethasone on response to the adrenocorticotropic hormone stimulation test in dogs. Am J Vet Res 50:1914, 1989.
245. Kemppainen RJ, Peterson ME: Regulation of α-melanocyte-stimulating hormone secretion from the pars intermedia of domestic cats. Am J Vet Res 60:245, 1999.
246. Kemppainen RJ, Boehrend E: Adrenal physiology. Vet Clin North Am 27:173, 1997.
247. Kemppainen RJ, et al: Preservative effect of aprotinin on canine plasma immunoreactive adrenocorticotropin concentrations. Domest Anim Endocrinol 11:355, 1994.
248. Kerl ME, et al: Evaluation of a low-dose synthetic adrenocorticotropic hormone stimulation test in clinically normal dogs and dogs with naturally developing hyperadrenocorticism. J Am Vet Med Assoc 214:1497, 1999.
249. Kintzer PP, Peterson ME: Mitotane (o,p'-DDD) treatment of 200 dogs with pituitary-dependent hyperadrenocorticism. J Vet Intern Med 5:102, 1991.
250. Kintzer PP, Peterson ME: Mitotane treatment of 32 dogs with cortisol-secreting adrenocortical neoplasms. J Am Vet Med Assoc 205:54, 1994.
251. Kipperman BS, et al: Diabetes mellitus and exocrine pancreatic neoplasia in two cats with hyperadrenocorticism. J Am Anim Hosp Assoc 28:415, 1992.
252. Kipperman BS, et al: Pituitary tumor size, neurologic signs, and relation to endocrine test results in dogs with pituitary-dependent hyperadrenocorticism: 43 cases (1980–1990). J Am Vet Med Assoc 201:762, 1992.
253. Kooistra HS, et al: Correlation between impairment of glucocorticoid feedback and the size of the pituitary gland in dogs with pituitary-dependent hyperadrenocorticism. J Endocrinol 152:387, 1997.
254. LaRue MJ, Murtaugh RJ: Pulmonary thromboembolism in dogs: 47 cases (1986–1987). J Am Vet Med Assoc 197:1368, 1990.
254a. Lusson D, Billiemaz B: Un cas d'hypercorticisme spontané chez un chat. Point Vét 31:57, 2000.
255. Mack RE, Feldman EC: Comparison of two low-dose dexamethasone suppression protocols as screening and discriminating tests in dogs with hyperadrenocorticism. J Am Vet Med Assoc 197:1603, 1990.

256. Mack RE, et al: Diagnosis of hyperadrenocorticism in dogs. Comp Cont Educ 16:311, 1994.
257. Mackedanz R, Struckmann B: Bericht über einem Fall von Hypercortisolismus bei einer Katze. Kleintier Praxis 37:843, 1992.
258. Mauldin GN, Burk RL: The use of diagnostic computerized tomography and radiation therapy in canine and feline hyperadrenocorticism. Probl Vet Med 2:557, 1990.
259. Mbugua SW, et al: Adrenocortical suppression by a glucocorticoid: Effect of a single I. M. injection of betamethasone depot versus placebo given prior to orthopaedic surgery in dogs. Acta Vet Scand 29:415, 1988.
260. Meij BP, et al: Alterations in anterior pituitary function of dogs with pituitary-dependent hyperadrenocorticism. J Endocrinol 154:505, 1997.
261. Meij BP, et al: Assessment of pituitary function after transsphenoidal hypophysectomy in beagle dogs. Domest Anim Endocrinol 14:81, 1997.
262. Meij BP, et al: Residual pituitary function after transsphenoidal hypophysectomy in dogs with pituitary-dependent hyperadrenocorticism. J Endocrinol 155:531, 1997.
263. Meij BP, et al: Results of transsphenoidal hypophysectomy in 52 dogs with pituitary-dependent hyperadrenocorticism. Vet Surg 27:246, 1998.
264. Meyer DJ, et al: Effect of otic medications containing glucocorticoids in liver function tests in healthy dogs. J Am Vet Med Assoc 196:743, 1990.
265. Moore GE, Hoenig M: Effect of orally administered prednisone on glucose tolerance and insulin secretion in clinically normal dogs. Am J Vet Res 54:126, 1993.
266. Moore GE, Hoenig M: Duration of pituitary and adrenocortical suppression after long-term administration of anti-inflammatory doses of prednisone in dogs. Am J Vet Res 53:716, 1992.
267. Muller PB, et al: Effects of phenobarbital treatment on adrenal function tests in dogs. Proc Annu Meet Am Coll Vet Intern Med 16:700, 1998.
268. Murphy CJ, et al: Iatrogenic Cushing's syndrome in a dog caused by topical ophthalmic medication. J Am Anim Hosp Assoc 26:640, 1990.
269. Nelson RW, et al: Hyperadrenocorticism in cats. Seven cases (1978–1987). J Am Vet Med Assoc 193:245, 1988.
270. Nelson RW, Feldman EC: Hyperadrenocorticism. In: August JR (ed): Consultations in Feline Internal Medicine. W.B. Saunders Co., Philadelphia, 1991, p 267.
271. Nelson RW, et al: Pituitary macroadenomas and macroadenocarcinomas in dogs treated with mitotane for pituitary-dependent hyperadrenocorticism: 13 cases (1981–1986). J Am Vet Med Assoc 194:1612, 1989.
272. Nelson RW, et al: Topics in the diagnosis and treatment of canine hyperadrenocorticism. Comp Cont Educ 13:1797, 1991.
273. Nichols R: Problems associated with medical therapy of canine hyperadrenocorticism. Probl Vet Med 2:551, 1990.
274. Nichols R: Concurrent illness and complications associated with hyperadrenocorticism. Probl Vet Med 2:565, 1990.
275. Norman EJ, et al: Dynamic adrenal function testing in eight dogs with hyperadrenocorticism associated with adrenocortical neoplasia. Vet Rec 144:551, 1999.
276. Ortega TM, et al: Systemic arterial blood pressure and urine protein/creatinine ratio in dogs with hyperadrenocorticism. J Am Vet Med Assoc 209:1724, 1996.
277. Penninek DG, et al: Radiographic features of canine hyperadrenocorticism caused by autonomously functioning adrenocortical tumors: 23 cases (1978–1986). J Am Vet Med Assoc 192:1604, 1988.
278. Peterson ME, et al: Immunocytochemical study of the hypophysis in 25 dogs with pituitary-dependent hyperadrenocorticism. Acta Endocrinol 101:15, 1982.
279. Peterson ME, et al: Adrenal function in the cat: comparison of the effects of cosyntropin (synthetic ACTH) and corticotropin gel stimulation. Res Vet Sci 37:331, 1984.
280. Peterson ME: Canine hyperadrenocorticism. In: Kirk RW (ed): Current Veterinary Therapy IX. W.B. Saunders Co., Philadelphia, 1986, p 963.
281. Peterson ME, Steele P: Pituitary-dependent hyperadrenocorticism in a cat. J Am Vet Med Assoc 189:680, 1986.
282. Peterson ME, et al: Plasma immunoreactive ACTH peptides and cortisol in normal dogs and dogs with Addison's disease and Cushing's syndrome: Basal concentrations. Endocrinology 119:720, 1986.
283. Peterson ME, Kemppainen RJ: Dose-response relationship between plasma concentrations of corticotropin and cortisol after administration of incremental doses of cosyntropin for corticotropin stimulation testing in cats. Am J Vet Res 54:300, 1983.
284. Peterson ME, Kemppainen RS: Comparison of immunoreactive plasma corticotropin and cortisol response to two synthetic corticotropin preparations (tetracosactrin and cosyntropin) in healthy cats. Am J Vet Res 53:1752, 1992.
285. Peterson ME, et al: Effects of synthetic ovine corticotropin-releasing hormone on plasma concentrations of immunoreactive adrenocorticotropic, α-melanocyte-stimulating hormone and cortisol in dogs with naturally acquired adrenocortical insufficiency. Am J Vet Res 53:1636, 1992.
286. Peterson ME, et al: Effect of spontaneous hyperadrenocorticism in endogenous production and utilization of glucose in the dog. Dom Anim Endocrinol 3:117, 1986.
287. Pinard SA, et al: Traitement de hypercorticisme spontane du chien par le kétoconazole: A propos de treize cas. Prat Méd Chirurg Anim Cie 30:319, 1995.
288. Poffenbarger EM, et al: Gray-scale ultrasonography in the diagnosis of adrenal neoplasia in dogs: Six cases (1981–1986). J Am Vet Med Assoc 192:228, 1988.
289. Randolph JF, et al: Use of urine cortisol-to-creatinine ratio for monitoring dogs with pituitary-dependent hyperadrenocorticism during induction treatment with mitotane (o,p'-DDD). Am J Vet Res 59:258, 1998.
290. Regnier A, Garnier F: Growth hormone responses to growth hormone-releasing hormone and clonidine in dogs with Cushing's syndrome. Res Vet Sci 58:169, 1995.
291. Reusch CE, Feldman EC: Canine hyperadrenocorticism due to adrenocortical neoplasia. J Vet Intern Med 5:3, 1991.
292. Reusch CE, et al: The efficacy of l-deprenyl in dogs with pituitary-dependent hyperadrenocorticism. J Vet Intern Med 13:291, 1999.
293. Rijnberk A, Belshaw BE: An alternative protocol for the medical management of canine pituitary-dependent hyperadrenocorticism. Vet Rec 122:406, 1988.
294. Rijnberk AD, Belshaw BE: o,p'-DDD treatment of canine hyperadrenocorticism: An alternative protocol.

In: Kirk RW, Bonagura JD (eds): Kirk's Current Veterinary Therapy XI. W.B. Saunders Co., Philadelphia, 1992, p 345.
295. Roberts SM, et al: Effect of ophthalmic prednisolone acetate on the canine adrenal gland and hepatic function. Am J Vet Res 45:1711, 1984.
296. Robson M, et al: Adrenal gland function in the cat. Comp Cont Ed 17:1205, 1995.
297. Rothuizen J, et al: GABAergic inhibition of the pituitary release of adrenocorticotropin and the α-melanotropin is impaired in dogs with hepatic encephalopathy. Domest Anim Endocrinol 13:59, 1996.
298. Rothuizen J, et al: Aging and the hypothalamus-pituitary-adrenocortical axis, with special reference to the dog. Acta Endocrinol (Copenh) 125:73, 1991.
299. Ruehl WW, et al: Adrenal axis dysfunction in geriatric dogs with cognitive dysfunction. Proc Annu Meet Am Coll Vet Intern Med 15:119, 1997
300. Sarfaty D, et al: Neurologic, endocrinologic, and pathologic findings associated with large pituitary tumors in dogs: Eight cases (1976–1984). J Am Vet Med Assoc 193:854, 1988.
301. Scavelli TD, et al: Results of surgical treatment for hyperadrenocorticism caused by adrenocortical neoplasia in the dog: 25 cases (1980–1984). J Am Vet Med Assoc 189:1360, 1986.
302. Schaer M, Ginn PE: Iatrogenic Cushing's syndrome and steroid hepatopathy in a cat. J Am Anim Hosp Assoc 35:48, 1999.
303. Scholten-Sloof BE, et al: Pituitary-dependent hyperadrenocorticism in a family of Dandie-Dinmont terriers. J Endocrinol 135:535, 1992.
304. Schulman J, Johnston SD: Hyperadrenocorticism in two related Yorkshire terriers. J Am Vet Med Assoc 182:524, 1983.
305. Schwedes CS: Mitotane (o,p'-DDD) treatment in a cat with hyperadrenocorticism. J Small Anim Pract 38:520, 1997.
306. Scott DW: Dermatologic use of glucocorticoids: Systemic and topical. Vet Clin North Am 12:19, 1982.
307. Scott DW, et al: Iatrogenic Cushing's syndrome in the cat. Feline Pract 12:30, 1982.
308. Scott DW: Cutaneous phlebectasias in cushingoid dogs. J Am Anim Hosp Assoc 21:351, 1985.
309. Simpson JW, van den Brock AHM: Assessment of fat absorption in normal dogs and dogs with hyperadrenocorticalism. Res Vet Sci 48:38, 1990.
310. Smith MC, Feldman EC: Plasma endogenous ACTH concentrations and plasma cortisol responses to synthetic ACTH and dexamethasone sodium phosphate in healthy cats. Am J Vet Res 48:1719, 1987.
311. Solter PF, et al: Assessment of corticosteroid-induced alkaline phosphatase isoenzyme as a screening test for hyperadrenocorticism in dogs. J Am Vet Med Assoc 203:534, 1993.
312. Stolp R, et al: Results of cyproheptadine treatment in dogs with pituitary-dependent hyperadrenocorticism. J Endocrinol 101:311, 1984.
313. Syakalima M, et al: The age dependent levels of serum ALP isoenzymes and the diagnostic significance of corticosteroid-induced ALP during long-term glucocorticoid treatment. J Vet Med Sci 59:905, 1997.
314. Theon AP, Feldman EC: Megavolt irradiation of pituitary macrotumors in dogs with neurologic signs. J Am Vet Med Assoc 213:225, 1998.
315. Valentine RW, Silber A: Feline hyperadrenocorticism: A rare case. Feline Pract 24:6, 1996.
316. Vandenbergh AGGD, et al: Haemorrhage from a canine adrenocortical tumour: A clinical emergency. Vet Rec 131:539, 1992.
317. van den Broek AHM, Stafford WL: Epidermal and hepatic glucocorticoid receptors in cats and dogs. Res Vet Sci 52:312, 1992.
318. van Liew CH, et al: Comparison of results of adrenocorticotropic hormone stimulation and low-dose dexamethasone suppression tests with necropsy findings in dogs: 81 cases (1985–1995). J Am Vet Med Assoc 211:322, 1997.
319. van Sluijs FJ, et al: Results of adrenalectomy in 36 dogs with hyperadrenocorticism caused by adrenocortical tumour. Vet Q 17:113, 1995.
320. van Vonderen IK, et al: Influence of veterinary care on the urinary corticoid:creatinine ratio in dogs. J Vet Intern Med 12:431, 1998.
321. van Wijk PA, et al: Molecular screening for somatic mutations in corticotropic adenomas of dogs with pituitary-dependent hyperadrenocorticism. J Endocrinol Invest 20:1, 1997.
322. van Wijk PA, et al: Effects of corticotropin-releasing hormone, vasopressin and insulin-like growth factor-I on proliferation of and adrenocorticotropic hormone secretion by canine corticotropic adenoma. Eur J Endocrinol 138:309, 1998.
323. Vollset I, Jakobsen G: Feline endocrine alopecia-like disease probably induced by medroxyprogesterone acetate. Feline Pract 16:16, 1986.
324. von Dehn BJ, et al: Pheochromocytoma and hyperadrenocorticism in dogs: Six cases (1982–1992). J Am Vet Med Assoc 207:322, 1995.
325. Voorhout G, et al: Computed tomography in the diagnosis of canine hyperadrenocorticism not suppressible by dexamethasone. J Am Vet Med Assoc 192:641, 1988.
326. Voorhout G, et al: Nephrotomography and ultrasonography for the localization of hyperfunctioning adrenocortical tumors in dogs. Am J Vet Res 51:1280, 1990.
327. Voorhout G, et al: Assessment of survey radiography and comparison with x-ray computed tomography for detection of hyperfunctioning adrenocortical tumors in dogs. J Am Vet Med Assoc 196:1799, 1990.
328. Ward DA, et al: Band keratopathy associated with hyperadrenocorticism in the dog. J Am Anim Hosp Assoc 25:583, 1989.
329. Watson ADJ, et al: Systemic availability of o,p'-DDD in normal dogs, fasted and fed, and in dogs with hyperadrenocorticism. Res Vet Sci 43:160, 1987.
330. Watson ADJ, et al: Plasma cortisol responses to three corticotropic preparations in normal dogs. Aust Vet J 76:255, 1998.
331. Watson PJ, Herrtage ME: Hyperadrenocorticism in six cats. J Small Anim Pract 39:175, 1998.
332. White SD: Facial dermatosis in four dogs with hyperadrenocorticism. J Am Vet Med Assoc 188:1441, 1986.
333. White SD, et al: Cutaneous markers of canine hyperadrenocorticism. Comp Cont Educ 11:446, 1989.
334. Widmer WR, Guptill, L: Imaging techniques for facilitating diagnosis of hyperadrenocorticism in dogs and cats. J Am Vet Med Assoc 206:1857, 1995.
335. Willard MD, et al: Ketoconazole-induced changes in selected canine hormone concentrations. Am J Vet Res 47:2504, 1986.
336. Willard MD, et al: Effects of long-term administration of ketoconazole in cats. Am J Vet Res 47:2510, 1986.

337. Willemse T, Mol JA: Comparison of *in vivo* and *in vitro* corticotropin releasing hormone-stimulated release of proopiomelanocortin derived peptides in cats. Am J Vet Res 55:1677, 1994.
338. Wilson SM, Feldman EC: Diagnostic value of the steroid-induced isoenzyme of alkaline phosphatase in the dog. J Am Anim Hosp Assoc 28:245, 1992.
339. Yamini B, et al: Ovarian steroid tumor resembling luteoma associated with hyperadrenocorticism (Cushing's disease) in a dog. Vet Pathol 34:57, 1997.
340. Young DW, Kemppainen RJ: Molecular forms of ß-endorphin in the canine pituitary gland. Am J Vet Res 55:567, 1994.
341. Zenoble RD, Kemppainen RJ: Adrenocortical suppression by topically applied corticosteroids in healthy dogs. J Am Vet Med Assoc 191:685, 1987.
342. Zerbe CA, et al: Hyperadrenocorticism in a cat. J Am Vet Med Assoc 190:559, 1987.
343. Zerbe CA, et al: Effect of nonadrenal illness on adrenal function in the cat. Am J Vet Res 48:451, 1987.
343a. Zerbe CA: The hypothalamic-pituitary-adrenal axis and pathophysiology of hyperadrenocorticism. Compend Cont Educ Pract Vet 21:1134, 1999.
343b. Zerbe CA: Screening tests to diagnose hyperadrenocorticism in cats and dogs. Compend Cont Educ Pract Vet 22:17, 2000.
343c. Zerbe CA: Differentiating tests to evaluate hyperadrenocorticism in dogs and cats. Compend Cont Educ Pract Vet 22:149, 2000.

Growth Hormone Physiology and Disease

344. Aribat T, et al: Growth hormone response induced by synthetic human growth hormone-releasing factor (1–44) in healthy dogs. J Am Vet Med Assoc 36:367, 1989.
345. Bell AG, et al: Growth hormone responsive dermatosis in three dogs. N Z Vet J 41:195, 1993.
346. Bercu BB, Diamond FB: Growth hormone neurosecretory dysfunction. Clin Endocrinol Metab 15:537, 1986.
347. Bourdin M, et al: Exploration functionnelle biochimique des troubles de la sécrétion de GH. Proc Gr Etud Dermatol Anim Comp 7:20, 1991.
348. Cornegliani L, Fabbrini F: Use of l-thyroxine and medicated shampoo in three cases of canine pituitary dwarfism. In: Kwochka KW, et al (eds): Advances in Veterinary Dermatology III. Butterworth-Heinemann, Oxford, 1998, p 483.
349. DeBowes LJ: Pituitary dwarfism in a German shepherd puppy. Comp Cont Educ 9:931, 1987.
350. Dicks P, et al: The localization and characterization of insulin-like growth factor-1 receptors and the investigation of melatonin receptors on the hair follicles of seasonal and nonseasonal fibre-producing goats. J Endocrinol 151:55, 1996.
351. Dubreuil P, et al: Long-term growth hormone-releasing factor administration on growth hormone, insulin-like growth factor-1 concentrations, and bone healing in the beagle. Can J Vet Res 60:7, 1996.
352. Eigenmann JE, et al: Panhypopituitarism caused by a suprasellar tumor in a dog. J Am Anim Hosp Assoc 19:377, 1983.
353. Eigenmann JE, et al: Elevated growth hormone levels and diabetes mellitus in a cat with acromegalic features. J Am Anim Hosp Assoc 20:747, 1984.
354. Eigenmann JE: Disorders associated with growth hormone oversecretion: Diabetes mellitus and acromegaly. In: Kirk RW (ed): Current Veterinary Therapy IX. W.B. Saunders Co., Philadelphia, 1986, p 1006.
355. Eigenmann JE: Growth hormone-deficient disorders associated with alopecia in the dog. In: Kirk RW (ed): Current Veterinary Therapy IX. W.B. Saunders Co., Philadelphia, 1986, p 1015.
356. Hamann F, et al: Pituitary function and morphology in two German shepherd dogs with congenital dwarfism. Vet Rec 144:644, 1999.
357. Klesty C, et al: Ein ungewöhnlicher Fall von extremen Hautwuchserungen bei einer jungen Rauhhaardackel-hundin während des Diöstrus ein Fall von Akromegalie? Kleintier Praxis 40:527, 1995.
358. Kooistra HS, et al: Progestin-induced growth hormone (GH) production in the treatment of dogs with congenital GH deficiency. Domest Anim Endocrinol 15:93, 1998.
359. Lothrop CD, Schmeitzel LP: Growth hormone-responsive alopecia in dogs. Vet Med Rep 2:82, 1990.
360. Lund-Larsen TR, Grondalen J: Atelioic dwarfism in the German shepherd dog: Low somatomedin activity associated with apparently normal pituitary function (two cases) and with panadenopituitary dysfunction (one case). Acta Vet Scand 17:298, 1976.
361. Morrison WB, et al: Orally administered clonidine as a secretagogue of growth hormone and as a thymotropic agent in dogs of various ages. Am J Vet Res 51:65, 1990.
362. Nixon AJ, et al: Localization of insulin-like growth factor receptors in the skin follicles of sheep (*Ovis aries*) and changes during an induced growth cycle. Comp Biochem Physiol A Physiol 118:1247, 1997.
363. Ramsey IK, et al: Concurrent central diabetes insipidus and panhypopituitarism in a German shepherd dog. J Small Anim Pract 40:271, 1999.
364. Randolph JF, et al: Delayed growth in two German shepherd dog littermates with normal serum concentrations of growth hormone, thyroxine, and cortisol. J Am Vet Med Assoc 196:77, 1990.
365. Randolph JF, Peterson ME: Acromegaly (growth hormone excess) syndromes in dogs and cats. In: Kirk RW, Bonagura JD (eds): Kirk's Current Veterinary Therapy XI. W.B. Saunders Co., Philadelphia, 1992, p 322.
366. Randolph JF, Peterson ME: Growth hormone therapy in the dog. In: Bonagura JD (ed): Kirk's Current Veterinary Therapy XIII. W.B. Saunders Co., Philadelphia, 1999, p 376.
367. Randolph JF: Personal communication, 1999.
368. Rijnberk A, et al: Disturbed release of growth hormone in mature dogs: A comparison with congenital growth hormone deficiency. Vet Rec 133:542, 1993.
369. Rosenkrantz W, Griffin CE: Lysodren therapy in suspect adrenal sex hormone dermatosis. Proc Annu Meet Wld Cong Vet Dermatol 2:121, 1992.
370. Roth JA, et al: Thymic abnormalities and growth hormone deficiency in dogs. Am J Vet Res 41:1256, 1980.
371. Roth JA, et al: Improvement in clinical condition and thymus morphologic features associated with growth hormone treatment of immunodeficient dwarf dogs. Am J Vet Res 45:1151, 1984.
372. Schmeitzel LP, Lothrop CD: Hormonal abnormalities in Pomeranians with normal coat and in Pomeranians with growth hormone-responsive dermatosis. J Am Vet Med Assoc 197:1333, 1990.
373. Schmeitzel LP, Parker W: Growth hormone and sex hormone alopecia. In: Ihrke PJ, et al (eds): Advances in Veterinary Dermatology, Vol 2. Pergamon Press, New York, 1993, p 451.

374. Schmeitzel LP, et al: Congenital adrenal hyperplasia-like syndrome. In: Bonagura JD (ed): Kirk's Current Veterinary Therapy XII. W.B. Saunders Co., Philadelphia, 1995.
375. Scott DW, Concannon PW: Gross and microscopic changes in the skin of dogs with progestogen-induced acromegaly and elevated growth hormone levels. J Am Anim Hosp Assoc 19:523, 1983.
376. Scott DW, Walton DK: Hyposomatotropism in the mature dog: A discussion of 22 cases. J Am Anim Hosp Assoc 22:467, 1986.
377. Selman PJ, et al: Progestins and growth hormone excess in the dog. Acta Endocrinol 125:42, 1991.
378. Selman PJ, et al: Progestin treatment in the dog 1. Effects on growth hormone, insulin like growth factor 1 and glucose homeostasis. Eur J Endocrinol 131:413, 1994.
379. Selman PJ: Progestins and mammary growth hormone production in the dog. Vet Q 19:S39, 1997.
380. Shanley KJ, Miller WH: Adult-onset growth hormone deficiency in sibling Airedale terriers. Comp Cont Educ 9:1076, 1987.
381. Trotot V, et al: Effets des conditions de conservation du sang total et du plasma de chien sur la concentration plasmatique en hormone de croissance. Rev Méd Vét 144:909, 1993.
382. van Garderen E, et al: Expression of growth hormone in canine mammary tissue and mammary tumors: Evidence for a potential autocrine/paracrine stimulatory loop. Am J Pathol 150:1037, 1997.
383. Yokoyama S, et al: Case of growth hormone responsive dermatosis in a Pomeranian caused by o,p'-DDD inhibition of adrenal cortical hormones. J Vet Med 51:27, 1998.

Sex Hormone Physiology and Disease

384. Allan FJ, et al: Endocrine alopecia in a miniature poodle. N Z Vet J 43:110, 1995.
385. Ashley PF, et al: Effect of oral melatonin administration on sex hormone, prolactin, and thyroid hormone concentration in adult dogs. J Am Vet Med Assoc 215:1111, 1999.
386. Barsanti JA, et al: Diethylstilbestrol-induced alopecia in a dog. J Am Vet Med Assoc 182:63, 1983.
387. Bruinsma DL, Ackerman LA: Male pseudohermaphroditism in a Miniature Schnauzer. Vet Med Small Anim Clin 78:1568, 1983.
388. Carlson RA: Endocrine alopecia in a dog showing response to FSH administration. J Am Anim Hosp Assoc 21:735, 1985.
389. Curtis CF, et al: Investigation of the reproductive and growth hormone status of dogs affected by idiopathic recurrent flank alopecia. J Small Anim Pract 6:162, 1996.
390. Eigenmann JE: Estrogen-induced flank alopecia in the female dog: Evidence for local rather than systemic hyperestrogenism. J Am Anim Hosp Assoc 20:621, 1984.
391. England GCW, et al: Evaluation of the testosterone response to hCG and the identification of a presumed anorchid dog. J Small Anim Pract 30:441, 1989.
392. England GCW: Ultasonographic diagnosis of nonpalpable Sertoli cell tumors in infertile dogs. J Small Anim Pract 36:476, 1995.
393. Fadok VA, et al: Hyperprogesteronemia associated with Sertoli cell tumor and alopecia in a dog. J Am Vet Med Assoc 188:1058, 1986.
394. Fayrer-Hosken RA, et al: Follicular cystic ovaries and cystic endometrial hyperplasia in a bitch. J Am Vet Med Assoc 201:107, 1992.
395. Feldman SR: Androgen insensitivity syndrome (testicular feminization): A model for understanding steroid hormone receptors. J Am Acad Dermatol 27:615, 1992.
396. Fiorito DA: Hyperestrogenism in bitches. Comp Cont Educ 14:727, 1992.
397. Fourrier P, Lepesant V: Dysendocrinie sexuelle chez un caniche mâle agé de 5 ans. Prat Méd Chir Anim Comp 22:395, 1987.
398. Griffin C: Linear prepucial erythema. Proc Annu Memb Meet Am Acad Vet Dermatol Am Coll Vet Dermatol 2:35, 1986.
399. Grossman CJ: Regulation of the immune system by sex steroids. Endocrinol Rev 5:435, 1984.
400. Hammerling R, et al: Is there a role for estradiol in the etiology of dermatoses in the male dog? Proc Annu Memb Meet Am Acad Vet Dermatol Am Coll Vet Dermatol 10:82, 1994.
401. Herrtage ME, Evans, H: The effect of progestogen administration on insulin-like growth factor concentrations in two pituitary dwarfs. Proc Am Coll Vet Intern Med 16:702, 1998.
402. Hubert B, Olivry T: Dermatologie et hormones sexuelles chez les carnivores domestiques 1re partie: physiopathologie. Prat Méd Chir Anim Comp 25:477, 1990.
403. Hubert B, Olivry T: Dermatologie et hormones sexuelles chez les carnivores domestiques 2e partie: Étude clinique. Prat Méd Chir Anim Comp 25:483, 1990.
404. Johnson GR, et al: Ultrasonographic features of testicular neoplasia in dogs: 16 cases (1980–1988). J Am Vet Med Assoc 198:1779, 1991.
405. Ladds PW: The male genital system. In: Jubb KV, et al (eds): Pathology of Domestic Animals, 4th ed, Vol 3. Academic Press, New York, 1993, p 471.
406. Laing EJ, et al: Spermatic cord torsion and Sertoli cell tumor in a dog. J Am Vet Med Assoc 183:879, 1983.
407. Lanore D, et al: Métastase sécrétante d'un sertolinome. Prat Méd Chir Anim Comp 27:727, 1992.
408. Lecomte R: Hyperoestrogenisme spontané ou iatrogène et ses répercussions cliniques et hématologiques. Prat Méd Chir Anim Comp 24:73, 1989.
409. Leyva-Ocariz H: Effect of hyperadrenocorticism and diabetes mellitus on serum progesterone concentrations during early metoestrus of pregnant and nonpregnant cycles induced by pregnant mares' serum gonadotrophin in domestic dogs. J Reprod Fert Suppl 47:371, 1993.
410. Mann FA, et al: Serum testosterone and estradiol 17-ß concentrations in 15 dogs with perineal hernia. J Am Vet Med Assoc 194:1578, 1989.
411. Medleau L: Sex hormone-associated endocrine alopecias in dogs. J Am Anim Hosp Assoc 25:689, 1989.
412. Miller WH Jr: Sex hormone-related dermatoses in dogs. In: Kirk RW (ed): Current Veterinary Therapy X. W.B. Saunders Co., 1989, p 595.
413. Morris BJ: Fatal bone marrow suppression as a result of Sertoli cell tumor. Vet Med Small Anim Clin 78:1070, 1983.
414. Nemzek JA, et al: Cystic ovaries and hyperestrogenism in a canine female pseudohermaphrodite. J Am Anim Hosp Assoc 28:402, 1992.
415. Nuttall T: What is your diagnosis? J Small Anim Pract 39:509, 1998.

416. Paradis M: Melatonin therapy for canine alopecia. In: Bonagura JD (ed): Kirk's Current Veterinary Therapy XIII. W.B. Saunders Co., Philadelphia, 1999, p 546.
417. Pluhar GE, et al: Granulosa cell tumor in an ovariohysterectomized dog. J Am Vet Med Assoc 207:1063, 1995.
418. Schmeitzel LP, Lothrop CD: Sex hormones and skin disease. Vet Med Rep 2:28, 1990.
419. Scott DW, Reimers TJ: Tail gland and perianal gland hyperplasia associated with testicular neoplasia and hypertestosteronemia in a dog. Canine Pract 13:15, 1986.
420. Suess RP, et al: Bone marrow hypoplasia in a feminized dog with an interstitial cell tumor. J Am Vet Med Assoc 200:1346, 1992.
421. Watson ADJ: Oestrogen-induced alopecia in a bitch. J Small Anim Pract 26:17, 1985.
422. Weaver AD: Survey with follow-up of 67 dogs with testicular Sertoli cell tumours. Vet Rec 113:105, 1983.

Miscellaneous

423. Bond R, et al: Metabolic epidermal necrosis in two dogs with different underlying diseases. Vet Rec 136:466, 1995.
424. Bruskiewicz KA, et al: Diabetic ketosis and ketoacidosis in cats: 42 cases (1980–1995). J Am Vet Med Assoc 211:188, 1997.
425. Bussiéras J, et al: Intérêt possible du minoxidil dans le traitement de certaines alopécies canines. Prat Méd Chir Anim Comp 22:25, 1987.
426. Camy G: Alopécie endocrinienne associée à un diabète chez un chien. Point Vét 20:501, 1988.
427. Carpenter JL, et al: Cutaneous xanthogranuloma and viral papilloma on an eyelid of a cat. Vet Dermatol 3:1987, 1992.
428. Chastain CB, Graham CL: Xanthomatosis secondary to diabetes mellitus in a dog. J Am Vet Med Assoc 172:1209, 1978.
429. Denerolle PJ: Three cases of feline cutaneous xanthomas. Proc Wld Cong Vet Dermatol 2:84, 1992.
430. Foster AP, et al: Recognizing canine hepatocutaneous syndrome. Vet Med 92:1050, 1997.
431. Grieshaber TL, et al: Spontaneous cutaneous (eruptive) xanthomatosis in two cats. J Am Anim Hosp Assoc 27:509, 1991.
432. Gross TE, et al: Glucagon-producing pancreatic endocrine tumors in two dogs with superficial necrolytic dermatitis. J Am Vet Med Assoc 197:1619, 1990.
433. Gross TL, et al: Superficial necrolytic dermatitis (necrolytic migratory erythema) in dogs. Vet Pathol 30:75, 1993.
434. Haitjema H: Metabolic epidermal necrosis associated with hepatopathy in a dog. Aust Vet Practit 25:20, 1995.
435. Harvey RG: The use of minoxidil (Loniten, Upjohn), in selected cases of canine alopecia: A report of an open trial. Vet Dermatol Newsl 12:36, 1990.
436. Huntley AC: The cutaneous manifestations of diabetes mellitus. J Am Acad Dermatol 7:427, 1982.
437. Jones BR, et al: Cutaneous xanthomata associated with diabetes mellitus in a cat. J Small Anim Pract 26:33, 1985.
438. Jones BR, et al: Inherited hyperchylomicronemia in the cat. Feline Pract 16:7, 1986.
439. Kimura T, Doi K: The effect of topical minoxidil treatment on hair follicular growth of neonatal hairless descendants of Mexican hairless dogs. Vet Dermatol 8:107, 1997.
440. Kwochka KW, Short BG: Cutaneous xanthomatosis and diabetes mellitus following long-term therapy with megestrol acetate in a cat. Comp Cont Educ 6:185, 1984.
441. Latimer KS, Mahaffey EA: Neutrophil adherence and movement in poorly and well-controlled diabetic dogs. Am J Vet Res 45:1498, 1984.
442. McNeil PE: The underlying pathology of the hepatocutaneous syndrome: A report of 18 cases. In: Ihrke PJ, et al (eds): Advances in Veterinary Dermatology, Vol 2. Pergamon Press, New York, 1993, p 113.
443. Miller WH Jr, et al: Necrolytic migratory erythema in dogs: A hepatocutaneous syndrome. J Am Anim Hosp Assoc 26:573, 1990.
444. Miller WH Jr, et al: Necrolytic migratory erythema in a dog with a glucagon-secreting endocrine tumor. Vet Dermatol 2:179, 1991.
445. Nara T, et al: Necrolytic migratory erythema in a dog. J Vet Med Tokyo 49:464, 1996.
446. Niemand HG: Bildbericht. Kleintierpraxis 16:193, 1971.
447. Patel A, et al: A case of metabolic epidermal necrosis in a cat. Vet Dermatol 7:221, 1996.
448. Price VH (ed): Rogaine (topical minoxidil, 2%) in the management of male pattern baldness and alopecia areata. J Am Acad Dermatol 16(3 Part 2), 1987.
449. Power HT: What's up about the hepatocutaneous syndrome? Dermatology Dialogue, Winter 1999, p 13.
450. Taboada J, Merchant SR: Superficial necrolytic dermatitis and the liver. Proc Am Coll Vet Intern Med 15:534, 1997.
451. Torres SMF, et al: Resolution of superficial necrolytic dermatitis following excision of a glucagon-secreting pancreatic neoplasm in a dog. J Am Anim Hosp Assoc 33:313, 1997.
452. Torres S, et al: Superficial necrolytic dermatitis and a pancreatic endocrine tumor in a dog. J Small Anim Pract 38:246, 1997.
453. Vitale CB, et al: Diet induced alterations in lipid metabolism and associated cutaneous xanthoma formation in 5 cats. In: Kwochka KW, et al (eds): Advances in Veterinary Dermatology III. Butterworth-Heinemann, Oxford, 1998, p 243.
454. Walton DK, et al: Ulcerative dermatosis associated with diabetes mellitus in the dog: A report of four cases. J Am Anim Hosp Assoc 22:79, 1986.
455. Wilkinson JS: Spontaneous diabetes mellitus. Vet Rec 72:548, 1960.

Chapter 11
Acquired Alopecias

An acquired alopecia is a hair loss that develops sometime during the life of an animal. The hereditary alopecias (see Chap. 12) and hair losses that develop as a result of specific disease processes, such as dermatophytosis, endocrine abnormalities, immunologic diseases, or self-inflicted hair loss from hypersensitivity or parasitism are discussed elsewhere in this book. The conditions presented here include a potpourri of acquired disorders characterized predominantly by noninflammatory alopecia. In most instances, the etiopathogenesis of these disorders is poorly understood.

• CANINE ACQUIRED ALOPECIAS

Canine Pinnal Alopecia

Pinnal alopecia is most common in dachshunds but has also been observed in other breeds, such as Chihuahuas, Boston terriers, Whippets, and Italian greyhounds.[43] The pinnal alopecia is seldom noticed in animals less than 1 year of age. If it is, a genetic alopecia is likely. At first, the haircoat is thinner and the hairs become smaller than normal on the pinnae. Progressive diminution of the hairs makes the alopecia more prevalent as the dog ages. With close observation, however, the clinician notes that very small vellus hairs are still present (Fig. 11-1A). Uncommonly, the condition may progress to total pinnal alopecia when the dog reaches 8 to 9 years of age. The remainder of the dog's coat is normal. Diagnosis is facilitated by dermatopathologic examination, which helps rule out other diseases. Changes similar to those of pattern baldness may be seen; these changes include hair follicles that are often in anagen but are reduced in length and diameter (miniaturized) (Fig. 11-2). No treatment is required, because this is a benign problem. However, some owners may wish to try therapy. Melatonin is being tried for a number of alopecia syndromes (see Chap. 3) and anecdotal reports suggest that it may be helpful in this condition.[29, 30] Topical minoxidil was reported effective in stimulating hair growth in genetically hairless dogs (see Chap. 12).[21]

It is important to differentiate such spontaneous alopecias from dermatoses that cause hair loss on the pinnae. Hair follicle dysplasias, estrogen-responsive dermatosis, rare cases of hypothyroidism, hyperadrenocorticism, dermatophytosis, and alopecia areata may also cause pinnal alopecia. Topical steroid-induced alopecia may be seen on the convex surface of the pinnae, even though the otic glucocorticoid-containing preparation may only be applied to the concave surface of the pinnae or to the ear canal (Fig. 11-3). This has been seen by the authors in dachshunds wherein it also aggravated the pinnal alopecia present previously. However, these other differentials do not feature miniaturization of hairs and hair follicles. Vasculitis or ischemic dermatitis can occur on the pinnae and cause alopecia with severe erythema, scaling, crusting, and eventually, ulceration and tissue loss at the pinnal margin. Other inflammatory diseases may cause alopecia and are differentiated by the history of inflammation or previous pruritus.

turely enter telogen and hair loss begins within 3 to 5 weeks (e.g., drug effects; periods of physiologic stress); (2) *delayed anagen release*, a common form, wherein follicles remain in prolonged anagen and their "release" results in increased shedding in 2 to 3 months (e.g., postpartum hair loss); (3) *short anagen*, a very speculative form, wherein an idiopathic shortening of anagen results in increased shedding and decreased hair length; (4) *immediate telogen release*, wherein normal telogen is shortened and hair loss begins in a few days or weeks (e.g., drug effects, such as minoxidil); and (5) *delayed telogen release*, wherein telogen is prolonged (e.g., irregularities in photoperiod).

Diagnosis is based on history, physical examination, and direct hair examination. Telogen hairs are characterized by a uniform shaft diameter and a slightly clubbed, nonpigmented root end that lacks root sheaths (see Fig. 2–28B). Anagen defluxion hairs are characterized by irregularities and dysplastic changes. The diameter of the shaft may be irregularly narrowed and deformed, and breaking often occurs at such structurally weakened sites, resulting in ragged points (see Fig. 2–28F). Skin biopsy is only rarely helpful. When the alopecia due to telogen defluxion begins, histopathologic examination shows only normal skin. In anagen defluxion, the characteristic changes are usually most evident in the affected hairs, and these are usually lost when the skin is clipped for biopsy. Typical histopathologic findings in anagen defluxion include apoptosis and fragmented cell nuclei in the keratinocytes of the hair matrix of anagen hair follicles, and eosinophilic dysplastic hair shafts within the pilar canal.[58]

Both anagen and telogen defluxion spontaneously resolve when the inciting factor is relieved.

Excessive Shedding

Owners often ask "Why does my dog (or cat) shed so much?" They are naturally concerned about large amounts of hair getting on their rugs, furniture, and clothing.[43] The shedding of hair is reported as the biggest disadvantage of pet ownership.[9] When owners perceive shedding hair as excessive, it compounds this feeling. If excessively shed hairs are not associated with gross alopecia, the condition may cause inconvenience to the owner, but it is probably normal or at least causes no problem for the animal. The hair growth cycle is controlled by a number of factors (see Chap. 1), and the questions about shedding are often difficult to answer. Very little information about it is available in the literature. In the northern hemisphere, many outdoor dogs and cats shed to varying degrees in spring and fall; indoor pets may shed all year long. When animals are shedding excessively, many hairs can be easily epilated, but areas of actual alopecia *cannot* be created. In contrast, the clinician can usually create alopecia by gentle manual epilation in animals with hair loss due to endocrine disorders and follicular dysplasias. When there is no obvious clinical disease, modification of behavior, diet, or adjustment of light and temperature can be considered treatment. Hyperexcitable or nervous animals seem to shed more excessively than their calm counterparts. Behavior modification programs or antianxiety treatments may be beneficial. If no abnormal conditions can be discovered, the only treatment is to remove the dead telogen hairs from the animal by combing, brushing, or in some cases, vacuuming. Loshed (A.B.S.) is marketed in a spray, wipe-on sheet, and shampoo formulation for dogs and cats. The spray and wipe-on formulations contain keratin, amino acids, vitamins, essential unsaturated fatty acids, and herbal extracts, and the manufacturer claims that regular use will reduce excessive shedding. Detailed studies on its efficacy or mode of action are unavailable.

Traction Alopecia

Traction alopecia has been described in dogs that have had barrettes, rubber bands, or other methods used to tie up their hair.[35, 58] When these devices have been applied too tightly or for too much time, alopecia may result. Initially, an inflammatory plaque may occur, but it progresses to an atrophic scarred patch. Invariably, lesions are present on the top or lateral aspects of the cranium. If the disease is allowed to progress too long, the alopecia becomes permanent (see Fig. 11–1C).

Diagnosis is based on the characteristic history and physical examination findings. In the late stages, there are few differentials because of the atrophic nature and location of the alopecia. Early lesions should be differentiated from alopecia areata, pseudopelade, and dermatophytosis. Biopsy findings depend on the stage of the lesion that is sampled.[35, 58] Early lesions may show variable mononuclear cell infiltrates, edema, and vasodilatation. Hydropic degeneration of epidermal basal cells and apoptosis of keratinocytes may be seen. Chronic cases may be characterized by fibrosing dermatitis and scarring alopecia or a "cell-poor" hydropic interface dermatosis with marked pilosebaceous atrophy ("faded" follicles).

Treatment consists of instructing the owner regarding proper placement of hair-holding devices. Atrophic scars do not respond to medical therapy; if treatment is desired for cosmetic purposes, surgical excision is required.

Trichorrhexis Nodosa

Trichorrhexis nodosa appears along the hair shaft as small, beaded swellings associated with a loss of cuticle.[22, 56] The expanded areas are composed of frayed cortical fibers through which the hair readily fractures. The basic cause is trauma, and a contributing factor is inherent weakness of the hair shaft. Examples of physical trauma include excessive brushing, back combing, application of heat, and prolonged ultraviolet light exposure. Sources of chemical trauma include bathing in excessively salty water or chlorinated swimming pools, shampooing, and insecticidal or acaricidal dips.[47] Trichorrhexis nodosa has also been reported in association with amitriptyline therapy.[47]

Clinical signs include multifocal or generalized hypotrichosis, wherein affected areas show broken, stubby hairs (Fig. 11–8). A trichogram reveals hairs with nodular areas of cortical splitting that resemble two brooms pushed together (see Fig. 11–19).

Treatment requires eliminating the source of physical or chemical trauma.

Medullary Trichomalacia

Medullary trichomalacia results in patchy alopecia, especially in German shepherd dogs (see Chap. 12).[54]

Trichoptilosis

Trichoptilosis ("split ends") is a common hair shaft abnormality associated with the cumulative effects of chemical and physical trauma. A severe form, resulting in patchy alopecia, has been described in Golden retrievers (see Chap. 12).[46]

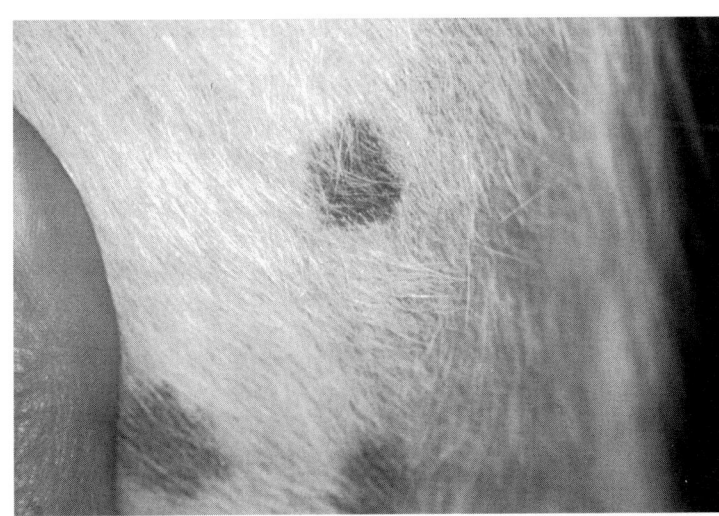

FIGURE 11–8. Trichorrhexis nodosa in a Greyhound associated with amitriptyline therapy. Note broken hairs and patchy alopecia. (Courtesy C. Tieghi.)

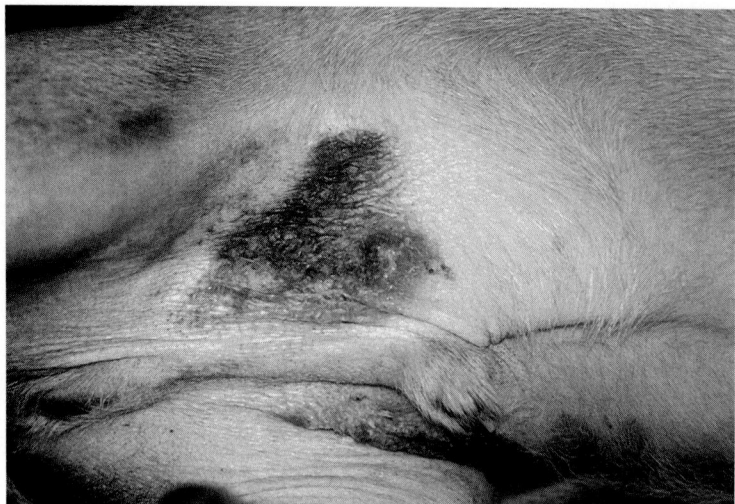

FIGURE 11-9. Topical steroid–induced erythema, hyperpigmentation, and flaccid bullae in groin of a dog.

Injection Reactions

Injection reactions may induce focal areas of alopecia.[47] Two types may be seen. In the first, there is an inflammatory reaction that is usually either a panniculitis or a vasculitis. Rabies vaccines (particularly those licensed for subcutaneous use) are most commonly associated with the vasculitic type of reaction.[38, 57, 58] In the second type, there is no gross inflammation and the hair just falls out. There may be associated pigment changes and dermal and epidermal atrophy. This form of reaction most commonly occurs with subcutaneous injections of glucocorticoid or progestational compounds.

Lesions are most commonly seen over the shoulders, back, and posterolateral thighs, which are sites where injections are given. The inflammatory reactions initially present as a circular to oval erythematous plaque. It is firm when palpated and may extend into the deeper tissues. In some cases, the skin is not erythematous but just thickened and firm. In other cases, there is an initial subcutaneous swelling (panniculitis). Chronically, the alopecic area becomes hyperpigmented and shiny, with or without mild scaling. The noninflammatory form presents as an atrophic, hypopigmented, oval-to-circular patch. With both forms, the first signs of the lesions usually occur 2 to 4 months after an injection.

Diagnosis is based on the presence of typical lesions with a compatible history. Differential diagnoses are dermatophytosis, folliculitis, cellulitis, demodicosis, alopecia areata, pseudopelade, and localized scleroderma. Dermatopathologic examination is useful for establishing the diagnosis and ruling out the other differentials. In the inflammatory form, varying degrees of panniculitis are present, and lymphoid nodules are often prominent.[14, 58] Vasculitis may or may not be evident. The overlying hair follicles are telogenized, atrophic, and occasionally, miniaturized. In the noninflammatory form, varying degrees of dermal and pilosebaceous atrophy are present.

Treatment is not usually required, although it may take months to over a year before hair regrowth occurs. In some cases, the alopecia is permanent. When hair regrowth does occur, the new hairs are often a different color. When hair growth does not recur, surgical excision is effective. For the inflammatory form, intralesional or systemic glucocorticoids may be beneficial. Pentoxifylline and dapsone have been used in the vasculitic form (see Chap. 9).

Topical Glucocorticoid Reactions

Topical products containing potent glucocorticoids may cause focal alopecia. Concurrent dermal atrophy, pyoderma, flaccid subepidermal bullae, comedones, or milia-like lesions may also be present in some cases (Fig. 11–9).[18] The most common history is the initial effective use of a topical glucocorticoid-containing product for the treatment of localized pruritus or papular dermatitis. With time, the reaction to the topical starts to induce lesions seen by the client, which are not attributed to the topical product. The topical product is then used more frequently, for a prolonged period of time, and sometimes on an increasingly larger area of skin. Lesions are most often seen on the groin or convex base of the pinnae (see Fig. 11–3).

Short Hair Syndrome of Silky Breeds

Yorkshire terriers and silky terriers normally have long, silky hair coats. The luxurious coat was achieved by many generations of selective breeding, and it is a source of great pride to the pet's owner. Occasionally, an apparently normal-coated mature dog loses its coat, and the coat is replaced with hairs that never grow to their former full length (see Fig. 11–1D).[26, 43] The owner is distressed by this and seeks help, often after unsuccessfully trying vitamin and mineral supplements or coat conditioners containing fatty acids. The affected dogs have no itching, erythema, or scaling of the skin. Onset occurs when the dog is 1 to 5 years of age. There are no broken or bitten hairs. Because the long silky hairs are gone, the remaining haircoat would be adequate for a mixed-breed dog or a purebred dog with shorter hair. The condition also occurs in younger dogs. In such cases, the puppy coat is normal, but it is replaced with a permanent shorter coat. The abnormal new coat is apparent when the dog is 5 months of age. The hair on the head is of normal length; however, the posterior abdominal area, hind legs, and chest have hairs that are shorter than normal. There is no scaliness or inflammation of the skin.

It can only be theorized that the hair cycle has been shortened by some unknown factor, such that the hairs are shed before they reach their normal full length. The most important differential diagnoses are hair follicle dysplasias, endocrine (especially hypothyroidism) and genetic disorders, and psychogenic alopecia. There is no known treatment.

Postclipping Alopecia

Failure to regrow hair following clipping has been termed *post-clipping alopecia* or *follicular arrest*.[14, 43] The hairs may not regrow for up to 24 months, but they usually regrow within 1 year. Although this condition has been described as relatively common, the authors consider it uncommon in their clinical experiences and discussion with groomers and surgeons. It is seen more often in breeds with long, thick coats, such as Siberian huskies and Chow Chows, but it may occur in any dog (see Figs. 11–1E, 11–10, and 11–11). The condition is most commonly seen following clipping for surgical procedures or for the removal of mats. The clinical appearance is typical; in the affected areas, the coat looks exactly as it did after it was clipped several months previously. The rest of the coat is usually normal. It has been proposed that this syndrome may occur as the result of vascular perfusion changes in response to cutaneous temperature changes.[14] Another possibility, however, is that these dogs are in their normal catagen stage of hair growth, between losing and growing a new haircoat. This theory is supported by the discovery of similar histologic changes in biopsies from normal-haired and affected areas[12]; both can show catagen arrest. Most of these dogs regrow hair in the clipped area after they go through a heavy shedding or so-called blowing of their coat.[12]

Cicatricial Alopecia

A variety of diseases may result in a scarring alopecia. Once adnexal units are replaced by scar tissue, hair loss becomes permanent.[10] In addition to the scarring diseases, deep physical, thermal, and chemical injury may result in scarring alopecia.

Chronic Radiant Heat Dermatitis

This syndrome, also referred to as erythema ab igne, was recently described in two dogs.[7] Erythema ab igne occurs in humans from prolonged and repetitive exposure to moderate

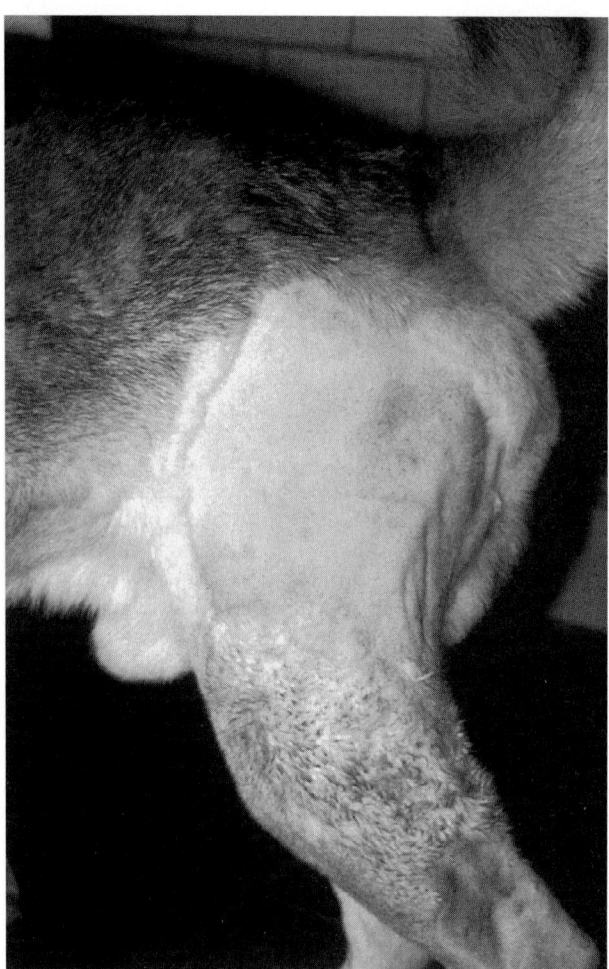

FIGURE 11-10. Postclipping alopecia in an Akita. Absence of hair regrowth at site of fracture repair 13 months after surgery.

FIGURE 11-11. Postclipping alopecia in an English bulldog. Absence of hair regrowth at site of intradermal skin testing 1 year later.

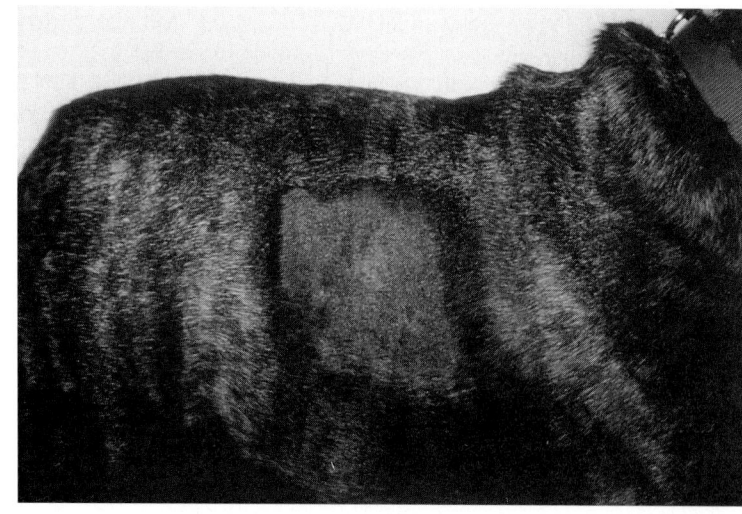

heat and results in erythema and hyperpigmentation. In the two dogs reported, the major findings were sharply marginated, irregular, asymmetric, alopecic patches. Variable degrees of erythema, central hypopigmentation, peripheral hyperpigmentation, crusts, and ulceration were seen. The dorsolateral thorax was most affected. Both dogs would lay by heating sources (infrared lamp, burning stove). Histopathology differs depending on the stage biopsied. Acute lesions were characterized by epidermal atrophy, focal basal cell vacuolation, and epithelial apoptosis, which may involve the adnexal epithelium. These apoptotic cells had enlarged, irregular, hyperchromatic nuclei. Scarring alopecia remained following removal of the source of the heat (see Chap. 16).

Follicular Lipidosis of Rottweilers

This recently recognized syndrome occurs in young Rottweilers of either sex. Although the etiology is unknown, the exclusive occurrence in Rottweilers suggests genetic predisposition (see Chap. 12).[17] All reported dogs and most seen by the authors were younger than 1 year of age. Hypotrichosis of the red-colored points is seen. The degree of alopecia may vary, and black hairs within the affected areas may be spared (Fig. 11–12). One reported case had concurrent thyroid atrophy and chronic renal disease. One author (CEG) has seen five cases, two of which also tested low on thyroid screens, but thyroid-stimulating hormone (TSH) response tests were not done. In all dogs followed, the disease improves or completely resolves clinically. Histopathology of affected skin shows hair matrix cells to be swollen and vacuolated (Fig. 11–13). Special stains and electron microscopy revealed lipid within the vacuoles (see Chap. 12).[17]

Alopecia Mucinosa

A 10-year-old Labrador retriever was reported with an 11-month history of progressive alopecia that started on the head and progressed to involve the limbs and patches on the trunk.[2] Periodic patchy hair growth would occur intermittently. Generalized scaling was also noted. A normocytic normochromic anemia, hyperglobulinemia and positive antinuclear antibody test (ANA > 1:32) were present. A total serum thyroxine was normal. Histopathology revealed orthokeratotic hyperkeratosis, acanthosis, hydropic degeneration of basal cells, sparse apoptosis of keratinocytes, pigmentary incontinence, and mononuclear perivascular dermatitis. The striking changes were perifollicular lymphohistiocytic inflammation with infiltration of lymphocytes into the follicular and sebaceous epithelium, epithelial degeneration, and cystic spaces within the follicular epithelium. These spaces stained positive for mucin.

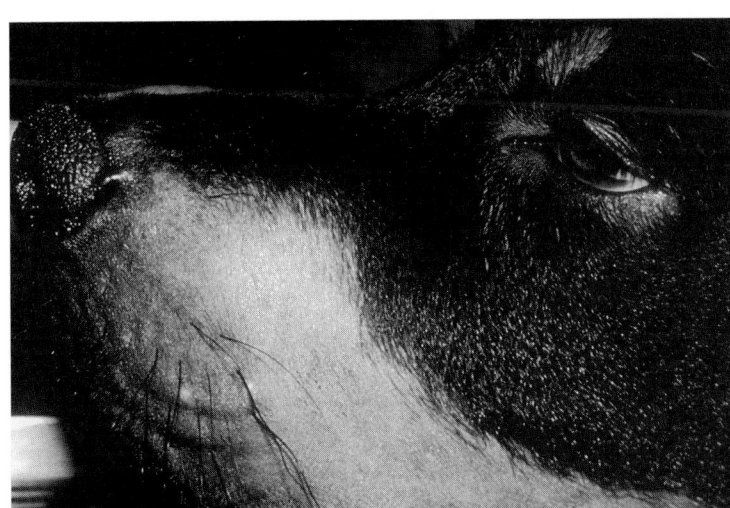

FIGURE 11–12. Rottweiler with follicular lipidosis; note the thinning alopecia of the red-haired areas and the unaffected black hair on the face.

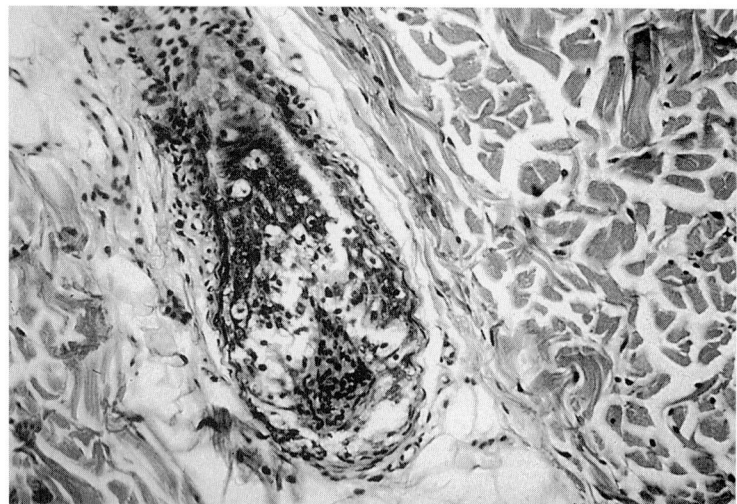

FIGURE 11–13. Follicular lipidosis. Note the vacuolar changes of the hair bulbs.

• FELINE ACQUIRED ALOPECIAS

Feline Pinnal Alopecia

Some Siamese cats develop a spontaneous periodic alopecia of the ears (see Fig. 11–1F).[40] Lesions are typically present on both pinnae. The alopecia may be patchy or involve most of the pinnal surface, and the affected skin is clinically normal. After several months, the hair regrows without treatment. The cause is unknown.[40] Histopathologic findings have not been reported.

Feline Preauricular Alopecia

The temporal region between the ear and eye of cats is more sparsely haired than are other parts of the head (see Fig. 11–1G).[40] This is a physiologic, not a pathologic, condition.[40] In long-haired or densely coated cats, this area is not noticeable; however, in cats with short or less dense haircoats, it can look like alopecia. When cat owners ask their veterinarians about the condition, they can be told that the condition is normal and neither requires nor would respond to treatment. In typical cases, skin scrapings, fungal cultures, and biopsies are totally unnecessary. If inflammation, excessive scale, or follicular casts are present, diagnostic tests for other diseases should be considered.

Feline Acquired Symmetric Alopecia

Feline acquired symmetric alopecia (formerly feline endocrine alopecia) is a rare acquired bilaterally symmetric hypotrichosis of unknown origin.[24, 39, 51]

CAUSE AND PATHOGENESIS

The exact cause and pathogenesis of feline acquired symmetric alopecia are unknown. The original name of feline endocrine alopecia was changed because no true endocrine cause had been proved.[26] However, there has been a study that suggests there may be abnormal thyroid function, and 73% of affected cats responded to liothyronine (T_3) therapy.[51, 52] One theory suggested that these cats may have had a decreased thyroid reserve. The results were based on basal changes in group averages. Individual cases can have normal total thyroxine (TT_4) or TT_3 levels or a normal response to TSH. However, as groups, these cats had a depressed response to TSH.[52] It has also been observed that an identical pattern of alopecia can be self-inflicted. Because cats are sometimes secret groomers, the owners may not be aware that they are licking or pulling excessively at the hairs. Hair regrowth that occurs with gonadal or thyroid hormones in these cats may be due to psychologic or other changes not related to treatment of a true deficiency. In this syndrome, placement of an Elizabethan collar or bucket on the cat's head for several weeks will demonstrate whether the alopecia was self-inflicted. If hair regrowth does not occur, traumatic causes can be excluded and this syndrome should then be considered. When hair does not regrow, demodicosis, hyperglucocorticoidism, hyperprogesteronism, and paraneoplastic alopecia should be considered.

CLINICAL FEATURES

Feline acquired symmetric alopecia is a rare disease seen mostly in neutered male and female cats. No breed predilection has been reported, but purebred cats are rarely affected. The age of affected cats ranges from 2 to 12 years, with an average of 6 years.

Feline acquired symmetric alopecia is characterized by bilaterally symmetric hypotrichosis, which begins in the genital and perineal regions (see Fig. 11–1H). Diffuse thinning of the hair, rather than complete baldness, affects the anogenital region, proximal tail, caudomedial thighs, and ventral abdomen. Long-standing cases may have hypotrichosis of the lateral thorax and flanks, but the dorsum is spared. Hairs in the affected areas are easily epilated. Pruritus and skin lesions are usually absent.

DIAGNOSIS

The first diagnostic question is whether the cat has bitten or licked the hairs, and thereby caused the alopecia, or the hairs have fallen out by themselves. Close examination by rolling the skin reveals normal numbers of hairs in cats that lick off the hair. A trichogram helps because the distal hair tips are intact and pointed, and the proximal (bulbar) ends are telogenized in this syndrome. If the distal end of the hair shows a broken or chewed off edge, the cat is creating the hair loss. It must be emphasized here that most cats with a symmetric alopecia that appears noninflammatory *are* causing it by licking and chewing and do not have acquired symmetric alopecia.[24]

The differential diagnosis includes the pruritic causes of alopecia such as flea bite hypersensitivity, atopy, food hypersensitivity, dermatophytosis, feline demodicosis (rare), and ectoparasites such as *Otodectes cynotis* and *Cheyletiella blakei*. Nonpruritic causes of alopecia include hypothyroidism (extremely rare), hyperglucocorticoidism (rare), hyperprogesteronism (extremely rare), paraneoplastic alopecia (rare), excessive shedding, trichorrhexis nodosa, telogen and anagen defluxion (rare), and psychogenic alopecia (rare). Lymphocytic and plasmacytic gastroenteritis has also been associated with symmetric alopecia of the cervical or inguinal region in 28.6% of the cases. It was suggested that this condition could have been a type of food hypersensitivity, but no pruritus or description of short stubby hairs was reported. Two of four affected cats resolved their alopecia as the gastroenteritis improved with prednisone and diet change.[8] Definitive diagnosis is based on history, physical examination, results of laboratory studies, and response to therapy. Hemogram, serum chemistries, urinalysis, and tests of thyroid and adrenal function are normal. Skin biopsy reveals telogenization of hair follicles.[43, 58]

CLINICAL MANAGEMENT

The client should be counseled about the benign nature of this condition and informed that treatment may not be necessary. If treatment is elected, T_3 should be tried initially. T_3—initially given orally at 20 μg/cat q12h, then slowly increased to 50 μg/cat—should be administered for 12 weeks.[51] The most significant side effects to consider are cardiac arrhythmias, including premature ventricular beats.

Alternatively, combined androgen-estrogen therapy appears to be more effective than either sex hormone alone.[40] Excellent results have been obtained with intramuscular

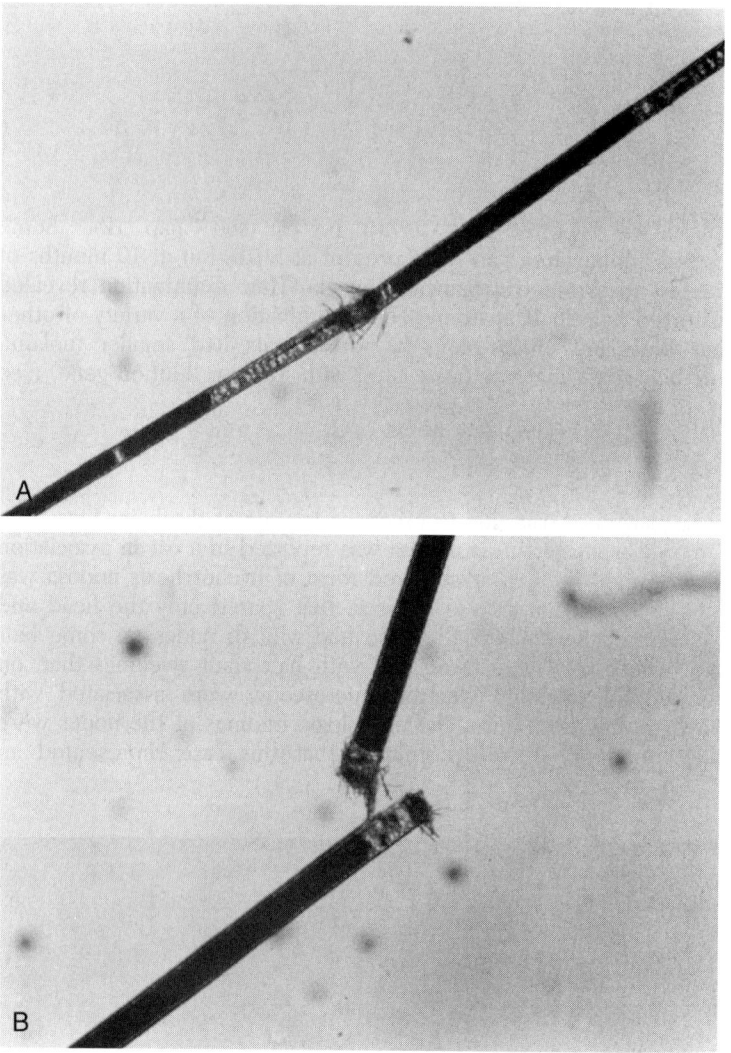

FIGURE 11–19. *A*, Trichorrhexis nodosa. Hair from the cat in Figure 11–18. Note the nodular area in the center of the hair shaft, where breakage will occur. *B*, Trichorrhexis nodosa. Hair from the cat in Figure 11–18. This hair has fractured at a nodule, giving the appearance of two brooms end to end.

acquired form of the disease secondary to excessive trauma associated with excessive grooming from fleas and possibly a hair keratin defect to explain the uncommon fragility of the hairs in this cat. Discontinuation of the flea shampoo or treatment of the flea bite hypersensitivity cured these two cats.

Idiopathic Lymphocytic Mural Folliculitis

Mural folliculitis is a reaction pattern that is characterized by inflammation that targets the hair follicle outer root sheath epithelium.[6, 14–16, 58] This reaction pattern may be seen with a variety of diseases, including dermatophytosis, demodicosis, early prodromal epitheliotropic T-cell lymphoma (see Fig. 11–24A), pseudopelade, sebaceous adenitis, food hypersensitivity, and drug reaction.[12, 14–16, 27, 33, 58] In one severe form of mucinous degenerative mural folliculitis there may be an association with feline immunodeficiency virus (FIV) infection, high-dose glucocorticoid therapy, epitheliotropic lymphoma, severe illness, and debilitation (Fig. 11–20). Pseudopelade is believed to have an immune-mediated etiology and is discussed in Chapter 9. Mural folliculitis as a manifestation of cutaneous adverse drug reaction (see Chap. 9) and sebaceous adenitis (see Chap. 18) are discussed elsewhere.

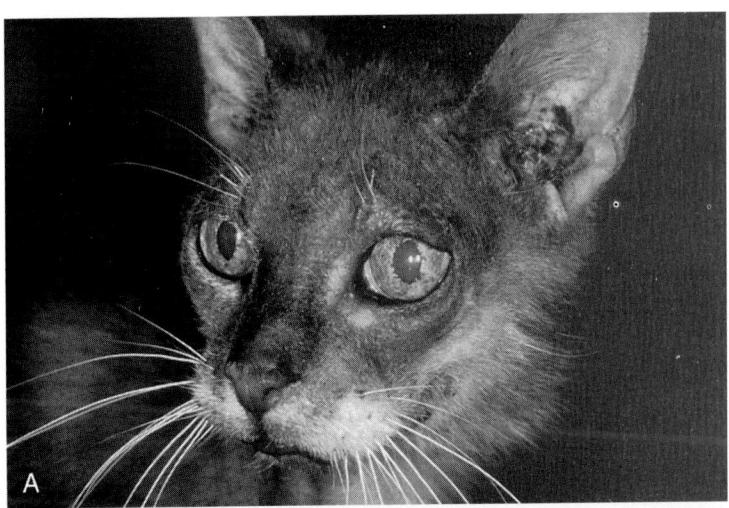
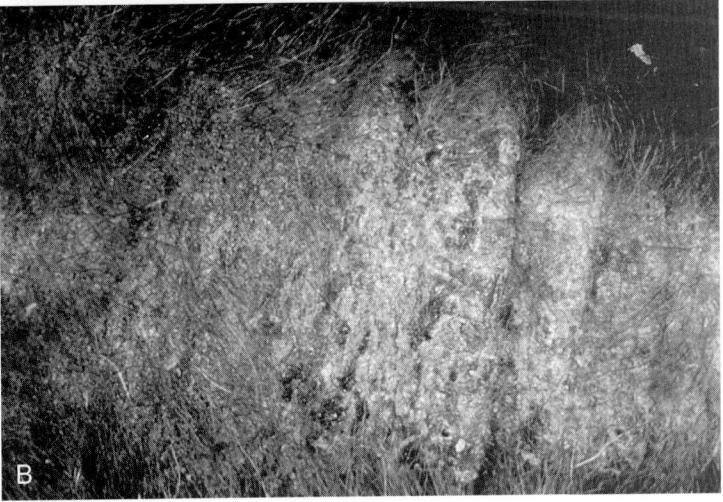

FIGURE 11–20. *A*, Facial alopecia in a cat with mucinous degenerative mural folliculitis. *B*, Close-up view of the trunk showing alopecia and scaling. (Courtesy Dr. T. Olivry.)

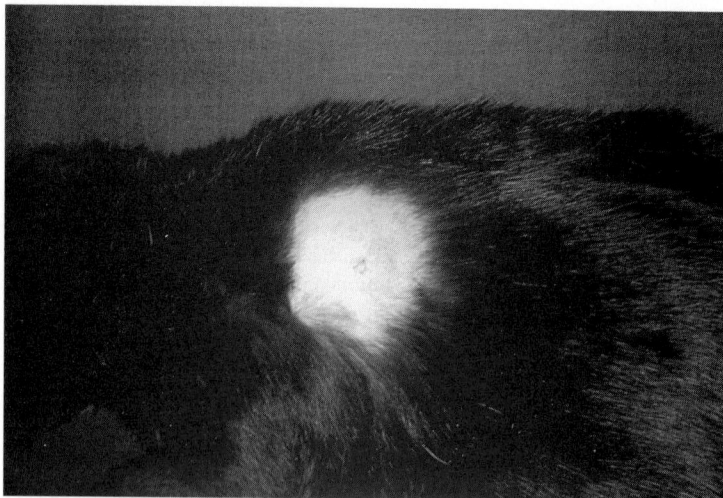

FIGURE 11–21. Idiopathic feline lymphocytic mural folliculitis. Annular area of alopecia and fine scaling over shoulder.

Idiopathic forms of lymphocytic mural folliculitis have been described.[6, 14–16, 27, 34] Idiopathic cases have been described in middle-aged to old cats, and may have one or more well-circumscribed, annular areas of alopecia (Fig. 11–21) or a diffuse partial alopecia (Fig. 11–22). Scaling is variable. The head, limbs, and trunk are most commonly involved. Pruritus is variable.

Although lymphocytic mural folliculitis is a reaction pattern seen in a number of feline dermatoses, careful histologic studies may allow separation of specific syndromes in the future. The presence of fungal elements or mites will, of course, document these diagnoses. Fungal elements may be quite sparse in cats with dermatophytosis and this reaction pattern. Fungal culture by a brush technique may be required. In cats with pseudopelade, the lymphocytic infiltrate targets the isthmus of the hair follicle, with sebaceous glands being spared early but often infiltrated or obliterated late in the disease. In sebaceous adenitis, the sebaceous glands are targeted, but the hair follicle isthmus and infundibulum may be less intensely infiltrated. Early or prodromal epitheliotropic lymphoma may require sequential biopsies over many months before it can be reliably differentiated from a non-neoplastic lymphocytic mural folliculitis.[6] Severely inflammatory

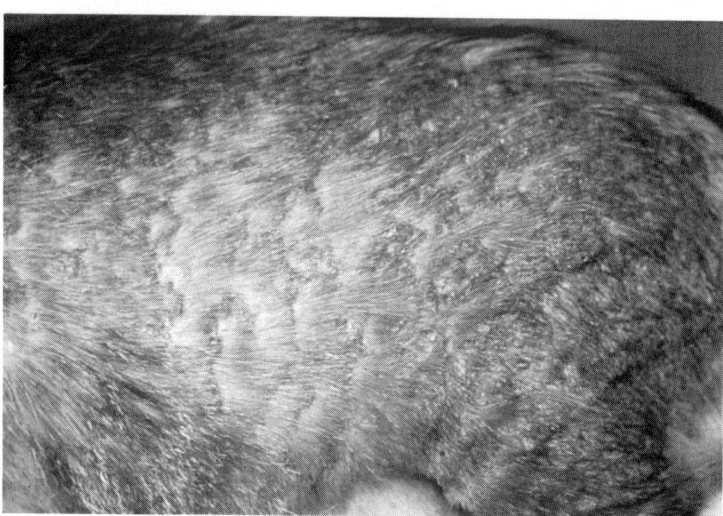

FIGURE 11–22. Idiopathic feline lymphocytic mural folliculitis. Marked exfoliation over trunk. (Courtesy J. Guillot.)

lymphocytic mural folliculitides—associated with histiocytes, fewer eosinophils and neutrophils, follicular mucinosis, and follicular destruction—may be associated with FIV infection or epitheliotropic lymphoma.[6, 34] Cats with idiopathic lymphocytic mural folliculitis and those with drug-induced or food-induced forms have the hair follicle infundibulum targeted (Fig. 11–23). Cats with drug- or food-induced reaction also seem to have a concurrent hydropic interface dermatitis and folliculitis (Fig. 11–24B).

Reports of therapeutic responses are anecdotal and confusing. Part of the confusion undoubtedly is generated by the failure to recognize that this follicular reaction pattern has numerous etiologies. Idiopathic cases have responded, and failed to respond, to glucocorticoids or systemic retinoids.[6, 34] The authors and others[6, 6a] have seen some cases resolve on a novel protein diet and relapse with dietary challenge. Other cases have resolved when concurrent drug therapy was discontinued. Still other cases have been reported to spontaneously resolve.[34]

Alopecia Mucinosa

In humans, alopecia mucinosa (follicular mucinosis) is characterized by well-demarcated areas of alopecia, fine scaling, and prominent hair follicle orifices, with or without slightly raised and mildly erythematous papules or plaques.[43] There are three clinical patterns. The first and most common is seen in young adults; it is restricted to the head and neck,

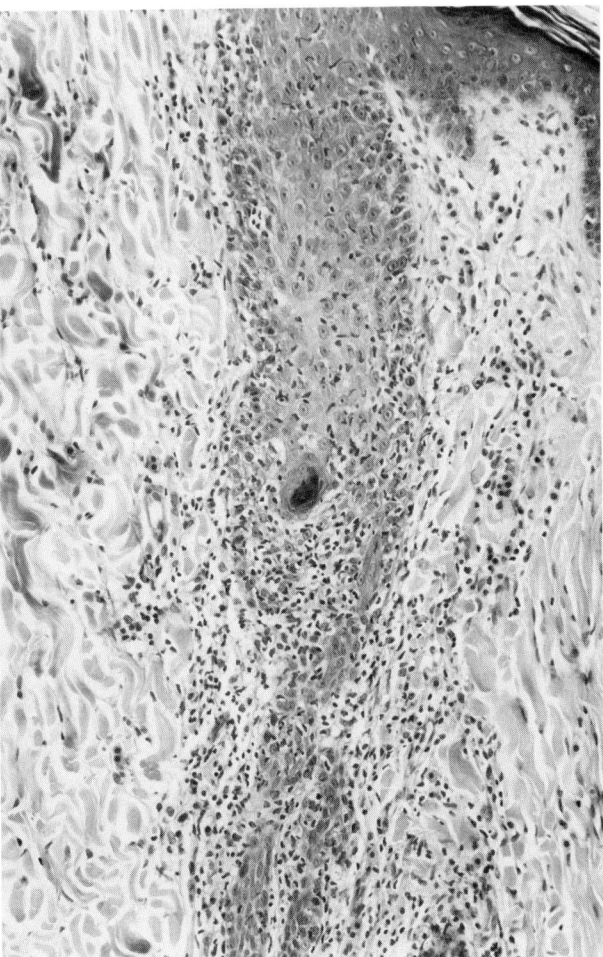

FIGURE 11–23. Idiopathic lymphocytic mural folliculitis in a cat. Entire infundibulum of hair follicle is infiltrated by lymphocytes.

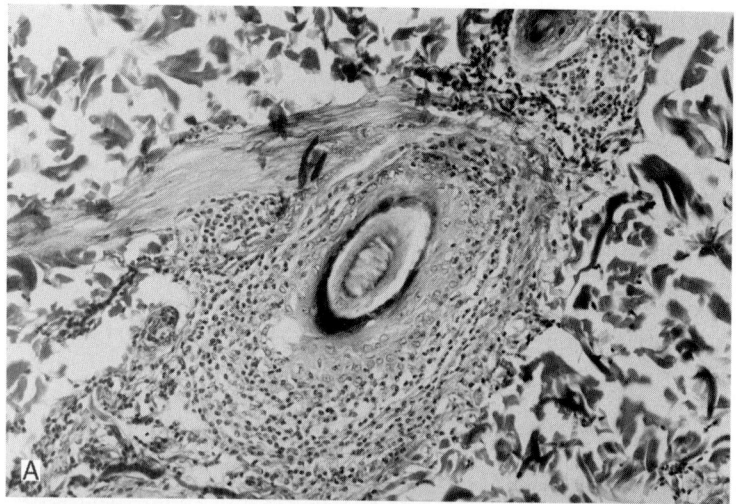
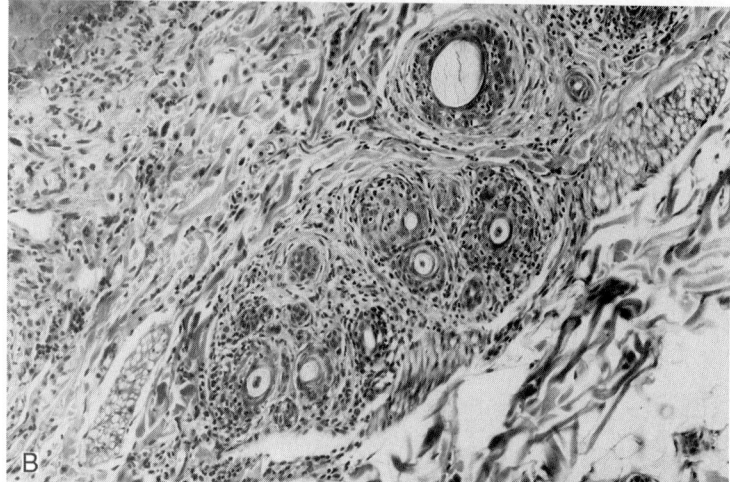

FIGURE 11-24. *A*, Early epitheliotropic lymphoma in a cat. Note mural and perifollicular infiltration of neoplastic lymphocytes. *B*. Adverse cutaneous reaction to food. In addition to interface folliculitis, the epidermal interface *(top left)* is similarly involved.

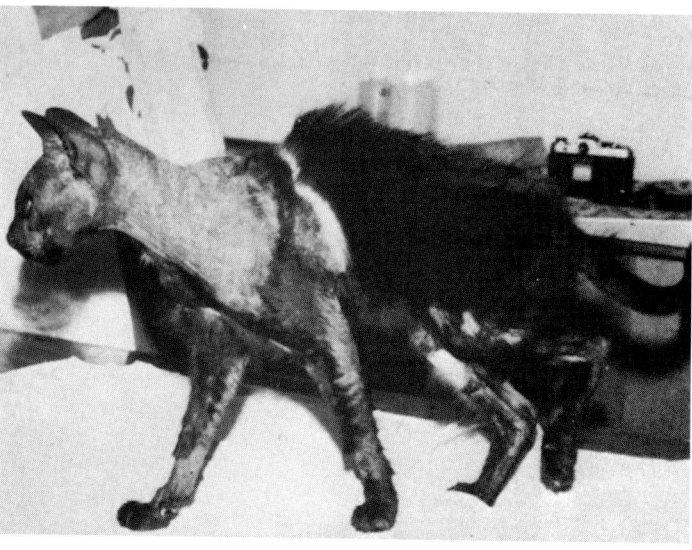

FIGURE 11-25. Feline alopecia mucinosa. Alopecia and scaling of head, neck, and front legs. (Courtesy V. Studdert.)

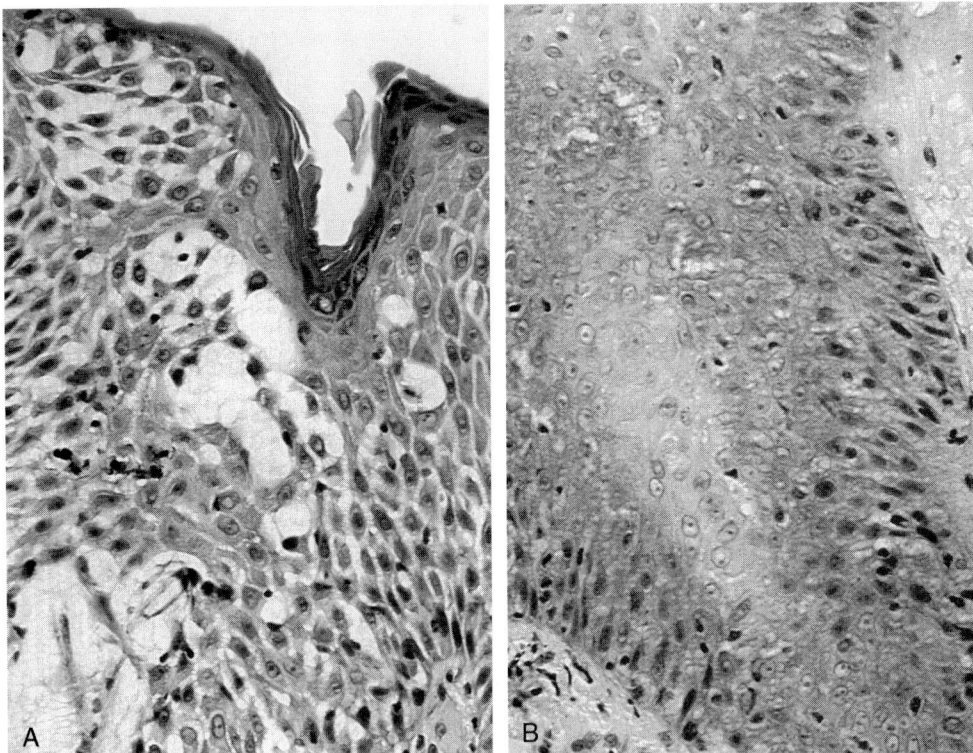

FIGURE 11–26. Feline alopecia mucinosa. *A*, Epidermal mucin appears as clear vacuolar areas and exaggerated intercellular spaces in H & E–stained sections. *B*, Epidermal vacuoles and intercellular spaces are filled with mucin and alcian blue–stained section.

and it resolves in about 2 years. The second form is seen in a slightly older age group, and lesions are more generalized and resolution takes longer. The third form is seen in aged people, and plaques of mycosis fungoides eventually develop within the areas of alopecia. The pathogenic mechanism of alopecia mucinosa is unknown.

Alopecia mucinosa was recognized in two adult cats with asymptomatic, well-demarcated alopecia and fine scaling on the head, ears, and neck (Fig. 11–25).[41] Biopsy specimens initially revealed mucinosis of the epidermis and the hair follicle's outer root sheath (Fig. 11–26). Several months later, both cats had plaques in the areas of alopecia. Biopsy results at this time were typical of epitheliotropic lymphoma (mycosis fungoides). Both cats were lost to follow-up.

• REFERENCES

1. Alhaidari Z, et al: Acquired feline hair shaft abnormality resembling trichorrhexis nodosa in humans. Vet Dermatol 7:235, 1996.
1a. Barrs VR, et al: What is your diagnosis? J Small Anim Pract 40:559, 1999.
2. Bell A, Oliver F: Alopecia mucinosa (follicular mucinosis) in a dog. Vet Dermatol 6:221, 1995.
3. Brooks DG, et al: Pancreatic paraneoplastic alopecia in 3 cats. J Am Anim Hosp Assoc 30:557, 1994.
4. Cieslowski D, Paradis M: Alopécie saisonnière canine. Méd Vét Québec 24:98, 1993.
5. Curtis CF, et al: Investigation of the reproductive and growth hormone status of dogs affected by idiopathic recurrent flank alopecia. J Small Anim Pract 37:417, 1996.
6. Declercq J: Lymphocytic mural folliculitis in two cats. Vlaams Diergeneeskd Tijdschr 64:177, 1995.
6a. Declercq J: A case of diet-related lymphocytic mural folliculitis in a cat. Vet Dermatol 11:75, 2000.
7. Declercq J, Vanstapel MJ: Chronic radiant heat dermatitis (Erythema ab igne) in two dogs. Vet Dermatol 9:269, 1998.
8. Dennis JS, et al: Lymphocytic/plasmacytic gastroenteritis in cats: 14 cases (1985–1990). J Am Vet Med Assoc 200:1712, 1992.
9. Endenburg N, Knol BW: Behavioural, household, and

9. social problems associated with companion animals: opinions of owners and nonowners. Vet Quart 16:130, 1994.
10. Fadok VA: The dynamics of hair growth and development. Dermatol Rep 4:1, 1985.
11. Godfrey DR: A case of feline paraneoplastic alopecia with secondary *Malassezia*-associated dermatitis. J Small Anim Pract 39:394, 1998.
12. Griffin CE: Personal observation, 1993.
13. Griffin CE: Open forum. Etretinate, how is it being used in veterinary dermatology? Derm Dialogue, Spring/Summer 1993, p 4.
14. Gross TL, et al: Veterinary Dermatopathology. Mosby–Year Book, St. Louis, 1992.
15. Gross TL, et al: Infiltrative mural folliculitis. Dermatopathology Session, Am Coll Vet Pathol, Albuquerque, 1997.
16. Gross TL, et al: An anatomical classification of folliculitis. Vet Dermatol 8:147, 1997.
17. Gross TL, et al: Follicular lipidosis in three rottweilers. Vet Dermatol 8:33, 1997.
18. Gross, T. L., et al.: Subepidermal bullous dermatosis due to topical corticosteroid therapy in dogs. Vet. Dermatol. 8:127, 1997.
19. Headington JT: Telogen effluvium. New concepts and review. Arch Dermatol 129:356, 1993.
20. Hodson S, et al: Resolution of paraneoplastic alopecia following surgical removal of a pancreatic carcinoma in a cat. Proc Eur Soc Vet Dermatol Eur Coll Vet Dermatol 14:107, 1997.
21. Kimura T, Kunio D: The effect of topical minoxidil treatment on hair follicular growth of neonatal descendants of Mexican hairless dogs. Vet Dermatol 8:107, 1997.
22. Kral F, Schwartzman RM: Veterinary and Comparative Dermatology. J. B. Lippincott Co, Philadelphia, 1964.
23. Kwochka KK, et al: Advances in Veterinary Dermatology, Vol 3. Butterworth Heinemann, Boston, 1998, p 511.
24. Miller WH, Jr: Symmetrical truncal hair loss in cats. Comp Cont Educ 12:461, 1990.
25. Miller MA, Dunstan RW: Seasonal flank alopecia in boxers and airedale terriers: 24 cases (1985–1992). J Am Vet Med Assoc 203:1567, 1993.
26. Muller GH, et al (eds): Small Animal Dermatology, 3rd ed. W. B. Saunders Co, Philadelphia, 1983.
27. Olivry T: Newly recognized feline syndromes: Selected topics. Proc. DVM Spring Seminar, Key West, 1998, p. 29.
28. Paradis M: Canine recurrent flank alopecia: Treatment with melatonin. Proc Annu Memb Meet Am Acad Vet Dermatol Am Coll Vet Dermatol 11:49, 1995.
29. Paradis M: Melatonin therapy in canine alopecia. In: Bonagura J (ed): Current Veterinary Therapy XIII. W. B. Saunders Co, Philadelphia, 2000, p 546.
30. Paradis M: Melatonin in the treatment of canine pattern baldness. In: Kwochka KW, et al (eds): Veterinary Dermatology III. Butterworth-Heinemann, Boston, 1998, p 511.
31. Pascal-Tenorio A, et al: Paraneoplastic alopecia associated with internal malignancies in the cat. Vet Dermatol 8:47, 1997.
32. Power H: Personal communication, 1993.
33. Power HT, et al: Novel feline alopecia areata-like dermatosis: cytotoxic T-lymphocytes target the follicular isthmus. Proc. World Cong Vet Dermatol 3:74, 1996.
34. Power, H. T.: Newly recognized feline skin diseases. Proc. Annu. Memb. Meet. Am. Acad. Vet. Dermatol. Am. Coll. Vet. Dermatol. 14:27, 1998.
35. Rosenkrantz WS, et al: Traction alopecia in the canine: four case reports. Calif Vet 43:7, 1989.
36. Rosenkrantz WS, Griffin CE: Unpublished observations, 1999.
37. Rothstein E, et al: A retrospective study of dysplastic hair follicles and abnormal melanization in dogs with follicular dysplasia syndromes or endocrine skin disease. Vet Dermatol 9:235, 1998.
38. Schmeitzel LP, et al: Focal cutaneous reactions at vaccination sites in a cat and four dogs. Proc Annu Memb Meet Am Acad Vet Dermatol Am Coll Vet Dermatol 2:39, 1986.
39. Scott DW: Thyroid function in feline endocrine alopecia. J Am Anim Hosp Assoc 11:98, 1975.
40. Scott DW: Feline dermatology, 1900–1978: A monograph. J Am Anim Hosp Assoc 16:331, 1980.
41. Scott DW: Feline dermatology 1983–1985: "The secret sits." J Am Anim Hosp Assoc 23:255, 1987.
42. Scott DW: Seasonal flank alopecia in ovariohysterectomized dogs. Cornell Vet 80:187, 1990.
43. Scott DW, et al: Muller and Kirk's Small Animal Dermatology, 5th ed. W. B. Saunders Co, Philadelphia, 1995.
44. Scott DW, et al: Exfoliative dermatitis in association with thymoma in 3 cats. Feline Pract 23:8, 1995.
45. Scott DW: Les agrégats de mélanine dans l'appareil pilo-sébacé: signification en dermatohistopathologie du chat. Méd Vét Québec 28:38, 1998.
46. Scott DW, Rothstein E: Trichoptilosis in three golden retrievers. Canine Pract 23:14, 1998.
47. Scott DW, Miller WH Jr: Idiosyncratic cutaneous adverse drug reactions in the dog: Literature review and report of 101 cases (1990–1996). Canine Pract 24:16, 1999.
48. Scott DW, Miller WH Jr: Idiosyncratic cutaneous adverse drug reactions in the cat: literature review and report of 14 cases (1990–1996). Feline Pract 26:10, 1998.
49. Scott DW: What's new in feline dermatology. Proc Br Small Anim Vet Assoc, 1999, p 128.
50. Tasker S, et al: Resolution of paraneoplastic alopecia following surgical removal of a pancreatic carcinoma in a cat. J Small Anim Pract 40:16, 1999.
51. Thoday KL: Differential diagnosis of symmetrical alopecia in the cat. In Kirk RW (ed): Current Veterinary Therapy IX. W. B. Saunders Co., Philadelphia, 1986, p 545.
52. Thoday KL: Aspects of feline symmetric alopecia. In: von Tscharner C, Halliwell REW (eds): Advances in Veterinary Dermatology I. Baillière-Tindall, Philadelphia, 1990, p 47.
53. Thompson DL, et al: Prolactin administration to seasonally anestrous mares: Reproductive, metabolic, and hair-shedding responses. J Anim Sc. 75:1092, 1997.
54. Tieghi C, et al: Medullary trichomalacia: A retrospective study of 6 cases in German shepherd dogs. (Submitted for publication 1999).
55. Waldman L: Seasonal flank alopecia in affenpinschers. J Small Anim Pract 36:271, 1995.
56. Whiting DA: Structural abnormalities of the hair shaft. J Am Acad Dermatol 16:1, 1987.
57. Wilcock BP, Yager JA: Focal cutaneous vasculitis and alopecia at sites of rabies vaccination in dogs. J Am Vet Med Assoc 188:1174, 1986.
58. Yager JA, Wilcock BP: Color Atlas and Text of Surgical Pathology of the Dog and Cat. Dermatopathology and Skin Tumors. Wolfe Publishing, London, 1994.

Chapter 12
Congenital and Hereditary Defects

Congenital and hereditary defects appear to be becoming more common. Some of this apparent increase in frequency no doubt reflects an enhanced ability to diagnose these conditions. However, this does not explain all cases. Many of the disorders discussed have an unproven mode of inheritance or are transmitted as recessive traits. Breeding of apparently normal parents or siblings of an affected dog or cat distributes the gene more widely, with the eventual production of new cases. Breeders of animals with suspected or proven genodermatoses should be instructed to avoid breeding of all close relatives of the affected animal.

• DISORDERS OF THE SURFACE AND FOLLICULAR EPITHELIUM

A variety of disorders of keratinization or cornification are recognized in dogs and cats. Those with a known or suspected inherited basis are discussed in this chapter, and the remainder are covered in Chapter 14. Also included here are developmental defects and inflammatory disorders with a hereditary basis.

Primary Seborrhea in Dogs

Primary seborrhea is used to describe animals with an inherited disorder of keratinization or cornification. The epidermis, the follicular epithelium, the hair cuticle, and the claw can all be involved.

CAUSE AND PATHOGENESIS

Primary seborrhea is most commonly recognized in the American Cocker spaniel, English springer spaniel, West Highland white terrier, and Basset hound.[5, 47, 71, 73, 80] Other breeds affected include the Irish setter, German shepherd dog, Dachshund, Doberman pinscher, Chinese Shar Pei, and Labrador retriever.[1, 3, 5, 9] Other seborrheic breeds (e.g., English bulldogs)[5] are seen in certain hospital populations because of breeding practices in the surrounding area. This disorder has been studied most extensively in the American Cocker spaniel[44-49] and the West Highland white terrier.[73, 75, 88] Data from these breeds may or may not apply to other breeds.

A variety of cellular kinetic studies have been performed in normal beagles, normal Cocker spaniels, and Cocker spaniels with primary seborrhea.[44-49] When the seborrheic Cocker spaniels were compared with normal dogs, their basal cell labeling indices were three to four times greater than normal values. The epidermis, the hair follicle infundibulum, and the sebaceous glands were all hyperproliferative, but the hair root matrix was normal.[44, 45] The calculated epidermal cell renewal time for these dogs was approximately 8 days[45] as compared with 21 days for normal Cocker spaniels.[46] Similar kinetic abnormalities have been demonstrated in seborrheic Irish setters.[9] The hyperproliferative nature of the Cocker spaniels' skin appears to be due to some as yet uncharacterized primary

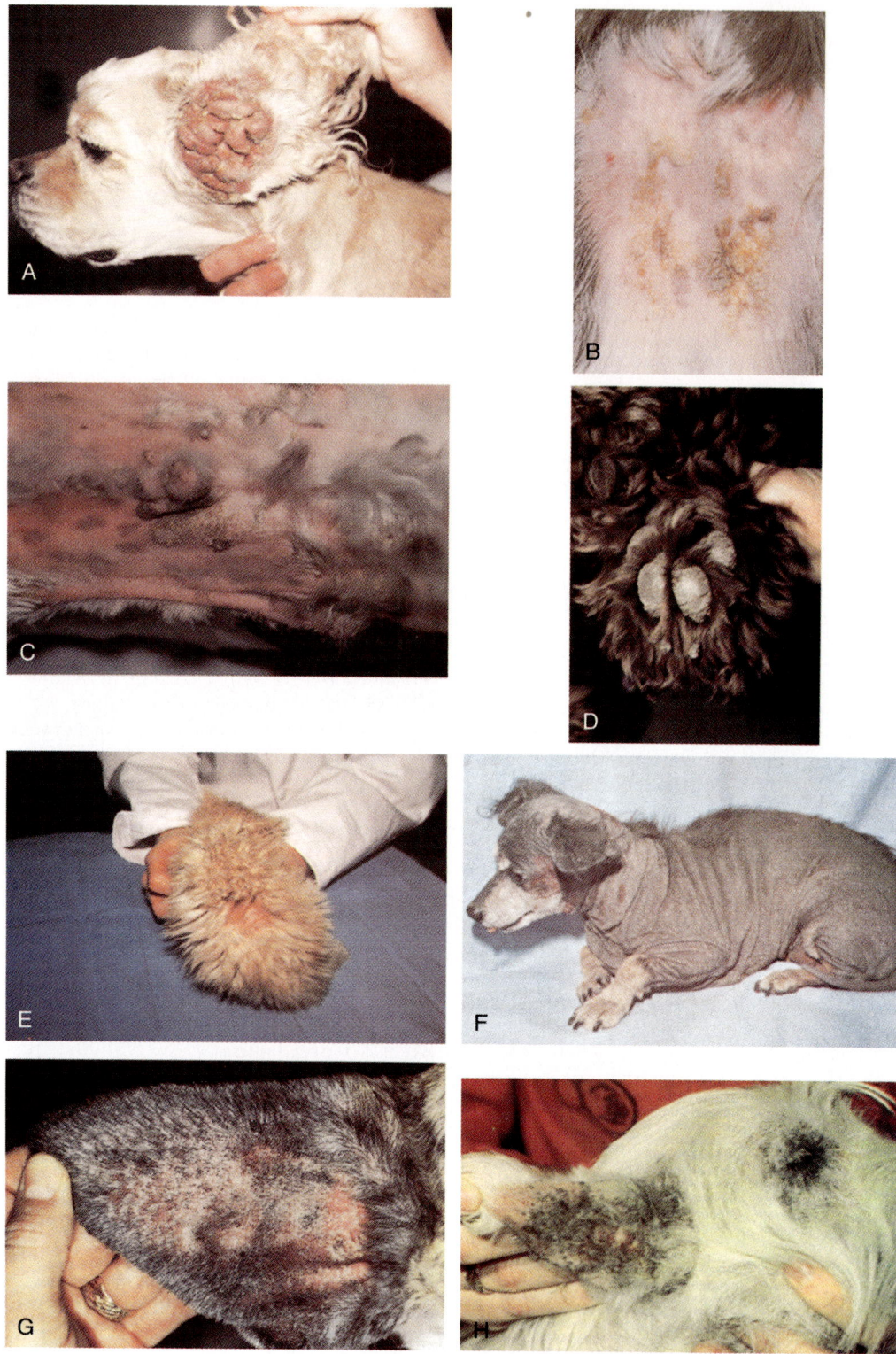

FIGURE 12-1. *A*, Primary seborrhea in a Cocker spaniel. Hyperplastic ceruminous otitis externa. *B*, Primary seborrhea in a Cocker spaniel. Seborrheic plaques in the intertriginous area of the ventral neck. *C*, Primary seborrhea in a Cocker spaniel. Erythema, apolecia, and seborrheic plaques on the abdomen. *D*, Primary seborrhea in a Cocker spaniel. Hyperkeratosis of the footpads and dystrophic claws in a 1-year-old dog. *E*, Primary

Legend continues on opposite page

cellular defect because the hyperproliferation remains in cell culture and persists when seborrheic skin is grafted onto normal dogs.[45, 48, 49]

In an extensive study of 100 West Highland white terriers over 12 generations, the inheritance of primary seborrhea was proved and it was probably transmitted as an autosomal recessive trait.[75] This mode of inheritance probably applies to other breeds because single affected dogs can be recognized in litters of clinically normal parents. Although labeled index studies were not performed in the seborrheic West Highland white terriers, histologic and ultrastructural studies indicated epidermal hyperproliferation.

CLINICAL FEATURES

Because of the inherited basis of the disease, signs occur early in life and become more severe with advancing age. Affected West Highland white terriers demonstrate clinical changes at 10 weeks of age.[75] In most dogs, early changes such as mild flaking or dullness of the coat are overlooked or attributed to intestinal parasites, inadequate nutrition, or other puppyhood problems. Usually by 12 to 18 months of age, the dog is presented for its seborrhea.

The presenting complaint varies from dog to dog. Common seborrheic findings include ceruminous, hyperplastic otitis externa (Fig. 12–1A); a dull coat with excessive flaking of the skin; greasy malodorous skin, which is marked in body folds or intertriginous areas; follicular casts; multiple discrete to coalescent, scaly or crusty pruritic patches (seborrheic dermatitis) (see Fig. 12–1B and C); digital hyperkeratosis (see Fig. 12–1D); and dry, brittle claws. Lesions of seborrheic dermatitis tend to be most severe around the eyes and mouth, on the pinna, or in the intertriginous areas of the feet, axillae, or groin.

Most seborrheic dogs have all of the seborrheic abnormalities described previously, but the severity of each varies from case to case. Irish setters and Doberman pinschers tend to have dry flaky skin, whereas Cocker spaniels, Springer spaniels, West Highland white terriers, Basset hounds, Chinese Shar peis, and Labrador retrievers usually exhibit otitis, greasy seborrhea, seborrheic dermatitis, or typically some combination of these. The greasiness and seborrheic dermatitis involve most or all of the body, but are most pronounced on the face, the ventral neck, the feet (especially interdigitally), the perineum, and the ventral body. Basset hounds and Chinese Shar peis also have signs of the disorder in their various body folds. The caudodorsum of these greasy dogs is often dry and flaky.

Aside from the visual and olfactory findings, pruritus occurs in many of these dogs. This is especially true when the dog is greasy or has seborrheic dermatitis. The pruritus follows the development of skin lesions, although it precedes the skin lesions in many secondarily seborrheic dogs. Dogs with seborrhea are prone to secondary bacterial infections and *Malassezia* dermatitis (see Chap. 14). When dogs with primary seborrhea have either condition, their skin lesions worsen rapidly and their pruritus increases dramatically, especially when *Malassezia* dermatitis is present. In some cases, the lesions of the secondary infections are so severe and widespread that the seborrheic lesions cannot be appreciated until the staphylococcal or *Malassezia* component is resolved.

DIAGNOSIS

The clinical lesions in primary or secondary seborrhea (see Chap. 14) are identical; thus, the diagnosis of primary seborrhea is made by exclusion. In dogs younger than 1 year, the list of differential diagnostic possibilities is short and includes demodicosis, cheyletiellosis,

---

FIGURE 12–1. Continued seborrhea in a Persian cat. Kitten with a greasy, matted haircoat and patchy alopecia. *F*, Canine icthyosis in a terrier-cross with generalized dry, hyperkeratotic, alopecic skin. The dog has appeared this way since birth. *G*, Congenital ichthyosis in a dog. Marked hyperkeratosis and mild erythema in a pinna. *H*, Pinna and periocular region of a dog with epidermal dysplasia. Chronic alopecia, hyperpigmentation, and lichenification.

nutritional deficiency, ichthyosis, epidermal dysplasia, and food hypersensitivity. In adult dogs, the list is much longer.

The diagnosis of primary seborrhea is supported by biopsy. In noninfected flaky or greasy areas, hyperplastic superficial perivascular dermatitis is visible. There is usually a marked keratinization defect, characterized by orthokeratotic or parakeratotic hyperkeratosis, follicular keratosis, and variable apoptosis of keratinocytes (Fig. 12–2). In many cases, the epidermis is normal to slightly increased in thickness. In mildly inflamed lesions, the perivascular cellular infiltrate is mild and consists of lymphocytes and plasma cells. In inflamed lesions, the perivascular inflammation becomes more intense, and papillomatosis and focal areas of parakeratotic hyperkeratosis (parakeratotic "caps") overlie edematous dermal papillae (papillary "squirting") (Fig. 12–3). This capping is common at the follicular ostia.[3] The follicular hyperkeratosis is typically orthokeratotic unless secondary infections are present. Bacteria are numerous in the surface, and follicular debris and yeast may also be present. Evidence of secondary bacterial infection (e.g., intraepidermal pustular dermatitis or folliculitis) is common.

CLINICAL MANAGEMENT

Primary seborrhea cannot be cured, and the ease of control varies from dog to dog. The seborrheic changes in these dogs worsen significantly with dietary inadequacies, external parasites, or endocrine or metabolic diseases, so these dogs should be monitored carefully for the development of any intercurrent disease. Seborrheic dogs are prone to secondary staphylococcal infections or *Malassezia* dermatitis. Administration of an appropriate antibiotic or ketoconazole is often necessary at the onset of antiseborrheic therapy to resolve pre-existing infections. During maintenance therapy, a sudden worsening of the dog's seborrhea may indicate that the infection has returned and the dog should be examined.

The mainstay of treatment involves the use of antiseborrheic shampoos and moisturizers. The shampoo selection and the vigor of treatment depend on the nature of the seborrhea.[42] Dry, uninflamed skin is easier to manage than greasy skin. Many dogs are

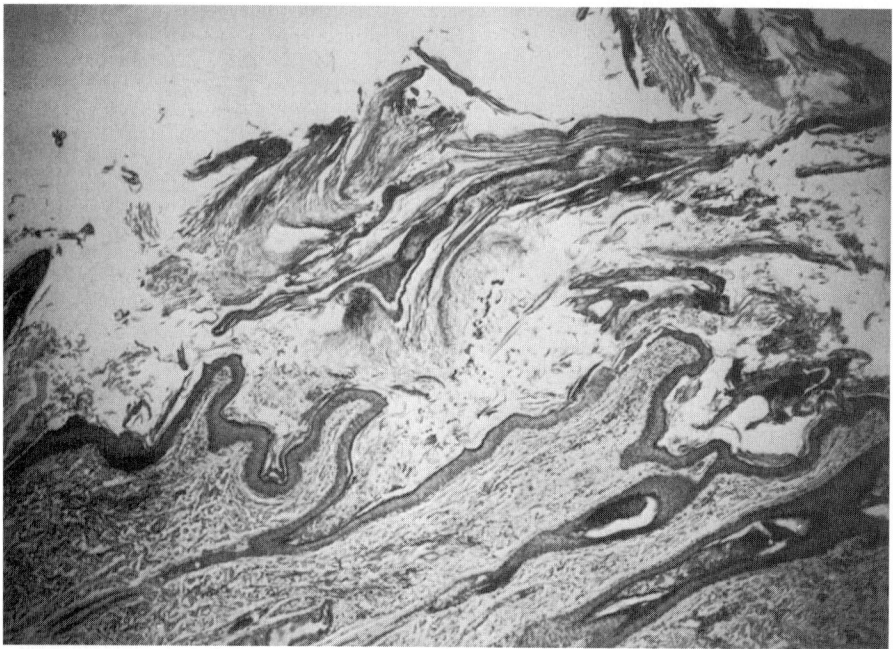

FIGURE 12–2. Canine seborrheic dermatitis. Hyperplastic superficial perivascular dermatitis with a marked keratinization defect and parakeratotic capping.

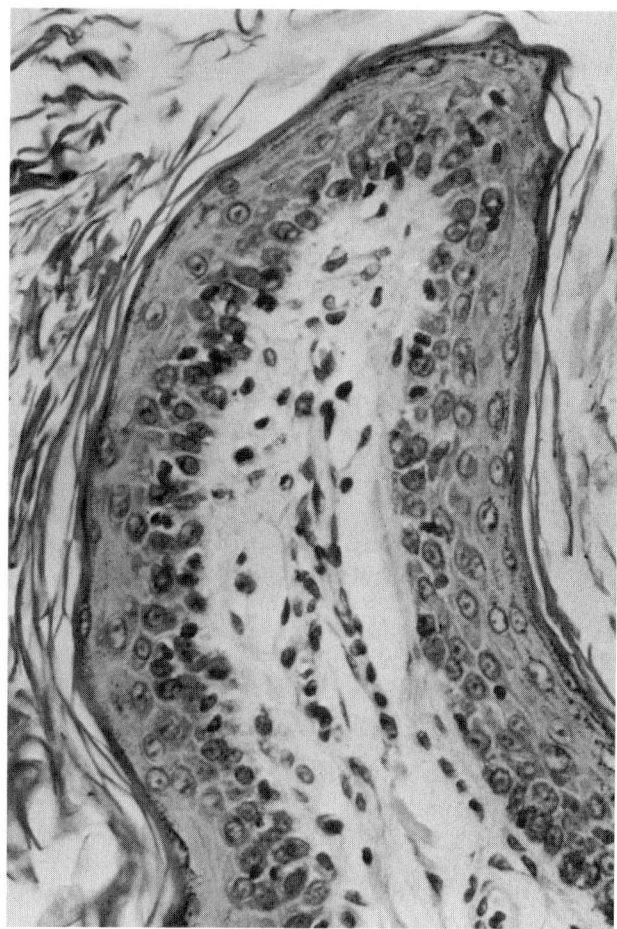

FIGURE 12–3. Close-up of Figure 12–2. Papillary squirting.

both dry and greasy, and greasiness is especially prominent in the intertriginous regions and between the toes and the pads. Long hair impedes the thorough cleaning of the skin, especially when the area is greasy, so owners should be encouraged to keep the coat cut short.

Dogs with dry skin with mild to moderate scaling usually require a bath once or twice weekly to return the skin to near-normal condition. Dogs with heavy scaling need to be bathed two or three times a week. This intense bathing is done for 2 to 3 weeks to reduce the corneocyte count to near normal,[24] and then the frequency of bathing is gradually decreased to some maintenance level. Some investigators set a frequency (e.g., once weekly), whereas other clinicians allow the client to decide on the basis of the individual dog's needs. As long as the dog is not prone to secondary bacterial infections, the latter method is most appropriate. Overbathing any dog, but especially one with dry seborrhea, can result in increased scaling.

A large number of grooming or antiseborrheic shampoos are appropriate for the bathing of dry skin. Product selection depends on client and veterinarian preference. It is advisable to start with the mildest product and change to a stronger one only if the initial product is unsatisfactory. For mildly flaky skin, moisturizing hypoallergenic shampoos (HyLyt°efa hypoallergenic moisturizing shampoo, DVM Pharmaceuticals; Allergroom shampoo, Virbac; MicroPearls Advantage Hydra-Pearls shampoo, EVSCO; DermaPet All Natural Conditioning Shampoo, DermaPet), colloidal oatmeal shampoos (Epi-Soothe, Virbac), or emollient-based chlorhexidine products (ChlorhexiDerm shampoo, DVM Pharmaceuticals; Nolvasan shampoo, Fort Dodge Animal Health; Hexadene shampoo, Virbac) are commonly used. For more severe flaking, sulfur and salicylic acid products (MicroPearls Advantage Seba-Moist Moisturizing Shampoo, EVSCO; DermaPet Seborrheic Shampoo, DermaPet; Sebolux shampoo, Virbac; SebaLyt shampoo, DVM Pharmaceuticals) are appropriate. For recalcitrant cases, mild tar products (MicroPearls Advantage Tar Moisturizing Shampoo, EVSCO; Nusal-T shampoo, DVM Pharmaceuticals; T-Lux shampoo, Virbac) might be appropriate but, because all tar products are degreasing agents, they should be used cautiously.

When there is secondary *Malassezia* dermatitis, products with both an antiseborrheic and antimycotic activity (Dermazole, Virbac; DermaPet Malacetic shampoo, DermPet; MicroPearls Advantage Miconazole or Seba-Hex shampoos, EVSCO) are useful. Even though the skin of seborrheic dogs is greasy, it is easy to irritate it, so caution should be used when strong shampoos (e.g., benzoyl peroxides, selenium sulfides) are to be used.

If the dog's coat is dirty, a rapid shampooing with a nonmedicated grooming product is indicated before the antiseborrheic bath. After the dog is lathered with the antiseborrheic product, the shampoo must remain in contact with the skin for 10 to 15 minutes for maximal effect. Gentle manipulation of the dog's skin during this waiting period tends to keep the dog happy and increases the cleaning action of the shampoo. After 10 to 15 minutes, the dog is rinsed thoroughly. Rinsing should take two to three times longer than lathering. Prolonged rinsing not only removes the debris and shampoo but aids in hydration of the skin. The dry skin of many of these dogs becomes flaky again soon after the bath, especially when the humidity is low. The application of an afterbath rinse or conditioner helps to provide a barrier to transepidermal water loss and its associated drying. Most manufacturers offer cream rinses for each shampoo they market, and one typically uses the rinse that matches the shampoo. Although any afterbath rinse can be effective, studies have shown that those containing oils, especially linoleic acid, are most effective in decreasing transepidermal water loss.[15] If the client keeps some diluted product in a misting bottle and sprays it on the dog as needed, the frequency of bathing can often be reduced.

For dogs with greasy skin, the shampoos must be stronger and need to be used more often. These dogs are prone to bacterial or yeast infections and often have to be treated with antibiotics or antifungal agents to control these secondary problems. Dogs with mildly to moderately greasy skin can be treated with sulfur and salicylic acid or mild tar products. Dogs with very greasy skin are often bathed with stronger tars (LyTar shampoo, DVM Pharmaceuticals; Allerseb-T, Virbac), selenium sulfides (Selsun Blue dandruff shampoo, Abbott), or benzoyl peroxides (OxyDex shampoo, DVM Pharmaceuticals; Pyoben shampoo, Virbac; MicroPearls Advantage Benzoyl-Plus, EVSCO). All these products are excellent degreasers and create a dry seborrhea if used excessively. After the presenting greasiness is resolved, many investigators switch to a less potent product or alternate between a strong and a mild product. Greasy dogs often need an afterbath rinse, especially if the dog's environment has low humidity. Most strong shampoos can disrupt the epidermal barrier and increase transepidermal water loss, with resultant worsening of the seborrhea.[16] An afterbath rinse can prevent this, but it may make the dog too greasy, so each case must be approached on its own merits.

Seborrheic dogs usually have ceruminous otitis externa, which must be treated routinely and regularly. Instead of antiseborrheic shampoos, ceruminolytic ear flushes are employed (see Chap. 19). The frequency of maintenance use is best determined by having the client smell the ears. When the waxy odor is first noticed, the ears should be cleaned. Despite vigorous cleaning, many of these dogs experience recurrent secondary bacterial or yeast infections. These infections are heralded by the sudden need to clean the ears frequently, otic pruritus, otic malodor, or combinations of these. Appropriate medications should be dispensed promptly and used for 2 to 3 weeks. Ear surgery should be considered for dogs that have frequent infections.

If the client is unable or unwilling to bathe the seborrheic dog, it becomes an unacceptable house pet. Some dogs, especially those that are greasy, have recurrent bacterial or yeast infections despite the most diligent efforts of their owners. These dogs are candidates for systemic treatment. Although omega-3 and omega-6 fatty acid supplements can be beneficial in these dogs,[5] they rarely provide complete control and should be used as an adjunct to other treatments. Because primary seborrhea is a hyperproliferative disorder, drugs that inhibit cell replication may be beneficial. Corticosteroids and cytotoxic drugs are applicable in such circumstances. Because these drugs have severe side effects and are needed for life, they should be reserved for cases in which all other measures have failed.

Retinoic acids have been used extensively in seborrheic dogs, with varying results from dog to dog and investigator to investigator. Although isotretinoin works in some cases (1 to 3 mg/kg q12h orally), results are usually disappointing.[20] Most favorable results have been obtained with etretinate. When 16 Cocker spaniels with severe seborrhea were given etretinate at a dosage of 1 mg/kg every 24 hours orally for 120 days, 15 dogs had a moderate to excellent response.[73] In moderately affected dogs, improvement was marked by day 60 of treatment. Severely affected dogs required longer courses of treatment for maximal responses. This treatment has no effect on the hyperplastic otitis of these dogs, and this must be managed by other means.[4] Five West Highland white terriers and four Basset hounds also studied showed no response to treatment.[73] Ten of the 25 dogs treated experienced side effects, including increased pruritus, reluctance to eat hard food, vomiting, stiff gait, conjunctivitis, and exfoliative dermatitis. The side effects disappeared with withdrawal of drug administration and did not recur with alternate-day drug administration.

Etretinate has been removed from the market and was replaced by acitretin. Anecdotal information suggests equal efficacy in the treatment of seborrheic dogs when administered at 1 mg/kg q24h. Data on treatment with lower doses are not available. The high cost of this agent will preclude its use in many dogs. Some investigators have returned to the use of retinol (see Chap. 17). Because retinol is much more toxic than the retinoic acids, the daily dosage should not exceed 400 IU/kg/day and the animal should be monitored carefully for signs of toxicity.

If there is a response to retinol or a retinoic acid, treatment should be for life. Alternate-day treatment is usually not satisfactory, and suggested regimens include administration for 5 of 7 days; 1 week on, 1 week off; or daily use during alternate months.[4] With long-term administration, some dogs may experience keratoconjunctivitis sicca and should be monitored for this condition. If it occurs, drug withdrawal may result in the regaining of tear function. Topical cyclosporine is usually effective if the etretinate administration cannot be stopped.[4] Both isotretinoin and etretinate can alter fat metabolism and liver function. Alterations usually occur early in treatment and are mild and transitory.[4] Long-term administration of etretinate has not resulted in severe metabolic changes in normal dogs, but cases should be monitored periodically.

Vitamin D analogs are receiving much attention in the treatment of psoriasis (see Chap. 15). These agents alter epidermal proliferation and terminal differentiation and significantly improve the skin lesions in psoriatic patients. When calcitriol (1,25-dihydroxyvitamin D_3) was given at 10 ng/kg q24h to Cocker spaniels with primary seborrhea, over 60% experienced significant improvement[50] and all dogs showed decreased cell proliferation in labeling studies. Because calcitriol can decrease PTH, electrolyte levels should be checked.

Seborrheic dogs unresponsive to bathing or retinoid administration are usually destroyed by their owners. Most of those dogs have greasy seborrhea, which predisposes them to near-constant bacterial or yeast infections. Maintenance treatment with antibiotics or ketoconazole often makes these dogs more acceptable to their owners and less malodorous. The expense of these drugs often precludes their use in all but small dogs. As a last resort, long-term corticosteroid or cytotoxic treatment is considered. Corticosteroids can be beneficial in greasy dogs because of their atrophic effects on the epidermis and sebaceous glands. Prednisolone is administered daily at 1 to 2 mg/kg until the greasiness is controlled and then adjusted slowly to the lowest alternate-day dosage that is effective. Some dogs require daily treatment.

Because these dogs are already prone to secondary infections and corticosteroids aggravate that predisposition, these patients must be examined frequently. Most of these dogs have signs of iatrogenic hyperadrenocorticism at some point in treatment. If the corticosteroids administration is stopped, a severe rebound in the seborrhea can be expected. Although we are aware of cases apparently well controlled with methotrexate,[5] specific details on protocols, efficacy, and side effects are not available. Because this drug is used in hyperproliferative disorders of humans,[2] it should be of some benefit in dogs. One of us (WHM) used azathioprine for pemphigus foliaceus in a seborrheic Cocker spaniel. While the dog was receiving maintenance treatment (2.2 mg/kg q48h), its seborrhea improved markedly. This suggests that drugs other than methotrexate may be beneficial. No details are available to support or refute that supposition.

Primary Seborrhea in Cats

Seborrhea is rare in cats, and primary seborrhea has been recognized in Persian, Himalayan, and exotic shorthaired cats.[69, 71] An autosomal recessive mode of inheritance was demonstrated in Persian cats. Cats of either sex or any coat color can be affected. Among affected cats, the severity of the seborrheic signs varies. Severe seborrhea is obvious in affected kittens by 2 to 3 days of age because their hairs paste together and they look dirty (see Fig. 12–1E). Breeders usually euthanize these animals. With time, the whole body becomes scaly and greasy and hair is lost (Fig. 12–4). Waxy debris accumulates in the face folds and ears (Fig. 12–5), and the cats have a rancid waxy odor. Mildly affected cats have similar signs, which are much milder and do not appear until about 6 weeks of age.

Biopsy of noninfected skin shows a marked keratinization defect, characterized by orthokeratotic hyperkeratosis and papillomatosis (Fig. 12–6). The perivascular cellular infiltrate is mild and consists predominantly of lymphocytes.

No effective treatment has been reported for severely affected cats. Retinoic acids have been used safely in cats[4] but are untried in primary seborrhea. A commercial product containing omega-3 and omega-6 fatty acids (DVM Derm Caps) was used unsuccessfully in two cats.[5] Mildly affected cats can be kept fairly normal by good grooming, periodic clipping, and occasional bathing with antiseborrheic shampoos. Tar products should not be used on cats.

Idiopathic Facial Dermatitis of Persian and Himalayan Cats

An idiopathic and presumably hereditary facial dermatosis of young Persian and Himalayan cats has been described.[11, 74] Cats of either sex can be affected, and the median age at

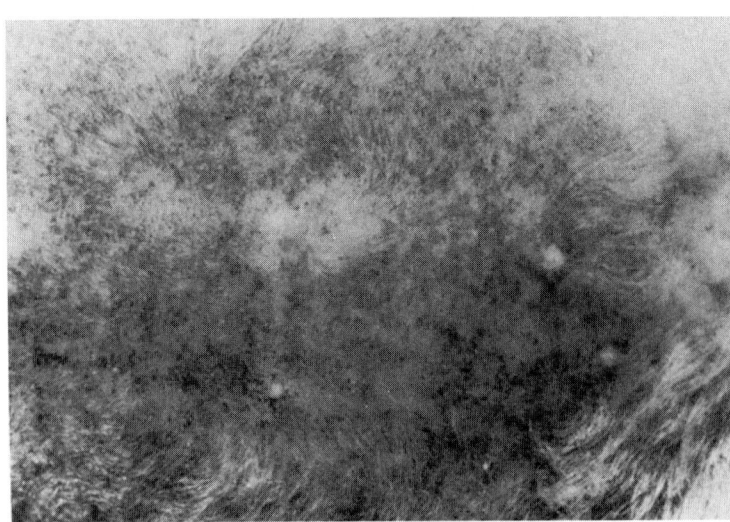

FIGURE 12–4. Primary seborrhea in a Persian kitten. Alopecia and marked comedone formation on the ventral thorax and abdomen.

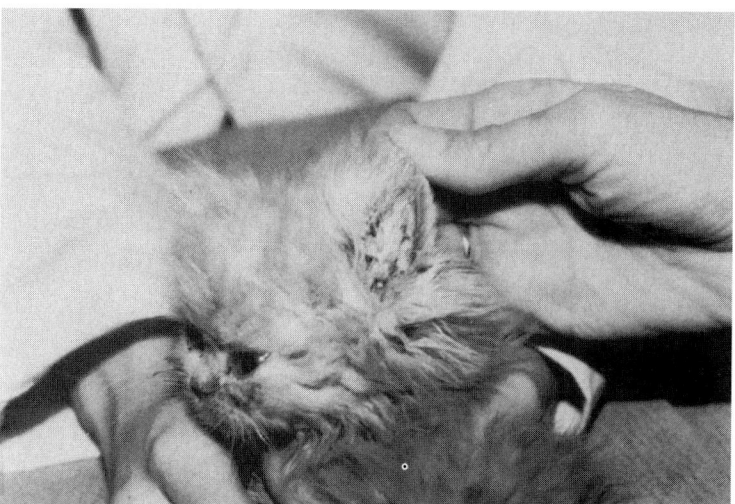

FIGURE 12–5. Primary seborrhea in a Persian kitten. Marked accumulation of cerumen on a pinna.

onset is 12 months. Skin lesions are confined to the head, especially the periocular, perioral, and chin regions (Figs. 12–7 and 12–8) and the neck, and are not caused by the cat. With time, the lesions often become pruritic, which increases their severity and distribution. Secondary bacterial or *Malassezia* infection also increases the symptoms and severity of the lesions.

Affected cats have a dirty face with an adherent black exudate on skin and distal portions of the hair shafts. The subjacent skin is inflamed, and the severity of the inflammation increases with time, pruritus, or secondary infection. Most cats also have accumulations of black, waxy materials in the ears. Histopathologic findings are nondiagnostic and include orthokeratotic hyperkeratosis, crusting, and hyperplasia of the epidermis and mixed-cell superficial perivascular to interface dermatitis. Eosinophils, neutrophils, and mast cells may be prominent, and pigmentary incontinence is usually present. Epidermal microabscesses containing eosinophils and neutrophils are occasionally seen.

No effective treatment has been identified. Topical and/or systemic treatments remove the exudate, but it reforms quickly after treatment is discontinued.

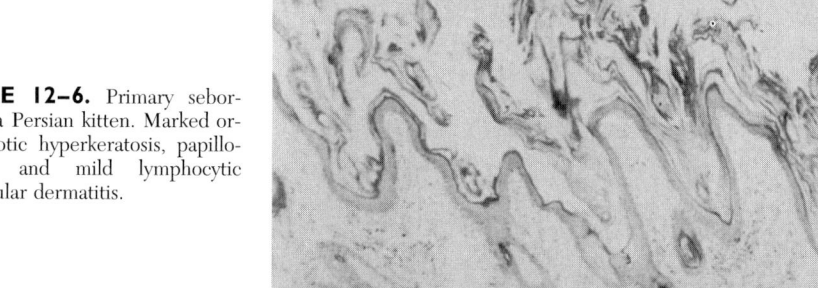

FIGURE 12–6. Primary seborrhea in a Persian kitten. Marked orthokeratotic hyperkeratosis, papillomatosis, and mild lymphocytic perivascular dermatitis.

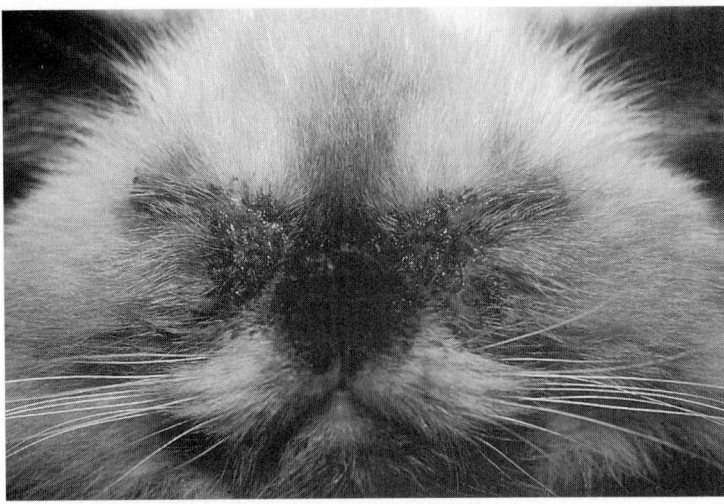

FIGURE 12-7. Idiopathic facial dermatitis of Persian and Himalayan cats. Accumulation of keratosebaceous debris around the eyes of a Himalayan cat.

Ichthyosis

Ichthyosis (fish scale disease) is a rare congenital skin disease and has been reported in dogs and cats. It is characterized by excessive hyperkeratosis on all skin surfaces including the digital, carpal, and tarsal pads.

CAUSE AND PATHOGENESIS

Ichthyosis in animals[1, 8, 34, 51, 57, 78] resembles but is not identical to ichthyosis in humans. Humans are affected by over a dozen ichthyosiform dermatoses. Most are inherited disorders with the onset of signs at or near birth, but some appear in childhood or adulthood. The skin disease can be accompanied by other developmental defects such as mental retardation and short stature. Various classification schemes have been used to describe the various ichthyosiform dermatoses, but none is ideal. Classifications focusing on the clinical, genetic, and biochemical data overlook the histopathologic abnormalities, whereas those revolving around ultrastructural alterations (e.g., epidermolytic and nonepidermolytic) probably are too narrowly focused. No classification system has been adopted

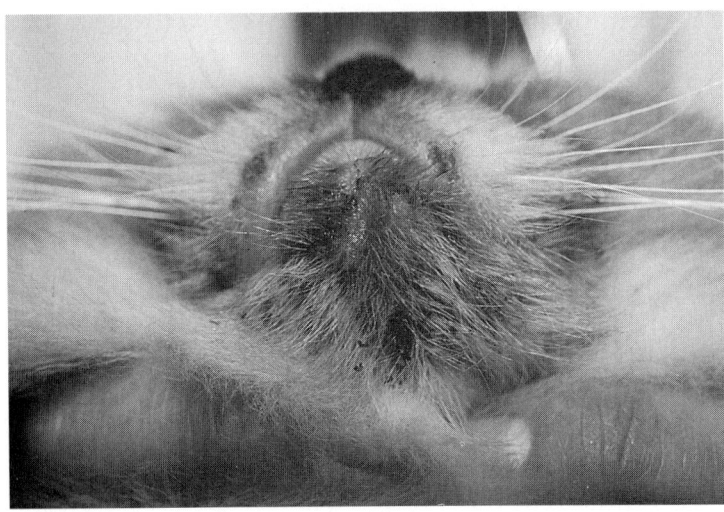

FIGURE 12-8. Idiopathic facial dermatitis of Persian and Himalayan cats. Exudation and crusting on the chin of the cat in Fig. 12-7.

for animals, but pathologists who have studied the disorder most intensively use the epidermolytic/nonepidermolytic scheme.[65]

Too few dogs and cats with ichthyosis have been reported in veterinary medicine to characterize the disorder. Because the parents of affected dogs have been normal, cases have been recognized in both sexes, and single cases have occurred in litters of five puppies or more, an autosomal recessive mode of inheritance is most likely.[5, 6] Beyond histopathology, labeled index and ultrastructural studies have been performed in a small number of dogs and one cat. Epidermal kinetic data have been gathered from one Jack Russell terrier[51] and three West Highland white terrier puppies.[5] In these dogs, the epidermal cell renewal time was approximately 3.6 days, which is 6 and 2 times faster than normal dogs (23.4 days) or dogs with primary seborrhea (7.9 days), respectively. Ultrastructural studies in two Cavalier King Charles spaniels[6] and one soft-coated Wheaten terrier[34] showed changes (e.g., increased DNA and RNA synthesis) that are also indicative of epidermal hyperproliferation in these, and probably most, dogs with ichthyosis. Additional ultrastructural irregularities in dogs include altered numbers and morphologic atypia of keratohyalin granules, curvilinear structures in the stratum corneum, and alteration in the intercorneocyte spaces.[6, 34, 51, 65] Ultrastructural studies in the cat showed sparse keratohyalin granules and abnormal tonofilament morphology in the stratum corneum.[65] The stratum corneum lipid layer of the Jack Russell terrier puppy showed decreased free fatty acids and acylceramide levels and increased ceramide III levels.[51]

CLINICAL FEATURES

Ichthyosis appears to be most common in West Highland white terriers but has also been recognized in many other breeds.* Either sex may be involved, and all dogs are abnormal at birth. Affected West Highland white terriers or Yorkshire terriers tend to be born with black skin, which cracks and peels off at about 2 weeks of age.[5, 18]

Much of the body of these dogs is covered with tightly adhering, verrucous, tannish gray scales (see Fig. 12–1F) and feathered keratinous projections, which give a rough texture to the skin (Fig. 12–9). Although some of these projections adhere to the skin, others constantly flake off, often riding up hair shafts in large sheets (see Fig. 12–1G). Large quantities of scaly, seborrheic-smelling debris accumulate on the skin surface. Scaly, erythematous dry patches are particularly prominent in the flexural creases and intertriginous areas. The horny layer of the nasal planum and digital pads thickens (Fig. 12–10). Masses of hard keratin accumulate at the margins of the pads and often extend upward from the margin in winglike projections. The entire paw of some patients appears grossly enlarged, and the whole foot can seem heavier than normal. Hyperkeratosis may surround the mucocutaneous junctions of the face. Some dogs have severe erythroderma or hair loss.[78] Insufficient details have been given about affected cats, but a striking cornification defect is present from birth.[5, 18] One kitten also had pronounced ectropion and eclabium.[5]

DIAGNOSIS

If the dog is presented in early puppyhood, no other diagnoses are appropriate. If the dog is presented as an adult with no prior history, all causes of seborrhea or exfoliative dermatitis must be considered (see Chap. 14). The diagnosis is confirmed by biopsy, which usually reveals characteristic histopathologic changes, especially the prominent granular layer and the presence of many mitotic figures in keratinocytes. Marked orthokeratotic hyperkeratosis (Fig. 12–11) and focal digitate projections of hyperkeratosis may occur. Follicular orthokeratotic keratosis and plugging are common. The epidermis may or may not be hyperplastic. One of the most characteristic histopathologic changes is marked hypergranulosis, but this layer may be normal,[3] thin,[78] or irregular.[6] Mitotic figures may be numerous. The superficial epidermis may contain numerous vacuolated keratinocytes,

---

*See references 1, 3, 5, 18, 34, 51, 65.

CLINICAL FEATURES

Like dogs with ichthyosis, these dogs experience a generalized seborrheic condition at or near birth that worsens with advancing age. Unlike the case with ichthyosis, the skin of the nasal planum and footpads of these dogs remains normal (Fig. 12–12) and there is minimal involvement of the glabrous skin of the abdomen, groin, and medial thighs. Pruritus is uncommon unless there is a secondary bacterial or *Malassezia* infection. Early on, the involved skin is scaly, but becomes thickened and crusted with time with numerous comedones. Hairs are often clumped together in a brownish-to-yellowish-to-blackish waxy material (Fig. 12–13). In two Rottweilers, bands of hyperkeratotic, hyperpigmented, often verrucous papules and plaques followed the lines of Blashko (Fig. 12–14). Advanced cases have a marked body odor.

DIAGNOSIS

With the widespread seborrheic lesions present near birth, the diagnosis of a congenital disorder of cornification is straightforward. With normal skin on the planum nasale and footpads, other seborrheic disorders can be discounted, but skin biopsy is needed for absolute confirmation of the diagnosis. Skin biopsies reveal a prominent surface and follicular keratinization disorder with a mild-to-moderate superficial perivascular dermati-

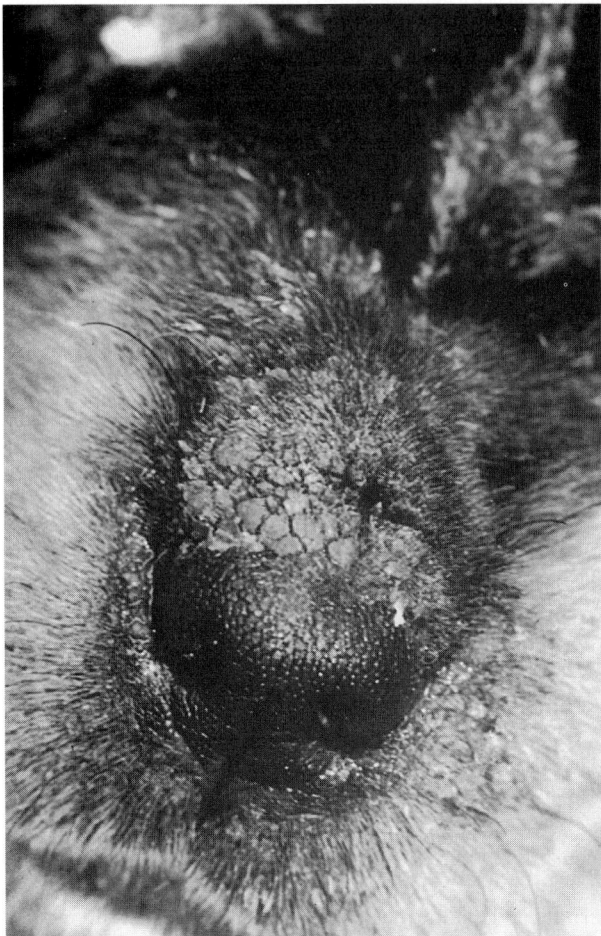

FIGURE 12–12. Follicular cornification disorder. Accumulation of keratosebaceous debris on the muzzle and bridge of the nose of a Rottweiler puppy. Note the sparing of the nasal planum.

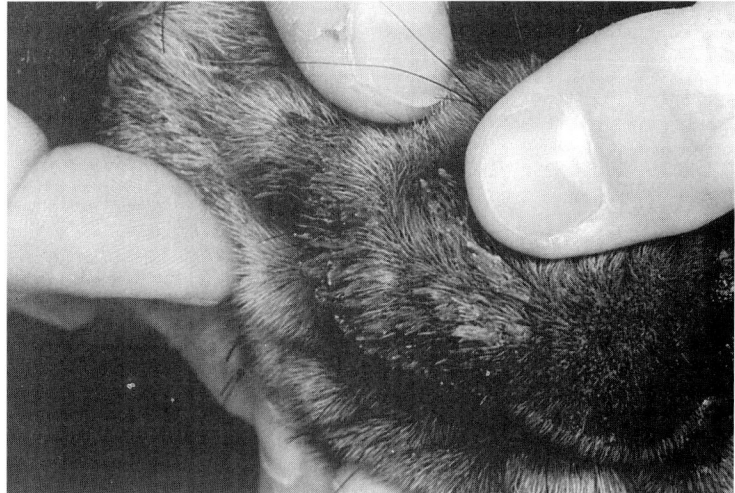

FIGURE 12–13. Follicular cornification disorder. Hairs on the muzzle are pasted together into large clumps.

tis. The surface epithelium is mildly affected and is hyperplastic and covered with a basket-weave orthokeratotic hyperkeratosis. The infundibular epithelium is hyperplastic, and the pilar canal is filled with a densely packed parakeratotic hyperkeratosis that projects above the skin surface in a conical fashion (Fig. 12–15A). Numerous lipid vacuoles are visible in the parakeratotic debris (Fig. 12–15B). A secondary suppurative bacterial folliculitis or *Malassezia* dermatitis may be visible. Ultrastructural studies performed in one dog detected abnormalities in keratinization only of the follicular epidermis. The cells in involved follicles had flattened nuclei, a less homogeneous interior, and course bundles of tonofilaments. Numerous lipid vacuoles are present within involved keratinocytes.

CLINICAL MANAGEMENT

No effective treatment for these dogs has been described. Bathing with strong antiseborrheic shampoos provides very short-term improvement; oral supplementation with zinc, retinoic acids, or calcitriol has been unrewarding.

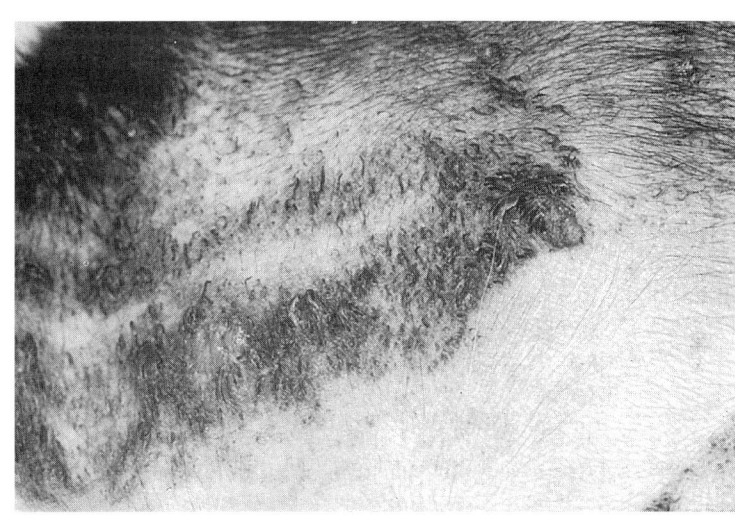

FIGURE 12–14. Follicular cornification disorder. Abdominal skin showing bandlike hyperkeratosis and follicular casting along the lines of Blachko.

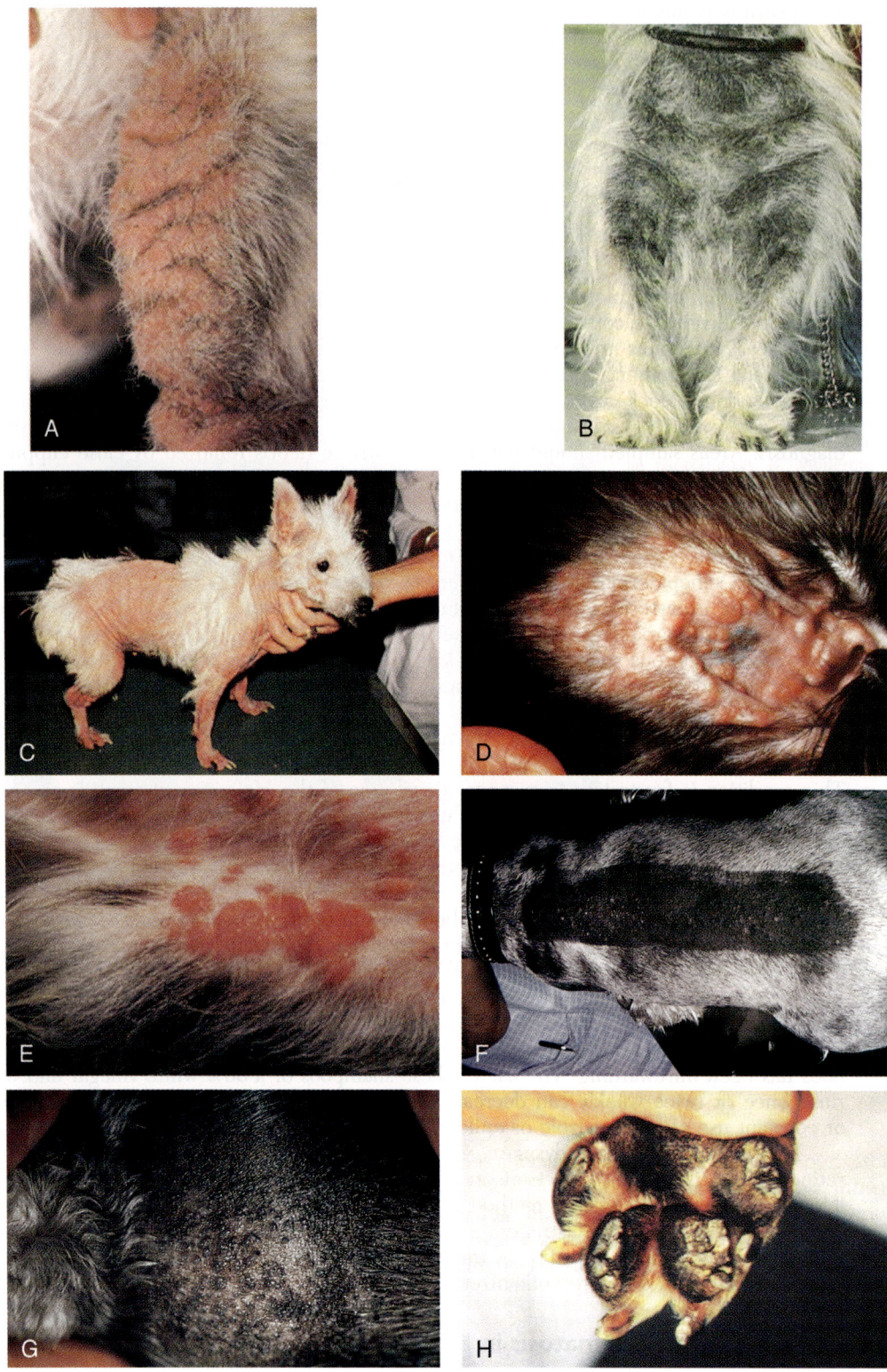

FIGURE 12–16. *A*, Epidermal dysplasia. Marked thickening and folding of erythematous, alopecic skin on a limb. *B*, Epidermal dysplasia. Chronic alopecia, hyperpigmentation, and lichenification. *C*, Epidermal dysplasia in a West Highland white terrier. Early erythroderma. *D*, Psoriasiform-lichenoid dermatosis in an English Springer
Legend continued on opposite page

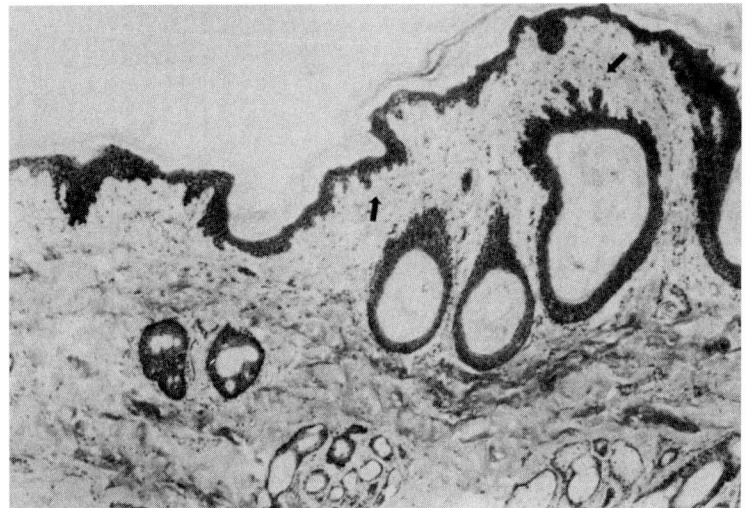

FIGURE 12–17. Epidermal dysplasia and *Malassezia pachydermatis* infection in a West Highland White terrier. Note marked epithelial budding of the epidermis and the hair follicle's outer root sheath *(arrows)*.

tially visible on the pinnae (see Fig. 12–16D), in the external ear canal, and in the inguinal region (see Fig. 12–16E). With time, lesions become increasingly hyperkeratotic (some almost papillomatous) and spread to involve the face, the ventral trunk, and the perineal area. Chronic cases resemble severe seborrhea. The exclusive occurrence of this dermatosis in English springer spaniels suggests a genetic predilection. It has been proposed that affected dogs have a distinct and exaggerated reaction to a superficial staphylococcal infection.[14]

Skin biopsy reveals superficial perivascular to interstitial dermatitis with psoriasiform epidermal hyperplasia and areas of lichenoid interface dermatitis, intraepidermal microabscesses (containing eosinophils and neutrophils), and Munro's microabscesses (Figs. 12–21 and 12–22).[3] Chronic hyperkeratotic lesions frequently show papillated epidermal hyperplasia and papillomatosis.

This dermatosis is characterized by a waxing and waning course for 1 to 3 years. Spontaneous remissions are not reported. Various medicaments, including anti-inflammatory doses of glucocorticoids, oral vitamin A, levamisole, dapsone, autogenous vaccine, and antiseborrheic shampoos, are of little or no help. In four cases treated with cephalexin (20 mg/kg q12h), response was excellent with complete resolution of lesions.[14]

Schnauzer Comedo Syndrome

The Schnauzer comedo syndrome affects the backs of some Miniature Schnauzer dogs and is typified by multiple comedones that may become crusted, nonpainful papules.

CAUSE AND PATHOGENESIS

This condition has been observed exclusively in Miniature Schnauzers. It seems to be a seborrheic or acneiform disorder and occurs in only certain predisposed individuals. The exclusive occurrence in Schnauzers and the clinicopathologic similarity to nevus comedonicus in humans[2] suggest that this syndrome may be a developmental dysplasia of hair

---

FIGURE 12–16. Continued spaniel. Erythematous lichenoid plaques on a pinna. (Courtesy of K. Mason.) *E*, Same dog as in *D*. Erythematous lichenoid papules and plaques on prepuce. (Courtesy of K. Mason.) *F*, Miniature Schnauzer whose back has been clipped to expose the area affected with lesions. *G*, Prominent, soft comedones on the skin of another Schnauzer. *H*, Marked hyperkeratosis of the footpads in a Dogue de Bordeaux. (Courtesy of M. Paradis.)

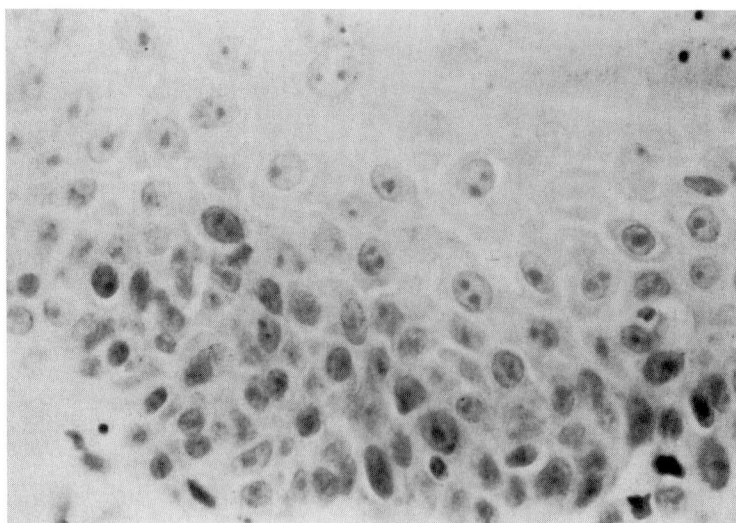

FIGURE 12–18. Close-up of Figure 12–17. Epidermal dysplasia. Increased mitosis, crowding, and loss of polarity of basilar keratinocytes.

follicles with an inherited basis. After it is recognized, Schnauzer comedo syndrome can usually be treated and easily controlled, but recurrences are common. However, there is much variability, with some cases responding more favorably to therapy than others.

CLINICAL FEATURES

In the predisposed individual, comedones (blackheads) tend to form over the back. These can be felt as sharp, crusted, papular projections above the surface of the skin. Some comedones are soft and waxy.

The lesions are most numerous at the midspinal area of the back, fanning out laterally and extending from the neck to the sacrum (see Fig. 12–16F). Schnauzer comedo syndrome is seldom noted in the early stage before the comedo extrudes from the follicular orifice. At that stage, there is no pain or discomfort. In some individuals, the comedo changes into a soft, small, acne-like pustule and causes slight irritation (see Fig. 12–16G). Dogs do not usually display visible pain or itching. In some dogs, the plugged follicles become infected. In these cases, the number of papular lesions increases rapidly;

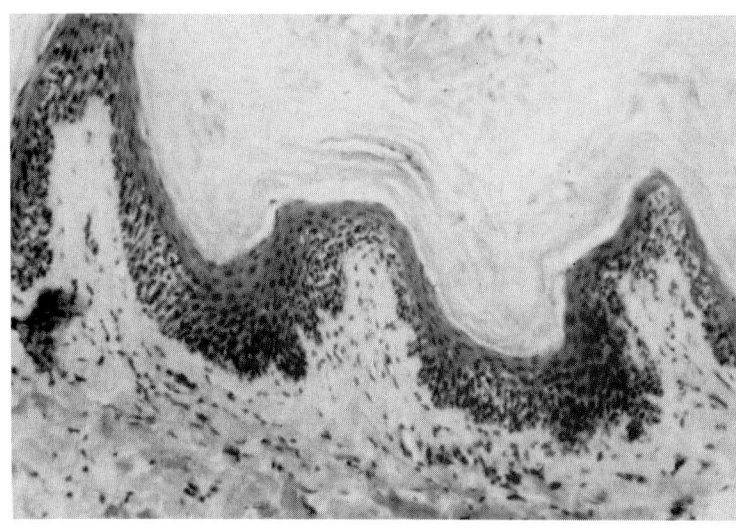

FIGURE 12–19. Close-up of Figure 12–17. Note diffuse spongiosis, lymphocytic exocytosis, and focal parakeratotic hyperkeratosis.

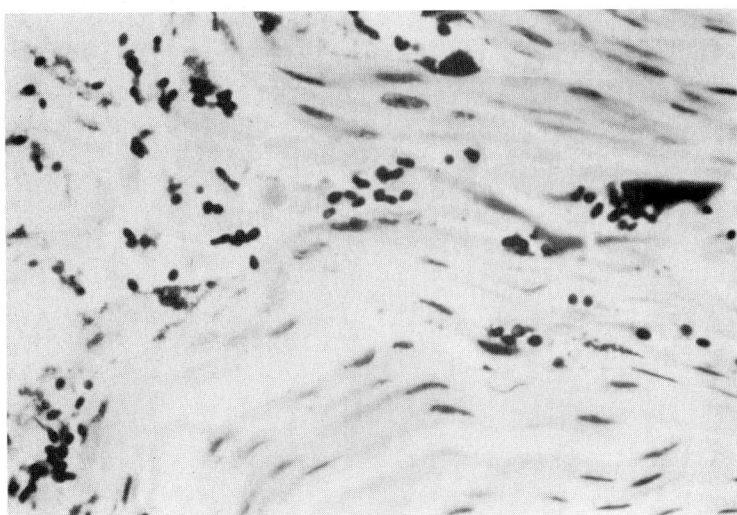

FIGURE 12–20. Close-up of Figure 12–17. Numerous yeasts in parakeratotic follicular keratin.

they become much more widespread and can involve the entire trunk. If secondary staphylococcal infection occurs, especially when it is widespread, the lesions tend to be pruritic or painful.

DIAGNOSIS

Clipping a small spot on the back exposes the skin so the individual comedones and papules can be seen. The restriction of these lesions to the caudal dorsum of a Schnauzer with no other signs of disease is virtually pathognomonic of the condition. The diagnosis can be confirmed by biopsy in which a section through one of the noninfected comedones reveals a keratinous plug blocking the hair follicle and sebaceous gland. A small cystic cavity is formed, lined by thin, stretched follicular epithelium and filled with keratin and sebum (Fig. 12–23). Sebum secretion accumulates behind the plug, which further dilates the cyst. If the follicle ruptures, a perifollicular inflammatory infiltrate appears. If a secondary bacterial infection is present, perifolliculitis, folliculitis, or furunculosis may be visible.

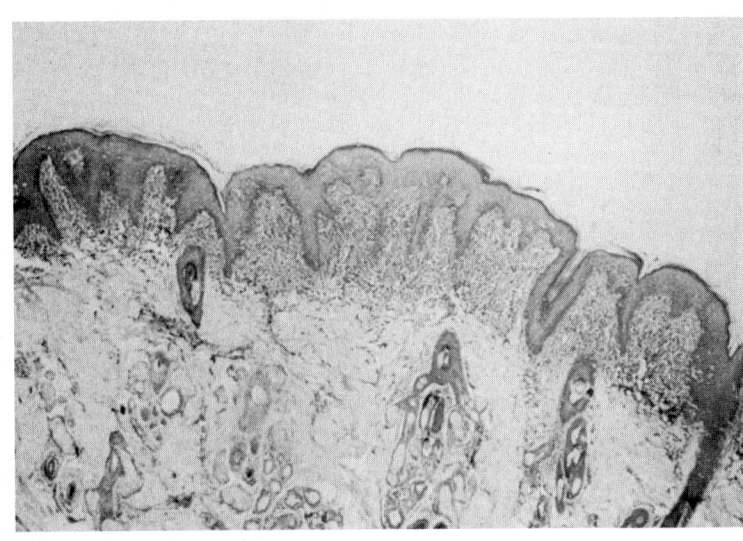

FIGURE 12–21. Psoriasiform-lichenoid dermatosis in an English Springer spaniel. Psoriasiform epidermal hyperplasia and lichenoid cellular infiltrate. (Courtesy of K. Mason.)

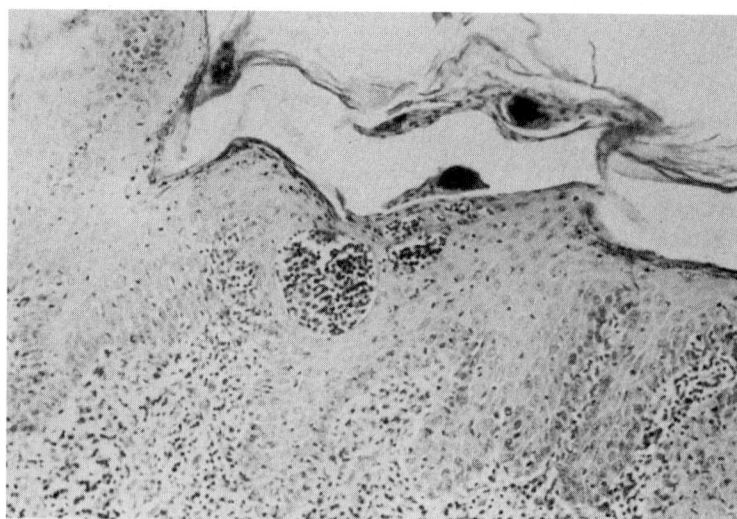

FIGURE 12–22. Psoriasiform-lichenoid dermatosis in an English Springer spaniel. Epidermal microabscess containing neutrophils and eosinophils. (Courtesy of K. Mason.)

CLINICAL MANAGEMENT

The owner should be informed that, because of its genetic basis, the condition can be controlled but not cured. Mild cases require no treatment and become apparent only when the coat is clipped or plucked. If the owner finds the lesions objectionable or they bother the dog or become infected repeatedly, topical antiseborrheic therapy should be instituted. If a secondary infection is present, systemic antibiotics should be administered for 3 to 4 weeks.

In mild cases, daily or alternate-day wiping of the area with various human acne cleaning pads, alcohol, or Listerine antiseptic (contains 0.06% thymol, 0.09% eucalyptol, 0.06% methyl salicylate, and 0.04% menthol) loosens or dissolves the comedones. Benzoyl

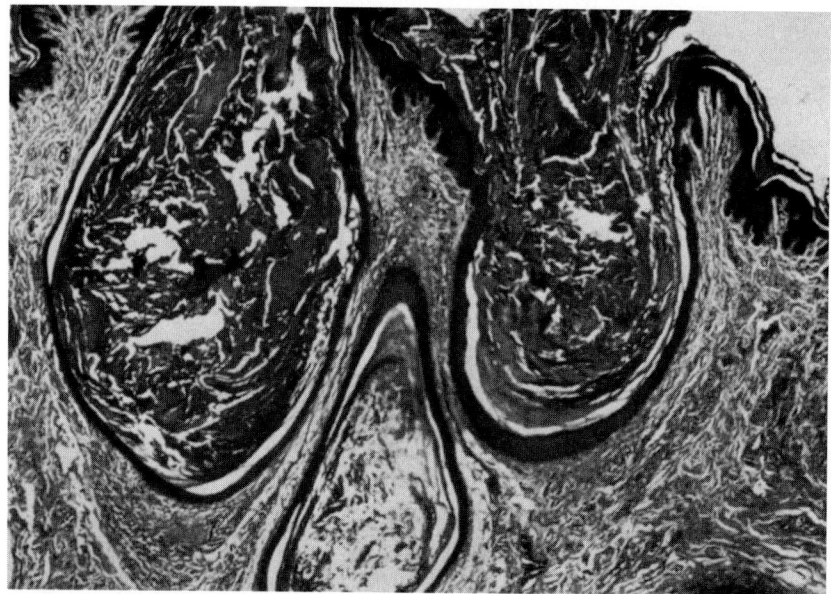

FIGURE 12–23. Schnauzer comedo syndrome. Dilation and plugging of hair follicles with compact keratin (comedones).

peroxide gel also can be used but may be irritating with repeated application. In more severe cases, antiseborrheic shampoos are indicated. Because these plugged follicles are easily inflamed by harsh agents, the mildest shampoo should be used first and only replaced by a stronger one if the first product is ineffective. Sulfur, tar and sulfur, benzoyl peroxide, and benzoyl peroxide plus sulfur shampoos are most commonly used. Bathing the dorsum twice weekly for 1 to 3 weeks removes the comedones, and then the frequency is adjusted to the patient's needs. The rare case that is refractory to topical therapy may benefit from the administration of isotretinoin at a dosage of 1 mg/kg every 12 hours.[4] One case was treated every-other day for 4 months after remission was achieved, and then therapy was discontinued.[29] No relapse was noted within a 1-year follow-up period.

Footpad Hyperkeratosis

Familial footpad hyperkeratosis has been reported in Irish terriers[10a, 41] and the Dogue de Bordeaux.[70] Single cases have been recognized in several related Kerry blue terriers,[5] the Labrador retriever, the Golden retriever, and mongrels.[5] Studies in Irish terriers suggested an autosomal recessive inheritance.[10a]

All cases experience severe hyperkeratosis by 6 months of age. All pads of all feet are involved. The entire surface of the pad is involved, but the keratin is more compacted in certain regions and forms horns (see Fig. 12–16H).[5, 70] With severe hyperkeratosis, fissures and secondary infection can occur and cause lameness. In Irish terriers, claws grow faster and their transverse profile is round rather than U-shaped.[10a] No other skin lesions are present.

Histopathologic findings include moderate to severe epidermal hyperplasia with marked papillated and diffuse orthokeratotic hyperkeratosis (Fig. 12–24).[70] Some fusion of the conical papillae by keratin can occur. Electron microscopic studies in Irish terriers were normal.[10a]

Treatment is symptomatic. Daily soaks in 50% propylene glycol cause significant improvement within 5 days, but treatment must be continued to maintain the re-

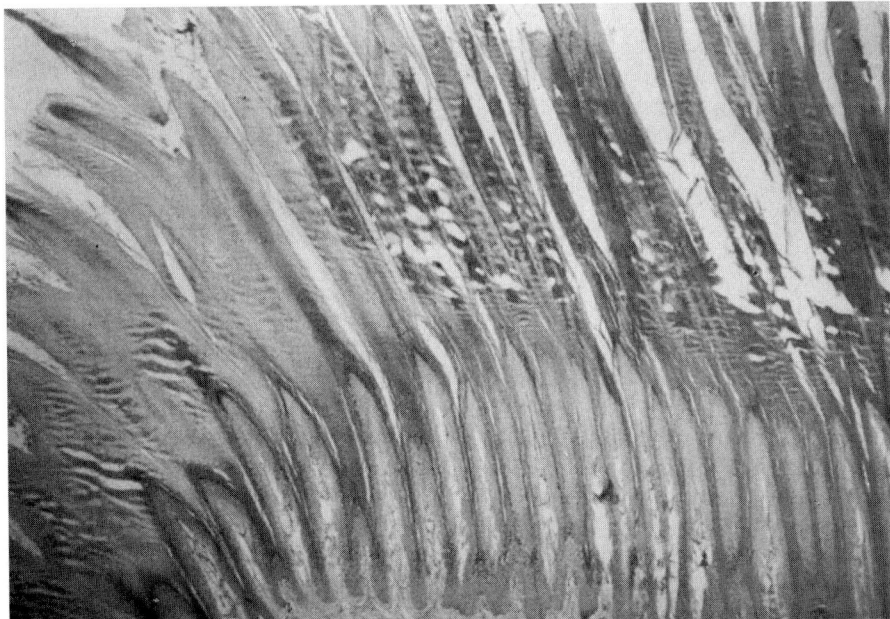

FIGURE 12–24. Digital hyperkeratosis in an Irish terrier. Marked papillated hyperplasia and orthokeratotic hyperkeratosis.

sponse.[10a, 70] Treatment with retinoic acids has been proposed but not tested. The mode of inheritance has not been established.

Nasal Hyperkeratosis

An apparently hereditary nasal hyperkeratosis has been described in Labrador retrievers.[67] Because the sires and dams of affected dogs were clinically normal, the condition was hypothesized to be autosomal recessive. The condition was recognized in males and females between 6 and 12 months of age. It mostly affected the dorsal nasal planum and was characterized by dry, rough, grayish, or brownish keratinous accumulations. Fissures developed occasionally. The lesions were stable over time, and the dogs were otherwise healthy. Histopathologic findings included mild to marked parakeratotic hyperkeratosis, moderate lymphocytic and neutrophilic exocytosis, and multifocal serous lakes within the upper epidermis. A superficial interstitial-to-interface dermatitis is present. No response occurred with antibiotic or zinc therapy. Improvement was marked with the topical application of 60% propylene glycol, 2 to 3 times daily, but the hyperkeratosis rapidly reappeared when treatment was stopped.

Aplasia Cutis

Aplasia cutis (epitheliogenesis imperfecta) is a congenital inherited discontinuity of squamous epithelium.[28, 35, 58] It is considered an autosomal recessive trait in cattle, horses, sheep, and pigs, but little is known of its inheritance in dogs and cats. The condition is characterized by areas of abrupt absence of epithelium, with resultant ulcers. Histologically, the ulcerated areas are distinguished by the complete absence of epidermis, hair follicles, and glands. The lesions of aplasia cutis in the newborn rapidly become infected, and septicemia soon results in death. With supportive therapy, small lesions may heal by scar formation. Skin grafting may be beneficial.

Dermal Dysplasia

A case of generalized dermal dysplasia was reported in a young mongrel dog.[61] The dog had multiple papules to nodules that had both epidermal and follicular abnormalities. The epidermis was hyperplastic with irregular keratinization, and basal cells were absent in some regions. Clusters of immature epithelial cells were present along the basement membrane zone of the epidermis or hair follicles. The hair follicles were deformed and surrounded by mucin.

Dermoid Sinus

A dermoid sinus is a neural tube defect resulting from incomplete separation of the skin and neural tube during embryonic development. The sinus is a tubular indentation of skin extending from the dorsal midline as a blind sac ending in the subcutaneous tissue or extending through the spinal canal to the dura mater. The lumen becomes filled with sebum, keratin debris, and hair. It may become cystic and is often inflamed. If infected, it may produce meningomyelitis and neurologic clinical abnormalities. Rarely, dermoid sinuses may be associated with spina bifida–type lesions, hemivertebrae, and vertebral fusions.[21]

Dermoid sinus has been reported in multiple Rhodesian ridgeback dogs and their crosses.[1, 7, 23, 50a, 53, 54, 82] Individual cases in a Boxer, English bulldog, Shih Tzu, Chow Chow, Boerboel, Yorkshire terrier, Great Pyrenees, English springer spaniel, and Siberian husky have also been reported.[5, 12, 14a, 17, 21, 72, 74a, 82] The dermoid sinus of Rhodesian ridgeback dogs may be caused by a gene complex. The only available data concerning inheritance of the dermoid sinus suggest that the factor may be inherited as a simple recessive gene.[54] If so, complete eradication of the problem can be achieved by only a program of progeny testing. However, by not breeding from affected animals, the incidence can be rapidly reduced. When additional cases occur, breeders should extend that policy by not using either parent or any sibling of an affected pup for breeding. The problem is complicated further because dermoid sinus is not always easy to detect in a young pup.

CLINICAL FEATURES

Lesions are often noted in young dogs. Whorled hair may be seen along the topline (normal in the Rhodesian ridgeback), or isolated whorls may appear at the dorsal midline at the cervicothoracic or lumbothoracic junction. A tuft of hair may protrude from single or multiple small openings in the skin and a cord of tissue may be palpated, descending from the skin toward the spine (Fig. 12–25). In densely coated dogs, the lesions are not visible and go unnoticed until the sinus becomes infected or ruptures and induces a draining pyogranulomatous dermatitis.[12, 17] In one dog, neurologic disease was precipitated when the owner attempted to squeeze material out of the sinus.[74a]

Diagnosis can be suspected on the basis of the anamnesis and the clinical appearance, but it is confirmed by a fistulogram. A tract may be delineated from the skin to the dorsal processes of the thoracic vertebrae. Lumbar myelograms may demonstrate attenuation of the subarachnoid space near the termination of the fistula.

CLINICAL MANAGEMENT

Sinuses that are quiescent need no treatment other than observation. If drainage or neurologic signs are present, surgical dissection is the treatment of choice, but because of the deep attachments of the dermoid sinus, complete removal is not always possible. The tissue at the base is often fibrous, and careful blunt dissection is needed. Meningitis may complicate these cases; therefore, extreme care should be taken to ensure an aseptic technique during surgery. Successful surgery often results in complete recovery. Affected patients should not be bred.

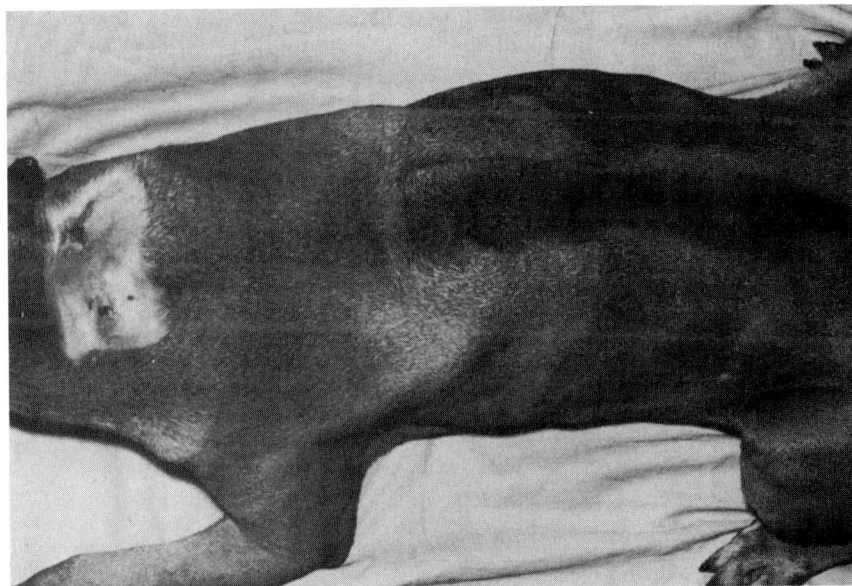

FIGURE 12–25. Dual fistulae opening on either side of the midline in the cervical region of the Rhodesian Ridgeback dog are typical lesions of a dermoid sinus. (Neck has been clipped.) Notice the whorled ridge of hair on the lower back from which the breed derived its name.

Table 12–1. TYPES OF EPIDERMOLYSIS BULLOSA (EB)

TYPE OF EB	STRUCTURE AFFECTED	DEFICIENT PROTEIN
EB simplex		
Dowling-Meara, Weber-Cockayne, Koebner	Intermediate filaments	Keratin 5 or 14
With muscular dystrophy	Hemidesmosomes	Plectin
Junctional EB		
With pyloric atresia	Hemidesmosomes	Integrins α_6 or β_4
Nonlethal	Anchoring filaments/lamina densa	Type XVIII collagen or laminin 5
Lethal	Anchoring filaments/lamina densa	Laminin 5
Dystrophy EB		
Dominant	Anchoring fibrils	Type VII collagen
Recessive	Anchoring fibrils	Type VII collagen

Epidermolysis Bullosa

In humans, the term epidermolysis bullosa refers to a group of mechanobullous diseases.[2] Most have a hereditary basis and are a result of a structural irregularity of the anchoring complexes of the epidermis (Table 12–1). One disorder, epidermolysis bullosa acquisita, is a nonfamilial autoimmune disorder targeting collagen type VII of the anchoring fibrils (see Chap. 9). The hereditary forms are divided into three major categories, namely epidermolysis bullosa simplex, junctional epidermolysis bullosa, and dystrophic epidermolysis bullosa. All forms have been reported in animals.

Epidermolysis bullosa simplex is the most superficial disorder, with clefting occurring in the basal layer of the epidermis. The first reports of epidermolysis bullosa simplex in dogs were in Collies[77] and Shetland sheepdogs.[56] Those dogs may have had dermatomyositis because the skin lesions mimicked those of dermatomyositis. We and others[193] have examined multiple Collies and Shetland sheepdogs with the classic skin lesions of dermatomyositis but have been unable to demonstrate muscle disease by electromyography (EMG) or multiple biopsies. These cases may be dermatomyositis without muscular involvement[31, 84] or epidermolysis bullosa simplex.

In junctional epidermolysis bullosa, blisters form within the lamina lucida (Fig. 12–26) of the dermoepidermal basement membrane. Multiple clinical subtypes are recognized in humans, and lethal and nonlethal variants are described in the dog. Junctional epidermolysis bullosa occurs in very young animals (e.g., at birth to 6 weeks of age) and has

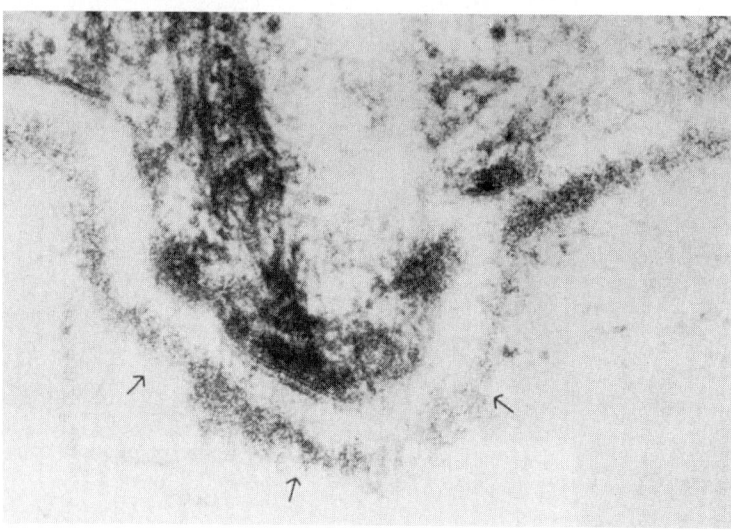

FIGURE 12–26. Junctional epidermolysis bullosa in a puppy. Electron microscopy reveals smaller than normal hemidesmosomes and decreased electron density in the underlying lamina lucida *(arrows)*. (Courtesy of R. Dunstan.)

been reported in a mongrel, Toy poodle, multiple Beaucerons, two German shorthaired pointer littermates,[19, 22, 26, 60, 63, 65] and multiple Siamese cats.[39] In the dogs, erosive-to-ulcerative lesions are most marked over bony prominences of the face, on the pinna, pressure points on the limbs, and/or the footpads (Fig. 12–27). Lesions can also be in the oral cavity, and the claws may be dystrophic. In the Beaucerons and German shorthaired pointers, an autosomal recessive mode of inheritance was suspected.

The cats were presented for shedding of all claws with secondary bacterial paronychia at 5 weeks of age. The sire of the kittens was affected. An autosomal recessive mode of inheritance was suggested.

Histologically, animals with junctional epidermolysis bullosa show a subepidermal separation with little or no subjacent dermal inflammation (Fig. 12–28). There was no expression of type XVII collagen in the German shorthaired pointers, and there was no abnormal expression of laminin 5, BPAG2 (type XVII collagen), integrin-α_6, and type VII collagen in the mongrel.

Dystrophic (dermatolytic) epidermolysis bullosa has been described in a domestic shorthaired cat,[93] a Persian cat,[66a] an Akita,[59] and multiple Beaucerons.[40] The domestic shorthaired cat had disease from 3 months of age, which included paronychia and claw loss on all feet; ulceration of the gums, tongue, palate, and oropharynx (Fig. 12–29A); and ulceration with crusting of the metacarpus, metatarsus, and digital pads (see Fig. 12–29B). The Persian cat had juvenile-onset ulceration of oral mucosa and footpads, onychomadesis, and fragile skin at sites of mechanical trauma. The Akita experienced its first skin lesions around 1 year of age. Footpad fissures and ulcers were the first lesions recognized, followed by claw dystrophy and alopecia and scarring of the ear margins, tail tip, and pressure points on the distal limbs. Multiple Beauceron pups from three separate litters were examined for the early development of erosive crusty lesions around mucocutaneous junctions and over pressure points and sloughing of claws. The dogs also had defects in tooth enamel, retarded growth, and an abnormal stance. In all animals, skin biopsy showed a sub-basilar dermoepidermal separation. Ultrastructurally, the separation occurs

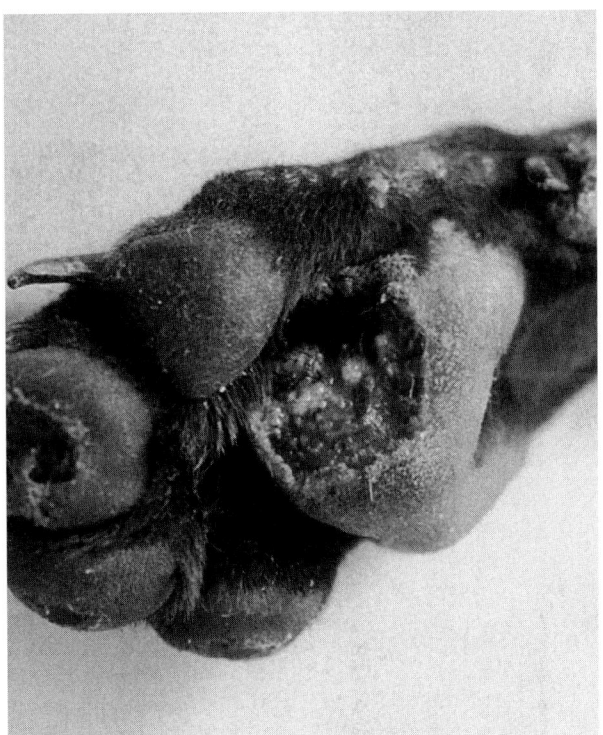

FIGURE 12–27. Junctinal epidermolysis bullosa. Full-thickness ulceration of the digital and main carpal pads. (Courtesy of T. Olivry.)

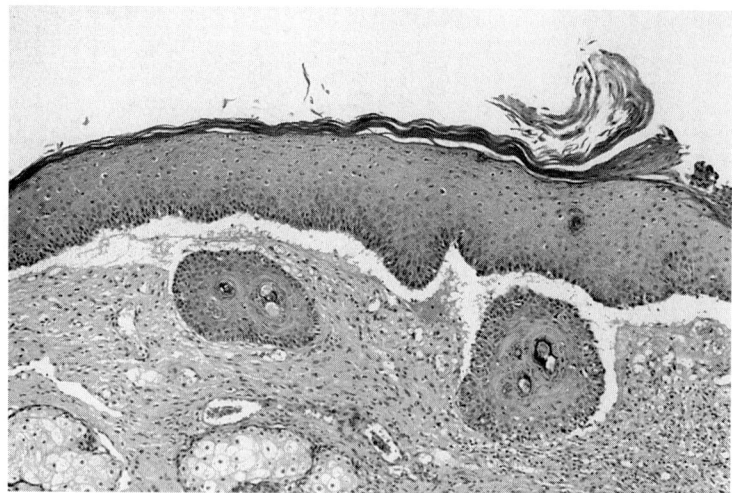

FIGURE 12–28. Junctional epidermolysis bullosa. Subepidermal separation with minimal dermal inflammation. (Courtesy of T. Olivry.)

beneath the lamina densa, with a reduction in the number of anchoring fibrils. There is decreased to absent expression of type VII collagen.[66a]

To date, only one case of epidermolysis bullosa acquisita has been described in animals (see Chap. 9).[64] With the clinical, histologic, and immunofluorescence similarities between this disease and bullous pemphigoid, it is possible that more cases exist but have gone unrecognized. The one case reported involved a 1-year-old Great Dane with acute-onset vesiculobullous disease involving the oral cavity, footpads, and truncal skin. Treatment with high levels of prednisone did little for the dog. On skin biopsy, the superficial dermis had a bandlike, neutrophilic, lymphocytic, and histiocytic infiltrate with an overlying dermoepidermal separation. Immunologic studies demonstrated circulating autoantibodies to the NCl domain of type VII collagen.

Aside from topical and/or systemic antibiotics or antifungals, no treatments help these animals. Management changes to minimize trauma may allow mildly affected dogs to lead a reasonably comfortable life.

Familial Canine Dermatomyositis

Familial canine dermatomyositis is a hereditary, idiopathic inflammatory condition of the skin and muscles of young Collies, Shetland sheepdogs, and Beauceron shepherds.[10, 21a, 27, 30, 31] It has also been reported in the Welsh corgi, Lakeland terrier, Chow Chow, German shepherd dog, and Kuvasz[3, 62, 92] and has been recognized in other purebred dogs. The familial basis in these other breeds is unproven.

CAUSE AND PATHOGENESIS

The cause of dermatomyositis in humans or dogs is unknown.[1, 13, 31] A genetically determined immune-mediated pathogenesis is suspected because of detectable immunologic abnormalities,[32] but it is unclear whether this immunologic reaction causes all of the changes or is in response to some pre-existing muscle or skin damage. Although dermatomyositis could be induced by drugs, vaccines, infections (especially viral ones), toxins, or internal malignancies, their causal relationship in dermatomyositis remains unproven.[2]

A familial history is rare in humans but common in Collies and Shetland sheepdogs. Breeding studies in Collies support an autosomal dominant mode of inheritance with variable expressivity.[31] Studies in the Shetland sheepdog conducted by one of us (WHM) and others[37] suggest a similar mode of inheritance in this breed.

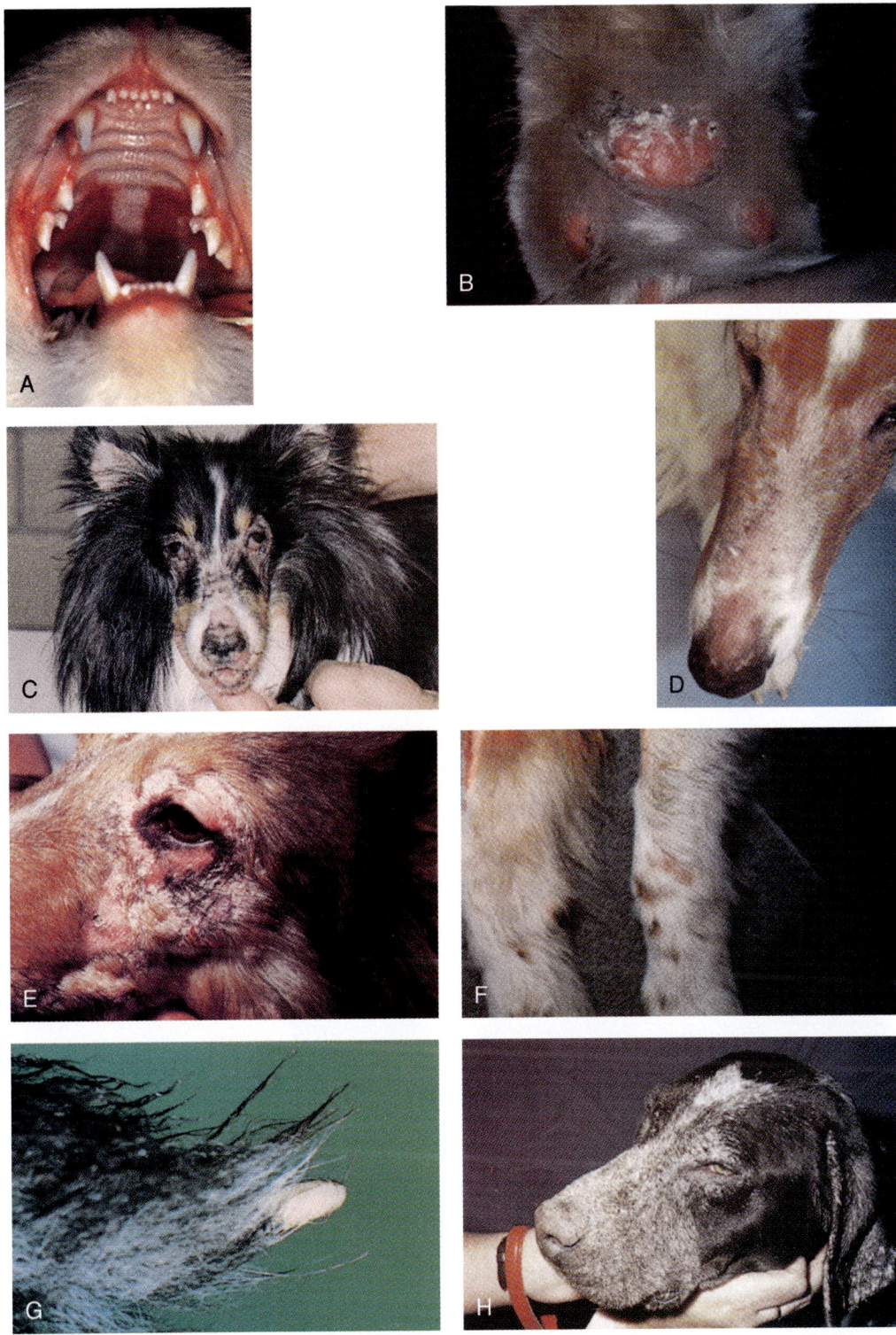

FIGURE 12–29. *A*, Dystrophic epidermolysis bullosa in a kitten. Oral ulceration. (Courtesy of S. White.) *B*, Dystrophic epidermolysis bullosa in a kitten. Ulcerated carpal footpad. (Courtesy of S. White.) *C*, Shetland sheepdog with dermatomyositis. Severe facial scarring and drop jaw. *D*, Dermatomyositis in a collie. Chronic case with scarring alopecia on the bridge of the nose. *E*, Shetland sheepdog with severe, typical lesions on cheek and eyelids. *F*, Dermatomyositis in a collie. Patchy alopecia and erythema over the cranial aspect of the carpi. *G*, Collie with dermatomyositis. Alopecia of the tip of the tail. *H*, Hereditary lupoid dermatosis in a German shorthaired pointer. Marked scaling and hyperkeratosis of the face and pinna. (Courtesy of M. Song.)

CLINICAL FEATURES

In Collies and Shetland sheepdogs, no coat color or coat length is associated with dermatomyositis. Either sex can be affected. Because of the familial predisposition, lesions occur early in life, typically before 6 months of age. Signs in some dogs appear as early as 7 to 11 weeks of age. The progression of lesions varies. Some mildly affected dogs have few lesions, which heal rapidly without scarring. Most dogs have new lesions after the first ones are recognized, but the rate of progression is variable. The extent of the skin lesions is known by 1 year of age. Unless management changes occur, lesions usually decrease in number and severity from that point on.

Skin lesions occur in areas of mechanical trauma and are common on the face (see Fig. 12–29C and D), especially around the eyes (see Fig. 12–29E) and muzzle (Fig. 12–30); on the tips of the ears; on carpal and tarsal regions (see Fig. 12–29F); on the digits; and on the tip of the tail (see Fig. 12–29G). Oral and footpad lesions are common but especially occur in the Beauceron. Although intact vesicles can occur in some dogs, primary lesions are usually absent. Typical skin lesions are characterized by alopecia, erythema, scaling, and mild crusting. Ulceration can occur in severely affected dogs. Skin lesions are usually not pruritic unless a secondary staphylococcal infection has occurred. Cutaneous pain seems to be prevalent in Beaucerons. In mildly to moderately affected dogs, large areas of normal skin remain, whereas in severely affected dogs, the entire face, distal limbs, and tail can be involved. Some dogs have onychorrhexis (Fig. 12–31), onychoschizia, or onychomadesis.

The myositis typically occurs months after the skin lesions are recognized and correlates with the severity of the skin lesions. Mildly affected dogs have no clinical muscle disease; convincing evidence of this may not be found on EMG testing or muscle biopsy. These patients may have epidermolysis bullosa simplex, dermatomyositis with focal but undetected myositis, or dermatomyositis without the myositis.[84] In humans, the diagnosis of amyopathic dermatomyositis can be confirmed only when no muscle changes are detected for 4 years or longer after the skin lesions have occurred. To our knowledge, this type of follow-up testing has not been performed in dogs. The rare dog related to dogs with classic dermatomyositis has EMG changes of myositis with no skin lesions. The significance of these findings is unknown.

Clinical signs of myositis vary. A common finding is a dirty water bowl that contains food particles. These dogs do not have trouble chewing their food, but do not swallow it completely, so residual pieces are washed from the mouth during drinking. Some dogs

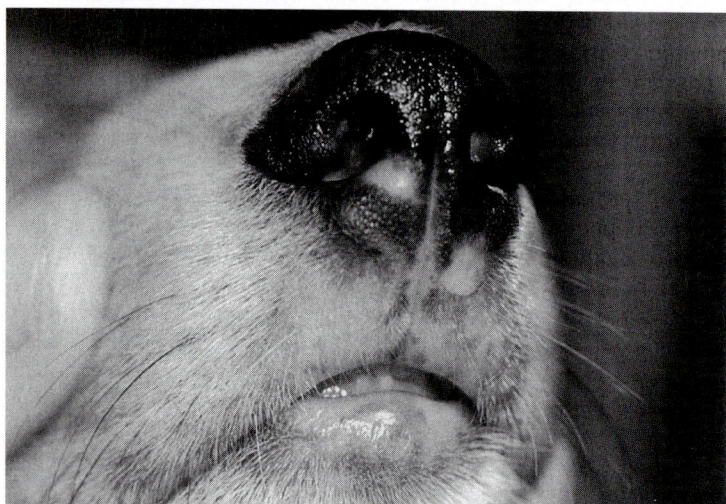

FIGURE 12–30. Dermatomyositis. Patchy depigmentation and scarring of the nasal planum. The lips are also scarred.

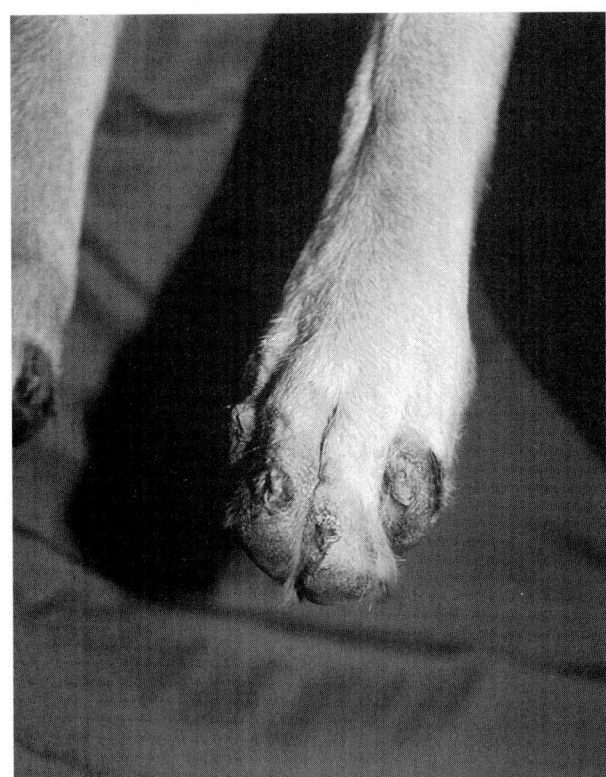

FIGURE 12–31. Dermatomyositis. Onychorrhexis of all claws on all four feet.

have a peculiar high-stepping gait. Severely affected dogs drink, chew, and swallow with difficulty; have a stiff gait; have megaesophagus; and often have secondary aspiration pneumonia. The most common sign of the myositis is asymptomatic atrophy, especially of the muscles of mastication and distal limbs. The rare dog has skin lesions only in adulthood.[21a, 31, 92]

DIAGNOSIS

The differential diagnostic considerations should include demodicosis, staphylococcal folliculitis, dermatophytosis, discoid lupus erythematosus, and epidermolysis bullosa simplex. The latter might be considered if there are no muscle signs or lesions and if vesicles are present.

Diagnosis is confirmed by history, physical examination findings, biopsy of affected skin and muscle, EMG, and laboratory tests to rule out other conditions. Biopsy of affected skin shows scattered hydropic degeneration of the surface and follicular basal cells (Fig. 12–32).[3] Apoptotic basal cells (Civatte's bodies) occasionally are visible. With confluent hydropic change, intrabasal or subepidermal clefting may be apparent (Fig. 12–33). Dermal inflammation can be absent. Most cases show a mild perivascular to interstitial dermatitis in which lymphocytes, plasma cells, and histiocytes predominate. Mild pigmentary incontinence may be present in the superficial dermis. Follicular atrophy and perifollicular fibrosis are common findings (Figs. 12–34 and 12–35) and may be the only findings in chronic lesions. Vasculitis occasionally is present in the skin. Muscle biopsy may show mixed inflammatory exudates accompanied by muscle fiber necrosis and atrophy.[31] Needle EMG abnormalities include positive sharp waves and fibrillation potentials in muscles of the head and of distal extremities.

Hemograms and serum chemistry profiles are usually unremarkable, but creatine

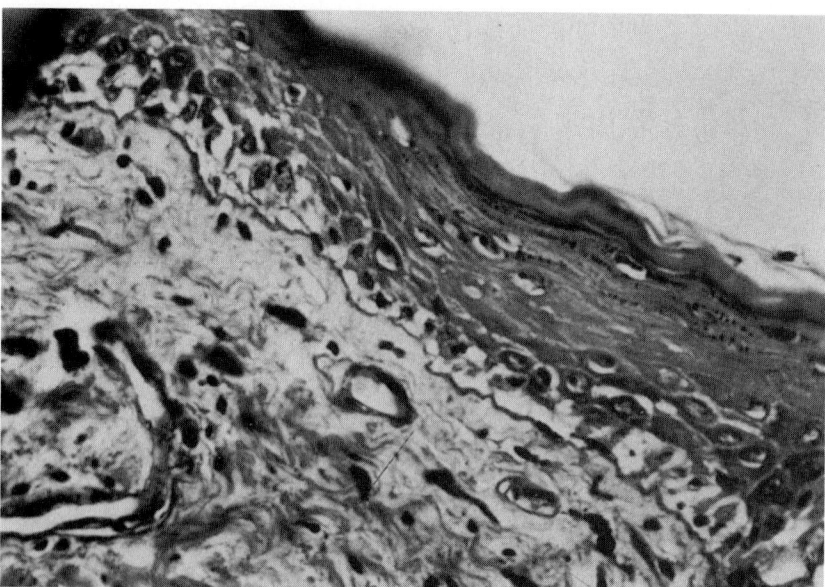

FIGURE 12–32. Dermatomyositis (epidermolysis bullosa simplex) in a collie. Marked hydropic degeneration of epidermal basal cells without inflammation. (From Scott DW, Schultz RD: Epidermolysis bullosa simplex in the collie dog. JAVMA 171:172, 1977.)

kinase levels can be increased. Neurologic examination and nerve conduction studies are usually normal. Elevated concentrations of immunoglobulin G and circulating immune complexes may be found in active disease.[32] The magnitude of the elevations in immunoglobulin G and circulating immune complex levels correlates with the severity of the skin disease.[31]

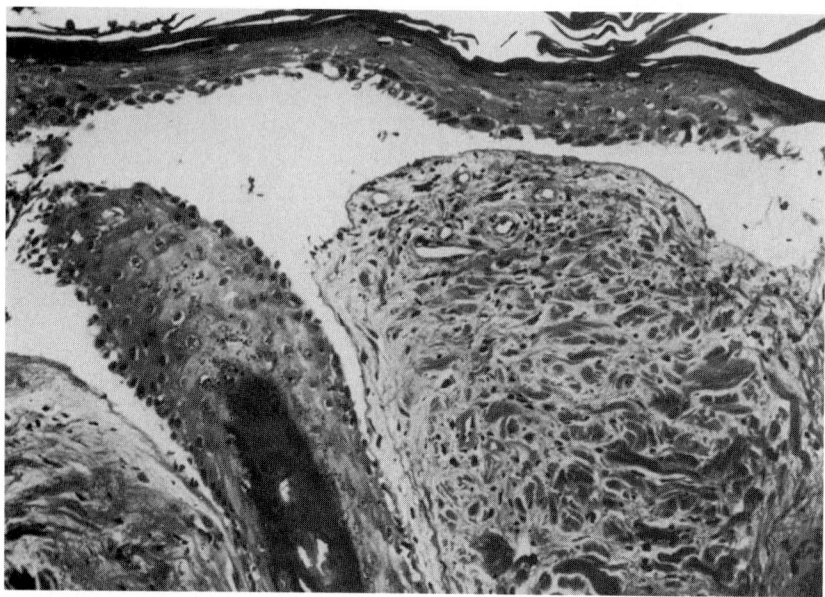

FIGURE 12–33. Dermatomyositis (epidermolysis bullosa simplex) in a collie. Subepidermal vesicle due to hydropic degeneration of epidermal basal cells. (From Scott DW, Schultz RD: Epidermolysis bullosa simplex in the collie dog. JAVMA 171:172, 1977.)

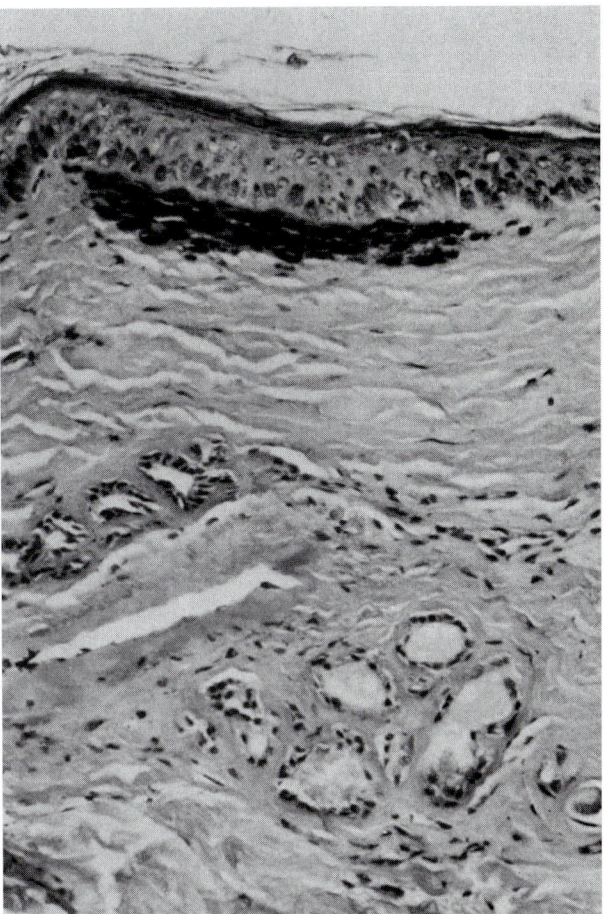

FIGURE 12-34. Canine dermatomyositis. Fibrosing dermatitis, with orphaned apocrine glands and pigmentary incontinence.

CLINICAL MANAGEMENT

The skin lesions of dermatomyositis are worsened by trauma and prolonged solar exposure. Management changes to avoid these secondary insults should be instituted. Mildly affected dogs usually require no additional treatment because their skin lesions heal spontaneously. Some of these dogs have permanently alopecic, hyperpigmented, and scarred areas where the most severe active lesions were. Severely affected dogs are difficult to care for. These dogs have widespread skin lesions and generalized myopathy, which results in lameness and difficulty in drinking and eating. These dogs often have aspiration pneumonia. Although large doses of prednisolone (1 to 2 mg/kg q24h) improve the skin lesions, it is difficult to maintain the animal on safe levels of the drug and the steroid-associated muscle changes compound the pre-existing changes. Humane euthanasia should be encouraged.

Mildly to moderately affected dogs can usually be maintained as acceptable pets for extended periods. Some skin lesions remain and muscle atrophy, especially of the muscles of mastication, is apparent. Oral doses of vitamin E (200 to 800 IU/day) or marine lipid supplements (e.g., DVM Derm Caps) appear to be beneficial for the skin but not for the muscle lesions. Some dogs require episodic courses of treatment with prednisolone (1 mg/kg q24h) to control traumatic or solar flares. Other dogs, especially those with moderately severe disease, need near-constant corticosteroid treatments. In these animals, pentoxifylline (Trental, Hoechst-Roussel) should be added to the corticosteroid regimen in the hope

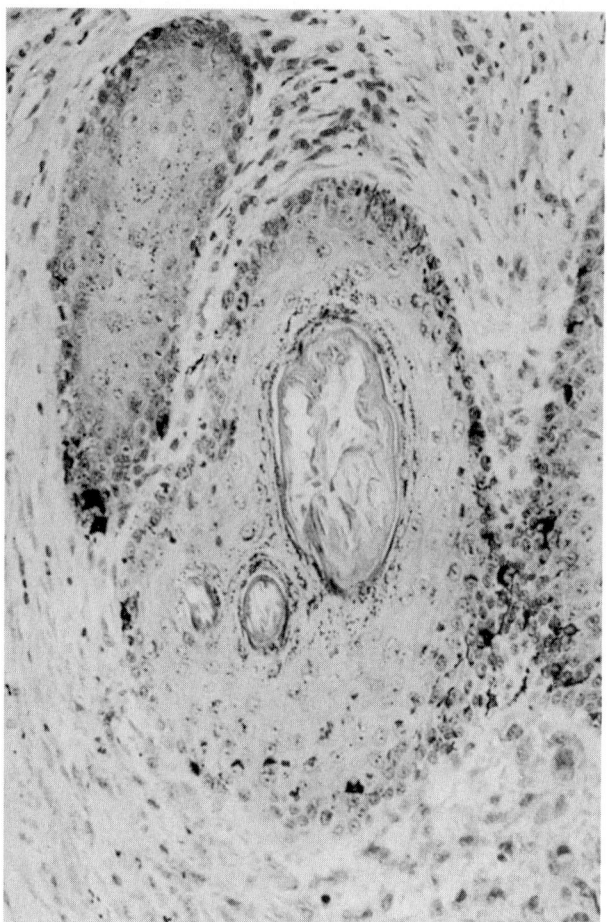

FIGURE 12-35. Canine dermatomyositis. Perifollicular fibrosis.

of significantly reducing or eliminating the corticosteroid. The drug is given with food at dosages of 200 to 400 mg q24h–q48h.[27, 31, 36, 62] Response time is slow, with 2 to 3 months of treatment needed before efficacy can be determined.

These treatments usually minimize the development of new skin lesions, and those that do occur tend to be milder. Muscle disease progresses, and old dogs have profound atrophy of the muscles of the head, the distal limbs, and sometimes the body. With severe atrophy, the animal's ability to eat and drink can be compromised and dietary manipulations become necessary. The limb and body atrophy can cause an abnormal gait, but locomotion is still possible. Amyloidosis occurs in some chronically affected dogs.[33]

Idiopathic Ulcerative Dermatosis in Shetland Sheepdogs and Collies

The ulcerative dermatosis described in Shetland sheepdogs and Collies is of unknown etiology. It was originally hypothesized to be a variant of dermatomyositis.[36] Results of a clinicopathologic study of five Shetland sheepdogs and two Collies with this syndrome led the authors to conclude that it is distinct from dermatomyositis and should be renamed *vesicular cutaneous lupus erythematosus* (see Chap. 9).[38]

CLINICAL FEATURES

Lesions occur in middle-aged to older dogs with no antecedent history of skin disease. The disease appears to be more prevalent in Shetland sheepdogs. No sex predilection is noted, but relapses or exacerbations can occur with estrus. In all dogs, there can be cyclic recrudescence, which often occurs in summer.

The initial lesions are vesiculobullous and are visible in the groin and then the axillary regions. The bullae tend to be flaccid and centered in areas of figurate erythema. Lesions coalesce and ulcerate to form large serpiginous lesions with distinct borders between normal and abnormal skin. In some cases, lesions can be found on the eyelids, the pinnae, the oral mucosa, the external genitalia, the anus, and the footpads. The lesions are painful, especially if secondarily infected.

DIAGNOSIS

The differential diagnostic considerations include bullous pemphigoid, erythema multiforme, systemic lupus erythematosus, and pemphigus vulgaris. Skin biopsy shows hydropic degeneration of basal cells and extensive individual keratinocyte apoptosis, which can extend into the stratum spinosum.[3, 38] In severe cases there may be extensive blister formation at the dermoepidermal junction. In the dermis, there is a superficial perivascular to partially lichenoid dermatitis. Interface folliculitis is often present. There is no follicular atrophy. Direct immunofluorescence and antinuclear antibody test results are negative. Some dogs have EMG abnormalities typical of dermatomyositis. Hemograms, serum chemistry profiles, and ANA test results are usually unremarkable or negative.

CLINICAL MANAGEMENT

Because lesions may be triggered or worsened by trauma, management changes to minimize trauma are appropriate. The photosensitive nature of the lesions makes photoprotection an important management consideration. Antibiotic therapy is indicated in cases with secondary infections. Glucocorticoids, with or without azathioprine, the combination of tetracycline and niacinamide, and vitamin E and pentoxifylline are reported to be effective. The cyclic nature of the disease can make maintenance management more difficult.

Canine Benign Familial Chronic Pemphigus

In humans, benign familial pemphigus (Hailey-Hailey disease) is an autosomal dominant disorder of cellular cohesion among keratinocytes.[2] The exact nature of the defect is unknown but probably lies between desmosomal protein 3 and desmosomal glycoproteins. In the early stages of lesion formation, the intracellular components of desmosomes are primarily disrupted.[85] There are reduced quantities of desmoglein and plakoglobin in normal-appearing epidermis.[85] Because of the defect, the epidermis cannot withstand trauma and vesiculobullous lesions develop in response to friction or infection. The disease is a genetic weakness in desmosomes. A similar disorder has been reported in English setters and their crosses.[83, 84a] The disorder has also been recognized in a Doberman pinscher.[5] The disorder in English setters and their crosses was inherited in an autosomal dominant fashion.[84a]

CLINICAL FEATURES

Lesions occur in dogs at about 6 months of age and occur over pressure points on the limbs,[83] on the ventral chest,[84a] or on the pinnae (Fig. 12–36).[5] Lesions are first characterized by alopecia, erythema, and slight scaling. Increased scaling and crusting occur later as the lesions become plaquelike. Vesicopustules are rare. Lesions remain localized and cannot be easily induced.

DIAGNOSES

The differential diagnosis is limited and includes pressure point irritation and superficial bacterial folliculitis. Skin biopsy shows acanthosis with orthokeratotic and parakeratotic hyperkeratosis and marked, diffuse, multifocal areas of acantholysis of the lower and middle portions of the epidermis and follicular outer root sheath.[83] The acantholysis is

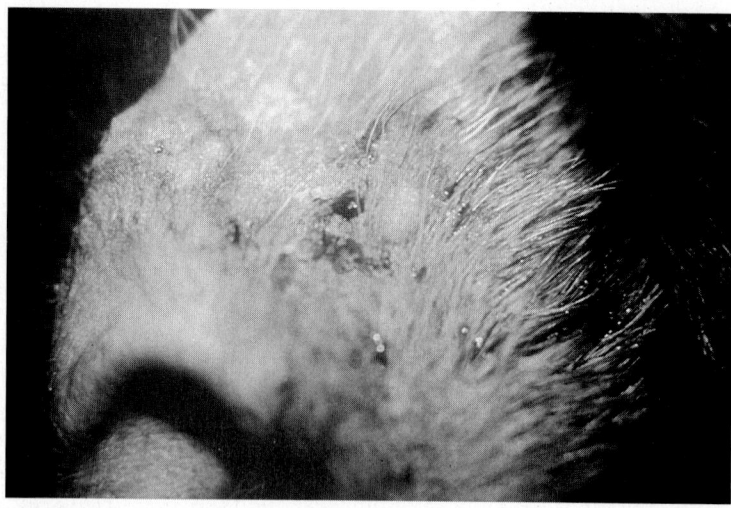

FIGURE 12-36. Benign familial chronic pemphigus. Multiple vesicular lesions on the inner pinnal surface of a Doberman pinscher.

often so marked that the appearance of the affected epidermis is likened to that of a dilapidated brick wall. Acantholytic dyskeratotic keratinocytes (corps ronds) may be visible (Fig. 12-37). Immunofluorescence testing yields negative results.

CLINICAL MANAGEMENT

In humans, treatment of infections with or without the use of topical corticosteroids and avoidance of trauma usually provide good results.[2] Severe patients can be helped by the administration of systemic glucocorticoids, methotrexate, dapsone, cyclosporine, and retinoids. Because the lesions in dogs are asymptomatic and localized, no treatment has been attempted.

Hereditary Lupoid Dermatosis of German Shorthaired Pointers

The lupoid dermatosis of German shorthaired pointers is an uncommon disorder. Cases have been recognized worldwide.[76, 86, 87, 89-91] Aside from a familial predisposition, no cause of the dermatosis has been determined. Results of immunopathologic studies led

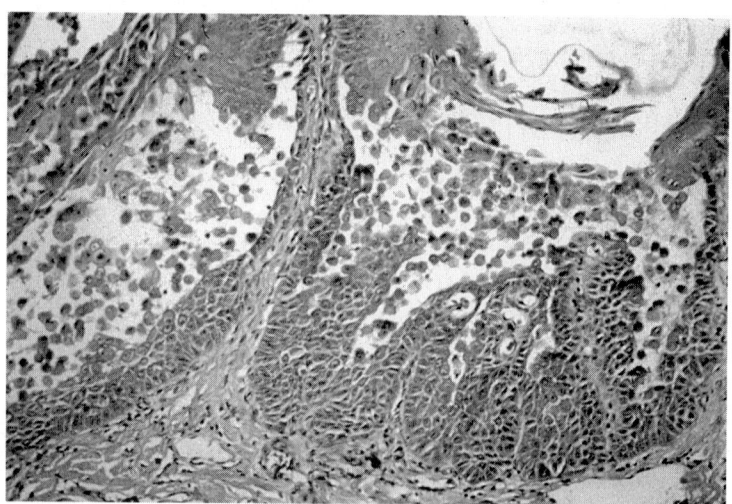

FIGURE 12-37. Benign familial chronic pemphigus. Suprabasalar acantholysis with numerous dyskeratotic cells (corp ronds).

the authors to conclude that this syndrome should be renamed *exfoliative cutaneous lupus erythematosus*.[66]

CLINICAL FEATURES

Typically, exfoliative skin lesions are first noted at about 6 months (3 to 36 months) of age. Scaling and crusting appear first on the face, the ears, and the back and then in a more generalized distribution (see Fig. 12-29H). The hocks and the scrotum may be severely involved. The lesions are variably painful or pruritic. Pyrexia and lymphadenopathy may accompany the skin lesions. Lesions may have a waxing and waning course or be persistent.

DIAGNOSIS

The differential diagnostic possibilities include nutritional disorders, a primary keratinization disorder, drug eruption, sebaceous adenitis, and systemic lupus erythematosus. The rare dog has laboratory evidence (proteinuria and positive antinuclear antibody titer) of systemic lupus erythematosus.[91] Skin biopsy shows mild to moderate acanthosis, orthokeratotic and parakeratotic hyperkeratosis, hydropic degeneration of basal cells, and extensive individual keratinocyte apoptosis with occasional satellitosis (Fig. 12-38).[91] The individual keratinocyte apoptosis is found throughout the stratum spinosum and may be confluent. Basilar clefting may be present. Interface folliculitis accompanies the interface dermatitis. The dermis shows a mixed cellular mild to moderate interface dermatitis, and sebaceous glands may be normal, small, or absent (in about half the cases). Ultrastructural studies in one dog showed decreased numbers of hemidesmosomes along the basal layer.[87] Immunopathologic studies have revealed the following: epitheliotropic/folliculotropic/sebotropic lymphocytes exhibited a unique $CD3^+$, $CD8\alpha^+$, $\gamma\delta TCR1^+$ phenotype; IgG, IgA, IgM, and C3 were detected at the epidermal and infundibular basement membrane zone in 97%, 3%, 18%, and 13% of the sections, respectively; and circulating antinuclear antibodies were not detected.[66]

CLINICAL MANAGEMENT

To date, no uniformly successful treatment has been reported. Antiseborrheic baths and immunosuppressive doses of corticosteroids have given poor results. Fatty acid supplements may be beneficial,[86, 89] but some cases show no response to this treatment. A small number of dogs have been treated with retinol or retinoic acids with no benefit.[87, 90]

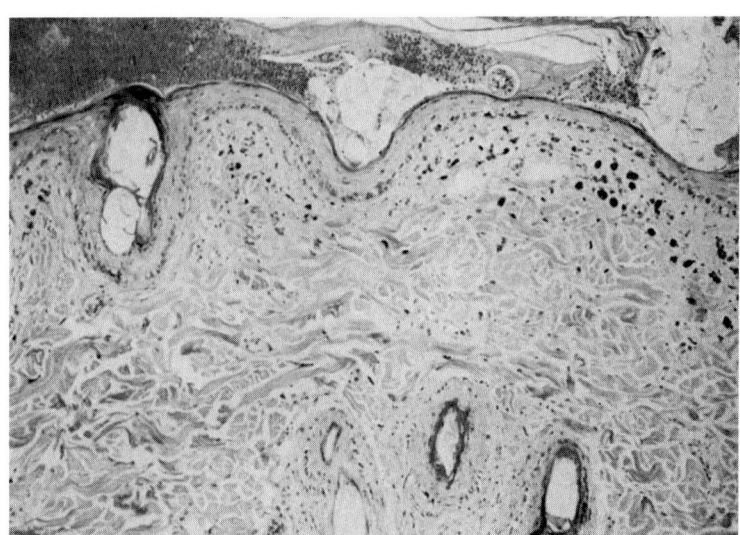

FIGURE 12-38. Hereditary lupoid dermatosis of German shorthaired pointer. Hydropic interface dermatitis. (Courtesy of T. Gross.)

• DISORDERS OF HAIRS AND HAIR GROWTH

A variety of inherited disorders of the hair shaft or hair growth are reported in dogs and cats.[1, 117] Congenital conditions are easily recognized because they occur near birth, when they are easy to differentiate from endocrine and other acquired alopecias. Inherited disorders with tardive onset are more difficult and can mimic a variety of other disorders. Careful inspection of hairs via a trichogram or a skin biopsy differentiates inherited disorders from other acquired alopecias. These tests should be performed routinely in animals with abnormal hairs, for hair loss early in life, or for hair loss with an unusual distribution.

Inherited hair disorders have no specific treatment. Nutritional supplements, special diets, and so forth, as espoused by some breeders, are of minimal benefit. Good gentle grooming is imperative to minimize secondary infections and seborrhea. Without the normal protection of their coat, affected animals are susceptible to frostbite, sunburn, the effects of low environmental humidity, and other environmental insults. With appropriate management changes, these animals can lead nearly normal lives.

Structural Defects of the Hair Shaft

In humans, a variety of inherited or acquired conditions affect the shape, composition, and strength of the hair shafts.[2] Depending on the condition, the defect can be recognized because the scalp hairs are unmanageable or unusual in appearance or because the hairs break easily with routine brushing or combing. Diagnosis is confirmed by light and scanning electron microscopic examination of affected hairs.

Coat abnormalities are common in veterinary medicine, but only six hair shaft defects have been reported. Undoubtedly, more occur but have gone unrecognized because microscopic examination of hair shafts was not a routine part of the clinical evaluation of patients with abnormal coats.

TRICHORRHEXIS NODOSA

In humans and animals, trichorrhexis nodosa is most often an acquired defect in which external insults damage the cuticle and weaken the hair shaft (see Chap. 11). In humans, some cases have an inherited basis.[2] Two of us (WHM and DWS) have examined two unrelated young Golden retrievers for a poor coat. At examination, there was no hair loss, but the hairs were uneven in length. Trichograms showed nodular hair fracture typical of trichorrhexis nodosa (Fig. 12–39). No systemic or topical cause of the problem could be identified, and the condition persisted. These cases suggest that inherited trichorrhexis nodosa may occur in animals.

TRICHOPTILOSIS

Trichoptilosis, the longitudinal splitting of the distal end of a hair ("split ends," "frizzies") is probably a very common condition in dogs and cats who are repeatedly bathed, sprayed, or otherwise treated topically with "mild" products or who have received one or more harsh treatments. If the animal's hairs are weaker than normal because of some congenital or acquired structural defect, the fracture will occur with minimal to no insult. Because the shaft fracture occurs at the tip of the hair, the area involved is not hairless, but is covered by hairs of unequal length. No other abnormalities should be detected.

Trichoptilosis was reported in three male Golden retrievers.[149] Two of the dogs were siblings. One dog had no history of topical treatments; the other two were treated with flea sprays. All dogs had widespread disease with poor feathering on the limbs (Fig. 12–40) and patchy hypotrichosis on the trunk (Fig. 12–41). Because one dog had disease that arose spontaneously and the extent of the disease in the other two seemed to be disproportionally severe, a hereditary hair shaft hyperfragility was proposed.

The diagnosis of trichoptilosis can only be confirmed by trichography (Fig. 12–42). The hair shaft distal to the fracture should be examined carefully for additional abnormali-

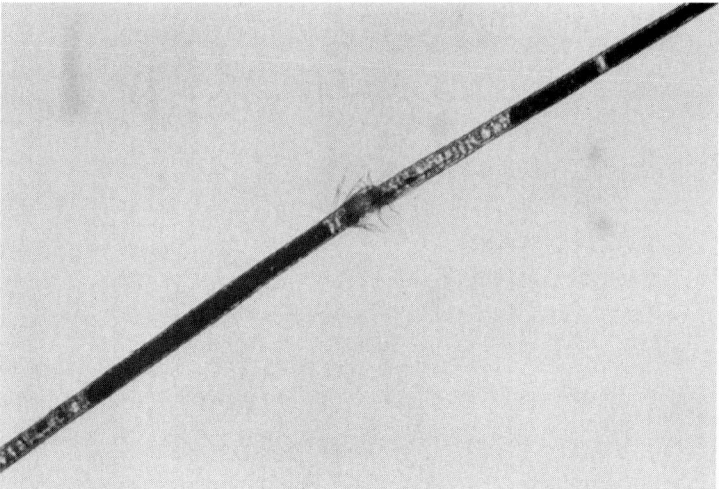

FIGURE 12-39. Trichorrhexis nodosa. Discrete splintering of hair.

ties that might explain the shaft fracture. If the shafts above and below the fracture point are normal, a detailed history of topical treatments should be taken and suspected treatments should be stopped. Once the trauma is discontinued, the coat should return to normal. If no insult can be found, it is unlikely that the coat will improve.

MEDULLARY TRICHOMALACIA

Medullary trichomalacia is an unusual hair shaft disorder wherein the medulla vacuolates spontaneously. The disorder has been studied in detail in six German shepherd dogs,[155] and a familial hyperfragility of hairs secondary to a disorder of keratinization is suspected in this breed. Because this disorder has also been recognized in several other breeds, an acquired, rather than congenital, etiology is also likely, but no cause was determined in those dogs.

The German shepherds had multiple patches of involvement over the dorsum. Prior to hair loss, the patches could be identified because the hairs lost their flexibility and stood away from the rest of the coat. On close inspection, the hairs appeared thicker than

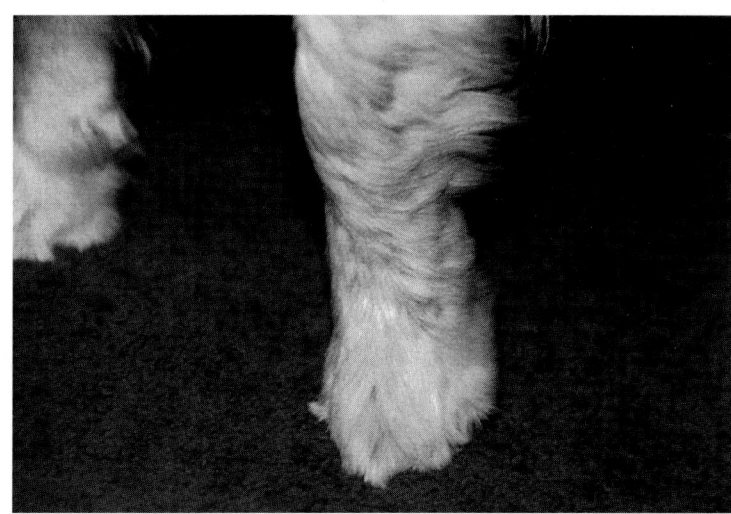

FIGURE 12-40. Trichoptilosis. Shaft fracture at different points along the hairs gives a disheveled and uneven look to the coat.

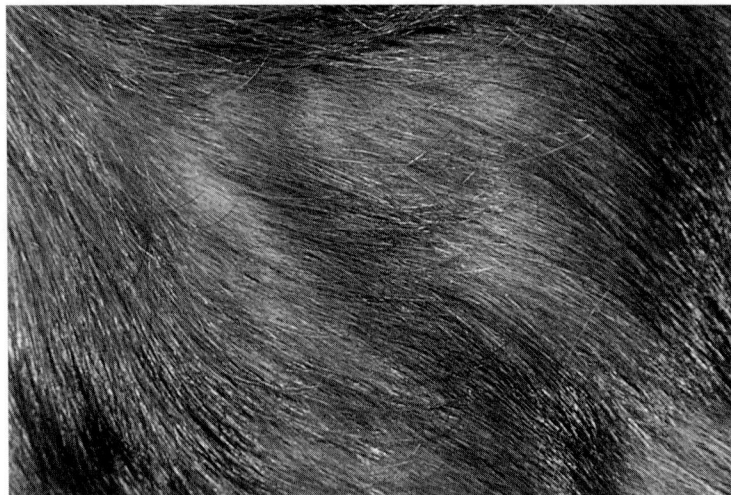

FIGURE 12–41. Trichoptilosis. Same dog as in 12–40 with involvement of the hairs over the chest wall.

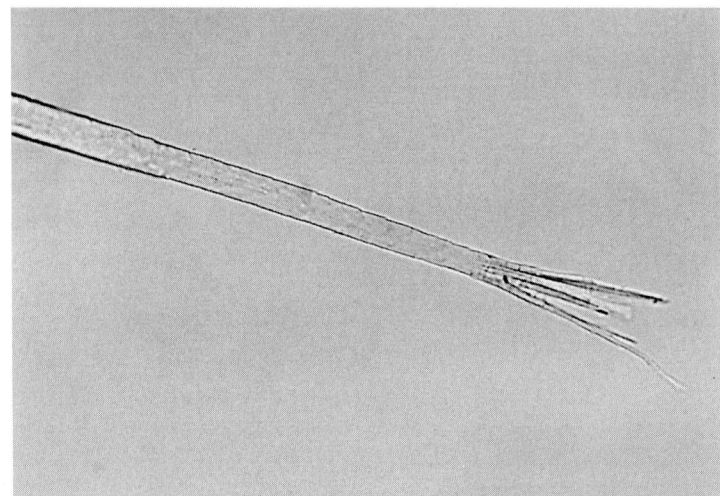

FIGURE 12–42. Trichoptilosis ("split ends") in a dog.

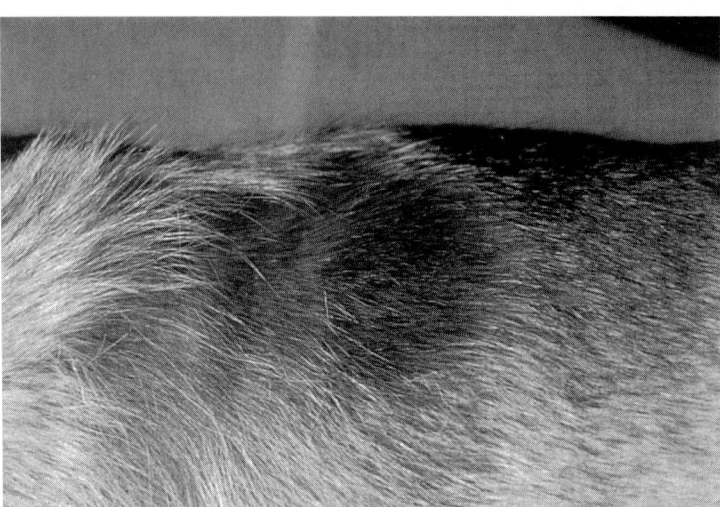

FIGURE 12–43. Medullary trichomalacia. Patch of hair fracture over the shoulder region of a German shepherd dog.

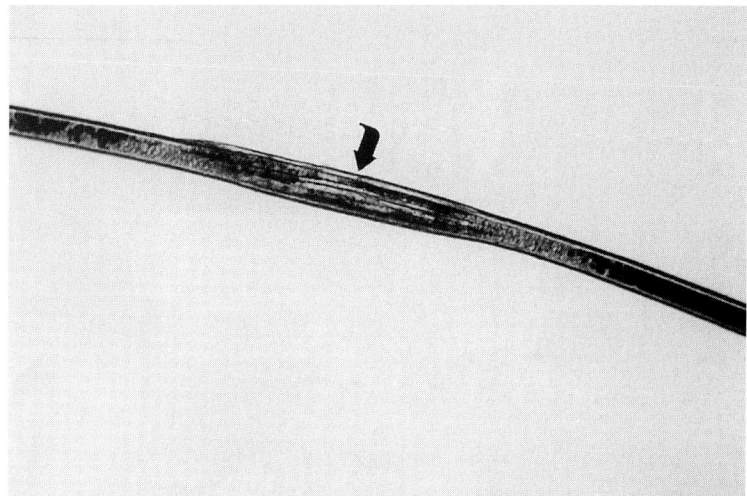

FIGURE 12-44. Medullary trichomalacia in a dog.

normal, were stiff to the touch, and broke with minimal trauma (Fig. 12-43). The hair loss in the other breeds was also patchy but not confined to the dorsum.

On trichography, the involved hairs have longitudinally split in the middle of the hair shaft and the medulla is depigmented and vacuolated (Fig. 12-44). Skin biopsies from affected areas show catagenization of most hair follicles, some of which contained increased numbers of apoptotic outer root sheath keratinocytes. Biopsies from normal areas or involved areas that had returned to normal showed no abnormalities.

In all cases, normal hairs regrow spontaneously at the next shed cycle. Relapses are uncommon. If a relapse occurs, the new patches can be more or less numerous and will be in the same region but not necessarily in the same location.

PILI TORTI

Pili torti is a condition in which curvature of the hair follicle leads to flattening and rotation of the hair shaft (Fig. 12-45). In humans, most cases have a hereditary basis and the patients often experience other cutaneous and systemic abnormalities.[2] Localized acquired pili torti can result from follicular inflammation.

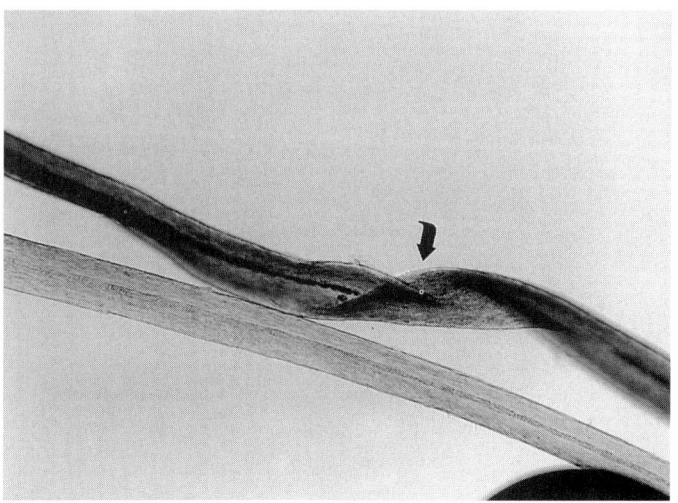

FIGURE 12-45. Pili torti. Note 360-degree twist of hair shaft on its long axis (*arrow*).

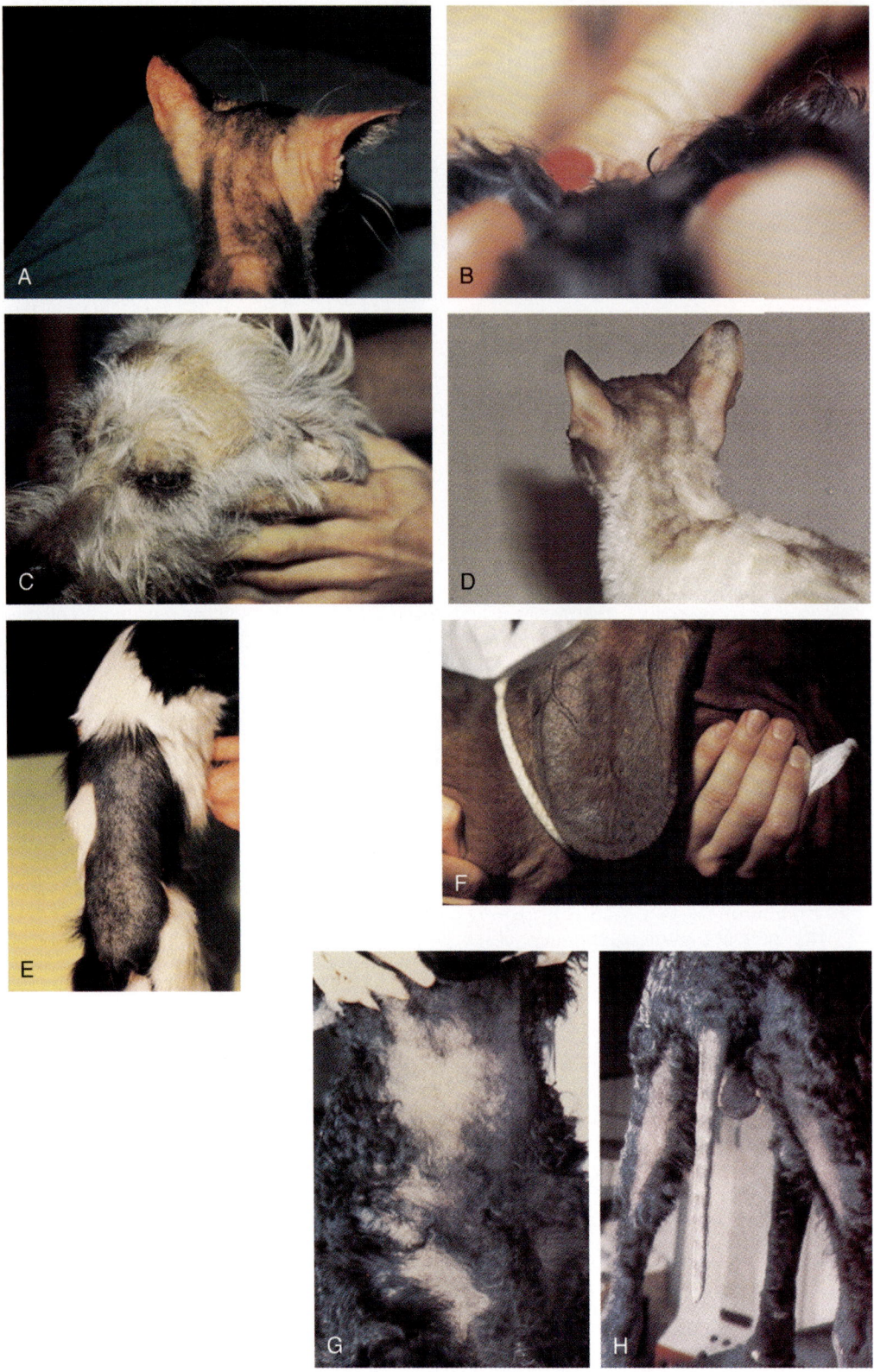

FIGURE 12-46. *A*, Pili torti in a cat. (Courtesy of C. Foil.) *B*, Spiculosis in a Kerry blue terrier. (Courtesy of H. Raue.) *C*, Congenital hypotrichosis in a dog. *D*, Congenital hypotrichosis in a Devon Rex cat. *E*, Black hair follicular dysplasia. Note the marked hypotrichosis over the dorsum that spares white-coated areas. (Courtesy of C. Foil.) *F*, Pattern baldness on the pinna of a 7-year-old dachshund. *G*, Pattern baldness on the ventral neck of an Irish water spaniel. *H*, Pattern baldness on the tail and thighs of an Irish water spaniel.

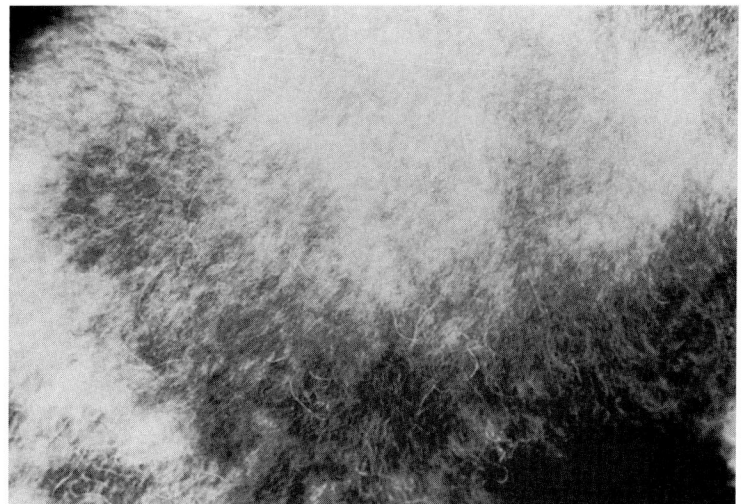

FIGURE 12–47. Pili torti in a cat. Note hypotrichosis and twisted hairs. (Courtesy of C. Foil.)

Pili torti has been reported in a litter of kittens[112] and in some Bull terriers with acrodermatitis.[215] In the dogs, most hairs were normal, suggesting that the affected hairs resulted from follicular inflammation. In the cats, all hairs were affected by 10 days of age (Fig. 12–46A). In addition to the generalized hair loss, the kittens had periocular and pedal dermatitis and paronychia. All secondary hairs showed the flattening and rotation typical of pili torti (Fig. 12–47), but primary hairs were not involved. On biopsy, follicular hyperkeratosis with occasional cystic dilatation was the only notable finding.

SHAFT DISORDER OF ABYSSINIAN CATS

Shaft disorder is an uncommon to rare condition of Abyssinian cats.[157] Only whiskers and primary hairs are affected. These hairs are rough and lusterless and have an onion-shaped swelling visible with the naked eye, usually at the tip of the hair (Fig. 12–48). Hair fracture can occur at the swelling. Skin biopsy shows no follicular abnormalities. The cause of the condition is unknown, but because of its restriction to Abyssinian cats, it must be considered an inherited disorder. No details on treatment are available.

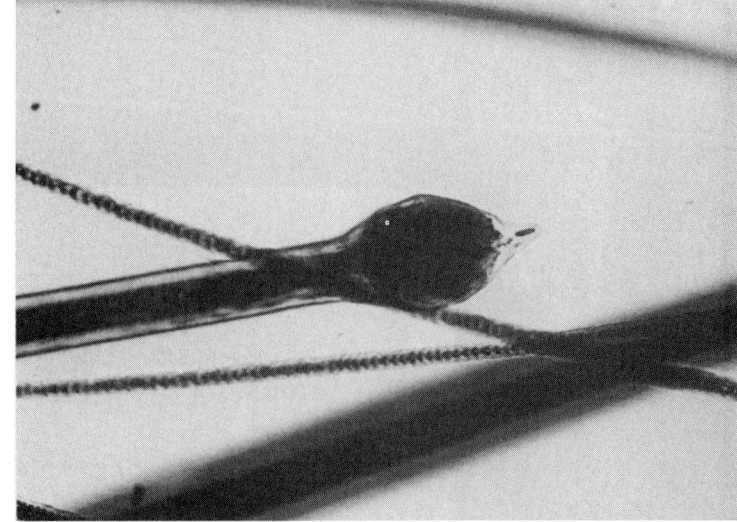

FIGURE 12–48. Shaft disorder of Abyssinian cats. Note the onion-shaped swelling at the tip of the hair.

SPICULOSIS

Spiculosis is a rare disorder of young intact male Kerry blue terriers.[130] Affected dogs have multiple, hard, brittle follicular spicules (see Fig. 12–46B), which are 1 to 2.5 mm in diameter and 0.5 to 3 cm in length. The spicules can be found on any haired surface but are most common over the lateral hock region. Although the spicules can be asymptomatic, most dogs lick or chew at them.

Biopsy shows follicular dysplasia with premature keratinization.[130] This defect results in an amorphous mass of keratin, which is shaped into the spicule by the outer root sheath and the follicular wall (Fig. 12–49).

In asymptomatic dogs, no treatment is indicated and the spicules persist. In pruritic animals, the only effective treatment has been with isotretinoin (1 mg/kg orally q24h). After 3 to 4 months of treatment, the spicules disappear. With discontinuation of the drug regimen, the dog may remain normal or the spicules may redevelop. In the latter case, maintenance therapy with isotretinoin is indicated.

Congenital Hypotrichosis or Alopecia

With congenital hair loss, hypotrichosis or alopecia is obvious at birth or develops during the first 2 to 4 weeks of life. Some animals have only hair follicle disease, whereas other animals also have involvement of other skin appendages. Additional ectodermal defects such as abnormal dentition or tear production may also be noted. To categorize these

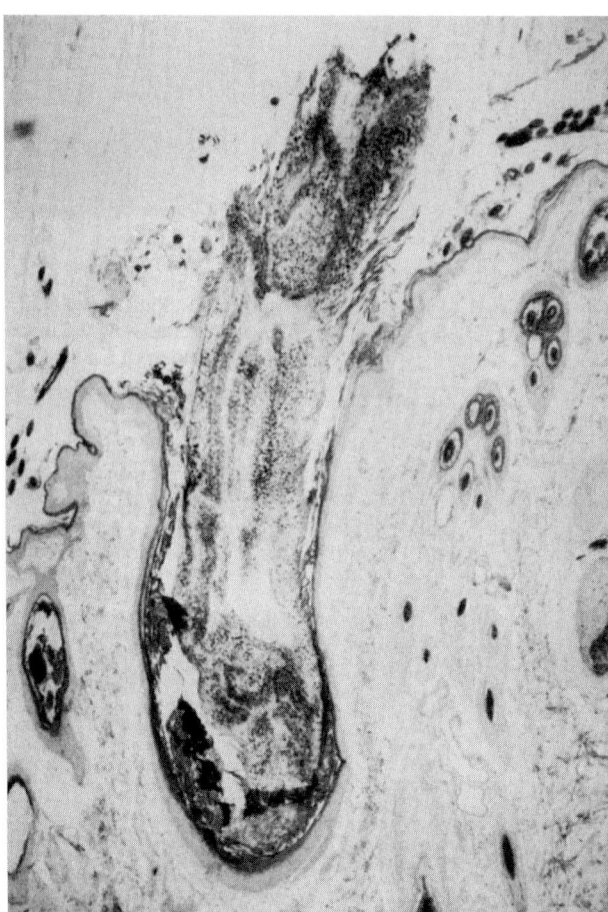

FIGURE 12–49. Spiculosis in a Kerry blue terrier.

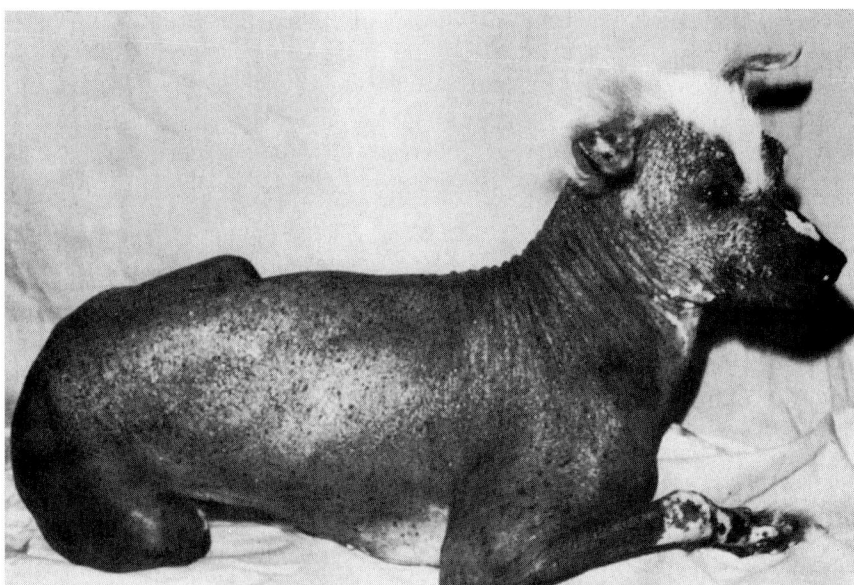

FIGURE 12–50. Chinese crested dog, a recognized breed.

animals accurately, Foil[1] proposed a numeric classification scheme, noting changes in hair, teeth, claws, adnexal glands, or other ectodermal structures. Classification of newly recognized cases according to this scheme should help to categorize these disorders and remove some of the confusion or misclassification in the veterinary literature.

ALOPECIC BREEDS

The best known examples of hairless dog breeds are the Mexican hairless dog and the Chinese crested dog (Fig. 12–50). Other hairless breeds include the Inca hairless dog, Peruvian Inca Orchid, and American hairless terrier.[1, 119, 122, 124] In cats, the Sphinx (Canadian hairless) is bred for its hairlessness (Fig. 12–51).[144]

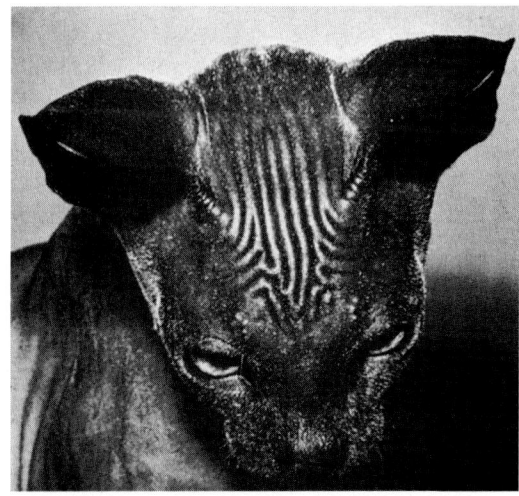

FIGURE 12–51. Feline alopecia universalis. (From Scott DW: Feline dermatology 1900–1978: A monograph, JAAHA 16:331, 1980.)

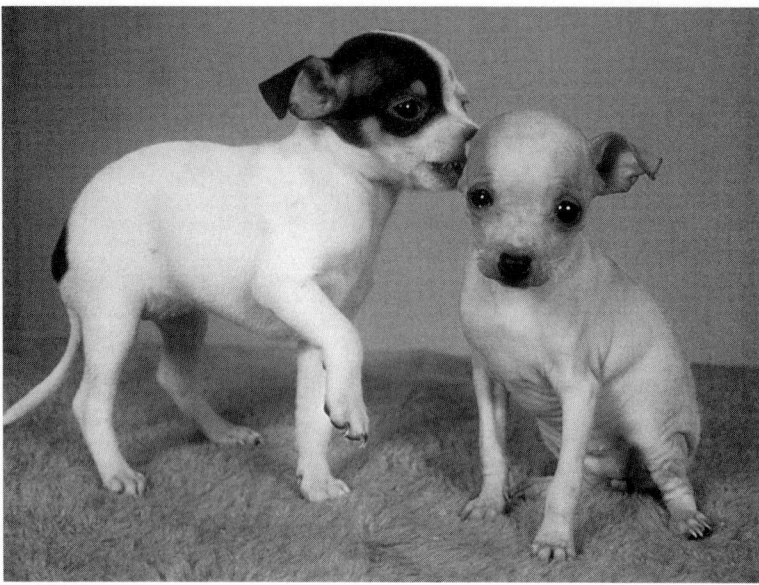

FIGURE 12–52. American hairless terrier and its normally haired littermate, an American rat terrier. (Courtesy of C. Foil.)

These hairless breeds resulted from the intentional breeding of animals with a spontaneous mutation. Aside from pets, these animals are useful in the study of sunscreens (see Chap. 16), topical glucocorticoids,[39a] and topical hair growth stimulators such as minoxidil.[123] Interestingly, minoxidil only stimulates hair growth in neonatal dogs. In the Mexican hairless, an autosomal dominant mode of inheritance has been demonstrated.[122] The American hairless terrier (Fig. 12–52) was developed from American rat terriers with an autosomal recessive hairless trait.[1] The hairless Mexican hairless dogs have a shorter survival time than their haired relatives.[119, 124] This decreased survival may be due to a familial immunoincompetence linked to the hairlessness.[111b, 119]

CONGENITAL HYPOTRICHOSIS

Congenital hypotrichosis is the term used to describe animals born without their normal pelage or who experience non–color-linked hair loss within the first month of life. Some animals have only hair follicle involvement, whereas other animals have additional ectodermal defects. Many cases are not well characterized.

Dogs

Congenital hypotrichosis has been described in the American Cocker spaniel, Belgian shepherd, German shepherd, Toy and Miniature poodles, Whippet, Beagle, French bulldog, Rottweiler, Yorkshire terrier, Labrador retriever, Bichon Frisé, Lhasa apso, and Basset hound.° We have recognized it in Cocker spaniel–Miniature poodle crossbreeds.[5] Most cases have been recognized in male animals, suggesting some sex linkage. The X-linkage was proven in the German shepherd.[101] Most affected animals are born with noticeable hair loss, which progresses over the next month or so. Some dogs are born

---

°See references 1, 3, 5, 101, 104, 105, 110, 113, 120, 126, 128, 133, 151, 154.

normally haired but lose it shortly thereafter.[1, 110] The hair loss is symmetric in distribution and typically involves the temporal regions, the ear pinnae, the caudal dorsum, and the entire ventrum (Figs. 12–53 and 12–54; also see Fig. 12–46C). Some patients are born nearly bald[120, 151] or experience near-total hair loss by 12 to 14 weeks of age.[110] When the hair loss is regionalized, it is well delineated from the adjacent normal skin. Early on, the hairless skin is clinically normal, but it can become hyperpigmented and seborrheic with time. If the dog is examined after its puppy teeth have been replaced by adult teeth, abnormalities in dentition may be recognized.

Cats

Congenital hypotrichosis has been reported in Birman,[102] Burmese,[97] Devon Rex,[153] and Siamese[148] cats. Multiple kittens in the litter are involved, and no sex linkage has been described. In Birman and Siamese cats, the condition is an autosomal recessive trait.

Affected cats either are born hairless (Fig. 12–55) or have a thin downy coat that is lost in the first weeks of life (see Fig. 12–46D). Affected Burmese cats have no whiskers, claws, or papillae on the tongue.[97] At necropsy of affected Birman kittens, no thymus was found.[102]

The tentative diagnosis of congenital hypotrichosis in dogs or cats is straightforward and is confirmed by skin biopsy (Figs. 12–56 to 12–58). In all cases, hair follicle involvement is marked. In some cases, there is complete absence of follicles,[101, 102] whereas hair follicles are hypoplastic and decreased in number in other cases.[96, 148] Adnexae (sebaceous glands, sweat glands, and arrector pili muscles) are reduced in number, hypoplastic, or absent.

BLACK HAIR FOLLICULAR DYSPLASIA

Black hair follicular dysplasia is an uncommon disorder in which dogs with bicolor or tricolor coats lose hairs in the black areas only at an early age.

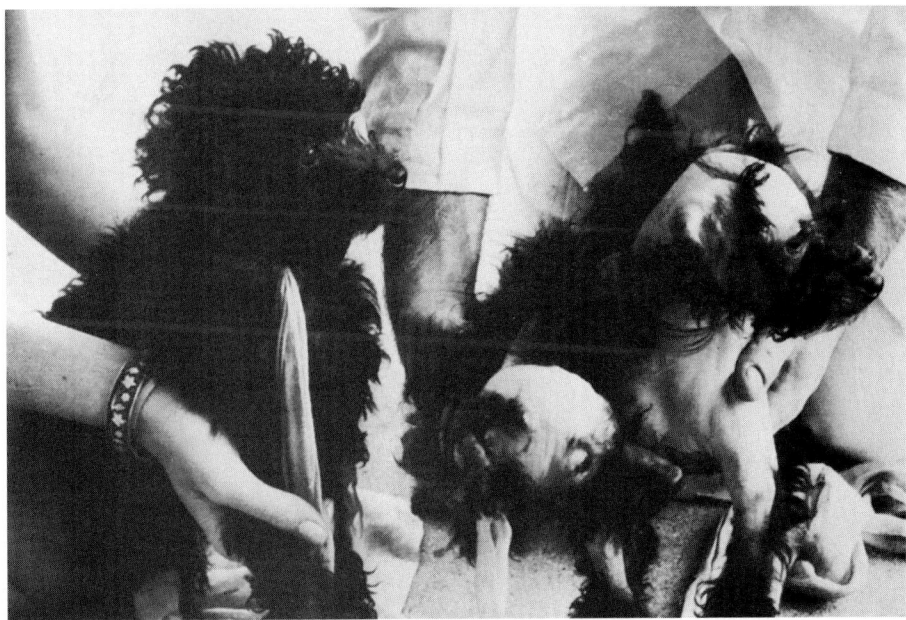

FIGURE 12–53. The partially alopecic males compared with a full-coated sister. The pattern of alopecia, which is bilaterally symmetric and includes about two thirds of the body surface, is the same in both males. (From Selmanowitz VJ, et al: Congenital ectodermal defect in miniature poodles. J Hered 61:196, 1970.)

960 • Congenital and Hereditary Defects

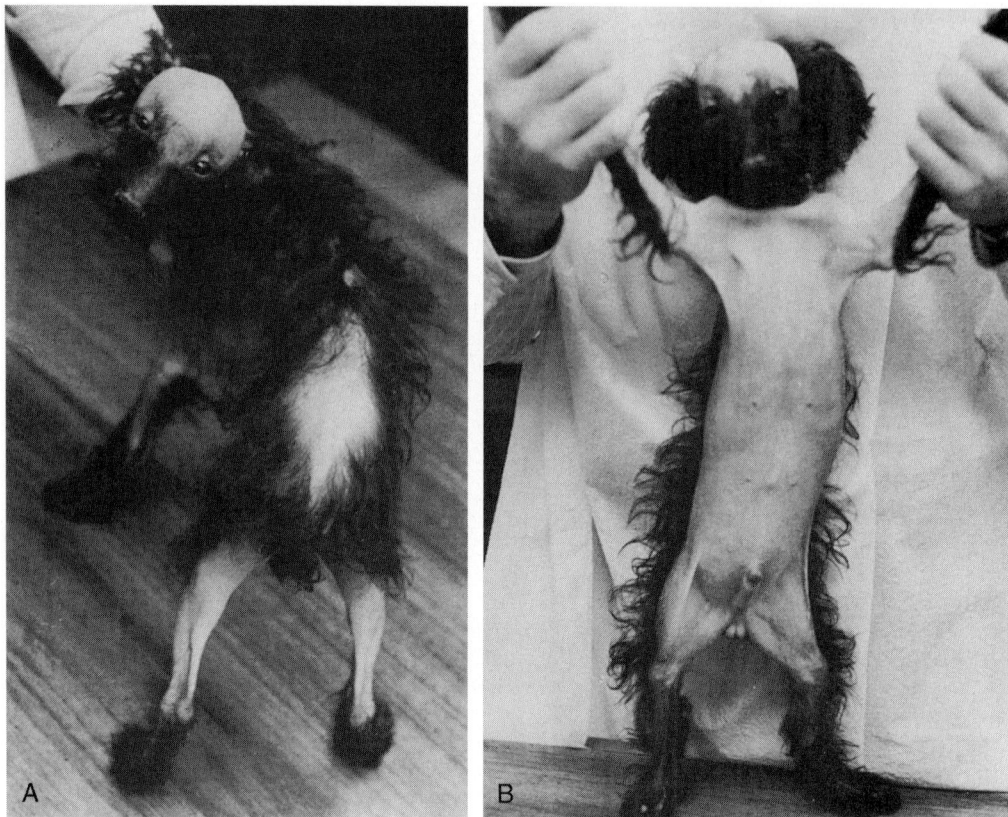

FIGURE 12–54. *A*, Diamond-shaped alopecic region over the dorsal pelvis and alopecia of the head and limbs. *B*, Ventral view of affected male, showing the pattern of alopecia on the trunk and legs. (From Selmanowitz VJ, et al: Congenital ectodermal defect in miniature poodles. J Hered 61:196, 1970.)

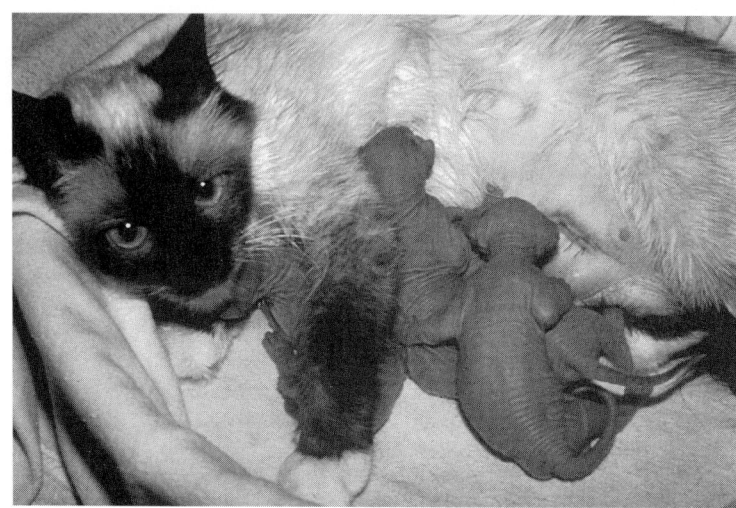

FIGURE 12–55. A Birman cat with her hypotrichotic kittens. (Courtesy of J. King.)

Congenital and Hereditary Defects • 961

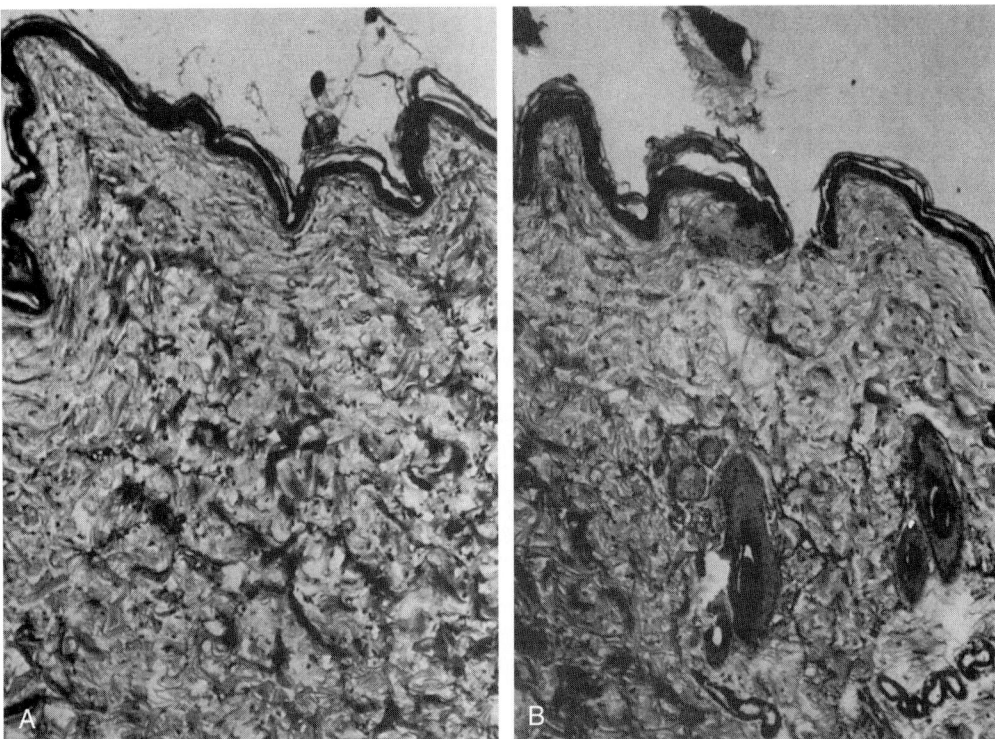

FIGURE 12–56. *A*, Appendage-free skin from the head; hair follicles, sebaceous glands, and sweat glands are absent. (Acid orcein elastica stain ×70.) *B*, Transition zone of appendage-free and appendage-containing skin. Hair follicles, sweat glands, and sebaceous gland cells (near the upper portion of the section of the follicle in the center of the photograph) appear normal. The portion of dermis lacking appendages marks the beginning of a large area of alopecia. There is no overt difference in the appearance of the epidermis and connective tissue on either side of the transition. (From Selmanowitz VJ, et al: Congenital ectodermal defect in miniature poodles. J Hered 61:196, 1970.)

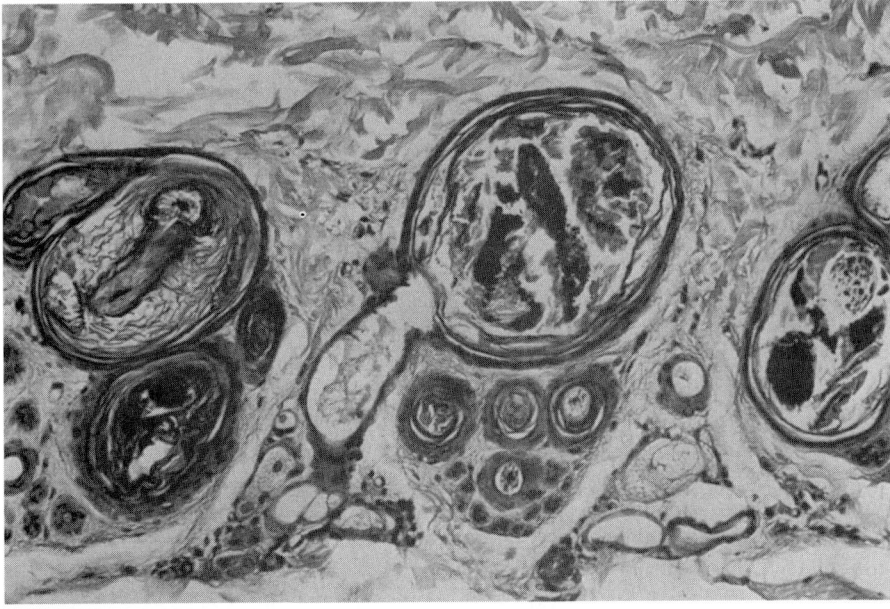

FIGURE 12–57. Canine hypotrichosis. Dystrophic hair follicles and abortive hair shafts.

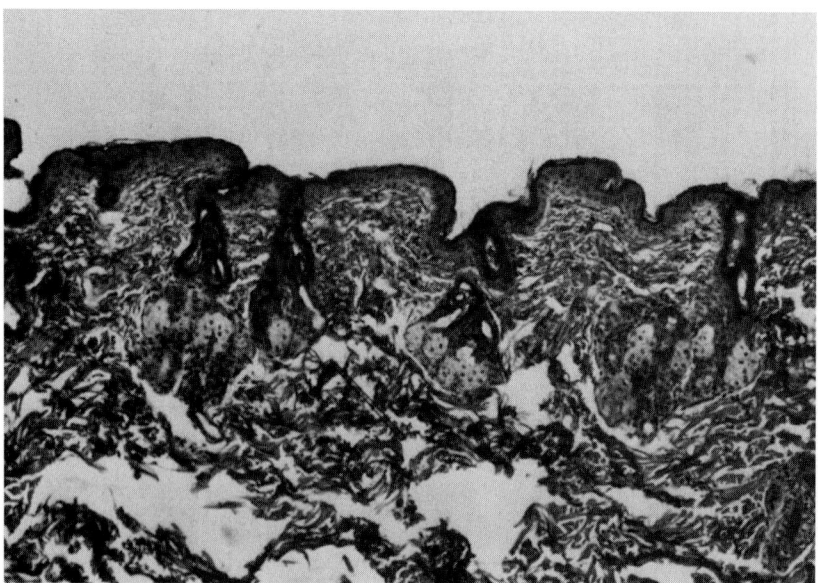

FIGURE 12–58. Hereditary hypotrichosis in a Siamese cat. The poorly developed hair follicles are devoid of hair shafts. (From Scott DW: Feline dermatology 1900–1978: A monograph. JAAHA 16:331, 1980.)

Cause and Pathogenesis

Black hair follicular dysplasia is a familial disorder with near-uniform involvement of the puppies with black coats. In one study, the condition was thought to be autosomal recessive.[147] Histologic and ultrastructural studies show disorders of pigment transfer and cuticular abnormalities of the affected and some normal hairs.[118] The early age at onset suggests that the defect in hair formation plays a significant role in the hair loss. With disorderly proliferation of hair matrix cells, normal pigment transfer to the developing hairs is not expected and the hairs are weakened even further. Some undetermined coat color genetic influence or possibly a deficiency in melanocyte-stimulating hormone could contribute to the pigmentary changes.[100]

Clinical Features

Black hair follicular dysplasia has been recognized in mongrels and purebred dogs of many breeds, including the Bearded collie, Border collie, Basset hound, Papillon, Saluki, Beagle, Jack Russell terrier, American Cocker spaniel, Schipperke, Cavalier King Charles spaniel, Dachshund, Gordon setter, large Munsterlander, and Pointer.° Dogs are born normal but show coat changes by 4 weeks of age. Only the black hairs are affected (see Fig. 12–46E). The first noticeable change in most dogs is loss of luster of the black hairs, followed by progressive hair loss until all black hairs are lost. In large Munsterlanders, dogs destined to lose hair are born with a gray and white, instead of a black and white, coat.[147] Because these dogs are born with a gray coat, this syndrome may more appropriately be called color dilution alopecia. Because the hair loss is due to shaft fracture, stubble can remain. Excessive scaliness occurs in the involved areas. The rate of hair loss is variable, but near-total alopecia occurs by 6 to 9 months of age.

Diagnosis

The color-linked nature and early age at onset of the hair loss make the diagnosis straightforward. Biopsy specimens from nonblack areas are normal, whereas black areas

---

°See references 1, 3, 5, 100, 108, 109, 118, 125, 129, 143, 147, 152.

Congenital and Hereditary Defects • 963

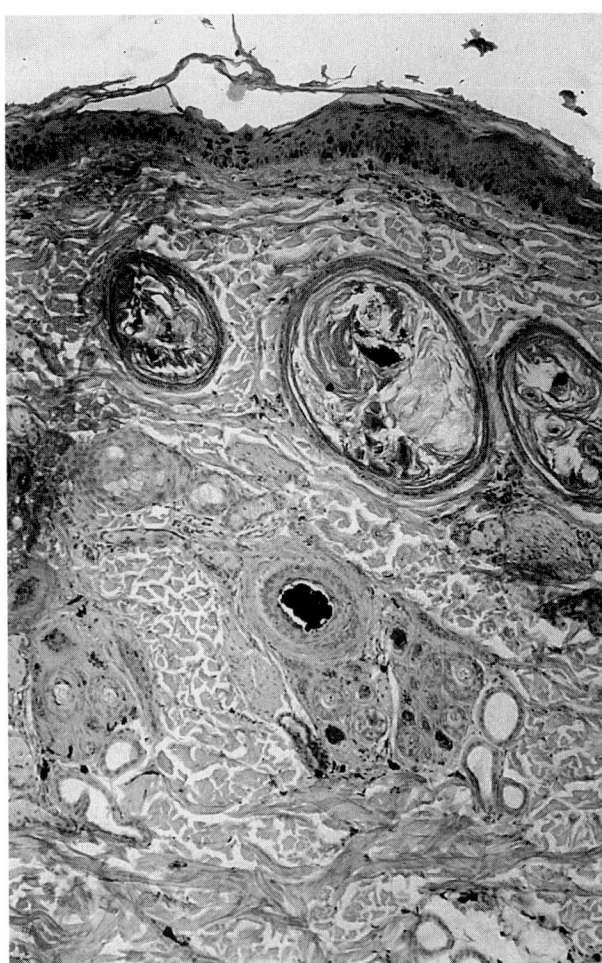

FIGURE 12–59. Black hair follicular dysplasia. Follicular dilatation with the accumulation of keratin and large clumps of free melanin.

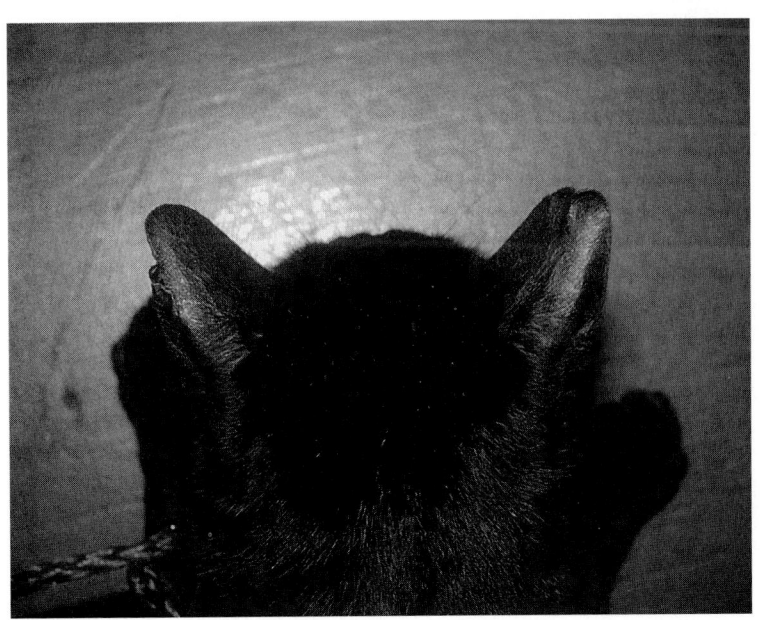

FIGURE 12–60. Patterned pinnal baldness. A 12-year-old cat with hair loss restricted to the pinnae. The hair loss began early in adulthood.

964 • Congenital and Hereditary Defects

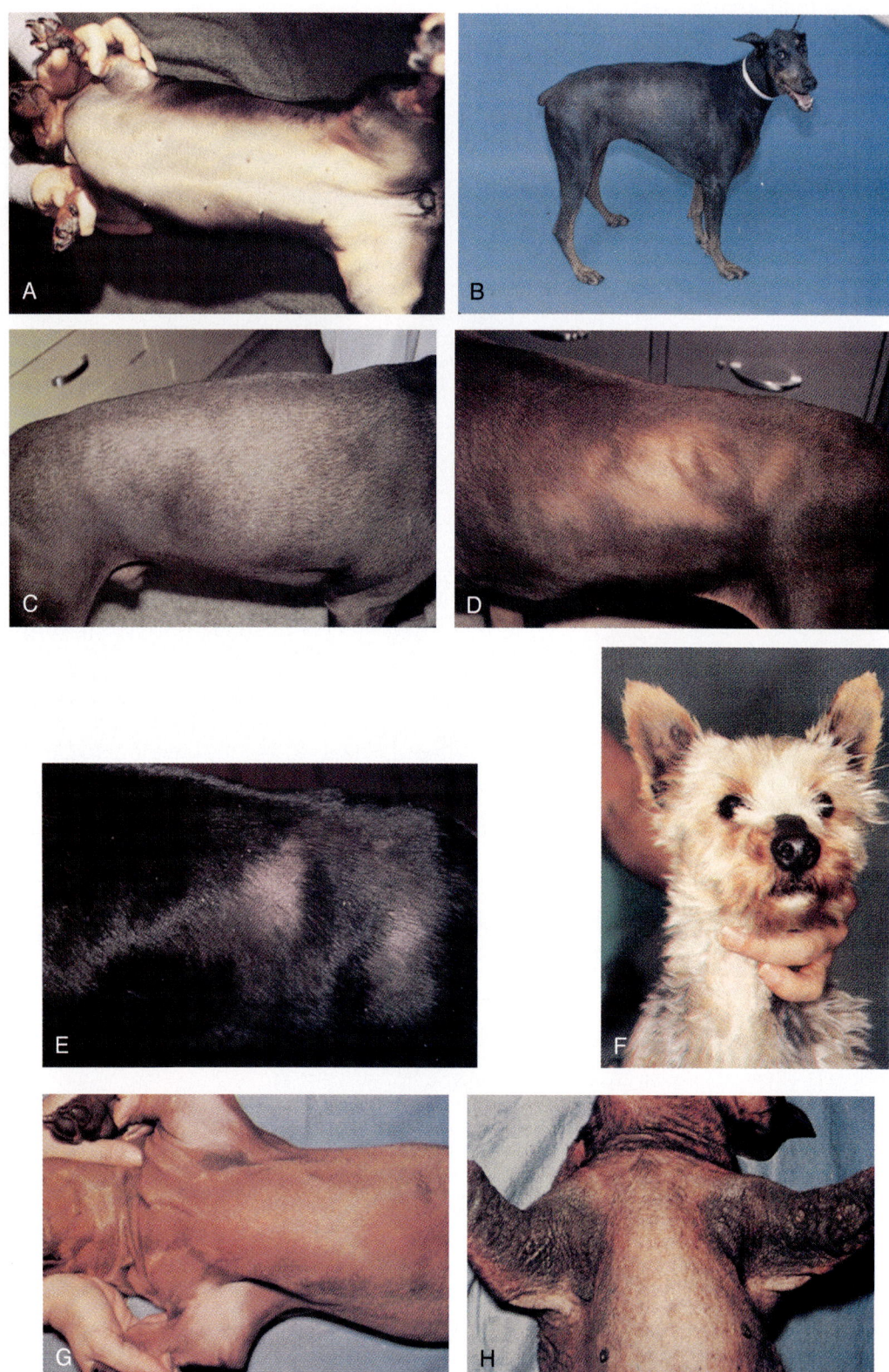

FIGURE 12-61. *Legend on opposite page*

show clumped melanin in epidermal and follicular basal cells and hair matrix cells.[3, 118] Large melanin granules (macromelanosomes) are visible within hair shafts, and the follicles are irregular, are dilated, and are filled with keratin, fragments of hair shafts, and large clumps of free melanin (Fig. 12–59). The normal architecture of hair shafts is often obscured, with unclear definition between cuticle, cortex, and medulla. Hair shaft outline is irregular and focally bulging, and severely affected shafts may be rather amorphous eosinophilic structures containing irregular clumps of melanin. Numerous peribulbar melanophages occur in the dermis. The pigmentary changes are less pronounced than they are in color dilution alopecia.

Tardive Hypotrichosis or Alopecia

Animals with tardive hypotrichosis or alopecia are born with normal coats. Focal, regionalized, or generalized hair loss occurs either about the time when the puppy coat is replaced by the adult coat or when the animal is a young adult.

PATTERN BALDNESS

Pattern baldness has been reported in only dogs, and four syndromes are recognized. The first is pinnal alopecia of male and, rarely, female Dachshunds. We have also recognized this disorder in dogs of other breeding and in the cat (Fig. 12–60). Affected dogs slowly start to lose hair from both pinnae at about 6 to 9 months of age, and the hair loss progresses slowly to complete pinnal alopecia (see Fig. 12–46F). Complete baldness usually occurs by 8 or 9 years of age. As the hair loss progresses, the exposed skin hyperpigments. Aside from the pinnal hair loss, the animals have normal coats.

The second syndrome occurs in American water spaniels and Portuguese water dogs. Hair loss in these dogs typically is noted at about 6 months of age and is restricted to the ventral neck, the caudomedial thighs, and the tail (see Fig. 12–46G and H). Recognition of this problem by the respective breed clubs has sharply reduced the frequency of occurrence.

The third syndrome occurs in Greyhounds, and affected dogs experience hair loss on the caudal thighs as might occur in early endocrine alopecia. Thyroid and sex hormone testing shows no endocrine basis for the hair loss, and the loss stays restricted to the caudal thighs.[106] This condition must be differentiated from the bald thigh syndrome of Greyhounds.[147a] In the bald thigh syndrome, the hair loss is on the lateral thighs and probably has an endocrine basis.

The last and most common syndrome is seen primarily in Dachshunds but also is recognized in Boston terriers, Chihuahuas, Whippets, Manchester terriers, Greyhounds, and Italian greyhounds.[1, 3] The condition is recognized almost exclusively in female animals. At approximately 6 months of age, affected dogs gradually begin to lose hair in the postauricular regions and along the ventral neck, on the entire ventrum (Fig. 12–61A), and on the caudomedial thighs. Hair loss is gradual over the next 12 months but remains restricted to the described areas. Close inspection of the hairless skin reveals multiple small fine hairs. The primary differential diagnosis for this syndrome is estrogen-responsive dermatosis (see Chap. 10). In estrogen-responsive dermatosis, the hair loss begins later in life and leaves no residual hairs.

Histologically, pattern baldness is characterized by a decrease in size (miniaturization)

FIGURE 12–61. A, Pattern baldness on the ventrum of a 2-year-old dachshund. B, Color dilution alopecia in a blue Doberman pinscher. C, Color dilution alopecia in a fawn Doberman pinscher. D, Follicular dysplasia in an adult red Doberman pinscher. E, Follicular dysplasia in an adult black Doberman pinscher. F, Facial and pinnal hyperpigmentation and alopecia in a Yorkshire terrier. G, Acanthosis nigricans, juvenile stage. Note the small hyperpigmented patches in the axillae of this 6-month-old dachshund. H, Acanthosis nigricans, severe hyperpigmentation, and lichenification in a 5-year-old dachshund.

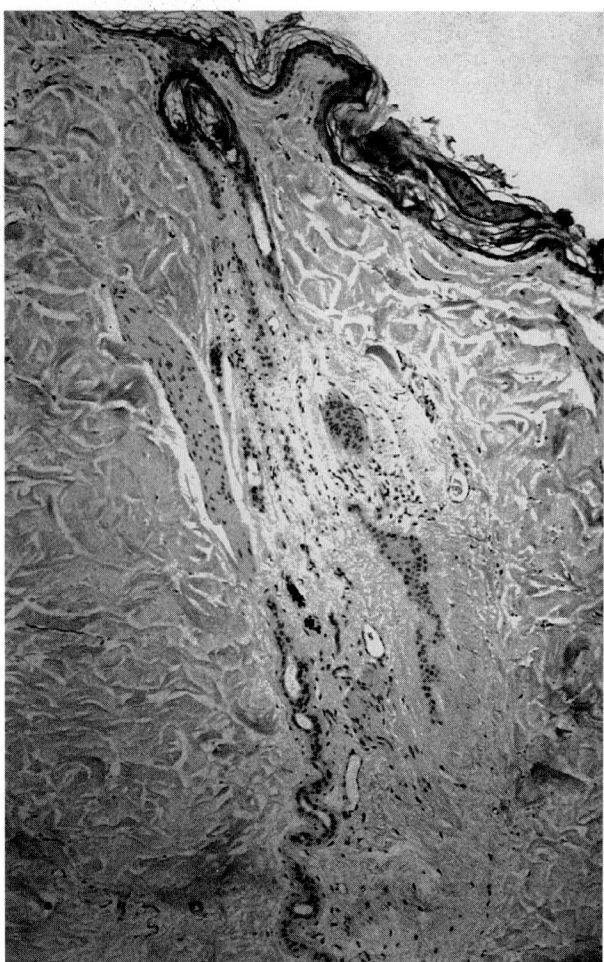

FIGURE 12-62. Patterned baldness. Involution and miniaturization of the hair follicles.

of the hair follicles and hair shafts with normal adnexal structures (Fig. 12-62).[3] The follicles are shorter and thinner, have smaller hair bulbs, and produce fine hair shafts.

When several dogs with recurrent flank alopecia and intercurrent pattern baldness received melatonin, hair regrew in all locations. These surprising results led to larger studies in which 11 dogs were either given oral melatonin (5 mg q24h) or 1 to 3 constant-release 12-mg implants. All dogs experience significant hair growth within 45 days.[139] Peak response occurred after 3 to 4 months of treatment. Melatonin has a short half-life in dogs when given by mouth or injection, and its bioavailability is dose dependent.[121, 127, 139] Oral dosages of 3 to 6 mg q8h have been suggested.[139] Because all oral formulations in the United States are nonprescription, potency and bioavailability may vary considerably from product to product. If no change occurs within 30 days, a dosage increase may be indicated.

COLOR DILUTION ALOPECIA

Color dilution alopecia (color mutant alopecia) occurs in some dogs with blue or fawn coat colors. These colors are dilutions of black or brown, respectively, and result from the influence of coat color genes at the D locus and possibly others.[136, 137] Color dilution alopecia does not occur in all dogs with blue or fawn coats, and the frequency within affected breeds varies.

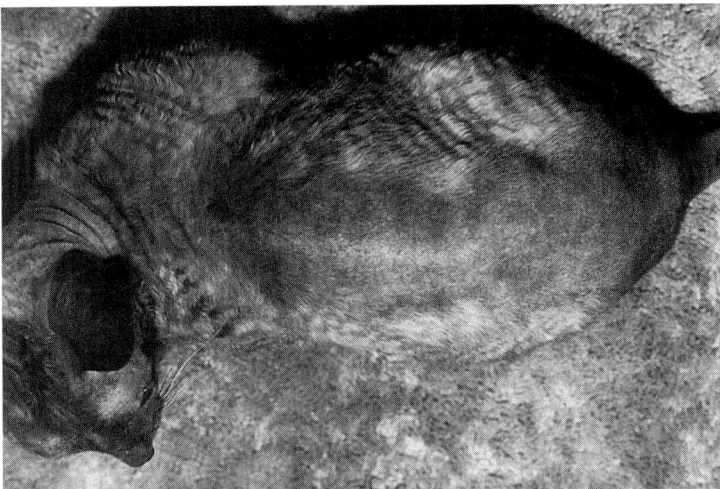

FIGURE 12-63. Follicular dysplasia. A symmetric, nonpruritic alopecia in a tricolored Cornish Rex.

Cause and Pathogenesis

The cause of color dilution alopecia is unknown, but coat color genes play a significant role in the condition. Under the influence of genes at the D locus and possibly others, dilute hairs have larger pigment granules (macromelanosomes) than their nondilute counterparts. Although the hairs are lighter in color, they contain as much or more melanin than nondilute black or brown hairs. Only one allele, d, is recognized at the D locus in dogs.[136, 137] If this gene were solely responsible for color dilution alopecia, all dogs with dilute coat colors would lose hair, but they do not. Unrecognized, deleterious alleles may be present within certain breeds and cause lethal pigmentary changes, which result in the hair loss.

All affected dogs have irregularities in melanin transfer and storage. Mature or stage IV melanosomes are stored irregularly in hairs, and epidermal keratinocytes and vacuolization of melanocytes in some hair bulb cells suggests a degenerative process.[116] Various ultrastructural studies have been undertaken to determine whether concurrent structural defects exist, and some conflicting results have been published. In the Doberman pinscher, the cuticle of affected hairs is normal except at the point of pigmentary clumping, whereas cuticular defects were detected in affected and normal hairs from Yorkshire terriers and Dachshunds.[96, 98, 145] All of these data suggest that the dilution genes may express themselves differently in different breeds and that a coincidental structural defect may exist in certain breeds.

Clinical Features

Color dilution alopecia is most widely recognized and reported in blue or fawn Doberman pinschers.[116, 136] It also has been reported in Dachshunds, Great Danes, Whippets, Italian greyhounds, Chow Chows, Standard poodles, miniature Doberman pinschers, Yorkshire terriers, Silky terriers, Chihuahuas, Boston terriers, Salukis, Newfoundlands, German shepherds, Shetland sheepdogs, Schipperkes, Bernese Mountain dogs, and mongrels with dilute coat colors.* It has also been reported in cream Chow Chow and blond Irish setters, but these cases may represent some other condition.[5] The frequency of the disease in blue or fawn Doberman pinschers can be as high as 93% in blues and 75% in fawns.[136] Incidence figures for other breeds are unknown but are probably much lower

---

*See references 1, 3, 5, 96, 98, 100, 102a, 132, 137

than they are in Doberman pinschers. Some breeds with a dilute coat color (e.g., Weimaraners) do not lose hair.

Color dilution alopecia can be first manifested by dorsally oriented, recurrent bacterial folliculitis or hypotrichosis. Only hairs or hair follicles in the dilute areas are involved. The onset of signs is tardive, and the starting point depends on management factors and the depth of the coat color. Dogs with light-blue (e.g., gray) coats are usually affected at approximately 6 months of age, whereas dogs with less dilution (e.g., steel blue) may not have noticeable signs until 2 to 3 years of age or later. Vigorous grooming can accelerate the process.

In the recurrent folliculitis form, papules and pustules occur and disappear with appropriate antibiotic treatment. The involved follicles tend to remain hairless or regrow hair slowly. With repeated bouts of infection, the hypotrichosis becomes more widespread and persistent. In the hair loss form, secondary pyodermas can also occur but the history and physical examination findings clearly show that hair loss preceded the infection. Dogs with the hair loss form typically lose hairs first over the dorsum and then from the rest of the body (see Fig. 12-61B and C). The rate of hair loss is variable, but most light-colored dogs are almost completely alopecic by 2 to 3 years of age.

The initial hair loss in these dogs is due to shaft fracture, and some broken hairs regrow. With time, the tendency to regrow decreases. Exposed skin is subject to environmental insults, and scaliness is common. One report suggests that these dogs may be more susceptible to skin tumors.[131] Because these dogs have no hair to protect against the mutagenic effects of the sun, they should be photoprotected.

Cats with a blue or cream-colored coat carry the Maltese dilution gene. As in the dog, this gene is expressed by clumping of melanin in the follicular epithelium and hair shafts but rarely is associated with dysplastic changes in the hair follicles and hairs themselves.[150] We have recognized the pathologic changes of color dilution alopecia in the skin biopsies of several other cats. The involved cats spontaneously experience symmetric truncal hypotrichosis to alopecia without a history or trichographic evidence of excessive grooming or harsh topical treatments.

Diagnosis

The differential diagnosis varies with the age at onset. In the young animal, only other inherited hair defects or demodicosis should be investigated. With onset at 2 to 3 years or later, endocrine disorders, especially hypothyroidism, are considered for dogs with just hair loss. All causes of superficial folliculitis should be considered in that presentation. In the cat, all causes of excessive grooming need to be considered (Fig. 12-63).

Microscopic examination of plucked hairs shows numerous macromelanosomes, of irregular shapes and sizes, unevenly distributed along the shaft. In some cases, the macromelanosomes are huge and distort the hair shaft (Fig. 12-64). The cuticle may be absent or fractured over the bulging pigment clumps (Fig. 12-65). Histopathologic study initially shows sebaceous melanosis; melanin clumping in epidermal and follicular basal cells (Fig. 12-66) and hair matrix cells; numerous macromelanosomes in hair shafts; hair follicles in various stages of growth with follicular hyperkeratosis, fractured hair shafts, and free clumps of melanin (Fig. 12-67); and numerous peribulbar melanophages.[3, 95, 136, 146] As mentioned before, the presence of melanin clumping indicates the action of dilution genes and does not necessarily mean the animal has color dilution alopecia. Microscopic examination of hairs from normal-coated color diluted dogs and cats reveals melanin clumping, but the normal architecture of the hair shaft is preserved. Other changes of follicular dysplasia, especially the presence of dysplastic hair shafts, must be present to confirm the diagnosis.[146] With time, all follicular activity ceases and the follicles become dilated and cystic.

Clinical Management

Early on, hair loss is due to shaft fracture, so every effort should be made to avoid the use of harsh shampoos and topical agents and vigorous grooming techniques. These

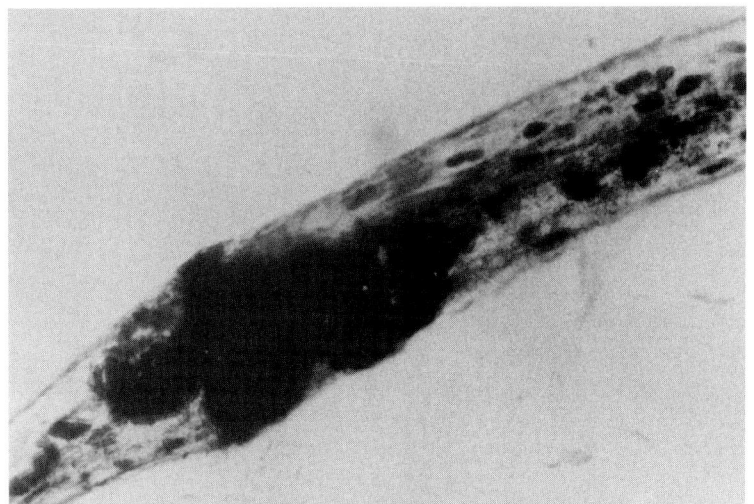

FIGURE 12–64. Color dilution alopecia. Marked melanin clumping and distortion of cuticular-cortical anatomy.

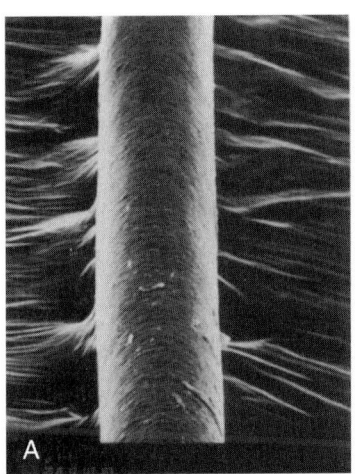 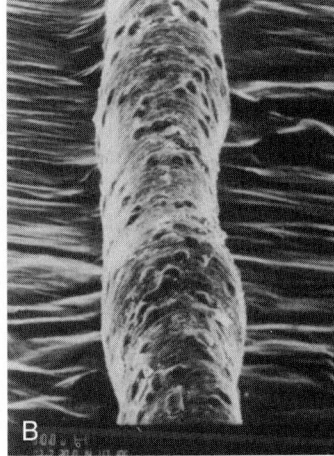

FIGURE 12–65. Color dilution alopecia. Scanning electron microscopic views (SEMs) of hairs from a normal black (A) and affected blue (B) Doberman pinscher. The cortical irregularities in B are due to macromelanosomes. (Courtesy of D. Prieur.)

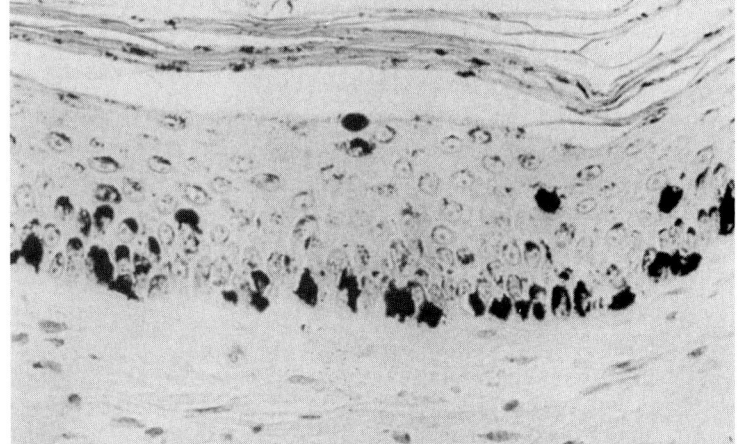

FIGURE 12–66. Color dilution alopecia. Melanin clumping in surface epidermis.

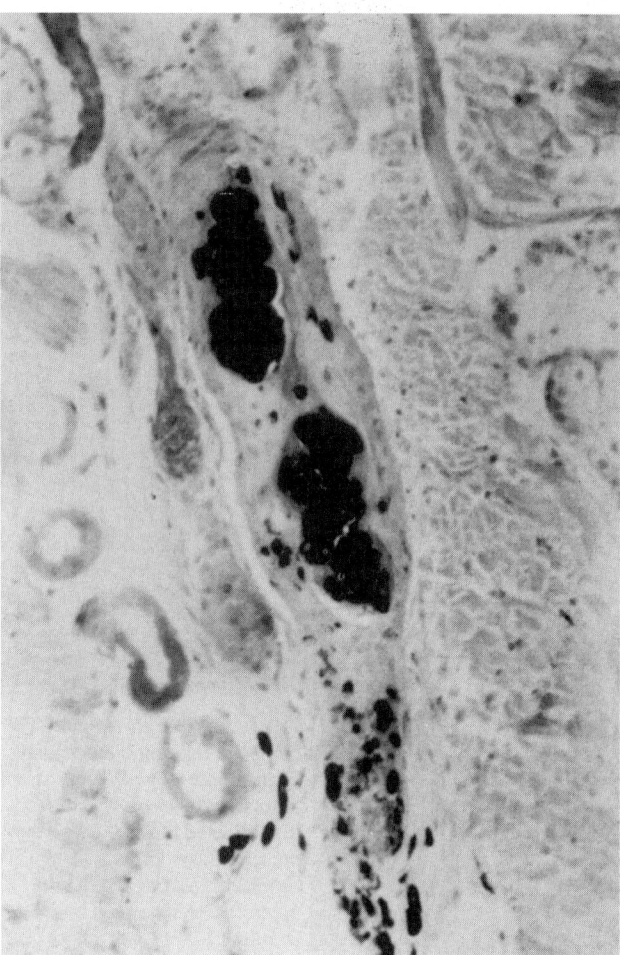

FIGURE 12–67. Color dilution alopecia. Marked clumping of melanin ("melanotic mush") in the pilar canal of a hair follicle.

measures should slow but not prevent hair loss. Anecdotal reports suggest that treatment with oral retinoic acids can be of benefit, but specific details are unavailable.[4] Etretinate was reported to occasionally help dogs with color dilution alopecia, resulting in decreased scaling and decreased frequency and severity of bacterial pyoderma.[114] However, any hair regrowth was partial and characterized by fine hairs.

FOLLICULAR DYSPLASIA

Non–color-linked follicular dysplasia has probably existed in veterinary dermatology for decades but went unrecognized. The diagnosis in affected dogs typically was idiopathic or nonresponsive endocrine skin disease because they had a spontaneous, symmetric, asymptomatic truncal alopecia. The dysplastic process was first reported in the Siberian husky in 1988[142] and has been recognized in many different breeds since then. With the high frequency of disease within certain breeds, genetic predisposition is most likely. Features of the disorder vary somewhat with the breed involved.

Both cyclic and structural follicular dysplasia are recognized. As the name suggests, cyclic follicular dysplasia is an interruption of the normal hair cycle, and affected animals experience hair loss that spontaneously disappears in the next one to four shed periods. The most common cyclic dysplasia is seasonal flank alopecia wherein affected dogs experience geographic flank and/or saddle area alopecia and hyperpigmentation. The hair loss usually occurs in the late fall or early spring, and regrowth is complete by late spring or early fall, respectively.[107, 111, 140, 156] Other less common cyclic dysplasias are postclipping alopecia and catagen arrest wherein spontaneous regrowth occurs, but in a much less predictable fashion. In all of these disorders, skin biopsies show alteration in the hair cycle, sebaceous melanosis, and the presence of dysplastic hair follicles.[95] All of these disorders are described in detail elsewhere (see Chap. 11).

In the structural dysplasias, the clinical picture (e.g., age at onset, distribution of hair loss) varies with the breed. In addition to the presence of sebaceous melanosis and dysplastic hair follicles, these dogs have other structural changes that weaken the hairs. Fracture of these weakened hairs is the initial cause of the hair loss, and it occurs in areas that have been too vigorously groomed or subjected to trauma (e.g., collar region). Because the structural changes are mild initially, the hairs continue to grow and the hair loss disappears spontaneously. However, the hair that regrows often is weaker than the hair that was lost and the hair loss will recur because trauma is unavoidable. With each and every episode, the structural changes become more pronounced, and eventually the hair loss becomes more or less permanent.

Siberian Husky and Malamute

Multiple dogs in a litter can be affected.[141, 142] At 3 to 4 months of age, the guard hairs on the trunk are lost in a slowly progressive fashion and the coat turns a reddish color. In Malamutes, the onset of signs may not be seen until 3 to 4 years of age. The head and the distal limbs are spared. Areas clipped for biopsy do not regrow hair. Secondary hairs are less frequently involved.

Doberman Pinschers, Miniature Pinschers, and Manchester Terriers

Black or red dogs can be affected, and the hair loss is noted between 1 and 4 years of age.[135] Hair loss begins in the flank region and progresses slowly to involve the caudal dorsum and entire flank region (see Fig. 12–61*D* and *E*). Complete truncal hair loss has not been recognized.

Airedale Terrier, Boxer, English Bulldog, Staffordshire Terrier, Wirehaired Griffons, and Affen Pinschers

Hair loss begins between 2 and 4 years of age and is restricted to the flank and/or saddle regions.[134] In some dogs, the hair loss persists, whereas cyclic loss and regrowth occurs in other dogs (see Chap. 11).

Irish Water Spaniels, Portuguese Water Dogs, and Curly-Coated Retrievers

The hair loss in these dogs is due to hair fracture.[3, 103, 138] Alopecia is usually not recognized until 2 to 4 years of age, but excessive hairs in grooming tools is recognized from an early age. Hair loss occurs first over the caudal dorsum and spreads slowly to involve most of the trunk. Early on, spontaneous hair regrowth can occur, but the new hairs are not of normal quality and texture. These and other hairs, are lost eventually, and the hair loss persists (Fig. 12–68). A dominant mode of inheritance has been suggested in the Irish water spaniel.[103]

Other Dogs

In recent years, we and other investigators have recognized one to several cases of follicular dysplasia in the Shetland sheepdog, Labrador retriever, Chihuahua, German shepherd dog, Bull mastiff, Pekingese, Australian shepherd, Rhodesian ridgeback, English springer spaniel, German shorthaired and wirehaired pointer, Rottweiler, Chesapeake Bay retriever, Miniature schnauzer, Bouvier de Flanders, and French bulldog. Undoubtedly, many other breeds could be added to the list if pathology records were carefully reviewed. Because too few cases within a specific breed have been published, details of the clinical patterns are not available.

Follicular dysplasia has been recognized in a tricolored Cornish Rex cat.[150] The symmetric hair loss affected the blue, beige, and cream-colored hairs (see Fig. 12–63).

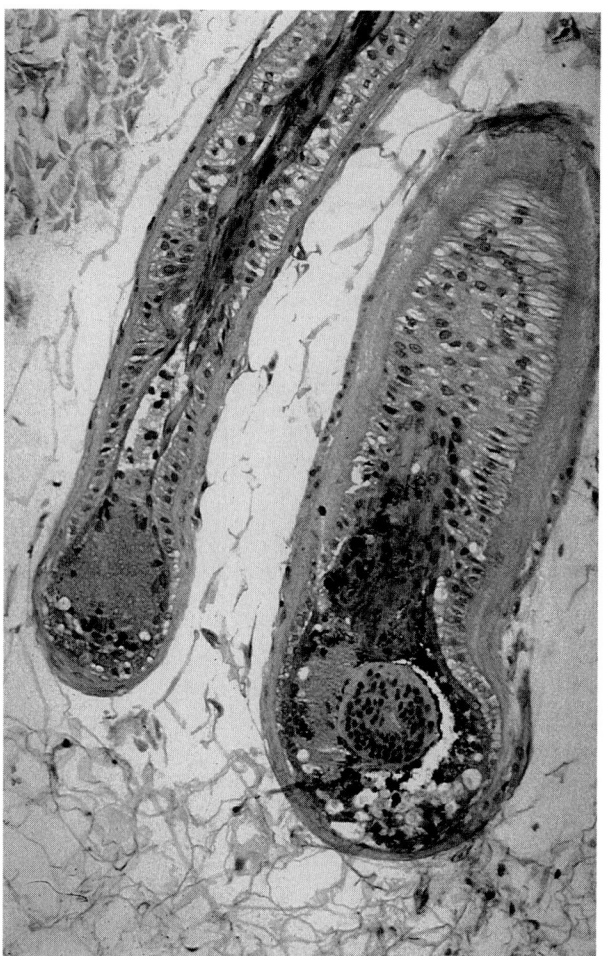

FIGURE 12–70. Follicular dysplasia of the Portuguese Water dog. Vacuolar alteration and dissolution of the hair matrix.

Treatment

Detailed long-term follow-up is not available, but it appears that the hair loss can resolve or persist, but remains confined to the mahogany points of the face and feet.

Melanoderma and Alopecia in Yorkshire Terriers

Melanoderma and alopecia in Yorkshire terriers is a well-recognized but poorly studied syndrome,[5, 94, 99] which appears to be decreasing in incidence. It is probably a genetic dermatosis, but the mode of inheritance is unknown. The cause is unknown, but one investigator demonstrated decreased dermal elastin and abnormal growth hormone response to clonidine administration in eight dogs.[99] Typically, the syndrome affects Yorkshire terriers of either sex, beginning at 6 months to 3 years of age.

The dogs have symmetric alopecia and marked hyperpigmentation over the bridge of the nose (see Fig. 12–61F), on the pinnae (Fig. 12–71), and occasionally on the tail and feet. Affected skin is smooth and shiny. There is no pruritus or pain, and affected dogs are otherwise healthy.

Skin biopsy specimens are reported to show orthokeratotic hyperkeratosis of the epidermal surface and of the hair follicles and epidermal melanosis.

Some dogs with mild lesions appear to recover spontaneously. Most dogs remain

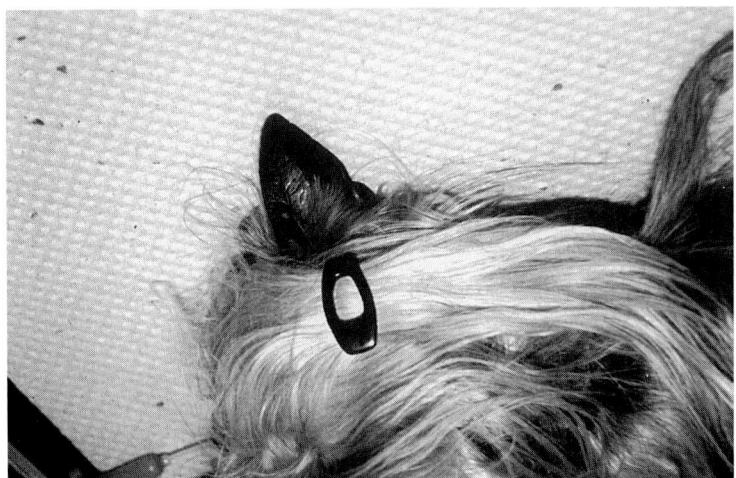

FIGURE 12–71. Melanoderma and alopecia in Yorkshire terriers. Total alopecia and marked hyperpigmentation of the pinna.

affected throughout their lifetime. Three dogs treated with growth hormone regrew hair but lost it again.[99]

• DISORDERS OF PIGMENTATION

Hypopigmentary Disorders

Loss of skin pigment (leukoderma) or hair pigment (leukotrichia) has a variety of inflammatory or metabolic causes. Idiopathic cases occur with some regularity and have been reported in dogs of various breeds.[3] The high frequency of these changes in the Belgian Tervurens, German shepherd dog, Rottweiler, and Doberman pinscher suggests a hereditary influence in these breeds (see Chap. 13).

Hyperpigmentary Disorders

Aside from lentigines (see Chap. 13) or macular melanosis associated with testicular neoplasia (see Chap. 10), hyperpigmentation in dogs and rarely in cats is poorly demarcated, involves large areas, and has a variety of inflammatory or endocrine causes. Acanthosis nigricans in some Dachshunds probably has a hereditary basis.

ACANTHOSIS NIGRICANS

Canine acanthosis nigricans is an uncommon cutaneous reaction pattern characterized by axillary hyperpigmentation, lichenification, and alopecia in association with various known and unknown causes.

Cause and Pathogenesis

Canine acanthosis nigricans is best thought of as a cutaneous reaction pattern with multiple causes.[1, 5, 158, 165] The pathogenesis of the reaction pattern is poorly understood. Canine acanthosis nigricans may be divided into primary (idiopathic) and secondary types.

Primary (idiopathic) canine acanthosis nigricans is almost exclusively a disease of Dachshunds. The striking breed predilection and early age at onset strongly suggest that this type of canine acanthosis nigricans is a genodermatosis. Indeed, one form of acanthosis nigricans in humans is known to be inherited.[2]

Secondary canine acanthosis nigricans is associated with underlying disorders, including (1) friction or intertrigo (conformational abnormalities, obesity, or both resulting in excessive axillary friction and dermatitis) with a secondary bacterial or *Malassezia* infection, (2) endocrinopathy (e.g., underlying hypothyroidism, hyperadrenocorticism, sex hormone imbalances), and (3) hypersensitivity (chronic axillary pruritus and dermatitis associated with atopy, food hypersensitivity, or contact dermatitis). In humans, acanthosis nigricans has been associated with tissue resistance to insulin, drugs (e.g., nicotinic acid, diethylstilbestrol, and glucocorticoids), and internal malignancy (especially of the gastrointestinal or female reproductive tract).[2, 162] Drug-induced acanthosis nigricans has not been reported in animals, and the cases in dogs associated with malignancy may have had other causes.[164]

Clinical Features

Although primary canine acanthosis nigricans has been reported in several breeds, Dachshunds are overwhelmingly the breed at risk. Primary canine acanthosis nigricans occurs in either sex and begins in dogs younger than 1 year. Secondary canine acanthosis nigricans may occur in any breed and is more commonly recognized in those predisposed to the various underlying diseases described previously. Secondary canine acanthosis nigricans generally mimics any sex or age predilection inherent in the underlying diseases.

The earliest sign of primary canine acanthosis nigricans is usually bilateral axillary hyperpigmentation (see Fig. 12–61G). With time, lichenification, alopecia, and seborrheic changes develop (see Fig. 12–61H). In severe cases, the dermatosis may spread to involve the forelimbs, the ventral neck, the chest, the abdomen, the groin, the perineum, the hocks, the periocular area, and the pinnae. Seborrheic skin disease (greasy with rancid odor) and secondary bacterial pyoderma or *Malassezia* dermatitis are common complicating factors. Pruritus is variable and is usually most severe when seborrheic changes, bacterial pyoderma, or *Malassezia* dermatitis is present.

Diagnosis

The differential diagnosis of canine acanthosis nigricans includes the previously mentioned causes of primary and secondary disease. Definitive diagnosis is based on history, physical examination findings, laboratory tests that rule out other conditions, skin biopsy, and response to therapy. Juvenile-onset acanthosis nigricans in a Dachshund is most likely to be primary and genetic. Thyroid function is usually normal in Dachshunds with acanthosis nigricans. Histopathologic examination is nondiagnostic, revealing hyperplastic superficial perivascular dermatitis with focal parakeratotic hyperkeratosis, epidermal melanosis, pigmentary incontinence, and follicular keratosis. The perivascular inflammatory infiltrate is usually mixed mononuclear cells and neutrophils. A similar histopathologic pattern may occur with many chronic inflammatory dermatoses.[3]

Clinical Management

The prognosis for cure in canine acanthosis nigricans varies with the underlying cause. When the acanthosis nigricans is due to some definable and correctable disorder, the lesions need no specific treatment and resolve spontaneously as the primary disease is treated. Response may be slow. Primary canine acanthosis nigricans in the Dachshund is a controllable, but not a curable, disease.

Early cases of acanthosis nigricans need no treatment. As the lesions become more widespread and hyperplastic, the resultant seborrheic changes necessitate treatment. Antiseborrheic bathing and the frequent application of talc to the intertriginous areas is beneficial, but provides only short-term improvement. When the lesions are confined to small areas, the application of a potent topical glucocorticoid (e.g., betamethasone valerate ointment) can be beneficial for some time. Eventually, the lesions become too widespread for the safe use of these topical products. Advanced cases can be treated with melatonin,[163] systemic glucocorticoids, or vitamin E.

Systemic glucocorticoids are effective in the treatment of canine acanthosis nigricans,[158] presumably via their anti-inflammatory, antiseborrheic, and anti-MSH effects. Prednisolone or prednisone is given orally at 1 mg/kg every 24 hours for 7 to 10 days, and then on an alternate-morning regimen. Vitamin E acetate (dl—tocopherol acetate), 200 IU given orally every 12 hours as the only treatment, produced improvement within 30 to 60 days in eight cases of primary acanthosis nigricans.[165] Hyperpigmentation was not reduced, but inflammation, lichenification, pruritus, greasiness, and objectionable odor all subsided. There were no side effects, and improvement was maintained while treatment continued.

Disorders of Atypical Coloration

Coat color is controlled by multiple genes with various known or presumed alleles at each locus. In mice, in which coat color genetics is best known, certain coat colors are external markers for serious internal disease. The importance of coat color in certain dermatologic or systemic illnesses in pets is of increasing interest.

CONGENITAL DISORDERS

Animals born with a dilute coat color (e.g., blue or beige) are at risk for color dilution alopecia. The best known examples of linkage of coat color with internal disease are cyclic hematopoiesis and the Chédiak-Higashi syndrome.

Chédiak-Higashi Syndrome

The Chédiak-Higashi syndrome is an inherited disorder of Persian cats, white tigers, Hereford cattle, Aleutian minks, and humans.[65, 160] In cats, it is an autosomal recessive disorder occurring only in Persian cats with blue-smoke hair color and yellow eyes. Microscopic examination of unstained hairs reveals multiple large, elongated, irregular clumps of melanin (macromelanosomes).[161] Affected cats have giant lysosomes in the cytoplasm of various cells, including neutrophils and macrophages.[159] On blood smears, these lysosomes appear as large eosinophilic granules.

Chédiak-Higashi syndrome is characterized by increased susceptibility to infection, partial oculocutaneous albinism, photophobia, and bleeding disorders. The cats have red fundic light reflection instead of yellow-green. Because of the immunologic deficiency, affected cats are at increased risk for infection. Most cases of dermatophytic pseudomycetoma have occurred in smoke-colored Persian cats.

There is no specific treatment. Affected animals should not be used for breeding.

Canine Cyclic Hematopoiesis

Cyclic hematopoiesis (gray Collie syndrome, or canine cyclic neutropenia) is a lethal autosomal recessive syndrome in which Collie puppies are born with a silver-gray haircoat that differs from the normal sable or tricolor coat.[160, 167] In some of these puppies, a slight yellow pigmentation may be present, which produces a mixture of light-beige and light-gray hair. The light-colored nose is a characteristic and diagnostic feature.

In addition to the hair color change, gray Collie puppies are usually smaller and weaker than their littermates, a difference observable by 1 week of age. By 8 to 12 weeks of age, signs of clinical illness appear, including fever, diarrhea, lymphadenopathy, infections, conjunctivitis, and arthralgia. The term *cyclic neutropenia* reflects the appearance of neutropenia alternating with rebounding neutrophilia. This cycle continues at 10- to 12-day intervals until death. Other hematologic abnormalities include nonregenerative anemia as well as cyclic reticulocytosis, monocytosis, and thrombocytosis.[5, 167] Other clinicopathologic abnormalities include hyperglobulinemia, depressed mitogenic responses of lymphocytes, and cyclic hormonogenesis.[4]

There is no effective treatment, and parents and littermates should not be used for breeding. Affected animals usually die before 6 months of age without supportive care. Even with optimal care, most die before 2 years of age because of hepatic or renal failure associated with amyloidosis. Bone marrow transplantation is effective but impractical.[167] In differential diagnosis, this syndrome must not be mistaken for the dominant or Maltese gray collie and a transient dilution called *powder puff*.

Coat Color Dilution and Cerebellar Degeneration in Rhodesian Ridgeback Dogs

An autosomal recessive trait in a family of Rhodesian ridgeback dogs has been described.[158a] Affected pups were born with a diluted coat color, and neurologic abnormalities were recognized at 2 weeks of age. The affected pups' coat color was bluish, and they were ataxic, had difficulty in crawling and nursing, opened their eyes later than their normal littermates, and did not grow normally. Most were euthanized at 4 to 6 weeks of age. At necropsy, the dogs had Purkinje's cell degeneration and cutaneous abnormalities typical of color dilution alopecia.

ACQUIRED DISORDERS

Coat color change in adult animals can be focal, regionalized, or generalized. Change can be due to reversion to puppy coloration after trauma or endocrine disorders, temperature effects, topical insults (e.g., sunlight and bleaching shampoos), nutritional disorders, drugs, and endocrine diseases (especially hyperadrenocorticism and sex hormone imbalances). Most of these conditions can occur in any breed. A peculiar gilding syndrome has been described in Miniature schnauzers.

Acquired Aurotrichia in Miniature Schnauzers

This syndrome was first reported in 1991 and appears to be uncommon.[166] Dogs of either sex can be affected, and the disorder is recognized in young adult dogs, typically between 2 and 3 years of age. More than half of the reported cases started in warm weather, but the condition can start in periods with minimal solar exposure. The cause of the alteration in hair color is unknown, but because of the restriction to the Miniature schnauzer breed, there must be some genetic influence.

Affected dogs typically have patchy color change of the hairs over the dorsal thorax and along the abdomen (see Chap. 13).[166] The affected hairs are golden in color. In a few dogs, the color change is diffuse in those areas and may involve the periocular region or ears. Concomitant with the gilding, the number of secondary hairs in the area is decreased. The dogs are otherwise healthy. Aside from some pigmentary changes in the guard hairs, there is no histologic explanation for the gilding.

No treatment is indicated or should be effective. The condition resolves spontaneously in 6 to 24 months. Both the coloration and the density of the undercoat return to normal. Relapses are uncommon.

• DISORDERS OF COLLAGEN

The best known example of a congenital disorder of collagen is Ehlers-Danlos syndrome in which abnormal production or degradation results in abnormally fragile skin. The other conditions discussed are less clear cut. They have a high incidence in certain breeds, which suggests an inherited predisposition, and abnormalities in dermal collagen are visible in biopsy specimens. However, it is not clear whether the collagen changes are primary or secondary to some as yet described condition. Because of the striking breed predisposition, the conditions are considered here.

Ehlers-Danlos Syndrome

Ehlers-Danlos syndrome, cutaneous asthenia, and dermatosparaxis are all terms used to describe group of inherited connective tissues diseases characterized by excessive fragility and hyperextensibility of the skin.[65, 176, 189] In humans, the term *cutaneous asthenia* is reserved for cases wherein abnormalities in both collagen and elastin (cutis laxa) exist. The cutis laxa syndromes are no longer included with the Ehlers-Danlos syndromes and have not been definitively documented in animals. The term *dermatosparaxis* literally means "torn skin" and is used to describe patients with one specific subtype, type VIIC, of Ehlers-Danlos syndrome in which the skin is extraordinarily fragile.

CAUSE AND PATHOGENESIS

The Ehlers-Danlos syndromes in humans continue to undergo reclassification as the molecular basis for the various clinical entities is identified. Currently, 10 subtypes, based on the clinical features, mode of inheritance, and nature of the biochemical defect, are defined; however, not all patients can be categorized in this scheme (Table 12-2).[2, 173] The molecular basis for all subtypes is not known. Where known, mutations in the genes coding fibrillar collagen or the enzymes that catalyze their post-translational modifications have been identified.[2] All forms have a genetic basis, and six are inherited as an autosomal dominant trait, three as an autosomal recessive trait, and one as an X-linked recessive trait.

Because of the collagen defects, the skin of affected animals often tears easily, resulting in large, gaping "fish mouth" wounds (Fig. 12-72A). These lacerations heal readily but leave thin, highly visible "cigarette paper" scars (see Fig. 12-72B). The tensile strength of the skin of affected dogs is reduced 40-fold, whereas that of affected cats is reduced tenfold.[177, 181] Ehlers-Danlos syndrome has been reported in sheep, cattle, mink, dogs, and cats.[171, 177, 179, 181, 194, 196a] Cases have been reported in various purebred and mongrel dogs and cats with varying modes of inheritance.[180]

Recessive cutaneous asthenia has been absolutely confirmed in only cats,[170-172, 175, 187, 193, 195] but the occurrence of the disease in a mongrel dog with apparently normal parents suggests a recessive form in dogs.[169] Affected collagen forms twisted ribbons rather than cylindric fibrils and fibers (Figs. 12-73 and 12-74). These structural changes are due to abnormalities in formation or maintenance of collagen fibrils and fibers.[172, 182, 187] Biochemical studies have demonstrated a procollagen processing defect in which there is decreased activity of procollagen peptidase and an accumulation of partially processed type I procollagen containing N-terminal propeptides.[187] Collagenase activity typically is increased 2½ times above normal levels.[187]

Dominant cutaneous asthenia is a simple autosomal trait in dogs and cats. Changes

● Table 12-2 **TYPES OF EHLERS-DANLOS SYNDROME**

TYPE	TISSUES AFFECTED	ABNORMALITY
I	Skin, joints	?
II	Skin, joints	Collagen V
III	Skin, joints	?
IV	Skin, blood vessels, intestine	Collagen III
V	Skin, joints, heart	Procollagen (lysyl oxidase deficiency)
VI	Skin, joints, bone, eyes	Procollagen (lysyl hydroxylase deficiency)
VIIa, b	Skin, joints	Procollagen
VIIc	Skin, joints	Procollagen (procollagen peptidase deficiency)
VIII	Skin, joints, teeth	?
IX	Skin, bones	Copper deficiency (lysyl oxidase deficiency)
X	Skin, joints, platelets	Fibronectin
XI	Joints	?

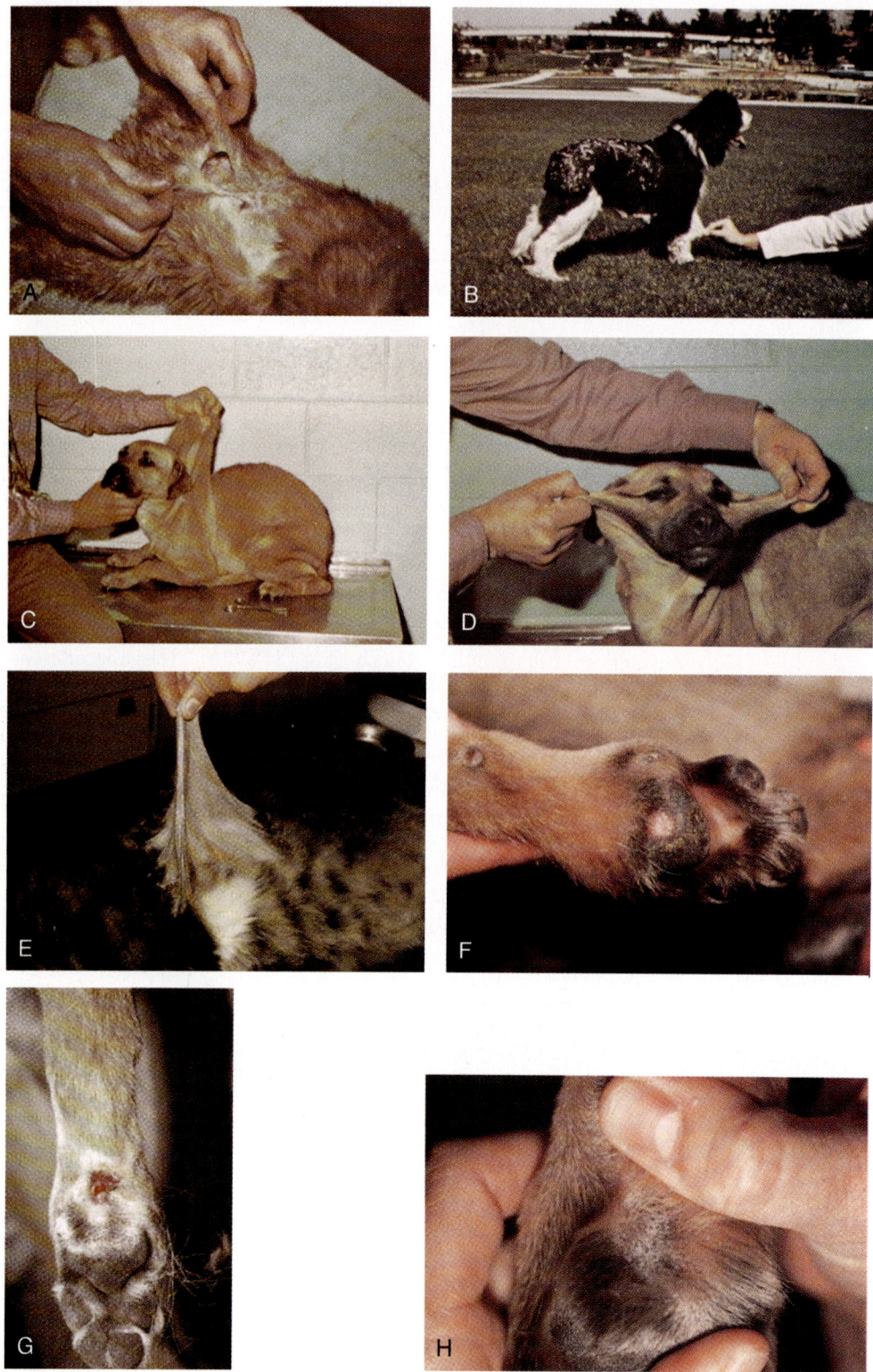

FIGURE 12-72. *A*, Cutaneous asthenia in a cat. Hyperfragility of the skin. *B*, Typical appearance of a Springer spaniel with cutaneous asthenia. Note the numerous scars on the back. (Courtesy of G.A. Hegreberg.) *C*. Cutaneous asthenia in a dog. Hyperextensibility of the skin. (Courtesy of G. Ackland.) *D*, Cutaneous asthenia in a dog. Same dog as in C. (Courtesy of G. Ackland.) *E*, Cutaneous asthenia in a cat. Hyperextensibility of the skin. (Courtesy of P. McKeever.) *F*, Collagen disorder of the footpads of a German shepherd. *G*, Solitary fistula on the caudal metatarsal area of a German shepherd. *H*, Fluctuant swelling on the caudal metatarsal area of a German shepherd.

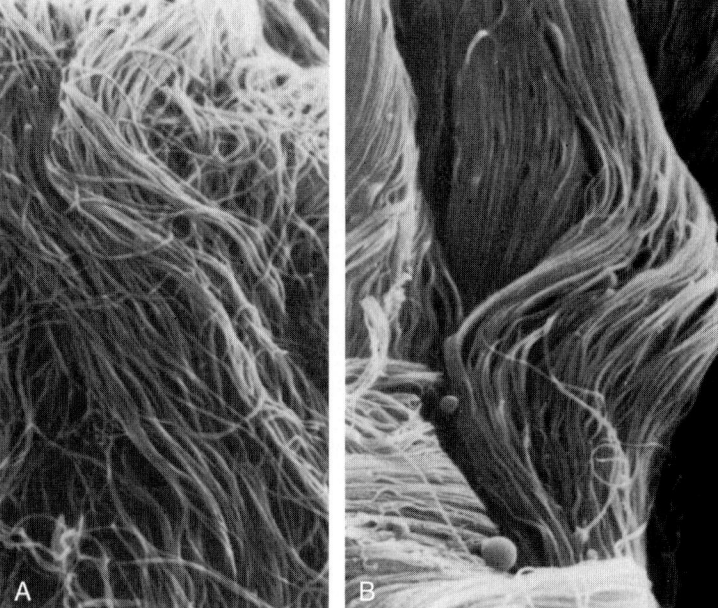

FIGURE 12–73. SEMs of collagen fibrils in a fiber bundle from the dermis of a dermatosparactic cat (A), and a normal cat (B) (×6000). (From Holbrook KA, et al: Dermatosparaxis in a Himalayan cat: II. Ultrastructural studies of dermal collagen. J Invest Dermatol 74:100, 1980.)

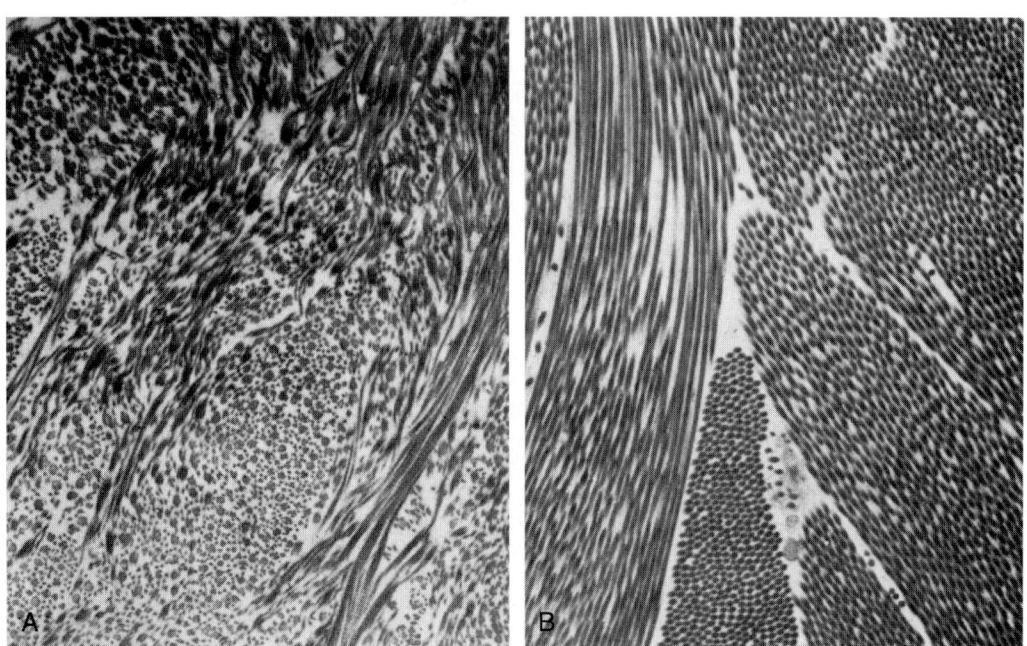

FIGURE 12–74. A, Transmission electron microscopic view (TEM) of a collagen fiber bundle from the dermis of the dermatosparactic cat showing fibers and fibrils in various planes of a section within the bundle (×10,000). B, TEM of a dermal collagen fiber bundle from the normal control cat. All fibrils within a fiber are organized in the same plane (×6200). (From Holbrook KA, et al: Dermatosparaxis in a Himalayan cat: II. Ultrastructural studies of dermal collagen. J Invest Dermatol 74:100, 1980.)

are recognizable in the fetus, and the trait is probably lethal in the homozygous state.[186, 196] The defect can cause focal or diffuse changes in the dermal collagen and results from abnormalities in the packing of collagen into fibrils and fibers owing to mutations of structural proteins. Unlike normal fibers in which the fibrils are uniform in diameter, cylindric, and packed in uniform parallel arrays, the fibers here are severely disorganized with many larger-than-normal fibrils.[187] A mixture of abnormal and normal fibers occurs in heterozygous animals. Biochemical studies show a decrease in proteodermatan sulfate levels, an increase in hyaluronic acid levels, and an altered iduronic acid/glucuronic acid ratio.[187]

Dermal thickness in dogs can be thinner than normal (1.21 mm versus 1.71 mm)[177] or normal.[173] The dermis in cats can also be thinned (0.25 mm versus 1.71 mm)[173] or normal.[5] Normal dermal thickness is usually a result of an increased thickness of individual collagen bundles.

Ehlers-Danlos syndrome has been reported in the Beagle, Dachshund, Boxer, St. Bernard, German shepherd dog, English springer spaniel, Greyhound, Manchester terrier, Welsh corgi, Red kelpi, soft-coated Wheaten terrier, Garafiano shepherd, Fila brasiliero, and mongrels.[1, 169, 182a, 194, 197] We have recognized it in the Irish setter, Keeshond, Toy poodle, and English setter.[5] Most cases in the cat occur in domestic shorthaired or longhaired breeds or Himalayan cats.

CLINICAL FEATURES

The skin is soft, pliable, and thin. It may or may not be loosely attached to underlying tissues or be hyperextensible. It has decreased elasticity and a moist, blanched appearance. The skin usually can be stretched to extreme lengths (see Fig. 12–72C to E) and may hang loosely in folds, especially on the legs and the throat. In long-coated dogs, the excessive folding may be noticed on only the face and may result in the need for repeated eyelid surgeries. Minimal trauma from traction or scratching may produce skin tears, with little or no bleeding. Healing is rapid, but irregular thin white scars are prominent disfiguring features (see Fig. 12–72B). Widening of the bridge of the nose, subcutaneous hematomas, elbow hygromas, coincidental umbilical and inguinal hernias in a puppy, and epicanthal folds are additional signs in some affected animals. Some animals manifest only cutaneous hyperextensibility or only fragility, whereas other animals exhibit both features. Some animals may have concurrent joint laxity and ocular changes (microcornea, sclerocornea, lens luxation, and cataracts).[169, 185]

DIAGNOSIS

The clinical syndromes of excessively folded skin, hyperextensible skin, easily torn skin, or excessively scarred skin in a young animal with no history of severe trauma are highly suggestive of cutaneous asthenia. Complete documentation may necessitate biopsies for ultrastructural and biochemical study. The skin extensibility index devised by Patterson and Minor[192] is helpful. Extensibility is quantified by manually extending a fold of dorsolumbar skin to the maximal distance above the spine that can be attained without pain. This distance is measured, as is the body length from the base of the tail to the occipital crest. Extensibility is calculated as follows:

$$\text{Extensibility index} = \frac{\text{Vertical height of skin fold}}{\text{Body length}} \times 100$$

In affected dogs, the skin extensibility index is greater than 14.5%; in affected cats, it is greater than 19%.[177]

Skin biopsy may reveal striking dermal abnormalities or normal skin. The inability to detect histologic changes is common in the cat.[174] When changes are present, the collagen fibers may be more eosinophilic than normal and blurred in appearance, fragmented, shortened, and disoriented (Fig. 12–75). Additionally, collagen fibers may form irregularly

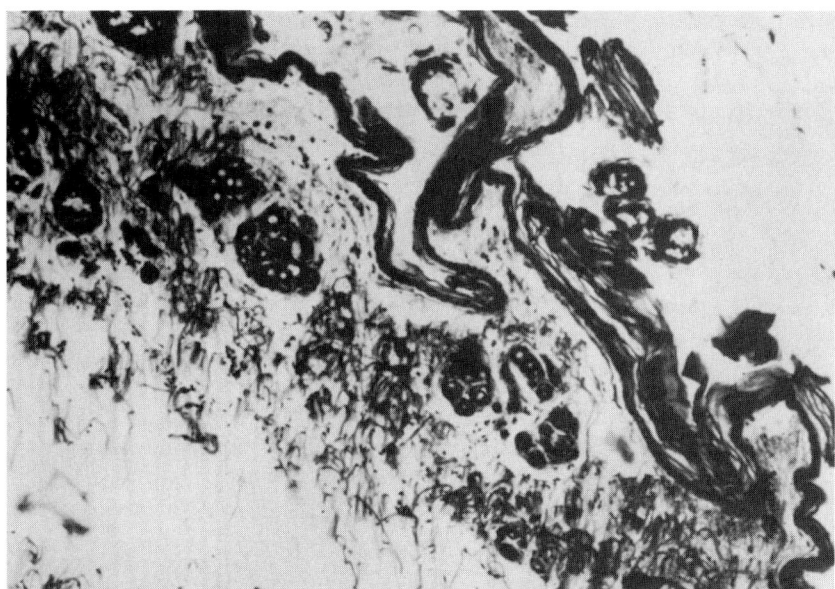

FIGURE 12-75. Cutaneous asthenia. Histopathologic view showing fragmented collagen fibrils that are shortened and disoriented.

sized bundles, may demonstrate improper interweaving, and may be surrounded by mucinosis.[181] Alternatively, the collagen may appear normal on light microscopy.[192] Masson's trichrome stain is useful in the light-microscopic evaluation of animals with collagen disorders. In a study of normal cats and diseased cats with either Ehlers-Danlos syndrome or the acquired fragility syndrome, the normal cats showed no staining abnormalities whereas 11 of the 12 diseased cats showed trichrome abnormalities of varying severity.[174] All 8 cats with Ehlers-Danlos syndrome showed staining abnormalities, even though light-microscopic abnormalities were absent in 6 cats evaluated with hematoxylin-and-eosin stain. The cat with no trichrome abnormalities had the acquired fragility syndrome. However, this technique is not foolproof because one cat with Ehlers-Danlos syndrome had no trichrome abnormalities.[171]

CLINICAL MANAGEMENT

The clinician should inform the owner of the nature, heritability, and chronic incurable course of the disease. The animal should not be used for breeding. Most affected animals are euthanized.

With appropriate lifestyle and housing modifications and prompt veterinary attention to wounds and intercurrent skin diseases, pets without joint laxity can lead long lives. Cats should be declawed to prevent wounding during grooming or scratching. The affected animal cannot play with other animals and must be leash-walked away from woody trees and shrubs. All visitors to the pet's household must be aware of the defect lest a sudden grab for restraint results in a large skin wound. Households contain numerous items with sharp corners or rough surfaces, which can rip the affected pet's skin. These must be removed or padded. Because these animals are prone to hygromas, floors and all resting places should be well padded. Any skin disease, especially conditions that result in pruritus, must be addressed and resolved quickly. Wounds should be sutured promptly.

Because vitamin C is necessary in collagen synthesis, two of us (WHM and DWS) treated three dogs and two cats with oral vitamin C. The cats were given 50 mg twice daily, whereas 500 mg twice daily was used in dogs. No change occurred in the cats, whereas two of the three dog owners were convinced that their dog's skin was less

984 • Congenital and Hereditary Defects

stretchy and less fragile with the vitamin supplementation. Further investigations with vitamin C are indicated to support or refute these findings.

Disorder of the Footpads in German Shepherd Dogs

The cause of this condition is unknown. Signs occur early in life, and multiple dogs of a litter are typically affected. The condition shows some clinical and histologic features of the familial vasculopathy of German shepherd dogs, suggesting some common etiopathogenesis.

CLINICAL FEATURES

German shepherd dogs of either sex are affected at a few weeks to a few months of age.[5, 168, 178] One case in an 11-month-old dog has been reported.[168] Usually, multiple dogs in the litter are involved. The pads of all feet are softer than normal. Swelling, depigmentation, ulceration, and crusting can develop on one or more pads (see Fig. 12–72F), especially the metacarpal and metatarsal pads. When ulcerated, the pads are tender and can cause lameness. The dogs are otherwise healthy.

DIAGNOSIS

In the absence of a drug history to induce a drug eruption or skin lesions elsewhere, the clinical signs are typical of this disorder. Diagnosis is confirmed by biopsy, which reveals deep diffuse dermatitis focused around multifocal areas of collagenolysis (Fig. 12–76). The inflammation can be neutrophilic[5] (Fig. 12–77) or lymphoplasmacytic.[168]

CLINICAL MANAGEMENT

Treatment with antibiotics, glucocorticoids, and topical agents has been unrewarding. With foot protection and good wound care, the ulcers heal spontaneously by 1 year of age. The pad softness remains. Long-term follow-up of most dogs has not been reported, but some dogs have developed renal amyloidosis and died by 2 to 3 years of age.[5, 178]

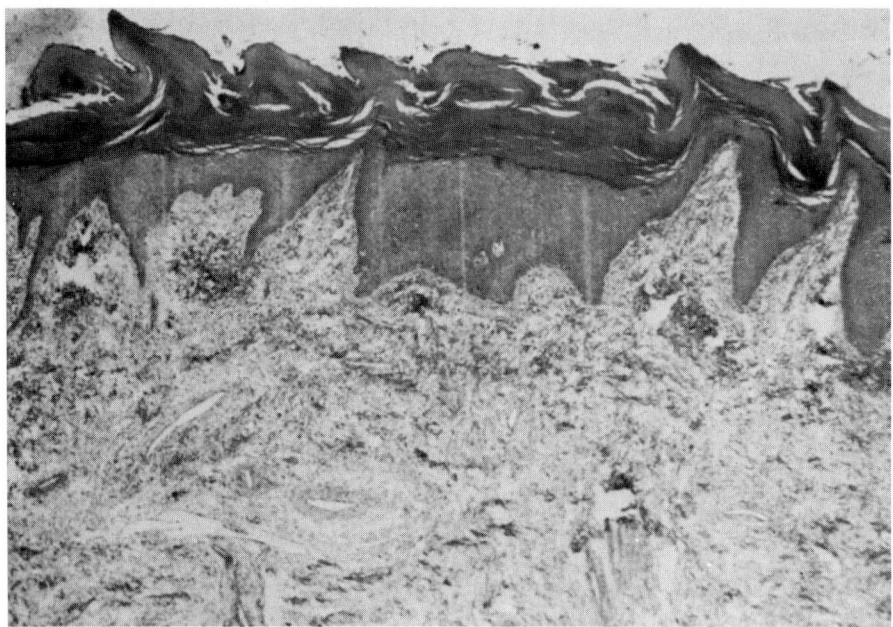

FIGURE 12–76. Collagen disorder of the footpads of German shepherds. Diffuse to nodular dermatitis.

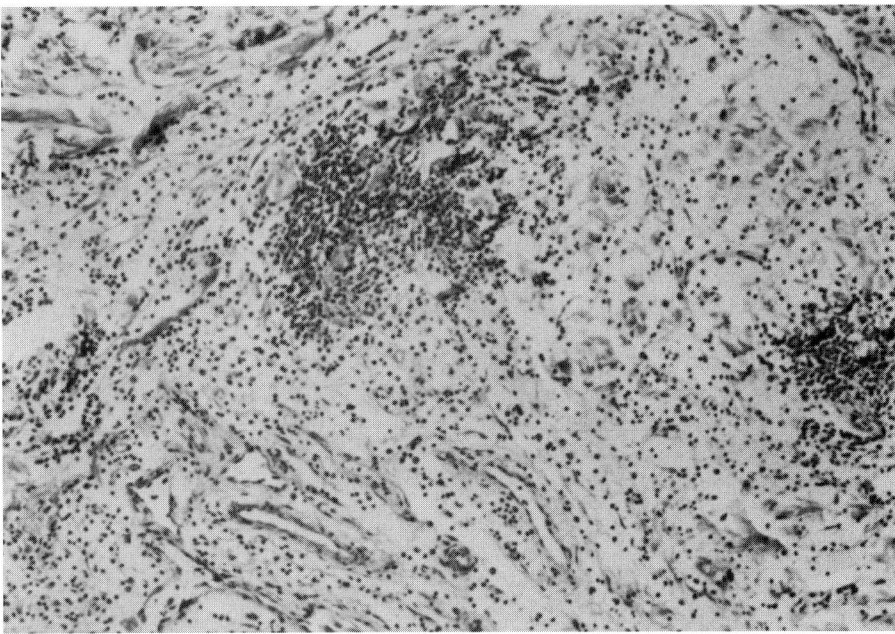

FIGURE 12-77. Close-up of Figure 12-76. Focal accumulations of neutrophils and mononuclear cells around degenerate collagen.

Focal Metatarsal Fistulation of German Shepherd Dogs

Metatarsal fistulation (deep metatarsal/metacarpal tortis, sterile pedal panniculitis) is an uncommon disorder of German shepherd dogs, one of unknown etiology.[183, 184, 190, 191] The condition appears to be most common in dogs of direct German ancestry.[5] All affected dogs that have been studied have had significantly elevated antibody levels against type I and II collagen.[5, 188] These latter findings suggest some familial disorder of collagen.

CLINICAL FEATURES

With the exception of one German shepherd dog crossbred, all cases have occurred in German shepherd dogs between the ages of 2 and 8 years.[5, 183, 184] In two reports on 55 dogs, 45 were males.[183, 190] The dogs that we have examined have all been of direct German ancestry and are low at the carpi and tarsi (flat-footed). Lesions are initially asymptomatic, and the owners become aware of them only because the dog licks the area or because bloody spots are seen on the floor.

Lesions occur on the central plantar surface of the metatarsus just proximal to the metatarsal pad (see Fig. 12–72G). Both hind legs are involved in most dogs, and the occasional dog has similar lesions above one or both metacarpal pads.[183, 184] At examination, a well-demarcated fistula with serosanguineous discharge is visible. Palpation identifies a fibrous tract to deeper tissues. Early lesions have an intact epithelium, with fluid accumulating beneath the surface, yielding a smooth, rounded, fluctuant cystic structure (see Fig. 12–72H). No other skin lesions may be identified, or those lesions may coexist in dogs with German shepherd pyoderma (see Chap. 4) or other infections.[183]

DIAGNOSIS

With a single lesion, the differential diagnostic considerations include a foreign body or focal bacterial or fungal infection. Bilaterally symmetric lesions in a German shepherd dog are pathognomonic.

Cytologic evaluation of the draining fluid shows pyogranulomatous inflammation with or without intracellular bacteria. Closed lesions are sterile, whereas open lesions may be secondarily infected by staphylococci. Biopsy shows deep nodular to diffuse dermatitis with fibrosis and fistulous tracts (Fig. 12–78). The cellular infiltrate is predominantly pyogranulomatous. Hair follicle rupture with endogenous foreign body reaction to follicular keratin and hair shafts is common.

Routine laboratory evaluations are noncontributory, and antinuclear antibody titers are negative. Titers of circulating antibodies to type I and II collagen were significantly elevated in 11 dogs.[188] Because nonaffected German shepherd dogs were not tested, the significance of these anticollagen antibodies is unknown.

CLINICAL MANAGEMENT

If the dog has other skin lesions, all must be treated simultaneously for good results. Surgical removal of the fistula and deep tissues provides temporary improvement, but new lesions re-form weeks to months later. Systemic antibiotic treatment improves secondarily infected lesions, but has no effect on early lesions. Prednisolone administration at 1.1 to 2.2 mg/kg every 24 hours results in resolution of the lesions in most dogs in 14 to 28 days. Vitamin E given at 200 to 300 IU q12h has resolved the lesion in one dog and reduced the maintenance of glucocorticoid dosage in two others.[191] Spontaneous resolution in one dog has been reported.[184] After resolution, the lesions may never recur[184] or relapses may be episodic. In these cases, repeated treatments with prednisolone are effective, but can induce signs of iatrogenic hyperadrenocorticism. Treatment with vitamin E or a topical corticosteroid may be beneficial. The twice-daily application of a 0.01% fluocinolone acetonide in dimethyl sulfoxide solution (Synotic, Syntex) to early lesions has prevented fistulation and has been satisfactory for long-term control in many dogs.[5] The combination of tetracycline and niacinamide is also effective (see Chap. 3).

Multiple Collagenous Nevi

Solitary collagenous nevi (see Chap. 20) can occur in any breed of dog. In some German shepherd dogs, multiple collagenous nevi develop between 3 to 5 years of age. These skin lesions are a cutaneous marker for renal cystadenocarcinomas or uterine leiomyomas. This trait appears to have an autosomal dominant mode of inheritance.

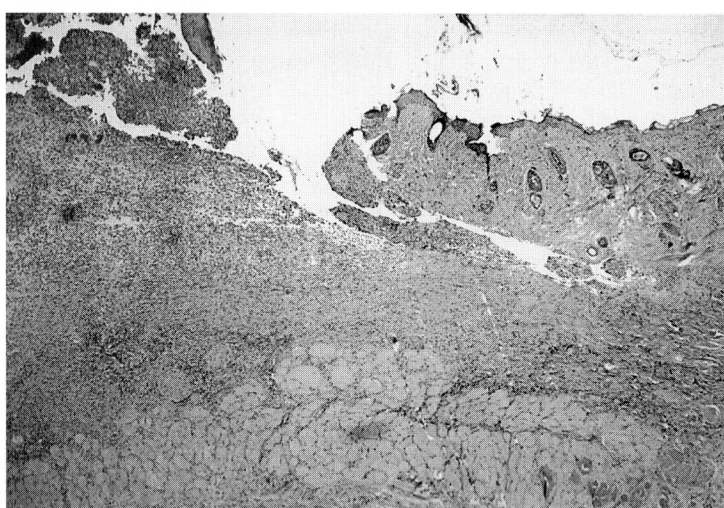

FIGURE 12–78. Metatarsal fistula in a German shepherd. Deep dermal pyogranulomatous inflammation with fisulation.

• DISORDERS OF ELASTIN

Cutis Laxa

Cutis laxa (dermatochalasis, elastolysis) is a hereditary disorder of elastic fibers in humans characterized clinically by skin that is pendulous, flaccid, hanging in folds, and seemingly excessive compared with the individual's body size. Cutaneous fragility is not present. The disorder is characterized histologically by a progressive loss of elastic fibers.

Cutis laxa has been anecdotally described in a Mâtin de Naples in France.[176] No histopathologic documentation of the diagnosis was supplied.

• DISORDERS OF VESSELS

Aside from the rare case of congenital hemangioma or arteriovenous fistula, inherited disorders of blood vessels are rare. Most cases of vascular disease are due to an acquired vasculitis (see Chap. 9), but an idiopathic and apparently familial vasculopathy has been described in five breeds of dogs.

Familial Vasculopathy

BEAGLES

A systemic necrotizing vasculitis of small to medium-sized arteries is well described in colony-bred Beagles.[212] No sex predilection is noted, and signs occur early in life (4 to 10 months of age). Signs are cyclic and include fever, lethargy, unwillingness to move, and a hunched stance. No skin lesions have been described.

GERMAN SHEPHERDS

Affected dogs have signs at 4 to 10 weeks of age, and the signs often occur 7 to 10 days after the first immunization.[200, 210, 214] No sex predilection is noted. The dogs are lethargic and pyrexic and have a peripheral lymphadenopathy and skin lesions. The bridge of the nose is swollen and crusted, ulcerated lesions occur on the ear margins, the nasal planum, and the tail tip. All footpads are soft and swollen with variable depigmentation. In severe cases, the central portion of the pads can ulcerate. One dog experienced generalized demodicosis.[200]

Skin biopsy shows nodular to diffuse lymphohistioplasmacytic dermatitis around degenerated collagen bundles and subtle vascular alteration, especially of postcapillary venules.[214] Depigmented lesions have a hydropic interface dermatitis with pigmentary incontinence. Necropsy reveals collagenolysis of footpads, peritendinous sheaths and deep fascia of the distal limbs, and ventrum.

Treatment with antibiotics or glucocorticoids causes minimal to no improvement. Dogs recover spontaneously by 5 to 6 months of age, with residual scarring at points of ulceration. The pads remain soft. Pyrexia, lethargy, or panosteitis can occur at each subsequent immunization.

To date, no cause of the condition has been defined. It is unclear whether there is some systemic immunologic abnormality that results in the vasculitis or whether the vessels are abnormal. The condition appears to have an autosomal recessive mode of inheritance.

GREYHOUNDS

Large numbers of racing Greyhounds have manifested this condition (see Chap. 9).[198] No sex predilection is noted, and signs can occur in dogs 6 to 72 months of age. Approxi-

988 • Congenital and Hereditary Defects

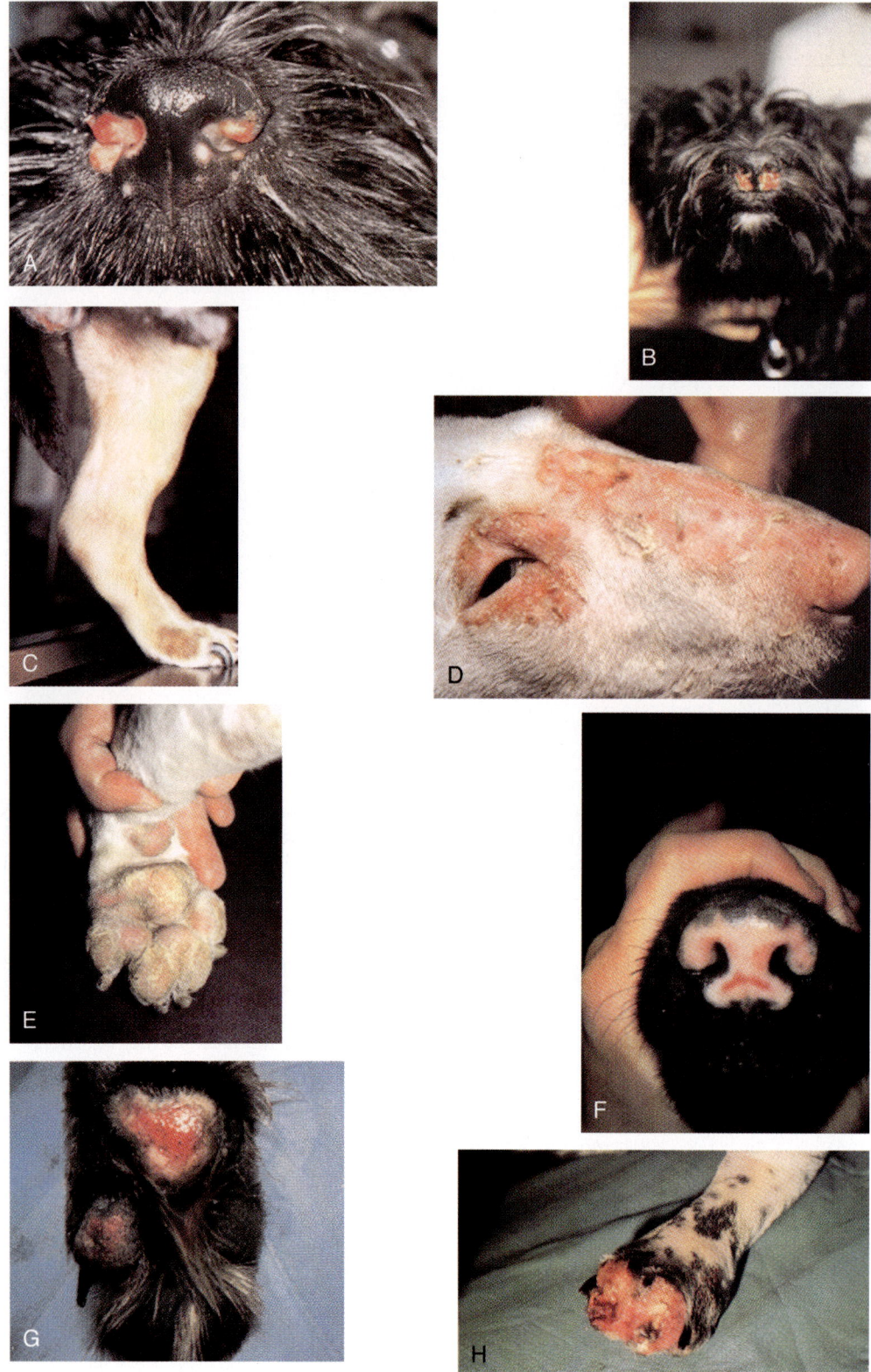

FIGURE 12–79. *Legend on opposite page*

mately 75% of cases have only skin lesions, whereas the remainder have renal plus cutaneous signs. In the latter situation, signs of renal disease are typically noted when the skin lesions are found, but they can precede or follow the skin lesions.

Skin lesions occur primarily over the tarsus, the stifle, or the inner thigh. Occasionally, the forelimb is involved. The first sign noted is swelling and tenderness, followed by sharply demarcated deep ulcerations. Lesions vary from 1 mm to 10 cm in diameter. Lesions heal slowly but spontaneously with routine wound care.

Skin biopsy shows thrombosis of arterioles, venules, and capillaries in the superficial or deep dermis.[198] There is speculation that this disorder is similar to the hemolytic uremic syndrome in humans.[197a, 199] That syndrome is most typically caused by a verotoxin (shiga-like toxin) that damages the vascular endothelium. Most racing Greyhounds eat raw meats, which likely contain the toxin producing *Escherichia coli*. It remains to be seen whether a familial vascular predisposition also exists.

SCOTTISH TERRIERS

This condition has been reported in five Scottish terrier puppies, and no additional cases have been reported with the withdrawal of their parents from the breeding program.[209] Affected dogs first experienced a bilateral nasal discharge at 3 to 4 weeks of age, followed by progressive ulceration and destruction of the nasal planum, the nostrils, and the nasal mucosa by 5 to 6 months of age (Fig. 12–79A and B). No treatments were effective. Skin biopsy showed nodular to diffuse pyogranulomatous dermatitis with leukocytoclastic vasculitis (Fig. 12–80). The condition probably had an autosomal dominant mode of inheritance.

JACK RUSSELL TERRIERS

Five cases of cutaneous vasculitis have been reported in the Jack Russell terrier, and we and others have examined additional cases in this breed.[207] Although the cases recognized in the mature adult dog may have a familial basis, the disorder recognized in dogs less than 1 year of age is more convincingly a genetically influenced condition.

Typical of the lesions occurring with small vessel vasculitis, these dogs have alopecic and discretely ulcerated and crusted skin lesions of the bony prominences of the head and extremities, V-shaped necrotic areas of the pinnae (see Fig. 9–51), and punctate ulcers of the footpads. The lesions in three of the five reported cases arose 2 to 3 weeks after routine vaccination. Treatment with dapsone (1 mg/kg q8h), prednisolone (1 mg/kg q24h), vitamin E (200 to 400 IU q24h), or combinations thereof resolved the lesions in the dogs, but relapses typically followed drug withdrawal.

Skin biopsy findings vary from case to case but typically show apoptosis of the basal layer of the epidermis, pigmentary incontinence, leukocytoclastic vasculitis, and ischemic degeneration of the hair follicles. These changes are more typical of canine systemic lupus erythematosus or dermatomyositis than primary vasculitis. If these findings are coupled with the postvaccinal onset of lesions in three of the five dogs, other causes of vasculitis should be considered before attributing the disorder to a genetic abnormality (see Chap. 9).

FIGURE 12–79. *Continued* *A*, Hereditary pyogranulomatous disease with vasculitis in Scottish terriers. Bilateral ulceration of the nostrils. *B*, Hereditary pyogranulomatous disease with vasculitis in Scottish terriers. Focal ulcerated granulomas, depigmentation, and loss of the surface architecture of the nasal planum. *C*, Congenital lymphedema in a dog. The hindleg is swollen and edematous, and pits easily. *D*, Lethal acrodermatitis in a bull terrier. Erythema, alopecia, and peeling skin on the face. *E*, Lethal acrodermatitis in a bull terrier. Hyperkeratotic footpads and pedal erythema. *F*, Canine tyrosinemia. Depigmentation and ulceration of the nose. (Courtesy G.A. Kunkle.) *G*, Canine tyrosinemia. Ulceration of footpads. (Courtesy of G. A. Kunkle.) *H*, Acral mutilation in an English pointer.

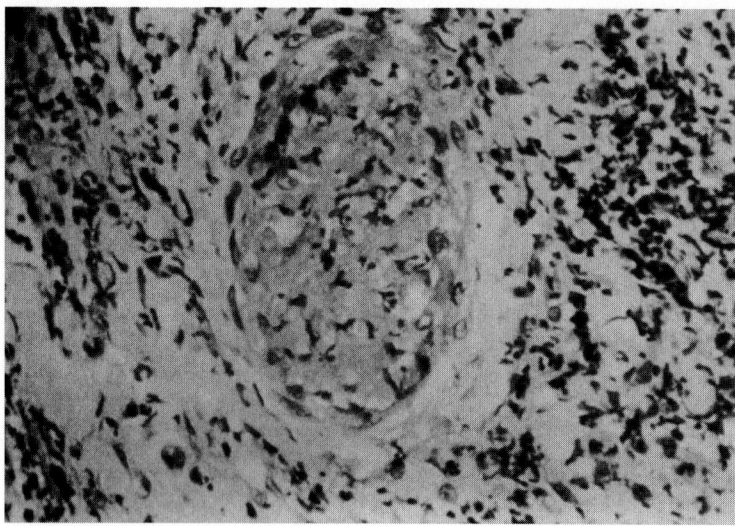

FIGURE 12-80. Hereditary pyogranulomatous disease with vasculitis in Scottish terriers. Leukocytoclastic vasculitis surrounded by pyogranulomatous dermatitis.

Lymphedema

Lymphedema is swelling of some part of the body due to abnormal lymph flow.

CAUSE AND PATHOGENESIS

Lymphedema can be primary or secondary.[201, 203, 206] Primary lymphedema is caused by developmental defects in lymphatics and lymph nodes. Secondary lymphedema results from the obstruction of lymphatics or lymphatic flow by inflammatory or neoplastic disease, surgery, or trauma. In some dogs, primary lymphedema has been shown to be inherited as an autosomal dominant trait with variable expressivity.[201, 205, 206, 208] Canine primary lymphedema has been classified by lymphangiography and histopathologic study into two basic structural defects: (1) lymphatic hypoplasia, with or without hypoplasia or absence of the regional lymph nodes, and (2) lymphatic hyperplasia and dilatation.[201, 202, 205]

Decreased transport capacity of the lymphatic system leads to an increase in protein-rich interstitial fluid.[211] Such lymphostasis affects the other two members of the dermal microcirculation as well, so that arterial and venous blood vessels are damaged (lymphostatic hemangiopathy). The tissues become infiltrated by inflammatory cells; the activated vascular endothelial cells and the dermal inflammatory cells release mediators acting on epidermal and dermal structures; the dermal connective tissue elements, ground substance, microfilaments, collagen, and elastic fibers are damaged; and angiogenic factors from vascular endothelial cells and inflammatory cells contribute to vascular proliferation.

CLINICAL FEATURES

Primary lymphedema has been recognized in the cat[203] and in several breeds of dogs, including the English bulldog (Fig. 12-81), German shepherd, Borzoi, Belgian Tervuren, Old English sheepdog, Labrador retriever, Great Dane, Poodle, and Old English sheepdog-Labrador retriever crosses.[201, 204] There appears to be no sex predilection. The onset of disease is usually within the first 12 weeks of life.

The hind limbs are the most commonly affected, although the front limbs, the ventrum, the tail, and the pinnae may be involved.[202] Affected skin is usually normal in surface appearance but is thickened and spongy and pits with digital pressure (see Fig. 12-79C). The swollen skin is not warm, tender, or inflamed. Regional lymph nodes may not be palpable, and the animals are usually healthy otherwise. Disturbed antigen recognition and pathways into lymphatics results in altered immunosurveillance, thus predisposing

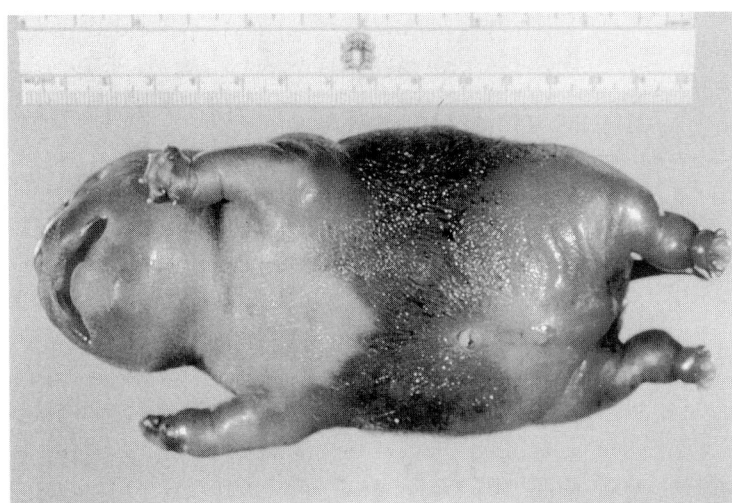

FIGURE 12–81. Congenital lymphedema in an English bulldog. (Courtesy of J. King.)

to infections and malignancy.[211] Because lymphedema predisposes affected tissues to secondary bacterial infection and delayed healing, these complications may be clinically apparent.

DIAGNOSIS

Differential diagnosis includes other causes of obstructive, inflammatory, and hypoproteinemic edema. Definitive diagnosis is based on history, physical examination findings, laboratory tests to rule out other conditions, skin biopsy, patent blue violet dye test, and lymphangiography.[202] In the dye test, the solution is injected subcutaneously into the foot of the affected limb. In animals with primary lymphedema, the purplish discoloration persists for extended periods of time.[203] Skin biopsy reveals variable degrees of subcutaneous and dermal edema.[213] Lymphatics may be dilated (Fig. 12–82) and hyperplastic, or they may be hypoplastic. Perilymphatic fibroblasts are increased, extravasated erythrocytes and their remnants are visible, and fragmentation and degeneration of collagen and elastic fibers ensues with chronic lymphedema. Chronic cases may involve variable degrees of fibrosis and epidermal hyperplasia. Inflammatory cells are usually few and include lympho-

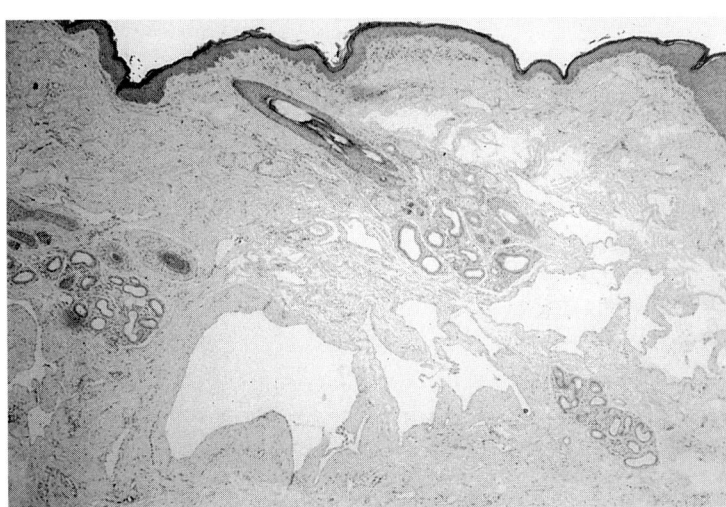

FIGURE 12–82. Lymphedema. Note the marked dilatation of the superficial-, mid-, and deep-dermal lymphatics.

cytes, macrophages (often containing lipid droplets), plasma cells, and mast cells. Changes of secondary infection may be present (Fig. 12-83).

CLINICAL MANAGEMENT

The prognosis and the indicated therapy vary with the severity of the lymphedema.[202] Mild cases may wax and wane, spontaneously regress, or persist indefinitely with no adverse consequences to the patient. More severe cases may require (1) frequent bandaging (e.g., modified Robert Jones splint) to reduce the lymphedema,[213] (2) surgical extirpation of the edematous tissues, (3) reconstructive surgery, or (4) amputation of the affected part. No successful form of medical management has been reported for dogs. The benzopyrene group of drugs has proven benefit in humans.[202] Good attention to skin care and hygiene and control of infections is essential. Dogs with severe primary lymphedema often die shortly after birth because of pleural and abdominal effusions.[204]

• ENDOCRINE, METABOLIC, AND IMMUNOLOGIC DISORDERS

Endocrine, metabolic, or immunologic diseases can occur in any animal. Certain breeds or specific families within a breed are at greater risk for a particular disease, suggesting a heritable influence. The reader is referred to Chapters 8, 9, and 10 for a complete discussion of these disorders. The disorders discussed subsequently have each been recognized in only one breed of dog and therefore are included in this chapter.

Acrodermatitis

Acrodermatitis has been reported as an inherited, autosomal recessive trait that produces a lethal syndrome in Bull terriers.[216, 218, 221] The clinical, pathologic, and genetic features of the syndrome resemble acrodermatitis enteropathica in humans, lethal trait A46 in Black Pied Danish cattle, and experimental zinc deficiency in dogs. Although affected Bull terriers had significantly lowered serum and liver concentrations of zinc and copper, they did not respond to high-dose zinc replacement therapy.[216, 221, 222] The specific cause of the condition is as yet incompletely defined, but affected dogs have defective zinc and copper metabolism.[220, 221] It is unknown whether both trace mineral deficiencies exist independent of each other or whether one causes the other.[222]

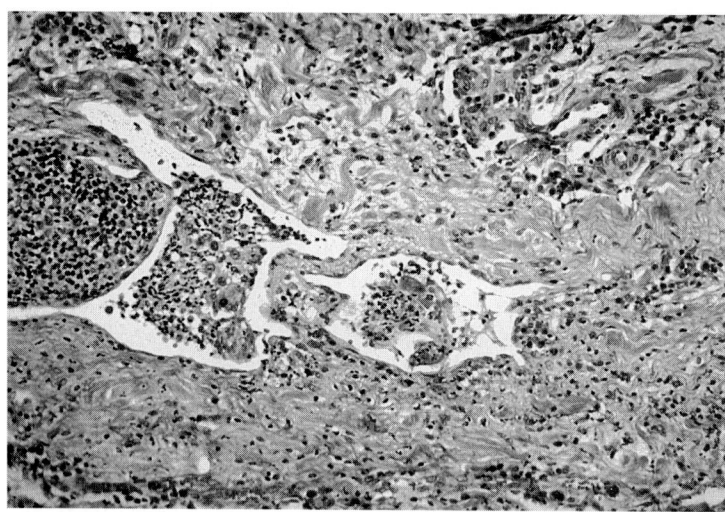

FIGURE 12-83. Lymphedema with a secondary lymphangitis.

CLINICAL FEATURES

At birth, affected pups have skin pigmentation that is lighter than normal, and the coat in some dogs is dull, brittle, and fluffy.[215] The pups are weaker than their normal littermates, and they cannot chew or swallow well because of their high-arched hard palate. Their growth is retarded.[206] By 6 weeks of age, their feet are splayed, the footpads are cracked, and crusted skin lesions appear between the toes. Ulcerated, exudative crusted lesions are also found on the ears and the muzzle (see Fig. 12–79D). Papular or pustular dermatitis may be found around all body orifices but most notably around those of the head. The foot lesions (see Fig. 12–79E) progress rapidly to severe interdigital pyoderma and paronychia. Later, there is onychodystrophy[219a] and frondlike keratinization of the noncontact areas of the footpads. Generalized bacterial folliculitis may develop, being most severe in areas prone to frictional trauma, such as the elbows and the hocks. Affected animals may have diarrhea and respiratory infections with chronic nasal discharges. At weaning time, they appear especially aggressive, but by 14 to 16 weeks, they become less active, less responsive to external stimuli, and sleep a great deal. Many have ocular abnormalities. The average survival time is 7 months, but conventional treatments may prolong this time.

DIAGNOSIS

If multiple puppies are presented at one time, no other differential diagnoses are appropriate. In individual cases, drug eruption, pemphigus foliaceus, and staphylococcal or *Malassezia* infection secondary to some congenital immunodeficiency may be considered. There is a high incidence (75% to 100%) of secondary yeast infection in Bull terriers with acrodermatitis.[215, 219] Skin biopsies should be performed in all cases.

Histopathology shows diffuse parakeratotic hyperkeratosis with focal crusting and intraepidermal pustules.[3] The superficial epidermis may show laminar pallor as occurs in necrolytic migratory erythema (see Chap. 10), but the keratinocytes are viable and not degenerating. Lymphocytes are severely reduced in T-cell areas of lymphoid tissues.

Routine laboratory tests show no consistent abnormalities specific for this disorder.[216, 221] Serum or liver levels of zinc and copper may be low or normal.[216, 220, 221] *Malassezia* yeasts can be isolated in most cases by scraping, on acetate tape preparations, or by biopsy.[215, 219]

CLINICAL MANAGEMENT

Efforts to return these dogs to normal status with oral or parenteral zinc supplementation have been unrewarding.[216, 221] Treatment with systemic antibiotics resolves cutaneous and systemic infections, but provides no long-term solution because infections return. If *Malassezia* infection is present, the administration of ketoconazole (10 mg/kg q12h) results in marked improvement.[138] One animal has been maintained well for nearly 2 years with ketoconazole.

Parents of affected dogs are carriers for the disorder, as are more than half of the clinically normal siblings of affected dogs. No relatives of the affected dogs should be used for breeding. Some of the apparently normal littermates may experience zinc-responsive dermatitis (see Chap. 17).

Tyrosinemia

A single case of congenital tyrosinemia in a young dog has been reported.[217] It appeared to be similar to tyrosinemia type II in humans or pseudodistemper in mink. Tyrosinemia, inherited as an autosomal recessive trait, is a group of distinct metabolic diseases with five phenotypes in humans.[2] The case reported in the dog was characterized by early-onset characteristic eye and skin lesions with varying degrees of mental retardation.

CAUSE AND PATHOGENESIS

The tyrosinemia in the dog was apparently hereditary because both parents had elevated serum tyrosine levels. The serum tyrosine levels were elevated because of the deficiency of cytosolic hepatic tyrosine aminotransferase. The pathophysiologic change is considered an inflammatory response to tyrosine crystals deposited in tissues. This appears to be the case with the corneal lesions, but many skin lesions have no crystals. Instead, there may be increased numbers of highly condensed tonofibrils and increased numbers of keratohyaline granules in the granular layer. Tyrosine is known to influence the number of microtubules in the tonofibrils.

CLINICAL FEATURES

The 7-week-old German shepherd puppy was small for its age when it first had conjunctivitis and cloudy corneas. The globes were small, and cataracts and corneal granulation were present, but there was no ulceration. There was ulceration of the nose, tongue, and central portions of the footpads (see Fig. 12–79F and G). As the disease progressed, ulcers involved the metatarsal pads and the claw folds, and claws were broken. Erythematous bullae were found on the abdomen. The nasal planum was affected by erythema, focal ulceration with marginal crusting, and hypopigmentation.

DIAGNOSIS

Diagnosis of a metabolic defect was suspected because of the historical and physical examination findings and confirmed by metabolic screening tests. High levels of tyrosine in the serum and urine were identified.

Histopathologic examination of ulcerated skin lesions revealed pyogranulomatous inflammation associated with large, dark-brown granules (110 to 170 mm in diameter) of tyrosine (Fig. 12–84) surrounded by an eosinophilic, amorphous material, which resembled the Splendore-Hoeppli reaction. The granules gave a positive orange reaction when stained with Millon's reaction for tyrosine.

CLINICAL MANAGEMENT

The prognosis for a cure is not good. In humans, dramatic reduction of plasma tyrosine levels with subsequent clearing of skin and eye lesions occurs in patients receiving diets

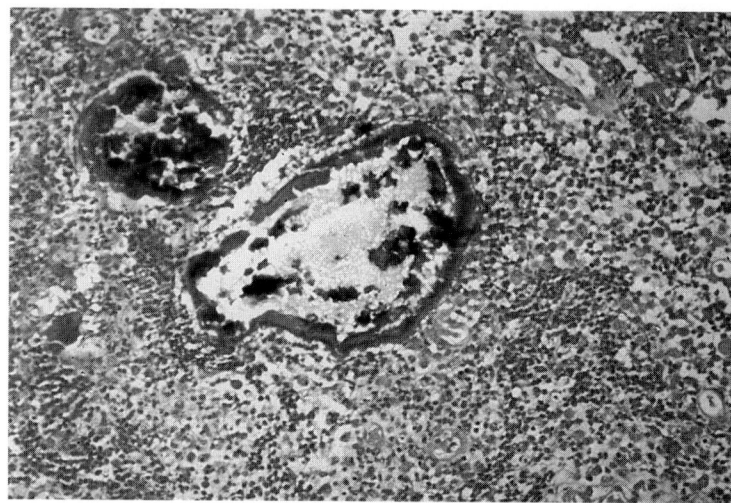

FIGURE 12–84. Tyrosinemia. Tyrosine granules surrounded by pyogranulomatous inflammation.

low in tyrosine and phenylalanine. Symptoms recur when a regular diet is resumed. Dietary manipulation also resulted in clearing of the dog's skin lesions.

• MISCELLANEOUS DISORDERS

Acral Mutilation Syndrome

Acral mutilation and analgesia is an unusual hereditary sensory neuropathy of dogs that results in progressive mutilation of the distal extremities.

CAUSE AND PATHOGENESIS

The disorder has been reported in German shorthaired pointers,[224] English springer spaniel,[227] and English pointer dogs. It is probably inherited in an autosomal recessive manner.[226, 227] Pathologic lesions are identified at the level of the primary sensory neuron. Necropsy changes occur grossly as a decrease in prominence of the spinal ganglia and dorsal roots. The nerve cell bodies of the subcapsular mantle zone are decreased in number (by 22% to 50%), and the neuron mantle is decreased in thickness. The number of small neurons (20 μm or less) in the affected ganglia is disproportionately increased in affected dogs. The spinal cord changes occur in the dorsolateral fasciculus, where reduced fiber density correlates well with the loss of pain perception that is clinically apparent. Light- and electron-microscopic examinations of spinal roots, ganglia, and peripheral nerves show myelinated and unmyelinated fiber degeneration. Neuronal degeneration does not account for the deficiency of sensory cell bodies. This mutilation acropathy is a manifestation of a sensory neuropathy in which the neuronal deficiency results from insufficient development and slowly progressive postnatal degeneration.[224]

CLINICAL FEATURES

The syndrome appears first in affected pups at 3 to 5 months of age. Both sexes and more than one pup per litter may be affected. The pups may be smaller than littermates. They begin to bite and lick their paws. There is total loss of temperature and pain sensation in the toes and sometimes in the proximal legs and trunk. Usually, the hind legs are most severely involved, and occasionally only the toes of the rear legs are affected.

The toes and feet become swollen, and the skin of the footpads, the plantar surface, and the area over the tuber calcis may be ulcerated. Paronychia is present, and autoamputation of the toes may be noted. The puppies walk unflinchingly on the mutilated feet (see Fig. 12-79H). Proprioception is normal, tendon reflexes are intact, and no motor or autonomic impairment is present. EMG studies reveal no denervation potentials.

DIAGNOSIS

History and a thorough clinical examination of puppies of predisposed breeds provides a presumptive diagnosis. Histopathologic examination of nerve tissues at necropsy establishes a definitive diagnosis.

CLINICAL MANAGEMENT

Attempts to prevent further mutilation by means of bandages, restraint collars, or sedation are of little benefit, and euthanasia is usually requested by the owners.

The hereditary aspects of this syndrome are important because it has been seen in several strains of English pointers.[5] Parents of affected pups should not be used as breeders. Siblings should not be used either until the mode of inheritance is firmly established. Even then, the breeding of siblings should probably be discouraged unless some test is developed to identify carriers of the disorder.

Persistent Scratching in Cavalier King Charles Spaniels

A neurogenic pruritus has been described in young adult Cavalier King Charles spaniels. Magnetic resonance imaging studies showed cerebellar tonsil herniation with syringohydromyelia.[231, 232, 232a] The disorder has been likened to the Chiari type I malformation in humans. With the young age at onset and apparent uniqueness of this condition to this breed, a familial basis is probable.

CLINICAL FEATURES

Affected dogs are presented for pruritus of the shoulder or neck region starting between 6 and 24 months of age. One or both sides may be involved. The pruritus interferes with normal activity and can be triggered or exacerbated by excitement, wearing of a collar, or manipulation of the area. On physical examination, no primary skin lesions are visible and the dog has lower motor neuron deficits of the ipsilateral thoracic limb.

TREATMENT

Surgical procedures to alleviate the herniation should be beneficial. Medications to reduce cerebrospinal fluid production can be useful; response has occurred in some dogs treated with dexamethasone (0.25 mg/dog q24h) and acetazolamide (3 mg/kg q8h). Clinical signs improve but do not disappear. Some dogs are stable over long periods of time with no treatment.[232a]

Cutaneous Mucinosis

Mucin is a component of the normal dermal ground substance.[2] Excessive accumulation, be it focal, regionalized, or generalized, can occur in hypothyroidism, acromegaly, alopecia mucinosa, dermatomyositis, or discoid lupus erythematosus,[228] or it can be idiopathic.[223] The Chinese Shar pei is prone to the latter (see Chap. 18).[225, 229]

Shar peis have more dermal mucin than do other breeds.[110, 225] Some dogs have exaggerated amounts and exhibit pronounced folding (see Fig. 18–58A), mucinous vesiculation (see Fig. 18–58B), or both. The exaggerated folding is most pronounced on the head, the ventrum, and the distal extremities, and some of these dogs snore and snort owing to involvement of tissues in the oropharynx. The vesicles vary in size and can occur in normal-appearing or edematous skin.

Recent studies in Shar peis with idiopathic mucinosis show that distorted lymphatics, massive accumulations of hyaluronic acid, and mast cells of the chymase–carboxypeptidase subtype are features of this disorder (see Chap. 18).

DIAGNOSIS

The tentative diagnosis of diffuse mucinosis is based on clinical findings of exaggerated folds and is confirmed by skin biopsy, in which the dermis contains excessive mucin with no other abnormalities.[110, 223, 228] Visually, the vesicles mimic those of the various autoimmune and immune-mediated disorders, but clinical evaluation of the vesicles' contents quickly identifies the mucinous nature of the fluid. Mucinous vesicles do not discharge fluid with puncture by a small-gauge needle. The fluid must be expressed by digital pressure and then is thick, clear, and sticky. Biopsy of these lesions shows focal accumulation of mucin in the superficial dermis. To date, the mucinosis in Shar peis has occurred in euthyroid dogs. Because this breed is prone to hypothyroidism,[229] an intercurrent thyroid abnormality could lead to severe mucinosis.

CLINICAL MANAGEMENT

In most cases, the excessive mucinosis in Shar peis is a cosmetic problem only. Most animals seem to outgrow it by 2 to 5 years of age.[225] Dogs with oropharyngeal involvement may warrant treatment because they can experience respiratory arrest with anesthesia.[229] High levels of prednisolone (2.2 mg/kg) for 6 days, followed by a slow reduction to no medication in 30 days, should reduce the amount of mucin.[225] Most animals remain normal after only one course of treatment. A few dogs require repeated or continuous treatment. These dogs should be evaluated for hypothyroidism.

Urticaria Pigmentosa

In humans, a mastocytosis syndrome is recognized wherein mast cell hyperplasia occurs in the skin and virtually all other organ systems.[2] Urticaria pigmentosa is the most common cutaneous manifestation of mastocytosis and is characterized by variably symptomatic, small, yellow-tan to reddish-brown macules or papules. Urticaria pigmentosa has been recognized in the dog, described in detail in three related Sphinx cats,[233] briefly described in young (younger than 1 year old) Himalayan cats,[5] reported in two unrelated Devon Rex cats,[230] and seen in a young Siamese cat by one of the authors (DWS).

CLINICAL FEATURES

All three Sphinx cats had the same grandsire and started their disease early in life (see Chap. 13). The cats had a multifocal, partially coalescing macular and crusted papular rash on the head and neck, ventrum (Fig. 12–86), and extremities. Some of the lesions were dark brown. Dermatographism could not be elicited in any cat.

The Himalayan cats had asymptomatic macular erythema and hyperpigmentation around the mouth, chin, neck, and eyes. The condition resolved spontaneously after several months.

The Siamese cat had erythema, hyperpigmentation, scaling, crusting, and pruritus involving the face and pinnae (Fig. 12–85).

DIAGNOSIS

In the absence of a familial history, all causes of crusted papular lesions in cats (miliary dermatitis—see Chap. 8) must be considered. Skin biopsies show moderate-to-severe, perivascular-to-diffuse dermal and subcutaneous infiltrate of well-differentiated mast cells with small numbers of eosinophils and neutrophils. Epidermal melanosis may be prominent. All three Sphinx cats had peripheral eosinophilia and basophilia, but no internal organ involvement could be identified.

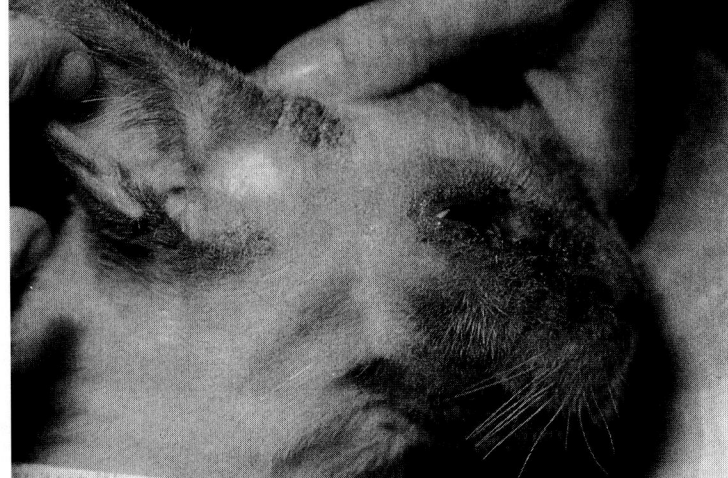

FIGURE 12–85. Urticaria pigmentosa. Siamese cat with facial crusted papular rash.

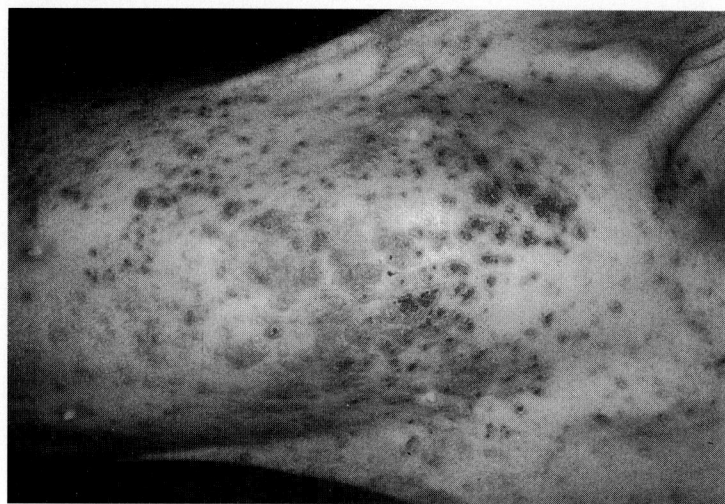

FIGURE 12–86. Urticaria pigmentosa. Ventral papular rash on a Sphinx cat. (Courtesy of C. Vitale.)

TREATMENT

Because the mast cell hyperplasia in urticaria pigmentosa has either a familial or an idiopathic basis, cure cannot always be expected. Treatment with corticosteroids with or without antihistamines controls the lesions in Sphinx and Siamese cats while the drugs are being administered.

• REFERENCES

General References

1. Foil CS: The skin. In Hoskins JD (ed): Veterinary Pediatrics, 2nd ed. W.B. Saunders Co, Philadelphia, 1995.
2. Freedberg IM, et al: Fitzpatrick's Dermatology in General Medicine, 5th ed. McGraw Hill Book Co, New York, 1999.
3. Gross TL, et al: Veterinary Dermatopathology. Mosby Year Book, St. Louis, 1992.
4. Power HT, Ihrke PJ: The use of synthetic retinoids in veterinary medicine. In Bonagura JD (ed): Kirk's Current Veterinary Therapy XII. W.B. Saunders Co, Philadelphia, 1995, p. 585.
5. Scott DW, et al: Muller and Kirk's Small Animal Dermatology, 5th ed. W.B. Saunders Co, Philadelphia, 1995.

Disorders of the Surface and Follicular Epithelium

6. Alhaidari Z, et al: Congenital ichthyosis in two Cavalier King Charles spaniel littermates. Vet Dermatol 5:117, 1994.
7. Antin IP: Dermoid sinus in a Rhodesian Ridge-back dog. J Am Vet Med Assoc 157:961, 1970.
8. August JR, et al: Congenital ichthyosis in a dog: Comparison with the human ichthyosiform dermatoses. Comp Cont Educ 10:40, 1988.
9. Baker BB, Maibach HI: Epidermal cell renewal in seborrheic skin of dogs. Am J Vet Res 48:726, 1987.
10. Bensignor E: A propos d'une observation de dermatomyosite chez un beauceron. Rec Méd Vét 173:125, 1997.
10a. Binder H, et al: Palmoplantar hyperkeratosis in Irish terriers: Evidence of autosomal recessive inheritance. J Small Anim Pract 41:52, 2000.
11. Bond R, et al: An idiopathic facial dermatitis of Persian cats. Vet Dermatol 11:35, 2000.
12. Booth MJ: Atypical dermoid sinus in a chow show dog. Tydskr S Afr Vet Ver 69:102, 1998.
13. Bourdeau P: La dermataomyosite familiale canine. Point Vét 28:553, 1996.
14. Burrows A, Mason KV: Observations of the pathogenesis and treatment of lichenoid-psoriasiform dermatitis of springer spaniels. Proc Annu Memb Meet Am Acad Vet Dermatol Am Coll Vet Dermatol 10:81, 1994.
14a. Camacho AA, et al: Dermoid sinus in a Great Pyrenees dog. Braz J Vet Res Anim Sci 32:170, 1995.
15. Campbell KL, Kirkwood AR: Effect of topical oils on transepidermal water loss with seborrhea sicca. In Ihrke PJ, et al (eds): Advances in Veterinary Dermatology, Vol 2. Pergamon Press, New York, 1993, p 157.
16. Campbell KL, et al: Effects of four anti-seborrheic shampoos on transepidermal water losses, hydration of the stratum corneum, skin surface lipid concentration, skin surface pH, and corneocyte counts in dogs. Proc Annu Memb Meet Am Acad Vet Dermatol Am Coll Vet Dermatol 10:85, 1994.
17. Cornegliani L, Ghibaudo G: A dermoid sinus in a Siberian husky. Vet Dermatol 10:47, 1999.
18. Credille KM, et al: Heterogeneity in nonepidermolytic ichthyosis in a cat and two dogs. In Kwochka KW,

et al (eds): Advances in Veterinary Dermatology III. Butterworth-Heinemann, Boston, 1998, p 529.
19. Dunstan RW, et al: A disease resembling junctional epidermolysis bullosa in a toy poodle. Am J Dermatopathol 10:442, 1988.
20. Fadok VA: Treatment of canine idiopathic seborrhea with isotretinoin. Am J Vet Res 47:1730, 1986.
21. Fatone G, et al: Dermoid sinus and spinal malformations in a Yorkshire terrier: Diagnosis and follow-up. J Small Anim Pract 36:178, 1995.
21a. Ferguson EA, et al: Dermatomyositis in five Shetland sheepdogs in the United Kingdom. Vet Rec 146:214, 2000.
22. Fontaine J, et al: Familial junctional epidermolysis bullosa in Beauceron dogs. Vet Dermatol (In press).
23. Gammie JS: Dermoid sinus removal in a Rhodesian ridgeback dog. Can Vet J 27:250, 1986.
24. Gordon JG, Kwochka KW: Corneocyte counts for evaluation of antiseborrheic shampoos in dogs. Vet Dermatol 4:57, 1993.
25. Gross TL, et al: Psoriasiform lichenoid dermatitis in the springer spaniel. Vet Pathol 23:76, 1986.
26. Guaguère E, et al: Epidermolyse bulleuse jonctionelle familale associée à une absence d'expression de collagène XVII (BPAG2, BP180) chez le Brague Allemand: À propos de deux case. Prat Méd Chir Anim Comp 32:471, 1997.
27. Guaguère E, et al: Familial canine dermatomyositis in 8 Beauceron shepherds. In Kwochka KW, et al (eds): Advances in Veterinary Dermatology III. Butterworth-Heinemann, Boston, 1998, p 527.
28. Gupta BN: Epitheliogenesis imperfecta in a dog. Am J Res 34:443, 1973.
29. Hannigan MM: A refractory case of Schnauzer comedo syndrome. Can Vet J 38:238, 1997.
30. Hargis AM, et al: A skin disorder in three Shetland sheepdogs: Comparison with familial canine dermatomyositis of Collies. Comp Cont Educ 7:306, 1985.
31. Hargis AM, Mundell AC: Familial canine dermatomyositis. Comp Cont Educ 14:855, 1992.
32. Hargis AM, et al: Complement levels in dogs with familial canine dermatomyositis. Vet Immunol Immunopathol 20:95, 1985.
33. Hargis AM, et al: Severe secondary amyloidosis in a dog with dermatomyositis. J Comp Pathol 100:427, 1989.
34. Helman RG, et al: Ichthyosiform dermatosis in a soft-coated wheaten terrier. Vet Dermatol 8:53, 1997.
35. Hewitt MP, et al: Epitheliogenesis imperfecta in a black Labrador puppy. Can Vet J 16:371, 1975.
36. Ihrke PJ, Gross TL: Ulcerative dermatosis of Shetland sheepdogs and Collies. In Bonagura JD (ed): Kirk's Current Veterinary Therapy XII. W.B. Saunders Co, Philadelphia, 1995, p 639.
37. Iwasaki T, et al: Canine familial dermatomyositis in a family of Shetland sheepdogs. Proc Annu Memb Meet Am Acad Vet Deramtol Am Coll Vet Dermatol 15:15, 1999.
38. Jackson HA, Olivry T: Cutaneous lupus erythematosus (ulcerative dermatitis) in the Shetland sheepdog and collie: A review and revelation of the clinical and histological features. Proc Annu Memb Meet Am Acad Vet Dermatol Am Coll Vet Dermatol 15:31, 1999.
39. Johnstone I, et al: A hereditary junctional mechanobullous disease in the cat. Proc Wld Cong Vet Dermatol 2:111, 1992.
39a. Kimura T, Doi K: Dorsal skin reactions of hairless dogs to topical treatment with corticosteroids. Toxicol Pathol 27:528, 1999.
40. Koch H, Walder E: Epidermolysis bullosa dystrophia in Beaucerons. In von Tscharner C, Halliwell REW (eds): Advances in Veterinary Dermatology, Vol 1. Baillière Tindall, Philadelphia, 1990, p 441.
41. Kral F, Schwartzman RM: Veterinary and Comparative Dermatology. J.B. Lippincott Co, Philadelphia, 1964.
42. Kwochka KW: Shampoos and moisturizing rinses in veterinary dermatology. In Bonagura JD (ed): Kirk's Current Veterinary Therapy XII. W.B. Saunders Co, Philadelphia, 1995, p 590.
43. Kwochka KW: Keratinization abnormalities: Understanding the mechanism of scale formation. In Ihrke PJ, et al (eds): Advances in Veterinary Dermatology, Vol 2. Pergamon Press, New York, 1993, p 91.
44. Kwochka KW: Cell proliferation kinetics in the hair root matrix of dogs with healthy skin and dogs with idiopathic seborrhea. Am J Vet Res 51:1570, 1990.
45. Kwochka KW: In vivo and in vitro examination of cell proliferation kinetics in the normal and seborrheic canine epidermis. Proc Annu Memb Meet Am Acad Vet Dermatol Am Coll Vet Dermatol 7:46, 1991.
46. Kwochka KW, Rademakers AM: Cell proliferation of epidermis, hair follicles, and sebaceous glands of beagles and Cocker spaniels with healthy skin. Am J Vet Res 50:587, 1989.
47. Kwochka KW, Rademakers AM: Cell proliferation kinetics of epidermis, hair follicles, and sebaceous glands of Cocker spaniels with idiopathic seborrhea. Am J Vet Res 50:1918, 1989.
48. Kwochka KW, Smeak DD: The cellular defect in idiopathic seborrhea of Cocker spaniels. In von Tscharner C, Halliwell REW (eds): Advances in Veterinary Dermatology, Vol 1. Ballière Tindall, Philadelphia, 1990, p 265.
49. Kwochka KW, et al: Development and characterization of an in vitro cell culture system for the canine epidermis. Proc Annu Memb Meet Am Acad Vet Dermatol Am Coll Vet Dermatol 3:9, 1987.
50. Kwochka KW: Advances in the management of canine scaling. Proceedings of the Third World Congress of Veterinary Dermatology, 1996, p 69.
50a. Lanore D, et al: Sinus dermöide chez une chienne rhodesian ridgeback. Point Vét 30:575, 1999.
51. Lewis DT, et al: Characterization and management of a Jack Russell terrier with congenital ichthyosis. Vet Dermatol 9:111, 1998.
52. Lewis DT, et al: A hereditary disorder of cornification and multiple congenital defects in 5 Rottweiler dogs. Vet Dermatol 9:61, 1998.
53. Lumbrechts N: Dermoid sinus in a crossbred Rhodesian ridgeback dog involving the second cervical vertebra. J S Afr Vet Assoc 67:155, 1996.
54. Mann GE, Stratton J: Dermoid sinus in the Rhodesian ridgeback. J Small Anim Pract 7:631, 1966.
55. Mason KV, et al: Characterization of lichenoid-psoriasiform dermatosis of springer spaniels. J Am Vet Med Assoc 189:897, 1986.
56. Miller WH Jr: Canine facial dermatoses. Comp Cont Educ 1:640, 1979.
57. Muller GH: Ichthyosis in two dogs. J Am Vet Med Assoc 169:1313, 1976.
58. Munday BL: Epitheliogenesis imperfecta in lambs and kittens. Br Vet J 126:47, 1970.
59. Nagata M, et al: Dystrophic form of inherited epider-

molysis bullosa in a dog (Akita Inu). Br J Dermatol 133:1000, 1995.
60. Nagata M, et al: Mitis junctional epidermolysis bullosa in a dog. In Kwochka KW, et al (eds): Advances in Veterinary Dermatology III. Butterworth-Heinemann, Boston, 1998, p 528.
61. Nakayama H, et al: Systemic dermal dysplasia with perifollicular mucinosis in a dog. Vet Pathol 34:5, 1997.
62. Nuttall TJ: What is your diagnosis? J Small Anim Pract 39:317, 1998.
63. Olivry T, et al: Absent expression of collagen XVII (BPAG2, BP180) in canine familial localized junctional epidermolysis bullosa. Vet Dermatol 8:203, 1997.
64. Olivry T, et al: Canine epidermolysis bullosa acquisita: Circulating autoantibodies target the aminoterminal noncollagenous (NC1) domain of collagen VII in anchoring fibrils. Vet Dermatol 9:19, 1998.
65. Olivry T, Mason IS: Genodermatoses: inheritance and management. In Kwochka KW, et al (eds): Advances in Veterinary Dermatology III. Butterworth-Heinemann, Boston, 1998, p 365.
66. Olivry T, et al: Interface dermatitis and sebaceous adenitis in exfoliative cutaneous lupus erythematosus ("lupoid dermatosis") of German shorthaired pointers. Proc Annu Memb Meet Am Acad Vet Dermatol Am Coll Vet Dermatol 15:41, 1999.
66a. Olivry T, et al: Reduced anchoring fibril formation and collagen VII immunoreactivity in feline dystrophic epidermolysis bullosa. Vet Pathol 36:616, 1999.
67. Pagé N, et al: Hereditary nasal hyperkeratosis in Labrador retrievers. Proc Annu Memb Meet Am Acad Vet Dermatol Am Coll Vet Dermatol 15:41, 1999.
68. Palshof P, Christoffersen E: *Malassezia pachydermatis* on the skin of normal and seborrheic West Highland white terriers. Proc Eur Soc Vet Dermatol 10:269, 1993.
69. Paradis M, Scott DW: Hereditary primary seborrhea oleosa in Persian cats. Feline Pract 19:17, 1990.
70. Paradis M: Footpad hyperkeratosis in a family of Dogues de Bordeaux. Vet Dermatol 3:75, 1992.
71. Paradis M: Les séborrhées primaires héréditaires. Point Vét 28:559, 1996.
72. Penrith ML: Dermoid sinus in a Boerboel bitch. J S Afr Vet Assoc 65:38, 1998.
73. Power HT, et al: Use of etretinate for treatment of primary keratinization disorders (idiopathic seborrhea) in Cocker spaniels, West Highland white terriers, and Basset hounds. J Am Vet Med Assoc 201:419, 1992.
74. Power HT: Newly recognized feline skin diseases. Proc Annu Meet Am Acad Vet Dermatol Am Coll Vet Dermatol 14:27, 1998.
74a. Pratt JN, et al: Dermoid sinus at the lumbosacral junction in an English springer spaniel. J Small Anim Pract 41:24, 2000.
75. Raczkowski JJ: Pathogenetic Studies of Canine Seborrheic Skin Disease in the West Highland White Terrier Breed. Masters thesis, Kansas State University, 1984.
76. Rest JR, Theaker AJ: Lupoid dermatosis in a German shorthaired pointer. Proc Eur Soc Vet Dermatol 10: 271, 1993.
77. Scott DW, Schultz RD: Epidermolysis bullosa simplex in a collie dog. J Am Vet Med Assoc 171:721, 1977.
78. Scott DW: Congenital ichthyosis in a dog. Compan Anim Pract 19:7, 1987.
79. Scott DW, Miller WH Jr: Epidermal dysplasia and *Malassezia pachydermatis* infection in West Highland white terriers. Vet Dermatol 1:25, 1989.
80. Scott DW, Miller WH: Primary seborrhoea in English springer spaniels: A retrospective study of 14 cases. J Small Anim Pract 37:173, 1996.
81. Scott DW, Miller WH Jr: Congenital follicular parakeratosis in a Rottweiler and Siberian husky. Canine Pract (in press, 1999).
82. Selcer EA, et al: Dermoid sinus in a Shih tzu and a boxer. J Am Anim Hosp Assoc 20:634, 1984.
83. Shanley KJ, et al: Canine benign familial chronic pemphigus. In Ihrke PJ, et al (eds): Advances in Veterinary Dermatology, Vol 2. Pergamon Press, New York, 1993, p 353.
84. Stonecipher MR, et al: Cutaneous changes of dermatomyositis in patients with normal muscle enzymes. Dermatomyositis sine myositis? J Am Acad Dermatol 28:951, 1993.
84a. Sueki H, et al: Dominantly inherited epidermal acantholysis in dogs, simulating human benign familial chronic pemphigus. Br J Dermatol 136:190, 1996.
85. Tada J, Hashimoto K: Ultrastructural localization of cell junctional components (desmoglein, phakoglobin, E-cadherin, and ß-catenin) in Hailey-Hailey disease, Darier's disease, and pemphigus vulgaris. J Cutan Pathol 25:106, 1998.
86. Theaker AJ: A case of lupoid dermatosis in a German short-haired pointer. Proc Br Vet Dermatol Study Grp 16:5, 1994.
87. Vercelli A, Schiavi S: A case report of lupoid dermatosis in a German short-haired pointer. In Kwochka KW, et al (eds): Advances in Veterinary Dermatology III. Butterworth-Heinemann, Boston, 1998, p 466.
88. Vroom MW: A retrospective study of 43 West Highland white terriers. Proc Wld Cong Vet Dermatol 2:70, 1992.
89. Vroom MW: Three cases with hereditary lupoid dermatosis of the German shorthaired pointer. Proc Eur Soc Vet Dermatol 10:67, 1993.
90. Vroom MW, et al: Lupoid dermatosis in 5 German short-haired pointers. Vet Dermatol 6:93, 1995.
91. White SD, Gross TL: Hereditary lupoid dermatosis of the German shorthaired pointer. In Bonagura JD (ed): Kirk's Current Veterinary Therapy XII. W.B. Saunders Co, Philadelphia, 1995.
92. White SD, et al: Dermatomyositis in an adult Pembroke Welsh corgi. J Am Anim Hosp Assoc 28:398, 1992.
93. White SD, et al: Dystrophic (dermolytic) epidermolysis bullosa in a cat. Vet Dermatol 4:91, 1993.

Disorders of Hairs and Hair Growth

94. Allen LSS: Skin condition in Yorkshire terriers. Canine Pract 12:29, 1985.
95. Bagladi MS, et al: Sebaceous gland melanosis in dogs with endocrine skin disease or follicular dysplasia: A retrospective study. Vet Dermatol 7:85, 1996.
96. Beco L, et al: Color dilution alopecia in seven Dachshunds: A clinical study and the hereditary, microscopical, and ultrastructural aspect of the disease. Vet Dermatol 7:91, 1996.
97. Bourdeau P, et al: Alopécie héréditaire généralisée féline. Rec Med Vet 164:17, 1988.
98. Brignac M, et al: Microscopy of color mutant alopecia. In von Tscharner C, Halliwell REW (eds): Advances in Veterinary Dermatology, Vol 1. Baillière Tindall, Philadelphia, 1990, p 448.

99. Carlotti D: A propos des alopécies auriculaires. Point Vét 25:8, 1993.
100. Carlotti DN: Canine hereditary black hair follicular dysplasia and color mutant alopecia: Clinical and histopathological aspects. In von Tscharner C, Halliwell REW (eds): Advances in Veterinary Dermatology, Vol 1. Baillière Tindall, Philadelphia, 1990, p 43.
101. Casal ML, et al: X-linked ectodermal dysplasia in the dog. J Heredity 88:513, 1997.
102. Casal ML, et al: Congenital hypotrichosis with thymic aplasia in nine Birman kittens. J Am Anim Hosp Assoc 30:600, 1994.
102a. Castellano MC: Colour dilution alopecia in a German shepherd dog. Canine Pract 24:6, 1999.
103. Cerundolo R, et al: Studies on the inheritance of hair loss in the Irish water spaniel. Proc Am Acad Vet Dermatol Am Coll Vet Dermatol 14:95, 1998.
104. Chastain CB, Sawyer DE: Congenital hypotrichosis in male Basset hound littermates. J Am Vet Med Assoc 187:845, 1985.
105. Conroy JD: Hypotrichosis in miniature poodle siblings. J Am Vet Med Assoc 166:697, 1975.
106. Cowan LA, et al: Thyroid hormone and testosterone concentrations in racing greyhounds with and without bald thigh syndrome. J Vet Int Med 11:142, 1997.
107. Curtis CF, et al: Investigation of the reproductive and growth hormone status of dogs affected by idiopathic recurrent flank alopecia. J Small Anim Pract 37;417, 1966.
108. Delmage D: Black hair follicular dysplasia. Vet Rec 137:79, 1995.
109. Dunn KA, et al: Black hair follicular dysplasia in dogs. Vet Rec 137:412, 1995.
110. Dunstan RW, Rosser EJ: Newly recognized and emerging genodermatoses in domestic animals. Curr Probl Dermatol 17:216, 1987.
111. Fontaine J, et al: Alopécie récidivante des flances: Étude de douze cas chez le griffon "Korthals." Point Vét 29:445, 1998.
111a. Fontaine J, Olivry T: Alopécie évoquant une lipidose folliculaire chez un Rottweiler. Prat Méd Chir Anim Comp 34:681, 1999.
111b. Fukata K, et al: Microscopic observation of skin and lymphoid organs in the hairless dog derived from the Mexican hairless. Exper Anim 40:69, 1991.
112. Geary MR, Baker KP: The occurrence of pili torti in a litter of kittens in England. J Small Anim Pract 27:85, 1986.
113. Grieshaber TL, et al: Congenital alopecia in a Bichon frisé. J Am Vet Med Assoc 188:1053, 1986.
114. Griffin CE: Etretinate—how is it being used in veterinary dermatology? Derm Dialogue, Spring/Summer 1993, p 4.
115. Gross TL, et al: Follicular lipidosis in three Rottweilers. Vet Dermatol 8:33, 1997.
116. Guaguère E: Aspects histopathologiques et ultrastructuraux de l'alopécie des robes diluées: A propos d'un cos chez un Doberman pinscher bleu. Prat Med Chirurg Anim Cie 26:537, 1991.
117. Guaguère E: Les alopécies d'origine génétique chez le chien. Point Vét 28:543, 1996.
118. Hargis AM, et al: Black hair follicular dysplasia in black and white Saluki dogs. Vet Dermatol 2:69, 1991.
119. Hirota Y, et al: Immunologic features in hairless descendants derived from Mexican hairless dogs. Jpn J Vet Sci 52:1217, 1990.
120. Ihrke PJ, et al: Generalized congenital hypotrichosis in a female Rottweiler. Vet Dermatol 4:65, 1993.
121. Johnson PD, et al: Coat color darkening in a dog in response to a potent melanotropic peptide. Small Anim Clin Endocrinol 5:1, 1995.
122. Kimura T, et al: The inheritance and breeding results of hairless descendants of Mexican hairless dogs. Lab Anim 27:55, 1993.
123. Kimura T, Doi K: The effect of topical minoxidil treatment on hair follicular growth of neonatal hairless descendants of Mexican hairless dogs. Vet Dermatol 8:107, 1997.
124. Kimura T, Doi K: Age-related changes in skin color and histologic features of hairless descendants of Mexican hairless dogs. Am J Vet Res 55:480, 1994.
125. Knottenbelt CM, Knottenbelt MK: Black hair follicular dysplasia in a tricolour Jack Russell terrier. Vet Rec 138:475, 1996.
126. Kral F, Schwartzman RM: Veterinary and Comparative Dermatology. J.B. Lippincott Co, Philadelphia, 1964.
127. Krishnaswamy Y, et al: Pharmacokinetics and oral bioavailability of exogenous melatonin in preclinical animal models and clinical implications. J Pineal Res 22:45, 1997.
128. Kunkle GA: Congenital hypotrichosis in two dogs. J Am Vet Med Assoc 185:84, 1984.
129. Lewis CJ: Black hair follicular dysplasia in UK bred salukis. Vet Rec 137:294, 1995.
130. McKeever PJ, et al: Spiculosis. J Am Anim Hosp Assoc 28:257, 1992.
131. Madewell BR, et al: Multiple skin tumours in a Doberman pinscher with colour dilution alopecia. Vet Dermatol 8:59, 1997.
132. Malik R, France MP: Hyperpigmentation and symmetrical alopecia in three Silky terriers. Aust Vet Pract 21:135, 1991.
133. Marks A, et al: Congenital hypotrichosis in a French bulldog. J Small Anim Pract 33:450, 1992.
134. Miller MA, Dunstan RW: Seasonal flank alopecia in boxers and Airedale terriers: 24 cases (1985–1992). J Am Vet Med Assoc 203:1567, 1993.
135. Miller WH Jr: Follicular dysplasia in adult black and red Doberman pinschers. Vet Dermatol 1:181, 1990.
136. Miller WH Jr: Color dilution alopecia in Doberman pinschers with blue or fawn coat colors: A study on the incidence and histopathology of this disorder. Vet Dermatol 1:113, 1990.
137. Miller WH Jr: Alopecia associated with coat color dilution in two Yorkshire terriers, one Saluki, and one mix-breed dog. J Am Anim Hosp Assoc 27:39, 1991.
138. Miller WH Jr, Scott DW: Follicular dysplasia of the Portuguese water dog. Vet Dermatol 6:67, 1995.
139. Paradis M: Melatonin in veterinary dermatology. Proc Annu Meet Can Vet Med Assoc Acad Can Med Vet 50:46, 1998.
140. Paradis M: Quel est votre diagnostic? Méd Vét Québec 26:103, 1996.
141. Post K, et al: Clinical and histopathologic changes as seen in Siberian husky follicular dysplasia. In von Tscharner C, Halliwell REW (eds): Advances in Veterinary Dermatology, Vol 1. Baillière-Tindall, Philadelphia, 1990, p 446.
142. Post K, et al: Hair follicle dysplasia in a Siberian husky. J Am Anim Hosp Assoc 24:659, 1988.
143. Rest JR, et al: Dark hair follicle dystrophy in a border collie. Vet Rec 136:607, 1994.

144. Robinson R: The Canadian hairless or sphinx cat. J Hered 64:47, 1973.
145. Roperto F, et al: Colour dilution alopecia (CDA) in ten Yorkshire terriers. Vet Dermatol 6:171, 1995.
146. Rothstein E, et al: A retrospective study of dysplastic hair follicles and abnormal melanization in dogs with follicular dysplasia syndromes or endocrine skin disease. Vet Dermatol 9:235, 1998.
147. Schmutz SM, et al: Black hair follicular dysplasia, an autosomal recessive condition in dogs. Can Vet J 39:644, 1998.
147a. Schoning PR, Cowan LA: Bald thigh syndrome of Greyhound dogs: gross and microscopic findings. Vet Dermatol 11:49, 2000.
148. Scott DW: Feline dermatology 1900–1978: A monograph. J Am Anim Hosp Assoc 16:313, 1980.
149. Scott DW, Rothstein E: Trichoptilosis in three golden retrievers. Canine Pract 23:14, 1998.
150. Scott DW: Les agrégats de mélanine dans l'appareil pilo-sébacé: Signification en dermatohistopathologie du chat. Méd Vét Québec 28:38, 1998.
151. Selmanowitz VJ, et al: Congenital ectodermal defect in poodles. J Hered 61:196, 1970.
152. Selmanowitz VJ, et al: Black hair follicular dysplasia in dogs. J Am Vet Med Assoc 171:1079, 1977.
153. Thoday K: Skin diseases of the cat. In Pract 3:21, 1981.
154. Thomsett LR: Congenital hypotrichia in the dog. Vet Rec 73:915, 1961.
155. Tieghi C, et al: Medullary trichomalacia: a retrospective study of 6 cases in the German shepherd. (In preparation, 1999).
156. Waldman L: Seasonal flank alopecia in affenpinschers. J Small Anim Pract 36:272, 1995.
157. Wilkinson GT, Kristensen TS: A hair abnormality in Abyssinian cats. J Small Anim Pract 30:27, 1989.

Disorders of Pigmentation

158. Anderson RK: Canine acanthosis nigricans. Comp Cont Educ 1:466, 1979.
158a. Chieffo C, et al: Cerebellar Purkinje's cell degeneration and coat color dilution in a family of Rhodesian Ridgeback dogs. J Vet Intern Med 8:112, 1994.
159. Colgan SP, et al: Defective in vitro motility of polymorphonuclear leukocytes of homozygote and heterozygote Chédiak-Higashi cats. Vet Immunol Immunopathol 31:205, 1992.
160. Halliwell REW, Gorman NT: Veterinary Clinical Immunology. W.B. Saunders Co, Philadelphia, 1989.
161. Prieur DJ, Collier LL: Morphologic basis of inherited coat-color dilutions of cats. J Hered 72:178, 1981.
162. Rendon MI, et al: Acanthosis nigricans: A cutaneous marker for tissue resistance to insulin. J Am Acad Dermatol 21:461, 1989.
163. Rickards RA: A new treatment for canine melanosis. Mod Vet Pract 47:38, 1966.
164. Schwartzman RM, Orkin M: A Comparative Study of Skin Diseases of Dog and Man. Charles C Thomas, Springfield, IL, 1962, pp 313–318.
165. Scott DW, Walton DK: Clinical evaluation of oral vitamin E for the treatment of primary acanthosis nigricans. J Am Anim Hosp Assoc 21:345, 1985.
166. White SD, et al: Acquired aurotrichia ("gilding syndrome") of miniature schnauzers. Vet Dermatol 3:37, 1991.
167. Yang T: Gray collie syndrome. J Am Vet Med Assoc 191:390, 1987.

Disorders of Collagen

168. Affolter V: Collagen disorder of the footpads of three German shepherd dogs. In Ihrke PJ, et al (eds): Advances in Veterinary Dermatology, Vol 2. Pergamon Press, New York, 1993, p 418.
169. Barnett KC, Cottrell BD: Ehlers-Danlos syndrome in a dog: Ocular, cutaneous and articular abnormalities. J Small Anim Pract 28:941, 1987.
170. Collier LA, et al: A clinical description of dermatosparaxis in a Himalayan cat. Feline Pract 10:25, 1980.
171. Colombo S, et al: Congenital collagenopathy in a kitten. Proc Annu Meet Eur Soc Vet Dermatol Eur Coll Vet Dermatol 14:190, 1997.
172. Counts DF, et al: Dermatosparaxis in a Himalayan cat. I. Biochemical studies of dermal collagen. J Invest Dermatol 74:96, 1980.
173. Ducatelle R, et al: A morphometric classification of dermatosparaxis in the dog and cat. Vlaams Diergeneesk Tudschr 56:107, 1987.
174. Fernandez CJ, et al: Staining abnormalities of dermal collagen in cats with cutaneous asthenia or acquired skin fragility as demonstrated with Masson's trichrome stain. Vet Dermatol 9:49, 1998.
175. Fontaine J, et al: Anomalie du collagene dermique: Dermatosparaxie chez un chat europeén. Point Vét 24:255, 1992.
176. Fontaine J, Olivry T: Les asthénies cutanées héréditaires. Point Vét 28:549, 1996.
177. Freeman LJ, et al: Ehlers-Danlos syndrome in dogs and cats. Semin Vet Med Surg 2:221, 1987.
178. Gruys E: Inflammatory syndrome of footpads in puppies and AA-amyloidosis. Vet Rec 138:264, 1996.
179. Hegreberg GA, Padgett GA: Ehlers-Danlos syndrome in animals. Bull Pathol 8:247, 1967.
180. Hegreberg GA, et al: A heritable connective tissue disease of dogs and mink resembling the Ehlers-Danlos syndrome of man. II: Mode of inheritance. J Hered 60:249, 1969.
181. Hegreberg GA, et al: A heritable connective tissue disease of dogs and mink resembling the Ehlers-Danlos syndrome of man. III: Histopathologic changes of the skin. Arch Pathol 90:159, 1970.
182. Holbrook KA, et al: Dermatosparaxis in the Himalayan cat. II: Ultrastructural studies of dermal collagen. J Invest Dermatol 74:100, 1980.
182a. Jelínek F, Karban J: Cutaneous asthenia in one dog. Acta Vet Brno 67:109, 1998.
183. Kristensen F: Deep metatarsal/metacarpal toritis in German shepherds. Proc Annu Meet Eur Soc Vet Dermatol Eur Coll Vet Dermatol 14:194, 1997.
184. Kunkle GA, et al: Focal metatarsal fistulas in five dogs. J Am Vet Med Assoc 202:756, 1993.
185. Matthews BR, Lewis GT: Ehlers-Danlos syndrome in a dog. Can Vet J 31:389, 1990.
186. Minor RR: Animal models of heritable diseases of the skin. In Goldsmith EL (ed): Biochemistry and Physiology of Skin. Oxford University Press, New York, 1982.
187. Minor RR, et al: Genetic diseases of connective tissues in animals. Curr Probl Dermatol 17:199, 1987.
188. Neibauerer GW, et al: Antibodies to canine collagen types I and II with spontaneous cruciate ligament rupture and osteoarthritis. Arthritis Rheum 30:319, 1987.
189. Olivry T: Congenital and acquired collagen degeneration in dogs and cats. Proc Annu Meet Eur Soc Vet Dermatol Eur Coll Vet Dermatol 14:139, 1997.
190. Pagé N, Paradis M: Quel est votre diagnostic? Méd Vét Québec 26:147, 1996.

191. Paterson S: Sterile idiopathic pedal panniculitis in the German shepherd dog—clinical presentation and response to treatment of four cases. J Small Anim Pract 36:498, 1995.
192. Patterson DF, Minor RR: Hereditary fragility and hyper-extensibility of the skin of cats. Lab Invest 37:170, 1977.
193. Rest JR: Pathology of two possible genodermatoses. J Small Anim Pract 30:230, 1989.
194. Rodriguez F, et al: Collagen dysplasia in a litter of Garafiano shepherd dogs. J Vet Med A 43:509, 1996.
195. Scott DW: Cutaneous asthenia in a cat. Vet Med (SAC) 69:1256, 1974.
196. Scott DW: Feline dermatology: Introspective retrospections. J Am Anim Hosp Assoc 20:537, 1984.
196a. Sequeira JL, et al: Collagen dysplasia (cutaneous asthenia) in a cat. Vet Pathol 36:603, 1999.
197. Sousa C: Soft-coated Wheaten terriers and E.D.S. Derm Dialogue 1:3, 1982.

Disorders of Vessels

197a. Burkett G: Skin disease in greyhounds. Vet Med 95:115, 2000.
198. Carpenter JL, et al: Idiopathic cutaneous and renal glomerular vasculopathy of greyhounds. Vet Pathol 35:401, 1988.
199. Cowan LA, et al: Clinical and clinicopathologic abnormalities in greyhounds with cutaneous and renal glomerular vasculopathy: 18 cases (1992–1994). J Am Vet Med Assoc 210:789, 1997.
200. Fondati A, et al: Familial cutaneous vasculopathy and demodicosis in a German shepherd dog. J Small Anim Pract 39:137, 1998.
201. Fossum TW, Miller MW: Lymphedema—etiopathogenesis. J Vet Intern Med 6:238, 1992.
202. Fossum TW, Miller MW: Lymphedema—clinical signs, diagnosis and treatment. J Vet Intern Med 6:312, 1992.
203. Jacobsen JOG, Egges C: Primary lymphoedema in a kitten. J Small Anim Pract 38:18, 1997.
204. Ladds PW, et al: Lethal congenital edema in bulldog pups. J Am Vet Med Assoc 155:81, 1971.
205. Luginbuhl H, et al: Congenital hereditary lymphedema in the dog, part II: Pathological studies. J Med Genet 4:153, 1967.
206. Neu H, et al: Primäre kongenitale lymphödeme bei sieben Labarador-, einem Deutschen Schäferhund- und einem Kanadischen Wolfswelpen. Kleintierpraxis 39:S383, 1994.
207. Parker WM, Foster RA: Cutaneous vasculitis in five Jack Russell terriers. Vet Dermatol 7:109, 1996.
208. Patterson DF, et al: Congenital hereditary lymphedema in the dog, part I: Clinical and genetic studies. J Med Genet 4:145, 1967.
209. Pedersen K, Scott DW: Idiopathic pyogranulomatous inflammation and leukocytoelastic vasculitis of the nasal planum, nostrils, and nasal mucosa in Scottish terriers in Denmark. Vet Dermatol 2:85, 1991.
210. Rest JR, et al: Familial vasculopathy of German shepherd dogs. Vet Rec 138:144, 1996.
211. Ryan T, Mortimer PS: Cutaneous lymphatic system. Clin Dermatol 13:417, 1995.
212. Scott-Moncrieff JCR, et al: Systemic necrotizing vasculitis in nine young beagles. J Am Vet Med Assoc 201:1553, 1992.
213. Takahashi JL, et al: Primary lymphedema in a dog: A case report. J Am Anim Hosp Assoc 20:849, 1984.
214. Weir JAM, et al: Familial cutaneous vasculopathy of German shepherd dogs: Clinical, genetic, and preliminary pathological and immunologic studies. Can Vet J 35:763, 1994.

Endocrine, Metabolic, and Immunologic Disorders

215. Bettenay SV: Acrodermatitis of bull terriers—long term management. Proc Wld Cong Vet Dermatol 2:69, 1992.
216. Jezyk PF, et al: Lethal acrodermatitis in bull terriers. J Am Vet Med Assoc 188:833, 1986.
217. Kunkle GA, et al: Tyrosinemia in a dog. J Am Anim Hosp Assoc 20:615, 1984.
218. McEwan NA: Confirmation and investigation of lethal acrodermatitis of bull terriers in Britain. In Ihrke PJ, et al (eds): Advances in Veterinary Dermatology, Vol 2. Pergamon Press, New York, 1993, p 151.
219. McEwan NA: Isolation of yeasts from bull terriers suffering from lethal acrodermatitis. Proc Eur Soc Vet Dermatol 10:277, 1993.
219a. McEwan NA: Nail disease, zinc deficiency and lethal acrodermatitis. Proc Br Vet Dermatol Study Grp, Spring: 29, 1999.
220. Mundell AC: Mineral analysis in bull terriers with lethal acrodermatitis. Proc Annu Memb Meet Am Acad Vet Dermatol Am Coll Vet Dermatol 4:22, 1988.
221. Smits B, et al: Lethal acrodermatitis in bull terriers: A problem of defective zinc metabolism. Vet Dermatol 2:91, 1991.

Miscellaneous Disorders

222. Uchida Y, et al: Serum concentrations of zinc and copper in bull terriers with lethal acrodermatitis and tail-chasing behavior. Am J Vet Res 58:808, 1997.
223. Beale KM, et al: Papular and plaque-like mucinosis in a puppy. Vet Dermatol 2:29, 1991.
224. Cummings JF, et al: Acral mutilation and nociceptive loss in English Pointer dogs. Acta Neuropathol 53:119, 1981.
225. Griffin CE, Rosenkrantz WS: Skin disorders of the Shar pei. In Kirk RW, Bonagura JD (eds): Kirk's Current Veterinary Therapy XI. W.B. Saunders Co, Philadelphia, 1991, p 519.
226. Hutt FB: Necrosis of the toes. In Genetics for Dog Breeders. W.H. Freeman, San Francisco, 1979.
227. Mason LT: The occurrence and pedigree analysis of a hereditary sensory neuropathy in the English springer spaniel. Proc Annu Memb Meet Am Coll Vet Dermatol Am Coll Vet Dermatol 15:23, 1999.
228. Miller WH Jr, Buerger RG: Cutaneous mucinous vesiculation in a dog with hypothyroidism. J Am Vet Med Assoc 196:757, 1990.
229. Miller WH Jr, et al: Dermatologic disorders of Chinese Shar-Peis: 58 cases (1981–1989). J Am Vet Med Assoc 200:986, 1992.
230. Noli C, Scarampella F: Feline urticaria pigmentosa-like disease in two unrelated Devon Rex cats. Proc Annu Memb Meet Am Acad Vet Dermatol Am Coll Vet Dermatol 15:65, 1999.
231. Rusbridge C: Persistent scratching in Cavalier King Charles spaniels. Vet Rec 140:239, 1997.
232. Rusbridge C: Persistent scratching in Cavalier King Charles spaniels. Vet Rec 141:179, 1997.
232a. Rusbridge C, et al: Syringohydromyelia in Cavalier King Charles spaniels. J Am Anim Hosp Assoc 36:34, 2000.
233. Vitale CB, et al: Feline urticaria pigmentosa in three related Sphinx cats. Vet Dermatol 7:227, 1996.

Table 13-1 TERMINOLOGY USED TO DESCRIBE PIGMENT CHANGES

TERM	DEFINITION
Hypopigmentation	General term meaning less pigment
Leukoderma	Lack of pigment in the skin
Leukotrichia	Lack of pigment in the hair
Graying	Decreased pigment of the hair
Hyperpigmentation	General term meaning increase in pigment
Melanoderma	Increased skin pigment
Melanotrichia	Increased pigment of the hair
Poliosis	Premature grayness of hair

HYPERPIGMENTATION

Hyperpigmentation or melanoderma is associated primarily with increased melanin in the epidermis and corneocytes. Histologically, there may also be dermal pigment, but when the majority of the pigment is in the dermis, a slate or steel blue coloration is present. Hyperpigmentation in animals may be genetic, acquired, or associated with pigmented tumors.

Genetic

LENTIGO

Lentigo is a macular melanosis that is intensely black and usually occurs as multiple lesions that are most common on the ventrum. Lentigines appear in mature dogs. They often increase in number and size over a period of several months; subsequently, they become static and remain unchanged for the life of the dog. The lesions are sometimes grouped in clusters or may spread rather diffusely over the ventral surface of the body. These sharply circumscribed macules do not itch and are of no consequence to the patient. They should not have a rough surface nor be palpably thickened. When a hyperkeratotic surface or thickening is present, other diseases such as epidermal nevi or papillomavirus-induced lesions must be considered. Lentigines have been referred to as "tar spots" (Fig. 13–1).

A hereditary form of lentigo called *lentiginosis profusa* has been reported in Pugs and was thought to have an autosomal dominant mode of inheritance.[4] Many of the lesions described in these dogs were clinically and histologically hyperplastic,[31] however, so it is likely that the authors were actually describing pigmented epidermal nevi[10] or papilloma-induced lesions.[20] Similarly, generalized lentigines—probably epidermal nevi—were reported in a cat.[21]

Histologically, early lentigines are characterized by a sharply localized increase in the number of melanocytes and melanosomes.[6, 28] The epidermal pigmentation is greatly increased, because almost every keratinocyte contains melanosomes. Usually, no structural changes or only mild structural changes occur in the epidermis. As the lesion develops, the epidermis may thicken slightly, mild orthokeratotic hyperkeratosis may occur, and slight rete ridge formation may be present.

This is a cosmetic lesion with no known significance in dogs and cats, because none have been reported to become malignant. The only significance is that this lesion may need to be differentiated from pigmented tumors, especially melanomas, papillomavirus-induced lesions (which may have a premalignant potential), and pigmented nevi.

LENTIGO SIMPLEX IN ORANGE CATS

Lentigo simplex has been described in orange cats.[26, 28] The condition is characterized by asymptomatic macular melanosis, usually beginning in cats younger than 1 year of age.

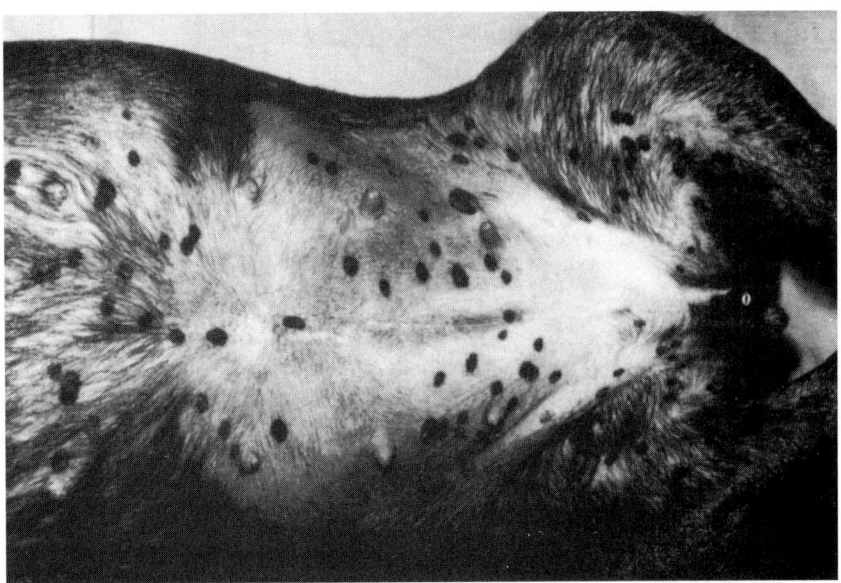

FIGURE 13–1. Close-up view of a 7-year-old French bulldog with multiple lentigines. Note the intensity of the pigmentation and the sharply demarcated borders.

The lesions start on the lips and begin as tiny, black, asymptomatic spots that gradually enlarge and become more numerous with time. There can be lesions on the nose, gingiva, and eyelids in addition to the lip. Well-circumscribed, generally circular areas of intense, uniform macular melanosis, ranging from 1 to 9 mm in diameter and occasionally coalescent, are present in variable numbers (Fig. 13–2 A). The surrounding tissue is normal. The lesions do not vary in the intensity of hyperpigmentation with the time of year. They are asymptomatic, do not develop into melanoma, and have no identified cause.

Histopathologic findings include marked hypermelanosis, predominantly of the basal cell layer of the epithelium, that is caused by the increased numbers of melanocytes and by hypermelanosis of the neighboring basal keratinocytes (Fig. 13–3). Occasionally, melanophages are seen in the superficial dermis.

Lentigo simplex is a cosmetic defect. These lesions do not require treatment, but if it is desired, surgical excision is the only way to eliminate them.

EPIDERMAL NEVUS

Nevi are developmental defects in the skin and, in some cases, have been hereditary in nature (see Chap. 20). They may have a relationship to dermatomes or peripheral nerves and can appear in a linear fashion.[34] Most epidermal and all melanocytic nevi are associated with increased pigmentation, but with epidermal nevi, the degree of pigmentation is variable. Comedo nevi are often pigmented but appear as peppered macules or plaques.

These lesions are often cosmetic, although secondary infections may occur and some may be pruritic or inflammatory. Surgical excision or laser surgery ablation is curative. Etretinate has been helpful in some nonsurgical lesions of epidermal or comedo nevi.

CANINE ACANTHOSIS NIGRICANS

This disease is seen most commonly in Dachshunds, and this has led to the belief that the primary (idiopathic) form is genetic in origin (see Chap. 12). Similar lesions may be acquired and occur secondary to a variety of chronic inflammatory diseases. Thus, the

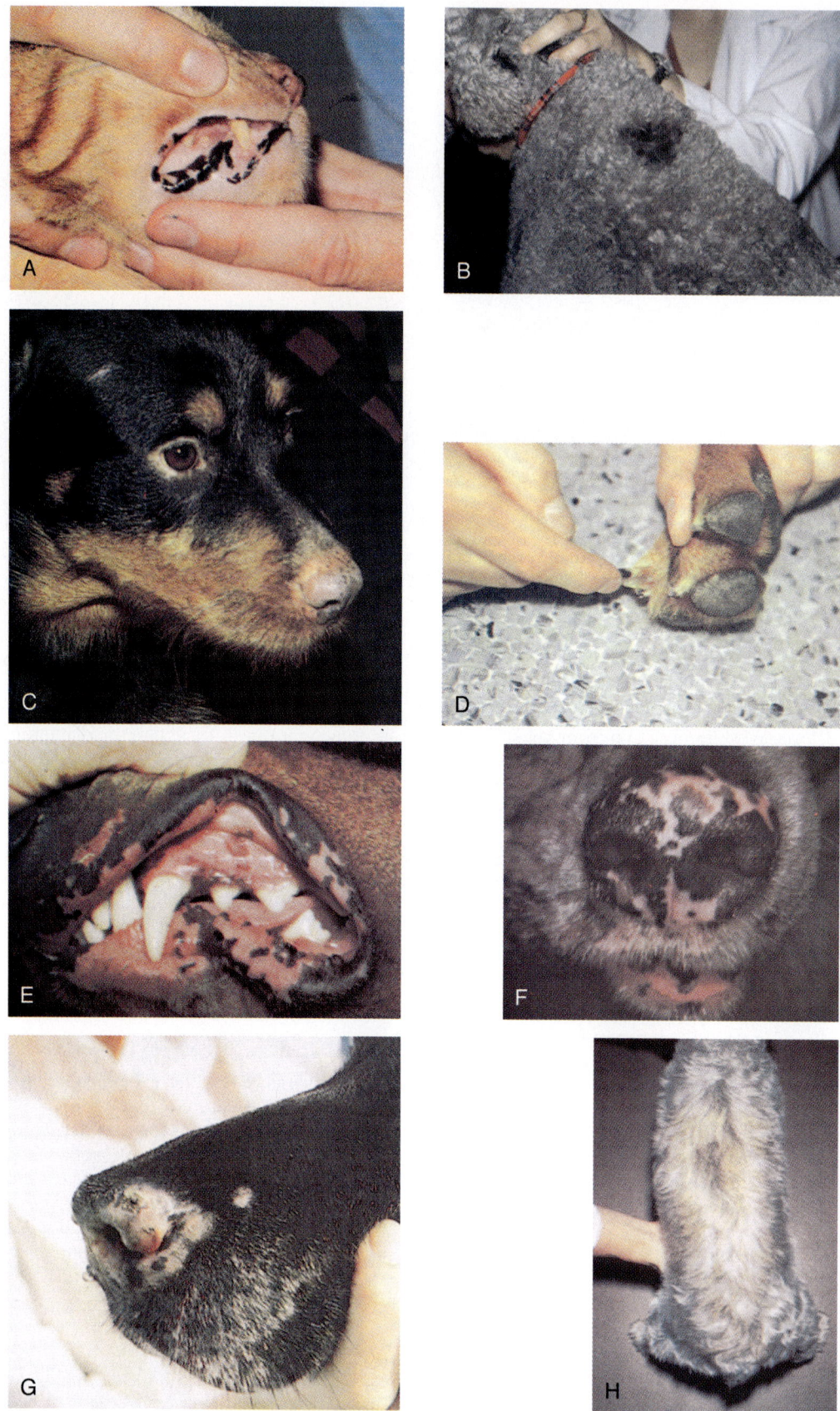

FIGURE 13–2. Legend on opposite page

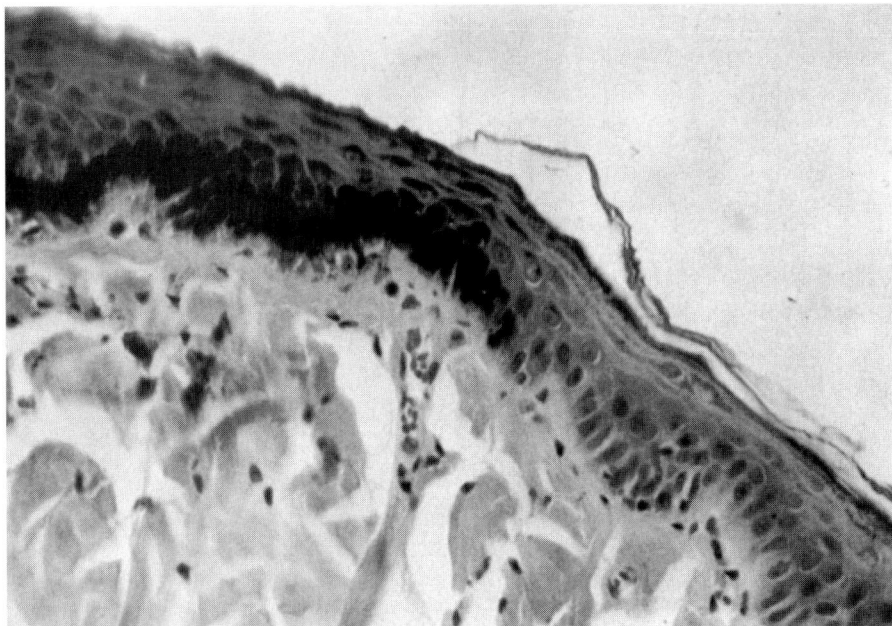

FIGURE 13-3. Feline lentigo simplex. Note the abrupt transition between the melanotic area *(left)* and normal epithelium *(right)*.

term has also been described as a reaction pattern associated with things such as friction (Fig. 13-4), hypersensitivity diseases, and seborrhea with *Malassezia*.

URTICARIA PIGMENTOSA

This disease has been reported in Sphinx cats and may have a genetic basis, as some cats were related.[32] Multifocal to generalized flat-topped papules and plaques can be seen (Fig. 13-5). These may have a dark brown color. The lesions are usually pruritic and may exhibit a distribution associated with previous trauma. Diagnosis is confirmed by histopathology revealing mast cell infiltration with no malignant features. Treatment with antihistamines and systemic glucocorticoids has been reported to be beneficial (see Chaps. 12 and 20).

Acquired

POSTINFLAMMATORY

The most common form of hyperpigmentation is postinflammatory. Many dogs and some cats produce more pigment in or around areas of inflammation. Many diseases characterized by chronic erythematous papular lesions may undergo hyperpigmentation. Often, this type of postinflammatory hyperpigmentation has a lattice-like appearance and is most commonly seen with superficial bacterial pyodermas.[17] Many other chronic inflammatory

---

FIGURE 13-2. Pigment abnormalities. *A*, Lentigo simplex in an orange cat with marked macular melanosis of the lips. *B*, Melanotrichia patches in a poodle with sebaceous adenitis. *C*, Vitiligo in a Rottweiler. Note the nasal and eyelid depigmentation and patch leukotrichia on the head. *D*, Vitiligo of the claws concurrent with onychodystrophy. *E*, Patchy hypopigmentation present from birth on the lips of a mature Doberman pinscher. *F*, A 2-year-old Newfoundland that had a normal black color at birth but gradually developed patchy hypopigmentation evident in skin and hairs. *G*, Epitheliotropic lymphoma affecting the nasal planum. *H*, Acquired aurotrichia in a miniature schnauzer. (Courtesy S. White.)

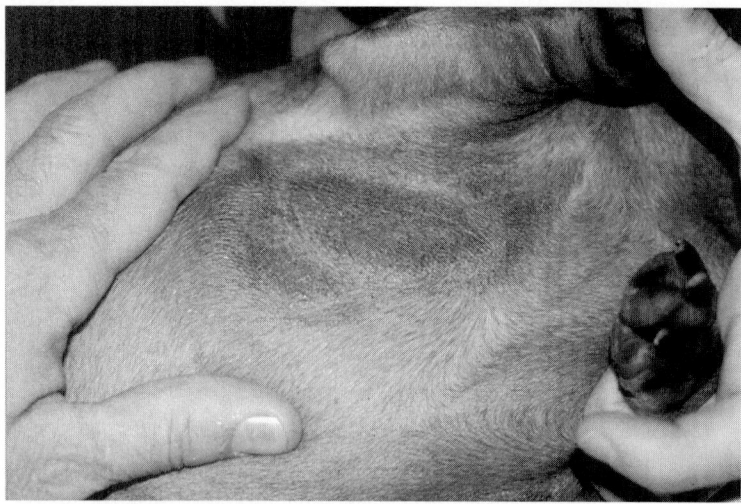

FIGURE 13-4. Hyperpigmented lichenified plaque in the axilla of a dachshund that developed after the dog gained several pounds.

diseases also result in hyperpigmentation; examples include the chronic or healing lesions of canine demodicosis, canine scabies, and the center of healing annular dermatophytosis. Occasionally, a patch of pigmented comedones appears as a hyperpigmented patch or plaque. These patches or plaques may be from slate blue to gray in color and should raise the suspicion of demodicosis, hyperadrenocorticism, or comedo nevus (Fig. 13–6).

More diffuse hyperpigmentation may result from the chronic diffuse inflammation that may be associated with such things as exposure to ultraviolet light of skin that has lost hair or from chronic irritation due to cutaneous friction. Most pruritic diseases may be incriminated because both friction and inflammation may lead to hyperpigmentation. It is common to see hyperpigmentation in dogs with hypersensitivity diseases.

Melanotrichia may also occur in animals after the healing of areas of deep inflammation (e.g., panniculitis, vaccine reaction). This is seen more commonly in certain breeds such as the Yorkshire terrier, Silky terrier, Bedlington terrier, Old English sheepdog, and Poodle. In some dogs, especially Poodles with sebaceous adenitis, multifocal areas of melanotrichia may be seen (see Fig. 13–2B). Because the inflammatory lesions of sebaceous adenitis occur even in areas without melanotrichia, it is possible that this alteration

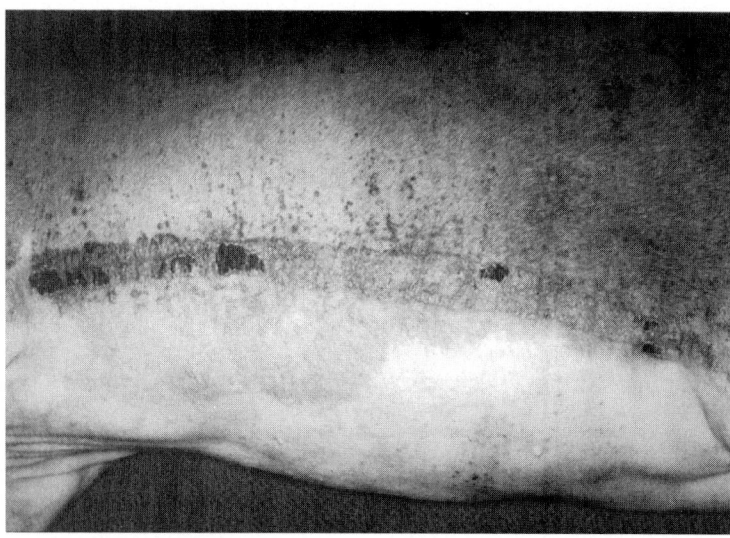

FIGURE 13-5. Urticaria pigmentosa in a Sphinx cat. (Courtesy C. Vitali). Several papules, many of which are coalesced to form a linear plaque on the lateral thoracoabdominal area.

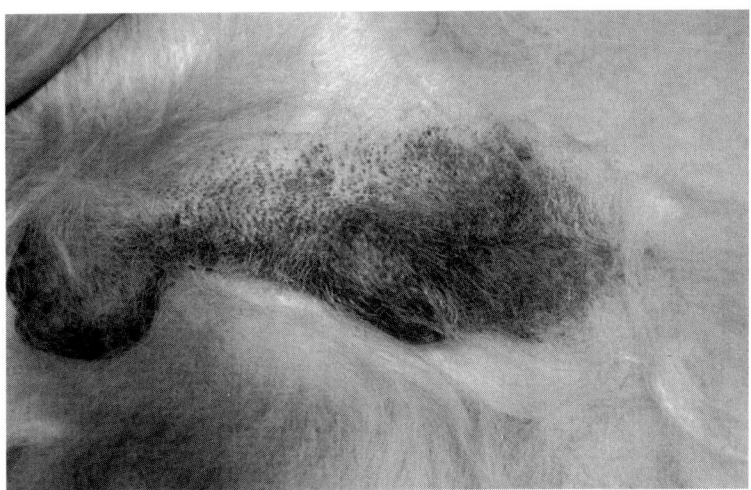

FIGURE 13–6. Hyperpigmentation in the prepucial area due to comedones in a case of demodicosis.

is not due to inflammation but occurs as a result of some other pathomechanism. Multifocal areas of melanotrichia have been seen in Poodles following bouts of intervertebral disk disease.

The exact mechanism of hyperpigmentation in these inflammatory diseases is unknown. Studies suggest that keratinocytes may be able to locally stimulate melanogenesis by releasing melanocyte stimulating factors. It is possible that these factors are present at low levels in the normal epidermis, but their levels and activity are increased in response to stimulation or keratinocyte stress.[37] The focal postinflammatory melanotrichia seen in adult dogs with silver or gray haircoats may be the result of reversion to a puppy coat under the influence of genes at the graying (G) locus. Silver dogs are usually born with dark coats that lighten when the adult hairs develop. If the melanotrichia is due to G locus influences, the hairs revert to their normal adult color at the next shedding. In other dogs, the melanotrichia may be due to the influence of melanocyte-stimulating factors such as LTB4.

HORMONE-ASSOCIATED

Diffuse hyperpigmentation may also result from some metabolic or hormonal disorders such as hyperadrenocorticism, hypothyroidism, and the sex hormone dermatoses (see Chap. 10). The mechanism is unknown, although it has been suggested that the hyperpigmentation may result from direct effects of the hormonal changes on the melanocytes. ACTH and other pituitary lipotrophic hormones stimulate melanogenesis, and this factor may be why some hyperadrenocorticism and adrenal sex hormone cases become hyperpigmented. However, the direct actions of other hormones on the melanocytes have not been well defined. In some cases, it also appears that ultraviolet exposure may play a role. When alopecia precedes the hyperpigmentation, skin is exposed to light, which can contribute to the pigment changes that occur. Protection of the skin decreases the hyperpigmentation in some animals.

Melanotrichia may also occur following the resolution of metabolic or hormonal disorders; it is commonly noted in dogs with hyperadrenocorticism that are treated with mitotane (o,p'-DDD) (Fig. 13–7). The mechanism is unknown, but G locus influences are probably important in dogs with silver coats.

DRUG-INDUCED

Hyperpigmentation due to drug administration is rare. o,p'-DDD therapy (or the control of the disease being treated) may be associated with hypermelanosis and melanotrichia. Because this change is usually temporary, even when o,p'-DDD therapy is continued, it is

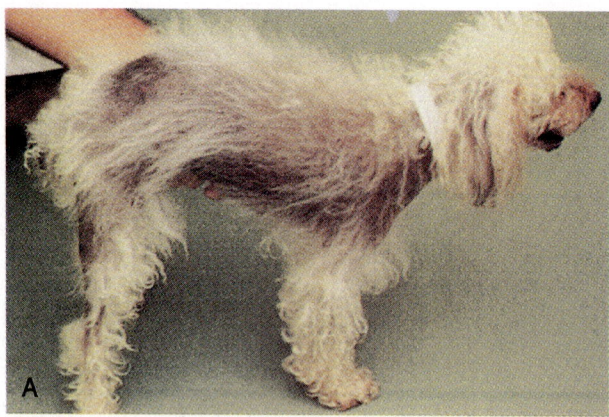
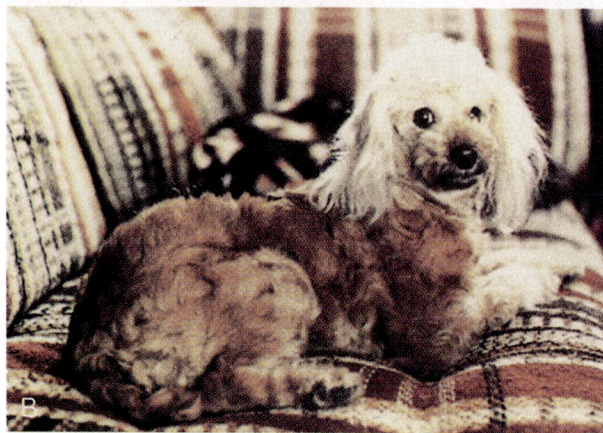

FIGURE 13–7. Apricot Poodle that developed melanotrichia following treatment of its Cushing's disease with mitotane (o,p'-DDD.) A, Before treatment. B, After treatment. Usually the normal coat color returns, even with continued o,p'-DDD maintenance therapy.

possibly caused by hormonal changes and not by the drug. Experimentally, the drug minocycline has been shown to cause hyperpigmentation in dogs,[1a] and the effect was believed to be attributable to iron deposition. In humans, a variety of other metallic substances may cause cutaneous pigment changes; for example, changes may be acquired by parenteral or topical absorption of metals such as silver, gold, and mercury.[2]

PAPILLOMAVIRUS-ASSOCIATED

Canine papillomaviruses induce at least two syndromes that may have pigmented lesions. Cutaneous exophytic papillomas usually occur in older dogs and more commonly in male dogs.[28] They appear as cauliflower-like nodules or keratinous plaques, mainly on the head, eyelids, and paws. The lesions may appear flesh tone, pink, brown, or black in color. These lesions may regress on their own. Papillomavirus-associated canine pigmented plaques have been compared with epidermodysplasia verruciformis.[20] This disease is seen mainly in young Pugs, miniature Schnauzers, and Shar peis and may have a genetic basis. The lesions are often slightly rough black pigmented macules to plaques. They occur mostly on the groin, abdomen, ventral thorax, and neck. They do not spontaneously regress and often are slowly progressive. They have been reported to transform into squamous cell carcinoma (see Chap. 20) (Fig. 13–8).

FELINE ACROMELANISM

Siamese, Himalayan, Balinese, and Burmese kittens are born white and develop points as adults owing to the influence of external temperature[28]; high environmental temperatures

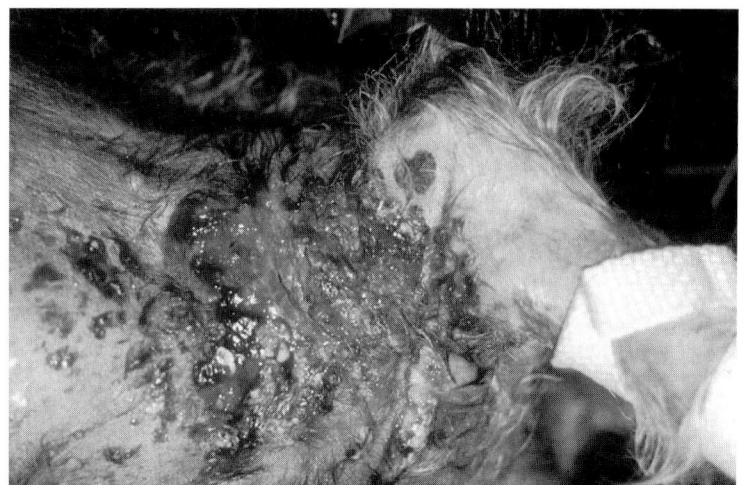

FIGURE 13-8. Pigmented viral papillomas that developed into a squamous cell carcinoma in the axillary area of a dog.

produce light hairs, and low temperatures produce dark hairs. Coat color also appears to be affected by physiologic factors that determine heat production and loss (e.g., inflammation, alopecia) (Fig. 15-9). These color change phenomena appear to be associated with a temperature-dependent enzyme involved in melanin synthesis. The changes in coat color are usually temporary, and the normal color returns with the next hair cycle, if the temperature influences are remedied.

PIGMENTED TUMORS

Many tumors have pigmentation different from the surrounding skin. This color difference may reflect the type of tissue and its associated color or other pigments. Vascular tumors may appear red, port wine, or red-blue. Histiocytic, lymphocytic, and plasmacytic tumors often appear pink, red, or purple. The common hyperpigmented (black) tumors are the melanocytoma and melanoma; however, a variety of tumors may occur with hyperpigmentation. Basal cell tumors, trichoblastomas, fibromas, epidermal nevi, and epithelial nevi may also commonly occur as hyperpigmented lesions. The lesions of squamous cell carcinoma in situ (Bowen's disease) in the cat may also be dark brown to black (Fig. 13-9).

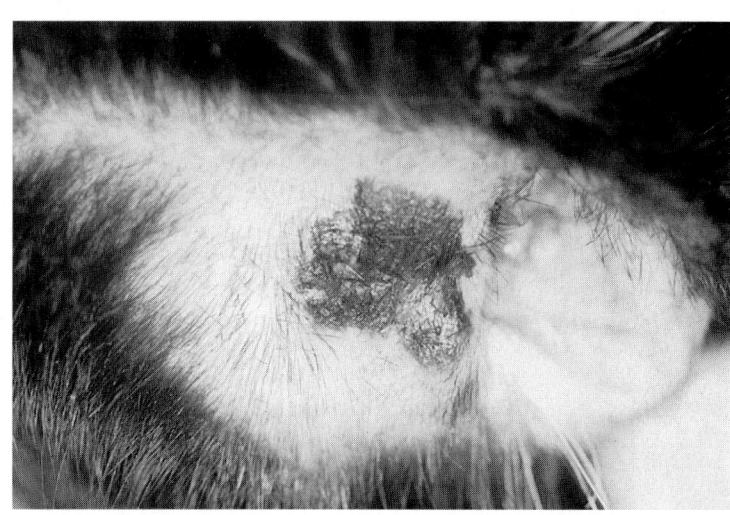

FIGURE 13-9. Pigmented plaque in a cat from Bowen's disease.

• HYPOPIGMENTATION

Hypopigmentation *(hypomelanosis)* refers to a lack or decrease of pigment in the skin or haircoat in areas that should normally be pigmented. Hereditary hypomelanoses have been divided into melanocytopenic (absence of melanocytes) and melanopenic (decreased melanin) forms.[1] Pigment loss may occur from melanocyte destruction, dysfunction, or abnormal dispersion of melanosomes as a result of abnormal melanosome transfer or from inflammation. Lack of or decrease in melanosome production may also be a cause. The disorder may be congenital or acquired.

Genetic

CHÉDIAK-HIGASHI SYNDROME

Chédiak-Higashi syndrome is an autosomal recessive disorder reported in Persian cats with yellow eyes and a blue smoke haircoat color.[1] It is characterized by partial oculocutaneous albinism and is discussed in Chapter 12.

ALBINISM

Albinism is a hereditary lack of pigmentation that is transmitted as an autosomal recessive trait.[1, 7, 11] Albino individuals have a normal complement of melanocytes, but they lack tyrosinase for melanin synthesis and, therefore, have a biochemical inability to produce melanin. Therefore, histopathologic studies reveal a normal epidermis with no pigment, but clear basal cells representing melanocytes are still seen. Skin, hair, and mucous membranes are amelanotic. Although humans have unpigmented (pink) irides, dogs typically have milder ocular changes, with blue eyes.[12] These dogs should not be used as breeders.

PIEBALDISM

Genetically determined white spotting is referred to as piebaldism.[1] It is common in dogs and is transmitted as a completely dominant trait. Melanocytes are absent or incompletely differentiated in affected sites.

WAARDENBURG-KLEIN SYNDROME

Waardenburg-Klein syndrome has been described in cats, Bull terriers, Sealyham terriers, Collies, and Dalmatians. In addition to blue eyes and amelanotic skin and hair, the affected animals are deaf and have blue or heterochromic irides.[1, 12] The defect is in the migration and differentiation of melanoblasts. Therefore, the affected skin has no melanocytes present. The syndrome is transmitted as an autosomal dominant trait with incomplete penetrance, so these animals should not be used for breeding.

CANINE CYCLIC HEMATOPOIESIS

Canine cyclic hematopoiesis (also known as gray collie syndrome and canine cyclic neutropenia) is a lethal autosomal recessive syndrome wherein collie puppies are born with a silver-gray haircoat that differs from the normal sable or tricolor coat (see Chap. 12). In some of these puppies, a slight yellow pigmentation may be present, which produces a mixture of light beige and light gray hair. The light-colored nose is a characteristic and diagnostic lesion.

Breed-Associated, Suspect Genetic

GRAYING

Graying results from a reduction in melanocyte replication through senescence. It appears to be age and genetically related as certain breeds are more prone. German shepherd dogs, Irish setters, Labrador retrievers and golden retrievers appear to be more likely to develop gray muzzles and chin at a relatively younger age (Fig. 13–10).

VITILIGO

A presumptive hereditary vitiligo has been described in Belgian Tervuren dogs, German shepherds, collies, Siamese cats, Rottweilers, Doberman pinschers, and giant Schnauzers. It has also been described in a Bull mastiff, Newfoundlands, Old English sheepdogs, and a Dachshund with adult-onset diabetes mellitus.[1, 11, 18, 24a, 27, 28, 30] Interestingly it has been reported in only female Siamese cats.[16] It appears that, as in humans, vitiligo in dogs and cats is inherited in a multifactorial genetic pattern.[15]

Although the exact cause of vitiligo is unknown, several theories have been proposed.[15] The *autoimmune theory* is a favored one, and antimelanocyte antibodies have been demonstrated in the serum of humans, dogs, and cats with active vitiligo.[22] Antimelanocyte antibodies were demonstrated in the serum of all 17 Belgian Tervuren dogs with vitiligo and in none of 11 normal Belgian Tervuren dogs tested.[22] Also, three affected Siamese cats had autoantibodies, but four normal Siamese cats did not. One Siamese cat had negative immunostaining for vimentin suggesting a destruction of dendritic cells.[16] The *autotoxicity theory* proposes an increased melanocyte susceptibility to melanin precursor molecules (such as dopachrome) or an inhibition of thioredoxin reductase, a free-radical scavenger located on the melanocyte membrane. The *neural theory* proposes nerve injury to explain dermatomally distributed vitiligo. A viral association has been suggested.[9] It is important to consider that multiple mechanisms could be responsible for the same phenotype.

The animals develop somewhat symmetric macular leukoderma and leukotrichia, especially of the nose, lips, buccal mucosa, and facial skin (see Fig. 13–2C and D). The footpads (Fig. 13–11) and claws, as well as the haircoat, may be affected. The authors have seen Rottweilers develop onychomadesis and leukonychia concurrently with vitiligo (Fig. 13–12). The onset of the condition is usually in young adulthood. In some cases, pigment returns to affected areas; in others, however, the depigmentation is permanent.

Diagnosis is based on history, physical examination, and histopathologic evaluation. Late lesions of vitiligo are characterized by a relatively normal epidermis and dermis, except that no melanocytes are seen (Fig. 13–13). In some cases (possibly early lesions), a mild lymphocytic interface dermatitis and occasional lymphocyte exocytosis may be seen.[10] Electron microscopy studies of melanocytes at the periphery of lesions demonstrate degenerative changes (cytoplasmic vacuolization, aggregation of melanosomes, autophagic vacuoles, fatty degeneration, and pyknosis).[15]

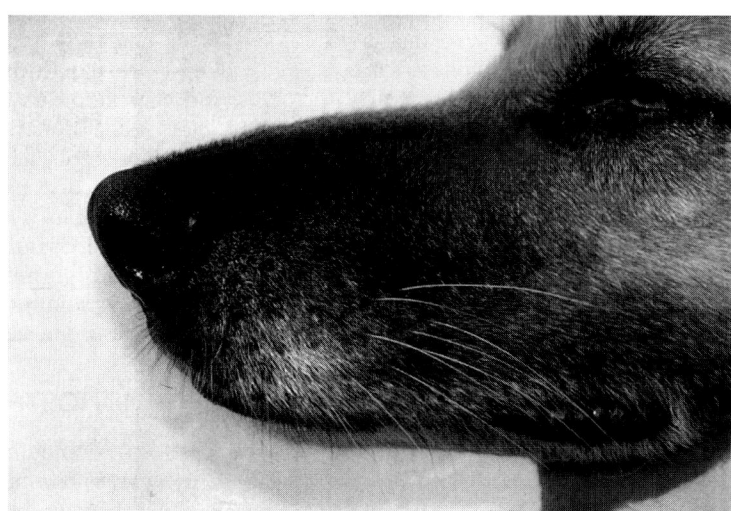

FIGURE 13–10. Gray muzzle in a German Shepherd dog.

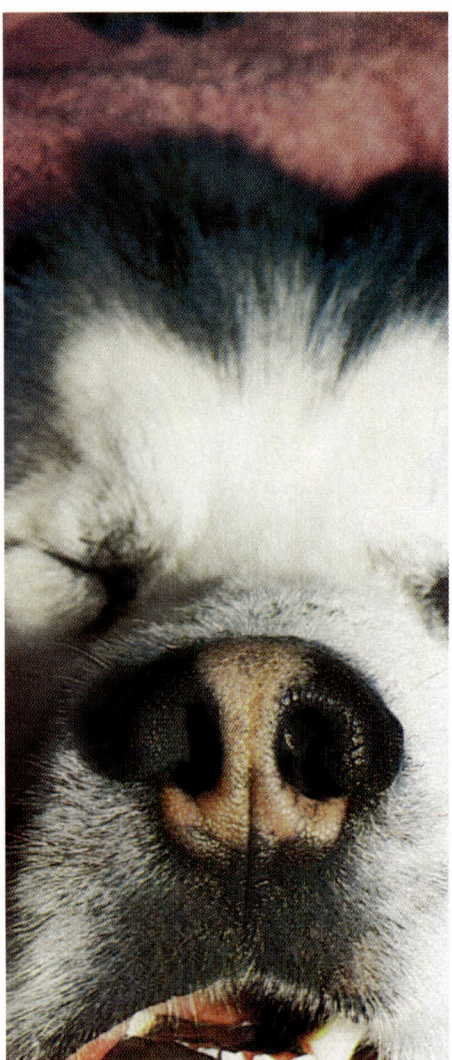

FIGURE 13-14. Canine snow nose.

Labrador retrievers. Some of these dogs also have seasonal nasal hypopigmentation. Although they have lightly pigmented noses, there is still enough pigment to prevent sunburn. Dogs with complete leukoderma of the nasal planum are prone to sunburn, which may develop into nasal solar dermatitis.

Hypopigmentation of the lips and nose occurs as a congenital condition in Doberman pinschers, Rottweilers, and occasionally, other breeds[7] (see Fig. 13-2E). It is present from birth and is static in contrast to vitiligo, which is acquired in mature dogs and often progresses or changes over time. The cause of congenital hypopigmentation is unknown. Many owners object to the cosmetic appearance, but no treatment is effective.

TYROSINASE DEFICIENCY

Tyrosinase deficiency has been reported in Chow Chows, but the condition is extremely rare. Puppies with this condition exhibit a dramatic color change. The normally bluish black tongue turns pink, and portions of the hair shafts turn white. The buccal mucosa may also rapidly depigment.

The change in color is the result of a deficiency of tyrosinase, the enzyme necessary to produce melanin. Tyrosinase deficiency can be confirmed by skin biopsy. After tyrosine is added to histologic preparations, the specimen is incubated, and the melanin is measured after tissue staining.[5] There is no effective treatment; however, melanin reappears spontaneously in 2 to 4 months. Chow Chow breeders have claimed success with the use of vitamins, unsaturated oils, and dietary changes, but the improvement was probably spontaneous.

Acquired

Acquired hypopigmentation of previously normal skin and hair can result from many factors that destroy melanocytes or inhibit melanocyte function.[3, 24] Trauma, burns, infections, and ionizing irradiation may have potent local effects. It may also be idiopathic. Dogs that sunbathe frequently or swim in chlorine pools and dry themselves in the sun may develop lighter and coarser haircoats.

POSTINFLAMMATORY

Inflammation may cause hypopigmentation. This postinflammatory hypopigmentation is less common than hyperpigmentation. Postinflammatory hypopigmentation is most evident in the groin and inguinal region following folliculitis. Multiple circular hypopigmented macules may be seen, or they can coalesce into variably shaped macules. Other infections, such as blastomycosis, sporotrichosis, and leishmaniasis, may cause hypopigmentation.[11, 18] One infectious disease in particular to consider with leukoderma without obvious swelling or infectious lesions is leishmaniasis (Fig. 13–15). Acquired hypopigmentation of the nose and lips can result from contact dermatitis from plastic or rubber food dishes. A red Irish setter puppy that had severe pustular dermatitis developed white bands around the hair shafts, presumably a result of the effects on pigment production in the hair bulb during the infection.[28]

A number of inflammatory diseases may begin with nasal hypopigmentation or depigmentation of the nose and occasionally lips. Discoid lupus erythematosus most commonly starts on the nasal planum, but occasionally, systemic lupus erythematosus, pemphigus

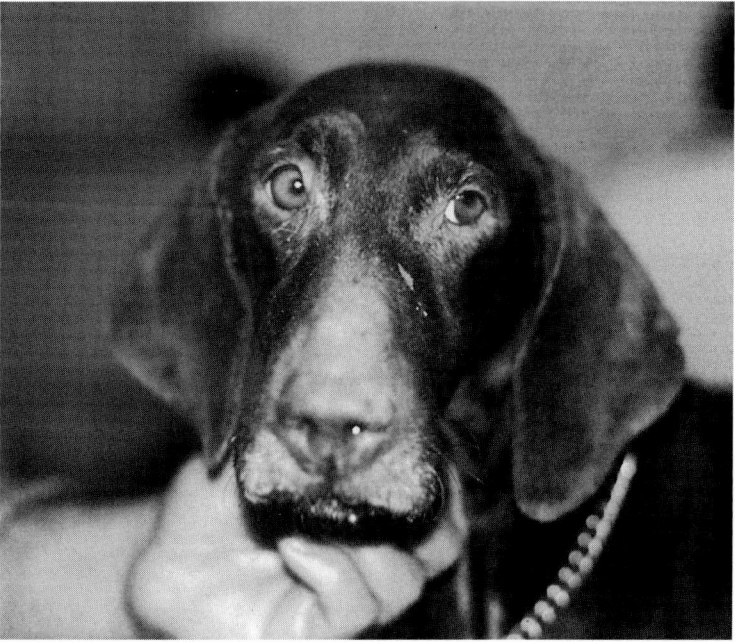

FIGURE 13–15. Nasal depigmentation associated with leishmaniasis (Courtesy A. Koutinas).

erythematosus and foliaceus, uveodermatologic syndrome, drug eruption, and bullous pemphigoid may also start on the nose.

DRUG-RELATED

Hypomelanosis due to drugs has been seen with subcutaneous injections of glucocorticoids and progestational drugs and with topical glucocorticoids. Some dogs that receive ketoconazole for mycotic infections or procainamide for cardiac disease develop diffuse lightening of their coats (Fig. 13–16). Chemical hypomelanosis may occur following the administration of potent antioxidants such as dihydroquinone and monobenzyl ether.[11, 18] One tricolor collie with lupus erythematosus developed leukotrichia following vitamin E therapy. A cause for the leukotrichia was not determined, although it was speculated that there was an association with vitamin E because the mucocutaneous depigmentation attributed to lupus was reversed with therapy before the leukotrichia developed.

METABOLIC

Some chronic metabolic diseases may affect haircoat color. This cause appears to be particularly prominent in the sex hormone dermatoses of male dogs. Deficiencies of nutrients such as zinc, pyridoxine, pantothenic acid, and lysine have produced graying of the hair. Copper deficiency is said to cause black hair to develop a reddish brown hue.

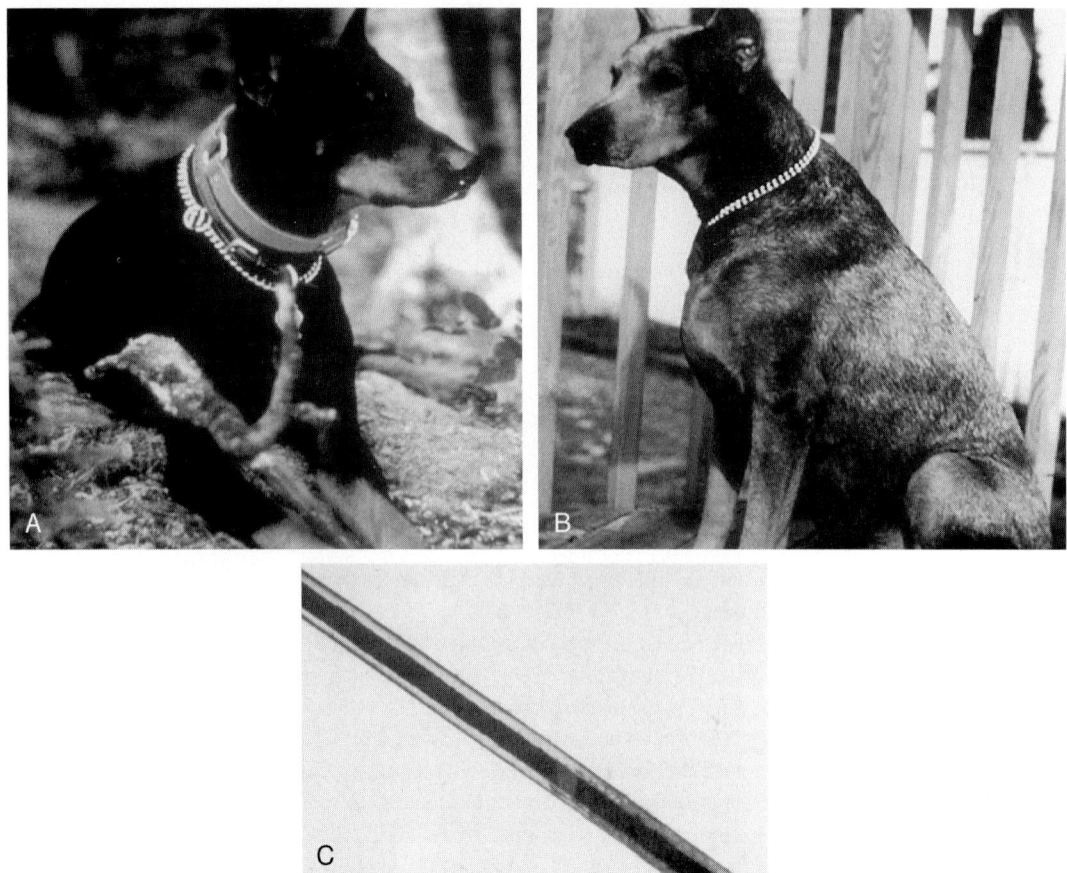

FIGURE 13–16. *A*, Doberman pinscher before therapy. *B*, Same dog during procainamide therapy. *C*, Abrupt alteration in hair pigmentation from a dog taking procainamide. The drug caused lightening of the coat color.

NEOPLASIA

Hypomelanosis associated with neoplastic conditions has been seen in dogs. Leukoderma or leukotrichia, especially of the nasal planum, lips, and face, may occur as an early sign of epitheliotropic lymphoma (mycosis fungoides and pagetoid reticulosis) (Fig. 13–2G).[18] Nasal depigmentation has also been seen with squamous cell carcinoma.[11] A peritumoral amelanotic halo has been seen around basal cell tumors.[11] Leukoderma or leukotrichia may be seen with mammary adenocarcinoma or gastric carcinoma.[11]

IDIOPATHIC

Normal black Newfoundlands, at about 18 months of age, may develop patches of depigmentation on the nose, lips, and eyelids (see Fig. 13–2F). The lesions steadily progress, affecting the hair follicles in a diffuse manner. The animals become "gray roans." Supplementation with trace minerals, vitamins, and zinc produces no improvement.

A litter of chocolate Labrador retriever puppies developed idiopathic leukotrichia that was reversible.[33] In this litter, 7 of 10 puppies were affected with varying degrees of leukotrichia, which was initially noted at 8 weeks of age on the face but then spread. By the time the puppies were 14 weeks of age, one owner reported that pigmentation was returning. Eventually, all of the affected puppies developed normal coat colors, and no recurrences were noted over the following 18 months.

Idiopathic, widespread but patchy leukotrichia is occasionally seen in adult black or chocolate Labrador retrievers (Fig. 13–17). The condition appears to be permanent.

PERIOCULAR LEUKOTRICHIA

Bilateral periocular leukotrichia (goggles) occurs in Siamese cats.[25] There is no apparent age predilection, but the condition is seen more commonly in females. Commonly recognized precipitating factors include pregnancy, dietary deficiency, and systemic illnesses. The condition is characterized by patchy or complete lightening of the hairs of the mask in a halo-like appearance around both eyes (Fig. 13–18). The condition is transient and usually resolves within the succeeding two hair cycles.

A syndrome of unilateral periocular depigmentation, called Aguirre's syndrome, has been described in Siamese cats. This condition is associated with Horner's syndrome, or corneal necrosis with uveitis, and upper respiratory tract infections.[13]

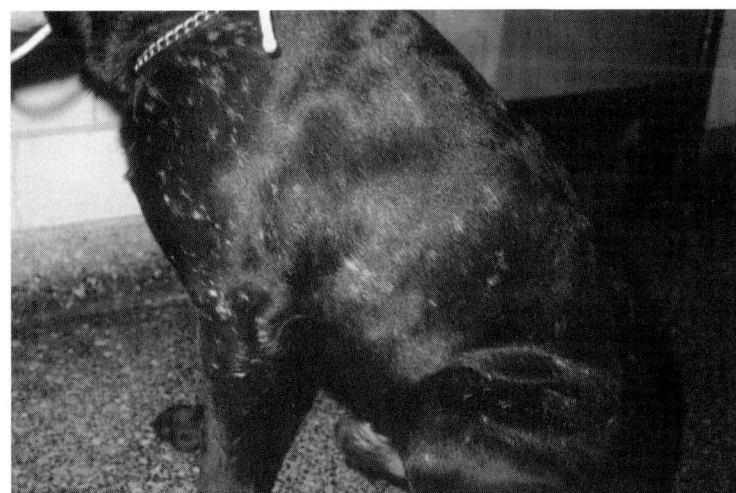

FIGURE 13–17. Idiopathic leukotrichia in an adult black Labrador retriever.

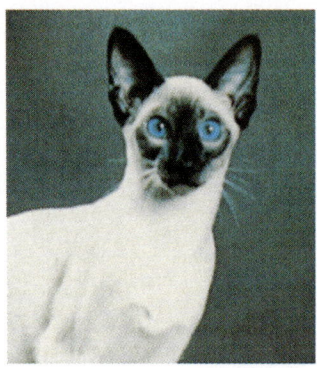

FIGURE 13–18. Periocular leukotrichia (goggles) in a Siamese cat after estrus.

• MISCELLANEOUS PIGMENT CHANGES

Acquired Aurotrichia

This syndrome occurs in miniature Schnauzers of either sex.[35] The primary guard hairs turn from silver or black to gold (see Fig. 13–2H). These gold hairs occur primarily in patches on the dorsal thorax and abdomen, although periocular and pinnal involvement occurs in some cases. An associated thinning of the secondary hair in the affected areas may be noted (see Chap. 12).

Red Hair

A variety of conditions can cause hair to become reddish in color. Lightly colored hair exposed to saliva or tears becomes stained by porphyrins. When seen in areas other than around the oral cavity or ventral to the eyes, this change usually indicates excessive licking. Poor-quality protein diets have been associated with the development of red hair; the condition resolves when a proper diet is followed.[8] This color change was associated with indicanuria and indicanemia. Diets deficient in copper may also cause red hair.

A variety of endocrinopathies may cause lightening of the haircoat or result in dark hair turning red. Although it is reported with hypothyroidism and hyperadrenocorticism, this change seems especially common with Sertoli cell tumors and in cases of hyperestrogenism or hyperprogesteronism. Some dogs with Sertoli cell tumors fail to shed their coat normally, and hairs are actually retained in catagen or telogen. The hairs remain for years; the lightened, red, dry, frizzy coat may be partly caused by chronic ultraviolet and environmental exposure. The potential effects of sun, chlorine, detergents, and environmental factors should be considered any time the coat color has changed.

Red/Brown Claws

Claws may turn a brown or red color. This problem can result from licking and salivary staining. *Malassezia* dermatitis has also been associated with this change, and less frequently, bacterial paronychia may also cause this discoloration (see Chap. 19).

Flushing

Cutaneous flushing, in which the skin turns varying shades of red, is due to vasodilatation of cutaneous blood vessels. Flushing can be persistent or paroxysmal; it is caused by emotional, autonomic, or endocrine influences, or by the direct action of vasoactive compounds in the blood vessels.[6, 28] In humans, widespread flushing can be caused by a variety of physiologic and pathologic conditions, especially the carcinoid syndrome, systemic mastocytosis, Zollinger-Ellison syndrome, or pheochromocytoma. In dogs, persistent flushing has been attributed to drug reactions and mast cell tumors. Paroxysmal flushing has been associated with pheochromocytoma and mast cell tumors.[19]

Drug-Induced Color Changes

Some drugs may induce color changes in the skin. Rifampin, ß carotene, and clofazamine are known in people to cause reddish orange discoloration of the skin. A cat treated with clofazamine developed reddish orange skin and mucus membranes, which resolved following discontinuation of therapy.[14] Pinnal erythema has been reported in cats in association with enrofloxacin or ciprofloxacin administration.[29]

• REFERENCES

1. Alhaidari Z, et al: Melanocytogenesis and melanogenesis: Genetic regulation and comparative clinical diseases. Vet Dermatol 10:3, 1999.
1a. Benitz KF, et al: Morphologic effects of minocycline in laboratory animals. Toxicol Appl Pharmacol 11:150, 1967.
2. Bergfeld WF, McMahon JT: Identification of foreign metallic substances inducing hypopigmentation of skin. Light microscopy, electron microscopy, and x-ray energy spectroscopic examination. In: Callen JP, et al (eds): Advances in Dermatology—Vol 2. Year Book Medical Publishers, Chicago, 1987, p 171.
3. Bolognia JL, Pawelek JM: Biology of hypopigmentation. J Am Acad Dermatol 19:217, 1988.
4. Briggs OM: Lentiginosis profusa in the pug: Three case reports. J Small Anim Pract 26:675, 1985.
5. Engstrom D: Tyrosinase deficiency in the Chow Chow. In: Kirk RW (ed): Current Veterinary Therapy II. WB Saunders Co., Philadelphia, 1966, p 352.
6. Fitzpatrick TB, et al: Dermatology in General Medicine, 4th ed. McGraw-Hill Book Co, New York, 1993.
7. Foil CS: Comparative genodermatoses. Clin Dermatol 3:175, 1985.
8. Griess D, Guaguère E: Variations de l'indicanémie et de l'indicanurie dans le syndrome rubra-pilaire du chien. Rev Méd Vé. 132:12, 1981.
9. Grimes PE, et al: Cytomegalovirus DNA identified in skin biopsy specimens of patients with vitiligo. J Am Acad Dermatol 35:21–26, 1996.
10. Gross TL, et al: Veterinary Dermatopathology: Gross and Microscopic Pathology of Skin Diseases. Mosby–Year Book, St. Louis, 1992.
11. Guaguère E, Alhaidari Z: Disorders of melanin pigmentation in the skin of dogs and cats. Proc Wld Small Anim Vet Assoc 8:47, 1991.
12. Guaguère E, Alhaidari Z: Pigmentary disturbances. Adv Vet Dermatol 1:395, 1990.
13. Holzworth J: Diseases of the Cat: Medicine and Surgery, Vol I. W.B. Saunders Co, Philadelphia, 1987.
14. Kaufman AC, et al: Treatment of localized *Mycobacterium avium* complex infection with clofazamine and doxycycline in a cat. J Am Vet Med Assoc 207:457, 1995.
15. Kovacs SO: Vitiligo. J Am Acad Dermatol 38:647, 1998.
16. Lopez R, et al: A clinical, pathological and immunopathological study of vitiligo in a siamese cat. Vet Dermatol 5:27, 1994.
17. MacDonald JM: Hyperpigmentation. In: Griffin CE, et al (eds): Current Veterinary Dermatology. Mosby–Year Book, St. Louis, 1993, p 234.
18. MacDonald JM: Nasal depigmentation. In: Griffin CE, et al (eds): Current Veterinary Dermatology. Mosby–Year Book, St. Louis, 1993, p 223.
19. Miller WH Jr: Cutaneous flushing associated with intrathoracic neoplasia in a dog. J Am Anim Hosp Assoc 28:217, 1992
20. Nagata M, et al: Pigmented plaques associated with papillomavirus infection in dogs: Is this epidermodysplasia verruciformis? Vet Dermatol 6:179, 1995.
21. Nash S, Paulsen D: Generalized lentigines in a silver cat. J Am Vet Med Assoc 196:1500, 1990.
22. Naughton GK, et al: Antibodies to surface antigens of pigmented cells in animals with vitiligo. Proc Soc Exp Biol Med 181:423, 1986.
23. Ortonne JP, Prota G: Hair melanins and hair color: Ultrastructural and biochemical aspects. J Invest Dermatol 101:82S, 1993.
24. Pawelek J, et al: New regulators of melanin biosynthesis and the autodestruction of melanin cells. Nature 286:617, 1980.
24a. Peterson A, et al: Progressive leukotrichia and leukoderma in a Newfoundland dog. In: Kwochka KW, et al (eds): Advances in Veterinary Dermatology III. Butterworth-Heinemann, Boston, 1998, p. 443.
25. Scott DW: Feline dermatology 1983–1985: The secret sits. J Am Anim Hosp Assoc 23:255, 1987.
26. Scott DW: Lentigo simplex in orange cats. Comp Anim Pract 1:23, 1987.
27. Scott DW: Vitiligo in the Rottweiler. Canine Pract 15:22, 1990.
28. Scott DW, et al: Muller and Kirk's Small Animal Dermatology, 5th ed. W.B. Saunders Co, Philadelphia, 1995.
29. Scott DW, Miller WH Jr: Idiosyncratic cutaneous adverse drug reactions in the cat: Literature review and report of 14 cases (1990–1996). Feline Pract 26(4):10, 1998.
30. Scott DW, Randolph JF: Vitiligo in two old English sheepdog littermates and a dachshund with juvenile onset diabetes mellitus. Comp Anim Pract 19:18, 1989.
31. VanRensburg IBJ, Briggs OM: Pathology of canine lentiginosis profusa. J S Afr Vet Assoc 57:159, 1986.

32. Vitale CB, et al: Feline urticaria pigmentosa in three related Sphinx cats. Vet Dermatol 7:227–233, 1996.
33. White SD, Butch S: Leukotrichia in a litter of Labrador retrievers. J Am Anim Hosp Assoc 26:319, 1990.
34. White SD, et al: Inflammatory linear verrucous epidermal nevus in four dogs. Vet Dermatol 3:107, 1993.
35. White SD, et al: Acquired aurotrichia ("Gilding syndrome") of miniature schnauzers. Vet Dermatol 3:37, 1992.
36. Yaar M, Gilchrest BA: Human melanocyte growth and differentiation: A decade of new data. J Invest Dermatol 97:611, 1991.
37. Yohn JJ, et al: Cultured human keratinocytes synthesize and secrete endothelin-1. J Invest Dermatol 100:23, 1993.

Chapter 14
Keratinization Defects

Keratinization defects are those that alter the surface appearance of the skin. The epidermis of animals is being replaced constantly by new cells. The epidermal cell renewal time in normal dogs is approximately 22 days.[32] Despite this high turnover rate, the epidermis maintains its normal thickness, has a barely perceptible surface keratin layer, and loses its dead cells invisibly into the environment. If the delicate balance between cell death and renewal is altered, the epidermal thickness changes, the stratum corneum becomes noticeable, and the normally invisible sloughed cells of the stratum corneum become obvious. The causes of keratinization defects are numerous; they produce clinical signs by altering proliferation, differentiation, desquamation, or some combination of these.[33, 62] Alterations in epidermal lipid formation and deposition can accompany these other changes.[36]

The keratinization defects include hyperkeratosis, hypokeratosis, and dyskeratosis. Hyperkeratosis is common in chronic dermatoses. It is further distinguished histopathologically into *parakeratotic* (nucleated) and *orthokeratotic* (anuclear) types.[27, 59] Hypokeratosis is not as common, but it is seen histologically in some cases, presumably as a result of very rapid exfoliation. Another fault in epidermopoiesis is dyskeratosis, which is seen in neoplastic skin diseases (such as squamous cell carcinoma).

Keratinization defects can be congenital or acquired. The congenital defects (e.g., primary seborrhea, ichthyosis, epidermal dysplasia of West Highland White terriers, psoriasiform-lichenoid dermatosis of English Springer spaniels, and Schnauzer comedo syndrome) are discussed in Chapter 12. The most common acquired keratinization defect is the callus, which is discussed in Chapter 16. The remainder are considered here.

A characteristic of healthy skin is that the relationship between transepidermal water loss and hydration remains directly proportional.[4] Following skin damage or a decrease in efficiency of the water barrier, a dissociation between hydration (water-holding capacity) and transepidermal water loss occurs. In pathologic skin, the correlation between transepidermal water loss and stratum corneum water content shows an inverse relationship due to a damaged skin barrier or alterations in keratinization, or both. Hence, there is increased transepidermal water loss and decreased hydration.

Dryness (xerosis) of the skin is caused by decreased water content, which must be more than 10% for skin to appear and feel normal.[18] Moisture loss occurs through evaporation to the environment under low humidity conditions and must be replenished by water from lower epidermal and dermal layers. In xerotic skin, the stratum corneum is thickened, disorganized, and fissured. An important part of the stratum corneum barrier is the presence of three intercellular lipids: sphingolipids, free sterols, and free fatty acids. Lamellar bodies are an essential part of this barrier to both trap and prevent excess water loss. The optimal stratum corneum water concentration to promote softness and pliability is 20% to 35%.

• ANTISEBORRHEIC TREATMENTS

Antiseborrheic agents are available as ointments, creams, gels, lotions, and shampoos.[57] In veterinary medicine, seborrheic lesions are usually widespread in nature and occur in haired skin, thus making the shampoo vehicle the most appropriate.[16] For the most part, veterinary shampoo formulations are not patented and "identical" products can be marketed by one or more generic manufacturers. The reader is advised to approach these products carefully. Although the active ingredients may be identical in name and concentration, the purity, stability, and irritability of the active and inert ingredients may be very different and the shampoo may perform poorly.[56] If a change from one brand of the "same" shampoo to another is contemplated, it is best to give the new product to the clients who have been using the shampoo to be replaced. If they believe that the new product is equally as good or better than the old one, the change can be made.

Antiseborrheics are commercially available in various combinations.[16, 35] The clinician must decide which combination of drugs to use and needs to know each drug's actions and concentrations. Ideal therapeutic response depends on the correct choice, but variations among individual patients do occur. For dry and scaly seborrhea (seborrhea sicca), a different preparation is needed than for oily and greasy seborrhea (seborrhea oleosa). Sulfur, for instance, is useful in dry seborrhea, but is not a good degreaser. Benzoyl peroxide, on the other hand, degreases well, but can be too keratolytic and drying for dry, brittle skin. The following discussion may help the clinician understand the differences and uses, and help distinguish the correct medication from among the myriad of commercially available pharmaceuticals.

Antiseborrheic drugs include keratolytic and keratoplastic ingredients. Keratolytic agents facilitate decreased cohesion among corneocytes, desquamation, and shedding, resulting in a softening of the stratum corneum with easy removal of scale. They do not dissolve keratin. Keratoplastic agents attempt to renormalize the keratinization and abnormal epithelialization that is present in keratinization disorders. The complete mechanism of these effects is not known, although some keratoplastic agents (particularly tar) are believed to normalize epidermal proliferation by decreasing deoxyribonucleic acid (DNA) production with a resultant decrease in the mitotic index of the epidermal basal cells. Follicular flushing is a term used to describe agents that help remove follicular secretions, remove bacteria, and decrease follicular hyperkeratosis. The most common major ingredients in antiseborrheic shampoos include tars, sulfur, salicylic acid, benzoyl peroxide, and selenium sulfide. Other commonly included active agents are urea, glycerine, and lactic acid. In an ultrasonographic biomicroscopic study of the ability of shampoos to remove scale from the skin of dogs,[44] selenium sulfide and colloidal oatmeal were the most effective, tar and sulfur-salicylic acid were moderately effective, and benzoyl peroxide, ethyl lactate, and chlorhexidine were ineffective.

Sulfur is both keratoplastic and keratolytic, probably through the interaction of sulfur with cysteine in keratinocytes. It is a mild follicular flushing agent, but not a good degreaser. Sulfur is also antibacterial, antifungal, and antiparasitic, and these actions are attributed to the formation of pentathionic acid and hydrogen sulfide. The smaller the sulfur particles are (colloidal are smaller than precipitated), the greater the efficacy. The best keratolytic action occurs when sulfur is incorporated in petrolatum. This is in sharp contrast to the findings with salicylic acid, which produces its effect faster when employed in an emulsion base. The keratolytic effect of sulfur results from its superficial effect on the horny layer and the formation of hydrogen sulfide. The keratoplastic effect is caused by the deeper action of the sulfur on the basal layer of the epidermis and by the formation of cystine.

In the shampoos marketed in North America by the well-recognized manufacturers of dermatologicals, a pure sulfur product cannot be purchased. Because of the synergistic activity between sulfur and salicylic acid, all "sulfur" shampoos contain both ingredients. Popular sulfur shampoos include DermaPet Seborrheic shampoo (DermaPet), SebaLyt (DVM Pharmaceuticals), SeboRx (DVM Pharmaceuticals), Micro Pearls Advantage SebaMoist shampoo (EVSCO), Micropearls Advantage SebaHex shampoo (EVSCO), and Sebolux (Virbac).

Salicylic acid (0.1% to 2%) is keratoplastic and exerts a favorable influence on the new formation of the keratinous layer. It is also mildly antipruritic and bacteriostatic. In stronger concentrations (3% to 6%), it solubilizes the intercellular "cement," thus acting as a keratolytic agent, causing shedding and softening of the stratum corneum. When salicylic acid is combined with sulfur, it is believed that a synergistic effect occurs. A common combination is a 2% to 6% concentration of each drug. In human dermatologic practice, a 40% salicylic acid plaster is used to treat calluses and warts.

Tar preparations are derived from destructive distillation of bituminous coal or wood. Birch tar, juniper tar, and coal tar are crude products listed in order of increasing capacity to irritate. Coal tar solution (5%, 10%, or 20%) produces a milder, more readily managed effect. Coal tar solution contains only 20% of the coal tar present in coal tar extract or refined tar. Most pharmaceutical preparations for dermatologic use have been highly refined to decrease the staining effect and the strong odor. In this refining process, some of the beneficial effects of tar are lost, and its potential carcinogenic danger is also decreased. Unadulterated tar products have no place in small animal practice because of their toxicity and tendency to cause local irritation. Cats are especially sensitive to coal tar. All tars are odiferous, potentially irritating and photosensitizing, and carcinogenic. Some tars may stain light-colored coats. In one of the author's (DWS) experience, tars are the most irritating topical antiseborrheic medications in veterinary dermatology, and he does not use tar-containing topical preparations.

Tar shampoos are widely used, however, and seem to be helpful in managing seborrhea. They are keratolytic, keratoplastic, and mildly degreasing. As with sulfur shampoos, tar products usually contain other ingredients, usually sulfur and salicylic acid. Two pure tar products are marketed: Clear Tar shampoo (VRx) and Micro Pearls Advantage Tar Moisturizing shampoo (EVSCO). Popular combination products include LyTar (DVM Pharmaceuticals), NuSal T (DVM Pharmaceuticals), Mycodex High Potency Tar and Sulfur shampoo (Pfizer), Mycodex Tar and Sulfur Pet shampoo (Pfizer), Allerseb-T (Virbac), and T-Lux (Virbac).

Benzoyl peroxide (2.5% to 5%) is keratolytic, antibacterial, degreasing, antipruritic, and follicular flushing. It is metabolized in the skin to benzoic acid, which lyses intercellular substance in the horny layer to account for its keratolytic effect. It is not a stable ingredient and should not be repackaged, diluted, or mixed with other products. Benzoyl peroxide is drying, can induce a contact dermatitis (in less than 10% of patients), and bleaches hair, clothing, and furniture. Skin tumor–promoting activity has been documented in laboratory rodents, but no such activity has been documented in any other species.[55]

Benzoyl peroxide is available as a 5% gel (OxyDex, DVM Pharmaceuticals) and (Pyoben, Virbac) and as a 2.5% to 3% shampoo (DermaPet Benzoyl Peroxide shampoo, DermaPet; OxyDex, DVM Pharmaceuticals; Micro Pearls Advantage Benzoyl-plus shampoo, EVSCO; Mycodex Benzoyl Peroxide Pet shampoo, Pfizer; and Pyoben, Virbac). Two products are available that also contain sulfur (DermaPet Benzoyl Peroxide Plus shampoo, DermaPet; SulfOxyDex, DVM Pharmaceuticals). Only reputable benzoyl peroxide products should be used, because poor products have short shelf lives, little activity, or increased irritation potential. Because of its potent degreasing action, benzoyl peroxide excessively dries out normal skin with prolonged use, and it is generally contraindicated in the presence of dry skin or significant irritation, or both.[56] A study showed that benzoyl peroxide combined with a liposome-based (Novasome microvesicles) humectant (Micro Pearls Advantage Benzoyl Peroxide shampoo) eliminates or minimizes this drying effect.[55] Pyoben, because of its spherulite formulation, should also be minimally drying.

Selenium sulfide alters the epidermal turnover rate and interferes with the hydrogen bond formation in keratin. It is keratolytic, keratoplastic, and very degreasing. At this writing, there are no selenium sulfide shampoos marketed specifically for veterinary use in North America. The human product that contains 1% selenium sulfide (Selsun Blue, Abbot Laboratories) is effective in dogs and usually is not too irritating.

In human medicine, there are dozens of keratolytic and keratoplastic agents marketed in the cream, gel, or ointment formulation. Very few are marketed in veterinary medicine, and most are generic products, e.g. 10% sulfur ointment, ichthammol ointment, zinc oxide, and thuja or those marketed for other purposes, for example, petroleum jelly, udder balm. KeraSolv Gel (DVM Pharmaceuticals) contains 6.6% salicylic acid, 5% sodium lactate, and 5% urea in a propylene glycol gel and is an effective local treatment for hyperkeratotic lesions, for example, nasal hyperkeratosis.

In the process of removing the excessive scale or grease, antiseborrheic products can damage the stratum corneum and alter the hydration of the epidermis.[10-13] Excessively low humidity can cause similar alterations. Emollients and moisturizers are used to counteract these effects.

Emollients are agents that soften or soothe the skin, whereas moisturizers increase the water content of the stratum corneum. Both types of drugs are useful in hydrating and softening the skin. Many of the occlusive emollients are actually oils (safflower, sesame, and mineral oil) or contain lanolin. These emollients decrease transepidermal water loss and cause moisturization. These agents work best if they are applied immediately after saturation of the stratum corneum with water. For maximal softening, the skin should be hydrated in wet dressings, dried, and covered with an occlusive hydrophobic oil. The barrier to water loss can be further strengthened by covering the local lesion with plastic wrap under a bandage. Nonocclusive emollients are relatively ineffective in retaining moisture. Examples of emollients include vegetable oils (olive, cottonseed, corn, and peanut oil), animal oils (lard, whale oil, anhydrous lanolin, and lanolin with 25% to 30% water), silicones, hydrocarbons (paraffin and petrolatum [mineral oil]), and waxes (white wax [bleached beeswax], yellow wax [beeswax], and spermaceti). Hygroscopic (humectant) agents are moisturizers that work by being incorporated into the stratum corneum and attracting water. These agents draw water from the deep epidermis and dermis, and from the environment *if* the relative humidity is greater than 70%.[18] These agents, such as propylene glycol, glycerin, colloidal oatmeal, urea, sodium lactate, and lactic acid, may also be applied between baths. Both occlusive and hygroscopic agents are found in a variety of veterinary spray and cream rinse formulations, which are matched to a corresponding shampoo, for example, HyLyt*efa cream rinse and shampoo (DVM Pharmaceuticals).[10-13]

The addition of novasomes or spherulites to veterinary antiseborrheics has increased the efficacy of the products while decreasing the labor intensity of the treatments. As discussed in Chapter 3, these are tiny capsules incorporated into shampoos that adhere to the skin and hair and remain there after rinsing. In a time-dependent fashion, some of the capsules disintegrate and release either water and lipids (novasomes) or active ingredients with or without moisturizers (spherulites). Because of the newness of these products, the number of studies documenting their efficacy is limited. In one study, Micro Pearls Advantage Hydra-Pearls Cream Rinse (EVSCO) was shown to be superior to a traditional humectant emollient (Humilac, Virbac) for the treatment of dry skin in dogs.[54] In a study on epidermal hydration, nine dogs had areas of their skin treated with water or Sebolux (Virbac), a sulfur/salicylic acid shampoo with spherulites. The shampoo-treated area had greater hydration than either the control or water-treated areas.[23] These preliminary data suggest that these modified shampoos have prolonged periods of action, and that cream rinses may be an unnecessary step in many treatment protocols.

Systemic antiseborrheic agents are used primarily in the treatment of the congenitohereditary seborrheic disorders (see Chapter 12). Because most of the generalized secondary seborrheas are due to altered environmental conditions, dietary deficiency, metabolic abnormalities, or other correctable disorders, systemic treatments are rarely considered and probably would be of little value. These agents might be of some value in those idiopathic conditions in which the defect appears to be due to altered keratinization, for example, feline acne.

Retinoids are the most commonly used systemic antiseborrheic agents in veterinary medicine. Retinoids refer to all the chemicals, natural or synthetic, that have vitamin A activity. Synthetic retinoids are primarily retinol, retinoic acid, or retinal derivatives or analogs. They have been developed with the intent of amplifying certain biologic effects while being less toxic than their natural precursors. More than 1500 synthetic retinoids have been developed and evaluated.[37,46] Different synthetic drugs, all classed as synthetic retinoids, may have profoundly different pharmacologic effects, side effects, and disease indications.

Naturally occurring vitamin A is an alcohol, all-*trans* retinol. It is oxidized in the body to retinal and retinoic acid. Each of these compounds has variable metabolic and biological activities, although both are important in the induction and maintenance of normal growth and differentiation of keratinocytes. Only retinol has all of the known functions of vitamin A. The two most widely used retinoids in veterinary dermatology were isotretinoin (13-cis-retinoic acid; Accutane, Roche), synthesized as a natural metabolite of retinol, and etretinate (Tegison, Roche), a synthetic retinoid. Etretinate is no longer available because tissue residues in humans can persist for years after drug withdrawal and might result in fetal defects.[45] It was replaced with acitretin (Soriatane, Roche), a free-acid metabolite of etretinate. Acitretin appears to be comparable to etretinate in efficacy and acute toxicity, but because it has a much shorted terminal elimination half-life (2 days versus etretinate's 100 days), its long-term safety should be better. It is available in 10- and 25-mg liquid-filled capsules, which come in prescription packs of 30 capsules. At this writing, each capsule costs between $8.00 and $10.00. To date, the only information available on its efficacy in dogs comes from anecdotal reports on the Internet. It appears to be as safe and effective as etretinate when given at 1 mg/kg q24h. Unless it is shown that lower dosages are equally as effective, the expense of acitretin will preclude its use.

The biological effects of retinoids are numerous and diverse, but their ability to regulate proliferation, growth, and differentiation of epithelial tissues is their major benefit in dermatology. They also affect proteases, prostaglandins, humoral and cellular immunity, and cellular adhesion and communication.[45] Isotretinoin is usually given in a dose of 1 to 3 mg/kg q12 to 24h hours and appears to be indicated in diseases that require alteration or normalization of adnexal structures, although some epidermal diseases may respond.[37] Diseases in which isotretinoin has been reported to be effective in veterinary dermatology include Schnauzer comedo syndrome,[37] sebaceous adenitis (particularly early in the disease in Poodles and Vizslas or shorthaired breeds),[37, 46, 61] ichthyosis,[37] feline acne,[37] epitheliotropic lymphoma,[37, 46, 65] keratoacanthoma,[26, 37, 46, 61] and sebaceous gland hyperplasias and adenomas.[46] Isotretinoin has been ineffective for primary idiopathic seborrhea of Cocker spaniels and Basset hounds, and epidermal dysplasia of West Highland White terriers.[21, 37, 46] It was also ineffective in the treatment of preneoplastic and squamous cell carcinoma lesions in cats.[20]

Toxicity of isotretinoin in the dog and cat appears to be less of a problem than in humans.[37, 46] In the dog, conjunctivitis, hyperactivity, pruritus, pedal and mucocutaneous junction erythema, stiffness, vomiting, diarrhea, and keratoconjunctivitis may be noted. Laboratory abnormalities that are generally not associated with clinical signs include hypertriglyceridemia, hypercholesterolemia, and increased levels of alanine aminotransferase, aspartate aminotransferase, and alkaline phosphatase.[37, 46] In cats, conjunctivitis, diarrhea, anorexia, and vomiting have been the major side effects noted.[37, 46, 59] These side effects may be transient or self-limited with discontinuation or decrease in dose of the drug. With long-term use, skeletal abnormalities, including cortical hyperostosis, periosteal calcification, and long bone demineralization, are a concern.[19, 37, 45, 46] All retinoids are potent teratogens.

Etretinate or acitretin are indicated in disorders of epithelial or follicular development or keratinization.[25] Most commonly, etretinate is given at 1 mg/kg every 24 hours. Etretinate is reportedly effective for primary idiopathic seborrhea of Cocker and Springer spaniels,[37, 46, 59] Golden retrievers, Irish setters, and some mixed breeds. It has not been effective in most West Highland White terriers, Basset hounds, or collies,[37, 46] but exceptions have been noted.[59] Etretinate can also be effective in the treatment of ichthyosis, solar dermatitis, squamous cell carcinoma, keratoacanthomas, and sebaceous adenitis.[26, 40, 46, 59] Dogs with follicular dysplasias such as color dilution alopecia may also respond with less scaling and partial hair growth.[26]

Toxicity with etretinate is similar to that seen with isotretinoin. In humans, etretinate is considered safer for long-term use because of a lower propensity for producing skeletal abnormalities. However, it is considered more of a teratogen and should be used only in spayed females, nonbreeding males, or female dogs that will not be used for breeding. Teratogenicity may persist even 2 years after cessation of therapy.[45, 46] Monitoring for both synthetic retinoids includes pretreatment measurement of tear production, hemogram, chemistry profile, and urinalysis. This is repeated in 1 to 2 months and, if no problems are detected, then repeated only as deemed necessary.[46] Because experience with increased triglyceride levels shows that they normalize when animals are receiving low-fat diets, it is recommended that dogs being given etretinate may benefit from changing to such a diet.[46]

A topical (calcipotriene or calcipotriol) or systemic vitamin D analog, especially 1,25-dihydroxyvitamin D_3 (calcitrol), is used in the treatment of psoriasis in humans[15, 25, 39, 47, 48] and a preliminary clinical trial was conducted in a small number of Cocker spaniels with primary seborrhea.[38] These agents were developed to maintain the positive impact of vitamin D on keratinization but minimize the hormonal influence on calcium and phosphorus metabolism. Vitamin D analogs inhibit keratinocyte proliferation, induce terminal differentiation of keratinocytes, and decrease immunologic reactivity by reduced production or transcription of various cytokines and reduced antigen-presenting function of Langerhans cells.[15, 25, 39] When calcitrol was given at 10 ng/kg q24h to seborrheic Cocker spaniels, significant improvement was noted in approximately two thirds of the dogs.[38] No adverse reactions were noted, but because these compounds influence calcium metabolism and accidental overdosing can be fatal,[7] the patient should have its PTH, calcium, and phosphorus levels monitored at least weekly.

Cytostatic or cytotoxic drugs have received wide usage in humans with psoriasis.[15] The most recent addition to the armamentarium is oral cyclosporine, which improves the clinical lesions by downregulating the proinflammatory epidermal cytokines.[47] Because cytotoxic treatments have anecdotal efficacy in the treatment of primary seborrhea in dogs[59] and cyclosporine is receiving wider usage in this species, cyclosporine might have some place in the treatment of serious disorders of keratinization.

• CANINE SEBORRHEA

Seborrhea is a chronic skin disease of dogs that is characterized by a defect in keratinization with increased scale formation, excessive greasiness of the skin and haircoat, and sometimes by secondary inflammation. Some patients are both flaky and greasy, depending on the region of the body involved. Ingrained in the veterinary literature are the terms seborrhea sicca, seborrhea oleosa, and seborrheic dermatitis. *Seborrhea sicca* denotes dryness of the skin and coat. There is focal or diffuse scaling of the skin with the accumulation of white to gray nonadherent scales, and the coat is dull and dry (Fig. 14–1A). *Seborrhea oleosa* is the opposite; the skin and hairs are greasy (see Fig. 14–1B). The greasy keratosebaceous debris is best appreciated by touch and smell. The malodor of dogs with severe seborrhea oleosa is tremendous. *Seborrheic dermatitis* is characterized by scaling and greasiness, with gross evidence of local or diffuse inflammation (see Fig. 14–1C). It is often associated with folliculitis. Animals with seborrhea oleosa or seborrheic dermatitis should be examined carefully for *Malassezia* yeast. The lipolytic nature of this organism worsens an already greasy skin condition. In addition, *Malassezia* yeast increase the proliferation rate of keratinocytes,[63] creating a vicious circle. The initial seborrheic condition encouraged yeast overgrowth, and then the yeast continue to stimulate seborrheic change. In advanced cases, the initial seborrheic condition could have been resolved, but the patient's clinical condition will remain the same until the yeast are eliminated. Classic *localized* seborrheic dermatitis has circular lesions with alopecia, erythema, marginal epidermal scaling, and later hyperpigmentation (see Fig. 14–1D). This condition must be differentiated from other disorders that cause similar lesions.

These three terms appropriately describe the dog's clinical appearance and aid in initial shampoo selection, but they cannot be used to direct the diagnostic effort to find the cause of the seborrhea. Individuals respond to the same seborrheic insult in different manners. Although most fatty acid–deficient dogs have dull, dry, and flaky coats, some are greasy, and a dog with early generalized demodicosis may be either flaky or greasy. Regardless of the nature of the seborrhea, all causes of seborrhea should be considered and excluded only by the appropriate testing.

Etiologically, seborrhea is classified into primary and secondary types. Primary sebor-

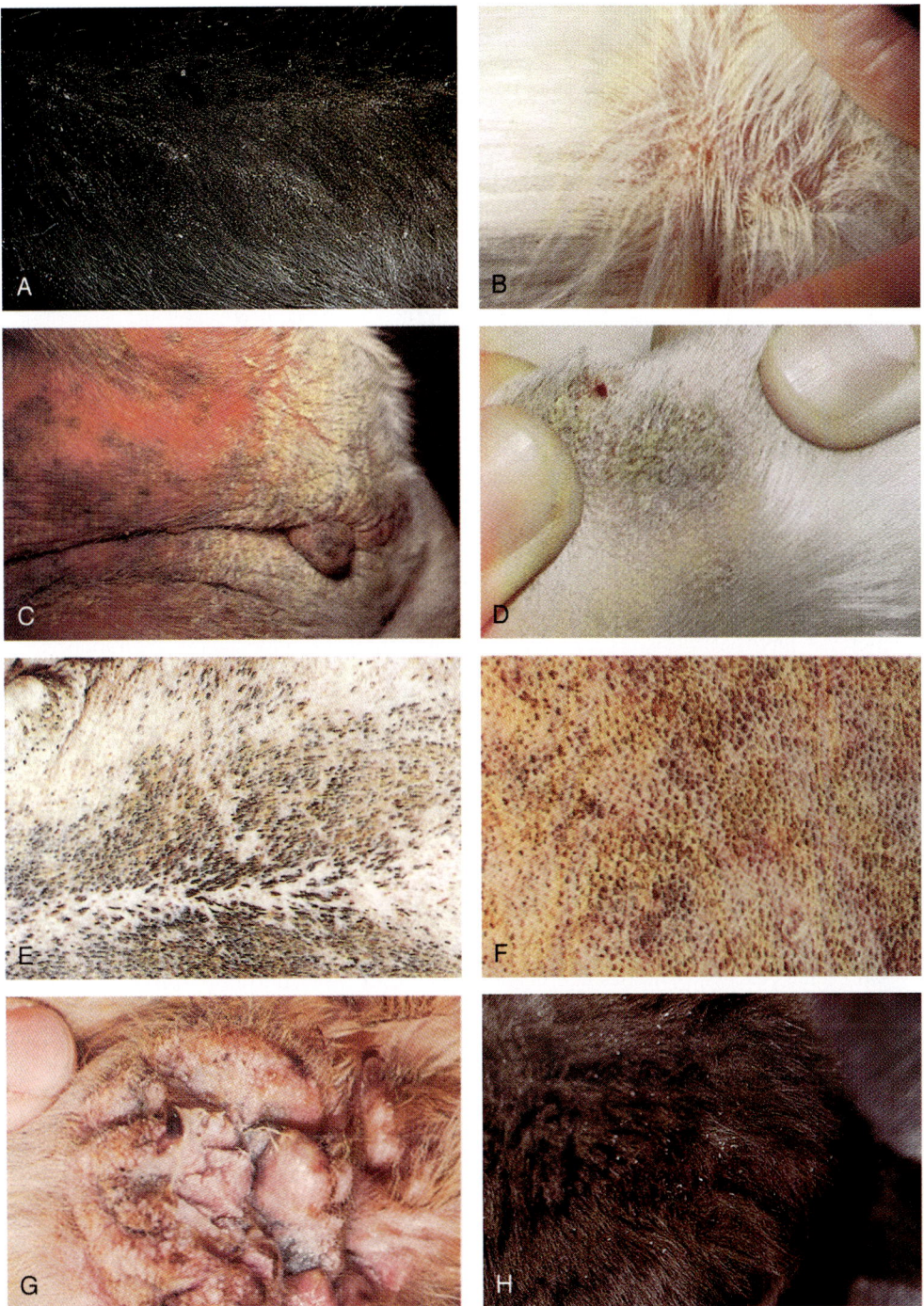

FIGURE 14–1. *A*, Severe flaking in a dog with a fatty acid deficiency. *B*, Greasy seborrhea in a dog with chronic liver disease. Note that the greasy material adheres to the hairs and stains them. *C*, Diffuse seborrheic dermatitis in a hypothyroid dog. *D*, Focal seborrheic dermatitis in a dog with vitamin A–responsive dermatosis. *E*, Vitamin A–responsive dermatosis in a Cocker spaniel. Marked comedo formation on the abdomen. *F*, Vitamin A–responsive dermatosis. Same dog as in *E*. Close-up of follicular plugging. *G*, Vitamin A–responsive dermatosis. Same dog as in *E* and *F*. Severe ceruminous otitis externa. *H*, Flaking in a cat caused by too low an environmental humidity level.

rhea is an inherited disorder of epidermal hyperproliferation and is discussed in Chapter 12. It is most commonly seen in American Cocker spaniels, English Springer spaniels, West Highland White terriers, and Basset hounds, but Irish setters, Doberman pinschers, Chinese Shar peis, dachshunds, Labrador retrievers, and German shepherds are at increased risk.[34, 59] However, not all individuals within those breeds are affected. A veterinarian does the owner and animal a great injustice if seborrheic signs in a dog of those breeds are immediately classified as primary seborrhea. The diagnosis of primary seborrhea is tenable only if the signs started early in life and appropriate diagnostic tests have failed to reveal a cause for the keratinization defect.

Secondary seborrheas are those caused by some external or internal insult that alters the proliferation, differentiation, or desquamation of the surface and follicular epithelium.[33] Virtually any disorder discussed in this textbook can result in seborrheic signs during the acute or healing phase of the disease.

Cause and Pathogenesis

Any disorder that alters cellular proliferation, differentiation, or desquamation produces seborrheic signs. In most instances, the mechanisms by which the following seborrhea-inducing factors cause their changes are incompletely understood.

- **Inflammation.** Inflammatory skin diseases are typically characterized by epidermal hyperplasia,[27] which probably results from the release or production of dermal eicosanoids, histamine, and cytokines. Leukotriene B4 (LTB_4) concentrations have been reported to be increased in the skin lesions of dogs with seborrhea.[31] Both LTB_4 and prostaglandin E_2 increase DNA synthesis in the basal layer and stimulate epidermal proliferation.[36, 62] If the inflammation is mild, seborrheic signs can develop in the absence of pruritus. Examples include grooming that is too vigorous,[2] demodicosis, dermatophytosis, cheyletiellosis, lice, low-grade contact dermatitis, and early epitheliotropic lymphoma.

- **Endocrine Factors.** Hormones influence cellular proliferation[59] and serum and cutaneous lipid profiles.[9, 60] Although all hormonal imbalances can cause seborrhea, spontaneous or iatrogenic hyperadrenocorticism and hypothyroidism are the most common causes (see Chap. 10). In hyperadrenocorticism, other signs of the disease are usually present; in contrast, some hypothyroid dogs are perfectly normal aside from the seborrhea.

- **Nutritional Factors.** Glucose, protein, essential fatty acids,[9, 14] and various vitamins and trace minerals are necessary for normal cellular proliferation and differentiation. Deficiency, excess, or imbalance in one or more of these nutrients can produce seborrhea (see Chap. 17). Because the vast majority of pets in developed countries eat high-quality, balanced diets, nutritional seborrheas are very uncommon.[9] When they do occur, they usually are secondary to malabsorption or maldigestion[29] or metabolic disease, especially hypothyroidism.[8]

- **Environmental Factors.** The water and lipid content of the skin is important to maintain normal invisible desquamation.[9-11, 33] If transepidermal water loss increases, desquamation changes and the squames (packets of dead cells) become visible. Low environmental humidity, excessive bathing (especially with harsh products), and fatty acid deficiency can produce this change.

As can be seen from the above-mentioned factors, virtually any disease can cause seborrhea and can do so by many different mechanisms.

Clinical Features

The clinical signs of secondary seborrhea include flakiness, greasiness, seborrheic dermatitis, ceruminous otitis externa, or some combination of these. The nature, distribution, and severity of the signs depend on the cause of the seborrhea and the individual patient. In general, systemic causes (e.g., endocrine disease, dietary deficiency, hepatic or gastrointestinal disease, and primary or secondary lipid abnormalities) result in generalized signs that

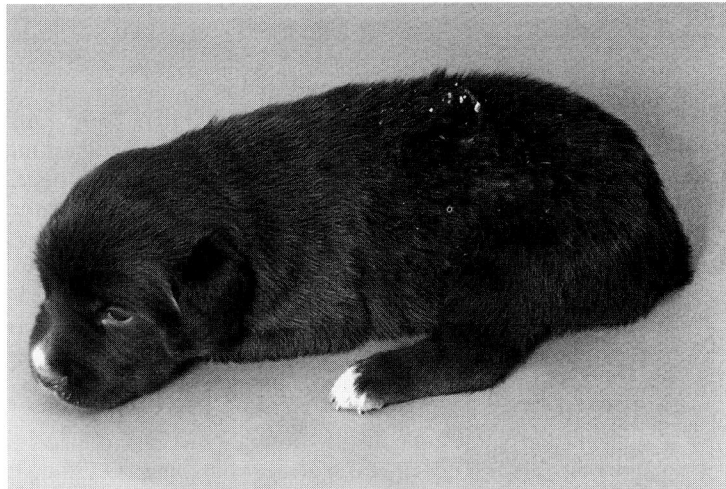

FIGURE 14–2. Secondary seborrhea. Dishevelment of the coat with seborrheic change in the saddle and flank region of a puppy.

are not pruritic at their onset. These animals can become pruritic, however, as the seborrhea worsens or if there is a secondary staphylococcal or *Malassezia* overgrowth. They often have more pronounced seborrheic changes around the face, feet (especially interdigitally), intertriginous areas, and perineum. Allergic disorders, although systemic diseases, tend to cause regionalized seborrheic changes, and pruritus precedes the seborrheic changes.

Except for low environmental humidity and overzealous or inappropriate topical treatments (e.g., excessive bathing, dipping, or powdering, contact dermatitis to a shampoo), external causes (e.g., cheyletiellosis, demodicosis, dermatophytosis) result in focal, multifocal, or regionalized signs of secondary seborrhea (Figs. 14–2 and 14–3). At examination, these dogs have areas of normal skin. Sebaceous adenitis, a disorder that results in the destruction of most, if not all, sebaceous glands often is initially regionalized to the face and dorsum of the trunk.

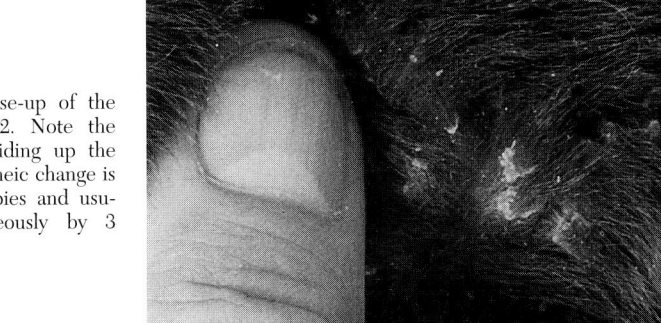

FIGURE 14–3. Close-up of the puppy in Figure 14–2. Note the large flakes of scale riding up the hair shafts. This seborrheic change is fairly common in puppies and usually resolves spontaneously by 3 months of age.

thus allows better contact of the antiseborrheic product with the skin. In general, the sulfur and salicylic acid products are less potent than the pure tar products, and those are less potent than the tar combination products. Benzoyl peroxide, with or without sulfur, and the selenium sulfide shampoos are the most potent and can remove a tremendous amount of scale and grease with just one bath. In addition to decreasing the surface lipids, strong tars, selenium sulfide, and benzoyl peroxide shampoos increase transepidermal water loss and must be used cautiously.[10, 12, 55]

After the quick cleansing bath, the antiseborrheic product should be applied. Owners should be cautioned not to apply a heavy strip of shampoo down the animal's back. This all too common technique wastes shampoo and can irritate the skin on the dorsum because it is difficult to rinse all of the product from the skin. With concentrated shampoos, the client should be instructed to put an ounce or so of the shampoo into a container of warm water. This shampoo solution is then sparingly poured over the dog. Shampoos marketed in spray bottles are also designed to more evenly disperse the shampoo.

After the dog has been lathered with the antiseborrheic product, the shampoo must remain in contact with the skin for 10 to 15 minutes for maximum effect. Gentle manipulation of the dog's skin during this waiting period tends to keep the dog content and increases the cleansing action of the shampoo. After 10 to 15 minutes, the dog should be rinsed thoroughly. It should take two to three times longer for the rinsing than it did for the lathering. Prolonged rinsing not only removes the debris and shampoo but also aids in hydration of the skin. Many dry dogs become flaky again soon after the bath, especially when the environmental humidity is low. The application of an after-bath cream rinse or emollient spray helps provide a barrier to transepidermal water loss and its associated drying.[54] Although any after-bath rinse can be effective, studies have shown that those containing oils, and especially linoleic acid, are most effective in decreasing transepidermal water loss.[11] If the client keeps some diluted product in a misting bottle and sprays it on the dog as needed, the frequency of bathing can often be reduced.

For greasy dogs, the shampoos used are stronger.[24, 35] Greasy dogs often need an after-bath rinse, especially if the humidity level is low. All strong shampoos can disrupt the epidermal barrier and increase transepidermal water loss, with resultant worsening of the seborrhea.[11] An afterbath rinse can prevent this, but it may make the dog too greasy. Each case must be approached on its own merits.

In occasional cases, the cause of the secondary seborrhea can be identified but not corrected; common examples include low winter humidity and intentional fatty acid deficiency for weight loss or control of pancreatitis or abnormalities in lipid metabolism. In these cases, bathing and moisturizing must be continued at some maintenance level. The application of moisturizers containing fat can be beneficial in these animals.[10]

• VITAMIN A–RESPONSIVE DERMATOSIS

A vitamin A–responsive dermatosis has been described primarily in Cocker spaniels, but it has also been recognized in a Labrador retriever and a miniature Schnauzer.[28, 30, 43, 51, 52] In these dogs, the condition is characterized by an adult-onset, medically refractory seborrheic skin disease, wherein marked follicular plugging and hyperkeratotic plaques with surface fronds are typically seen (see Fig. 14–1E and F). The follicular plugging and hyperkeratotic plaques are especially prominent on the ventral and lateral chest and abdomen. Other lesions include varying degrees of focal crusting, scaling, alopecia, and follicular papules. A ceruminous otitis externa is usually present (see Fig. 14–1G). A generally dry, dull, disheveled, easily epilated haircoat is present, along with a rancid skin odor and mild to moderate pruritus. Except for the skin disease, the dogs are generally healthy.

K. W. Kwochka (personal communications) and the authors have recognized a group of Gordon setters with a vitamin A–responsive condition that differs in its clinical presentation. Instead of a seborrheic presentation, these dogs have a pruritic disorder, especially over their dorsums, with a papular dermatitis in the pruritic regions. Treatment with antibiotics resolves the papular dermatitis and lessens the pruritus but a relapse can be expected when the antibiotic is withdrawn. Allergy testing is inconclusive, and skin biopsies show the disproportionate follicular hyperkeratosis of vitamin A–responsive dermatosis. Treatment with vitamin A alcohol results in resolution of the rash and pruritus, and the dog remains normal with continued treatment.

The marked follicular plugging that occurs in these dogs is highly suggestive of this disease. In the absence of systemic signs of hyperadrenocorticism, only sebaceous adenitis (see Chap. 18), true vitamin A deficiency or hypervitaminosis A (see Chap. 17), atypical generalized demodicosis (see Chap. 6), and follicular dysplasia (see Chaps. 11 and 12) produce such profound follicular changes. The clinical lesions are characterized histologically by profound, disproportionately marked follicular orthokeratotic hyperkeratosis (Fig. 14–5). At present, the final diagnosis of vitamin A–responsive dermatosis can be confirmed only by response to treatment.

Treatment consists of 10,000 U vitamin A (retinol) given orally, once daily with a fatty meal. Improvement can be expected in 3 weeks, with complete clinical remission in 8 to 10 weeks. Treatment should be continued for life because the lesions and symptoms reappear when treatment is discontinued.

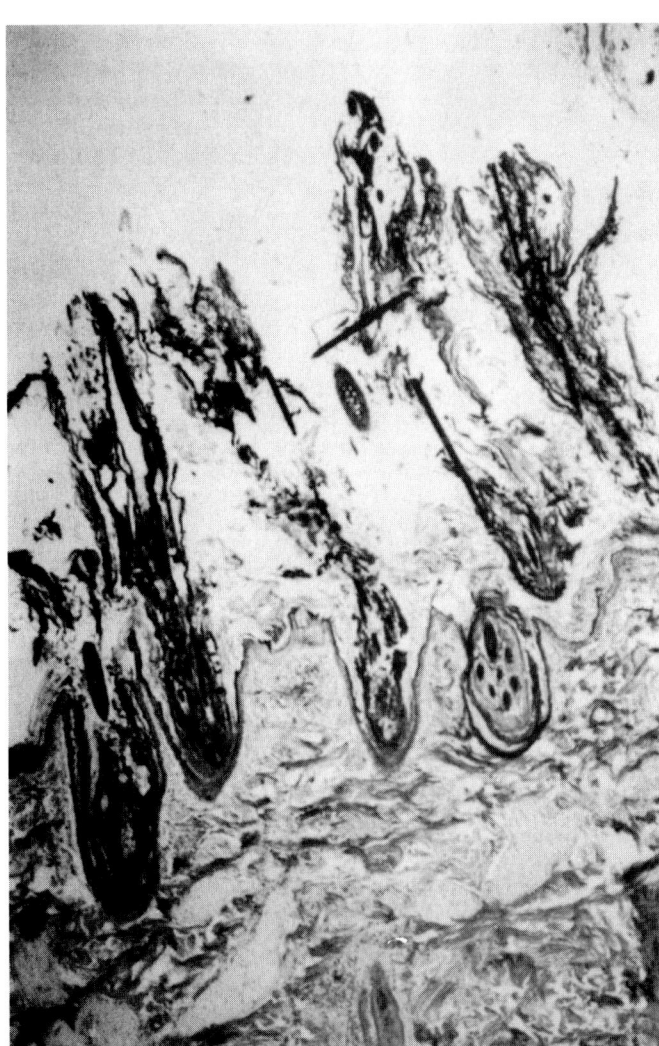

FIGURE 14–5. Vitamin A–responsive dermatosis. Disproportionate orthokeratotic hyperkeratosis of multiple hair follicles.

• FELINE SEBORRHEA

Primary seborrhea is very rare in cats (see Chap. 12). Although cats suffer from many of the disorders that cause secondary seborrhea in dogs,[51] seborrheic signs are uncommon in this species. Cats' fastidious grooming habits, which remove scales quickly, may be partially responsible for this lower incidence.

When cats do become seborrheic, they usually have seborrhea sicca, with fine white or gray flakes and scales in the coat (see Fig. 14–1H). When the signs are fairly generalized and the cat is not pruritic, dietary deficiency, intestinal parasitism, low environmental humidity, diabetes mellitus, hyperthyroidism, cheyletiellosis, and pediculosis are the primary differentials.[51, 59] Contact dermatitis and overzealous shampooing or powdering could be added to the list, but these causes are easily excluded through the history. With pruritus or more localized lesions, demodicosis, dermatophytosis, lymphocytic mural folliculitis (see Chap. 11), and allergy must be considered. Greasy seborrheic signs (seborrhea oleosa) (Fig. 14–6A) are extraordinarily rare in the cat and usually indicate severe chronic hepatic, pancreatic, or intestinal disease, drug eruption, or systemic lupus erythematosus.[51, 59] As in dogs, some cats with the disorders just mentioned will have dry flaky skin (Fig. 14–7), so any one disease cannot be included or excluded just on the nature of the seborrheic change.

As in dogs, correction of the cause for the seborrhea results in spontaneous resolution of the signs. Bathing can help hasten the cat's response but is not widely done because most cats are intolerant of repeated bathing. With the exception of products that contain tar, selenium, quaternary ammonium compounds, or phenol, shampoos used on dogs can also be used on cats. Caution is warranted with benzoyl peroxide, because it can cause variable degrees of irritation in about 25% of the cats treated.

• NASODIGITAL HYPERKERATOSIS

Nasodigital hyperkeratosis is characterized by increased amounts of horny tissue originating from and tightly adherent to the epidermis of the footpads or nasal planum.

Cause and Pathogenesis

Hyperkeratosis of the nose, footpads, or both can occur as a congenitohereditary disorder, an idiopathic entity, or as a coexistent feature of a variety of disorders. The idiopathic form occurs most commonly in old dogs. It shows no breed or sex predilection and is probably a senile change.[27, 34, 59]

Nasodigital hyperkeratosis can be seen in a variety of disorders but especially in the congenitohereditary disorders of keratinization (see Chap. 12), distemper or leishmaniasis (see Chap. 7), pemphigus foliaceus, drug reaction, or systemic lupus erythematosus (see Chap. 9), zinc-responsive and generic dog food dermatosis (see Chap. 17), necrolytic migratory erythema (see Chap. 10) and cutaneous lymphoma (see Chap. 20). With nasal hyperkeratosis only, discoid lupus erythematosus and pemphigus erythematosus (see Chap. 9) must be considered. If lesions are restricted to the pads, familial pad hyperkeratosis[42] (see Chap. 12) and papillomavirus infection (see Chap. 7) enter the list of differential diagnoses. Except for familial pad hyperkeratosis and papillomavirus, all of the aforementioned disorders usually have lesions in the haired skin and often produce systemic signs of illness. However, some cases have lesions restricted to the nose, footpads, or both, either at their onset or during their entire course.

Clinical Features

The hyperplastic keratin that develops in senile nasodigital hyperkeratosis grows in a variety of shapes, depending on its location, its stage of development, and the variation among individual animals. At times, small verrucous keratin growths appear in a regular

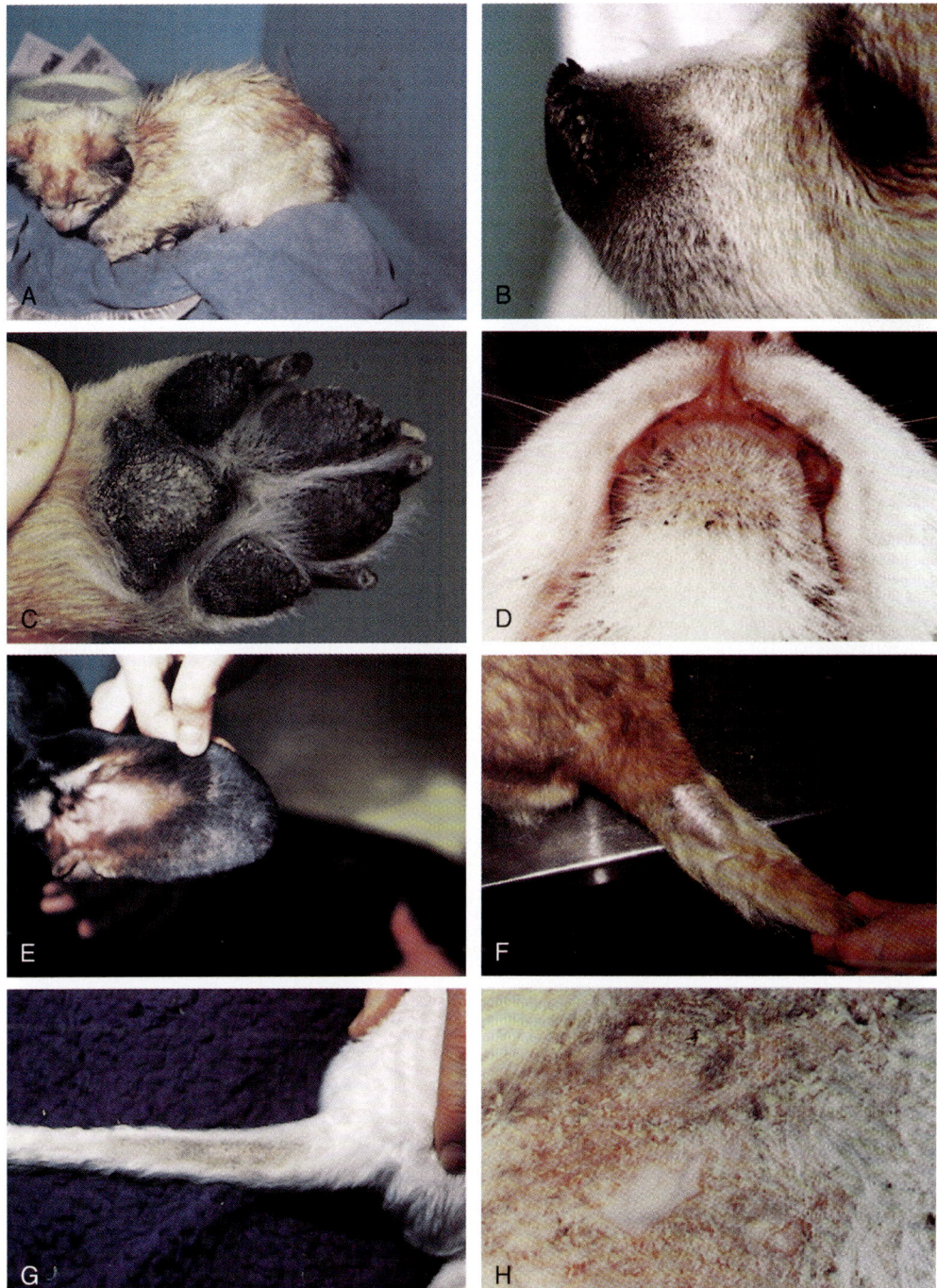

FIGURE 14-6. *A*, Greasy seborrhea in a cat with pancreatic insufficiency. *B*, Nasodigital hyperkeratosis. Note the frondlike hyperkeratosis on the dorsum of the nasal planum. *C*, Nasodigital hyperkeratosis. Same dog as in *B*. Keratin accumulation is most marked at the edges of the pads. *D*, Feline acne. Multiple comedones on the chin. *E*, Ear margin dermatosis with marginal hypotrichosis and scaling. *F*, Canine tail galnd hyperplasia. *G*, Feline tail gland hyperplasia. *H*, Parapsoriasis. Coalescent erythematous, scaly plaques on the abdomen of a dog. A small island of normal skin is visible.

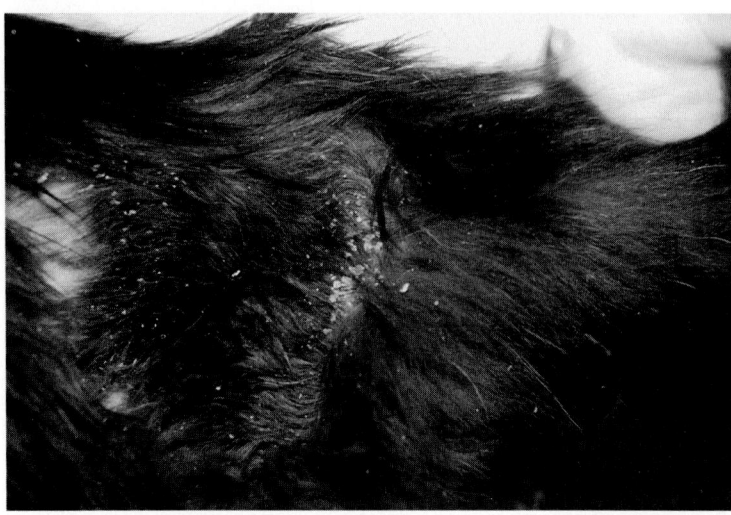

FIGURE 14–7. Dishevelment of the coat with seborrhea sicca in a cat with hepatitis.

pattern. At other times, the keratin is ridged, grooved, or feathered. Dryness is the characteristic common to all lesions. The nasal planum, which is moist, black, soft, and shiny in normal dogs, becomes hard, dry, rough, and hyperkeratotic, especially on the dorsum of the nose (see Fig. 14–6B). Fissures, erosions, and ulcers develop in the dry epidermal tissue.

The digital hyperkeratosis involves the entire surface of all pads but is most pronounced at the edges of weightbearing pads (see Fig. 14–6C) and on the accessory carpal and tarsal pads. The contact surfaces of weightbearing pads are less involved because friction during walking wears down the keratin. The hard, cracked pads contain excess keratin tissue, which makes walking painful, especially for heavy dogs. Fissures and erosions add significantly to the discomfort. Corns form in the feet of some individuals because excess keratin develops into deep, circular plaques.[59] These plaques press into the surrounding footpad and cause pain when pressure is created as the animal walks.

Diagnosis

The diagnosis of simple nasodigital hyperkeratosis can be straightforward or very complicated. If the typical lesions occur in an old dog with no other skin or systemic problems, the diagnosis can be made on the basis of the clinical findings. If the nasodigital hyperkeratosis is present along with other skin lesions in a young to middle-aged dog, or if it occurs with nasal or pedal depigmentation, erythema, erosion, and crusting, all of the disorders mentioned previously must be considered and excluded by means of the appropriate testing.

The diagnosis is confirmed by a biopsy that reveals the characteristic features of idiopathic nasodigital hyperkeratosis and none of the features for the other differential diagnoses. Histopathologic findings in idiopathic nasodigital hyperkeratosis include irregular to papillated epidermal hyperplasia and marked orthokeratotic to parakeratotic hyperkeratosis.

Clinical Management

Because the formation of excess keratin cannot be stopped, treatment must be lifelong and directed toward the softening and removal of the excessive keratin. Because these measures are time consuming and somewhat messy, they are usually reserved for patients in which the hyperkeratosis causes discomfort or fissuring.

Dogs with profound hyperkeratosis should have the excess keratin removed with scissors or a razor blade. After appropriate instruction, many clients can perform the trimming at home and may choose to use it as the sole method of treatment for asymptomatic dogs. In most cases, the trimming is necessary only at the onset of treatment because further keratin buildup is minimized by the application of hydrating and softening agents.

Topical treatment must include hydration and the application of a keratolytic agent. Hydration of the pads is easily accomplished by soaking the feet in water and applying wet compresses to the nose. After 5 to 10 minutes of hydration, the areas are covered with keratolytic agent. Petroleum jelly, ichthamnol ointment, various human dry skin lotions, 50% propylene glycol, 6.6% salicylic acid, 5% sodium lactate, and 5% urea in propylene glycol gel (KeraSolv gel, DVM Pharmaceuticals, Inc.), and tretinoin gel (Retin-A, Ortho) can all be effective.[34, 41, 59] If petroleum jelly or ichthammol are used, the animal must be confined to a crate or the feet must be bandaged so that floors, carpets, and furniture are not stained. When the nose or pads are fissured, ointments containing antibiotics and corticosteroids are indicated.

Typically, daily hydration and softening must be performed for 7 to 10 days to return the nose and pads to near normal. The owners should be warned not to try to remove all of the keratin, because overzealous treatment can remove the normal protective keratin layer and predispose the nose and pads to lacerations and frictional ulcers. When the nose and pads are near normal, some clients prefer to stop all treatments until significant buildup occurs; others prefer to continue treatment once or twice weekly to prevent buildup. Each case must be managed on its own merits. When topical treatment is impossible, isotretinoin or etretinate therapy may be of some benefit, but their efficacy remains unproven.[46]

• ACNE

In humans, acne is a multifactorial disease of the pilosebaceous unit.[22] Acne-prone individuals have an alteration in the pattern of follicular keratinization and produce more sebum than do their normal counterparts. The levels of linoleic acid in sebum from an acne patient are low. Bacteria *(Propionibacterium acnes, Propionibacterium granulosum,* and micrococci) and yeast *(Pityrosporum ovale)* play an important contributory role through their lipolytic action on sebum to produce free fatty acids, the production of inflammatory enzymes (e.g., proteases), and the induction of follicular inflammation. Because androgens stimulate sebum production, patients with systemic hormonal imbalances can have severe acne. Acne patients have increased 5α-reductase activity in their skin. Because this enzyme system converts testosterone to dihydrotestosterone, local hormone influences are probably very important.

Acne in dogs and cats is uncommon and has not been thoroughly studied.[5, 50] Pets with acne have abnormal follicular keratinization; beyond that, however, there probably is little pathomechanistic similarity to human acne. For example, the comedonal lipid profiles from hairless dogs showed a predominance of free sterols, ceramides, and free fatty acids.[3] These lipids are of epidermal rather than sebaceous origin and suggest that the sebaceous glands are minimally important in acne in dogs.

Canine Acne

Although skin lesions are fairly common in the skin of the chin and lips of young dogs, it is doubtful that this is a true acne in which the defect in follicular keratinization arises de novo. Careful inspection of the involved skin rarely reveals comedones; instead, sterile or secondarily infected papules or furuncles are the primary lesions seen. In all likelihood, canine acne is due to a traumatic follicular insult with resultant folliculitis. The subject is discussed in detail under muzzle folliculitis and furunculosis in Chapter 4.

Feline Acne

Feline acne is an uncommon condition that affects cats of any breed or gender and is not confined to adolescence.

CAUSE AND PATHOGENESIS

Feline acne is an idiopathic disorder of follicular keratinization.[5, 50, 51] Although some cats experience only one episode during their lives, many affected cats have cyclic or near-constant disease. Poor grooming habits, an underlying seborrheic predisposition, the production of abnormal sebum, hair cycle influences, stress, direct viral influences, and immunosuppression have all been considered in the pathogenesis.[49, 50, 66] Although each of these would be an aggravating factor, none has been proven causal. Hormonal influences probably play little or no role in the pathogenesis because cases are recognized with equal frequency in males and females.[59]

CLINICAL FEATURES

The earliest lesions are crusts and comedones on the chin, the lower lip, and occasionally, the upper lip (see Fig. 14–6D).[66] At this stage, there are no symptoms associated with the lesions, so they are often overlooked or ignored by the client. Some cases remain in the comedonal stage, but others progress and develop papules and pustules. In severe cases, a suppurative folliculitis, furunculosis, or cellulitis may develop (see Fig. 4–10A) (*Pasteurella multocida*, ß-hemolytic streptococci, staphylococci, *Malassezia*, dermatophytes).[66] In severe cases, the chin and lips can become edematous and thickened, and the cat often scratches or rubs the chin on furniture or other rough surfaces. Regional lymphadenopathy may be prominent. Follicular cysts of variable sizes and scarring are commonplace in chronic cases.

DIAGNOSIS

In most cases, the diagnosis of feline acne is straightforward and is based on the presence of classic lesions on the chin and lips. In the comedonal stage, demodicosis, dermatophytosis, and *Malassezia* infection should be excluded by the appropriate tests. With furuncular lesions, primary or secondary bacterial or fungal infections should be considered and documented by appropriate cytologic and cultural techniques. With pronounced chin edema (the so-called fat chin), an eosinophilic granuloma with collagen flame figures must be considered (see Chap. 18).

Histopathologic findings in feline acne include follicular keratosis, plugging, and dilatation (comedo).[27] In advanced cases, perifolliculitis, folliculitis, and furunculosis with an associated pyogranulomatous dermatitis may be seen (Fig. 14–8).

CLINICAL MANAGEMENT

The need for treatment and intensity of treatment vary from case to case. If the owner does not object to the presence of asymptomatic comedones, no treatment is required. If the lesions are visually objectionable or if they progress to sterile or secondarily infected papules or furuncles or induce pruritus, treatment is required.

Topical therapy is beneficial in all cases and is directed toward the dislodgement and dissolution of the comedone. In many cases, the ease and efficacy of treatment can be increased by clipping the area before treating it. If draining papules and furuncles are admixed with the comedones, the area should be hot packed in a magnesium sulfate (Epsom salt) solution (2 tbsp/quart or 30 ml/L warm water) for 5 to 10 minutes. Soaking promotes drainage and softens the surrounding comedones. Because drainage typically indicates secondary bacterial infection, appropriate antibiotics should be administered orally for 14 to 21 days. Antibiotic selection depends on the invading organism, but clavulanated amoxicillin, a fluoroquinolone, or a cephalosporin are good empiric choices.

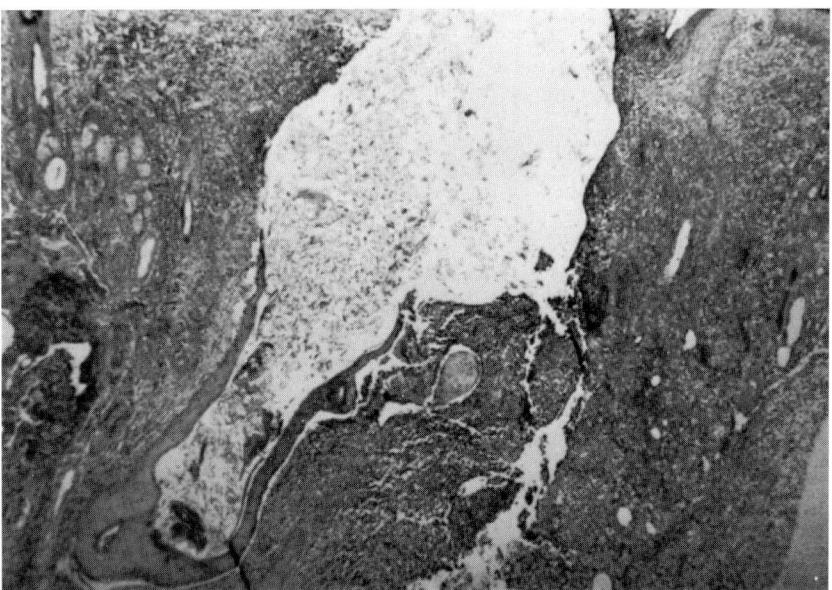

FIGURE 14-8. Feline acne. ruptured comedo (follicular plug) with surrounding pyogranulomatous dermatitis.

Topical treatment with mupirocin (see later) may alleviate the need for systemic antibiotics.

Although alcohol, various human acne cleaning pads, or Listerine antiseptic can be effective comedolytic agents in cats, most investigators dispense antiseborrheic shampoos for daily to twice-weekly use. Sulfur-salicylic acid, ethyl lactate, or benzoyl peroxide products are used.[5, 50] Benzoyl peroxide has pronounced follicular flushing properties but may be too irritating for some cats. Other topical products used in cats include vitamin A acid (Retin-A 0.05% cream) and topical clindamycin, tetracycline, or erythromycin solutions or ointments.[50] Topical metronidazole 0.75% gel has been reported to be useful, perhaps through its combined antibacterial and anti-inflammatory properties.[6] Mupirocin ointment applied twice daily can be very effective.[66] When 25 cats were treated, 24 had a good to excellent response.

After all the papules and comedones have been eliminated, treatment should be discontinued gradually over several weeks. Some cats remain free of lesions for extended periods and others relapse. Once the amount of time that passes before relapse is known, a maintenance cleaning program can be instituted. Those cats with recurrent acne may benefit from fatty acid supplementation.[50]

Aside from antibiotics and fat supplements, systemic therapy is rarely indicated. In cats with severe inflammation, a 10- to 14-day course of oral prednisolone (1 to 2 mg/kg q24h) can be beneficial and may reduce scar tissue formation. Any bacterial infection should be resolved before the corticosteroid is administered. Cats that do not allow topical treatment or are refractory to it may benefit from the oral administration of isotretinoin (2 mg/kg/day).[46, 50] If response is to occur, it should be seen in 30 days. Approximately one third of treated cats respond.[50] Responders require long-term treatment, but the frequency of administration can often be reduced to every 2 or 3 days.

● CANINE EAR MARGIN DERMATOSIS

Marginal seborrhea affecting the pinna of the ear is characterized by numerous small, greasy plugs (follicular casts) adhering to the skin and hairs of the medial and lateral margins. It is most common in Dachshunds but also occurs in other breeds with pendulous ears (see Fig. 14–6E). Sleeping next to a forced air duct or wood stove seems to increase the frequency or severity of disease. The small particles can easily be removed for diagnosis with the thumb nail or a flat instrument. These particles are soft, irregular, and greasy. With time, the scaling becomes more confluent and can involve the entire ear margin, and the condition can be accompanied by partial alopecia of the pinna. In chronic cases, the seborrheic debris on the ear margins, especially at the tips, can become very thick and hard. With head shaking, scratching, or blunt trauma, the hard crust and its subjacent viable tissues can crack and result in an ear fissure (see Chap. 19). The fissure is painful and causes the dog to shake its head, which accelerates the fissuring.

In early cases, the diagnosis of ear margin dermatosis is straightforward. Seborrheic changes are restricted to the ear margin of a dog with pendulous ears. Pruritus and pain are absent. With heavy crusting and fissures, all the causes of vasculitis (Fig. 14–9) must be considered (see Chap. 9). Histopathologic examination shows marked surface and follicular orthokeratotic or parakeratotic hyperkeratosis (Fig. 14–10).

Ear margin dermatosis is an incurable condition that can be controlled with antiseborrheic treatments. Coupled with these treatments, management changes should be considered. Affected dogs should not be allowed to sleep near forced air heating ducts, wood stoves, or other dry heat sources.[59] In addition, the dog's diet should be reviewed and improved if necessary.

Because of the follicular nature of the seborrhea, sulfur-salicylic acid, benzoyl peroxide, or benzoyl peroxide-sulfur shampoos are most commonly used to remove the accumulated debris. In chronic cases in which the debris is hard, the areas should be soaked in warm water for 5 to 10 minutes before the shampoo is applied. The areas are shampooed every 24 to 48 hours until the debris is completely removed. Severe cases can take 10 to 14 days for this to occur. After the cleaning, a moisturizer should be applied to minimize transepidermal water loss. When the ears are near normal, the frequency of shampooing is reduced to an as-needed basis.

In some cases, removal of the debris results in pinnal inflammation. In most instances, however, this inflammation is mild and requires no treatment. Moderately inflamed lesions benefit from the application of a 1% hydrocortisone cream or ointment.[19]

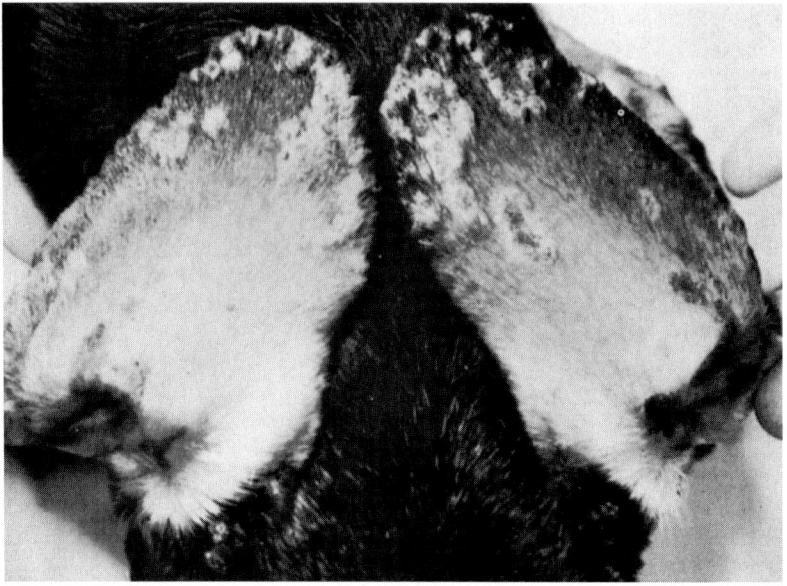

FIGURE 14–9. Ear margin scaling and crusting in a Dachshund. Lesions away from the ear margins suggest an underlying vasculopathy.

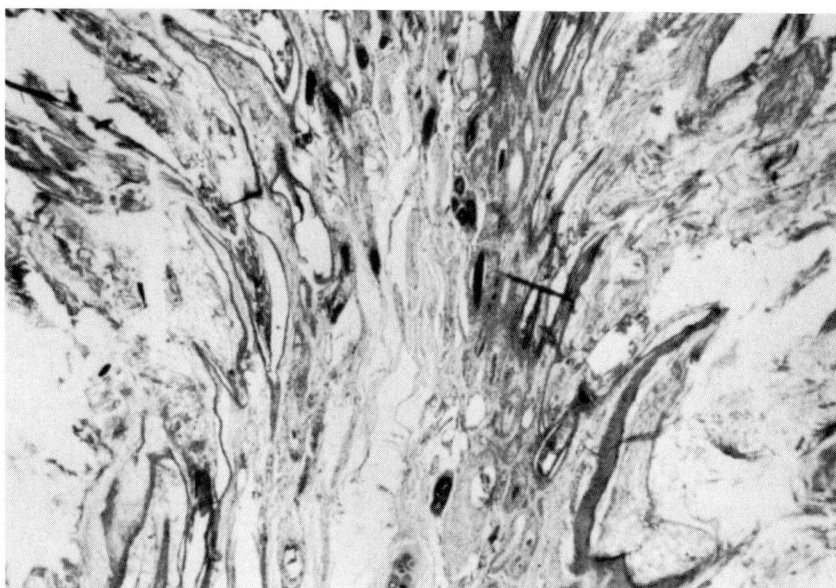

FIGURE 14–10. Histopathologic section of ear margin dermatosis. Tangential section shows a papillated epidermis with orthokeratotic hyperkeratosis.

With severe inflammation or early fissures, prednisolone (1 mg/kg q24h orally) or a potent steroid-antibiotic topical product is needed for 7 to 10 days. With extensive fissuring, pinnal surgery is required. With multiple fissures, a cosmetic ear crop should be performed. Appropriate diagnostic tests should be performed before surgery to ensure that the fissure was not caused by some underlying vasculitic process.

• CANINE TAIL GLAND HYPERPLASIA

All dogs have an oval spot on the dorsal surface of the tail, about 2.5 to 5 cm distal to the anus, that is different from other skin. The area has simple instead of compound hair follicles and numerous large sebaceous and circumanal (perianal or hepatoid) glands (Figs. 14–11 and 14–12).

Some dogs with primary or secondary seborrhea, or with relative or absolute elevated blood androgen levels develop hyperplasia of the sebaceous glands, circumanal glands in the tail gland, or both. When the androgen levels are elevated, the circumanal glands around the anus and elsewhere are also typically hyperplastic. Early tail gland hyperplasia usually goes unnoticed because the overlying hairs hide the defect. With time, however, the area becomes hairless because of friction and compression of the hair follicles by the hyperplastic glands. At this stage, the owner notices an oval, bulging, hairless area on the tail (see Fig. 14–6F). The overlying skin may be scaly, greasy, hyperpigmented, or some combination thereof. In advanced cases, the area can have a nodular appearance because of nonuniform glandular hypertrophy and cystic dilatation or secondary infection.

The area of the tail gland hyperplasia may become infected, although this is uncommon. Grouped or single pustules may develop, with each pustule representing an acne-like sebaceous or circumanal gland infection. Puncturing the pustules, expressing the contents, and administering systemic antibiotics usually provide relief. In some cases, the infection may recur.

Tail gland hyperplasia is usually a strictly cosmetic defect requiring no treatment. Because many cases are caused by hyperandrogenism, castration should be offered to prevent further enlargement. When castration is performed, a beneficial response usually

1046 • Keratinization Defects

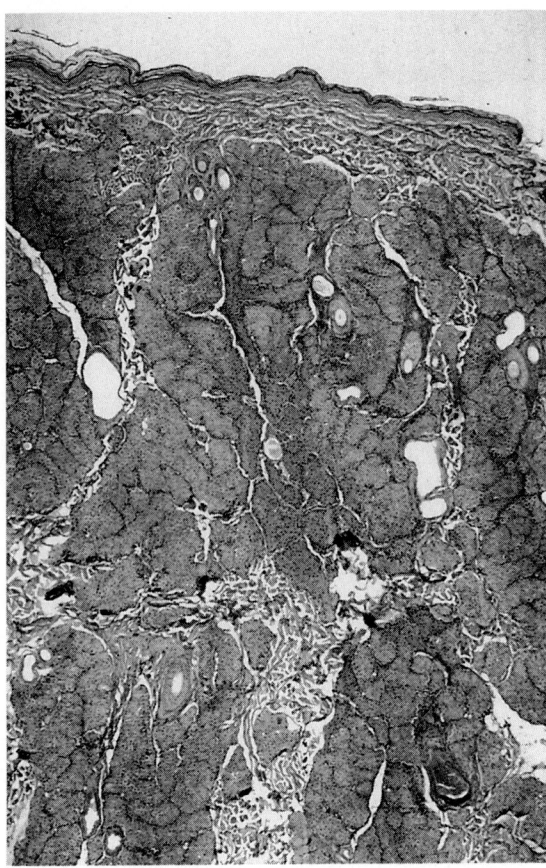

FIGURE 14-11. Canine tail gland hyperplasia. Marked hyperplasia of the circumanal glands. Compression of the hair follicles disrupts the hair cycle and results in alopecia.

occurs within 2 months. The owner should be warned that castration may not lead to complete resolution of the existing lesion. Although the glands should become less hyperplastic, the alopecia may be permanent as a result of prolonged glandular pressure on the hair follicles. In the past, medical treatment with estrogens or progestational compounds has been recommended because of their antiandrogenic effects. As a result of their potential serious side effects, however (e.g., bone marrow suppression, diabetes mellitus), these agents are no longer suggested.

Animals that do not respond sufficiently to castration or are not neutered may benefit from surgery. An elliptic piece of skin is removed from the dorsal area of the tail over the enlargement. Blunt dissection and curettage are then performed to remove the excess glandular material under and lateral to the incision. Before the wound is sutured, additional loose skin can usually be removed to provide a normal conformation of skin around the tail. The area should be bandaged to prevent self-damage or suture removal by the dog. Excellent cosmetic correction usually results, with only a small scar remaining visible. Without castration, recurrence can be expected in 1 to 3 years.

• FELINE TAIL GLAND HYPERPLASIA

Cats have the same tail gland area as dogs, but it is located in a line along the dorsal aspect of the tail and is commonly called the supracaudal organ. As in dogs, this area is rich in sebaceous and epitrichial sweat glands (Fig. 14–13), and a waxy secretion accumulates on the surface.

In some cats, especially those kept in catteries or small enclosures, unusually large

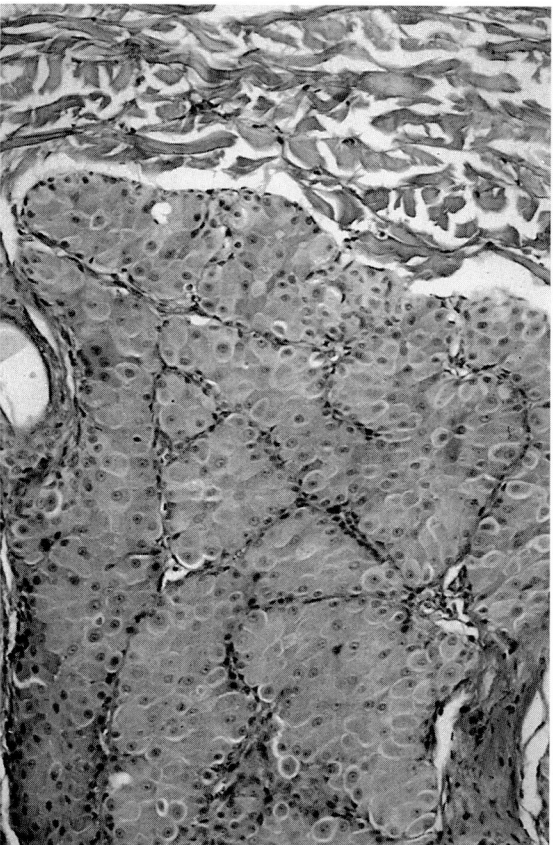

FIGURE 14–12. Close-up of the circumanal (perianal or hepatoid) glands in the tail gland.

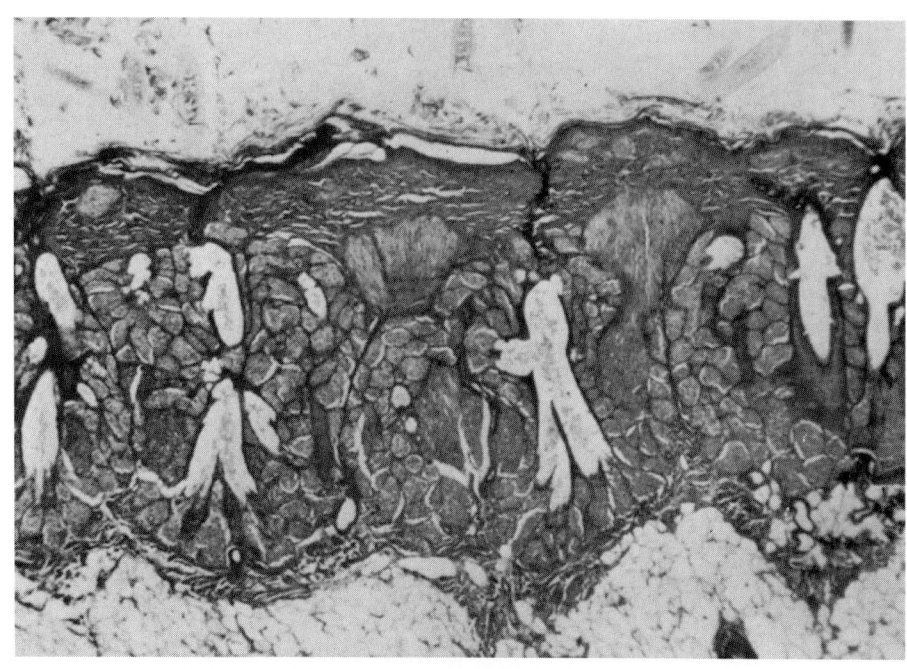

FIGURE 14–13. Feline stud tail. Marked sebaceous gland hyperplasia.

1048 • Keratinization Defects

amounts of excess secretions accumulate and cause matting of the hair and the formation of scales and crusts (Fig. 14–14). In some cases, the overlying haircoat is thinned, and the skin may become hyperpigmented (see Fig. 14–6G). Rarely, secondary bacterial folliculitis and furunculosis complicate the condition. This condition is of great concern to owners of uncastrated male show cats, which accounts for the popular name stud tail[51]; however, it has also been observed in females and altered males. Castration does not resolve the condition but may help stop its progression.[59]

Treatment consists of clipping the affected area and washing it with antiseborrheic shampoos. Benzoyl peroxide shampoo can be very useful. This treatment can be followed by daily cleaning with alcohol or a milder antiseborrheic shampoo (e.g., sulfur-salicylic acid). It is advisable to provide affected cats with as little confinement as possible, because fresh air and sunshine may help prevent recurrence. The unconfined cat usually resumes cleaning itself and the tail gland area with the customary fastidiousness characteristic of healthy, well-adjusted cats. Progestational compounds may be helpful; because of their common side effects, however, their advisability as therapy for a benign, asymptomatic disease is questionable. Retinoids have not been used in this condition, but they may be of some value in recalcitrant cases.

If the cat fails to care for the problem, the owner must carefully and frequently comb and groom the area to prevent recurrence.

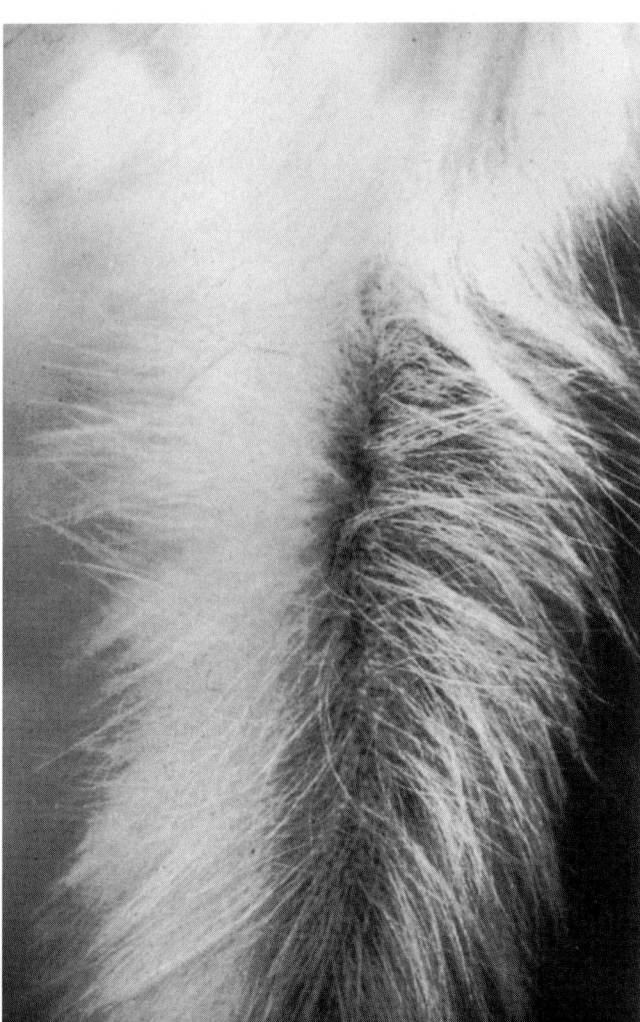

FIGURE 14–14. Feline tail gland hyperplasia with accumulation of greasy material in the hairs.

• EXFOLIATIVE DERMATOSES

Virtually every surface or superficial follicular skin lesion in dogs and cats exfoliates (falls off in scales and layers) during its development, maturation, or involution. With the coalescence of adjacent lesions, large areas of exfoliation can occur, making the list of possible exfoliative dermatoses large indeed. True exfoliative dermatoses, however, are characterized by generalized severe desquamation with or without generalized erythema (erythroderma). Although affected animals may have some unaffected areas on the body, those that are involved are uniformly affected, with no visible normal skin.

In animals receiving no medications for a systemic or skin disease, the following must be considered as causes of the exfoliative dermatitis: ichthyosis, contact dermatitis to a topical agent (shampoo, dip, and so forth), pemphigus foliaceus, feline leukemia virus (FeLV) or feline immunodeficiency virus (FIV) dermatitis, systemic lupus erythematosus, erythema multiforme or toxic epidermal necrolysis, epitheliotropic lymphoma, the disorders that cause cutaneous flushing, and parapsoriasis.[1, 41, 53, 59] When an animal is receiving medications, drug eruption and unexpected physiologic response to the drug must be added to the list. Corticosteroids from internal (e.g., hyperadrenocorticism) or external sources increase the number of possibilities. In these animals, widespread superficial bacterial folliculitis, dermatophytosis, *Malassezia* dermatitis, demodicosis, cheyletiellosis, and occasionally scabies must be considered. Idiopathic cases are reported.[1]

With careful consideration of the history, physical findings, and routine in-office diagnostic tests (e.g., skin scrapings, trichography, cytologic tests), the list of differential diagnoses for an exfoliative dermatosis becomes considerably shorter. Definitive diagnosis is often made by skin biopsy. Most causes of exfoliative dermatosis are covered elsewhere in this textbook. Parapsoriasis, cutaneous flushing, thymoma, and physiologic response to a drug are considered here.

• THYMOMA

A generalized exfoliative dermatitis has been described in a small number of cats with thymoma.[17, 49a, 58] Affected cats were middle-age to old, with an exfoliative dermatitis first noted on the head and pinna. Pruritus usually is minimal or absent, but may be intense. Despite treatment with steroids, antibiotics, or other agents, lesions spread and involve the entire body in a matter of weeks to several months. Hair loss can accompany the exfoliation (Fig. 14–15), and seborrheic debris accumulates in the interdigital spaces and

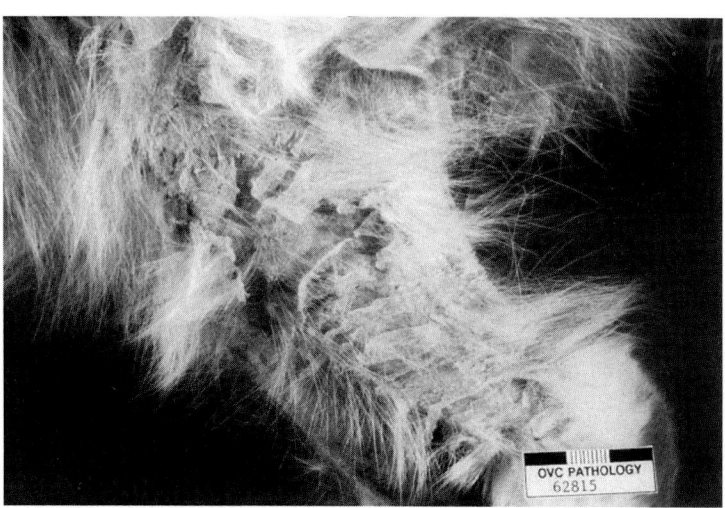

FIGURE 14–15. Hair loss and seborrheic change in a cat with a thymoma. Note how the epithelium exfoliates in large sheets.

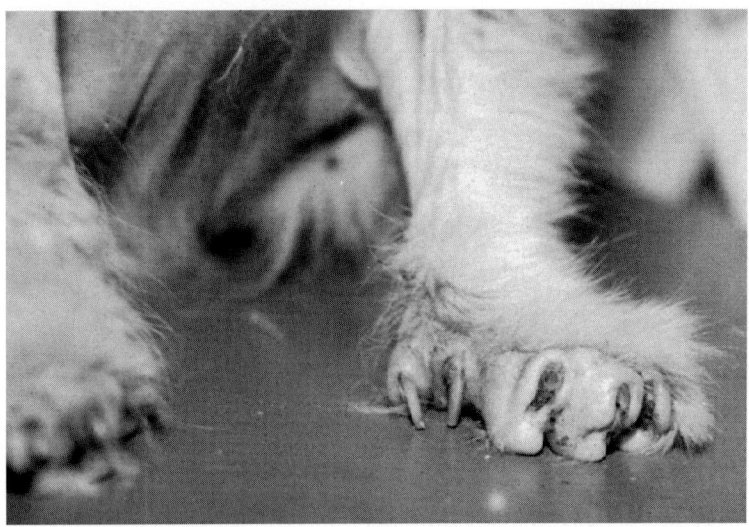

FIGURE 14–16. Hair loss and seborrheic paronychia in a cat with a thymoma.

around the clawbeds (Fig. 14–16). Some affected cats lose hair pigment and turn white. Beyond the skin lesions, the cats appear otherwise healthy.

The differential diagnosis includes systemic lupus erythematosus, FeLV or FIV dermatitis, drug reaction, demodicosis, or hyperadrenocorticism with secondary bacterial, dermatophyte, or *Malassezia* involvement. On skin biopsy, a cell-poor hydropic interface dermatitis of the surface and follicular epithelium is seen (Fig. 14–17). Apoptotic keratinocytes are seen in the basal layer and, to a lesser extent, in the stratum spinosum. In one case, the infiltrating lymphocytes were CD8+, and sebaceous glands were also infiltrated.[49a]

Most thymomas are benign, and surgical removal will result in permanent resolution of the skin lesions.

• PARAPSORIASIS

In humans, parapsoriasis (resembling psoriasis) is grouped into three major entities, each of which has several morphologic variants.[22] To date, only large plaque parapsoriasis has

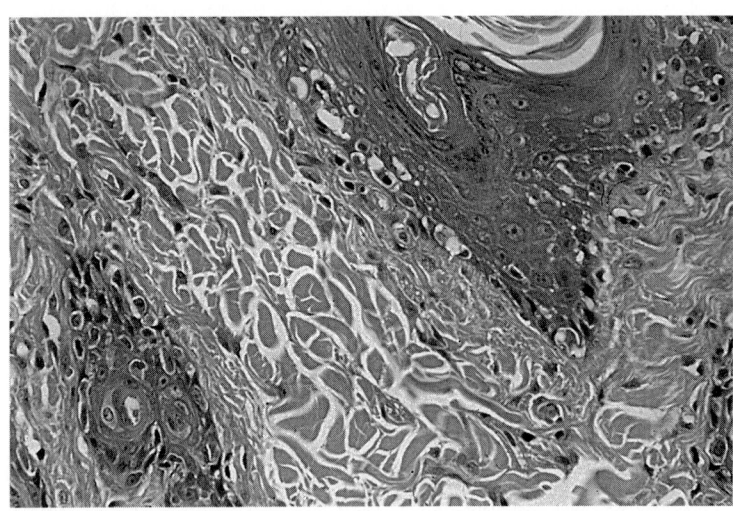

FIGURE 14–17. Thymoma. A cell-poor hydropic interface dermatitis.

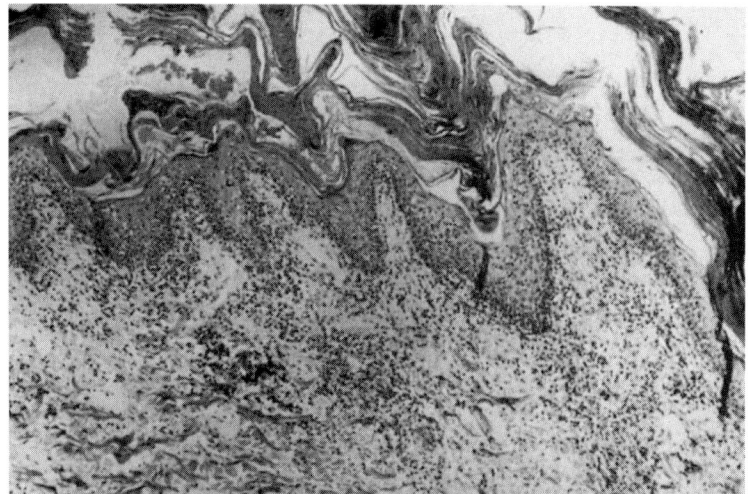

FIGURE 14–18. Parapsoriasis. Superficial perivascular to lichenoid dermatitis with parakeratotic hyperkeratosis and diffuse exocytosis of lymphocytes.

been reported in animals and only in one dog and one cat.[53] The dermatoses were characterized by widespread erythematous, scaly plaques that spared the head, pinnae, and distal limbs (see Fig. 14–6H). Irregular hair loss occurred in the involved areas. In the dog, many of the plaques were studded with large, superficial, flaccid, yellow pustules, annular erosions, and epidermal collarettes that were a result of a secondary staphylococcal infection.

Biopsy of affected skin showed a focally parakeratotic, regularly hyperplastic, superficial perivascular to lichenoid interface dermatitis with diffuse exocytosis of normal lymphocytes (Fig. 14–18). A striking finding was a diffuse accumulation of lymphocytes arranged in a line within the basal cell layer of the epidermis and hair follicle outer root sheaths (Fig. 14–19).

Both animals were treated with high levels of corticosteroids, the dog with oral prednisolone (2.2 mg/kg q24h) and the cat with methylprednisolone acetate injections (5 mg/kg q2wk). Marked healing occurred in 8 to 10 days, with complete resolution of all lesions in 6 to 10 weeks. Both cases required maintenance therapy to prevent relapse.

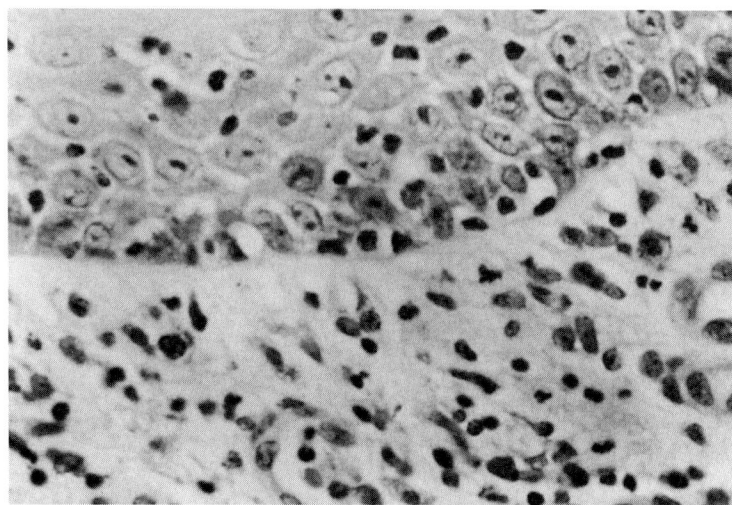

FIGURE 14–19. Parapsoriasis. Diffuse spongiosis and exocytosis of lymphocytes. Note the row of lymphocytes within the basal layer.

• CUTANEOUS FLUSHING

Cutaneous flushing is due to vasodilation of the cutaneous blood vessels and is manifested by the skin turning various shades of red.[22] The flushing can be regionalized or generalized and paroxysmal or persistent. Pathologic flushing is due to the direct action of vasoactive compounds on the blood vessels. Because some vasoactive compounds (e.g., histamine) are pruritogenic, some flushing disorders can be pruritic, but the flushing precedes the pruritus.

In dogs, persistent, widespread erythema (erythroderma) can be a feature of systemic lupus erythematosus, demodicosis, drug reaction, thallium toxicosis, mast cell tumor, cutaneous lymphoma, or systemic mastocytosis.[41, 64] Paroxysmal flushing has been associated with pheochromocytoma, drug reaction, mast cell tumor, and the carcinoid syndrome.[41]

In humans, the carcinoid syndrome refers to an uncommon condition associated with slow-growing malignant carcinoid tumors derived from enterochromaffin cells, which produce a variety of vasoactive compounds.[22] In most instances, the tumor is located in the gastrointestinal tract, but it can also be found in the ovary, testis, skin, or bronchus. In dogs, the carcinoid syndrome has been reported in association with pulmonary adenocarcinoma[41] and has been recognized in several dogs with intestinal lesions.[59]

At their onset, flushing disorders in dogs have no associated exfoliation. In chronic cases, especially when the flushing is persistent, desquamation occurs but remains overshadowed by the erythroderma. All animals with such a presentation should have a thorough evaluation for an internal malignancy.

• PHYSIOLOGIC RESPONSE TO DRUGS

As mentioned earlier, virtually all surface or superficial follicular skin lesions exfoliate at some point, especially during their involution. Accordingly, the drugs used to treat the lesions cause exfoliation in effect. If the skin lesions are widespread and numerous, an exfoliative dermatosis will result. Because clients are aware of the initial lesions, most recognize that the exfoliation is a sign of healing and are not concerned by it.

Drugs that influence epidermal turnover (e.g., hormones, cytotoxic agents, retinoic acids) can cause an exfoliative dermatitis near the onset of treatment or after discontinuation of the drug. Exfoliation at the termination of treatment with a cytostatic agent should be expected, and the client should be made aware of this expectation. The most common example is the profound scaling that occurs when an animal is withdrawn from a chronic

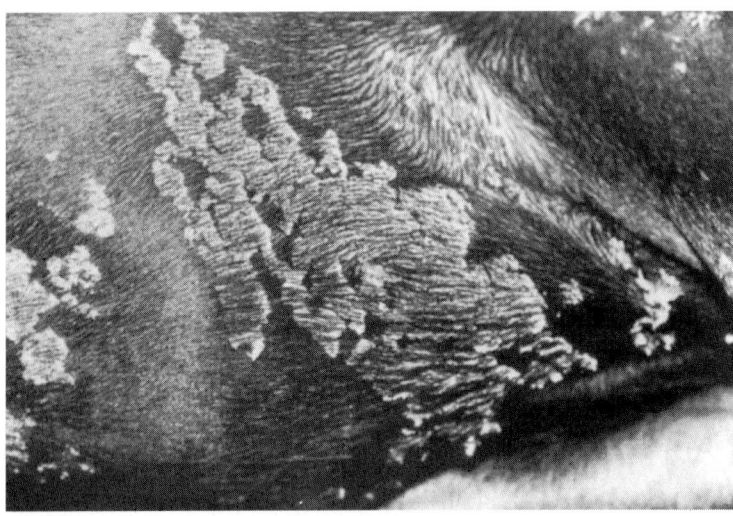

FIGURE 14–20. Exfoliative dermatosis in a hypothyroid Doberman pinscher resulting from the institution of thyroid hormone replacement therapy.

course of treatment with moderate to high doses of a corticosteroid. Similar changes can occur in dogs with spontaneous hyperadrenocorticism that are being treated with mitotane (o,p'-DDD) and in hypothyroid dogs within the first few weeks of treatment with thyroid hormone. Much more problematic is the exfoliation that occurs 1 to 2 weeks after treatment with a nonsteroidal agent is instituted (Fig. 14–20). The basic quandary is whether the exfoliation represents a drug eruption or clinical evidence of increased epidermal turnover. If the pharmacology of the drug allows this change and the animal is showing no clinical or laboratory evidence of systemic illness, the question can be answered by observing the animal carefully for 7 to 10 days. Pharmacologic exfoliation will lessen or stop within this time, but a drug eruption will persist or worsen.

• REFERENCES

1. Anderson RK: Exfoliative dermatitis in the dog. Comp Cont Educ 3:885, 1981.
2. Baker BB, et al: Epidermal cell renewal in dogs after clipping the hair. Am J Vet. Res 35:445, 1974.
3. Bedford CJ Young JM: A comparison of comedonal and skin surface lipids from hairless dogs showing clinical signs of acne. J Invest Dermatol 77:341, 1981.
4. Berardesca E, Borroni G: Instrumental evaluation of cutaneous hydration. Clin Dermatol 13:323, 1995.
5. Bond R: Canine and feline acne. Vet Ann 33:230, 1993.
6. Breen P, Jeromin A: Practice tips. Derm Dialogue, Winter 93/94, p 7.
7. Campbell A: Calcipotriol poisoning in dogs. Vet Rec 141:27, 1997.
8. Campbell KL, Davis CA: Effects of thyroid hormones on serum and cutaneous fatty acid concentrations in dogs. Am J Vet Res 51:752, 1990.
9. Campbell KL, et al: Effects of oral sunflower oil on serum and cutaneous fatty acid concentration profiles in seborrheic dogs. Vet Dermatol 3:29, 1992.
10. Campbell KL, Schaeffer DJ: Effects of four veterinary shampoos on transepidermal water losses, hydration of the stratum corneum, skin surface lipid concentrations, and corneocyte counts in dogs. Proc Annu Memb Meet Am Acad Vet Dermatol Am Coll Vet Dermatol 9:96, 1993.
11. Campbell KL, Kirkwood AR: Effect of topical oils on transepidermal water loss in dogs with seborrhea sicca. In: Ihrke PJ, et al (eds): Advances in Veterinary Dermatology, Vol. 2. Pergamon Press, Oxford, 1993, p 157.
12. Campbell KL, et al: Effects of four anti-seborrheic shampoos on transepidermal water losses, hydration of the stratum corneum, skin surface lipid concentration, skin surface pH, and corneocyte counts in dogs. Proc Annu Memb Meet Am Acad Vet Dermatol Am Coll Vet Dermatol 10:85, 1994.
13. Campbell KL, et al: Effects of four topical humectant/emollient solutions on the skin of dogs. Proc Annu Meet Am Acad Vet Dermatol Am Coll Vet Dermatol 12:49, 1996.
14. Campbell KL, Bibus D: Effect of α-linolenic acid on the skin and plasma phospholipids of beagle puppies. Proc Am Acad Vet Dermatol Am Coll Vet Dermatol 15:105, 1999.
15. Christophers E, Mrowietz U: Psoriasis. In: Freedberg IM, et al (eds): Fitzpatrick's Dermatology in General Medicine, 5th ed. McGraw-Hill Book Co., San Francisco, 1999, p 495.
16. Curtis C: Use and abuse of topical dermatological therapy in dogs and cats. Part 1. Shampoo therapy. In Pract 20:244, 1996.
17. Day MJ: Review of thymic pathology in 30 cats and 36 dogs. J Small Anim Pract 38:393, 1997.
18. Draelos ZD: New developments in cosmetics and skin care products. Adv Dermatol 12:3, 1997.
19. Ellis CN, Voorhees JJ: Etretinate therapy. J Am Acad Dermatol 16:267, 1987.
20. Evans AG, et al: A trial of 13-*cis*-retinoic acid for treatment of squamous cell carcinoma and preneoplastic lesions of the head in cats. Am J Vet Res 46:2553, 1985.
21. Fadok VA: Treatment of canine idiopathic seborrhea with isotretinoin. Am J Vet Res 47:1730, 1986.
22. Freedberg IM, et al: Fitzpatrick's Dermatology in General Medicine, 5th ed. McGraw-Hill Book Co., New York, 1999.
23. Gardey L, et al: Hydrating effect of a shampoo on the skin of healthy dogs. Proc Am Acad Vet Dermatol Am Coll Vet Dermatol 15:27, 1999.
24. Gordon JG, Kwochka KW: Corneocyte counts for evaluation of antiseborrheic shampoos in dogs. Vet Dermatol 4:57, 1993.
25. Gottlieb SL, et al: Cellular actions of etretinate in psoriasis: Enhanced epidermal differentiation and reduced cell-mediated inflammation are unexpected outcomes. J Cutan Pathol 23:404, 1996.
26. Griffin CE: Open forum—Etretinate—How is it being used in veterinary dermatology? Derm Dialogue, Spring/Summer 1993, p 4.
27. Gross TL, et al: Veterinary Dermatopathology. Mosby–Year Book, St. Louis, 1992.
28. Guaguère E: Cas clinique: Séborrhée primaire répondant à l'administration de vitamine A. Point Vét 16:689, 1984.
29. Guaguère E: Quel est votre diagnostic? Point Vét 18:245, 1986.
30. Ihrke PJ, Goldschmidt MH: Vitamin A–responsive dermatosis in the dog. J Am Vet Med Assoc 182:682, 1983.
31. Kietzmann M: Eicosanoid levels in canine inflammatory skin diseases. In: von Tscharner C, Halliwell REW (eds): Advances in Veterinary Dermatology I. Baillière-Tindall, London, 1990, p 211.
32. Kwochka KW, Rademakers AM: Cell proliferation of epidermis, hair follicles, and sebaceous glands of Beagles and Cocker spaniels with healthy skin. Am J Vet Res 50:587, 1989.
33. Kwochka KW: Keratinization abnormalities: Understanding the mechanism of scale formation. In: Ihrke

PJ, et al (eds). Advances in Veterinary Dermatology, Vol. 2. Pergamon Press, Oxford, 1993, p 91.
34. Kwochka KW: Keratinization disorders. Current Veterinary Dermatology. Mosby–Year Book, St. Louis, 1993, p 167.
35. Kwochka KW: Shampoos and moisturizing rinses in veterinary dermatology. In: Bonagura JD (ed): Kirk's Current Veterinary Therapy XII. W. B. Saunders Co, Philadelphia, 1995, p 590.
36. Kwochka KW: The structure and function of epidermal lipids. Vet Dermatol 4:151, 1993.
37. Kwochka KW: Retinoids and vitamin A therapy. In: Griffin CE, et al (eds): Current Veterinary Dermatology. Mosby–Year Book, St. Louis, 1993, p 203.
38. Kwochka KW: Advances in the management of canine scaling. Proc 3rd World Cong Vet Dermatol 1996, p. 99.
39. Lu I, et al: Modulation of epidermal differentiation, tissue inflammation, and T-lymphocyte infiltration in psoriatic plaques by topical calcitriol. J Cutan Pathol 23:419, 1996.
40. Marks SL, et al: Clinical evaluation of etretinate for the treatment of canine solar induced squamous cell carcinoma and preneoplastic lesions. J Am Acad Dermatol 27:11, 1992.
41. Miller WH Jr: Cutaneous flushing associated with intrathoracic neoplasia in a dog. J Am Anim Hosp Assoc 28:217, 1992.
42. Paradis M: Footpad hyperkeratosis in a family of Dogues de Bordeaux. Vet Dermatol 3:75, 1992.
43. Parker W, et al: Vitamin A–responsive seborrheic dermatitis in the dog: A case report. J Am Anim Hosp Assoc 19:546, 1983.
44. Paterson S, et al: Ultrasonographic biomicroscopy to assess changes in the skin after shampoo therapy. In: Kwochka KW, et al (eds): Advances in Veterinary Dermatology, Vol 3. Butterworth-Heinnemann, Boston, 1999, p 523.
45. Peck GL, Di Giovanna JJ: Retinoids. In: Freedberg IM, et al (eds): Fitzpatrick's Dermatology in General Medicine, 5th ed. McGraw-Hill Book Co., San Francisco, 1999.
46. Power HT, Ihrke PJ: The use of synthetic retinoids in veterinary medicine. In: Bonagura JD (ed): Kirk's Current Veterinary Therapy XII. W. B. Saunders Co, Philadelphia, 1995, p 585.
47. Prens EP, et al: Effects of cyclosporine on cytokines and cytokine receptors in psoriasis. J Am Acad Dermatol 33:947, 1995.
48. Reichrath J, et al: Biologic effects of topical calcipotriol (MC 903) treatment in psoriatic skin. J Am Acad Dermatol 36:19, 1997.
49. Reister M: Ask the vet: Feline acne problem. Cat Fancy 39:16, 1996.
49a. Rivierre C, Olivry T: Dermatite exfoliative paranéoplasique associée à un thymome chez un chat: Résolution des symptômes après thymectomie. Prat Méd Chir Anim Comp 34:531, 1999.
50. Rosenkrantz WS: The pathogenesis, diagnosis, and management of feline acne. Vet Med 86:504, 1991.
51. Scott DW: Feline dermatology 1900–1978: A monograph. J Am Anim Hosp Assoc 16:331, 1980.
52. Scott DW: Vitamin A–responsive dermatosis in the Cocker spaniel. J Am Anim Hosp Assoc 22:125, 1986.
53. Scott DW: Exfoliative dermatoses in a dog and a cat resembling large plaque parapsoriasis in humans. Comp Anim Pract 2:22, 1986.
54. Scott DW, et al: A clinical study on the efficacy of two commercial veterinary emollients (Micropearls and Humilac) in the management of wintertime dry skin in dogs. Cornell Vet 81:419, 1991.
55. Scott DW, et al: A clinical study on the effect of two commercial veterinary benzoyl peroxide shampoos in dogs. Canine Pract 19:7, 1994.
56. Scott DW: Clinical assessment of topical benzoyl peroxide in treatment of canine skin diseases. Vet Med 74:808, 1979.
57. Scott DW: Topical cutaneous medicine, or "Now what should I try?" Proc Am Anim Hosp Assoc 46:89, 1979.
58. Scott DW, et al: Exfoliative dermatitis in association with thymoma in three cats. Feline Pract 23:8, 1995.
59. Scott DW, et al: Muller and Kirk's Small Animal Dermatology, 5th ed. W. B. Saunders, Co., Philadelphia, 1995.
60. Simpson JW, van den Brock AHM: Fat absorption in dogs with diabetes mellitus or hypothyroidism. Res Vet Sci 50:346, 1991.
61. Stewart LJ, et al: Isotretinoin in the treatment of sebaceous adenitis in two vizslas. J Am Anim Hosp Assoc 27:65, 1991.
62. Suter MM, et al: Keratinocyte biology and pathology. Vet Dermatol 8:67, 1997.
63. von Tscharner C, et al: Proliferation characteristics of canine keratinocyte cultures infected with *Malassezia pachydermatis*. Proc Am Acad Vet Dermatol Am Coll Vet Dermatol 15:107, 1999.
64. White SD: The skin as a sensor of internal medical disorders. In: Ettinger SJ (ed): Textbook of Veterinary Internal Medicine, 3rd ed. W. B. Saunders Co, Philadelphia, 1989, p 5.
65. White SD, et al: Isotretinoin and etretinate in the treatment of benign and malignant cutaneous neoplasia and in sebaceous adenitis of longhaired dogs. Proc Annu Memb Meet Am Acad Vet Dermatol Am Coll Vet Dermatol 7:101, 1991.
66. White SD, et al: Feline acne and results of treatment with mupirocin in an open clinical trial: 25 cases (1994–1996). Vet Dermatol 8:157, 1997.

Chapter 15
Psychogenic Skin Diseases

Psychodermatology, also known as psychocutaneous medicine and dermatopsychosomatics, is a growing field of interest in human medicine.[7, 24] Workers in this field believe that the body (soma) and mind (psyche) have been treated separately for too long and that they constitute a single unit. It is believed that the role of emotional factors in diseases of the skin is of such significance that if emotional factors are ignored, effective management of at least 40% of the patients who come to departments of dermatology is impossible. One exploratory model for these mind-body relationships is the neuro-immuno-cutaneous-endocrine (NICE) network, in which these four organ systems are intimately linked and share a language of neuropeptides, cytokines, glucocorticoids, and other effector molecules.[18] Research in laboratory animals and humans indicates that the central nervous system (CNS), through the effects of neurohormones, can significantly modulate immune responses and pruritus. The relationship between the hypothalamus and the immune system seems to involve neurohormones secreted by the hypothalamus (thyrotropin releasing factor, prolactin releasing factor, gonadotropin releasing hormone); the neurotransmitters norepinephrine, serotonin, dopamine, acetylcholine, γ-aminobutyric acid; and the polypeptide neuroregulators somatostatin, vasoactive intestinal peptide, substance P, calcitonin gene-related peptide, pituitary adenylate cyclase activating peptide, α-melanocyte-stimulating hormone, neurotensin, neurokinin A, neuropeptide γ, enkephalins, and endorphins.[18, 24] These factors are known to have vasomotor, immunomodulatory, chemotactic, and cellular growth effects.[18]

The role of neurotransmitters and neuroregulators in veterinary dermatology is unknown. The field of behavior is rapidly expanding in veterinary medicine, and the use of behavioral pharmacotherapy is rapidly growing.[22, 41, 42] Many of the drugs in use act on the monoamine neurotransmitters, which include dopamine, serotonin, and norepinephrine. Recent studies with drugs that block serotonin reuptake, norepinephrine reuptake, or endorphin actions suggest that they play some role. Part of the effect may be related to the decrease in the effects of endorphin-induced histamine release.

Studies in laboratory animals have shown that the CNS can interact with the immune system. Guinea pigs sensitized to bovine serum albumin were conditioned by repeatedly being exposed to the allergen and an odor simultaneously.[34] They eventually experienced the allergic reaction when exposed to the odor alone, without the allergen.

In humans, psychodermatologic conditions are divided into psychophysiologic disorders in which there is a bona fide skin disorder (allergy, urticaria) that can be exacerbated by emotional stress; primary psychiatric disorders in which there is anxiety, depression, delusion, and obsessive-compulsive behavior; and secondary psychiatric disorders.[7, 14]

Most lesions of psychogenic dermatoses in animals are the result of self-induced damage. There is good clinical evidence that psychological disturbances are the cause.[3, 8, 22, 31, 47] Obsessive-compulsive disorders are characterized by repetitive, stereotypic, ritualistic behaviors in excess of what is required for normal function; the execution of these behaviors interferes with normal daily activities and functioning.[3, 8, 22, 31] Behavioral conditions that can be present in obsessive-compulsive animals include boredom, attention-seeking, hyperactivity, and anxiety. Three general factors are involved in the etiopathogenesis:

1. Breed predisposition. Breeds that are emotional and nervous develop more psychogenic dermatoses. Oriental breeds of cats (Abyssinian, Siamese, Burmese, and Oriental) are especially at risk.[35, 37] Among dogs, the predisposed breeds include Doberman pinschers, Great Danes, Irish setters, Labrador retrievers, and German shepherds.[21, 38, 48]
2. The lifestyle of the animal can be causative or contributory. When individuals not of predisposed breeds are forced into stressful, isolated, or boring situations and are without human or canine companionship, they may develop psychogenic dermatoses. Long confinement in crates, continual chain restraint, small-pen housing, or domination by a forceful or inconsiderate owner may precipitate problems. A rival animal in the same house or an aggressive neighborhood animal can trigger a psychogenic disturbance.
3. The individual animal, regardless of breed or lifestyle, can be particularly nervous, hyperesthetic, fearful, or shy.

The diagnosis of a psychogenic dermatosis is by exclusion and generally cannot be well documented. The diagnosis is also occasionally used for those frustrating cases that do not respond to treatment, even when a thorough work-up has not been performed. Physical causes must always be eliminated before a diagnosis of psychogenic dermatosis is made. This includes ruling out such causative factors as trauma, neuropathy, local pain, parasites, allergy, bacterial or fungal infections, and internal diseases. The problem of accurate diagnosis can be compounded by the fact that psychogenic factors may play a partial role in a disease; a work-up may reveal an organic disease, but the psychological component may be significant enough that such treatment becomes necessary for adequate control of the whole condition.

Dermatoses thought to be psychogenic in origin or to have a significant psychogenic component include acral lick dermatitis (lick granuloma), tail dock neuroma, feline psychogenic alopecia and dermatitis, and miscellaneous psychogenic manifestations such as tail sucking (feline), tail biting (canine), flank sucking, foot licking, self-nursing, and anal licking.

● PSYCHOLOGICAL DRUG THERAPY

A variety of drugs that affect CNS neurotransmitters or endorphins or that have other sedative, antidepressant, or antianxiety effects may be beneficial in diseases characterized by self-destructive behavior, abnormal licking or chewing, and pruritus.* In general, these drugs are tried when the disease is believed to have a significant psychological component in its cause. These drugs, which work by a variety of mechanisms, include antidepressants, antipsychotics, opiate antagonists, anxiolytics, and mood stabilizers.

The drugs that have been evaluated the most are the heterocyclic (tricyclic) antidepressants (amitriptyline, clomipramine, doxepin) and fluoxetine, another antidepressant that is structurally different from the heterocyclic antidepressants but that has a similar mechanism of action.† These drugs act primarily by increasing neurotransmitter levels of serotonin. They work primarily by blocking the reuptake of serotonin by the presynaptic neuronal membrane, which effectively increases the activity of serotonin. Doxepin, clomipramine, and amitriptyline also increase the effect of norepinephrine, which is responsible for arousal and stimulating the behavioral focus.[30] Clomipramine and fluoxetine are more potent at increasing the synaptic levels of serotonin. Amitriptyline and doxepin are potent H_1 blockers, and this may be helpful in some cases as well. These other effects may help to make these drugs useful in allergic diseases as well, especially when a psychogenic component to the pruritus is present. Amitriptyline hydrochloride at 1 mg/kg every 12 hours was effective in 16% of the allergic dogs treated,[17] whereas doxepin hydrochloride

---

*7, 10, 13, 22, 31, 41, 42: see References.
†10, 11, 17, 20, 22, 31, 33, 35, 40, 41: see References.

at 1 mg/kg every 8 hours was ineffective.[26] However, one author (CEG) has seen excellent responses to doxepin in some animals. Anecdotal reports indicate that the serotonin reuptake inhibitor fluoxetine hydrochloride at 1 mg/kg q24h is effective in 30% of dogs with allergic pruritus.[25, 40] All these drugs at the following dosages have been reported effective for a variety of psychogenic dermatoses in dogs and cats to be described.[22]

- Fluoxetine (Prozac), 1 mg/kg q24h, can be used.[22, 31, 33, 40] The problem is that it is very expensive.
- Clomipramine (Clomicalm, Anafranil), 2 to 4 mg/kg daily given q24h or divided q12h for dogs, and 0.5 to 1.5 mg/kg daily given q24h for cats.[5, 10, 11, 27, 29, 31, 35] Clomipramine is available as a veterinary drug (Clomicalm), now licensed for use in dogs with separation anxiety. In dogs, clomipramine has a short elimination half-life and marked interdog variability.[11] It should be given with food to minimize vomiting.[10] Absorption following oral administration is similar when clomipramine is given with or without meals.[12a]
- Amitriptyline (Elavil), 1 to 3 mg/kg q12h,[13, 17, 22] although less expensive, may not be as effective as clomipramine or fluoxetine.
- Doxepin (Sinequan, Adapin), 0.5 to 2 mg/kg q12h with higher doses used more in psychogenic dermatoses, also has the advantage of being less expensive.
- Imipramine (Tofranil), 2 to 4 mg/kg q24h.

In general, the potentially more serious side effects of these drugs are induction of cardiac arrhythmias, such as promotion of heart block by slowing of cardiac conduction, and anticholinergic effects including dry mouth, urine retention, and reduced tear production.[7, 17, 41] They also lower the seizure threshold, and they enhance monamine oxidase inhibitor toxicity in addition to having the metabolic results and side effects that are inherent to first-generation antihistamines. Up to 30% of animals treated may show varying combinations and variably severe degrees of vomiting, diarrhea, lethargy, hyperexcitability, polydipsia, increased frequency of urination and/or defecation, urinary retention, aggression, personality changes, and anorexia.[10, 29, 30, 31, 40]

Endorphins may also play a role in perpetuating or inducing pruritic behavior such as excessive grooming. The opiate antagonists bind competitively to opiate receptors in the CNS and block the binding of endogenous endorphins that may be produced or released from self-destructive behavior.[22, 30] This prevents or inhibits the euphoric state that the endorphins would induce, helping to alleviate the desire to be self-destructive. Feline psychogenic alopecia and canine acral lick dermatitis are two syndromes characterized by excessive self-licking. Studies using endorphin blockers demonstrated some efficacy. In cats with feline psychogenic alopecia, naloxone (Narcan) injected subcutaneously (1 mg/kg) resulted in improvement in four of five treated cats.[50] Another study in dogs with acral lick dermatitis showed that the endorphin blocker naltrexone (Trexan) (2.2 mg/kg q24h) was helpful in 70% of the cases treated.[49] Adverse reactions are considered quite uncommon, although there is a report of a dog with naltrexone-induced pruritus.[36] Naltrexone (Nemexin) administered orally successfully suppressed pruritus in various internal and dermatologic diseases in humans, wherein traditional therapeutic modalities had failed.[16a]

Anxiolytic oral drugs (especially benzodiazepines and antihistamines) that may be helpful are phenobarbital, 2.2 to 6.6 mg/kg q12h; diazepam (Valium), 0.2 mg/kg q12h in cats; 0.25 to 1.1 mg/kg q12h in dogs; hydroxyzine (Atarax), 2.2 mg/kg q8h; buspirone (BuSpar) 2.5 to 10 mg q8 to 12h for dogs; 2.5 to 7.5 mg q8–12h for cats.[22, 42] The mechanism of action of this class of drugs is not well known. Possible mechanisms include increased γ-aminobutyric acid activity and antagonism of serotonin activity. Buspirone blocks serotonin presynaptic and postsynaptic receptors and has dopamine agonist activity.[7, 42] Adverse effects include mild sedation, appetite stimulation, personality changes, and paradoxical excitation. In cats, diazepam causes an idiosyncratic hepatotoxicosis that is often fatal.[2] This drug must be discontinued if cats become unduly sedated, lethargic, or anorectic or begin vomiting. Baseline screening serum biochemistry is recommended prior to initiating therapy and after 3 to 5 days of treatment. Special attention is paid to serum alanine aminotransferase (ALT) and aspartate aminotransferase (AST).

• CANINE PSYCHOGENIC DERMATOSES

Acral Lick Dermatitis

Acral lick dermatitis, also known as lick granuloma, results from an urge to lick the lower cranial portion of a leg, producing a thickened, firm, oval plaque. The condition may be organic or psychogenic in origin.[38, 43, 48] In the past, many authors thought that most cases that presented with lesions and a history compatible with acral lick dermatitis were of psychogenic origin; today, however, it is believed that organic disease is commonly present (see Chap. 4, Acral Lick Furunculosis). Potential organic causes should always be excluded. At the very minimum, bacterial or fungal disease, demodicosis, previous trauma, allergy (inhalant, food, flea), and underlying joint disease should be ruled out before diagnosing a case as purely psychogenic in origin. If readily available, electromyography (EMG) may be a valuable tool to identify cases with abnormal paraspinal muscle activity suggesting a neurological origin.[43]

CAUSE AND PATHOGENESIS

Boredom or separation anxiety may cause a dog to develop the habit of licking its leg. A careful history may reveal that the dog is alone much of the day. The classic patient is a large, active dog whose owners work and have no children at home. Either there is no companion dog or another dog in the household provides no play activity. Unusual restrictions on the dog's freedom can be a causative factor. Dogs kept in crates for long periods or dogs that are chained can become bored and relieve their frustrations by constantly licking a leg. In other dogs, a preexisting focal dermatosis (e.g., an infection, neoplasm, or wound) precipitates a vicious circle. The constant licking produces an eroded area on the skin that itches exquisitely. An itch-lick cycle is established until a firm, ulcerated lesion results. Possibly, a wound may initiate the licking, or the licking may occur in response to stress or boredom. The licking of the erosion or wound leads to ulceration and to the exposure of deeper skin layers. The licking prevents the ulcer from healing and predisposes the animal to secondary infection. Epidermal hyperplasia and dermal fibrosis account for the nodular plaque that is characteristic of the disease. The lesion at this stage used to be called a granuloma or tumor, but it is neither neoplastic nor granulomatous.

Excessive licking may cause the production and release of endorphins, making the animal feel better (euphoric) and at the same time producing an analgesic effect that decreases the animal's pain perception. This process essentially addicts the dog to the compulsive licking.

Electrophysiologic studies have suggested that a mild distal sensory axonal polyneuropathy may be present in some cases of acral lick dermatitis,[46] although these abnormalities may be a result and not the cause of the disease. EMG studies of paraspinal muscles demonstrated abnormal spontaneous activity in 56% of the cases, suggesting a possible lesion in ventral motor nerve roots, which is not likely to be a result of the licking in a peripheral area.[43] No cases of primary sensory neuropathy were demonstrated in this study.

On the basis of the phenomenology of the condition and the pharmacologic response, it has been proposed that canine acral lick dermatitis is an animal model of obsessive-compulsive disorder.[19, 22, 31]

CLINICAL FEATURES

Predisposed breeds include the Doberman pinscher, Great Dane, Labrador retriever, Irish setter, golden retriever, and German shepherd.[21, 31, 38, 48] Other breeds, including smaller dogs, can also develop acral lick dermatitis. It can occur at any age, although most dogs are older than 5 years of age when presented for treatment. Males with the disorder outnumber females two to one.

In almost all cases, the lesion is single and unilateral (Fig. 15–1A). In some cases, multiple legs may be affected, and these cases may respond poorly to treatment because there is often an organic disease, such as staphylococcal furunculosis, or an allergy that must be addressed. One clue that there may be a psychogenic component to the condition is the development of a newly licked area when the original lesion has been covered by a bandage or wrap. The most common site for a lesion is the cranial carpal or metacarpal area (see Fig. 15–1B and C). The next most frequent sites are the cranial radial, metatarsal, and tibial regions. Chronic lesions become hard, thickened plaques or nodules that have an ulcerated surface and a hyperpigmented halo (see Fig. 15–1D). Extremely large lesions on the joints that have been present for years may be associated with arthritis or ankylosis of the underlying joint.

DIAGNOSIS

A tentative diagnosis can usually be made from the clinical examination and history. A definitive diagnosis requires ruling out the other differential diagnoses, which include neoplasia, pressure point granulomas, calcinosis circumscripta, bacterial furunculosis, demodicosis, dermatophytosis, mycotic or mycobacterial granulomas, and underlying hypersensitivity disorders. Histiocytomas and mastocytomas may be mistaken for acral lick dermatitis if they occur on the cranial surface of the leg. Fungal cultures confirm the diagnosis of lesions induced by mycoses; exfoliative cytological findings and biopsy samples provide the basis for diagnosis. However, hypoallergenic diets and intradermal tests are often indicated to detect a causative or concurrent allergic disease.

Histopathologically, the lesions usually show features that are characteristic of the disorder but are not diagnostic by themselves.[38] An ulcerated surface is bordered by irregular epidermal hyperplasia, which may be papillated and is usually marked (Fig. 15–2). A mild perivascular accumulation of neutrophils and mononuclear cells is usually present. The dermis shows varying degrees of fibroplasia, and dermal papillae often show vertical streaking of fibroblasts and collagen fibrils (Fig. 15–3). Common findings include moderate-to-marked numbers of plasma cells around the epitrichial sweat glands (Fig. 15–4) and inferior segments of hair follicles and sebaceous gland hyperplasia. Folliculitis or furunculosis may coexist.

Radiographs usually reveal a secondary periosteal reaction of bones that underlie large, chronic, acral lick dermatitis lesions.[38] Joint disease is not induced by the licking; if present, joint disease may be the cause of the excessive licking.

CLINICAL MANAGEMENT

Psychological counseling with the client should be the first step in the management of acral lick dermatitis of psychogenic origin. The client needs to understand that the dog's problem is in its head and not just on the leg. Together, the clinician and client must become psychological detectives to find what caused the dog to lick its leg. Examples of causes include the following:

1. The dog is left alone all day.
2. The dog is confined for long periods to a crate, kennel, cage, or run.
3. There is a new pet in the home.
4. There is a new baby in the home.
5. A female dog is in heat nearby but not accessible to the male dog.
6. A new dog has come to the neighborhood.
7. A death has occurred in the family.
8. A long-time companion of the dog has died.
9. Children or other family members have moved away.

The first step in treatment is to recognize the cause and eliminate it, if possible. Sometimes a change in the dog's lifestyle is the answer. Each situation differs, but the following are examples of successful corrective measures:

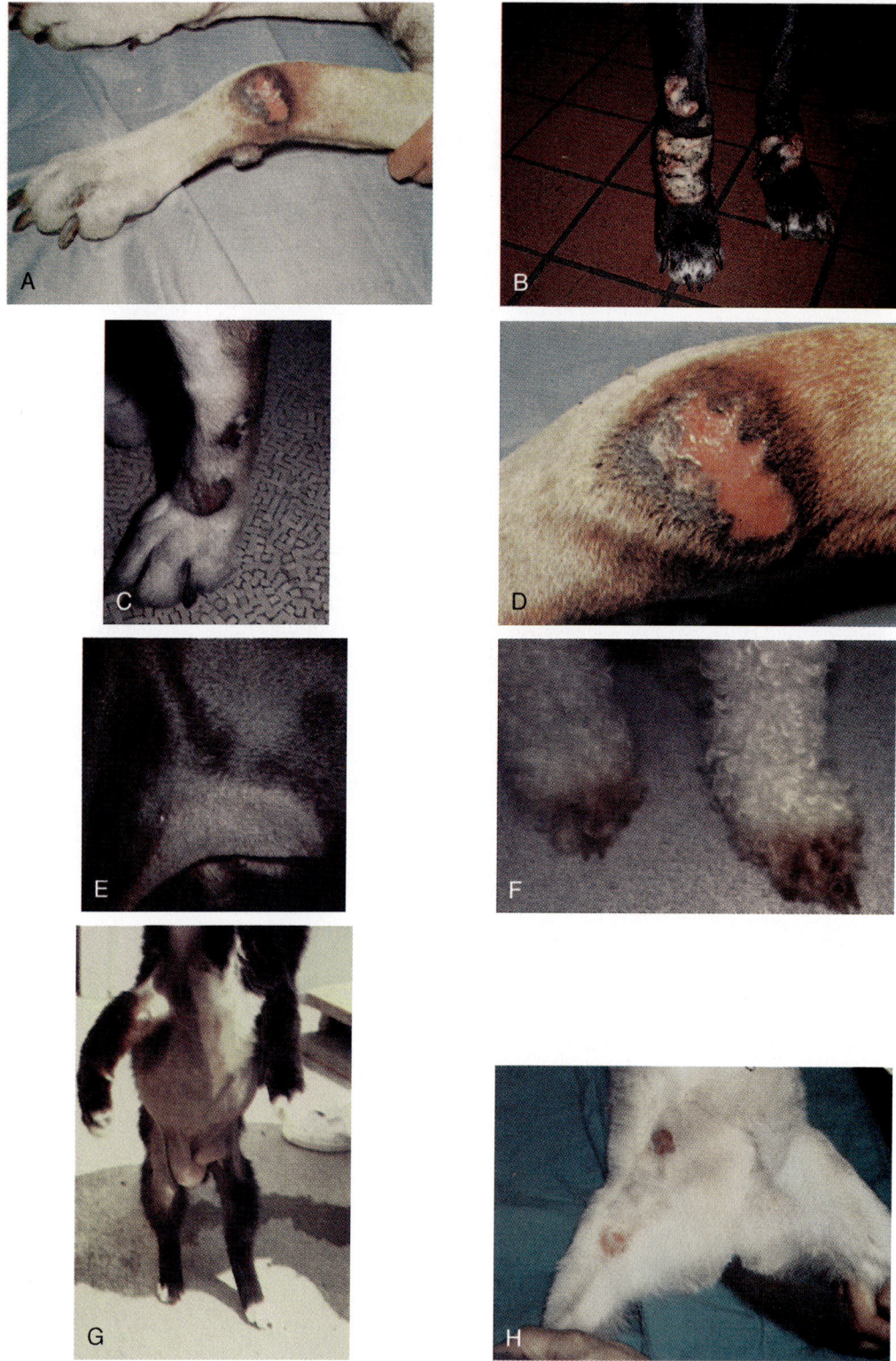

FIGURE 15–1. *A*, Acral lick dermatitis. The carpal area is commonly affected. *B*, Bilateral acral lick dermatitis in a Great Dane. *C*, Metatarsal acral lick dermatitis demonstrating characteristic location and appearance. *D*, Close-up of *A* shows the thickened nodule with the characteristic ulcerated epidermis surrounded by a hyperpigmented halo. *E*, Flank sucking. Focal area of alopecia, lichenification, and hyperpigmentation in the flank of a

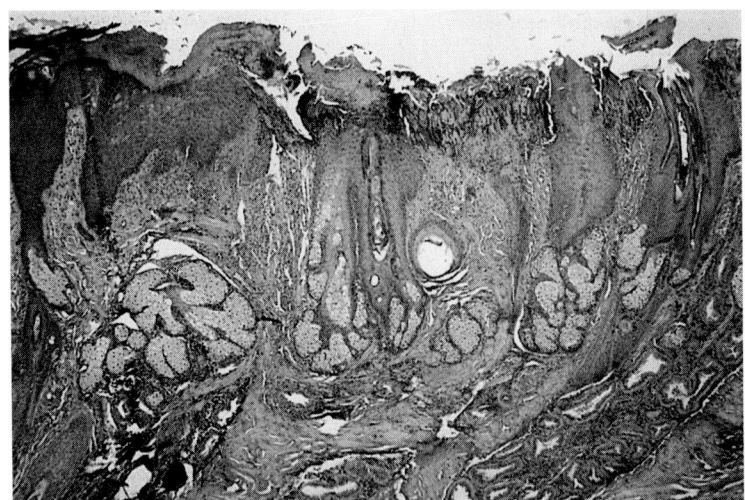

FIGURE 15-2. Canine acral lick dermatitis. Fibrosing dermatitis with marked epidermal and sebaceous gland hyperplasia, and surface ulceration.

1. More walks and human companionship are very helpful. Some owners can take their dog to work if they own a small shop or business.
2. For a kennel dog, avoidance of confinement to cages, kennels, or runs can be beneficial. The owner can make a house pet of the afflicted dog. Even nightly confinement to a cage may cause enough frustration to trigger acral lick dermatitis.
3. A new puppy as a companion can act as a diversion that may discourage further licking. The success of this method depends on the extent to which a friendship develops between the two dogs. For a male dog, a spayed female is very suitable. The owner should be aware, however, that obtaining a companion dog is not a guaranteed cure.
4. Freedom to leave the house and premises can enable the dog to develop a life of its own in the neighborhood. This suggestion is suitable for some rural areas but is usually impossible in suburban or urban areas where leash laws are in effect.

Once the lesion is present, therapy for the psychological component alone may not be effective. Systemic, topical, and surgical treatment may be required along with psychotherapy. One or more of the following approaches may be useful.[20–22]

- **Psychological Drug Therapy.** The psychological drugs may be needed for only a short while, until the habit is broken by behavior modification or the underlying boredom or stress is eliminated. In other cases, long-term treatment may be required. *Antidepressants* are the most effective. Doxepin and amitriptyline are less expensive and can be used when long-term treatment is required. In some cases, a more expensive drug such as fluoxetine or clomipramine may be needed initially, but maintenance with a less expensive drug may be possible. For difficult cases, fluoxetine and clomipramine have been the most effective treatments. In a double-blind, placebo-controlled study, clomipramine was effective for the treatment of canine acral lick dermatitis.[10] However, stressors were not removed, and all dogs relapsed when clomipramine therapy was stopped. Others have also had success with clomipramine.[27]

Anxiolytic oral drugs (especially benzodiazepines and antihistamines) that may be helpful but less effective than the antidepressants are phenobarbital and diazepam. Hy-

---

FIGURE 15-1. *Continued* Doberman pinscher. *F*, Salivary staining of the paws associated with *Malassezia* pododermatitis in an atopic dog. *G*, Typical pattern in feline psychogenic alopecia with self-inflicted alopecia of the abdomen, groin, and inguinal regions. Note the alopecia on the medial forelegs and the mammary enlargement in this cat that were caused by megestrol acetate. *H*, Erosive plaque of dermatitis in a cat from self-licking. Alopecia is also present.

1062 • Psychogenic Skin Diseases

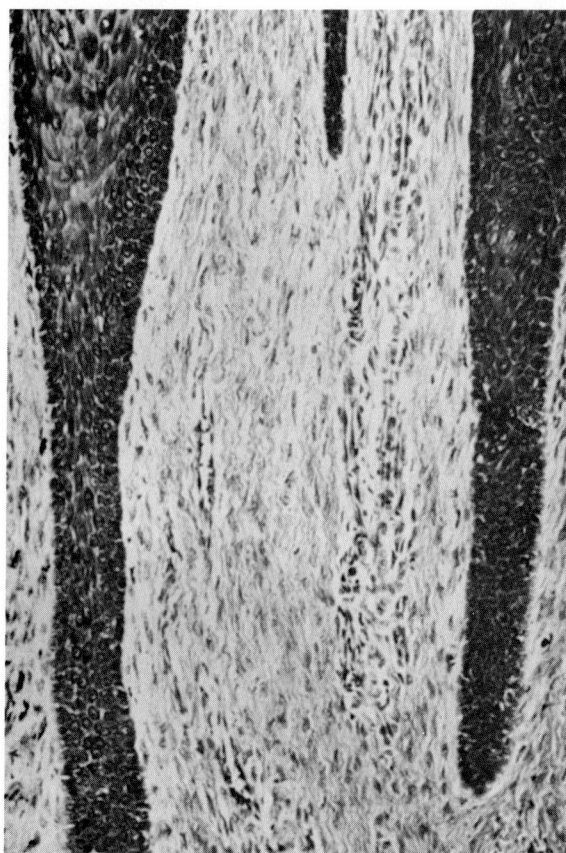

FIGURE 15–3. Canine acral lick dermatitis. Vertical streaking of collagen fibrils between rete ridges.

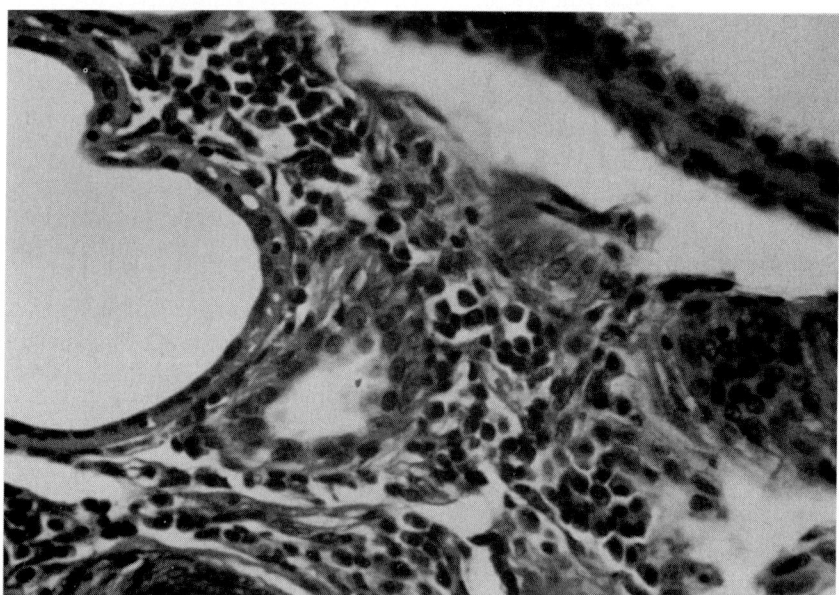

FIGURE 15–4. Canine acral lick dermatitis. Periepitrichial sweat gland accumulation of plasma cells.

droxyzine (Atarax), 2.2 mg/kg q8h, is a piperazine-derivative antihistamine with other effects that has been helpful in some cases, especially those associated with allergy.

Endorphin blockers may also be effective. Naltrexone (Trexan) has been used in dogs with severe chronic acral lick dermatitis.[3, 49] Dogs were treated with 2.2 mg/kg orally every 24 hours. Of 10 dogs, 7 responded well, but 4 dogs relapsed when the drug was discontinued. Long-term control may be accomplished with reduced doses or longer intervals between doses. No significant side-effects have been seen. The drug is very expensive.

Endorphin substitution by the administration of an exogenous source of opiate may decrease dogs' desire to stimulate the release of endorphins. Hydrocodone (Hycodan) at 0.25 mg/kg q8h improved 3 dogs within 3 weeks.[1] Two were 100% better after 16 weeks of treatment.

Progestagens have a calming effect, especially on male dogs. An injection of repositol progesterone (Depo-Provera, 20 mg/kg every 3 weeks) has been successful in selected cases.[28] Megestrol acetate (Megace, Ovaban) has been used orally at 1 mg/kg q24h, then tapered to minimal maintenance doses and frequencies. These agents have to be continued for several months and should not be used in intact female dogs.

- **Treating the Lesion.** At the same time as the psychological treatment, the skin lesion should be treated until it is healed; treatment of the lesion alone yields disappointing results. Attempts at preventing licking mechanically by the use of Elizabethan collars, buckets, muzzles, bandages, casts, and wire-cloth devices may be helpful in allowing initial healing but are usually unsuccessful alone. Repellent liquids and creams have shown only limited success and usually only with early and mild lesions.

  - *Topical Applications.* Topical corticosteroids may be helpful, but their use is limited to the mild early lesion. One commercially available product, Synotic, contains fluocinolone acetonide 0.01% in 60% dimethyl sulfoxide (DMSO). This product is applied twice a day. Dissolved in DMSO, corticosteroids can penetrate the lesion. One homemade formula uses equal parts of 90% DMSO solution and a solution of 1% hydrocortisone acetate and 2% Burrow's solution in propylene glycol (Hydro B-1020, Hydro-Plus). This solution is applied to the lesion twice a day for several weeks. Rubber gloves should be worn by the dog's owner when handling this and all other products containing DMSO. A combination of fluocinolone in DMSO (Synotic) and flunixin meglumine (Banamine) has been reported to be effective in many cases.[38] Three milliliters of flunixine meglumine are added to an 8-ml vial of Synotic. This solution is applied twice a day until the lesion has healed. The treatment time varies from 3 to 8 weeks. The *analgesic* capsaicin (HEET) mixed with bitter apple (isopropyl alcohol, water, bitter extract)—one part HEET (capsaicin 0.25%, methyl salicylate 15%, camphor 3.6%, acetone, alcohol) to two parts bitter apple—has also been reported to be effective in early lesions.[9] This solution is applied initially two to three times per day, then tapered as needed.

  - *Intralesional Injections.* Triamcinolone acetonide (Vetalog) or methylprednisolone acetate (Depo-Medrol) injections have also been recommended. These agents are helpful in lesions smaller than 3 cm in diameter. They are useless in large chronic lesions.

  - *Surgical Removal.* In some cases, surgical excision of the entire lesion is the treatment of choice. This is easily and quickly accomplished if the lesion is small enough to allow surgical repair without undue skin tension. The clinician should always close the incision with mattress sutures and use bandages or protective devices to prevent removal of the sutures or self-inflicted trauma by the dog before healing is complete, which requires at least 2 to 3 weeks. If the animal traumatizes the surgical site before complete healing has occurred, the resulting wound will be very difficult to manage. Systemic antibiotics should always be prescribed postoperatively. In extreme cases, excision of the lesion and replacement with a full-thickness skin graft can be performed.

- *Laser Therapy.* Some cases may respond to laser therapy, which has the advantages of sterilizing the lesion as the tissue is vaporized and less postoperative pain.
- *Radiation Therapy.* The occasional effectiveness of radiation therapy has, in general, been shown to correlate with the duration and size of the lesion.[16, 23, 32] Large chronic lesions are much less likely to respond favorably. Only 35% of the cases have sustained excellent responses to radiation therapy.[32]
- *Cryosurgery.* Cryosurgery may be used as a last resort for lesions that are so large they cannot be removed surgically, cannot be grafted with a full-thickness skin flap, and have not responded to other treatment. When properly performed, the hardened mass of tissue is frozen and sloughs over several weeks. New healthy skin begins to grow from the wound margins. Freezing destroys nerve endings, thereby blocking the itch-lick cycle. The procedure must usually be repeated two or three times. It should be attempted only by those familiar with cryosurgical techniques.
- *Acupuncture.* Acupuncture has been reported to be effective, but its usefulness must be documented further.[15]
- *Electroshock.* Good responses were reported in a few dogs with the use of remote punishment, using precisely controlled momentary shock from an electronic training collar.[4]

In summary, a guarded prognosis should be given to the client before beginning any treatment. Acral lick dermatitis is one of the most obstinate skin disorders, but at least it is not life-threatening.

Miscellaneous Psychogenic Manifestations

There is a group of six psychogenic manifestations (obsessive-compulsive disorders) that involves sucking or licking a specifically selected anatomic area.[22, 47] The animal concentrates on one area to which it habitually returns. The treatment regimens that can be tried are those discussed for canine acral lick dermatitis and feline psychogenic alopecia and dermatitis.

TAIL BITING

Tail biting is seen mostly in young, long-tailed, long-haired dogs. These dogs chase their tail and then bite the tip (Fig. 15–5). Many of the afflicted dogs stop this habit when they

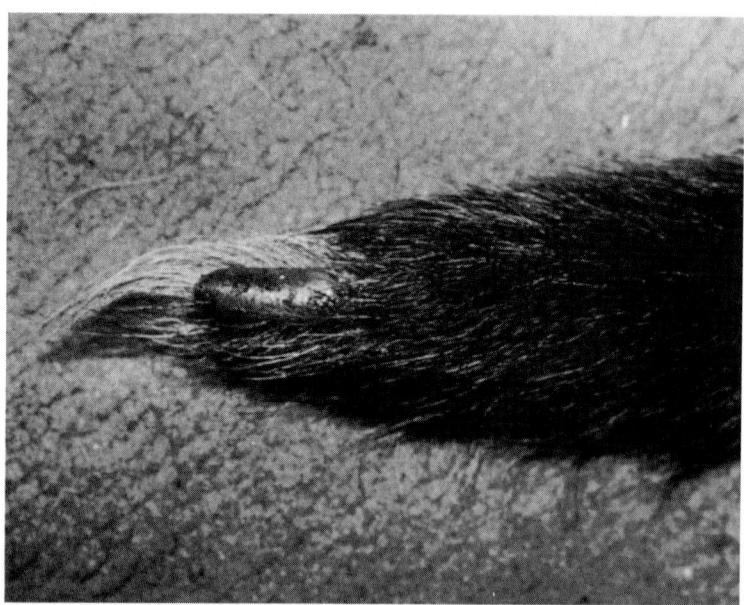

FIGURE 15–5. Tail biting in a dog. Notice the alopecia and excoriation on the tip of the tail.

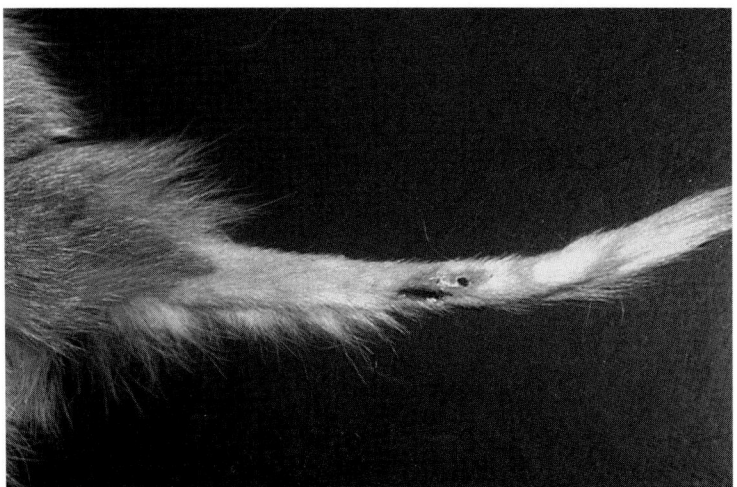

FIGURE 15-6. Excessive tail grooming in a cat with a sacral vertebral anomaly.

get older. These tail-chasers must be differentiated from the dog and occasional cat (Fig. 15-6) that traumatizes the tail tip when it becomes infected and pruritic or when the tail's normal sensations are altered by lumbosacral stenosis, cauda equina syndrome, or tail dock neuroma.

TAIL DOCK NEUROMA

This is a rare disorder that follows some tail dockings.[6] Cocker spaniels may be predisposed. The nerves attempt to regrow in a haphazard fashion, and a neuroma develops. This is palpable as a firm, deep nodule that usually adheres to the skin in the scarred tail tip. Histologically, the nodule is characterized by fibrous tissue with thick collagen bundles and multiple small nerve bundles randomly located throughout the nodule (see Chap. 20). This neuroma appears to stimulate pain or some sensation that causes the dog to lick or chew at its tail. Surgical removal of the neuroma is the treatment of choice.

FLANK SUCKING

Flank sucking in dogs is similar, in most respects, to tail sucking in cats, but it is more common and is especially prevalent in Doberman pinschers (see Fig. 15-1E). At one time, trichuriasis was thought to be a cause of the disorder, but this has not been documented. In fact, treatment for whipworms or surgical removal of the cecum (typhlectomy) was rarely successful. It has been suggested that tail biters and flank suckers may have a form of psychomotor epilepsy. This condition should be differentiated from localized folliculitis, which is pruritic. Folliculitis is usually associated with inflammation and alopecia, and it may demonstrate hyperpigmentation and lichenification. These conditions respond to antibiotics. Atopy and food hypersensitivity should also be ruled out. Biopsies should be performed before a diagnosis of psychogenic flank sucking is made because the presence of dermatopathological abnormalities suggests that an underlying organic disease is present. Therapy with phenobarbital or primidone may be helpful. One investigator has suggested a single intramuscular injection of medroxyprogesterone acetate (20 mg/kg) as possible therapy.[28]

SELF-NURSING

This is largely restricted to female dogs and cats but can occasionally be seen in males. Usually the self-nursing is confined to one nipple, and the animal repeatedly suckles that nipple. The nipple may become enlarged through inflammation and lichenification. Spaying the animal seems to be helpful in correcting this annoying habit. Sedation and psychological training to break the habit may also be useful.

ANAL LICKING

This habit, which is almost impossible to break, occurs only in dogs, and a breed predilection exists for Poodles. Many dogs, and particularly Poodles, lick the anal area because of anal sac disease, *Malassezia* anal sacculitis, and even perianal *Malassezia* dermatitis. However, if these causes, atopy, and food hypersensitivity are ruled out, the possibility of psychogenic anal licking becomes much more likely. Removal of the anal sacs is not curative in this syndrome. Anorectal disease, particularly inflammation of the lower colon and rectal mucosa, should also be ruled out. Neurotic Poodles that lick the anal area cause their owners much anguish. When this condition is chronic, the perianal skin becomes thickened, hyperpigmented, verrucous, and lichenified (Fig. 15–7). Secondary bacterial pyoderma or *Malassezia* dermatitis is likely, and some response to antibiotics or antiyeast medication occurs. The specific therapy is to try to identify and remove the cause or to administer antianxiety or antidepressant drugs as for acral lick dermatitis.

FOOT LICKING

This condition is usually associated with atopy, other hypersensitivities, or *Malassezia* dermatitis (see Fig. 15–1F); foot licking is rarely seen alone. It is a difficult habit to break, but therapy with heterocyclic antidepressants may be helpful.

• FELINE PSYCHOGENIC DERMATOSES

Psychogenic Alopecia and Dermatitis

Psychogenic alopecia or dermatitis *(neurodermatitis)* is an alopecia or a chronic skin inflammation produced by constant licking. When dermatitis is not present, the complaint may be of excessive grooming.[12, 37] The dermatic form results from more severe grooming.

CAUSE AND PATHOGENESIS

The primary abnormality is thought to be excessive grooming that may result from an anxiety neurosis. The anxiety may be caused by psychological factors such as displacement phenomena (e.g., a new pet or baby in the household, a move to new surroundings, boarding, hospitalization, loss of a favorite bed or companion, or competition for a social hierarchy position with other pets in the household or in response to other cats entering the affected cat's territory). There is a breed predilection for the more emotional breeds, such as Siamese and Abyssinian, although all the Oriental breeds may be predisposed.[35, 37] Feline psychogenic alopecia has been proposed as an animal model of obsessive-compulsive disorder.[8, 22, 35]

Feline psychogenic alopecia and dermatitis may be expressed in many ways. Some cats lick vigorously at a particular area until the sharp barbs on the tongue produce alopecia, abrasion, ulceration, and secondary infection. Other cats lick and chew more gently or over a more widespread area so that alopecia is the predominant lesion. Some cats actually chew at their hair or skin, whereas others chew and pull their hair out.

It has been proposed that the stress may induce an elevation in the levels of adrenocorticotropic hormone and melanocyte-stimulating hormone, which then causes increased endorphin production.[50] The endorphins protect the animal from abnormalities associated with chronic stress. However, their narcotic, addictive-like effect may act to reinforce the abnormal grooming behavior. Agents with dopaminergic or opioid effects may decrease excessive grooming.[51]

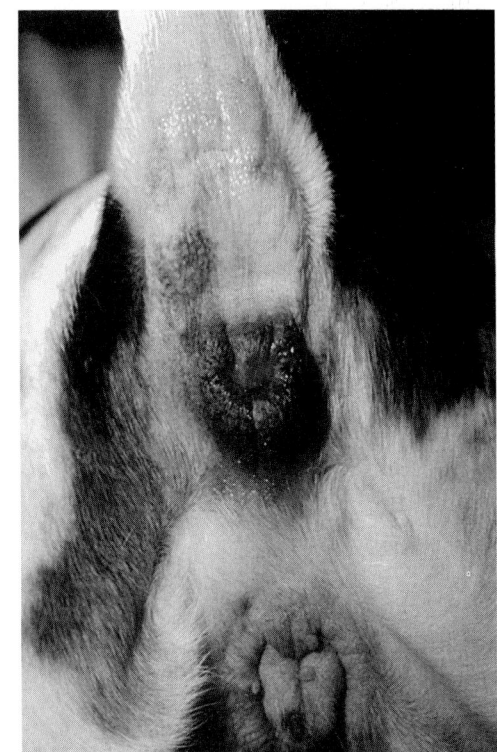

FIGURE 15–7. Anal licking in a dog. The perianal area is erythematous, lichenified, and hyperpigmented.

CLINICAL FEATURES

There are no age or sex predilections.[35, 37] Areas that the cat can lick easily are the most common sites: medial forelegs, the inside of the thigh, the caudal abdomen, and the inguinal region (Fig. 15–8; see also Fig. 15–1G). Less commonly, the dorsal lumbar, sacral, or tail regions may be involved. This pattern should raise one's index of suspicion about flea bite hypersensitivity. A symmetric alopecia may also involve the caudomedial thighs and ventrum. The characteristic lesion of the dermatitic form is a bright red, elongated, oval plaque or red streak (see Fig. 15–1 H). Eosinophilic plaques may result. Animals with chronic cases develop lichenification and hyperpigmentation. The course is long and progresses slowly, sometimes remaining static for months. Siamese or Siamese-cross cats often lick out the hair in a localized area of the back, the ventral abdomen, or a leg without causing a skin reaction. Because the temperature-labile enzymes that convert melanin precursors into melanin are active (high temperatures produce white hair, low temperatures produce pigmented hair, and the hairless area is cool), the hair becomes dark (Fig. 15–9). After the next shedding, the hair is usually replaced by normal-colored hair.

DIAGNOSIS

Lesions of the dermatitic form may be confused with or possibly develop into eosinophilic plaques. The alopecic forms may be confused with dermatophytosis, demodicosis, atopy, food or flea bite hypersensitivity, and feline acquired symmetric alopecia. Because cats are often reclusive groomers, owners may not know that the cat is licking or chewing excessively. Several helpful techniques are available to answer the question, "Does the cat groom excessively?" Tufts of hair may have been found in the cat's favorite hiding places. Alternatively, the cat may be vomiting hairballs, or hair may be visible in the feces. With cats that use litter boxes, the client can inspect the feces over the next several days and

1068 • Psychogenic Skin Diseases

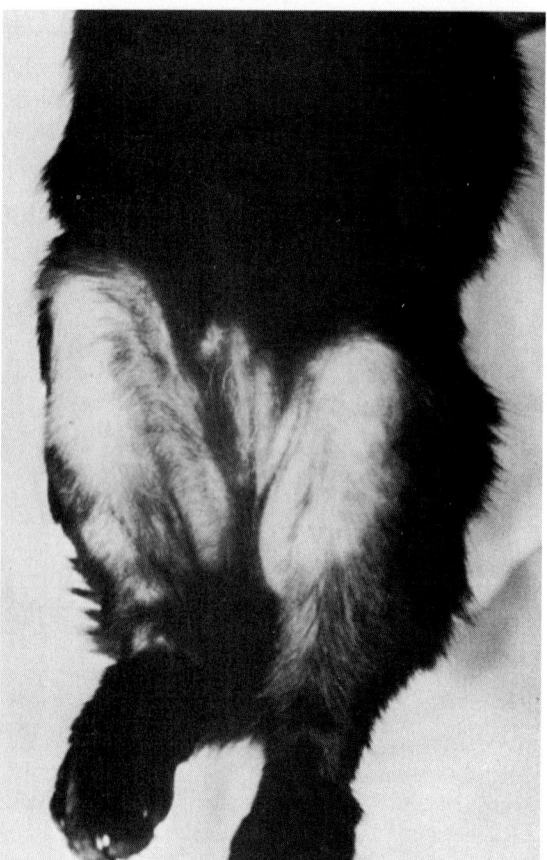

FIGURE 15-8. Feline psychogenic alopecia. Hair has been removed from the inguinal area by the cat's licking and biting.

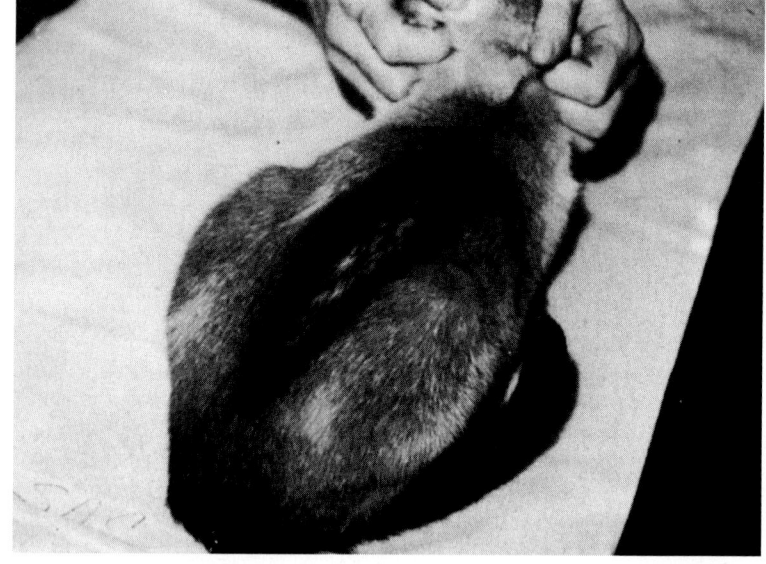

FIGURE 15-9. Constant licking removed hair from the back, reducing the skin temperature and causing the hair to grow in dark in color.

find that they contain hair. Physical examination reveals short stubby hairs that are readily palpated by rubbing the fingertips against the normal angle of hair growth. Another method is to roll the skin and view the folded skin perpendicularly to reveal numerous shorn-off hairs (Fig. 15–10). Placing an Elizabethan collar on the cat will result in hair growth in areas that cannot be groomed. This time-consuming procedure is rarely needed to establish excessive grooming as a cause of the hair loss. A simple laboratory test for differentiating between self-induced hair loss and spontaneous alopecia is the epilation and microscopic examination of hairs from the affected areas. In psychogenic alopecia, hairs do not epilate easily; they appear to be broken off when examined microscopically (see Fig. 2–28G), and the hairs regrow while the cat is wearing an Elizabethan collar. In addition, cats that are fur-mowing as a result of a hypersensitivity often respond to an injection of methylprednisolone acetate, whereas cats with psychogenic disease do not.

Because feline psychogenic alopecia is diagnosed primarily by ruling out other differential diagnoses, an accurate diagnosis involves a complete work-up. Skin scrapings, fungal cultures, biopsies (which should show normal skin in nondermatitic areas), and a complete blood cell count constitute the minimal database that should be obtained. If an eosinophilia is present or the biopsy reveals an inflammatory or endocrine appearance, the diagnosis of psychogenic alopecia is not warranted. Further tests should include hypoallergenic diet trials; trial ectoparasite therapy for *Cheyletiella*, *Otodectes*, and the superficial *Demodex gatoi* mite (see Chap. 6); intradermal allergen testing; and endocrine function testing. An initial alternative to the endocrine function test may be a 30-day trial with an Elizabethan collar. Cats that respond to liothyronine supplementation do not regrow their hair when grooming is prevented.[45]

CLINICAL MANAGEMENT

Many of the treatments for psychogenic dermatoses have potential side effects, require frequent administration, and are expensive. Therefore, cats with the alopecic form of the disease may best be served by no treatment other than attempts at relieving the stressful situation.

Cats are such territorial creatures that a change in the pecking order of animals in the territory has tremendous anxiety potential. One needs to look for a new cat that entered the household or that invaded the cat's territory. Other factors are barking dogs, a new baby, moving to a new home, or major changes in the present home. If these problems can be modified or removed, the cat may improve without any therapy or with just a 30-day course of antianxiety drugs to break the habit. If potential stressors cannot be eliminated, the cat may have to be maintained on medication continuously.[35]

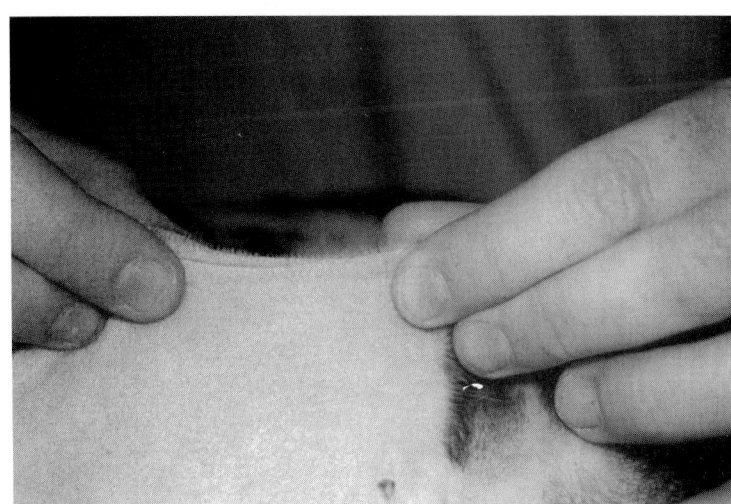

FIGURE 15–10. "Fur-mowing" in a cat. By rolling the skin one can see the short broken hairs still present.

Topical medications are of little value because the cat immediately licks them off. The alopecic form may be successfully managed with phenobarbital (2.2 to 6.6 mg/kg q12h orally) or diazepam (total dose of 1 to 2 mg orally q12h to q24h). Some authors have reported occasional success with 12.5 to 25 mg of primidone administered orally q8h to q24h.[12]. Treatment with the endorphin blocker naloxone 1 mg/kg subcutaneously has been shown to have some efficacy, with one injection lasting up to several weeks.[50, 51] Fluoxetine at 1 mg/kg q24h has been reported effective in two cats with behaviorally induced symmetrical alopecia.[8, 33] In a study of 11 cats with psychogenic alopecia, 5 of 5 responded to clomipramine at 1.25 to 2.5 mg PO q24h; 2 of 3 responded to amitriptyline at 5 mg PO q12h, and 1 of 4 responded to buspirone at 5 mg PO q12h.[35] Others have also had success with clomipramine.[39, 44] If a thorough diagnostic work-up was not performed or if previous treatments proved ineffective, trial therapy with chlorpheniramine 2 mg/cat q12h or systemic glucocorticoids is warranted. A response may be seen in some cases of psychogenic alopecia; however, allergic dermatitis may also respond. Aggressive flea control may help in cats that are not intradermally test-positive to fleas. Whether this response to flea control reflects an undetected flea allergy or that the presence of fleas stresses the cat is unknown. In cases of dermatitis, if cytologic tests reveal intracellular bacteria, concurrent antibiotic therapy is indicated. Progestational compounds (a total dose of 2.5 to 5.0 mg megestrol acetate [Ovaban] administered orally every other day, then weekly, or 100 mg medroxyprogesterone acetate [Depo-Provera] administered subcutaneously as needed) have also been recommended. Again, the side effects of these drugs can be striking, so one must weigh the gravity of the disease against the possible drug toxicities.

Tail Sucking

Tail sucking occurs mostly in cats and specifically in Siamese cats. It is easily recognized by a wetness of the distal 2 to 3 cm of the tail (Fig. 15–11). Close examination of the

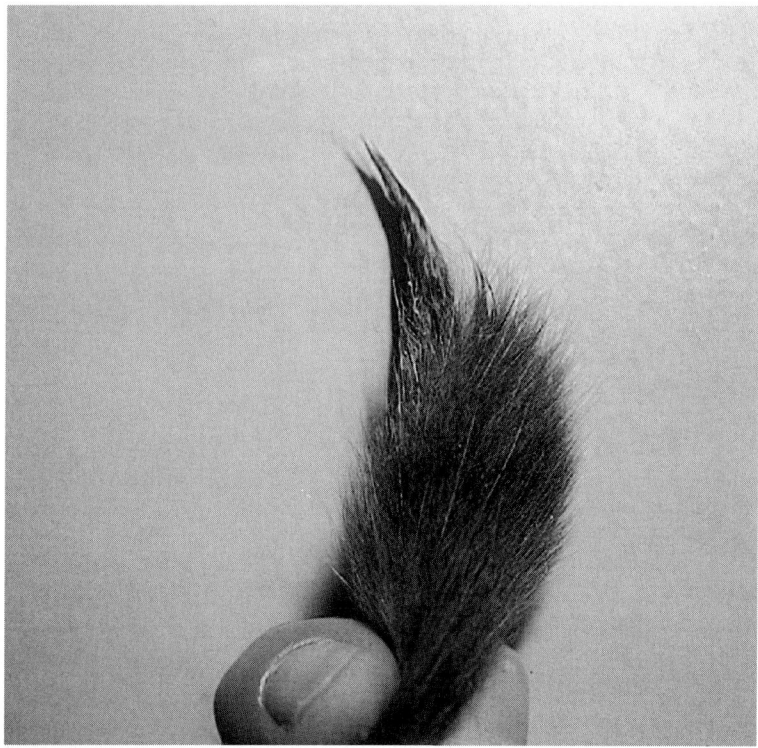

FIGURE 15–11. Tail sucking in a cat. The tip of the tail is wet and matted.

skin reveals normal skin without inflammation or scaling. Whenever the cat ceases to lick the tail and the hair dries, the condition can no longer be detected. Drying occurs when the cat's attention is focused on interesting activities; when bored, the cat resumes licking its tail. Treatment is not successful until the cat's boredom is relieved, possibly by changes in its lifestyle.

• REFERENCES

1. Brignac MM: Hydrocodone treatment of acral lick dermatitis. Proc World Congress Vet Dermatol 2:50, 1992.
2. Center SA, et al: Fulminant hepatic failure associated with oral administration of diazepam in 11 cats. J Am Vet Med Assoc 209:618, 1996.
3. Dodman NH, et al: Use of narcotic antagonists to modify stereotypic self-licking, self-chewing, and scratching behavior in dogs. J Am Vet Med Assoc 193:815, 1988.
4. Eckstein RA, Hart BL: Treatment of canine acral lick dermatitis by behavior modification using electronic stimulation. J Am Anim Hosp Assoc 32:225, 1996.
5. Goldberger E, Rapoport JL: Canine acral lick dermatitis: Response to the antiobsessional drug clomipramine. J Am Anim Hosp Assoc 27:179, 1991.
6. Gross TL, Carr SH: Amputation neuroma of docked tails in dogs. Vet Pathol 27:61, 1990.
7. Gupta MA, Gupta AK: Psychodermatology: An update. J Am Acad Dermatol 34:1030, 1996.
8. Hartmann L: Cats as possible obsessive-compulsive disorder and medication models. Am J Psychiatry 152:1236, 1995.
9. Helton-Rhodes K: Bitter apple: HEET combination topical therapy in the dog. Dermatol Spring/Summer 1993, p 5.
10. Hewson CJ, et al: Efficacy of clomipramine in the treatment of canine compulsive disorder. J Am Vet Med Assoc 213:1760, 1998.
11. Hewson CJ, et al: The pharmacokinetics of clomipramine in dogs: Parameter estimates following a single oral dose and 28 consecutive daily oral doses of clomipramine. J Vet Pharmacol Ther 21:214, 1998.
12. Holzworth J: Diseases of the Cat: Medicine and Surgery, vol. I. W.B. Saunders Co, Philadelphia, 1987.
12a. King JN, et al: Pharmacokinetics of clomipramine in dogs following single-dose intravenous and oral administration. Am J Vet Res 61:74, 2000.
13. Koblenzer CS: Pharmacology of psychotropic drugs useful in dermatologic practice. Int J Dermatol 32:162, 1993.
14. Koo JYM, Pham CT: Psychodermatology: Practical guidelines in pharmacotherapy. Arch Dermatol 128:381, 1992.
15. Looney AL, Rothstein E: Use of acupuncture to treat psychodermatosis in the dog. Canine Pract 23:18, 1998.
16. MacDonald JM: Personal communication, 1991.
16a. Metze D, et al: Efficacy and safety of naltrexone, an oral opiate receptor antagonist, in the treatment of pruritus in internal and dermatological diseases. J Am Acad Dermatol 41:533, 1999.
17. Miller WH Jr, et al: Nonsteroidal management of canine pruritus with amitriptyline. Cornell Vet 82:53, 1992.
18. O'Sullivan RL, et al: The neuro-immuno-cutaneous-endocrine network: Relationship of mind and skin. Arch Dermatol 134:1431, 1998.
19. Overall KL: Recognition, diagnosis, and management of obsessive-compulsive disorders: Part 1. Canine Pract 17:40, 1992.
20. Overall KL: Recognition, diagnosis, and management of obsessive-compulsive disorders: Part 2—a rational approach. Canine Pract 17:25, 1992.
21. Overall KL: Recognition, diagnosis, and management of obsessive-compulsive disorders: Part 3—a rational approach. Canine Pract 17:39, 1992.
22. Overall KL: Clinical Behavioral Medicine for Small Animals. Mosby, St. Louis, 1997.
23. Owen LN: Canine lick granuloma treated with radiotherapy. J Small Anim Pract 30:454, 1989.
24. Panconesi E: Stress and skin diseases: Psychosomatic dermatology. Clin Dermatol 2:4, 1984.
25. Paradis M, Bettenay S: Nonsteroidal antipruritic drugs in small animals. In: Ihrke PJ, et al (eds): Advances in Veterinary Dermatology II. Pergamon Press, New York, 1993, p 429.
26. Paradis M, et al: Further investigations on the use of nonsteroidal anti-inflammatory agents in the management of canine pruritus. J Am Anim Hosp Assoc 27:44, 1991.
27. Paterson S: A placebo-controlled study to investigate clomipramine in the treatment of canine acral lick dermatitis. In: Kwochka KW, et al (eds): Advances in Veterinary Dermatology III. Butterworth-Heinemann, Oxford, 1998, p 436.
28. Pemberton PL: Canine and feline behavior control: Progestin therapy. In: Kirk RW (ed): Current Veterinary Therapy VIII. W.B. Saunders Co, Philadelphia, 1983, p 62.
29. Pfeiffer E, et al: Clomipramine-induced urinary retention in a cat. Can Vet J 40:265, 1999.
30. Plumb DC: Veterinary Drug Handbook, 3rd ed. Iowa State University Press, Ames, 1999.
31. Rapoport JL, et al: Drug treatment of canine acral lick: An animal model of obsessive-compulsive disorder. Arch Gen Psychiatr 49:517, 1992.
32. Rivers B, et al: Treatment of canine acral lick dermatitis with radiation therapy: 17 cases (1979–1991). J Am Anim Hosp Assoc 29:541, 1993.
33. Romatowski J: Two cases of fluoxetine-responsive behavior disorders in cats. Feline Pract 26:14, 1998.
34. Russell M, et al: Learned histamine release. Science 225:733, 1984.
35. Sawyer LS, et al: Psychogenic alopecia in cats: 11 cases (1993–1996). J Am Vet Med Assoc 214:71, 1999.
36. Schwartz S: Naltrexone-induced pruritus in a dog with tail-chasing behavior. J Am Vet Med Assoc 202:278, 1993.
37. Scott DW: Feline dermatology 1900–1978: A monograph. J Am Anim Hosp Assoc 16:331, 1980.
38. Scott DW, Walton DK: Clinical evaluation of a topical

treatment for canine acral lick dermatitis. J Am Anim Hosp Assoc 20:562, 1984.
39. Seksel K, Linderman MJ: Use of clomipramine in the treatment of anxiety-related and obsessive-compulsive disorders in cats. Aust Vet J 76:317, 1998.
40. Shoulberg N: The efficacy of fluoxetine (Prozac) in the treatment of acral lick and allergic-inhalant dermatitis in canines. Proc Annu Member Meeting Am Acad Vet Dermatol Am Coll Vet Dermatol 6:31, 1990.
41. Simpson BS, Simpson DM: Behavioral pharmacotherapy: Part I—antipsychotics and antidepressants. Comp Continuing Education Pract Vet 18:1067, 1996.
42. Simpson BS, Simpson DM: Behavioral pharmacotherapy: Part II—anxiolytics and mood stabilizers. Comp Continuing Education Pract Vet 18:1203, 1996.
43. Steiss JE, et al: Letters to the editor—High incidence of EMG abnormalities in canine acral lick dermatitis. Vet Dermatol 6:115,1995.
44. Swanepoel N, et al: Psychogenic alopecia in a cat: Response to clomipramine. J S Afr Vet Assoc 69:22, 1998.
45. Thoday KL: Aspects of feline symmetric alopecia. In: von Tscharner C, Halliwell REW (eds): Advances in Veterinary Dermatology I. Baillière Tindall, London, 1990, p 47.
46. van Nes JJ: Electrophysiological evidence of sensory nerve dysfunction in 10 dogs with acral lick dermatitis. J Am Anim Hosp Assoc 22:157, 1986.
47. Voith VL: Behavioral disorders. In: Davis LE (ed): Handbook of Small Animal Therapeutics. Churchill Livingstone, New York, 1985, p 519.
48. Walton DK: Psychodermatoses. In: Kirk RW (ed): Current Veterinary Therapy IX. W.B. Saunders Co, Philadelphia, 1986, p 557.
49. White SD: Naltrexone for treatment of acral lick dermatitis in dogs. J Am Vet Med Assoc 196:1075, 1990.
50. Willemse T, et al: Feline psychogenic alopecia and the role of the opioid system. In: von Tscharner C, Halliwell REW (eds): Advances in Veterinary Dermatology I. Baillière Tindall, London, 1990, p 195.
51. Willemse T, et al: The effect of haloperidol and naloxone on excessive grooming behavior of cats. Eur Neuropsychopharmacol 39:45, 1994.

Chapter 16

Environmental Skin Diseases

• PHOTODERMATITIS

Electromagnetic radiation comprises a continuous spectrum of wavelengths varying from fractions of angstroms to thousands of meters. The ultraviolet (UV) spectrum is of particular importance in dermatology.[37] UVC (less than 290 nm) is damaging to cells but does not typically reach the earth's surface because of the ozone layer.[27] UVB (290 to 320 nm) is often referred to as the sunburn, or erythema, spectrum and is about 1000 times more erythemogenic than UVA. UVA (320 to 400 nm) penetrates deeper into the skin than UVB and is the spectrum associated with photosensitivity reactions.[27]

Incident ultraviolet light (UVL) is partially reflected, absorbed, and transmitted inward. Absorbed light raises the energy level of light-absorbing molecules (chromophores), resulting in various biochemical processes that can damage virtually any component of a cell. This damage can result in cellular hyperproliferation, mutagenesis, alteration of cell surface markers, and toxicity. Chromophores in the skin include keratin proteins, blood, hemoglobin, porphyrin, carotene, nucleic acids, melanin, lipoproteins, peptide bonds, and aromatic amino acids, such as tyrosine, tryptophan, and histidine.[66] Natural barriers to UVL damage include the stratum corneum, melanin, blood, and carotenes. Melanins absorb UVL and scavenge free radicals produced during the burning but release other free radicals that can be equally or more damaging.[27] These barriers can easily be overcome by prolonged, repeated exposure to sunlight.

Photodermatology is an ever-expanding field in human medicine and includes photodynamic mechanisms and various specific diseases not recognized in veterinary medicine.[37, 67] Phototoxicity and photosensitivity are of primary concern to veterinary clinicians.[96] Phototoxicity is the classic sunburn reaction and is a dose-related response to light exposure. Photosensitivity occurs when the skin has increased susceptibility to the damaging effects of UVL because of the production, ingestion, and injection of or contact with a photodynamic agent. Photosensitivity is most prevalent in farm animals, but cases are recognized in dogs.[30, 51]

• SOLAR DERMATITIS

Solar dermatitis occurs from an actinic reaction on white skin, light skin, or damaged skin (e.g., depigmented or scarred areas) that is not sufficiently covered by hair.[7, 35, 96] The condition develops when such skin is exposed to direct or reflected sunshine. The rapidity of onset and the severity of the reaction depend on various factors related to the animal, the duration of sun exposure, and the intensity of the sunlight. The sun's rays are most intense during the summer months from 9 AM to 3 PM but especially from 11 AM to 2 PM. Altitude influences solar intensity. For every 300-m (1000-ft) increase in elevation, the sun's intensity increases by 4%.[37] The dermatitis is purely a phototoxic reaction (sunburn) and has no apparent relationship to a hypersensitivity state. The pathogenesis of phototoxicity is incompletely understood, but it involves the epidermis and blood vessels of the superficial and deeper vascular plexus. Exposure to UVB and UVC results in the formation of clusters of vacuolated keratinocytes in the superficial epidermis (so-called sunburn cells), as well as apoptotic keratinocytes, vascular dilatation and leakage, and depletion of Langerhans' and mast cells, with an increase in tissue levels of histamine, prostaglandins, leukotrienes, other vasoactive compounds, inflammatory cytokines, adhesion molecules, and reactive oxygen species.[7, 37, 46, 59, 60] These latter changes could be the direct result of the UVB or could be mediated by cytokines released by the epidermal cells.

Oxygen intermediates—superoxide radical (O_2^-), hydrogen peroxide (H_2O_2), and hydroxyl radical ($HO\cdot$)—may be particularly important in the pathogenesis of solar damage.[19a] These substances deplete antioxidants, recruit neutrophils, and can destroy and degrade all components of connective tissue. Natural defenses (antioxidants) include superoxide dismutase, catalase, glutathione peroxidase, vitamin E, vitamin C, and ubiquinones. A biphasic apoptosis can occur. Some apoptotic keratinocytes are seen within 4 hours of exposure due to UVA's direct damaging effect on the cell membrane. Other apoptotic cells appear about 24 hours after exposure. This delayed damage is a result of DNA alteration.[27] Solar dermatitis in companion animals is divided into canine nasal solar dermatitis, feline solar dermatitis, and canine solar dermatitis of the trunk and extremities. The nasal and feline forms are the most common entities and therefore are discussed in the greatest detail.

Canine Nasal Solar Dermatitis

Canine nasal solar dermatitis is an actinic reaction in poorly pigmented nasal skin of dogs.[8, 35, 53, 83, 96]

CAUSE AND PATHOGENESIS

This is a phototoxic reaction occurring in poorly pigmented skin. Affected dogs may be born without pigment, or the nose may have undergone spontaneous noninflammatory depigmentation (see Chap. 13). Australian shepherds appear to be at increased risk.[78, 96] Any dog with an active or resolved traumatic or inflammatory condition that causes hair loss, depigmentation, or scarring of the nasal area is also susceptible to this photodermatitis. The condition is more frequently seen in sunny climates.

CLINICAL FEATURES

The lesions are found principally at the junction of the haired and hairless skin of the nose (Fig. 16–1A), but any area on the nasal planum or the face can be affected if it is sparsely haired and lightly pigmented. Initially, the area that was devoid of pigment becomes erythematous and scaly. If sun exposure continues, perilesional hair loss occurs, with resultant involvement of the newly exposed skin. Exudation and crusting follow, and ulceration may be seen, especially if the dog rubs the area. If intense photoprotection is started early, the area can heal completely. In most cases, these measures are adopted too late, and the lesion heals by scarring. The healed area is larger than the original lesion, and the scarred skin is more susceptible to solar and traumatic damage. Progression and enlargement of the lesions are evident with the passage of each year, but are especially rapid during periods of prolonged exposure to intense sunlight. This usually occurs during the summer months, but may be seen during the winter as a result of reflection from snow. In chronic cases, deep ulcers form and tissues of the nares and nasal tip disappear, exposing unsightly nasal tissues that bleed easily. Sometimes, vertical fissures occur at the nasal tip, dorsal to and involving the nares. After they are established, these fissures are often permanent. Although rare, squamous cell carcinomas can occur.

DIAGNOSIS

The diagnosis of nasal solar dermatitis can be straightforward or complicated, depending on the chronicity of the condition. The key features of the diagnosis are the restriction of

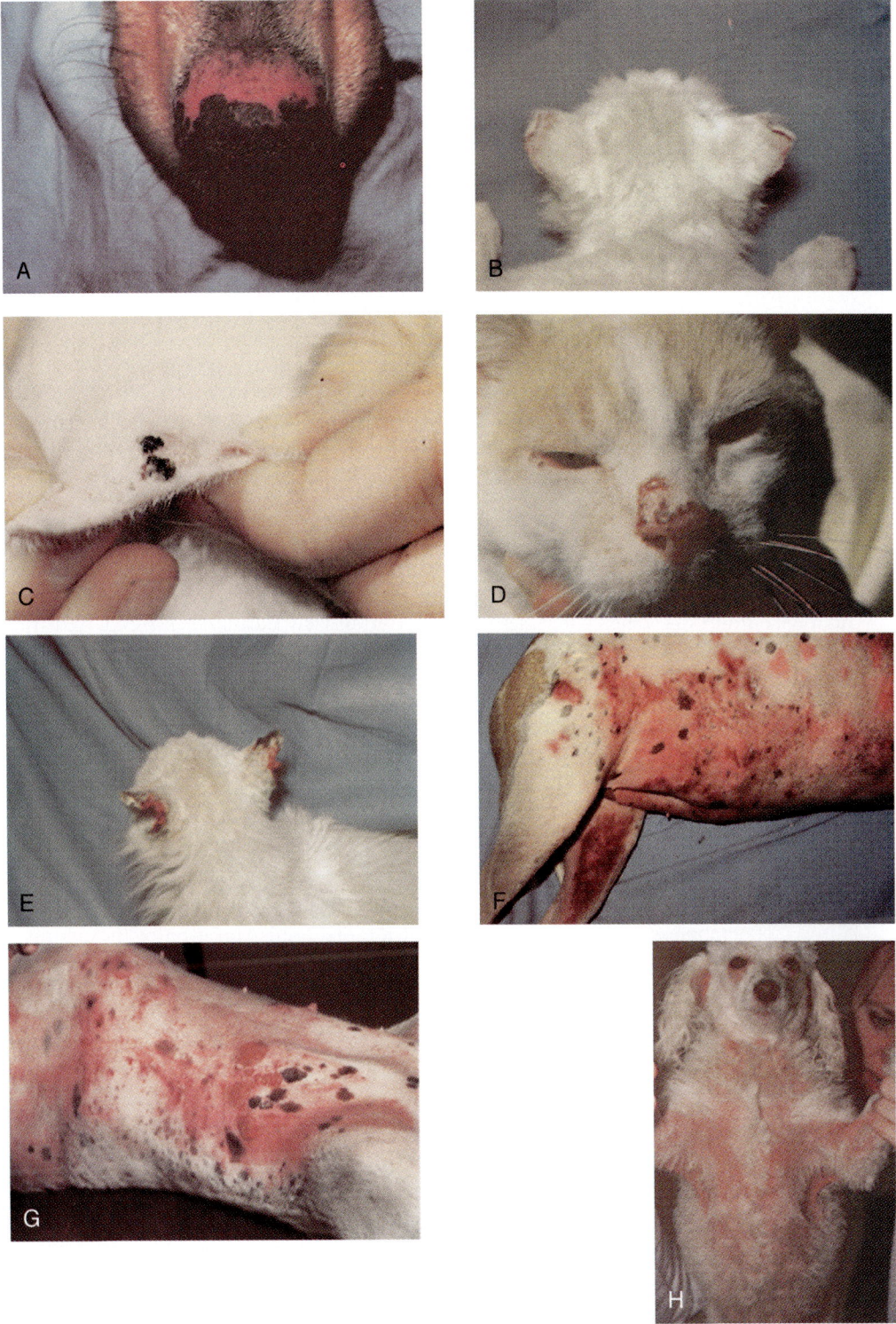

FIGURE 16-1. *A*, Nasal solar dermatitis. Note sharp margin of erythematous, sunburned depigmented area. Negative direct immunoflourescent test. *B*, Feline solar dermatitis. Sunburned, erythematous margins of the pinnae precede the more serious stage of the disease. Note the characteristic curling of the tips. *C*, Actinic keratoses on the pinnal margin. *D*, Actinic keratoses on the nasal area. *E*, This 14-year-old cat had the disease for several years until a squamous cell carcinoma developed on both ears. *F*, Truncal solar dermatitis. Squamous cell carcinoma has developed on the posterior abdomen of sun-loving brown and white Staffordshire terrier. *G*, Close-up of the same dog as in *F*. *H*, Contact dermatitis due to a carpet deodorizer.

lesions to sun-exposed, nonpigmented, sparsely haired skin; the onset of signs after solar exposure; the absence of skin lesions in the affected area before the current condition began; and the complete or near-complete resolution of the lesions with removal from sunlight. In early cases, the affected area is red and scaly, but the architecture should be normal and adjacent areas of black skin should be perfectly normal. If all of the above-mentioned factors are true, the diagnosis of solar dermatitis is warranted.

Because of the scarring nature of solar dermatitis, the diagnosis of chronic cases is more problematic. These cases start with abnormal skin from previously unrecognized or unreported episodes and do not heal completely with strict photoisolation. The basic quandary here is whether the dog has chronic solar dermatitis or some other nasal skin disease with a secondary photodermatitis. If the animal has identical lesions in areas that are not exposed to sun or lesions that are heavily pigmented, the latter case is true. However, many dogs with underlying disease have lesions restricted to the face.

The list of facial dermatoses (those that start on, remain confined to, or have their most pronounced lesions on the face) is extensive. The ones germane to this discussion are discoid lupus erythematosus, systemic lupus erythematosus, dermatomyositis and epidermolysis bullosa, pemphigus foliaceus, pemphigus erythematosus, drug reaction, and infectious folliculitis and furunculosis due to bacterial, dermatophyte, *Demodex*, yeast, or leishmanial infection. Except for discoid lupus erythematosus (see Chap. 9), which tends to start on and remain restricted to the perinasal area, these diseases tend to start in the haired skin on the bridge of the nose and work toward the nasal planum. They also tend to involve the pinnae and the mucocutaneous junctions and have no predilection for nonpigmented skin. When the nasal planum is extensively ulcerated, fissured, and friable, vasculitis, neoplasia (especially basal cell tumors, squamous cell carcinomas, fibrosarcomas, and lymphomas), and granulomatous diseases (especially sterile pyogranuloma syndrome) must be considered.

The diagnosis of solar dermatitis is confirmed by biopsy. The early depigmented areas of the nose show fewer melanocytes and less melanin pigment than are seen in normal skin. After exposure to solar radiation, epidermal hyperplasia with intraepidermal edema is observed. Vacuolated (sunburn cells) and apoptotic keratinocytes may be seen.[60] Perivascular accumulations of inflammatory cells are seen in the upper dermis, and vascular dilatation is noted in the lower dermis. Solar elastosis (basophilic degeneration of elastin) usually is not seen (Fig. 16–2),[35, 36] and requires special stains (e.g., periodic acid–Schiff [PAS] stain) for best visualization. A more common change is bandlike superficial dermal fibrosis. Ulceration can cause disappearance of the epidermis and even of the dermis and underlying cartilages. In rare advanced cases, activity in the cells of the basal layer is increased, and large, polyhedral tumor cells that invade the dermis and subcutaneous

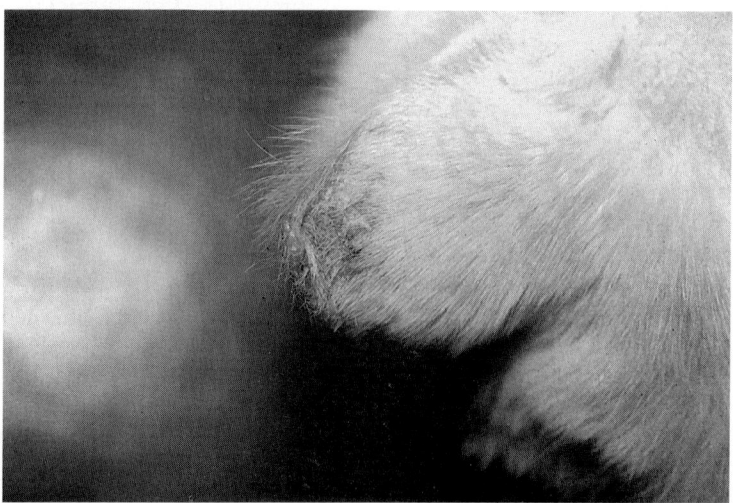

FIGURE 16–2. Feline solar dermatitis. Chronic exposure has resulted in dysplastic changes characterized by alopecia, scaling, thickening, and curling of the pinnae.

tissue are formed. A squamous cell carcinoma forms, and cords of neoplastic cells invade the tissue to the level of the nasal cartilage.

CLINICAL MANAGEMENT

After the diagnosis is confirmed, the pre-existing lesions must be treated, and, most important, new lesions must be prevented. In early cases, photoprotection allows the lesions to heal spontaneously. In more advanced cases, corticosteroids are necessary to decrease the inflammation. Although topical products are most beneficial, many dogs resent their thorough application, and thus the oral route is commonly used. Prednisolone (1.1 mg/kg q24h) administered for 7 to 10 days should be sufficient. If the lesions shows cytologic evidence of bacterial infection, antibiotics should be administered.

Avoidance of direct or reflected sunlight is paramount, especially in chronic cases in which solar sensitivity is extreme.[96] During the summer, the most dangerous photoperiod is from 9 AM to 3 PM, with the peak from 11 AM to 2 PM. Affected dogs should be kept indoors or in the shade during these times. When indoors, the dog can sunbathe beneath a closed window because glass effectively filters UVB, but open windows or doors defeat the purpose of the animal's being kept indoors.[37] Reflections from white concrete sidewalks or run flooring must also be avoided.

Strict photoisolation is usually impossible, and sunblocks or sunscreens can allow some sun exposure.[37] Sunblocks are opaque agents that reflect and scatter incident light. White or colored zinc oxide preparations are most commonly used in humans and may be of benefit in dogs that do not lick the area. Most clients prefer sunscreens that are clear and absorb incident light. Most products absorb only UVB, but some agents contain ingredients to screen UVA as well. Waterproof products with a sun protective factor (SPF) of 15 or higher should be used.[96] SPF 15 products absorb more than 92% of the incident UVB and are sufficient to protect most animals.[60] For maximal efficacy, the product should be applied and gently rubbed into the area 15 to 30 minutes before sun exposure. When solar exposure is unpredictable, the sunscreen should be applied twice daily on a regular basis.[96]

The addition of artificial pigmentation to the area can be beneficial, but does not negate the need for other measures, because black skin can still absorb some sunlight and be burned.[44] Black ink can be applied to the skin's surface with felt-tipped markers or by a cotton-tipped applicator (Q-tip) with permanent laundry or stamp pad ink. Markers are easiest to use, but the solvents can be irritating. Permanent coloring can be achieved by tattooing. Tattooing was popular in the past, but poor early results, the expense of the equipment, the need for multiple treatments under general anesthesia,[89] and rare adverse reactions to the tattoo ink[79] have limited its use. Most of the early treatment failures were because skin with an active immune-mediated disorder (e.g., discoid lupus erythematosus) but not true solar dermatitis was tattooed. Tattooing should be considered when other photoprotection measures are ineffective.

Although some benefit may be seen with the administration of ß-carotene,[75] treatment with systemic agents usually is unrewarding. Preliminary work has shown that topically applied vitamin C can help protect pig skin against UVL damage when the vitamin C is applied after irradiation.[19] This treatment or the oral administration of vitamin C may or may not be beneficial in dogs.

When the solar dermatitis progresses to an actinic keratosis or squamous cell carcinoma or results in massive tissue destruction, treatments with retinoic acid, hyperthermia, cryosurgery, surgical excision, photochemotherapy, or radiotherapy may be of some benefit, but efficacy data are limited.[96] Patients requiring these treatments have a poor prognosis.

Feline Solar Dermatitis

Feline solar dermatitis is a chronic actinic dermatitis of the white ears and, occasionally, the eyelids, the nose, and the lips of cats, which is caused by repeated sun exposure.[8, 83, 96, 102] It can develop into an actinic keratosis or true squamous cell carcinoma.[77]

CAUSE AND PATHOGENESIS

The disease occurs in white cats or in colored cats with white-haired areas on the face or ears. Blue-eyed, white cats are most susceptible. Actinic damage to the ear tip occurs from repeated exposure to UVB light. Early lesions are often ignored or unrecognized, but the damage makes the area more susceptible to further actinic insults. The disease occurs mostly in warm, sunny climates such as those of California, Florida, Hawaii, Australia, and South Africa. Sixteen cats with solar dermatitis were examined for heme biosynthesis abnormalities, but none were demonstrated.[54]

CLINICAL FEATURES

The earliest sign is erythema and fine scaling of the margin of the pinna. The hair is lost in this area, making it even more accessible to solar radiation. There is almost no discomfort to the cat at this stage. In susceptible cats, the first lesions can occur as early as 3 months of age. Lesions become progressively more severe each summer. The advancing lesions consist of severe erythema of the pinna, peeling of the skin, and formation of marginal crusts (see Fig. 16–1B and 16–2). At this stage, many cats demonstrate that they are in pain and further damage their ears by scratching. The margins of the pinnae may be curled. The margins of the lower eyelids, nose, and lips may be affected, especially in white, blue-eyed cats. An actinic keratosis or invasive squamous cell carcinoma can develop in some cases on the ears, the nose, or other areas (see Fig. 16–1C and D). Carcinomatous change may occur, usually after 6 years of age, but sometimes as early as 3 years. The squamous cell carcinoma appears as an ulcerating, hemorrhagic, and locally invasive lesion. It is partially crusted and, in advanced cases, destroys the pinna (see Fig. 16–1E).

DIAGNOSIS

A tentative diagnosis of feline solar dermatitis can be made from the clinical appearance, the color of the cat, and the history. As in the dog, the question remains as to whether the cat has a primary or secondary solar dermatitis. For pinnal lesions, the primary differential diagnostic considerations include dermatophytosis, early notoedric mange, fight wounds, vasculitis, and possibly frostbite or cryoglobulinemia. Discoid or systemic lupus erythematosus and pemphigus erythematosus or foliaceus may have to be considered. The differential diagnostic possibilities are excluded by skin biopsy, which also detects dysplastic or neoplastic changes.

Histopathologic study shows that, in the early stages, superficial perivascular dermatitis (spongiotic, hyperplastic changes) is present. Vacuolated (sunburn cells) or apoptotic keratinocytes may be seen. Solar elastosis may be noted in the superficial dermal connective tissue. With the formation of squamous cell carcinoma, the epidermal surface is ulcerated and the dermis is invaded by nests of polyhedral epithelial tumor cells. In a disorganized manner, these cells resemble the stratum spinosum. Their nuclei vary moderately in size, and mitotic figures are frequent. In advanced cases, the masses of tumor tissue extend to the level of the cartilage.

CLINICAL MANAGEMENT

Affected cats should be kept indoors from 9 AM to 3 PM and should not be allowed to sunbathe by open doors or windows. During the summer, the ears should be protected with a waterproof sunscreen. ß-Carotene and canthaxanthin (25-mg doses of active carotenoids) are administered orally to treat feline solar dermatitis.[54] Only the most severely affected cats fail to respond. Carotenoids are thought to quench the triplet state of singlet oxygen and free radicals and possibly to form a lipid-carotene complex in skin that absorbs the damaging solar radiation.

After early irreversible lesions develop, serious consideration should be given to a cosmetic amputation of the ear tips. This merely rounds off the ears, removes the thinly haired tips, and allows hair to cover and protect the pinna. Results are usually excellent, cosmetically and prophylactically. Photoprotection is necessary to prevent new lesions.

Cats with actinic keratoses who are not candidates for surgery may benefit from treatment with retinoic acids. Although isotretinoin at 3 mg/kg was ineffective,[28] more recent studies with etretinate (10 mg per cat q24h) have shown some promise.[92] Etretinate is no longer available in the United States, but acetretin could be used at 5 to 10 mg per cat q24h. If retinoid treatment is ineffective, superficial irradiation (plesiotherapy) with a hand-held strontium probe can be beneficial. If all of the above-mentioned therapies fail or the cat has advanced disease at presentation, radical amputation of the pinna (pinnectomy) is necessary.

Canine Solar Dermatitis of the Trunk and Extremities

Although the nose and the ears are the areas most exposed and, therefore, are most susceptible to actinic damage, other regions of the body can also be affected. A solar glossitis is recognized in sled dogs.[2] A combination of factors is necessary for sun damage to occur. First, the skin must be unpigmented or poorly pigmented. Second, only a sparse haircoat covers the skin, allowing the ultraviolet rays of the sun to reach the epidermis. Third, the areas so predisposed must be exposed to the sun. This occurs in dogs that like to sunbathe or that are confined to areas where no sun shelter is available during the middle of the day, especially if the ground cover is highly reflective. As is true of the other types of solar dermatitis, the chance of actinic disease is increased in sunny climates.

Breeds predisposed to truncal solar dermatitis include the Dalmatian, American Staffordshire terrier, German shorthaired pointers, white Boxers, Whippets, Beagles, and white Bull terriers.[8, 74, 75, 83, 86, 96] The flank and the abdomen are the areas most severely affected (see Fig. 16–1F and G). In dogs who sunbathe in right or left lateral recumbency, the flanks and the ventrolateral abdomen are most commonly affected, but lesions can be seen on the nose, the ears, the tail tip, or the distal limbs. Dogs that sunbathe on their back or that are caged on wire above white concrete can have the entire ventrum involved. The duration of exposure influences the damage done. A single prolonged exposure as might occur in cool weather or with a strong breeze results in full-thickness necrosis.[74] At first, regular sunburning occurs and the affected areas are erythematous and scaly. One to three days later, the site becomes extremely tender and will become necrotic. With repeated but episodic exposure, the initial sun burning is followed by an actinic folliculitis, actinic follicular cyst formation, or dermal fibrosis.[74] Running a hand over affected areas of skin may produce a bumpy feeling, because the white areas of skin are thickened, whereas the black areas are normal. At this stage, biopsy reveals variable degrees of superficial perivascular dermatitis and folliculitis. Superficial dermal fibrosis may be prominent. Solar elastosis may be seen (Fig. 16–3).

With chronic exposure, the sunburned areas become thicker and develop erosion, ulceration, crusting, and comedones, and they occasionally develop necrosis, fistulae, and scarring. At this stage, a skin biopsy may reveal follicular cysts, pyogranulomatous inflammation, and premalignant actinic keratosis. Finally, a squamous cell carcinoma can develop, especially if the dog continues to be exposed to direct sunlight. Such squamous cell carcinomas should be removed surgically, and the procedure should be repeated, if necessary. There is always a danger of metastasis to the regional lymph nodes and internal structures. Skin with solar damage is also more likely to develop a hemangioma or hemangiosarcoma.[96]

Therapy involves photoprotection by keeping the animal out of the sun and by using topical sunscreens and T-shirts if practical. It has been reported that ß-carotene (30 mg orally q12h for 30 days, then q24h for life), in combination with anti-inflammatory doses of prednisone or prednisolone, is effective in early cases.[75] Etretinate at 1 mg/kg every 24 hours or divided every 12 hours is effective when dysplastic change has occurred.[92] Etretinate is no longer available in the United States, but acetretin could be used at 0.5 to 1 mg/kg q24h.

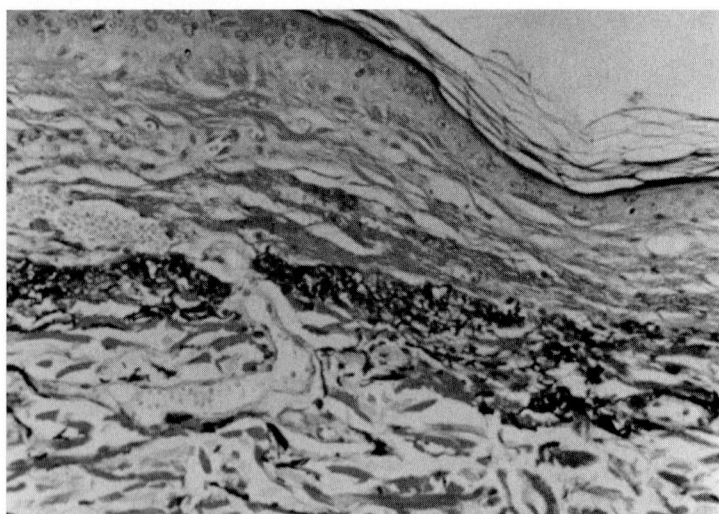

FIGURE 16–3. Solar elastosis. Degeneration of elastin fibers. (Courtesy A. Hargis.)

Photosensitivity

Photosensitivity occurs when the skin has an increased susceptibility to nonburning doses of UVL. The increased susceptibility is due to the production of (e.g., congenital or acquired porphyria),[47, 108] ingestion of (e.g., drugs), or contact with a photodynamic agent.[26] Photosensitization is uncommon in dogs and cats.

Unlike solar dermatitis, lesions of photosensitivity occur in well-haired regions of the body. The hairs must be light in color. Most cases are recognized in the white regions of black-and-white-coated dogs or cats,[31, 32, 51] but generalized disease has been reported in a Siamese cat and yellow Labrador retriever with acquired porphyria.[47]

In black-and-white animals, the tentative diagnosis of photosensitization is straightforward. The white-haired areas are involved, whereas the immediately adjacent black-haired skin is normal. Early on, the affected skin is red and can return to normal once the animal is removed from the sun. In more sensitive animals, the skin ulcerates and becomes necrotic. In porphyric animals, systemic signs (e.g., hyperthermia) can accompany the skin lesions.

As in all solar diseases, the animal should be removed from sunlight immediately and should be bathed if a contactant is likely. Every effort should be made to identify the sensitizing agent, but most cases defy diagnosis.

Actinic Keratosis

Actinic keratoses may be seen in dogs and cats and are premalignant epithelial dysplasias (see Chap. 20).

Miscellaneous Effects of Solar Exposure

Exposure to UVL is an important factor in precipitating or potentiating a number of skin lesions and may also exacerbate generalized systemic disease activity.[8, 66, 67] Although the role of UVL is clearly defined in some conditions, its pathogenic role in other disorders is less well understood. For example, UVL exposure may induce or exacerbate the lesions of discoid lupus erythematosus, systemic lupus erythematosus, pemphigus (especially pemphigus erythematosus),[56] and pemphigoid (see Chap. 9).

In addition, UVL exposure of skin has important local and systemic immunologic consequences (photoimmunologic changes).[66] For example, exposure to UVB or UVA changes Langerhans' cell morphologic features and function, and influences cutaneous cytokine production. Impaired antigen recognition and processing and impaired immune responses may influence susceptibility to cutaneous neoplasms and infections. The damaging effects on cutaneous immunity of low-dose UVB are genetically determined in mice.[105] This UVB susceptibility is mediated almost exclusively by tumor necrosis factor-α (TNF-α), and the trait appears to be a risk factor for the development of squamous cell carcinoma and basal cell carcinoma.

• IRRITANT CONTACT DERMATITIS

Contact dermatitis is an inflammatory skin reaction caused by direct contact with an offending substance.[37, 82, 83]

CAUSE AND PATHOGENESIS

The disease is divided into two types: primary irritant contact dermatitis and contact hypersensitivity[21] (see Chap. 8). Newer information blurs the distinction between immunologic and nonimmunologic events, and makes the distinction between these two entities problematic.[95a]

Primary irritant contact dermatitis causes cutaneous inflammation in most exposed dogs and cats without any antecedent period of sensitization. The rapidity of onset and the intensity of the reaction depend on the nature of the contactant, its concentration, and the duration of the contact. Corrosive substances such as strong acids and alkalies injure the skin immediately and produce lesions of varying severity. Severe reactions should be classified as chemical burns. Less potent contactants need prolonged or repeated contact to produce irritation. A number of primary irritants such as soaps, detergents, disinfectants, hair-coloring agents, weed and insecticidal sprays, fertilizers, strong acids and alkalies, and flea collars are potential causative agents.[1, 10, 81-83] Although most primary irritants are chemicals, similar skin lesions can be produced by thermal injuries, solar overexposure, and contact with living organisms and plants.

In humans, irritant contact dermatitis is more common in the young and in atopic individuals.[75b] The authors believe this to also be true in dogs and cats.

CLINICAL FEATURES

Irritant contact dermatitis can affect any animal of any age. Whereas atopic dogs, German shepherd dogs, Poodles, and several other breeds appear to be at an increased risk for contact hypersensitivity, no breed predisposition is recognized in irritant contact dermatitis.[113] However, animals with skin disease have lost one or more protective layers (e.g., hair) of their defense system and probably are at increased risk as a secondary phenomenon.

Environmental irritants such as fertilizers and carpet cleaners typically produce dermatitis in areas where the haircoat is thin or missing. The abdomen, the chest, the axillae, the flanks, the interdigital spaces, the legs, the perianal area, and the ventral surface of the tail are the most susceptible areas (Fig. 16–4A and B; also see Fig. 16–1H). When the offending agent is a liquid (e.g., shampoo and flea dip solution) or a topical medication (see Fig. 16–4C) or is bound to a collar (see Fig. 16–4D and E), the reaction occurs where the substance touches the skin. Licking of the contactant can cause oral lesions (Fig. 16–4F) and spread the agent to other areas of the body.

Patches of erythema and papules represent primary lesions (see Fig. 16–4A). Vesicles are rarely present in dogs and cats (see Fig. 16–4C). As the disease progresses, crusts, excoriations, hyperpigmentation, and lichenification occur. Intense pruritus may promote severe scratching and biting. Pyotraumatic dermatitis and eventual ulceration may obliterate primary lesions.

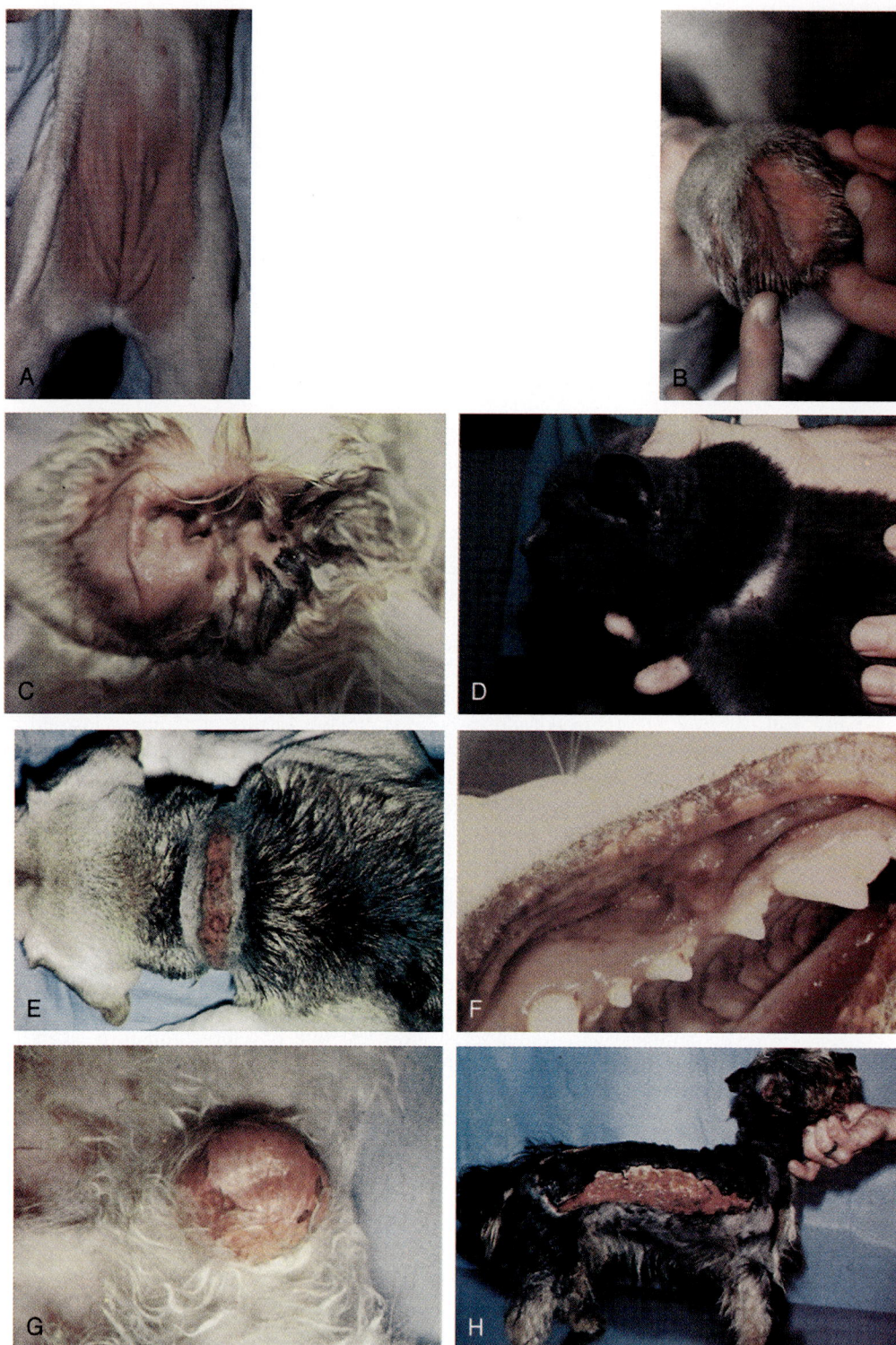

FIGURE 16-4. *A,* Contact dermatitis due to a floor cleaner. *B,* Contact dermatitis caused by a caustic cage cleaner. *C,* Acute vesicular eruption due to an ear medication. *D,* Contact dermatitis caused by a leather collar. *E,* Acute erythema and erosion due to flea collar dermatitis. *F,* Cheilitis and gingivitis due to contact with a lawn fertilizer. *G,* Irritant contact dermatitis affecting the delicate scrotal skin. *H,* Full-thickness thermal burn in a Silky terrier, with sloughing and infection.

Single episodes are common in primary irritant contact dermatitis, as in scrotal involvement from soap that is not rinsed off (see Fig. 16-4G). Seasonal recurrence results from exposure to plants, lawn fertilizer, herbicides, and ice-melting substances.

DIAGNOSIS

The tentative diagnosis of contact dermatitis is based on historical and physical findings. If multiple animals in a household are affected, primary irritant contact dermatitis is much more likely than contact hypersensitivity. When the contactant is harsh and produces immediate reactions or is applied intentionally (e.g., medication), the diagnosis is straightforward. With low-grade environmental contactants, identification is more difficult, and atopy, food hypersensitivity, drug reaction, *Malassezia* dermatitis, and early scabies must be considered.

In most clinical cases, the histopathologic changes of primary irritant contact dermatitis consist of nondiagnostic superficial perivascular dermatitis (spongiotic, hyperplastic changes).[113] The exact appearance depends on the stage of contact dermatitis and the effects of secondary infection and excoriation. Neutrophils or mononuclear cells may predominate in a given case.

The confirmation of irritant contact dermatitis can be made by provocative exposure testing, in which the agent is applied to normal and diseased skin. With low-grade irritants, one application to normal skin may not be sufficient to cause irritation, so diseased skin should also be challenged. With harsh irritants, which cause ulceration and necrosis, provocative exposure testing should be avoided. Patch testing is of unproven value in the diagnosis of irritant contact dermatitis.

CLINICAL MANAGEMENT

The difficult task of discovering and eliminating offending substances depends on the correlation of a detailed history and a careful examination of the environment of the dog. Soap, flea collars, grasses, pollens, insecticides, petrolatum, paint, wool, carpets, rubber, and wood preservatives are examples of contact irritants. If the location of the initial inflammation can be correlated with an agent that came in contact with that area, the cause can sometimes be found. With removal of the irritant, the lesions should heal spontaneously. For pruritic patients, a 5- to 7-day course of prednisone or prednisolone (1.1 mg/kg q24h) can be beneficial.

When the contactant cannot be found, relief depends on systemic and topical therapy. The involved areas should be bathed frequently with plain water or a mild, nonirritating shampoo. Drying must be complete, because macerated tissue is more susceptible to the irritant. For localized lesions, topical corticosteroids may be beneficial in controlling the inflammation. For animals with widespread lesions, repeated 7- to 10-day courses or alternate-day administration of oral steroids is necessary. Pentoxifylline (10 mg/kg q12h) is beneficial in the treatment of contact hypersensitivity.[72] It may be of benefit in irritant dermatitis as well.

● BURNS

Superficial and deep burns are painful, often produce scarring, and are an important cause of sepsis. Burn management is long and arduous.

CAUSE AND PATHOGENESIS

Burns can be caused by strong chemicals, electric currents, solar and microwave radiation, and heat.[10, 18, 83, 94, 97, 106] Most cases in small animals are caused by heat from fires, boiling liquids, electric heating pads, animal driers, and hot metals (e.g., mufflers and wood stoves). The length of exposure and the temperature of the heat source are key in determining the extent of the burn. In pigs, water at 44°C (111.2°F) needed 6 hours of contact to cause a burn, whereas temperatures of 70°C (158°F) or greater caused transepidermal necrosis in less than 1 second.[106] The temperature of flames, boiling liquids, and common hot metal sources greatly exceeds 70°C (158°F), and burns occur instantaneously with exposure.

Electric heating pads are a common unexpected cause of burns in small animals. Heat output can vary from pad to pad and can fluctuate during use. At the lowest setting, temperatures as high as 44°C (111.2°F) can be achieved, whereas temperatures of 56°C (132.8°F) can be obtained at the medium setting.[106] The burn potential of these pads is modified by the padding surrounding the unit, the nature of the animal's coat, and several other factors, but clearly, animals kept on these pads for prolonged periods are at great risk. Large volumes of subcutaneous fluids may increase the animal's sensitivity and allow burning at very low settings.

As discussed in the section on solar dermatitis, sunlight does most of its damage in nonpigmented or lightly pigmented skin. However, black skin absorbs nearly 50% more solar radiation than does white skin and intense solar exposure can cause thermal burns in darkly pigmented dogs. This is demonstrated in the report of two Dalmatians who developed ulcerative, necrotic, crusted, plaquelike lesions in their black spots.[44] Lesions developed 7 days after exposure of 4 hours or more to intense sunlight. Because solar burns are rare in darkly pigmented skin, the animal should be evaluated for an underlying irregularity in thermoregulation.

Burns of dogs and cats have been categorized into two types: partial-thickness burns and full-thickness burns.[83] Partial-thickness burns involve the epidermis and the superficial dermis. Healing of the burned area can be complete with little or no scarring because of re-epithelialization from the hair follicles and sebaceous glands.[34] In full-thickness burns, there is complete destruction of all cutaneous structures. Without surgical intervention, healing occurs via second intention with extensive scarring.

The cause of the burn and the percentage of body involvement have great impact on the patient's survival. Patients burned by fire are at great risk for damage to the respiratory tract, and chemicals can burn the mouth or other tissues if they are spread by licking or careless handling by the owner.[97] Heat causes capillary leakage at and distant to the burn site. Patients with large burns experience fluid and electrolyte imbalances, and can die rapidly if not treated appropriately.[37, 97]

Loss of the skin as a protective barrier opens the underlying tissue to invasive infection. Although microcirculation is restored within 48 hours to areas of partial-thickness injury, the full-thickness burn is characterized by complete occlusion of the local vascular supply. The avascular, necrotic tissue of the full-thickness burn, with impaired delivery of humoral and cellular defense mechanisms, provides an excellent medium for bacterial proliferation, with the ever-present potential for life-threatening sepsis. Initial colonization of the burn wound surface by gram-positive organisms shifts by the third to fifth day after the burn to an invasive gram-negative flora (especially *Pseudomonas aeruginosa*).

CLINICAL FEATURES

Burns caused by fire or contact with hot metal are obvious from the outset but may not reach their full extent for 24 to 48 hours. Burns from microwave radiation, electric currents, chemicals, and electric heating pads or cage driers can be more insidious, because the haircoat may hide the trauma and the owner may be aware of only the animal's apparent pain and its accompanying behavioral changes.[18, 94, 106] When the animal is presented for treatment of skin burned by heating pads or cage driers, the affected skin is usually hard and dry. Chemical, electric, solar, or microwave burns are erosive to necrotic in nature.[10, 18, 94] These burns may also not be maximally expressed for an additional 24 to 48 hours. Infection causes a purulent discharge and sometimes an unpleasant odor. Large areas of necrotic skin may slough and reveal a deep, suppurating wound (see Fig. 16–4H). If the skin is débrided and sutured, temporary closure may be achieved. However, the sutured area almost always sloughs, leaving a large, raw surface.

If 25% of the body is involved in the burn, there are usually systemic manifestations, including septicemia, shock, renal failure, and anemia.[34, 97]

DIAGNOSIS

The diagnosis is straightforward if the client has observed the accidental burning. If the burn was not observed or was malicious, the diagnosis can be more difficult, especially if the burn is superficial. The histologic findings of a gradually tapering coagulation necrosis of the epidermis and deeper tissues confirm a thermal or chemical burn. Superficial burns produce full-thickness epidermal necrosis and resultant subepidermal vesicle formation (Fig. 16–5). With microwave burns, there is full-thickness coagulation necrosis.[94] Electric burns may show a diagnostic histologic feature of a fringe of elongated, degenerated cytoplasmic processes that protrudes from the lower end of the detached basal cells into the space separating the epidermis and the dermis. The nuclei of the basal cells and often of the higher-lying epidermal cells appear stretched in the same direction as the fringe of cytoplasmic processes. This gives the image of keratinocytes that are "standing at attention" (see Fig. 2–32).

CLINICAL MANAGEMENT

For minor and major burns, the initial wound management, after evaluation and stabilization as needed, is the same.[34, 83, 97] For extensive burns, prompt attention to the patient's fluid and electrolyte balance is crucial for survival. Patients with chemical burns should be bathed when possible to remove any residual agent. After the patient is stabilized, wound management can begin. The best treatment of burns is the prompt surgical excision of the diseased tissue with sutured wound closure. Except for small burns, this is impractical in pets. Regardless of the location or the depth of the wound, removal of all debris, loose skin, and necrotic tissue is imperative. The wound is thoroughly cleaned with povidone-iodine or some other suitable antiseptic cleaner and is débrided as needed. Daily hydrotherapy is used for complete cleaning of all burn wounds. Suturing is seldom necessary, because the sutured area almost always sloughs. After all burn wounds have been adequately cleaned and débrided, local care consists of the application of topical antimicrobial agents. Occlusive burn wound dressings are avoided because of their tendency to produce a closed wound with bacterial proliferation and to delay healing. Nonocclusive dressings,

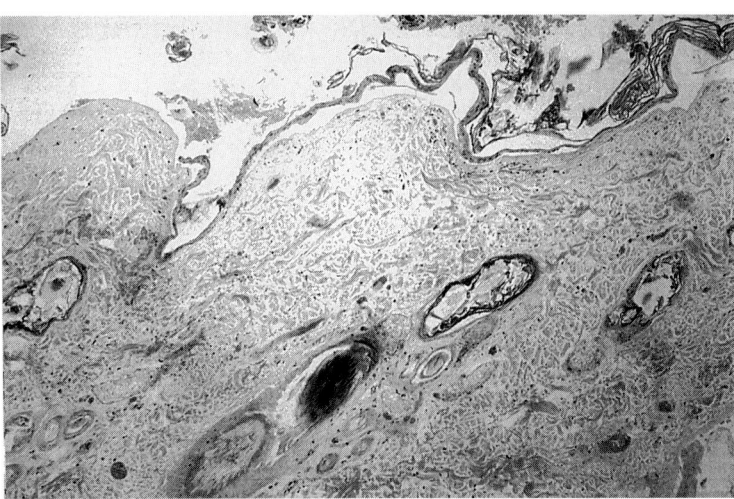

FIGURE 16–5. Thermal burn. Superficial dermal edema and epidermal necrosis resulting in epidermal separation. Follicular necrosis is also visible.

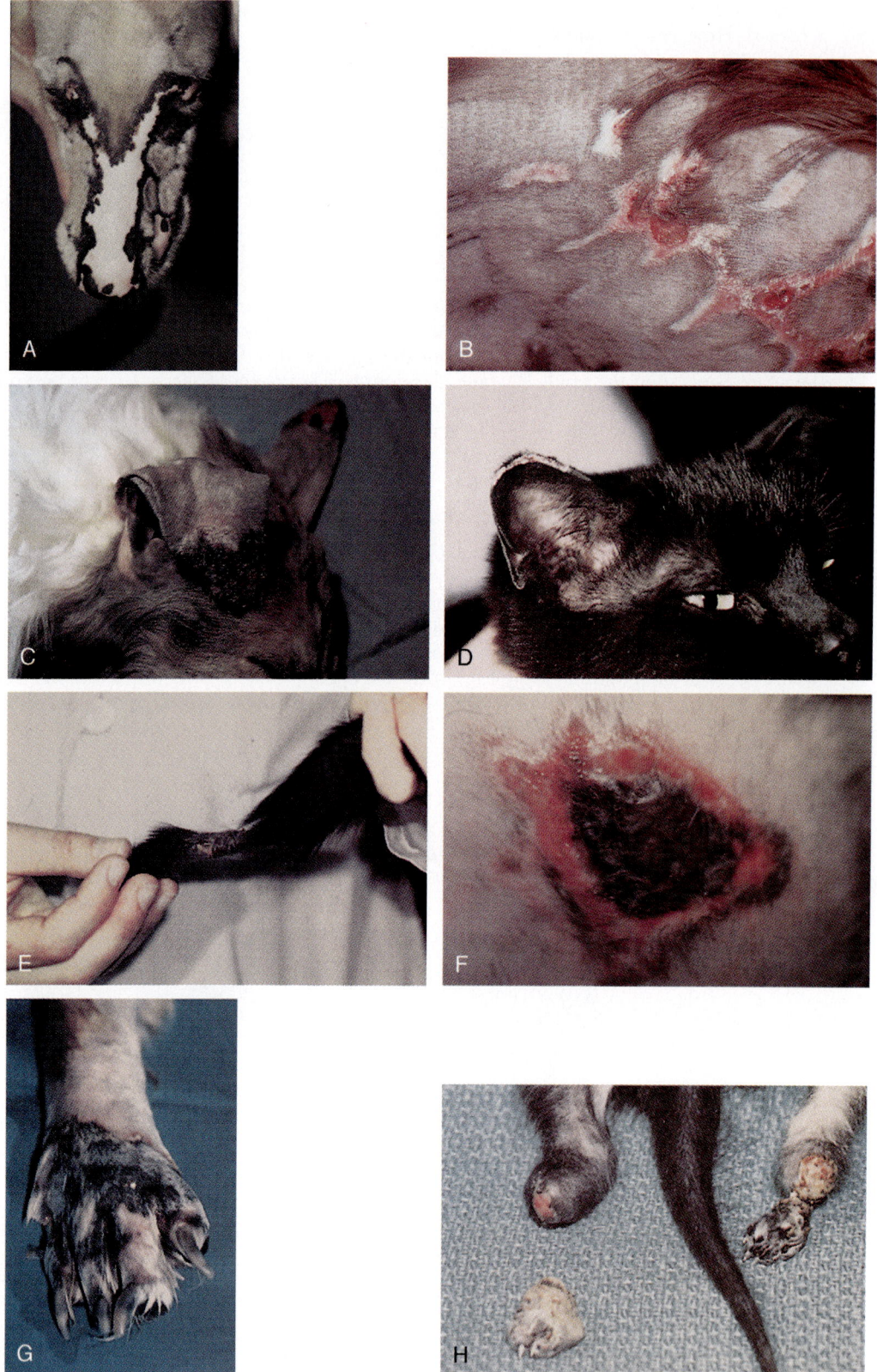

FIGURE 16–6. *Legend on opposite page*

changed frequently, can be useful in certain cases. The wound should be cleaned two or three times daily and the topical product should be reapplied.

In human patients with burns, a 0.5% silver nitrate solution, silver sulfadiazine, mafenide acetate (Sulfamylon) cream, and iodophors receive wide use.[37] The silver nitrate solution is used as a wet dressing and is considered effective. Because most veterinary patients do not tolerate wet dressings, silver sulfadiazine is probably the most commonly used burn cream.[78, 83] It is nonstaining, painless, and has fair penetration of an eschar. Practitioners report excellent results with mupirocin ointment (Bactoderm, Pfizer Animal Health).[78] The technical information on this product warns of nephrotoxicity due to absorption of the polyethylene glycol in the base. Treatment of large deep burns could result in renal failure. Systemic antibiotics are not effective in preventing burn wound infection and may allow invasion by resistant organisms.

Burn healing is slow, with weeks to months of treatment. Most burns that receive veterinary attention are full thickness and heal as hairless areas with scarring (Fig. 16–6A). In some cases, the scarring impedes function and various plastic surgical procedures must be performed. After all of these obstacles are overcome, most patients lead a normal life. Because the scarred skin is hairless and often nonpigmented, solar exposure should be limited. Burn scar malignancies have been reported in dogs, so the areas should be examined periodically.[40]

• RADIANT HEAT BURNS

Prolonged, repetitive exposure to hot radiant heat sources (e.g., wood stoves, infrared lamps) can result in thermal burns.[19, 22] Considering the frequent use of wood stoves in the colder climates and the tendency for dogs and cats to lie extremely close to them, radiant burns should be considered rare.

Unlike a conduction burn, which occurs in areas of contact with a known high temperature heat source, radiant burns occur over the dorsum and lateral chest walls without a history of exposure. Because the owner never sees the dog touch the stove, they do not associate the skin disease with heat source and will not volunteer that history.

Radiant burns occur in a driplike configuration with hair loss, erythema, and ulceration (see Fig. 16–6B). Adjacent haired skin can be hyperpigmented. With dorsally oriented, well-established lesions, as shown in the figure, the differential diagnosis is limited to a caustic or malicious thermal burn. The diagnosis can be confirmed by skin biopsy. Nonulcerated lesions are hyperplastic with surface and infundibular hyperkeratosis. There is focal hydropic degeneration of the basal cells with pigmentary incontinence. Occasional apoptotic cells can be seen scattered in the suprabasilar layers. Superficial dermal mucinosis is a consistent finding.

Once the animal is removed from exposure, the lesions heal spontaneously and relapses are prevented by management changes.

• RADIATION INJURY

Skin changes are an expected consequence of radiation therapy and are somewhat dose dependent. With treatment, the mitotic activity of the epidermis, melanocytes, hair follicles, and sebaceous glands stops. After a 2- to 3-week lag period, the treated area becomes

FIGURE 16–6. *A,* Permanent scarring and depigmentation from a healed burn. The dog is now susceptible to solar dermatitis. *B,* Radiant heat burn. Erythema, erosion and ulceration, and crusting in a driplike fashion on the chest wall. Area was clipped. *C,* Frostbite. Pinnal necrosis and ulceration. *D,* Frostbite. The tip of the pinna has sloughed. *E,* Frostbite. Necrosis of the distal tail. *F,* Tissue slough secondary to deep vascular occlusion. *G,* Pedal necrosis secondary to disseminated intravascular coagulation. *H,* Pedal necrosis in a kitten fed an inappropriate milk replacement.

chogenic carcinoma or follicular lymphoma, respectively.[5] Necrosis and sloughing of the digits have been reported as sequelae of hepatitis in dogs.[73] Necrosis and sloughing of the digits have also been seen in puppies and kittens (see Fig. 16–6H) fed highly concentrated formulas containing evaporated milk.[55, 78] Neonatal isoerythrolysis was suspected as a cause of tail tip necrosis in kittens (see Chap. 9). Necrosis has been associated with sensory nerve damage either because it induces self-trauma (e.g., cauda equina syndrome and so-called chilblains)[57, 62] or because it interferes with proprioception (e.g., trophic ulcer of the footpad).[52]

• SUBCUTANEOUS EMPHYSEMA

Subcutaneous emphysema is characterized by free gas in the subcutis. Possible causes include air entering through a cutaneous wound, a lung punctured by a fractured rib, internal penetrating wounds, extension from pulmonary emphysema, extension from tracheal rupture, and gas gangrene infections. With deep ulcers over active joints, air may be "pumped" into the subcutis. It can also occur secondary to alveolar rupture associated with positive-pressure ventilation[15] and following gastrostomy tube placement.[75a]

Subcutaneous emphysema is characterized by soft, fluctuant, crepitant, subcutaneous swellings. The lesions are usually not painful, and the animals are not acutely ill, except in the case of gas gangrene.

Diagnosis is based on history and physical examination. Treatment is directed at the underlying cause. Sterile subcutaneous emphysema requires no treatment, unless it is extensive and incapacitating, wherein multiple skin incisions may be necessary.

• SUBCUTANEOUS CHYLE

The subcutaneous accumulation of chyle has been reported subsequent to thoracic duct ligation,[33] and secondary to lymphangiectasis and lymphangioma.[33a] The subcutaneous swellings are fluctuant, nonpainful, and often occur in the groin and/or pelvic limb. Aspiration cytology reveals chyle (triglyceride, cholesterol, protein, lymphocytes). Therapy is directed at the underlying cause.

• SNAKE BITE

Two subfamilies of venomous snakes are indigenous to the United States: Crotalidae and Elapidae. Crotalidae, commonly called pit vipers, include the copperhead, the cottonmouth moccasin, and the rattlesnake. One or more species of this subfamily are found in virtually all of the 48 contiguous states. Elapidae are represented in this country by two genera of coral snakes, which are found in only the southeastern and southwestern United States. In Germany, common vipers (*Vipera berus*) are most problematic.[64] In Australia, brown, tiger, and black snakes account for most bites.[80] *Vipera xanthina palestinae* is the major culprit in the Middle East.[3]

Snake venoms contain over 25 toxic polypeptides, low-molecular-weight proteins, and enzymes.[63, 70, 71, 91, 98, 104] Venoms vary in their toxicity between species of snake and within a species depending on the habitat of the snake and season of the year.[48, 49] In general, venoms produce alterations in the resistance and integrity of blood vessels, changes in blood cells and blood coagulation mechanisms, direct or indirect changes in cardiac dynamics, alterations of nervous system function, depression of respiration, and necrosis at the site of envenomation.[16] Necrosis is much more common with pit viper bites than with coral snake bites.[63, 71] The severity of a poisonous snake bite depends on the type and size of the snake, the amount of venom injected in relation to the victim's weight, the site of venom injection, and the time interval between the venom injection and the onset of medical therapy.[91]

Most snake bites occur during spring and summer, and animals in rural areas (especially near rodent burrows) are most at risk. In one study,[3] young medium-to-large breed dogs were at increased risk, especially German shepherds and Rottweilers (guard dogs, trained to attack). The face and legs are most commonly involved. If there is no pain or swelling at the bite site within 1½ hours of the bite, no venom was injected. Bites around the face are potentially serious because of rapid swelling and respiratory embarrassment (Fig. 16–9A). Cutaneous manifestations of snake bites with venom injection include rapid, progressive edema, which usually obliterates the fang marks (see Fig. 16–9B); pain; and, occasionally, local hemorrhage. Ecchymosis and discoloration become apparent several hours later, and this area often becomes necrotic and sloughs.

All snake bites are potentially lethal, especially in small dogs or cats, and specific wound treatments should be postponed until the patient is stable. Although there can be some benefit to removal of local venom by suction, the stress to the dog or cat can outweigh any potential benefits. Antivenin should be administered when available.[63, 71, 91] In one study, the survival rate of dogs and cats treated with antivenom was 75% and 91%, respectively.[50] The survival rate of those not treated was approximately 30% lower. For maximum efficacy, the antivenom should be administered within 2 hours of the bite. When administration is delayed for 8 hours or more, the antivenom is of little use. Because these antisera contain horse serum, the patient should undergo skin testing with the product before administration. Even with a negative test, reactions can occur, so the patient should be monitored carefully for signs of anaphylaxis. Because snake bites are contaminated by the oral flora, which often includes *Pseudomonas* sp. and *Clostridium tetani*,[91] broad-spectrum antibiotics and tetanus toxoids should be administered.

Beyond the above-mentioned measures, treatment recommendations vary. Some investigators administer antihistamines or corticosteroids, whereas other researchers do not.[63, 71, 91] With pit viper bites, tissue slough can be expected, and the resulting wound should be managed similarly to a burn.[63]

• FOREIGN BODIES

Foreign bodies occasionally cause skin lesions in dogs and cats. Although porcupine quills (Fig. 16–10; also see Fig. 16–9C), suture materials (Figs. 16–11 and 16–12),[23] air rifle pellets, and road gravel are common foreign bodies, most are of plant origin (seeds and awns, wood slivers). One of the most notorious plants in the United States in this regard is the foxtail (*Hordeum jubatum*). A related plant (*Hordeum murinum*) causes problems in France.[9]

In a retrospective study of 182 cases of grass awn migration in dogs and cats in California, younger dogs (with increased activity) and hunting and working breeds (with increased exposure) were at greater risk.[14] The most common site of grass awn localization was the external ear canal (51% of cases), with the other common cutaneous sites being the interdigital webs (see Fig. 16–9D). Lesions consist of nodules, abscesses, and draining tracts. Secondary bacterial infection is exceedingly common.

Another common plant foreign body in the United States is the burdock (*Arctium* sp.).[39] The burs of these common weeds become trapped in the haircoat, where they often cause local irritation and mat formation. Dogs generally do not tolerate the burs well, and chew and lick them from their fur. In doing so, the dogs may produce focal skin lesions (see Fig. 16–9E) or, more commonly, oral lesions. The lesions of typical burdock stomatitis are seen as (1) multiple 2- to 3-mm, whitish, shiny papules along the junction of the upper buccal and gingival mucosa or (2) multiple, erythematous, granular papules and plaques on the dorsal surface of the tongue (see Fig. 16–9F). Some dogs with burdock stomatitis are remarkably asymptomatic, whereas other animals show typical signs of stomatitis. Biopsies reveal the burdock (Fig. 16–13) and a nodular to diffuse pyogranulomatous inflammation containing numerous eosinophils and centered on plant material (Fig. 16–14).

Free hair shafts are a common endogenous foreign body in the dog. The hair can

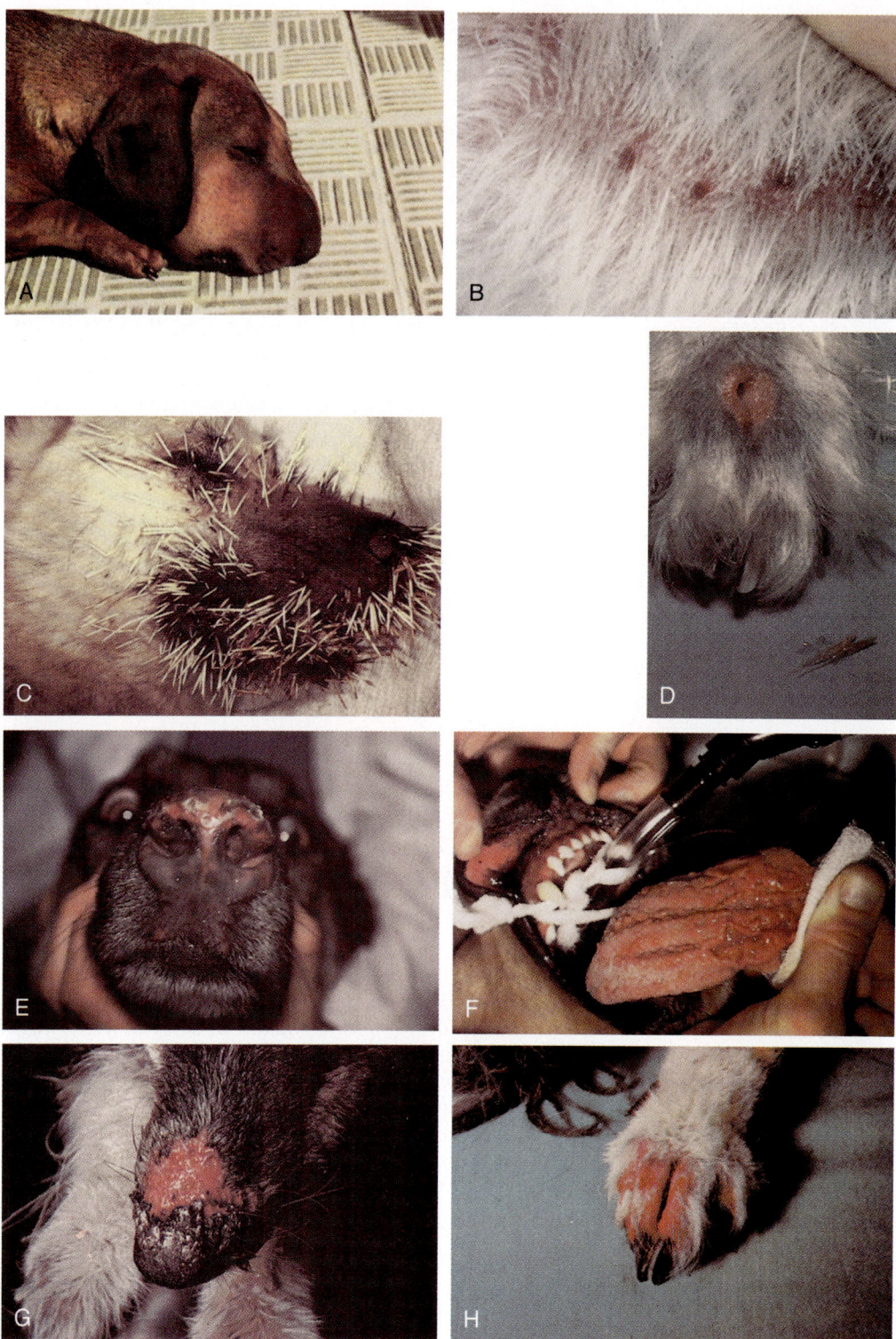

FIGURE 16-9. *A*, Profound facial edema secondary to a puff adder bite. (Courtesy P. Bland.) *B*, Snake fang marks. (Courtesy D. Carlotti.) *C*, Porcupine quills. *D*, Digital draining tract secondary to foxtail penetration. (Courtesy S. White.) *E*, Burdock dermatitis of the nose and muzzle. *F*, Burdock glossitis. *G*, Thallium intoxication. Severe ulceration and crusting of the skin of the nasal region. A purulent exudate is present. *H*, Thallium intoxication. Erythema, alopecia, and erosion of the digits and interdigital spaces.

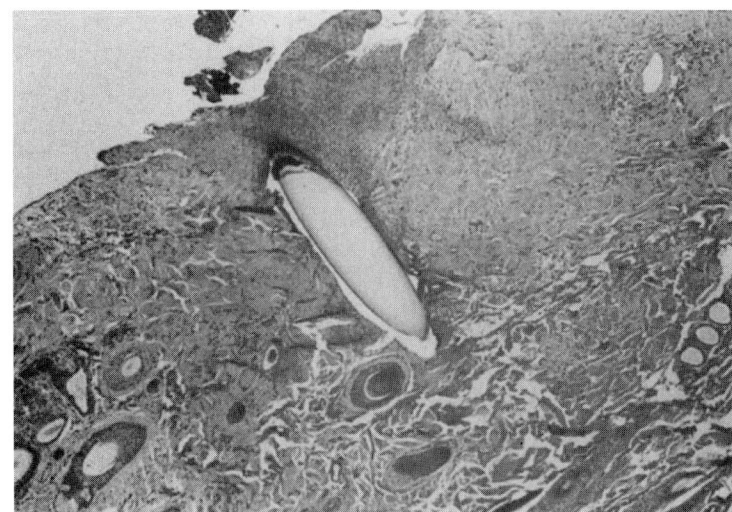

FIGURE 16–10. Porcupine quill lodged in a necrotic dermatitis.

reach the dermis either by being pushed through a normal hair follicle wall by constant licking or when the inflamed follicle ruptures (Fig. 16–15). The rupture of the inflamed follicle is most common and is a frequent sequela to bacterial folliculitis and furunculosis. The foreign body reaction around the hair shaft (Fig. 16–16) complicates the treatment of the primary follicular disease because it is difficult to determine what part of the patient's symptoms and tissue inflammation is due to infection or the sterile reaction to the hair shaft. Although exceptions can be found, it is best to assume that infection is still present

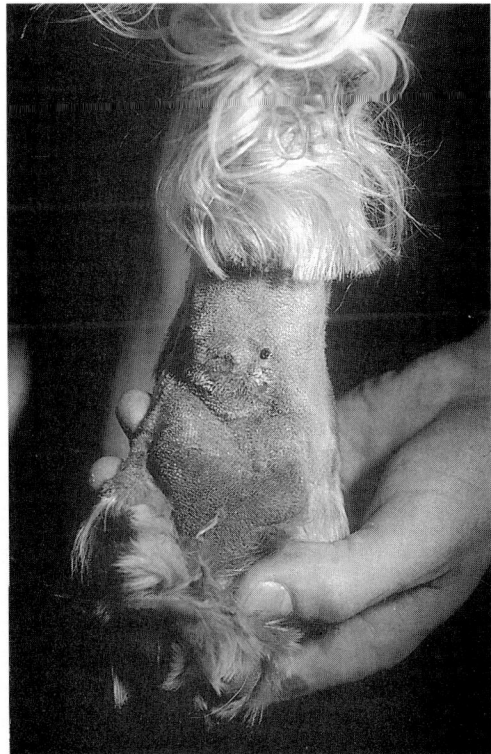

FIGURE 16–11. Large, tender granulomatous mass surrounding buried sutures at the site of a laceration repair.

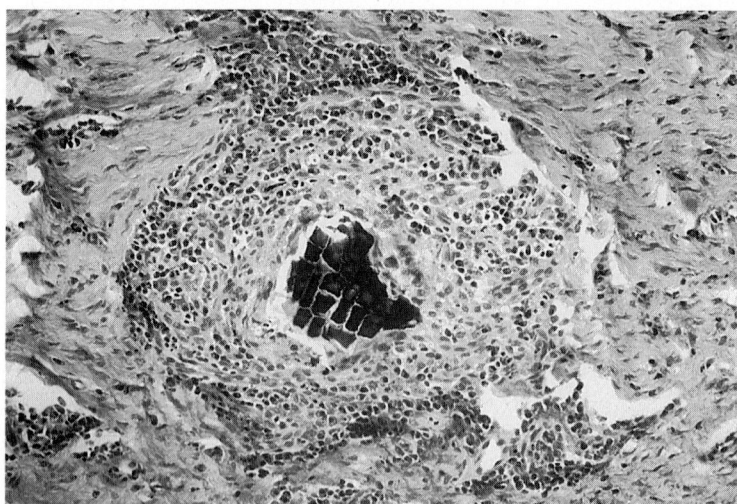

FIGURE 16–12. Fragments of chromic gut suture surrounded by pyogranulomatous inflammation.

when the lesion is tender to palpation. Clinically, significant foreign body disease is suspected by: (1) the persistence of palpable, hard, painless dermal papules ("BBs") after concurrent infection has been adequately treated, and (2) the recurrence of infection at frequent intervals in these sites. Predilected areas of skin include the chin, interdigital spaces, and periocular region. The treatment of choice of persistent hair shaft pyogranulomas or other foreign body reactions is surgical removal. When surgery is impossible, topical glucocorticoid therapy is often useful.

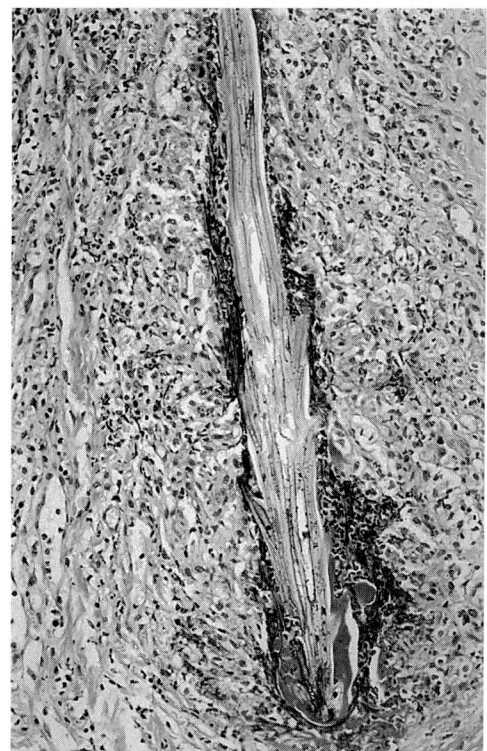

FIGURE 16–13. Burdock fragment buried in the skin. Note the visible barbing on the sides which prevents easy removal and encourages inward migration.

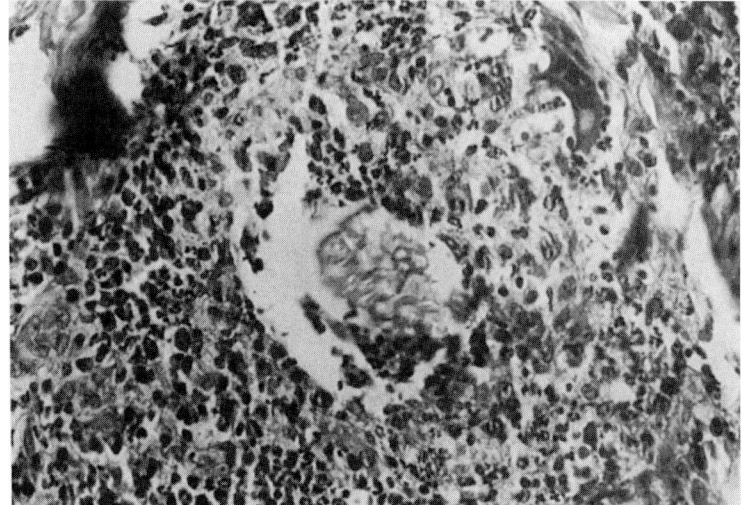

FIGURE 16–14. Burdock surrounded by mixed inflammatory infiltrate.

• ARTERIOVENOUS FISTULA

An *arteriovenous fistula* is a vascular abnormality, defined as a direct communication between an adjacent artery and a vein that bypasses the capillary circulation.[45] Arteriovenous fistulae may be congenital or acquired and are rarely reported in dogs and cats.[12, 17, 42, 45, 83, 110] Most clinically relevant cutaneous arteriovenous fistulae are acquired, and most of these result from penetrating wounds or blunt trauma, although they may also be secondary to infection, neoplasia, and iatrogenic factors (surgical declaw procedures and extravascular injections of irritating substances). Recurrent peripheral arteriovenous fistula has been reported in a cat with hyperthyroidism.[42]

Acquired arteriovenous fistulae most commonly involve the paws (after declaw procedures or injury) and the neck (secondary to neoplasms), but they have involved the temporal region, the pinnae, the legs, the flank, the prepuce, and the tongue. Affected areas show persistent or recurrent edema, pain, and occasionally, secondary infection and hemorrhage. Superficial blood vessels proximal to the fistula may be distinct and tortuous. Arteriovenous fistulae are generally characterized by pulsating vessels, palpable thrills, and

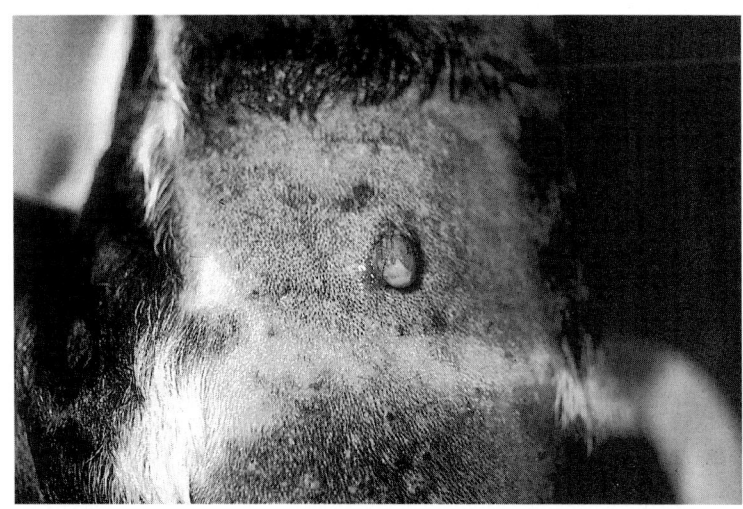

FIGURE 16–15. Multiple residual papules and a nodule on the back of a dog successfully treated for bacterial furunculosis. The lesions were sterile pyogranulomas surrounding free hair shafts.

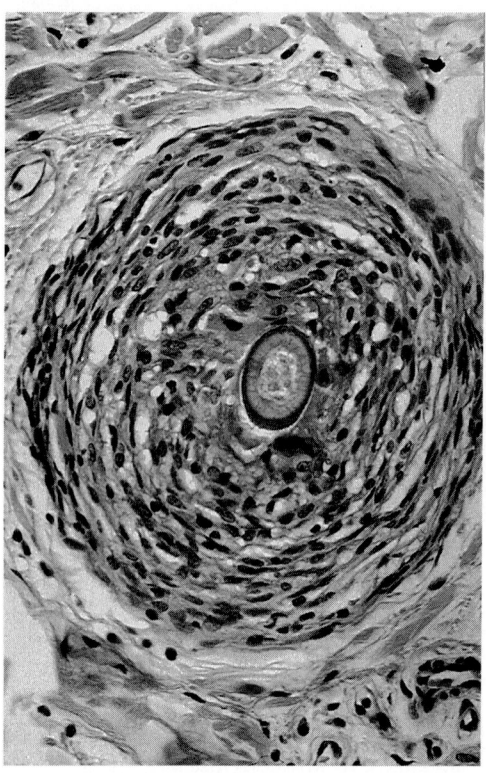

FIGURE 16–16. Granulomatous reaction around a fragment of hair shaft.

continuous machinery murmurs. Occlusion of the artery proximal to the fistula results in a sudden decrease in heart rate and disappearance of the murmur and thrill.[45]

Diagnosis is based on the history, physical examination findings, and demonstration of the arteriovenous fistula by contrast radiography. Therapy includes surgical extirpation of the fistula or, in some instances, amputation of the affected part.

• MYOSPHERULOSIS

Myospherulosis is a rare granulomatous reaction thought to be due to the interaction of ointments, antibiotics, endogenous fat, or oily contents of cysts with erythrocytes.[43, 90, 114] It is associated with small saclike structures (parent bodies) filled with endobodies (spherules) and has been reported in humans and dogs. The condition has been induced experimentally in laboratory animals. Myospherulosis is most commonly reported after injections of oil medicaments or after the topical application of oily products to open wounds. Because muscle is not always involved, it has been suggested that *spherulocytosis* or *spherulocytic disease* might be a better designation for this entity.[68]

Patients are usually presented for solitary subcutaneous or dermal nodules, which may or may not be discharging and are tender.[43, 78] Histologic examination reveals several solid and cystic masses. The walls of the cystic area and most solid areas are composed of histiocytes with abundant vacuolated cytoplasm. Histiocytes surround parent bodies (30 to 350 m) composed of thin eosinophilic walls and filled with homogeneous eosinophilic, 3- to 7-m spherules (Fig. 16–17). Parent bodies and spherules do not stain with periodic acid-Schiff, Grocott-Gomori methenamine-silver, or Ziehl-Neelsen stains but are positive for endogenous peroxidase (diaminobenzidine reaction) and hemoglobin, indicating that the spherules are erythrocytes.[114]

The only effective treatment is surgical excision.

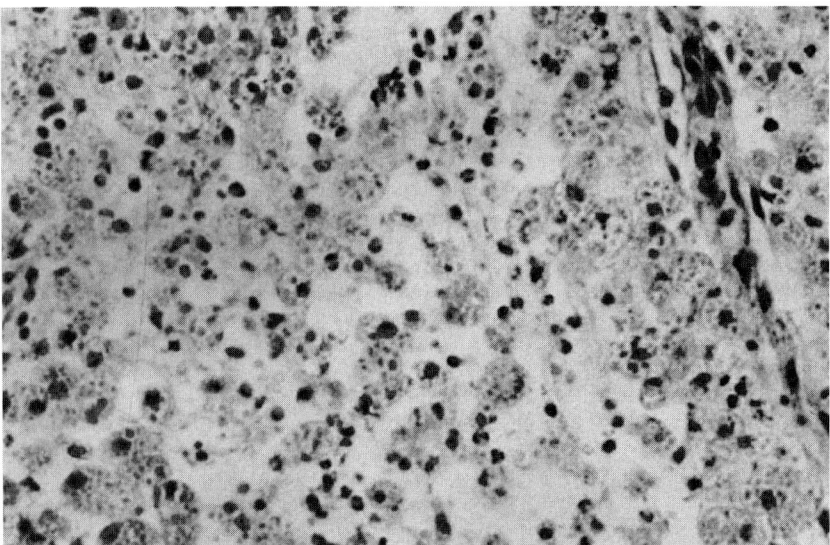

FIGURE 16–17. Myospherulosis. Macrophages containing many intracytoplasmic inclusions (fragments of erythrocytes).

• THALLIUM TOXICOSIS

Thallium is a cumulative, general cell poison that may produce skin lesions or systemic toxicity.[87, 109, 115]

Cause and Pathogenesis

The use of thallium as a rodenticide and roach poison in the United States was banned more than 25 years ago because of its toxicity. Despite the unavailability of thallium for all these years, cases of thallium toxicosis are still occasionally recognized in the United States from baits found in house walls, garages, and barns.[109, 115] With doses of more than 20 mg/kg of body weight, the fatality rate is 100%, and the clinical signs are those of damage to the central nervous system and circulatory system.[87] Nervousness, convulsions, tremors, salivation, weakness, and paralysis, together with a rapid, weak pulse, are seen. Reliable early signs of less acute toxicity include vomiting, hemorrhagic gastroenteritis, polydipsia, pyrexia, and brick red mucous membranes. Colic and dyspnea are often apparent. Smaller doses of thallium may be cumulative and may produce the subacute or a chronic syndrome. Even with the best of care, the mortality rate can be extremely high (70%); therefore, the prognosis is poor. Thallium is rapidly absorbed through the oral and intestinal mucosa and through the skin. It is mainly excreted in the urine, but it may persist in various tissues for up to 3 months. Thallium and potassium move together through cell walls and are excreted together in the urine. Therefore, increased turnover of one substance increases the secretion of the other. In rats, cystine and methionine seem to protect against the alopecic and toxic effects of thallium.

Researchers emphasize that thallium poisoning may be commonly unrecognized in cats that do not show cutaneous involvement.[83] Although the syndrome with skin lesions is classic and highly suggestive, cases of poisoning without skin lesions exhibit multisystemic problems that necessitate a detailed case work-up and laboratory support for accurate diagnosis. Even with intensive supportive care, only 19% of the feline patients in one study recovered; thus, a poor prognosis must be given.[83] Many of the antidotal drugs suggested for other species are highly toxic to cats, and consequently, the clinician is further handicapped in treating this species.

Clinical Features

Thallium poisoning is divided into two syndromes. In acute toxicity, the onset of signs is delayed by 12 to 96 hours after ingestion, but the length of the course until death is only 4 to 5 days. Skin lesions are not seen in acute intoxication. If the animal ingests smaller amounts or survives the peracute signs, severe gastrointestinal signs occur, which necessitate intensive supportive care. With ingestion of small amounts over some time, chronic intoxication occurs. Signs may not develop for 7 to 21 days after ingestion and may not reach their peak for an additional 21 days. Chronically intoxicated animals have hyperemic mucous membranes, mild to moderate gastrointestinal signs, and skin lesions characterized by erythema and hair loss. The hair loss is first noted in frictional areas, and ulceration may follow the hair loss. Advanced cases have involvement of the face (see Fig. 16–9G), the ears, the ventrum, the perineum, the feet (see Fig. 16–8H), and the mucocutaneous junctions (Fig. 16–18A). The footpads become hyperkeratotic and ulcerated. Signs of other organ involvement are common.

Diagnosis

Because thallium intoxication is rare, it often is not suspected. The primary differential diagnostic possibilities to explain the systemic and cutaneous signs include drug eruption, systemic lupus erythematosus, necrolytic migratory erythema, toxic epidermal necrolysis, erythema multiforme major, lymphoreticular neoplasia, and the various rickettsial and protozoal diseases. The diagnosis is confirmed by the detection of thallium in the urine by a rapid colorimetric spot test (Gabriel-Dubin test) or absorption spectrophotometry.[87] The spot test is inexpensive and more readily available than absorption spectrophotometry, but is less sensitive, with both false-positive and false-negative reactions reported. In most cases, these urine tests are performed after skin biopsy results suggest thallotoxicosis.

Thallium exerts a local toxic effect on epidermal cells in the process of differentiation leading to keratin formation. Degenerative changes are evident in the hair follicle and in the surface epidermis.[101] The direct insult to the hair follicle is especially noteworthy in anagen hairs; the hair shaft is converted to an amorphous mass, the bulb degenerates, and the hair is lost (Fig. 16–19). Follicular plugging and parakeratosis are prominent. The surface epidermis shows massive parakeratotic hyperkeratosis and apoptosis with vacuolar degeneration of keratinocytes (Fig. 16–20). Multiple spongiform microabscesses are present in the superficial epidermis and the hair follicle's outer root sheath. The superficial dermis shows edema, vascular dilatation, and extravasation of erythrocytes.

Clinical Management

The prognosis in all cases of thallitoxicosis is grave, and most animals die. In mildly intoxicated cases, supportive care with the administration of appropriate fluids, electrolytes, antibiotics, and so forth is paramount and may be the only treatment needed, because the thallium is slowly eliminated from the body via the bile and urine. Various specific treatments have been suggested, but none is without hazard. Aside from specific adverse reactions for each agent, all can precipitate a thallium crises by drawing thallium from tissues into the blood. Because of this rebound, chelators such as dithizone (diphenylthiocarbazone) (70 mg/kg q8h) or dithiocarb sodium (diethyldithiocarbamate sodium) (30 mg/kg q8h) are no longer recommended.[109, 115] Gastrointestinal trapping of the thallium with Prussian blue or activated charcoal may be of some benefit. The charcoal appears to be more effective. Potassium chloride supplementation (1 to 2 g q8 to 12h) promotes renal elimination by competing with thallium for distal tubular reabsorption. Patients should be monitored for signs of cardiac and renal toxicity. Combination treatment with charcoal and potassium chloride has been suggested.[109, 115]

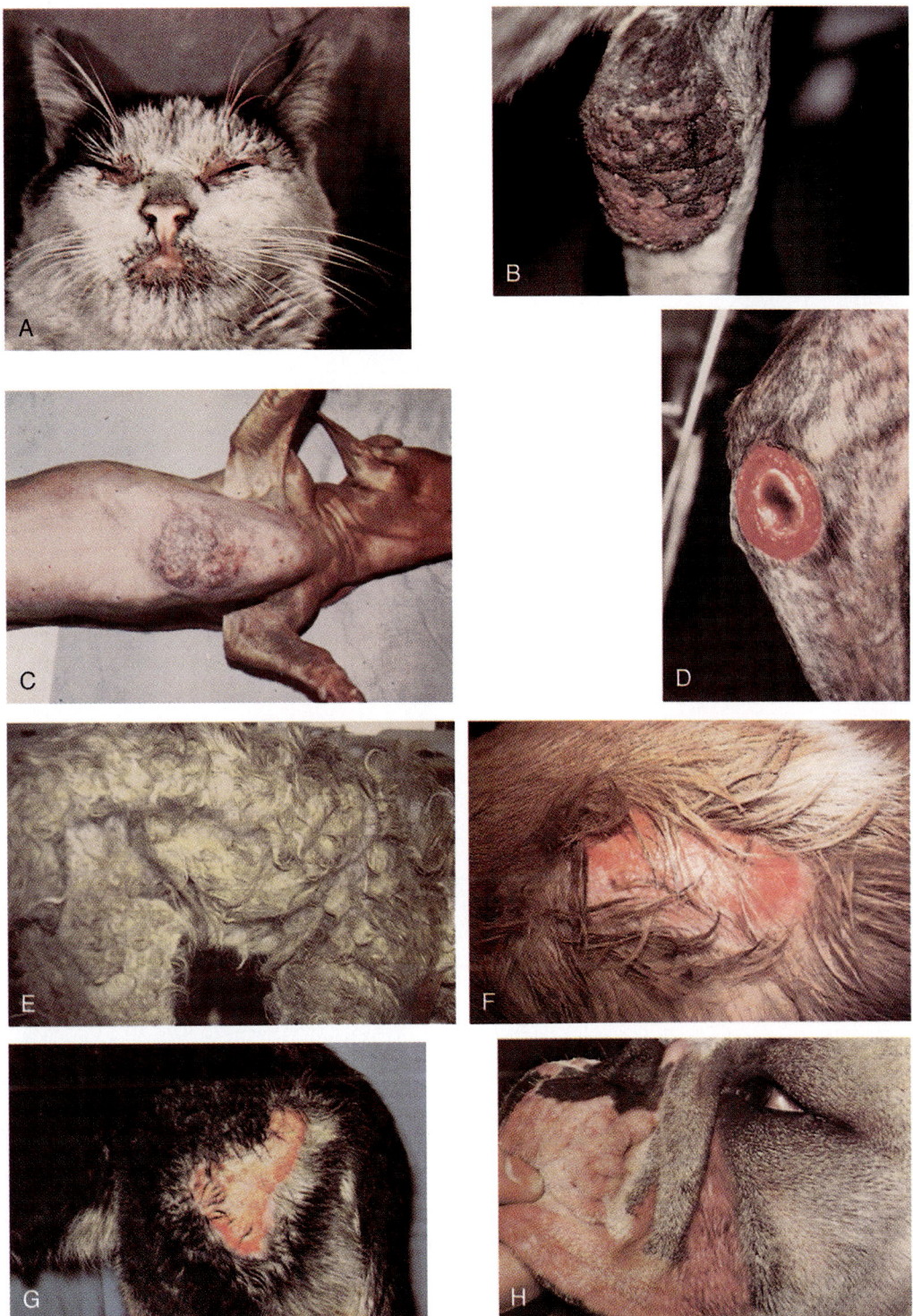

FIGURE 16-18. *A*, Early inflammation and crusting of the eyelids and lips of a cat with thallium poisoning. (From Zook BD, et al: Thallium poisoning in cats. JAVMA 153:285, 1968.) *B*, Callus dermatitis. Note intertriginous folds in the thick, rugose callus. *C*, Sternal callus in a dachshund. *D*, Pressure sore in the hock region. *E*, Severe matting predisposes the animal to pyotraumatic dermatitis. *F*, Pyotraumatic dermatitis with sharp margins. *G*, Pyotraumatic dermatitis typically develops rapidly into a glistening, suppurative, hairless lesion bordered by a band of erythematous skin. *H*, Facial fold intertrigo. The thumb is pulling the lip forward to expose the erythematous, infected crevice hidden in the fold.

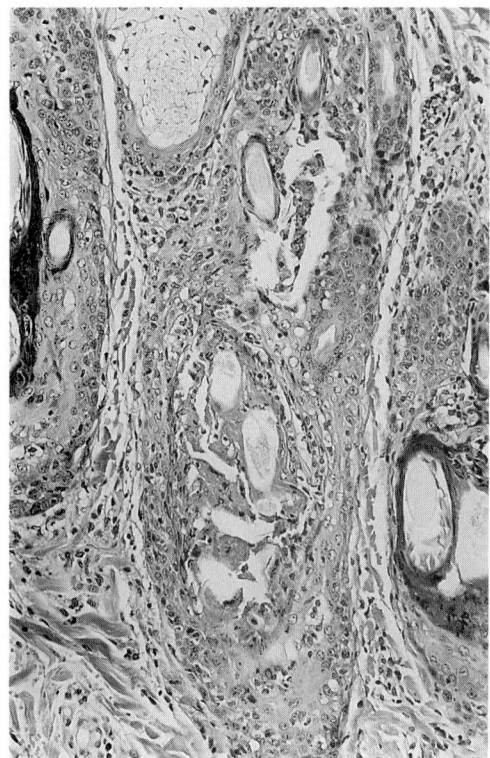

FIGURE 16-19. Thallium toxicosis. Follicular necrosis and degeneration of hair shafts.

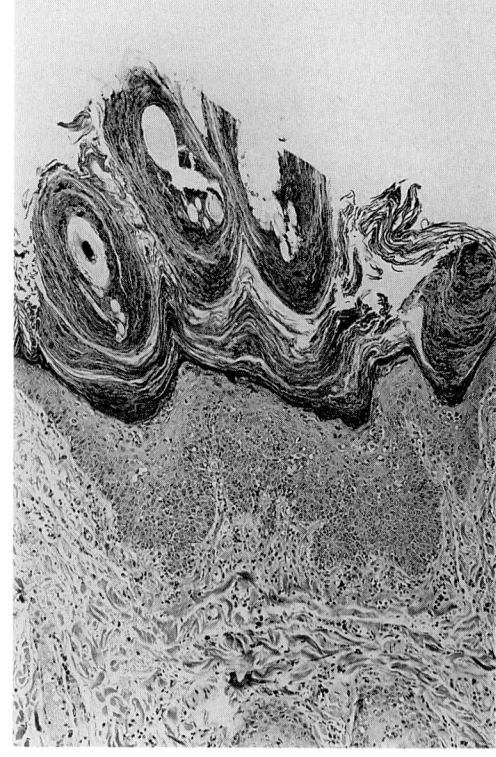

FIGURE 16-20. Thallium toxicosis. Marked parakeratotic hyperkeratosis overlying epidermal hyperplasia and vacuolar degeneration of keratinocytes.

If the animal survives the intoxication, the skin lesions heal spontaneously with complete hair regrowth. Bathing with mild shampoos or hydrotherapy can accelerate the skin's healing but may unduly stress the animal.

• MISCELLANEOUS TOXICOSES

Veterinary textbooks on toxicology mention skin changes for many compounds.[87] Most cases involve farm animals, but pets can be equally as susceptible. The agents can cause skin lesions by direct action on the skin, by altering levels of vital nutrients, or by altering the function of other organs. The number of cases of reported cutaneous toxicoses in small animals is small, but these cases are probably underreported.

Arsenic is a general tissue poison that combines with and inactivates sulfhydryl groups in tissue enzymes.[29, 85] Sources of arsenic include herbicides, rodenticides, pesticides, and arsenical medicaments. Signs of arsenic toxicosis vary according to the dose, the physical form, the route of administration, and the composition (organic or inorganic).

Arsenic toxicosis was reported in a mature dog presented for listlessness, anorexia, weight loss, rough coat, swollen muzzle, and necrosis and ulceration of the pinnae, feet, lips, and prepuce.[29] A container of liquid insecticide (44% sodium arsenite) was found to be leaking into the dog's house. Arsenic concentrations were found at toxic levels in urine, blood, feces, and hair. Bathing the dog and cleaning up its environment resulted in complete remission within 1 month. Chronic arsenic toxicosis is a known cause of Bowen's disease in humans.[37] Although cases in animals (see Chap. 20) do not appear to be associated with arsenic poisoning, it should be considered, especially when the animal has intercurrent gastrointestinal signs.

Mycotoxins are toxic metabolites produced by molds. Intoxication occurs by ingestion of spoiled grain or grain products. Ergotism was the first recognized mycotoxicosis and has been reported to cause necrotizing skin lesions in dogs.[30] A case of necrolytic migratory erythema (see Chap. 10) was reported in a dog that ate moldy biscuit meal containing ochratoxin A, citrinin, and sterigmatocystin.[69] Because most owners do not feed obviously spoiled foods, this may be an isolated case. However, it does demonstrate that agents that produce no direct skin signs can do so by altering the function of other organs.

• CALLUS AND HYGROMA

A *callus* is a round or oval hyperkeratotic plaque that develops on the skin, typically over bony pressure points. The elbow and the hock are the most common sites. Dogs with deep chests often develop sternal lesions. Large breeds are especially susceptible if the dog sleeps on cement, brick, or wood. Many adult dogs develop varying degrees of callus. Dogs that sleep in unusual positions because of orthopedic disease or that are hypothyroid can have calluses in unusual locations. Callosities are a normal, protective response to pressure-induced ischemia and inflammation.[83] The callus is hairless and gray, and has a wrinkled surface (see Fig. 16–9B). Histologically, there is irregular to papillated epidermal hyperplasia and orthokeratotic to parakeratotic hyperkeratosis. Small follicular cysts are seen in the dermis.

Although calluses, especially those in unusual locations, can be mistaken for lesions of ringworm, demodicosis, or other inflammatory disorders, diagnosis in most cases is straightforward. Most callosities need no treatment, but some calluses necessitate treatment because the owner finds them objectionable or because they are extremely hyperplastic and become ulcerated or easily infected. Environmental modification is mandatory.

Padding (e.g., foam rubber pads, air mattresses, and straw bedding) must be provided, and the dog must use it consistently. Padding efforts often frustrate the client because the dog avoids the padding or destroys it. If the environment cannot be padded, the individual lesions can be protected by making pads for affected areas (e.g., elbow pads). With some ingenuity, virtually any callus can be padded. Again, the dog can frustrate the effort by removing the pad. After padding is provided, the callus can be softened with any good hand cream. In extreme cases, the callus can be removed surgically. This has to be performed carefully because there can be excessive hemorrhage and sutures often do not hold. Wound dehiscence is a possible complication of surgery.

Hygroma is a false or acquired bursa that develops subcutaneously over bony prominences.[83] Hygromas develop after repeated trauma-induced necrosis and inflammation over pressure points. They are initially soft to fluctuant (fluid filled) but may become abscesses or granulomas with or without fistulous tracts, especially if they are secondarily infected.

Histologically, hygromas are characterized by cystic spaces surrounded by dense walls of granulation tissue, the inner layer of which is a flattened layer of fibroblasts. Early lesions usually respond well to loose, padded bandages applied for 2 to 3 weeks and corrective housing. More severe lesions may necessitate extensive drainage, extirpation, or skin grafting procedures.

• CALLUS DERMATITIS AND PYODERMA

Callus dermatitis is a secondary infection of a callus subjected to repeated trauma or softened without the obligatory environmental modifications.

Cause and Clinical Features

The callus is the initial response to trauma. Continued trauma and the proliferative skin reaction that follows produce crevices in the callus and intertriginous areas, which results in a fold dermatitis. Additional trauma causes epidermal breakdown, ulceration of pressure points, and fistulae. The lesions are most common over the hock and elbow joints of giant breeds such as Great Danes, St. Bernards, Newfoundlands, and Irish wolfhounds (see Fig. 16–17*B*). Sternal calluses on the chest of Dachshunds, setters, Pointers, Boxers, and Doberman pinschers may also become secondarily ulcerated and infected (see Fig. 16–17*C*). Often, there are no specific bacterial flora involved in this infection, although staphylococci are commonly isolated. Pressure point granulomas, which contain free hair shafts, may develop.

Ulcerated or fistulated lesions may be deeply infected, and exudative cytologic examination should be performed in all cases. The surface should be scrubbed, and the lesion should be squeezed firmly before samples are collected. In many cases, pieces of hair shafts pop to the surface. Infection usually results in a pyogranulomatous inflammation.

Clinical Management

Primary attention must be given to relieving the trauma so the tissue can heal. This can be accomplished through the use of waterbeds, special bedding, pads for various body parts, or a combination of these measures. In severe cases, surgical excision of the callus may be indicated. This is major surgery with a difficult postoperative course, and the reader is referred to texts on soft tissue surgery for details of treatment.

Mild surface inflammation and fold dermatitis can be relieved by daily whirlpool baths in warm water. Distal lesions may be amenable to soaking in a bucket. With imbedded hair shafts, a mildly hypertonic drawing solution of magnesium sulfate (Epsom salts) (30 ml/L or 2 tbsp/qt of warm water) can be beneficial. In noninfected lesions, hydrotherapy is typically sufficient to cause healing. When this is not possible, the topical application of an antibiotic cream or Preparation H, a human hemorrhoid preparation containing live yeast extract and shark liver oil, can be beneficial.

Infected lesions necessitate a prolonged course with antibiotics. Six weeks or longer of treatment is usually necessary. Because the infected tissue cannot return to normal condition with antibiotic treatment, the client is not able to determine when the infection is resolved. Cytologic examinations should be performed every second week. When no sign of infection is present, treatment should be continued for an additional 7 to 14 days. Relapses are prevented by management changes.

• VENTRAL COMEDONE SYNDROME

This is common in Greyhounds.[16a] Friction and pressure-point contact with the ground result in comedone formation on the sternum. Secondary bacterial infection produces papules and pustules. Treatment includes comedolytic and antibacterial topical applications, and management changes.

• PRESSURE SORES

Pressure sores (decubital ulcers) result from prolonged application of pressure concentrated over a bony prominence in a relatively small area of the body. The pressure is sufficient to compress the capillary circulation, causing tissue damage or frank necrosis.[30, 37, 83] The severity of pressure sores is variable, and as expected, more severe lesions are difficult to treat. Grade I lesions affect the epidermis and superficial dermis, whereas Grade IV lesions extend to the underlying bone.[107] Grade II lesions stop at the subcutis, and Grade III lesions involve the deep fascia. Pressure sores almost invariably become infected with a variety of pathogenic bacteria. Within 24 to 48 hours, the edges of the ulcerated area are undermined. Because of the area of capillary and venous congestion at the base of the ulcer and tissue margins, systemic antibiotics do not penetrate well.

Animals that are recumbent for prolonged periods on hard surfaces are at increased risk for pressure sores. Emaciation increases the susceptibility. Lesions are initially characterized by an erythematous to reddish purple discoloration. This progresses to oozing, necrosis, and ulceration. The resultant ulcers tend to be deep, to be undermined at the edges, to be secondarily infected, and to heal slowly (see Fig. 16–17D).

Prevention is paramount. All recumbent animals should be kept on a waterbed or eggcrate foam rubber pad, be turned frequently, and receive a daily whirlpool bath. If a pressure sore develops, additional padding should be supplied in that area. The wound should be cleaned frequently with an appropriate antiseptic solution. If the patient recovers from its disease fairly quickly, the pressure sore should heal spontaneously but slowly. Application of Preparation H, raw honey,[11] mupirocin,[58] or hydrogen peroxide may accelerate healing. Although hydrogen peroxide at high concentrations is cytotoxic, low concentrations (1.5% to 3%) stimulate fibroblasts and angiogenesis, and can increase wound healing.[111] In Grade II to IV lesions, surgery often is necessary to close the defect.[107] Surgery must be postponed until the animal is ambulatory, otherwise the wound dehiscence can be expected. Presurgical application of agents that encourage a healthy bed of granulation tissue (e.g., Granulex, Pfizer Animal Health) can be beneficial.

• TUG-OF-WAR BLISTERS

Dogs who play tug-of-war vigorously, especially with another dog, can develop blisters on the digital and main pads of the front feet. Dogs who are tug-of-war fanatics and have a high tolerance for pain are most at risk. Dr. Eve Brown, a practitioner in the Cornell area, sees the condition often enough that she encourages her clients not to let their dogs play tug-of-war.

The onset of signs is acute and is characterized by lameness. At examination, classic frictional blisters are seen on one or more pads. Most of the blisters are ruptured, and examination of the floor of the blister shows normal pad epithelium. This is in contrast to more typical pad ulcers seen in dogs with mechanobullous diseases (see Chap. 12), immune-mediated disorders (see Chap. 9), or those subject to severe, acute trauma (e.g., drag injuries). In the case of dogs with mechanobullous diseases or acute trauma, the ulcers are sharply marginated and the dermis is visible.

With the appropriate history, the diagnosis is straightforward. In a puppy, in which there can be concern for an underlying hyperfragility of the pads, biopsies may be needed to rule out other disorders. Treatment is simply palliative and involves cutting the separated pad away and protective bandaging. Because an intact epithelium exists at the bottom of the blister, the dog should return to normal function quickly.

• PYOTRAUMATIC DERMATITIS

Pyotraumatic dermatitis (acute moist dermatitis, or "hot spots") is produced by self-induced trauma as the patient bites or scratches at a part of its body in an attempt to alleviate some pain or itch.[83] The majority of cases are complications of flea bite hypersensitivity, but allergic skin diseases, other ectoparasites, anal sac problems, inflammations such as otitis externa, foreign bodies in the coat, irritant substances, dirty unkempt coats (see Fig. 16–17E), psychoses, and painful musculoskeletal disorders may be underlying causes. These factors initiate the itch-scratch cycle, which varies in intensity with individuals. The intense trauma produces severe large lesions in a few hours. Animals particularly disposed to this problem are those with a heavy pelage that has a dense undercoat, such as Golden and Labrador retrievers, Collies, German shepherds, and St. Bernards. The problem is much more common in hot, humid weather and may be related to lack of ventilation in the coat.

A typical lesion is red, moist, and exudative. There is a coagulum of proteinaceous exudate in the center of the area surrounded by a red halo of erythematous skin. The hair is lost from the area, but the margins are sharply defined from the surrounding normal skin and hair (see Fig. 16–17F). The lesion progresses rapidly if appropriate therapy is not started at once (see Fig. 16–17G). Much pain is associated with the local area, and this may eventually deter the animal from further self-trauma. Lesions are often located in close proximity to the primary painful process (e.g., near infected ears, anal sacs, and flea bites on the rump).

True hot spots have bacteria colonizing the surface of the lesion but are not skin infections. This is in contrast to pyotraumatic folliculitis (see Chap. 4) in which the dog traumatizes the skin over a staphylococcal folliculitis or furunculosis.[95] Without clipping and palpating the lesion, it can be difficult (if not impossible) to differentiate pyotraumatic dermatitis from pyotraumatic folliculitis.

Diagnosis is made by the history of acute onset, the physical appearance, and some association with a primary cause. True pyotraumatic dermatitis is a relatively flat, eroded to ulcerated lesion. Histologically (Fig. 16–21), the tissue reaction is acute, exudative, and involves the surface epithelium only. Lesions that are thickened, are plaquelike, and are bordered by papules or pustules (satellite lesions) should always suggest a primary eruptive process, especially a staphylococcal infection, which the dog has traumatized.[95]

Therapy is effective if applied promptly and vigorously. Application of pramoxine spray or conditioner, sedation, or anesthesia may be needed to allow thorough cleaning of the area. Cleaning with povidone-iodine or chlorhexidine is the first and most important

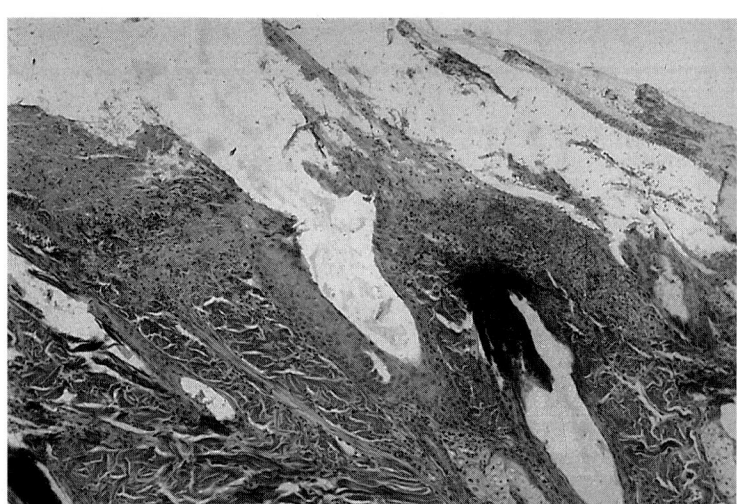

FIGURE 16–21. Pyotraumatic dermatitis. Traumatic erosion of the epidermis with marked serum exudation. The hair follicles and mid- to-deep dermal tissues are normal.

step in local therapy. Cleaning is more rapid and effective when the hair is clipped, but clipping is not always possible in show dogs. In unclipped areas, the shampoo formulation of the antiseptic should be used, whereas solutions are applied on clipped lesions.

After the wound is cleaned, the nature of additional treatments depends on the dog and the investigator. A few dogs lose all interest in the lesion after they create it and only require the application of a drying agent. A 2% aluminum acetate solution (Domeboro solution), an aluminum acetate and 1% hydrocortisone solution, or a menthol and *Hamamelis* solution (Dermacool, Virbac) are commonly used products and can be effective.[4] The solution is applied two to three times daily until a healthy scab develops. Herbal extracts are also reported to be effective, but detailed studies are lacking.[112]

Because the lesion is inflamed and tender, most dogs need treatment with a corticosteroid. If oral corticosteroids are not contraindicated, prednisolone or prednisone (1.1 mg/kg q24h) is most useful because the owner does not have to manipulate a tender lesion. If oral drugs are contraindicated or the lesion is not severe enough to warrant systemic treatment, topical agents can be used. Although many dogs have been successfully treated with a topical steroid (e.g., betamethasone valerate cream) alone, a recent study showed that a neomycin-prednisolone combination was more effective than either individual ingredient.[100] The prednisolone alone gave the poorest results. The duration of treatment depends on the severity of the lesion and the agent used, but 7- to 14-day courses are typical.

At the time of the initial treatment, it is most important to find the predisposing factor and to eliminate or modify it to stop the patient's reflex self-trauma. The treatment to accomplish this goal varies, depending on the primary cause. Some unfortunate dogs have repeated problems. There is no simple prophylaxis. Constant attention to grooming, hygiene, baths, and parasite control and periodic cleaning of the ears and anal sacs helps. Owners should be particularly vigilant during periods of hot, humid weather. Although diet (e.g., high protein content) is often suggested as a cause, except for severe fatty acid deficiency or food hypersensitivity, this has never been proved.

• INTERTRIGO

Intertrigo (skin fold dermatitis) is a frictional dermatitis that occurs in areas where two skin surfaces are intimately apposed. The apposition results from the intentional breeding of certain dogs (e.g., English bulldog and Chinese Shar pei) or cats (e.g., Persians) for pronounced folding, congenital, or acquired anatomic defects; it may also result from thickening of the dermis or subcutis caused by obesity, hormonal influences, or inflammatory skin disease. Skin rubbing against skin is irritating, and the areas where this occurs have poor air circulation. If moisture, sebum, glandular secretions, and excretions such as tears, saliva, and urine are present, these areas provide an environment that favors skin maceration and bacterial or *Malassezia* yeast overgrowth. Although bacteria or yeast play a central role in the pathogenesis of fold dermatitis, they rarely invade viable tissues, so the old designation of fold pyoderma is inaccurate.[38] The surface organisms act on the trapped secretions and sebum, and produce breakdown products, which are irritating and odoriferous. As the irritants are rubbed on the apposed surface, inflammation results and produces the clinical signs of the disease and causes the increased production of more irritants. A vicious cycle is created.

Satisfactory treatment of an intertrigo necessitates resolution of the inflammation and exudation and elimination of the tissue apposition that triggered the intertrigo. If the folding cannot be eliminated because the anatomic defect is uncorrectable or would destroy the desired appearance of the animal, cure cannot be achieved and a long-term control regimen should be instituted. In some animals, control measures do not work and surgery is needed.[76] When the folding can be eliminated, only a short course of treatment is necessary to resolve the dermatitis.

Removal of the surface organisms and the entrapped debris is essential and necessitates the use of antiseborrheic products. Benzoyl peroxide–based or sulfur-based prod-

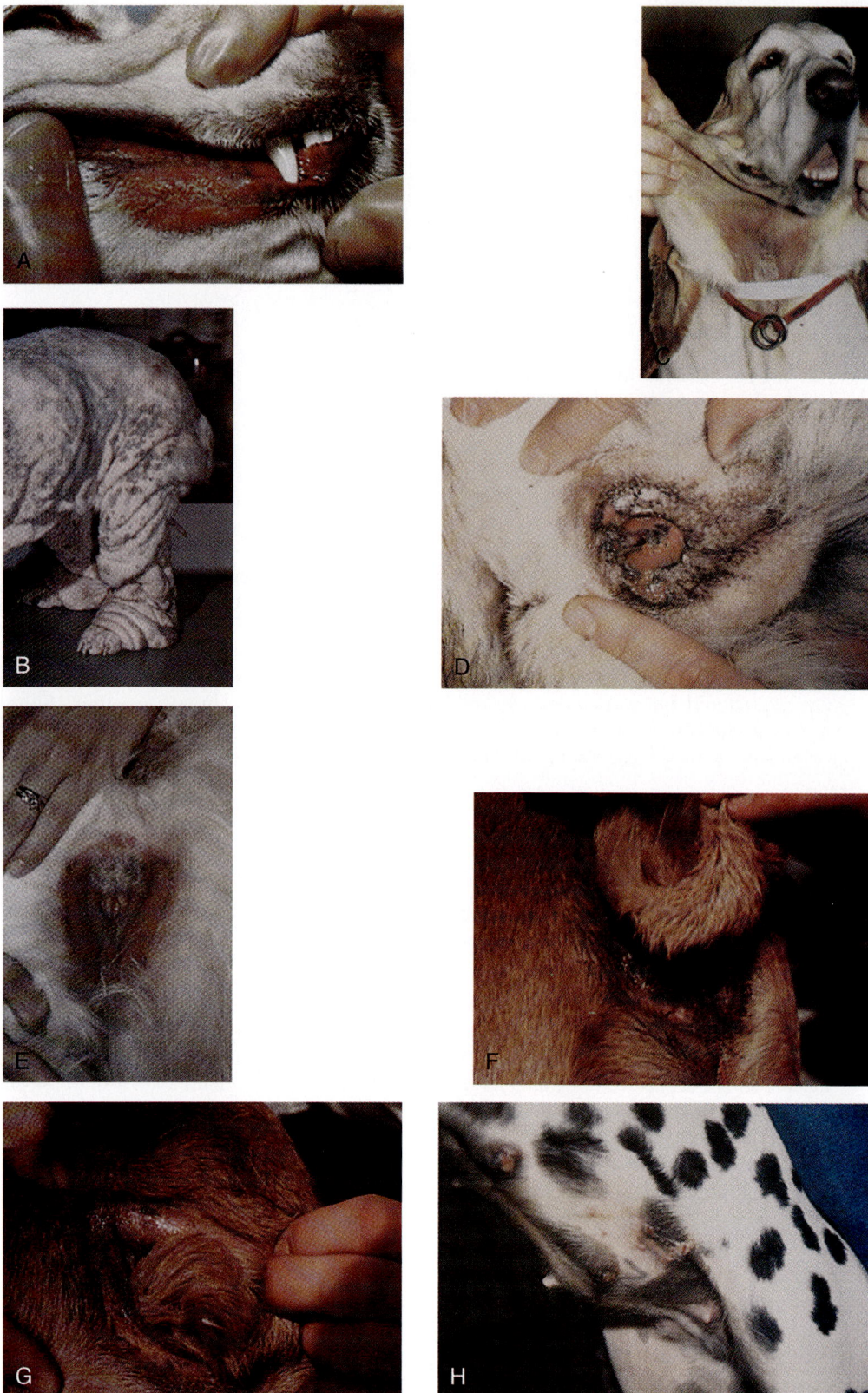

FIGURE 16–22. *A,* Lip fold intertrigo characterized by erythema, exudation, and fetid odor. *B,* Profound folding predisposes this Shar pei to fold dermatitis. *C,* Neck fold intertrigo. *D,* Vulvar fold intertrigo with erosion. *E,* Vulvar fold intertrigo. Severe dermatitis due to constant licking. *F,* Tail fold intertrigo in a dog with screw tail conformation. (Courtesy P. Ihrke.) *G,* Close-up of the dog in *F*. (Courtesy P. Ihrke.) *H,* Calcinosis cutis secondary to percutaneous penetration of calcium carbonate.

ucts, in gel, ointment, or shampoo formulations, are most commonly used. Although the gels and ointments have better residual activity, they can be irritating and worsen the inflammation if used at the onset of treatment. Most investigators use shampoos to gain control and reserve the other formulations for maintenance treatments.

After the surface debris is removed, tissue inflammation can be eliminated by the topical application of a corticosteroid cream or the oral administration of prednisolone (1.1 mg/kg q24h). A 5- to 7-day course of treatment should be sufficient. In mild cases, an aluminum acetate and hydrocortisone solution is very effective.

If the skin apposition cannot be eliminated (e.g., by surgery or weight loss), the dermatitis recurs unless maintenance cleaning with an antiseborrheic product is instituted. For folds of the face, the body, or the vulva, the daily application of a plain or medicated talc can be beneficial and reduce the amount of bathing required. Lip, vulvar, and tail folds are usually not amenable to talcing. The talc is applied carefully to the crevice of each fold. Before the next application, the previous day's dose must be removed by brushing with a dry cloth or by washing. If the area is washed, it should be dried completely before the talc is reapplied. In many cases, the talcing can reduce the frequency of washing from once daily to once or twice weekly. When talcing is ineffective, prophylactic application of a benzoyl peroxide gel can be extremely beneficial. When *Malassezia* yeast predominate, commercial or homemade acetic acid products are beneficial.[61]

Facial fold intertrigo is seen in brachycephalic breeds, especially Pekingese, English bulldogs, and Pugs (see Fig. 16–17H).[83] It is also occasionally seen in Persian and Himalayan cats. The fold may rub on the cornea and cause severe keratitis and ulceration. The breed standards in some cases require a facial fold, so even though its presence may damage the eye, one should be careful to explain the ramifications of surgical correction to owners and should obtain their approval before ablating the folds.

Lip fold intertrigo is primarily an aesthetic problem to owners, because it produces severe halitosis.[83] Owners may need to be convinced that the small lip fold can produce all that odor. This problem is prevalent in dogs with a large lip flap, such as spaniels and St. Bernards (Fig. 16–22A). *Malassezia* overgrowth is extremely common in this area and acetic acid treatments once to twice daily can be beneficial. Cheiloplasty is curative.

Body fold intertrigo occurs primarily in obese individuals, and in certain Basset hounds and Chinese Shar pei dogs (see Fig. 16–22B and C).[83] It is most common in Shar pei puppies that have an increased number of folds and in those with a tendency to seborrhea. As the puppies mature, they do grow out of their folds on parts of the body, and therefore fold dermatitis in the adult Shar pei is more concentrated on the head and face, where the folds persist. It may also be seen on the ventral midline of female dogs and cats with intertrigo between pendulous mammary glands or with rolls of body fat.

Vulvar fold intertrigo is common in obese older female animals that have infantile vulvae as a result of spaying at a young age (see Fig. 16–22D).[83] The vulva is recessed, and vaginal secretions and drops of urine may accumulate in the folds of the perivulvar region. This is a special stimulus to ulceration and bacterial growth, and the odors produced are especially unpleasant. Licking is a near-constant feature and worsens the dermatitis (see Fig. 16–22E). Ascending bacterial urinary tract infections are a common sequela to vulvar fold intertrigo. Several methods of management may help. Because obesity is usually present, weight reduction is indicated. Estrogenic treatments can cause vulvar enlargement with reduction of the folds, but the potential danger of such endocrine therapy must be considered. Surgical vulvopasty (episioplasty), with fixation of the dorsal vulvar commissure to elevate the vulva out of the crevice, is curative. Squamous cell carcinoma has been reported to arise from chronic vulvar fold dermatitis.[83]

Tail fold intertrigo results from pressure of corkscrew tails on the skin of the perineum (see Fig. 16–22F and G). It is seen in English bulldogs, Pugs, Boston terriers, and other breeds with that type of tail.[83] In addition, a rump fold intertrigo may be seen in certain Manx cats. In some cases, the tail may partially obstruct the anus, so that feces, anal sac secretions, and other skin gland products enhance the skin maceration from the intertrigo. Amputation resolves the problem, but the surgery is complicated.

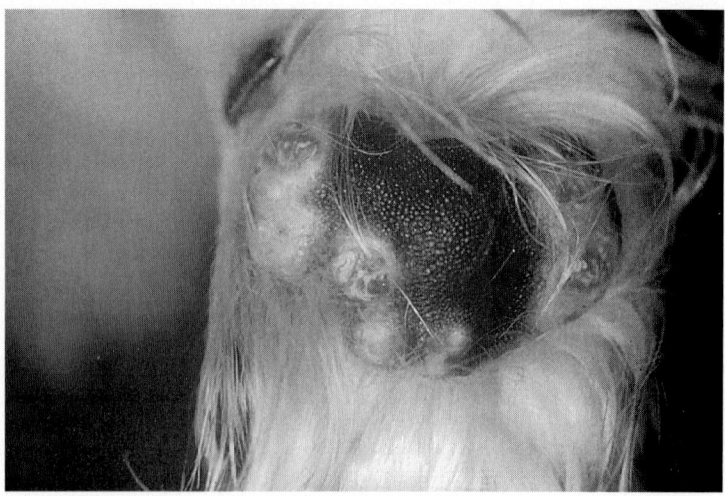

FIGURE 16–23. Calcinosis cutis. Coalescing papular lesions on the edge of the main carpal pad of dog that walked over a calcium-containing ice melter.

• CALCINOSIS CUTIS

Calcinosis cutis involves the deposition of calcium salts in dermal tissues. Lesions can be localized and secondary to trauma in normal or metabolically abnormal dogs (see Chap. 20) or widespread.[20, 41] In dogs, widespread calcinosis cutis typically occurs in spontaneous or iatrogenic hyperadrenocorticism (see Chap. 10), but several reports describe ventral calcinosis caused by percutaneous penetration of calcium carbonate or calcium chloride.[88, 99] Lesions consisted of multiple erythematous, crusted, ulcerated papules and plaques on the glabrous skin of the ventral abdomen, the inguinal region, and the medial thighs (see Fig. 16–11H). The authors have also seen pedal lesions (Fig. 16–23) associated with calcium-containing ice melters.

When calcinosis cutis is recognized in glabrous areas or other areas of contact, the owner should be questioned carefully about possible exposure to bone meal, landscaping products, or barn dusts before adrenal function tests are performed. Once exposure to the calcium is stopped, the lesions should resolve spontaneously. Treatment with DMSO gel may hasten resolution of the lesions.[6] A thin film should be applied once to twice daily.

• REFERENCES

1. Al-Bagdadi FK, et al: Hair dye effects on the hair coat and skin of the dog: A scanning electron microscopic study. Anat Histol Embryol 17:349, 1988.
2. Arnold P, et al: Solare glossitis bei Schlittenhunden. Schweiz Arch Tierheilk 140:328, 1998.
3. Aroch I, Harrus S: Retrospective study of the epidemiological, clinical, haematological, and biochemical findings in 109 dogs poisoned by *Vipera xanthina palestinae*. Vet Rec 144:532, 1999.
4. Ascher F, et al: Intérêt d'une solution topique non antibiocorticoïde dans le traitement de la dermatite pyotraumatique du chien. Prat Méd Chir Anim Comp 30:345, 1995.
5. Ashley PF, Bowman LA: Symmetric cutaneous necrosis of the hind feet and multicentric follicular lymphoma in a cat. J Am Vet Med Assoc 214:211, 1999.
6. Beale KM, Morris DO: Treatment of canine calcinosis cutis with dimethylsulfoxide gel. Proc Annu Memb Meet Am Acad Vet Dermatol Am Coll Vet Dermatol 14:97, 1998.
7. Bensignor E: Soleil et peau chez les carnivores domestiques 1—effets des rayonnements solaires sur les structures cutanées. Point Vét 30:225, 1999.
8. Bensignor E: Soleil et peau chez les carnivores domestiques 2—affections photoinduites et photoaggravées. Point Vét 30:229, 1999.
9. Bergeaud P: Pathologies liées aux épillets. Point Vét 26:105, 1994.
10. Bilbrey SA, et al: Chemical burn caused by benzalkonium chloride in eight surgical cases. J Am Anim Hosp Assoc 25:31, 1989.
11. Borum T: Management of decubital ulcers with the topical application of raw honey. Mississippi Vet J Summer:16, 1986.
12. Bouayad H, et al: Peripheral acquired arteriovenous fistula: Report of four cases and literature review. J Am Anim Hosp Assoc 23:205, 1987.

13. Bradley DM, et al: Biochemical and histopathological evaluation of changes in sled dog paw skin associated with physical stress and cold temperatures. Vet Dermatol 7:203, 1996.
14. Brennan KE, Ihrke PJ: Grass awn migration in dogs and cats: A retrospective study of 182 cases. J Am Vet Med Assoc 182:1201, 1983.
15. Brown DC, Holt D: Subcutaneous emphysema, pneumothorax, pneumomediastinum, and pneumopericardium associated with positive-pressure ventilation in a cat. J Am Vet Med Assoc 206:997, 1995.
16. Brown DE, et al: Echinocytosis associated with rattlesnake envenomation in dogs. Vet Pathol 31:654, 1994.
16a. Burkett G: Skin diseases in greyhounds. Vet Med 95:115, 2000.
17. Butterfield AB, et al: Acquired peripheral arteriovenous fistula in a dog. J Am Vet Med Assoc 176:445, 1980.
18. Coyne BE, et al: Thermoelectric burns from improper grounding of electrocautery units: Two case reports. J Am Anim Hosp Assoc 29:7, 1993.
19. Darr D, et al: Protection against UVB damage to porcine skin with topical application of vitamin C. In: von Tscharner C, Halliwell REW (eds): Advances in Veterinary Dermatology, Vol 1. Baillière Tindall, London, 1990, p 463.
19a. Darr D, Fridovich I: Free radicals in cutaneous biology. J Invest Dermatol 102:671, 1994.
20. Davidson EB, et al: Calcinosis circumscripta of the thoracic wall in a German shepherd dog. J Am Anim Hosp Assoc 34:153, 1998.
21. Day MJ: Expression of major histocompatibility complex class II molecules by dermal inflammatory cells, epidermal Langerhans' cells and keratinocytes in canine dermatological disease. J Comp Pathol 115:317, 1996.
22. DeClercq J, Vanstapel M-J: Chronic radiant heat dermatitis (*Erythema ab igne*) in two dogs. Vet Dermatol 9:269, 1998.
23. DeNardo GA, et al: Comparison of seven different suture materials in the feline oral cavity. J Am Anim Hosp Assoc 32:164, 1996.
24. Dernell WS, Wheaton LG: Surgical management of radiation injury—Part I. Comp Cont Ed 17:181, 1995.
25. Dernell WS, Wheaton LG: Surgical management of radiation injury—Part II. Comp Cont Ed 17:499, 1995.
26. Dolowy WC: Giant hogweed photodermatitis in two dogs in Bellevue, Washington. J Am Vet Med Assoc 209:722, 1996.
27. Dunstan RW, et al: The light and the skin. In: Kwochka KW, et al (eds): Advances in Veterinary Dermatology III. Butterworth-Heinemann, Boston, 1998, p 3.
28. Evans AG, et al: A trial of 13-*cis*-retinoic acid for treatment of squamous cell carcinoma and preneoplastic lesions of the head in cats. Am J Vet Res 46:2553, 1985.
29. Evinger JV, Blakemore JC: Dermatitis in a dog associated with exposure to an arsenic compound. J Am Vet Med Assoc 184:1281, 1984.
30. Fadok VW: Necrotizing skin diseases. In: Kirk RW (ed): Current Veterinary Therapy VIII. W.B. Saunders Co, Philadelphia, 1983, p 473.
31. Fairley RA: Photosensitivity dermatitis in two collie working dogs. N Z Vet J 30:61, 1982.
32. Fairley RA, MacKenzie IS: Photosensitivity in a kennel of Harrier hounds. Vet Dermatol 5:1, 1994.
33. Farnsworth R, Birchard S: Subcutaneous accumulation of chyle after thoracic duct ligation in a dog. J Am Vet Med Assoc 208:2016, 1996.
33a. Fossum TW, et al: Generalized lymphangiectasis in a dog with subcutaneous chyle and lymphangioma. J Am Vet Med Assoc 197:231, 1991.
34. Fox SM: Management of thermal burns—Part I. Comp Cont Educ 7:631, 1985.
35. Frank LA, Calderwood-Mays MB: Solar dermatitis in dogs. Compend Cont Educ 16:465, 1994.
36. Frank LA, et al: Distribution and appearance of elastic fibers in the dermis of clinically normal dogs and dogs with solar dermatitis and other dermatoses. Am J Vet Res 57:178, 1996.
37. Freidberg IM, et al: Fitzpatrick's Dermatology in General Medicine 5th ed. McGraw-Hill Book Co, New York, 1999.
38. Garny G: Cas clinique: Pyodermite des plis. Point Vét 18:411, 1986.
39. Georgi ME, et al: Pappus bristles: The cause of burdock stomatitis in dogs. Cornell Vet 72:43, 1982.
40. Gourley IM, et al: Burn scar malignancy in a dog. J Am Anim Hosp Assoc 180:109, 1982.
41. Gross TL: Calcinosis circumscripta and renal dysplasia in a dog. Vet Dermatol 8:27, 1997.
42. Harari J, et al: Recurrent peripheral arteriovenous fistula and hyperthyroidism in a cat. J Am Anim Hosp Assoc 20:759, 1984.
43. Hargis AM, et al: Myospherulosis in the subcutis of a dog. Vet Pathol 21:248, 1984.
44. Hargis MM, Lewis TP II: Full-thickness cutaneous burn in black-haired skin on the dorsum of the body of a Dalmatian puppy. Vet Pathol 10:39, 1999.
45. Hosgood G: Arteriovenous fistulas: Pathophysiology, diagnosis and treatment. Comp Cont Educ 11:625, 1989.
46. Hruza LL, Pentland AP: Mechanisms of UV-induced inflammation. J Invest Dermatol 100:35S, 1993.
47. Hubert BM: Porphyries: Cutaneous manifestations in a cat and a dog. In: Kwochka KW, et al (eds): Advances in Veterinary Dermatology III. Butterworth-Heinemann, Boston, 1998, p 461.
48. Hudelson S, Hudelson P: Pathophysiology of snake envenomization and evaluation of treatments—Part I. Comp Cont Ed 17:889, 1995.
49. Hudelson S, Hudelson P: Pathophysiology of snake envenomization and evaluation of treatments—Part II. Comp Cont Ed 17:1035, 1995.
50. Hudelson S, Hudelson P: Pathophysiology of snake envenomization and evaluation of treatments—Part III. Comp Cont Ed 17:1385, 1995.
51. Hudson WE, Florax MJH: Photosensitization in foxhounds. Vet Rec 128:618, 1991.
52. Hunt GB, Chapman BL: "Trophic" ulceration of two digital pads. Aust Vet Pract 21:196, 1991.
53. Ihrke P: Nasal solar dermatitis. In: Kirk RW (ed): Current Veterinary Therapy VII. W.B. Saunders Co, Philadelphia, 1981, p 440.
54. Irving RA, et al: Porphyrin values and treatment of feline solar dermatitis. Am J Vet Res 43:2067, 1982.
55. Israel E, et al: Microangiopathic hemolytic anemia in a puppy: Grand Rounds Conference. J Am Anim Hosp Assoc 14:521, 1978.
56. Iwasaki T, Maeda Y: The effect of ultraviolet (UV) on the severity of canine pemphigus erythematosus. Proc Annu Memb Meet Am Acad Vet Dermatol Am Coll Vet Dermatol 13:86, 1997.
57. Jepson PGH.: Chilblain syndrome in dogs. Vet Rec 108:392, 1981.

58. Kanj LF, et al: Pressure ulcers. J Am Acad Dermatol 38:517, 1998.
59. Kimura T, Doi K: Responses of the skin over the dorsum to sunlight in hairless descendants of Mexican hairless dogs. Am J Vet Res 55:199, 1994.
60. Kimura T, Doi K: Protective effects of sunscreens on sunburn and suntan reactions in cross-bred Mexican hairless dogs. Vet Dermatol 5:175, 1994.
61. Knevitt R: Lip fold pyoderma. Cont Therap Series 187:829, 1995.
62. Komarek JV: Fallbericht: Verfolgung der Rute beim Hund-Cauda-equina-syndrome. Kleintier-Prax 33:25, 1988.
63. Kostolich M: Reconstructive surgery of a snakebite wound. Canine Pract 16:15, 1990.
64. Kraft W, et al: Schlangenbisse bei Hunden. Tierärztl Prax 26:104, 1998.
65. Kral, F., Schwartzman, R. M.: Veterinary and Comparative Dermatology. J.B. Lippincott Co, Philadelphia, 1964.
66. Ledo E: Photodermatosis. Part I: Photobiology, photoimmunology, and idiopathic photodermatoses. Int J Dermatol 32:387, 1993.
67. Ledo E: Photodermatoses. Part II: Chemical photodermatoses and dermatoses that can be exacerbated, precipitated, or provoked by light. Int J Dermatol 32: 480, 1993.
68. Lazarov A, et al: Dermal spherulosis (myospherulosis) after topical treatment for psoriasis. J Am Acad Dermatol 30(Part 1):265, 1994.
69. Little CJL, et al: Hepatopathy and dermatitis in a dog associated with the ingestion of mycotoxins. J Small Anim Pract 32:23, 1991.
70. Mansfield PD: The management of snake venom poisoning in dogs. Comp Cont Educ 6:988, 1984.
71. Marks SL, et al: Coral snake envenomation in the dog: Report of four cases and review of the literature. J Am Anim Hosp Assoc 26:629, 1990.
72. Marsella R, et al: Use of pentoxifylline in the treatment of allergic contact reaction to plants of the Commelinceae family in dogs. Vet Dermatol 8:121, 1997.
73. Mason BJE: Necrosis of a dog's toes following hepatitis. Vet Rec 101:286, 1977.
74. Mason K: Actinic dermatosis in dogs and cats. Proc Annu Meet Eur Soc Vet Dermatol Eur Coll Vet Dermatol 12:67, 1997.
75. Mason KV: The pathogenesis of solar induced skin lesions in bull terriers. Proc Annu Memb Meet Am Acad Vet Dermatol Am Coll Vet Dermatol 4:12, 1987.
75a. Mason NJ, Michel KE: Subcutaneous emphysema, pneumoperitoneum, and pneumoretroperitoneum after gastrostomy tube placement in a cat. J Am Vet Med Assoc 216:1096, 2000.
75b. McAlvany JP, Sherertz EF: Contact dermatitis in infants, children, and adolescents. Adv Dermatol 9: 205, 1994.
76. Messinger LM: Treatment of skin fold dermatitis affecting a cat's perineal urethrostomy site. J Am Anim Hosp Assoc 30:341, 1994.
77. Miller WH Jr: Epidermal dysplastic disorders of dogs and cats. In: Bonagura JD (ed): Kirk's Current Veterinary Therapy XII. W.B. Saunders Co, Philadelphia, 1995.
78. Miller WJ Jr, Scott DW: Unpublished observations, 1999.
79. Mills BC: Feline deaths following tattooing with Indian ink. Univ Sydney Post-Grad Comm Vet Sci Control Therapy 134:2355, 1987.
80. Mirtschin PJ, et al: Snake bites recorded by veterinary practices in Australia. Aust Vet J 76:195, 1998.
81. Mulcahy J, Rand J: Oral and dermal ulceration in a cat exposed to a quaternary ammonium compound. Aust Vet Pract 26:194, 1996.
82. Muller GH: Contact dermatitis in animals. Arch Dermatol 96:423, 1967.
83. Muller GH, et al: Small Animal Dermatology IV. W.B. Saunders Co, Philadelphia, 1989.
84. Nagata M, et al: Cryoglobulinaemia and cryofibrinogenaemia: A comparison of canine and human cases. Vet Dermatol 9:277, 1998.
85. Neiger RD: Arsenic poisoning. In: Kirk RW (ed): Current Veterinary Therapy X. W.B. Saunders Co, Philadelphia, 1989, p 159.
86. Nikula KJ, et al: Ultraviolet radiation, solar dermatoses, and cutaneous neoplasia in beagle dogs. Radiat Res 129:11, 1992.
87. Osweiler GD, et al: Clinical and Diagnostic Veterinary Toxicology, 3rd ed. Kendall/Hunt Publishing Co, Dubuque, IA, 1985.
88. Paradis M, Scott DW: Calcinosis cutis secondary to percutaneous penetration of calcium carbonate in a Dalmatian. Can Vet J 30:57, 1989.
89. Patterson JM: Nasal solar dermatitis in the dog—a method of tattooing. J Am Anim Hosp Assoc 14:370, 1978.
90. Patterson JW, Kannon GA: Spherulocystic disease ("myospherulosis") arising in a lesion of steatocystoma multiplex. J Am Acad Dermatol 38:274, 1998.
91. Peterson ME, Meerdink GL: Bites and stings of venomous animals. In: Kirk RW (ed): Current Veterinary Therapy X. W.B. Saunders Co, Philadelphia, 1989, p 177.
92. Power HT, Ihrke PJ: The use of synthetic retinoids in veterinary medicine. In: Bonagura JD (ed): Kirk's Current Veterinary Therapy XII. W.B. Saunders Co, Philadelphia, 1995.
93. Purkayastha SS, et al: Efficacy of pentoxifylline with aspirin in the treatment of frostbite. Indian J Med Res 107:239, 1998.
94. Reedy LM, Clubb FJ: Microwave burn in a Toy Poodle: A case report. J Am Anim Hosp Assoc 27:497, 1991.
95. Reinke SI, et al: Histopathologic features of pyotraumatic dermatitis. J Am Vet Med Assoc 190:57, 1987.
95a. Rietschel RL: Irritant contact dermatitis. Mechanisms in irritant contact dermatitis. Clin Dermatol 15: 557, 1997.
96. Rosenkrantz WS: Solar dermatitis. In: Griffin CE, et al: Current Veterinary Dermatology. Mosby–Year Book, St. Louis, 1993, p 309.
97. Saxon WD, Kirby R: Treatment of acute burn injury and smoke inhalation. In: Kirk RW, Bonagura JD (eds): Kirk's Current Veterinary Therapy XI. W.B. Saunders Co, Philadelphia, 1992, p 146.
98. Schaer M: Eastern diamondback rattlesnake envenomation of 20 dogs. Comp Cont Educ 6:997, 1984.
99. Schick MP, et al: Calcinosis cutis secondary to percutaneous penetration of calcium chloride in dogs. J Am Vet Med Assoc 190:207, 1987.
100. Schroeder H, et al: Efficacy of a topical antimicrobial—anti-inflammatory combination in the treatment of pyotraumatic dermatitis in dogs. Vet Dermatol 7: 163, 1996.

101. Schwartzman RM, Kirschbaum JO: The cutaneous histopathology of thallium poisoning. J Invest Dermatol 39:169, 1962.
102. Scott DW: Feline dermatology, 1900–1978: A monograph. J Am Anim Hosp Assoc 16:331, 1980.
103. Shakespeare AC, et al: Infarction of the digits and tail secondary to disseminated intravascular coagulation and metastic hemangiosarcoma in a dog. J Am Anim Hosp Assoc 24:517, 1988.
104. Springer TR, Bailey WJ: Snake bite treatment in the United States. Int J Dermatol 25:479, 1986.
105. Streilein JW: Sunlight and skin-associated lymphoid tissues (SALT). J Invest Dermatol 100:47S, 1993.
106. Swaim SF, et al: Heating pad and thermal burns in small animals. J Am Anim Hosp Assoc 25:156, 1989.
107. Swain SF, et al: Pressure wounds in animals. Comp Cont Ed 18:203, 1996.
108. Tennant BC: Lessons from the porphyrias of animals. Clin Dermatol 16:307, 1998.
109. Thomas ML, et al: Chronic thallium toxicosis in a dog. J Am Anim Hosp Assoc 29:211, 1993.
110. Trower ND, et al: Arteriovenous fistula involving the prepuce of a dog. J Small Anim Pract 38:455, 1997.
111. Tur E, et al: Topical hydrogen peroxide treatment of ischemic ulcers in the guinea pig: Blood recruitment in multiple skin sites. J Am Acad Dermatol 33:217, 1995.
112. Vedros NA, Steinberg K: *In vitro* and *in vivo* activity of plant extracts for use on canine pyotraumatic dermatitis. Canine Pract 19:8, 1994.
113. Walder EJ, Conroy JD: Contact dermatitis in dogs and cats: Pathogenesis, histopathology, experimental induction, and case reports. Vet Dermatol 5:149, 1994.
114. Waldman JS, et al: Subcutaneous myospherulosis. J Am Acad Dermatol 21:400, 1989.
115. Water CB, et al: Acute thallium toxicosis in a dog. J Am Anim Hosp Assoc 201:883, 1992.

Chapter 17
Nutritional Skin Diseases

Dermatoses may result from numerous nutritional deficiencies, excesses, or imbalances, but the skin responds with only a few types of clinical reactions and lesions. These include scaling, crusting, alopecia, comedones, erythema, and a dry, dull or greasy haircoat. Consequently, physical examinations alone can seldom reveal a specific nutritional cause.

It is useful to know the nutritional requirements of dogs and cats[1, 26] but it is difficult to prove that a specific deficiency causes a specific skin disease. Since the 1980s, a few new skin diseases were described that were definitely connected to nutritional factors, and it became fashionable to name them in terms of their response to a nutrient rather than in terms of a deficiency. Notable examples of these are the zinc-responsive dermatoses and the vitamin A–responsive dermatoses (rather than zinc deficiency and vitamin A deficiency). In many instances, these entities may represent genetically related inabilities to absorb or metabolize the nutrients rather than true nutritional deficiencies; in others, the response obtained may be the result of presently unknown effects of supraphysiologic doses of the nutrients.

Major nutritional problems of concern are deficiencies of essential fatty acids, protein, the minerals zinc and copper, and vitamins A, B, and E, as well as excessive levels of vitamin A.[25] Food hypersensitivity may also produce dermatoses (see Chap. 8).

• FATTY ACID DEFICIENCY

Fatty acid deficiency is uncommon to rare and is seen only in animals that are fed dry rations, commercial food that has been poorly preserved (storage, temperature, preservative problems), or homemade foods.[1, 16, 26, 37] A deficiency may occur because fat was left out of the food to save costs, because it leaked from the bag during storage, or because it became rancid. Fatty acid deficiency also may occur from diets that contain fat but have inadequate antioxidants, such as vitamin E. Signs of fatty acid deficiency can be seen in dogs that are fed high-quality reducing dog foods in which the fat content has been lowered.

Dog food should have a minimum of 3% fat in canned food and 7% to 8% fat in dry food. Cats usually have 35% to 40% of their calories provided by fat—a much higher amount—because they need a dense caloric formula. The oxidation of fat during storage is a great concern because when fat becomes rancid, the essential fatty acids as well as vitamins D, E, and biotin are destroyed. Oxidation may occur in canned food after 1 year and in dry food after 6 months, especially if the food is stored at high temperatures. Animals may also develop fatty acid deficiency in association with intestinal malabsorption, pancreatic disease, and chronic hepatic disease.

Animals must be on a diet deficient in essential fatty acids for several months before skin problems become evident.* There is an early decrease in lipid production with resultant fine scaling of the skin and loss of the luster and sheen of the hair (Fig. 17–1A).

---

*See references 6, 13, 14, 16, 26, 38, 39.

This dry phase can last for months and can have associated hair loss and secondary bacterial infections. Eventually, the skin thickens and becomes greasy, especially in the ears, in the intertriginous areas, and between the toes. The dryness of the coat is replaced by greasiness, and many animals become pruritic. Secondary bacterial or *Malassezia* infections can occur, with intensification of the seborrheic changes and pruritus.

Fatty acid deficiency in a number of species produces abnormal keratinization, resulting in epidermal hyperplasia, hypergranulosis, and orthokeratotic or parakeratotic hyperkeratosis (Fig. 17–2). This abnormal keratinization is thought to result from arachidonic acid deficiency with resultant prostaglandin E deficiency, which causes aberrations in the ratios of epidermal cyclic adenosine monophosphate (cyclic AMP) to cyclic guanosine monophosphate (cyclic GMP) and in DNA synthesis.

The polyunsaturated fatty acid linoleic acid is essential in the diet of all animals. Arachidonic and linolenic acids are also required; however, with the exception of arachidonic acid in the cat, these acids can be synthesized from linoleic acid. Cats seems to lack an active Δ-6-desaturase to initiate the conversion of linoleic acid to arachidonic acid and thus are obligate carnivores.[1, 16, 27]

Therapy produces visible responses after 3 to 8 weeks of fatty acid supplementation if the dermatosis is indeed an essential fatty acid deficiency. In such cases, the coats may develop more luster. Fatty acid deficiency can be corrected by changing the dog's ration to one of higher quality and fat content, through the administration of various veterinary fatty acid supplements, or by the addition of household fats to the diet. Because fat supplements have a high caloric density, might trigger an episode of pancreatitis in a predisposed dog, and need to be supplemented with at least vitamin E, this old route of treatment is no longer used routinely.

It is more beneficial to upgrade the basic diet or to use balanced nutritional supplements. If the fatty acid deficiency is compounded by intercurrent vitamin or mineral imbalances, household supplements will not correct them and may aggravate a vitamin E deficiency. Most prescription supplements contain all the necessary vitamins and minerals for the skin in addition to the essential fatty acids. Although most supplements are reasonably priced, the cost of using them continually in a normal dog or cat usually exceeds the cost of a better quality pet food.

Excessive fat supplementation is contraindicated in cases in which the fatty acid deficiency is intentional, such as in the management of obesity, pancreatic disease, or hyperlipidemia disorders. In these cases, treatment with balanced omega-6 and omega-3 fatty acid supplements (Derm Caps, DVM Pharmaceuticals; EFA Caps, Virbac; Efa Vet, Efamol Vet) may be of some benefit.[29] These supplements contain linoleic acid plus the marine lipids, eicosapentaenoic and docosahexaenoic acid. They are thought to modulate arachidonic acid metabolism with the production of various leukotrienes and prostaglandins, which can alter the inflammatory cascade and epidermal proliferation.[5] These products have received the most attention in the treatment of allergic disorders (see Chaps. 3 and 8), but those reports indicate that improvement in coat quality also occurs with their use. It is unknown whether the improvement is due to the modulation of epidermal proliferation or to some other mechanism. The products supply high-quality fats in small volumes with low caloric density (fewer than 5 calories for every 9.1 kg of body weight); therefore, their use in obese animals should not significantly slow the weight loss. No data are available on the safety and efficacy of these supplements in dogs with pancreatitis or other disorders of lipid metabolism. The authors are aware of cases of flare-ups in pancreatitis when the full recommended dosage was initiated suddenly; with gradual introduction over 2 weeks, however, some dogs with pancreatitis have been able to tolerate the supplement.

When dietary fat supplementation is impossible, topical application of essential fatty acids may be of some benefit. Studies in mice have shown that topically applied fats can correct the cutaneous changes of fatty acid deficiency.[29] No data are available to support or refute this mechanism in dogs. Some of these dogs do very well when bathed with shampoos containing fatty acids (e.g., HyLyt°efa, DVM Pharmaceuticals) or rinsed with after-bath products containing fatty acids (e.g., Alpha-Sesame Oil-V Rx). The response

1114 • Nutritional Skin Diseases

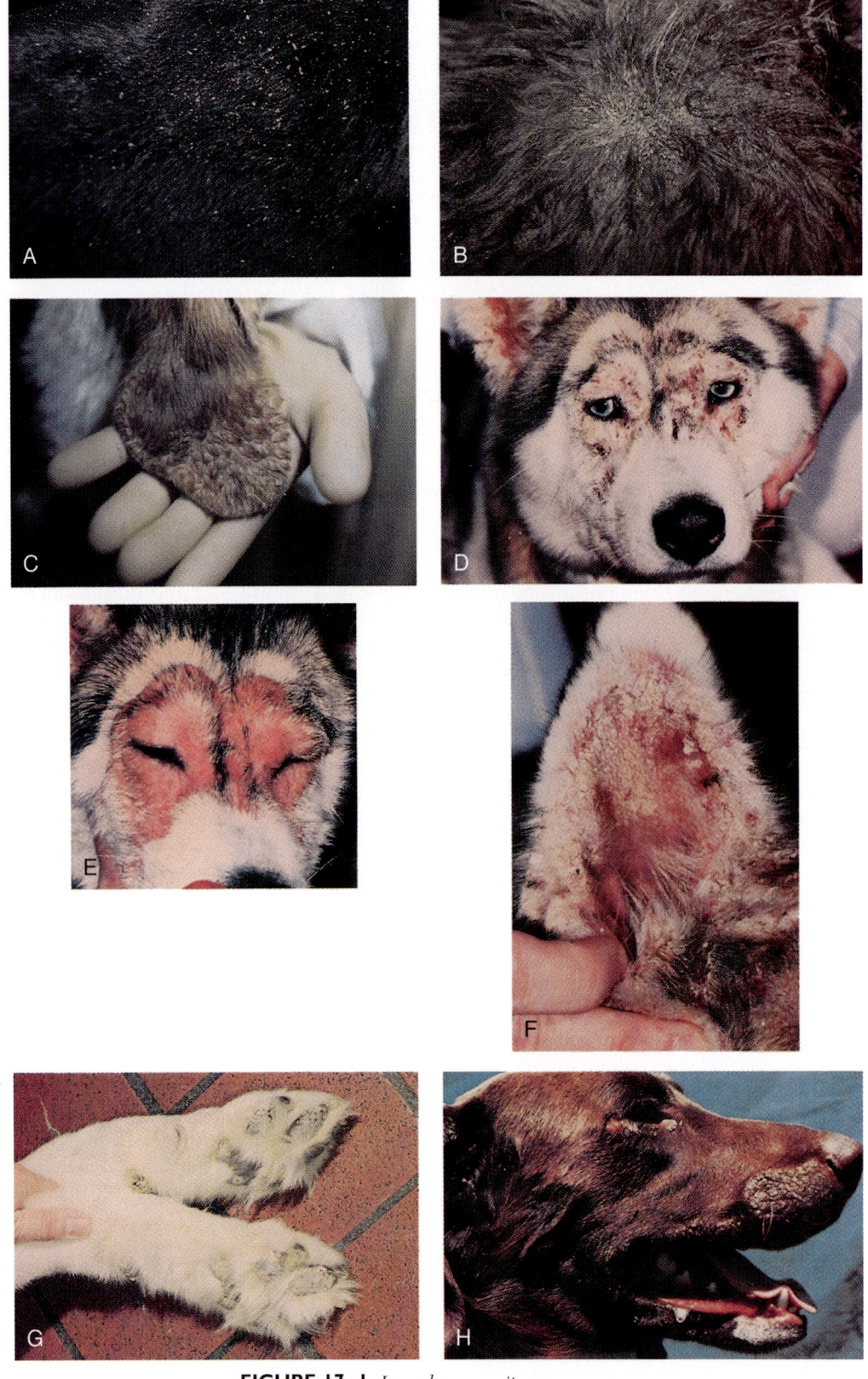

FIGURE 17–1. *Legend on opposite page*

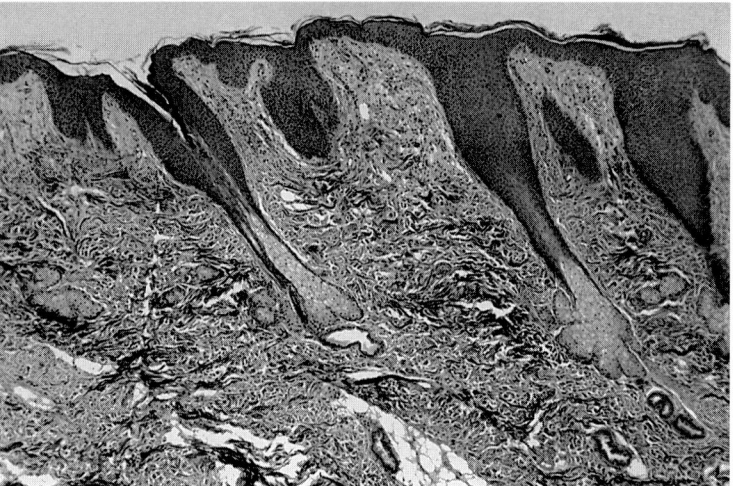

FIGURE 17–2. Essential fatty acid deficiency in a dog. Epidermal and follicular hyperplasia with a mild, mononuclear perivascular dermatitis.

seen in these animals may be due to mechanisms other than transepidermal fat absorption.

Fatty acid deficiency responds gradually to supplementation. Mild cases should return to normal in 4 to 8 weeks, but severe cases can take up to 6 months. Shampooing with antiseborrheic products hastens the clinical improvement, but these products should be used only when absolutely necessary. There is no specific laboratory test for fatty acid deficiency; the diagnosis is confirmed by response to treatment. If seborrheic changes are controlled by bathing, it may be impossible to determine whether the supplementation is of any benefit.

• PROTEIN DEFICIENCY

Protein deficiency may be produced by inanition, starvation, feeding kittens commercial dog food, or feeding dogs special or very low-protein diets. Many commercial pet foods are actually extremely high in protein; as a result, protein deficiency is rare.

Hair is 95% protein with a high percentage of amino acids that contain sulfur. The normal growth of hair (the sum of growth in all follicles of the dog being 100 feet per day) and the keratinization of skin require 25% to 30% of the animal's daily protein requirement.[16, 26, 27] Animals with protein deficiency have hyperkeratosis, epidermal hyperpigmentation, and loss of hair pigment. There is patchy alopecia in which hairs become thinner, rough, dry, dull, and brittle. They are easily broken and grow slowly; shedding is prolonged. These lesions, together with scales and crusts, may appear symmetrically on the head, back, thorax, and abdomen, and on the feet and legs. Lesions are more prominent in young, growing dogs whose protein requirements are higher. Because adequate protein is needed for wound healing, there is a high rate of wound dehiscence in protein-depleted dogs.[33, 44] In humans, a mean hair root diameter of less than 0.06 mm suggests protein deficiency, but no similar specifications are available for animals. An

---

FIGURE 17–1. *A,* Fatty acid deficiency in a dog. Dull, dry, brittle haircoat and diffuse scaling. *B,* Vitamin A deficiency in a dog. Marked follicular hyperkeratosis and follicular casts. *C,* Vitamin E deficiency in a dog. Marked exfoliative erythroderma on the pinna. *D,* Zinc-responsive dermatosis. Facial crusting. *E,* Same dog as in *D,* Severe erythema underlying crusts. *F,* Same dog as in *D* and *E.* Erythematous, crusted pinna. *G,* Same dog as in *D, E,* and *F.* Hyperkeratosis of footpads. *H,* Generic dog food dermatosis. Hyperkeratotic, crusted plaques with peripheral erythemas in a mucocutaneous distribution. (Courtesy of P. Ihrke.)

analysis of the diet and the provision of protein on a dry matter basis (25% for dogs and 33% for cats) should be therapeutic. High-quality protein from eggs, meat, or milk is important in supplementation.

• VITAMIN DEFICIENCIES

Vitamin A

This vitamin functions to maintain healthy skin and epithelial cells; therefore, deficiency and toxicity signs, which are similar, are manifested cutaneously.[16, 26, 27, 37] There is hyperkeratinization of the epithelial surfaces. Hyperkeratosis occurs in the sebaceous glands, occluding their ducts and blocking secretion. Localized or generalized firm papular eruptions with a firm center are formed. A poor coat, alopecia, scaling of the skin, and an increased susceptibility to bacterial infection are also observed. Wound healing is impaired.[19] A single injection of 6000 IU aqueous vitamin A solution per kg of body weight is adequate therapy for a serious deficiency.

True vitamin A deficiency has been recognized in a mongrel dog.[41] The dog had severe seborrheic skin lesions, nyctalopia, and diarrhea since puppyhood. The skin was thickened, hyperpigmented, and alopecic, with marked follicular hyperkeratosis (see Fig. 17–1B). Antiseborrheic shampoos were of no benefit, and the dog responded only partially to low-dose supplementation of vitamin A.

Because vitamin A is stored so well, toxicity may be of greater concern than deficiency. There is real danger of oversupplementation or toxicity from excess liver in the diet. A level 30 times the requirement for 2 to 3 months can produce toxicity. The dosage of retinol for dogs and cats should not exceed 400 IU/kg/day orally. Retinoids are derivatives of retinol with an increased therapeutic index but decreased toxicity.[19] In human medicine, they are used in skin cancer, photoaging, acne, lichen planus, discoid lupus erythematosus, and disorders of keratinization. In veterinary dermatology, isotretinoin and etretinate have received widest use in disorders of keratinization. Both of these agents are safe in dogs and cats, but their expense precluded prolonged use in most cases. Etretinate is no longer marketed and has been replaced by one of its major metabolites, acitretin. The new product is of unproven efficacy in animals but is so expensive that it will probably receive little use. The high cost of the retinoids has prompted some to return to treatment with retinol. These animals should be monitored carefully for signs of intoxication.

Hypervitaminosis A is best described in cats fed large amounts of liver.[22] Among their other signs, these cats have disheveled, seborrheic coats probably as a result of their inability to groom themselves properly. Reports of this condition in dogs are rare.[22, 41] Affected dogs show pain when manipulated owing to vertebral changes, and they have seborrheic skin lesions identical to those seen in animals with hypovitaminosis A or vitamin A–responsive dermatosis.

Vitamin A–Responsive Dermatosis

Some cases of severe seborrhea in Cocker spaniels and several other breeds have responded to vitamin A supplementation[17] and are discussed in detail in Chapter 14.

Vitamin D

Vitamin D is produced in the skin and has its major impact in calcium homeostasis. Naturally occurring excess or deficiency has not been reported in animals. In addition to its role in calcium homeostasis, 1,25-dihydroxy vitamin D_3 impacts keratinocyte proliferation and differentiation.[3, 15, 21] With this activity, various topical or systemic analogs are being investigated in the treatment of psoriasis. Because primary seborrhea (see Chap. 12) is a hyperproliferative disorder, vitamin D analogs are being studied in dogs.

Vitamin E

Vitamin E, selenium, and fatty acids have a balanced relationship. Experimental vitamin E deficiency in dogs also results in severe suppression of in vitro lymphocyte blastogenesis.[24] In cats, a similar imbalance produces pansteatitis.[16, 20, 37] This syndrome results when high-fat foods, such as canned red tuna, are fed almost exclusively. If food processing or fat oxidation has inactivated the vitamin E, the imbalance results. Cats show pain on gentle palpation and are anorectic, lethargic, and irritable. They may die in several weeks. There are large, firm lumps in the subcutaneous tissues and abdominal cavity. Diagnosis can be made at biopsy or autopsy by finding yellow fat and steatitis. Biopsy reveals lobular panniculitis and ceroid within lipocytes, macrophages, and giant cells (Fig. 17–3). Ceroid is a pink to yellow homogenous material on H & E stain and is deep crimson on acid-fast stain.

Naturally occurring vitamin E deficiency has not been reported in dogs, but experimentally induced vitamin E deficiency has been studied.[40] Researchers showed that skin lesions can be produced. They consisted of an early keratinization defect (seborrhea sicca), and a later greasy and inflammatory stage (erythroderma and seborrhea oleosa) (see Fig. 17–1C); in addition, the dogs tended to develop secondary bacterial pyoderma. The dermatohistopathologic findings in dogs with experimentally produced vitamin E deficiency are nondiagnostic. Morphologically, the findings are characterized by hyperplastic superficial perivascular dermatitis (Fig. 17–4). This is a common reaction pattern in canine skin, one most commonly seen in hypersensitivity reactions, ectoparasitisms, and seborrheic disorders. When the experimental dogs that had been fed a vitamin E–deficient diet were provided a vitamin E supplement equal to or double the National Research Council recommendations, the dermatosis responded dramatically. The erythema and greasiness subsided within 3 to 6 weeks, and the scaling resolved within 8 to 10 weeks.

Vitamin E deficiency induces T cell dysfunction in dogs and has been associated as a causal factor in generalized demodicosis in dogs.[9, 10] Research has not been able to substantiate this claim. Megadose vitamin supplementation, although of some probable benefit, has not been curative.[12]

Vitamin E is an antioxidant, stabilizes lysosomes, reduces prostaglandin E_2 (PGE_2) synthesis, and increases interleukin 2 (IL-2) production with resultant anti-inflammatory and immunostimulatory effects.[19] Alone or in combination with vitamin A where it has synergistic effects, it has been used to treat dystrophic epidermolysis bullosa, discoid lupus erythematosus, granuloma annulare, or benign familial pemphigus in humans. In dogs, some cases of discoid lupus erythematosus, dermatomyositis, or acanthosis nigricans re-

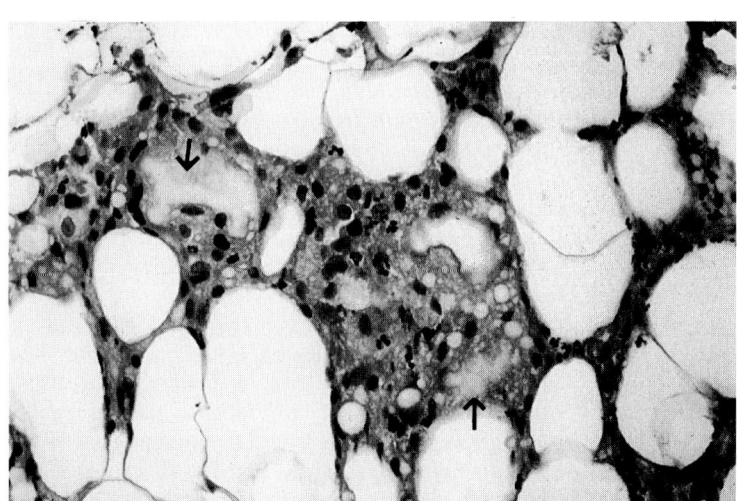

FIGURE 17–3. Steatitis in a cat. Pyogranulomatous, lobular panniculitis. Amorphous material (*arrows*) is ceroid.

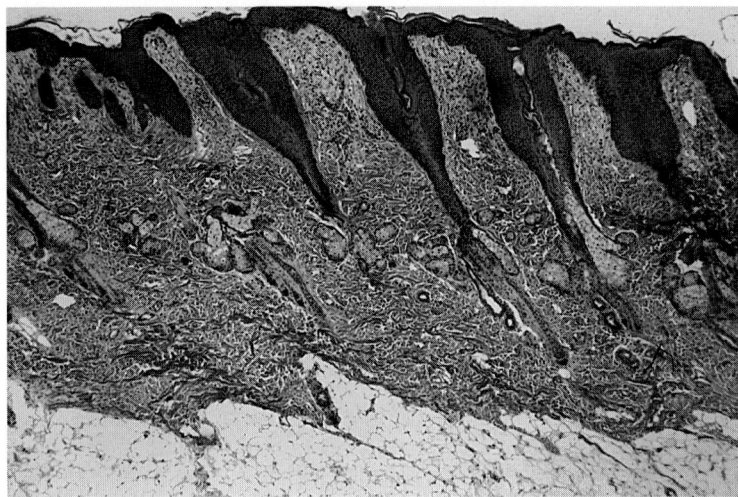

FIGURE 17–4. Experimental vitamin E deficiency in a dog. Epidermal and follicular hyperplasia is the most marked feature and mimics that seen in essential fatty acid deficiency (see Fig. 17–2).

spond to treatment with vitamin E.[41] It is unlikely that vitamin E deficiency would occur in dogs on commercial diets. It would enter into the differential diagnosis of a dog with seborrhea or erythroderma. Diagnosis would be based on dietary history, physical examination, the ruling out of more common canine dermatoses, compatible skin biopsy results, and response to vitamin E therapy.

Vitamin E, d- and α-tocopherol being the most biologically active form, is used in doses of 10 mg (13.5 IU)/kg/day as an antioxidant and for the therapy of pansteatitis in cats (resulting from excess tuna or fat in the diet). In severe cases, it is mandatory to use systemic corticosteroids during the painful period of treatment (2 to 3 weeks).[20] Vitamin E in doses of 400 to 800 IU q12h has been used successfully in discoid lupus erythematosus and systemic lupus erythematosus, and in disorders involving the basement membrane zone.

Vitamin B

B-complex vitamins are considered as a group because deficiencies of single B vitamins are very rare and the clinical syndromes are similar.[16, 26, 27] These vitamins are synthesized by intestinal bacteria; because they are water soluble and not stored, a constant supply is needed, and toxicities do not occur. It is possible for biotin, riboflavin, niacin, and pyridoxine deficiencies to have clinical ramifications.

Biotin can be inactivated by feeding the animal a diet high in uncooked eggs.[16, 26, 27] The whites contain avidin, which binds biotin so that it cannot be absorbed. Biotin deficiency can also result from prolonged oral antibiotic therapy. The most striking sign is a "spectacle eye" of alopecia around the face and eyes. Biotin deficiency should be differentiated from demodicosis, dermatophytosis, and other facial dermatoses (discoid lupus erythematosus, pemphigus, dermatomyositis, epidermolysis bullosa). In severe cases, crusted lesions of the face, neck, body, and legs are present. There may also be lethargy, emaciation, and diarrhea. Biotin deficiency has been shown to cause a widespread papulocrustous dermatitis in cats.[16]

Riboflavin deficiency may produce a dry, flaky dermatitis (seborrhea), especially around the eyes and ventrum; the outstanding sign, however, is cheilosis.[26, 27] The deficiency also produces alopecia on the head of cats.[16] Riboflavin deficiency is all but impossible if any meat or dairy products are present in the diet.

Niacin deficiency is manifested as pellagra and is characterized by ulcerated mucous membranes, diarrhea, and emaciation. It may produce a pruritic dermatitis of the rear legs and abdomen.[26, 27] For a deficiency to be produced, the diet must be low in animal protein and high in corn. Corn and all cereals are low in tryptophan, which is converted to niacin by all animals except cats. Commercial pet foods contain more than enough niacin; therefore, supplementation is not needed.

Pyridoxine deficiency, produced experimentally in cats, causes a dull, waxy, unkempt haircoat with generalized and fine white scales.[31] In some experimental cats, it caused multiple areas of alopecia in the temporal and periauricular area, on the dorsum of the muzzle, periorally, and on the extremities. When these experimental pyridoxine-deficient cats were fed a balanced diet, all of the skin lesions resolved. This condition has not been observed clinically and remains a laboratory phenomenon.

The most common signs of B-complex deficiencies are a dry, flaky seborrhea with alopecia, anorexia, and weight loss. Effective treatment consists of brewer's yeast, B-complex injections, or both. Supplementation may be needed only if the animals are anorectic or have problems that cause excess water turnover.

When 119 dogs with dull coat, brittle hair, loss of hair, scaly skin, pruritus, or dermatitis were given biotin (0.5 mg/10 kg body weight/day) for 3 to 5 weeks, 108 (91%) were cured or improved significantly.[11] Insufficient data were supplied to determine whether these dogs were truly deficient in biotin or responded by some other therapeutic effect. This report highlights the need for broad-based vitamin supplementation when a nutritional deficiency is suspected or when fatty acids are added to a seborrheic dog's diet.

● MINERAL IMBALANCES

Zinc, copper, and calcium are three minerals that influence iodine metabolism and each other; abnormal levels of any one of them may be reflected in the skin. Because of the great variation among individuals, only one or several of a group of animals may develop lesions, even though all have been fed and managed alike.

Copper deficiency should appear as a balance problem only if excess zinc is added to the diet.[26, 27] Copper is needed by enzymes that convert L-tyrosine to melanin and by the follicular cells in the conversion of prekeratin to keratin. A deficiency is manifested by hypopigmentation and faulty keratinization of the skin and hair follicles, with the hair becoming dull and rough. Because commercial pet foods have adequate copper levels, supplements are not needed. Bull terriers with lethal acrodermatitis, a zinc deficiency disorder, are also copper deficient.[45] Dogs with zinc-responsive disorders may also have irregularities in their copper balance.

● ZINC-RESPONSIVE DERMATOSIS

Zinc is an important cofactor and modulator of many critical biological functions.[30, 34] Although zinc deficiency was thought to play a role in many dermatoses of the dog, recent work[28] indicates that zinc deficiency is rare in the dog. Zinc deficiency has been documented in Bull terriers with acrodermatitis (see Chap. 12), and relative or absolute deficiency is suspected in two other dermatologic syndromes.[8, 23, 32]

Syndrome I occurs in Siberian huskies and Alaskan malamutes primarily, but Bull terriers may also be affected.[23, 28] Although a familial history is lacking in many cases, the striking breed predilection strongly supports a genetic linkage and affected dogs should not be used for breeding.[7] Skin lesions in these breeds develop despite well-balanced diets with sufficient zinc. Lesions develop early in adulthood (at 1 to 3 years of age) and progress at a variable rate. Most dogs develop their lesions in September through January.[7] Over one-half of the dogs have lesional pruritus, and pruritus in "normal" skin can be the hallmark of a pending relapse during maintenance. There is early erythema followed by alopecia, crusting, scaling, and underlying suppuration around the mouth, chin, eyes, and ears (see Fig. 17–1D to F). Other body openings and the scrotum, prepuce, and vulva may be affected. Although the coat is dull, there is excess sebum production. Thick crusts may appear on the elbows and other pressure points. The skin may be inelastic and the legs stiff, as a result of hardened crusts. Secondary bacterial or *Malassezia* infections are common, especially when there is pruritus. The footpads may become hyperkeratotic (see Fig. 17–1G), and claw disease, especially onychomalacia, may be observed.[28a] In chronic cases, hyperpigmentation occurs in the area of the lesions. There may be a decreased sense of smell (hyposmia) and taste (hypogeusia). Clinical signs may be precipitated or intensified by stress and estrus.

It has been shown that malamutes have a genetic defect of decreased capability for zinc absorption from the intestines.[23, 27] In some Siberian huskies, hypothyroidism and a decreased serum zinc level have been reported, but the significance of these conditions is unknown.[23] Dogs on high-calcium or high-cereal diets, which have high levels of phytate, show poor zinc absorption, owing to binding of the zinc. High levels of iron—occasionally found in well water or the water in houses with old plumbing—may interfere with zinc absorption. Prolonged enteritis and diarrhea also prevent normal absorption. A severe deficiency may cause poor growth and weight loss in young puppies and poor wound healing in any animal.[35, 36]

Syndrome II occurs in rapidly growing puppies or young adult dogs that are fed zinc-deficient diets, diets high in phytates or minerals such as calcium (which interfere with zinc absorption), or diets that are oversupplemented with minerals and vitamins. Many breeds may be abnormal, but Great Danes, Doberman pinschers, Beagles, German shepherds, German shorthaired pointers, Labrador retrievers, Rhodesian ridgebacks, and standard Poodles have been reported.[2, 17, 23, 32, 46] The severity of lesions can vary greatly within a litter. Some animals may be normal, whereas others are stunted, depressed, and anorectic. The skin lesions are hyperkeratotic plaques over areas of repeated trauma or where calluses might normally occur. The footpads and nasal planum may be affected, and any thickened area may have deep fissures. There may be secondary infection of the crusts and an associated lymphadenopathy. Severely affected dogs can look as though they have canine distemper.

In both syndromes, serum or hair zinc levels may be abnormal. Proper analysis for zinc is difficult and can be unreliable, however, because samples may be contaminated by zinc in glassware or rubber stoppers, and by the influences of various environmental, physiologic, and disease-related factors.[28, 46, 49]

Diagnosis may be made by history taking, physical examination, and skin biopsy. Hyperplastic superficial perivascular dermatitis, with marked diffuse and follicular parakeratotic hyperkeratosis, is suggestive of zinc deficiency (Figs. 17–5 and 17–6). Papillomatosis and mild diffuse spongiosis are also common findings. Eosinophils and lymphocytes are often prominent in the perivascular cellular infiltrate. Intraepidermal pustular dermatitis and suppurative folliculitis reflect secondary bacterial infection. Histologic features of secondary *Malassezia* infection may be present (see Chap. 5).

Treatment involves the inspection and correction of any inadequacy in the diet, including the base diet, water, and any treats or supplements given to the animal. Secondary bacterial or *Malassezia* infections must be appropriately treated. In Syndrome II, dietary adjustments alone can resolve the skin lesions in 2 to 6 weeks. Zinc supplementation is necessary in Syndrome I and can hasten the animal's response in Syndrome II. In the latter case, the supplement need be given for only a few weeks to restore the zinc stores in the animal. In Syndrome I, approximately 25% of dogs can have the zinc supplementation stopped without an immediate relapse in the condition. For the remainder, supplementation must be lifelong but the dosage may have to be adjusted.

Oral zinc supplementation at a dose of 1 mg of elemental zinc/kg/day should be sufficient for most dogs.[7] Zinc sulfate (10 mg/kg/day), zinc gluconate (5 mg/kg/day), or zinc methionine (1.7 mg/kg/day) are commonly used preparations. If zinc sulfate is used, the tablets should be crushed and mixed with food to enhance absorption and decrease gastric irritation. In Syndrome II, the supplement can be withdrawn when the skin has returned to normal, if the nutritional problem has been corrected. In Syndrome I, zinc administration typically is lifelong. If little or no response is seen within 4 weeks of initiating treatment, the dosage should be increased by 50%. In both syndromes, existing skin lesions can be improved by hydrating the crusts with wet dressings or whole-body

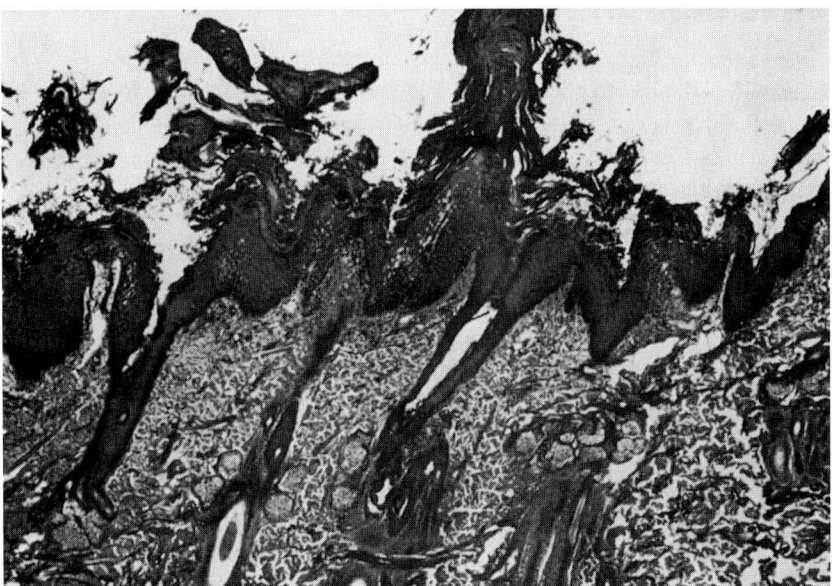

FIGURE 17–5. Zinc-responsive dermatosis in a Siberian husky. Hyperplastic perivascular dermatitis with marked diffuse parakeratotic hyperkeratosis.

warm water soakings for 5 to 10 minutes and then bathing the animal with an antiseborrheic shampoo. Lesions on the face and elsewhere improve with the application of petrolatum or an ointment-based topical agent. Topical agents are less messy, and the active ingredient—an antibiotic or keratolytic agent—provides additional benefits. Once the dog returns to normal, it is not unusual to be able to decrease the dosage of zinc, especially in the warm months. Relapses during the cool months or later in life may occur but should respond to dosage increase.

Some dogs, especially Siberian huskies, do not respond to oral zinc supplementation. Intravenous injection with sterile zinc sulfate solutions at dosages of 10 to 15 mg/kg has been effective.[47] Weekly injections for at least 4 weeks are necessary to resolve the lesions, and maintenance injections every 1 to 6 months are necessary to prevent relapses.

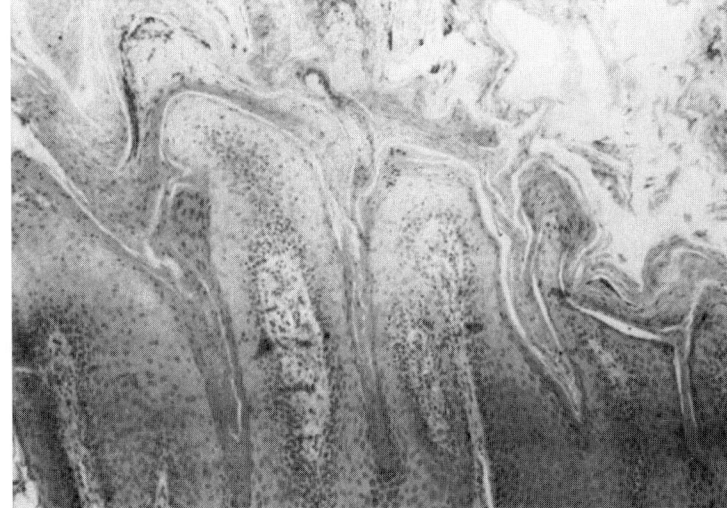

FIGURE 17–6. Close-up of Figure 17–5. Papillomatosis and diffuse parakeratotic hyperkeratosis that also involves hair follicles.

Intravenous treatment is expensive and cardiac arrhythmias can occur if the drug is administered too fast. A recent study documents the place of low-dose corticosteroids in the treatment of dogs who do not respond to zinc alone.[4] Corticosteroids are known to increase zinc absorbtion from the gastrointestinal tract by induction of metallothionein, but they may also have some direct effect on the skin in these dogs. In these dogs, discontinuation of the corticosteroid lowers the serum zinc levels and results in a clinical relapse. Some dogs seem to respond better to zinc when they are also treated with omega-6/omega-3 fatty acids.

In kittens, dietary zinc deficiency was reported to cause thinning of the haircoat, slow hair growth, scaly skin, and ulceration of the buccal margins.[18] The cat's requirement for dietary zinc was estimated at between 15 and 50 ppm.

• GENERIC DOG FOOD SKIN DISEASE

Dogs fed only generic dog foods marketed in the late 1980s developed bilateral symmetric scaling and crusting dermatoses.[43, 46] The lesions developed within a month of eating the food and involved the bridge of the nose, mucocutaneous junctions, pressure points, and distal extremities (see Fig. 17–1H). Well-demarcated, older lesions had erythematous borders with scales, crusts, and variable hyperpigmentation and lichenification. A few dogs had alopecia, focal erosions, papules, and pustules; most had fever, depression, lymphadenopathy, and pitting edema of dependent areas.

Skin biopsies showed hyperplastic superficial perivascular dermatitis with diffuse parakeratotic hyperkeratosis, prominent focal keratinocyte apoptosis, and a mixed dermal cellular infiltrate (Fig. 17–7). Although the clinical and histopathologic findings are similar to those seen in the zinc-responsive dermatoses, the acuteness of onset and the frequent occurrence of systemic illness suggest that other nutritional imbalances may play a role.

The differential diagnosis should include relative or absolute zinc deficiency, immune-mediated skin diseases (especially pemphigus foliaceus and systemic lupus erythematosus), staphylococcal folliculitis, and necrolytic migratory erythema. Treatment with antibiotics or corticosteroids was unsuccessful, but rapid response occurred 1 week after simply chang-

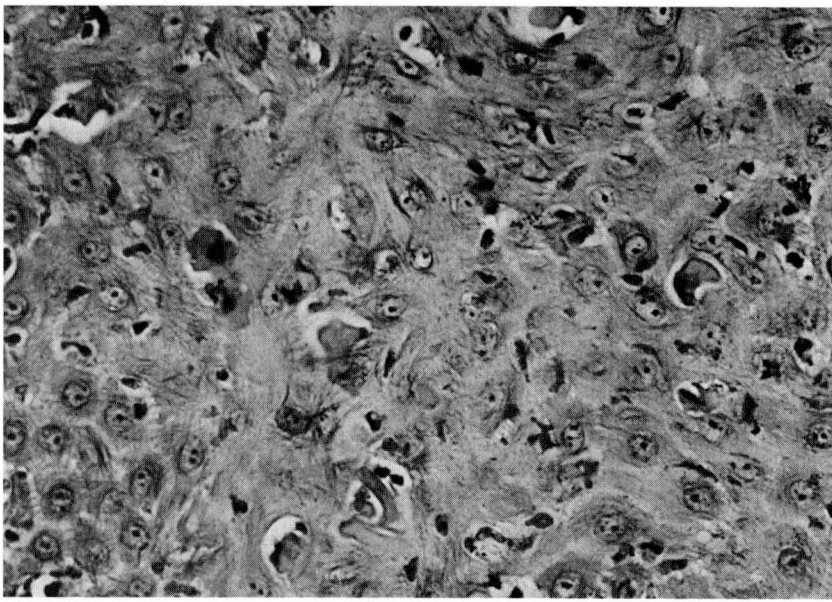

FIGURE 17–7. Generic dog food dermatosis. Multiple apoptotic keratinocytes.

ing the dogs' diet to a national brand of dog food that met National Research Council requirements.

Since the original reports on this disorder, no additional cases have been reported. Improvements in the formulation of generic pet foods must have been made, because they are still marketed.

• NUTRITIONAL SUPPLEMENTS

Pets that are fed high-quality commercial foods typically receive no benefits from additional supplements. When disease results from the animal eating low-quality food or from inherent metabolic defects that alter the digestion or absorption of one or more nutrients, one can choose to supplement the existing diet or upgrade the base diet with a higher quality food. It is more appropriate and cost effective to upgrade the base diet because all nutrients should be in the correct proportion. If the owners are reluctant to change foods without absolute proof of the benefit of doing so, or if the animal refuses to eat anything different, a supplement proposed by Lewis can be beneficial.[26, 27] For every 9 to 14 kg of body weight, the dog should be given 1 teaspoon (5 ml) of corn oil or safflower oil, 2 ounces (56 g) of cooked liver, 100 mg of zinc sulfate, and 1 drop of tincture of iodine. Most owners find it convenient to make large batches of the supplement. Problems with thorough mixing of the ingredients and giving the dog the correct amount can be overcome by making a puree of the mixture in a blender and freezing the supplement in ice cube trays. At each meal, the owner can thaw the appropriate number of cubes and add them to the diet. Because this supplement provides fat, protein, vitamins A and E, biotin, riboflavin, niacin, iodine, and zinc, it should resolve all nutritional dermatoses unless they have a genetic basis (e.g., Syndrome I zinc-responsive dermatoses) or are secondary to severe gastrointestinal disorders. If no change is seen after 8 weeks of supplementation, nutritional causes can be discounted; if a good response is seen, the supplement can be continued or a new base diet can be selected.

• REFERENCES

1. Anderson RW (ed): Nutrition of the Dog and Cat: Proceedings of an International Symposium. Elmsford, New York, Pergamon Press, 1980, p 67.
2. Bensignor E: Dermatose améliorée par le zinc chez un caniche. Point Vét 28:741, 1996.
3. Bikle DD: Vitamin D: A calciotropic hormone regulating calcium-induced keratinocyte differentiation. J Am Acad Dermatol 37:S42, 1997.
4. Burton G, Mason KV: The possible role of prednisolone in "zinc-responsive dermatosis" in the Siberian husky. Aust Vet Pract 28:20, 1998.
5. Campbell KL: Fatty acid supplementation and skin disease. Vet Clin North Am (Small Anim Pract) 20:1475, 1990.
6. Campbell KL, et al: Effects of animal and soy fats and proteins in the diet on fatty acid concentrations in the serum and skin of dogs. Am J Vet Res 56:1465, 1995.
7. Colombini S, Dunstan RW: Zinc-responsive dermatosis in northern-breed dogs: 17 cases (1990–1996). J Am Vet Med Assoc 211:451, 1997.
8. Fadok VA: Nutritional therapy in veterinary dermatology. In: Kirk RW (ed): Current Veterinary Therapy IX. W.B. Saunders Co, Philadelphia, 1986, p 591.
9. Figueiredo C: Vitamin E serum contents, erythrocyte and lymphocyte counts, PCV and Hg determination in normal dogs, dogs with scabies, and dogs with demodicosis. Proc Annu Memb Meet Am Acad Vet Dermatol 1:1, 1985.
10. Figueiredo C, et al: Clinical evaluation of the effect of vitamin E in the treatment of generalized canine demodicosis. Adv Vet Dermatol 2:247, 1993.
11. Frigg M, et al: Clinical study on the effect of biotin on skin conditions in dogs. Schweiz Arch Tierheilk 131:621, 1989.
12. Gilbert PA, et al: Serum vitamin E levels in dogs with pyoderma and generalized demodicosis. J Am Anim Hosp Assoc 28:407, 1992.
13. Hansen AE, Weise HF: Fat in the diet in relation to nutrition of the dog. I. Characteristic appearance and gross changes of animals fed diets with and without fat. Tex Rep Biol Med 52:205, 1951.
14. Hansen AE, Weise HF: Studies with dogs maintained on diets low in fat. Proc Soc Exp Biol Med 52:205, 1943.
15. Holick MF, et al: Clinical uses for calciotropic hormones 1,25-dihydroxyvitamin D_3 and parathyroid hormone–related peptide in dermatology: A new perspective. J Invest Dermatol Symp Proc 1:1, 1996.
16. Holzworth J: Diseases of the Cat: Medicine and Surgery. W.B. Saunders Co, Philadelphia, 1987.
17. Ihrke PJ, Goldschmidt MH: Vitamin A–responsive dermatosis in the dog. J Am Vet Med Assoc 182:687, 1983.
18. Kane E, et al: Zinc deficiency in the cat. J Nutr 111:488, 1981.
19. Keller KL, Fenske NA: Use of vitamins A, C, and E

and related compounds in dermatology: A review. J Am Acad Dermatol 39:611, 1998.
20. Koutinas AF, et al: Pansteatitis (steatitis, "yellow fat disease") in the cat: A review article and report of 4 spontaneous cases. Vet Dermatol 3:101, 1993.
21. Kragballe K: The future of vitamin D in dermatology. J Am Acad Dermatol 37:S72, 1997.
22. Kronfeld DS: Vitamin and Mineral Supplementation for Dogs and Cats. Veterinary Practice Publishing Co, Santa Barbara, CA, 1989.
23. Kunkle GA: Zinc-responsive dermatoses in dogs. In: Kirk RW (ed): Current Veterinary Therapy VII. W.B. Saunders Co, Philadelphia, 1980, p 472.
24. Langweiler M, et al: Effect of vitamin E deficiency on the proliferative response of canine lymphocytes. Am J Vet Res 42:1681, 1981.
25. Leibetseder J: Ernährungsbedingte Erkrankungen der Haut bei Hund und Katze. Wien Tierärztl. Mschr 83:19, 1998.
26. Lewis LD: Cutaneous manifestations of nutritional imbalances. Proc Am Anim Hosp Assoc 48:263, 1981.
27. Lewis LD, Morris ML Jr: Small Animal Clinical Nutrition, 2nd ed. Mark Morris Associates, Topeka, KS, 1984.
28. Logas DL, et al: Comparison of serum zinc levels in healthy, systemically ill, and dermatologically diseased dogs. Vet Dermatol 4:61, 1993.
28a. McEwan NA: Nail disease, zinc deficiency and lethal acrodermatitis. Proc Brit Vet Dermatol Study Grp, Spring 1999, p. 29.
29. Miller WH Jr: Nutritional considerations in small animal dermatology. Vet Clin North Am 19:497, 1989.
30. Norris D: Zinc and cutaneous inflammation. Arch Dermatol 121:985, 1985.
31. Norton A: Skin lesions seen in cats with vitamin B (pyroxidine) deficiency. Proc Annu Memb Meet Am Acad Vet Dermatol Am Coll Vet Dermatol 3:24, 1987.
32. Ohlen B, Scott DW: Zinc responsive dermatitis in puppies. Canine Pract 13:2, 1986.
33. Rhoads JE, et al: The mechanism of delayed wound healing in the presence of hypoproteinemia. J Am Med Assoc 118:21, 1942.
34. Russell RM, et al: Zinc and the special senses. Ann Intern Med 99:227, 1983.
35. Sanecki RK, et al: Tissue changes in dogs fed a zinc-deficient ration. Am J Vet Res 43:1642, 1982.
36. Sanecki RK, et al: Extracutaneous histologic changes accompanying zinc deficiency in pups. Am J Vet Res 46:2119, 1985.
37. Scott DW: Feline dermatology 1900–1978: A monograph. J Am Anim Hosp Assoc 17:331, 1980.
38. Scott DW: Feline dermatology 1979–1982: Introspective retrospections. J Am Anim. Hosp Assoc 20:537, 1984.
39. Scott DW: Feline dermatology 1983–1985: "The secret sits." J Am Anim Hosp Assoc. 23:255, 1987.
40. Scott DW, Sheffy BE: Dermatosis in dogs caused by vitamin E deficiency. Comp Anim Pract 41:42, 1987.
41. Scott DW, et al: Muller & Kirk's Small Animal Dermatology V. W.B. Saunders, Philadelphia, 1995, p 891.
42. Sousa CA, et al: Dermatosis associated with feeding generic dog food: 13 cases (1981–1982). J Am Vet Med Assoc 192:676, 1988.
43. Sousa CA: Nutritional dermatoses. In: Nesbit GH (ed): Dermatology: Contemporary Issues in Small Animal Practice. Churchill Livingstone, Inc., New York, 1987.
44. Thompson W, et al: The effect of hypoproteinemia on wound disruption. Arch Surg 26:500, 1938.
45. Uchida Y, et al: Serum concentrations of zinc and copper in bull terriers with lethal acrodermatitis and tail-chasing behavior. Am J Vet Res 8:808, 1997.
46. van den Broek AHM, Thoday KL: Skin disease in dogs associated with zinc deficiency: A report of 5 cases. J Small Anim Pract 27:313, 1986.
47. Willemse, T.: Zinc-responsive disorders of the dog. In: Kirk RW, Bonagura JD (eds): Kirk's Current Veterinary Therapy XI. W.B. Saunders Co, Philadelphia, 1992, p 532.
48. Wolf AM: Zinc-responsive dermatosis in a Rhodesian ridgeback. Vet Med 80:37, 1985.
49. Wright RP: Identification of zinc-responsive dermatoses. Vet Med 80:37, 1985.

Chapter 18

Miscellaneous Skin Diseases

• CANINE SUBCORNEAL PUSTULAR DERMATOSIS

Subcorneal pustular dermatosis is a very rare, idiopathic, sterile, superficial pustular dermatosis of dogs.[3, 8, 9]

Cause and Pathogenesis

The cause of subcorneal pustular dermatosis is unknown. In humans, it has been postulated that immunologic mechanisms play a role.[1, 8, 10] Immune complexes and immunoglobulin (Ig)A that could be chemoattractant to neutrophils have been demonstrated in vivo in the stratum corneum. Elevated levels of tumor necrosis factor-α (TNF-α) have been demonstrated in the serum and pustules of a human with subcorneal pustular dermatosis.[7] Some cases of human subcorneal pustular dermatosis are associated with the presence or development of paraproteinemia (usually the IgA type), with or without myeloma, but this condition has not been reported in dogs.[8]

IgA myelomas and intraepidermal IgA deposits have been described in humans.[10]

Clinical Features

No apparent age (6 months to 14 years old) or sex predilection exists. Although many breeds have been affected, Miniature schnauzers have accounted for about 40% of the cases.

Affected dogs usually have a multifocal to generalized, pustular to seborrhea-like dermatitis. The head and trunk, particularly, are affected in a symmetric fashion. Intact pustules are usually nonfollicular, greenish yellow, and transient, persisting for only 2 to 4 hours at a time (Fig. 18–1A and B). Thus, the affected dogs often have only circular areas of alopecia, erosion, scaling, crusting, and epidermal collarettes. Lesions tend to heal centrally, often with hyperpigmentation, and to spread peripherally, producing annular and serpiginous configurations. Rarely, the footpads are affected and peel superficially. Pruritus varies from nonexistent to extreme. The course of the dermatosis is often to erupt and regress. Usually, the dogs are otherwise healthy. Occasional dogs have peripheral lymphadenopathy; rarely, they have pyrexia, anorexia, and depression.

Diagnosis

Because this dermatosis is diagnosed by the exclusion of other conditions, improved diagnostic techniques should make it rare.

The differential diagnosis includes bacterial folliculitis, pemphigus foliaceus, linear IgA pustular dermatosis, systemic lupus erythematosus, sterile eosinophilic pustulosis, seborrheic skin disease, scabies, atopy, and food hypersensitivity. Definitive diagnosis is based on history, physical examination, exclusion through laboratory testing, and response to therapy. Subcorneal pustular dermatosis responds poorly to systemic antibiotics, systemic glucocorticoids, and topical agents. Direct smears from intact pustules usually reveal numerous nondegenerate neutrophils, occasional acantholytic keratinocytes, and no micro-

1126 • Miscellaneous Skin Diseases

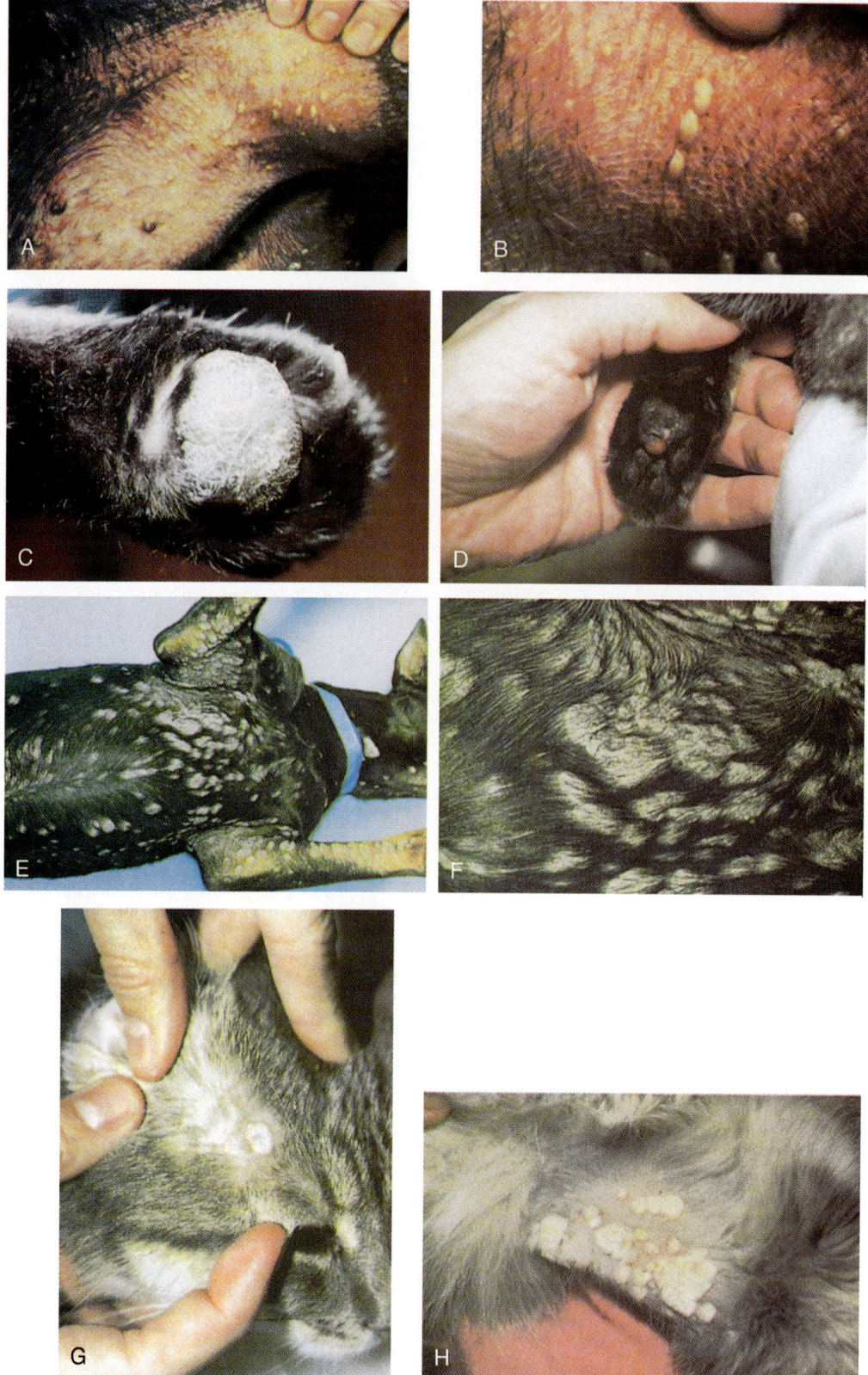

FIGURE 18–1. *See legend on opposite page*

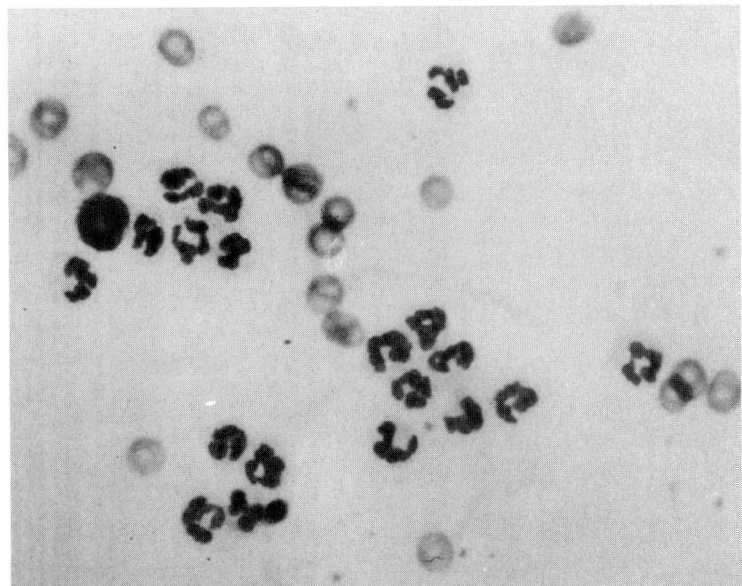

FIGURE 18–2. Canine subcorneal pustular dermatosis. Cytologic examination reveals nondegenerate neutrophils and no microorganisms.

organisms (Fig. 18–2). Carefully performed cultures from intact pustules are usually negative, but a few colonies of coagulase-negative or coagulase-positive staphylococci are occasionally isolated. Immunofluorescence testing results are negative. Skin biopsy reveals intraepidermal (subcorneal) pustular dermatitis.[3, 8] Acantholysis is usually minimal, but it is occasionally marked. Neutrophils do not show degenerative changes. Hair follicles are rarely involved (Figs. 18–3 and 18–4).

Up to one half of affected dogs may have mild to moderate mature neutrophilia (13.8 to 21.1 × 10^3/ml).[8] Serum protein electrophoresis occasionally reveals increased amounts of α_1, α_2, and β globulins.[8]

Clinical Management

The drug of choice in subcorneal pustular dermatosis is dapsone (see Chap. 9), which is given orally at 1 mg/kg q8h. A beneficial response usually occurs in 1 to 4 weeks. In a minority of cases, the therapy can be stopped and long-term remission may result; more often, however, the drug is tapered to maintenance levels, with the dosage varying from dog to dog (1 mg/kg, q24h to twice a week).

In dogs, the major side effects of dapsone have been hematologic and hepatic. Many dogs experience mild nonregenerative anemia and leukopenia as well as mild to moderate elevations of serum alanine aminotransferase during induction therapy. If these laboratory abnormalities are not associated with clinical signs, it is not necessary to stop therapy; the levels will return to normal when maintenance doses are achieved. Dapsone has also caused fatal thrombocytopenia in one dog, profound leukopenia in one dog, occasional vomiting and diarrhea, and generalized, pruritic erythematous maculopapular skin eruptions.[8] Dapsone is not licensed for use in dogs.

FIGURE 18–1. *A*, Multiple nonfollicular pustules on the abdomen of a dog with subcorneal pustular dermatosis. *B*, Close-up view of *A*. *C*, Feline plasma cell pododermatitis. Swollen footpad with cross-hatched white striae. *D*, Feline plasma cell pododermatitis. Ulcerated nodule projecting from a footpad. *E*, Lichenoid dermatitis on the chest and forelegs of a dog. *F*, Same dog as in *E*. Lichenoid papules and plaques on the chest. *G*, Idiopathic lichenoid dermatitis in a cat. Cluster of lichenoid papules in the preauricular area. *H*, Same cat as in *G*. Cluster of lichenoid papules and plaques in the axillary area.

1128 • Miscellaneous Skin Diseases

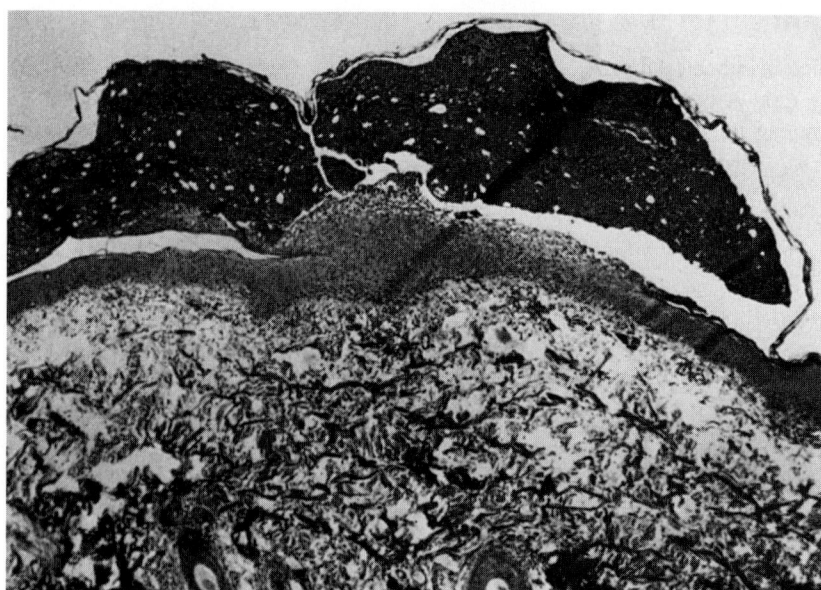

FIGURE 18-3. Canine subcorneal pustular dermatosis. A large subcorneal pustule.

Very rarely, dogs have apparently become resistant to dapsone. These dogs may or may not benefit from the oral administration of sulfasalazine (Azulfidine, Pharmacia & Upjohn), 10 to 20 mg/kg q8h, until the dermatosis is controlled, and then as needed. Chronic administration of sulfasalazine may be associated with keratoconjunctivitis sicca. One dog that did not respond to dapsone was successfully treated with injectable gold salts.[6]

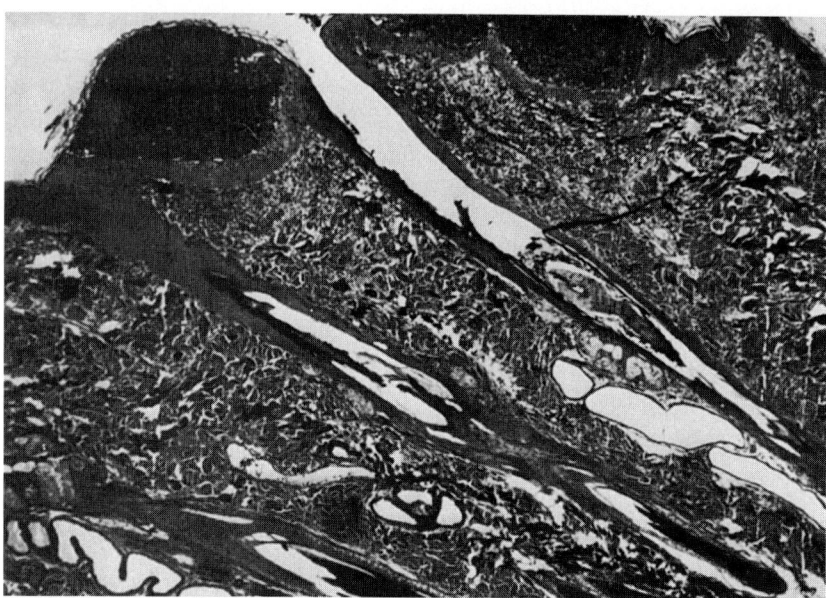

FIGURE 18-4. Canine subcorneal pustular dermatosis. Subcorneal pustules that do not involve hair follicles.

• FELINE PLASMA CELL PODODERMATITIS

Plasma cell pododermatitis is a rare cutaneous disorder of cats.[3, 16, 17]

Cause and Pathogenesis

The cause and pathogenesis of this disorder are unknown. The tissue plasmacytosis, the consistent hypergammaglobulinemia, and the beneficial response to immunomodulating drugs suggest an immune-mediated pathogenesis. However, the localization to pads and favorable response to surgery suggest a structural component to the etiology. In addition, some cases have recurred seasonally, suggesting that the condition is an allergic response.

In one study, 50% of the cats with plasma cell pododermatitis had concurrent feline immunodeficiency virus (FIV) infection.[14] In the latter study, four of six cats with FIV infection had plasma cell pododermatitis.[18] In this study, immunohistochemical examination of an affected footpad from one cat demonstrated FIV-immunoreactive cells within the inflammatory infiltrate.

Clinical Features

No age, breed, or sex predilections are apparent. Clinically, plasma cell pododermatitis begins as a soft, painless swelling of multiple footpads on multiple paws (see Fig. 18–1C). Rarely, a single footpad is involved. The central metacarpal or metatarsal pads are usually affected. Lightly pigmented pads may take on a violaceous hue. The surface of affected pads is cross-hatched with white scaly striae. Affected pads are swollen and feel mushy or flaccid. Initially, the cat is usually asymptomatic.[12] The cats are usually otherwise healthy. In some cases, one or more pads may become ulcerated and secondarily infected, which occasionally results in pain, lameness, and regional lymphadenopathy. Cats occasionally experience recurring hemorrhage from ulcerated or nodular areas of a footpad (see Fig. 18–1D).[19]

A minority of cats with plasma cell pododermatitis also have plasma cell stomatitis, which is characterized by ulceroproliferative gingivitis and symmetric vegetative plaques at the palatine arches.[16] In addition, a cat occasionally has immune-mediated glomerulonephritis or renal amyloidosis.[17]

Diagnosis

The differential diagnosis includes infectious or sterile granulomas and pyogranulomas, eosinophilic granuloma, mosquito or insect bite reaction, or neoplasia, all of which typically affect only one footpad. A tentative diagnosis may be based on history, physical examination, and aspiration cytologic study wherein plasma cells are numerous. Definitive diagnosis is based on culture and biopsy. Neutrophilia and lymphocytosis may be visible, and hypergammaglobulinemia is typical.

Serum protein electrophoresis reveals polyclonal gammopathy. Carefully performed cultures are negative. Aspiration cytologic study reveals numerous plasma cells with smaller numbers of lymphocytes and neutrophils. Antinuclear antibody test results are occasionally positive, and direct immunofluorescence testing rarely reveals Ig at the basement membrane zone. However, these latter two immunologic findings are nondiagnostic. Most cats in the original reports were feline leukemia virus (FeLV)-negative and FIV-negative.[16, 17, 19] In another study, 50% of cats were FIV-positive.[14]

Skin biopsy of early lesions is characterized by superficial and deep perivascular dermatitis, with plasma cells predominating. Later lesions are characterized by diffuse plasmacytic dermatitis (Figs. 18–5 and 18–6).[3, 4] Many plasma cells contain Russell's bodies (Mott's cells). Numbers of neutrophils are variable, reflecting the absence or presence of ulceration and secondary infection. Rarely, leukocytoclastic vasculitis is also present.

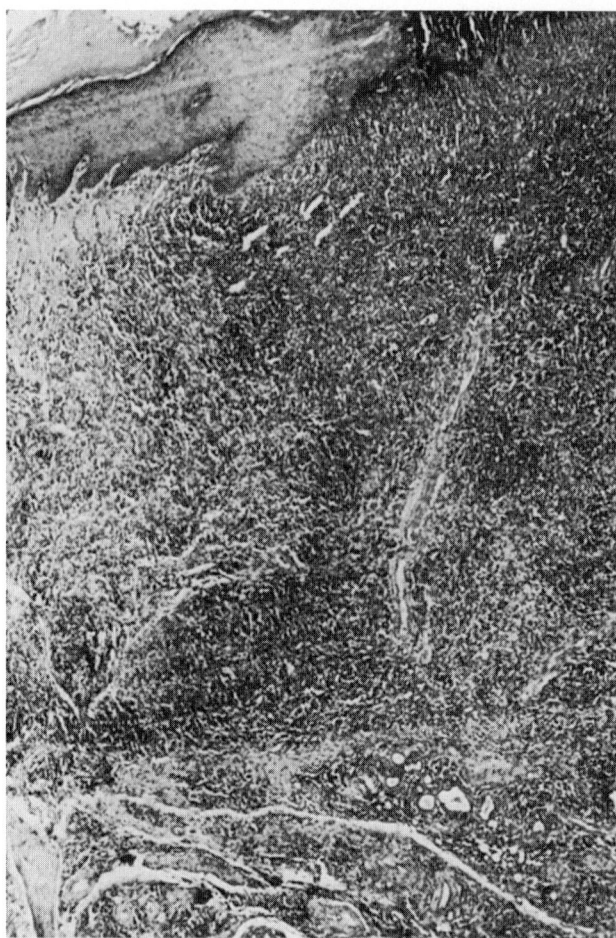

FIGURE 18–5. Feline plasma cell pododermatitis. Diffuse plasmacytic dermatitis.

Clinical Management

The therapy of choice is not clear. Because plasma cell pododermatitis is usually asymptomatic and may spontaneously regress, treatment may not be indicated in most cases. When treatment is necessary, both large doses of systemic glucocorticoid (prednisone or prednisolone administered orally at 4.4 mg/kg q24h) or chrysotherapy (see Chap. 9) may be effective.[13, 15–17, 19] Triamcinolone acetonide, 0.4 to 0.6 mg/kg q24h, or dexamethasone, 0.5 mg q24h, as initial treatments may be effective in cases refractory to prednisone. Once effective, the dose of glucocorticoids is reduced. A clear response to therapy is evident in 2 to 3 weeks, and maximum improvement occurs in 10 to 14 weeks. Footpads may remain slightly enlarged. Focal ulcers or nodules that hemorrhage usually require surgical correction.[11, 19] Surgical excision of the fatty footpad has also been described as beneficial, with no recurrence of disease in the surgically treated pads with follow-up periods of 2 years.[11, 14, 19a]

• LICHENOID DERMATOSES

Lichenoid dermatoses are rare, usually idiopathic skin disorders of dogs and cats.[21–26]

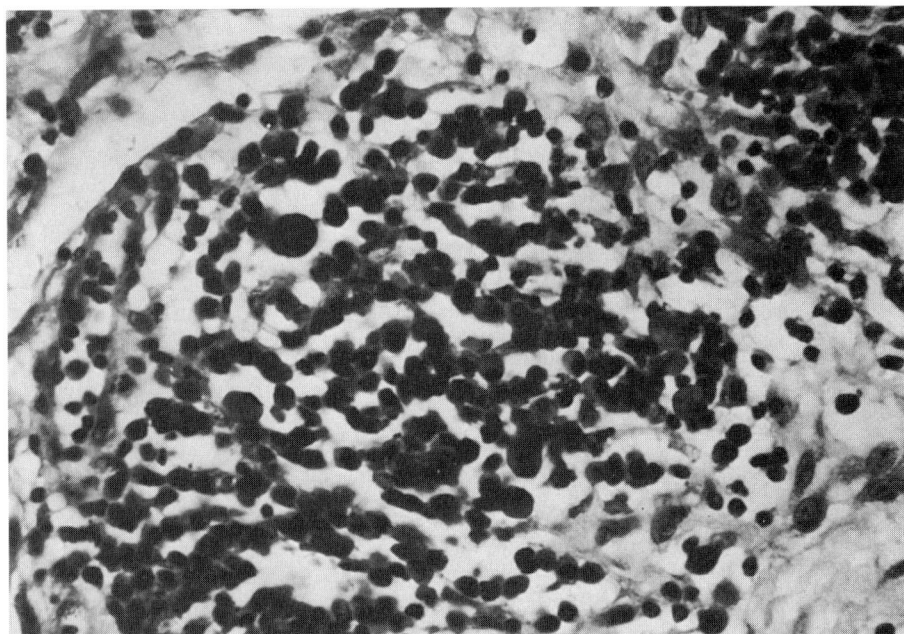

FIGURE 18–6. Feline plasma cell pododermatitis. Numerous plasma cells.

Cause and Pathogenesis

The cause and pathogenesis of most of these dermatoses are unclear; their clinical and histopathologic features suggest an immune-mediated pathomechanism.[1]

Clinical Features

There are no confirmed age, breed, or sex predilections. However, Doberman pinschers have accounted for several of the published cases.[22, 23, 26] Lichenoid dermatoses are characterized by the usually asymptomatic, symmetric onset of grouped, angular, flat-topped papules that develop a scaly to markedly hyperkeratotic surface (see Fig. 18–1E to H). Lesions may coalesce to form hyperkeratotic, alopecic plaques, and they may occur anywhere on the body. Lesions may appear anywhere, though we find that the concave surface of the pinnae and ventral thorax and abdomen are commonly affected. Lesions may be limited to the pinnae.[20] Affected animals are usually otherwise healthy.

Diagnosis

These lesions are usually visually diagnostic. The differential diagnosis includes psoriasiform lichenoid dermatosis of English Springer spaniels, staphylococcal folliculitis, and dermatophytosis. Various granulomatous and neoplastic conditions (especially the plaque-like forms of viral papillomas) rarely enter into the differential diagnosis. Definitive diagnosis is based on history, physical examination, exclusion through laboratory testing, and skin biopsy. Carefully performed cultures are negative. Skin biopsy reveals hyperkeratotic and hyperplastic lichenoid and hydropic interface dermatitis (Fig. 18–7). The inflammatory infiltrate is characteristically lymphoplasmacytic. If intraepidermal pustular dermatitis, suppurative folliculitis, or both are present, one should suspect a lichenoid tissue reaction in response to staphylococcal infection. Such cases respond to appropriate systemic antibiotic therapy. If eosinophilic microabscesses are present, one should suspect a

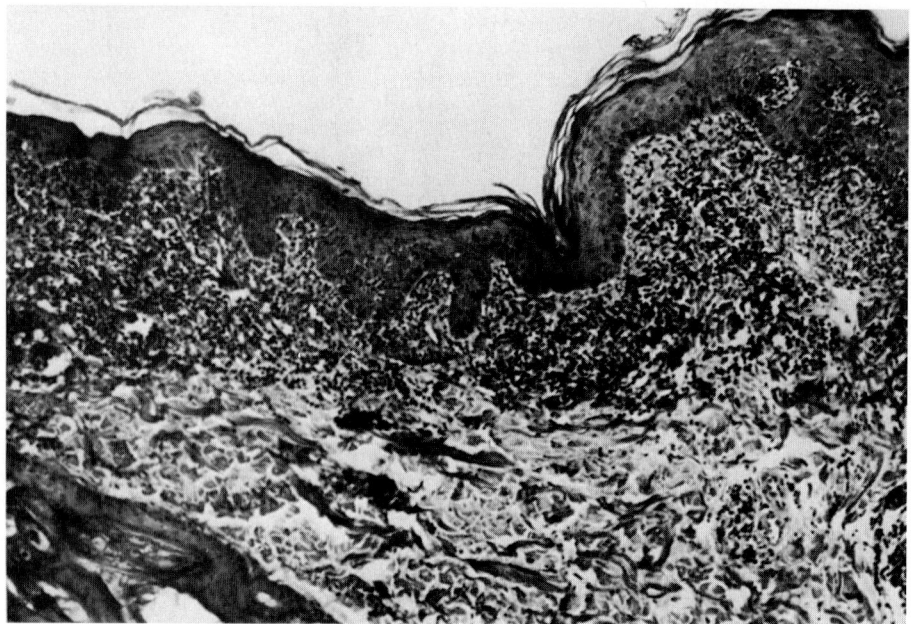

FIGURE 18-7. Canine idiopathic lichenoid dermatitis. Lichenoid interface dermatitis.

lichenoid tissue reaction in response to an ectoparasite (especially scabies or cheyletiellosis) or *Malassezia*.

Clinical Management

The prognosis for canine and feline idiopathic lichenoid dermatoses appears to be good. All cases have undergone spontaneous remission after a course of 6 months to 2 years. No form of therapy has been shown to be beneficial. In humans, oral retinoids have been useful in many cases.[1] Focal lesions have responded to surgical excision, and laser therapy may be beneficial. Antibiotic therapy has improved some lesions, though recurrences are possible.

• CANINE STERILE EOSINOPHILIC PUSTULOSIS

Sterile eosinophilic pustulosis is a rare idiopathic dermatosis of dogs.[28, 29, 32, 33, 35]

Cause and Pathogenesis

The cause and pathogenesis are unknown. The peripheral eosinophilia, sterile tissue eosinophilia, and responsiveness to systemic glucocorticoids that characterize this syndrome suggest that it may be immune mediated. However, intradermal skin testing, hypoallergenic diets, and immunopathologic studies have not been helpful in elucidating the etiopathogenesis. The cause in humans is unknown, though an association with human acquired immunodeficiency syndrome has been reported.[4] The condition in one human was thought to represent an adverse cutaneous reaction to indeloxazine.[30] Cats also rarely experience a clinical and pathologic sterile eosinophilic folliculitis; the clinical presentation is different, however, and the lesions are associated with an underlying hypersensitivity such as atopy, food hypersensitivity, flea bite hypersensitivity, and mosquito bite hypersensitivity (see Chap. 8).[34]

Clinical Features

No apparent age, breed, or sex predilections exist. The onset of clinical signs is often acute, and the distribution of lesions is multifocal (especially involving the trunk) or generalized. Pruritic, erythematous, follicular and nonfollicular papules and pustules evolve into annular erosions with epidermal collarettes (Fig. 18–8A and B). Peripheral spread, central healing, and hyperpigmentation of lesions result in numerous target lesions. Although most dogs are otherwise healthy, fever, anorexia, depression, and peripheral lymphadenopathy may be present.

Diagnosis

The differential diagnosis includes staphylococcal folliculitis, pemphigus foliaceus, drug reaction, and subcorneal pustular dermatosis. Definitive diagnosis is based on history, physical examination, hemogram, direct smears, cultures, and skin biopsy. Most dogs have peripheral eosinophilia (up to 5.6×10^3/ml). Direct smears reveal numerous eosinophils, nondegenerative neutrophils, occasional acantholytic keratinocytes, and no microorganisms (Fig. 18–9).[33] Carefully performed cultures are negative. Biopsy reveals intraepidermal eosinophilic pustular dermatitis and eosinophilic folliculitis and furunculosis (Fig. 18–10).[33] Flame figures are occasionally visible in the surrounding dermis. Direct and indirect immunofluorescence results are negative.[33] Serum α, β, and γ globulins may be elevated.[33]

Clinical Management

Most dogs respond well to systemic glucocorticoids (oral prednisone or prednisolone, 2.2 to 4.4 mg/kg q24h) in 5 to 10 days; however, stopping treatment consistently results in relapses. Thus, long-term, alternate-morning therapy is indicated, and cure is unlikely. In two dogs that could not be treated with glucocorticoids, we had good success with dapsone or the combination of an antihistamine (diphenhydramine) and an omega-6 and omega-3 fatty acid supplement (Derm Caps, DVM Pharmaceuticals). Isotretinoin and interferon-α_{2b} were successful in treating two humans with eosinophilic pustular folliculitis.[27, 31]

• FELINE HYPEREOSINOPHILIC SYNDROME

The hypereosinophilic syndrome is a rare disorder of cats.[37, 39] It is characterized by persistent idiopathic eosinophilia associated with a diffuse infiltration of various organs by mature eosinophils.

Cause and Pathogenesis

The cause and pathogenesis of this syndrome are unknown. It represents a leukoproliferative process likely caused by a number of disorders, all of which are marked by sustained overproduction of eosinophils.[42]

Clinical Features

The disease is more common in middle-aged female cats.[37, 39] Tissue infiltration with mature eosinophils results in multisystemic organ dysfunction. The bone marrow, lymph nodes, liver, spleen, and gastrointestinal tract are typically involved. Rarely, cardiac abnormalities are found; in one cat, restrictive cardiomyopathy was a clinical feature.[40] The most common clinical signs include diarrhea, weight loss, vomiting, and anorexia.[39] Physical examination often reveals thickened bowel loops, lymphadenopathy, and hepatosplenomegaly. Rarely, affected cats have dermatosis characterized by generalized maculopapular

1134 • Miscellaneous Skin Diseases

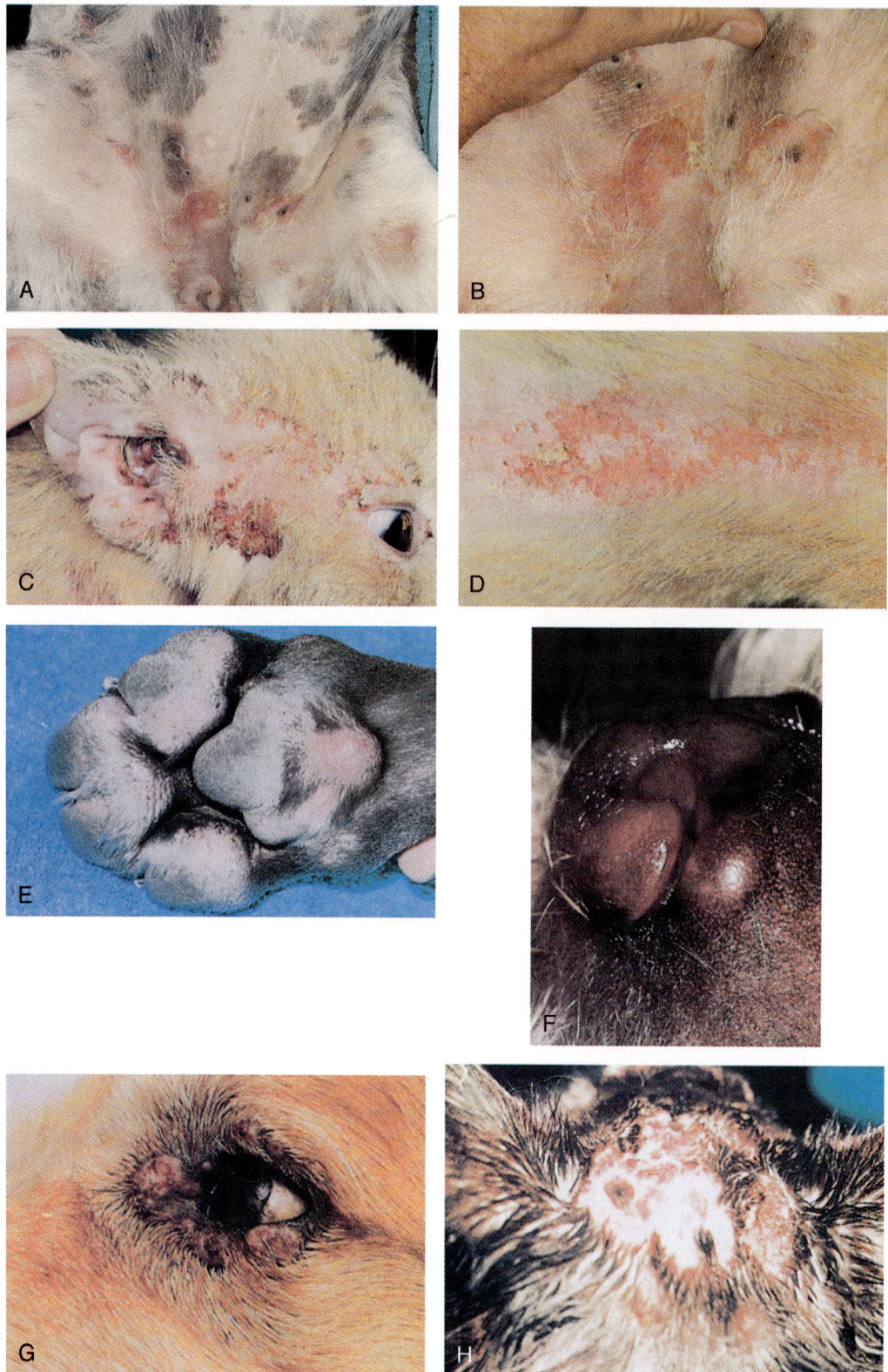

FIGURE 18–8. *See legend on opposite page*

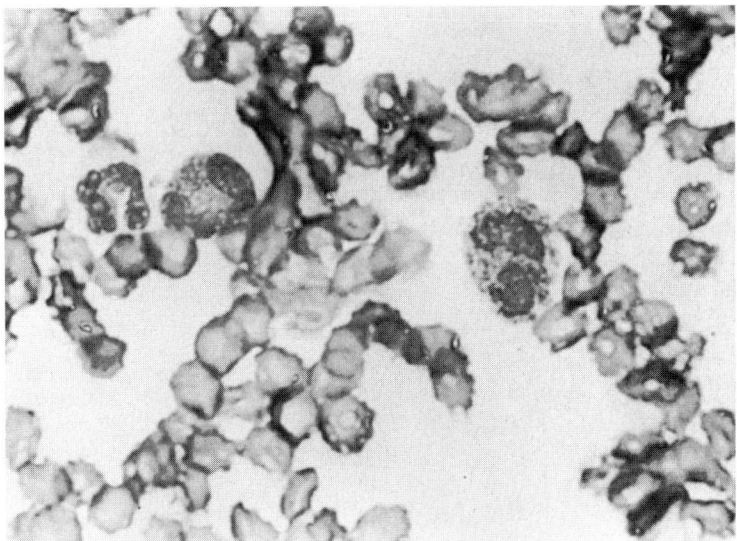

FIGURE 18-9. Canine sterile eosinophilic pustulosis. Cytologic examination reveals numerous eosinophils.

erythema, severe pruritus, marked excoriation, and possibly wheals and soft tissue swellings of the limbs (see Fig. 18–8C and D).[36, 38, 41]

Diagnosis

Diagnosis is based on history, physical examination, exclusion through laboratory testing, and skin biopsy. There are no specific tests for this syndrome: Rather, the syndrome is defined by a combination of unexplained prolonged eosinophilia and evidence of multiorgan involvement.[1, 5, 42] Flea bite hypersensitivity, eosinophilic granuloma complex, food hypersensitivity, asthma, eosinophilic gastroenteritis, endoparasitic infections, and mast cell tumor should be ruled out. The other consideration is eosinophilic leukemia, which is very similar but may show abnormal cells and an increased M/E ratio greater than 10:1 on bone marrow examination.[37] Moderate to marked peripheral eosinophilia (average, 42.6×10^3/ml) is characteristic in cats. Direct smears of skin lesions reveal a predominance of eosinophils and basophils. Skin biopsy reveals variable degrees of superficial and deep perivascular-to-interstitial dermatitis, with eosinophils predominating.

Clinical Management

The prognosis is poor; in most cases, survival times are short and patients do not respond to any treatment. Cats with cutaneous lesions may have slowly progressive disease and longer survival times (2 to 4 years).[36, 41] These cats may have a favorable, but transient, response to high doses of glucocorticoids. Interferon-α has been beneficial in treating some humans.[1, 42]

FIGURE 18-8. *A*, Canine sterile eosinophilic pustulosis. Pustules and annular erosions on the abdomen. *B*, Close-up of the dog in *A*. Annular erosion with epidermal collarettes. *C*, Feline hypereosinophilic syndrome. Erythema and excoriation of the face and pinna. *D*, Same cat as in *C*. Erythema, alopecia, and excoriation over the back. *E*, Canine sterile pyogranuloma. Erythematous nodules bordering footpads. *F*, Canine sterile pyogranuloma. Erythematous nodules bordering nostrils. *G*, Canine sterile pyogranuloma. Multiple erythematosus, ulcerated, crusted papules around the eye. *H*, Idiopathic sterile pyogranulomas in a cat. Violaceous papules and nodules on the top of the head (the area has been clipped).

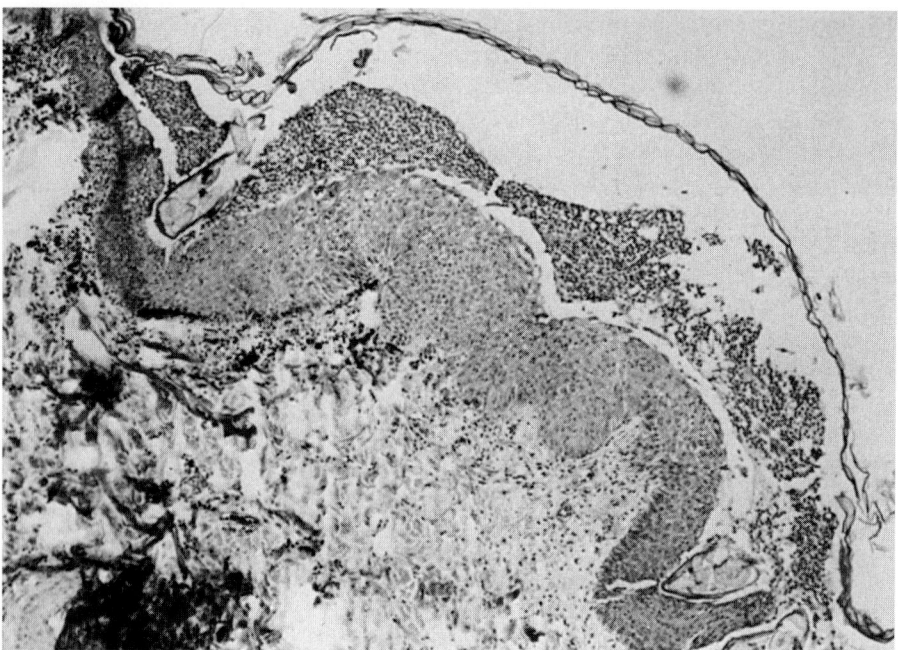

FIGURE 18-10. Canine sterile eosinophilic pustulosis. Subcorneal eosinophilic pustular dermatitis and eosinophilic luminal folliculitis.

• IDIOPATHIC STERILE GRANULOMA AND PYOGRANULOMA

Idiopathic, sterile, granulomatous to pyogranulomatous skin disease is uncommon in dogs and very rare in cats.[44, 46, 48]

Cause and Pathogenesis

The cause and pathogenesis of these conditions are unknown. The characteristic granulomatous histopathologic appearance, absence of microbial agents and foreign material, and good response to systemic glucocorticoids suggest an aberrant inflammatory histiocytic response. The favorable response of some dogs to tetracycline/doxycycline and niacinamide also supports an immune dysfunction. It has been proposed that this syndrome is due to immune dysfunction in response to a chronic antigenic stimulus and is related to cutaneous histiocytosis.[45]

In human sarcoidosis, a classic "sterile" granulomatous disease, polymerase chain reaction (PCR) technology has shown that mycobacterial (multiple species) DNA is present in most lesions.[45a] Similar studies in canine and feline sterile granulomatous dermatoses are awaited.

Clinical Features

DOG

The disorder may occur in dogs of all ages, breeds, and sexes, but collies, Weimaraners, Great Danes, Boxers, and Golden retrievers may be predisposed.[46] Lesions are usually multiple and typically affect the head (especially the bridge of the nose, the muzzle, and the periocular region), the pinnae, and the paws. Firm, painless, nonpruritic, dermal papules, plaques, and nodules are present (see Fig. 18-8E to G). The lesions may become alopecic, ulcerated, and secondarily infected, especially on the paws. Animals are usually otherwise healthy. One dog with sterile pyogranuloma syndrome had associated hypercalcemia.[43]

CAT

In cats, two clinical syndromes have been described.[3, 48] Some animals have pruritic papules and nodules on the head and pinnae (see Fig. 18–8H). Lesions are usually erythematous to violaceous in color. Other cats present with pruritic, symmetric, preauricular plaques (preauricular xanthogranulomas) (Fig. 18–11).[3, 48] Papules and wheal-like lesions coalesce to form orange-yellow, friable, well-circumscribed plaques. These plaques become reddish purple on palpation.

Diagnosis

The differential diagnosis includes other granulomatous and pyogranulomatous (bacterial, mycotic, foreign body) and neoplastic disorders. Definitive diagnosis is based on history, physical examination, cultures, and biopsy. The major differential diagnoses are the infectious diseases. Cytologic examination reveals pyogranulomatous or granulomatous inflammation with no microorganisms (Fig. 18–12). In rare cases of mycobacterial diseases, direct smears from lesions reveal mycobacteria; formalin-fixed tissue samples are negative. Direct smears stained with acid-fast stains for mycobacteria should be examined cytologically. Cultures (aerobic, anaerobic, mycobacterial, and fungal) are best grown from tissue taken by aseptic surgical biopsy techniques, and they are negative. In dogs, biopsy usually reveals nodular to diffuse, granulomatous to pyogranulomatous dermatitis.

Early lesions show a characteristic vertical orientation of oblong (sausage-shaped) perifollicular granulomas or pyogranulomas that track, but do not initially involve, the hair follicles (Figs. 18–13 to 18–15).[46] In later, larger lesions, the pyogranulomatous-to-granulomatous process becomes diffuse, often severely attenuating or obliterating adnexae and even extending into the subcutis. Special stains and polarization reveal no microorganisms or foreign material. Rarely, dogs have diffuse sarcoidal granulomatous dermatitis (Fig. 18–16).[49] PCR testing for infectious agents may also be considered.

In cats, biopsy of the papulonodular lesions on the head and pinnae reveals perifollic-

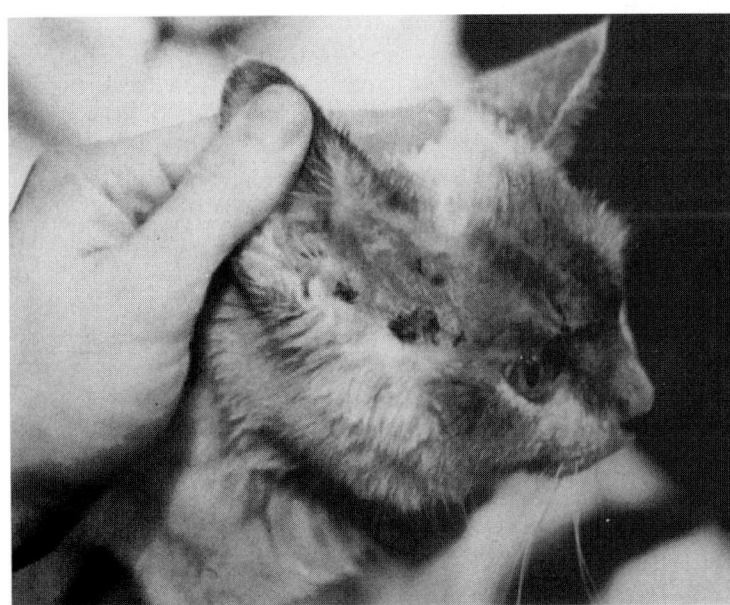

FIGURE 18–11. Idiopathic sterile granulomas in a cat. Preauricular plaque.

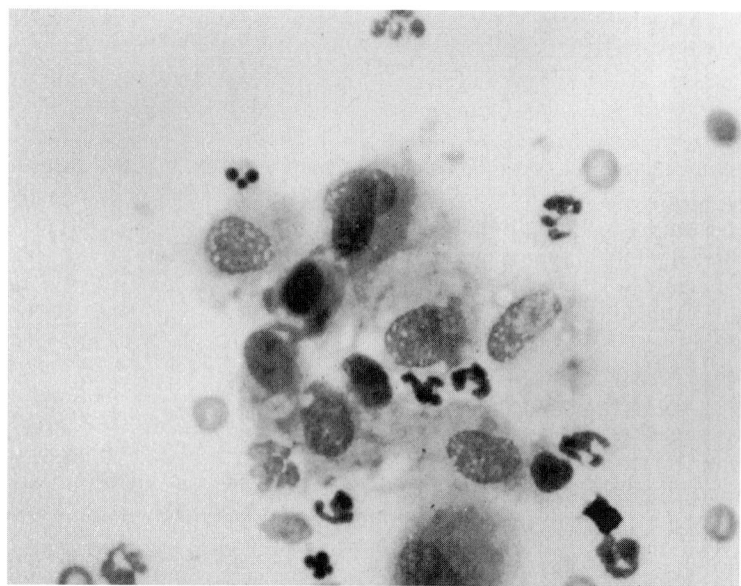

FIGURE 18–12. Canine sterile pyogranuloma. Cytologic examination reveals macrophages, nondegenerate neutrophils, and no microorganisms.

ular pyogranulomatous dermatitis.[48] Biopsy of the preauricular plaques reveals diffuse granulomatous dermatitis that is separated from epithelial structures by a narrow Grenz zone, contains numerous multinucleated histiocytic giant cells, and exhibits unexplained purpura (Figs. 18–17 and 18–18).[3, 48]

Clinical Management

Therapy may consist of surgical excision of solitary lesions, if feasible, or of systemic glucocorticoids if multiple lesions are present or surgery is impractical.[46] Some cases may

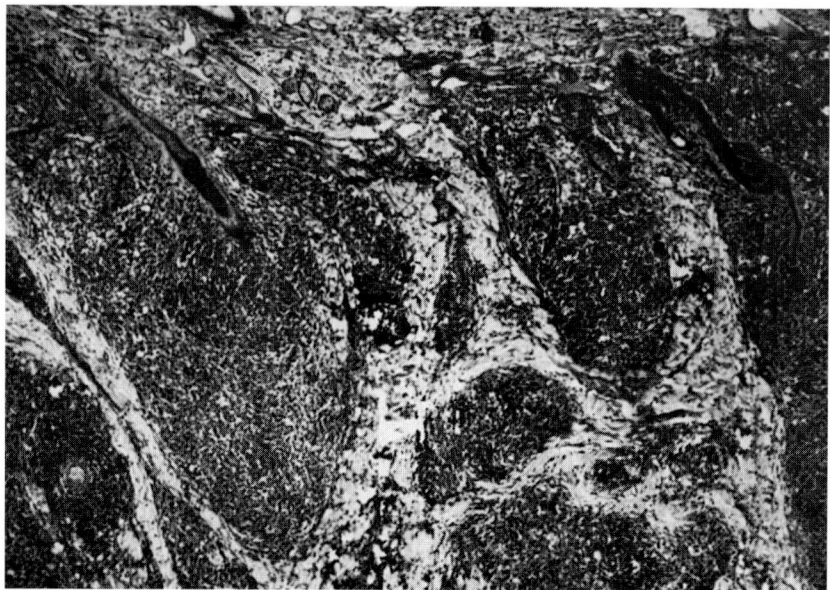

FIGURE 18–13. Canine idiopathic sterile granuloma. Granulomatous dermatitis that tends to track appendages (AOG stain).

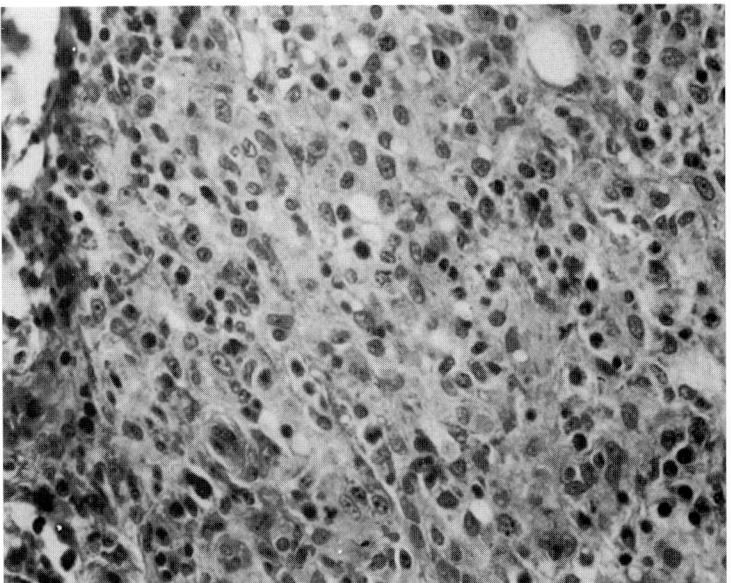

FIGURE 18–14. Canine sterile granuloma. Granulomatous dermatitis.

respond to tetracycline/niacinamide, even when glucocorticoids are ineffective (see Chap. 3).[47] Doxycycline and niacinamide may also be effective. Tetracycline and niacinamide are dosed at 250 mg q8h in dogs under 10 kg and 500 mg q8h in dogs over 10 kg. In dogs, prednisone or prednisolone is administered orally at 2.2 to 4.4 mg/kg q24h until the lesions have regressed in 7 to 14 days. About 60% of dogs then require prolonged alternate-morning glucocorticoid therapy.[46]

Occasionally, cases in dogs are unresponsive to glucocorticoids or become refractory after variable periods of remission. Azathioprine (Imuran, Glaxo Wellcome) is useful in such cases and is administered orally at 2.2 mg/kg q24h until remission, then on alternate days. Once remission has been maintained for several months, therapy may be successfully

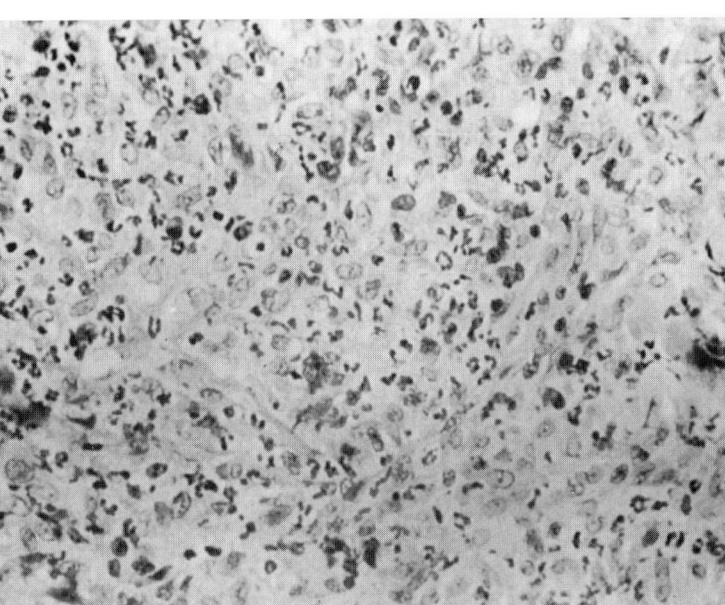

FIGURE 18–15. Canine sterile pyogranuloma. Pyogranulomatous dermatitis.

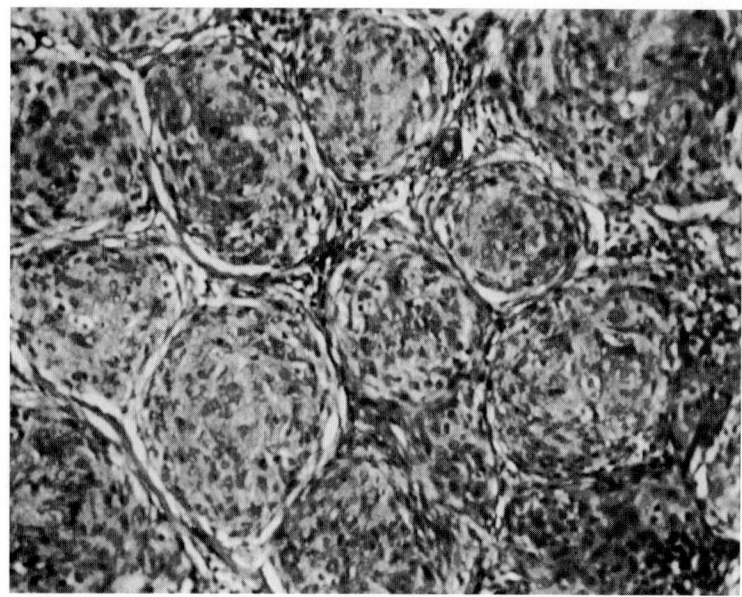

FIGURE 18–16. Canine sterile sarcoidal granuloma. Confluent sarcoidal (naked epithelioid) granulomas.

discontinued in some cases. Others may require long-term low-dose therapy. We have occasionally been able to reduce the dosage and frequency of administration of azathioprine to 0.25 mg/kg once weekly. The oral administration of sodium iodide has been reported useful in some cases[4] but not in others.[46] In cats, lesions often spontaneously resolve after about 9 months.[48]

● GRANULOMATOUS SEBACEOUS ADENITIS

Granulomatous sebaceous adenitis is an uncommon idiopathic dermatosis of dogs and is rare in cats.[2, 53, 60, 62–66] Since the description of this condition in the dog, a histopathologically similar disease has been recognized in humans.[55, 59]

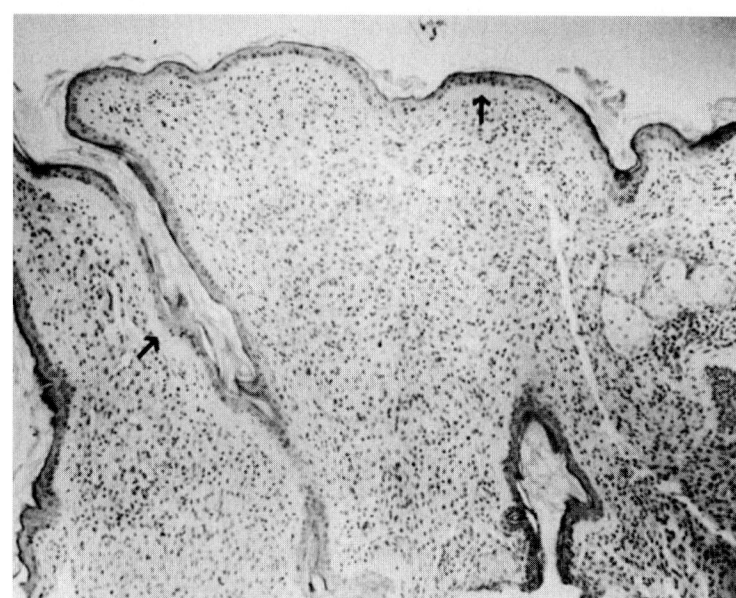

FIGURE 18–17. Feline preauricular granuloma. Diffuse granulomatous dermatitis with narrow Grenz zone (*arrows*).

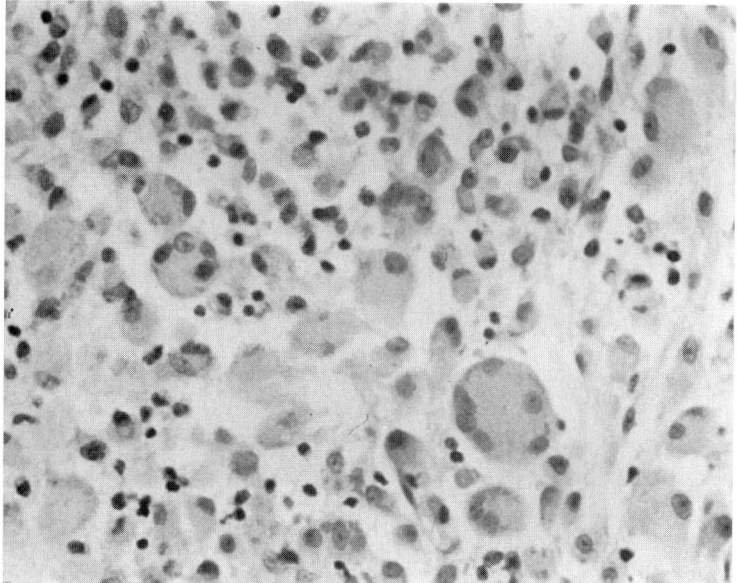

FIGURE 18–18. Feline preauricular granuloma. Numerous histiocytes and multinucleated histiocytic giant cells.

Cause and Pathogenesis

The cause and pathogenesis of the disorder are unknown, but speculations include the following: (1) sebaceous gland destruction is a developmental and inherited defect; (2) sebaceous gland destruction is due to a cell-mediated immunologic reaction directed against a component of the gland; (3) the initial defect is a keratinization abnormality with subsequent obstruction of the sebaceous ducts, resulting in inflammation of the glands; and (4) the sebaceous adenitis and keratinization defects are the result of an abnormality in lipid metabolism.[2, 51, 61, 64] Studies in rodents suggest that primary sebaceous gland disease and destruction can result in follicular plugging and inadequate dissociation of the internal root sheath from the hair shaft, which results in hair shafts perforating the bulbar area of the hair follicle and causing inflammation.[64a]

Preliminary pedigree analysis of affected and related Standard Poodles suggests an autosomal recessive mode of inheritance.[51] However, because over 25% of affected dogs may have subclinical disease, breeding studies are being undertaken to confirm the mode of inheritance.

Clinical Features

DOG

There is no apparent sex predilection, and the disorder tends to appear in young adult to middle-aged dogs. Although many breeds and mongrels may be affected, there are breed predilections for Standard Poodles, Akitas, Vizslas, Samoyeds, and Belgian sheepdogs.[2, 54, 64, 66] In general, the dermatologic abnormalities are bilaterally symmetric; prominent on the face, head, pinnae, and trunk; and dominated by abnormal keratinization (see Fig. 18–20B). Initial lesions usually occur on the dorsal surfaces of the body, particularly the head and cervical region. Some dogs have severe involvement of the tail ("rat-tail").[66] Secondary pyoderma may be present and can be superficial folliculitis or deep folliculitis and furunculosis. In one study, 43% of patients had concurrent pyoderma.[66] Ceruminous otitis externa is common.[58] In Belgian sheepdogs, bilateral suppurative otitis externa was a constant finding.[54] In addition, the disease in Belgian sheepdogs seemed to be photoaggravated.[54] The cutaneous changes are somewhat dependent on haircoat type and breed.

In short-coated dogs, such as Vizslas and Dachshunds, lesions begin as generally annular areas of scaling and alopecia that tend to enlarge peripherally, to become polycyclic, and occasionally to coalesce (Fig. 18–19A). The surface scales are usually fine, white,

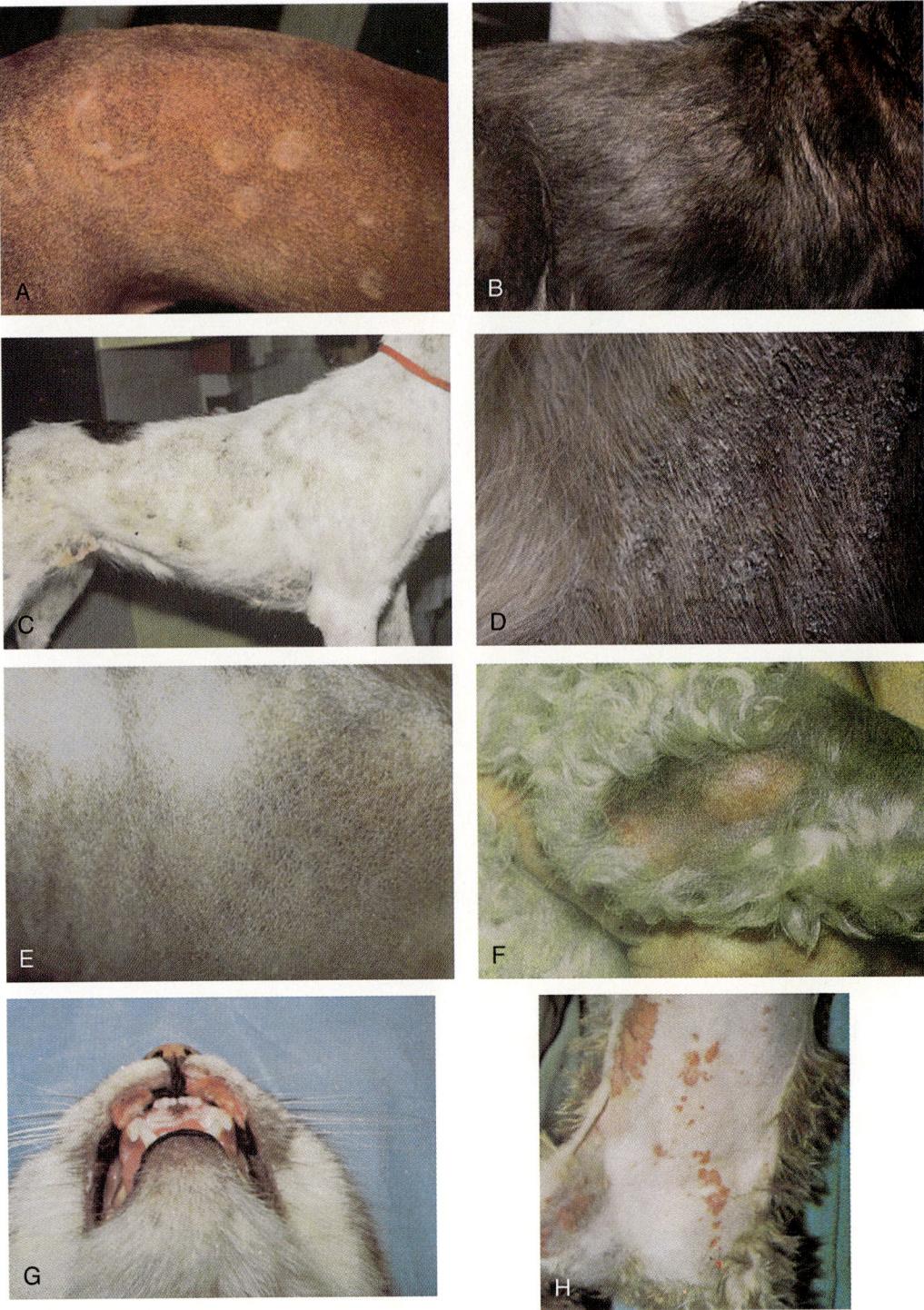

FIGURE 18-19. *A*, canine granulomatous sebaceous adenitis. Annular and arciform areas of alopecia and scaling in a Vizsla. *B*, Canine sebaceous adenitis. Early disease in an Akita with a thin, broken, dishevelled haircoat. *C*, Canine sebaceous adenitis. Advanced disease in an Akita, with pronounced hair loss, hyperkeratosis, and dermatitic areas. *D*, Canine sebaceous adenitis. Marked hyperkeratosis, follicular casting, and broken hairs. *E*, Feline sebaceous adenitis. Marked follicular hyperkeratosis, broken hairs, and alopecia over the trunk. *F*, Canine morphea, Alopecic, shiny plaque on lateral elbow. *G*, Feline indolent ulcer. Bilateral lip ulcers that are chronic and necrotic. *H*, Eosinophilic plaque in scattered patches on the cat's abdomen and chest. Hair has been clipped away. Lesions are well demarcated, red, moist, and raised and have been licked incessantly.

and nonadherent. Hair casts are prominent. Lesions are usually asymptomatic, unless secondary staphylococcal infection occurs. Intermittent edematous swelling of the muzzle, lips, and eyelids occurs occasionally.[56, 65, 66]

The Standard Poodle manifests marked hyperkeratosis followed by alopecia. The hairs are dull and brittle, with tightly adherent, silver-white scales that incorporate small tufts of matted hairs. Hair casts are prominent. In some cases, the initial changes may be a loss of the tight curls as the hair straightens and coat color changes (Fig. 18–20A). Lesions often begin on the face and pinnae but progressively involve the neck and dorsal trunk.

Akitas tend to have fairly generalized, erythematous and greasy skin changes (see Fig. 18–19B to D). Papules, pustules, scales, matting of the hair, and yellow-brown greasy keratosebaceous debris are usually prominent. Hair casts are often prominent (Fig. 18–20C). Severe hair loss, especially of the undercoat, is often present. Secondary pyoderma is common and often more severe in this breed when sebaceous adenitis is present. Some animals may show signs of systemic illness, such as fever, malaise, and weight loss.

Samoyeds experience moderate to severe, predominantly truncal alopecia and scaling. Hairs are dull, brittle, and broken. Hair casts are prominent.

In German shepherds, lesions may begin on the tail and progress cranially on the body.

Dogs with granulomatous sebaceous adenitis are generally nonpruritic. However, secondary staphylococcal infection is a frequent complication, and affected animals may then become pruritic. In the breeds that are not predisposed, sebaceous adenitis may occur as acute-onset generalized exfoliative erythroderma that may be intensely pruritic. As these cases progress, the erythroderma and pruritus ceases and alopecia results. At this point, these cases are easily confused with endocrinopathies.

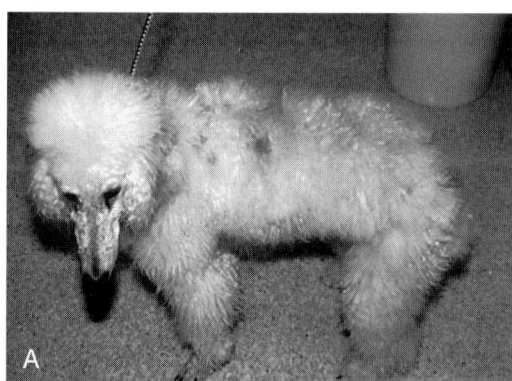
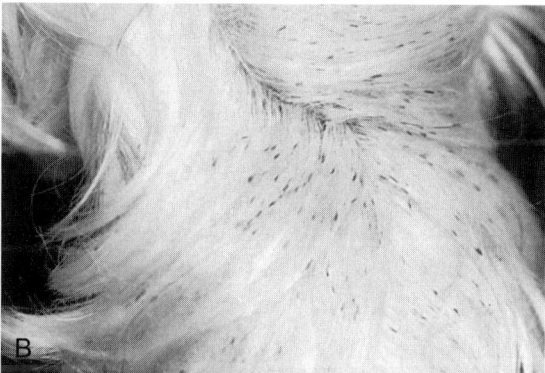
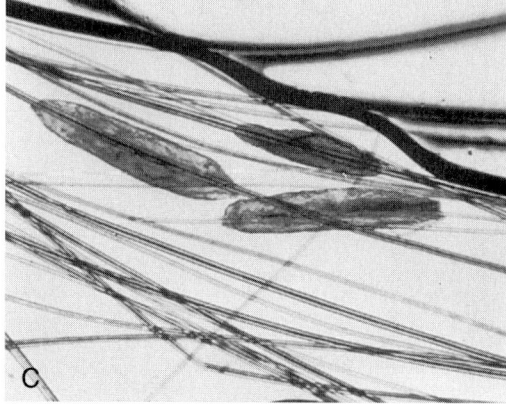

FIGURE 18–20. *A*, Sebaceous adenitis in a Poodle showing hair with loss of tight curls. *B*, Sebaceous adenitis in a Miniature Schnauzer. Note the numerous hair casts. *C*, Canine sebaceous adenitis. Trichogram reveals prominent casts of keratosebaceous debris surrounding numerous hair shafts.

CAT

Lesions consist of multifocal annular areas of scales, crust, broken hairs, hair casts, and alopecia (see Fig. 18–19E).[57, 63, 64] Lesions begin on the head, pinnae, and neck, then spread caudally on the body.

Diagnosis

The differential diagnosis includes staphylococcal folliculitis, demodicosis, dermatophytosis, keratinization defects (especially seborrhea and ichthyosis), follicular dysplasia, and endocrinopathies. Skin scrapings and carefully performed cultures are negative. Prominent hair casts are most likely associated with granulomatous sebaceous adenitis, seborrhea, vitamin A–responsive dermatosis, demodicosis, and follicular dysplasia. Microscopic examination of affected hairs reveals casts or collars of yellow-brown keratosebaceous material surrounding hair shafts at varying intervals (see Fig. 18–20C).

Dermatohistopathologic findings are variable in intensity. They vary with the chronicity of the lesion and, to some extent, with the haircoat type and breed of animal.[2, 3, 52, 64] In general, early lesions are characterized by variable degrees of sebaceous adenitis (granulomatous to pyogranulomatous). In most cases, sebocytes are no longer visible within the granulomas and the diagnosis is based on the finding of discrete perifollicular granulomas in areas in which sebaceous glands are normally found (Figs. 18–21 and 18–22). The other adnexae are spared. Short-coated dogs (e.g., Vizslas) often have large granulomatous lesions, some of which extend into the subcutis.

Chronic lesions are characterized by hyperplastic superficial perivascular dermatitis with prominent orthokeratotic or parakeratotic hyperkeratosis of epidermis and hair follicles and variable degrees of perifollicular fibrosis and follicular atrophy. Sebaceous glands are absent. Standard Poodles may have only a scanty lymphocytic inflammation at the level of the sebaceous duct, but no sebaceous glands are present. Nonpredisposed breeds may have a noninflammatory, endocrine-like histologic pattern, but without sebaceous glands. Complete absence of sebaceous glands is *not* a feature of endocrine disorders.

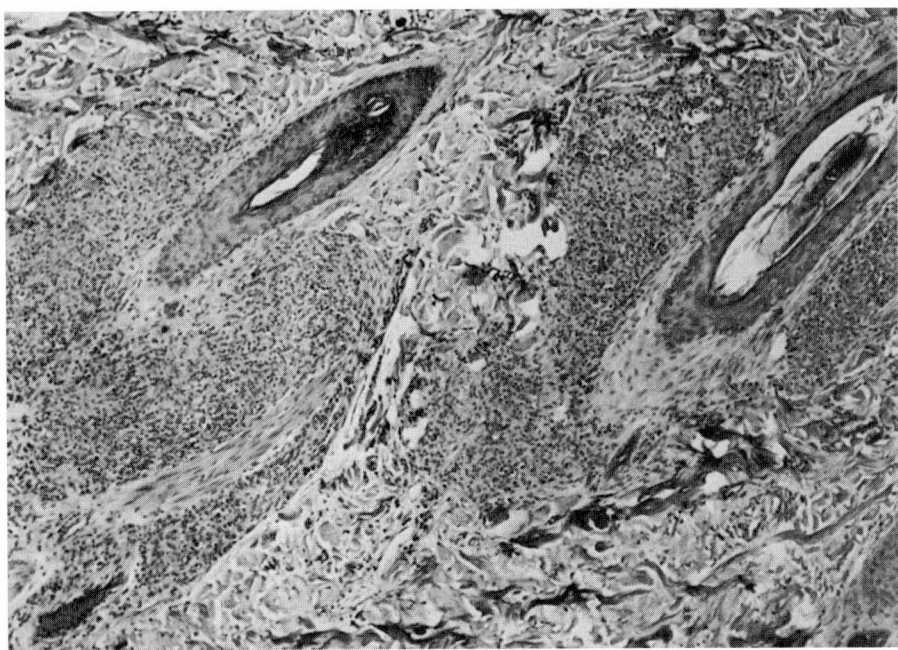

FIGURE 18–21. Sebaceous adenitis. Perifollicular granulomas where sebaceous glands should be.

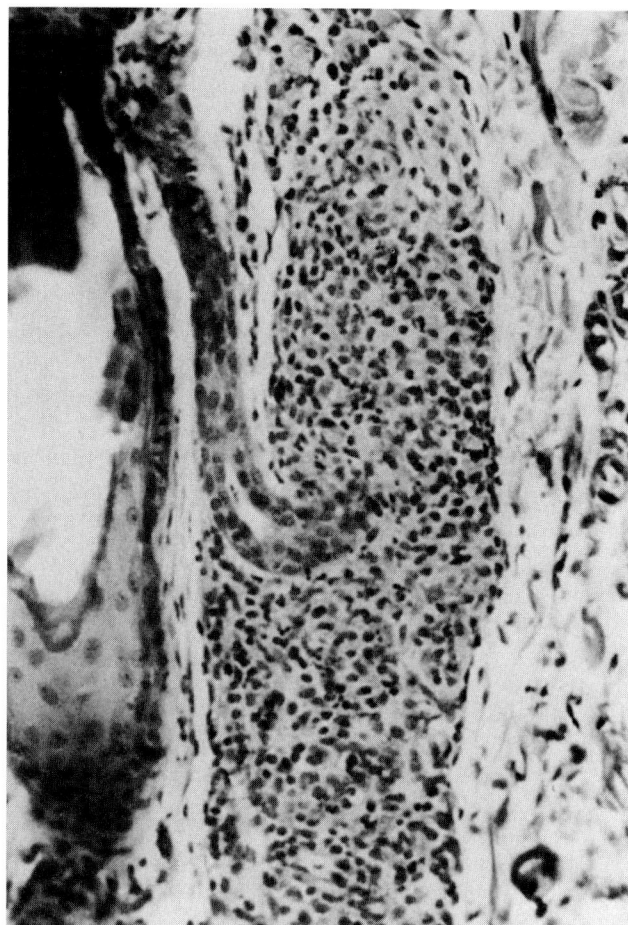

FIGURE 18–22. Canine granulomatous sebaceous adenitis. Sebaceous duct exiting a granuloma.

It has been reported that biopsies from clinically normal standard Poodles that were still normal 2 years later may contain focal areas of mild granulomatous sebaceous adenitis.[51, 64] Animals with secondary staphylococcal infections may have areas of neutrophilic intraepidermal pustular dermatitis, suppurative folliculitis and furunculosis, and nodular to diffuse pyogranulomatous dermatitis or panniculitis.

An immunohistologic study revealed that $CD1c^+$, $CD11c^+$ dendritic cells, neutrophils, and $CD3^+$ T lymphocytes dominated the cellular infiltrate.[61] The majority of T lymphocytes were TCR-$\alpha\beta^+$, $CD8^+$, and $CD4^+$. $CD21^+$ B lymphocytes and plasma cells were uncommon. Indirect immunofluorescence results for circulating autoantibodies were negative.

Clinical Management

Many authors have found that response to therapy varies somewhat, depending on the severity or chronicity of the disease and on the breed of animal.[2, 53, 54, 58, 64] Further confusion is created by the fact that some dogs have cyclic patterns of spontaneous improvement and worsening that are independent of any therapy.[2] However, White and colleagues reported that response to therapy could not be predicted on the basis of breed, clinical signs, histopathologic findings, or presence or absence of sebaceous glands in skin biopsy specimens.[66] Mild cases may be satisfactorily controlled with keratolytic shampoos and emollient rinses.[58] More stubborn cases may benefit from the topical application of 50% to 75% propylene glycol in water as a spray or rinse once daily, then two to three times weekly as needed.[2, 64] Some dogs respond to oral administration of products containing omega-6 and omega-3 fatty acids; others do not.[2, 56, 58, 64] We are aware of anecdotal reports of beneficial effects from baby oil soaks (undiluted or diluted 1:1 with water; let stand 1 to 6 hours) followed by shampooing out the excess oil as a treatment for Poodles. These applications are repeated weekly until maximum improvement is achieved, then every 3 to 4 weeks as needed.

Systemic glucocorticoids are not efficacious, though they may help to decrease the pruritus that may occur in generalized exfoliative cases.[54] They do not alter the course of the disease because sebaceous gland destruction and alopecia still occur.

In severe or refractory cases, synthetic retinoids (see Chap. 3) may be useful, though their expense has severely limited their use. Synthetic retinoids were reported to be effective in 60% of the dogs treated.[66] "Effective" was defined as greater than 50% reduction in scaling and alopecia. It was interesting to note that some dogs in which the initial choice of retinoid (either isotretinoin or etretinate) failed did respond to the second retinoid.

In the past, it was suggested that certain breeds respond more favorably to a particular type of retinoid (e.g., Vizslas and Poodles to isotretinoin; Akitas to etretinate).[56, 64, 65] However, this was not detected in the study by White and associates.[66] In Belgian sheepdogs, response to etretinate was minimal but response to isotretinoin was good.[54] Isotretinoin (1 to 2 mg/kg/q24h orally) and etretinate (1 to 2 mg/kg/q24h orally) have been evaluated the most. Acitretin has replaced etretinate and is dosed at 0.5 to 2 mg/kg q24h.[54a] Responses to synthetic retinoids generally require 4 to 8 weeks of therapy, and therapy must usually be continued for life. The potential side effects of synthetic retinoids are legion (see Chap. 3), but they are uncommon and are usually mild when they do occur.[56]

Cyclosporine (Sandimmune, Novartis, 5 mg/kg q12h orally) has been reported to be effective in dogs in which synthetic retinoids failed.[2, 50] Cyclosporine commonly produced side effects in dogs: gastrointestinal irritation, gingival hyperplasia, hirsutism, nephrotoxicity, hepatotoxicity, papillomatosis, increased frequency of bacterial and viral infections, and lymphoplasmacytic dermatitis, when dosed at 20 to 30 mg/kg/day (see Chap. 3). These side effects appear to be uncommon at the lower doses.

Rarely, dogs and cats undergo spontaneous remission.[53, 57, 58, 64] Still other dogs respond to none of the currently recommended treatments.[58] One of the authors (DWS) has treated a Standard Poodle that had failed to respond to multiple medicaments (topicals, vitamin A, isotretinoin, etretinate, omega-6/omega-3 fatty acids) with tetracycline and niacinamide (see Chap. 3). The keratinization abnormality gradually improved over a 4-month period, and recurrent bacterial folliculitis ceased. Because of the possible hereditary nature of granulomatous sebaceous adenitis in certain breeds, it would be wise to discourage the use of affected animals for breeding purposes. No information on the treatment of granulomatous sebaceous adenitis in cats has been published.

• LOCALIZED SCLERODERMA

Localized scleroderma (morphea) is a rare disease of dogs and cats.[67, 68, 70]

Cause and Pathogenesis

In humans, the cause and pathogenesis of localized scleroderma are unknown.[1] Three predominant theories on pathogenesis have emerged: (1) the vascular theory (early endothelial injury, perivascular fibrosis, hypoxia, and abnormal vascular reactivity); (2) the abnormal collagen metabolism theory (increased production of collagen and reduced collagenase activity); and (3) the immunologic theory (humoral and cell-mediated autoimmunity). There are reports of *Borrelia burgdorferi* playing a role in the development of morphea lesions in humans.[1]

Clinical Features

In dogs and cats, no age, breed, or sex predilections are apparent. Localized scleroderma is characterized by asymptomatic, well-demarcated, sclerotic plaques that are alopecic, smooth, and shiny (see Fig. 18–19F). Hypopigmentation may occur. Lesions tend to be linear and to occur on the trunk and limbs. Affected animals are otherwise healthy.

Diagnosis

The diagnosis is based on history, physical examination, and skin biopsy. Histopathologic examination reveals fibrosing dermatitis. The overlying epidermis is unremarkable (Fig. 18–23A and B). The entire dermis and subcutis are replaced by collagenous tissue. The

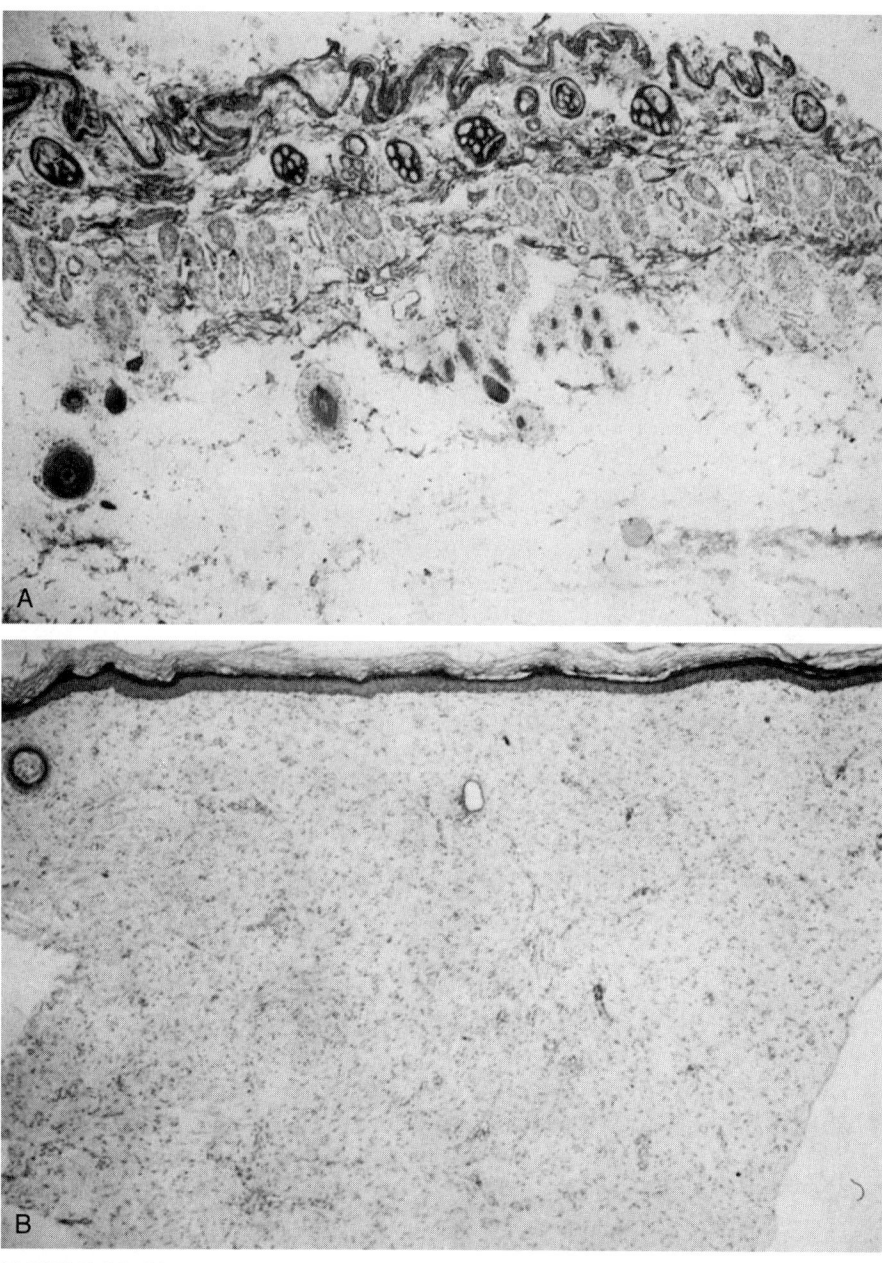

FIGURE 18–23. A, Canine morphea. Normal skin peripheral to a lesion. B, Canine morphea. Lesional skin. Fibrosing dermatitis.

normal loosely woven, fine-fibered appearance of the superficial dermis is replaced by dense collagen bundles. Pilosebaceous units are essentially absent. Mild superficial and deep perivascular accumulation of lymphohistiocytic cells is present.

Clinical Management

The prognosis appears to be good. Spontaneous remission may occur over a course of several weeks,[67, 68] or permanent scarring may result.[70] When regrowth occurs, the hair is usually thinner and finer than normal, and it may be a slightly different color.[70] In humans, no forms of topical or systemic therapy are known to be of regular benefit to patients with localized scleroderma. In humans, pentoxifylline has been recommended for morphea.[69]

• FELINE EOSINOPHILIC GRANULOMA COMPLEX

The eosinophilic granuloma complex includes a group of lesions that affect the skin, mucocutaneous junctions, and oral cavity of cats. The term itself is often used as a final diagnosis; in fact, there is another primary cause. It is essential to realize that the eosinophilic granuloma complex is nothing more than a mucocutaneous reaction pattern in cats—not a specific disease.

Three lesions have traditionally been recognized: (1) the indolent ulcer, (2) the eosinophilic plaque, and (3) the eosinophilic granuloma. These lesions are common and are most common in cats that have hypersensitivities (allergies) to inhalants, foods, or insects, especially to fleas and mosquitoes (see Chap. 8).[2, 4, 5, 71, 72, 78, 79, 81] In a group of 88 cats with pruritus due to allergic skin diseases, 31% had one or more lesions of the eosinophilic granuloma complex.[78] In another study of 25 cats with suspected allergic skin disease, only 12% had lesions compatible with eosinophilic granuloma complex: Intradermal testing results were positive for housedust mite in all three cats, for pollen in two cats, and for flea antigen in one cat.[71] The latter cat was still tentatively considered atopic. Bacterial involvement occasionally is a factor because antibiotic therapy resolves or markedly improves some lesions.[2, 80]

In some instances, these lesions may be heritable.[2, 77] Eosinophilic granulomas and indolent ulcers occurred in a colony of specific pathogen–free cats and other cats with limited genetic diversity.[57] A genetic dysregulation of eosinophil signaling and/or regulation was suspected. These cats typically "outgrew" their disease at 2 to 3 years of age. Therefore, when no hypersensitivity can be documented, a heritable form of the disorder should be considered. In contrast with what had been reported in earlier veterinary literature, more recent attempts to transmit eosinophilic plaques by autologous tissue techniques have been unsuccessful.[73]

It has been postulated that some oral eosinophilic granulomas result from imbedded, swallowed insect parts.[74]

Feline Indolent Ulcer

Indolent ulcer (eosinophilic ulcer, rodent ulcer) is a common cutaneous, mucocutaneous, and oral mucosal lesion of cats. Clinically, most indolent ulcers occur unilaterally on the upper lip (see Fig. 18–19G). However, lesions also occur in the oral cavity, in other areas of the skin, and bilaterally. The lesions are usually well circumscribed, red-brown, alopecic, and glistening; they have a raised border. Pruritus and pain are rare, and peripheral lymphadenopathy may be present. There are no age or breed predilections, but females may be predisposed. Lip ulcers appear to be precancerous and rarely undergo malignant transformation into squamous cell carcinoma (see Chap. 20). Cats with indolent ulcers may also have eosinophilic plaques, eosinophilic granulomas, or both.

The differential diagnosis includes infectious ulcers (bacterial, fungal, FeLV-associated), trauma, and neoplasia (squamous cell carcinoma, mast cell tumor, lymphoma).

Carefully performed cultures are negative. Biopsy is nondiagnostic, revealing hyperplastic, ulcerated, superficial perivascular to interstitial dermatitis (with neutrophils and mononuclear cells usually predominating) and fibrosing dermatitis (Fig. 18–24). Blood eosinophilia and tissue eosinophilia are rare. Chronic, recurrent, medically refractory cases should be evaluated for underlying flea bite hypersensitivity, atopy, and food hypersensitivity.

Therapy with systemic glucocorticoids is often effective. Prednisone or prednisolone is administered orally (4.4 mg/kg q24h) until the lesions are healed. Alternatively, methylprednisolone acetate (Depo-Medrol, Pharmacia & Upjohn) may be administered subcutaneously at 20 mg/cat every 2 weeks until the lesions are healed, or either dexamethasone (0.4 mg/kg q24h) or triamcinolone (0.8 mg/kg q24h) may be administered orally. Recurrent lesions may be managed with alternate-evening oral glucocorticoids or repeated subcutaneous injections of methylprednisolone (never more frequently than every 2 months).

Medically refractory lesions should be evaluated for underlying hypersensitivity disorders and managed appropriately. Some refractory lesions respond to systemic antibiotics (e.g., amoxicillin clavulanate, cefadroxil, enrofloxacin) or topical mupirocin.[2, 74, 80] Antibiotic-responsive lesions contain numerous neutrophils on cytologic and histopathologic examination. Other methods of treatment reported to be occasionally successful in feline indolent ulcer include radiotherapy, cryosurgery, laser therapy, surgical excision, mixed bacterial vaccines, and immunomodulating drugs such as levamisole, thiabendazole, interferon-α (60 to 300 units/day, orally or subcutaneously, for 30 days [see Chap. 3]), and aurothioglucose (Solganal, Schering-Plough).[2, 4, 5, 74] Progestational compounds, such as megestrol acetate (Ovaban, Schering-Plough) have also been effective in many cases of feline indolent ulcer. However, these drugs are not recommended because of their side effects.

Feline Eosinophilic Plaque

Eosinophilic plaque is a common cutaneous lesion of cats. Clinically, most eosinophilic plaques occur on the abdomen and medial thighs (Fig. 18–25A; see Fig. 18–19H).

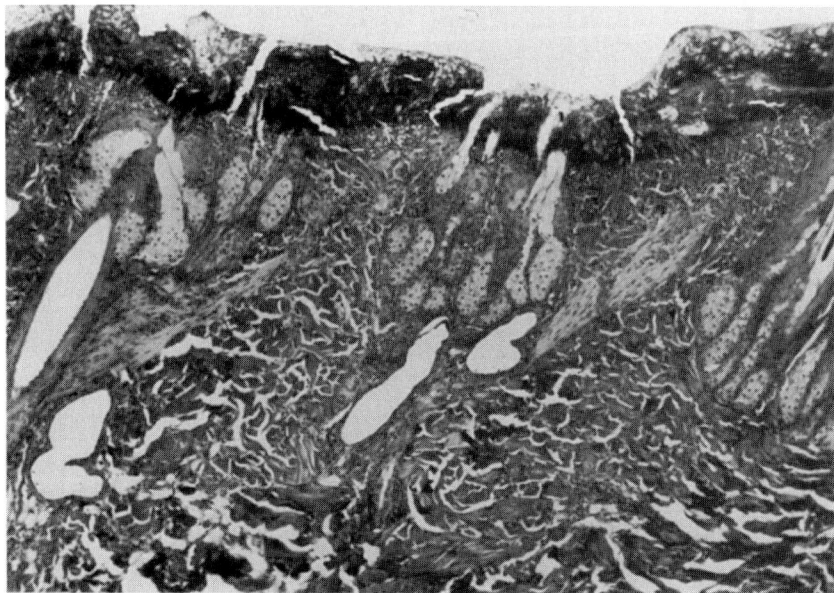

FIGURE 18–24. Histologic section of indolent ulcer. There is surface ulceration with fibrin covering the necrotic surface and a dense mononuclear cellular infiltrate in the dermis. Note the ulcerative perivascular dermatitis. (From Scott, DW: Feline dermatology 1900–1978: A monograph. J Am Anim Hosp Assoc 16:331, 1980.)

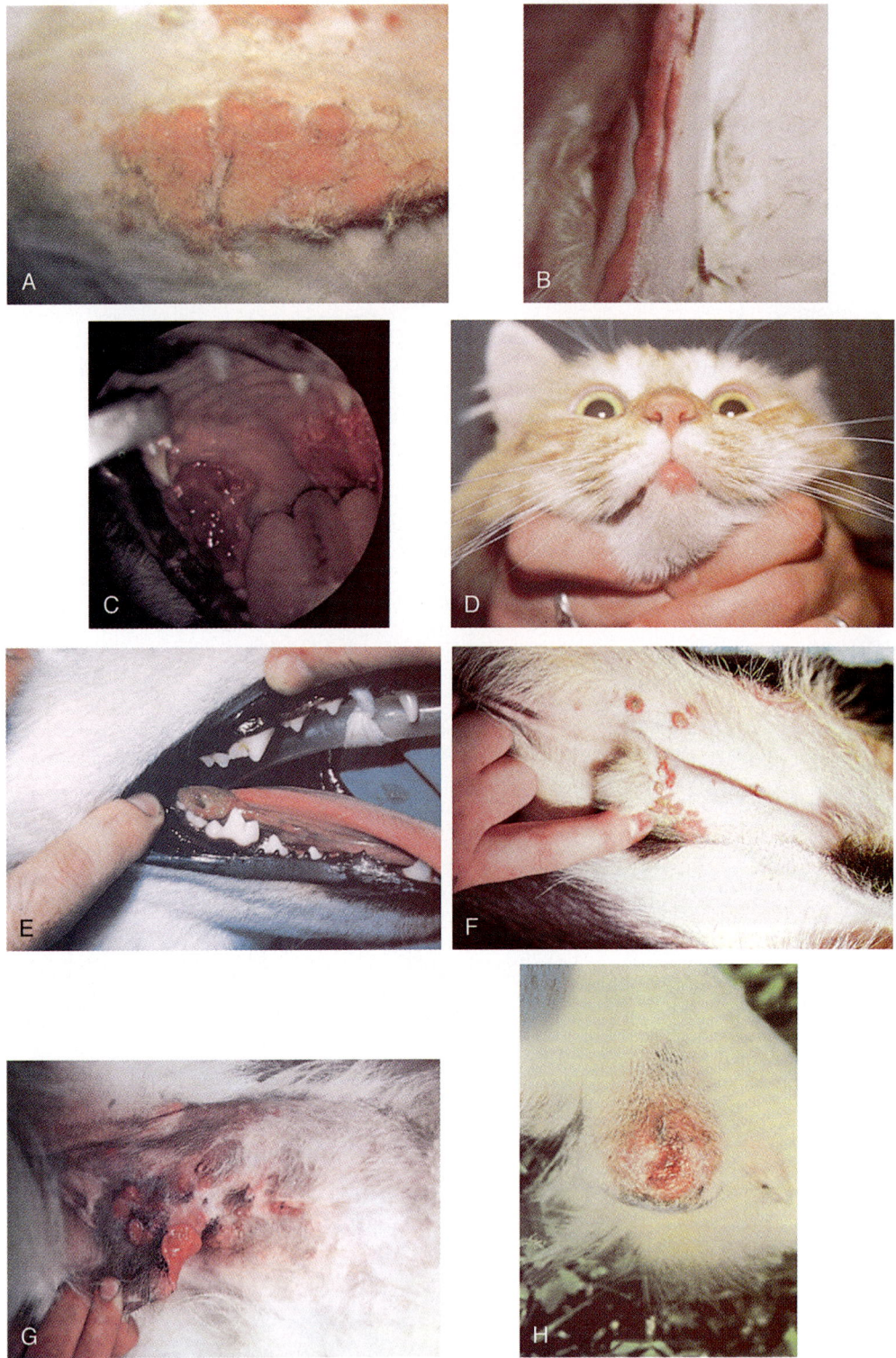

FIGURE 18–25. *A*, Feline eosinophilic plaque. Raised, erythematous abdominal plaque. *B*, Typical eosinophilic granuloma on a white cat's rear leg with hair clipped away. The firm cordlike masses are slightly pink and not ulcerated, painful, or pruritic. *C*, Eosinophilic granuloma bilaterally located at the angles of the jaw behind
Legend continued on opposite page

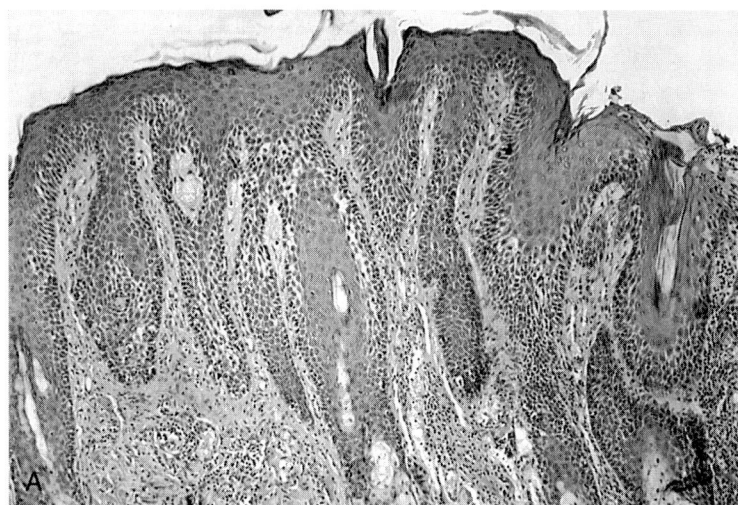
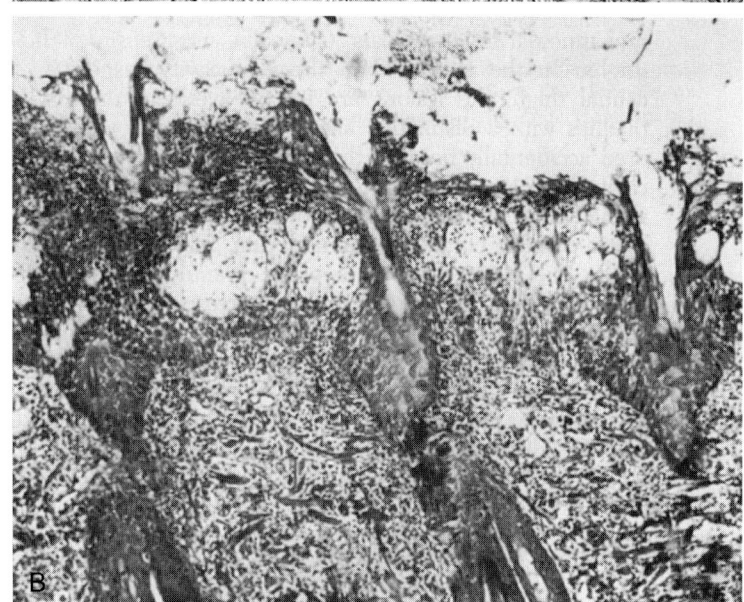

FIGURE 18–26. *A*, Feline eosinophilic plaque. Diffuse spongiosis of epidermis and hair follicle outer root sheaths. *B*, Feline eosinophilic plaque. Diffuse spongiosis and microvesicle or microvesicopustule formation in the epidermis.

Lesions may be single or multiple, and they may also occur on mucocutaneous junctions or in other areas of the skin. Eosinophilic plaques are well circumscribed, raised, round to oval, red, oozing, often ulcerated, and 0.5 to 7 cm in diameter. Pruritus is usually severe. Peripheral lymphadenopathy may be present. Cats with eosinophilic plaque may also have indolent ulcers, eosinophilic granulomas, or both. Lesions that are histologically similar to eosinophilic plaques occasionally occur in the conjunctiva[76] and cornea.[75] There are no age or breed predilections, but females may be predisposed.

FIGURE 18–25 *Continued.* the last molars. A metal mouth gag and plastic endotracheal tube can be seen. The ulcerated lesions have a fibronecrotic surface. Radiation therapy caused prompt remission. *D*, Feline eosinophilic granuloma. Pinkish nodule on the lower lip. *E*, Canine eosinophilic granuloma. Greenish brown mass on the ventrolateral aspect of the tongue near the commissure of the lips. (Courtesy of J. O. Noxon.) *F*, Canine eosinophilic granuloma. Erythematous papules and nodules on the abdomen. *G*, Canine eosinophilic granuloma. Ulcerated nodule on prepuce. *H*, Canine eosinophilic granuloma. Ulcerated nodule on a foot.

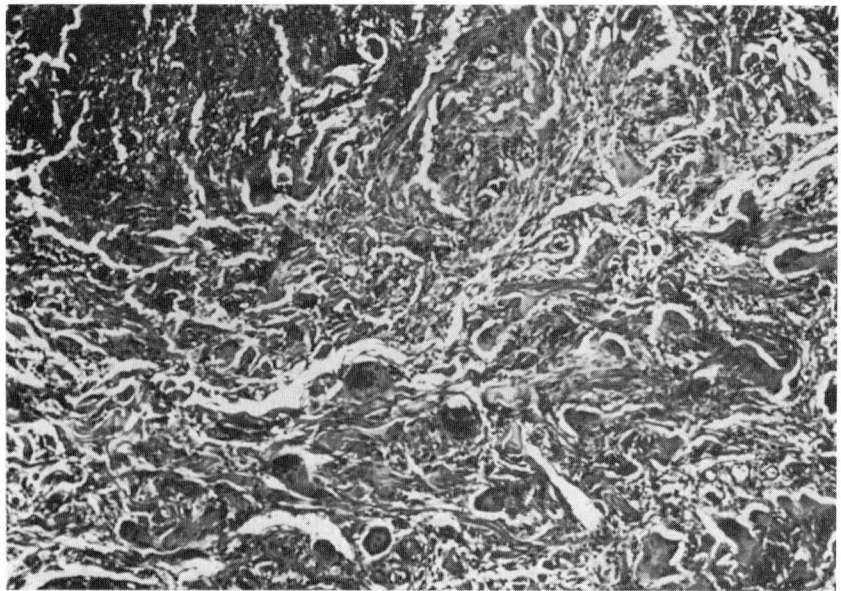

FIGURE 18–29. Feline eosinophilic granuloma. Granulomatous dermatitis associated with flame figures and foreign-body giant cells. (High-power view of Fig. 18–28B.)

of fibrinolysis, disorder of phagocytic function, disorder of catabolic enzyme release, and cell-mediated immune response. In dogs, no antecedent trauma or disease has been recognized, and cultures for bacteria, fungi, and viruses are negative. Macerated tissue from lesions produces no lesions in dogs that have been injected. The tissue eosinophilia, occasional blood eosinophilia, and glucocorticoid responsiveness of lesions have prompted speculation regarding a hypersensitivity state. In addition, the tendency of the oral form of the disease to occur in Siberian huskies and Cavalier King Charles spaniels has suggested a genetic basis for the disease. Some authors have reported the seasonal recurrence of cutaneous eosinophilic granulomas in dogs, suggesting that the condition may be a hypersensitivity reaction to pollens, molds, and insects.

Clinical Features

Although any age, breed, or sex of dog may be affected, eosinophilic granulomas are most common in dogs less than 3 years of age (80% of cases), Siberian huskies (76%), and males (72%). Eosinophilic granulomas occur most commonly in the oral cavity as ulcerated palatine plaques and vegetative lingual masses. The lingual masses often have a greenish brown hue (see Fig. 18–25E). In Cavalier King Charles spaniels, lesions may be solitary on the soft palate or bilateral near the tonsils.[82] Less commonly, they occur as multiple cutaneous papules, nodules, and plaques over the ventral abdomen, prepuce, digits, flanks, and cheek (see Figs. 18–25F to H and 18–30A). The cutaneous lesions are usually nonpruritic and painless, and the dogs are otherwise healthy. Rarely, solitary lesions occur in the external ear canal.[87] There has been one report of a tracheal lesion.[83]

Diagnosis

The differential diagnosis includes granulomatous and neoplastic disorders. Diagnosis is based on biopsy. Characteristic histopathologic findings include variably sized foci of flame figure formation, eosinophilic and histiocytic cellular infiltration, and palisading granulomas (Figs. 18–30B and 18–31). Properly performed cultures are negative, and blood eosinophilia occurs occasionally.

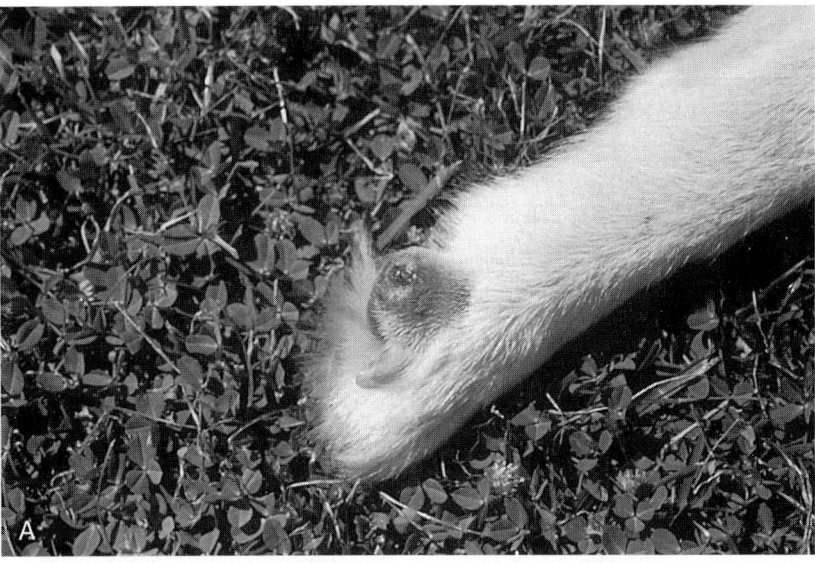
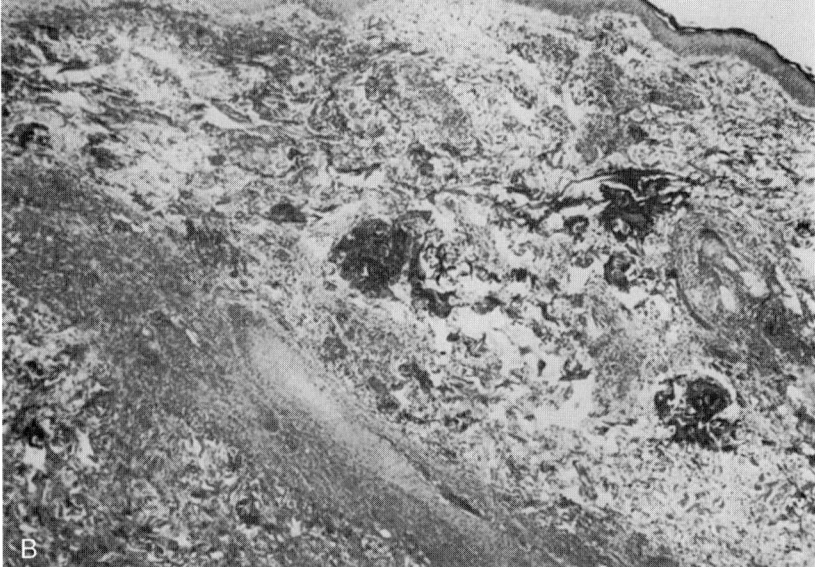

FIGURE 18–30. *A*, Nodule of eosinophilic granuloma on the digit of a Siberian husky. *B*, Canine eosinophilic granuloma. Granulomatous dermatitis associated with flame figures.

Clinical Management

Canine eosinophilic granulomas are usually very glucocorticoid responsive. Seventy-eight percent of cases were treated with prednisolone or prednisone orally (0.5 to 2.2 mg/kg/day); lesions regressed in 10 to 20 days, and no further therapy was needed. Some lesions undergo spontaneous remission, and some lesions are seasonally or chronically recurrent.

• EOSINOPHILIC DERMATITIS AND EDEMA IN DOGS

A syndrome of eosinophilic dermatitis and edema has been described in dogs and compared with eosinophilic cellulitis (Wells' syndrome) in humans.[89a] Four of the 9 dogs were

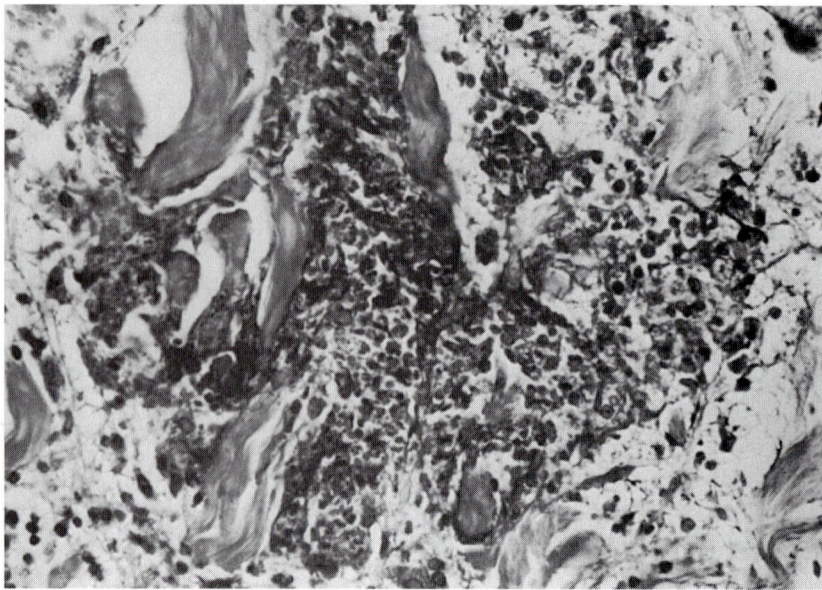

FIGURE 18-31. Canine eosinophilic granuloma. Focal flame figures and accumulation of eosinophils.

Labrador retrievers. All dogs had an acute onset of erythematous macules that progressed and coalesced into arciform and serpiginous plaques, especially on the pinnae and ventral abdomen and thorax. Edema varied from facial to generalized and pitting. Numerous possible triggering events were identified: drugs, new diets, arthropods, and concurrent allergic or immune-mediated diseases.

Histopathologic findings included superficial and deep perivascular to interstitial dermatitis with marked dermal edema and vascular dilatation. Eosinophils were numerous, and flame figures were seen in about half the specimens.

Seven of the 9 dogs were treated with glucocorticoids or hydroxyzine and recovered in 1 to 3 weeks. Two dogs received no treatment: one recovered in 1 week, the other continued to wax and wane.

• PANNICULITIS

Panniculitis is a multifactorial inflammatory condition of the subcutaneous fat, characterized by deep-seated cutaneous nodules that often become cystic and ulcerated and develop draining tracts. The disorder is uncommon in dogs and cats.[101]

Cause and Pathogenesis

The lipocyte (fat cell, adipocyte) is particularly vulnerable to trauma, ischemia, and neighboring inflammatory disease. In addition, damage to lipocytes results in the liberation of lipid, which undergoes hydrolysis into glycerol and fatty acids. Fatty acids are potent inflammatory agents, and they incite further inflammatory and granulomatous tissue reactions.

Multiple etiologic factors are involved in the genesis of panniculitis in human beings (Table 18-1). Many of these factors have yet to be recognized in dogs and cats, but this fact may only reflect lack of awareness. Hereditary deficiency of α_1-antitrypsin predisposes humans to panniculitis in response to various stimuli.[97] α_1-Antitrypsin protects the body

● Table 18–1 **DIFFERENTIAL DIAGNOSIS OF HUMAN PANNICULITIS**

INFECTIOUS
Bacterial,° myobacterial,° actinomycetic,° fungal,° chlamydial, viral
IMMUNOLOGIC
Lupus erythematosus,° rheumatoid arthritis, drug eruption,° erythema nodosum,° arthropod bite°
PHYSICOCHEMICAL (FACTITIAL)
Trauma,° pressure, cold, foreign body° (e.g., postsubcutaneous injection of vaccines or bulky, oily, or insoluble liquids)
PANCREATIC DISEASE
Inflammation,° neoplasia°
POSTGLUCOCORTICOID THERAPY
VASCULITIS*
Leukocytoclastic, periarteritis nodosa, thrombophlebitis, embolism°
NUTRITIONAL
Vitamin E deficiency°
ENTEROPATHIES
HEREDITARY
α_1-Antitrypsin deficiency
IDIOPATHIC*

°Recognized in dogs and cats.

against connective tissue degradation by the neutrophil proteases, elastase and cathepsin G. Serum concentrations of α_1-antitrypsin were found to be normal (1.62 to 2.43 mg/dl) in nine dogs with sterile panniculitis.[97] Infectious and nutritional causes of canine and feline panniculitis are discussed elsewhere (see Chaps. 4, 5, and 17) and are therefore not addressed here. This discussion concentrates on sterile forms of panniculitis.

Nodular panniculitis refers to sterile subcutaneous inflammatory nodules and is not a specific disease. It is a purely descriptive term, clinically representing the end result of several known and unknown etiologic factors.[101] Weber-Christian panniculitis has been a frequently misused term and does not exist as a specific disease. In dogs and cats, the majority of cases of sterile nodular panniculitis are solitary lesions of idiopathic origin. A few cases of lupus erythematosus panniculitis and erythema nodosum have been recognized in dogs (see Chap. 9).[4, 101] Panniculitis has also been described in dogs and cats in association with pancreatic disease (carcinoma, necrosis).[92, 97, 99, 100] Eosinophilic panniculitis in humans has been associated with arthropods, injection reactions, and lymphoma.[90] Eosinophilic panniculitis is rarely described in dogs and cats[96, 101] and could be associated with arthropods and injections.

Clinical Features

Panniculitis is manifested clinically as deep-seated cutaneous nodules. The lesions may occur singly or in crops; they are either localized to specific areas or generalized, and they vary from a few millimeters to several centimeters in diameter. Nodules may be firm and well circumscribed or soft and ill defined (Fig. 18–32A). They are initially subcutaneous but may fix the overlying skin as they progress. The lesions may become cystic, ulcerate, and develop draining tracts that discharge an oily, yellowish brown to bloody substance (see Fig. 18–32B and C). The lesions may or may not be painful and often heal with depressed scars. Hyperpigmentation may also occur around the lesions or at the site of healing lesions. A report of pedal panniculitis in German shepherd dogs describes localized panniculitis proximal to the tarsal and carpal pads.[98] We believe that these cases are identical to *metatarsal fistulation* (see Chap. 12).

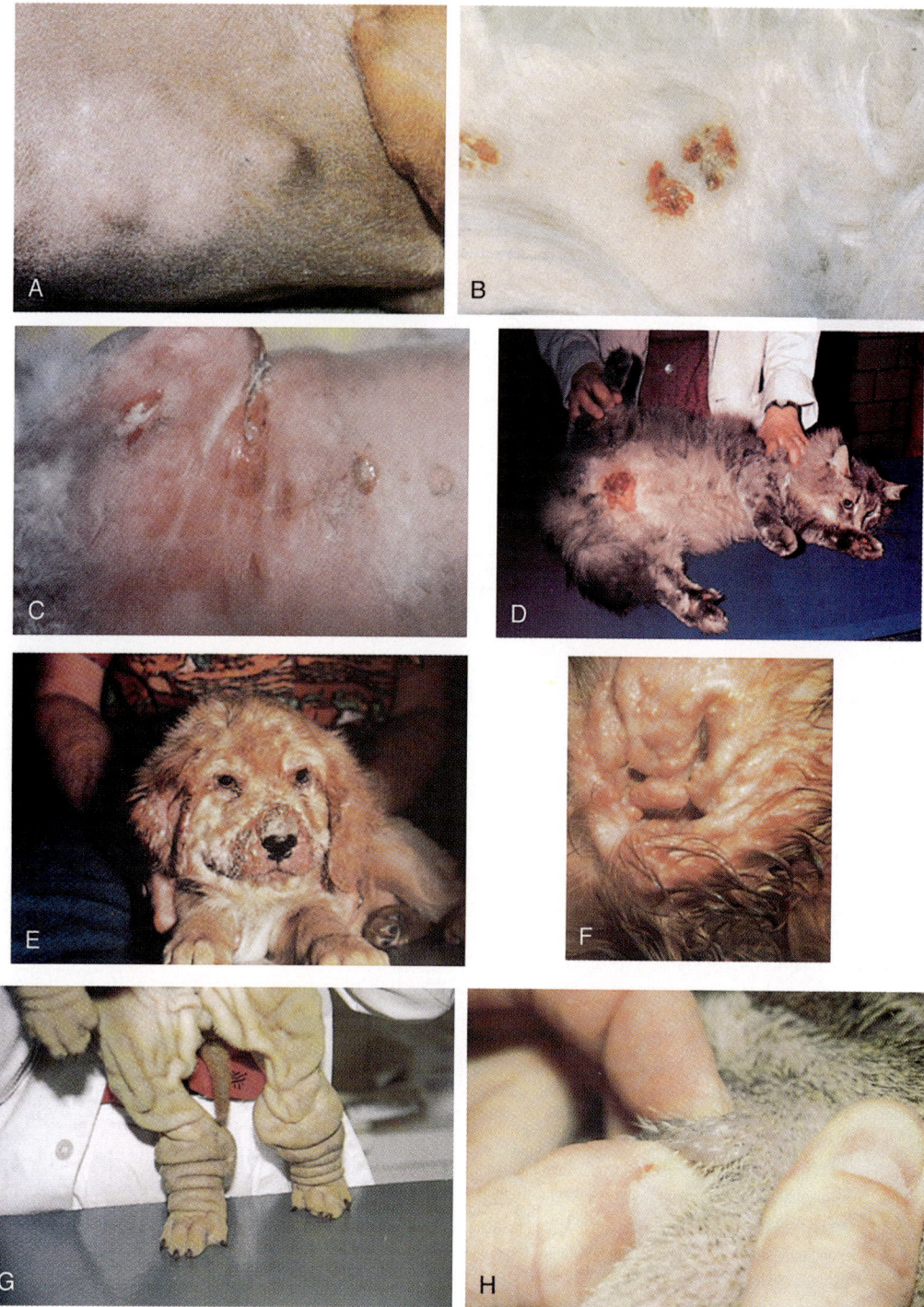

FIGURE 18–32. *A*, Idiopathic sterile panniculitis in a Dachshund. Two subcutaneous nodules on the trunk. *B*, Canine idiopathic sterile panniculitis. Subcutaneous nodule with multiple draining tracts. *C*, Feline panniculitis. Multiple fistulae on the ventral abdomen. *D*, Idiopathic sterile panniculitis in a cat. Ulcerated nodule in the groin. *E*, Juvenile cellulitis in a Golden retriever. Erythema, edema, exudation, crusting, and alopecia on the face and pinnae. *F*, Same dog as in *E*. Multiple pustules in the ear canal and on the pinna. *G*, Idiopathic mucinosis in a Chinese Shar pei. Marked thickening and folding of the skin. *H*, Idiopathic mucinosis in a Chinese Shar pei. Close-up of a mucinous vesicle.

DOG

The majority (80%) of dogs have a solitary lesion, most commonly over the ventrolateral chest, neck, and abdomen.[101] No age, breed, or sex predilections are apparent in dogs with solitary lesions.

Dogs with multiple lesions often have constitutional signs, including poor appetite, depression, lethargy, and pyrexia.[91, 95, 101, 102] These signs are sometimes intermittent, heralding a new crop of skin lesions. A rare dog has arthralgias, abdominal pain, vomiting, or hepatosplenomegaly.[91, 95, 97] In dogs with multiple skin lesions, the trunk is most commonly involved. There is no age predilection, but female dogs may be over-represented. Although all breeds and mongrels may be affected, Dachshunds and Poodles appear to be predisposed.[2, 5, 97]

Dogs with pancreatic panniculitis have severe systemic signs (fever, anorexia, depression, vomiting, abdominal pain) and concurrent necrotizing steatitis (abdominal, mesenteric, pleural).[92, 92a, 99]

CAT

The majority (95%) of cats have a solitary lesion, most commonly over the ventral abdomen and ventrolateral thorax (see Figs. 18–32D and 18–33A).[101] Cats with multiple lesions often have constitutional signs as described for dogs.[95, 100, 101] No age, breed, or sex predilections are evident.

Diagnosis

Sterile nodular panniculitis is most commonly misdiagnosed as deep pyoderma, cutaneous cysts, or cutaneous neoplasms. Aspirates from intact lesions usually reveal numerous neutrophils, foamy macrophages, and no microorganisms (see Fig. 18–33B).[94] The presence of numerous eosinophils suggests arthropod- or injection-induced lesions. Sudan stains may reveal extracellular and intracellular lipid droplets. Animals with multiple lesions and systemic illness often have mild to moderate leukocytosis and neutrophilia, mild nonregenerative anemia, and elevated α_2, β_1, and β_2 globulin fractions on serum protein electrophoresis.[95] Direct immunofluorescence testing may reveal the deposition of Ig and complement at the basement membrane zone.[95] Animals with pancreatic panniculitis may have increased serum concentrations of amylase and lipase.

Panniculitis can be diagnosed only by biopsy, and excision biopsy is the only biopsy technique that is satisfactory for subcutaneous nodules.[3, 5] Punch biopsies fail to deliver tissue sufficient to be of diagnostic value in about 75% of cases. Panniculitis may be lobular, septal, or diffuse, or it may have a combination of these characteristics.[101] In addition, panniculitis may be granulomatous, pyogranulomatous, suppurative, eosinophilic, necrotizing, or fibrosing.[101] Thrombosis of subcuticular blood vessels, lymphoid nodules, and radial fat crystals may occur.[101] The histopathologic pattern and cytomorphologic picture of the reactions have little diagnostic, therapeutic, or prognostic significance (Figs. 18–34 to 18–37). Lipid-laden macrophages (lipophages) are often prominent (see Fig. 18–37B). It is imperative to realize that most panniculitides, regardless of cause, look histologically identical. Thus, one cannot diagnose sterile nodular panniculitis from a biopsy specimen. Special stains and cultures are always indicated to rule out infectious agents, and polarized light examination is indicated to rule out foreign bodies. Tissue cultures for aerobic, anaerobic, and mycobacterial cultures are negative prior to a diagnosis of sterile nodular panniculitis.

If the panniculitis is predominantly lymphohistioplasmacytic, with or without concurrent neutrophilic vasculitis or interface dermatitis, or if other clinical signs suggest lupus erythematosus, other diagnostic tests may include antinuclear antibody and direct immunofluorescence testing of lesional skin (see Chap. 9). If vasculitis is present, the diagnostic tests indicated may reflect the differential diagnosis of vasculitis (see Chap. 9). If panniculitis is persistent and refractory or if the patient shows concurrent signs of gastrointestinal disease, pancreatic disease should be ruled out.

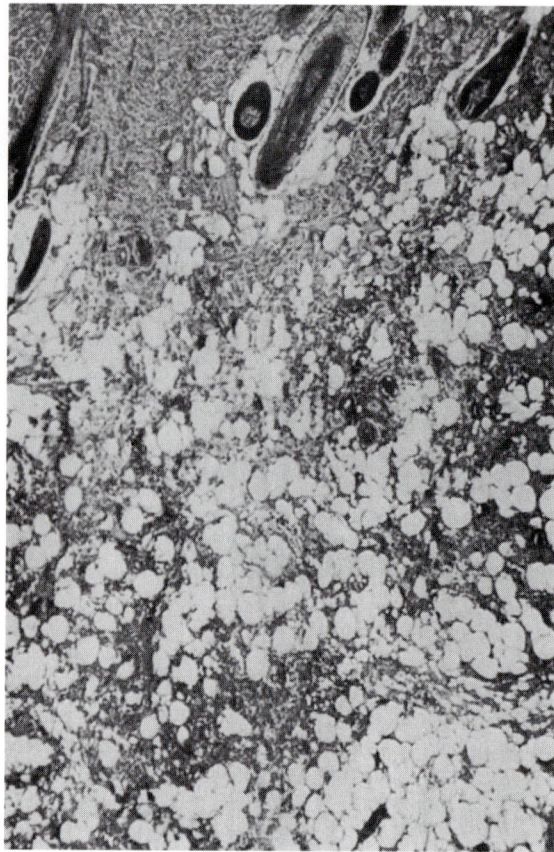

FIGURE 18-36. Feline idiopathic sterile panniculitis. Marked lobular panniculitis and fat necrosis. (From Scott DW: Feline dermatology 1900-1978: A monograph. J Am Anim Hosp Assoc 16:331, 1980.)

Prednisolone or prednisone may be administered orally (2 mg/kg q24h in dogs, 4 mg/kg q24h in cats) until the lesions have regressed (in 3 to 8 weeks). Therapy should be stopped at that point because many dogs, especially young dogs, experience long-term or permanent remission. In recurrent cases, alternate-day steroid therapy may be required for prolonged periods.

In a few canine and feline cases, good results have been obtained with oral vitamin E (dl-α-tocopherol acetate), 400 IU q12h.[4, 101] The vitamin E must be given at least 2 hours before or after a meal for maximum effectiveness. In humans, oral potassium iodide has been used successfully in cases of sterile nodular panniculitis; one of us (D.W.S.) has used this agent successfully in two dogs. One case of pedal panniculitis responded to only vitamin E therapy; vitamin E therapy had a steroid-sparing effect in two others.[98] We have had success with tetracycline and niacinamide in a few dogs (see Chap. 3).

● SUBCUTANEOUS FAT SCLEROSIS

Subcutaneous fat sclerosis has been described in a 1-year-old male domestic shorthaired cat.[104] An inguinal abscess had been treated by surgical drainage and antibiotics 5 weeks prior to the appearance of a rapidly growing abdominal subcutaneous mass. The mass was a firm, painless subcutaneous plaque that extended from the xiphoid process to the pelvic inlet and laterally to the lumbar processes. The borders were raised and distinct, and the normal overlying skin was cool, indurated, and adherent. The mass was large enough to restrict movement of the legs. Differential diagnosis included neoplasia, panniculitis, and nutritional steatitis. Results of a hemogram and serum chemistry profile were normal. Bacterial and fungal cultures were negative. Oral treatment with prednisolone was not

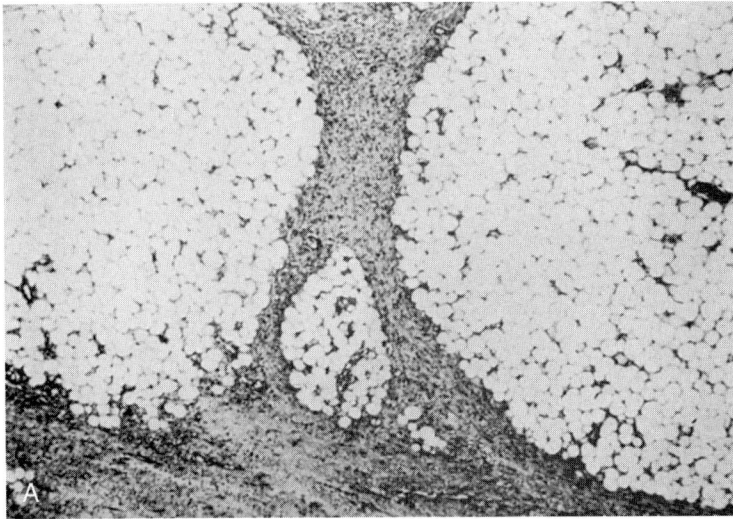
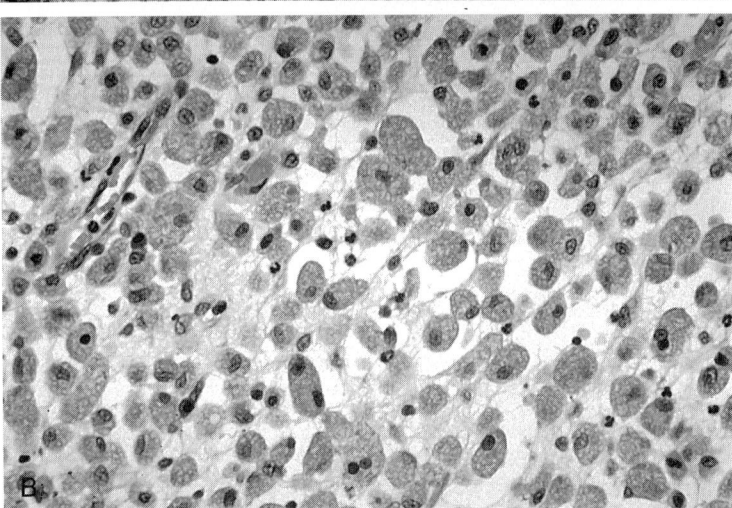

FIGURE 18-37. *A*, Septal panniculitis in a cat. *B*, Numerous lipophages in a postinjection panniculitis in a cat.

effective. Later, small subcutaneous satellite nodules could be palpated on the chest wall cranial to the mass.

On necropsy, the abdominal subcutaneous tissues were thickened, fibrous, and adherent to the dermis. Histopathologic findings revealed extensive subcutaneous fibrosis with minimal fat necrosis and inflammation. Within the subcutaneous fat, or within the fat-rich interstitial tissues of abdominal muscles, were bands of septal fibrosis, fat cells of increased size (fat micropseudocyst formation), and lipocytes containing needle-shaped fat clefts (fat crystals) (Fig. 18-39). Although a few scattered lymphocytes, histiocytes, and multinucleated histiocytic giant cells were found, and although there were isolated foci of neutrophils, the process was largely noninflammatory.

These findings are similar to two rare human disorders: sclerema neonatorum and subcutaneous fat necrosis of the newborn.[1] The latter is indistinguishable from poststeroid panniculitis, but this cat had no history of corticosteroid administration.

• CANINE JUVENILE CELLULITIS

Juvenile cellulitis (juvenile pyoderma, puppy strangles, juvenile sterile granulomatous dermatitis and lymphadenitis) is an uncommon granulomatous and pustular disorder of the face, pinnae, and submandibular lymph nodes, usually of puppies.[3, 107-109]

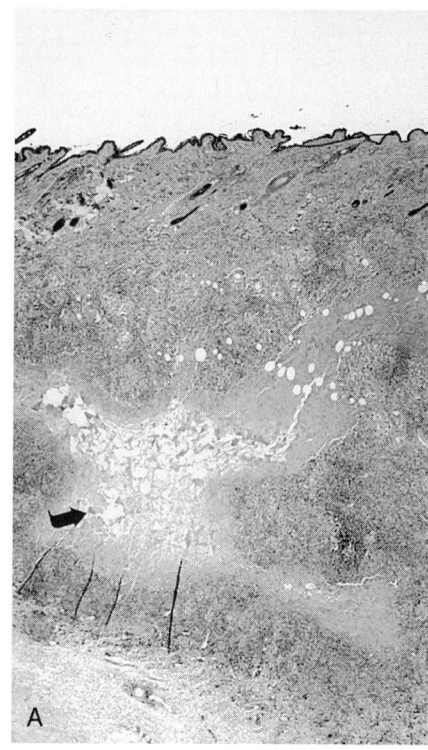
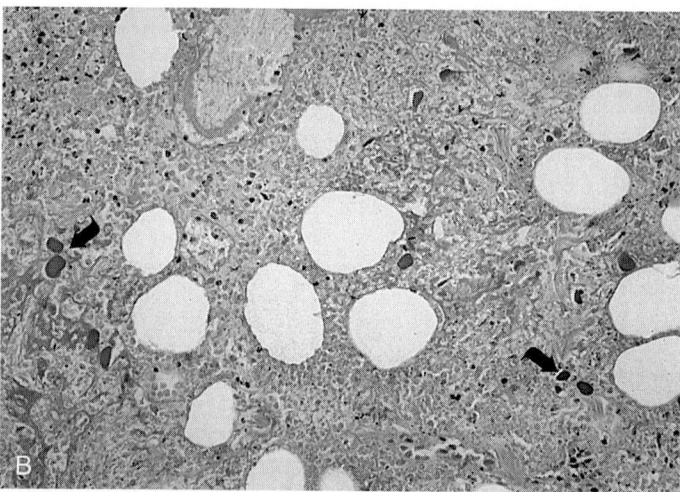

FIGURE 18–38. Postinjection panniculitis (rabies vaccine) in a cat. A, Granulomatous nodule surrounding central area of necrosis and flocculent foreign material (*arrow*). B, Close-up of A. Note shiny, amorphous deposits of vaccine-related material (*arrows*).

Cause and Pathogenesis

The cause and pathogenesis are unknown. Heritability is supported by an increased occurrence in certain breeds and by familial histories of disease.[3, 107–109] The occurrence of sterile granulomas and pustules that respond dramatically to glucocorticoids suggests an underlying immune dysfunction. Special stains and electron microscopic examination of tissues do not reveal microorganisms, and cultures are negative.[108] Attempts to transmit the disease with lesional tissues have been unsuccessful.[108]

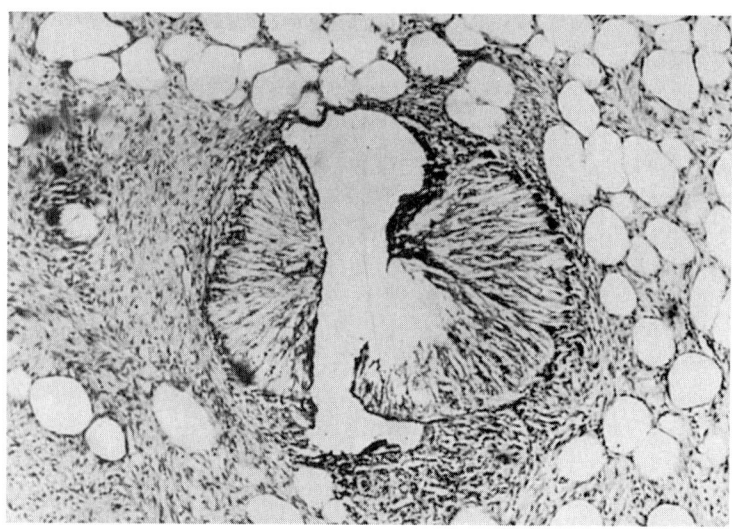

FIGURE 18–39. Sclerosing panniculitis in a cat. Fat crystal with radial configuration.

Clinical Features

Puppies are affected between the ages of 3 weeks and 4 months, and one or several puppies in a litter may have the condition. A 2-year-old Lhasa apso experienced adult-onset juvenile cellulitis; we have also seen this in young adult dogs.[106] Although numerous breeds have experienced the disorder, Golden retrievers, Dachshunds, and Gordon setters appear to be predisposed.[3, 4, 107–109] The initial abnormality noticed by most owners is an acutely swollen face, especially the eyelids, lips, and muzzle. Physical examination at this time reveals striking submandibular lymphadenopathy. Within 24 to 48 hours, papules and pustules develop rapidly, especially on the lips, muzzle, chin, bridge of the nose, and periocular area. Lesions typically fistulate, drain, and crust (see Fig. 18–32E). A marked pustular otitis externa is common (Fig. 18–32F), and the pinnae frequently are thickened and edematous. Affected skin is usually painful but not pruritic. About 50% of affected puppies are lethargic. Anorexia, pyrexia, and joint pain (sterile suppurative arthritis) are present in up to 25% of cases.

Puppies occasionally have concurrent sterile pyogranulomatous panniculitis with firm to fluctuant subcutaneous nodules that may be painful or fistulate. These nodules especially occur on the trunk or in the preputial or perianal areas.[3, 4, 107–109] Two Shetland sheepdog puppies with panniculitis had neurologic signs consistent with spinal cord lesions.

Diagnosis

In very early cases, the differential diagnosis is angioedema (see Chap. 8). However, angioedema is not accompanied by marked regional lymphadenopathy or systemic illness. After the dramatic inflammatory lesions have appeared, the differential diagnosis includes staphylococcal dermatitis, demodicosis, and adverse cutaneous drug reaction.

Cytologic examination of papulopustular lesions reveals pyogranulomatous inflammation with no microorganisms (Fig. 18–40). Carefully performed cultures are negative. Biopsies of early lesions reveal multiple discrete or confluent granulomas and pyogranulomas consisting of clusters of large epithelioid macrophages with variably sized cores of neutrophils (Fig. 18–41).[3, 5, 108] Sebaceous glands and epitrichial sweat glands may be obliterated. In later severe lesions, suppurative changes in the superficial dermis, in and

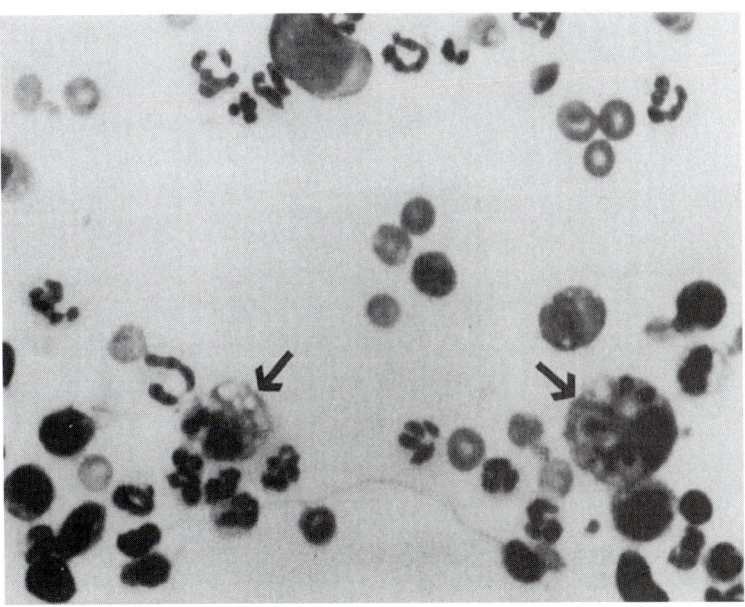

FIGURE 18–40. Juvenile cellulitis. Cytologic examination reveals pyogranulomatous inflammation wherein neutrophils appear nondegenerate and no microorganisms are seen. Note neutrophagocytosis by two macrophages (*arrows*).

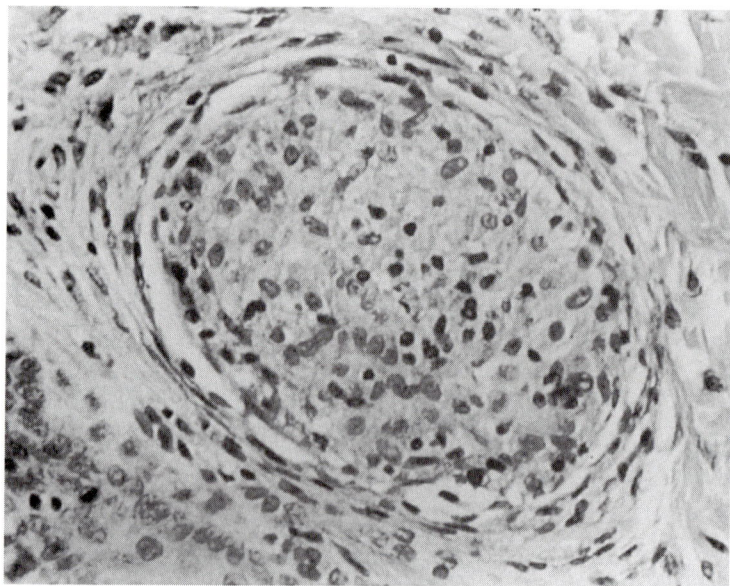

FIGURE 18-41. Juvenile cellulitis. Well-demarcated dermal granuloma from an early case.

around ruptured hair follicles, and in the subjacent panniculus are predominant (Fig. 18-42).

Total globulin levels and results of serum electrophoresis, immunoelectrophoresis, and bactericidal assays are normal.[5] Lymphocyte blastogenic responses to phytomitogens are suppressed in association with a serum suppressor factor.[4, 105]

Clinical Management

Early and aggressive therapy is indicated because scarring can be severe. Large doses of glucocorticoids are the treatment of choice. Prednisone or prednisolone (2 mg/kg q24h

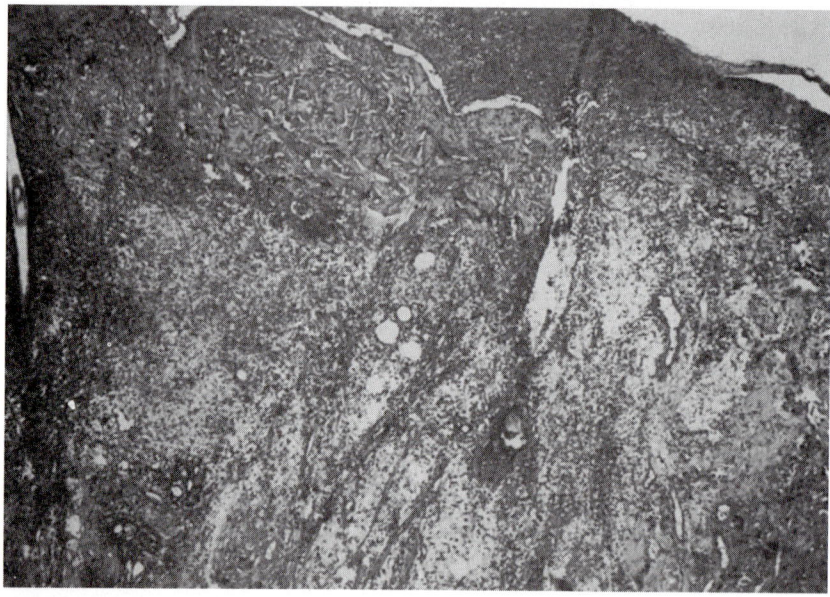

FIGURE 18-42. Juvenile cellulitis in a dog. Note diffuse cellulitis.

orally) is administered daily until the disease is inactive (usually in 10 to 14 days). Dogs with intercurrent truncal panniculitis may require a longer course of treatment to resolve all lesions. Some dogs respond much better to dexamethasone (0.2 mg/kg q24h orally). If there is cytologic or clinical evidence of secondary bacterial infection, bactericidal antibiotics (cephalexin, cefadroxil, amoxicillin clavulanate) should be given simultaneously. Topical therapy, especially wet soaks with aluminum acetate or magnesium sulfate (see Chap. 3) are useful, but puppies often find the restraint and pain undesirable, and the struggling and stress associated with the topical therapy become counterproductive. Relapses are virtually unheard of.

● FELINE ULCERATIVE DERMATITIS WITH LINEAR SUBEPIDERMAL FIBROSIS

This is an uncommon feline dermatosis.[3, 110]

Cause and Pathogenesis

The cause and pathogenesis of this disorder are unknown. Trauma, injections, foreign bodies, and infectious agents do not appear to play a role.

Clinical Features

Any age, breed, or sex of cat may be affected. Typically, lesions are solitary and occur over the dorsal neck and shoulder area (Fig. 18–43). Crusted ulcers, 0.2 cm to 1 cm in diameter, enlarge slowly over a period of weeks to months. No pruritus and pain are

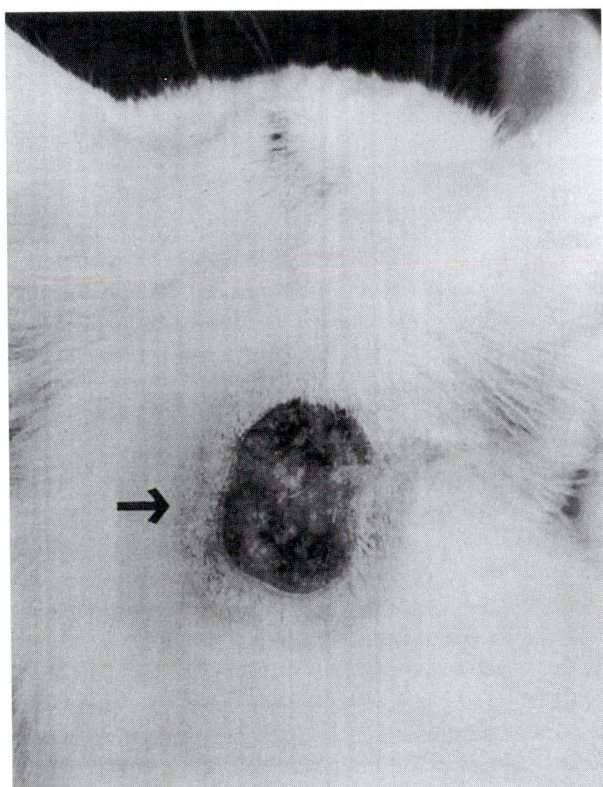

FIGURE 18–43. Feline ulcerative dermatitis with linear subepidermal fibrosis. Chronic nonhealing ulcer over the dorsal neck. Note the rim of thickened skin that surrounds the ulcer (*arrow*; area has been clipped).

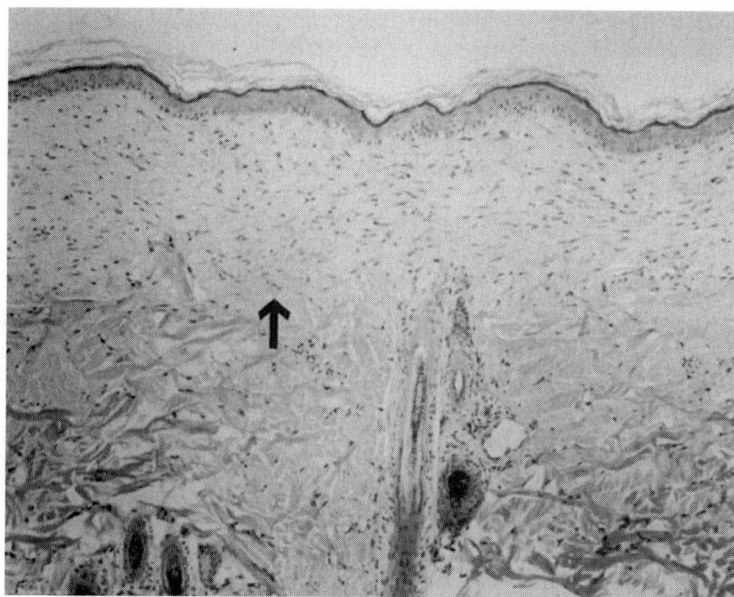

FIGURE 18-44. Feline ulcerative dermatitis with linear subepidermal fibrosis. Note the bandlike area of subepidermal fibrosis of the superficial dermis (*arrow*).

present, and affected cats are otherwise healthy. These nonhealing ulcers typically have a thick, adherent, brown crust, and a rim of firm, thickened skin surrounds the ulcer.

Diagnosis

The differential diagnosis includes trauma, injection reactions, burns, infections, panniculitis, and neoplasia (especially squamous cell carcinoma). Biopsy reveals ulcerative dermatitis with rather mild, subjacent superficial perivascular to interstitial dermatitis. Eosinophils are not a prominent inflammatory cell type. The characteristic finding is a linear subepidermal band of superficial dermal fibrosis (Fig. 18-44) that extends peripherally from the ulcer to a distance of several pilosebaceous units.

Clinical Management

Either surgical excision or aggressive glucocorticoid therapy is usually curative. The recommended glucocorticoid protocol is 20 mg of methylprednisolone acetate/cat subcutaneously, every 2 weeks, until the cat is cured.

• PERFORATING DERMATITIS

An unusual perforating dermatitis has been described in cats.[111, 112] Multiple firm, conical, hyperkeratotic, yellowish brown lesions, 2 to 7 mm in diameter, are present over various areas of the body (Fig. 18-45). The lesions tend to cluster and form linear configurations. The lesions cannot easily be scraped or pulled off. In one cat,[112] pruritus and pain were not features. In another cat,[111] lesions occurred wherever the animal excoriated itself and at the sites of suture placement after skin biopsy.

The differential diagnosis is that of a cutaneous horn (see Chap. 20). Biopsy reveals superficial interstitial dermatitis, rich in eosinophils and mast cells, underlying a conical, exophytic projection from the skin surface (Fig. 18-46). The exophytic mass consists of necrotic cellular debris, strands of keratin, and numerous collagen fibers in varying degrees of degeneration. There is transepidermal elimination of collagen fibers, often vertically oriented, into the base of the surface mass (Fig. 18-47). Superficial and middle

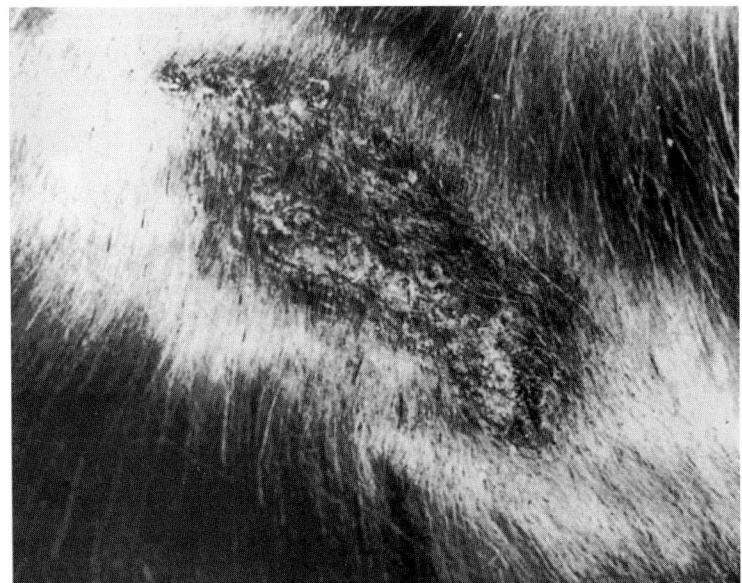

FIGURE 18–45. Perforating dermatitis over the hip of a cat. Note the linear arrangement of hyperkeratotic papules.

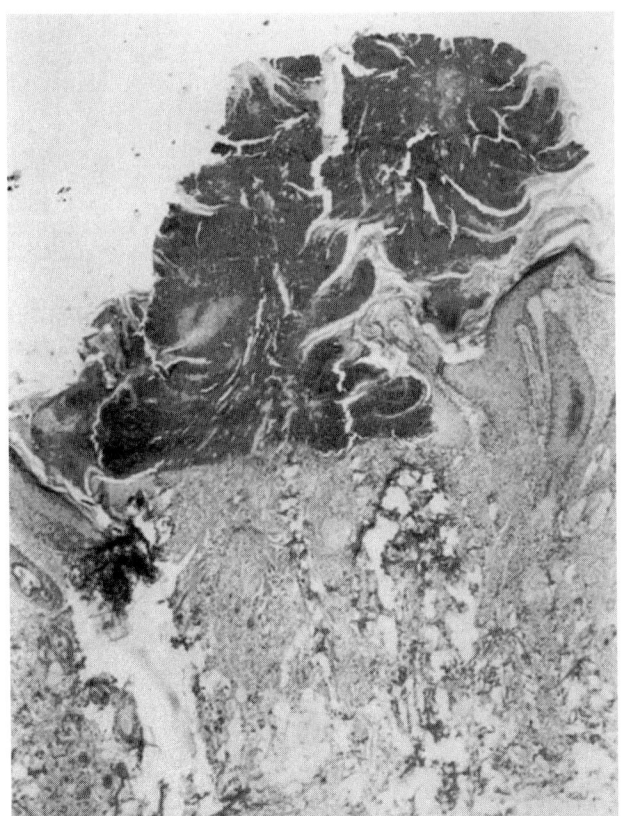

FIGURE 18–46. Perforating dermatitis in a cat. Exophytic conical mass containing degenerate collagen, inflammatory cells, and keratin.

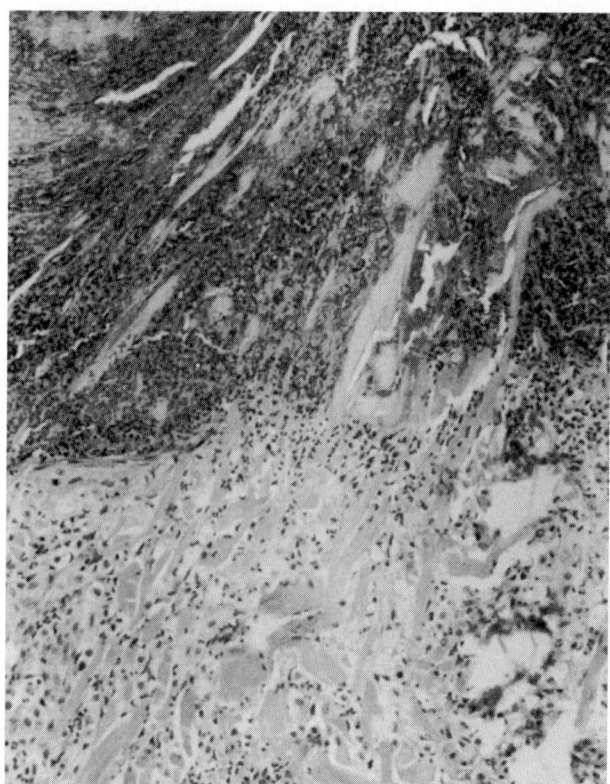

FIGURE 18-47. Perforating dermatitis in a cat. Vertical orientation of degenerate collagen fibers projecting into the exophytic surface mass.

dermal collagen fibers show a segmental staining abnormality in sections stained with Masson's trichrome. With this stain, collagen fibers stain homogeneously blue. In perforating dermatitis, the collagen fibers show segmental red bands. This staining abnormality has been described in animals with cutaneous asthenia and acquired skin fragility; it presumably indicates some kind of abnormality in collagen metabolism (synthesis, packing, degradation).

Clinical Management

In one cat,[112] treatment with ascorbic acid (vitamin C), 100 mg q12h orally, resulted in resolution of the lesions within 30 days. However, when therapy was stopped, the lesions recurred within 8 months. In another cat, successful treatment also necessitated controlling the concurrent allergic skin disease.[111]

• FELINE ACQUIRED SKIN FRAGILITY

This is a rare disorder with multiple etiologic factors. It is characterized by markedly thin and fragile skin in the absence of hyperextensibility.[3, 113–116]

Cause and Pathogenesis

The pathogenesis of the cutaneous changes is unknown, and the cause appears to be multifactorial. Most reported cases have been associated with spontaneous or iatrogenic Cushing's syndrome (see Chap. 10), diabetes mellitus, or the excessive use of progestational compounds.[3, 114, 116] However, isolated cases have been reported in association with liver disease (lipidosis, cholangiohepatitis, or cholangiocarcinoma), phenytoin administration, feline dysautonomia, or nephrosis.[113–116] In some cats, serum biochemical profiles and

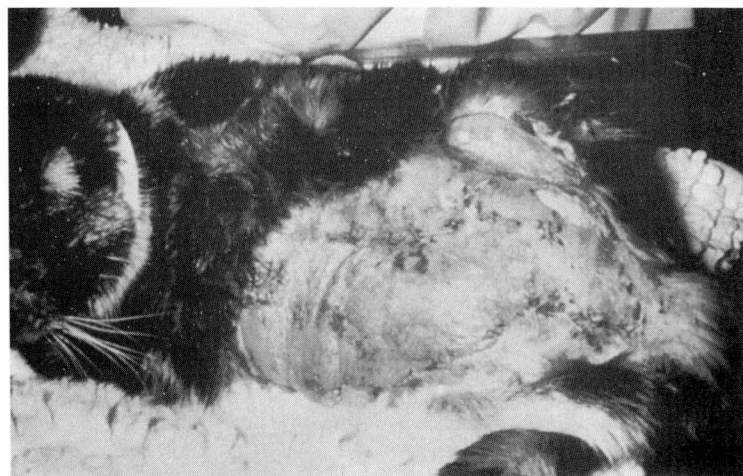

FIGURE 18–48. Feline acquired skin fragility. Extensive area of full-thickness skin loss over the trunk of a cushingoid cat. (Courtesy of R. Rosychuk.)

adrenal function test results have been normal, and no associated diseases were found at necropsy.[3, 114]

Clinical Features

Most affected cats are middle-aged or older. The skin becomes markedly thin and is damaged readily by minor trauma. Extreme cutaneous friability leads to irregular tears and the shedding of large sheets of skin (Figs. 18–48 to 18–50). The skin may become so thin that it takes on a translucent quality. Partial alopecia may occur. The skin is not hyperextensible.

Diagnosis

The differential diagnosis includes spontaneous and iatrogenic Cushing's syndrome and diabetes mellitus; appropriate laboratory tests should be performed. Similar signs occur in

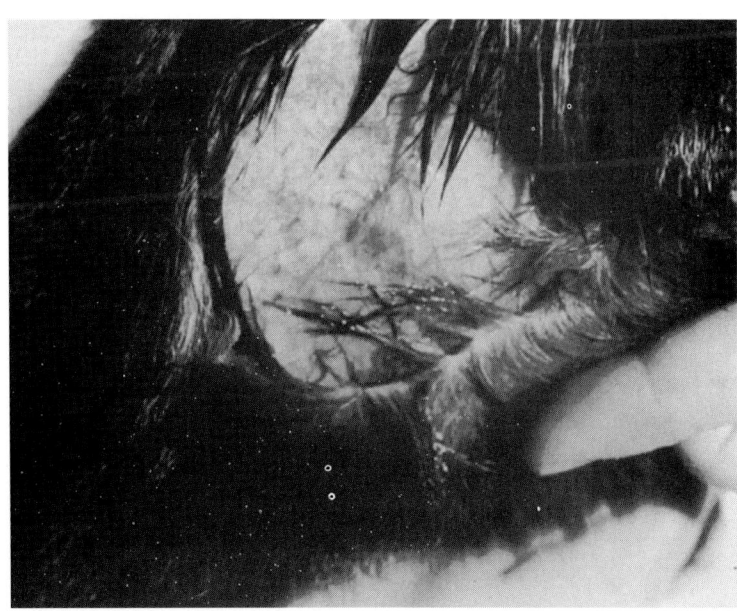

FIGURE 18–49. Feline acquired skin fragility. Large, full-thickness tear over the thorax of a cat with cholangiohepatitis.

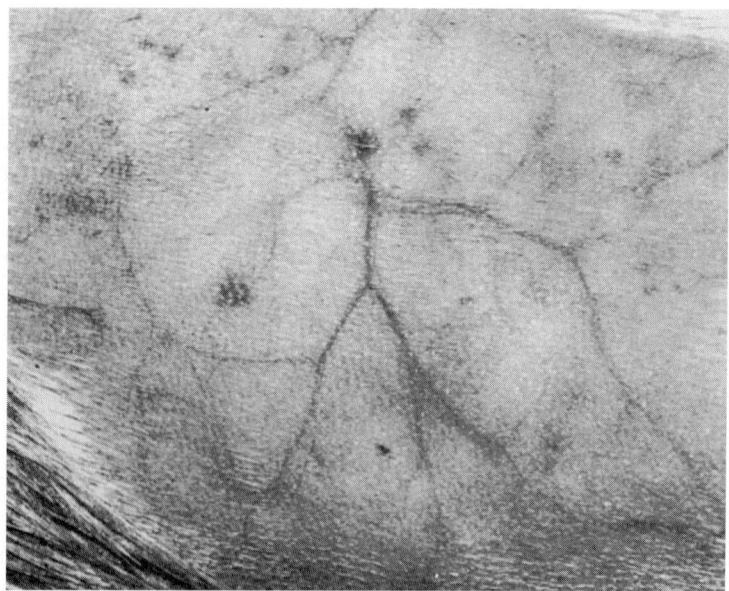

FIGURE 18–50. Feline acquired skin fragility. Remarkable thinning of truncal skin with resultant easy visualization of the underlying blood vessels in a cat with megestrol acetate-induced diabetes mellitus.

some cats with cutaneous asthenia; in these cases, however, the abnormalities are present from birth. Whereas the skin extensibility index is a useful clinical tool for the documentation of cutaneous asthenia (see Chap. 12), its use is contraindicated in acquired skin fragility.

Because of the extreme attenuation of the skin, biopsy is difficult. The tissue often folds and twists as wet tissue paper does, and the dermis is severely atrophic. Dermal collagen fibers are very thin and disorganized (Fig. 18–51).[3, 114] Panniculus is usually not present in biopsy specimens. The epidermis and hair follicles may be atrophied. Masson's trichrome–stained sections may show the segmental staining abnormality of collagen seen in cutaneous asthenia (see Chap. 12), but to a much milder degree.[114] Electron microscopic findings may be impossible to distinguish from those of severe cases of cutaneous asthenia (see Chap. 12).[114]

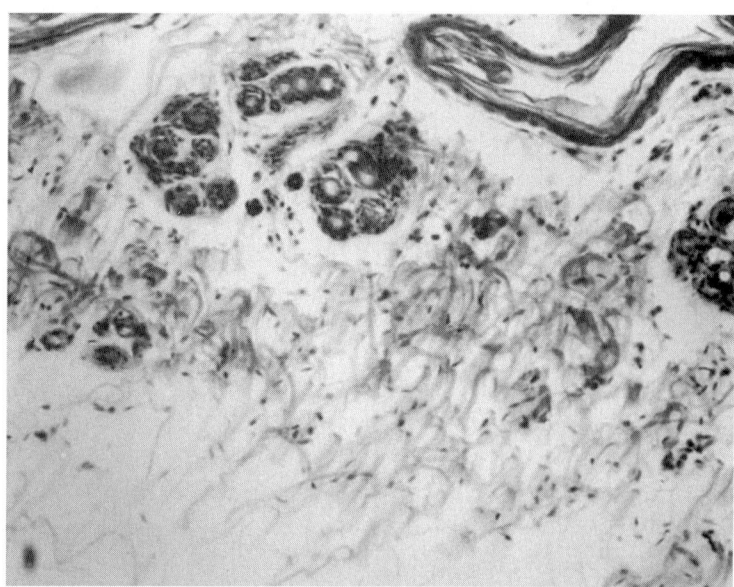

FIGURE 18–51. Feline acquired skin fragility. Note attenuated, disorganized, and wispy collagen fibers.

Clinical Management

Regardless of the underlying cause demonstrated, the prognosis is grave. Affected cats are very difficult to handle without skinning them. Surgical repair is usually unsuccessful and leads to more extensive damage. Early cases in association with spontaneous or iatrogenic Cushing's syndrome have resolved when the inciting cause was eliminated.

• IDIOPATHIC DIFFUSE LIPOMATOSIS

This condition is extremely rare in dogs and cats.[3, 5, 117] Adult animals are presented for progressively enlarging skin folds, especially over the neck and trunk. The cutaneous abnormalities are symmetric, but may be more severe on one side of the body than on the other (Fig. 18–52). The skin folds are pendulous, thick, heavy, and blubbery. Skin overlying larger folds may be thin, hypotrichotic, and traumatized from contact with the environment.

Biopsy reveals a remarkable diffuse thickening of the panniculus (Fig. 18–53). Proliferating fat may resemble mature adipose tissue, with mucinosis only of interlobular septae and with small numbers of primitive mesenchymal cells and lipoblasts around blood vessels. In other cases, the normal anatomy of the panniculus is lost in a proliferative mixture of normal-appearing and dysplastic lipocytes (Fig. 18–54).

There is no effective therapy.

• IDIOPATHIC ACQUIRED CUTANEOUS LAXITY

An unusual dermal collagen disorder was reported in a 9-year-old male English setter[118] in which large folds of pendulous skin had recently developed on both sides of the head and under the neck. The folds were composed of thin skin with a jelly-like subcutis, whereas other areas of the dog's body were covered with normal skin. On necropsy, the dermis in the affected areas was found to be only two thirds of the normal thickness, and the dermal collagen bundles were smaller than normal in diameter, fragmented, and widely separated by ground substance. The elastin was normal. The affected tissues contained areas of necrotic subcutaneous fat and vessels with endothelial swelling and a decreased lumen. No inflammation was observed. Vascular insufficiency was proposed as the cause.

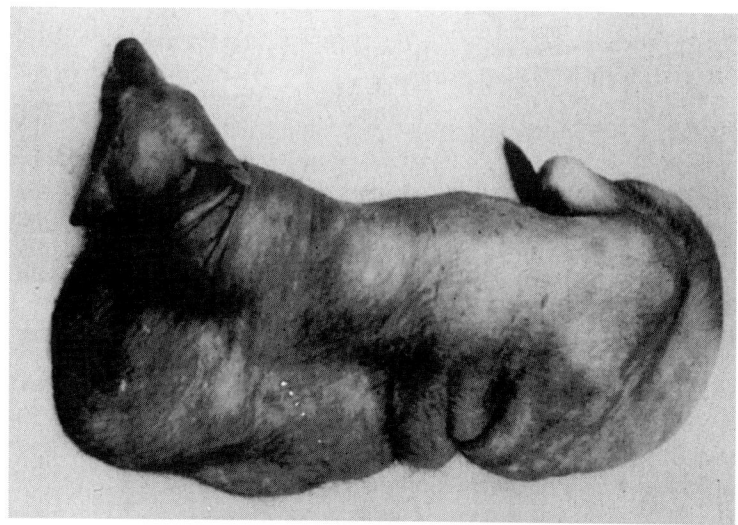

FIGURE 18–52. Idiopathic diffuse lipomatosis. Remarkable irregular proliferation of subcutaneous fat with resultant distortion of the body. (Courtesy of L. A. Lima.)

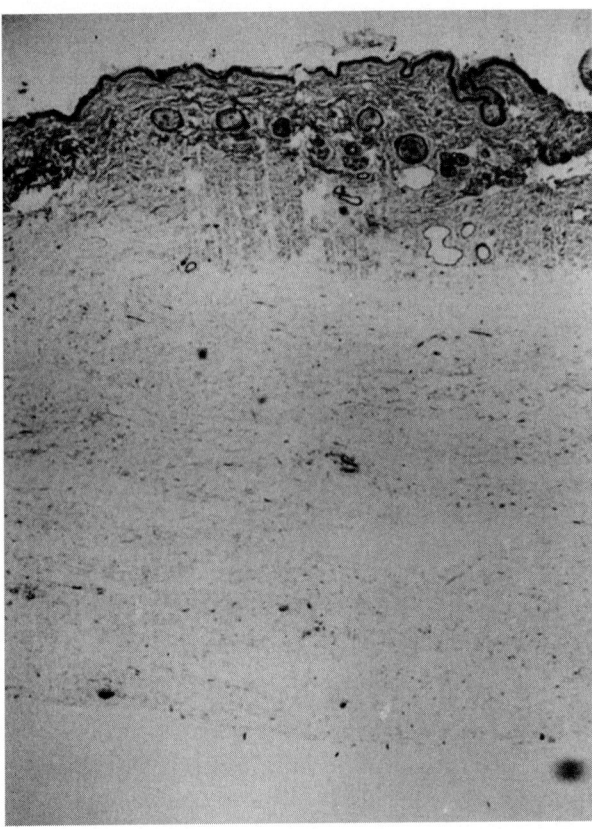

FIGURE 18-53. Idiopathic diffuse lipomatosis. The skin is markedly thickened because of the abnormal proliferation of lipocytes. Note the complete loss of the normal lobular-septal anatomy of the panniculus.

• IDIOPATHIC MUCINOSIS

Idiopathic mucinosis is rare in dogs and occurs almost exclusively in the Chinese Shar pei (see Chap. 12).[3, 120, 122a, 126, 127] The incidence varies from 4.8% to 5% (in Shar peis presenting to a veterinary teaching hospital) to 12.6% (in Shar peis presenting to a dermatology specialty practice).[122, 123, 125] Abnormal deposition of mucin may be focal or diffuse and may vary from mild to severe. Gross deformity of a leg occurred in one case.[123]

Clinically, mucinosis may be manifested as generalized, thickened, puffy, nonpitting skin. Thickened folds are often most prominent over the face, neck, and limbs (Figs. 18-55A and see 18-32G). Severe focal mucinosis is usually associated with some degree of generalized mucinosis. Multiloculated vesicles or bullae may occur with the thickened skin or as the only lesions (see Figs. 18-32H and 18-55B). When ruptured, these lesions yield an acellular, clear, viscid, sticky, and stringy fluid (Fig. 18-55C). Affected dogs are not pruritic, do not have clinically inflamed skin, and are otherwise healthy.

An unusual type of focal mucinosis was reported in a 5-week-old Chow Chow cross puppy.[119] The puppy had pruritic, crusted, papular, and plaquelike lesions on the head and pinnae.

Idiopathic mucinosis occurs in young Chinese Shar peis that do not have pruritus or clinically evident inflammation. Diagnosis is straightforward in such cases. A diagnosis may be supported by pricking or puncturing the skin with a hypodermic needle. Stringy, sticky, clear fluid oozes from the puncture site (see Fig. 18-55C).[122] Confirmation is by biopsy, which reveals marked diffuse dermal mucinosis and mild perivascular accumulations of mast cells and eosinophils (Figs. 18-56 and 18-57). One study of Shar peis with idio-

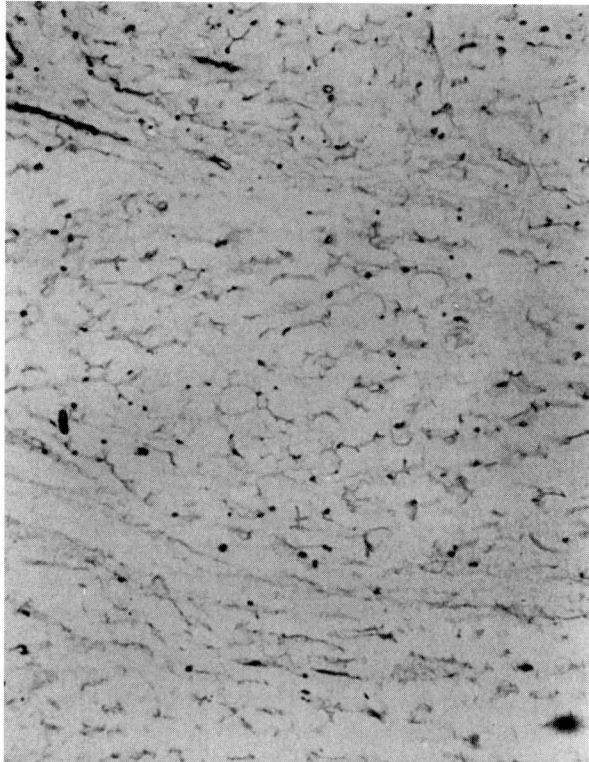

FIGURE 18–54. Idiopathic diffuse lipomatosis. Proliferation of often misshapen lipocytes.

pathic mucinosis and mucinous vesicles indicated that dilated, distorted lymphatics (factor VIII–related antigen-positive) were a characteristic finding in most cases.[124] Whether the lymphatic changes are the cause or an effect of the condition is unknown. The mucinosis of Shar peis results from the massive accumulation of hyaluronic acid and, to a lesser extent, of chondroitins 4 and 6 sulfate and dermatan sulfate.[121]

Thirteen Shar peis with mucinosis and 13 normal dogs underwent cutaneous mast cell density and mast cell subtype studies based on protease content.[127a] In sections stained with toluidine blue, normal dogs had a median mast cell density of 31.2/mm^2, compared with 9.1 mm^2 in Shar peis with mucinosis. The predominant mast cell subtype in normal dogs was the tryptase-chymase-carboxypeptidase-cathepsin G subtype, whereas in Shar peis with mucinosis it was the chymase-carboxypeptidase subtype.

Chinese Shar peis also experience localized and generalized mucinosis in conjunction with hypersensitivities (e.g., atopy, food hypersensitivity, flea bite hypersensitivity) and hypothyroidism. In these cases, typical signs of the primary disease are also apparent.

Some cases of idiopathic mucinosis in Chinese Shar peis spontaneously resolve, or deflate, as the dogs age. Remarkable deflation also follows the administration of glucocorticoids.[120, 122a, 126, 127] Triamcinolone has been effective in some cases with poor response to prednisone. Pentoxifylline, 10 mg/kq q8h, was effective in a case that had been glucocorticoid-responsive but required chronic therapy.

• WATERLINE DISEASE OF BLACK LABRADOR RETRIEVERS

Waterline disease is a poorly understood condition of black Labrador retrievers of either sex.[4, 5] Affected dogs present with severe pruritus, secondary seborrhea, and alopecia of

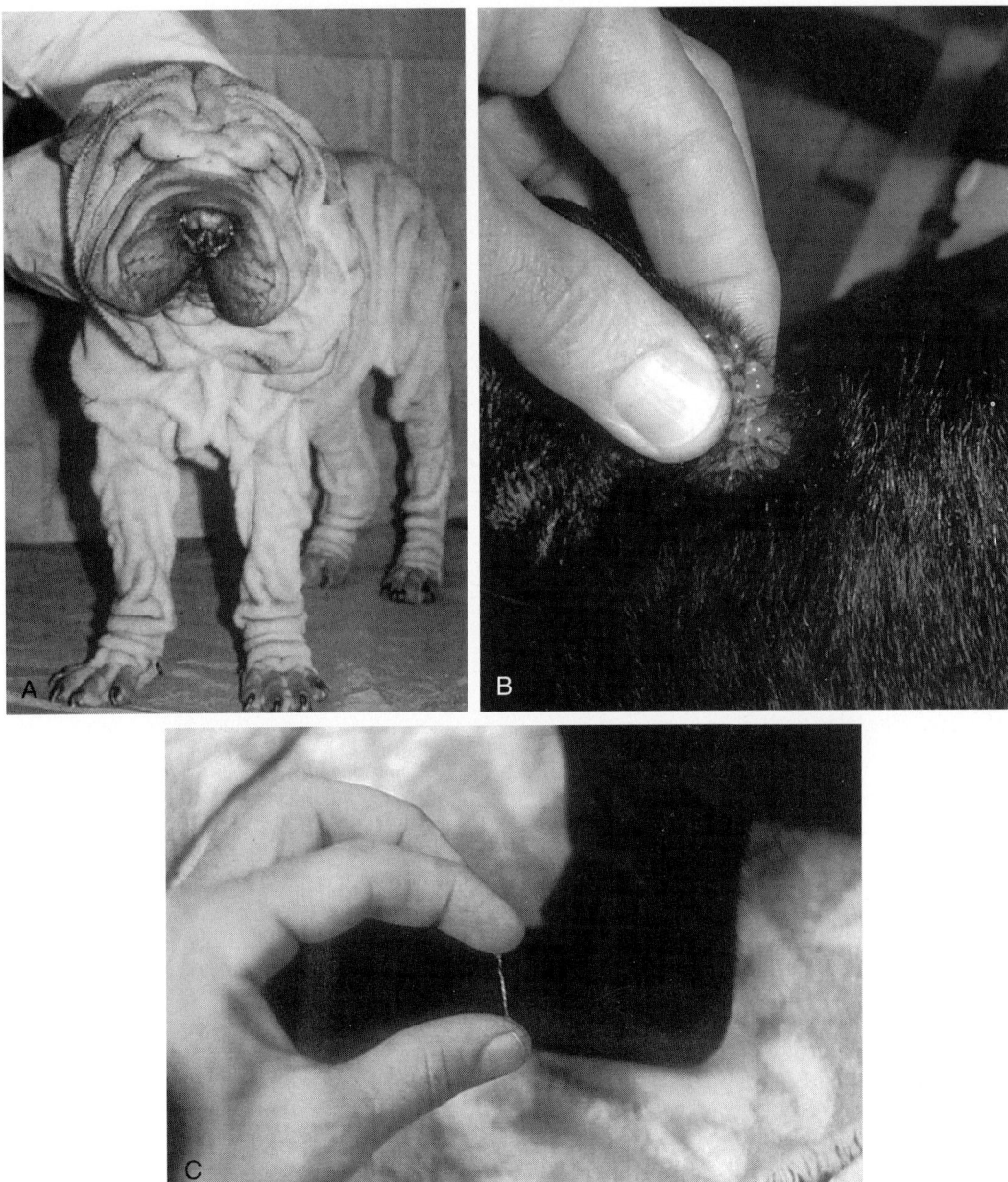

FIGURE 18–55. *A*, Idiopathic mucinosis of the Chinese Shar pei. Note the remarkable thickening and folding of the skin. (Courtesy M. Paradis.) *B*, Multiple mucin containing vesicles on a Chinese Shar pei. *C*, Note string of mucin between the fingertips that was expressed from a small hypodermic needle puncture.

the legs and ventrum (Fig. 18–58) and, occasionally, of the head. Scrapings and cultures are negative, as are responses to intradermal skin tests and hypoallergenic diets. The disorder is poorly responsive to systemic glucocorticosteroids. Our recent cases of this "syndrome," whether in Labrador retrievers or other breeds, have involved *Malassezia* dermatitis and responded to ketoconazole administration (see Chap. 5). We seriously doubt the existence of "waterline disease."

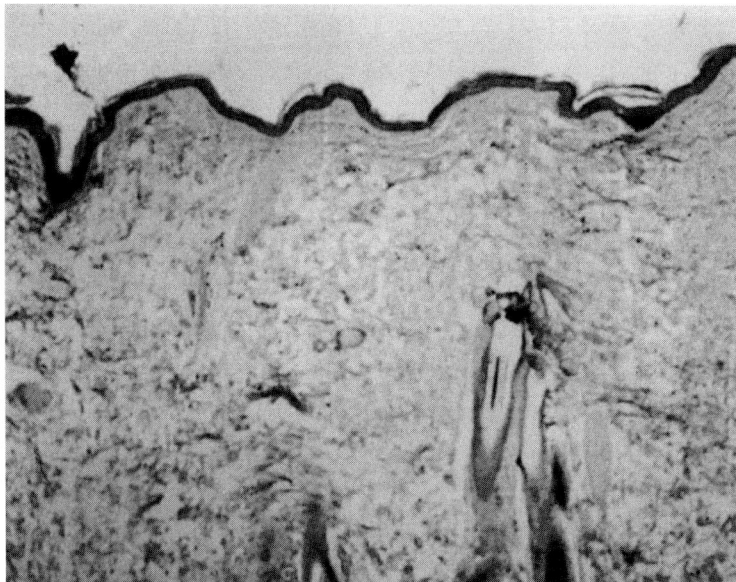

FIGURE 18–56. Idiopathic mucinosis of the Chinese Shar pei. Diffuse dermal mucinosis with minimal inflammation.

• IDIOPATHIC PREAURICULAR ULCERATIVE DERMATITIS OF CATS

A pruritic, unilateral to bilateral, preauricular ulcerative dermatitis was reported in a 3-month-old kitten and two of its littermates.[128] The condition was unresponsive to glucocorticoids, antihistamines, fatty acids, antibiotics, and hypoallergenic diets. Isotretinoin (10 mg q24h orally) resulted in healing after 3 weeks. Further details were not given.

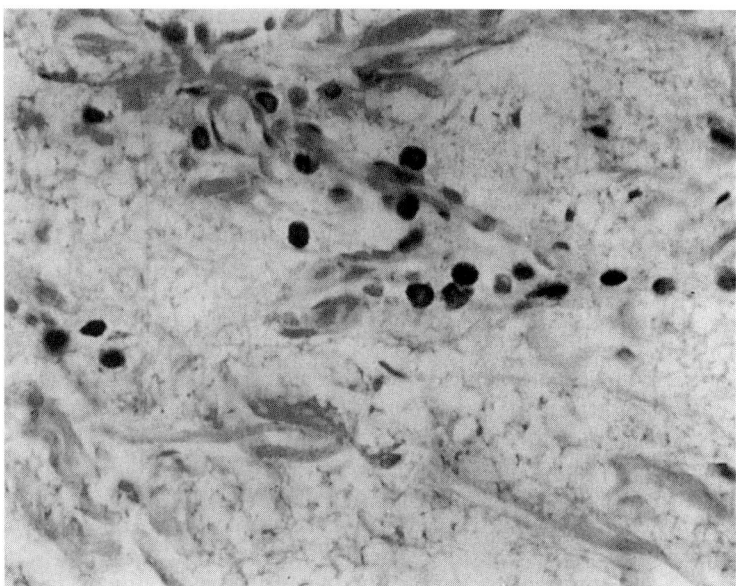

FIGURE 18–57. Idiopathic mucinosis of the Chinese Shar pei. Close-up of mucinosis and perivascular mast cells.

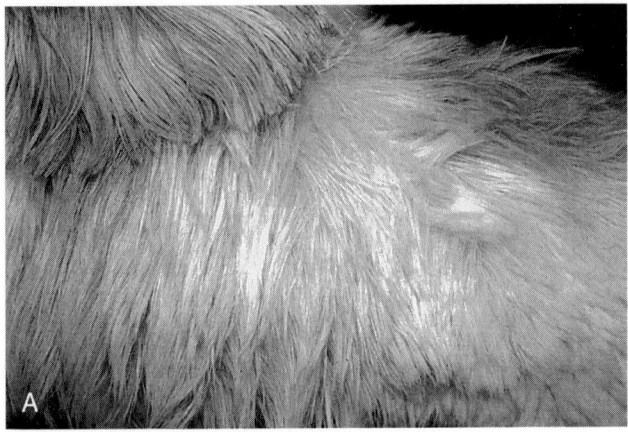
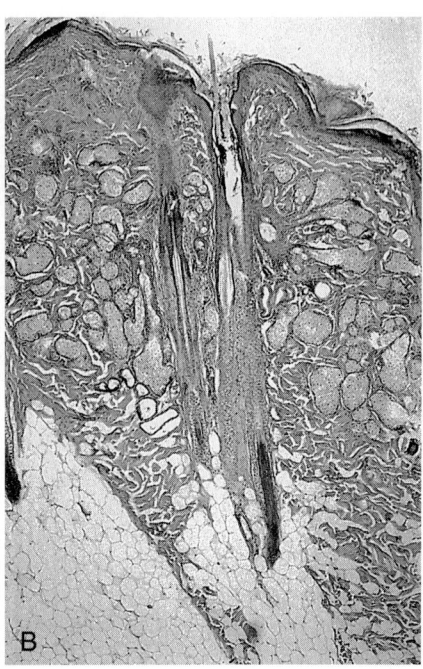

FIGURE 18–60. Idiopathic greasy skin and hair coat with sebaceous gland hyperplasia in a dog. *A*, The hair coat is clumped and matted with grease. *B*, Biopsy reveals hyperplastic sebaceous glands in otherwise normal skin.

thy, and bone marrow plasmacytosis.[130] The condition is unresponsive to therapy, and the course is invariably chronic, but asymptomatic for years.

Systemic plasmacytosis was diagnosed in a 9-year-old Keeshond with waxing and waning, ventral pitting edema and variable erythema.[130] The dog also had abnormal claw growth, mild lethargy, and gradual weight loss. Skin biopsy revealed a severe, deep perivascular and periadnexal accumulation of mature plasma cells and a superficial leukocytoclastic vasculitis. Serum protein electrophoresis revealed a polyclonal gammopathy and elevated IgG levels. Five months of treatment with prednisone, cyclophosphamide, and melphalan was of no benefit. The condition remained unchanged over a 3-year period.

• REFERENCES

General References

1. Freedberg IM, et al: Fitzpatrick's Dermatology in General Medicine, 5th ed. McGraw-Hill, Inc., New York, 1999.
2. Griffin CE, et al: Current Veterinary Dermatology. Mosby-Year Book, St. Louis, 1993.
3. Gross TL, et al: Veterinary Dermatopathology. Mosby-Year Book, St. Louis, 1992.
4. Muller GH, et al: Small Animal Dermatology, 4th ed. W.B. Saunders Co., Philadelphia, 1989.
5. Scott DW, et al: Muller and Kirk's Small Animal Dermatology, 5th ed. W.B. Saunders Co., Philadelphia, 1995.

Canine Subcorneal Pustular Dermatosis

6. Clasper M: Successful use of gold in the treatment of a case of canine sub-corneal pustular dermatosis. N Z Vet J 39:65, 1991.
7. Grob JJ, et al: Role of tumor necrosis factor-α in Sneddon-Wilkinson subcorneal pustular dermatosis. J Am Acad Dermatol 25:944, 1991.
8. Kalaher KM, Scott DW: Subcorneal pustular dermatosis in dogs and in human beings: Comparative aspects. J Am Acad Dermatol 22:1023, 1990.
9. McKeever PJ, Dahl MV: A disease in dogs resembling human subcorneal pustular dermatosis. J Am Vet Med Assoc 170:704, 1977.
10. Takata M, et al: Subcorneal pustular dermatosis associated with IgA myeloma and intraepidermal IgA deposits. Dermatology 189:111, 1994.

Feline Plasma Cell Pododermatitis

11. Canonge F, et al: Pododermatite lymphocytaire quadripodale chez un chat. Point Vét 29:753, 1998.
12. Foil CS: Facial, pedal and other regional dermatoses. Vet Clin North Am Small Anim Pract 25:923, 1995.
13. Gisseleire Y: Preliminary results of a study of the comparative efficacy of corticosteroids and chrysotherapy in the management of feline plasma cell pododermatitis. Proc Br Small Anim Vet Assoc 1994.
14. Guaguère E, et al: Feline pododermatitis. Vet Dermatol 3:1, 1992.
15. Nuttall T: What is your diagnosis? J Small Anim Pract 39:459, 1998.

16. Scott DW: Feline dermatology 1979–1982: Introspective retrospections. J Am Anim Hosp Assoc 20:537, 1984.
17. Scott DW: Feline dermatology 1983–1985: "The secret sits." J Am Anim Hosp Assoc 23:255, 1987.
18. Simon M, et al: Plasma cell pododermatitis in immunodeficiency virus-infected cats. Vet Pathol 30:477, 1993.
19. Taylor JE, Schmeitzel LP: Plasma cell pododermatitis with chronic footpad hemorrhage in two cats. J Am Vet Med Assoc 197:375, 1990.
19a. Yamamura Y, et al: A surgically treated case of feline plasma cell pododermatitis. J Jpn Vet Med Assoc 51:669, 1998.

Lichenoid Dermatoses

20. Anderson WI, et al: Idiopathic benign lichenoid keratosis on the pinna of the ear in four dogs. Cornell Vet 79:179,89.
21. Buerger RM, Scott DW: Lichenoid dermatitis in a cat: A case report. J Am Anim Hosp Assoc 24:55, 1988.
22. Gill PA, Purvis-Smith G: Idiopathic lichenoid dermatosis in a Doberman bitch. Aust Vet Practit 25:144, 1995.
23. Guaguère E, Mialot M: Dermatite lichénoide idiopathique chez un Doberman. Prat Méd Chir Anim Comp 26:355, 1991.
24. Scott DW: Lichenoid reactions in the skin of dogs: Clinicopathologic correlations. J Am Anim Hosp Assoc 20:305, 1984.
25. Scott DW: Lichenoid dermatoses in dogs and cats. In: Kirk RW (ed): Current Veterinary Therapy X. W.B. Saunders Co., Philadelphia, 1989, p 614.
26. Scott DW: Idiopathic lichenoid dermatitis in a dog. Canine Pract 11:22, 1984.

Canine Sterile Eosinophilic Pustulosis

27. Berbis P, et al: Eosinophilic pustular folliculitis (Ofuji's disease): Efficacy of isotretinoin. Dermatologica 179:214, 1989.
28. Carlotti D, et al: La maladie d'Ofugi (pustulose éosinophilique stérile). Prat Méd Chir Anim Comp 24:131, 1989.
29. Craig JM: A case of sterile eosinophilic pustulosis in a dog. Vet Dermatol Newsl 15:11, 1993.
30. Kimura K, et al: A case of eosinophilic pustular folliculitis (Ofuji's disease) induced by patch and challenge tests with indeloxazine hydrochloride. J Dermatol 23:479, 1996.
31. Mohr C, et al: Eosinophilic pustular folliculitis: Successful treatment with interferon-α. Dermatology 191:257, 1995.
32. Scott DW: Sterile eosinophilic pustulosis in the dog. J Am Anim Hosp Assoc 20:585, 1984.
33. Scott DW: Sterile eosinophilic pustulosis in dog and man: Comparative aspects. J Am Acad Dermatol 16:1022, 1987.
34. Scott DW, et al: Sterile eosinophilic folliculitis in the cat: An unusual manifestation of feline allergic skin disease? Comp Anim Pract 19:6, 1989.
35. Thomsen MK, et al: Impairment of neutrophil functions in a dog with an eosinophilic dermatosis. Acta Vet Scand 32:519, 1991.

Feline Hypereosinophilic Syndrome

36. Harvey RG: Feline hypereosinophilia with cutaneous lesions. J Small Anim Pract 31:453, 1990.
37. Huibregtse BA, Turner JL: Hypereosinophilic syndrome and eosinophilic leukemia: A comparison of 22 hypereosinophilic cats. J Am Anim Hosp Assoc 30:591, 1996.
38. Muir P, et al: Hypereosinophilic syndrome in a cat. Vet Rec 132:358, 1993.
39. Neer TM: Hypereosinophilic syndrome in cats. Comp Cont Educ 13:549, 1991.
40. Saxon B, et al: Restrictive cardiomyopathy in a cat with hypereosinophilic syndrome. Can Vet J 32:367, 1991.
41. Scott DW, et al: Hypereosinophilic syndrome in a cat. Feline Pract 15:22, 1985.
42. Weller PF: The idiopathic hypereosinophilic syndrome. Arch Dermatol 132:583, 1996.

Idiopathic Sterile Granuloma and Pyogranuloma

43. Barnett SJ, et al: Challenging cases in internal medicine: What's your diagnosis? Vet Med 93:35, 1998.
44. Houston DM, et al: A case of cutaneous sterile pyogranuloma/granuloma syndrome in a golden retriever. Can Vet J 34:121, 1993.
45. Kramer L, et al: Sterile granuloma/pyogranuloma syndrome and cutaneous histiocytosis in a dog: An immunohistochemical report. Proc Annu Congr Eur Soc Vet Dermatol/Eur Coll Vet Dermatol 14:193, 1997.
45a. Li N, et al: Identification of mycobacterial DNA in cutaneous lesions of sarcoidosis. J Cutan Pathol 26:271, 1999.
46. Panich R, et al: Canine cutaneous sterile pyogranuloma/granuloma syndrome: A retrospective analysis of 29 cases (1976 to 1988). J Am Anim Hosp Assoc 27:519, 1991.
47. Rothstein E, et al: Tetracycline and niacinamide for the treatment of sterile pyogranuloma/granuloma syndrome in a dog. J Am Anim Hosp Assoc 33:540, 1997.
48. Scott DW, et al: Idiopathic sterile granulomatous and pyogranulomatous dermatitis in cats. Vet Dermatol 1:129, 1990.
49. Scott DW, Noxon JO: Sterile sarcoidal granulomatous skin disease in three dogs. Canine Pract 15(3):11, 1990.

Granulomatous Sebaceous Adenitis

50. Carothers MA, et al: Cyclosporine-responsive granulomatous sebaceous adenitis in a dog. J Am Vet Med Assoc 198:1645, 1991.
51. Dunstan RW, Hargis AM: The diagnosis of sebaceous adenitis in standard poodle dogs. In: Bonagura JD (ed): Kirk's Current Veterinary Therapy XII. W.B. Saunders Co., Philadelphia, 1995.
52. Gross TL, et al: An anatomical classification of folliculitis. Vet Dermatol 8:147, 1997.
53. Guaguère E, et al: Adénite sébacée granulomateuse: A propos de trois cas. Prat Méd Chir Anim Comp 25:169, 1990.
54. Guaguère E, et al: Granulomatous sebaceous adenitis in 7 Belgian sheepdogs. Proc Annu Congr Eur Soc Vet Dermatol Eur Coll Vet Dermatol 14:191, 1997.
54a. Guaguère E: Adénite sébacée granulomateuse chez un Akita Inu. Prat Méd Chir Anim Comp 35:47, 2000.
55. Martins C, et al: Sebaceous adenitis. J Am Acad Dermatol 36:845, 1997.
56. Power HT, Ihrke PJ: Synthetic retinoids in veterinary dermatology. Vet Clin North Am Small Anim Pract 20:1525, 1990.
57. Power HT: Newly recognized feline skin diseases.

58. Prost C: Adénite sébacée granulomateuse: Étude rétrospective de 13 cas. Proc GEDAC 12:255, 1997.
59. Renfro L, et al: Neutrophilic sebaceous adenitis. Arch Dermatol 129:910, 1993.
60. Rosser EJ Jr, et al: Sebaceous adenitis with hyperkeratosis in the standard poodle: A discussion of 10 cases. J Am Anim Hosp Assoc 23:341, 1987.
61. Rybnicek J, et al: Sebaceous adenitis: An immunohistochemical examination. In: Kwochka KW, et al (eds): Advances in Veterinary Dermatology III. Butterworth-Heinemann, Boston, 1998, p 539.
62. Scott DW: Granulomatous sebaceous adenitis in dogs. J Am Anim Hosp Assoc 22:631, 1986.
63. Scott DW: Adénite sébacée pyogranulomateuse stérile chez un chat. Point Vét 21:107, 1989.
64. Scott DW: Sterile granulomatous sebaceous adenitis in dogs and cats. Vet Ann 33:236, 1993.
64a. Stenn KS, Sundberg JP: Hair follicle biology, the sebaceous gland, and scarring alopecia. Arch Dermatol 135:973, 1999.
65. Stewart LJ, et al: Isotretinoin in the treatment of sebaceous adenitis in two Vizslas. J Am Anim Hosp Assoc 27:65, 1991.
66. White SD, et al: Sebaceous adenitis in dogs and results of treatment with isotretinoin and etretinate: 30 cases. J Am Vet Med Assoc 207:197, 1995.

Localized Scleroderma

67. Bensignor E, et al: Morphea-like lesion in a cat. J Small Anim Hosp 39:538, 1998.
68. Bourdeau P, et al: Observation d'un cas de sclérodermie localisée (morphée) chez un chien. Rev Méd Vét 167:1121, 1990.
69. Samlaska CP, Winfield EA: Pentoxifylline. J Am Acad Dermatol 30:603, 1994.
70. Scott DW: Localized scleroderma (morphea) in two dogs. J Am Anim Hosp Assoc 22:207, 1986.

Feline Eosinophilic Granuloma Complex

71. O'Dair H, et al: An open prospective investigation into aetiology in a group of cats with suspected allergic skin disease. Vet Dermatol 7:193, 1996.
72. Mason KV, Evans AG: Mosquito bite-caused eosinophilic dermatitis in cats. J Am Vet Med Assoc 198:2086, 1991.
73. Moriello KA, et al: Lack of autologous tissue transmission of eosinophilic plaques in cats. Am J Vet Res 51:995, 1990.
74. Moriello KA: Diseases of the skin. In: Sherding RG (ed): The Cat: Diseases and Clinical Management II, Vol II. Churchill-Livingstone, New York, 1994, p 1907.
75. Paulsen ME, et al: Feline eosinophilic keratitis: A review of 15 clinical cases. J Am Anim Hosp Assoc 23:63, 1987.
76. Pentlarge VW: Eosinophilic conjunctivitis in five cats. J Am Anim Hosp Assoc 27:21, 1991.
77. Power HT: Eosinophilic granuloma in a family of specific pathogen-free cats. Proc Annu Memb Meet Am Acad Vet Dermatol/Am Coll Vet Dermatol 6:45, 1990.
78. Prost C: Diagnosis of feline allergic diseases: A study of 90 cats. In: Kwochka KW, et al (eds): Advances in Veterinary Dermatology III. Butterworth-Heinemann, Boston, 1998, p 516.
79. Scott DW, et al: Miliary dermatitis: A feline cutaneous reaction pattern. Proc Ann Kal Kan Semin 2:11, 1986.
80. Song MD: Diagnosing and treating feline eosinophilic granuloma complex. Vet Med 89:1141, 1994.
81. von Tscharner C, Bigler B: The eosinophilic granuloma complex. J Small Anim Pract 30:228, 1989.

Canine Eosinophilic Granuloma

82. Bredal WP, et al: Oral eosinophilic granuloma in three Cavalier King Charles spaniels. J Small Anim Pract 37:499, 1996.
83. Brovida D, Castagnaro M: Tracheal obstruction due to an eosinophilic granuloma in a dog: Surgical treatment and clinicopathological observations. J Am Anim Hosp Assoc 28:8, 1992.
84. da Silva Curiel JM, et al: Eosinophilic granuloma of the nasal skin in a dog. J Am Vet Med Assoc 193:566, 1988.
85. Fontaine J, et al: Deux cas de granulomes éosinophiliques oraux chez un Husky Sibérien et un Malamute. Ann Méd Vét 134:223, 1990.
86. Norris JM: Cutaneous eosinophilic granuloma in a crossbred dog: A case report and literature review. Aust Vet Practit 24:74, 1995.
87. Poulet FM, et al: Focal proliferative eosinophilic dermatitis of the external ear canal in four dogs. Vet Pathol 28:171, 1991.
88. Scott DW: Cutaneous eosinophilic granulomas with collagen degeneration in the dog. J Am Anim Hosp Assoc 19:529, 1983.
89. van Duijn HE: Drie gevallen van een oraal eosinofiel granuloom bij Siberische huskies. Tijdschr Diergeneesk 120:712, 1995.

Eosinophilic Dermatitis and Edema in Dogs

89a. Holm KS, et al: Eosinophilic dermatitis with edema in nine dogs, compared with eosinophilic cellulitis in humans. J Am Vet Med Assoc 215:649, 1999.

Panniculitis

90. Adame J, Cohen PR: Eosinophilic panniculitis: Diagnostic considerations and evaluation. J Am Acad Dermatol 34:229, 1996.
91. Aoki S, et al: Nodular nonsuppurative panniculitis in a dog. J Jpn Vet Med Assoc 41:659, 1988.
92. Brown PJ, et al: Multifocal necrotizing steatitis associated with pancreatic carcinoma in three dogs. J Small Anim Pract 35:129, 1994.
92a. Campbell KL, et al: Cutaneous markers of hepatic and pancreatic diseases in dogs and cats. Vet Med 95:306, 2000.
93. Dahl PR, et al: Pancreatic panniculitis. J Am Acad Dermatol 33:413, 1995.
94. DeManuelle TC, Stannard AA: Difficult dermatologic diagnosis. J Am Vet Med Assoc 213:356, 1998.
95. Guaguère E, et al: Panniculite nodulaire stérile chez le chien: A propos de trois cas. Rev Méd Vét 164:195, 1988.
96. Hendrick MJ, Dunagan CA: Focal necrotizing granulomatous panniculitis associated with subcutaneous injection of rabies vaccine in cats and dogs: 10 cases (1988–1989). J Am Vet Med Assoc 198:304, 1991.
97. Hughes D, et al: Serum α_1-antitrypsin concentration in dogs with panniculitis. J Am Vet Med Assoc 209:1582, 1996.
98. Patterson S: Sterile idiopathic pedal panniculitis in the German shepherd dog—clinical presentation and response to treatment of four cases. J Small Anim Pract 36:498, 1995.

99. Patterson S: Panniculitis associated with pancreatic necrosis in a dog. J Small Anim Pract 35:116, 1994.
100. Ryan CP, Howard EB: Systemic lipodystrophy associated with pancreatitis in a cat. Feline Pract 11:31, 1981.
101. Scott DW, Anderson WI: Panniculitis in dogs and cats: A retrospective analysis of 78 cases. J Am Anim Hosp Assoc 24:551, 1988.
102. Shibayta K, et al: Idiopathic nodular panniculitis with systemic signs in a dog. Jpn J Vet Dermatol 5:10, 1999.
103. Stanley RG, Jabara AG: Chronic skin reaction to a combined feline rhinotracheitis virus (herpesvirus) and calicivirus vaccine. Aust Vet J 65:128, 1988.

Subcutaneous Fat Sclerosis
104. Buerger RG, et al: Subcutaneous fat sclerosis in a cat. Comp Cont Educ 9:1198, 1987.

Canine Juvenile Cellulitis
105. Barta O, Oyekan PP: Lymphocyte transformation test in veterinary clinical immunology. Comp Immunol Microbiol Infect Dis 4:209, 1981.
106. Jeffers JG, et al: A dermatosis resembling juvenile cellulitis in an adult dog. J Am Anim Hosp Assoc 31:204, 1995.
107. Mason IS, Jones J: Juvenile cellulitis in Gordon setters. Vet Rec 124:642, 1989.
108. Reimann KA, et al: Clinicopathologic characteristics of canine juvenile cellulitis. Vet Pathol 26:499, 1989.
109. White SD, et al: Juvenile cellulitis in dogs: 15 cases (1979–1988). J Am Vet Med Assoc 195:1609, 1989.

Feline Ulcerative Dermatitis With Linear Subepidermal Fibrosis
110. Scott DW: An unusual ulcerative dermatitis associated with linear subepidermal fibrosis in eight cats. Feline Pract 18(3):8, 1990.

Perforating Dermatitis
111. Haugh PG, Swendrowski MA: Perforating dermatitis exacerbated by pruritus. Feline Pract 23(6):8, 1995.
112. Scott DW, Miller WH Jr: An unusual perforating dermatitis in a Siamese cat. Vet Dermatol 2:173, 1991.

Feline Acquired Skin Fragility
113. Diquelou A, et al: Lipoïdose hépatique et syndrome de fragilité cutanée chez un chat. Prat Méd Chir Anim Comp 26:151, 1991.
114. Fernandez CJ, et al: Staining abnormalities of dermal collagen in cats with cutaneous asthenia or acquired skin fragility as demonstrated with Masson's trichrome stain. Vet Dermatol 9:49, 1998.
115. Regnier A, Pieraggi MT: Abnormal skin fragility in a cat with a cholangiocarcinoma. J Small Anim Pract 30:419, 1989.
116. Zur G: Feline skin fragility syndrome in a cat with hepatic lipidosis. In: Kwochka KW, et al (eds): Advances in Veterinary Dermatology III. Butterworth-Heinemann, Boston, 1998, p 495.

Idiopathic Diffuse Lipomatosis
117. Gilbert PA, et al: Diffuse truncal lipomatosis in a dog. J Am Anim Hosp Assoc 26:586, 1990.

Idiopathic Acquired Cutaneous Laxity
118. Pieraggi MT, et al: An unusual dermal collagen disorder in a dog. J Comp Pathol 96:289, 1986.

Idiopathic Mucinosis
119. Beale KM, et al: Papular and plaque-like mucinosis in a puppy. Vet Dermatol 2:29, 1991.
120. Bomhard DV, Kraft W: Idiopathische Mucinosis Cutis beim Chinesichen Shar Pei: Epidemiologie, klinisches Bild, histopathologische Befunde und Behandlung. Tierärztl Praxis 26:189, 1998.
121. Delverdier M, et al: Les mucinoses cutanées du chien et du chat: Étude histologique et histochimique à partir de 106 cas. Rev Méd Vét 146:333, 1995.
122. Griffin CE, Rosenkrantz WS: Skin disorders of the Shar Pei. In: Kirk RW, Bonagura JD (eds): Kirk's Current Veterinary Therapy XI. W.B. Saunders, Philadelphia, 1992, p 519.
122a. López A, et al: Cutaneous mucinosis and mastocytosis in a shar-pei. Can Vet J 40:881, 1999.
123. Madewell BR, et al: Cutaneous mastocytosis and mucinosis with gross deformity in a shar pei dog. Vet Dermatol 3:171, 1992.
124. Mauldin EA, et al: More than mucin? Proc Annu Memb Meet Am Acad Vet Dermatol Am Coll Vet Dermatol 14:67, 1998.
125. Miller WH, et al: Dermatologic disorders of Chinese Shar Peis: 58 cases (1981–1989). J Am Vet Med Assoc 200:986, 1992.
126. Rosenkrantz WS, et al: Idiopathic mucinosis in a dog. Comp Anim Pract 1:39, 1987.
127. Schäfer H, Spieth K: Fallbericht: Idiopathische Muzinose bei einem Shar Pei. Kleintierpraxis 37:403, 1992.
127a. Welle M, et al: Mast cell numbers and subtypes in the skin of Shar Peis with cutaneous mucinosis. Proc Annu Congr Eur Soc Vet Dermatol Eur Coll Vet Dermatol 14:179, 1997.

Idiopathic Preauricular Ulcerative Dermatitis of Cats
128. Breen PT, Jeromin AM: A case of feline idiopathic ulcerative dermatosis responding to isotretinoin. Dermatol Dialogue, Spring/Summer, 1993, p 6.

Idiopathic Ulcerative Dermatitis of the Upper Lip in Dogs
128a. Rosenbaum M: Cyclosporine. Derm Dialogue, Summer: 1999.

Colloid Milium
129. Touart DM, Sau P: Cutaneous deposition diseases: Part I. J Am Acad Dermatol 39:149, 1998.

Systemic Plasmacytosis
130. Gookin JL, et al: Systemic plasmacytosis and polyclonal gammopathy in a dog. J Vet Intern Med 12:471, 1998.

Chapter 19

Diseases of Eyelids, Claws, Anal Sacs, and Ears

• EYELID DISEASES

The eyelids are complex folds of skin that are susceptible to many structural and functional disorders. This discussion is limited to diseases that affect eyelids and not the eyeball, the conjunctiva, and the third eyelid, which are purely in the realm of the ophthalmologist.

Anatomy

Canine and feline eyelids consist of an upper eyelid, a lower eyelid, a row of cilia in the upper lid only, and a number of glands.[6] Meibomian glands (tarsal glands) are modified, large sebaceous gland units that produce a viscous, oily secretion. Zeis' glands are sebaceous glands associated with cilia. Moll's glands are modified epitrichial sweat glands associated with cilia. In addition, accessory lacrimal glands in the eyelids discharge tears into the conjunctival sac and contribute to the precorneal film. The largest of these in the dog is the superficial gland of the membrana nictitans, also known (erroneously) as the Harder gland (or harderian gland).

The bacterial and fungal flora of the eyelids of normal dogs has been studied.[11, 14] The bacteria most commonly isolated include *Staphylococcus intermedius*, coagulase-negative staphylococci, and *Corynebacterium* spp. These are similar to the bacteria found on normal canine skin in many other locations (see Chap. 1). However, fungi were rarely isolated from eyelids, whereas they are commonly isolated from other areas of the skin.

Diseases

Because of the thin and delicate nature of the skin on the eyelid, its loosely attached subcutis, and the presence of a mucocutaneous junction at the eyelid margin, the eyelid and periocular area demonstrate exaggerated responses to numerous dermatologic conditions.[13] Because a normal eyelid margin is necessary for maintenance of tear film and protection of the cornea, abnormalities of the eyelid margin often produce signs of ocular discomfort and discharge. In addition, eyelid disease may result in abnormal tear composition, which may result in qualitative tear film disease.[19] This may lead to keratoconjunctivitis and corneal ulcers. These signs can be the primary reason that the owner seeks veterinary care.

BLEPHARITIS

Inflammation of the eyelid is termed blepharitis.[6, 7] Often, a mucous discharge is apparent. Many dermatoses may cause blepharitis or may be limited to the lids (Table 19–1).[2, 5] Some of these diseases are more likely to present with blepharitis only. In young dogs, localized *Demodex* infestation may appear on the lids (Fig. 19–1A). Usually, only one eye and only part of the eyelid are involved. Alopecia with minimal inflammation may be seen. Periocular noninflammatory alopecia may also occur with topical ocular steroid reactions but is usually diffuse. Every year, the authors see a number of cases referred from

Table 19-1. DISEASE LIMITED TO OR THAT MAY FIRST PRESENT AS EYELID OR PERIOCULAR DERMATOSES

Demodicosis	Self-trauma resulting from ocular disease
Dermatophytosis	Lupus erythematosus
Malassezia dermatitis	Vitiligo
Bacterial folliculitis	Periocular leukotrichia (especially in Siamese cats)
Atopy	Solar dermatitis
Food hypersensitivity	Distemper
Zinc-responsive dermatosis	Topical steroid alopecia
Juvenile cellulitis	Drug eruption
Idiopathic periocular alopecia	

ophthalmologists because of chronic conjunctivitis and blepharitis due to atopy and, less commonly, food hypersensitivity. Varying combinations of blepharitis with periocular alopecia, hyperpigmentation, and lichenification may result from chronic pruritus. Although other symptoms may be found on close examination, they often go unrecognized by the owner.

An idiopathic periocular crusting, occasionally associated with *Malassezia* or feline acne, may be seen in cats, particularly Persians.[21] Idiopathic facial dermatitis has been described in primarily Persian cats and is characterized by scale and crust, and is often periocular (see Chap. 12).[4] Idiopathic seborrhea and bacterial folliculitis in dogs, and dermatophytosis in dogs and cats (see Fig. 19–1B to D) may also cause scaling and crusting periocularly. Immune-mediated dermatoses have a mucocutaneous predilection and often involve the eyelids (see Fig. 19–1E to G). Other diseases are known for their periocular distribution, although they are not limited to that area (see Fig. 19–1H) (Table 19–2).[2]

An idiopathic chronic ulcerative blepharitis, localized to the medial canthal region, has been described in Dachshunds, German shepherds, and Poodles.[1] Biopsy reveals a diffuse lymphoplasmacytic dermatitis. Response to topical or systemic glucocorticoids is excellent, but therapy must often be maintained for life.

Ulcers and nodules were seen on the eyelids of a dog with neosporosis.[7] A proliferative mass at the lateral canthus was described in a malamute that was histologically a pyogranuloma associated with *Onchocerca* sp.[9]

ENTROPION AND ECTROPION

Entropion (inversion, or turning in) and ectropion (eversion, or turning out) of the lid margins are best corrected by surgery. Chronic conjunctivitis or other diseases of the eye that may result in distortion of the lids should also receive attention.

HORDEOLUM (STYE)

This is an acute, painful pyogenic infection of a sebaceous gland of the eyelid. Two types are recognized. The external hordeolum (zeisian stye) involves the glands of Zeis and the cilia on the outer eyelid. The internal hordeolum (meibomian stye) involves the meibomian gland in the inner surface of the eyelid. The internal type is the most common hordeolum in dogs. Treatment consists of incising the abscess and applying an antibiotic ointment. Appropriate systemic antibiotics are useful when the hordeolum is caused by staphylococci.

CHALAZION

A chronic inflammation of a meibomian gland, a chalazion appears externally on the skin surface of the lid as a painless nodule and internally on the palpebral conjunctiva as a yellow, smaller nodule. The irritation from the inner swelling causes conjunctivitis. Treat-

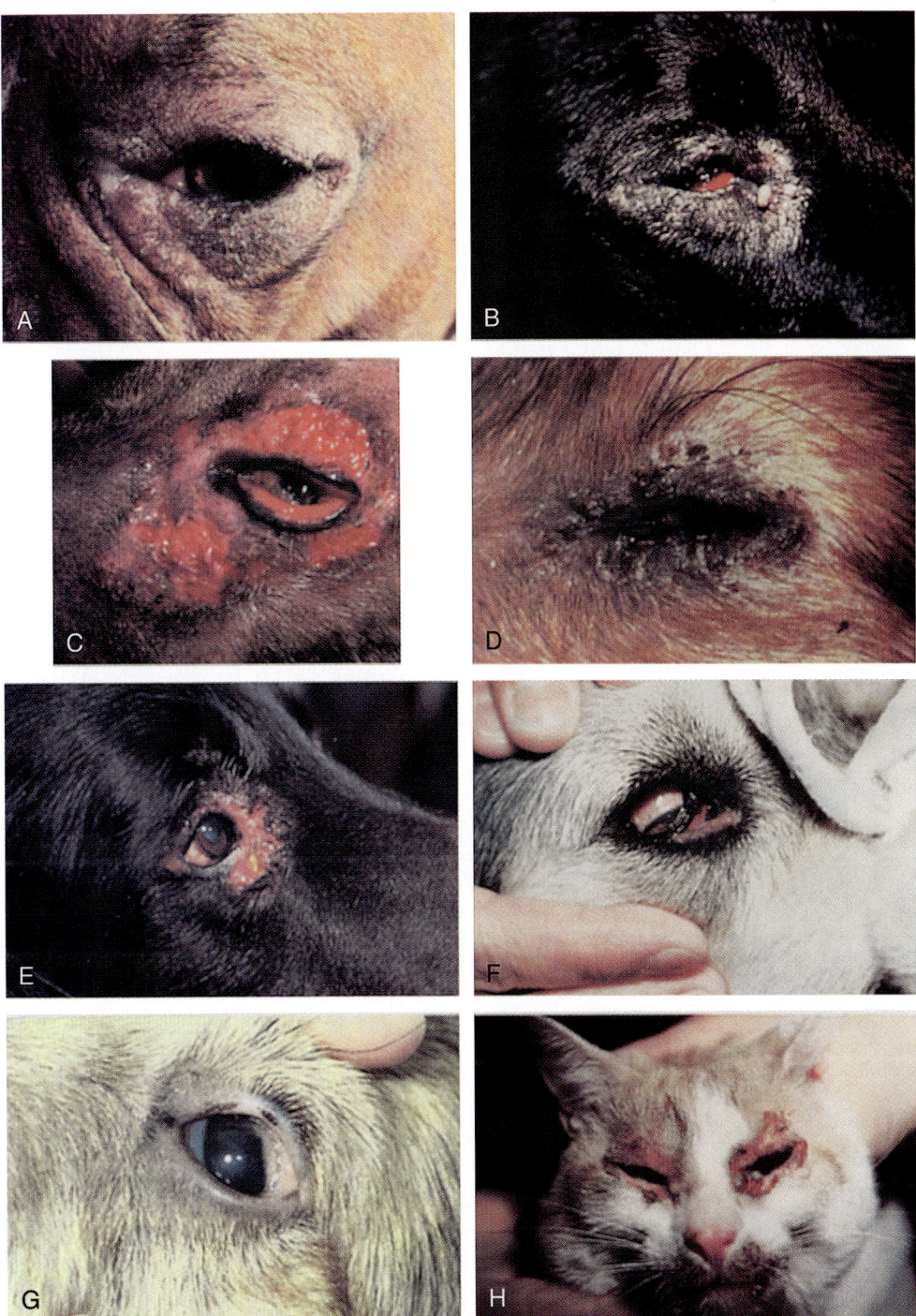

FIGURE 19–1. *A*, Marked focal alopecia due to demodectic blepharitis. *B*, Hypothyroid dog with staphylococcal blepharitis. *C*, Ulcerative blepharitis in a dog with mucocutaneous staphylococcal pyoderma. *D*, Dog with mycotic blepharitis due to *Trichophyton terrestre*. *E*, Ulcerative blepharitis in a dog with bullous pemphigoid. *F*, Ulcerative blepharitis in a dog with discoid lupus erythematosus. *G*, Depigmentation of eyelids in a dog with uveodermatologic syndrome. *H*, Severe blepharitis in a cat with hypereosinophilic syndrome.

Table 19-2 DISEASES THAT AFFECT THE EYELID OR PERIOCULAR AREA IN ADDITION TO OTHER SITES	
Pemphigus foliaceus	Solar dermatitis
Pemphigus erythematosus	Vitiligo
Systemic lupus erythematosus	Hypereosinophilic syndrome
Discoid lupus erythematosus	Drug eruption
Uveodermatologic syndrome	Leishmaniasis
Canine familial dermatomyositis	Vasculitis
Canine necrolytic migratory erythema	Pemphigus vulgaris
Erythema multiforme	Bullous pemphigoid

ment consists of incision and curettage of accumulated sebaceous material. Large chalazia may be excised completely to prevent recurrence.

TRICHIASIS

This disorder is an abnormal position or direction of the cilia, resulting in epiphora, mucous ocular discharge, and sometimes corneal vascularization and even corneal ulceration. Treatment consists of meticulous electroepilation of the involved cilia.

DISTICHIASIS

Animals with distichiasis display aberrant cilia on the lid. They may emerge from the openings of the meibomian glands or the inner lid margin. Electroepilation is the treatment of choice. Distichiasis has been reported in Poodles, Boxers, Pekingese, German shepherds, Cocker spaniels, Shetland sheepdogs, and Bedlington and Yorkshire terriers, as well as in the Shih tzu, Pug, and St. Bernard.[15-17]

EPIPHORA

Epiphora is common in Poodles (Fig. 19–2A). The cause may be atresia, blockage of the nasal lacrimal system, or lid or membrana nictitans deformities.[3] Surgical correction of the lid problem or deepening of the lacrimal lake frequently permits improved function of the lower puncta. Correction of possible causes of chronic lacrimation from ocular irritation should also be implemented. In some cases of white dogs, the chief complaint is the brown staining that may represent oxidized tears on the hair. Besides white Poodles, this is a problem in Maltese and Bichon frise. Bacteria may play a role because the administration of tetracycline or other antibiotics decrease the brown staining in some cases. In others, treatment with topical ointment blocks the chronic wetting or reaction of the tears with the hair. Topical applications of hydrogen peroxide are useful for reducing the staining of hairs.

TUMORS OF THE EYELIDS

These tumors are difficult to manage because of the problems with plastic repair after surgery, or with protection of the globe if radiation therapy is contemplated. In dogs, papillomas, sebaceous gland tumors, and melanocytic neoplasms are the most common (see Fig. 19–2B) (see Chap. 20). Basal cell tumors, mast cell tumors (see Fig. 19–2C), and epitheliotropic lymphoma (see Fig. 19–2D) are also found. A metastatic ocular tumor that was believed to arise from a primary eyelid epitrichial sweat gland tumor has been reported.[12] In cats, squamous cell carcinoma is, by far, the most common.[18] A histiocytoma of the eyelid of a 10-month-old Afghan that regressed spontaneously has been reported.[10] Other sterile granulomatous or pyogranulomatous nodules have also been reported in the eyelid.[8,20] In one case, the sterile pyogranuloma or granuloma was responsive to tetracycline and niacinamide therapy.[20]

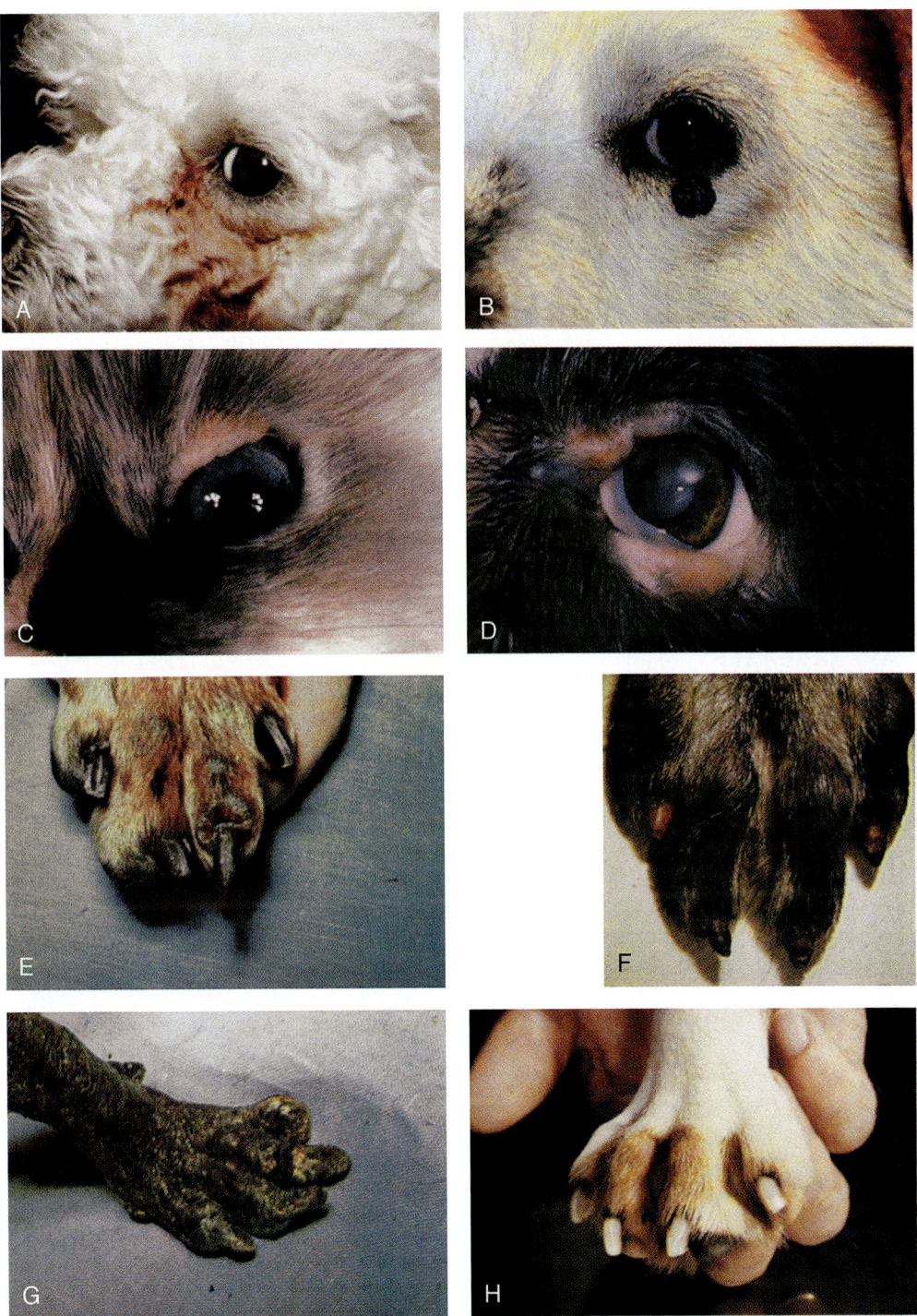

FIGURE 19–2. *A,* Epiphora. The chronic discharge of tears is common in poodles and results in brown staining of the wet hair. (This phenomenon is seen anywhere that white hair is constantly wet.) *B,* Verrucous, hyperpigmented sebaceous gland hyperplasia on the lower eyelid. *C,* Mast cell tumor. Alopecic pink plaque on the upper eyelid of a cat. (Courtesy M. Paradis.) *D,* Epitheliotropic lymphoma. Depigmentation and erythematous papules on the eyelid of a dog. *E,* Bacterial paronychia with ulceration of the claw fold. Note the purulent exudate at the base of the nail. *F,* Onychomadesis in a dog with bacterial paronychia and hypothyroidism. *G,* Onychomycosis in a dog caused by *Trichophyton mentagrophytes*. Claws are grossly deformed, and there is secondary paronychia in the central toe. *H,* Claw bed *Malassezia* in an atopic dog. Brown discoloration on the claws in a dog with *Malassezia* paronychia.

Table 19–3 NEOPLASTIC CONDITIONS THAT MAY AFFECT THE EYELID OR PERIOCULAR AREA	
Squamous cell carcinoma	Lymphoma
Actinic keratosis	Epitheliotropic lymphoma
Melanocytoma and melanoma	Papilloma
Sebaceous gland tumors	Mastocytoma
Fibrous histiocytoma	Histiocytoma
Dermoid	

In older dogs, eyelid tumors are common (Table 19–3).[2] These can be adenomas and adenocarcinomas of Zeis' and Moll's glands, as well as meibomian gland tumors. For treatment, surgical removal is indicated when the tumor is on the palpebral junction and touches the cornea. This can be accomplished by surgical excision, electrosurgery, or cryosurgery. Tumors that touch the conjunctiva and cause irritation (and sometimes ulceration) must be removed. It is important to remove the entire tumor; otherwise, it regrows. The surgery can be performed with a sedative (tranquilizer) plus local anesthesia. A small V-shaped incision exposes the entire tumor for removal and can be closed with one or two sutures. Animals with massive eyelid tumors that require removal of a large section of lid should be referred to an ophthalmologist, because correct plastic repair is necessary for proper lid function.

• CLAW DISEASES

Claws may be affected by many of the diseases described in this text. However, dogs and cats presenting with claw disorders as the only dermatologic manifestation of disease are rarely encountered. Such dogs and cats accounted for approximately 1.3% and 2.2%, respectively, of all dogs and cats examined for dermatologic disease at one university teaching hospital.[35, 36]

Claws and their disorders have received little attention in veterinary medicine.[34–36] Reviews on canine and feline claw diseases have been published.[35, 36] The most commonly reported types of claw diseases are asymmetric and result from known or presumed trauma with or without secondary bacterial infection and onychodystrophy. The normal microanatomy of the canine claw has been studied,[31] but no in-depth microanatomic study of claw disorders has been published. Further work is warranted, because chronic claw diseases are debilitating for affected animals and frustrating for both veterinarians and owners.

Anatomy

The claw is a specialized structure that is a direct continuation of the dermis and epidermis (Fig. 19–3A).[31, 36] The distal phalanx of each toe has a crescent-shaped dorsal process called the ungual crest. The dermis of adjacent skin is continuous with, and extends distally from, this bony process as the periosteum of the phalanx. It has a rich blood supply, which is the source of the profuse hemorrhage if the claw is trimmed too short. The structures constituting the claw are compressed laterally and may be divided into the coronary band, the ventral sole, and the lateral and medial walls. Most of the claw is formed from the coronary band and the dorsal ridge. In many areas, the dermis has fine papillae that project distally and interdigitate with soft epidermal lamellae.

The epidermis of adjacent skin is also continuous with that of the claw. The basal layer of the epidermis, supported by the dermis, is most active in the coronary band and dorsal ridge areas and causes growth in a circular fashion, producing a curved claw. This is why the claw may grow around into the volar surface of the footpad. The horny walls grow over the sole of the claw for the same reason. During the first 2 years of life, the

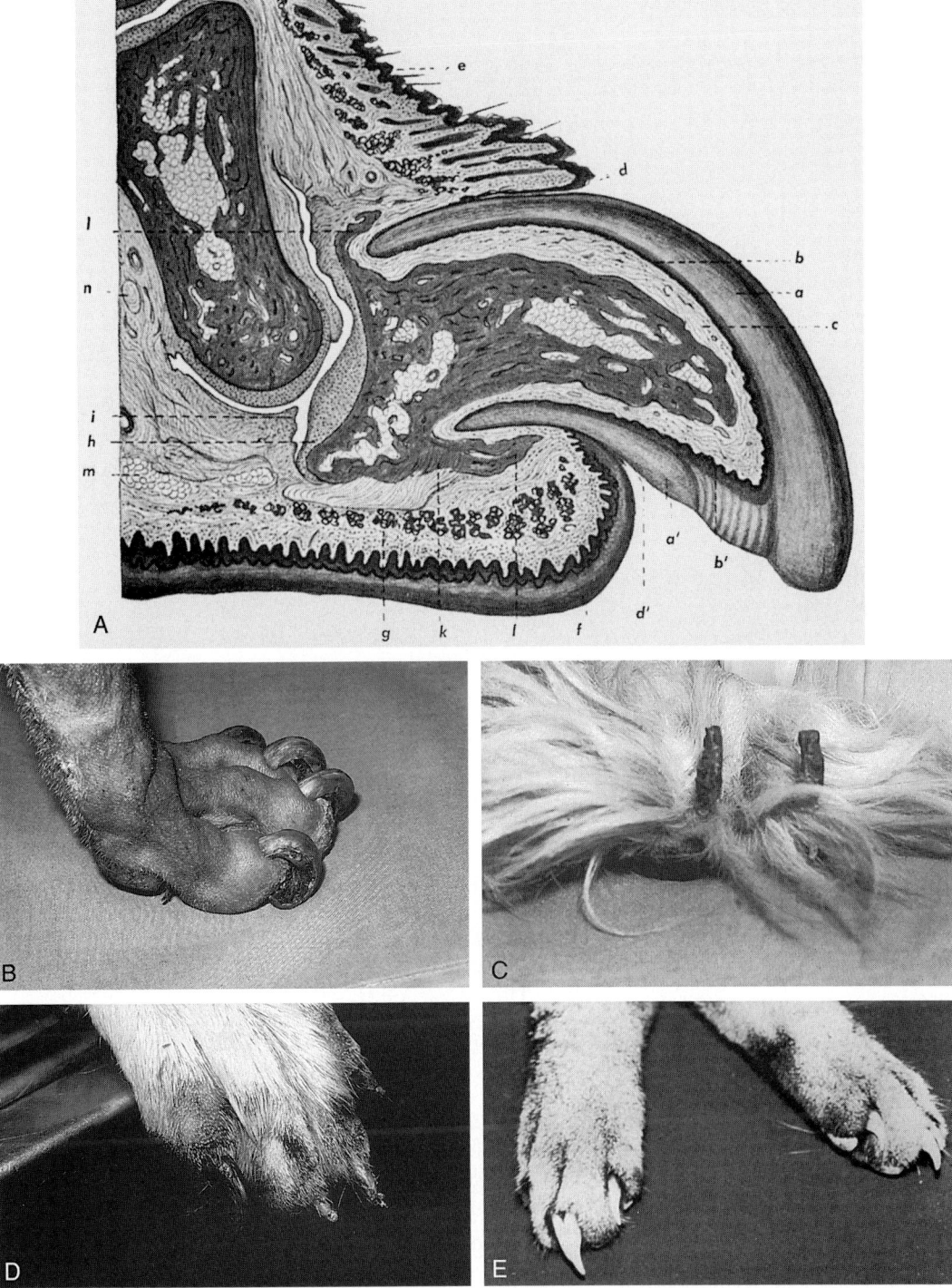

FIGURE 19-3. *A*, Midsagittal section through the claw of the dog: a, stratum corneum of the epidermis of the claw; a', stratum corneum of the epidermis of the sole; b,b', deep, noncornified epidermal layers of the dorsum and sole of the claw; c, corium (papillated in the area of the sole); d, claw fold; d', limiting furrow separating the sole from the digital pad; e, skin with hair and glands; f, epidermis of the digital pad with stratum granulosum and lucidum; g, tubular glands in the digital pad; h, articular cartilage of the third phalanx; i, meniscus; k, Sharpey's fibers from a tendon insertion; l, ungual crest; m, fat cushion within the digital pad; n, lamellar corpuscle. (From Trautmann A, Fiebiger J: Fundamentals of the Histology of Domestic Animals. Copyright 1952 by Cornell University. Reprinted by permission of Cornell University Press.) *B*, Onychocryptosis with the claw growing back into the pad. *C*, Onychomalacia with the claws soft and growing in the wrong direction. *D*, Onychorrhexis with longitudinal striations that have split the claw open, and another digit with onychomadesis, the sloughing of a claw. *E* Onychogryphosis in a cat with hyperthyroidism.

Figure continued on following page

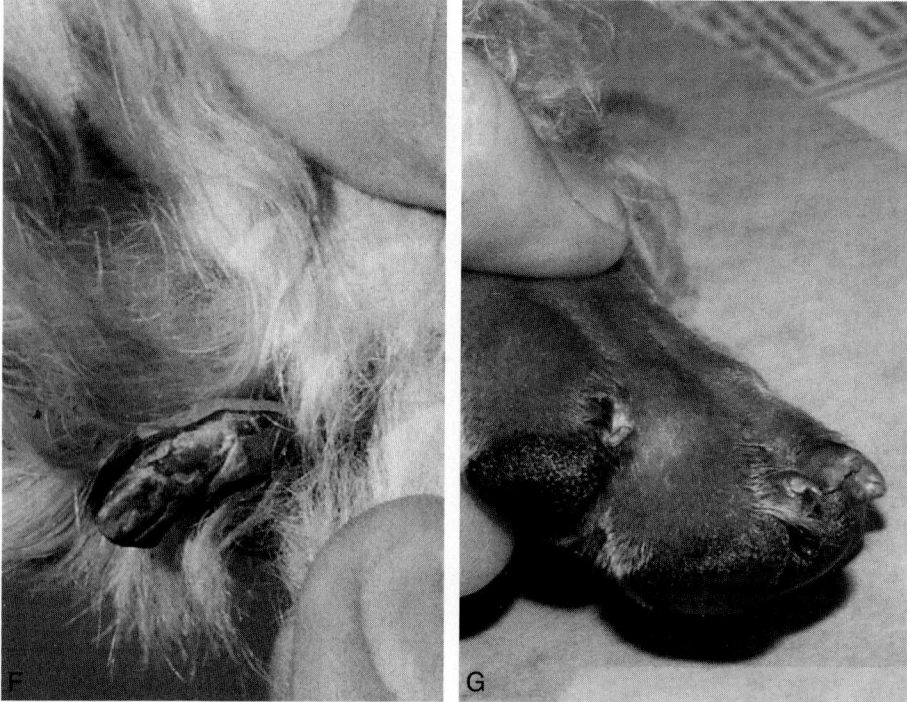

FIGURE 19-3 Continued. *F*, Onychoschizia with splitting and lamination, longitudinal striations, and breaking of the claw. *G*, Onychodystrophy, abnormal claw formation, may be seen following trauma, such as in dogs that regrow dystrophic claws following onychomadesis, or in dogs with no known previous damage such as this Welsh terrier.

claws of beagles grow an average of 1.9 mm per week, but this rate declines with age. Rates of growth as slow as 0.8 mm per week have been reported.[21, 36]

The epidermis of the claw sole has distinct granular and clear layers, as well as the usual structures. However, the epidermis of the rest of the claw is largely composed of a thick horny layer that consists of flat cornified epidermal cells fused into a horny plate, with an absent stratum granulosum. On the ventral surface, the claw is separated from the footpad by a distinct furrow. The sole is relatively soft and is compressible. A fold of modified skin hides the dorsal junction of hairy skin and claw. This claw fold is free from hair on its inner surface and produces the thin stratum tectorium that is the outer layer of the proximal claw.

The claws of animals have important functions as prehensile, locomotor, and offensive and defensive organs. A dog's claws should be kept properly trimmed for good foot health and normal locomotion. Abnormal claws predispose the feet to trauma, strains, and pododermatitis. Because of the long growth cycle, the correction of abnormalities may necessitate 6 to 8 months of treatment.

A study on the microanatomy of the normal canine claw revealed that numerous intranuclear vacuoles are present in the keratinocytes of the stratum basale and stratum spinosum.[31] Additionally, focal areas of subepidermal clefting were frequently seen. An evaluation of normal cat claws has shown a variety of artifacts.[37] Clefts were seen at dermo-epidermal junction as well as other levels. Intracytoplasmic vacuoles in keratinocytes (in contrast to intranuclear), pseudospongiosis (prominent interkeratinocyte spaces), and apoptotic keratinocytes (2 to 3 per high-power field [HPF] in dorsal and ventral matrices) were seen. It was suggested that the intracytoplasmic vacuoles may be an artifact of occlusion, as had been previously suggested in the human literature. These findings must be kept in mind when considering the diagnosis of inflammatory and interface dermatoses, and dystrophies of the claw.

Certain terms are used specifically when describing claw abnormalities (Table 19–4; see Figs. 19–3B to G).[36] Many of these abnormalities may be seen together in the same claw or in different claws of the same animal. Some conditions have little diagnostic specificity, although others may. For example, leukonychia with no other abnormalities is suggestive of vitiligo. Other changes that may affect claws include crusting or excessive keratinous, waxy deposits on the claws, staining of the claws (often to a brown or red color), and an abnormally rapid growth rate. Inflammation of the claw fold and distal digit (paronychia) often leads to an abnormally rapid growth rate, which, in some cases, is associated with onychogryphosis. Extension of all the claws and difficulty jumping to elevated surfaces was reported in a cat with polycythemia vera.[26] Varying degrees of lameness, pain on touch or palpation, pruritus, and regional lymphadenopathy may be present.

Because nomenclature has not been rigorously followed when various claw disorders have been reported, there is much confusing and relatively unuseful information in the literature. For instance, onychodystrophy is a common *sequelae* of many claw disorders (e.g., bacterial and fungal infections, autoimmune diseases, vasculitides, and "idiopathic" onychomadesis). It may be more useful to focus on the earliest signs of disease. For instance, dogs with symmetric lupoid onychodystrophy begin with onychomadesis, and usually respond to omega-6 or omega-3 fatty acids or tetracycline and niacinamide. However, dogs that develop onychodystrophy as a result of initial onycholysis do not respond to these medications.

Diseases

A wide variety of diseases were shown to be associated with claw diseases in dogs (Table 19–5) and cats (Table 19–6). In addition, idiopathic onychomadesis, food hypersensitivity, drug eruption, vaccination reaction, zinc-responsive dermatosis, and linear epidermal nevus have been described as causes of claw disease.[24, 28, 37]

TRAUMA

Trauma is the most common cause of claw disease seen in dogs and the second most common in cats.[35, 36] Usually, the trauma is physical, although chemical trauma due to

• Table 19–4 TERMINOLOGY FOR CLAW DISORDERS

Anonychia	Absence of claws (usually congenital)
Brachyonychia	Short claws
Leukonychia	Whitening of claws
Macronychia	Unusually large claws
Micronychia	Unusually small claws, often shorter or narrower than normal
Onychalgia	Claw pain
Onychauxis (hyperonychia)	Simple hypertrophy of claws
Onychia (onychitis)	Inflammation somewhere in the claw unit
Onychocryptosis (onyxis)	Ingrown claw
Onychodystrophy	Abnormal claw formation
Onychogryphosis (onychogryposis)	Hypertrophy and abnormal curvature of claws
Onycholysis	Separation of claw structure at distal attachment and progressing proximally
Onychomadesis (onychoptosis)	Sloughing of claws
Onychomalacia (hapalonychia)	Softening of claws
Onychomycosis	Fungal infection of claws
Onychopathy (onychosis)	Disease or abnormality of claws
Onychorrhexis	Fragmentation and horizontal separation in lamellae at the free edge
Onychoschizia (onychoschisis)	Splitting or lamination of claws, usually beginning distally
Pachyonychia	Thickening of claws
Paronychia (perionychia)	Inflammation or infection of claw folds
Platonychia	Increased curvature of claws in long axis

Modified from Leider M, Rosenblum M: A Dictionary of Dermatologic Words, Terms, and Phrases. McGraw-Hill Book Co, New York, 1968.

Table 19-5 CAUSES OF CLAW DISORDERS IN 196 DOGS

DIAGNOSIS	NUMBER OF CASES
Bacterial paronychia secondary to broken or torn claw	49
Bacterial paronychia, one paw, idiopathic	13
Bacterial paronychia, four paws, secondary to hypothyroidism	4
Bacterial paronychia, four paws, secondary to hyperadrenocorticism	2
Bacterial paronychia, front paws, secondary to atopy	1
Bacterial paronychia, four paws, recurrent, idiopathic	4
Broken or torn claw	44
Neoplasia	24
Demodicosis	3
Dermatophytosis (*Trichophyton mentagrophytes*)	3
Candidiasis secondary to diabetes mellitus	1
Blastomycosis	1
Geotrichosis	1
Cryptococcosis	1
Symmetric lupoid onychodystrophy	7
Pemphigus foliaceus	2
Pemphigus vulgaris	2
Bullous pemphigoid	1
Epidermolysis bullosa	1
Onychodystrophy, idiopathic	18
Onychodystrophy or onychoschizia secondary to seborrhea	4
Onychodystrophy or onychorrhexis, idiopathic	9
Onychomadesis, four paws, with atrial fibrillation	1

From Scott DW, Miller WH Jr: Disorders of the claw and clawbed in dogs. Comp Cont Educ 14:1448, 1992.

substances such as fertilizers may occur. Trauma most commonly affects one or just a few claws (asymmetric claw disease). Occasionally, all four paws have multiple claws affected (symmetric claw disease), owing to trauma such as that induced by excessive running on hard (asphalt, concrete) surfaces and gravel. The resulting embedment of debris in the distal ends of the claws may cause secondary bacterial infections. Clipping too closely can also lead to injury from embedded debris or predispose the claws to secondary infections. Contaminated clippers may also be a source for infection when clipping claws back to the quick and may affect multiple claws in cases in which many are intentionally cut back.

Table 19-6 CAUSES OF CLAW DISORDERS IN 65 CATS

DIAGNOSIS	NUMBER OF CASES
Onychodystrophy (idiopathic)	23
Bacterial paronychia secondary to broken or torn claws	9
Broken or torn claws	8
Bacterial paronychia secondary to feline leukemia virus infection	7
Pemphigus foliaceus	3
Bacterial paronychia (recurrent, idiopathic)	2
Squamous cell carcinoma	2
Systemic lupus erythematosus	2
Bacterial paronychia secondary to acquired arteriovenous fistula	1
Bacterial paronychia secondary to diabetes mellitus	1
Bacterial paronychia secondary to iatrogenic Cushing's syndrome	1
Dermatophytosis from *Microsporum canis*	1
Cryptococcosis	1
Sporotrichosis	1
Eosinophilic plaque (atopy, presumptive)	1
Hemangiosarcoma	1
Metastatic bronchogenic carcinoma	1

From Scott DW, Miller WH Jr: Disorders of the claw and clawbed in cats. Comp Cont Educ 14:449, 1992.

INFECTIONS

Infectious causes of claw diseases are also common. Bacteria are most often incriminated, and bacterial infections should always be considered secondary (see Fig. 19–2E). A search for an underlying cause should be made. If none is found, recurrences, especially when all four paws are involved, are likely and a guarded prognosis should be given. Trauma is the most common underlying cause. However, hypothyroidism, hyperadrenocorticism, diabetes mellitus, atopy, immune-mediated diseases, arteriovenous fistulae, other infectious agents, and dystrophy may be responsible (see Fig. 19–2F). Onychodystrophy and other diseases that scar and permanently damage the coronary band may result in defective claw growth that predisposes the animal to onychorrhexis and onychoschizia. These sites may break open and become readily infected. Purulent exudate within or under the claw is the preferred source of specimens for cytologic examination or culture and susceptibility testing.

Fungal infections, which are referred to as onychomycosis, may also occur (see Fig. 19–2G). Dermatophytosis, particularly *Trichophyton* infection in the dog, blastomycosis, cryptococcosis, geotrichosis, and sporotrichosis have all been reported, although rarely. Lesions are not usually confined to the claws. Dermatophytes invade the claw keratin and, therefore, are usually associated with onychomalacia. Claws may be brittle and easily broken or powdered. *Malassezia* infection may affect only the claws.[29] Generally, these cases have mild paronychia with a brown, dry to slightly moist claw fold exudate that attaches to the claw. The claw becomes discolored brown-red (see Fig. 19–2H). Often, these are atopic dogs, and the paw pruritus, due to *Malassezia* infection, may be the only symptom after successful control of the atopic disease.[30]

Parasites may also result in claw diseases. Demodicosis may be accompanied by a paronychia that stimulates abnormal claw growth. *Ascaris* infection, hookworm dermatitis, and leishmaniasis have been reported causes of claw disease. Leishmaniasis is most commonly associated with onychogryphosis. Hookworm dermatitis may produce rapid claw growth, onychogryphosis, and onychodystrophy.

IMMUNE-MEDIATED DISEASES

Immune-mediated diseases often involve the claw fold, resulting in paronychia. In some cases, other claw changes, especially onychomadesis, may occur, and less commonly, only claw disease is seen. Symmetric lupoid onychodystrophy appears to be the most common immune-mediated disease to cause abnormal claws (Fig. 19–4A).[34–36] When claw disease alone is seen, symmetric lupoid onychodystrophy, lupus erythematosus, bullous pemphigoid, and pemphigus vulgaris are the most likely immune-mediated causes. With paronychia or footpad involvement, pemphigus foliaceus is most likely the underlying condition in both the dog and the cat (see Fig. 19–4B). Cryoglobulinemia, drug reaction, and vasculitis have been reported to affect the claws.[34, 36] It has been suggested that vaccinations may induce sudden onset of onycholysis or onychomadesis, possibly due to vasculitis.[24] Claw disease may appear several days to several weeks post-vaccination. Vascular occlusion or ischemia may also result in claw abnormalities.

A form of vascular disease similar to Raynaud's disease in humans was recently described (see Fig. 19–4C).[25] Carlotti reported three middle-aged female dogs with this condition. The dogs developed onychalgia, onychogryphosis, and intermittent acrocyanosis of multiple digits and paws. Long-term therapy with the vasodilator, isoxsuprine, at a dose of 1 mg/kg/q24h PO, was very helpful in controlling the disease.[37]

SYMMETRIC LUPOID ONYCHODYSTROPHY

A symmetric lupoid onychodystrophy has been described in dogs.[34, 38] German shepherd dogs appear to be predisposed. The condition was reported in two sibling Rottweilers.[38a] The dogs' ages ranged from 3 to 8 years. Two other reports describe eight dogs with

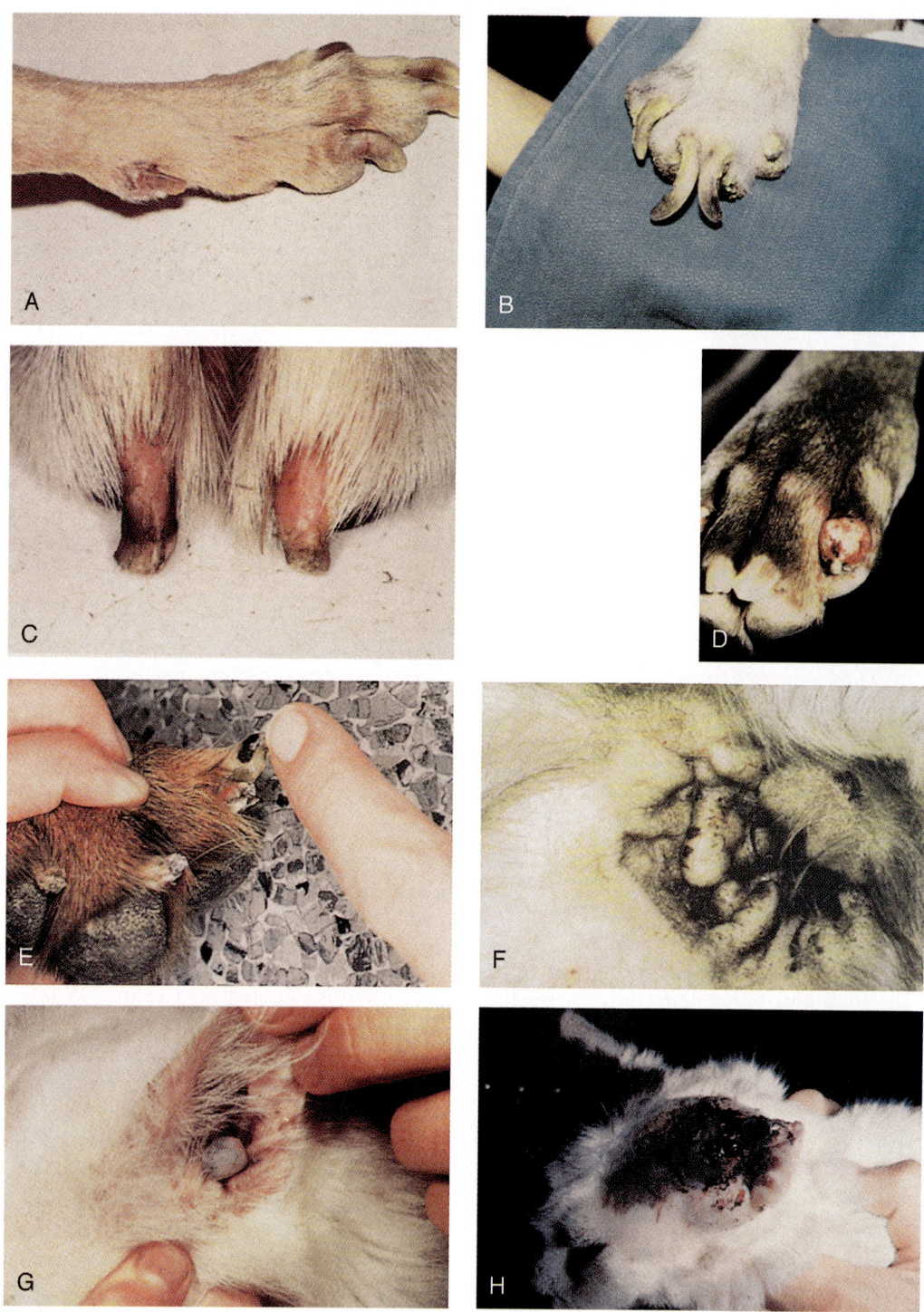

FIGURE 19–4. *A*, Onychogryphosis in a dog with discoid lupus erythematosus. (Courtesy D. Carlotti.) *B*, Onychogryphosis and onychomadesis in a dog with pemphigus foliaceus. (Courtesy D. Carlotti.) *C*. A case of Raynaud-like disease in a dog. *D*, Squamous cell carcinoma of the claw bed. *E*, A Rottweiler that developed concurrent claw dystrophy and vitiligo. Notice the depigmentation of the onycholytic claw. *F*, Idiopathic ceruminous otitis externa in a dog. *G*, Nasopharyngeal polyp. Blue polyp protruding from the ear of a cat with chronic otitis externa. *H*, Ceruminal gland carcinoma. Severe deformation and ulceration of the pinna of an aged cat.

Figure continued on opposite page

Diseases of Eyelids, Claws, Anal Sacs, and Ears • 1197

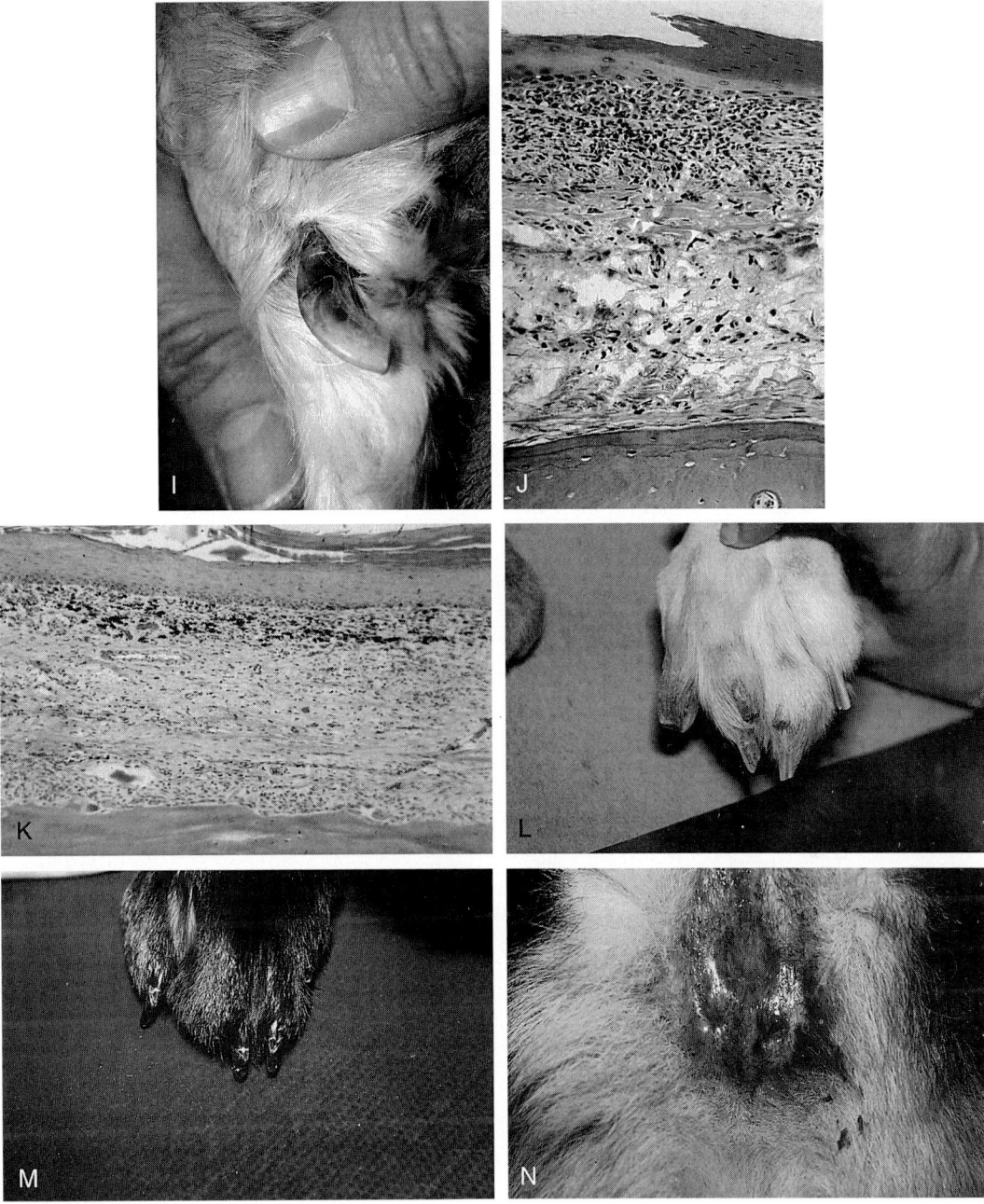

FIGURE 19-4 Continued. *I*, Subungual hemorrhage in a claw of a dog with symmetric lupoid onychodystrophy. This suggests vascular damage. *J*, Claw biopsy from a dog with symmetric lupoid onychodystrophy. Active lesions show lymphoplasmacytic hydropic and lichenoid dermatitis. *K*, Same dog as in *J*. Chronic lesions show pigmentary incontinence. *L*, Congenital supranumery claws on the hind paw of a yellow Labrador retriever. *M*, Horizontal band defects on the claws of a dog, coinciding with the prior presence of a portosystemic shunt. *N*, Anal sac abscess in a dog.

lupoid onychodystrophy, of which three were Rottweilers and three were giant or standard Schnauzers.[22, 24] All dogs were presented for claw disease and were otherwise healthy. Typically, owners first noticed a single abnormal claw on two paws or more. However, within 2 to 9 weeks, every claw on all four paws was affected. The initial clinical sign was usually a separation at the claw bed and sloughing of one or more claws. Subungual hemorrhage was seen in some dogs (see Fig. 19–4I). After the claws had been sloughed, regrowth was characterized by short, misshapen, dry, soft, brittle, often crumbling and discolored claws. About half of the dogs exhibit lameness or pain, or both, on palpation. Secondary bacterial infection may be seen. Histopathologically, the disorder is characterized by hydropic and lichenoid interface dermatitis (see Fig. 19–4J and K). Direct immunofluorescence testing did not reveal a lupus band. Although most cases have been idiopathic,[22, 38] Mueller reported cases that responded to antibiotic therapy and that resolved with an elimination diet.[33, 37] Lupoid onychodystrophy may be a reaction pattern of the claw, with several potential causes (e.g., food hypersensitivity, drug reaction, idiopathy).

Response to omega-3 and omega-6 fatty acids (Derm Caps, DVM Pharmaceuticals) or systemic glucocorticoids is usually good.[22, 38] A limited number of cases are not fatty acid responsive.[23, 36] The combination of tetracycline or doxycycline and niacinamide administered orally (see Chap. 3) is often effective, and has been used successfully when fatty acid therapy has failed.[34, 37] With successful therapy, clinical improvement is usually obvious within 3 to 4 months and maximal in 1 year. When treatment is stopped, the condition often relapses.[22, 38]

NEOPLASIA

Neoplasia may also involve the claw or the distal digit (see Chap. 20).[21] Usually, one claw is affected, although rarely multiple claws may be involved. Epithelial neoplasms are most common and include squamous cell carcinoma, subungual keratoacanthoma, inverted squamous papillomas, and atrichial sweat gland carcinomas (see Fig. 19–4D). Atrichial sweat gland carcinomas and squamous cell carcinomas in the claws of cats tend to be aggressive. Melanoma, mast cell tumors, fibrosarcoma, osteosarcoma, lymphosarcoma, hemangiosarcoma, metastatic carcinomas (especially from the lung), myxosarcoma, and neurofibrosarcoma have all been reported.[21, 25, 27, 35–37]

IDIOPATHIC ONYCHODYSTROPHY

Onychodystrophy is often diagnosed when multiple paws and claws are affected and other causes cannot be determined. Again, it is important to include in this category only those dogs that developed onychodystrophy as the initial clinical manifestation of their disease, *not* as a result of onychomadesis, onycholysis, and so forth. These animals often have secondary bacterial infections, so that improvement may be seen with aggressive antimicrobial therapy. However, recurrence after discontinuation of appropriate therapy is routine. Certain breeds appear predisposed and include Siberian huskies, Dachshunds, Rhodesian Ridgebacks, Rottweilers, and Cocker spaniels.[21, 22, 25, 27, 34, 36] In a report of seven dogs with claw disease, the three Rottweilers had symmetric lupoid onychodystrophy.[24] Cocker spaniels may have onychodystrophy as a manifestation of primary seborrhea. One of the authors (CEG) has also seen two cases in Welsh terriers (see Fig. 19–3G). One owner, a breeder, reported that a littermate had a similar problem, and other breeders, anecdotally, reported the same. Old dogs are prone to idiopathic onychodystrophy. Dogs with idiopathic onychodystrophy may respond to gelatin or biotin. Retinoids might be useful here, but the authors are unaware of any attempts to use these agents.

IDIOPATHIC ONYCHOMADESIS

Idiopathic onychomadesis is also described as a problem, particularly in the German shepherd, Whippet, and English Springer spaniels.[27, 28, 34, 36] This may also be a problem of the Rottweiler.[23] Most of these dogs have not had claw biopsies performed and, thus, could actually represent a number of different disorders. In one case, a Rottweiler had vitiligo and, concurrently, onycholysis (see Fig. 19–4E). These cases, besides having onychomadesis, are characterized by frequent secondary bacterial infections under the claw plate, onychoschizias, and onychorrhexis. The mineral composition of claws from 21 dogs with idiopathic onychomadesis (including 8 German shepherds) showed a significant increase in the concentrations of calcium, potassium, sodium, and phosphorus, and decreased concentrations of iron, manganese, and magnesium, as compared with 32 normal dogs (which also included 8 German shepherds).[28] The German shepherds with idiopathic onychomadesis had significantly decreased concentrations of iron, manganese, and magnesium. German shepherd dogs with idiopathic onychomadesis were significantly overrepresented compared with the reference hospital population. Anecdotal information[33] indicates that German shepherd dogs with idiopathic onychomadesis may benefit from treatment with pentoxifylline (see Chap. 3).

Miscellaneous Claw Disorders

Miscellaneous causes of claw disease reported or seen by the authors include epidermolysis bullosa, dermatomyositis, drug eruption, ergotism, thallotoxicosis, linear epidermal nevi, nutritional deficiencies, disseminated intravascular coagulation, and necrolytic migratory erythema. Carlotti reported two young malamutes with paronychia and onychorrhexis of all digits that had histopathologic findings suggestive of zinc-responsive dermatosis and a dramatic response to zinc sulfate therapy.[37] Carlotti also reported a linear epidermal nevus in a dog, which was present since birth, which extended from the groin to two digits of the paw.[37] The lesion responded to the oral administration of etretinate. Another situation that may occur is the development of permanent onychodystrophy after destruction of the basal cells of the germinative layers. Even though the infectious agent may be eliminated and the underlying or primary disease is cured or controlled, the claw continues to grow with a permanent deformity. If this area is prone to cracking, resultant infections may ensue.

Trachyonychia (lusterless, longitudinally ridged, and rough-surfaced claws) was diagnosed in an 8-year-old Rhodesian Ridgeback.[25a] The claw abnormality had begun at 1 year of age and affected all 20 claws. Pieces occasionally broke off the claws, resulting in bleeding. Over the years, the dog had lost many claws, but they always grew back. Claw biopsy revealed lymphocytic infiltration of the claw matrix.

Supranumery claws were present congenitally on the hind paws of a yellow Labrador retriever (see Fig. 19–4L). Horizontal bands were seen on all claws of a dog (see Fig. 19–4M). These bands appeared 1 month after the treatment of a portosystemic shunt, suggesting a disturbance in claw growth coincidental with the systemic disease.

Diagnosis

Because of the numerous causes of claw disease, it is obvious that a wide variety of diagnostic tests, or procedures, may be needed. These are often determined on the basis of history and physical examination findings. The history should include a thorough drug history including vaccinations. Claw disease may develop 2 to 8 weeks following a vaccination.[24] In these cases or those suspected of a vascular etiology, the biopsy and work-up should not be put off, because the diagnostic lesions may only be present early in the course of the disease. When only claw disease is present, a simpler approach may be warranted. In general, when only one or a few asymmetric claws are affected, the initial work-up may be limited to a complete history, physical examination, and cytologic evaluation of collected exudate or debris. Material from within the claw fold or under the claw should be obtained for evaluation. Cytologic examination is helpful in establishing the presence of bacterial or fungal infection (suppurative to pyogranulomatous to granulomatous inflammation, degenerate neutrophils, and phagocytosed microorganisms), pemphigus diseases (nondegenerate neutrophils or eosinophils and numerous acantholytic keratinocytes), and neoplasia.

If bacteria, yeast, or another cause is not identified, fungal cultures and skin scrapes are indicated. The presence of intracellular bacteria supports a diagnosis of bacterial disease, and trauma is the most likely inciting factor. If there is no evidence of neoplasia, initial trial antibiotic therapy is indicated. When multiple paws and claws are symmetrically affected, or when antibiotic therapy is ineffective, a work-up for underlying diseases should be begun. At this point, biopsy is often warranted.

Anal sac abscess occurs as the result of an infection, which is often associated with some degree of impaction. The ruptured sac releases the infection, and secretion into the surrounding tissue results in cellulitis and possible fistula formation (see Fig. 19–4N).

Anal sac neoplasia may also occur and most commonly is an adenocarcinoma (see Chap. 20). Older females are overrepresented. Clinical signs may be minimal or unapparent except for a mass or swelling in the perianal area.[47] Tenesmus, constipation, and polyuria and polydipsia are more commonly seen than typical signs of anal sac impaction or infection.[47]

Clinical Features

Abnormalities of the anal sacs cause scooting, licking, biting, or rubbing the anus, and pyotraumatic dermatitis from self-trauma may result in the surrounding region. These signs are not specific for anal sac disease and may be seen with any anal pruritic disease such as atopy, food hypersensitivity, psychogenic anal licking, vulvar fold dermatitis, tail fold dermatitis, vaginitis, proctitis and perianal fistulae.[40, 46] Cats rarely scoot but typically cause traumatic alopecia of the tailhead and/or caudal abdominal areas. Infected anal sacs may rupture, resulting in cellulitis with localized erythema, swelling, and pain, and a subsequent draining fistulous tract may occur 1 to 2 cm lateral to the anus. The abscess is usually unilateral, and the course is short (7 to 10 days). A foul-smelling odor may be noted by the owners or on examination without expressing the sacs. Infected anal sacs are a focus of infection that has the potential for several untoward results. Some veterinarians are convinced that dogs licking the anal region in such cases transfer infection to the mouth with resultant tonsillitis, pharyngitis, and gagging, and only treatment of both areas (anal sacs and pharynx) has produced good results. In other cases, anal sac infection may be the source of antigen in dogs with widespread bacterial hypersensitivity.[39]

Clinical Management

IMPACTIONS

Feline impactions usually occur without infection, and manual expression (by lateral external compression) usually relieves clinical signs for a relatively long time.[43, 48]

Canine impactions tend to recur. They should be gently but thoroughly expressed. This may have to be repeated several times at weekly intervals by gently placing a gloved finger in the posterior rectum and compressing the sac between the finger and the thumb (positioned lateral to the distended sac). A fetid brownish yellow or black discharge is expressed. If recurrence is frequent, irrigation should be performed as for chronically infected anal sacs.

INFECTED ANAL SACS

Chronically infected anal sacs should be treated as any infection—by drainage. This need not be surgical. Frequent expression of the purulent or bloody exudate followed by instillation of an antibiotic solution may be curative. Inferior results are often obtained with this method because the tenderness of the region precludes thorough treatment. It is preferable to anesthetize the patient lightly and to lavage both sacs thoroughly with lactated Ringer's solution, using a blunt needle or cannula attached to a syringe. Ceruminolytic agents such as hexamethyltetracosane (Cerumene, EVSCO) may also be useful as lavage fluids. After the sac is thoroughly flushed, it is important to instill an antibiotic cream, nitrofurazone solution, or a lotion containing antibiotic and corticosteroid in a ceruminolytic base (e.g., Liquichlor, EVSCO). This may be repeated in 5 to 7 days. If yeasts are involved, a solution containing nystatin (Panolog, Fort Dodge) or clotrimazole (Otomax, Schering-Plough) may be used. If recurrence develops after the initial response, surgical removal of the sacs is indicated.

An acutely infected anal sac (abscess) must be treated by liberal incision at the point of localization and by curettage and application of 5% to 7% iodine solution (Lugol's solution, Butler). Healing occurs by granulation. If the anal sac abscess does not heal with the above-mentioned treatments or if it recurs repeatedly, surgical excision of the anal sacs is indicated.

• EXTERNAL EAR DISEASES

Anatomy and Physiology

The primary purpose of the external ear canal and pinnae is to collect sound waves and transmit them to the tympanic membrane. In normal young dogs, air-conducted stimuli are detected at 0 to 10 decibels (dB) and bone-conducted stimuli are detected at 50 to 60 dB.[152] The pinnae and vertical canal is the part formed with the auricular cartilage. At the external orifice of the ear, the auricular cartilage begins to roll into a funnel shape, which becomes tube shaped as it reaches down into the lower portions of the ear canal. The external ear canal is variable in length (5 to 10 cm) and classically divided into the vertical and horizontal portions.[21] The vertical portion originates from the pinnae and extends in a rostral ventral direction before bending medially (horizontal canal) and continuing until it reaches the tympanic membrane. The lumen is 0.5 to 1 cm in diameter.[21] Shar peis have an ear canal of small diameter compared with other dog breeds.[147] This is especially true of the vertical ear canal. The cartilage structures and the bony external acoustic process are lined by skin (Fig. 19-5).

The skin lining the ear canal normally is a relatively smooth surface and, similar to

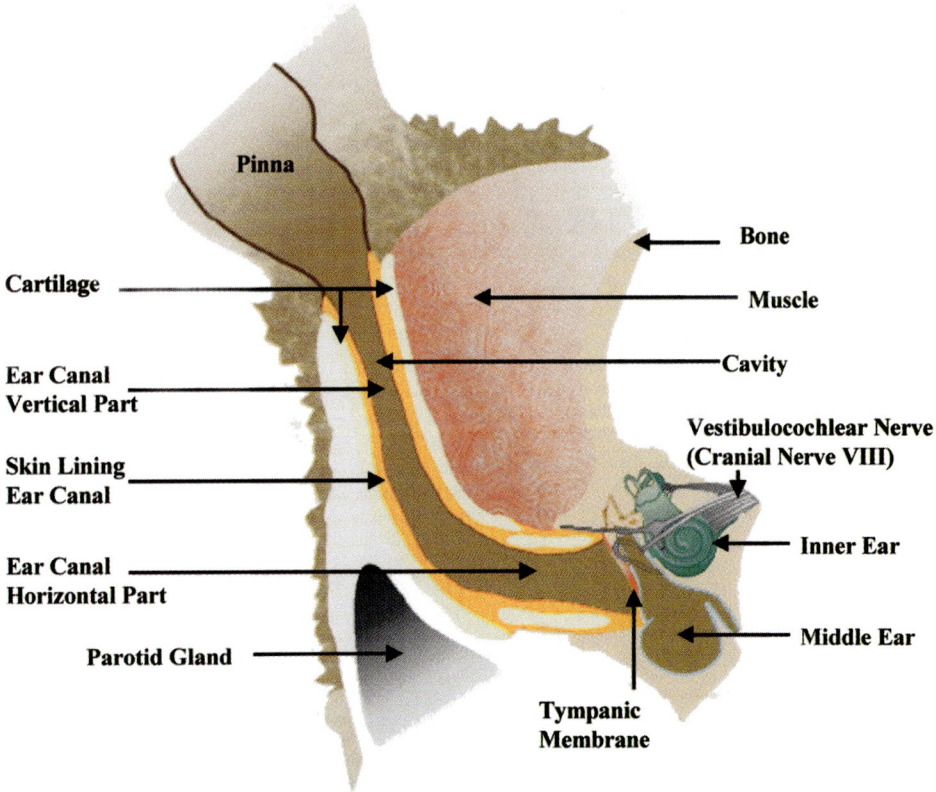

FIGURE 19–5. Schematic diagram of the anatomy of the ear. (Courtesy of CLIVE, Univ. of Edinburgh).

most body regions, has a thin epidermis and dermis that contains adnexa (hair follicles, and sebaceous and ceruminal glands). The vertical canal has relatively more adnexa than the horizontal canal. To date, breed differences in the amount of sebaceous glands have not been shown, although ceruminal (apocrine) gland and hair follicle density does differ.[144] An association between the development of otitis externa and ceruminal gland density has also been shown.[144]

The skin and adnexa are constantly producing exfoliating cells and glandular secretions. This material forms the earwax and cerumen that is believed to play some protective role. Canine immunoglobulins A, G, and M have been identified in canine cerumen.[86] IgG is the predominant immunoglobulin found in both normal and inflamed ears with its relative concentration significantly increasing in diseased ears. The ear canal has a clearing mechanism. The movement of the epidermis, epithelial cell migration, clears out the epithelial cells and glandular secretions (cerumen), and trapped dirt and debris.[91, 151a]

The tympanic membrane is an epithelial structure that separates the external ear laterally from the middle ear cavity located medially. The normal tympanic membrane when viewed from the external ear canal during an otoscopic examination is a concave, translucent membrane, although there is a white C-shaped area in the dorsal part (Fig. 19–6). This corresponds to the attachment of the manubrium of the malleus bone. For descriptive purposes, the tympanic membrane is divided into two parts: the pars flaccida and pars tensa. The pars flaccida is the smaller part that lies next to the manubrium. The pars tensa is the ventral portion that ends at the most distal point of the tympanic membrane. This region may be difficult to visualize by otoscopic examination.

The middle ear consists of the tympanic cavity and walls, medial wall of the tympanic membrane, the auditory ossicles and associated ligaments, muscles and nerves (chorda tympani and other smaller nerves), and the auditory tube. In the normal ear, the only communication from the middle ear to the outside environment is through the auditory tube, which opens into the nasal pharynx. The tympanic cavity is divided into three parts: dorsal, middle, and ventral. The dorsal is the smallest and contains the head of the malleus and the incus. The middle part, also called tympanic cavity proper, is adjacent to the tympanic membrane. The auditory tube opens in the middle portion of the tympanic cavity. The ventral portion is the tympanic bulla and is the largest portion. The tympanic bulla is somewhat egg shaped, with the dorsal aspect open to communicate with the middle part. When otitis media is present, this part acts as a reservoir to trap the debris and toxins. This portion also has the poorest access and, even with a ruptured tympanum, cannot be adequately examined by otoscopy. Structures running close to or in channels along the middle ear include the facial nerve, vagus nerve, and carotid and lingual arteries.

Otitis Externa

Otitis externa is inflammation of the ear canal, which may result from numerous causes. The most relevant classification scheme divides the causes of otitis externa into predisposing, primary, secondary, and perpetuating (Table 19–8).[61, 79, 118, 151a] In every case, the clinician should identify as many causes and factors as possible that may contribute to the otitis. Most chronic cases have at least one primary and several other causes or factors present. Failure to recognize and correct one or more of these causes may lead to treatment failures.

PREDISPOSING FACTORS

Predisposing factors increase the risk of developing otitis externa.[21, 52, 151a] They work in conjunction with primary causes, secondary causes, or perpetuating factors to cause clinical disease. The most successful management of otitis externa necessitates that they be recognized and controlled whenever possible.

Ear type has been reported to predispose the animal to otitis externa by altering the microclimate.[52, 84] Climatic factors do appear to play a role because the incidence of otitis

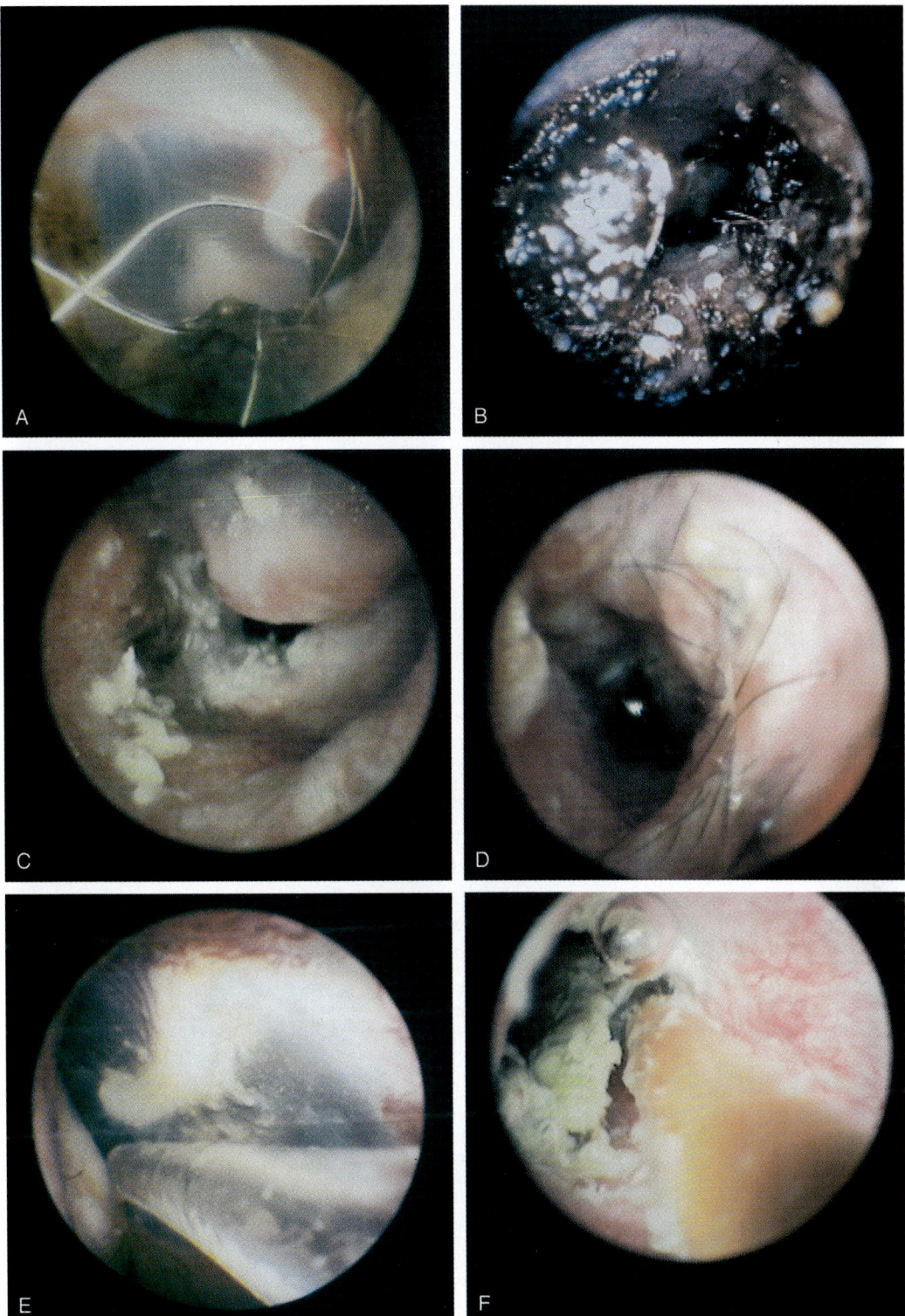

FIGURE 19-6. Fiberoptic videoscope views of ears. *A*, Normal tympanic membrane, some hairs, and cerumen. *B*, Ear mites and excessive cerumen. (Courtesy L. Gotthelf). *C*, Horizontal ear canal with proliferative changes seen as papules and folds in contrast to a normal smooth lining. *D*, Deep horizontal ear canal with proliferative changes, erythema, and multiple ulcers. The ability to make photographic records of a case is an advantage of the otic videoscope. *E*, Tympanic membrane and manubrium of the malleus clearly visible, and a catheter points to the highest level at which a myringotomy should be performed. *F*, Feeding tube down an exudative ear canal showing an accumulation of pus and debris and an air bubble being cleaned out of the canal.

Table 19–8 FACTORS AND CAUSES OF OTITIS EXTERNA

PREDISPOSING FACTORS

Conformation	Stenotic canals
	Hair in canals
	Pendulous pinnae
	Hairy concave pinnae
Excessive moisture	Swimmer's ear
	High-humidity climate
Excessive cerumen production	Overactive glands
Treatment effects	Trauma from cotton applicators
	Irritant topicals
	Superinfections by altering normal microflora
Obstructive ear disease	Neoplasms
	Polyps
	Granulomas (infections, foreign body, sterile)
Systemic disease	Immune suppression or viral disease
	Debilitation
	Catabolic states

PRIMARY CAUSES

Parasites	*Otodectes cynotis*
	Demodex canis, D. cati, Sarcoptes scabiei, Notoedres cati
	Chiggers (especially *Eutrombicula*)
	Flies (especially *Stomoxys calcitrans*)
	Ticks (especially *Otobius megnini*)
	Fleas (especially *Echidnophaga gallinacea* and *Spilopsylla cuniculi*)
Microorganisms	Dermatophytes
	Sporothrix schenckii
Hypersensitivity diseases	Atopy
	Food hypersensitivity
	Contact hypersensitivity
	Drug reactions
Keratinization disorders	Primary idiopathic seborrhea
	Hypothyroidism
	Sex hormone imbalances
	Lipid-related conditions
Foreign bodies	Plants (especially foxtails)
	Hair
	Sand, dirt
	Hardened medications and secretions
Glandular disorders	Ceruminal gland hyperplasia
	Sebaceous gland hyperplasia or hypoplasia
	Altered secretion rate
	Altered type of secretions
Autoimmune diseases	Lupus erythematosus
	Pemphigus foliaceus
	Pemphigus erythematosus
	Cold agglutinin disease
Viral diseases	Canine distemper
Miscellaneous conditions	Solar dermatitis
	Frostbite
	Vasculitis, vasculopathy
	Juvenile cellulitis
	Eosinophilic dermatitis or granuloma
	Sterile eosinophilic folliculitis
	Aural chondritis

SECONDARY CAUSES

Bacteria	*Staphylococcus intermedius*
	Proteus sp.
	Pseudomonas sp.
	Escherichia sp.
	Klebsiella sp.

Table continued on opposite page

● Table 19-8	**FACTORS AND CAUSES OF OTITIS EXTERNA** (Continued)
Yeast	*Malassezia pachydermatis*
	Candida albicans
Topical reactions	Abnormal skin required
Foreign bodies	Small or microscopic
PERPETUATING FACTORS	
Pathologic responses	Epidermal
	Altered epithelial cell migration
	Hyperkeratosis
	Hyperplasia
	Epithelial folds
	Dermal
	Edema
	Fibrosis
	Adnexal
	Ceruminal gland—hypertrophy or hyperplasia
	Hidradenitis
	Lumen
	Stenosis
	Cartilage
	Mineralization
Tympanic membrane changes	Opacity
	Dilation
	Diverticulum
Middle ear cavity	Epithelial changes
	Simple purulent
	Caseated or keratinous
	Cholesteatoma
	Proliferative
	Destructive osteomyelitis

Modified from Griffin CE et al: Otitis externa and media. Current Veterinary Dermatology: The Art and Science of Therapy. Mosby–Year Book, St. Louis, 1993, p 245.

externa is greater in the months with greater relative humidity and temperature.[84] Although increased temperature and relative humidity have been suggested, only one of these explanations still seems plausible. The temperature of the external ear canal is not different in erect versus pendulous eared dogs.[88] However, the pinnae have higher relative humidity at the skin surface than other body regions.[63] Therefore, increased relative humidity may be an important factor. Occasionally, dogs and cats present for chronic recurrent otitis that appears to have only excessive cerumen production as the underlying cause (see Fig. 19–4F). A variety of secondary bacterial or yeast infections occur. Workups reveal no underlying cause of these cases of idiopathic excessive cerumen production. In dogs with hairy ear canals prone to otitis externa, hair removal should be part of the management. However, in dogs without any ear disease or history of it, hair removal is not recommended by the authors. In fact, hair removal can precipitate or exacerbate otitis externa. Obstructive ear diseases often lead to otitis externa. Feline nasopharyngeal polyps and neoplasia in dogs are most often likely to cause this problem. Shar peis have ear canals of smaller diameter than those of other dog breeds and some individuals, especially those with mucinosis, have stenotic vertical ear canals and external orifices.

Feline Nasopharyngeal Polyps

Feline nasopharyngeal polyps is a relatively uncommon inflammatory disease in cats.[93, 126] They may originate from the pharyngeal mucosa, the auditory (eustachian) tube, or the middle ear (see Fig. 19–4G). Although their etiology is unknown, inflammatory polyps may be congenital or secondary to viral or bacterial infections. A congenital cause has been proposed because polyps occur primarily in young cats and because they have been seen in sibling kittens. Feline calicivirus has been recovered from the tissues of several cats.

Nasopharyngeal polyps should be considered in the differential diagnosis of unilateral, medically resistant otitis externa or otitis media with or without respiratory signs. Otorrhea (dark brown ceruminous or purulent exudate) without signs of inflammation of the ear canal lining, head-shaking behavior, and a mass in the horizontal ear canal are the most common signs of external ear involvement. Middle ear involvement may cause head tilt, nystagmus, and disequilibrium.

Diagnosis is confirmed by examination of the ear and upper airway under anesthesia. Histopathologically, the lesion is a loose mass of connective tissue containing numerous blood vessels and mononuclear leukocytes, covered by an epithelium that may be stratified, nonkeratinized squamous, or simple to bilayered ciliated columnar. Treatment includes surgical removal of the polyp and, often, bulla osteotomy. Postsurgical complications include regrowth, persistent discharge, and transient Horner's syndrome.

Ceruminal Gland Neoplasms

Neoplasms of the ear include those capable of affecting the skin elsewhere, as well as primary neoplasms of ceruminal glands (see Chap. 20).[21, 72, 135, 149] In the dog, the most common pinnal neoplasms are sebaceous gland tumors, histiocytomas, and mast cell tumors. In the cat, the most common pinnal neoplasms are squamous cell carcinoma, basal cell tumor, hemangiosarcoma, and melanocytic neoplasms.

The most common neoplasm of the ear canal is ceruminal gland in origin (see Fig. 19–4H).[100, 107, 108, 120] These neoplasms are more common in cats than in dogs. In the dog, the neoplasms are typically benign, whereas in the cat, they are malignant in about 50% of cases. *Ceruminal gland neoplasms* typically occur in older animals and in one ear. Clinical signs include variable degrees of head-shaking and ear-scratching behavior, otorrhea, an offensive necrotic odor, frequent secondary bacterial otitis externa, and even intermittent hemorrhage from the affected ear. Occasionally, ceruminal gland neoplasms present as bulging, ulcerative, draining masses below the ear in the parotid region (Fig. 19–7). Otoscopic examination usually reveals a small (less than 1 cm in diameter), well-circumscribed, pinkish white, dome-shaped mass, with frequent ulceration, hemorrhage, and secondary infection (Fig. 19–8). Ceruminal gland tumors are positive for cytokeratin.[100] The only effective therapy is surgical excision, usually by lateral ear resection or total ablation of the ear canal. The best results are achieved with ear canal ablation and

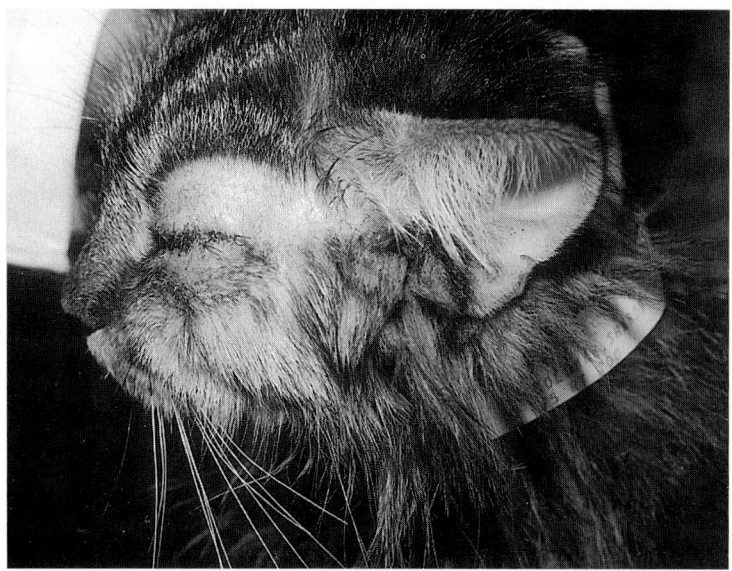

FIGURE 19–7. Ceruminal gland carcinoma in a cat presenting as a mass in the parotid area.

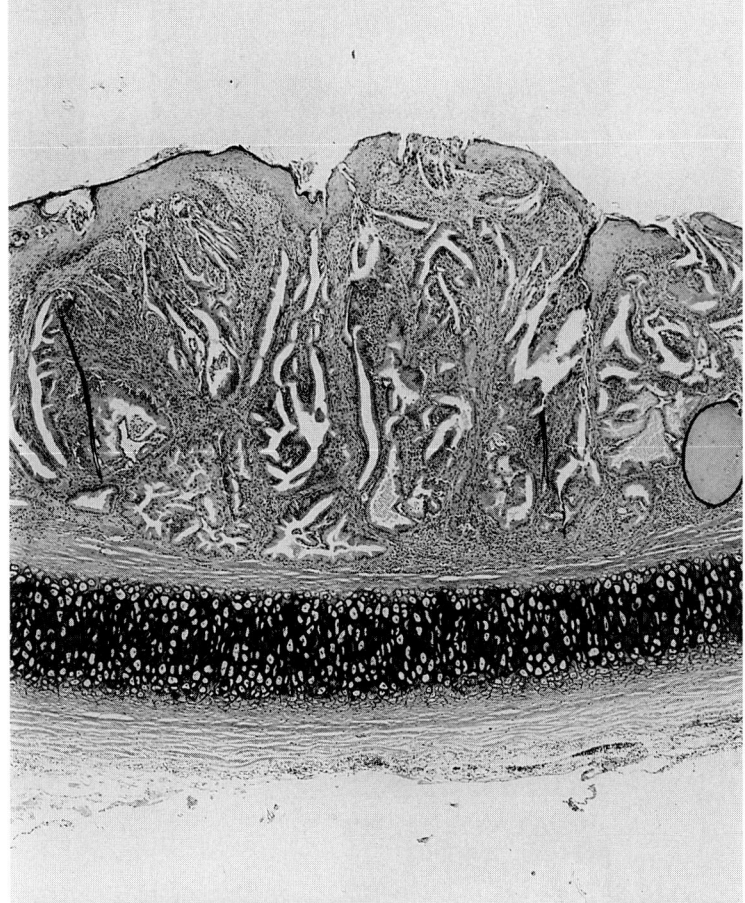

FIGURE 19-8. Nodular ceruminal gland carcinoma.

lateral bulla osteotomy.[107, 108] The recurrence rate is around 70% with lateral ear resection.[107, 108]

PRIMARY CAUSES

Primary causes directly induce otitis externa. The most common causes seen by the authors are atopy, food hypersensitivity, keratinization disorders, and ear mites. It is critical to successful long-term management that a primary cause be found and controlled.

Parasites

A number of parasites have been associated with otitis externa (see Table 19–8).[21] However, the ear mite *Otodectes cynotis* is most common (see Chap. 6), being responsible for up to 50% of the otitis externa cases diagnosed in cats and 5% to 10% of the cases in dogs (see Fig. 19–6B). Ear mites may initiate otitis externa but remain undetected. One reason is the difficulty that may occur in demonstrating the mites. As few as two or three mites can cause clinical otitis externa.[74] This may be explained by studies showing that ear mites can induce Arthus-type and immediate-type hypersensitivity reactions.[128, 151] Another explanation is that the mites initiate the otitis externa and then leave the canal or are destroyed by the inflammation or the secondary infection. In recurrent cases of parasitic otitis externa, the possibility of other in-contact animals being asymptomatic carriers should be considered. Owing to variations in the time necessary for transmission from carrier to affected patient, the time of onset of hypersensitivity reactions, and the develop-

Diseases of Eyelids, Claws, Anal Sacs, and Ears

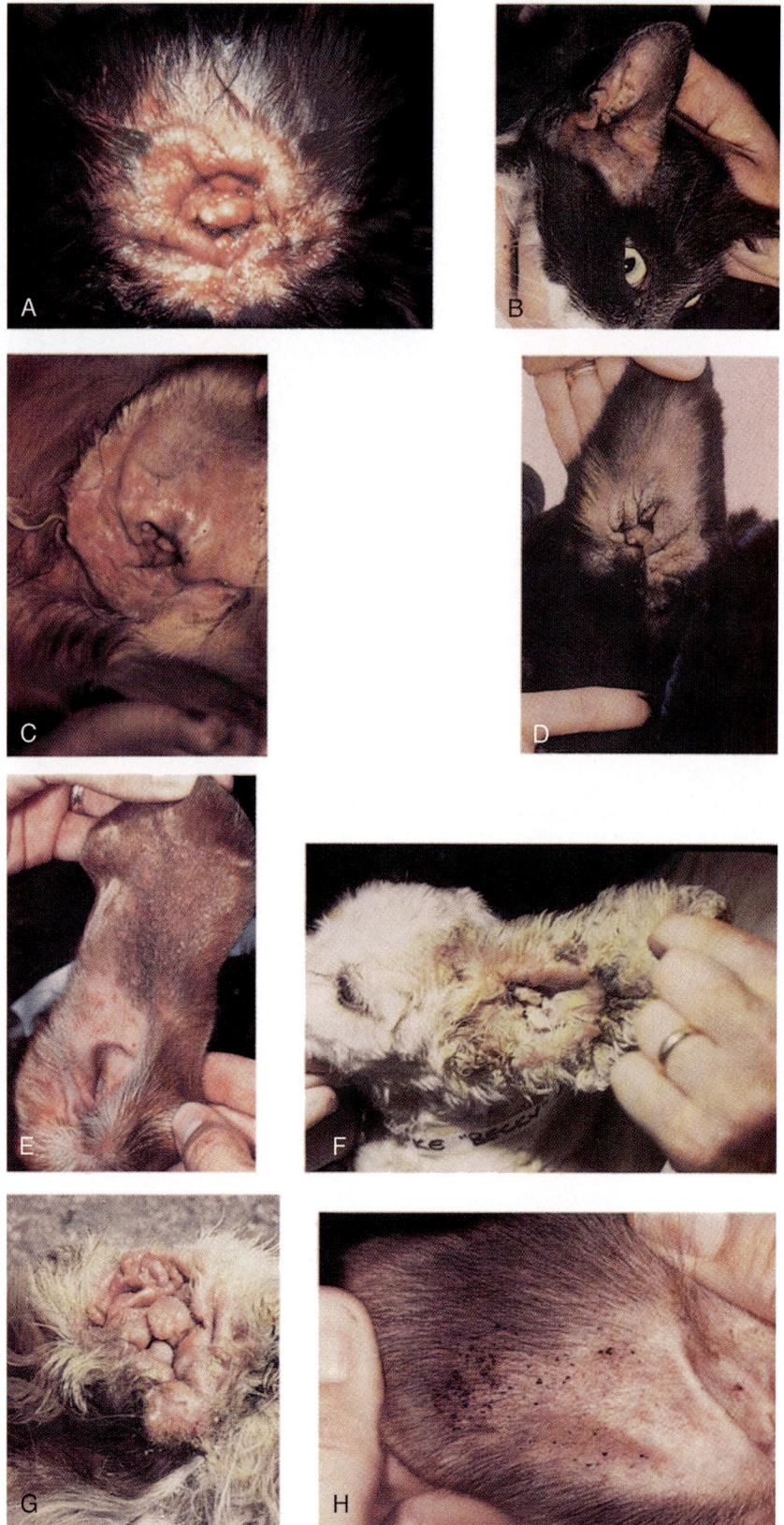

FIGURE 19–9. Legend on opposite page

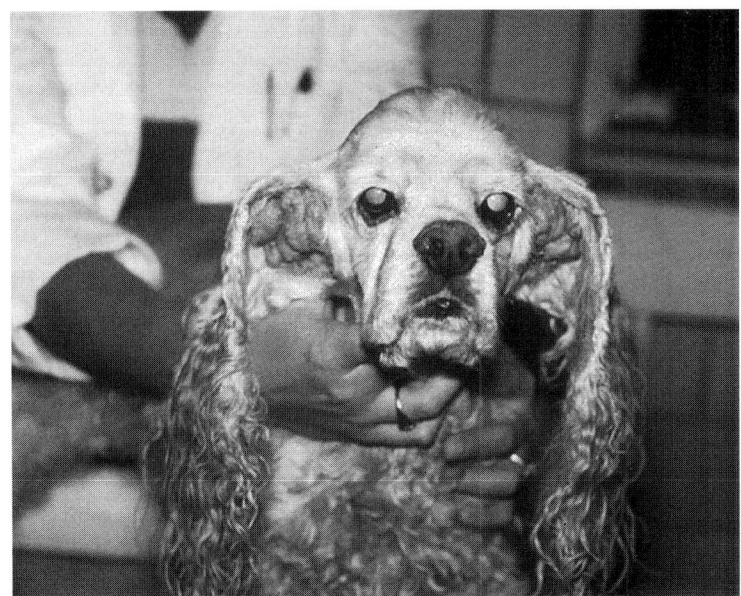

FIGURE 19–9 *Continued. I,* Idiopathic inflammatory and hyperplastic otitis externa in a Cocker spaniel. Both ear canals are mineralized, causing the pinna to extend out laterally.

ment of clinical signs noticeable by the owner, these diseases may present as rapidly or intermittently recurrent cases.[77]

Fly bites are a common cause of pinnal dermatitis during fly season (see Chap. 6). Pinpoint ulcers that are rapidly covered by a black-red crust are typical (see Fig. 19–6H).

Hypersensitivities

Atopy, food hypersensitivity, and contact hypersensitivity can cause otitis externa (see Chap. 8).[21, 61] The otitis externa may be secondary to self-trauma, or the hypersensitivity reaction may involve the external ear canal. Atopic dogs have otitis signs in 83% of the cases, with 24% having otic symptoms at the onset of their allergic disease.[122] Otitis may be the only symptom in some cases.[77, 78, 139] Atopy, as a result of its high incidence and the incidence of otitis in atopics, is more frequently associated with otitis externa than is food hypersensitivity. Erythema of the pinna and vertical canal is a common feature of allergic otitis externa (see Fig. 19–9A and B).[77] Chronic inflammation may eventually lead to secondary bacterial or yeast infections.

Ear disease is present in up to 80% of dogs and cats with food hypersensitivity, and food hypersensitivity is the second most common hypersensitivity reaction to affect the ear. Cocker spaniels and Labrador retrievers have been suggested as breeds more likely to present with otitis externa as the only symptom of food hypersensitivity.[81] Dogs younger than 6 months of age with acute bilateral otitis and no evidence of ear mites or foreign bodies should also be considered as more likely to have food hypersensitivity.

Contact hypersensitivity may result from medications (e.g., neomycin) used to treat otitis externa. In addition, vehicles such as propylene glycol can also be responsible for hypersensitive or irritant reactions in the ear.[77] Therefore, changing medications on the basis of major active ingredients may not alleviate a treatment reaction. Typically, these

---

FIGURE 19–9. *A,* Allergic otitis externa in a dog with atopy. *B,* Contact hypersensitivity in a cat due to a topical product that contained neomycin. *C,* Erythema multiforme in a dog with severe ulceration of the ear canal. *Candida albicans* was found in cytologic studies and in otic cultures. *D,* Seborrheic otitis externa in a hypothyroid dog. *E,* Sterile eosinophilic pinnal folliculitis in a dog. *F, Pseudomonas* otitis externa in a Cocker spaniel with atopy and primary seborrhea. *G,* Proliferative otitis externa with numerous folds resulting. Similar changes are present in the vertical and horizontal canal. *H,* Classic fly bites *(Stomoxys calcitrans)* on the pinna of a dog.

cases have a history of either (1) short-term response to therapy, and then as medication administration is continued, symptoms worsen; or (2) previous good responses to a product, but a worsening with the most recent course of treatment.[140, 141] Another clinical clue is the development of erythema dorsally and ventrally to the external orifice, because the medications usually contact these areas as well. Drug reactions may also involve the ear canal and the pinnae. This may be due to contact allergic or irritant effects. In other cases, systemic drug reactions, such as erythema multiforme, may affect the ear canal (see Fig. 19–9C).

Keratinization Disorders

The keratinization disorders generally present as chronic ceruminous otitis externa.[21] Breeds prone to primary idiopathic seborrhea tend to have ceruminous otitis externa (see Chap. 14). Endocrinopathies, such as hypothyroidism and sex hormone imbalances (see Chap. 10) may result in chronic ceruminous otitis externa, most likely by altering keratinization and, possibly, glandular function (see Fig. 19–6D). Hypothyroidism is the most commonly encountered endocrinopathy involving the ear. Many times, the primary cause of the otitis externa is a disease that has some other historical or physical examination findings as a clue.

Foreign Bodies

Foreign bodies that enter the ear canal and become lodged usually result in otitis externa.[21] Typically, it occurs unilaterally, although bilateral disease may occur. Most commonly, the dogs and cats have acute onset of head shaking and scratching at the ear or ears. There is no initial discharge; however, if immediate veterinary care is not sought, these cases may rapidly become secondarily infected and present with a purulent exudate. Examples of otic foreign bodies include plant awns, sand, and dried out medicaments.

Glandular Disorders

Glandular disorders are not well documented in the dog and cat. One study did show that Cocker spaniels with otitis had a greater surface area of glands in their ears than did Cocker spaniels without ear disease.[144] Cocker spaniels, English Springer spaniels, and Labrador retrievers have more ceruminal glands and hair follicles in their ear canals than do Greyhounds and mongrels.[144] In addition, one of the authors (CEG) has seen cases in dogs and cats that had chronic ceruminous otitis and also demonstrated histologic sebaceous gland hyperplasia. They had no other evidence of keratinization disorder or skin disease. Management necessitated that clients learn how to clean the ears on a routine basis.

Autoimmune Diseases

Autoimmune diseases may affect the ear canal, but most commonly cause pinnal disease.[21] Of the diseases listed in Table 19–8, the one most commonly seen is pemphigus foliaceus.

Viral Diseases

Viral diseases are known to cause otitis externa in humans but have rarely been incriminated in the dog. Canine distemper virus has been associated with otitis externa, but whether this is actually directly due to viral invasion of the ear or is secondary to debilitation, spread of respiratory infection, or immune suppression is unknown.

Miscellaneous Conditions

Idiopathic inflammatory or *hyperplastic otitis externa* is seen primarily in Cocker spaniels, initially at a relatively young age.[133] Over one to several years, these dogs develop marked proliferative otitis externa if they are not aggressively managed. Without treatment, they often progress to calcified ear canals. These cases usually do not have other skin disease, although it is imperative to rule out atopy, primary idiopathic seborrhea of Cocker spaniels, and food hypersensitivity. In the authors' experience, food hypersensitivity is the disease most often overlooked, because a diet trial alone will not reverse the perpetuating factors. Food hypersensitivity can only be ruled out with a diet trial and provocative exposure testing once the ears have been improved with therapy. The etiology of this disease is unknown but, considering the histopathologic glandular changes, it is attractive to consider that this may represent a primary glandular disorder.[144]

Juvenile cellulitis often involves the ear canal and occasionally initially starts with otitis externa and pinnal disease (see Chap. 18). These puppies have marked lymphadenopathy at presentation. This has also been described in a 2-year-old Lhasa apso.[90]

Canine sterile eosinophilic pinnal folliculitis is an uncommon idiopathic, nonseasonal, bilaterally symmetric pinnal dermatosis of dogs (see Fig. 19–9E).[136] Erythematous papules and crusts are present on the concave surface of the pinnae. Pruritus is variable. The ear canal is not involved. Cytologic examination of papules reveals numerous eosinophils and no microorganisms. Biopsy reveals eosinophilic folliculitis and furunculosis. Cultures are negative. The condition is responsive to topical or oral glucocorticoids but usually recurs.

Canine proliferative eosinophilic otitis externa is an uncommon idiopathic inflammatory disorder of the ear canal of dogs.[127] Affected dogs have a history of chronic unilateral otitis externa. Otoscopic examination reveals solitary or multiple polypoid masses attached to the ear canal lining by a slender stalk. The masses obstruct the canal. Biopsy reveals a papillomatous, proliferative eosinophilic dermatitis or eosinophilic granuloma. Intraepidermal eosinophilic microabscesses are found. Some lesions contain multifocal areas of degenerate collagen and flame figures, with or without an accompanying palisading granuloma. Surgical excision may be curative or be followed by recurrence.

SECONDARY CAUSES

Secondary causes contribute to or cause pathology only in the abnormal ear or in combination with predisposing factors. These same organisms or agents may be found in normal ears without disease. They are generally easy to manage with a specific drug once the diagnosis is made. In some cases, eliminating the concurrent predisposing factor or primary disease may result in the resolution of the secondary cause.

Bacteria

Bacteria are rarely primary causes; therefore, a diagnosis of bacterial otitis externa is usually not a complete diagnosis. *S. intermedius* and the gram-negative organisms *Pseudomonas* spp. (see Fig. 19–9F), *Proteus* spp., *E. coli*, and *Klebsiella* spp. are most commonly isolated as secondary pathogens (Table 19–9).[54, 59, 61, 64, 118] The four gram-negative organisms are not routinely cultured from normal ears. *Pseudomonas* spp. are more prevalent in chronic otitis. This may reflect that this organism is well adapted for the warm moist environment of ears occluded by hyperplasia of skin and ceruminal glands.[71] Scarification, moisture, and alkalinization were used to create *Pseudomonas aeruginosa* ear infections in normal dogs.[109] After these organisms establish infection, they significantly contribute to the inflammation, damage, and clinical signs.

Yeast

M. pachydermatis is the most common yeast that contributes to otitis externa as a perpetuating factor.[59, 61, 118] It is a budding yeast that has a peanut or bottle shape and may be found in as many as 36% of normal canine ears.[56] In otitis, it is found in up to 76% of the ears and frequently in combination with *Staphylococcus* sp.[56, 95] It has been proposed that *S. intermedius* produces a factor that stimulates the growth of *M. pachydermatis*.[56] It has also been shown that *M. pachydermatis* is a heterogeneous species, with at least two groups identified by a variety of biochemical characteristics.[94] Two strains were different in that one could not grow in the absence of nicotinic acid but grew well in the presence of staphylococci. Possibly, this is the factor that staphylococci supply. *M. pachydermatis* is a common complication with hypersensitivity disorders and may result in a

• Table 19-9 ORGANISMS ISOLATED FROM NORMAL EAR CANALS AND FROM EARS AFFECTED WITH OTITIS EXTERNA AND OTITIS MEDIA

ORGANISMS	CLINICALLY NORMAL				OTITIS EXTERNA					OTITIS MEDIA
	Ear Canals			Middle Ear	Ear Canals					
	Grono, Frost (1969) %	Sampson et al. (1973) %	Marshall et al. (1974) %	Matsuda et al. (1984) %	Grono (Data to be Published) %	Boyle, Grono (Data to be Published) %	Sampson et al. (1973) %	Marshall et al. (1974) %	Cole et al. (1998) HEC %	Cole et al. (1998) ME %
Gram-Positive										
Staphylococcus intermedius	—	—	—	2	—	—	—	—	60.5	36.8
Staphylococcus aureus	—	—	—	7	—	—	—	—	—	—
Staphylococcus xylosus	—	—	1.7	10	—	—	—	—	—	—
Staphylococcus	47.6	15	—	—	30.9	30.4	35.0	38.0	—	—
Pediococcus	—	—	—	2	—	—	—	—	—	—
Unidentified cocci	—	—	—	5	—	—	—	—	—	—
Corynebacterium spp.	—	—	—	0	—	—	—	—	15.8	13.2
β-hemolytic Streptococcus	—	—	—	—	—	—	—	—	7.9	18.4
α-hemolytic Streptococcus	—	—	—	—	—	—	—	—	5.3	NI
Bacillus spp.	—	—	—	0	—	—	—	—	—	—
Unidentified rod	—	—	—	0	—	—	—	—	—	—
Gram-Negative										
Aspergillus	0	—	—	—	0.8	1.1	—	—	—	—
Branhamella spp.	—	—	—	0	—	—	—	—	—	—
Escherichia coli	—	—	—	2	—	—	—	—	NI	5.3
Enterobacter aerogenes	—	—	—	0	—	—	—	—	—	—
Mycoplasma sp.*	—	—	—	2	—	—	—	—	—	—
Enterococcus spp.	—	—	—	—	—	—	—	—	15.8	13.2
Citrobacter spp.	—	—	—	0	—	—	—	—	2.6	2.6
Unidentified rod	—	—	—	—	—	—	—	—	—	—
Nongroup-D Streptococcus	—	—	—	—	—	—	—	—	NI	5.3
Anaerobes	—	—	—	—	—	—	—	—	NI	2.6
Lactobacillus spp.	—	—	—	—	—	—	—	—	NI	2.6
Yeasts and Fungi										
Malassezia spp.	37.9	6	28.3	—	35.9	44.3	23.0	86.2	65.8	34.2
Pseudomonas spp.	2.4	4	0	—	34.6	16.5	5.0	16.4	26.3	36.8
Proteus spp.	1.6	0	0	—	20.8	9.9	5.0	8.6	10.5	13.2
Streptococcus spp.	0	—	—	—	0.8	1.1	—	—	—	—
Culture negative ears	—	—	—	53	—	—	—	—	—	—

Data from Grono LR: Otitis externa. In: Kirk RW (ed): Current Veterinary Therapy VI. W. B. Saunders Co., Philadelphia, 1980; Cole LK, et al: Microbial flora and antimicrobial susceptibility patterns of isolated pathogens from the horizontal ear canal and middle ear in dogs with otitis media. J Am Vet Med Assoc 212:534, 1998; Matsuda H, et al: The aerobic bacterial flora of the middle and external ears in normal dogs. J Small Anim Pract 25:269, 1984.

*Examination for *Mycoplasma* was carried out in 20 ears.

ME = Middle ear. HEC = Horizontal ear canal. NI = Not isolated.

superinfection after antibiotic therapy. *M. pachydermatis* has been shown to be pathogenic when it or fluid is put in the ear canal.[105] Two major phenotypes (large and small colony types) of *M. pachydermatis* have been described, but the significance of these is unknown.[86, 94] Oleic and linoleic acids were shown to be mycostatic, and the common fatty acids found in canine cerumen are margaric, stearic, oleic, and linoleic.[86] The possibility of a public health significance for *M. pachydermatis* has been raised. It was reported in an intensive care nursery where 15 infants were culture positive over a period of approximately 15 months.[62] The culture-positive babies were at greater risk for lower weight and had greater severity of concomitant illness. It was speculated that the *M. pachydermatis* was introduced into the intensive care nursery from a health-care worker's hands after being colonized from pet dogs at home. Further studies to support or explain this association are anxiously awaited.

Topical Acquired Irritant Reactions

Various therapeutic ingredients may induce inflammation in the already damaged aural epidermis and dermis but have no effect on normal skin.[81] As a result, they are not typical topical allergic or irritant reactions. They may have a similar history as other topical irritant or allergic reactions, but often they will cause the ear canal to become ulcerated. Some of these ingredients, such as propylene glycol, are present in numerous topical products, even though active ingredients may be totally different. The continued use of those ingredients hinders the healing and beneficial effects that are expected.

PERPETUATING FACTORS

Perpetuating factors prevent the resolution of otitis externa or otitis media. They result from inflammation and the pathologic responses of the skin and otic structures. These changes occur from the effect of the predisposing factors, and primary and secondary causes. In chronic cases, one or more of these factors are present. In acute cases of otitis externa, treating the primary cause may be sufficient in controlling a case, but after the establishment of some perpetuating factors, treatment must be directed at them. Perpetuating factors may be the major reason for poor response to therapy, regardless of the predisposing factors and primary causes present.

Progressive Pathologic Changes

The microanatomy of the canine and feline ear canal have been studied.[68, 70, 144, 146] Chronic inflammation stimulates the skin lining the ear canal to undergo numerous changes, including epidermal hyperkeratosis and hyperplasia, dermal edema and fibrosis, ceruminal gland hyperplasia, and dilatation. Hidradenitis or inflammation of the ceruminal glands may also occur. A study found that sebaceous glands do not atrophy, as had been previously reported.[144] Morphometric analysis showed that breeds predisposed to otitis externa had an increased quantity of ceruminal glands compared with the number of sebaceous glands, and that dogs with otitis externa had an even greater area of ceruminal glands. An occasional animal may have sebaceous gland hyperplasia. Chronic inflammation can lead to permanent changes in the microanatomy and physiology of the ear canal.[103]

Abnormal epithelial cell migration may occur in response to inflammation.[151a] This mechanism, which is normally responsible for the removal of the waxes, lipids, exfoliating corneocytes, and associated commensal bacteria, is affected. Inflammation and stenosis may be responsible for slowing, stopping, and even reversing this migration pattern. Some evidence to support this in the dog is the finding that dogs with otitis media may have adnexa and stratified epidermis growing in the middle ear that is believed to have migrated in from the external ear canal.[102]

These progressive changes cause a thickening of the skin, which eventually extends to both sides of the auricular cartilage. The swelling leads to stenosis of the canal lumen. More important, the skin is thrown into numerous folds, which inhibit effective cleaning and application of topical medications (see Fig. 19–9G). These folds act as sites for the accumulation of secretions and exudates, and the perpetuation and protection of secondary microorganisms (see Fig. 19–6C). The epidermis becomes thickened, and the hyperkeratotic stratum corneum increases the keratin debris that is exfoliated into the canal lumen. The increased secretions and epithelial debris favor the proliferation of bacteria and yeast.

The combination of microbial metabolic byproducts, secretions, and debris trapped within the folds and ear canal from the stenosis further contribute to the pathologic changes. In a sense, regardless of the initial disease process, the clinician is now faced with numerous areas of *fold dermatitis*. Fibrosis and calcification complicate management by contributing to stenosis of the ear canal and by inhibiting the effective treatment of deep infections. It is interesting to note that the calcification occurs in the connective tissue outside of the auricular or annular cartilage. These changes have a major impact on therapeutic regimens and must be considered in the management of chronic cases.

Tympanic Membrane Alterations

The abnormal tympanic membrane thickens, becomes opaque or slightly colored, and loses its transparency. Additionally, the attachment to the manubrium cannot be seen. It may appear white, off-white, yellow, brown, or gray. Therefore, it can appear the same as impacted exudates or keratin plugs.[77, 81] This is a common problem when cases are referred to specialists and the referring veterinarian believes the tympanic membrane is intact, but it is not.

It has been theorized that the tympanic membrane may dilate and extend into the tympanic cavity. Because the tympanic membrane is capable of reepithelializing after rupture, it is common to have otitis media with an intact tympanic membrane.[151a] In one study in which 8 dogs were necropsied, ruptured tympanic membranes were identified in only 2 of 14 ears with otitis externa and media.[102] However, out of the 62 middle ear specimens examined, histologically definitive tympanic membrane could only be recognized in 26%. Tissue, including adnexal structures that originate from the external ear canal, may be found in the middle ear cavity, even when the tympanic membrane appears intact. The auditory tube was patent in all cases in which it was examined at necropsy. Commonly, the tympanic membrane thickens in response to inflammation and may develop polyploid extensions of granulation tissue into the middle ear cavity, which, in some cases, form adhesions with middle ear mucosa.

Aural cholesteatoma is a keratin-filled epidermoid cyst, located within the middle ear cavity. Aural cholesteatoma may occur in 11% of the animals with chronic otitis media.[102] It has been postulated that cholesteatomas result when a pocket of tympanic membrane forms within the middle ear cavity. One predisposing factor may be spontaneous occlusion of the external ear canal from chronic proliferative changes, leading to external ear canal stenosis.

Another response of the tympanic membrane is the development of a pocket (false middle ear) that allows the impaction and sequestration of material from topical therapy. This may explain why some dogs appear to regrow their tympanic membrane rapidly after flushing of the false middle ear.[77] In contrast to dogs with ruptured tympanic membranes, these animals cannot have their middle ear flushed through the eustachian tube and are less susceptible to ototoxicity.

Otitis Media

Otitis media is inflammation of the middle ear.[118] The normal middle ear cavity may contain some bacteria (staphylococci, streptococci) and occasional yeast,[110] but there is no exudate or inflammatory cells. The presence of exudate within the tympanic cavity is difficult to treat with topical therapy and often remains as a source for infections and proinflammatory toxins and debris to reach the external ear canal. In more advanced cases, the authors have found keratin plugs developing within the tympanic cavity (Fig. 19–10). The keratin may serve as a reservoir for bacteria and a source for inflammation. Eventually, calcification may occur, which may be observed radiographically. In some cases, osteomyelitis of the bony wall or within the newly proliferated bone occurs. Osteomyelitis is difficult to treat medically and often requires surgery to alleviate. Otitis media

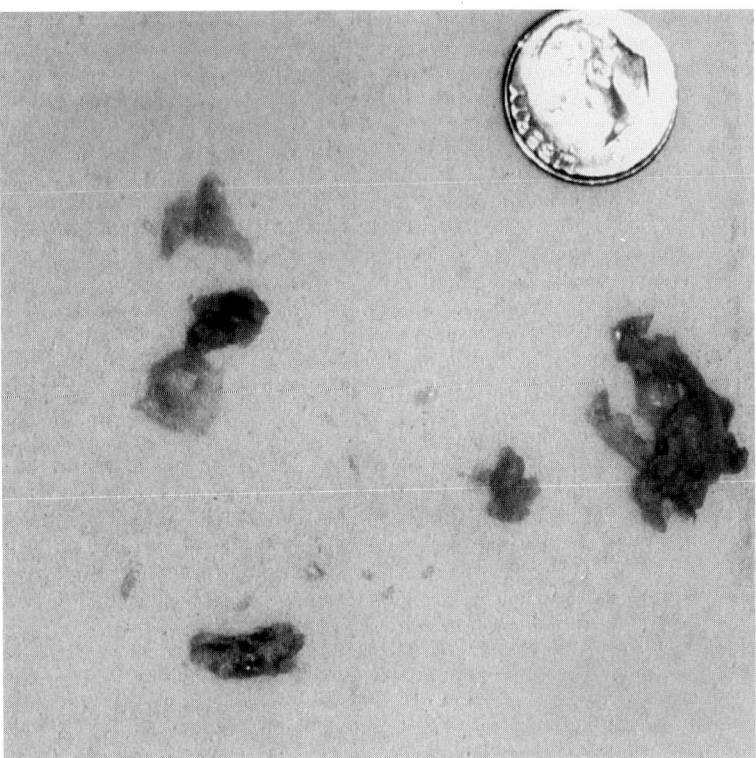

FIGURE 19-10. Keratinous plugs removed by flushing from a middle ear cavity (a dime is in the upper right corner).

occurs commonly with chronic otitis externa. Histologic changes in the middle ear may be present, even with an intact tympanic membrane.[102] The presence of adnexa in some of these cases also supports the idea that previous tympanic membrane rupture was present, but the tympanic membranes have since healed—possibly even while otitis externa or media is present. In one study, otitis media was diagnosed in 38 dog ears, and an intact tympanic membrane was present in 71% of the ears.[64]

Otitis media may occur from extension of otitis externa through the tympanic membrane, from ascending nasal or respiratory infections through the auditory tube, and from hematogenous spread. In dogs, only extension from otitis externa is considered a common cause of otitis media, but in cats, upper respiratory infections are known causes of otitis media. Otitis media has been reported to be present in 16% of dogs with acute otitis externa and 52% of dogs with chronic otitis externa.[143] Another study reported otitis media in 82.6% of chronic otitis externa ears and that the tympanic membranes were intact in 71% of the dogs with otitis media.[64] A difference in total microbial isolates or their susceptibility patterns between horizontal canal and middle ear samples were found in 89.5% of the ears.[64] Bilateral otitis media was present in 72.7% of the dogs.

An extremely rare complication of bacterial otitis media is meningoencephalitis.[141a]

One author (WHM) has examined two allergic dogs who presented for head shaking, head tilt, and Horner's syndrome. Both dogs had externally bulging, normal-appearing tympanic membranes, as is seen in serous otitis media in children, and both dogs responded completely to treatment with amitriptyline.

CLINICAL FEATURES

Otitis externa is a common condition in dogs, perhaps accounting for 15% of all the dogs presented for veterinary care.[51, 61, 115, 117] The true incidence of otitis externa is not known, and one study noted that 5.8% of supposedly normal dogs had a history of otic symptoms.[122] In cats, the incidence is much lower, perhaps 4%.[51, 115–117, 137] The lower incidence in cats may be partially attributable to the upright position of the pinna and the relatively hairless ear canal.

The most common indication of otitis externa is aural pruritus or head shaking. As otitis externa progresses, a mild to marked exudate or malodor may develop. This is usually when the client presents the pet to the veterinarian. It is imperative that a thorough history, both general and dermatologic, be taken. If that is not done, many patients are unnecessarily misdiagnosed. History taking should include questions regarding predisposing factors. Additionally, the majority of cases of chronic ear disease have historical or physical evidence of the primary disease. The common indications that the underlying problem is a hypersensitivity disorder are seasonality and pruritus in other body locations. Keratinization disorders may have changes in coat quality, color, and density or scale formation. Hearing loss may also occur and should always be assessed by asking questions about the dogs hearing as well as observing responses to sounds made during the examination. One study using brainstem auditory evoked response showed that hearing loss in otitis cases most commonly was a result of conductive hearing loss due to pathology in the external or middle ear and that only 2% were deaf.[66]

Clinical signs of otitis media are quite variable and not specific. Most commonly the symptoms mimic or occur because of concurrent otitis externa and include head shaking, aural discharge, or odor. Deafness with extension to inner ear disease may also occur. Pain when eating may be noticed in dogs with severe disease or in animals with otitis media that has progressed to involve the temporomandibular joint.[102]

PHYSICAL FINDINGS

Physical findings indicative of otitis externa include erythema, swelling, scaling, crusting, alopecia, broken hairs, head shyness, otic discharge (otorrhea), malodor, and pain on palpation of the auricular cartilage. Some animals attempt to scratch the ear with the ipsilateral hind paw or shake the head during or after palpation of the ear canal. Lesions may involve the pinna and the skin caudal to the pinna on the head, on the lateral face, and around the vertical canal. Pyotraumatic dermatitis of the lateral face and aural hematomas are the lesions most commonly associated with aural pruritus, although clinical otitis externa may not be noticeable. Head tilt may be seen with either otitis externa or otitis media. However, concurrent facial nerve abnormalities (e.g., facial palsy and hemifacial spasm) or Horner's syndrome indicates otitis media, although facial palsy may also be seen with hypothyroidism and concurrent ceruminous otitis.

Palpation of the external ear canal and tympanic bulla may provide additional information. The thickness, firmness, and pliability of the vertical and horizontal canal should be determined. Thicker, firmer, and less pliable canals are associated with proliferative changes and support a more guarded prognosis. Mineralized canals are rock hard and can rarely be returned to normal or successfully managed with medical therapy (see Fig. 19–9I).[77] Pain and palpable abnormalities of the tympanic bulla imply the presence of otitis media.

Erythema of the concave surface of the pinna with a normal convex surface is strongly suggestive of atopy or, less likely, food hypersensitivity. Early cases may have minimal erythema of the vertical canal with a normal horizontal canal. Cases that started with only ear canal disease and, after treatment, spread peripherally in rostral and ventral directions should make one suspect topical therapy reactions. Ulcerations of the external orifice and/or ear canal should make one consider the secondary causes *Pseudomonas* infection, *Candida* infection, and topical reactions.

Otoscopic Examination

The otoscopic examination is used to detect foreign bodies, to determine whether otitis media is present, and to assess what type of lesions, exudate, and progressive pathologic changes have occurred. If unilateral disease is present, the unaffected ear should be examined first. This decreases the possibility of the dog's experiencing pain and resisting examination of the second ear. Examining the unaffected ear first decreases the risk of spreading an infectious agent from the diseased ear to the unaffected ear. Having multiple otoscopic cones of varying sizes placed in cold sterilization containers allows one to use aseptic cones. One problem often encountered in practice is the extremely painful, ulcerated, swollen ear that one cannot adequately examine. Even with anesthesia, these cases may not be adequately examined, and it may be necessary to treat the animal and to reduce the swelling and inflammation, then have the patient return in 4 to 7 days so that an otoscopic examination can be properly performed.[77]

A record of lesions should be kept. Proliferative changes, the amount and type of discharge, and the presence of erythema or ulcers should be noted (see Fig. 19–6D). Assessment of the tympanic membrane should be made and recorded.

The degree of canal stenosis should be determined, because changes in lumen size can be used to help monitor treatment. Is proliferation the result of diffuse thickening, or does the canal epithelium have a cobblestone appearance? The location of the stenosis should also be noted. Does it involve the horizontal canal, the vertical canal, or both?

The type of discharge can be used to help determine what primary or perpetuating factors may be involved. Dry coffee ground–like debris is typical of ear mites. Moist brown discharge tends to be associated with staphylococcal and yeast infections. Purulent creamy to yellow exudates are often seen with gram-negative infections. Waxy, greasy, yellow to tan debris is typical of ceruminous otitis, sometimes with concurrent *Malassezia* infection. Ceruminous discharge is most often seen with keratinization, glandular conditions, and chronic hypersensitivity disorders.

Fiberoptic video–enhanced otoscopes are now available. These machines improve the visualization of the ear canal and tympanic membrane (see Figs. 19–6A to F). They allow photographic records to be taken, which are valuable for patient records as well as to show clients what is occurring in their pets' ear canals.

DIAGNOSIS

A diagnosis of otitis externa is easily made from the history and the physical examination. Otitis media is much more difficult to diagnose, because many patients present with symptoms of only otitis externa. Evidence of inflammation of the tissue surrounding the middle ear or the inner ear usually indicates that otitis media has occurred. Even with otoscopic examination, many cases of otitis media may not be detected, and in cases with apparently intact diseased tympanic membranes, otitis media may be present. The tympanic membrane becomes opaque and white, gray, pinkish, or brown owing to disease and thickening. When this occurs and it loses its characteristic opalescent, fish scale appearance, it may resemble a keratinous plug.[77] In addition, middle ear changes or the medial wall of the tympanic bulla may be interpreted as a diseased but intact tympanic membrane. The tympanum is rarely seen to bulge in canine otitis media, and when it does, it is usually associated with inspissated middle ear debris rather than fluid.[80] An evaluation of tympanometry, otoscopy, and palpation findings revealed that in inflamed ears, only tympanometry was accurate in determining the integrity of the tympanic membrane.[101] This study revealed that even after lavage of the ear canal, a satisfactory view of the tympanic membrane could be obtained in only 28% of cases otoscopically examined while under anesthesia.

Radiography is indicated in suspected cases of otitis media and especially before surgical procedures involving the middle ear. However, radiography is helpful only when it demonstrates middle ear pathologic changes (e.g., fluid lines or changes in the osseous bulla); normal radiographs do not rule out the presence of otitis media.[118, 131, 151a] Tympanometry appears valuable in the diagnosis of a ruptured tympanic membrane. Its value in clinically inflamed ears and ears with otitis media needs to be determined, although it appears preferable to previously described techniques.[101, 118]

Palpation of the tympanic membrane with a blunt instrument has been shown to be inaccurate and causes a statistically significant incidence of damage to the tympanic membrane.[101, 118] However, palpation and positioning of a soft feeding tube to help determine the presence or the location of the tympanic membrane is a valuable technique that may reveal false middle ear cavities.[77] The feeding tube is passed under visualization through a surgical otoscope head within the ear canal to the level where the tympanic membrane is expected to be located. In a normal ear, the tip of the tube remains visualized. In ears with false middle ear or ruptured tympanic membranes, the tube is passed beyond view and in a ventral direction below the normal plane of the horizontal canal.

Myringotomy has been promoted in the past as a technique to gain access to the middle ear for draining fluid, relieving pressure and instilling medication.[132] Though it is a useful technique for those indications, it is also considered the best way to detect otitis media when combined with cytology and culture.[64] The important aspect is that the tympanic membrane is incised or punctured in the ventral half, preferably the posterio-ventral quadrant, which is below the attachment to the manubrium.

Cytologic examination of discharge usually does not establish a definitive diagnosis, but it is valuable in determining what infectious agents, if any, are present. Cytologic study reveals any cocci (especially *Staphylococcus* and *Streptococcus*), rods (especially *Pseudomonas* and *Proteus*), other gram-positive or gram-negative organisms, budding yeasts (*Malassezia* and *Candida*), and mixed infections. The presence of white blood cells, as well as phagocytosis of bacteria, indicates that the body is responding to the infection and that treatment of the infection is warranted. The mere visualization of numerous bacteria in the absence of an inflammatory response and phagocytosis usually indicates only multiplication and colonization by the microorganism, not clinical infection. If there are toxic neutrophils, the ear canal must be flushed to remove the toxins.

Cytology is the most appropriate method to determine the importance of bacteria. In one study, 31.6% of ears were culture positive for *Staphylococcus* or *Streptococcus* but were cytologically negative for cocci.[64] When gram-negative organisms were cultured, only 20% were cytologically negative.[80] The criteria used for bacterial significance on cytology was four or more organisms per oil immersion field (OIF). Unfortunately, the significance of these findings is unclear, because the presence of inflammatory cells, phagocytosis, and response to antibiotic therapy directed against the cultured organisms were not recorded. One of the authors (C.E.G.) uses one bacterium/OIF as significant, especially if inflammatory cells are present.

Cytologic evaluation is the preferred method to ascertain the role of *Malassezia* in a particular case for two reasons. In one study, 18% of the cases that had *Malassezia* detected by cytologic examination were sterile on culture by a commercial laboratory culturing specifically for *Malassezia* at 37°C (98.6°F).[77] Another blinded study compared the sensitivity of cytologic study versus culture for detecting bacteria or yeast in normal and otitic canine ears.[87] The sensitivity of cytologic examination of cerumen for detection of gram-positive cocci, gram-negative rods, and yeasts was 84%, 100%, and 100%, respectively. However, the sensitivity of the culture for detection of these organisms was 59%, 69%, and 50%, respectively. It has been suggested that if *Malassezia* organisms are found in ear swab cytologic examination in numbers averaging 10 or more per HPF or 4 or more per OIF, the yeast should be considered to be an important pathogen.[64, 130]

Cytology should be done from the deep ear canal and, when appropriate, the middle ear cavity. The incidence of otitis media with an intact tympanic membrane is as high as 59% in dogs with chronic otitis.[64] Studies by Cole and colleagues have demonstrated that the findings from the external ear canal cytology and middle ear cytology may also vary greatly. Yeast were considered significant in 65.8% of ear canals and 34.2% of middle ears in 38 ears with otitis media and externa.[64] When otitis externa and media are both present, cytologic examination of both compartments reveals the same organisms in only 58.6% of the cases.[80] Any time a relatively normal tympanic membrane is not visualized in a chronic recurrent case of otitis externa, the middle ear should be sampled.

Histopathologic studies have been conducted on many dogs and cats with otitis externa.[69, 73, 149] Unfortunately, these have usually been animals with chronic disease in which the cause of the otitis externa was not specified. In general, there are variable degrees of epidermal, sebaceous gland, and ceruminal gland hyperplasia. The inflammation is usually interstitial, diffuse, or nodular in pattern, with lymphocytes, plasma cells, and mast cells usually predominating. Many cases show some degree of fibrosis and cystic dilatation of ceruminal glands. Suppurative epidermitis and hidradenitis may be seen.

CULTURE AND SUSCEPTIBILITY TESTING

The primary indication for culture and susceptibility testing is the presence of otitis media or severe otitis externa associated with rodlike bacteria when systemic therapy is going to be prescribed. Culture and susceptibility testing should not be done without cytologic evaluation, which demonstrates that bacteria and white blood cells (that are exhibiting degenerative changes and are phagocytosing the bacteria) are present in the discharge. However, the conclusion of one study, demonstrating the relatively inaccurate results for detecting bacteria with cytology versus culture of the middle ear, is that otitis media should be cultured.[64] They also found that bacteria isolated by culture from the external and middle ear of the same ear were usually not identical either in type or antibiotic susceptibility. Therefore, all cases of otitis media to be cultured should have both the ear horizontal canal and middle ear sampled.[64] It is common for otitis patients to have multiple types of bacteria isolated from an inflamed ear canal. In one study of 176 otitis cultures, 49.4% had two or more types of bacteria and 27.3% had three or greater different isolates per specimen.[96] Because numerous bacterial species may be cultured from tissues of the osseous bulla, a single antimicrobial agent to which all bacterial isolates are susceptible may not be identified.[149a] Individual specimens for culture should be obtained from both osseous bullae during bilateral total ear canal ablations, because different bacterial species may be isolated from each ear.[149a] Bacteria and yeasts usually multiply to large numbers in abnormal ear canals, and the mere ability to culture large numbers of one or more microorganisms does not demonstrate that these organisms are involved in the disease process. It is important to remember that resistance to a particular antibiotic in vitro may not correlate with clinical response, because direct application of medication to the ear canal results in a higher antibiotic concentration than with systemic medication. For some canine otic isolates—such as *P. aeruginosa*, β-hemolytic streptococci, and enterococci—disk diffusion techniques (Kirby-Bauer) indicate in vitro susceptibility, whereas minimum inhibitory concentration (MIC) testing indicates resistance.[65] When therapy will be limited to topical treatment, culture and susceptibility testing are rarely cost effective.

Depending on the primary diagnosis, many other tests may be needed to make a definitive diagnosis. Which tests are most cost effective and indicated depends on the history and complete physical examination findings.

TREATMENT

Therapy of otitis externa depends on identifying and controlling the predisposing factors and primary causes whenever possible. In addition, cleaning the ear canals and the middle ear, applying topical therapies, and administering systemic medications may be necessary for the effective elimination or control of primary and secondary causes as well as perpetuating factors.[61, 118, 151a]

The administration of sedatives such as xylazine or ketamine and diazepam may be needed to allow adequate examination or treatment in some cases. Other animals require a general anesthetic. Many clients are reluctant to have their dogs anesthetized but are often more understanding if the need for getting the ears cleaned and completely examined is explained in detail.

Cleaning

Thorough cleaning of the ear canals is extremely important for the effective management of otitis externa.[21, 77, 116, 118, 151a] In chronic cases of otitis media, or in animals with a false middle ear, management includes cleaning that area. Cleaning is valuable for several reasons. Besides preventing effective therapy, the exudate may interfere with adequate examination until it is cleaned out. Foreign bodies, especially small ones, are eliminated

Table 19-10 OTIC CLEANSERS, CERUMINOLYTICS, AND DRYING AGENTS

	CERUMINOLYTIC CLEANSERS	MILD CLEANSERS	DRYING AGENTS	DRYING CLEANSERS
Docusate Solution (Life Science)	X			
Clear$_x$ Ear Cleansing Solution (DVM)	X			
Panotic (Pfizer)	X			
Clear$_x$ Cleanser (DVM)	X			
Cerumenex (Purdue-Fredericks)	X			
Cerumene (EVSCO)	X			
Oticalm (DVM)		X		
Cerulytic (Virbac)		X		
Corium-20 (VRx)		X		
Nolva-Cleanse (Fort Dodge)		X		
Oti-Clens (Pfizer)		X		
Otipan (Harlman)		X		
Clear$_x$ Drying Solution (DVM)			X	
Bur-Otic Astringent Ear Drops (Virbac)			X	
Dermal Dry (Butler)			X	
Domeboro Otic (Dome)			X	
Otic-Care B Drying Cream (ARC Labs)				X
Alocetic Ear Rinse (DVM)				X
Epi-Otic (Virbac)				X
Oticlean A Ear Cleansing Lotion (ARC Labs)				X
Otic-Fresh (Pan American)				X
Nolvasan Otic (Fort Dodge)				X
Otocetic Solution (Vedco)				X
Chlorhexiderm Flush (DVM)				X

when ears are adequately cleaned. Pus and inflammatory debris can inactivate some medications (e.g., polymyxin). Thorough cleaning removes bacterial toxins, degenerating cellular debris, and free fatty acids, thus decreasing the stimulation for further inflammation. In proliferative conditions of the ear canals, thorough cleaning is one of the most valuable steps in management, just as it is in treating intertrigo (fold dermatitis).[77]

Ceruminolytic agents greatly facilitate and expedite the cleaning procedure (Tables 19-10 and 19-11). They include various types of surfactants, such as dioctyl sodium

Table 19-11 OTIC CLEANSING PREPARTIONS

PRODUCT (COMPANY)	INGREDIENTS
Adams Pan-Otic (Pfizer)	Isopropyl alcohol, aloe vera, urea, propylene glycol, dioctyl sodium sulfosuccinate
Alocetic Ear Rinse (DVM)	Acetic acid, aloe vera
Bur-Otic Astringent Ear Drops (Virbac)	Acetic acid, Burow's solution, propylene glycol
Cerulytic Ear Ceruminolytic (Virbac)	Benzoyl alcohol, propylene glycol
Cerumene (EVSCO)	Squalene
Chlorhexiderm Flush (DVM)	Chlorhexidine
Clear$_x$ Ear Cleansing Solution (DVM)	Dioctyl sodium sulfosuccinate, urea peroxide
DermaPet Ear/Skin Cleanser (DermaPet)	Acetic acid, boric acid
Epi-Otic Ear Cleanser (Virbac)	Lactic acid, salicylic acid, chitosanide, propylene glycol
Gent-L-Clens (Schering-Plough)	Lactic acid, salicylic acid, propylene glycol
Nolva-Cleanse (Fort Dodge)	Propylene glycol, surfactants
OtiCalm Cleansing Solution (DVM)	Benzoic acid, malic acid, salicylic acid, eucalyptus
Oti-Clens (Pfizer)	Malic acid, benzoic acid, salicylic acid, propylene glycol

sulfosuccinate (docusate, DSS) (Docusate solution, Life Science) or calcium sulfosuccinate, and detergents that act by emulsifying the waxes and lipids. Carbamide peroxide (Earoxide ear cleanser, Tomlyn) is a slightly less potent ceruminolytic agent that acts as a humectant by releasing urea when activated. It releases oxygen, creating a foaming action that helps to break down or dislodge large clumps of debris. Carbamide peroxide is particularly helpful with more purulent exudates. The ceruminolytic Clear$_X$ ear cleansing solution (DVM Pharmaceuticals) combines DSS and carbamide peroxide, thus possessing the surfactant, humectant, and oxygen-producing effects of both ingredients.

Some ear cleansers also have antimicrobial properties.[102a, 102b] Epi-Otic (Virbac) was reported to eliminate *S. intermedius*, *P. aeruginosa*, and *M. pachydermatis*.[102a]

Three ceruminolytic ear cleansers (Panotic, Pfizer; Clear$_X$ Cleanser, DVM Pharmaceuticals; Cerumenex, Purdue-Fredericks) with a variety of ingredients including propylene glycol, DSS, carbamide peroxide, or triethanolamine caused middle ear damage when administered directly into the middle ear of normal dogs and guinea pigs.[106] Squalene (Cerumene, EVSCO), a milder surfactant cleanser, caused no significant middle ear pathology when administered in the same way to normal dogs or guinea pigs.[106] The clinical significance of these findings is unknown, because labeled manufacturer's guidelines for the products were not used, and the products were not used as they would be in clinical practice (e.g., the products were injected into the middle ear and left there—no flushing was performed).[58]

Propylene glycol, glycerin, and mineral oil have mild ceruminolytic effects and are best used for the relatively normal, slightly dirty ear. Veterinary cleaners that are mild and can be sent home are listed in Table 19–10. Although these products are mild wax removers, they still have ingredients, such as propylene glycol, which may be ototoxic if they allowed to remain in the middle ear. For chronic control of excess cerumen, ceruminolytic agents administered two or three times weekly are usually effective.

Most ceruminolytics and detergents are contraindicated with a ruptured tympanum. Some disinfectant cleaners, such as chlorhexidine and iodophors, are also contraindicated with a ruptured tympanum.[75, 89] Frequently, the condition of the tympanic membrane cannot be determined until the ear canal has been cleaned. When a rupture is suspected, these agents should not be used. In some cases, a ruptured tympanic membrane is not detected until after these agents have already been used. The probability of ototoxicity may be decreased by thorough flushing with water or sterile physiologic saline. Additional detergents or disinfectants are not used in the flushing water or saline unless an intact tympanum is noted. The use of ear loops, flushing the ear with water or saline, or the use of a suction apparatus is the least ototoxic method of cleaning if a ruptured tympanum is suspected.

Several methods for removing the pus, debris, and emulsified waxes and lipids have been described. One of the easiest to set up, implement, and clean up is the use of a rubber ear bulb syringe. After the use of a ceruminolytic agent, repeated flushing with lukewarm water or saline removes most of the exudate. When the tympanic membrane is known to be intact, the use of a detergent or disinfectant solution may improve the results. A space should always be left between the rubber nipple and the canal orifice. This allows back flow and helps prevent excessive pressure on the tympanic membrane. This procedure is not effective for cleaning false middle ears or the tympanic bulla. Ear curets or loops are helpful in removing debris lodged deep near the tympanum in cases of milder, waxy, crusty accumulation with small foreign bodies or leftover waxy debris. For larger foreign bodies or keratin plugs in the middle ear, an alligator forceps may be used. However, in most situations, an ear curet is preferred. If the tympanum is ruptured, the animal may be noticed to swallow when flushing is performed or fluid may run out of the nose. Thus, if the animal is anesthetized, it is important to have a tracheal tube in place to prevent possible aspiration pneumonia.

The ear curet is gently pulled along the epidermis to break loose any debris. This is less traumatic than using cotton swabs. Ear curets are placed down the ear canal through a surgical otoscope head. Under visualization, the loop is passed along the epithelium of the canal until the wax to be removed is reached. The loop is then rolled over the debris and gently pulled out of the canal. This method minimizes the risk of damaging an intact tympanum.

A feeding tube and a 12-ml syringe are effective for flushing the ear canal. Feeding tubes of various diameters, cut to different lengths, can be kept in cold sterilization. The tube, attached to a syringe filled with water or saline, is passed through a surgical otoscope head and cone and passed down the ear canal under visualization. After the tip is located at the desired point of the ear canal, the solution can be infused and then aspirated back out, along with the debris that was broken up. In severe cases, and whenever the tympanum is ruptured, flushing with a syringe and feeding tube is the most effective and safe flushing technique and is usually the method of choice (see Fig. 19–6F).[77] This will allow retrograde flushing and, if the tube is placed into the middle ear cavity, allows flushing of the middle ear cavity. The tip of the tube should be directed toward the ventral aspect of the tympanic bullae as the more delicate structures are located in the middle and dorsal compartments of the middle ear cavity (see Fig. 19–6E). This is a preferred method for drying the ear out, as well, especially when there is no tympanum present.

Vestibular syndrome or deafness may occur after ear flushing, even when no ototoxic drugs are used. These side effects are rare and are usually transient when they do occur. In 105 otitic dog ears cleaned and examined, none had detectable damage to hearing as assessed by brainstem auditory evoked response testing, and cleaning actually produced measurable improvements in several dogs.[66] Ototoxicity is a much talked about subject.[103, 104, 118] However, the prevalence of ototoxicity secondary to the use of flushing solutions, cleaning, and medications when a ruptured tympanic membrane exists is unknown. Two separate studies have evaluated the effects of chlorhexidine[119] and gentamicin[145] in normal dogs with ruptured tympanic membranes. No cochlear or vestibular dysfunction was measurable after 3 weeks of otic application of these two agents. In clinical practice, ototoxicity following cleaning or treatment appears to be rare.[80]

A suction apparatus is possibly the most effective method of cleaning ears, especially when thick, inspissated pus or keratin plugs are left in the middle ear. A Frazier suction tip works well. The tip can be positioned to exactly the desired location before initiating suction. Suction may also be combined with tube flushing, and this is a very effective cleaning method and the treatment of choice when ceruminolytics must be avoided. The suction apparatus is effective in rapidly cleaning out the external ear canal and the middle ear cavity. The disadvantages are the limited access to the middle ear, the time needed to clean the equipment, and when used alone, the lack of infusion of liquid.

Some clinicians use a dental water propulsion device (Water Pik). These devices rapidly clean the ear with multiple rapid pulses of water. There is no suction, and the time needed to set up and clean the equipment eliminates some of the advantages they seem to offer. It is not as effective in cleaning the middle ear as are the syringe and feeding tube. Care must be taken to avoid directing the pulsating stream directly onto a damaged tympanic membrane. The use of a curved water current defuser (Anthony Products) helps avoid tympanic membrane damage.

After the flushing has been completed, the ear canal is dried, or in cases complicated by infection, a disinfectant may be applied to the canal. If the tympanum is ruptured, acetic acid at 2% to 5% is preferred. A 5% concentration of acetic acid may cause a burning sensation when it is applied to inflamed, eroded, or ulcerated epithelium and is best applied while the patient is still sedated.

After the ear is cleaned and relatively dry, topical medications or drying agents can be used. Most drying agents contain isopropyl alcohol and one or more of the following: boric acid, benzoic acid, salicylic acid, acetic acid, aluminum acetate, sulfur, and silicone dioxide. By reading the labels, the major ingredients and, therefore, activity of the products can be determined. Veterinary products of the drying or drying cleanser type include Clear$_x$ ear drying solution (DVM Pharmaceuticals), Bur-Otic Astringent ear drops (Virbac), Dermal Dry (Butler), Domeboro Otic (Dome), and Otic-Care B drying cream (ARC

Labs). These products can be used at home for prophylactic treatment of swimmer's ear and idiopathic excessive cerumen production and as a deodorizer. Alcohol and higher concentrations of the acids may be irritating or cause a burning sensation in ulcerated ears. For chronic control of moist ears, drying agents applied twice weekly are usually effective.

Modified drying products with less drying ingredients and more antimicrobial properties and mild ceruminolytic agents are available. Ingredients often combined with the drying agents achieve these effects and include propylene glycol, lanolin, glycerin, parachlorometaxylenol, and chlorhexidine. Some of the veterinary products in this group are listed in Table 19–10. These products are used most effectively in mildly dirty ears. Ears that have a mild objectionable odor to the client are helped by these products. They are not as helpful for clinical otitis externa, although they may be used for long-term management of milder cases of recurrent waxy otitis externa, after the inflammation is controlled. An advantage of these products is their lack of antibiotics or glucocorticoids, which may induce bacterial resistance or adrenal suppression, respectively.

In especially waxy or exudative ears, the client may need to clean the ears intermittently so that topical medications can be properly applied. In most chronic cases, the combination cleanser-dryers are not sufficient. In these cases, the client should be instructed in the use of the ear bulb syringe for home flushing and possibly the use of ceruminolytics.[77] These cases must be carefully selected. In general, the tympanum should be intact if ceruminolytics are going to be used. This is because the client may not be able to rinse adequately all residual drug, and repetitive application could be dangerous, especially if the agent is not being rinsed out. The client must be willing and able to try flushing, and the animal must be tolerant of the procedure. Many animals tolerate home flushing after the initial inflammation and pain are resolved. This procedure is rarely recommended in acutely inflamed or ulcerated ears. Detergents are not routinely used for home flushing and necessitate thorough rinsing. The clients use cotton balls or swabs only in areas that they can visualize, not down the ear canal.

Owners should rarely clean the ears more than once every 48 hours. With more frequent applications, the ears often do not have an opportunity to dry out, and the resultant increased humidity, epithelial maceration, and facilitation of microbial growth promote delayed healing, irritation, and secondary infection.

Topical Therapy

Numerous topical preparations for the external ear canal are available.[151a] Most of the ear products contain various combinations of glucocorticoids, antibiotics, antifungals, and parasiticides (Tables 19–12 to 19–15). Topical therapeutic agents are selected on the basis of the effects needed. As the case progresses, the patient should be monitored and products changed accordingly. Each of these types of ingredients is discussed, but the clinician should be aware of the vehicle.

The base or type of vehicle should be considered when selecting a treatment of otitis externa. In general, dry, scaly, crusty lesions are benefited by oil or ointment bases, which help moisturize the skin. Moist, exudative conditions should be treated with solutions or lotions and not occlusive ointments or oils. Creams are frequently poor choices because the client may have difficulty in getting the medication to the horizontal canal. In addi-

● Table 19–12 **OTIC GLUCOCORTICOID PREPARATIONS**

DRUG (COMPANY)	INGREDIENTS
Bur-Otic HC Ear Treatment (Virbac)	Hydrocortisone, acetic acid, Burow's solution, propylene glycol
Epi-Otic HC (Virbac)	Hydrocortisone, lactic acid
Hydro-10 Mist (Butler)	Hydrocortisone
Synotic Otic Solution (Fort Dodge)	Fluocinolone, dimethyl sulfoxide

Table 19-13 OTIC ANTIMICROBIAL—GLUCOCORTICOID PREPARATIONS

DRUG (COMPANY)	INGREDIENTS
Clear$_x$ Ear Drying Solution (DVM)	Acetic acid, colloidal sulfur, hydrocortisone
Forte-Topical (Pharmacia & Upjohn)	Penicillin, neomycin, polymyxin B, hydrocortisone
Gentocin Otic Solution (Schering-Plough)	Gentamicin, betamethasone
°Neo-Predef (Pharmacia & Upjohn)	Neomycin, isoflupredone
Otomax (Schering-Plough)	Gentamicin, betamethasone, clotrimazole
Panalog Ointment (Fort Dodge)	Nystatin, neomycin, thiostrepton, triamcinolone
Topagen Ointment (Schering-Plough)	Gentamicin, betamethasone
Tresaderm (Merial)	Thiabendazole, neomycin, dexamethasone
Tritop (Pharmacia & Upjohn)	Neomycin, isoflupredone, tetracaine

°Ophthalmic product, excellent for ears.

tion, many clients find the application of fluid drops aesthetically more pleasing compared with the application of viscous materials or the need to insert an applicator down the ear canal.

Topical glucocorticoids are beneficial in most cases of otitis externa (see Tables 19-12 and 19-13). Glucocorticoids have antipruritic and anti-inflammatory effects, decrease exudation and swelling, cause sebaceous gland atrophy, decrease glandular secretions, reduce scar tissue, and decrease proliferative changes, all of which help promote drainage and ventilation. Because pain and pruritus are alleviated, the animal becomes easier to medicate. There are different types and potencies of topical glucocorticoids available, which the clinician should become familiar with. The more potent topical glucocorticoids in ear products include betamethasone valerate (Gentocin Otic and Otomax, Schering-Plough), and fluocinolone acetonide (Synotic, Fort Dodge). Studies have shown that even the moderately potent glucocorticoids triamcinolone acetonide (Panalog, Fort Dodge) and dexamethasone (Tresaderm, Merial) are absorbed systemically (see Chap. 3).[121] Treated dogs have elevated levels of liver enzymes and suppressed adrenal response to corticotropin (adrenocorticotropic hormone [ACTH]) stimulation. The systemic absorption of more potent topical glucocorticoids should make the clinician cautious of long-term treatment. The initial therapy or acute exacerbations may necessitate a potent topical glucocorticoid (fluocinolone, betamethasone, dexamethasone, or triamcinolone) but, after the inflammation or allergic reaction is controlled, prophylactic or long-term therapy should use the least potent topical glucocorticoid possible, such as 0.5% or 1% hydrocortisone, contained in Hydro B-1020 (Butler), Bur-Otic HC and Epi-Otic HC (Virbac), Clear$_x$ ear drying solution (DVM Pharmaceuticals), and Cort/Astrin solution (Vedco). Stronger than these hydrocortisone products, but still milder than the potent glucocorticoids, are combination products such as Forte-Topical (Pharmacia & UpJohn) and Liquichlor (EVSCO). In cases of otitis externa due to atopy or food hypersensitivity, the pinna is frequently affected and

Table 19-14 OTIC ANTIMICROBIAL PREPARATIONS

DRUG (COMPANY)	INGREDIENTS
Betadine Solution (Purdue-Fredericks)	Povidone-iodine
Chloromycetin Otic (Parke-Davis)	Chloramphenicol
Ciloxan Ophthalmic (Alcon)°	Ciprofloxacin
Conofite Lotion (Schering-Plough)	Miconazole
Gentocin Ophthalmic (Schering-Plough)†	Gentamicin
Nolvasan Solution (Fort Dodge)	Chlorhexidine
Tobrex Ophthalmic (Alcon)°	Tobramycin
Xenodine (VPL)	Iodine

°Not a veterinary product, but useful.
†Ophthalmic product, but good in ears.

Table 19–15 OTIC ANTIPARASITIC PREPARATIONS

PRODUCT (COMPANY)	INGREDIENTS
Aurimite (Schering-Plough)	Pyrethrins, benzocaine, dioctyl sodium sulfosuccinate
Cerumite (EVSCO)	Pyrethrins, squalene
Ear Mitecide (Vedco)	Rotenone
Ear Mite Lotion (Durvet)	Rotenone
Eradimite (Fort Dodge)	Pyrethrins
Mita-Clear (Pfizer)	Pyrethrins
Nolvamite (Fort Dodge)	Pyrethrins
Otomite (Virbac)	Pyrethrins

should be treated. Antibiotic agents are present in many topical ear products. Uncomplicated cases of allergic or ceruminous otitis externa may be managed by topical glucocorticoid application alone, and inappropriate use of topical antibiotics may cause a secondary superinfection or sensitization. All other concerns about the use of topical glucocorticoids should be considered (see Chap. 3).

Topical antibacterial agents are indicated when infection is present (see Tables 19–13 and 19–14).[151a] The aminoglycosides—neomycin (Panolog, Fort Dodge; Tresaderm, Merial), neomycin-polymyxin (Forte-Topical, Pharmacia & Upjohn), and gentamicin (Gentocin Otic Solution and Otomax, Schering-Plough)—and chloramphenicol (Liquichlor, EVSCO) are potent topical antibiotics with good activity against pathogens usually found in otitis externa.[54, 55, 83, 142] Chloramphenicol (Liquichlor, EVSCO) is frequently effective, but may stimulate excessive granulation tissue in the middle ear.[77] Clients should also be careful not to come in contact with chloramphenicol owing to the possibility of idiosyncratic bone marrow suppression. Using topical antibiotics that are not likely to be needed as systemic drugs may decrease the occurrence of resistant cases of otitis externa and otitis media. The more potent broad-spectrum antibiotics (gentamicin and chloramphenicol) should not be used as first-choice treatments so that resistant strains of bacteria are not created. Therefore, neomycin-polymyxin is preferred by the authors as a first-line topical antibiotic. Most topical antibiotics contain a glucocorticoid, and its potency may not always be desirable.

Gram-negative, gentamicin-resistant infections are the bane of many practitioners. In Scotland, 81% of the *Pseudomonas* isolates from canine otitis externa are resistant to gentamicin and fluoroquinolones.[124] The typical response is to look for an antibiotic the organism is susceptible to. Multiple studies have shown that *Pseudomonas* is usually susceptible to polymyxin B, and this antibiotic is often overlooked in the treatment of difficult *Pseudomonas* cases.[64, 71, 95] One possible reason is that polymyxin B is inactivated by pus and should be used in only clean ears. Ticarcillin was shown to be effective either topically or topically and systemically in 11 of 12 dogs with *Pseudomonas* infections resistant to fluoroquinolones and gentamicin.[124] An injectable form or the equine uterine infusion (Ticillin, Pfizer Animal Health) may be used as ear drops.[82, 124] The Ticillin is reconstituted to 100 mg/ml and this is stable for one month if frozen. It may be divided into 10 to 15 ml vials, which are stable in the refrigerator for 3 days, so clients must freeze the vials and bring a new one out every 3 days for treatment. Other antibiotic regimens that are useful include injectable amikacin (50 mg/ml) applied at 3 to 5 drops in each ear every 12 hours, Tobramycin ophthalmic drops, and in-office formulated enrofloxacin drops.[71, 82, 133, 151a] Topical enrofloxacin is made by adding 4 ml of the 2.27% injectable enrofloxacin (20 mg/ml) (Baytril, Bayer) to 12 ml of a liquid base (such as propylene glycol and water; Epiotic, Virbac; or Clear$_X$ ear drying solution, DVM Pharmaceuticals; or 24 ml saline if the tympanic membrane may be ruptured).[71, 84] The risk of ototoxicity has not been evaluated, but none is reported.

Treatment options are available that do not depend on alternative antibiotics, but frequent cleaning should not be forgotten. Presoaking the ear with tromethamine-ethylenediaminetetraacetic acid (Tris EDTA, Derma Pet) for 5 to 10 minutes or mixing gentamicin at 3 mg/ml with Tris EDTA increases the efficacy against gram-negative organisms.[151a] Tris EDTA solution is made from the commercial preparation or from stock chemicals by mixing 4.8 g of EDTA (disodium salt), 24.2 g of Tris (Trizma) base, 3900 ml distilled water, and 100 ml white vinegar.[71] The pH of this mixture is then adjusted to 8.0 with additional vinegar. The pH-balanced solution should then be autoclaved so that sterilization is achieved. Tris EDTA has also been shown to be synergistic with amikacin, neomycin, cephaloridine, kanendomycin, and enrofloxacin.[67, 142] Tris EDTA can be valuable in long-term treatment and prevention of recurrence as part of an ear cleaning regimen or as a presoak before instillation of antibiotic (usually two to three times a week).

Topical antiseptics such as povidone-iodine, chlorhexidine, aluminum acetate, and acetic acid are helpful in the treatment of bacterial otitis externa (see Table 19-14).[151a] Acetic acid has been effective in the treatment of otitis externa in humans. It is believed that its activity is not completely due to the pH because other acidic products are not as effective in killing *Pseudomonas* and *Staphylococcus*. Acetic acid is most effective against *Pseudomonas*, with a 2% solution being lethal within 1 minute of contact.[71, 77] *Staphylococcus* and *Streptococcus* can be killed within 5 minutes of contact with 5% acetic acid solution. However, this concentration is occasionally irritating. In vitro studies indicated that mixtures of boric acid and acetic acid were effective antibacterial agents: 0.5% boric acid with 0.5% acetic acid was lethal for *P. aeruginosa*; 5% boric acid with 0.5% acetic acid was lethal for *S. intermedius*.[53] Aluminum acetate has also been shown to be as effective as polymyxin and hydrocortisone ear drops in a group of acute otitis externa cases in humans that were often associated with swimming, and 34% also had *Pseudomonas pyocyanea* infections.[98] Stinging from the aluminum acetate drops resulted in their being discontinued in 5% of the cases treated. Silver sulfadiazine at 1% has been reported to be an effective antimicrobial in cases of otitis externa.[61, 148] It is active against *P. aeruginosa*, *Proteus* spp., enterococci, and *S. intermedius*. It is made by mixing 0.1 g of silver sulfadiazine powder with 100 ml of distilled water or 1.5 ml (1/3 teaspoon) of silver sulfadiazine cream with 13.5 ml distilled water, and applying the solution at a dose of 0.5 ml per ear twice daily.[71] Another study showed that a 0.1% solution is also effective and is more liquid, allowing easier application and better dispersal in the ear canal.[123] Occasional erosive, severe inflammatory reactions can be seen in ears treated with silver sulfadiazine, but ototoxicity has not been reported.

Antifungal agents are required in any case complicated or caused by the yeasts *Malassezia* and *Candida* or by dermatophytes (see Tables 19-13 and 19-14).[151a] *Malassezia* and dermatophytes usually respond well to topical 1% miconazole (Conofite lotion, Schering-Plough) or clotrimazole (Otomax, Schering-Plough). In vitro testing has shown nystatin (Panolog, Fort Dodge) to be effective against *Malassezia*. Thiabendazole (Tresaderm, Merial), although not effective in vitro, may work in some cases. Again, povidone-iodine or chlorhexidine is also effective. When bacteria and *Malassezia* are present together, the combination of gentocin, clotrimazole, and betamethasone (Otomax, Schering-Plough) or neomycin, thiostrepton, nystatin, and triamcinolone (Panalog, Fort Dodge) is effective, as is povidone-iodine, chlorhexidine, or 5% acetic acid. For chronic, recurrent bacterial or yeast infections, antimicrobial agents used two or three times weekly may be effective.

Parasiticidal agents are indicated in ear products for *Otodectes* and, less commonly, *Demodex*, *Otobius*, and trombiculid infestations (see Table 19-15). Most cases respond to products containing pyrethrins (Otomite Plus, Virbac; Cerumite, EVSCO; Mita-Clear, Pfizer Animal Health; Otic-Care M, ARC Labs), rotenone (Ear Miticide, Phoenix; Ear Miticide, Vedco; Ear Mite Lotion, Durvet), and thiabendazole (Tresaderm, Merial). In addition to the use of an effective parasiticidal agent, two important points should be considered. First, many animals may be asymptomatic carriers of *Otodectes*. Because of this, all in-contact animals, both dogs and cats, must be treated. Second, *Otodectes* can be found on other body areas. Therefore, whole-body treatments with effective parasiticidals must be done. The life cycle of *Otodectes* necessitates that otic and body treatment be continued for at least 3 weeks, with a month being necessary in some cases. Some veterinarians recommend topical application of ivermectin (drops in the ears), especially in cats. Although this may be effective, one study showed that the recurrence rate was higher and the time to remission slower than with systemic ivermectin therapy.[76] Amitraz (1 ml of amitraz in 9 to 29 ml of mineral oil) is also effective when applied as otic drops.[21] Fipronil spray may eliminate ear mites both from the ear and the body with one application. Selamectin is reported to be effective after one or two applications.

Systemic Therapy

Systemic therapy is indicated if otitis externa is severe, marked proliferative changes are present, otitis media is present, when owners cannot administer topical treatments, and in cases in which topical adverse reactions are suspected. Appropriate antibiotics or antifungals should be used until at least 1 week after cure. Antibiotics that are known to penetrate bone or that have a good history of benefit in treating otitis media should be selected and given at doses that are at the high end of the recommended doses. Examples of antibiotics that are useful for otitis media and proliferative otitis include trimethoprim-sulfadiazine, 25 mg/kg every 12 hours; ormetoprim-sulfadimethoxine (Primor, Pfizer Animal Health), 55 mg/kg day 1 and 25 mg/kg every 24 hours subsequent days; clindamycin (Antirobe, Pharmacia & Upjohn), 7 to 10 mg/kg every 12 hours; cephalexin, 22 mg/kg every 12 hours; enrofloxacin (Baytril, Bayer Corporation), 5 to 20 mg/kg every 24 hours; and orbifloxacin (Orbax, Schering-Plough) 2.5 to 12.5 mg/kg q24h. In general, fluoroquinolones are needed at higher doses for *Pseudomonas aeruginosa* infections, such as 20 mg/kg enrofloxacin, 12.5 mg/kg orbifloxacin, or 20 mg/kg ciprofloxacin q24h.[71, 150] Marbofloxacin at 5 mg/kg every 24 hours has shown encouraging results for treating *Pseudomonas* otitis.[60] The use of acupuncture with conventional otitis therapy was shown in a blinded study to decrease the signs and symptoms of otitis more rapidly than conventional therapy alone.[134] However, the overall success and cure rate at 3 months was no different between groups. Ketoconazole (Nizoral, Janssen) at 10 mg/kg every 12 to 24 hours is given when otitis media is associated with *Malassezia*. In unresponsive cases, itraconazole (Sporanox, Janssen) may be effective. Otoscopic and cytologic examination is required before a patient can be considered cured.

Ivermectin, although not approved for this use in the United States, is an extremely effective systemic therapy for *Otodectes* infection (see Chap. 6). When given subcutaneously at 0.3 mg/kg and repeated three times at 10-day intervals, it eradicates the ear mites. This form of therapy treats the whole pet and eliminates a carrier state; therefore, it can be used to rule out *Otodectes* infection. In some recurrent cases related to ear mites the use of ivermectin in all the household pets was rewarding. Collies, Shetland sheepdogs, Old English sheepdogs, other herding breeds, and crosses of these breeds should not be treated with high-dose ivermectin. Systemic therapy with moxidectin at 0.2 to 0.4 mg/kg SQ or PO at 10 day intervals or every 72 hours for 7 treatments is also effective.[57]

Systemic glucocorticoid therapy is indicated when there is markedly inflamed edematous otitis and when chronic pathologic changes cause marked stenosis of the canal lumen.[151a] Oral prednisone or prednisolone, 1 to 2 mg/kg PO, or triamcinolone acetonide 0.1 to 0.2 mg/kg PO, may be given daily for 4 to 7 days, then tapered to alternate-day regimens. This treatment is continued until the proliferative tissue has resolved or has stopped improving. Some cases of allergic otitis externa may be treated with systemic glucocorticoids, allowing the initial topical therapy to be a low-potency glucocorticoid product. Injectable dexamethasone is useful if only 2 to 3 days' action is required. For the uncommon case of stenosis, primarily of the vertical canal, or when systemic glucocorticoids are ineffective in reducing the proliferative tissue, intralesional triamcinolone acetonide may be helpful.[77] Triamcinolone acetonide is particularly effective for inhibiting fibroblasts and reducing collagen production.

Isotretinoin (Accutane, Roche) and etretinate (Tegison, Roche) have been helpful in a limited number of cases of otitis externa. Isotretinoin was used in a few dogs and cats that had histologic evidence of sebaceous gland hyperplasia. Although it appeared to be helpful, its administration was stopped owing to side effects or expense. One study of etretinate in Cocker spaniels with primary keratinization disorders indicated that the ceruminous otitis externa in these dogs did not improve.[129] However, in these cases, other perpetuating factors were not adequately treated. Etretinate is no longer available in the United States. When the ears are repetitively cleaned and concurrent infections are treated, retinoids may be more beneficial. Further work and studies with synthetic retinoids are indicated (see Chap. 3).

Surgery

Surgical procedures that may promote drainage or ventilation are described in most surgical textbooks. It should be emphasized that surgical procedures do not replace a thorough diagnostic work-up and that case selection should be done carefully. In cases with marked proliferative changes of the medial wall, surgical debridement is indicated.

Surgery is also indicated to alleviate stenosis of the canal, to remove tumors or polyps, to improve ventilation and response to medical therapy, and to manage medically resistant otitis media. It is imperative for the best results that the primary diagnosis is determined before surgery. Many animals have undergone surgical procedures only to continue to experience otitis externa. Although these cases may sometimes be easier to treat after the procedure, clients not properly educated about expectations may be unsatisfied with the results. Even cases that have been successfully ablated may have persistent pruritus and inflammation of the pinna.[77, 97]

Lateral ear canal resection eliminates the lateral wall of the vertical canal. It is successful in approximately 50% of cases, and clients should be warned of the relatively high failure rate.[99] When the procedure is performed early in disease before the development of otitis media or other perpetuating factors, it is much more successful.[92] In one study, lateral resection failed in 86.5% of the Cocker spaniels, but Shar peis tended to have a better outcome than other breeds.[147] It is indicated when there is a stenotic vertical ear canal or when medical management is not effective and improvement of drainage and ease of topical application may help the medical management. It may decrease the humidity of the ear canal by up to 10%. Contraindications are stenotic horizontal ear canals, otitis media, and severe proliferative disease or mineralization of the auricular cartilage. The most important step is to make certain that the opening to the canal is as wide as possible and that there is skin-to-skin apposition to decrease scar tissue formation. The cartilage flap must be pulled ventrally, and skin-to-skin apposition should be obtained.

Vertical canal ablation may be indicated if the primary disease is limited to the vertical canal. This procedure removes a larger area of tissue and may reduce sensitivity that was associated with the medial wall of the vertical canal. A study reported improvement in 95% of cases so treated.[114] Elimination of signs occurred in only 23% of patients, with the other patients requiring continued medical therapy. However, medical therapy was easier to carry out or was needed less frequently.[114] It is not commonly recommended by the authors. When horizontal canal stenosis or otitis media is present, other procedures are indicated. One should not amputate at the horizontal canal but at the last centimeter of the vertical canal. It is better to leave two drain boards, both dorsal and ventral.

Total ear canal ablation is often recommended in dogs with end-stage ear disease that is poorly or completely unresponsive to aggressive cleaning and medical therapy. In some animals with significant hearing loss that require frequent cleanings, this salvage procedure is less expensive and often preferable as a long-term solution. It is often combined with a bulla osteotomy and curettage of the tympanic bulla, which decreases the incidence of postoperative infections and fistula formation.[77, 85, 108, 111] A major reason for not recommending total ablations has been the concern with hearing loss. Hearing loss is significant but not usually complete.[97, 112, 113] Although this may be a problem in normal dogs, this is a minor concern in dogs with chronic diseases.[111]

Dehiscence of the surgical wound after total ear canal ablation and lateral bulla osteotomy is common.[149a] Wound contamination may be an important contributing factor in postoperative dehiscence. One study demonstrated that during surgery, there is substantial contamination of subcutaneous tissue with bacteria (*E. coli* or *Streptococcus canis*

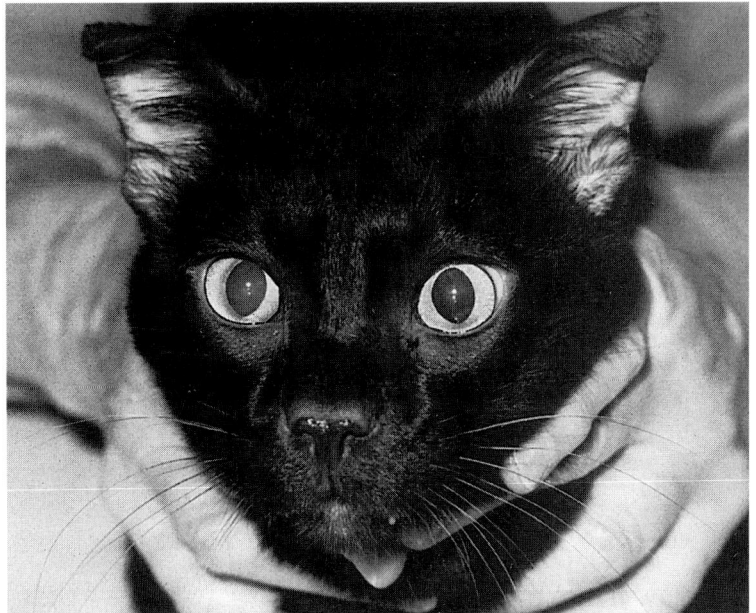

FIGURE 19–11. Acquired folding of the pinna in a cat with iatrogenic hyperglucocorticoidism.

contamination in 94% of the surgical procedures) from excised tissues of the osseous bulla.[149a]

Acquired Folding of the Pinna

Acquired folding of the pinnae ("flop-eared" cats) occurs in adult cats.[125, 138] A sudden, bilateral, lateral folding over of the distal one third of the pinnae is seen (Fig. 19–11). The folded portion of the pinna is cool, thin, and palpably devoid of cartilage. All cats have received long-term (8 months to 2 years) daily applications of glucocorticoid-containing otic preparations. Serum cortisol responses to ACTH are depressed, suggesting the presence of iatrogenic secondary adrenocortical insufficiency and iatrogenic Cushing's syndrome. Stopping the glucocorticoid therapy may or may not result in any improvement of the pinnal folding.

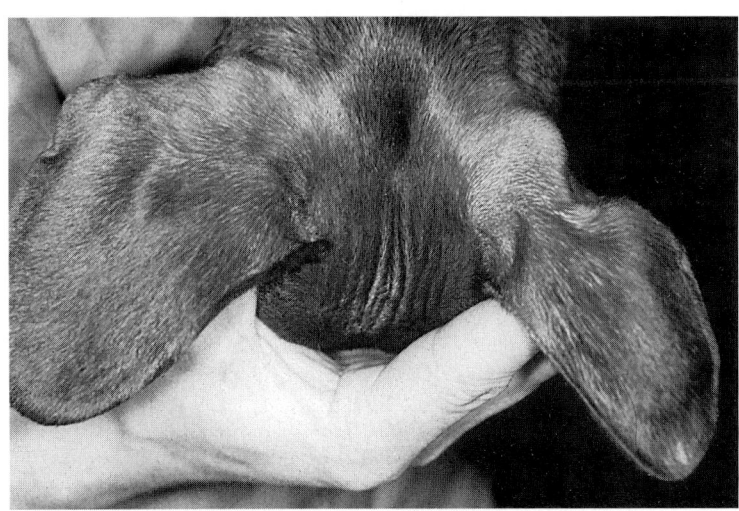

FIGURE 19–12. Congenital microtia in a Dachshund. Left pinna is smaller than the right pinna.

Miscellaneous

Congenital microtia was seen in a Dachshund (Fig. 19–12).

• REFERENCES

Eyelids

1. Abegneli PL: Pathologie des paupières chez les carnivores domestiques. Rev Méd Vét 165:217, 1989.
2. Angarano DW: Dermatologic disorders of the eyelid and periocular region. In: Kirk RW (ed): Current Veterinary Therapy X. W.B. Saunders Co, Philadelphia, 1986, p 678.
3. Bistner SI: Diseases of the nasolacrimal system. In: Kirk RW (ed): Current Veterinary Therapy V. W.B. Saunders Co, Philadelphia, 1974, p 488.
4. Bond R, et al: An idioipathic facial dermatitis of 13 persian cats. Proc Eur Soc Vet Dermatol Eur Coll Vet Dermatol 14:155, 1997.
5. Charbonne L, Clerc B: Les blepharites des carnivores domestiques. Point Vét 20:33, 1988.
6. de Geyer G: Dermatologie des paupières du chien et du chat. Première partie: Étude générale. Prat Méd Chir Anim Comp 28:605, 1993.
7. de Geyer G: Dermatologie des paupières du chien et du chat. Deuxième partie: Étude spéciale. Prat Méd Chir Anim Comp 28:613, 1993.
8. Dugan SJ, et al: Variant nodular granulomatous episclerokeratitis in four dogs. J Am Anim Hosp Assoc 29:403, 1993.
9. Gardiner CH, et al: Onchocerciasis in two dogs. J Am Vet Med Assoc 203:828, 1993.
10. Gelatt KN: Histiocytoma of the eyelid of a dog. Vet Med (Small Anim Clin) 70:305, 1975.
11. Gerdin PA, et al: Survey and topographic distribution of bacterial and fungal microorganisms in eyes of clinically normal dogs. Canine Pract 18:34, 1993.
12. Hirai T, et al: Apocrine gland tumor of the eyelid in a dog. Vet Pathol 34:232, 1997.
13. Johnson BW, Campbell KL: Dermatoses of the canine eyelid. Comp Cont Educ 11:385, 1989.
14. Kakoma I, et al: Identification of staphylococci and micrococci from eyes of clinically normal dogs: Relative frequency of isolation, β-lactamase production, and selected antimicrobial sensitivity profiles. Canine Pract 18:11, 1993.
15. Ketring KL: Diseases of the eyelids. In: Kirk RW (ed): Current Veterinary Therapy VII. W.B. Saunders Co, Philadelphia, 1980, p 546.
16. Lawson DD: Canine distichiasis. J Small Anim Pract 14:469, 1973.
17. Lenehan TA, Tarvin G: Personal communication, 1993.
18. McLaughlin, SA, et al: Eyelid neoplasms in cats: A review of demographic data (1979 to 1989). J Am Anim Hosp Assoc 29:63, 1993.
19. Moore CP: Qualitative tear film disease. Vet Clin North Am Small Anim Pract 20:565, 1990.
20. Rothstein E, et al: Tetracycline and niacinamide for the treatment of sterile pyogranuloma/granuloma syndrome in a dog. J Am Anim Hosp Assoc 33:540, 1997.
21. Scott DW, et al: Muller and Kirk's Small Animal Dermatology V. W.B. Saunders Co, Philadelphia, 1995.

Claws

22. Bergvall K: Treatment of symmetrical onychomadesis and onychodystrophy in five dogs with omega-3 and omega-6 fatty acids. Vet Dermatol 9:263, 1998.
23. Boord M: Personal communication, 1993.
24. Boord MJ, et al: Onychectomy as a therapy for symmetric claw and claw fold disease in the dog. J Am Anim Hosp Assoc 33:131, 1997.
25. Carlotti D: Nail diseases in the dog and cat: Differential diagnosis and treatment. Proceedings, William Dick Bicentenary, Edinburgh, July, 1993.
25a. De Jonghe SR, et al: Trachyonychia associated with alopecia areata in a Rhodesian Ridgeback. Vet Dermatol 10:123, 1999.
26. Evans LM, Caylor KB: Polycythemia vera in a cat and management with hydroxyurea. J Am Anim Hosp Assoc 31:434, 1995.
27. Foil CS, Conroy J: Dermatoses of claws, nails, and hoof. In: Von Tscharner C, Halliwell REW(eds): Advances in Veterinary Dermatology I. Baillière Tindall, Philadelphia, 1990, p 420.
28. Harvey RG, Markwell PJ: The mineral composition of nails in normal dogs and comparison with shed nails in canine idiopathic onychomadesis. Vet Dermatol 7: 29, 1996.
29. Griffin CE: Claw diseases. Presentation, European School of Advanced Veterinary Studies, Luxembourg, 1994.
30. Griffin CE: *Malassezia* paronychia in atopic dogs. J Vet Allergy Clin Immunol 5:78, 1997.
31. Mueller RS, et al: Microanatomy of the canine claw. Vet Dermatol 4:5, 1993.
32. Mueller R, Olivry T: Onychobiopsy without onychectomy: Description of a new biopsy technique for canine claws. Vet Dermatol 10:55, 1999.
33. Mueller RS, et al: Evaluation of the pathogenesis of canine claw disease—a prospective study of 24 dogs. Proc Ann Memb Meet Am Acad Vet Dermatol Am Coll Vet Dermatol 14:83, 1998.
34. Rosychuk RAW: Diseases of the claw and claw fold. In: Bonagura JD (ed): Kirk's Current Veterinary Therapy XII. W.B. Saunders Co, Philadelphia, 1995, p 641.
35. Scott DW, Miller WH: Disorders of the claw and clawbed in cats. Comp Cont Educ 14:449, 1992.
36. Scott DW, Miller WH: Disorders of the claw and clawbed in dogs. Comp Cont Educ 14:1448, 1992.
37. Scott DW, Foil CS: Claw diseases in dogs and cats. In: Kwochka KK, et al (eds): Advances in Veterinary Dermatology, Vol 3. Butterworth Heinemann, Boston, 1998, p 406.
38. Scott DW, et al: Symmetrical lupoid onychodystrophy in dogs: A retrospective analysis of 18 cases (1989–1993). J Am Anim Hosp Assoc 31:194, 1995a.
38a. Vicek T, et al: Symmetrical lupoid onychodystrophy in two sibling Rottweilers. Vet Pathol 34:5, 1997.

Anal Sacs

39. Anderson RK: Anal sac disease and its related dermatoses. Comp Cont Educ 6:829, 1984.
40. Duijkeren E: Disease conditions of canine anal sacs. J Small Anim Pract 36:12, 1995.
41. Greer WB, Calhoun ML: Anal sacs of the cat (*Felis domesticus*). Am J Vet Res 27:773, 1966.
42. Hajsig M, Lukman P: *Pityrosporum pachydermatis* (*P. canis*) in the inflamed canine anal sacs. Vet Arch 50:43, 1980.
43. Harvey CE: Incidence and distribution of anal sac disease in the dog. J Am Anim Hosp Assoc 10:573, 1974.
44. Lukman P: Nalazista glijvice *Pityrosporum canis* u organizuma zdravih i bolenith pasa. Vet Arch 52:37, 1982.
45. Montagna W, Parks H: A histochemical study of the glands of the anal sac of the dog. Anat Rec 100:297, 1948.
46. Muse R: Anal gland disease and anal pruritus. In: Griffin CE, et al (eds): Dermatology. Western Veterinary Conference, Las Vegas, 1998, p 186.
47. Ross JT, et al: Adenocarcinoma of the apocrine glands of the anal sac in dogs: A review of 32 cases. J Am Anim Hosp Assoc 27:349, 1991.
48. Seim HB: Diseases of the anus and rectum. In: Kirk RW (ed): Current Veterinary Therapy IX. W. B. Saunders Co, Philadelphia, 1986, p 916.
49. Titkemeyer C: Applied anatomy of the perianal region of the dog. Mich St Univ Vet 18:162, 1958.
50. Vercelli A: Perianal diseases in dogs. Proc Eur Soc Vet Dermatol Eur Coll Vet Dermatol 14:51, 1997.

Ear Canals

51. Ascher F, et al: Mise au point et étude expérimentale d'une formulation destinée au traitement des otites externes du chien et du chat. Partie 1. Epidémiologie et microbiologie. Prat Méd Chir Anim Comp 23:267, 1988.
52. August JR: Diseases of the ear canal. In: Complete Manual of Ear Care. Veterinary Learning Systems, Princeton Junction, NJ, 1986, p 37.
53. Benson CE: Susceptibility of selected otitis externa pathogens to individual and mixtures of acetic and boric acids. Proc Annu Memb Meet Am Acad Vet Dermatol Am Coll Vet Dermatol 14:121, 1998.
54. Blanco JL, et al: Microbiological diagnosis of chronic otitis externa in the dog. Zentralbl Veterinarmed 43:475, 1996.
55. Blue JL, Wooley RE: Antibacterial sensitivity patterns of bacteria isolated from dogs with otitis externa. J Am Vet Med Assoc 177:362, 1977.
56. Bornand V: Bacteriologie et mycologie de l'otite externe du chien. Schweiz Arch Tierheilkd 134:341, 1992.
57. Bourdeau P, et al: The probable role of environmental conditions in the efficacy of treatment of *Otodectes cynotis* infestation in dogs: An example with moxidectin (Cydectin) in 50 dogs. Proc Eur Soc Vet Dermatol Eur Coll Vet Dermatol 15:149, 1998.
58. Boyanowski KJ, et al: Ceruminolytic agents. J Am Anim Hosp Assoc 34:281, 1998.
59. Breitwieser F: Ergebnisse bakteriologischer und mykologischer Untersuchungen bei der Otitis externa des Hundes. Tierärztl Prax 25:257, 1997.
60. Carlotti DN, et al: Marbofloxacin for the systemic treatment of *Pseudomonas* spp. suppurative otitis externa in the dog. In: Kwochka KK, et al (eds): Advances in Veterinary Dermatology III. Butterworth Heinemann, Boston, 1998, p 463.
61. Carlotti DN, Taillieu-LeRoy S: L'otite externe chez le chien: Étiologie et clinique, revue biblographique et étude rétrospective portant sur 752 cas. Prat Méd Chir Anim Comp 32:243, 1997.
62. Chang HJ, et al: An epidemic of *Malassezia pachydermatis* in an intensive care nursery associated with colonization of health care workers' pet dogs. N Engl J Med 338:757, 1998.
63. Chesney CJ: The intimate envelope: Water and skin. In: Kwochka KK, et al (eds): Advances in Veterinary Dermatology III. Butterworth Heinemann, Boston, 1998, p 47.
64. Cole LK, et al: Microbial flora and antimicrobial susceptibity patterns of isolated pathogens from the horizontal ear canal and middle ear in dogs with otitis media. J Am Vet Med Assoc 212:5348, 1998.
65. Cole LK, et al: Kirby-Bauer and minimum inhibiting concentration susceptibility testing of enrofloxacin on isolated bacterial pathogens from dogs with chronic otitis externa and otitis media. Proc Annu Memb Meet Am Acad Vet Dermatol Am Coll Vet Dermatol 14:123, 1998.
66. Eger CE, Lindsay P: Effects of otitis on hearing in dogs characterized by brainstem auditory evoked response testing. J Small Anim Pract 38:380, 1997.
67. Farca AM, et al: Potentiating effect of EDTA-Tris on the activity of antibiotics against resistant bacteria associated with otitis, dematitis and cystitis. J Small Anim Pract 38:243, 1997.
68. Fernando SDA: A histological and histochemical study of the glands of the external auditory canal in the dog. Res Vet Sci 7:116, 1966.
69. Fernando SDA: Certain histopathologic features of the external auditory meatus of the cat and dog with otitis externa. Am J Vet Res 28:278, 1967.
70. Fernando SDA: Microscopic anatomy and histochemistry of glands in the external auditory meatus of the cat (*Felis domesticus*). Am J Vet Res 26:1157, 1965.
71. Foster AP, DeBoer DJ: The role of *Pseudomonas* in canine ear disease. Comp Cont Educ Pract Vet 20:909, 1998.
72. Franc M, et al: Tumeurs du conduit auditif externe des carnivores. Rev Méd Vét 132:733, 1981.
73. Fraser G: The histopathology of the external auditory meatus of the dog. J Comp Pathol 71:253, 1961.
74. Frost RC: Canine otoacariasis. J Small Anim Pract 2:253, 1961.
75. Gallé HG, Venker-van Haagen AJ: Ototoxicity of the antiseptic combination chlorhexidine/cetrimide (Savlon): Effects on equilibrium and hearing. Vet Q 8:56, 1986.
76. Gram D, et al: Treatment of ear mites in cats: A comparison of subcutaneous and topical ivermectin. Vet Med 89:1122, 1994.
77. Griffin CE: Otitis externa and media: In: Griffin CE, et al (eds): Current Veterinary Dermatology. Mosby–Year Book, St. Louis, 1993, p 245.
78. Griffin CE: Principles for treatment of the diseased ear canal. In: Complete Manual of Ear Care. Veterinary Learning Systems, Princeton Junction, NJ, 1986, p 61.
79. Griffin CE, et al: Otitis in dogs and cats. CD ROM, CLIVE, University of Edinburgh, 1998.
80. Griffin CE, Song MD: Management of otitis externa. In: Kwochka KK, et al (eds): Advances in Veterinary

81. Griffin CE: Etiology and pathogenesis of otitis. In: Griffin CE, et al (eds): Otology Medicine and Surgery. Western Veterinary Conference, Las Vegas, 1998, p 3.
82. Griffin CE: *Pseudomonas* otitis therapy. In: Bonagura JD (ed): Kirk's Current Veterinary Therapy XIII. W.B. Saunders Co, Philadelphia, 2000, p 586.
83. Grono LR: Otitis externa. In: Kirk RW (ed): Current Veterinary Therapy VII. W.B. Saunders Co, Philadelphia, 1980, p 461.
84. Hayes HM Jr, Pickle WJ: Effects of ear type and weather on the hospital prevalence of canine otitis externa. Res Vet Sci 42:294, 1987.
85. Holt D, et al: Lateral exploration of fistulas developing after total ear canal ablations: 10 cases. J Am Anim Hosp Assoc 32:527, 1996.
86. Huang HP, Little CJL: Effects of fatty acids on the growth and composition of *Malassezia pachydermatis* and their relevance to canine otitis externa. Res Vet Sci 55:119, 1993.
87. Huang HP, et al: The relationship between microbial numbers found on cytological examination and microbial growth density on culture of swabs from the external ear canal in dogs. Proc Eur Soc Vet Dermatol 10:81, 1993.
88. Huang HP, et al: The application of an infrared tympanic membrane thermometer in comparing the external ear canal temperature between erect and pendulous ears in dogs. In: Kwochka KK, et al (eds): Advances in Veterinary Dermatology III. Butterworth Heinemann, Boston, 1998, p 57.
89. Igarashi Y, Oka Y: Vestibular ototoxicity following intratympanic applications of chlorhexidine gluconate in the cat. Arch Otorhinolaryngol 242:167, 1985.
90. Jeffers JG, et al: A dermatosis resembling juvenile cellulitis in an adult dog. J Am Anim Hosp Assoc 31:204, 1995.
91. Johnson A, Hawke M: An Ink impregnation study of the migratory skin of the external auditory canal of the guinea pig. Acta Otolaryngol (Stockholm) 101:269, 1986.
92. Johnston DE: Early lateral drainage prodecure for chronic otitis externa in dogs. Proc Eur Coll Vet Surg 4:38, 1995.
93. Kapatkin AS, et al: Results of surgery and long-term follow-up in 31 cats with nasopharyngeal polyps. J Am Anim Hosp Assoc 26:387, 1990.
94. Kiss G, et al: Characteristics of *Malassezia pachydermatitis* strains isolated from canine otitis externa. Mycoses 39:313, 1996.
95. Kiss G, et al: New combination for the therapy of canine otitis externa. I. Microbiology of otitis externa. J Small Anim Pract 38:51, 1997.
96. Kowalski JJ: The microbial environment of the ear canal in health and disease. Vet Clin N Am Small Anim Pract 18:743, 1988.
97. Krahwinkel DJ, et al: Effect of total ablation of the external acoustic meatus and bulla osteotomy on auditory function in dogs. J Am Vet Med Assoc 202:949, 1993.
98. Lambert IJ: A comparison of the treatment of otitis externa with 'otosporin' and aluminium acetate: A Report from a services practice in Cyprus. J R Coll Gen Pract 31:291, 1981.
99. Layton CE: The role of lateral ear resection in managing chronic otitis externa. Semin Vet Med Surg Small Anim 8:24, 1993.
100. Leonardi L, et al: Neoplasia involving the ear canal of dogs and cats: Histological and immunohistochemical evaluation of 23 cases. Proc Eur Soc Vet Dermatol Eur Coll Vet Dermatol 14:195, 1997.
101. Little CJL, Lane JG: An evaluation of tympanometry, otoscopy, and palpation for assessment of the canine tympanic membrane. Vet Rec 124:5, 1989.
102. Little CJL, et al: Inflammatory middle ear disease of the dog: The clinical and pathological features of cholesteatoma, a complication of otitis media. Vet Rec 128:319, 1991.
102a. Lloyd DH, Lamport AI: Evaluation in vitro de l'activité antimicrobienne de topiques cutanés et auriculaires chez le chien. Prat Méd Chir Anim Comp 34:259, 1999.
102b. Lloyd DH, et al: Antimicrobial activity in vitro and in vivo of a canine ear cleanser. Vet Rec 143:111, 1998.
103. Logas DB: Diseases of the ear canal. Vet Clin N Am Small Anim Pract 24:905, 1994.
104. Mansfield PD: Ototoxicity in dogs and cats. Comp Cont Educ 12:331, 1990.
105. Mansfield PD, et al: Infectivity of *Malassezia pachydermatis* in the external ear canal of dogs. J Am Anim Hosp Assoc 26:97, 1990.
106. Mansfield PD, et al: The effects of four commercial ceruminolytic agents on the middle ear. J Am Anim Hosp Assoc 33:479, 1997.
107. Marino DJ, et al: Results of surgery and long-term follow-up in dogs with ceruminous gland adenocarcinoma. J Am Anim Hosp Assoc 29:560, 1993.
108. Marino DJ, et al: Results of surgery in cats with ceruminous gland adenocarcinoma. J Am Anim Hosp Assoc 30:54, 1994.
109. Mathison PT, et al: Development of a canine model for *Pseudomonas* otitis externa. Proc Annu Memb Meeting Am Acad Vet Dermatol Am Coll Vet Dermatol 11:21, 1995.
110. Matsuda H, et al: The aerobic bacterial flora of the middle and external ears in normal dogs. J Small Anim Pract 25:269, 1984.
111. Matthiesen DT, Scavelli T: Total ear canal ablation and lateral bulla osteotomy in 38 dogs. J Am Anim Hosp Assoc 26:257, 1990.
112. McAnulty JF, et al: Wound healing and brainstem and evoked potentials after experimental total ear canal ablation with lateral tympanic bulla osteotomy in dogs. Vet Surg 24:1, 1995.
113. McAnulty JF, et al: Wound healing and brainstem and evoked potentials after experimental ventral tympanic bulla osteotomy in dogs. Vet Surg 24:9, 1995.
114. McCarthy RJ, Caywood DD: Vertical ear canal resection for end-stage otitis externa in dogs. J Am Anim Hosp Assoc 28:545, 1992.
115. McKeever PJ, Richardson HW: Otitis externa, part 2: Clinical appearance and diagnostic methods. Companion Anim Pract 2:25, 1988.
116. McKeever PJ, Richardson HW: Otitis externa, part 3: Ear cleaning and medical treatment. Companion Anim Pract 2:24, 1988.
117. McKeever PJ, Torres S: Otitis externa, part 1: The ear and predisposing factors to otitis externa. Comp Anim Pract 2:7, 1988.
118. Merchant SR: Medically managing chronic otitis externa and media. Vet Med 92:518, 1997.
119. Merchant SR, et al: Ototoxicity assessment of a chlor-

hexidine otic preparation in dogs. Prog Vet Neurol 4:72, 1993.
120. Moisan PG, Watson GL: Ceruminous gland tumors in dogs and cats: A review of 124 cases. J Am Anim Hosp Assoc 32:448, 1996.
121. Moriello KA, et al: Adrenocortical suppression associated with topical otic administration of glucocorticoids in dogs. J Am Vet Med Assoc 193:329, 1988.
122. Muse R, et al: The prevalence of otic manifestations and otitis externa in allergic dogs. Proc Am Acad Vet Dermatol Am Coll Vet Dermatol 12:33, 1996.
123. Noxon JO, et al: Minimal inhibitory concentration of silver sulfadiazene on *Pseudomonas aeruginosa* and *Staphyloccus intermedius* isolates from the ears of dogs with otitis externa. Proc Am Acad Vet Dermatol Am Coll Vet Dermatol 13:72, 1997.
124. Nuttall TJ: Use of ticarcillin in the management of canine otitis externa complicated by *Pseudomonas aeruginosa*. J Small Anim Pract 39:165, 1998.
125. Pearson T: Floppy pinnae in Siamese cats. Vet Rec 143:456, 1998.
126. Pope ER: Feline inflammatory polyps. Companion Anim Pract 19:33, 1989.
127. Poulet FM, et al: Focal proliferative eosinophilic dermatitis of the external ear canal in four dogs. Vet Pathol 28:171, 1991.
128. Powell MB, et al: Reaginic hypersensitivity in *Otodectes cynotis* infestation of cats and mode of feeding. Am J Vet Res 41:877, 1980.
129. Power HT, Ihrke PJ: Synthetic retinoids in veterinary dermatology. Vet Clin North Am Small Anim Clin 20:1525, 1990.
130. Rausch FD, Skinner GW: Incidence and treatment of budding yeast in canine otitis externa. Mod Vet Pract 59:914, 1978.
131. Remedios AM, et al: A comparison of radiographic versus surgical diagnosis of otitis media. J Am Anim Hosp Assoc 27:183, 1991.
132. Rose WR: Surgery 1-myringotomy. Vet Med Small Anim Clin 72:1646, 1977.
133. Rosychuck RAW: Management of otitis externa. Vet Clin North Am 24:921, 1994.
134. Sanchez-Araujo M, Puchi A: Acupuncture enhances the efficacy of antibiotics treatment for canine otitis crises. Acupunct Electrother Res 22:191, 1997.
135. Schulte A: Neoplasien im Ohr der Katze. Kleintier-Praxis 33:407, 1988.
136. Scott DW: Canine sterile eosinophilic pinnal folliculitis. Comp Anim Pract 2:19, 1988.
137. Scott DW: Feline dermatology 1900–1978: A monograph. J Am Anim Hosp Assoc 16:331, 1980.
138. Scott DW: Feline dermatology 1986 to 1988: Looking to the 1990s through the eyes of many counsellors. J Am Anim Hosp Assoc 26:515, 1990.
139. Scott DW: Observations on canine atopy. J Am Anim Hosp Assoc 17:91, 1981.
140. Scott DW. Miller WH Jr: Idiopathic cutaneous adverse drug reactions in the cat: Literature review and report of 14 cases (1990–1996). Feline Pract 26:10, 1998.
141. Scott DW, Miller WH Jr: Idiosyncratic cutaneous adverse drug reactions in the dog: Literature review and report of 101 cases (1990–1996). Canine Pract 24:16, 1999.
141a. Spangler EA, Dewey CW: Meningoencephalitis secondary to bacterial otitis media/interna in a dog. J Am Anim Hosp Assoc 36:239, 2000.
142. Sparks TA, et al: Antimicrobial effect of combinations of EDTA-Tris and amikacin or neomycin on the microorganisms associated with otitis externa in dogs. Vet Res Comm 18:241, 1994.
143. Spruell JSA: Treatment of otitis media in the dog. J Small Anim Pract 5:107, 1964.
144. Stout-Graham M, et al: Morphologic measurements of the external horizontal ear canal of dogs. Am J Vet Res 51:990, 1990.
145. Strain GM, et al: Ototoxicity assessment of a gentamicin sulfate otic preparation in dogs. Am J Vet Res 56:532, 1995.
146. Strickland JH, Calhoun ML: The microscopic anatomy of the external ear of *Felis domesticus*. Am J Vet Res 21:845, 1960.
147. Sylvestre AM: Potential factors affecting the outcome of dogs with a resection of the lateral wall of the vertical ear canal. Can Vet J 39:157, 1998.
148. Thomas ML: Development of a bacterial model for canine otitis externa. Proc Annu Memb Meet Am Acad Vet Dermatol Am Coll Vet Dermatol 6:28, 1990.
149. van der Gaag I: The pathology of the external ear canal in dogs and cats. Vet Q 8:307, 1986.
149a. Vogel PL, et al: Wound contamination and antimicrobial susceptibility of bacteria cultured during total ear canal ablation and lateral bulla osteotomy in dogs. J Am Vet Med Assoc 214:1641, 1999.
150. Walker RD, et al: Pharmacokinetic evaluation of enrofloxacin administered orally to healthy dogs. Am J Vet Res 53:2315, 1992.
151. Weisbroth SH, et al: Immunopathology of naturally occurring otodectic otoacariasis in the domestic cat. J Am Vet Med Assoc 165:1088, 1974.
151a. White PD: Medical management of chronic otitis in dogs. Comp Cont Educ Pract Vet 21:716, 1999.
152. Wolschrijn CF, et al: Comparison of air and bone conducted brain stem auditory evoked responses in young dogs and dogs with bilateral ear canal obstruction. Vet Q 19:158, 1997.
153. Swaim SF, Bradley DM: Evaluation of a closed-suction drainage for treating auricular hematomas, J Am Anim Hosp Assoc 32:36, 1996.

Chapter 20

Neoplastic and Non-Neoplastic Tumors

• CUTANEOUS ONCOLOGY

Veterinary oncology has come into its own as a specialty. Detailed information on the etiopathogenesis and immunologic aspects of neoplasia is available in other publications[1-4, 6, 7] and therefore is not presented here. This chapter is an overview of canine and feline cutaneous neoplasia as well as non-neoplastic tumors.

The combined *incidence rates* (the number of new cases of a disease diagnosed in 1 year divided by the population at risk and expressed as cases per 100,000 of the population at risk) for benign and malignant neoplasms in dogs and cats were reported to be about 1077 and 188, respectively.[3, 6, 7, 32] Thus, dogs have about six times as many neoplasms as do cats. The incidence rates for canine and feline skin neoplasms are about 728 and 84, respectively.

The peak age period for neoplasm occurrence in dogs and cats is 6 to 14 years. The median ages for cutaneous neoplasm occurrence in dogs and cats are 10½ years and 12 years, respectively. The frequency of various skin neoplasms differs in dog and cat breeds (Table 20–1). Canine breeds that have the highest neoplasm incidence are the Boxer, Scottish terrier, Bull mastiff, Basset hound, Weimaraner, Kerry blue terrier, and Norwegian Elkhound.* Siamese and Persians appear to be at risk for certain cutaneous neoplasms in cats.[1] The overall incidence of neoplasia is greater in female dogs than in male dogs (56% versus 44%); in cats, however, male cats predominate (56% versus 44%) in most surveys.[3, 5, 6, 35]

There are no completely satisfactory criteria for distinguishing benign neoplasms from certain proliferative inflammatory lesions and hyperplastic processes and for distinguishing benign from malignant neoplasms.[3, 6, 7] In general, malignant neoplasms are usually characterized by sudden onset, rapid growth, infiltration, recurrence, and metastasis. The most important criterion of malignancy is metastasis. In dogs, the number of malignant neoplasms is only about half the number of benign neoplasms.[3, 6, 7, 32] However, in cats, there are about three times as many malignant neoplasms as benign neoplasms.[3, 6, 7, 32, 35]

The skin is the most common site of occurrence of neoplasms in the dog (about 30% of the total) and the second most common site in the cat (about 20% of the total).[3, 6-9, 12, 29, 32, 35-38, 41] The most common skin neoplasm in dogs and cats varies somewhat from one report to another. In general, canine skin neoplasms may be broadly categorized as about 55% mesenchymal, 40% epithelial, and 5% melanocytic in origin, and feline skin neoplasms as 50% epithelial, 48% mesenchymal, and 2% melanocytic. In the dog, the most common skin neoplasms, in approximate descending order, are lipoma, sebaceous gland hyperplasia, mast cell tumor, histiocytoma, and papilloma (squamous papilloma and fibropapilloma). In the cat, the approximate order is basal cell tumor, squamous cell carcinoma, mast cell tumor, and fibrosarcoma.

The key to appropriate management and accurate prognosis of cutaneous neoplasms is specific diagnosis. This can be achieved only by biopsy and histologic evaluation. Exfoliative cytologic techniques (aspiration and impression smear) are easy and rapid, and often

---

*See references 1, 3, 5–7, 11, 21, 32, 34.

● Table 20–1 **BREED PREDILECTIONS FOR CUTANEOUS NEOPLASMS AND NON-NEOPLASTIC LUMPS IN THE DOG AND CAT**

Papilloma	Cocker spaniel, Kerry blue terrier
Keratoacanthoma	Collie, German shepherd dog, Keeshond, Lhasa apso, Norwegian elkhound, Old English sheepdog, Yorkshire terrier
Squamous cell carcinoma	Scottish terrier, Pekingese, boxer, Poodle, Norwegian elkhound
Squamous cell carcinoma, glabrous, nonpigmented skin of trunk (actinic)	Dalmatian, bull terrier, American Staffordshire terrier, beagle
Squamous cell carcinoma, clawbed	Black Labrador retriever, Black Standard Poodle, Giant Schnauzer, dachshund, Bouvier de Flandres
Feline benign basal cell tumor	Persian, Himalayan
Basal cell carcinoma	Cocker spaniel, English Springer spaniel, Kerry blue terrier, Poodle, Shetland sheepdog, Siberian husky, Siamese cat
Trichoepithelioma	Cocker spaniel, English Springer spaniel, Basset hound, German shepherd dog, Golden retriever, Irish setter, Miniature Schnauzer, Standard Poodle, Persian cat
Tricholemmoma	Afghan hound
Pilomatrixoma	Kerry blue terrier, Old English sheepdog, Poodle
Trichoblastoma	Cocker spaniel, Poodle
Sebaceous gland tumors	Beagle, Cocker spaniel, dachshund, Irish setter, Lhasa apso, Malamute, Miniature Schnauzer, Poodle, Shih tzu, Siberian husky, Persian cat
Sweat gland tumors	Cocker spaniel, German shepherd dog, Golden retriever
Circumanal gland tumors	Beagle, Cocker spaniel, English bulldog, German shepherd dog, Lhasa apso, Samoyed, Shih tzu, Siberian husky, Afghan hound, dachshund
Fibroma	Boston terrier, boxer, Doberman pinscher, fox terrier, Golden retriever
Fibropruritic nodule	German shepherd dog
Fibrosarcoma	Cocker spaniel, Doberman pinscher, Golden retriever
Myxoma or myxosarcoma	Doberman pinscher, German shepherd
Schwannoma	Fox terrier
Hemangioma	Airedale terrier, boxer, English Springer spaniel, German shepherd dog, Golden retriever
Hemangioma, glabrous, nonpigmented skin (actinic)	American Staffordshire terrier, Basset hound, beagle, Dalmatian, English Springer spaniel, Greyhound, Saluki, Whippet
Hemangiosarcoma	Bernese Mountain dog, boxer, German shepherd dog, Golden retriever
Hemangiosarcoma, glabrous, nonpigmented skin (actinic)	See actinic hemangioma
Hemangiopericytoma	Beagle, Boxer, Cocker spaniel, Collie, Fox terrier, English Springer spaniel, German shepherd dog, Irish setter, Siberian husky
Lipoma	Cocker spaniel, Dachshund, Doberman pinscher, Labrador retriever, Miniature Schnauzer, Weimaraner, Siamese cat
Liposarcoma	Brittany spaniel, dachshund, Shetland sheepdog
Mast cell tumor	American Staffordshire terrier, Beagle, Boston terrier, Boxer, Bull terrier, Dachshund, English bulldog, Fox terrier, Golden retriever, Labrador retriever, Pug, Shar pei, Weimaraner, Siamese cat
Lymphoma	Basset hound, boxer, Cocker spaniel, German shepherd dog, Golden retriever, Irish setter, Scottish terrier, St. Bernard
Plasmacytoma	Cocker spaniel
Histiocytoma	American Staffordshire terrier, Boston terrier, boxer, Cocker spaniel, Dachshund, Doberman pinscher, English Springer spaniel, Great Dane, Labrador retriever, Miniature Schnauzer, Rottweiler, Scottish terrier, Shar pei, Shetland sheepdog, West Highland white terrier
Malignant histiocytosis	Bernese Mountain dog
Systemic histiocytosis	Bernese Mountain dog
Cutaneous histiocytosis	Collie, Shetland sheepdog
Benign fibrous histiocytoma	Collie, Golden retriever

Table continued on following page

Table 20-1	BREED PREDILECTIONS FOR CUTANEOUS NEOPLASMS AND NON-NEOPLASTIC LUMPS IN THE DOG AND CAT *Continued*
Melanocytic tumors	Airedale terrier, Boston terrier, boxer, Chihuahua, Chow Chow, Cocker spaniel, Doberman pinscher, English Springer spaniel, Golden retriever, Irish setter, Irish terrier, Miniature Schnauzer, Scottish terrier
Follicular cyst	Boxer, Doberman pinscher, Miniature Schnauzer, Shih tzu
Dermoid cyst	Boxer, Kerry blue terrier, Rhodesian Ridgeback
Collagenous nevus	German shepherd dog
Vascular nevus, scrotal	Airedale terrier, Kerry blue terrier, Labrador retriever, Scottish terrier
Epidermal nevus	Miniature Schnauzer, Pug
Actinic keratosis	American Staffordshird terrier, Basset hound, Beagle, Bull terrier, Dalmatian
Calcinosis circumscripta	Boston terrier, Boxer, German shepherd dog
Focal mucinosis	Doberman pinscher, Shar pei

provide valuable information about neoplastic cell type and differentiation. The techniques, methods, and interpretation used in cytologic studies have been beautifully described and illustrated (see Chap. 2).[42a–46a] However, exfoliative cytologic evaluation is inferior to and is no substitute for biopsy and histopathologic examination. Historical and clinical considerations often allow the experienced clinician to formulate an inclusive differential diagnosis on a cutaneous neoplasm but variability renders such "odds playing" unreliable. In short, "a lump is a lump" until it is evaluated histologically.

The detailed histopathologic description of canine and feline cutaneous neoplasms is beyond the scope of this chapter. Only the histopathologic essence of individual neoplasms is presented here. For in-depth information and photomicrographic illustrations, the reader is referred to other texts on cutaneous neoplasia[1–3, 42] and the individual references cited for each neoplasm.

The use of markers—enzyme histochemical and immunohistochemical methods for identifying specific cell types—has increased and has facilitated the diagnosis of many neoplastic conditions in dogs and cats.[47–64] Examples of these markers are presented in Chapter 2.

Clinical management of cutaneous neoplasms may include surgery, cryosurgery, electrosurgery, radiotherapy, laser therapy, chemotherapy, immunotherapy (Table 20–2), hyperthermia, phototherapy, and combinations of these. Detailed information on the various treatment modalities is available in a number of excellent references.[4, 6, 7, 25, 41a] Brief comments on treatment are included under clinical management for each tumor.

The crucial difference between normal and neoplastic cells stems from discrete changes in specific genes controlling proliferation and tissue homeostasis.[114] More than

Table 20-2	IMMUNOTHERAPY AGENTS USED IN CANINE AND FELINE NEOPLASIA		
PRODUCT NAME	ACTIVE INGREDIENT	INDICATIONS	TOXICITY
Acemannan Immunostimulant (Carrington Laboratories, Dallas, Texas)	Polymannose	Fibrosarcoma	Discomfort, decreased activity, vomiting, loose stools
ImmunoRegulin (Vetoquinol-Immunovet, Tampa, Florida)	*Propionibacterium acnes*	Neoplasia°	Fever, chills, anorexia, lethargy
Regressin-V (Vetrepharm Research, Athens, Georgia)	Nonpathogenic *Mycobacteria spp.*	Neoplasia°	

°Off-label.
Modified from VanKampen KR: Immunotherapy and cytokines. Sem Vet Med Surg 12:186, 1997.

100 such cancer-related genes have been discovered. Two principal types of growth-regulating genes have been associated with the pathogenesis of neoplasia: *oncogenes* encode proteins that convey various growth advantages, while *tumor-suppressor genes* encode proteins that restrict cell proliferation and differentiation.[107]

The p53 tumor-suppressor gene is the most striking and well-studied example, and mutations of this gene occur in about 50% of all cancer types in humans.[107, 114] Tumor-suppressor genes are vulnerable sites for critical DNA damage because they normally function as physiologic barriers against clonal expansion or genomic mutability, and they are able to hinder growth and metastasis of cells driven to uncontrolled proliferation by oncogenes. p53 participates in many cellular functions: cell cycle control, DNA repair, differentiation, genomic plasticity, and programmed cell death. p53 is an important component in a biochemical pathway or pathways central to carcinogenesis, and p53 mutations provide a selective advantage for clonal expansion of preneoplastic and neoplastic cells.

Overexpression of p53 is positively associated with gene mutation. Overexpression of p53 was detected in most canine squamous cell carcinomas and circumanal gland adenocarcinomas.[107] Mutations in p53 were found in most feline and canine squamous cell carcinomas.[138] In a recent study, p53 mutations were found in only 3 of 20 feline neoplasms.[181]

Cyclins are associated with and activate various cyclin-dependent kinases at various phases of the cell cycle.[101] In humans, overexpression of cyclin D and downregulation of cyclin E expression may be involved in keratinocyte carcinogenesis.[101]

The apoptotic index and mitotic index of various benign and malignant canine skin neoplasms were compared.[16a] In general, there was an inverse relationship between apoptotic index and mitotic index in benign neoplasms, and no correlation in malignant neoplasms. Thus, classification of canine skin neoplasms according to their apoptotic and mitotic indices did not reflect the clinical behavior of some tumor types.

• EPITHELIAL NEOPLASMS

Papilloma

CAUSE AND PATHOGENESIS

Since the mid-1980s, great advances have been made concerning the understanding and classification of papillomaviruses in animals and humans.[73, 77, 84] Differentiation of papillomavirus types by cleavage patterns produced by treating viral DNA with restriction endonucleases and the in vitro hybridization of viral DNA have emphasized the heterogeneity of papillomaviruses within animal genera. In dogs, at least five types of papillomaviruses tend to have site specificity on the animal as well as histologic specificity.[5, 84] It would appear that multiple feline papillomaviruses exist.[83, 83a] The papillomaviruses are transmitted by direct and indirect (via fomites) contact. In general, infection occurs in damaged skin. The incubation period varies from 1 to 2 months.[77]

No in vitro system for papillomavirus propagation is available. Detection methods differ dramatically in their sensitivity.[73] *Southern blot hybridization* is highly specific and sensitive, but it is time-consuming and does not allow detection of DNA segments of unknown types. *Dot blot* and *reverse blot hybridization* have good sensitivity and reasonable accuracy, but are also laborious. *In situ hybridization* is less sensitive than Southern blot, but does allow identification of cells harboring viral DNA. *Polymerase chain reaction* (PCR) is the most widely used technique, but it is not as sensitive as the others.

Papillomavirus is fairly stable in the environment and can survive for 63 days at 4 to 8°C or for 6 hours at 37°C.[77] Humoral immunity (neutralizing antibodies) protects against viral challenge but does not play a role in clearance of established lesions.[77] Cellular immunity is of key importance in papilloma regression.[77] Papillomavirus vaccines (live or formalin-inactivated) are effective preventives, but are of no known therapeutic benefit.[77]

There is great interest and much research in the role of papillomaviruses and oncogenesis.[73] The viral genome can be divided in parts labeled as L (later region), E (early region), and LCR (long control region). The L1 and L2 genes encode for viral capsid proteins, and E region consists of genes involved in regulation of viral DNA replication (E1 and E2) or cell proliferation and immortalization (E6 and E7). In addition, E2 protein is an important viral transcription factor regulating expression of E6 and E7 oncogenes. E4 protein binds keratins and facilitates production of virions by disrupting normal cell differentiation. E6 and E7 proteins have oncogene potential and can interfere with cellular factors involved in the control of cell proliferation and the prevention of cell immortalization. E6 and E7 oncogenes are capable of immortalizing cells, inducing cell growth, and promoting chromosomal instability in the host cell. E6 oncoprotein causes degradation of p53 protein by the cellular ubiquitin proteolysis system, leading to unblocking of cell division and host DNA synthesis, which results in chromosomal instability and accumulation of various mutations in affected cells.

Papillomaviruses appear to be involved in the etiology of certain forms of squamous cell carcinoma in dogs and cats (see Squamous Cell Carcinoma).[77]

Severe or unusual forms of papillomatosis have been seen in dogs with IgA deficiency or receiving glucocorticoids or cancer chemotherapy.[70, 72, 74, 82, 84, 85] It would appear that glucocorticoids and immunosuppression can exacerbate latent infections and cause expansion of the tissue tropism of the virus.

CLINICAL FINDINGS

Dog

Cutaneous papillomas (warts and verrucae) are common in the dog, and at least five syndromes are recognized clinically. *Canine oral papillomatosis* is common and affects young dogs with no apparent breed or sex predilection. Lesions are almost always multiple and affect the buccal mucosa, the tongue, the palate, the pharynx, the epiglottis, the lip, the nasal planum, the skin, the eyelids, the conjunctiva, and the cornea (Fig. 20–1A and C).[1, 5–7, 84] The lesions begin as white, flat, smooth, shiny papules and plaques of a few millimeters in diameter and progress to whitish gray, pedunculated or cauliflower-like hyperkeratotic masses up to 3 cm in diameter. The surface of well-developed lesions is covered by fronds of hyperkeratosis. Florid oral papillomatosis has been seen in Beagles in association with IgA deficiency.[82, 84] Severe oral papillomatosis with generalized cutaneous papillomas (same virus) was seen in a young Shar pei in association with glucocorticoid therapy.[82] Multiple papillomas were reported in the face, inguinal, and perineal region of a dog receiving cancer chemotherapy.[72]

Cutaneous papillomas occur uncommonly in older dogs and are more common in male dogs, Cocker spaniels, and Kerry blue terriers.[5–7, 12, 27, 31, 33] Cutaneous papillomas may be single or multiple, occurring mainly on the head, the eyelids, and the feet (Fig. 20–1B). They are usually pedunculated or cauliflower like, firm to soft, well circumscribed, alopecic, and smooth to keratinous; they are usually smaller than 0.5 cm in diameter. Papillomavirus has been identified in the lesions.[76, 77, 84, 86]

Cutaneous inverted papillomas are usually seen in dogs 8 months to 3 years of age, with no apparent breed or sex predilection.[66, 79] Lesions occur commonly on the ventral abdomen and the groin; are small (1 to 2 cm in diameter), raised, and firm; and contain a central pore opening to the surface of the skin (Fig. 20–2). DNA hybridization studies with a canine oral papillomatosis virus probe revealed that cutaneous inverted papillomas are due to a different papillomavirus from that causing canine oral papillomas.

Multiple pigmented, papular, cutaneous papillomas associated with a novel papillomavirus were seen in a 6-year-old boxer receiving long-term systemic glucocorticoids.[70] The lesions were black, rounded, had a waxy surface, and occurred on the ventrum. The papillomas spontaneously regressed 3 weeks after glucocorticoid administration was stopped.

Multiple pigmented plaques associated with papillomavirus infection has been reported in miniature Schnauzers and Pugs (Fig. 20–3).[75] The condition has been reported in an

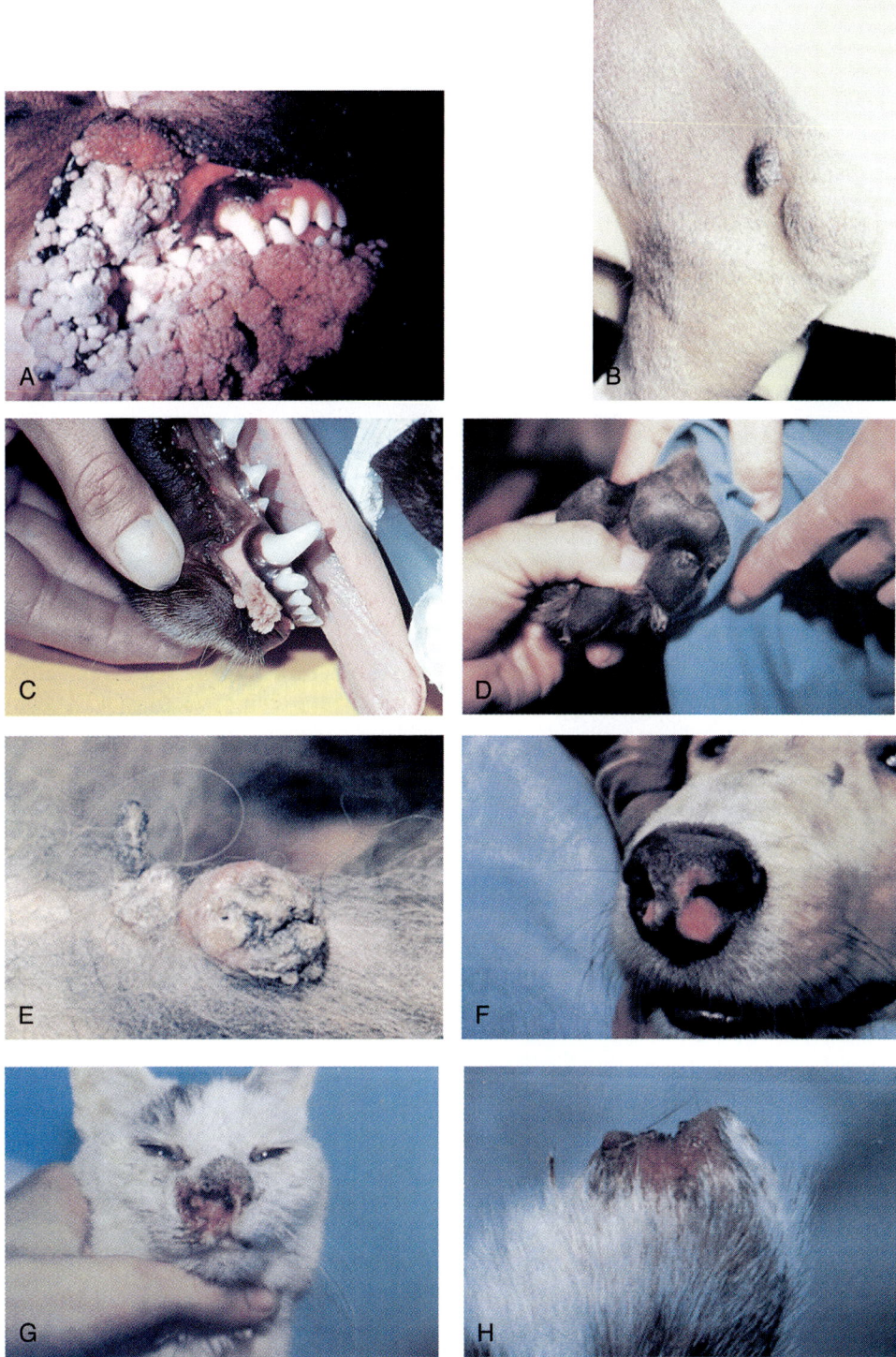

FIGURE 20–1. *A*, Severe oral viral papillomatosis in a young dog. *B*, Squamous papilloma on the hock of an old dog. *C*, Viral papilloma on the lip of a young dog. *D*, Multiple squamous papillomas on the footpads of a young dog. *E*, Two keratoacanthomas on the dorsal neck of an Old English sheepdog. The lesion at the left has an overlying cutaneous horn. *F*, Squamous cell carcinoma on the nose of a collie. *G*, Squamous cell carcinoma on the nose of a cat. *H*, Squamous cell carcinoma on the tip of the pinna of a white cat.

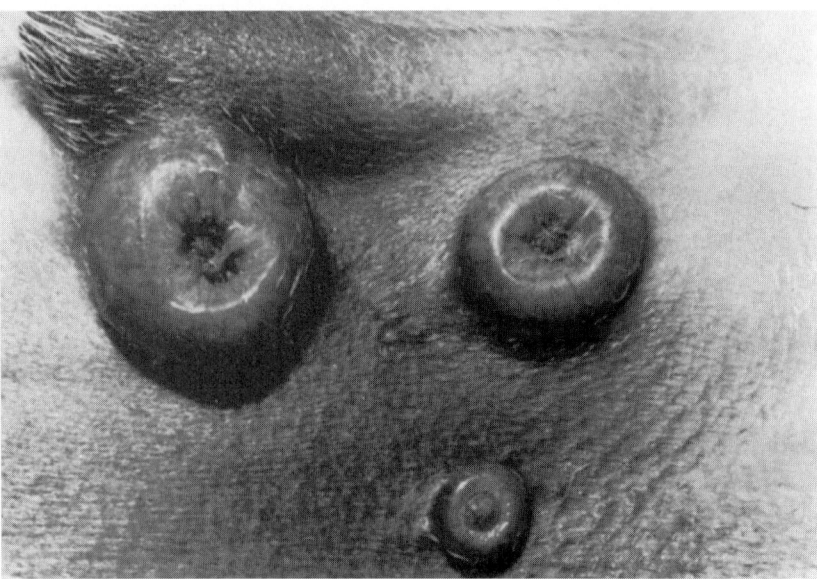

FIGURE 20–2. Inverted papillomas near the prepuce of a young dog.

English setter,[87] and the authors have seen cases in the Shar pei (Fig. 20–4). Lesions often begin at 2 to 4 years of age, and are most common on the ventrum and medial thighs. Melanotic macules and plaques become progressively more scaly and hyperkeratotic. This condition appears to be identical to that previously referred to as "pigmented epidermal nevi" and "lentigines."[2, 5] In miniature Schnauzers and Pugs, the condition appears to be inherited in an autosomal dominant fashion.[75] Some lesions may undergo malignant transformation into squamous cell carcinomas.[75, 87] This syndrome appears to be very similar to epidermodysplasia verruciformis in humans.[75]

Multiple papillomas have been recognized on the footpads of adult dogs.[5] Lesions were firm, hyperkeratotic, and often hornlike in appearance. They occurred on multiple footpads of two paws or more (see Fig. 20–1D). Larger lesions were associated with lameness. These papillomas have not been definitively shown to be caused by viruses.

Occasionally, cutaneous horns may overlie papillomas.

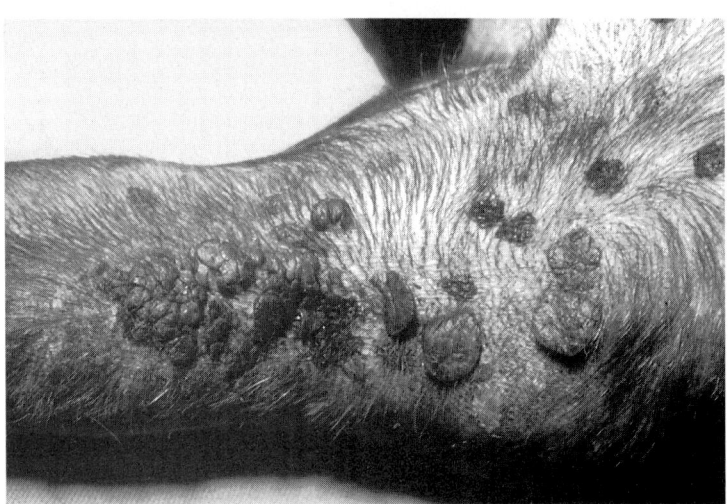

FIGURE 20–3. Pigmented viral papillomas on the leg of a Pug.

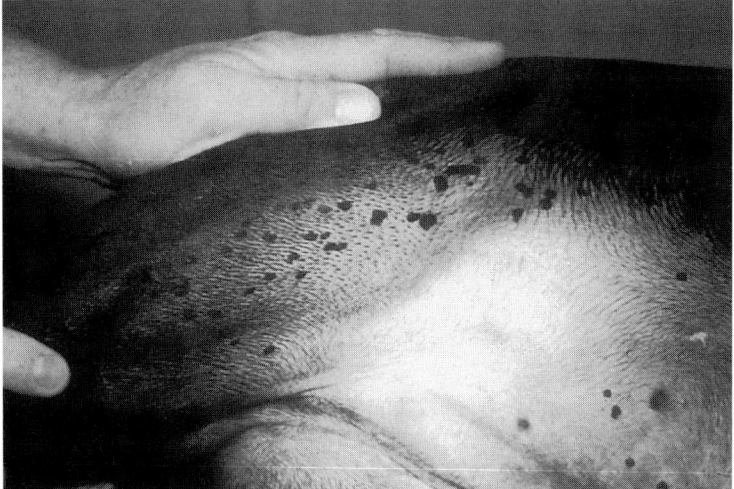

FIGURE 20-4. Multiple pigmented viral papillomas on the thigh and abdomen of a Shar pei.

Although cutaneous viral papillomas are usually benign, apparent transformation into squamous cell carcinoma has been recognized in some canine cases.[5, 6, 77, 84] Some dogs treated with a live virus vaccine that was made from papillomavirus isolated from naturally occurring oral papillomas experienced squamous cell carcinomas at the sites of vaccine inoculation.[65, 77, 84] This did not occur when formalin-inactivated vaccines were used.[77] Rare cases of viral papillomatosis have been completely unresponsive to treatment, perhaps owing to immunologic defects (Fig. 20-5).[74, 77]

Cat

There are at least two types of papillomaviruses in domestic cats: oral (FdPV-2) and skin (FdPV-1).[83a] Tongue lesions occur in 6-month to 9-year-old cats, and are multifocal, small (4 to 8 mm), soft, light pink, oval, slightly raised, and flat-topped. The ventral tongue is usually affected. Solitary cutaneous papillomas are rare in cats, and most are not known to be caused by papillomaviruses.[26, 27, 35, 39] Papillomavirus was identified in one eyelid papilloma of a cat.[68] Lesions are seen in adult cats with no apparent breed, sex, or site predilection. The papillomas are solitary, pedunculated to cauliflower like, well circumscribed, and hyperkeratotic; they are smaller than 0.5 cm in diameter.

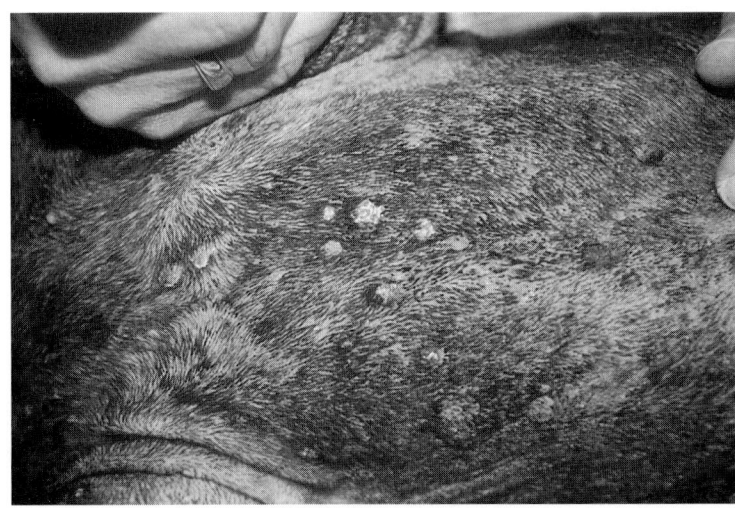

FIGURE 20-5. Multiple viral papillomas in an immunosuppressed, aged Shar pei.

Multiple viral papillomas were first reported in cats in 1990.[67] Affected cats are middle-aged to old, and no breed or sex predilections are reported.[67, 69, 71] Multiple lesions can occur anywhere on the body, especially the head, neck, dorsal thorax, ventral abdomen, and proximal limbs. The lesions vary from 3 mm to 3 cm in diameter, begin as melanotic macules, and evolve into plaques, which become progressively more scaly, hyperkeratotic, and occasionally, greasy. Recent information indicates that these viral papillomas are the precursors to feline multicentric squamous cell carcinoma (Bowen's disease) (see Squamous Cell Carcinoma).[20]

Occasionally, cutaneous horns overlie papillomas.[35]

DIAGNOSIS

The differential diagnostic considerations in dogs include keratoacanthoma, trichofolliculoma, cutaneous horn, lentigo, and melanocytic neoplasm, whereas in cats, they include mast cell tumor, cutaneous horn, dilated pore of Winer, and melanocytic neoplasm. Histologically, papillomas may be divided into squamous and fibrous types.[1, 2, 5-7] Squamous papillomas (the most common type) are characterized by papillated (exophytic papilloma) or plaquelike (verruca plana, or flat wart) epidermal hyperplasia and papillomatosis, with variable degrees of ballooning degeneration (koilocytosis) and giant, clumped, pleomorphic keratohyaline granules (Figs. 20–6 and 20–7).[1, 2, 5] Basophilic intranuclear inclusion bodies are variable findings. Inverted papillomas (endophytic papilloma) are cup-shaped lesions with a central core of keratin.[1, 66] The cup is lined by mature squamous epithelium with centripetal papillary projections, ballooning degeneration, abnormal keratohyaline granules, and variable intranuclear inclusion bodies. Keratoacanthomas are histo-

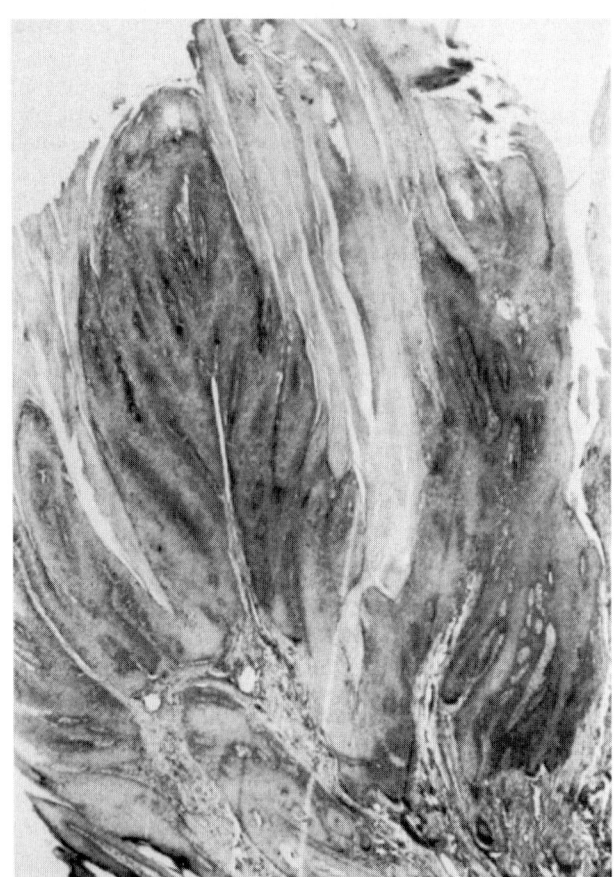

FIGURE 20–6. Canine viral squamous papilloma. Note papillomatosis and vacuolated keratinocytes.

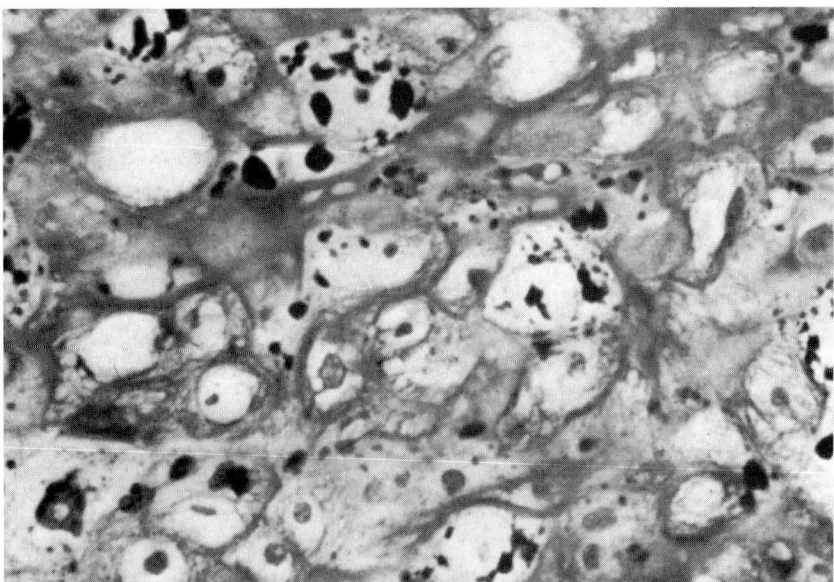

FIGURE 20–7. Canine viral squamous papilloma. Note ballooning degeneration and clumping of keratohyaline granules.

logically similar but lack evidence of viral infection. Idiopathic squamous papillomas are histologically identical to viral squamous papillomas, except that they lack evidence of virus infection (ballooning degeneration, abnormal keratohyaline granules, and intranuclear inclusion bodies).[2] Routine use of immunohistochemical or PCR techniques would greatly reduce the number of "idiopathic" cases. Fibropapilloma (fibrous polyp) is characterized by a fibroma-like proliferation of collagen with papillomatosis and papillated epidermal hyperplasia (Fig. 20–8). The recently reported pigmented papular papillomas have a unique, cup-shaped appearance with marked parakeratotic hyperkeratosis, angular baso-

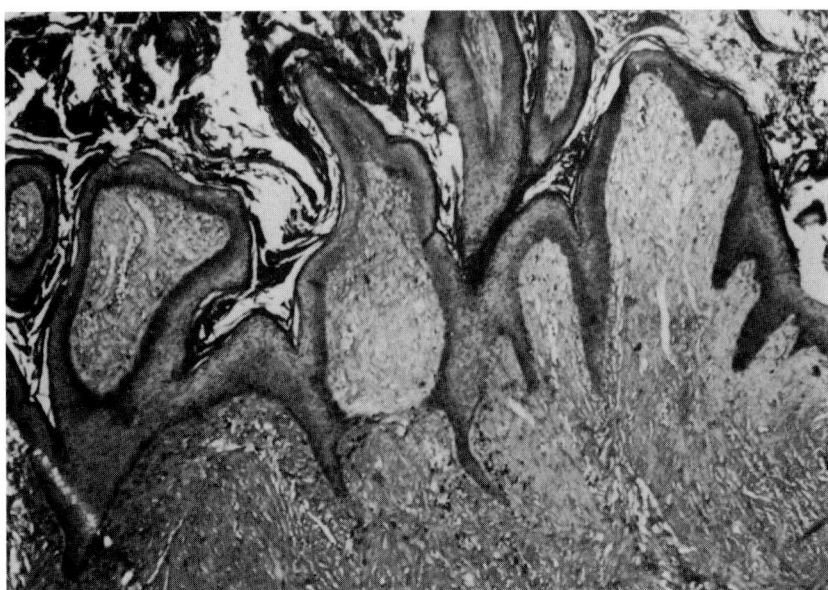

FIGURE 20–8. Canine fibropapilloma. Papillomatous proliferation of epidermis and fibroblasts.

philic intranuclear inclusion bodies, eosinophilic fibrillar cytoplasmic inclusions (modified keratin protein), and scarce keratohyalin granules (Figs. 20–9A and B).[70] The multiple macular and plaquelike papillomas show a typical squamous papilloma configuration with marked epidermal melanosis and giant keratohyalin granules (Figs. 20–10A and B).[75]

The feline multiple viral papillomas are characterized early by focal, abrupt, plaquelike epidermal and infundibular hyperplasia and orthokeratotic hyperkeratosis, hypermelanosis, ballooning degeneration, and abnormal keratohyaline granules (Fig. 20–11).[67, 69, 71, 83a] Basophilic intranuclear inclusions and gray intracytoplasmic inclusions (proliferating cytokeratin filaments) are variably present. Fine, coalescent, pink, fibrillar, intracytoplasmic masses first appear in the keratinocytes of the stratum spinosum and become irregular, solitary, large, and amphophilic in the stratum granulosum.

Papillomavirus antigen can be detected by immunohistochemical techniques in viral papillomas.[*] However, other techniques, such as PCR, are much more sensitive.[73] Papillomavirus has also been detected in some canine and feline squamous cell carcinomas[20, 78, 86] but not in canine basal cell tumors, hair follicle neoplasms, sebaceous gland tumors, or sweat gland neoplasms.[78] Papillomas are positive for cytokeratin.[50, 61]

---

*See references 66, 67, 69–71, 75–82, 84, 86.

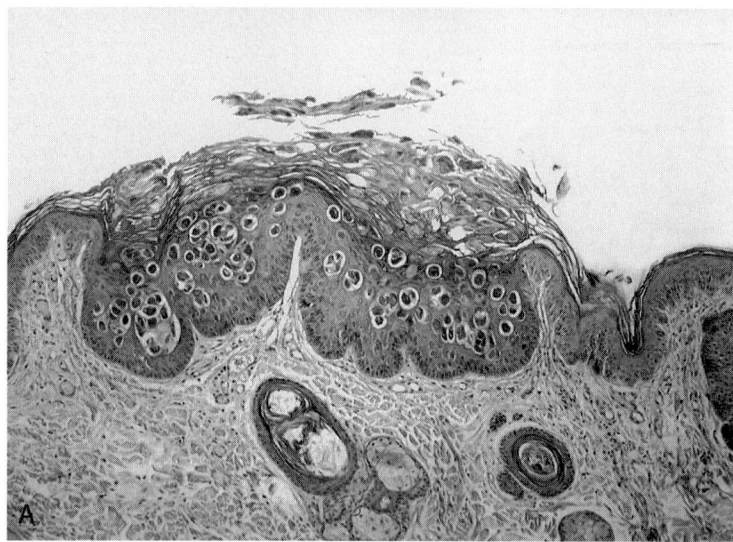
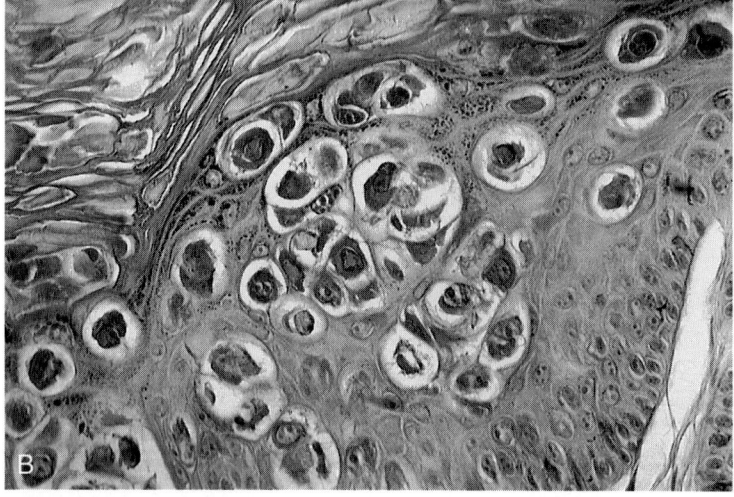

FIGURE 20–9. A, Pigmented papular viral papilloma from an immunosuppressed dog. B, Close-up of A. Koilocytosis, intranuclear, and intracytoplasmic inclusion bodies.

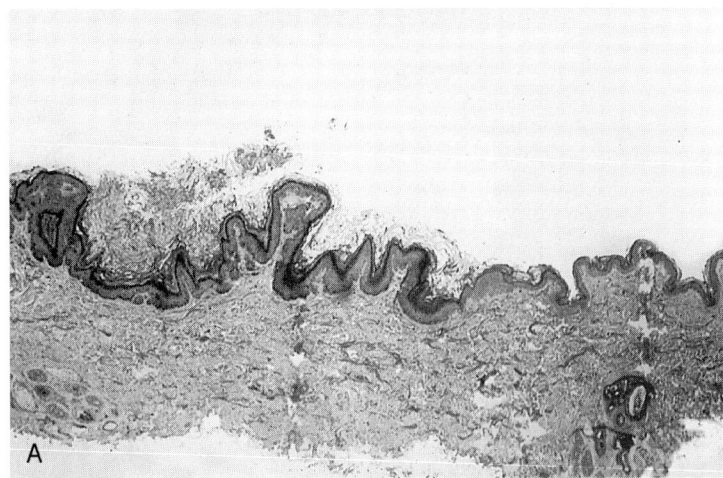
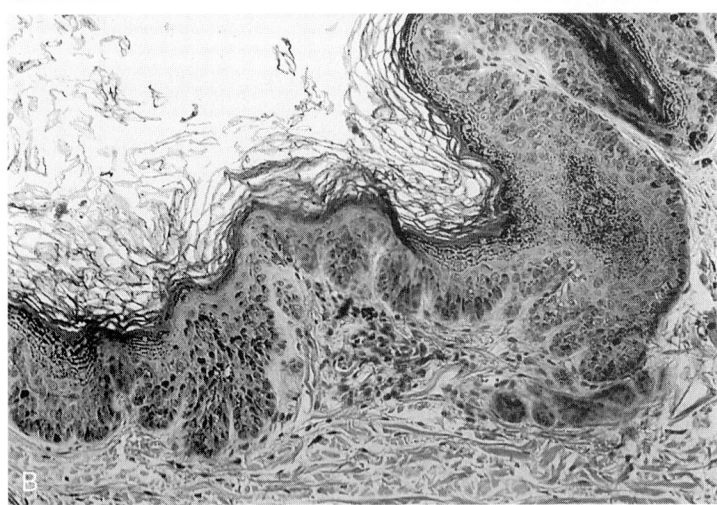

FIGURE 20–10. *A*, Pigmented viral papilloma from a Shar pei. Note sudden transition from normal skin *(right)* to papilloma *(left)*. *B*, Close-up of *A*.

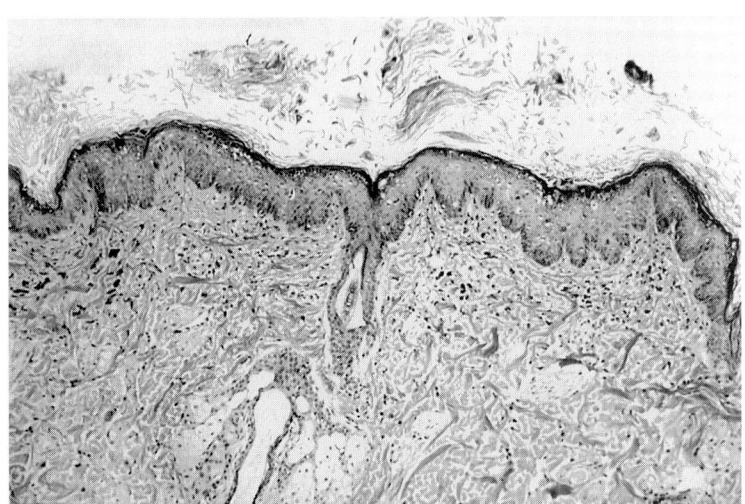

FIGURE 20–11. Feline viral papilloma. Note the "flat wart" appearance with hyperkeratosis and koilocytosis within the stratum granulosum.

CLINICAL MANAGEMENT

Clinical management of papillomas may include surgical excision, cryosurgery, electrosurgery, and observation without treatment.[4-7] Canine oral papillomatosis usually undergoes spontaneous regression within about 3 months, and solid immunity follows experimental or natural infection.[77, 85] Autogenous or commercially produced wart vaccines and immunomodulating drugs (e.g., levamisole and thiabendazole) are without documented therapeutic value. Live virus vaccines produced from canine oral papillomas are protective but have been associated with injection site squamous cell carcinomas.[65, 84, 85] Formalin-inactivated papillomavirus vaccine administered intradermally afforded complete protection against natural and experimental infection and produced no injection site squamous cell carcinomas.[77, 85] In certain cases with large masses of proliferating tissue, eating and maintaining oral hygiene may be facilitated by surgically removing some of the larger papillomas, which is usually performed by cryosurgery or electrosurgery. There is absolutely no evidence to suggest that the removal or crushing of some papillomas causes early regression of the others. Reports have indicated that intralesional injections of bleomycin, 5-fluorouracil, or interferon, as well as the oral administration of levamisole or retinoids, are beneficial to humans with recalcitrant papillomas.[73] Retinoids have been reported to be effective in the treatment of canine inverted papillomas.[333] Canine inverted papillomas have also been reported to regress spontaneously.[79] Anecdotal reports indicate that interferon (Roferon-A, Hoffman-LaRoche), 1.5 to 2 million units/m² BSA given subcutaneously 3 times a week, is effective for the treatment of severe cases of oral or cutaneous viral papillomatosis, or both (see Chap. 3).[88]

Keratoacanthoma

CAUSE AND PATHOGENESIS

Keratoacanthomas (intracutaneous cornifying epitheliomas, or infundibular keratinizing acanthomas) are uncommon benign neoplasms of the dog.[1, 4-7, 92] It has been suggested that these neoplasms are of hair follicle origin.[2] There are unsubstantiated references to the occurrence of keratoacanthomas in the cat. The cause of keratoacanthomas is unknown, although the generalized forms may have a hereditary basis in dogs and humans. Immunohistochemical studies failed to identify papillomavirus antigen.[66, 78, 80]

CLINICAL FINDINGS

Usually, these neoplasms occur in dogs 5 years of age or younger. Male dogs are more commonly affected than female dogs. The incidence is higher in purebred dogs and particularly in the Norwegian Elkhound and Keeshond, which are predisposed to the generalized form.[1, 4-7, 27, 92] However, the generalized form has also been recognized in the German shepherd dog and Old English sheepdog.[5, 6, 27] Collies, Lhasa apsos, and Yorkshire terriers are also reported to be at risk for the solitary form.[1, 5]

Although keratoacanthomas are usually solitary, they may be multiple in the Norwegian Elkhound, Keeshond, German shepherd dog, and Old English sheepdog (see Fig. 20-1E). Most tumors occur on the back, the neck, the thorax, and the limbs. There is considerable variation in the gross appearance of keratoacanthomas. Most of the tumors appear as firm to fluctuant, well-circumscribed dermal or subcutaneous masses varying from 0.5 to 4 cm in diameter, with a pore opening onto the skin surface that ranges from less than 1 mm to several millimeters in diameter. The opening usually contains a hard keratinized plug, varying from small and inconspicuous to large and hornlike. Superficial lesions with large keratinous plugs are easily mistaken for cutaneous horns. Some of the tumors are entirely dermal or subcutaneous, do not communicate with the surface of the skin, and are easily confused with cysts. Keratoacanthomas are not invasive or metastatic. However, in the generalized form (up to 50 lesions) a recurrent problem should be anticipated, because affected dogs tend to have new tumors at other sites throughout their lives.

DIAGNOSIS

The differential diagnostic considerations include papillomas, trichofolliculomas, cutaneous horns, and cysts. Histopathologically, keratoacanthomas are characterized by a keratin-filled crypt in the dermis that opens to the skin surface (Fig. 20–12).[1, 2, 33, 92] The wall of the crypt is composed of a thick, complex, folded layer of well-differentiated stratified squamous epithelium, with columns of squamoid cells projecting peripherally from the basal surface of the wall and forming small epithelial nests (Fig. 20–13). The major histopathologic differential is the inverted papilloma.[3, 66] However, the keratoacanthoma does *not* have ballooning degeneration, abnormal keratohyaline granules, or intranuclear inclusion bodies. Keratoacanthomas are positive for cytokeratin.[47]

CLINICAL MANAGEMENT

Clinical management of keratoacanthomas may include surgical excision, cryotherapy, electrotherapy, and observation without treatment.[4–7] Chemotherapy with cyclophosphamide and prednisone and immunotherapy with autogenous vaccine or levamisole have been ineffective in dogs.[5] The oral administration of retinoids or intralesional injections of 5-fluorouracil or methotrexate have provided good results in the treatment of keratoacanthomas in humans.[5] The oral administration of retinoids (isotretinoin or etretinate) has been successful for the treatment of multiple keratoacanthomas in some dogs (see Chap. 3).[7, 89, 90, 333] A good response is seen after 3 to 4 months of therapy, and treatment must be continued intermittently for life in most cases. Keratoacanthomas are also known to resolve spontaneously.[5, 91]

Squamous Cell Carcinoma

Squamous cell carcinomas (epidermoid carcinomas) are common malignant neoplasms of the dog and cat, arising from keratinocytes.[1, 2, 3–9, 12, 18, 24, 32, 35] The etiology of squamous cell carcinoma is not clear in all cases (Table 20–3). Squamous cell carcinoma occurs

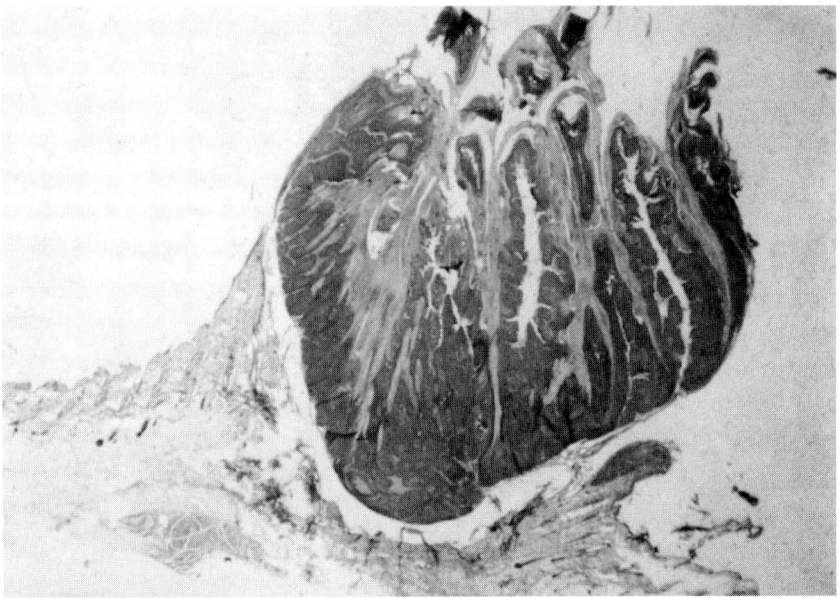

FIGURE 20–12. Canine keratoacanthoma. A central keratin-filled crypt opens to the skin surface.

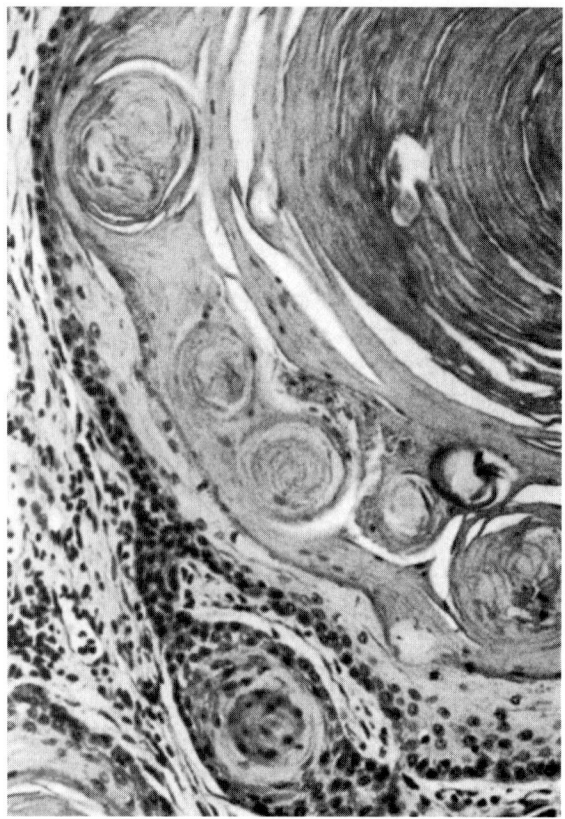

FIGURE 20–13. Canine keratoacanthoma. Note multiple horn cysts and projections of squamoid cells. (From Weiss E, Frese K: VII. Tumors of the skin. Bull World Health Organ 50:79, 1974.)

most frequently in sun-damaged skin and is usually preceded by actinic (solar) keratosis.* Thus, squamous cell carcinoma is seen more frequently in geographic areas characterized by long periods of intense sun exposure. Rarely, squamous cell carcinoma has been reported to arise from burn scars or chronic infectious processes.[5, 6, 109, 122] Squamous cell carcinoma was reported to arise in chronic discoid lupus erythematosus lesions[134] and in multiple infundibular cysts[133] in dogs. In humans, squamous cell carcinomas occasionally

---

*See references 1–9, 12, 18, 24, 32, 35.

● Table 20–3 **FACTORS CONTRIBUTING TO THE DEVELOPMENT OF SQUAMOUS CELL CARCINOMA**

Ultraviolet radiation
Ionizing radiation
Arsenic
Polycyclic aromatic hydrocarbons
Papillomaviruses
Tobacco (from second-hand smoke)
Lack/loss of pigment
Lack/loss of hair
Genodermatoses (albinism, piebaldism, epidermodysplasia verruciformis)
Chronic ulcer/sinus tract
Scar
Pre-existing chronic dermatitis
Immunosuppression

arise from burn and frostbite scars, radiation burns, and stasis dermatitis.[5] Papillomavirus structural antigens were demonstrated in up to 50% of the canine squamous cell carcinomas tested, suggesting an etiologic role for these viruses.[78, 81, 86] The results of similar studies were negative in the cat.[80, 81] However, a recent report indicated that 45% of the cats with multicentric squamous cell carcinoma in situ (Bowen's disease) had papillomavirus antigen in their lesions.[20] Squamous cell carcinomas occurred at the site of injection of a live canine oral papillomavirus vaccine in some dogs.[65, 84] Squamous cell carcinomas occurred in 24% of the feline immunodeficiency virus (FIV)–infected cats in one study.[116] Naturally occurring oral and conjunctival papillomas in dogs may rarely progress to squamous cell carcinoma.[85] A 1bp deletion was detected in codon 89 in exon 4 of tumor-suppressor gene p53 in a canine squamous cell carcinoma.[121a]

CLINICAL FINDINGS

Dog

Squamous cell carcinoma occurs at an average age of 9 years, with no sex predilection, although puppies are rarely affected.[115] In general, Scottish terriers, Pekingese, Boxers, Poodles, and Norwegian Elkhounds are predisposed.[4–7, 136] Squamous cell carcinomas with claw bed origin are seen most commonly in black-coated dogs of large breeds, especially Labrador retrievers, standard poodles, giant Schnauzers, Dachshunds, and Bouvier de Flandres.[1, 4–7, 124, 125, 132] Short-coated breeds with white or piebald ventral coat and skin color (Dalmatian, American Staffordshire terrier, Bull terrier, and Beagle) have the highest incidence of solar-induced squamous cell carcinoma.[2, 5, 7, 120, 121] These dogs usually spend many hours a day lying in the sun. Nasal squamous cell carcinomas may rarely occur as a sequela to depigmentation associated with conditions such as discoid lupus erythematosus (Fig. 20–14), pemphigus erythematosus, and vitiligo that result in increased susceptibility to actinic damage.[5, 134]

Lesions occur most commonly on the trunk, the limbs, the digits, the scrotum, the

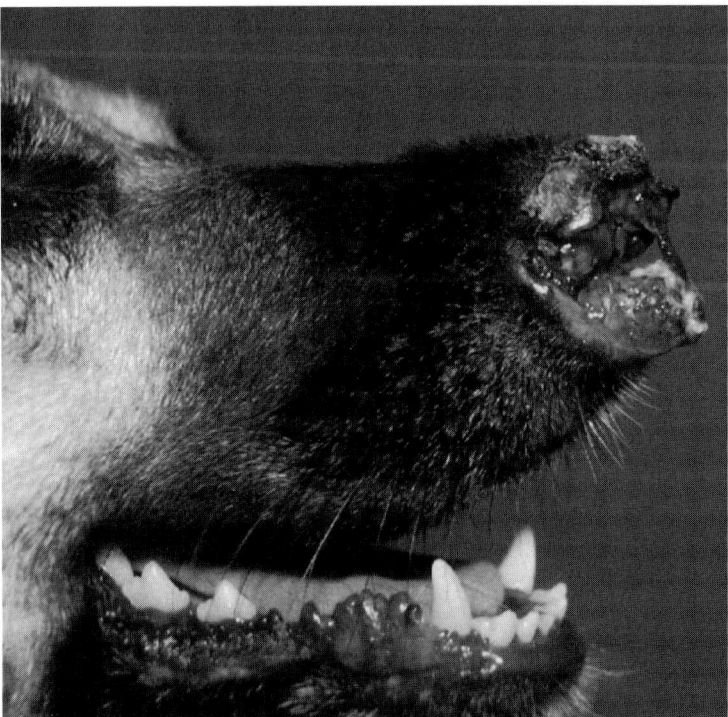

FIGURE 20–14. Squamous cell carcinoma arising from chronic, uncontrolled discoid lupus erythematosus.

lips, the anus, and the nose (see Fig. 20–1F) and may be proliferative or ulcerative. The proliferative types are papillary masses of varying size, many of which have a cauliflower-like appearance. The surface tends to be ulcerated and bleeds easily. Cutaneous horns may develop on the surface of such lesions. The ulcerative types initially appear as shallow, crusted ulcers that become deep and crateriform. Squamous cell carcinomas are usually solitary, but they may be multiple on the trunk of sunbathing dogs or in the claw beds of large, black-coated breeds. Dogs with claw bed (subungual) squamous cell carcinomas usually have a single affected digit (Fig. 20–15), which is swollen and painful with a misshapen or absent claw and paronychial discharge, and they may experience multiple neoplasms in other digits over a period of years (Fig. 20–16). Squamous cell carcinoma is the most common neoplasm of the digit of the dog.[28]

Cat

Squamous cell carcinoma occurs at an average age of 9 years, with no breed or sex predilection. White cats (short-haired or long-haired cats) have squamous cell carcinoma about 13 times as frequently as do other cats, owing to increased susceptibility to actinic damage.* The most common sites are the external nares (see Fig. 20–1 G) (about 80% to 90% of affected cats), the pinnae (Fig. 20–1H) (about 50%), the eyelids (Fig. 20–17) (about 20%), and the lips (Fig. 20–18A).[1, 103, 128, 130] Squamous cell carcinoma of the nasal planum is rare (Fig. 20–19).[119, 129] Lesions may be proliferative or ulcerative and may

---

*See references 4–7, 30, 35, 103, 104, 108a, 128, 130.

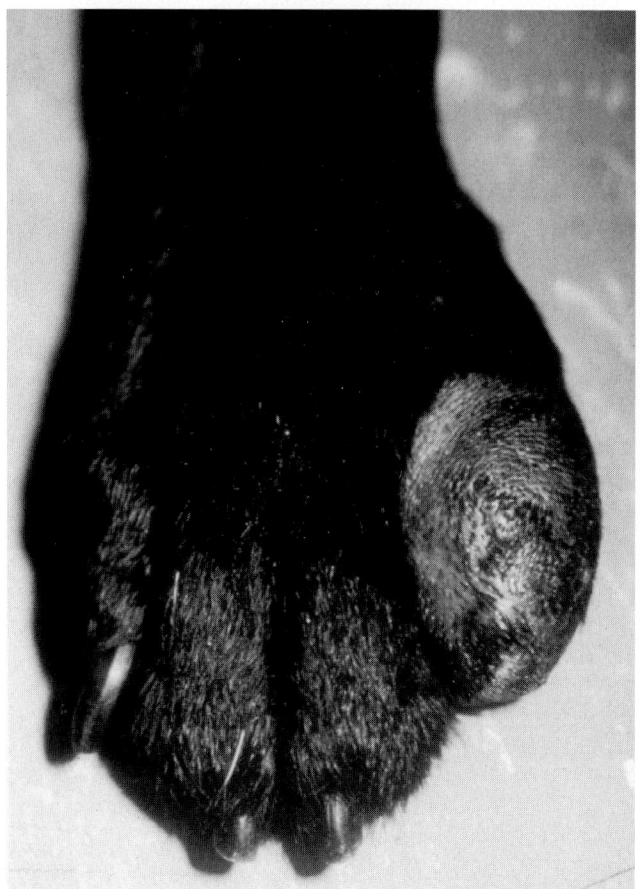

FIGURE 20–15. Subungual squamous cell carcinoma in a dog. Digit is enlarged, and claw has sloughed. (Courtesy C. Foil.)

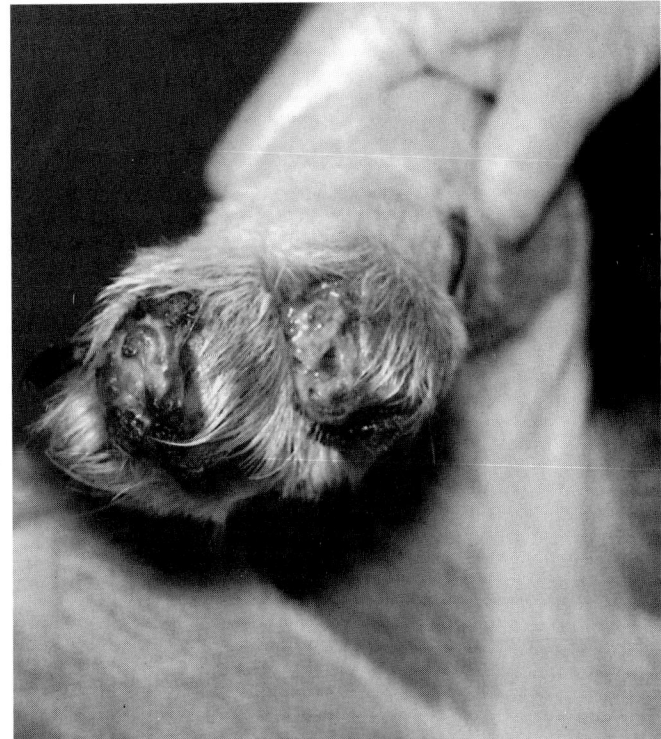

FIGURE 20–16. Multiple subungual squamous cell carcinomas in a dog.

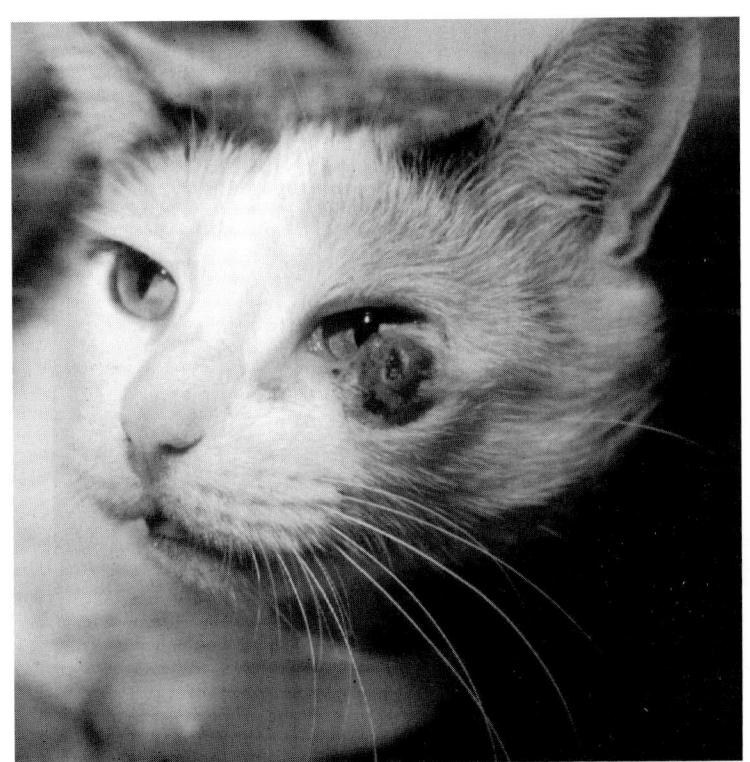

FIGURE 20–17. Squamous cell carcinoma on lower eyelid of a cat.

epinephrine produced a complete response in 64% of cats with nasal planum lesions, and no systemic toxicity was seen.[117] In cats with advanced-stage squamous cell carcinoma of the nasal planum, intratumoral administration of carboplatin in purified sesame oil produced complete remission in 67% of the cases with no systemic toxicity.[140] Recombinant feline interferon showed dramatic in vitro antitumor effect against squamous cell carcinoma.[137]

In all cases, avoidance of sunlight is an important part of prevention.[5, 128, 130] The development of new squamous cell carcinomas is common when ultraviolet light is not avoided.[103] It is important to remember that normal window glass does not totally block ultraviolet rays.[128, 130] Tattoos, magic markers, and sunscreens are not usually practical or effective.[129] In Australia, an anecdotal report indicated that "surfing gear" (full bodysuit Factor 40 fabric) has been modified for, well tolerated by, and effective for preventing truncal actinic dermatitis and squamous cell carcinomas in many Bull terriers.[105]

Multicentric Squamous Cell Carcinoma In Situ

CAUSE AND PATHOGENESIS

Multicentric squamous cell carcinoma in situ (Bowen's disease) is uncommon (in cats) to very rare (in dogs).[2, 5, 100, 110, 123] Exposure to ultraviolet light and arsenic are not causal factors.[123] Papillomavirus antigen has been demonstrated in 45% of the feline skin lesions by immunohistochemical methods.[20] Thus, these carcinoma in situ lesions probably represent a malignant transformation of the viral papillomas (see Papilloma). In one report, five old cats had *Demodex cati* infestation only in the squamous cell carcinomas.[111] All of the cats were feline leukemia virus (FeLV) negative, but three were FIV positive. The authors hypothesized that (1) the papillomavirus infection and squamous cell carcinomas created a local immunodeficiency state, allowing the demodicids to multiply excessively, or (2) the FIV infection and its associated immunodeficiency state predisposed the cats to both the papillomavirus infections and the *D. cati* proliferations.

CLINICAL FINDINGS

The condition is seen in older cats (10 years of age or older) and dogs. Lesions are multifocal, and in cats, they occur most commonly over the head, neck, dorsal thorax, abdomen, and proximal limbs.[100, 123] Most lesions have occurred in thickly haired and darkly pigmented skin. They are initially characterized by well-circumscribed, melanotic, hyperkeratotic macules and plaques, 0.5 to 3 cm in diameter (see Fig. 20–18B). Some lesions become almost verrucous. Cutaneous horns may develop on the surface of some lesions.[127] Later, the lesions become thick, crusted, ulcerated plaques that tend to bleed easily. In dogs, the oral mucosa and the genitalia may be involved, and nodules may be seen in addition to the lesions described earlier for cats.[2, 110]

DIAGNOSIS

Histopathologically, well-circumscribed areas of irregular epidermal and superficial follicular hyperplasia and dysplasia are seen (Figs. 20–23A and B).[2, 100, 123] Keratinocyte size and appearance are highly variable, and mitotic figures are common in all cell layers. Orthokeratotic to parakeratotic hyperkeratosis and hypermelanosis are common, and a lichenoid inflammatory infiltrate may be seen. In one study,[20] 27% of the cats had focal areas of invasive squamous cell carcinoma. Typical viral papilloma changes may be seen at the margins of the squamous cell carcinoma, and papillomavirus antigen is most commonly detected in these margins.[20]

In five cats, *Demodex cati* infestation was detected only in the squamous cell carcinomas (Fig. 20–24).[111]

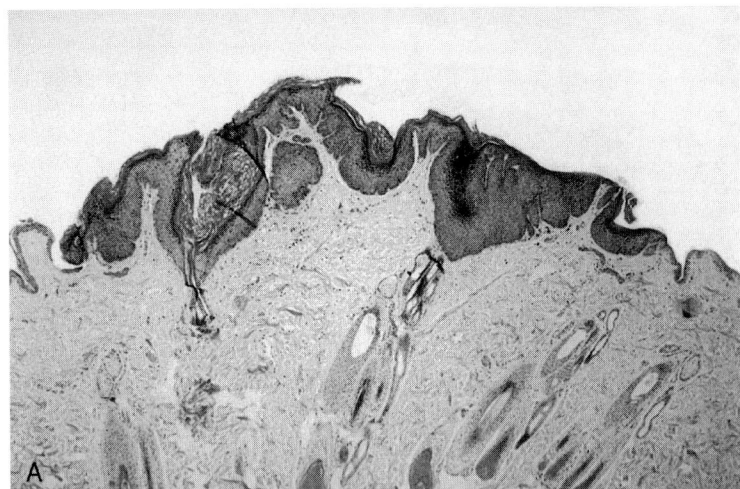
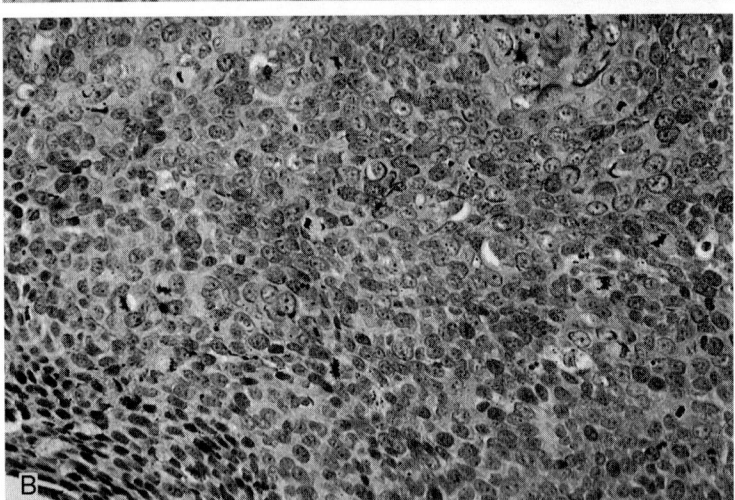

FIGURE 20–23. Squamous cell carcinoma in situ in a cat. *A*, marked irregular hyperplasia, hyperpigmentation, and dysplasia of epidermis and hair follicle infundibula. *B*, Close-up of *A*. Marked epidermal dysplasia and several mitoses.

CLINICAL MANAGEMENT

The mean course of disease, before animals are euthanized because of cosmetic concerns and owner frustration, is more than 2 years. No metastases have been recorded, although a footpad lesion invaded contiguous bone in one dog.[110] Lesions may wax and wane in size or, in some instances, individual lesions may disappear. However, multiple lesions are always present.

In dogs, the topical application of 5-fluorouracil caused regression of some lesions.[110] In cats, ^{90}Sr plesiotherapy (β-irradiation) is effective in healing thin lesions (less than 2 to 4 mm in thickness).[20, 123] However, new lesions continue to develop, and thicker plaques do not respond. The oral administration of isotretinoin was ineffective in one cat,[123] but other reports indicate that etretinate (2 mg/kg/day; no longer available) or acitretin (3 mg/kg/day) may be effective.[20, 111] In many instances, in otherwise healthy, asymptomatic animals, observation without therapy may be the most practical approach.

Basal Cell Tumors

The term *basal cell tumor* has been used in the veterinary literature to classify a large group of common neoplasms of dogs and cats presumed to be derived from basal

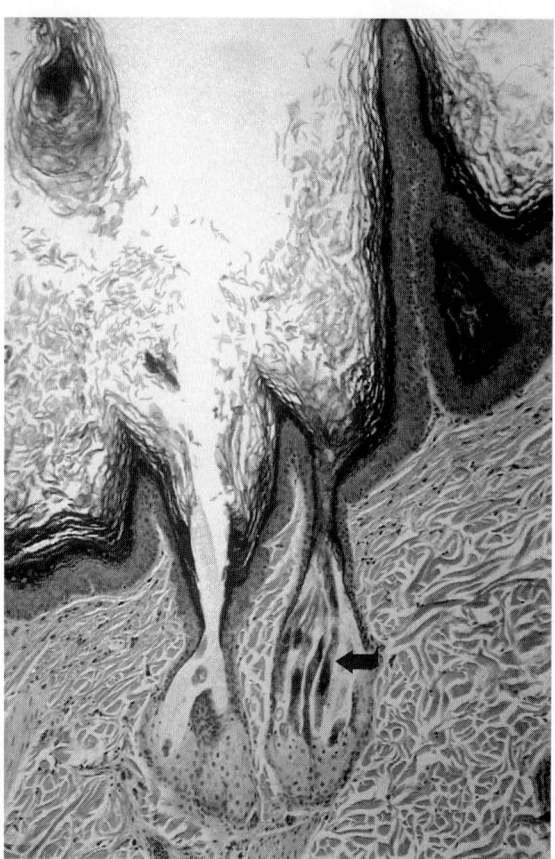

FIGURE 20–24. Numerous *Demodex cati (arrow)* in a squamous cell carcinoma in situ.

epithelial cells of both epidermal and adnexal origin. Numerous histopathologic subclassifications have been applied to these neoplasms: medusa head, garland or ribbon, trabecular, solid, cystic, adenoid, basosquamous, and granular cell. In general, these various histopathologic types are often found within the same neoplasm and offer no useful clinical, prognostic, or therapeutic information.[27] Most veterinary basal cell tumors are benign and are not contiguous with the basal cell layer of the epidermis (medusa head, garland or ribbon, trabecular, adenoid, and granular cell types); these lesions generally, show differentiation toward follicular structures and have been reclassified (see later).[2, 5, 142a] The subclassifications solid basal cell tumor and basosquamous basal cell tumor are reported to be biologically aggressive in some instances; most of these lesions are probably true basal cell carcinomas.[2, 5] The term basal cell tumor, borrowed from human dermatopathology, is now considered synonymous with basal cell carcinoma of low-grade malignancy. Some authors prefer the terms basal cell epithelioma and basaloma, both of which indicate the relatively good prognosis of the neoplasm.[2, 5]

In conclusion, the term basal cell tumor appears to have limited usage in veterinary medicine and is retained for an uncommon, true basal cell neoplasm of cats that has no obvious adnexal features.[2, 5]

BENIGN FELINE BASAL CELL TUMOR

• **Cause and Pathogenesis.** These tumors are uncommon benign neoplasms of the cat that are thought to arise from the basal cells of the epidermis. The entire basal cell tumor category accounted for 11% to 30% of all feline skin tumors in multiple surveys.* It

---

*See references 8, 12–15, 26, 30, 35, 39, 95.

is impossible to determine what proportion of these tumors represents benign feline basal cell tumor.[2, 5] The cause of basal cell tumors in cats is unknown. In humans, there is a strong correlation between exposure to ultraviolet light and the development of basal cell tumors.

- **Clinical Findings.** Basal cell tumors occur in adult cats with no sex predilection. Himalayan, Siamese, and Persian cats may be predisposed.[1, 7] Usually, basal cell tumors are solitary, but they may occasionally be multiple.[96] The most common sites of occurrence are the head, the neck (see Fig. 20–18C), the limbs, and the dorsal trunk.[1, 2, 5] Basal cell tumors are usually firm, rounded, elevated, and well circumscribed; they are situated at the dermoepidermal junction and are usually 1 to 2 cm in diameter. They are often melanotic (see Fig. 20–18D), may be cystic, and are frequently ulcerated and alopecic.

- **Diagnosis.** Histopathologically, basal cell tumors are characterized by a well-circumscribed, symmetric proliferation of basaloid cells that has a fairly broad zone of connection to the overlying epidermis (Fig. 20–25A and B).[1, 2] The tumor often has a lima bean–shaped silhouette, with the central indentation at the tumor surface. The basaloid cells are arranged in tightly packed lobules and trabeculae. Basal cell tumors are positive for cytokeratin.[49]

- **Clinical Management.** Clinical management of basal cell tumors may include surgical excision, cryotherapy, electrosurgery, and observation without treatment.[4–7]

BASAL CELL CARCINOMA

- **Cause and Pathogenesis.** Basal cell carcinomas are common (in cats) to uncommon (in dogs) low-grade malignancies arising from small, pluripotential epithelial cells within the basal cell layers of the epidermis and adnexa.[2, 5] Numerical incidence data are difficult to provide, because these neoplasms have been traditionally included in the broad category of basal cell tumor (see earlier). The cause of basal cell carcinomas in dogs and cats is unknown. In humans, there is a strong correlation between ultraviolet light exposure and the development of basal cell carcinomas. Despite high mitotic activity, basal cell tumors have a slow growth. A recent study suggested that this may be due to an increased duration of the entire cell cycle and increased apoptosis.[97]

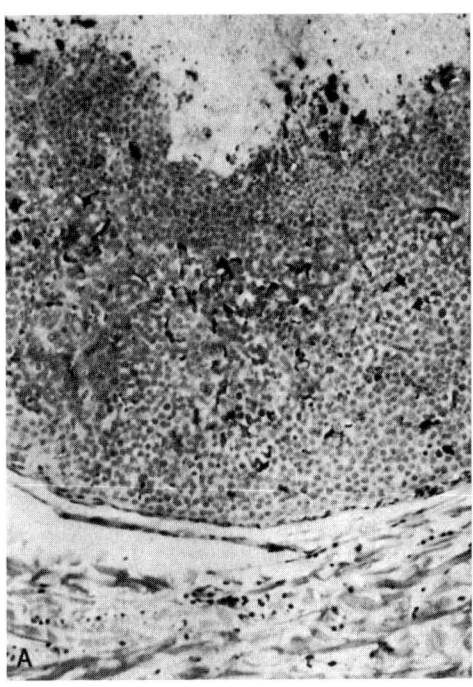

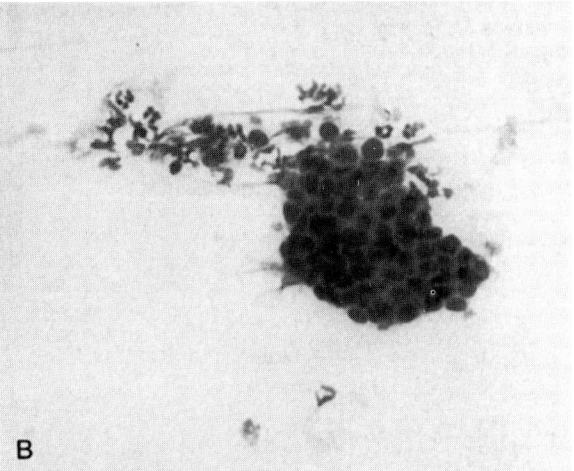

FIGURE 20–25. *A*, Feline basal cell tumor. Proliferation of basaloid cells and melanocytes. *B*, Feline basal cell tumor. Cytologic examination of aspirate shows typical clusters of monomorphic basaloid cells.

- **Clinical Findings.** Basal cell carcinomas occur in dogs and cats at an average age of 7 to 10 years and with no sex predilection.* Siamese cats, Cocker spaniels, Kerry blue terriers, Shetland sheepdogs, Siberian huskies, English Springer spaniels, and Poodles appear to be predisposed.† The tumors occur most commonly on the head, the neck, and the thorax. In cats, lesions occasionally occur on the nasal planum or the eyelids. Basal cell carcinomas are usually solitary, well circumscribed, firm to cystic, rounded, 0.5 to 10 cm in diameter, and commonly alopecic and ulcerated. Basal cell carcinomas are frequently melanotic (Fig. 20–26).
- **Diagnosis.** Three major histopathologic variants of basal cell carcinoma occur in dogs and cats: solid, keratinizing (basosquamous), and clear cell.[1, 2] *Solid basal cell carcinoma* is the most common subtype in cats and is characterized by circumscribed, irregular dermal masses comprising multiple basaloid cell aggregates embedded in a moderate stroma (desmoplasia). Mitotic activity is low to high, and atypical mitotic figures are common. Variable secondary features include cyst formation (necrosis), melanization, adnexal differentiation, mucinosis, artifactual cleft formation between stroma and neoplastic cells, and cartilaginous metaplasia.[2, 93]

Keratinizing basal cell carcinoma (basosquamous carcinoma) is the most common type in dogs and is characterized by an irregular dermal mass of basaloid cells having a plaquelike configuration, multifocal epidermal contiguity, and multiple areas of abrupt squamous differentiation and keratinization.[2]

Clear cell basal cell carcinoma is rare and is more commonly encountered in cats.[2] The overall architecture is identical to that of solid basal cell carcinoma, but the epithelial cells are large and polygonal and have water-clear or finely granular cytoplasm. Basal cell carcinomas are positive for cytokeratin.[47, 49, 50, 60, 61] Papillomavirus antigen was not detected in feline basal cell carcinomas.[80]

- **Clinical Management.** Clinical management of basal cell carcinomas may include surgical excision, electrosurgery, cryosurgery, and observation without therapy.[4–7] The

---

*See references 1, 2, 5–7, 12, 30, 35, 95.
†See references 1, 5–7, 12, 14, 95, 99.

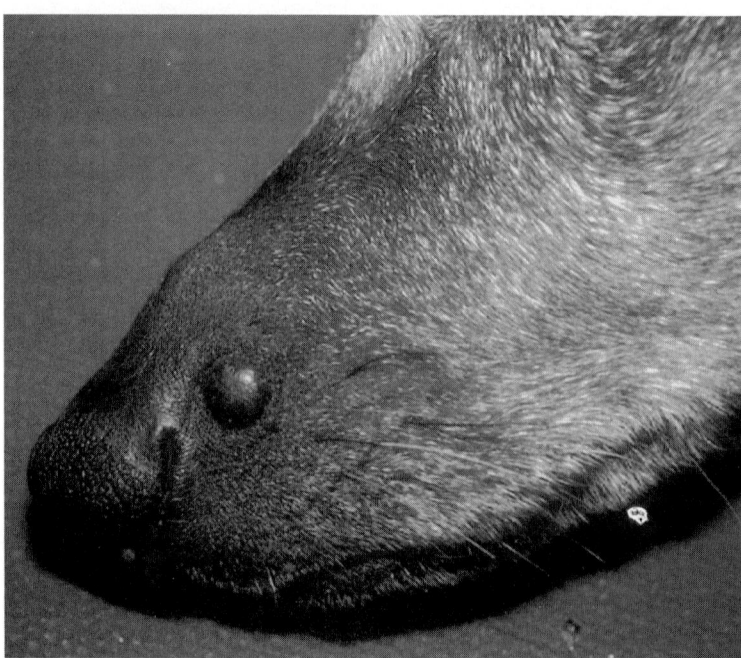

FIGURE 20–26. Melanotic basal cell tumor on muzzle of a dog.

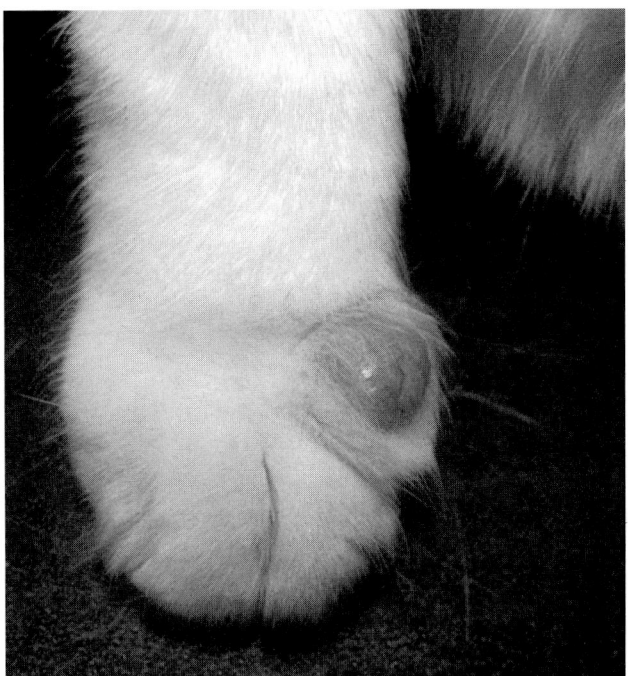

FIGURE 20–27. Trichoepithelioma on the paw of a cat.

incidence of recurrence and metastasis is very low.[94] In humans, intralesional injections of interferon have been used to treat basal cell carcinoma.

Hair Follicle Tumors

Previous surveys of hair follicle neoplasms in dogs and cats indicated that these neoplasms account for about 5% and 1%, respectively, of all skin neoplasms seen in these species.[*] The most common subtypes were trichoepithelioma and pilomatrixoma.[149] With the reclassification of so-called basal cell tumors (see earlier), it appears that the majority of previous reports of these neoplasms were examples of trichoblastoma.[2, 5, 142a] Thus, neoplasms of hair follicle origin are much more common than previous veterinary literature suggested. Hair follicle tumors are positive for cytokeratin.[47, 54, 61]

TRICHOEPITHELIOMA

• **Cause and Pathogenesis.** Trichoepitheliomas are uncommon benign neoplasms of dogs and cats that are thought to arise from keratinocytes that differentiate toward all three segments of the hair follicle.[1, 2, 5, 33, 149] The cause of trichoepitheliomas in dogs and cats is unknown. In humans, a syndrome of multiple trichoepitheliomas is hereditary.

Usually, trichoepitheliomas occur in dogs and cats older than 5 years of age. No sex predilection appears to exist in either species. In cats, there is a predilection for Persians, and the neoplasms occur most commonly on the head, the limbs (Fig. 20–27), and the tail.[1, 142a, 150] In dogs, there may be a predilection for the dorsal lumbar (see Fig. 20–18E) and lateral thoracic and limb areas, and Golden retrievers, Basset hounds, German shepherd dogs, Cocker spaniels, Irish setters, English Springer spaniels, miniature Schnauzers, and Standard Poodles may be predisposed.[1, 142a, 149]

Although these neoplasms are usually solitary, they may occasionally be multiple. They are solid or cystic, rounded, elevated, well circumscribed, and dermoepidermal in position,

---

*See references 12, 14, 26, 27, 33, 149, 150.

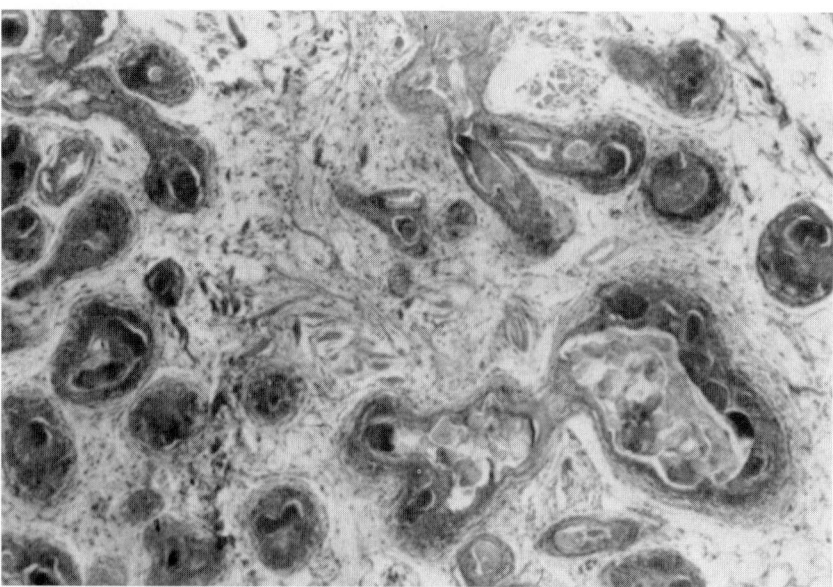

FIGURE 20-28. Canine trichoepithelioma. Disorganized proliferation of hair follicle–like structures and hairs.

ranging from 0.5 to 15 cm in diameter. Frequently, they become ulcerated and alopecic. Trichoepitheliomas are rarely invasive or metastatic.[5]

• **Diagnosis.** Histopathologically, trichoepitheliomas vary considerably, depending on the degree of differentiation and whether the tumor is primarily related to the follicular sheath or the hair matrix (Fig. 20-28).[1, 33, 149] Frequent characteristics include horn cysts, lack of intercellular bridges (desmosomes), differentiation toward hair follicle–like structures, formation of abortive or rudimentary hairs, desmoplasia, inflammation, melanization, and shadow (ghost) cells.[149] Dystrophic mineralization or malignant transformation may be seen in up to 18% of the cases.[149] A variant showing marked mucinosis is most common in Golden retrievers.[149]

• **Clinical Management.** Clinical management of trichoepitheliomas may include surgical excision, cryotherapy, electrosurgery, and observation without treatment.[4-7] Recurrence and metastasis are rare, in spite of histopathologic evidence of malignancy.[1, 7, 149]

TRICHOLEMMOMA

• **Cause and Pathogenesis.** Tricholemmomas are rare benign neoplasms of dogs and cats that arise from keratinocytes of the outer root sheath of hair follicles.[1, 2, 142a, 143, 149, 150] The cause of tricholemmomas is unknown. In humans, a syndrome of multiple tricholemmomas is hereditary.

• **Clinical Findings.** In dogs, tricholemmomas occur at 5 to 13 years of age. There appears to be no sex predilection, but Afghan hounds may be predisposed. These neoplasms occur most commonly on the head and neck and are usually firm, ovoid, and 1 to 7 cm in diameter.

• **Diagnosis.** Histopathologically, tricholemmomas are characterized by a nodular proliferation of keratinocytes, many of which are clear and have a positive reaction with periodic acid–Schiff (PAS) stain owing to their glycogen content (Fig. 20-29).[1, 2, 149] The tumor lobules are surrounded by a distinct, often thickened basement membrane zone.

• **Clinical Management.** Clinical management of tricholemmomas may include surgical excision, cryotherapy, electrosurgery, and observation without treatment.[4-7]

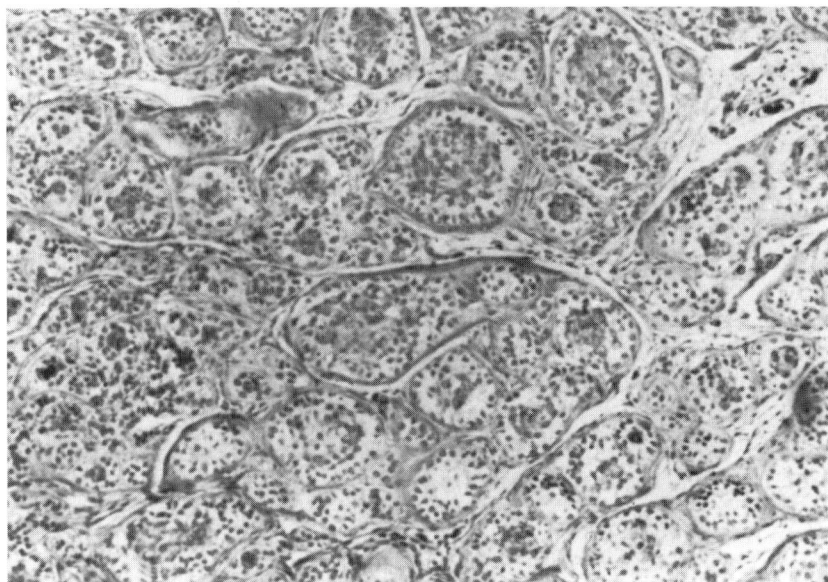

FIGURE 20–29. Canine tricholemmoma. Proliferation of predominantly clear, outer root sheath–like keratinocytes. Individual nodules are often surrounded by a distinct, thick basement membrane zone.

TRICHOFOLLICULOMA

- **Cause and Pathogenesis.** Trichofolliculomas are rare benign neoplasms of dogs that are highly structured hamartomas of the pilosebaceous unit.[2, 5, 149] The cause of trichofolliculomas is unknown.
- **Clinical Findings.** Trichofolliculomas occur in adult dogs, with no apparent age, breed, sex, or site predilections. The lesions are solitary, dome-shaped, firm papules or nodules, often containing a central depression or pore that may exude keratosebaceous material or contain a tuft of hairs.
- **Diagnosis.** Histopathologically, trichofolliculomas are characterized by a central large dilated or cystic follicle with smaller follicles or follicle-like structures that radiate outward from the central follicle into the surrounding connective tissue in an arborizing pattern (Fig. 20–30).[5, 149]
- **Clinical Management.** Clinical management may include surgical excision and observation without treatment.[5, 149]

DILATED PORE OF WINER

- **Cause and Pathogenesis.** Dilated pore of Winer is an uncommon benign follicular tumor of cats.[2, 142a, 146, 148] The cause of this lesion is unknown, although most evidence favors a developmental origin arising from the combined forces of obstruction and intrafollicular pressure leading to hair follicle hyperplasia.
- **Clinical Findings.** Dilated pore is seen in older cats, with no apparent breed or sex predilection. The lesions are solitary and occur most frequently on the neck, head, and trunk (see Fig. 20–18F).[142a, 146, 148] They are characterized by a well-demarcated, smooth, dermoepidermal cyst–like structure with a central, keratin-filled wide-mouthed pore.
- **Diagnosis.** Histopathologically, this disorder is characterized by a markedly dilated, keratinized, pilar infundibulum lined by an epithelium that is atrophic near the ostium but increasingly hyperplastic toward the base of the lesion (Fig. 20–31).[146, 148] The epithelium

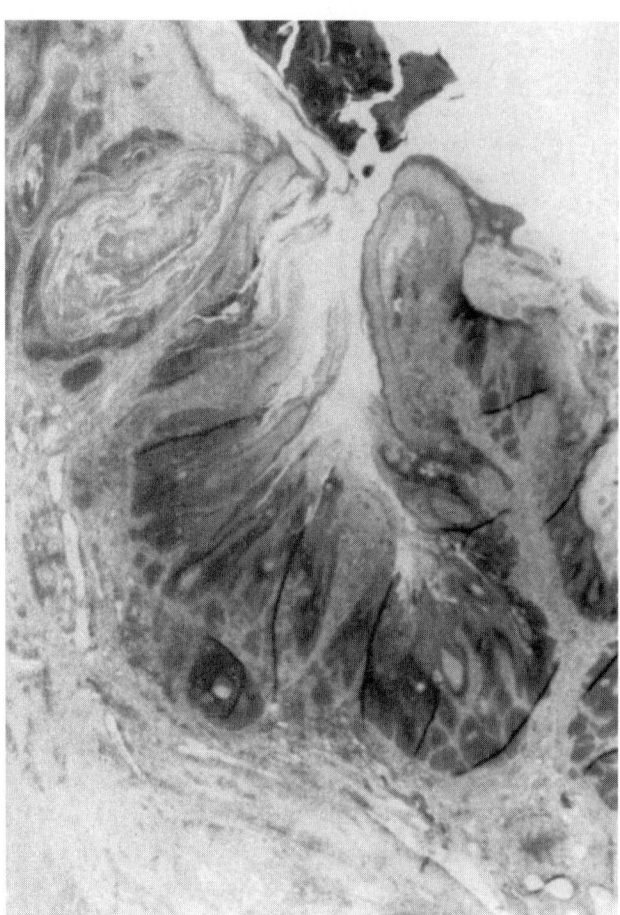

FIGURE 20–30. Canine trichofolliculoma. Central large hair follicle with numerous smaller abortive hair follicles radiating into the surrounding dermis.

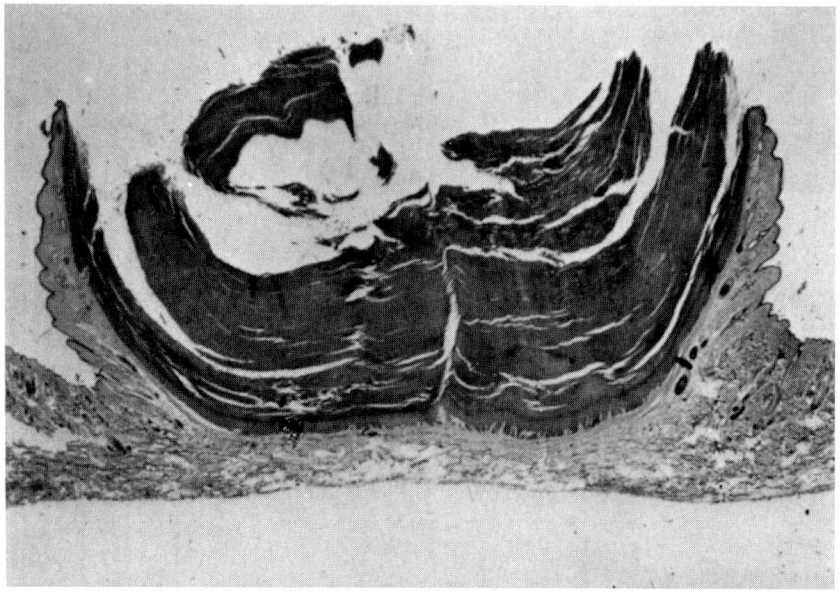

FIGURE 20–31. Feline dilated pore of Winer. Widely dilated, keratin-filled hair follicle.

at the base shows psoriasiform hyperplasia with rete ridges and irregular, thin projections into the surrounding dermis (Fig. 20–32).

- **Clinical Management.** Clinical management includes surgical excision and observation without treatment.[5, 148]

WARTY DYSKERATOMA

- **Cause and Pathogenesis.** Warty dyskeratoma is a rare, benign, epithelial proliferation of dogs.[5, 145] Although warty dyskeratoma is believed by many investigators to arise from pilosebaceous structures, its occurrence in the oral cavity of humans has challenged traditional interpretations.[5]
- **Clinical Findings.** Warty dyskeratoma occurs in dogs, but too few cases have been recognized to infer age, breed, sex, or site predilections. The lesions are solitary, wartlike papules or nodules with a hyperkeratotic umbilicated center.
- **Diagnosis.** Histopathologically, warty dyskeratoma is characterized by a cup-shaped invagination connected with the surface by a keratin-filled channel (Fig. 20–33).[5, 145] The large invagination contains numerous acantholytic, dyskeratotic cells (Fig. 20–34). The lower portion of the invagination is occupied by numerous villi (elongated dermal papillae lined with a single layer of basal cells) (Fig. 20–35). Typical corps rounds (dyskeratotic acanthocytes with a pyknotic nucleus surrounded by a clear halo) can usually be found.
- **Clinical Management.** Clinical management of warty dyskeratoma may include surgical excision and observation without treatment.[5]

PILOMATRIXOMA

- **Cause and Pathogenesis.** Pilomatrixomas (pilomatricomas, or calcifying epitheliomas [of Malherbe]) are uncommon (in dogs) to rare (in cats) neoplasms and are thought to arise from the hair matrix.[1, 2, 142a, 149, 150] The cause of pilomatrixomas is unknown.
- **Clinical Findings.** Pilomatrixomas usually occur in dogs and cats older than 5 years of age.[1, 2, 149, 150] There is no apparent sex predilection. Kerry blue terriers, Poodles, and Old English sheepdogs appear to be predisposed. Usually, pilomatrixomas are solitary.

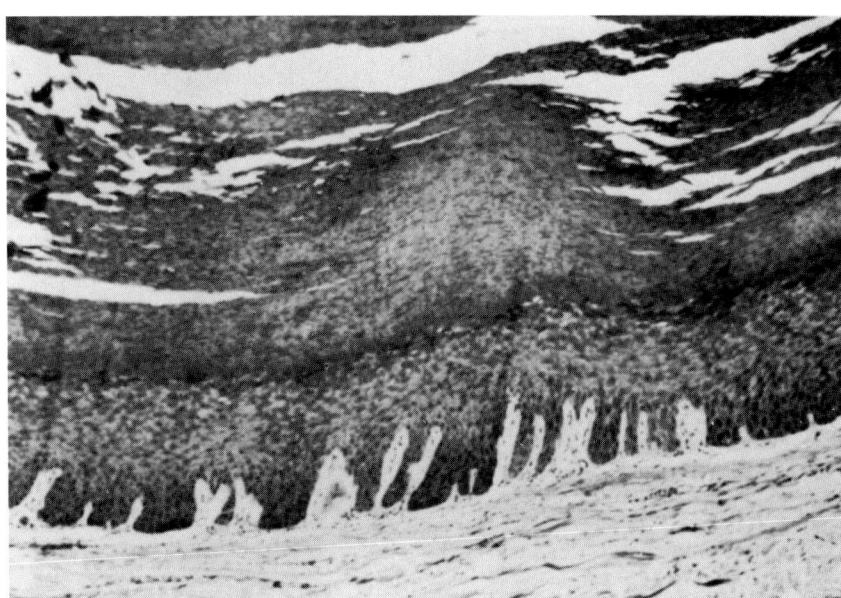

FIGURE 20–32. Close-up of Figure 20–31. The base of the lesion shows characteristic psoriasiform epithelial hyperplasia.

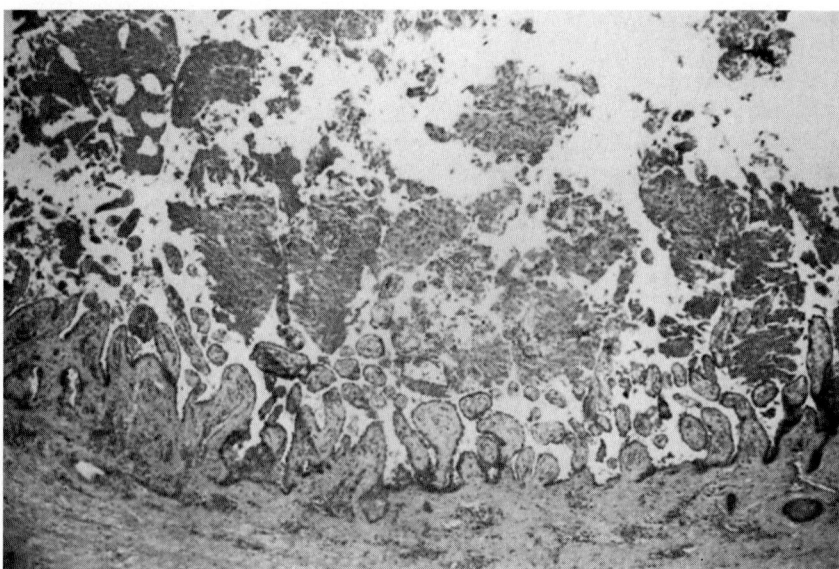

FIGURE 20–33. Canine warty dyskeratoma. The base of a keratin-filled mass shows multiple villi.

There may be site predilection to neck, shoulders, lateral thorax, and back. Pilomatrixomas are solid to cystic, rounded, elevated, well circumscribed, and dermal to subcutaneous in position, and they range from 1 to 10 cm in diameter. They frequently become ulcerated and alopecic. Pilomatrixomas are rarely invasive or metastatic (matrical carcinoma) to lymph nodes, lungs, nervous system, and bone.[1, 2, 5, 147, 149]

• **Diagnosis.** Histopathologically, pilomatrixomas are characterized by a well-circumscribed, cystic, multilobulated, deep dermal to subcutaneous proliferation of basophilic

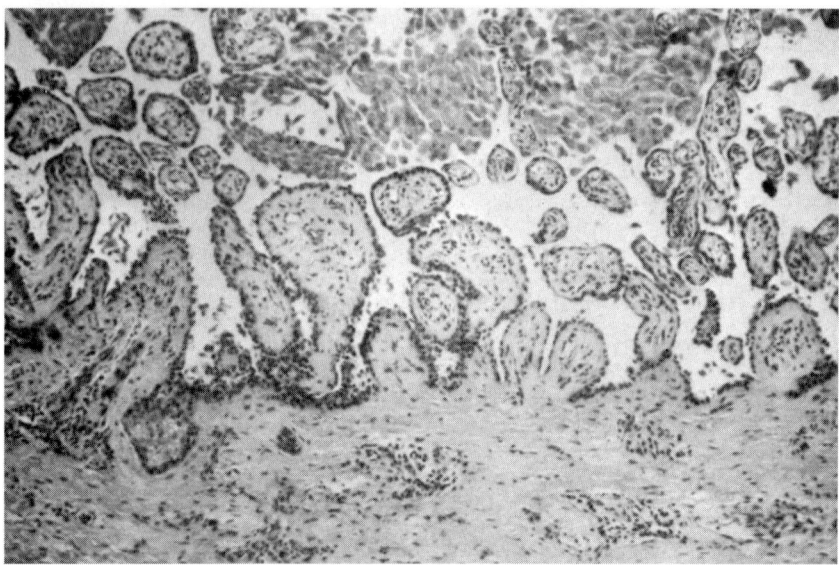

FIGURE 20–34. Close-up of Figure 20–33. Basal villi with a single layer of attached keratinocytes.

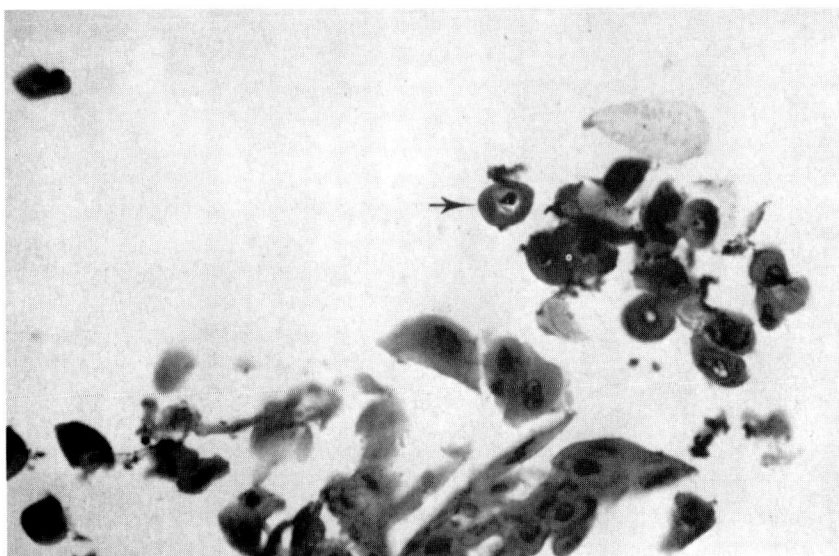

FIGURE 20–35. Close-up of Figure 20–33. Acantholytic cells and typical corps rounds (*arrow*).

cells (which resemble hair matrix cells) and shadow, or ghost, cells (fully keratinized, faintly eosinophilic cells with a central, unstained nucleus) (Fig. 20–36).[33, 149] Shadow cells are not pathognomonic, having been found in other hair follicle neoplasms, various keratinizing cysts, inflamed hair follicles, and chronic hyperkeratotic dermatoses.[5, 149] There is abrupt keratinization (no stratum granulosum), and the keratin is homogeneous, relatively amorphous, and nonfibrillar (tricholemmal keratin). A constant feature of pilomatrixomas is the occurrence of multiple dermal papilla–like structures within the basaloid cellular component (Fig. 20–37).[149] Other frequent but not constant features of pilomatrixomas are calcification within the areas of shadow cells, desmoplasia, and inflammation.[149]

- **Clinical Management.** Clinical management of pilomatrixomas may include surgical excision, cryotherapy, and observation without treatment.[4–7, 149, 150]

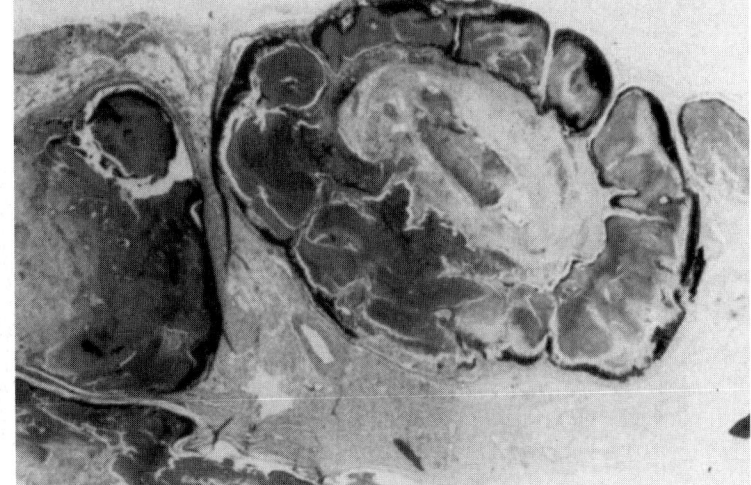

FIGURE 20–36. Canine pilomatrixoma. Multilocular mass consisting of deeply basophilic epithelial wall and brightly eosinophilic homogeneous central keratin.

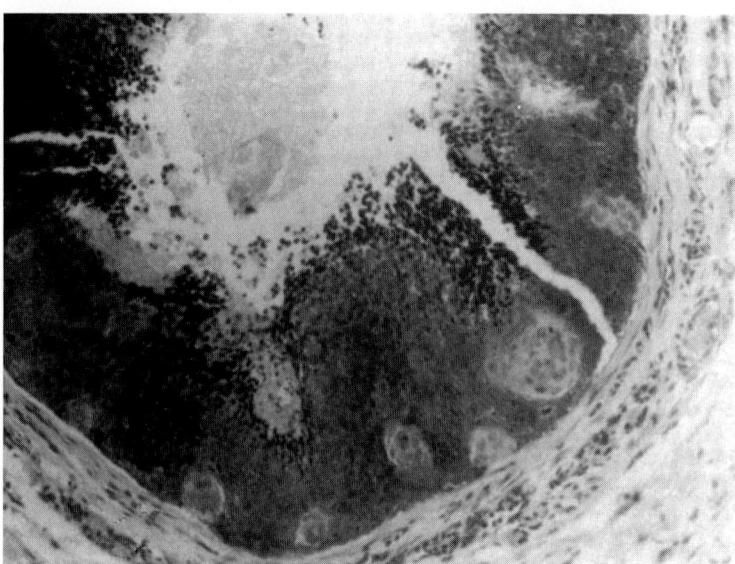

FIGURE 20-37. Close-up of Figure 20-36. Multiple dermal papilla-like structures within the basaloid wall of a neoplasm.

TRICHOBLASTOMA

- **Cause and Pathogenesis.** Trichoblastomas are common, usually benign neoplasms in dogs and cats, which are presumably derived from trichoblastic (primitive hair germ) epithelium.[2, 5, 142a] The incidence of these tumors in dogs is probably close to that previously reported under the term basal cell tumor (see earlier).[2, 5, 142a] The incidence in cats is more difficult to estimate because cats have several types of neoplasms that are composed of small basaloid epithelial cells (to include benign feline basal cell tumor, ductular epitrichial sweat gland neoplasms, and primitive hair follicle neoplasms).[2, 5] The cause of trichoblastomas is unknown.

- **Clinical Findings.** Trichoblastomas occur in dogs and cats older than 5 years of age.[2, 5, 142a] No sex predilection is evident, but Poodles and Cocker spaniels may be overrepresented. Lesions are usually solitary, dome shaped, firm, 1 to 2 cm in diameter, and often alopecic, ulcerated, and melanotic. In dogs, lesions occur most commonly on the head and the neck, especially the base of the ear. In cats, lesions occur most commonly on the cranial half of the trunk. Metastasis is extremely rare.[144]

- **Diagnosis.** Trichoblastomas occur in three basic histopathologic subtypes: ribbon (garland, or medusa head), trabecular, and granular cell.[2, 5] The ribbon type is most common in dogs and is characterized by basaloid cells arranged in branching, winding, and radiating columns with no epidermal contiguity (Fig. 20-38).[2, 5] The trabecular type is most common in cats and is characterized by lobules and broad trabeculae of basaloid cells with prominent peripheral palisading and no epidermal contiguity.[2, 5] The granular cell type is rare and is architecturally identical to the ribbon type of trichoblastoma, but many of the epithelial aggregates are composed entirely of larger cells with granular or vacuolated cytoplasm.[2, 5, 98]

- **Clinical Management.** Clinical management of trichoblastomas may include surgical excision, cryotherapy, and observation without treatment.[4-7]

Sebaceous Gland Tumors

CAUSE AND PATHOGENESIS

Sebaceous gland tumors are common (in dogs) to uncommon (in cats) epithelial growths arising from sebocytes.[1, 2, 14, 151-155] Their cause is unknown.

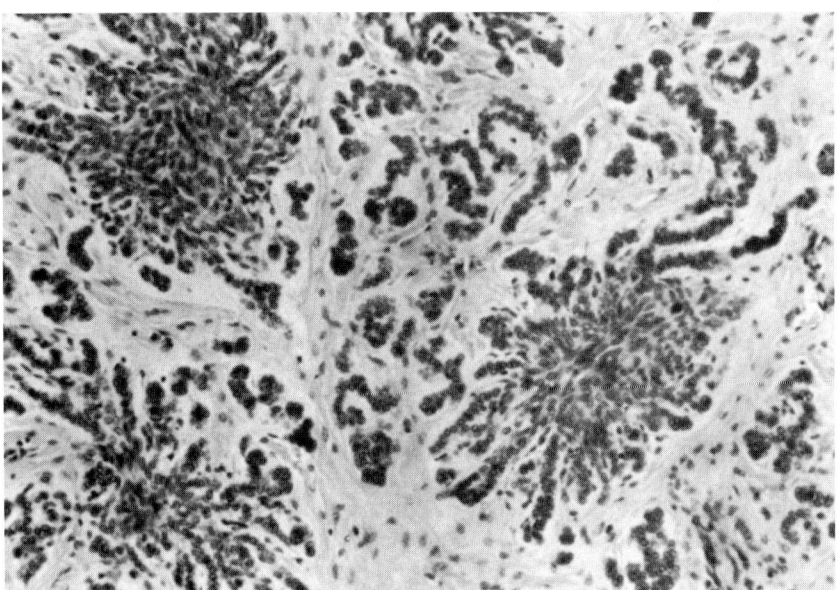
FIGURE 20–38. Canine trichoblastoma. Ribbon or medusoid type.

CLINICAL FINDINGS

Dog

Sebaceous gland tumors are common in dogs, accounting for 6% to 21% of all canine skin tumors in multiple surveys.[151, 152] Affected dogs average 9 to 10 years of age, and there is no sex predilection. Nodular sebaceous hyperplasias account for about 53% of the lesions and occur most commonly in Beagles, Cocker spaniels, Poodles, Dachshunds, and miniature Schnauzers.[1, 152] The lesions are usually solitary (about 70% of cases), well circumscribed, raised, smooth and greasy to hyperkeratotic, wartlike or cauliflower-like in appearance, pinkish to orangish, 3 mm to 7 cm in diameter, and frequently melanotic or ulcerated (see Fig. 20–18G).[152] They occur most commonly on the limbs, the trunk, and the eyelids.

Sebaceous epitheliomas (basal cell carcinoma with sebaceous differentiation) account for about 37% of sebaceous gland tumors and occur most commonly in Shih tzus, Lhasa apsos, Malamutes, Siberian huskies, and Irish setters.[152] The lesions are usually solitary (about 67% of cases), well circumscribed, raised, smooth, and greasy to hyperkeratotic, wartlike or cauliflower-like in appearance, pinkish to orangish, 5 mm to 5 cm in diameter, and frequently ulcerated or melanotic.[152] They occur most commonly on the eyelids and the head (see Fig. 20–18H).

Sebaceous adenomas account for about 8% of sebaceous gland tumors and occur most commonly on the eyelids and the limbs (Fig. 20–39A).[152] The appearance of the lesions is as described for sebaceous hyperplasia and sebaceous epithelioma (see earlier).

Sebaceous carcinoma accounts for only about 2% of the tumors.[152] Lesions are solitary, nodular, 2.5 to 7.5 cm in diameter, and frequently ulcerated (Fig. 20–39B). The head and the limbs are most commonly affected.[1] Cocker spaniels may be predisposed.[1]

Cat

Sebaceous gland tumors are uncommon in cats, accounting for about 3% of all feline skin tumors.[1, 14, 153] Affected cats are usually 10 years of age or older; there is no apparent sex predilection. Persians may be predisposed.[1] Lesions are usually solitary and occur most commonly on the head, the neck, and the trunk. They are well circumscribed, raised,

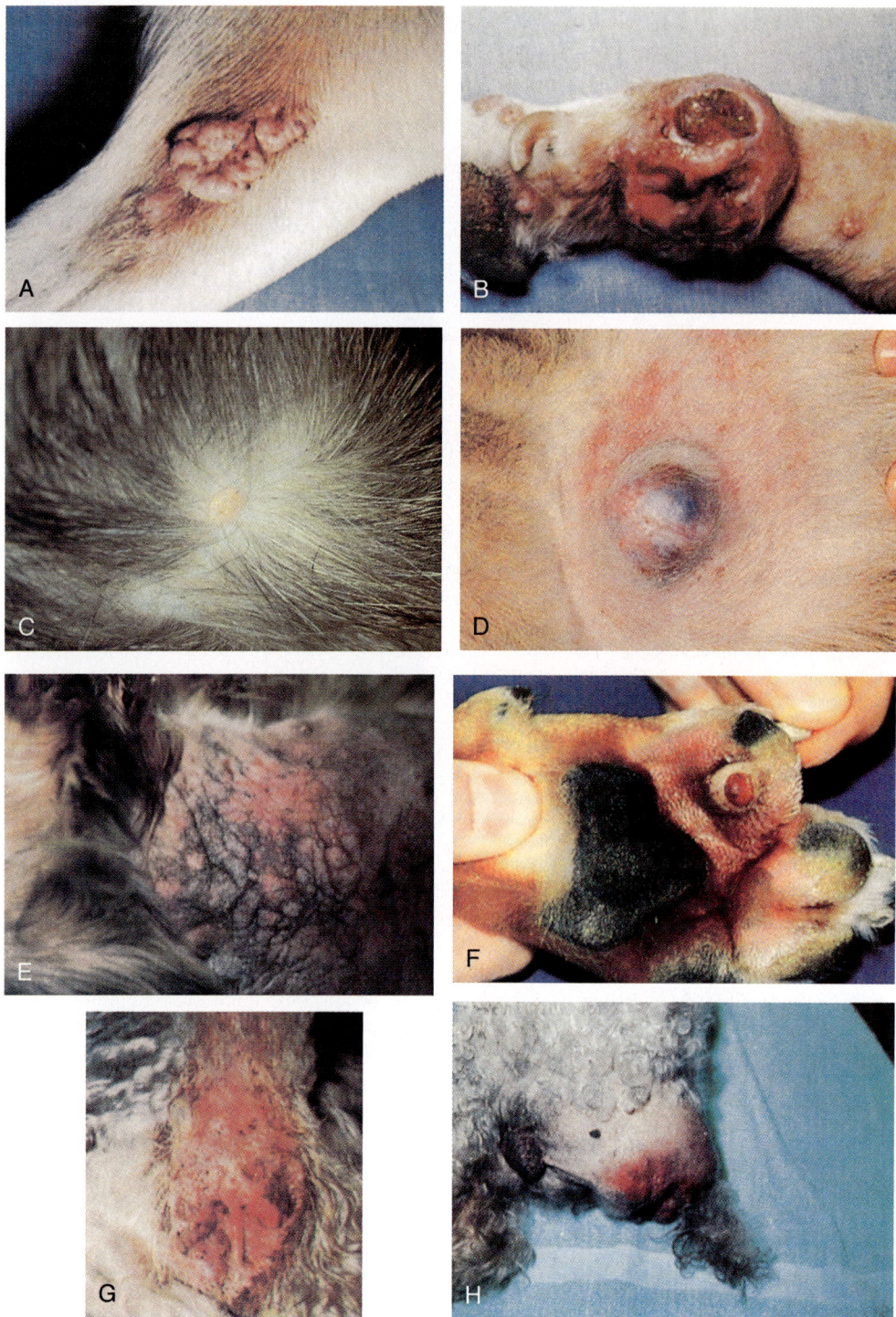

FIGURE 20–39. *A*, Sebaceous adenoma on the medial limb of a dog. *B*, Sebaceous carcinoma on the limb of a dog. *C*, Sebaceous gland hyperplasia on the thorax of a cat. Note striking resemblance to feline mast cell tumor in Figure 20–100C. *D*, Epitrichial sweat gland adenoma over the thorax of a dog. *E*, Epitrichial sweat gland carcinoma over the lateral neck and shoulder of a dog. *F*, Atrichial sweat gland adenoma on the footpad of a dog. *G*, Circumanal gland adenoma in the perianal region of a dog. *H*, Circumanal gland carcinoma in a dog.

smooth and greasy to hyperkeratotic, wartlike to cauliflower-like in appearance, pinkish to orangish, and 0.5 to 1 cm in diameter. Nodular sebaceous hyperplasia accounts for about 67% of all feline sebaceous gland tumors (Fig. 20–39C).[14, 153]

DIAGNOSIS

Cytologic examination reveals clustering of lipidized sebocytes (Fig. 20–40B). Histopathologically, sebaceous gland tumors are classified as nodular sebaceous hyperplasia (greatly enlarged sebaceous glands composed of numerous lobules grouped symmetrically around centrally located sebaceous ducts) (Fig. 20–40A); sebaceous adenoma (lobules of sebaceous cells of irregular shape and size, which are asymmetrically arranged and well

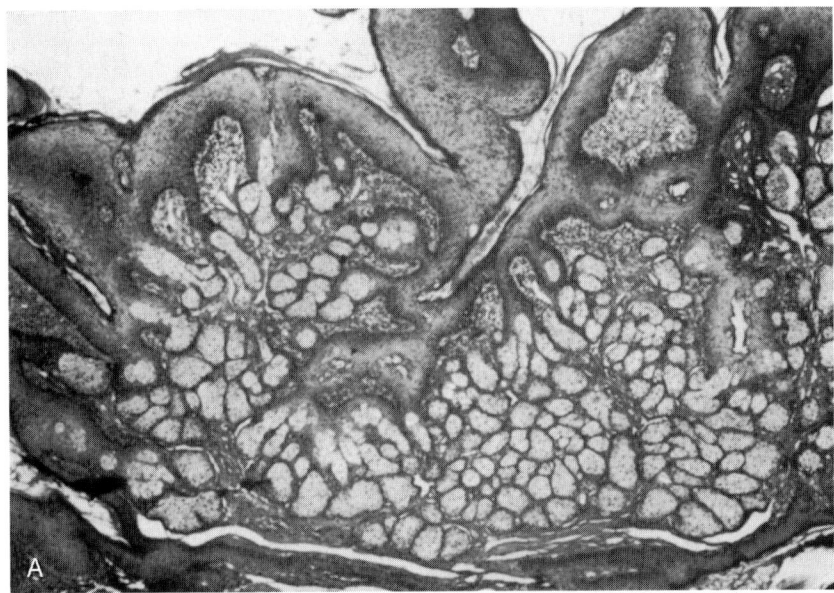

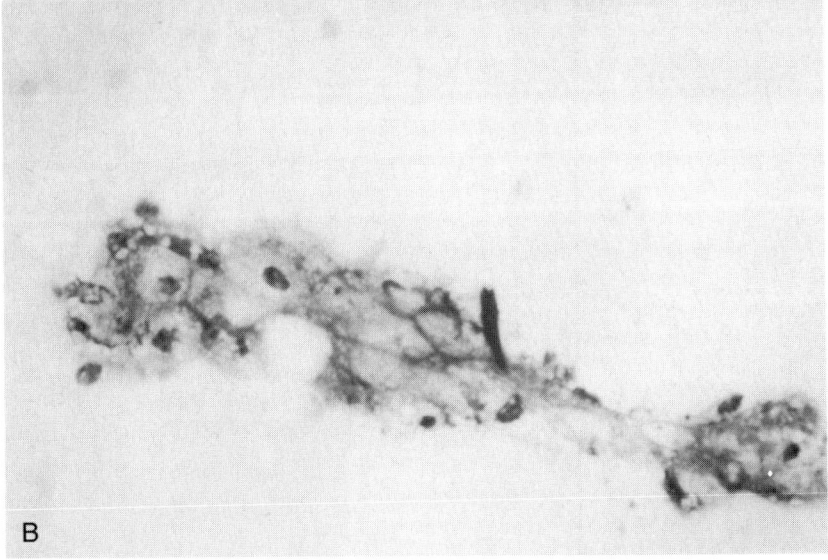

FIGURE 20–40. A, Nodular sebaceous hyperplasia in a dog. B, Nodular sebaceous hyperplasia in a dog. Cytologic examination of aspirate shows the typical clustering of highly lipidized sebocytes.

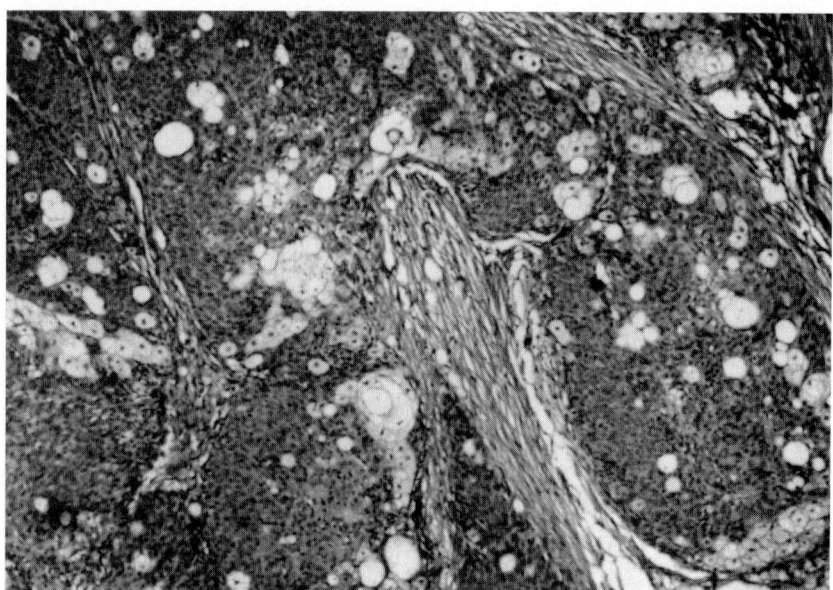

FIGURE 20-41. Canine sebaceous epithelioma. Proliferation of basaloid cells with frequent sebaceous differentiation.

demarcated from the surrounding tissue and contain mostly mature sebocytes and fewer undifferentiated germinative cells); sebaceous epithelioma (tumor similar to basal cell tumor but containing mostly undifferentiated germinative cells and fewer mature sebocytes) (Fig. 20-41); and sebaceous carcinoma (tumor with pleomorphism and atypia) (Fig. 20-42).[2, 33, 152, 153] In one study, about 81% of sebaceous epitheliomas and 54% of sebaceous adenomas in dogs had areas of sebaceous hyperplasia peripheral to and often phasing into epitheliomatous or adenomatous areas, suggesting that sebaceous hyperplasia

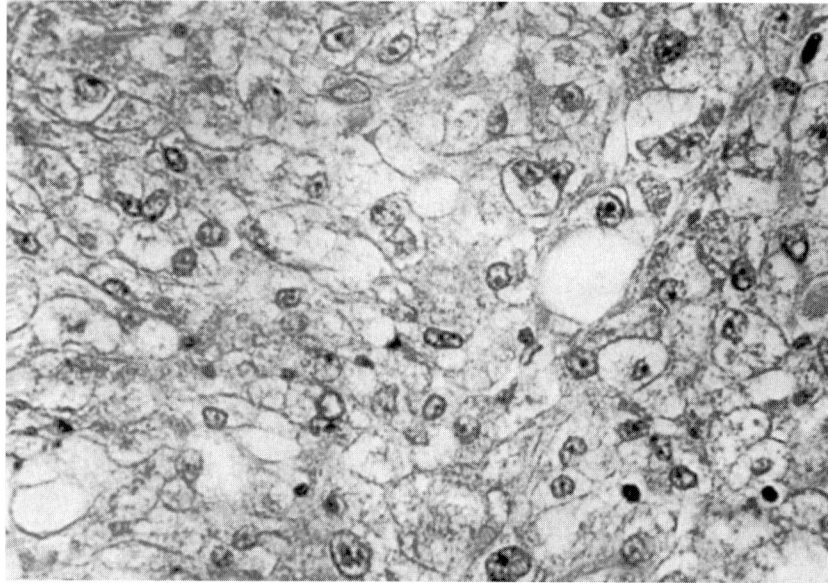

FIGURE 20-42. Canine sebaceous carcinoma. Proliferation of pleomorphic, atypical sebocytes.

may be a precursor to the other lesions.[152] Sebaceous gland tumors are positive for cytokeratin.[47, 49]

CLINICAL MANAGEMENT

Clinical management of sebaceous gland tumors may include surgical excision, cryotherapy, electrosurgery, and observation without treatment.[4-7] Sebaceous gland neoplasms rarely recur after surgery, and sebaceous carcinomas rarely metastasize.[152, 153] Oral retinoids have been an effective treatment of sebaceous hyperplasia in humans and a small number of dogs (see Chap. 3).[88, 89] Neither in dogs nor in cats were any clinical variables found to be useful predictors of the histopathologic type of sebaceous gland abnormality.[152, 153]

Sweat Gland Tumors

CAUSE AND PATHOGENESIS

Epitrichial (apocrine) sweat gland tumors are uncommon growths in the dog and cat arising from the glandular or ductular components of epitrichial sweat glands.[1, 2, 14, 27, 33, 158] Atrichial (eccrine) sweat gland tumors are rare in dogs and cats.[2, 14, 27, 33] The cause of sweat gland tumors is unknown. Cytogenetic analysis of two feline epitrichial sweat gland neoplasms revealed a loss of chromosome E3 or B2 and E3 in both.[160]

CLINICAL FINDINGS

Dog

Epitrichial sweat gland tumors may be benign or malignant in the dog.[1, 158] However, no clinical features are consistently helpful in distinguishing histologically benign from histologically malignant tumors.[158] These neoplasms generally occur in dogs that are 10 years of age or older, with no apparent sex predilection. Golden retrievers, Cocker spaniels, and German shepherd dogs may be predisposed.[1, 5, 158] Epitrichial sweat gland neoplasms are usually solitary (about 93% of cases), well circumscribed, firm, raised, 0.5 to 10 cm in diameter, and frequently ulcerated. Some tumors may be cystic and have a bluish or purplish tint when viewed through the overlying skin (see Fig. 20–39D). Lesions occur most commonly on the neck, the head, the dorsal trunk, and the limbs.[1, 2, 27, 33, 158] Some epitrichial sweat gland carcinomas are poorly circumscribed, infiltrative, plaquelike, or ulcerative growths (see Fig. 20–39E), especially in the ventral abdomen, proximal limb, or neck area, which may be misdiagnosed as pyotraumatic dermatitis or staphylococcal dermatitis.

Atrichial sweat gland tumors may be benign or malignant and are extremely rare.[2, 5, 27, 159] The lesions are solitary, firm, well to poorly circumscribed, frequently ulcerated, and 1 to 3 cm in diameter; they occur on the footpads (see Fig. 20–39F). Atrichial sweat gland carcinomas may present as a poorly defined swelling of the footpad and the digit.

Cat

Epitrichial sweat gland tumors may be benign or malignant in cats.[1, 158] However, no clinical features are consistently helpful in distinguishing histologically benign from histologically malignant neoplasms.[158] These neoplasms generally occur in cats that are 10 years of age or older, with no apparent breed or sex predilection. Epitrichial sweat gland carcinomas may be more frequent in the Siamese.[1] Epitrichial sweat gland tumors are usually solitary (about 100% of cases), well circumscribed, firm, raised, 0.3 to 3 cm in diameter, and frequently ulcerated. Some lesions may be cystic and have a bluish or purplish tint when viewed through the overlying skin. Lesions occur most commonly on the head (especially the cheek), the pinna, the neck, the axilla, the limb (Fig. 20–43), and the tail.[1, 5, 14, 27, 30, 158] Dry gangrene and sloughing of the claws and distal phalanges on all paws was reported in a cat with metastatic epitrichial sweat gland carcinoma.[161]

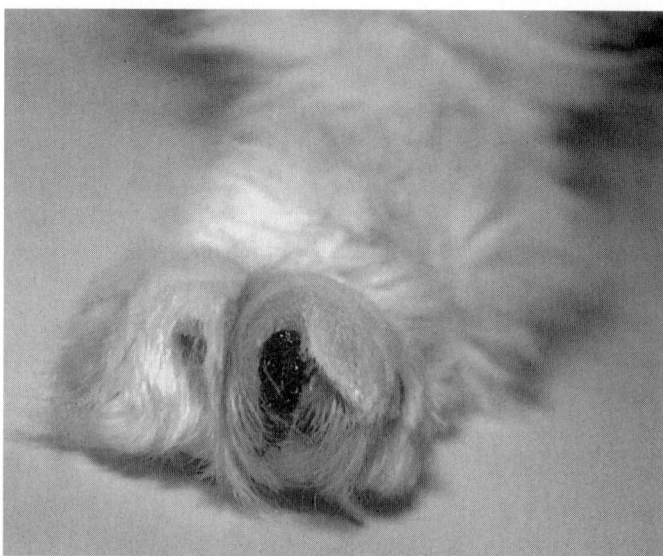

FIGURE 20–43. Epitrichial sweat gland carcinoma on the digit of a cat.

Atrichial sweat gland tumors are almost always malignant in cats and are extremely rare.[2, 14] Atrichial sweat gland carcinomas usually present as poorly defined swellings of the footpad and the digit and may affect multiple digits in cats. Ulceration is common.

DIAGNOSIS

Cytologic examination reveals clusters of epithelial cells containing secretory droplets (Fig. 20–44). The literature on histopathologic classification of sweat gland neoplasms is confusing and includes numerous subtypes: cystadenoma, glandular adenoma, ductular adenoma, syringoadenoma, spiradenoma, cylindroma, hidradenoma papilliferum, and carcinoma (solitary, papillary, tubular, glandular, ductular, mixed, clear cell, signet ring) (Figs. 20–45 to 20–48).* The clinical significance of these various histologic types is unknown. In one

---

*See references 1–3, 5, 6, 156–158.

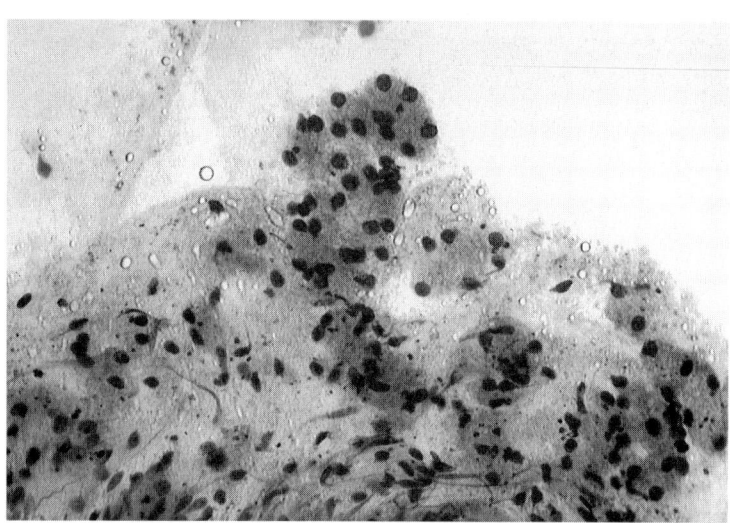

FIGURE 20–44. Epitrichial sweat gland adenoma in a dog. Cytologic examination of aspirate reveals clustered epitrichial sweat gland cells containing secretion material (sweat).

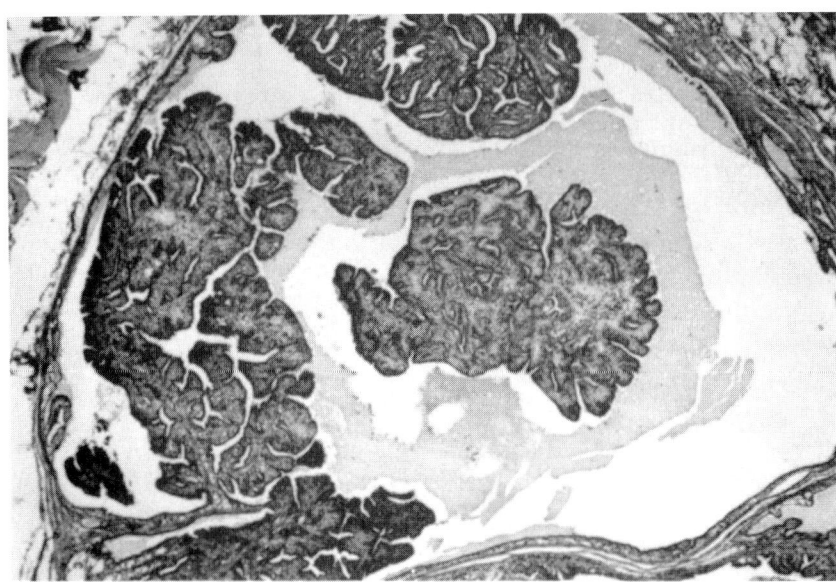

FIGURE 20–45. Feline papillary cystadenoma. Papillary processes, lined with a single row of cuboidal to epitrichial sweat gland cells, projecting into a cyst cavity containing amorphous secretory material.

retrospective study, most epitrichial sweat gland neoplasms in dogs (91 per cent) and cats (80 per cent) were histologically malignant.[158] Most carcinomas were the solid type, and there was no apparent relationship between the histopathologic subtype and clinical variables. In dogs, about 22 per cent of carcinomas showed lymphatic invasion (see Fig. 20–48), and cartilaginous or osseous metaplasia was rarely seen. Epitrichial sweat gland neoplasms (Fig. 20–49) are positive for cytokeratin.[47, 49, 52] Carcinomas, but not adenomas, were positive for carcinoembryonic antigen (in secretory cells) and vimentin (in myoepithelial cells).[52]

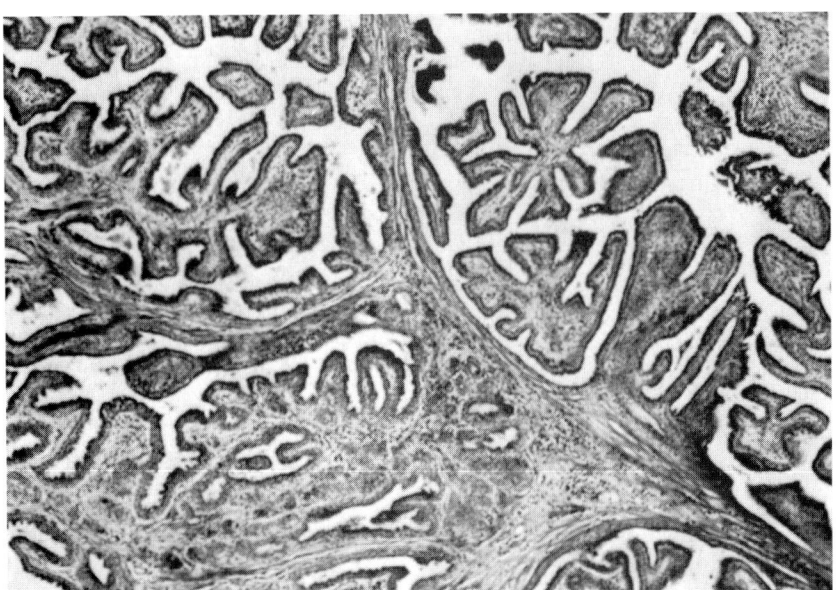

FIGURE 20–46. Canine papillary syringadenoma.

1278 • Neoplastic and Non-Neoplastic Tumors

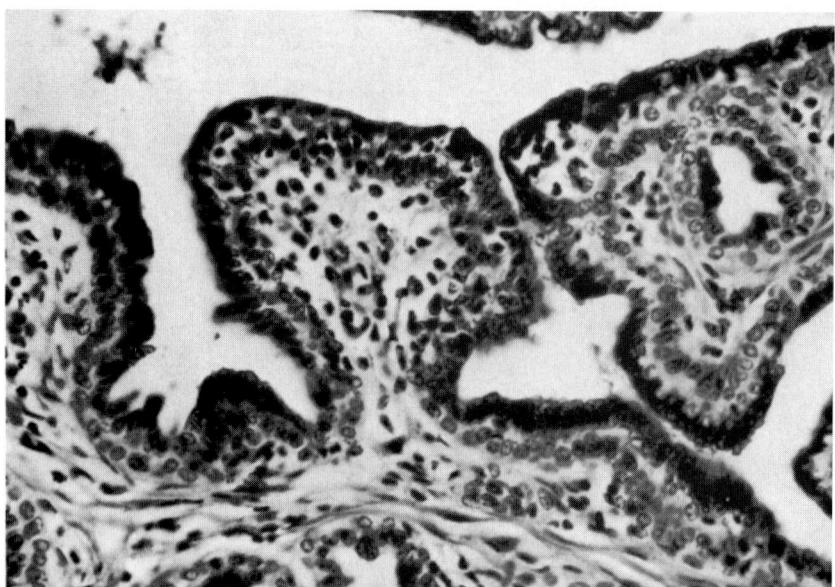

FIGURE 20–47. Close-up of Figure 20–46.

FIGURE 20–48. Canine epitrichial sweat gland carcinoma. Proliferation of atypical epitrichial sweat gland cells in cords and glandular structures, with lymphatic invasion *(right)*.

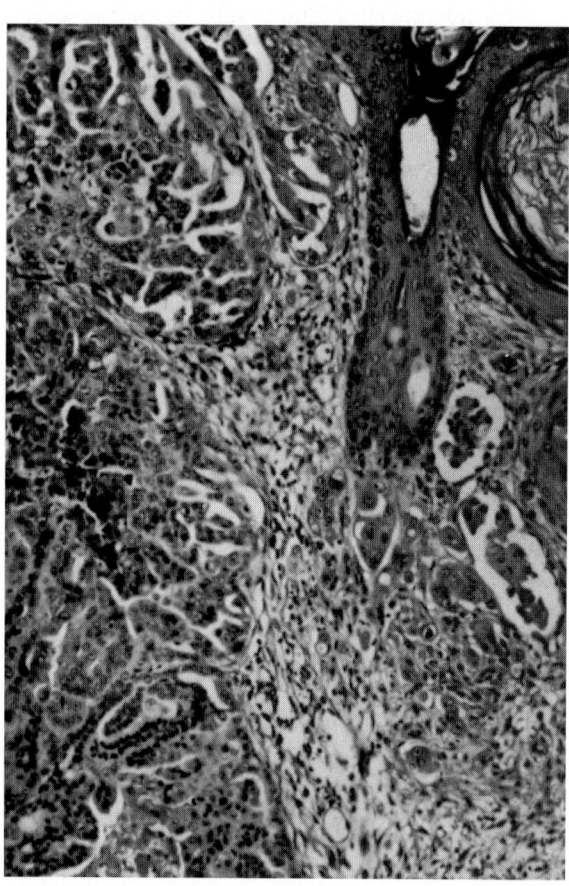

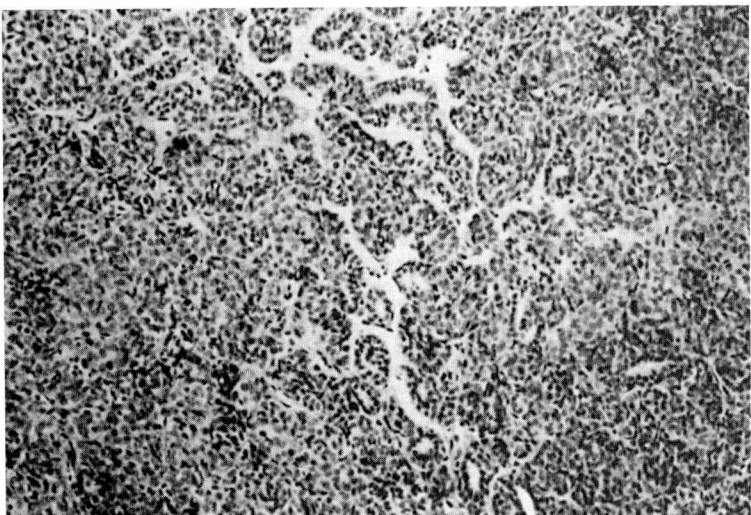

FIGURE 20-49. Canine atrichial sweat gland adenoma.

CLINICAL MANAGEMENT

Clinical management of sweat gland tumors may include surgical excision, cryosurgery, electrosurgery, and observation without treatment.[4-7] Although epitrichial sweat gland carcinomas are occasionally reported to be highly invasive and rapidly metastatic to lymph nodes, lungs, and bones,[6, 27, 33, 35, 158, 162] no instances of metastasis were documented in one retrospective study,[158] even though about 22% of cases had histologically evident lymphatic invasion. Atrichial sweat gland carcinomas are aggressive and exhibit rapid metastasis to regional lymph nodes and subcutaneous tissues of the affected limb.[2, 5]

Perianal Gland Tumors

CAUSE AND PATHOGENESIS

Perianal gland tumors, which are common in the dog, arise most frequently from circumanal glands (perianal or hepatoid glands and modified sebaceous glands) and less commonly from anal sac glands (apocrine glands of the anal sacs).* The cause of perianal gland tumors is unknown. However, the circumanal glands and their tumors are known to be modulated by sex hormones and contain both androgen and estrogen receptors.[165]

CLINICAL FINDINGS

Circumanal gland tumors occur in dogs at an average age of 11 years. Adenomas are about nine times more frequent in male than in female dogs. Carcinomas occur with equal frequency in male and female dogs. Cocker spaniels, English bulldogs, Samoyeds, Afghans, Dachshunds, German shepherd dogs, Beagles, Siberian huskies, Shih tzus, and Lhasa apsos are predisposed to the development of circumanal gland tumors. Apocrine neoplasms of anal sac origin are most common in old female dogs and are often associated with pseudohyperparathyroidism.[1, 4-7, 163] Circumanal gland neoplasms may be solitary or multiple. Most occur adjacent to the anus, but they may occur on the tail, perineum, prepuce, thigh, and dorsal lumbosacral area. The smaller (less than 1 cm in diameter) neoplasms are spherical or ovoid and tend to become multinodular and ulcerated as they

---

*See references 1, 2, 4, 6, 7, 10, 27, 33, 163, 164.

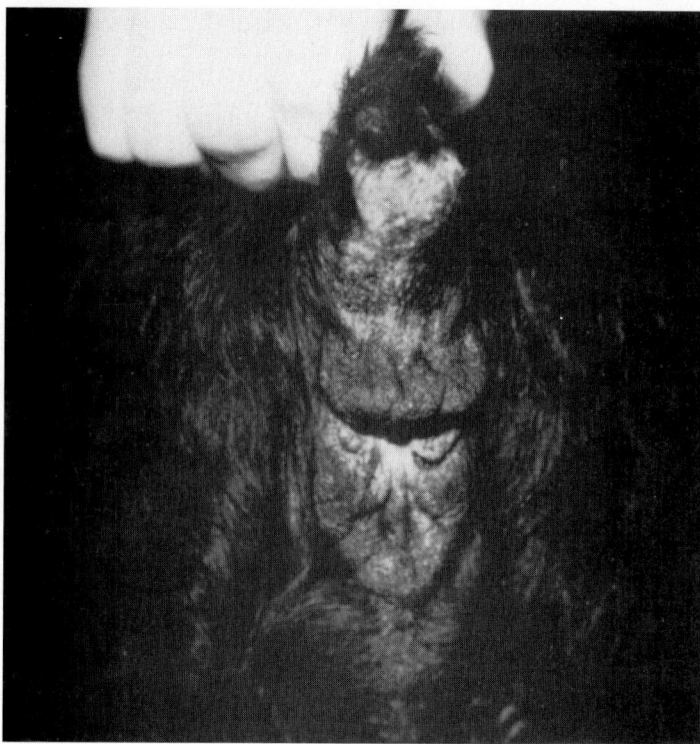

FIGURE 20–50. Diffuse circumanal gland hyperplasia around the anus of a dog.

become larger (up to 10 cm in diameter). Perianal neoplasms are usually firm, dermoepidermal in location, and well circumscribed to poorly circumscribed.

Nodular circumanal gland hyperplasia may occur as multiple discrete nodules of varying size that are impossible to distinguish from circumanal gland adenomas (see Fig. 20–39G) or as a diffuse bulging ring around the anus (Fig. 20–50). Most circumanal gland tumors are benign.

Circumanal gland carcinomas (see Fig. 20–39H) tend to grow more rapidly, attain a larger size, and ulcerate more extensively than do adenomas. Dogs with lesions larger than 5 cm in diameter have an 11-fold higher risk of dying of tumor-related causes.[164] Metastasis, especially to the sacral and sublumbar lymph nodes, occurs in up to 30% of cases.[1]

Apocrine tumors of anal sac origin are usually adenocarcinomas, present as a perineal mass (ventrolateral to the anus), and often produce pseudohyperparathyroidism. The tumors usually metastasize, especially to the sacral and sublumbar lymph nodes.[1, 163]

DIAGNOSIS

Histologically, perianal gland tumors are classified into two basic types: (1) circumanal gland tumors (hyperplasia [Fig. 20–51], adenoma, and carcinoma) and (2) apocrine tumors of anal sac origin.° Perianal gland neoplasms are positive for cytokeratin.[47, 166] Myoepithelial cells stained for neuron-specific enolase and synaptophysin.[166]

CLINICAL MANAGEMENT

Clinical management of circumanal gland tumors may include surgical excision, cryosurgery, electrosurgery, radiotherapy, castration, and the administration of estrogens.[4–7] Cas-

---

°See references 1, 2, 5, 7, 33, 163, 164.

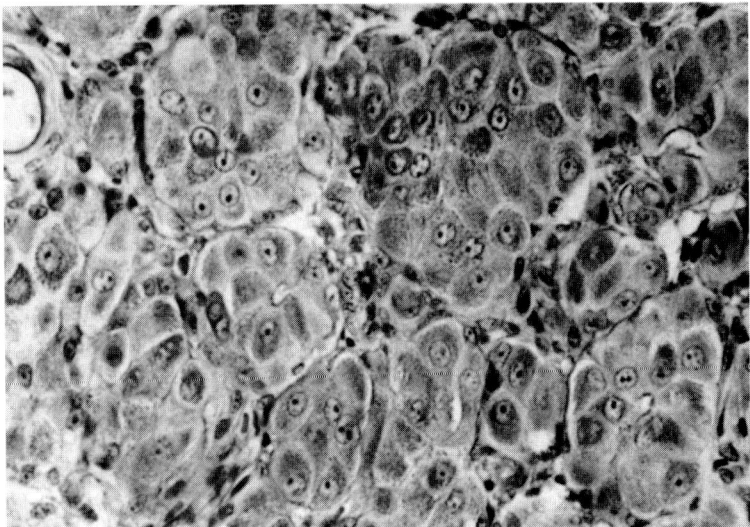

FIGURE 20–51. Canine circumanal gland hyperplasia.

tration is usually the treatment of choice for circumanal gland hyperplasias and adenomas, with 95% of dogs responding well. Concurrent surgical excision is usually needed only with ulcerated or recurrent neoplasms in male dogs but is usually mandatory for circumanal gland neoplasms in female dogs. Castration is not effective for carcinomas. Estrogen therapy is not usually recommended, because any tumor regressions induced are transient. Recurrence of circumanal hyperplasia or adenoma after surgical resection and castration, or occurrence of these lesions in female dogs, suggests that these animals should be evaluated for hyperadrenocorticism (elevated androgen levels, see Chap. 10).[5, 7] Apocrine neoplasms of anal sac origin have a poor prognosis, because local recurrence and metastasis are common.[163]

Salivary Gland Tumors

Salivary gland neoplasms are rare in dogs and cats.[167] There are no apparent breed or sex predilections, and neoplasms generally occur in animals 10 years of age or older. Typical presentations include an ulcerated mass near the lateral commissure of the mouth and a subcutaneous mass caudoventral to the angle of the mandible or below the ear. The majority (85%) of the neoplasms are malignant. Recurrence after surgery and metastasis are common.

• MESENCHYMAL NEOPLASMS

The classification of some mesenchymal neoplasms, especially the sarcomas, is controversial. Many authors lump fibrosarcomas, hemangiopericytomas, myxosarcomas, rhabdomyosarcomas, liposarcomas, malignant fibrous histiocytomas, undifferentiated sarcomas, and schwannomas into a "grab-bag" category called *soft tissue sarcoma*.[7, 23, 40, 182, 183] The histologic distinction between some of these neoplasms is often subtle, and there is inconsistency in the use of nomenclature for them. These neoplasms have similar clinical presentations and biological behaviors. A recent immunocytochemical study on canine cutaneous fibrosarcomas, hemangiopericytomas, and schwannomas suggested that these terms carry little precision in respect to tumor cell differentiation.[64] The authors of this study suggested that these three "tumors" merely reflect varieties of proliferative patterns that may be manifested by cells of varying lineage, and that they would support the use of the term spindle cell tumor of canine soft tissue to encompass this group of lesions.

Sarcomas are frequently characterized by a pseudocapsule of compressed neoplastic cells and stroma.[7, 40] Thus, simple lumpectomy is not likely to be curative and should always be followed with radiotherapy with or without hyperthermia. If surgery is to be successful, it must be aggressive (e.g., compartmental resection or amputation).[40]

Reports of the use of radiotherapy on animal sarcomas before the routine use of megavoltage radiation and the appreciation that more aggressive time-dose schemes would be necessary suggested that soft tissue sarcomas were relatively radioresistant (e.g., orthovoltage radiation resulted in 1-year local cure rates of only 17%[173]). With the use of megavoltage radiation (doses of 45 to 50 Gy), 1-year control rates of 48% to 67% have been achieved.[182, 183] However, the probability of long-term control of many soft-tissue sarcomas with radiation therapy remains low.[7, 40]

Tumors of Fibroblast Origin

FIBROMA

- **Cause and Pathogenesis.** Fibromas are uncommon benign neoplasms of the dog and cat arising from dermal or subcutaneous fibroblasts.[2, 4-7, 33] The cause of fibromas is unknown. In one canine fibroma, cytogenetic evaluation demonstrated trisomy 1.[210]
- **Clinical Findings.** These neoplasms usually occur in older dogs and cats. There is no breed or sex predilection in cats. In dogs, however, fibromas are reported to occur most commonly in Boxers, Boston terriers, Doberman pinschers, Golden retrievers, and Fox terriers.[1, 4-7, 12, 16] Female animals are predisposed. Usually, these lesions are solitary (Fig. 20–52A) and may be more common on the limbs, flanks, and groin. They are usually well circumscribed, firm (fibroma durum) to soft (fibroma molle), dome shaped to pedunculated, dermoepidermal to subcutaneous in location, and 1 to 5 cm in diameter. In dogs, fibromas may be melanotic (see Fig. 20–52B), have a pin-feathered appearance, or both. In France, an unusual fibroma has been reported on the bridge of the nose in dogs.[55] Although it is histologically benign, the neoplasm is locally aggressive, grows to a large size, and may invade the orbital cavity. Fibromas are usually noninvasive and are nonmetastatic.
- **Diagnosis.** Cytologic examination reveals small numbers of spindle-shaped fibroblasts (Fig. 20–53B). Histologically, fibromas are characterized by whorls and interlacing bundles of fibroblasts and collagen fibers (Fig. 20–53A).[2, 33] The neoplastic cells are usually fusiform, and mitoses are rare. Fibromas containing focal areas of mucinous or

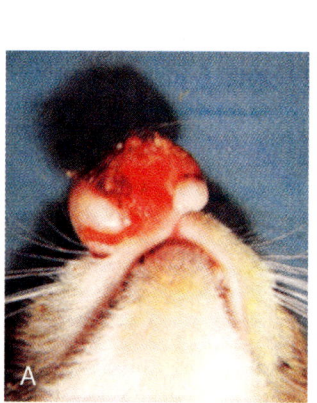
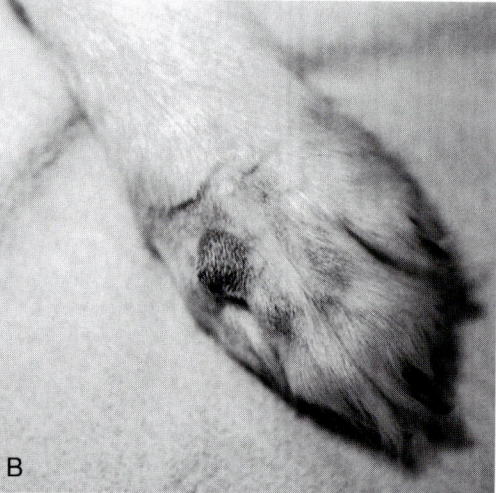

FIGURE 20–52. *A*, Fibroma, cat. *B*, Melanotic digital fibroma in a dog. Note resemblance to digital melanoma in Figure 20–147.

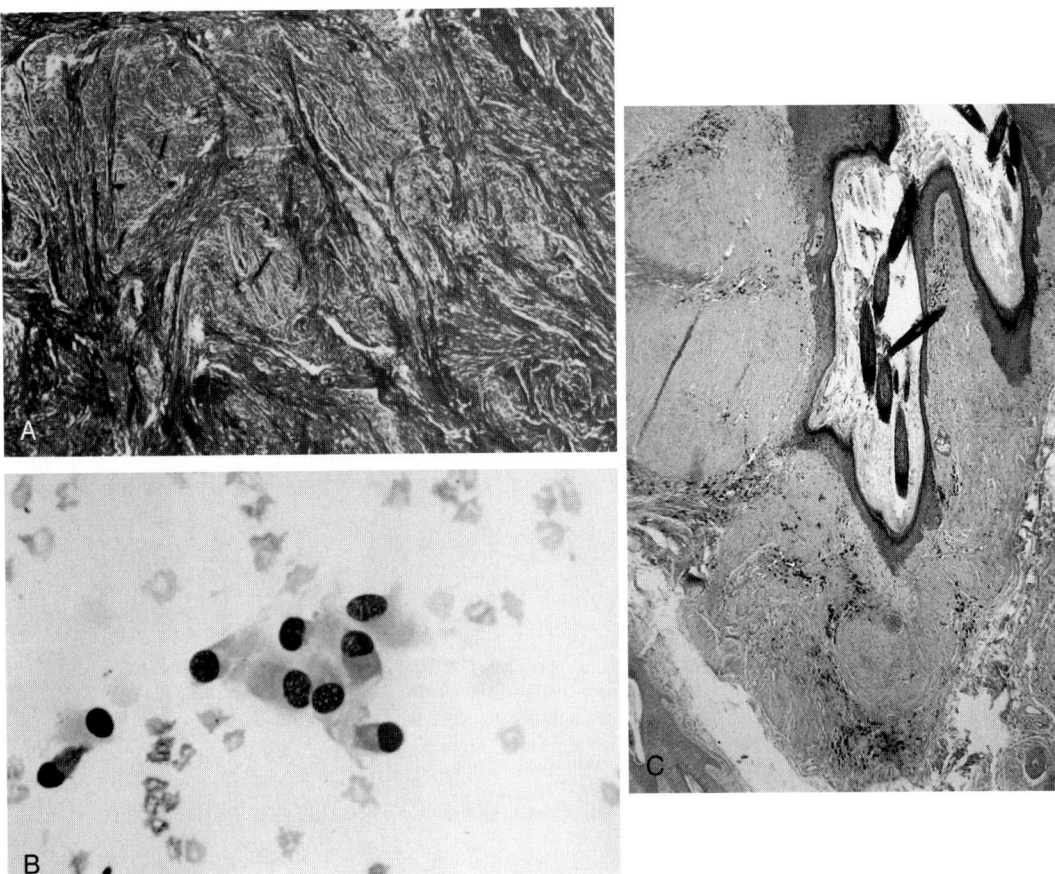

FIGURE 20–53. *A*, Canine fibroma. Interlacing proliferation of well-differentiated fibroblasts and collagen fibers. *B*, Canine fibroma. Cytologic examination of aspirate reveals small numbers of monomorphic fibroblasts. *C*, Perifollicular fibroma from a dog.

myxomatous degeneration are often called fibromyxomas. Some fibromas are distinctly perifollicular (Fig. 20–53C). Fibromas are positive for vimentin.[47]

• **Clinical Management.** Clinical management of fibromas may include surgical excision, cryosurgery, electrosurgery, and observation without treatment.[4–7]

DERMATOFIBROMA

• **Cause and Pathogenesis.** Dermatofibromas are rare fibrocytic tumors in dogs and cats.[2] The cause is unknown, and there is controversy about whether the lesion is neoplastic or reactive.

• **Clinical Findings.** Dermatofibromas appear as solitary, well-circumscribed, firm nodules that are usually less than 2 cm in diameter. The overlying epidermis is alopecic and thickened. Lesions occur most often on the head, and affected animals are usually younger than 5 years old.

• **Diagnosis.** Histopathologically, dermatofibromas are characterized by spindle and stellate fibrocytic cells arranged in haphazard bundles and small whorls, interspersed with a moderate stroma composed of collagen fibers and bundles of varying thickness.[2]

• **Clinical Management.** Clinical management of dermatofibromas may include surgical excision, cryosurgery, and observation without treatment.

FIBROVASCULAR PAPILLOMA

A fibrovascular papilloma (skin tag, keratin tag, skin polyp, acrochordon, fibroepithelial polyp, or soft fibroma) is an uncommon benign tumor of fibrovascular origin in dogs.[1, 2, 5] The cause of these growths is unknown, but they may be a proliferative response to trauma or focal furunculosis.

- **Clinical Findings.** No sex predilection is established, but large and giant breeds appear to be predisposed, especially the Doberman pinscher and Labrador retriever.[1] The lesions may be solitary or multiple, filiform to pedunculated, smooth or hyperkeratotic, soft, and 2 to 5 mm in diameter by 1 to 2 cm in length (Fig. 20–54). Fibrovascular papillomas occur most commonly on bony prominences, the trunk, and the sternum.
- **Diagnosis.** Histopathologically, fibrovascular papillomas are characterized by a fibrovascular core exhibiting papillomatosis and irregular hyperplasia of the overlying epidermis (Fig. 20–55).[2, 5]
- **Clinical Management.** Clinical management of fibrovascular papillomas may include surgical excision, cryosurgery, electrosurgery, and observation without treatment.[5]

FIBROPRURITIC NODULE

- **Cause and Pathogenesis.** The etiopathogenesis of fibropruritic nodules is unknown. However, they have been described only in conjunction with the chronic self-trauma of canine flea bite hypersensitivity (see Chap. 8).[2, 5]
- **Clinical Findings.** Fibropruritic nodules are most commonly seen in dogs older than 8 years of age and may be more common in German shepherd dogs and their crosses.[2, 5] Solitary to multiple firm, sessile or pedunculated, alopecic nodules develop, which vary in size from 1 to 2 cm in diameter (Fig. 20–56A). Lesions may be erythematous or hyperpigmented, or smooth or hyperkeratotic, and are occasionally ulcerated. Fibropruritic nodules are located predominantly over the dorsal lumbosacral area of dogs with chronic flea bite hypersensitivity.
- **Diagnosis.** The clinical presentation is characteristic. Histopathologically, fibropruritic nodules are characterized by nodular dermal fibrosis, inflammation, and often, marked papillated epidermal hyperplasia (Fig. 20–57).[2, 5] Eosinophils are usually a prominent inflammatory cell.

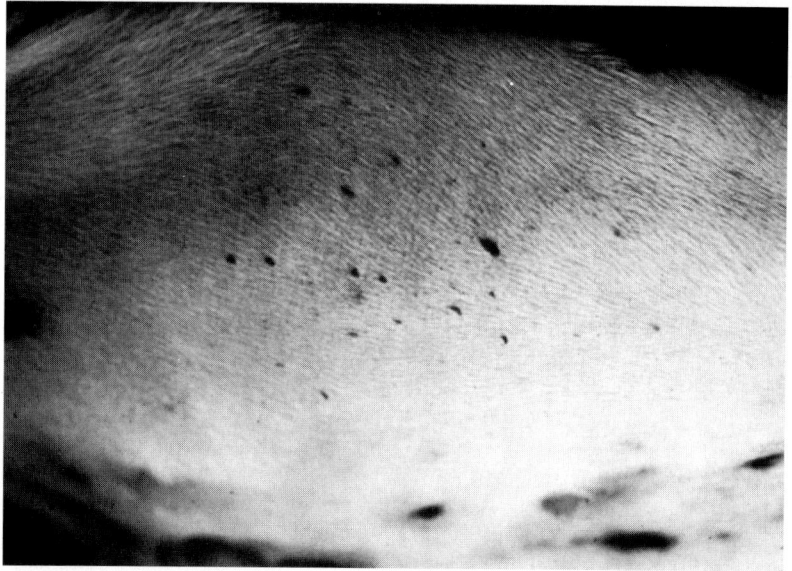

FIGURE 20–54. Multiple fibrovascular papillomas on the sternum of a dog.

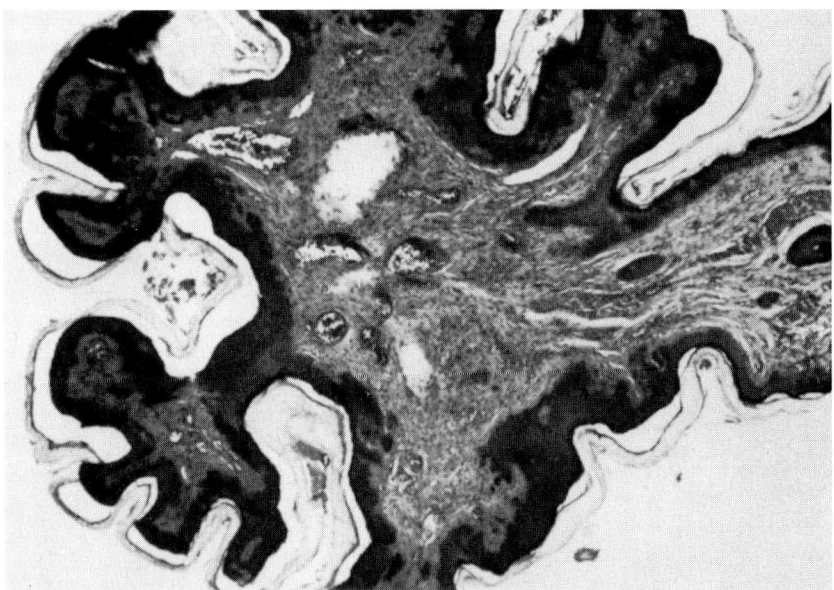

FIGURE 20-55. Canine fibrovascular papilloma. Papillomatous proliferation of epidermis and fibrovascular core.

• **Clinical Management.** The treatment of choice is surgical excision and controlling the associated flea bite hypersensitivity.

FELINE "SARCOID"

• **Cause and Pathogenesis.** The cause of this rare neoplasm is unknown. Because of its histologic resemblance to the equine sarcoid, immunohistochemical tests for bovine papillomavirus were performed but were negative.[20] In addition, immunohistochemical tests for FeLV and feline sarcoma virus (FeSV) were also negative.[20]

• **Clinical Findings.** Affected cats are often young (1 to 2 years of age) and spend time outdoors in rural areas. Single or multiple nodules, up to 2 cm in diameter, which are often ulcerated, occur most commonly on the nasal philtrum (Fig. 20-58).[20, 168] Lesions also occur on the external nares, upper lip, digits, pinnae, and tip of tail. The lesions are usually slow growing but often recur with markedly increased growth rate after surgical excision.

• **Diagnosis.** Histologically, nonencapsulated, poorly demarcated dermal nodules are characterized by a dense proliferation of fibroblastic cells with prominent swirling. The overlying epidermis forms long, pointed rete ridges (Fig. 20-59), and spindle cells may abut the epidermis in a picket fencelike configuration.

• **Clinical Management.** Good responses have been gained with cryosurgery, radiotherapy, or amputation (pinna, tail).[20]

FIBROSARCOMA

• **Cause and Pathogenesis.** Fibrosarcomas (fibroblastic spindle cell sarcomas) are common (in cats) to uncommon (in dogs) neoplasms arising from dermal or subcutaneous fibroblasts. The cause of fibrosarcomas in older animals is unknown. Some feline fibrosarcomas are virus induced.[4-7, 172] Such fibrosarcomas, and cell-free extracts derived from them, contain C-type virus particles. Cell-free extracts produce multicentric fibrosarcomas when they are injected into kittens and puppies. Cats older than 5 years appear to be more resistant to the oncogenic effects of FeSV and usually have no neoplasms or benign

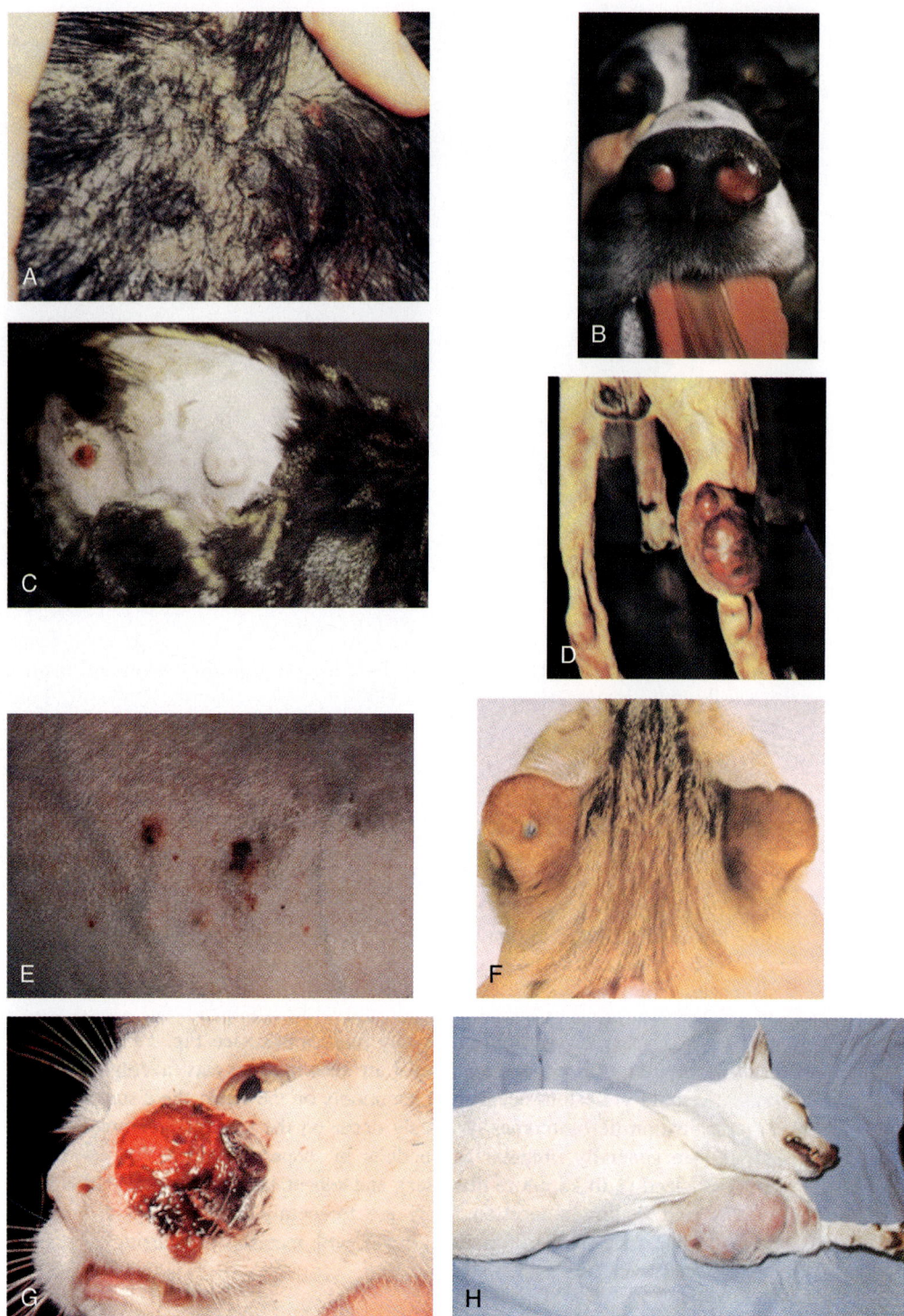

FIGURE 20-56. *A,* Multiple fibropruritic nodules over the rump of a dog with flea bite hypersensitivity. *B,* Fibrosarcoma. Fleshy masses involving both nostrils. (Courtesy J. Harvey.) *C,* Multiple fibrosarcomas over the trunk of a young, feline leukemia virus (FeLV)–positive cat. *D,* Schwannoma on the hock of a dog. *E,* Multiple solar-induced hemangiomas in a Saluki. (Courtesy A. Hargis.) *F,* Bluish hemangioma on the left pinna of a cat. *G,* Hemangiosarcoma on the face of a cat. *H,* Hemangiopericytoma on the proximal front limb of a dog.

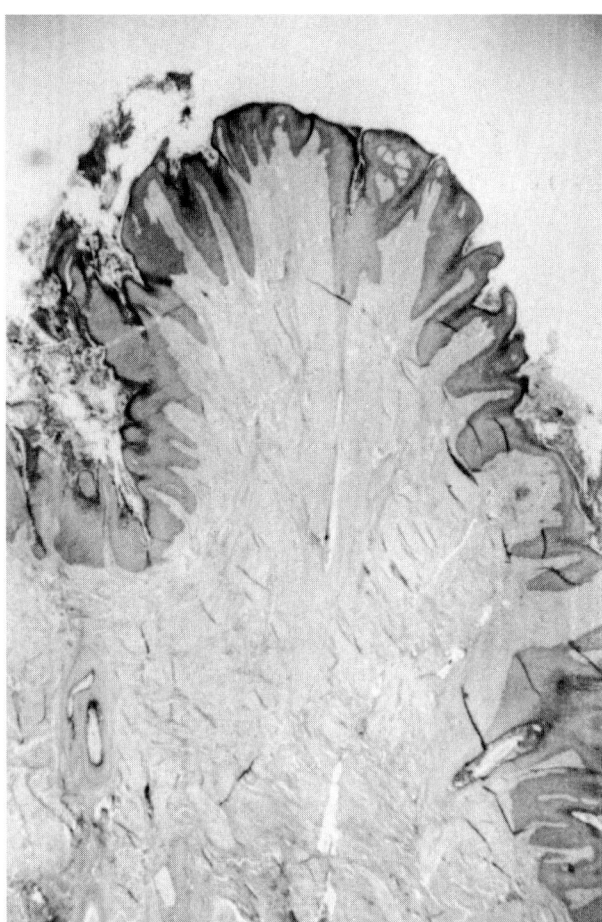

FIGURE 20–57. Canine fibropruritic nodule.

neoplasms that spontaneously regress. The FeSV is a mutant of FeLV, and cats with FeSV-induced fibrosarcomas are FeLV positive. FeSV is not associated with the solitary fibrosarcomas in old cats. It is believed that injection site reactions (especially with FeLV and rabies vaccines) may eventuate in fibrosarcomas in some cats, especially if vaccines are repeatedly given at the same site (cervical, interscapular) (see Postvaccinal Sarcomas).[253–257] Cytogenetic analysis of nine feline fibrosarcomas revealed heterogeneous karyotypic changes, including trisomy D1, marker F1, and nonrandom involvement of chromosome E1, as well as mutations in the tumor-suppressor gene p53.[177–180]

- **Clinical Findings**

Dog. Fibrosarcomas are uncommon in the dog.[1, 2, 4–7] They occur in older and female dogs, and Cocker spaniels, Doberman pinschers, and Golden retrievers may be predisposed.[1, 4–7, 12, 16] Fibrosarcomas are usually solitary, irregular and nodular in shape, firm to fleshy (see Figs. 20–56B and 20–60), poorly circumscribed, variably sized (1 to 15 cm in diameter), and subcutaneous in location. They are often ulcerated and alopecic. Lesions occur most commonly on the limbs and the trunk. Immune-mediated thrombocytopenia has been reported in association with canine fibrosarcoma.

Cat. Fibrosarcomas are common in the cat.° FeSV-associated fibrosarcomas are seen in cats younger than 5 years of age and are usually multicentric (see Fig. 20–56C).[1, 2, 4–7, 172] Fibrosarcomas that are not associated with FeSV are seen in older cats

---

°See references 1, 2, 4–7, 16, 26, 33, 35, 171.

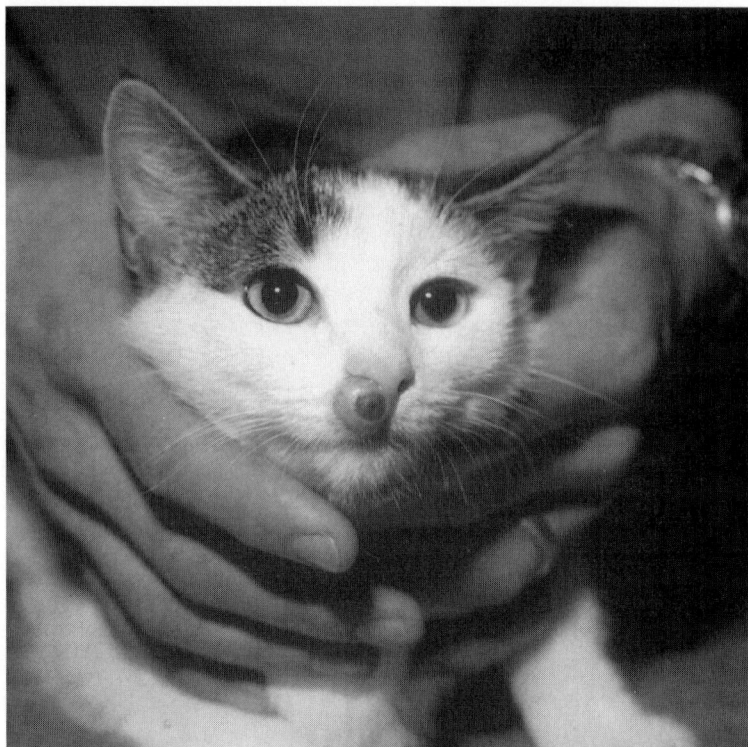

FIGURE 20-58. Feline sarcoid. Well-circumscribed, ulcerated nodule on muzzle.

(average age 12 years) and are typically solitary. Lesions occur most commonly on the trunk, the distal limbs, and the pinnae. Postvaccination fibrosarcomas obviously occur at the sites of previous injections.[253-257] The neoplasms are generally irregular and nodular in shape, firm to fleshy, poorly circumscribed, variably sized (1 to 15 cm in diameter), and subcutaneous (trunk and distal limbs) or dermal (pinnae and digits) in location. They are frequently alopecic and ulcerated. Most fibrosarcomas demonstrate rapid, infiltrative growth, with metastasis (regional lymph nodes, lung) occurring in less than 20% of the cases.[1, 4-7, 16, 23, 171]

- **Diagnosis.** Cytologic examination reveals pleomorphic, atypical fibroblasts (Fig. 20-61A). Histopathologically, fibrosarcomas are characterized by interwoven bundles of immature fibroblasts and moderate numbers of collagen fibers.[1, 2, 33, 171] The neoplastic cells are usually fusiform, mitotic figures are common, and cellular atypia is pronounced (Fig. 20-61B). Areas of necrosis or hemorrhage are not uncommon. Fibrosarcomas with focal areas of mucinous or myxomatous degeneration are often called fibromyxosarcomas. Fibrosarcomas are positive for vimentin.[47, 49, 50, 58] AgNOR counts and PCNA indices significantly correlated with the proliferative activity of fibrosarcomas but not with the mitotic indices.[174]

Fibrosarcomas arising in subcutaneous vaccination sites are accompanied by a lymphoid and granulomatous inflammatory response at the periphery, with epithelioid macrophages and multinucleate histiocytic giant cells, which have an amorphous gray-brown to bluish material within their cytoplasm (see Postvaccinal Sarcomas).[1, 253-257] FeLV antigen was demonstrated in feline multicentric fibrosarcomas but not in feline postvaccinal fibrosarcomas.[249]

- **Clinical Management.** The clinical management of choice for fibrosarcomas is wide surgical excision.[4-7, 19, 171] Radiotherapy, chemotherapy (with (Adriamycin), doxorubicin, cyclophosphamide, methotrexate, and vincristine), immunotherapy (with mixed bacte-

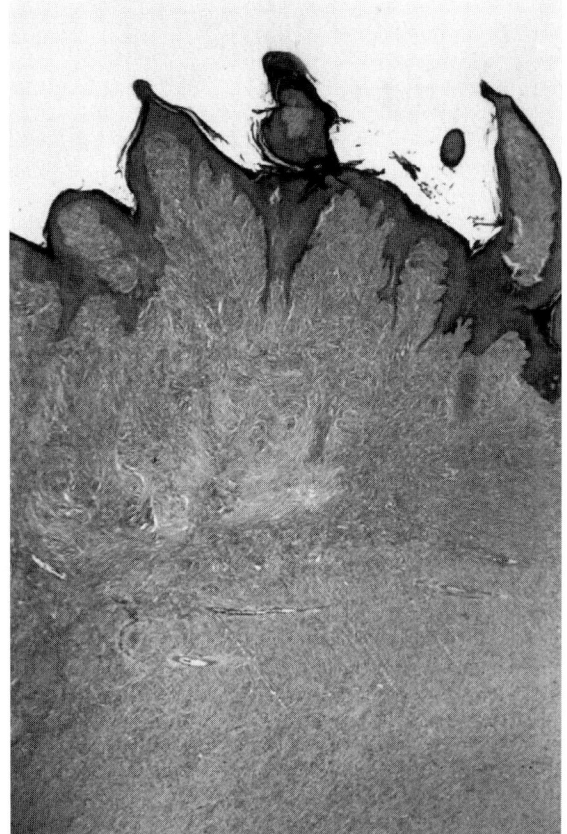

FIGURE 20–59. Feline sarcoid. Dense, swirling proliferation of fibroblasts underlying a papillated epidermis with long, pointed rete ridges.

rial vaccine and levamisole), and cryosurgery have been of limited benefit.° Acemannan (Acemannan Immunostimulant) is a carbohydrate moiety that enhances macrophage release of tumor necrosis factor-α (TNF-α), interleukin-1 (IL-1), interleukin-6 (IL-6), and interferon-γ (IFN-γ), increases natural killer cell activity, enhances T cell function, and enhances macrophage phagocytosis.[25, 175, 176] The product has been advocated (repeated intraperitoneal and intratumoral injections) for the treatment of fibrosarcoma in cats and dogs.[175] However, controlled studies are completely lacking, and the product is controversial.[7, 171]

In a study of 44 cats with fibrosarcomas, it was found that the mitotic index and tumor site correlated with prognosis, whereas histologic appearance, tumor size, and duration of tumor growth did not.[169] Cats with fibrosarcomas of the head, the back, or the limbs and with a mitotic index of 6 or greater had the poorest prognosis. In a study of 84 dogs with fibrosarcomas, the site of tumor occurrence, tumor size, and delay between detection of the tumor and surgical excision had little influence on the prognosis for recurrence or metastasis.[170] Mitotic index of the neoplasms has a significant predictive value for recurrence, postsurgical survival time, and metastasis.[23, 170]

MYXOMA AND MYXOSARCOMA

- **Cause and Pathogenesis.** Myxomas and myxosarcomas are rare neoplasms of the dog and cat arising from dermal or subcutaneous fibroblasts, the cause of which is

---

°See references 4–7, 23, 40, 171, 182, 183.

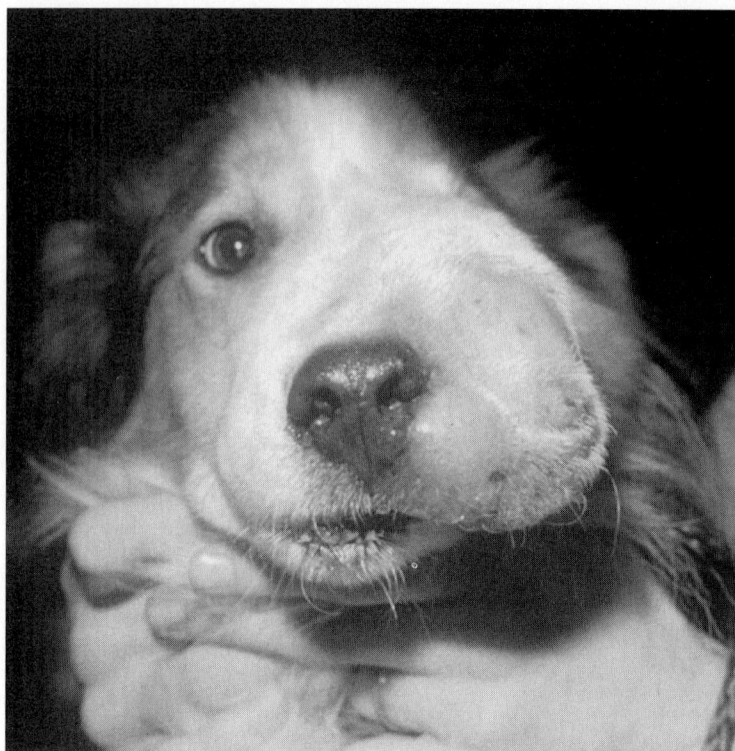

FIGURE 20-60. Fibrosarcoma, dog. (Courtesy H. Harvey.)

unknown.[1, 2, 4-7, 16, 33] Myxoma has been reported to develop at the site of a subcutaneous pacemaker in a dog.[184]

- **Clinical Findings.** These neoplasms usually occur in older dogs and cats, with no sex predilections. Doberman pinschers and German shepherd dogs may be predisposed.[1] These neoplasms may occur more frequently on the limbs, the back, or the groin.[1] They are usually solitary infiltrative growths that are soft, slimy, and poorly circumscribed and have no definite shape. Myxomas are benign. Myxosarcomas are malignant but apparently do not commonly metastasize. Both neoplasms frequently recur after surgery, owing to their infiltrative growth patterns.
- **Diagnosis.** Histopathologically, myxomas and myxosarcomas are characterized by stellate to fusiform cells distributed in a vacuolated, basophilic, mucinous stroma that may be partitioned by collagenous connective tissue septae (Fig. 20-62).[2, 33] Myxomas and myxosarcomas are positive for vimentin.[56]
- **Clinical Management.** In clinical management, the therapy of choice for myxomas and myxosarcomas is radical surgical excision.[4-7, 19]

NODULAR FASCIITIS

- **Cause and Pathogenesis.** Nodular fasciitis (pseudosarcomatous fasciitis) is a rare, benign, non-neoplastic growth of the dog and cat.[16, 33, 55] Nodular fasciitis is thought to represent a proliferative inflammatory process arising from the subcutaneous fascia and exhibiting a clinically aggressive behavior that suggests a locally invasive neoplasm.
- **Clinical Findings.** There are no age, breed, or sex predilections for dogs and cats. Nodular fasciitis can occur anywhere on the body but may favor the head, the face, and the eyelids. The masses are usually solitary, firm, poorly circumscribed, 0.2 to 5 cm in diameter, and subcutaneous in location. In humans, nodular fasciitis is self-limited, and thus, even if it is incompletely excised, it regresses. Cutaneous nodular fasciitis in dogs and cats is also benign, but spontaneous regression has not been reported.

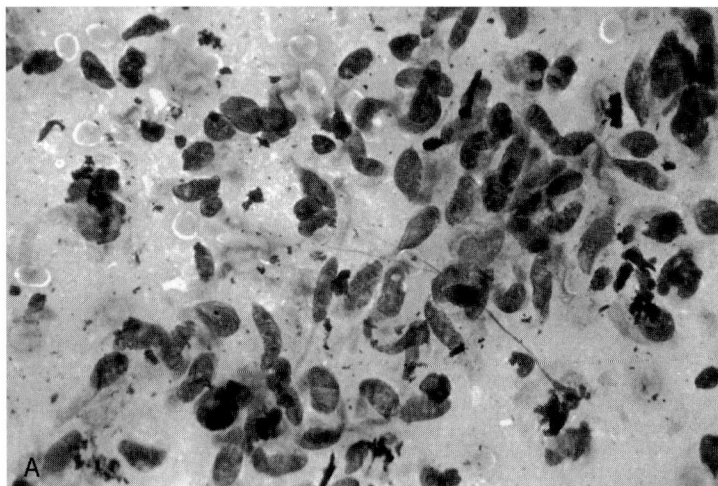
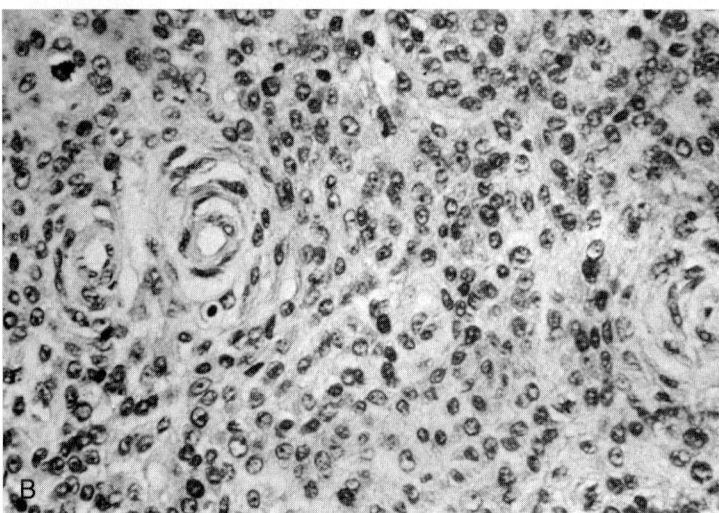

FIGURE 20–61. Canine fibrosarcoma. *A*, Cytologic examination of aspirate reveals pleomorphic, atypical fibroblasts. (Courtesy J. Blue.) *B*, Proliferation of pleomorphic, atypical fibroblasts.

- **Diagnosis.** Histopathologically, nodular fasciitis is characterized by a poorly circumscribed, infiltrative proliferation of pleomorphic fibroblasts growing haphazardly in a highly vascularized stroma with a varying amount of mucoid ground substance.[33] Mitoses and giant cells are common, and a chronic inflammatory infiltrate is often present.
- **Clinical Management.** The clinical management of nodular fasciitis in dogs and cats has consisted of surgical excision.

Tumors of Neural Origin

SCHWANNOMA

- **Cause and Pathogenesis.** Schwannomas (neurofibroma, neurilemoma, neurinoma, or perineural fibroblastoma) are rare neoplasms of the dog and cat arising from dermal or subcutaneous Schwann cells (nerve sheath).* The cause of schwannomas is unknown.

There is much confusion about terminology concerning these neoplasms in the veterinary literature. The lesions have been classified as neurinomas, neurilemomas, schwanno-

---

*See references 1, 2, 5–7, 16, 185, 189.

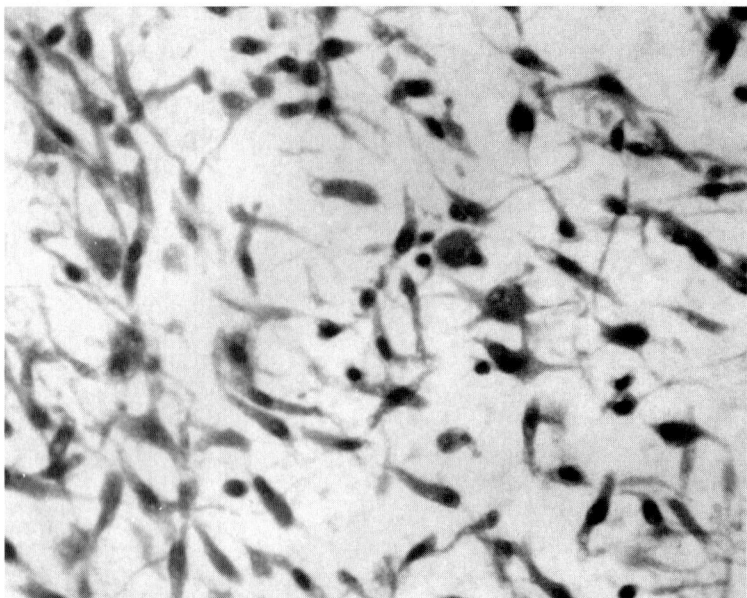

FIGURE 20–62. Feline myxosarcoma. Atypical fibroblasts (fusiform-to-stellate) with abundant ground substance (mucin).

mas, malignant schwannomas, neurofibromas, and neurofibrosarcomas.[173] Some authors have proposed the term *peripheral nerve sheath tumor* to include those neoplasms involving peripheral nerves and nerve roots, because of the presumed common cell of origin (Schwann cell) and similar biological behavior.[185, 189]

• **Clinical Findings.** Schwannomas usually occur in older dogs (average 9 years) and cats (average 12 years), with no sex predilection. In cats, no breed predilection exists, but in dogs, the Fox terrier may be predisposed.[5] Schwannomas are usually solitary. They occur most commonly on the limbs, the head, and the neck in cats, but they occur more commonly on the limbs, the head, and the tail in dogs (see Fig. 20–56D).[1, 2, 5–7, 185, 189] Schwannomas are firm (especially in dogs), well circumscribed to poorly circumscribed, often lobulated, variable in size, and dermal (especially in cats) to subcutaneous (especially in dogs) in location. They are often alopecic. Rarely, schwannomas may be plexiform (multinodular) (Fig. 20–63).[189] There may be obvious nerve involvement with or without

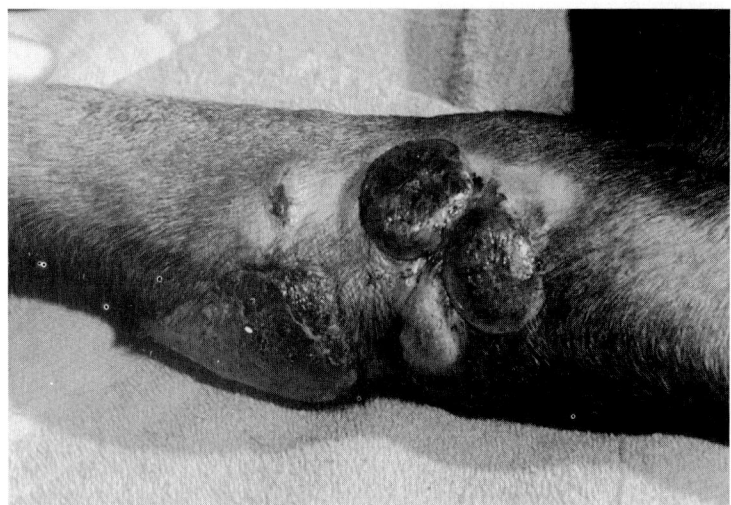

FIGURE 20–63. Multinodular schwannoma, dog.

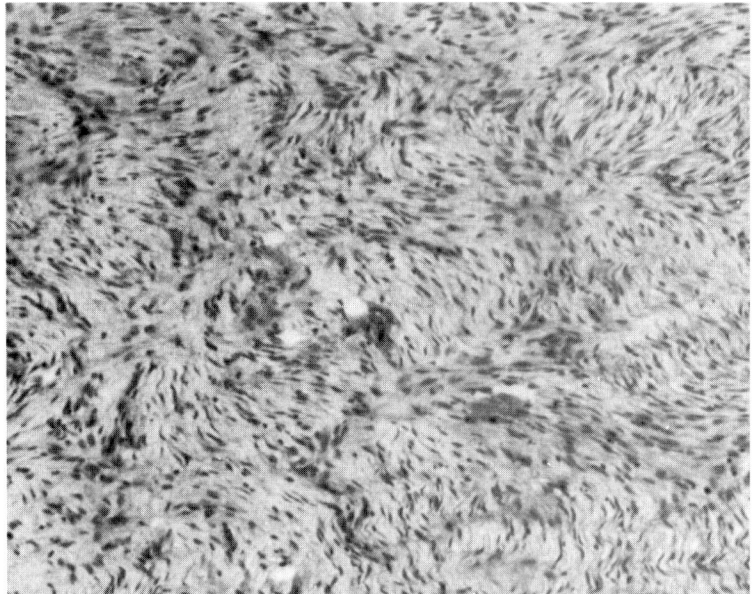

FIGURE 20–64. Canine schwannoma. Palisading spindle-shaped cells with fine, wavy fibers.

neurologic deficit. Some lesions are painful or pruritic (owing to paresthesias?) and may be complicated by acral lick dermatitis.[5, 189] Schwannomas are often malignant and even histologically benign lesions recur frequently after surgery.

• **Diagnosis.** Histopathologically, schwannomas are characterized by two patterns: (1) neurofibroma—faintly eosinophilic, thin, wavy fibers lying in loosely textured strands that extend in various directions, with spindle-shaped cells that may exhibit nuclear palisading (Fig. 20–64); and (2) neurilemoma—areas of spindle-shaped cells exhibiting nuclear palisading and twisting bands or rows (Antoni type A tissue), alternating with an edematous stroma containing relatively few haphazardly arranged cells (Antoni type B tissue) (Fig. 20–65).[1, 2, 5, 33] Benign and malignant histopathologic types are seen. These neoplasms can be extremely pleomorphic, with cells being arranged in fascicles, sheets, and whorls, and individual neoplastic cells being fusiform, ovoid to round, or multinu-

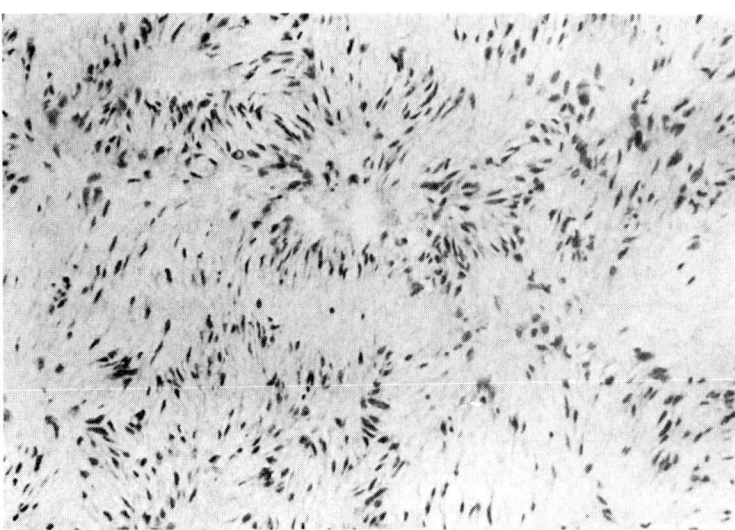

FIGURE 20–65. Canine schwannoma. Antoni A and B type tissue.

cleated all in the same neoplasm.[185] Schwannomas are positive for vimentin and S-100 protein.[16, 49, 58]

- **Clinical Management.** The therapy of choice is surgical excision.[4–7, 19, 185, 189] Amputation may occasionally be necessary. Radiotherapy, chemotherapy, immunotherapy, and cryosurgery appear to be of minimal benefit. Schwannomas recur frequently after surgery, which frequently results in euthanasia. Metastasis is rare.

NEUROTHEKEOMA

- **Cause and Pathogenesis.** Neurothekeomas are rare benign cutaneous neoplasms of Schwann cell origin.[2, 5] The cause of these neoplasms is unknown.
- **Clinical Findings.** Neurothekeomas occur in dogs[2, 5] but not enough cases have been seen to generate age, breed, or sex data. The lesions are solitary, firm, nodular, and subcutaneous to dermal in location. They occur on the legs and digits.
- **Diagnosis.** Histopathologically, neurothekeomas are characterized by nests and cords of cells in a variably mucinous matrix (Fig. 20–66). A close relationship to small nerves may be seen.[2, 5]
- **Clinical Management.** Clinical management includes surgical excision.

GRANULAR CELL TUMOR

- **Cause and Pathogenesis.** Granular cell tumors (granular cell myoblastoma, or granular cell schwannoma) are rare neoplasms of the dog and cat.[1, 5, 186, 190] Although the cell of origin is not established with certainty, current evidence suggests a neural source. In humans, granular cell tumors contain neuron-specific enolase and myelin basic protein.[5, 51] The cause of granular cell tumors is unknown.
- **Clinical Findings.** Granular cell tumors have been reported in dogs from 2 to 13 years old, with no breed or sex predilection. Most of the neoplasms occurred as solitary, firm, round, well-circumscribed masses within the tongue. Other dogs had a solitary subcutaneous neoplasm near the shoulder or on the lip or ear, and one dog had multiple dermoepidermal and subcutaneous malignant neoplasms with visceral metastasis (Fig. 20–

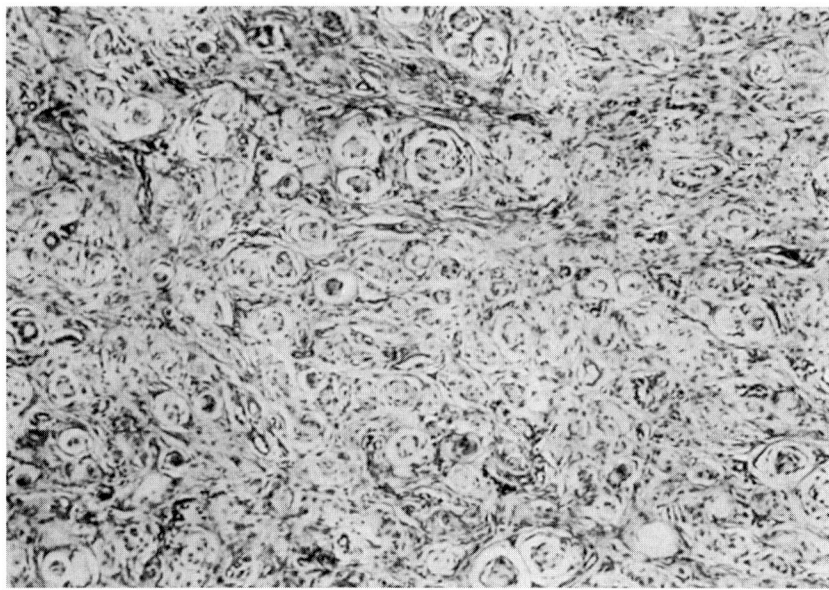

FIGURE 20–66. Canine neurothekeoma. Nests of neuroid tissue.

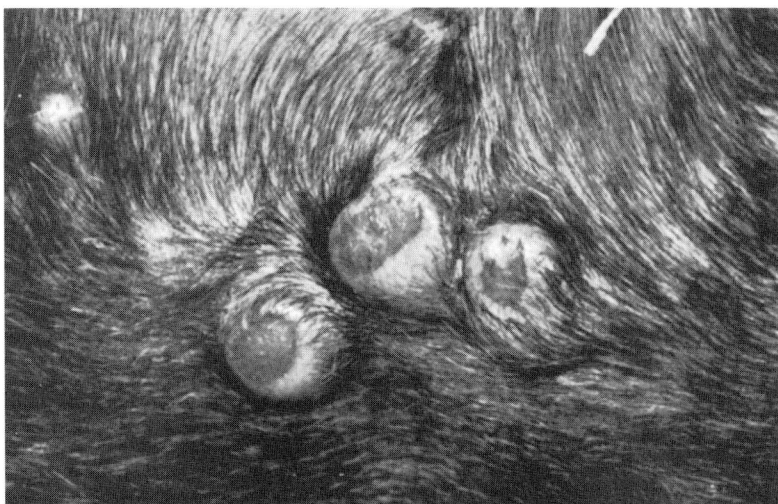

FIGURE 20–67. Malignant granular cell tumors on the thorax of a dog.

67).[5, 186, 190] Most canine granular cell tumors have been benign. In cats, granular cell tumors have been seen on the tongue, vulva, and digits.[190]

• **Diagnosis.** Histopathologically, granular cell tumors are characterized by a circumscribed mass of ovoid to polyhedral cells with central or eccentric nuclei and pale cytoplasm containing numerous small, faintly eosinophilic granules.[1, 5, 186, 190] The tumor cells may be arranged diffusely or in nests and rows (Fig. 20–68). The cytoplasmic granules are PAS positive. The pseudocarcinomatous hyperplasia that so frequently overlies granular cell tumors in humans is rarely seen in dogs and cats. Canine granular cell tumors are positive for neuron-specific enolase and variably positive for vimentin and S-100 protein.[186, 190]

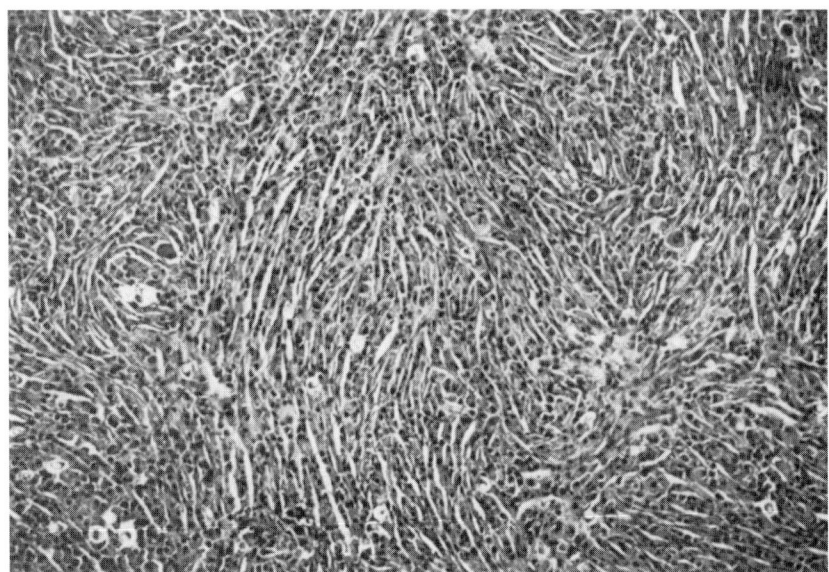

FIGURE 20–68. Canine malignant granular cell tumor. Cords and clusters of anaplastic cells with fine, eosinophilic cytoplasmic granules.

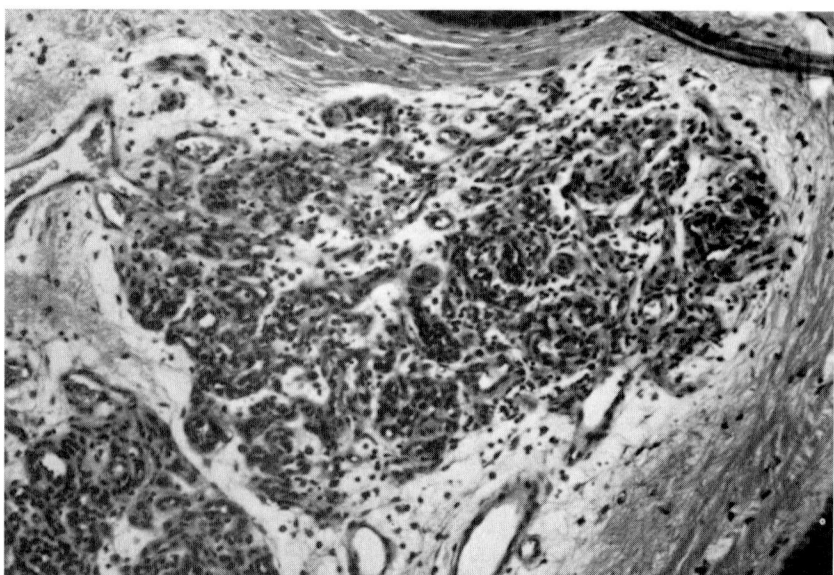

FIGURE 20–71. Canine capillary hemangioma. Superficial dermal proliferation of normal-appearing endothelial cells and blood vessels.

subcutaneous in location. Spontaneous or trauma-induced bleeding from these neoplasms may occur.

• **Diagnosis.** Histologically, hemangiomas are characterized by the proliferation of blood-filled vascular spaces lined by single layers of well-differentiated endothelial cells.[1, 2, 33] Hemangiomas are often subclassified as cavernous or capillary, depending on the size of the vascular spaces and the amount of intervening fibrous tissues (Figs. 20–71 and 20–72).[1, 2, 5, 33] Solar-induced lesions are often less well circumscribed, and solar

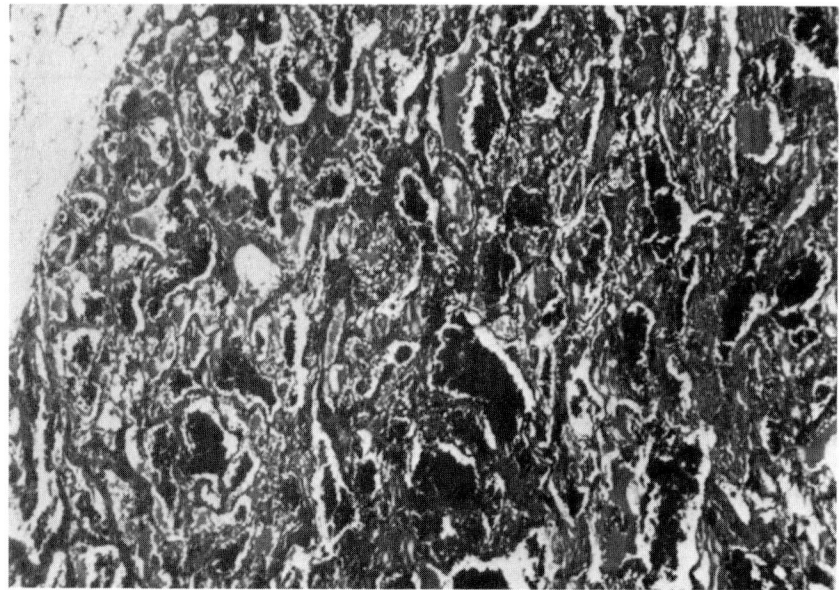

FIGURE 20–72. Canine cavernous hemangioma. Deep dermal proliferation of widely dilated, blood-filled vessels.

dermatitis and elastosis may be present.[2, 5, 205, 211] Electron microscopy may be beneficial in determining the vascular origin of a neoplasm, because Weibel-Palade bodies are a specific cytoplasmic marker for endothelial cells.[5] In addition, immunohistochemistry may be useful, because vimentin, factor VIII-related antigen (von Willebrand's factor [vWf]), and type IV collagen and laminin are found in vascular proliferations.[47, 50, 55, 62, 212] In a recent study,[198] vWf and CD31 (platelet endothelial cell adhesion molecule [PECAM]) both consistently marked normal vascular endothelium and all hemangiomas from dogs. Lectins (e.g., *Ulex europaeus* [UEA-1]) are not good markers for canine vascular neoplasms.[191, 198] Anemia, purpura, thrombocytopenia, hypofibrinogenemia, and findings associated with disseminated intravascular coagulation have been reported in conjunction with hemangiomas.[204]

- **Clinical Management.** Clinical management of hemangiomas may include surgical excision, cryosurgery, electrosurgery, and observation without treatment.[4–7]

HEMANGIOSARCOMA

- **Cause and Pathogenesis.** Hemangiosarcomas (angiosarcomas, or malignant hemangioendotheliomas) are uncommon malignant neoplasms of dogs and cats arising from the endothelial cells of blood vessels.[1, 2, 4–7, 194a, 211, 223] The cause of most hemangiosarcomas is unknown. In humans, they have been associated with exposure to thorium dioxide, arsenicals, and vinyl chloride.[5] Studies strongly suggest that chronic solar damage may be the cause of hemangiosarcomas in the ventral glabrous skin of lightly pigmented, sparsely coated dogs[2, 205] and on the pinnae of white-eared cats.[212]

- **Clinical Findings**

Dog. Hemangiosarcomas occur in dogs at an average of 10 years of age, with no apparent sex predilection. Typical hemangiosarcomas occur most commonly in German shepherd dogs, Golden retrievers, Bernese Mountain dogs, and Boxers.* Lesions are often rapidly-growing and are most commonly found on the trunk and the extremities. Whippets, Dalmatians, beagles, greyhounds, American Staffordshire terriers, Basset hounds, Salukis, English pointers, and other short-haired and light-skinned breeds are at increased risk for solar-induced hemangiosarcomas.[2, 204, 205]

Solar-induced hemangiosarcomas are often multiple and most common on the ventral thorax and the abdomen. Typical hemangiosarcomas are usually solitary, whereas solar-induced lesions may be multiple. Dermal hemangiosarcomas (usually solar induced) are well-to-poorly circumscribed, red to dark blue plaques or nodules that are usually less than 2 cm in diameter. Subcutaneous hemangiosarcomas (usually *not* solar-induced) are poorly circumscribed, dark red or blue-black, bruiselike, spongy masses that can measure up to 10 cm in diameter.[205, 223] Alopecia, thickened skin, hemorrhage, and ulceration are common features of dermal or subcutaneous hemangiosarcomas.

Cat. Hemangiosarcomas usually occur in male cats older than 10 years of age.† There is no breed predilection. White cats may be prone to cutaneous hemangiosarcoma owing to the role of ultraviolet light exposure in the development of lesions.[194a] Lesions are usually solitary, rapidly growing, and occur most commonly on the head (see Fig. 20–56G) and the pinna (especially in white-haired cats), on the limbs, and in the inguinal and axillary regions. Dermal hemangiosarcomas are poorly circumscribed, red to dark blue plaques or nodules that are usually less than 2 cm in diameter. Subcutaneous hemangiosarcomas are poorly circumscribed, dark red or blue-black, spongy masses that can measure up to 10 cm in diameter. Alopecia, thickened skin, hemorrhage, and ulceration are common features of dermal or subcutaneous hemangiosarcomas. In one study,[211] two thirds of the cats with cutaneous hemangiosarcoma eventually developed multicentric lesions. Proliferative vascular lesions of varying morphologic appearance are occasionally seen on the digits and distal limbs of older cats (Fig. 20–73).[201] These often have an

---

*See references 1, 4–7, 12, 16, 194a, 196, 219, 223.
†See references 1, 2, 4–7, 16, 30, 207, 211, 212.

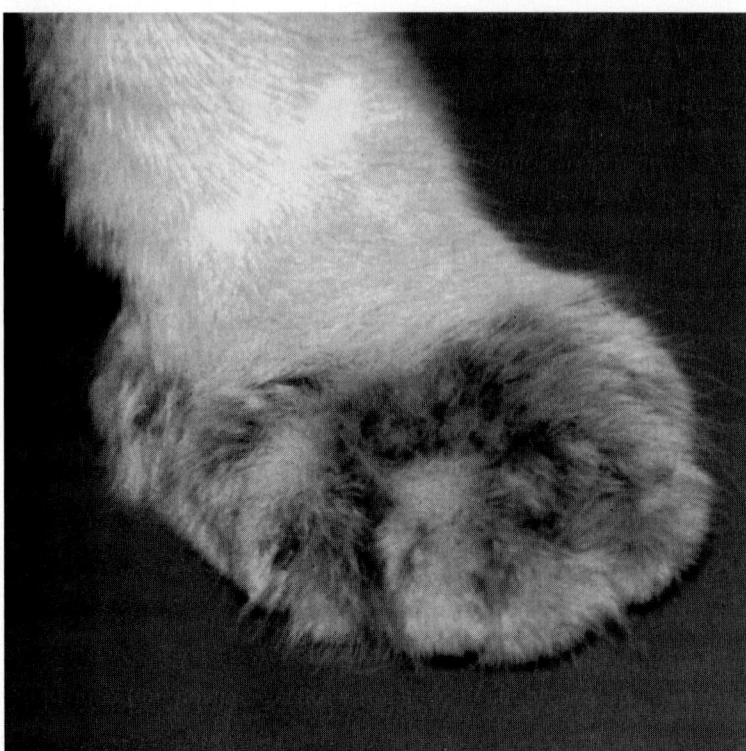

FIGURE 20-73. Feline hemangiosarcoma. Paw is swollen and studded with multifocal black crusts.

aggressive biological behavior and have been referred to as "progressive angiomatosis," "hemangiomatosis," "infiltrative hemangioma," or "low-grade hemangiosarcoma." We concur with others[201] and would prefer to call these lesions simply "hemangiosarcoma." A peripheral arteriovenous fistula was reported in a cat with a hemangiosarcoma of a limb.[208]

• **Diagnosis.** Histopathologically, hemangiosarcomas are characterized by an invasive proliferation of atypical endothelial cells with areas of vascular space formation (Figs. 20–74A and B).* Solar-induced lesions may have associated solar dermatitis and solar elastosis.[2, 205] Hemangiosarcomas are positive for vimentin, S-100 protein, factor VIII–related antigen (vWf), type IV collagen, and laminin.† In a recent study,[198] vWf marked 73% and CD31 (PECAM) marked 100% of the canine hemangiosarcomas investigated. vWf can be aberrantly expressed in some carcinomas and in macrophages.[198] CD31 also reacts with normal canine lymphatic vessel endothelium and is probably of little or no value in distinguishing between hemangiosarcomas and lymphangiosarcomas.[198] Lectins (e.g., *Ulex europaeus*, UEA-1) are not good markers for canine vascular neoplasms.[191, 198] Anemia, purpura, thrombocytopenia, hypofibrinogenemia, and findings associated with disseminated intravascular coagulation have been reported in conjunction with hemangiosarcomas.[5, 204]

Because visceral hemangiosarcomas can metastasize to the skin, it has been suggested that these skin tumors should be staged via hemogram, serum biochemistry, urinalysis, thoracic radiographs, echocardiography, and abdominal ultrasonography.[194a]

• **Clinical Management.** The therapy of choice for hemangiosarcomas is radical surgical excision.[4-7, 19, 197, 223] However, after any form of therapy, the prognosis for animals with hemangiosarcoma is poor, with local recurrence and metastasis being common. They are highly invasive and malignant in dogs, with an average survival time of 4

---

*See references 1, 2, 33, 205, 211, 212, 223.
†See references 47, 49–51, 55, 56, 62, 212.

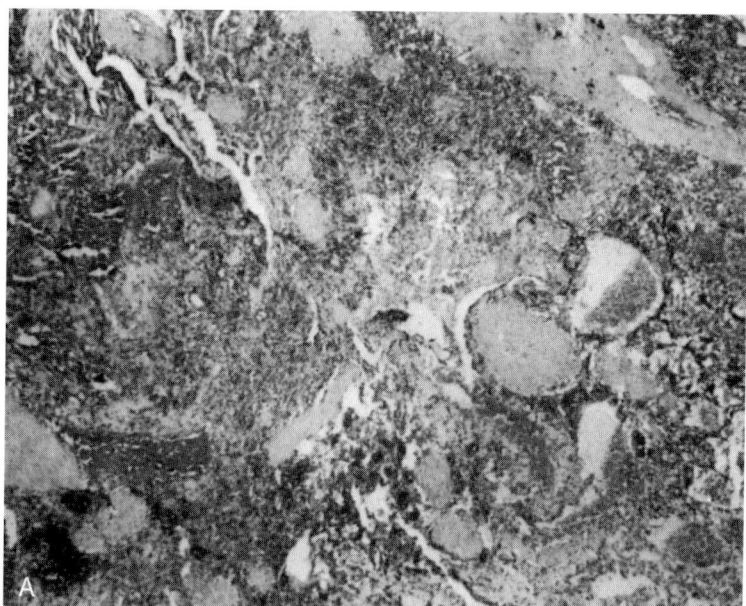
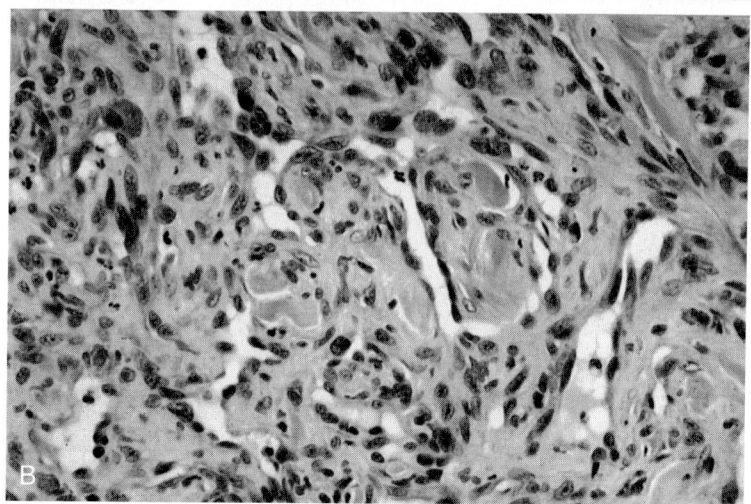

FIGURE 20–74. Canine hemangiosarcoma. A, Proliferation of atypical vascular structures associated with necrosis and hemorrhage. B, Close-up of A. Proliferation of atypical endothelial cells and abnormal vascular structures.

months after diagnosis.[182] In cats, hemangiosarcomas are reported to frequently recur after surgical excision but to metastasize rarely.[14, 211, 212, 217] However, in a recent report,[207] all cats with cutaneous hemangiosarcoma developed metastatic lesions. Early amputation is usually curative for feline hemangiosarcomas of the distal limbs and digits. Palliative responses have been obtained in dogs with the concomitant administration of doxorubicin and vincristine.[4, 5, 7]

Canine cutaneous hemangiosarcomas were staged based on the depth of histologic location: stage I (dermal), stage II (subcutis), and stage III (down to muscle).[223] Stage I lesions were small, raised, red-purple nodules; were commonly found on the ventral abdomen, prepuce, and pelvic limb; and had a median postsurgical survival of 780 days. Stage II and III lesions were larger, poorly circumscribed, soft to fluctuant, often bruise-like; had no anatomic site predilection, and had shorter postsurgical survival times (median 172 and 307 days, respectively, for stages II and III lesions). Six dogs with subcutaneous (stage II) hemangiosarcomas achieved a median postsurgical survival of 425 days with concurrent vincristine, doxorubicin, cyclophosphamide (VAC) chemotherapy.[203]

1302 • Neoplastic and Non-Neoplastic Tumors

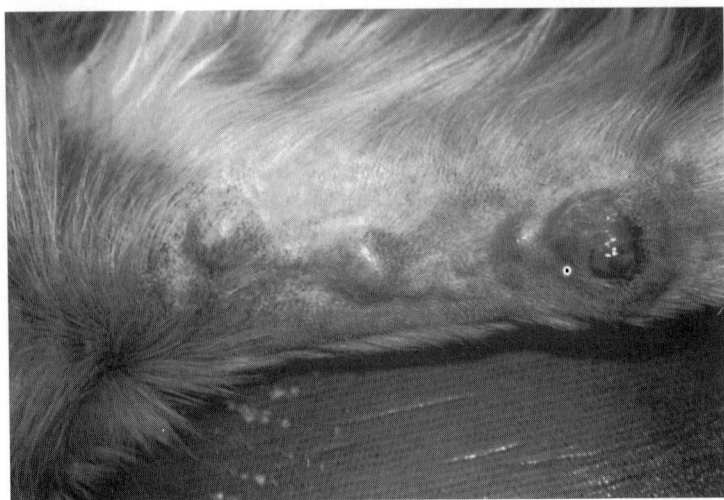

FIGURE 20–75. Multiple hemangiopericytomas on the front leg of a dog.

Ideally, the efficacy of single-agent chemotherapy should be determined before combination therapy is attempted.[194a] Some authors believe that combination chemotherapy has no strong survival advantage compared with single-agent chemotherapy and recommend a doxorubicin-based protocol adjuvant to surgery.[194a] Mixed bacterial vaccines are of no benefit.[194] Dogs receiving surgery, chemotherapy, and liposome-encapsulated muramyl tripeptide phosphatidylethanolamine had significantly longer survival times (median, 277 days) than did dogs treated with surgery and chemotherapy alone (median, 143 days).[221a]

HEMANGIOPERICYTOMA

- **Cause and Pathogenesis.** Hemangiopericytomas (pertheliomas) are common neoplasms of the dog arising from vascular pericytes.[*] Rare cases of hemangiopericytoma in cats have been reported.[5, 13, 14] The cause of hemangiopericytomas is unknown. Trisomy 2 (three copies of chromosome 2) has been reported in three cases of canine hemangiopericytoma.[209] In another three cases, cytogenetic evaluation revealed different abnormalities in all three: trisomy 9; trisomy 2 and 29; trisomy 2 and deleted chromosomes.[210]

- **Clinical Findings.** Hemangiopericytomas occur in dogs at a mean age of 7 to 10 years. Boxers, German shepherd dogs, Cocker spaniels, Springer spaniels, Irish setters, Siberian huskies, Fox terriers, Collies, and Beagles are predisposed.[1, 4–7, 16] There is no apparent sex predilection. Hemangiopericytomas are usually solitary and occur most commonly on the limbs (especially the stifle and elbow). They are usually firm, multinodular, well circumscribed, 2 to 25 cm in diameter, and dermal to subcutaneous in location (Fig. 20–75; see Fig. 20–56H). Alopecia, hyperpigmentation, and ulceration are common.

- **Diagnosis.** Several patterns are associated with the hemangiopericytoma, and one pattern may predominate or several patterns may be identified within the same mass. This variable histopathologic appearance is considered unique to the hemangiopericytoma.[1] The classic pattern is the perivascular whorls (fingerprint pattern) of spindle-shaped to ovoid cells (Fig. 20–76A and B).[†] Other patterns include storiform, myxoid, and epithelioid. Hemangiopericytomas are positive for vimentin[47, 56, 213] but negative for S-100[203a] and factor VIII–related antigen.[213] Fifty percent of the tumors coexpress muscle actin.[213]

- **Clinical Management.** The therapy of choice for hemangiopericytomas is surgical excision or amputation.[4–7, 19, 202, 215] Recurrent tumors have fewer whorls and look more

---

*See references 1, 2, 4–7, 16, 202, 215, 226.
†See references 1, 2, 4–7, 16, 33, 226.

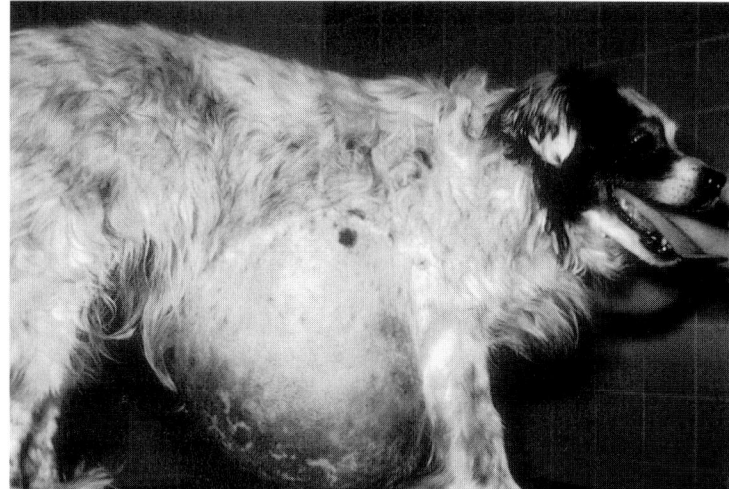

FIGURE 20–83. Huge lipoma on the ventral thorax of a dog.

ties, the thorax, and the neck. The neoplasms are large, poorly circumscribed, soft, deep subcutaneous masses that infiltrate adjacent muscle, fascia, tendon, joint capsule, and bone; they may cause dysfunction because of mechanical interference or pressure pain.[231]

• **Diagnosis.** Cytologic examination reveals an often acellular preparation containing numerous lipid droplets (Fig. 20–85). Histologically, lipomas are characterized by a well-circumscribed proliferation of normal-appearing lipocytes (Figs. 20–86 and 20–87).[1, 2, 33] Some neoplasms have a marked fibrous tissue component and are called fibrolipomas. Infiltrative lipomas are characterized by a poorly circumscribed proliferation of normal-appearing lipocytes that infiltrates surrounding tissues, especially muscle and collagen.[2, 228] Angiolipomas are characterized by mature adipose tissue with a complex, branching blood vascular component (Fig. 20–88).[5] Lipomas are positive for vimentin.[47, 50, 58]

• **Clinical Management.** The treatment of choice for all types of lipomas is surgical excision.[4–7] In obese animals, a restricted diet for a few weeks before surgery often reduces the size of the neoplasms and improves the definition from surrounding tissues. Small, asymptomatic lipomas are often merely observed, unless they grow large. Lipomas that are large can usually be easily peeled out, because they are well circumscribed and

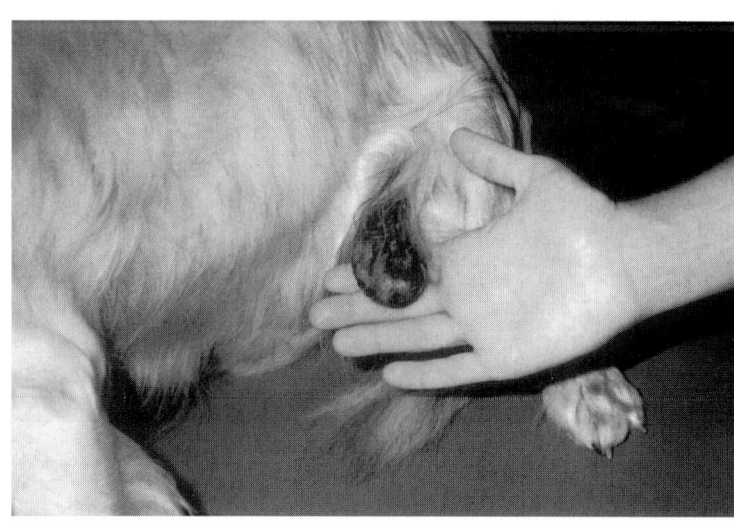

FIGURE 20–84. Pigmented lipoma in the flank of a dog.

1310 • Neoplastic and Non-Neoplastic Tumors

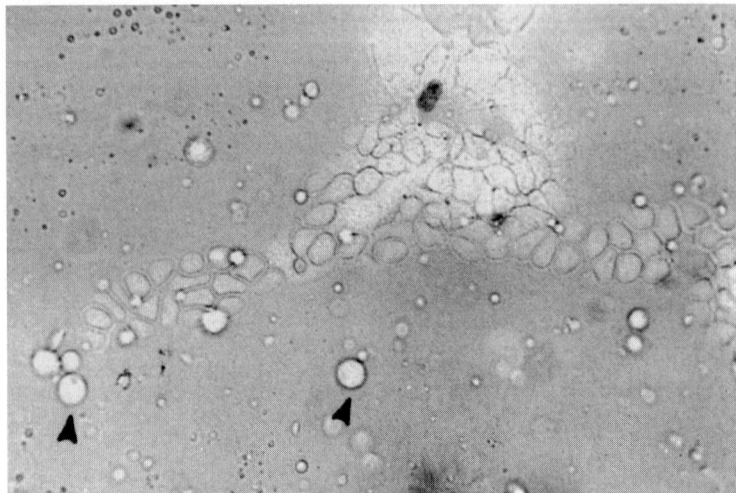

FIGURE 20-85. Canine lipoma. Cytologic examination of aspirate reveals fat droplets *(arrows)*.

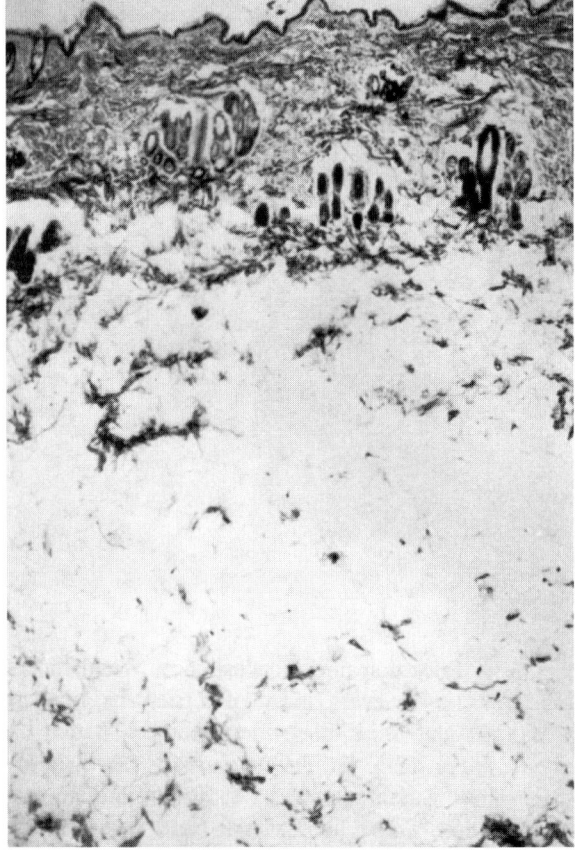

FIGURE 20-86. Feline lipoma. Proliferation of normal-appearing fat.

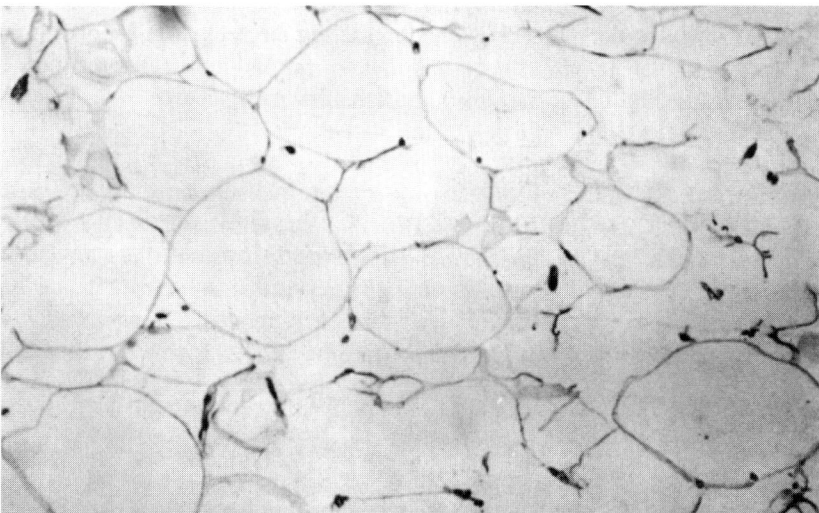

FIGURE 20–87. Close-up of Figure 20–86. Normal-appearing lipocytes.

have a poor blood supply. The intratumoral injection of 10% calcium chloride solution caused complete remission in 4 of 18 canine lipomas treated, with a 50% reduction in size of the other 14 treated tumors.[227] Although infiltrative lipomas are not malignant, they necessitate radical surgical excision to prevent local recurrence, which still may occur in 36% of the cases.[228] It is difficult to distinguish infiltrative lipoma from normal fat, thus surgical margins are hard to define.

LIPOSARCOMA

- **Cause and Pathogenesis.** Liposarcomas are rare malignant neoplasms of the dog and cat; they arise from subcutaneous lipoblasts.[1, 2, 5–7, 16] The cause of liposarcomas is

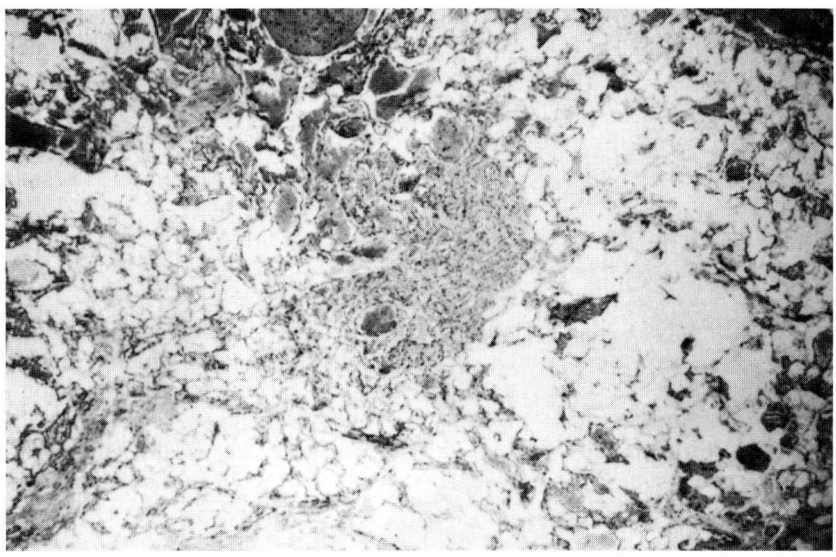

FIGURE 20–88. Canine angiolipoma. Proliferation of lipocytes with a central branching vascular component.

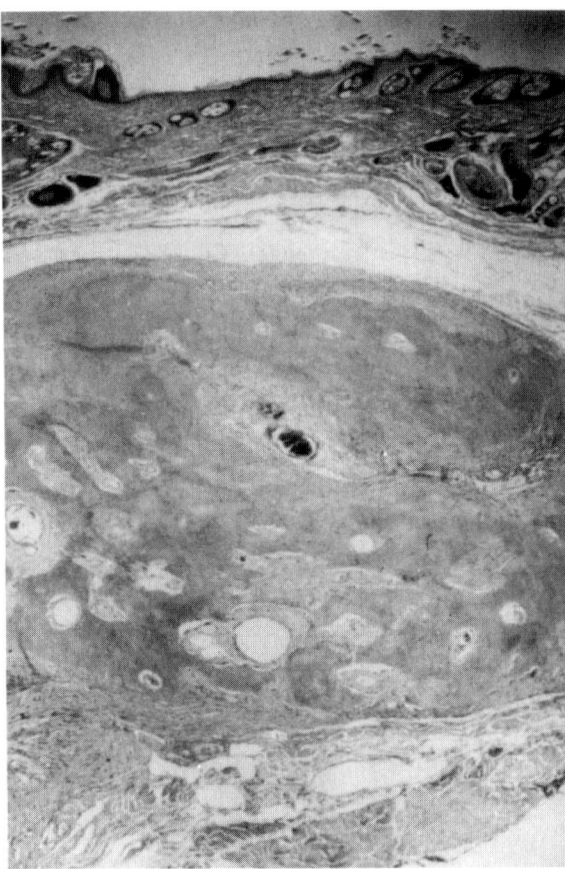

FIGURE 20-93. Feline osteoma. Bone formation in the subcutis.

occurred in the subcutaneous tissue of the neck, flank, groin, limb, and thorax. Histologically, malignant cells with chondroid differentiation (Fig. 20-95) formed nodules within the dermis and subcutis.

• **Clinical Management.** The treatment of choice is surgical excision.

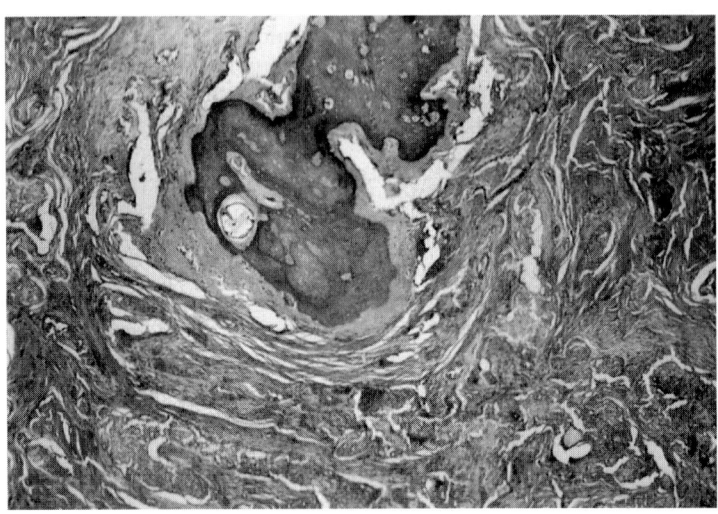

FIGURE 20-94. Canine osteosarcoma. Invasive proliferation of atypical osteoblasts and osteoid formation.

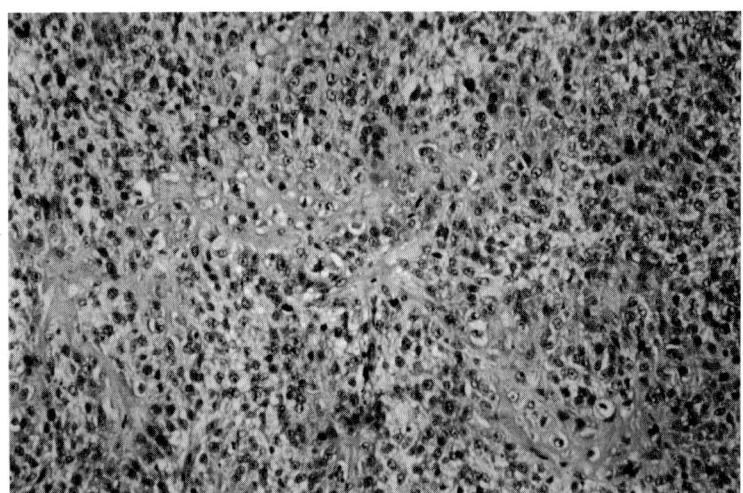

FIGURE 20–95. Canine chondrosarcoma. Proliferation of sarcoma cells with chondroid differentiation.

POSTVACCINAL SARCOMA

• **Cause and Pathogenesis.** The incidence of postvaccinal sarcomas in cats has increased in the last decade.[171, 247, 253–257, 261] Yearly prevalence estimates are 1 to 10 cases/ 10,000 cats.[247, 253] Epidemiologic studies have suggested that feline postvaccinal sarcomas occur most frequently: (1) if vaccines are repeatedly given at the same site, (2) following rabies or FeLV vaccines, and (3) when adjuvated vaccines are used.[247, 252, 253, 255, 261] However, cases have been reported in association with other killed, adjuvated vaccines (e.g., panleukopenia), with modified live vaccines (e.g., herpes-calici-parvo), and with the injection of three drugs (penicillin, metoclopramide, dexamethasone) in the same syringe.[246, 250a, 253, 257] There were no apparent differences in occurrence with different brands of rabies and FeLV vaccines.[247, 253] In one study,[254] the number of postvaccinal sarcomas declined abruptly when a switch was made to modified live virus vaccines.

The macrophages and multinucleated histiocytic giant cells associated with postvaccinal sarcomas contain granular to crystalline, gray-brown to bluish material within their cytoplasm. Electron probe x-ray microanalysis revealed that the material was composed of aluminum and oxygen, and aluminum hydroxide and aluminum phosphate are used as adjuvants in some feline vaccines.[253, 255, 257, 261] It has been hypothesized that the chronic inflammation that follows vaccine reactions, with resultant proliferation of resident fibroblasts and myofibroblasts, causes neoplastic transformation.[246, 251, 255, 257] Thus, postvaccinal granulomatous and necrotizing panniculitides could be viewed as premalignant lesions.[171]

A short-term (4 weeks) study was conducted on the local effects of various vaccines in cats.[260] Specific pathogen–free (SPF) cats were injected with FeLV, rabies, and rhinotracheitis-calicivirus-panleukopenia vaccines, and saline. Repeated physical and cytologic examinations were performed. Only rabies vaccine caused palpable lesions in all cats, and cytologic examination revealed increasing numbers of lymphocytes and macrophages with fewer eosinophils and neutrophils. The macrophages often contain granular to crystalline bluish material in their cytoplasm.

Immunohistochemical and PCR techniques detected FeLV antigen in multicentric feline fibrosarcomas but not in feline postvaccinal sarcomas.[249]

• **Clinical Findings.** Postvaccinal sarcomas develop in younger cats (average 8 years versus 11 years) and are larger (larger than 4 cm diameter) than nonvaccine-associated sarcomas.[248, 252, 261] No breed or sex predilections are known. Postvaccinal sarcomas necessarily occur at sites of vaccination: interscapular area, dorsal neck, shoulder, flank, and femoral area. Nonvaccine-associated sarcomas occur on the head, pinnae, and distal limbs. Postvaccinal sarcomas are usually preceded by postvaccinal panniculitis. The lesions are

1318 • Neoplastic and Non-Neoplastic Tumors

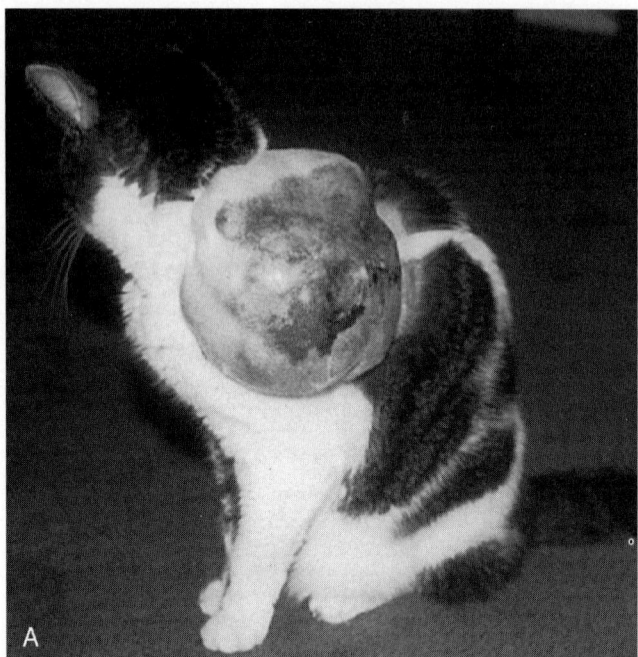

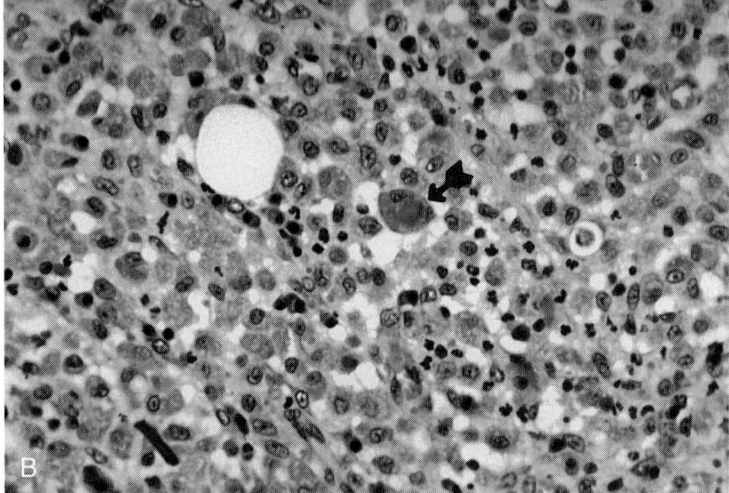

FIGURE 20-96. Feline postvaccinal sarcoma. *A*, Huge tumor over withers and left shoulder. *B*, Granulomatous reaction peripheral to sarcoma contains macrophages and multinucleated histiocytic giant cells (*arrow*) that have phagocytosed an amorphous substance.

irregular in shape, firm, multilobular, and large (larger than 4 cm diameter in over 50% of the cases).[246, 248, 252, 255, 261] They are poorly circumscribed, involve the subcutis (and often the underlying musculature; occasionally the dorsal spinous processes of the underlying vertebrae), and exhibit rapid growth (Fig. 20-96A).

• **Diagnosis.** The sudden occurrence of a tumor at an injection site, often preceded by postvaccinal panniculitis, is highly suggestive. Most masses that occur within 3 weeks following vaccination are granulomatous panniculitides, and these typically resolve within 1 to 3 months. Lesions that persist beyond this time, or show progressive enlargement after 4 weeks, should be aspirated for cytologic examination or biopsied.

Histopathologically, most postvaccinal sarcomas are fibrosarcomas.* Less common neoplastic types include malignant fibrous histiocytoma, rhabdomyosarcoma, osteosarcoma, chondrosarcoma, liposarcoma, myxosarcoma, and myofibroblastic sarcoma. A characteristic

---

*See references 171, 246, 248, 251, 252, 255, 257, 261.

finding with postvaccinal sarcoma is a peripheral granulomatous, often necrotizing, inflammatory response wherein macrophages and multinucleated histiocytic giant cells contain granular to crystalline gray-brown to bluish material within their cytoplasm (see Fig. 20–96B).[246, 248, 251, 252, 257, 261] Lymphoid nodules or eosinophils, or both, may be prominent.

- **Clinical Management.** Postvaccinal sarcomas are locally invasive, poorly demarcated, and recur frequently following surgical excision.[246, 252, 252a, 255–257, 261] Surgery alone, other than amputation where possible, is seldom curative. Recurrent sarcomas tend to be more difficult to excise. In one study,[252] postvaccinal sarcomas recurred in 86% of the cats within 6 months after excision. Twenty-two percent of the cats had two to four recurrences. In contrast, only 14% of nonvaccinal sarcomas recurred after surgical excision.[252] Radical first excision provides a significantly longer interval to first recurrence (325 days) than marginal first excision (79 days).[252a] Excision at a referral institution resulted in a significantly longer interval to first recurrence (274 days) than excision at a referring veterinary clinic (66 days).[252a]

Postvaccinal sarcomas were initially said to metastasize rarely.[252] However, several metastatic sarcomas have been reported.[171, 230, 245, 250, 258, 259] Most of these metastases have been from an interscapular sarcoma and have been of the fibrosarcoma histopathologic type. Metastases have involved lung, liver, mediastinum, and pericardium. More recent studies indicate metastatic rates of 22%[252a] to 24%,[247a] mostly to the lungs, which develop concurrently with or after recurrence of the primary tumor.

It appears that postvaccinal sarcomas are more radiosensitive than nonvaccinal sarcomas, and that radiotherapy may be a useful postsurgical adjunctive therapy.[171, 247a, 255] As a last resort, palliative control may be achieved in some cases with Adriamycin (1 mg/kg every 3 weeks for five or six treatments).[171, 255]

The following measures have been recommended to reduce the frequency of postvaccinal sarcomas in cats and to make epidemiologic studies more useful[252a, 254, 255, 261]:

1. Avoid unnecessary vaccines.
2. Use as little killed vaccines as possible.
3. Do not administer killed vaccines in the interscapular space (harder to excise, higher recurrence rates, decreased survival).
4. Standardize vaccination sites (caudal half of left side of body for FeLV, caudal half of right side of body for rabies).
5. Avoid previous vaccine sites.
6. Maintain detailed records about vaccinations (site, route, vaccine manufacturer, vaccine type, vaccine serial number).
7. Instruct owners to watch for postvaccinal reactions and document their occurrence.
8. If postvaccinal skin reactions (a) persist for more than 3 months, (b) are larger than 2 cm in diameter, or (c) are increasing in size 1 month post-vaccination, recommend biopsy or excision and biopsy. Fine-needle aspirates are *not* reliable.

UNDIFFERENTIATED SARCOMA

- **Cause and Pathogenesis.** Classification of some mesenchymal neoplasms may be difficult or impossible on histopathologic criteria.[5–7, 19] Such anaplastic sarcomas are usually called undifferentiated, or spindle cell, sarcomas. Employing electron microscopy or immunohistochemical (marker) techniques greatly reduces the incidence of such diagnoses, but these are not always available to practitioners, nor are they always economically feasible.

- **Clinical Findings.** Undifferentiated sarcomas usually occur in older dogs and cats and have the clinical features of fibrosarcomas, neurofibrosarcomas, and hemangiopericytomas. An aggressive undifferentiated sarcoma with widespread metastasis was reported in a 6-month-old Neapolitan Mastiff.[264] In cats, undifferentiated sarcoma has been reported to involve the footpads of one or more feet.[35] Affected cats are usually lame, and affected pads are soft, mushy, and painful, and may be ulcerated.

In dogs, an undifferentiated sarcoma has been reported to affect the digit.[262] Affected dogs were 11 to 15 years old and had solitary, soft to firm, variably ulcerated masses involving a digit. Lesions were described as growing out of an ulcerated digital pad or occurring around a claw bed. The tumors caused lameness. Histologically, the tumors appeared to arise in the area of dense collagenous trabeculae located proximal to the fat pad and atrichial sweat glands. The tumor cells had some features of histiocytes: nuclear and cytoplasmic pleomorphism, frequent mitoses, and multinucleate tumor giant cells. Although most of these tumors had neoplastic cells in vessels, no recurrences or metastases were recorded. Tumor cells were positive for vimentin, but negative for desmin, S-100 protein, and histiocyte markers. Electron microscopic examination revealed 200-nm to 400-nm intracytoplasmic secretory granules.

Undifferentiated sarcomas were reported in old dogs on the lower lip at the mucocutaneous junction.[263] The tumors were about 2 to 3 cm in diameter, frequently ulcerated, and metastases (regional lymph node, lung) were recorded in 75% of the cases. Histologically, the tumors were similar to the digit tumors described earlier.[262] Extensive electron microscopic and immunohistochemical studies failed to identify the neoplastic cells. The authors suspected a myelomonocytic origin.

• **Clinical Management.** Radical surgical excision is the treatment of choice for undifferentiated sarcomas.[5, 19] Radiotherapy or chemotherapy alone does not provide adequate control.[23] Radiotherapy plus hyperthermia may be more effective.[183]

Mast Cell Tumor

CAUSE AND PATHOGENESIS

Mast cell tumors (mastocytomas, mast cell sarcomas, or mastocytoses) are common neoplasms of the dog and cat that arise from mast cells.[°] The cause of mast cell tumors is unknown. In dogs (especially puppies), mast cell tumors have been experimentally transmitted using tissues and cell-free extracts, which suggests a viral cause. However, ultrastructural examination of mast cell tumors has only occasionally revealed viral particles. It has been theorized that Boxers and Boston terriers possess oncogenes that are transmitted to offspring and combine with a genetically determined deficiency of immune surveillance to result in an increased incidence of mast cell tumors in these breeds. Rarely, canine mast cell tumor has been thought to arise within scars and chronic dermatoses.[5, 292] Chromosomal fragile site expression, a phenomenon thought to predispose humans genetically to develop certain tumors, have been shown to be increased in boxers with mast cell tumors.[7] In the dog, it has been suggested that abnormalities in the c-kit/c-kit ligand system is involved in the pathogenesis of mast cell tumors.[283, 284b, 293] Mutations of the c-kit gene may lead to an activation of its product, the kit receptor, which leads to uncontrolled proliferation and maturation of mast cell precursors.[283a, 290a] In cats, transmission studies with various mast cell tumor extracts failed to produce neoplasms in normal individuals. Multiple histiocytic mast cell tumors have been described in 6- to 8-week-old Siamese kittens in which multiple kittens of two litters (sired by the same tom) were affected, suggesting a genetic influence.[274]

CLINICAL FINDINGS

Dog

Mast cell tumors occur in dogs at an average age of 8 years but are rarely reported in puppies.[†] There is no apparent sex predilection, but Boxers, Boston terriers, English bulldogs, Bull terriers, Fox terriers, Staffordshire terriers, Labrador retrievers, Dachshunds, Beagles, Pugs, Golden retrievers, Weimaraners, and Shar peis are at increased risk. Shar peis are often younger than other breeds when they develop mast cell tumors (average age, 4 years; 28% are younger than 2 years old).[289] They may also be more likely

---

°See references 1, 2, 4–7, 27, 30, 272, 282, 300.
†See references 1, 2, 4–7, 22, 28, 269, 275, 282, 289, 295.

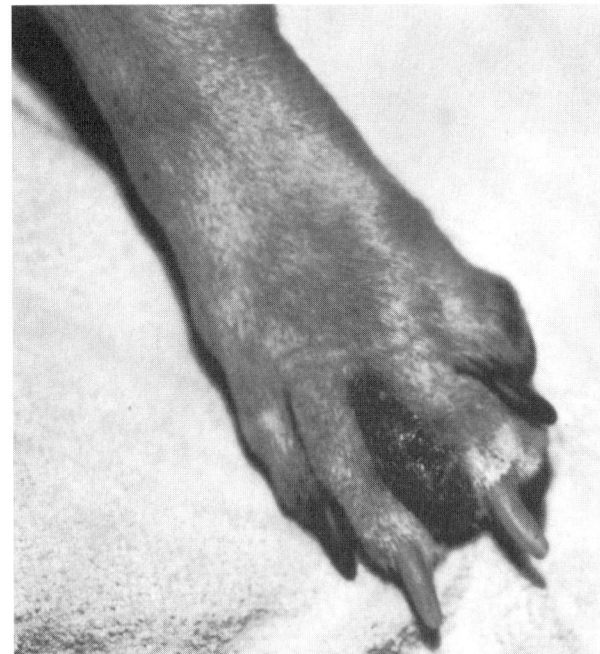

FIGURE 20-97. Canine mast cell tumor. Melanotic interdigital nodule.

to develop multiple lesions. The clinical appearance of mast cell tumors is variable. Lesions may be firm to soft (see Fig. 20–79F), papular to nodular to pedunculated, dermal to subcutaneous in location (see Fig. 20–79G), well to poorly circumscribed, and skin colored to erythematous (see Fig. 20–79H) to hyperpigmented (Fig. 20–97). They vary from a few millimeters to several centimeters in diameter. Some lesions may appear as urticarial swellings or diffuse areas of edema and inflammation resembling cellulitis (Fig. 20–98). Some neoplasms have a pin-feathered appearance (Fig. 20–99) or are

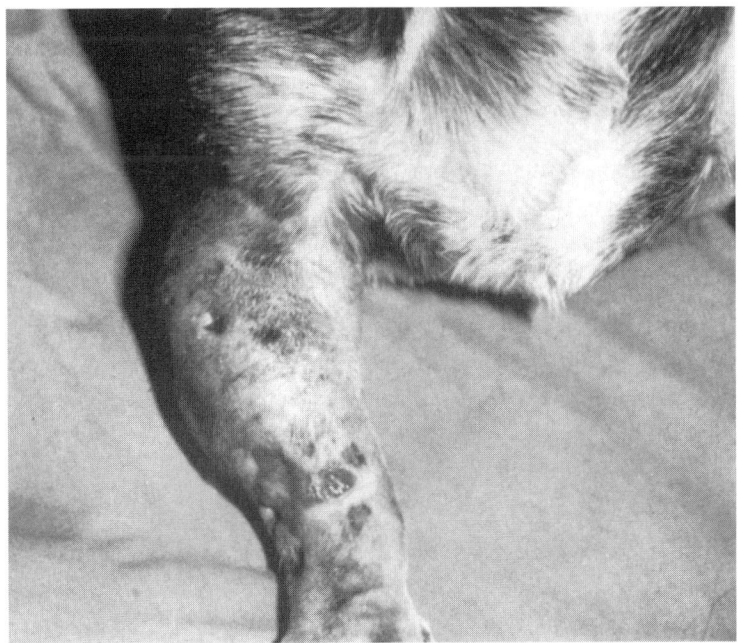

FIGURE 20-98. Canine mast cell tumor. Swollen, cellulitic-appearing forelimb. (Courtesy D. Angarano.)

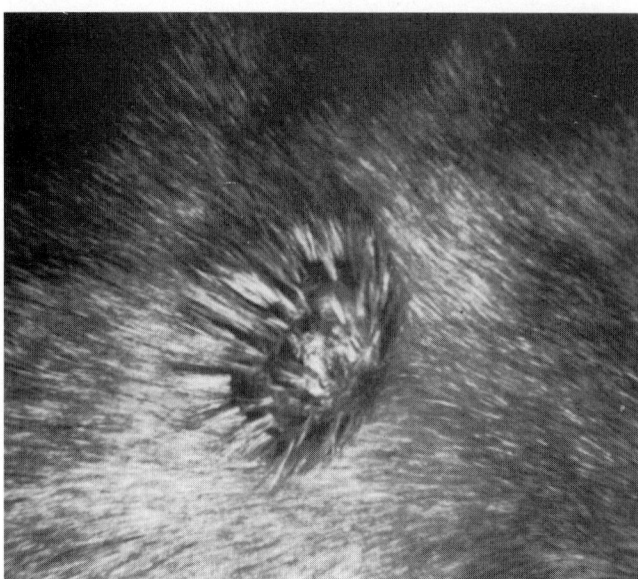

FIGURE 20–99. Canine mast cell tumor. Pin-feathered nodule over stifle region.

ulcerated. Palpation of some lesions may result in release of vasoactive substances and resultant local edema and inflammation (Darier's sign). Flushing (sudden, symmetric, diffuse reddening of large areas of skin) has been rarely reported in dogs with mast cell tumors. Mast cell tumors are usually solitary but may be multicentric either synchronously or sequentially. The neoplasms are distributed as follows: 50% on the trunk, 40% on the extremities, and 10% on the head. Some interesting breed-site predilections have been reported[1]: Boxer (hind limbs, multiple lesions), Boston terrier (hind limb), Rhodesian ridgeback (tail), American Staffordshire terrier (hind limb), Pug (hind limbs, multiple lesions), Weimaraner (multiple lesions), and English setter (head, hind limb). Diffuse mast cell tumor produced gross distention and deformity of the hind limbs in Shar peis.[284a, 285] Noncutaneous symptoms that can be associated with mast cell tumors include gastric and duodenal ulcers, defective blood coagulation, and immune-mediated thrombocytopenia.[4–7, 269, 282]

A case of cutaneous mastocytosis resembling *urticaria pigmentosa* was reported in a puppy.[276] At 3 weeks of age, the dog had multiple cutaneous papules and nodules, pruritus, and lethargy. The lesions were generally alopecic, raised, pink to red, slightly firm, 1 to 5 cm in diameter, and especially numerous on the head, neck, legs, and perineum. By the time the dog was 27 weeks old, the condition resolved spontaneously.

Urticaria pigmentosa–like disease was also reported in two adult dogs.[279] Both had been affected since 6 months to 1 year of age. Papules and nodules would come and go over many areas of the body. Biopsies revealed the accumulation of well-differentiated mast cells in the superficial dermis and very few eosinophils. Occasionally, erythematous rashes that would progress to wheals or bullae would appear and disappear within hours. Traumatizing the lesions could produce sudden increase in size (edema), and stroking normal skin could result in a wheal-and-flare response (Darier's sign). Both dogs were otherwise healthy and were followed for several years. The lesions were responsive to glucocorticoids, and to a combination of H_1- and H_2-blocking antihistamines.

Cat

Mast cell tumors occur in cats at an average age of 10 years, although kittens can be affected.[1, 30, 272, 284, 290, 300] Male and Siamese cats are apparently predisposed.[1, 282] Lesions occur most commonly on the head and the neck. The clinical appearance of mast cell tumors is variable: (1) multiple raised, soft, round, poorly demarcated, edematous, pinkish, variable-sized (0.5 to 5 cm in diameter) masses that are fixed to the overlying skin; (2) multiple raised, firm, round, well-circumscribed, white to yellow, small (2 to 10 mm in diameter) papules and nodules that are fixed to the overlying skin (Fig. 20–100A); (3) single or multiple raised, firm, erythematous, well-circumscribed, variable-sized (1 to 7 cm in diameter) plaques (Fig. 20–100B) that are frequently ulcerated and pruritic; and (4) solitary, firm to soft, well-circumscribed, variable-sized (0.3 to 3 cm in diameter), often alopecic dermal masses, some of which grossly mimic sebaceous gland tumors. Occasionally, solitary mast cell tumors may spontaneously resolve, only to be followed by a new tumor at a different location (Fig. 20–100C).[35, 272, 290, 300] A case of diffuse cutaneous mastocytosis in a 1-year-old cat was reported.[271] Generalized pruritus, papules, and erosions were present.

Urticaria pigmentosa is a proliferative mast cell disorder of humans.[5, 299] A syndrome with some clinicopathologic similarities to the human disorder has been seen in cats (see Chap. 12).

A histiocytic subtype of mast cell tumor occurs primarily in Siamese cats from 6 weeks to 4 years of age.[2, 30, 274, 300] Multiple firm, pinkish papules and nodules occur primarily on the head and pinnae (Fig. 20–101) and eventually spontaneously regress.

Noncutaneous symptoms that may be associated with feline mast cell tumors include gastric and duodenal ulcers (thought to be histamine induced) and defective blood coagulation (thought to be heparin induced).

DIAGNOSIS

This is one tumor in which stained impression smears or aspirates are useful in establishing a tentative immediate diagnosis (Fig. 20–102).[7, 43, 45] However, anaplastic and histiocytic mast cells may not contain the distinctive cytoplasmic granules. Hence, cytologic examination should not replace a complete histologic examination. Smears of cutaneous mast cell tumors in cats may reveal endocytosis of erythrocytes by the neoplastic mast cells.

Histologically, mast cell tumors are characterized by a diffuse to multinodular proliferation of mast cells (Figs. 20–103 and 20–104).[1, 2, 23] Frequent findings in canine mast cell tumors include tissue eosinophilia, focal areas of collagen degeneration, and a wide variety of vascular lesions (hyalinization, fibrinoid degeneration, and eosinophilic vasculitis) (Fig. 20–105). Even highly malignant tumors usually have a low mitotic index, making this an insensitive measure of tumor behavior.[295] In cats, special caution is warranted to avoid confusing mast cell tumors with other round cell tumors and eosinophilic plaques. However, the striking tissue eosinophilia and collagen degeneration seen commonly in canine mast cell tumors is rare in cats.[1, 30, 272, 300] The histiocytic mast cell tumor in cats (especially Siamese) often has a granulomatous appearance (Figs. 20–106A and B), and the diagnosis can be confirmed only by electron microscopic demonstration of mast cell granules in some cases.[1, 2, 300] Canine mast cell tumors were subjected to several special stains.[294] No stain was ideal, and all stains became less effective as tumor cells become less differentiated. Feline mast cell tumors were negative for tryptase and erratically positive for chymase.[267] Mast cell tumors are positive for vimentin, α_1-antitrypsin, chymotrypsin–like protease, and dipeptidyl peptidase II.[49, 54, 56, 59] Recent investigations suggest that c-kit can be used as a reliable immunohistochemical marker for canine mast cells and mast cell tumors.[293]

CLINICAL MANAGEMENT

Clinical management of mast cell tumors may include surgical excision, cryosurgery, electrosurgery, chemotherapy, radiotherapy, immunotherapy, and some combination of these.[4–7, 281, 282, 297, 298] In dogs, mast cell tumors should always be treated as potentially malignant neoplasms, because metastasis occurs in about 30% of cases (especially regional lymph nodes, spleen, liver, and bone marrow). Tumors arising from the perineum, the

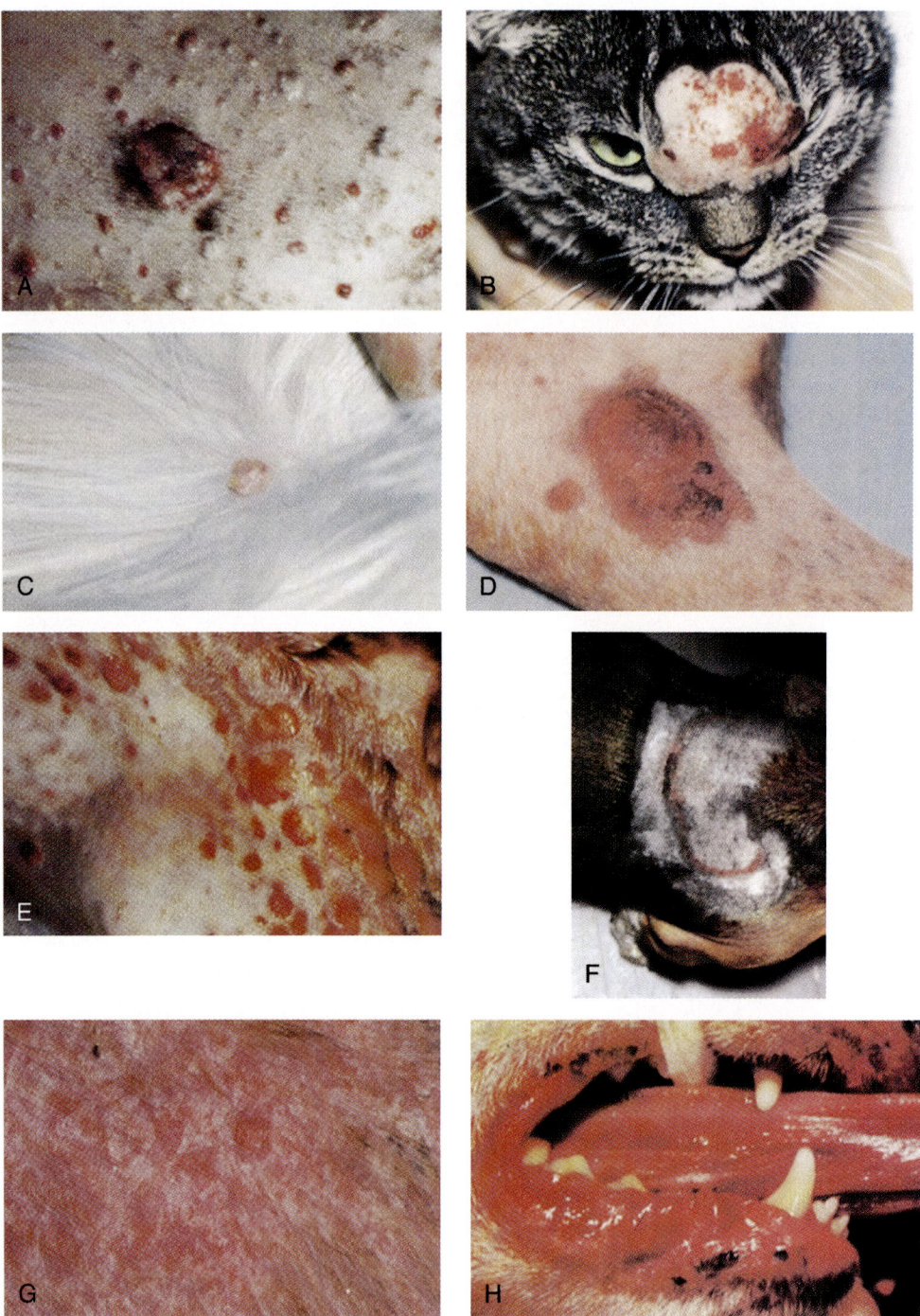

FIGURE 20-100. *A*, Feline mast cell tumor. Multiple papular-to-nodular lesions over the thorax (the area has been clipped). *B*, Feline mast cell tumor. Large, ulcerated nodule between the eyes. *C*, Feline mast cell tumor. Small, yellowish papule resembling a sebaceous gland tumor. *D*, Canine nonepitheliotropic lymphoma. Large erythematous plaques and multiple erythematous papules on a medial hind limb. *E*, Feline nonepitheliotropic lymphoma. Multiple erythematous plaques on the abdomen. *F*, Canine nonepitheliotropic lymphoma. Raised, erythematous lesion in the shape of an arc or **C** over the withers (the area has been shaved). *G*, Canine epitheliotropic lymphoma (mycosis fungoides). Erythroderma, alopecia, and scales. *H*, Canine epitheliotropic lymphoma (pagetoid reticulosis). Erythema, infiltration, and ulceration of the lips.

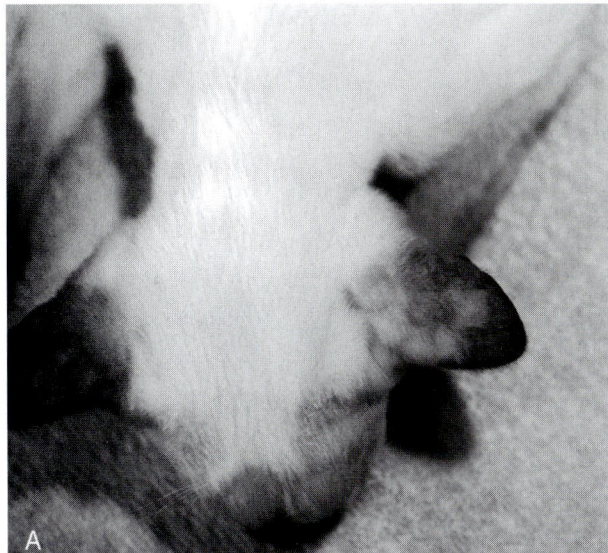
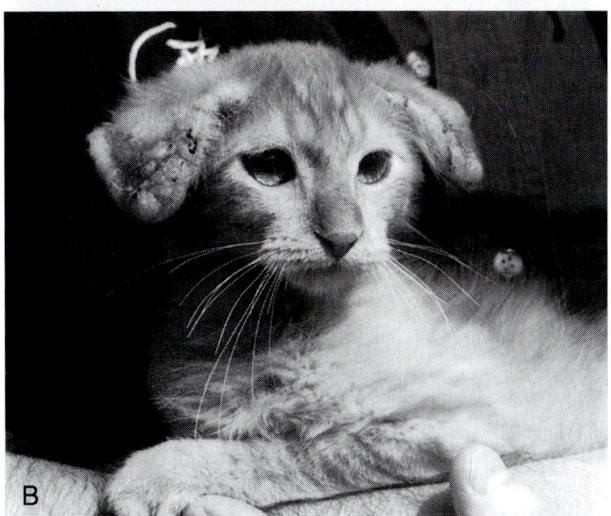

FIGURE 20-101. Feline histiocytic mast cell tumor. *A*, Siamese kitten with multiple papules and nodules on pinnae and forehead. *B*, Domestic shorthair kitten with multiple, coalescent lesions that have caused both pinnae to droop. (Courtesy B. Kieger.)

prepuce, the scrotum, mucocutaneous sites, and the digits are more commonly aggressive and malignant. Prognosis is based on tumor growth rate, tumor site, local tumor recurrence, systemic signs, tumor staging, previous chemotherapy, histologic grading, AgNOR frequency, and Ki-67 positivity.[264a, 269, 277b, 278a, 280, 282, 295, 295a] However, biological behavior is not always predictable. In general, Boxers have a better prognosis, mainly because they have significantly more well-differentiated mast cell tumors.[269, 282] In general, Shar peis have a worse prognosis, because they have more poorly differentiated mast cell tumors.[289] A histologic grading system (Table 20–4) and a clinical staging system (Table 20–5) have been developed for canine mast cell tumors. The recommended therapeutic approach for each canine mast cell tumor case is based on an amalgamation of these systems (Table 20–6). The clinical staging system is predicated on the results of studies of lymph node and bone marrow aspirates, as well as buffy coat examinations. However, mast cells may be found in lymph node and bone marrow aspirates from normal dogs, as well as buffy coat smears from dogs with allergic and ectoparasitic skin disease.[273] On the basis of results of quantitative buffy coat evaluations, the severity of mastocytemia in dogs without mast cell tumors often exceeds that during tumor staging in dogs with mast cell tumors,

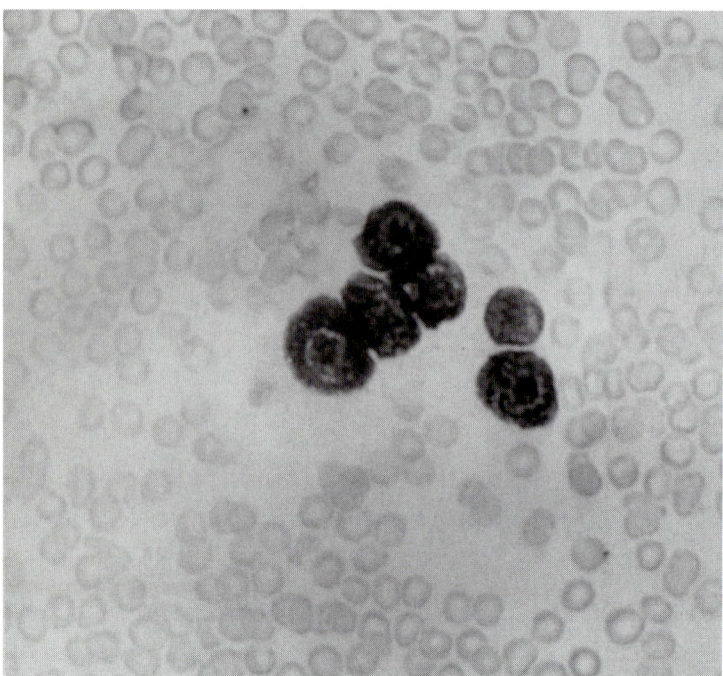

FIGURE 20–102. Canine mast cell tumor. Aspiration of a skin nodule reveals a clump of mast cells.

and random detection of mast cells in blood smears during hemogram determination in dogs is usually *not* secondary to mast cell tumor.[288a]

Early surgical excision is indicated in animals with a solitary neoplasm. Wide surgical margins, at least 3 cm between the palpable tumor and the incision, are recommended when possible. Approximately 50% of canine mast cell tumors recur, even after a wide

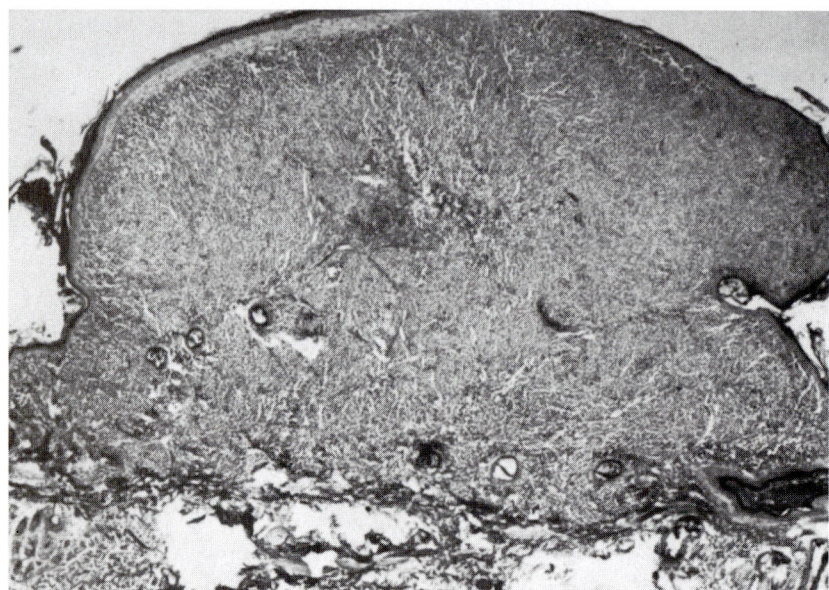

FIGURE 20–103. Feline mast cell tumor. Well-circumscribed, dome-shaped proliferation of mast cells.

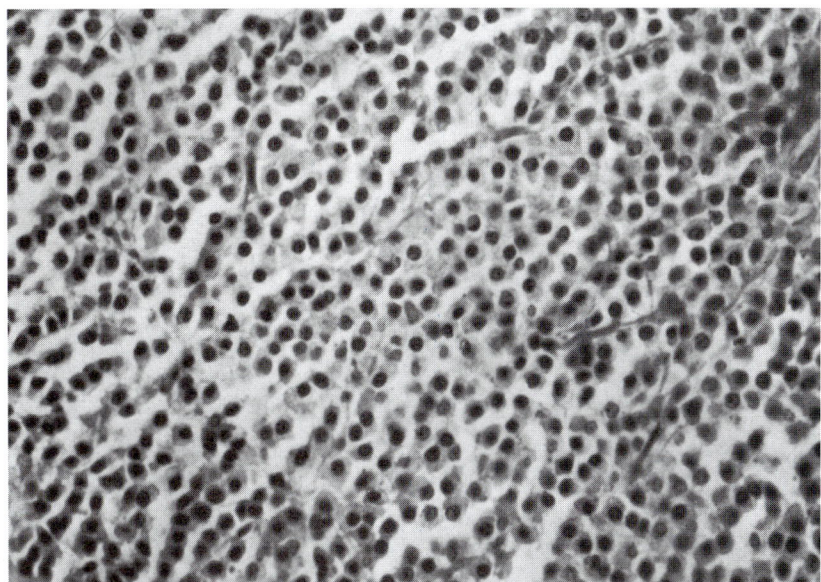

FIGURE 20–104. Close-up of Figure 20–103. Proliferation of monomorphous mast cells.

surgical excision, usually within 4 months.[4–7, 269, 270, 282, 295] Presurgical treatment with intralesional or systemic glucocorticoids, or both, may decrease tumor volume and local swelling and inflammation, thus helping to achieve adequate excision.[282] Presurgical radiotherapy or intralesional deionized water might accomplish this, as well.[282] In dogs with mast cell tumors, the survival time is related to the degree of histologic differentiation.[270, 282, 286, 291, 296] For animals with high-grade mast cell tumors, the mean survival time is 18 weeks after diagnosis; with intermediate-grade tumors, 28 weeks; and with low-grade tumors, 51 weeks. However, some veterinary pathologists believe that tumor grade is

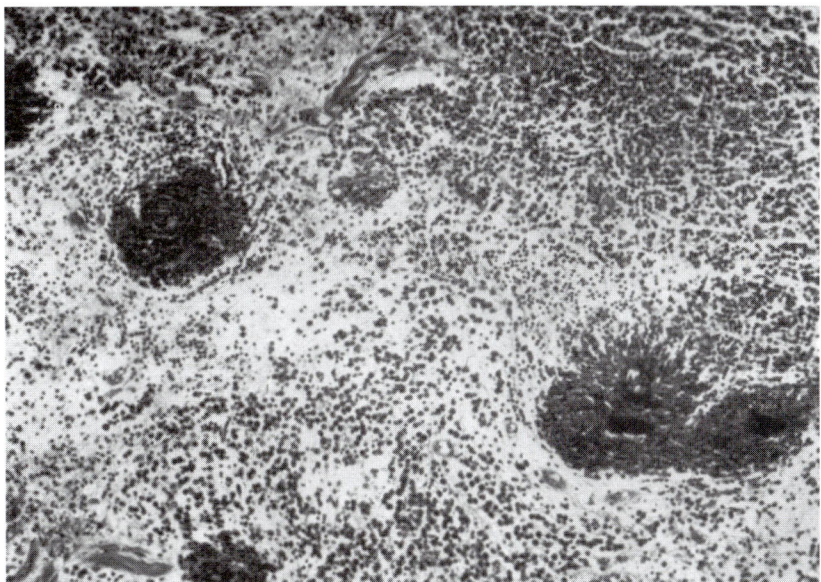

FIGURE 20–105. Canine mast cell tumor. Diffuse proliferation of mast cells, marked edema, and multifocal areas of collagenolysis.

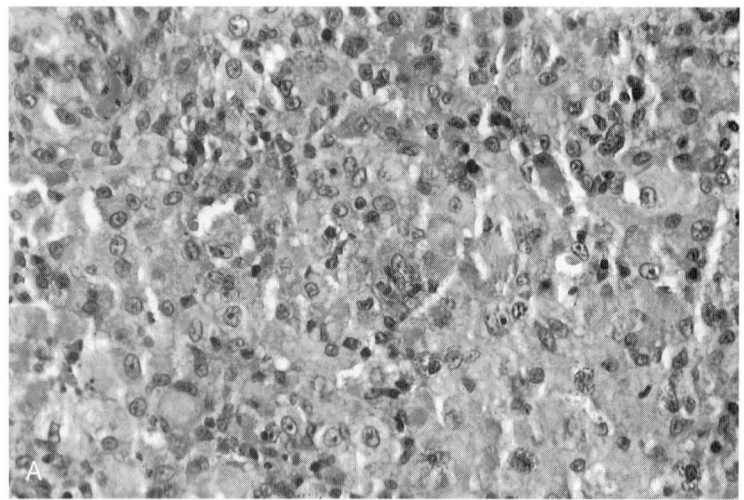
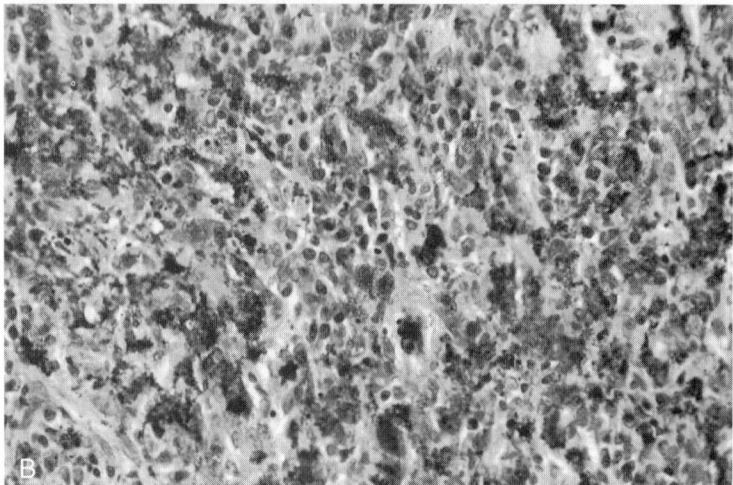

FIGURE 20-106. Feline histiocytic mast cell tumor. *A*, Mast cell cytoplasmic granules do not stain with H & E. *B*, Mast cell cytoplasmic granules stain with AOG.

● Table 20-4 **HISTOLOGIC CLASSIFICATION OF MAST CELL TUMORS**

GRADE	MICROSCOPIC DESCRIPTION
High (anaplastic, Grade I,[270] Grade III[291])	Highly cellular, indistinct cytoplasmic boundaries: irregular size and shape of nuclei, often frequent mitotic figures; low number of cytoplasmic granules
Intermediate (intermediate differentiation, Grade II,[270] Grade II[291])	Closely packed cells with indistinct cytoplasmic boundaries; nucleus to cytoplasm ratio lower than that of high grade; mitotic figures infrequent; more granules than in high-grade tumors
Low (well differentiated, Grade III,[270] Grade I[291])	Clearly defined cytoplasmic boundary with regular, spherical, or ovoid nucleus; mitotic figures rare; cytoplasmic granules large, deep staining, and plentiful

● Table 20–5 **CLINICAL STAGING SYSTEM FOR MAST CELL TUMORS**

Stage	
Stage I	One tumor confined to the dermis without regional lymph node involvement a. Without systemic signs b. With systemic signs
Stage II	One tumor confined to dermis with regional lymph node involvement a. Without systemic signs b. With systemic signs
Stage III	Multiple dermal tumors; large infiltrating tumors with or without regional lymph node involvement a. Without systemic signs b. With systemic signs
Stage IV	Any tumor with distant metastasis or recurrence with metastasis

From Tams TR, Macy DW: Canine mast cell tumors. Comp Cont Educ 3:873, 1981.

often an unreliable prognostic indicator and are reluctant to grade these neoplasms.[1, 295] Histologic grade does not always correctly predict biological behavior (benign versus malignant), especially in intermediate grades, which are the most frequent type.[264a]

DNA ploidy status of canine mast cells tumors was not found to be of prognostic significance.[266] In one study,[295] three methods were simultaneously evaluated for their prognostic significance in dogs: histologic grading, argyrophilic nucleolar organizer regions (AgNOR), and antiproliferating cell nuclear antigen (PCNA). A combination of the three methods was superior to any method alone, and these methods accurately predicted outcome in about 80% of the cases. PCNA was best at distinguishing between recurrent, nonrecurrent, and metastatic tumors. In another study,[264a] the number of Ki-67 positive nuclei was significantly and inversely associated with patient survival, whereas PCNA was less accurate. Immunohistochemical detection of p53 tumor-suppressor protein was not associated with histologic grade, tumor location, breed, tumor recurrence, or survival time.[277b, 278a] The AgNOR method was compared on fine-needle aspirate and biopsy specimens, and results correlated well.[280]

Radiotherapy is effective for mast cell tumors.[4–7, 298] When orthovoltage or megavoltage radiotherapy is given postsurgically for intermediate grade (grade II) mast cell tumors in dogs, 94% to 97% of the animals were disease free for 1 year, 93% for 3 years, and 86% for 5 years.[265, 277] Results are significantly worse for high-grade mast cell tumors.[277, 298]

In cats, the vast majority of cutaneous mast cell tumors are benign.[2, 30, 272, 282, 290, 300] A histologic grading system similar to that used in dogs was evaluated in feline mast cell tumors and found not to correlate with biological behavior.[272, 290] The authors have followed some cats with cutaneous mast cell tumors and positive buffy coats for years with no signs of systemic disease. In one study,[290] there was no significant difference between

● Table 20–6 **SUGGESTED TREATMENT OF MAST CELL TUMORS BASED ON CLINICAL STAGES**

STAGE	TREATMENT
I	Surgical excision only. (Surgery is defined as the excision of the tumor with a minimum margin of 3 cm between palpable tumor and the incision line; such excision should include regional lymph node when possible.)
II	Surgical excision plus radiation.
III	Intralesional steroids plus cimetidine. (Intralesional steroid is defined as the intralesional injection of 1 mg of triamcinolone for every centimeter diameter of tumor. This dose is to be administered every 2 weeks.)
IV	Systemic steroids° plus cimetidine.†

°A dose of 0.5 mg/kg of body weight of prednisolone to be administered every 24 to 48 hours.
†Cimetidine should be given daily at a dose of 4 mg/kg q6h.
From Tams TR, Macy DW: Canine mast cell tumors. Comp Cont Educ 3:876, 1981.

complete or incomplete surgical excision and recurrence! The histiocytic mast cell tumor of cats, which is often characterized clinically by multiple cutaneous nodules in Siamese cats younger than 4 years, undergoes spontaneous remission frequently.[2, 30, 274, 300] Adult, non-Siamese cats with widespread lesions are more likely to have visceral involvement.[268]

Chemotherapy has been advocated for disseminated mast cell tumors.[4–7] Administration of oral prednisolone or prednisone (0.5 mg/kg q24h) or intralesional triamcinolone (1 mg for every 1 cm of diameter of tumor) has been recommended (see Table 20–4). This treatment may cause temporary regression of the tumors that may last a few to several months. Only 20% of the dogs with mast cell tumors responded to 1 mg/kg/day prednisone administered for 28 days, and responses were transient.[287] Combination chemotherapy (glucocorticoids plus cyclophosphamide, vincristine, or vinblastine, for example) has been recommended by some investigators. A cyclophosphamide-vinblastine-prednisone combination produced a 78% response rate (all partial responses) with a median survival time of 150 days in dogs with metastatic mast cell tumors.[276a] A cyclophosphamide-vincristine-prednisone-hydroxyurea combination produced a 60% response rate (mostly partial responses) with a median response duration of only 53 days in dogs with measurable mast cell tumors.[277a] A vinblastine-prednisone combination produced a 47% response rate with a median response duration of 153 days.[295a] Lomustine produced predominantly partial and temporary responses (mean 109 days) in 42% of treated dogs.[293a] Only 7% of the dogs with mast cell tumors responded to vincristine, and all responses were only partial.[288]

Cimetidine (4 mg/kg orally q6h) has been recommended in dogs with evidence of systemic or lymph node involvement or with evidence of gastrointestinal hemorrhage. Cimetidine acts by competitively inhibiting the action of histamine on the H_2 receptors of gastric parietal cells, thus reducing gastric acid output and concentration.

Deionized (distilled) water is hypo-osmotic and oncolytic. It has been injected into the surgical margins following removal of canine mast cell tumors.[269, 278] The recurrence rate with surgery alone was 52.6%, whereas that with surgery plus deionized water was 26.2%.[278] In addition, small (smaller than 0.25 cm^3) mast cell tumors were injected intralesionally, and all regressed.[278] Injections are usually administered every 1 to 3 weeks for four treatments. In another study, deionized water was of no benefit, although none of the dogs received as many as four postsurgical treatments.[278b] The treatments are painful and usually require heavy sedation, local anesthesia, or general anesthesia.

In dogs, there is a frequent tendency for local hemorrhage during surgery and delayed wound healing at the site of tumor removal.[1, 4–7, 269, 395] Cryosurgery, hyperthermia, or manipulation may rarely precipitate a shocklike reaction in dogs that have not been pretreated with antihistamines.[1, 4–7, 269, 282]

LYMPHOHISTIOCYTIC NEOPLASMS

Tumors of Lymphocytic Origin

LYMPHOMA

Cutaneous lymphoma (malignant lymphoma, lymphosarcoma, lymphoreticular neoplasm, lymphomatosis, or reticulum cell sarcoma) is an uncommon malignant cutaneous neoplasm of the dog and cat.* In cats, the cause of most types of lymphoma is FeLV, although cats with cutaneous lymphoma are usually FeLV negative. Recently, it was reported that 40% of the feline cutaneous lymphomas tested were positive for FeLV antigen by immunohistochemical or PCR techniques.[315] In dogs, the cause of lymphoma is unknown, although (1) lymphoma can be transmitted to puppies by the injection of whole-cell preparations of malignant lymphocytes, (2) C-type viruses were found in neoplastic cells

---

*See references 1, 2, 4–7, 14, 35, 317.

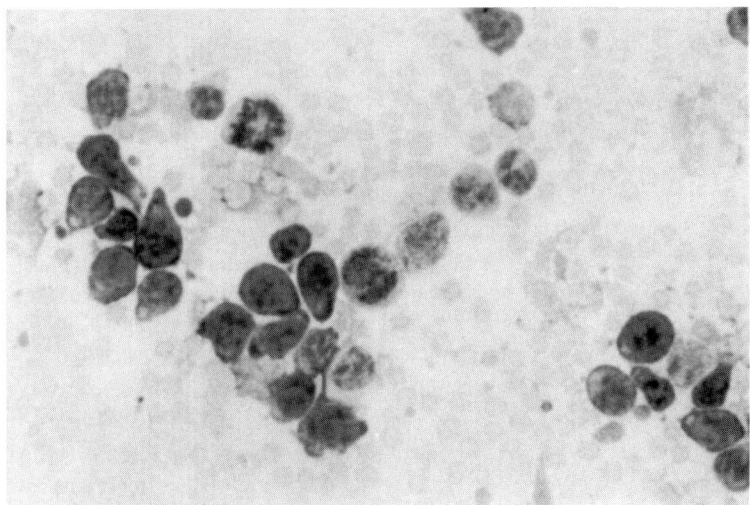

FIGURE 20–107. Canine epitheliotropic lymphoma. Aspirate from a skin nodule reveals pleomorphic, atypical lymphocytes.

from dogs with lymphoma, and (3) lymphoma has been induced in neonatal puppies by injections of FeLV.[4–7, 312, 312a]

Histologically, lymphoma can be divided into nonepitheliotropic and epitheliotropic forms.[57] The epitheliotropic lymphomas are a subset of cutaneous T cell lymphomas. Mycosis fungoides and its associated leukemia, the Sézary syndrome, account for the majority of cases of epidermotropic cutaneous T cell lymphoma. pagetoid reticulosis (Woringer-Kolopp and Ketron-Goodman types) is a T cell lymphoma in which the lymphoid infiltrate is almost entirely confined to the epidermis in the early stages of the disease. Nonepitheliotropic cutaneous lymphomas are large-cell lymphomas of the dermis and subcutis, and are a heterogeneous group with respect to immunophenotype. In humans, B cell lymphomas may rarely be epitheliotropic, thus mimicking clinically and histopathologically the T cell lymphomas.[307a] In addition, nonepitheliotropic cutaneous lymphomas may be of T cell origin.[304a] One study suggested that immunocytochemical studies of cytospin preparations of fine-needle aspirates provided a practical, economical, and accurate method for the diagnosis and phenotyping of canine lymphoma.[307]

Cytologic examination of aspirates reveals pleomorphic, atypical lymphocytes (Fig. 20–107).

Nonepitheliotropic Cutaneous Lymphoma

Nonepitheliotropic cutaneous lymphoma occurs in older dogs and cats with no sex predilection.* In dogs, Boxers, St. Bernards, Basset hounds, Irish setters, Cocker spaniels, German shepherd dogs, Golden retrievers, and Scottish terriers appear to be predisposed. Nonepitheliotropic cutaneous lymphoma is the most common form of cutaneous lymphoma in the cat but is the least common form in the dog.[57]

Nonepitheliotropic cutaneous lymphoma is usually generalized or multifocal and has a variety of cutaneous manifestations. Nodules are present in virtually all cases; they are firm, dermal or subcutaneous, often alopecic and red to purple (see Fig. 20–100D and E).[35, 304] Exfoliative erythroderma is present in about 20% of cases, but pruritus and oral mucosal involvement are rare.[304] Occasionally, lesions are present in bizarre, arciform, or serpiginous shapes (see Fig. 20–100F).[5, 303] Rarely, dogs and cats may have solitary skin lesions. Affected animals usually have signs of systemic involvement. Rarely, nonepitheliotropic cutaneous lymphoma is associated with monoclonal or biclonal gammopathies,

---

*See references 1, 2, 4–7, 14, 35, 306, 317.

1332 • Neoplastic and Non-Neoplastic Tumors

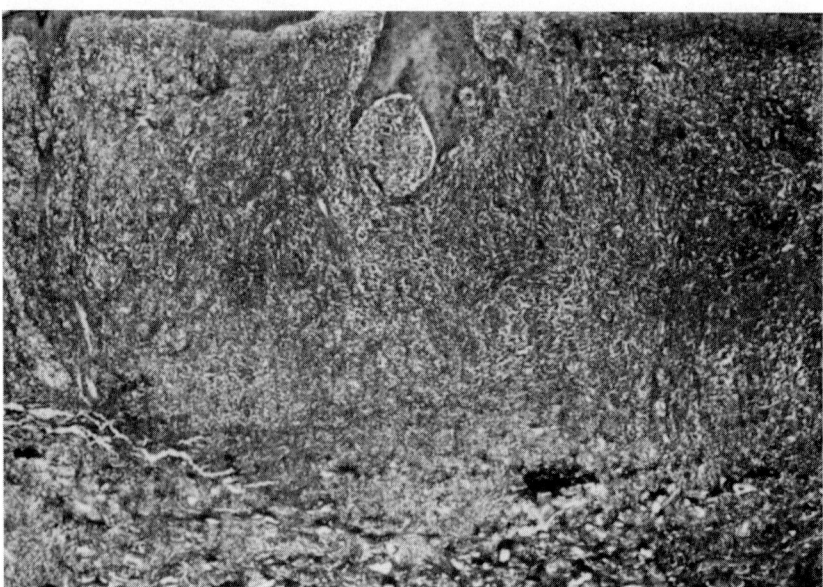

FIGURE 20–108. Feline nonepitheliotropic lymphoma. Diffuse dermal and subcutaneous infiltration of neoplastic lymphocytes.

serum hyperviscosity, or hypercalcemia.[4–7] Symmetric cutaneous necrosis and sloughing of the hind paws was seen in association with multicentric lymphoma in a cat.[301] Progression of the lesions is rapid, with lymph node and systemic metastasis.

Histologically, nonepitheliotropic cutaneous lymphomas are characterized by diffuse dermal and subcutaneous infiltration by malignant lymphocytes (Fig. 20–108). These malignant lymphocytes are lymphocytic (well differentiated or poorly differentiated), lymphoblastic, histiocytic (most common), or "clear cell" in cytologic form (Figs. 20–107 to 20–109).[1, 2, 4–7, 57] In dogs, most nonepitheliotropic cutaneous lymphomas are T cell

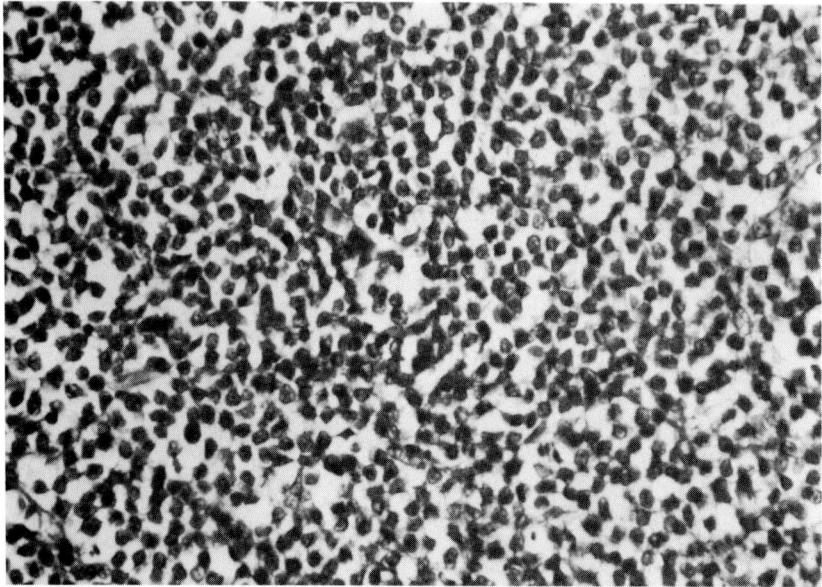

FIGURE 20–109. Close-up of Figure 20–108. Neoplastic lymphocytes.

lymphomas, often of a CD4 to CD8 phenotype.[57, 308] Some are classified as non-T, non-B cell cutaneous lymphomas (null cell lymphomas?).[57] Rarely, these lymphomas may be B cell lymphomas.[308] In cats, most nonepitheliotropic cutaneous lymphomas are T cell lymphomas,[308, 315] and 40% of those tested have been positive for FeLV antigen by immunohistochemical or PCR methodology.[315]

Clinical management of nonepitheliotropic cutaneous lymphoma is usually unsuccessful.[4–7, 57, 304] Traditional regimens of combined chemotherapy or chemoimmunotherapy may occasionally induce short-term (average, 8 months) remission. Rarely, surgical excision of a solitary cutaneous lymphoma lesion results in long-term remission or, perhaps, cure. The average survival from the onset of skin lesions to death (usually due to euthanasia) is about 4 months.[304]

Epitheliotropic Cutaneous Lymphoma

Epitheliotropic cutaneous lymphoma is an uncommon cutaneous malignancy of dogs and cats.° Epitheliotropic cutaneous lymphomas are usually of T lymphocyte origin.† In most instances, the cause of epitheliotropic lymphomas is unknown. There is controversy about whether human mycosis fungoides, the prototypic epitheliotropic (T cell) lymphoma, begins as a reactive process or as a neoplastic process.[5, 318] In human adult T cell leukemia-lymphoma, the causative factor is believed to be the human T cell lymphotrophic virus type I.[5] Epitheliotropic lymphoma of dogs and cats is of unknown etiology, and all affected cats have been serologically negative for FeLV. However, tumor DNA was extracted from a cat with epitheliotropic cutaneous T cell lymphoma, amplified for FeLV provirus by PCR, and shown to be positive.[330] This suggests that FeLV may be involved in the etiology of epitheliotropic cutaneous T cell lymphoma in cats, even when cats test negative with commonly used methods of detecting FeLV antigen in blood.

Epitheliotropic cutaneous lymphoma encompasses a spectrum of disease, including mycosis fungoides, Sézary syndrome, and pagetoid reticulosis.[57]

Mycosis Fungoides

In dogs and cats, mycosis fungoides usually affects older animals (average of 9 to 11 years), with no apparent breed or sex predilections. Four clinical presentations are described: (1) generalized pruritic erythema and scaling (exfoliative erythroderma) (see Fig. 20–100G), which is usually misdiagnosed as allergy, scabies, or seborrhea; (2) mucocutaneous erythema, infiltration, depigmentation, and ulceration (see Fig. 20–100H, Fig. 20–110A and B, and Fig. 20–111), which is usually misdiagnosed as immune-mediated disease (pemphigus vulgaris, bullous pemphigoid, or lupus erythematosus); (3) solitary or multiple cutaneous plaques or nodules (Fig. 20–110C and D); and (4) infiltrative and ulcerative oral mucosal disease, which is usually misdiagnosed as a non-neoplastic, chronic stomatitis (Fig. 20–110E).‡ Footpads may be hyperkeratotic, ulcerated, or depigmented (Fig. 20–112). Affected animals often have peripheral lymphadenopathy and signs of systemic illness. In cats, lesions may be initially well-circumscribed, annular areas of alopecia, erythema, and scaling (usually misdiagnosed as dermatophytosis or demodicosis) (Fig. 20–110F).[5, 302] Rarely, dogs have lesions isolated to the lips, nasal planum, nasal philtrum, or anus.[318, 319] Mycosis fungoides developed within the lesions of alopecia mucinosa in cats (see Chap. 11)

Histopathologically, mycosis fungoides is characterized by epitheliotropism, Pautrier microabscesses (focal accumulations of pleomorphic, atypical lymphocytes within the epithelium) (Figs. 20–113 and 20–114), and the presence of mycosis cells (large, 20μ to 30μ lymphocytes with hyperchromatic, indented or folded nuclei) and Sézary, or Lutzner, cells (smaller, 8μ to 20μ lymphocytes that have markedly hyperconvoluted nuclei with numerous finger-like projections, producing a classic cerebriform appearance).[1, 2, 5, 302, 328, 330]

°See references 1, 2, 5, 302, 317, 332, 334.
†See references 57, 302, 308, 309, 312, 313, 318, 319, 330.
‡See references 5, 57, 302, 304, 308, 319, 332, 334.

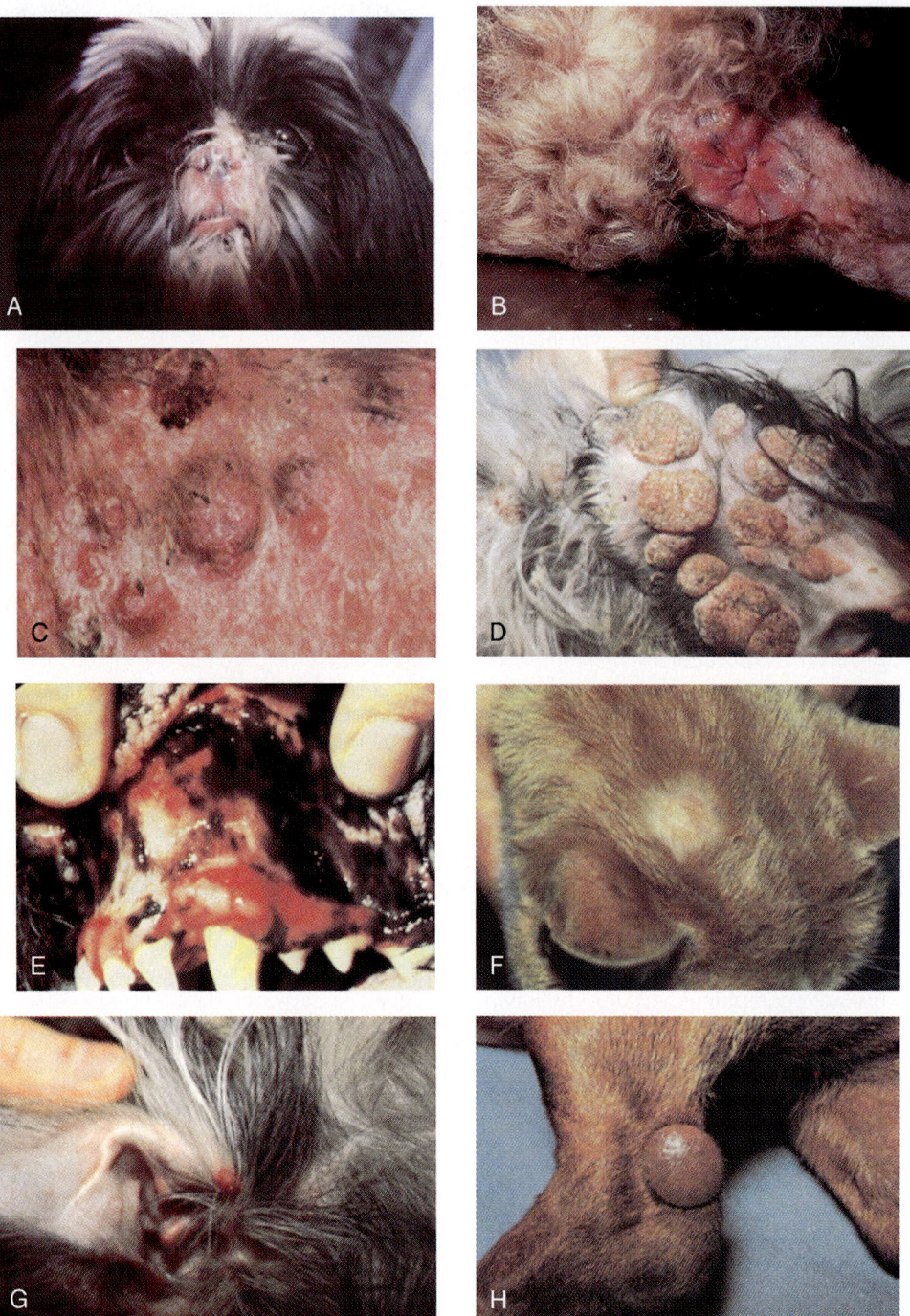

FIGURE 20–110. *A*, Canine epitheliotropic lymphoma. Depigmentation, infiltration, and mild erythema of the nose and lips. *B*, Canine epitheliotropic lymphoma. Anus is infiltrated and ulcerated. *C*, Canine epitheliotropic lymphoma. Numerous nodules, some of which are ulcerated and crusted, on a background of exfoliative erythroderma. *D*, Canine epitheliotropic lymphoma. Numerous cauliflower-like nodules on the pinna with background skin that appears normal. *E*, Canine epitheliotropic lymphoma. Infiltration and ulceration of the oral mucosa. *F*, Feline epitheliotropic lymphoma. Annular area of alopecia, scaling, and mild erythema on the head. *G*, Canine plasmacytoma. Erythematous papule at the base of the ear. *H*, Canine histiocytoma. Characteristic button tumor on the hock.

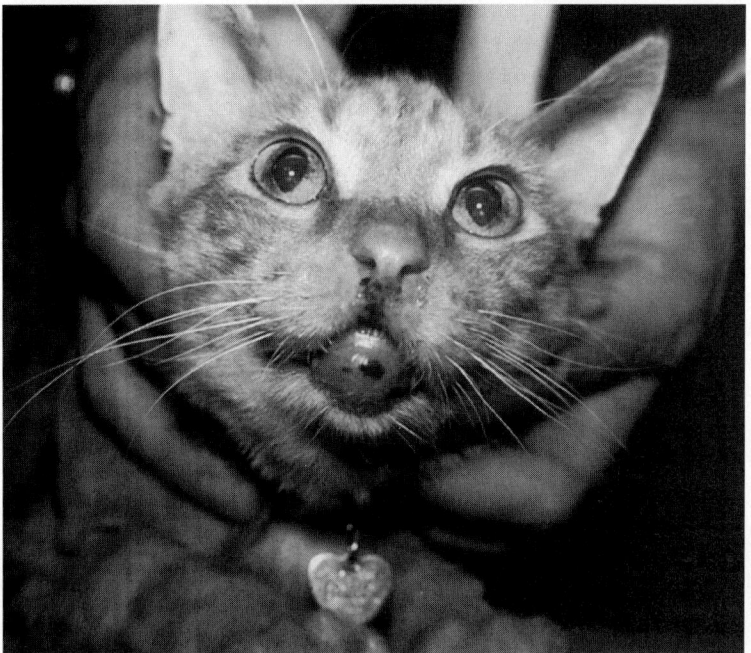

FIGURE 20–111. Feline epitheliotropic lymphoma. Alopecia and infiltration of muzzle and chin.

In dogs, the neoplastic lymphocytes are often more "histiocytic" in appearance than in humans.[318, 319] Often, a lichenoid band of pleomorphic lymphoid cells, with or without plasma cells, neutrophils, and eosinophils, is present in the superficial dermis and surrounding appendages. Epidermal mucinosis (acid mucopolysaccharides) and mild fibrosis of the immediate subepidermal superficial dermis may be seen. In dogs, there is a striking tropism for hair follicles and epitrichial sweat glands, unlike what is seen in humans.[318, 319] In addition, epidermotropism is still prominent in the tumor stage, unlike what is seen in humans.[318, 319]

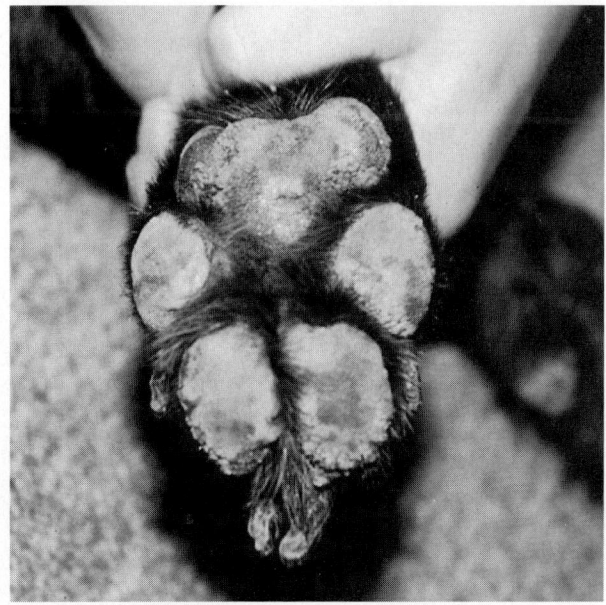

FIGURE 20–112. Canine epitheliotropic lymphoma. Hyperkeratotic, depigmented, infiltrated footpads.

1336 • Neoplastic and Non-Neoplastic Tumors

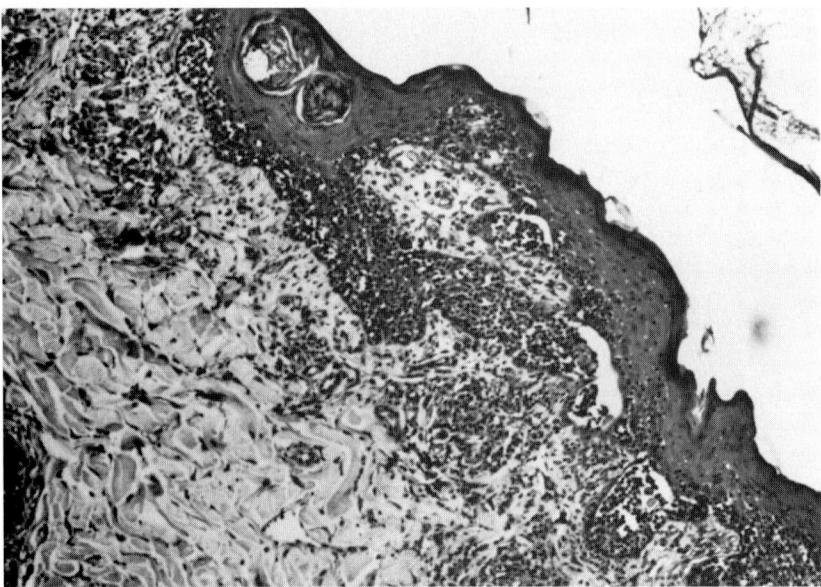

FIGURE 20–113. Canine epitheliotropic lymphoma. Infiltration of the lower portion of the epidermis with neoplastic lymphocytes.

The histopathologic distinction between mycosis fungoides and benign lymphocytic dermatoses can be difficult to impossible. Large studies in humans have shown that certain histopathologic findings—Pautrier microabscesses, markedly disproportionate epidermotropism, hyperconvoluted epidermal lymphocytes, haloed lymphocytes, epidermal lymphocytes larger than dermal lymphocytes—are significantly more common in mycosis fungoides.[325, 327] However, none of these findings is of sufficient sensitivity or specificity to serve as independent absolute diagnostic tools for mycosis fungoides. Unfortunately, even

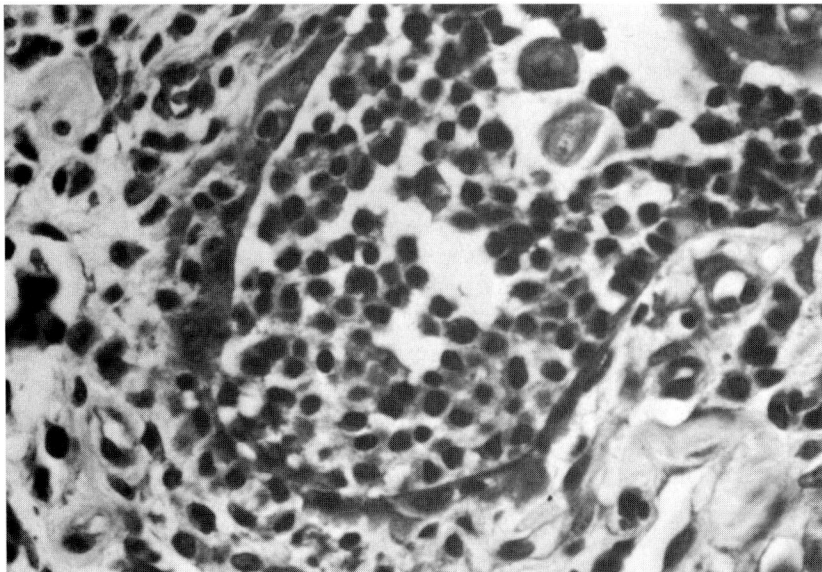

FIGURE 20–114. Close-up of Figure 20–113. Pautrier microabscess containing pleomorphic and atypical lymphocytes.

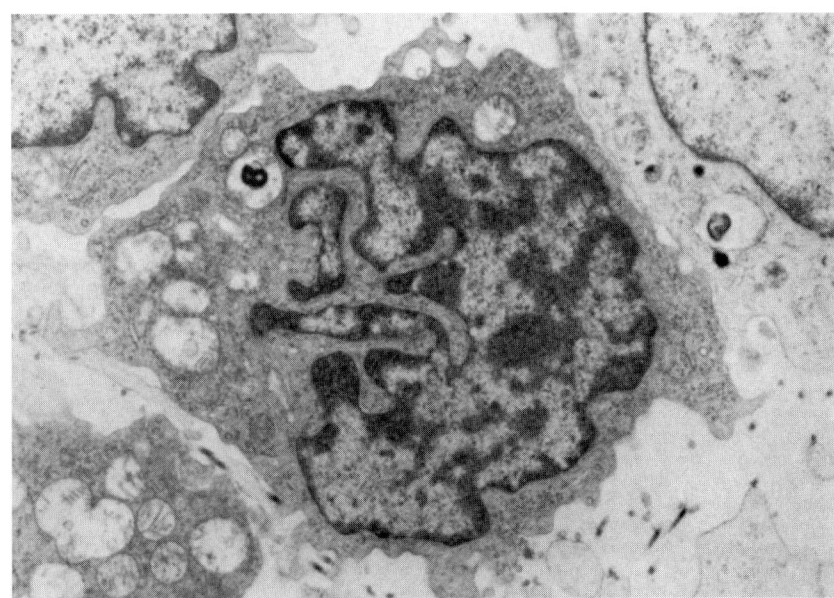

FIGURE 20–115. Feline epitheliotropic lymphoma. Typical Sézary cell.

lymphocyte immunophenotyping and genotyping (clonal T cell receptor chain gene rearrangements) are of poor sensitivity and specificity.[305, 331]

Electron microscopy reveals many tumor cells characterized by a high ratio of nucleus to cytoplasm, deep invaginations of the nuclear membrane (convoluted or cerebriform nucleus), a relatively wide rim of peripheral chromatin, a paucity of organelles, and peripheral cytoplasmic villi or projections (Fig. 20–115).[2, 5, 302, 328] Direct immunofluorescence testing may show the intercellular deposition of immunoglobulin in the epithelium, falsely suggesting a diagnosis of pemphigus.[5, 328]

In canine mycosis fungoides, the neoplastic T cells are typically CD3 and CD8 positive.[57, 313, 318] In humans, the cells are typically CD3 and CD4 positive. In the minority of canine cases, the T cells are CD4 and CD8 negative.[57, 318] The majority of cases of canine mycosis fungoides express T cell receptor (TCR) $\gamma\delta$, the rest express TCR α ß.[57] Discordant pan T cell antigen expression is frequently observed in canine mycosis fungoides.[57, 318] In dogs, no significant correlations were found between epithelial lymphocyte infiltration and keratinocyte ICAM-1 and lymphocyte LFA-1 expression.[321] Thy-1-, factor XIIIa-, MHCII-, CD4-, and CD18-positive dermal dendrocytes were seen in all cases of canine mycosis fungoides, especially in the superficial dermis.[310] Clonal TCR rearrangement was demonstrated in canine mycosis fungoides.[311] Epitheliotropic lymphomas may dedifferentiate or lose expression of various surface molecules.[308]

The prognosis for animals with canine and feline mycosis fungoides is grave.[5, 7, 302, 304, 332, 334] In dogs, the average survival time from the onset of skin lesions until death (usually due to euthanasia) is 5 to 10 months.[5, 304, 332, 334] Occasionally, dogs and cats with mycosis fungoides may live for longer than 2 years after a diagnosis is made, with or without treatment.[5, 318] Death is due to septicemia, metastatic lymphosarcoma, or euthanasia.

Therapy for mycosis fungoides in dogs and cats has usually been of little or no benefit.* Chemotherapy with various combinations of prednisolone, chlorambucil, vincristine, cyclophosphamide, doxorubicin, and methotrexate have occasionally produced some degree of clinical improvement for 1 to 5 months. Rarely, solitary nodules can be surgically excised, with long-term remissions or cures ensuing.[5, 332, 334]

---

*See references 5, 7, 302, 304, 317, 332–334.

The most commonly effective treatment of canine mycosis fungoides is the topical application of mechlorethamine (nitrogen mustard).[5, 317] Mechlorethamine hydrochloride, 10 mg, is dissolved in 50 ml of water or propylene glycol and applied to the clipped surface (total body) two or three times weekly until lesions have regressed. The solution is then applied as needed for maintenance (every 2 to 4 weeks). No signs of toxicity or drug hypersensitivity have been reported in dogs. Occasionally, dogs have experienced demodicosis. Because mechlorethamine is a potent sensitizing agent in humans, gloves should be worn when applying the drug, and the dog should not be handled for the first few hours after application. In addition, exposure to the powder form or vapors from the drug can produce burning of the eyes and throat. Although topical mechlorethamine appears to be useful for managing the "dermatitic" and plaque stages of mycosis fungoides, no evidence suggests that it alters in any way the ultimately fatal course of eventual systemic involvement. In addition, mechlorethamine is a topical carcinogen and cocarcinogen, and may be associated with the subsequent development of cutaneous epithelial malignancies (squamous cell carcinoma and basal cell carcinoma), colon cancer, and Hodgkin's disease in humans.[5]

In humans, topical carmustine (BCNU) has been reported to be effective in mycosis fungoides, with fewer toxicities and hypersensitivity reactions than seen with topical mechlorethamine and no development of secondary skin neoplasms.[5] Other therapies reported to be of benefit in humans with mycosis fungoides include the administration of oral retinoids or interferon, oral methoxsalen (8-methoxypsoralen) and subsequent exposure to ultraviolet A light (PUVA), cyclosporine, photophoresis, and electron beam therapy.[5]

Retinoids (isotretinoin at 1 to 8 mg/kg/day; etretinate at 1 to 8 mg/kg/day) have occasionally been useful in dogs and cats with mycosis fungoides.[5, 89, 90, 333] In one study, only about 50% of the dogs with epitheliotropic and nonepitheliotropic cutaneous lymphoma that were treated with oral retinoids had a clinical improvement of more than 50%.[333] Survival time in these dogs varied from 5 to 17 months (mean, 11 months). Acitretin (1 mg/kg q12h) was ineffective in a dog with nonepitheliotropic T cell lymphoma.[304a] Cyclosporine and omega-3 and omega-6 fatty acid–containing products have not been effective.[5] However, large doses of linoleic acid (3 ml/kg of safflower oil [76% linoleic acid] administered orally twice weekly) was reported to induce remissions in 7 of 10 dogs treated.[314, 322] About 50% of the dogs with mycosis fungoides treated with peg L-asparaginase (weekly or biweekly injections of 30 U/kg intramuscularly or intraperitoneally) experienced a reduction in erythema and scaling.[320] However, there was no effect on plaques and tumors, and no indication that the treatment prolonged survival time.

Anecdotal reports indicate that interferon (Roferon-A, Hoffman-LaRoche), 1 to 1.5 million units/m^2 BSA given subcutaneously three times/week, may be effective in dogs with epitheliotropic lymphoma (see Chap. 3).[88]

One dog with mycosis fungoides (plaque on chin, submandibular lymph nodes) was treated with dacarbazine (1000 mg/m^2 intravenously in fluid drip over a 2-hour period; three treatments at 3-week intervals).[316] The disease was still in remission 1 year later.

Sézary's Syndrome

Sézary's syndrome is an epitheliotropic T cell lymphoma characterized by erythroderma (generalized erythema), pruritus, peripheral lymphadenopathy, and the presence of Sézary, or Lutzner, cells (see Mycosis Fungoides in this chapter) in the cutaneous infiltrate and in the peripheral blood.[5, 57, 319] Histopathologically, the skin biopsy specimens are usually indistinguishable from those in mycosis fungoides. Most authors believe that Sézary's syndrome and mycosis fungoides are variants of the same T cell lymphoma.

Sézary's syndrome is extremely rare in dogs[5, 57, 312, 329] and cats.[324] The animals have generalized pruritus, exfoliative erythroderma, multiple skin plaques and nodules, and lymphocytic leukemia (Fig. 20–116). Skin biopsies reveal epitheliotropic lymphoma. Sézary-like cells are found in the peripheral blood and the skin. As in mycosis fungoides, the neoplastic lymphocytes in canine Sézary syndrome are CD3 and CD8 positive.[57, 312] Dogs and cats usually do not respond to chemotherapy.

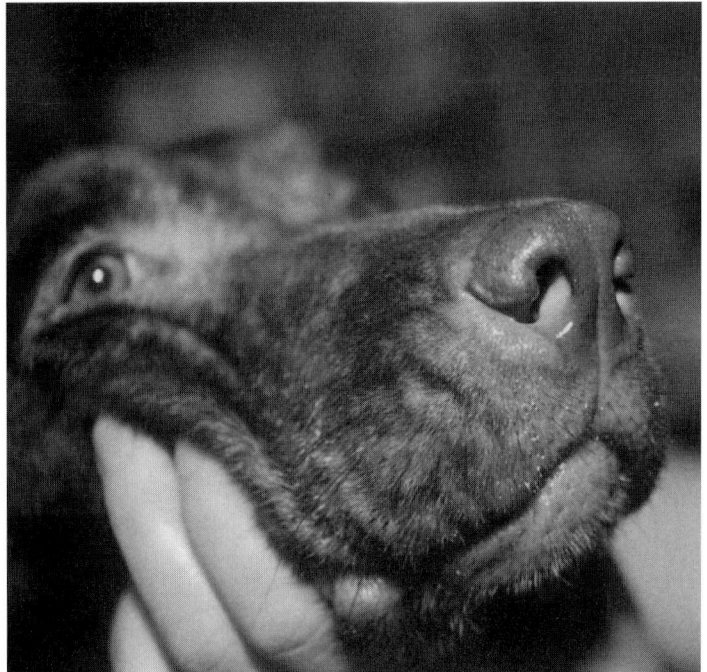

FIGURE 20–116. Sézary syndrome in a dog. Depigmentation, erythema, infiltration, and alopecia of nose, muzzle, chin, and periocular area.

Pagetoid Reticulosis

Pagetoid reticulosis occurs in two clinical forms: localized lesions (Woringer-Kolopp form) with a benign clinical course, and generalized lesions (Ketron-Goodman form) with a progressive clinical course.[57, 319, 323] Histologically, the disease exhibits early, almost exclusive invasion of epidermis and appendages by neoplastic lymphocytes. The neoplastic lymphocytes are CD3 and CD8 positive and exclusively γ/Δ T cells.[57, 323]

In the dog, most cases of pagetoid reticulosis are the Ketron-Goodman form.[57, 319, 323, 332] Erythematous papules, plaques (Fig. 20–117), erosions, and ulcers are seen on the mucocutaneous junctions, oral cavity, paws, and abdomen. Affected dogs become ill and metastases have been recorded.[57, 332] Cases of focal Woringer-Kolopp form have been reported in dogs, but no details were given.[2]

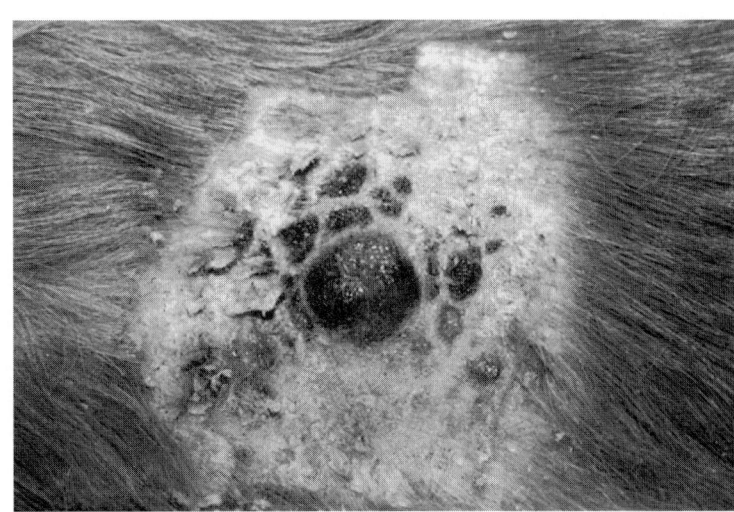

FIGURE 20–117. Pagetoid reticulosis in a dog. Alopecia, scaling, crusting, and several erythematous plaques and nodules on lateral thorax.

Early histopathologic findings included extreme epitheliotropism (epidermis and adnexae) and monomorphous, haloed neoplastic lymphocytes (Figs. 20–118 and 20–119).

LYMPHOMATOID GRANULOMATOSIS

Lymphomatoid granulomatosis is a rare lymphohistiocytic proliferative disorder in dogs.[2, 326] The atypical lymphohistiocytic cells that characterize this disease are variably CD3 positive, suggesting that this is an atypical T cell lymphoma.[326]

Most dogs have only visceral lesions (especially cardiopulmonary and skeletal muscle). Occasional cutaneous involvement has been characterized by multiple chronic, recurrent, punctate to crateriform ulcers that heal with scarring (Fig. 20–120). Subcutaneous plaques may be present. Lesions involve the face, the eyelids, the mucocutaneous junctions, the elbows, and the trunk.

Biopsy reveals abrupt foci of full-thickness epidermal necrosis and ulceration overlying wedge-shaped zones of dermal necrosis.[2, 326] There is a multicentric, angiodestructive, lymphohistiocytic proliferation. A polymorphous lymphohistiocytic infiltrate invades blood vessel walls in the deep dermis and panniculus (Fig. 20–121), resulting in ischemic necrosis. Atypical large lymphocytes with pale cytoplasm and mitotic figures increase in number during the course of the disease. Successful therapy has not been reported.

PSEUDOLYMPHOMA

Pseudolymphomas are a heterogeneous group of benign reactive T or B cell lymphoproliferative processes of diverse causes that simulate cutaneous lymphomas clinically or histo-

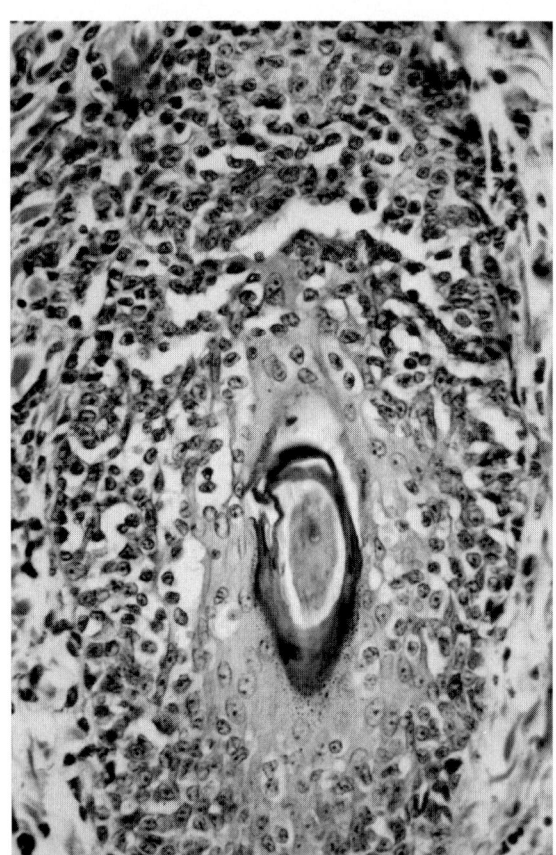

FIGURE 20–118. Pagetoid reticulosis in a dog. Neoplastic lymphocytes exhibit extreme folliculotropism.

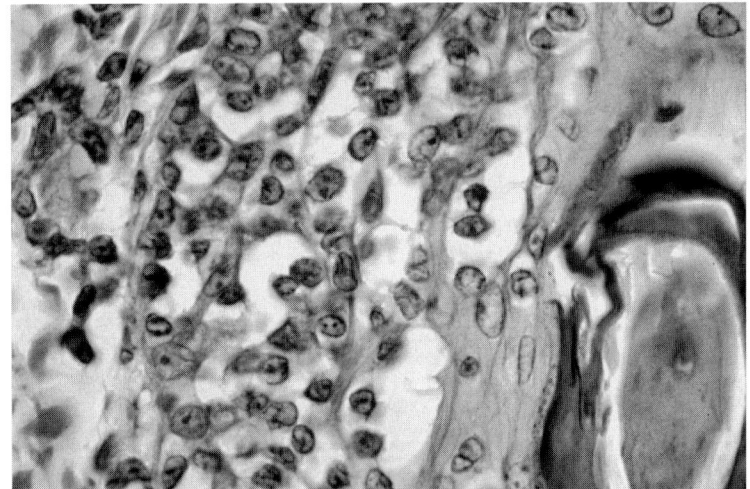

FIGURE 20–119. Pagetoid reticulosis in a dog. Close-up of Figure 20–118.

logically, or both.[335, 336] In humans, pseudolymphomas have been associated with reactions to sunlight, drugs (especially anticonvulsants), arthropods, viruses, foreign material (especially tattoo ink), and contactants, as well as with idiopathy.

Pseudolymphomas usually present as plaques or nodules, usually solitary, often erythematous, and occasionally ulcerated. Age, breed, sex, and site predilections are not clear in small animals. Animals with pseudolymphoma, regardless of the number of skin lesions or regional lymph node involvement, are typically otherwise healthy. Pseudolymphomas have been recognized in dogs and cats in association with arthropod (especially tick) bites, vaccinations, and drugs.[5] A case of pseudolymphoma resembling pseudo-Hodgkin's disease was reported in a dog.[335] The dog had multiple, widespread, discrete, firm nodules and plaques that were alopecic and red-purple (Fig. 20–122). Biopsy revealed a nodular to diffuse dermal and subcutaneous proliferation of pleomorphic and atypical lymphohistiocytic cells with numerous Reed-Sternberg cells (large cells with a multilobulated nucleus whose morphology is such that nuclear lobes appear to be "kissing," or "mirror images") (Fig. 20–123A and B). The disorder spontaneously resolved.

Histopathologically, the distinction between malignant lymphoma and pseudolymphoma of the skin is one of the most difficult problems in dermatopathology.[336] The

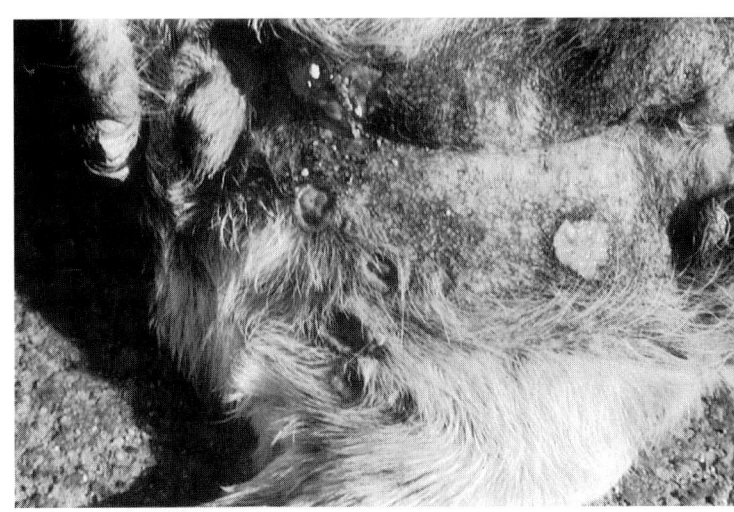

FIGURE 20–120. Lymphomatoid granulomatosis. Crateriform ulcers on ventral abdomen and medial thigh. (Courtesy W. Rosenkrantz.)

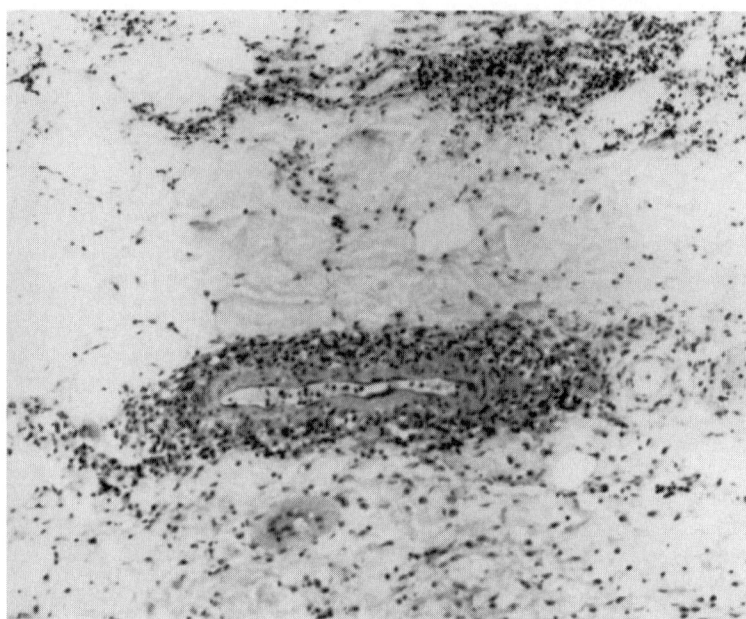

FIGURE 20–121. Canine lymphomatoid granulomatosis. Pleomorphic lymphohistiocytic cells infiltrating a deep dermal vessel. (Courtesy E. Walder.)

cellular infiltrate is usually bandlike, nodular, or diffuse, and is composed predominantly of lymphocytes. There is variable epitheliotropism, and usually little or no cellular atypia. However, some lesions may show marked cellular atypia.[335, 336] Major points of differentiation between lymphoma and pseudolymphoma are presented in Table 20–7.

Treatment of pseudolymphoma is best directed at the underlying cause. Surgical excision of solitary lesions is usually curative.

CUTANEOUS PLASMACYTOMA

• **Cause and Pathogenesis.** Cutaneous plasmacytomas (cutaneous extramedullary plasmacytomas) are common in the dog and extremely rare in the cat.° These neo-

---

°See references 1, 2, 5, 367, 368, 371–374.

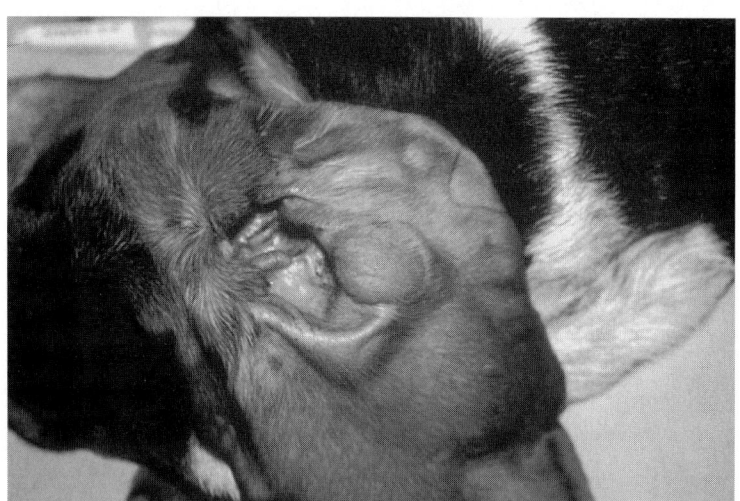

FIGURE 20–122. Pseudolymphoma in a dog. Multiple nodules on pinna.

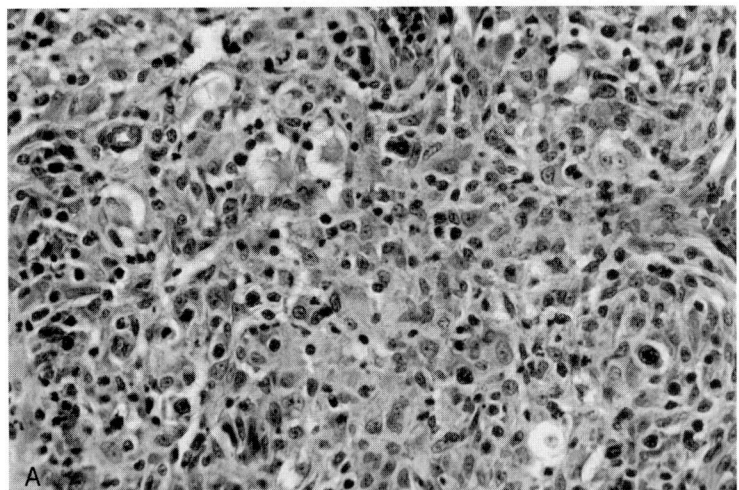
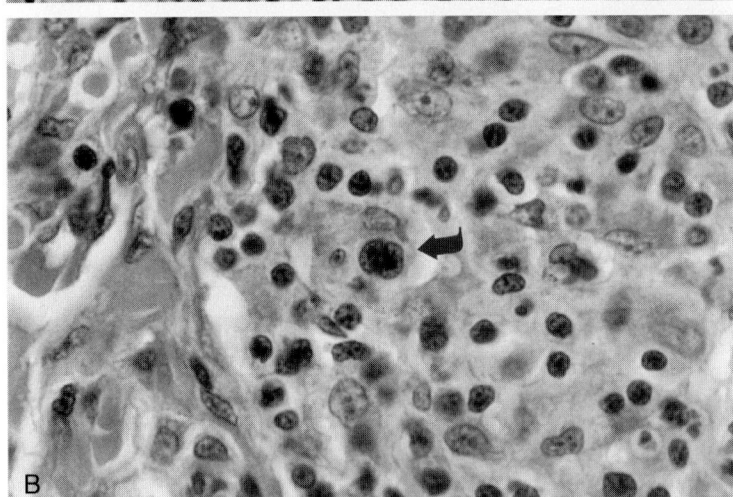

FIGURE 20–123. Pseudolymphoma in a dog. A, Pleomorphic, atypical lymphohistiocytic cells with numerous mitoses. B, Close-up of A. Reed-Sternberg–like cell with "kissing" nuclei (arrow).

● Table 20–7 **HISTOLOGIC CRITERIA FOR THE DIFFERENTIATION OF MALIGNANT LYMPHOMA FROM PSEUDOLYMPHOMA**

MALIGNANT LYMPHOMA	PSEUDOLYMPHOMA
Cellular infiltrate greater in deep dermis ("bottom heavy")	Cellular infiltrate greater in superficial dermis ("top heavy")
Monomorphous cellular infiltrate	Polymorphous (mixed cell) infiltrate
Medium-sized or large lymphocytes usually predominate	Small lymphocytes usually predominate
Germinal centers rare	Germinal centers common
Polychrome (tingible body) macrophages rare	Polychrome (tingible body) macrophages common
Necrosis en masse may be present	No necrosis en masse
Epithelial and vascular structures often involved	Epithelial and vascular structures spared
Cytologic atypia common	Cytologic atypia rare
Monoclonal immunocytologic pattern	Polyclonal immunocytologic pattern

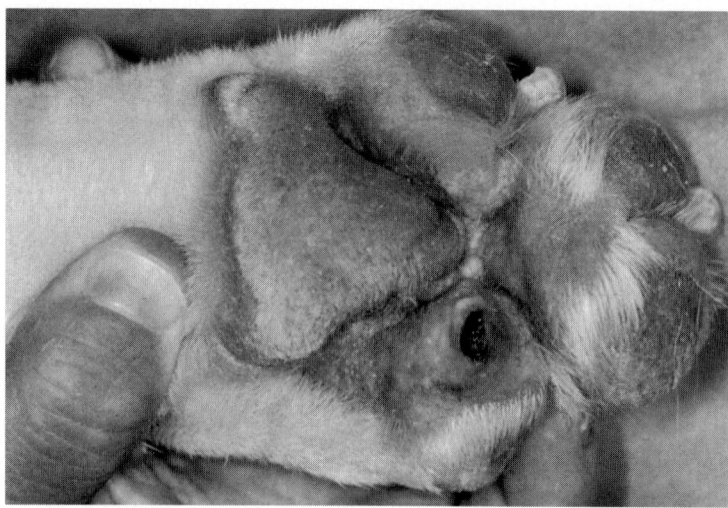

FIGURE 20–124. Canine plasmacytoma. Ulcerated nodule on digital pad. (Courtesy C. Foil.)

plasms are of plasma cell origin and are rarely associated with multiple myeloma. The cause of cutaneous plasmacytomas is unknown. Because canine plasmacytomas occur frequently in areas associated with chronic immune cell stimulation (e.g., gingiva in association with periodontal disease, pinna in association with otitis externa, chin and paws in association with chronic allergic dermatitis), it has been hypothesized that these neoplasms may arise due to chronic, prolonged B cell recruitment and cytokine stimulation.[377] It is likely that these neoplasms were previously reported as reticulum cell sarcoma, atypical histiocytoma, lymphoma, or neuroendocrine tumor.

• **Clinical Findings.** Cutaneous plasmacytomas occur in dogs at an average age of 10 years, there is no sex predilection, and Cocker spaniels may be predisposed.° They are usually solitary and occur most commonly on the digits (Fig. 20–124), the lips, the chin, and the ears (especially in the external ear canal) (see Figs. 20–110G and 20–125). Most plasmacytomas are well circumscribed, raised, smooth, firm to soft, pink to red, dermal in location, and 1 to 2 cm in diameter (range, 0.2 to 10 cm). Tumors in the ear canal are often polypoid, and those on digits are often ulcerated and hemorrhagic. Dogs with multiple cutaneous lesions are rarely seen.[5, 367]

Plasmacytomas are extremely rare in cats, being reported on the leg, lip, and gingiva of aged animals.[369, 372]

°See references 1, 2, 5, 367, 368, 371, 374.

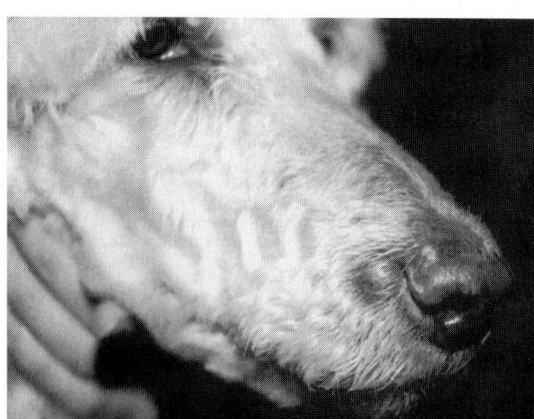

FIGURE 20–125. Canine plasmacytoma. Purplish nodule on muzzle.

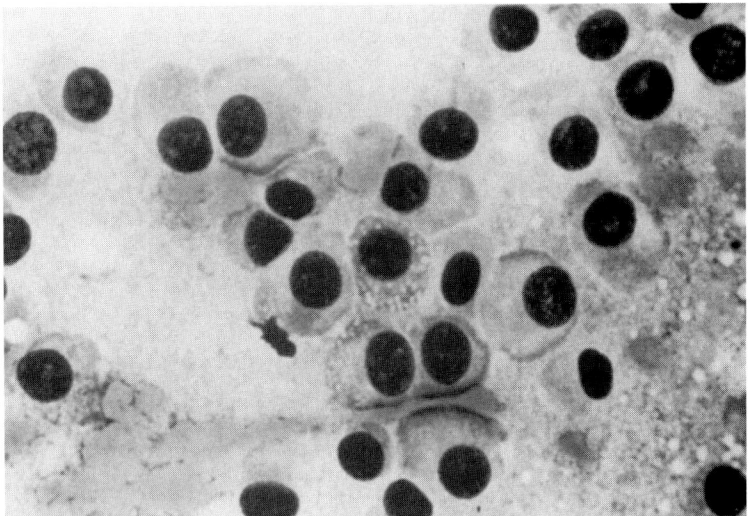

FIGURE 20–126. Canine plasmacytoma. Cytologic examination of aspirate shows pleomorphic plasma cells. (Courtesy T. French.)

• **Diagnosis.** Cytologic examination reveals sheets of variably differentiated plasma cells (Fig. 20–126). Histologically, plasmacytomas are characterized by sheets, packets, and cords of cells infiltrating the dermis and subcutis (Figs. 20–127 and 20–128).[2, 367, 368, 371–374] The neoplastic cells may be well differentiated or extremely pleomorphic and atypical. Amyloid is present in about 10% of lesions.[1, 2, 375] Electron microscopy or immunohistochemical techniques may be required to confirm the plasma cell origin of the

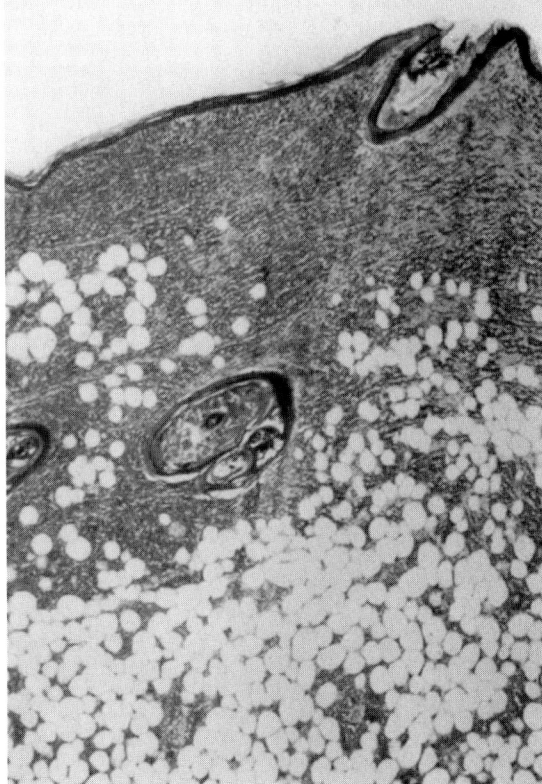

FIGURE 20–127. Canine plasmacytoma. Diffuse infiltration of dermis.

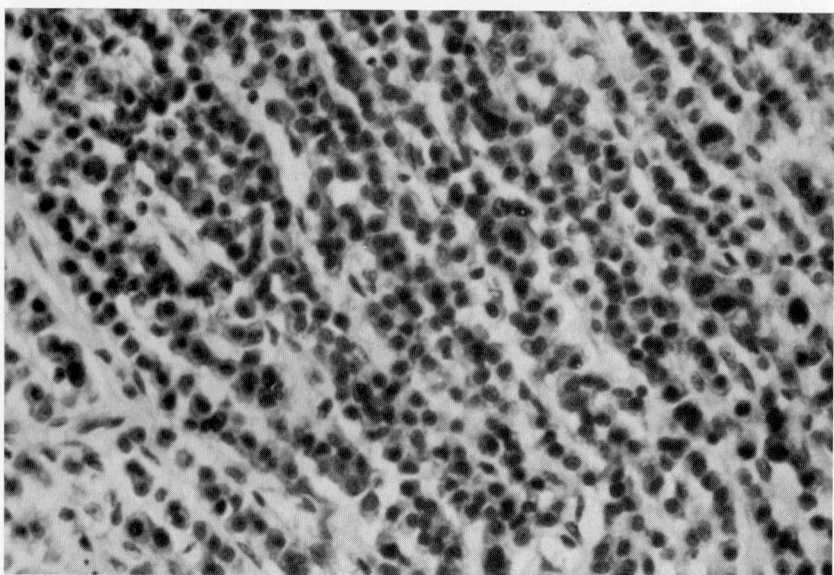

FIGURE 20–128. Close-up of Figure 20–127. Cordlike proliferation of pleomorphic, atypical plasma cells.

neoplastic cells. Immunohistochemical studies have shown that most plasmacytomas are positive for immunoglobulin G heavy chains and light chains.[308, 367, 368, 372, 375–377] Plasmacytomas are positive for vimentin, and most stain with thioflavine T.[5, 367, 377] In one study, 80% of the canine plasmacytomas were positive for CD79a.[377] In addition, CD3-positive T cells and CD18-positive dendritic cells were scattered throughout the neoplasms.[377] Attempts to correlate DNA aneuploidy and oncoprotein content with histopathologic appearance and biological behavior of canine plasmacytomas was fraught with false-positive and false-negative results.[370] A histologic grading system and determination of proliferation rate (immunohistochemical detection of Ki-67 antigen) were also found to be of minimal prognostic value.[373]

- **Clinical Management.** The treatment of choice is surgical excision. Local recurrence and metastasis are rare.[1, 7, 367, 368, 374] Some authors believe that plasmacytomas containing amyloid are more likely to recur after surgery.[1] A histologic grading system was of no benefit, because neoplasms exhibited benign biological behavior in spite of malignant histologic appearance.[1, 340, 341] Rarely, plasmacytomas may occur simultaneously with, or precede (by weeks to months), the development of multiple myeloma.[2, 5, 374]

Tumors of Histiocytic Origin

There are at least five defined histiocytic proliferative disorders that may involve the skin of the dog.[57, 337] These disorders can be a frustrating group of diseases because it can be difficult to impossible to differentiate them from granulomatous, reactive inflammatory disorders or from lymphoproliferative diseases in regular paraffin sections. The clinical presentation, behavior, and responsiveness to therapy vary tremendously between the syndromes. *Histiocytomas* usually occur as solitary lesions in younger dogs, and they spontaneously regress. *Cutaneous histiocytosis* presents with solitary or multiple lesions, which tend to wax and wane. Most cases respond to immunomodulatory therapy, and some may eventually spontaneously regress. *Systemic histiocytosis* is especially common in Bernese Mountain dogs, and it is a slowly progressive disease that requires continuous immunomodulatory therapy. *Malignant histiocytosis*, especially common in Bernese Mountain dogs, Rottweilers, and Golden retrievers, is a multicentric, rapidly progressive disease that responds poorly to treatment. *Histiocytic sarcoma* is a recently reported disorder—

especially common in Bernese Mountain dogs, Rottweilers, Golden retrievers, and Flat-coated retrievers—which requires early radical excision or amputation.

Extensive immunophenotyping has shown that these disorders are all proliferations of dendritic antigen-presenting cells.[57, 337] In all of these disorders, the proliferating cell is CD1a, b, c; CD11c; CD18; CD45; and MHC II positive.[20] However, histiocytomas lack expression of CD4 and CD90 (Thy-1), which distinguishes them from cutaneous histiocytosis and systemic histiocytosis.[57, 337] Similarly, malignant histiocytosis and histiocytic sarcoma are CD4 and Thy-1 negative.

It has been suggested that cutaneous histiocytosis and systemic histiocytosis not be considered to be separate entities but rather be considered to be within the spectrum of reactive Langerhans' cell histiocytosis.[57] However, breed predilections for the two syndromes are different, and immunophenotypically these disorders appear to represent a proliferation of the perivascular dermal dendritic antigen-presenting cells.[337] In the same way, it has been suggested that malignant histiocytosis and histiocytic sarcoma are within a spectrum of malignant Langerhans' cell histiocytosis, and that these two entities could be referred to as "disseminated and localized malignant histiocytosis."[57] More recently, it has been suggested that these two disorders be referred to as "localized histiocytic sarcoma" and "disseminated histiocytic sarcoma."[337] Because the breeds at risk for the two syndromes are identical, this seems reasonable.

Histiocytoma

- **Cause and Pathogenesis.** Histiocytomas are common benign neoplasms of the dog.[1, 2, 5-7, 27] There are rare anecdotal reports of histiocytomas in the cat.[13, 14, 26] Their cause is unknown, although they are more likely a unique proliferation or reactive hyperplasia rather than a true neoplasm. Immunohistochemical and electron microscopic studies have shown that the proliferating cell is the Langerhans' cell.[337, 340, 342] It has been suggested that the canine cutaneous histiocytoma might best be called an epidermotropic Langerhans' cell histiocytosis.[57, 342]

- **Clinical Findings.** Characteristically, histiocytomas affect young dogs, with about 50% of cases occurring in dogs younger than 2 years.[1, 2, 5-7] However, old dogs may also be affected. Boxers, Dachshunds, Cocker spaniels, Great Danes, Scottish terriers, Boston terriers, American Staffordshire terriers, Rottweilers, Shar peis, West Highland white terriers, Doberman pinschers, Labrador retrievers, miniature Schnauzers, English Springer spaniels, and Shetland sheepdogs are predisposed. There is no sex predilection. Histiocytomas are usually solitary and occur most commonly on the head, the pinnae, and the limbs (Fig. 20-129A; also see Fig. 20-110H and 20-130). They are usually small (less than 3 cm in diameter), firm, dome or button shaped, well circumscribed, dermal in location, and frequently ulcerated. Histiocytomas are fast growing but benign. Most of the rare reports of alleged generalized histiocytomas in older dogs were not confirmed ultrastructurally or immunohistochemically and probably represented histiocytic lymphosarcoma, cutaneous histiocytosis, or pseudolymphoma.[5, 3, 10] Rarely, cases of multiple histiocytomas, even with regional lymph node involvement, have been documented.[337, 342] This may be more common in Shar peis.[57, 337] It is possible that inappropriate systemic glucocorticoid therapy potentiated some of these.

- **Diagnosis.** Cytologic examination reveals sheets of pleomorphic "histiocytes" (Langerhans' cells) with variable numbers of lymphocytes and neutrophils, depending on the stage of growth or involution (Fig. 20-131). Histopathologically, histiocytomas are characterized by uniform sheets and cords of pleomorphic histiocytic cells infiltrating the dermis and subcutis, and displacing the collagen fibers and adnexae (Figs. 20-132 and 20-133).[1, 2, 33] A characteristic feature of this neoplasm is a high mitotic index. The overlying epidermis is typically hyperplastic, with prominent rete ridges and subjacent dermal edema. Epithelial invasion is frequent, and intraepithelial nests of Langerhans' cells resemble the Pautrier's microabscesses of epitheliotropic lymphoma.[57, 342] In fact, solitary or multiple histiocytomas in an older dog are a diagnostic dilemma, because the distinction from epitheliotropic lymphoma is often impossible histologically.[57, 337, 342] In

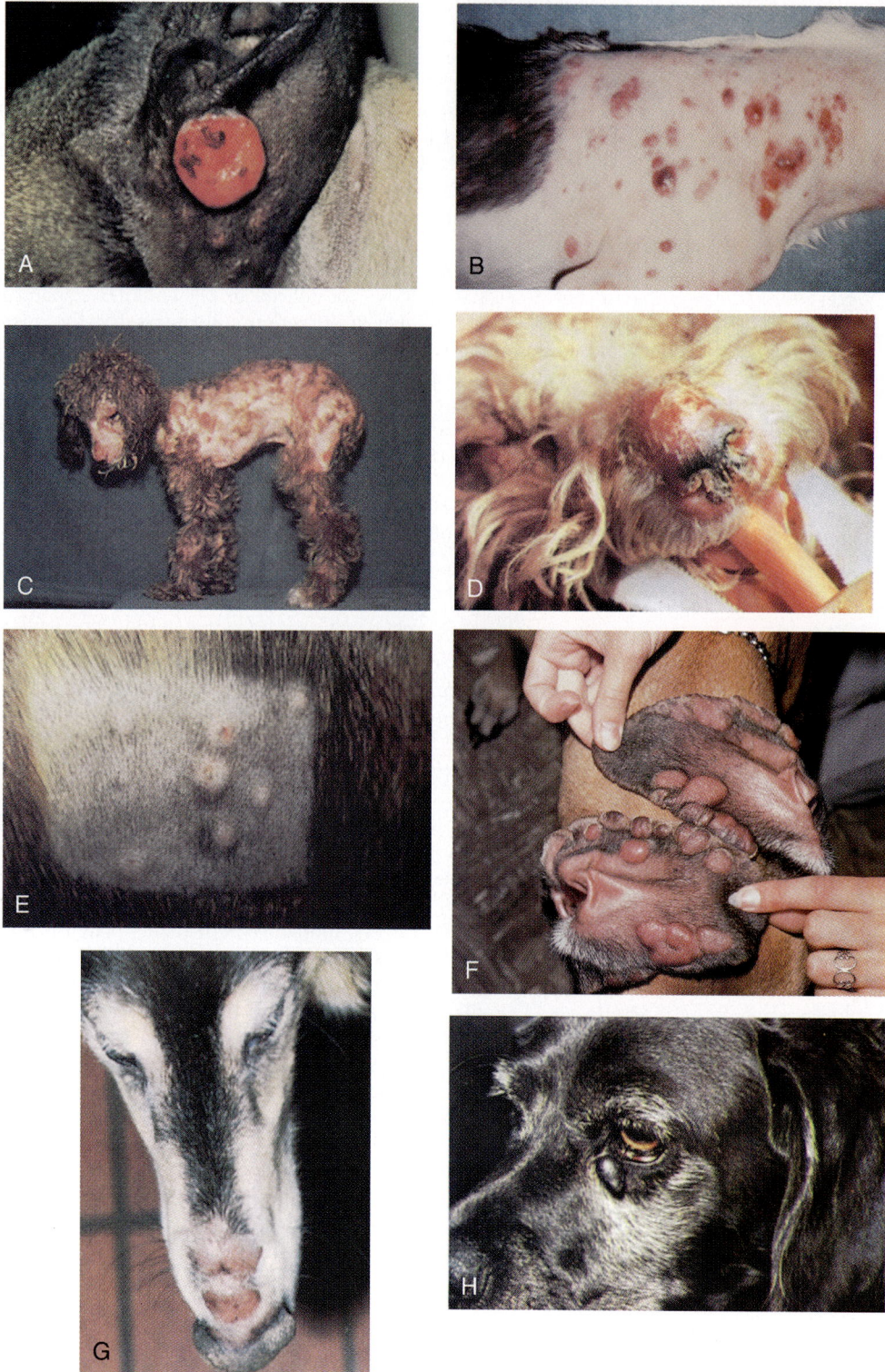

FIGURE 20–129. *A*, Canine histiocytoma. Ulcerated nodule on a pinna. *B*, Malignant histiocytosis. Multiple red-purple macules, papules, and nodules over shoulder and neck (area has been clipped). *C*, Canine systemic histiocytosis. Multiple erythematous papules, nodules, and plaques over the trunk (the area has been clipped). *D*, Same dog as in *C*. Infiltration, erythema, and depigmentation of the nose. *E*, Canine cutaneous histiocytosis. Multiple violaceous nodules over the lateral thorax (the area has been clipped). *F*, Cutaneous histiocytosis. Multiple red papules, nodules, and plaques on both pinnae. *G*, Canine malignant fibrous histiocytoma. Nodules on the bridge of the nose. *H*, Canine melanocytoma. Melanotic nodule on the lower eyelid.

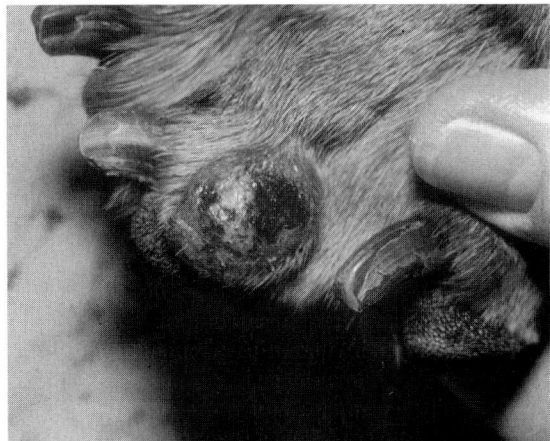

FIGURE 20–130. Ulcerated canine cutaneous histiocytoma on toe.

such cases, immunophenotyping is indispensable. Lymphocytic infiltration (CD8-positive cytotoxic T cells) and areas of necrosis develop in regressing neoplasms. Histiocytomas are CD1a, b, c; CD11a, c; CD18; CD45; ICAM-1; and MHC II positive.[337–342] Histiocytomas lack expression of CD4 and CD90 (Thy-1), which are consistently expressed in cutaneous and systemic histiocytosis.[57] Upregulation of expression of VLA-4, CD11b, CD44, and CD54 (ICAM-1) is observed in most histiocytomas.[57] In addition, they are often vimentin positive, occasionally lysozyme positive, and usually S-100 negative.[340]

- **Clinical Management.** Clinical management of histiocytomas may include surgical excision, cryosurgery, electrosurgery, and observation without treatment.[4–7] The majority of these neoplasms undergo spontaneous regression within 3 months. Even cases with multiple skin lesions and regional lymph node involvement undergo spontaneous resolution, although some lesions regress as new ones appear over a course of, perhaps, several months.[57, 342] Lesions that are causing problems (pruritus, ulceration, and secondary infec-

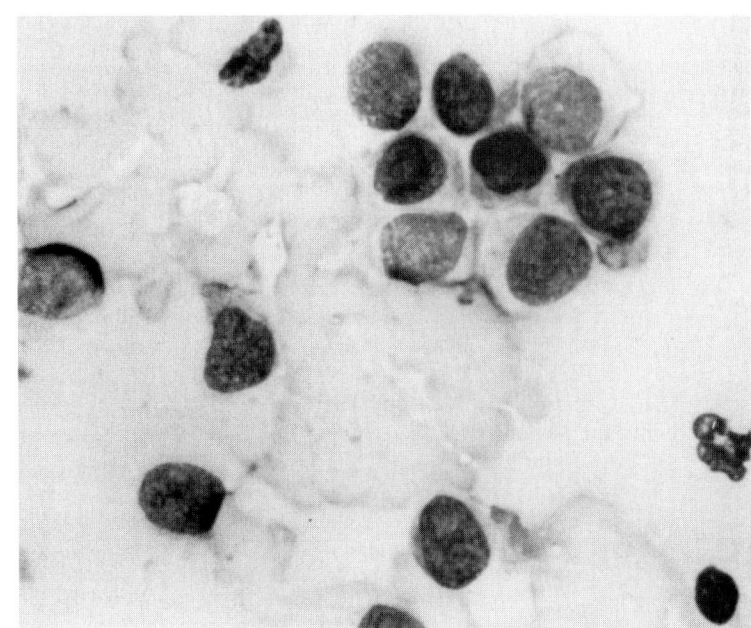

FIGURE 20–131. Canine histiocytoma. Aspirate of skin nodules shows numerous pleomorphic Langerhans' cells ("histiocytes"). (Courtesy J. Blue.)

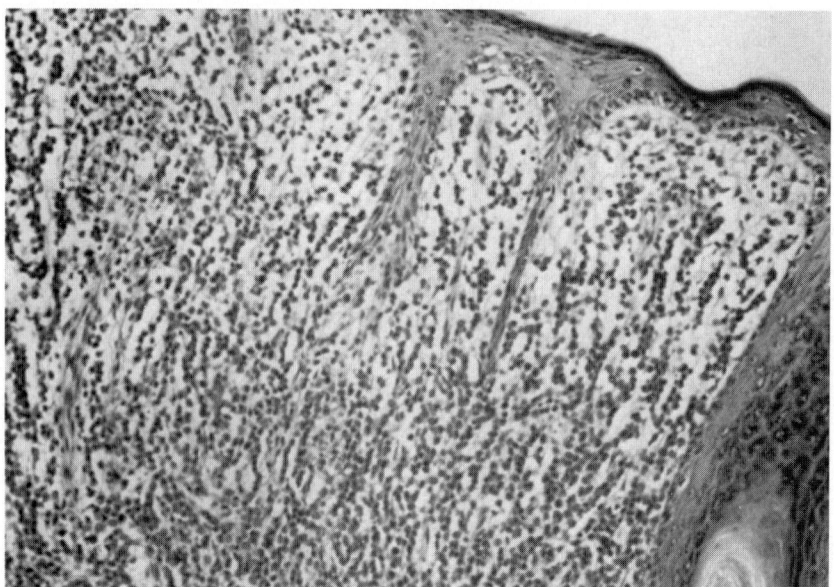

FIGURE 20–132. Canine histiocytoma. Diffuse infiltration of Langerhans' cells ("histiocytes") with edema of superficial dermis and hyperplasia of overlying epidermis.

tion), but are in areas where surgical excision is difficult, respond dramatically to the topical administration of a glucocorticoid in dimethyl sulfoxide.

Malignant Histiocytosis

- **Cause and Pathogenesis.** Malignant histiocytosis (disseminated histiocytic sarcoma) is a rare, malignant neoplasm of Langerhans' cell origin in dogs.* The cause of the neoplasm is unknown.
- **Clinical Findings.** Malignant histiocytosis has been recognized in several breeds of dogs with no sex predilection; typically, older animals are affected. This neoplasm has also been reported in closely related Bernese Mountain dogs, predominantly male dogs.[353] Other breeds that appear to be predisposed include the Rottweiler, Golden retriever, Labrador retriever, and Flat-coated retriever.[57, 337] Spleen, liver, lymph nodes, and lungs are most commonly involved. Cutaneous lesions are uncommon and are characterized by multiple, firm, dermal to subcutaneous nodules (Fig. 20–129B) or plaques anywhere on the body. Lesions may or may not be alopecic, erythematous, or ulcerated. Typical clinical signs of malignant histiocytosis include lethargy, weight loss, lymphadenopathy, hepatosplenomegaly, and pancytopenia. The course is rapidly progressive and invariably fatal.
- **Diagnosis.** Histopathologically, malignant histiocytosis is characterized by nodular to diffuse, deep dermal and subcutaneous infiltration, with cytologically atypical histiocytic cells exhibiting cytophagocytosis and high mitotic index (Fig. 20–134).[1, 351–356] The neoplastic cells may be in dense proliferations of pleomorphic, individualized round cells, more densely packed bundles of plump spindle cells, or both.[337] Large round or stellate multinucleated giant cells are common. Neoplastic cells are positive for CD1, CD11c, ICAM-1, and MHC II.[57] Unlike the cells, cutaneous and systemic histiocytosis, the cells of malignant histiocytosis are not CD4 and CD90 (Thy-1) positive.[57, 337] The neoplastic cells of malignant histiocytosis are also positive for lysozyme, α_1-antitrypsin, and cathepsin B.[5, 351, 353]

---

*See references 1, 5, 20, 57, 337, 351–356.

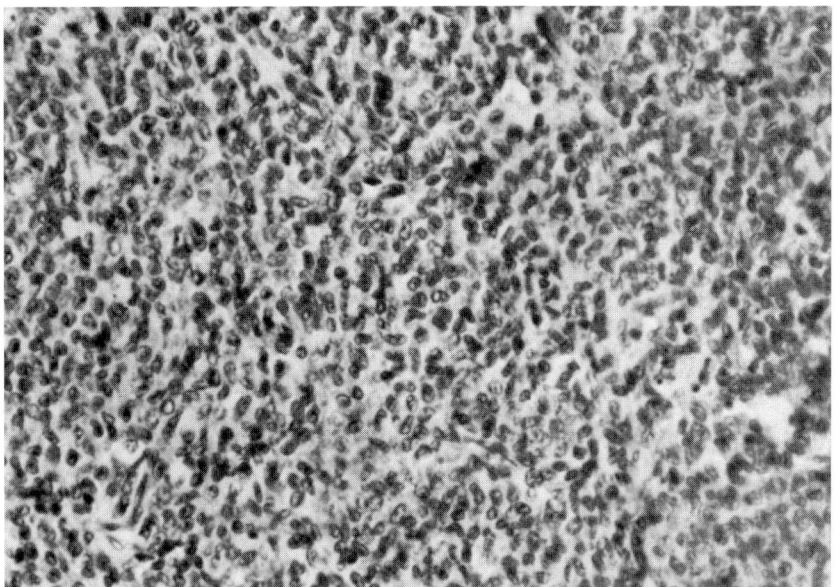

FIGURE 20–133. Close-up of Figure 20–132. Proliferation of pleomorphic, hyperchromatic Langerhans' cells ("histiocytes").

- **Clinical Management.** At present, there is no effective treatment. The disease usually progresses rapidly to death or euthanasia.

Histiocytic Sarcoma

- **Cause and Pathogenesis.** Histiocytic sarcoma ("localized histiocytic sarcoma") is a rare, malignant neoplasm of Langerhans' cell origin in dogs.[20, 57] The cause of the neoplasm is unknown.

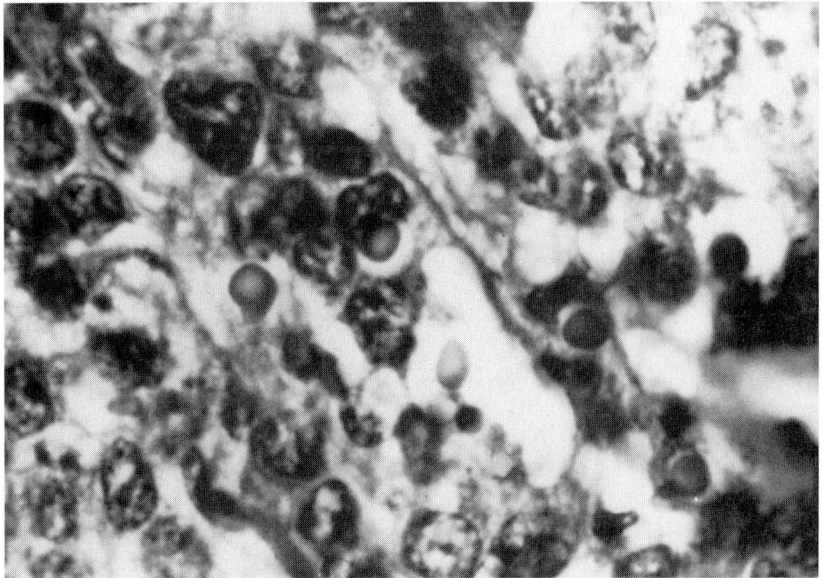

FIGURE 20–134. Canine malignant histiocytosis. Atypical "histiocytes" exhibiting erythrophagocytosis.

- **Clinical Findings.** Histiocytic sarcoma has been recognized in several breeds, and Bernese Mountain dogs, Rottweilers, Golden retrievers, Labrador retrievers, and Flat-coated retrievers appear to be predisposed.[20, 57, 337] It is seen in adult to aged animals with no sex predilection. Lesions are solitary or multiple, rapidly growing, dermal to subcutaneous nodules, and most occur around joints (especially elbow and stifle). Lesions may extend circumferentially around a joint, or actually infiltrate the joint, and involve tendons and muscles. Metastasis to regional lymph nodes has been documented in a few cases late in the course of the disease.
- **Diagnosis.** Histopathologically, histiocytic sarcoma is characterized by a dermal and subcutaneous proliferation of spindle cells forming bundles and whorls, large round cells arranged in sheets and arrows, individual pleomorphic round cells, or mixtures of these types.[20] Mitotic index ranges from 1 to 5/HPF. Multinucleated neoplastic giant cells are frequent. The neoplastic cells are CD1a, b, c; CD11c; CD18; ICAM-1; and MHC II positive.[20, 57, 337] Unlike the cells of cutaneous and systemic histiocytosis, the cells of histiocytic sarcoma are not CD4 and CD90 (Thy-1) positive.[57, 337]
- **Clinical Management.** Histiocytic sarcomas have been cured by early surgical excision,[20] often requiring amputation of the entire extremity.[337] Advanced cases have a poor prognosis, with no successful therapy reported.

Systemic Histiocytosis

- **Cause and Pathogenesis.** Systemic histiocytosis is a proliferative disorder of perivascular dermal dendritic antigen-presenting cells of dogs.[1, 57, 346, 348-350] The cause of the condition is unknown. It is thought to represent a "reactive histiocytosis."[337]
- **Clinical Findings.** Systemic histiocytosis occurs most commonly in closely related Bernese Mountain dogs of 2 to 8 years of age, with male dogs predominating.[346, 348, 349] Although an autosomal recessive mode of inheritance had been proposed,[346] an analysis of 127 cases ruled out autosomal recessive, autosomal dominant, and sex-linked modes of inheritance, and implicated a polygenic mode of inheritance.[348] In the Bernese Mountain dog, multiple cases can occur within the same litter, multiple cases can be produced by the same dams or sires, and there is a higher frequency in the offspring of affected parents compared with the offspring of normal parents that have produced the disease.[348] The disorder has rarely been recognized in other breeds of dogs.[347, 350]

Clinical signs vary with the severity of the disease and include anorexia; weight loss; respiratory stertor; marked conjunctivitis, episcleritis, and chemosis; peripheral lymphadenopathy; and multiple cutaneous or subcutaneous papules, plaques, and nodules over the entire body, especially the muzzle, the nasal planum, the eyelids, the dorsum, the flanks, and the scrotum (see Figs. 20–129C and D).[57, 345, 346, 348-350] The surface of the lesions may appear normal to erythematous to ulcerated, and the lesions may be asymptomatic or painful. The course is often prolonged and fluctuating, with alternating episodes of exacerbation and remission, or rapidly progressive and fatal. Ultimately, most dogs die or are euthanized and show histiocytic infiltration of multiple organ systems, especially lung, liver, spleen, bone marrow, and lymph nodes.

- **Diagnosis.** Histopathologically, systemic histiocytosis is characterized by predominantly deep perivascular, nodular, or diffuse dermal and subcutaneous infiltrations of cytologically normal histiocytic cells (Fig. 20–135).* Variable populations of lymphocytes, neutrophils, and eosinophils are present. Histiocytic cells frequently invade vascular walls, which may produce thrombosis and ischemic necrosis. The tumor cells express CD1a, b, c; CD11c; ICAM-1; and MHC II.[57, 337, 347] They also express CD4 and CD90 (Thy-1), which differentiates them from the cells in malignant histiocytosis, histiocytic sarcoma, and histiocytoma.[57, 337] Enzyme histochemical studies revealed that the cells were also positive for acid phosphatase, nonspecific esterase, and lysozyme.[5, 346]
- **Clinical Management.** In general, treatment with large doses of glucocorticoids

---

*See references 1, 2, 337, 345, 346, 349, 350.

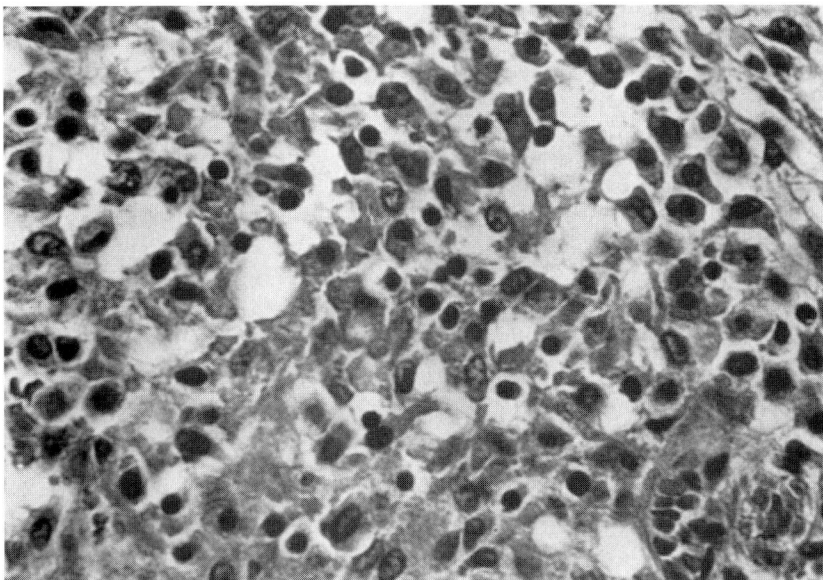

FIGURE 20–135. Canine systemic histiocytosis. Proliferation of normal-appearing "histiocytes" and occasional lymphocytes.

and cytotoxic drugs has been generally ineffective.[57] Early cases with less severe disease may occasionally respond.[57, 349] A preliminary report indicated that treatment with bovine thymosin fraction 5 may be beneficial,[346] but a subsequent report indicated that responses were very inconsistent.[57] Anecdotal reports suggest that cyclosporine and leflunomide are effective.[57, 337] Ocular lesions tend to be more difficult to treat and often require the application of cyclosporine-containing ophthalmic drops.[337]

Cutaneous Histiocytosis

- **Cause and Pathogenesis.** Cutaneous histiocytosis is a benign proliferation of perivascular dermal dendritic antigen-presenting cells of dogs.* The cause of the disorder is unknown. It is thought to represent a "reactive histiocytosis."[337]
- **Clinical Findings.** Cutaneous histiocytosis occurs in dogs, with no apparent age or sex predilections. Collies and Shetland sheepdogs may be predisposed.[2, 5, 57] Lesions occur as multiple, erythematous, dermal or subcutaneous plaques or nodules, 1 to 5 cm in diameter, anywhere on the body (see Figs. 20–129E and F). The lesions may occur in localized clusters or in a more generalized distribution. Some dogs have lesions limited to the nasal planum and nasal mucosa, producing a "clown nose" appearance.[2] Lesions often wax and wane and appear in new sites.[338a] Systemic involvement and lymphadenopathy are not reported.
- **Diagnosis.** Histopathologically, cutaneous histiocytosis is characterized by nodular to diffuse, predominantly deep dermal or subcutaneous infiltrations of cytologically normal histiocytes, lymphocytes, and neutrophils (Fig. 20–136A).[1, 2, 5, 337] Involvement of the superficial dermis is inconsistent, epidermotropism is not usually seen, but folliculotropism may be present (see Fig. 20–136B) and vessel wall invasion is not prominent.[57] The overlying epidermis usually lacks the prominent hyperplasia and rete ridge formation seen with histiocytoma. The histiocytic cells express CD1a, b, c; CD11c; ICAM-1; and MHC II.[57, 337] They also express CD4 and CD90 (Thy-1), which differentiates them from the cells in malignant histiocytosis, histiocytic sarcoma, and histiocytoma.[57, 337] Enzyme histochemical studies showed that the cells were positive for nonspecific esterase.[341]

*See references 1, 2, 57, 338, 341, 343, 344.

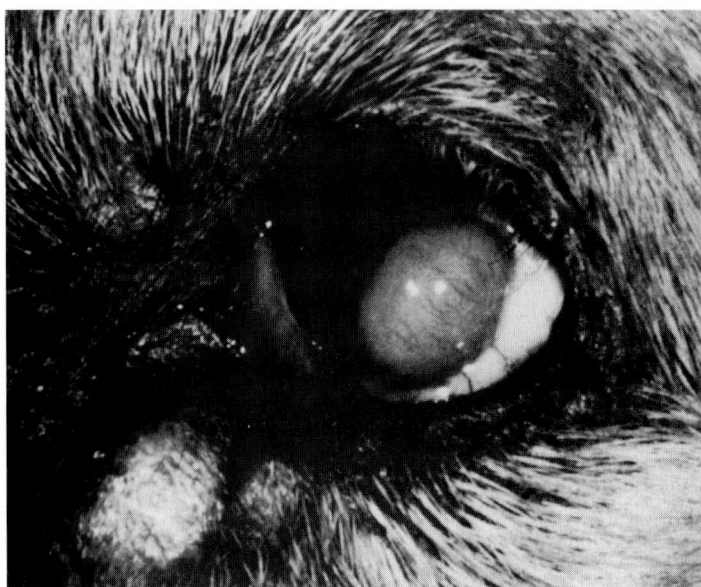

FIGURE 20–139. Canine benign fibrous histiocytoma. Nodule on the sclera of a collie.

to rare (in dogs) malignant neoplasms.* These neoplasms are believed to arise from undifferentiated mesenchymal cells. The cause of malignant fibrous histiocytomas is unknown. Malignant fibrous histiocytomas have occurred experimentally after radiotherapy.[359] Cytogenic analysis of four feline malignant fibrous histiocytomas revealed variable karyotypic changes and frequent nonrandom involvement of chromosome E1.[180, 362]

Some consider malignant fibrous histiocytoma not to be a single entity but rather a "grab-bag" diagnosis that includes pleomorphic forms of several soft tissue sarcomas.[360] In

---

*See references 1, 2, 5, 7, 16, 27, 30, 361–366.

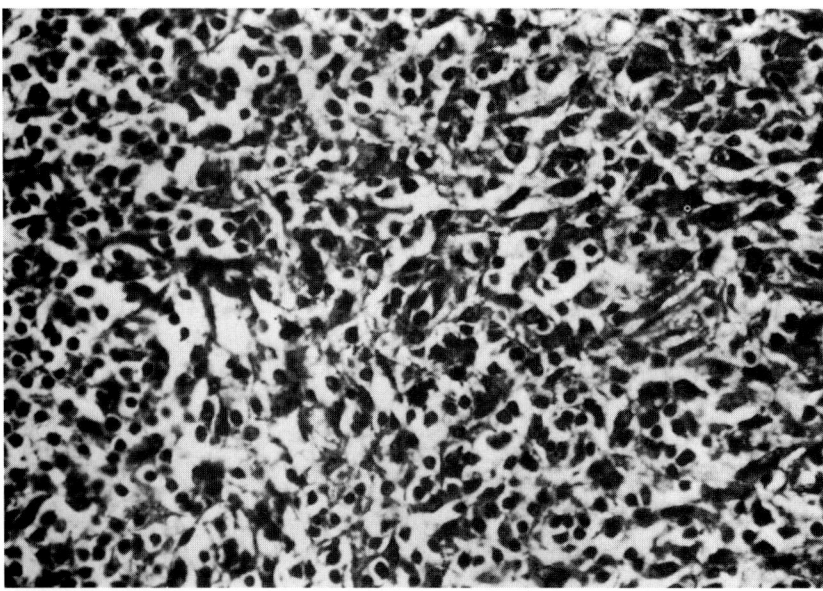

FIGURE 20–140. Canine benign fibrous histiocytoma. Proliferation of histiocytic and fibroblastic cells with intermingling lymphocytes.

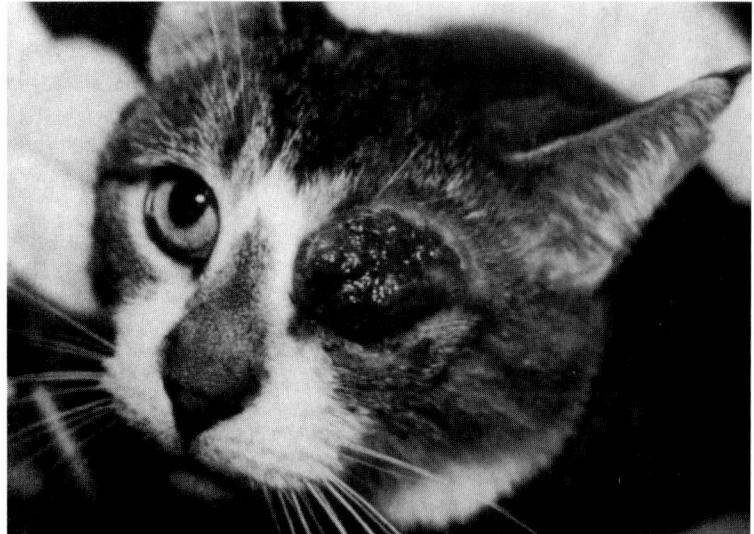

FIGURE 20–141. Feline malignant fibrous histiocytoma. Large, ulcerated mass originating in the periorbital region.

one study, histologically pure malignant fibrous histiocytoma, malignant histiocytosis, and hybrid lesions (diagnostic criteria for both present in same mass) were studied.[360] Age, breed, and lesion distribution data were remarkably similar. The authors offered two hypotheses: (1) these tumors are derived from the same undifferentiated precursor cell that differentiates toward one tumor type or the other with overlapping phenotypes; or (2) these tumors are derived from different cell types, at least one of which can differentiate toward the phenotype of the other.

- **Clinical Findings.** Malignant fibrous histiocytomas occur in older cats and dogs, with no apparent breed or sex predilection. In one report,[364] a 4-month-old puppy was affected. They are usually solitary, firm, poorly circumscribed, variable in size and shape, and dermal and subcutaneous in location (Fig. 20–141; also see Fig. 20–129F). There is a predilection for the leg (especially the paw) and the shoulder.* These neoplasms are locally invasive (to muscle and bone). Early reports indicated that these tumors were slow to metastasize, but 9 of 10 dogs in a recent report developed metastasis, usually widespread.[366] The mean survival after diagnosis in these 10 dogs was 61 days.

- **Diagnosis.** Histologically, malignant fibrous histiocytomas are characterized by an infiltrative mass composed of varying mixtures of pleomorphic histiocytes, fibroblasts, and multinucleate tumor giant cells (Figs. 20–142A and B).[1, 2, 361, 363, 365, 366] Mitotic figures and a storiform ("cartwheel") arrangement of fibroblasts and histiocytes are common features. Recognized histologic subtypes include giant cell type, storiform-pleomorphic type, and dermatofibrosarcoma type.[2, 366] Malignant fibrous histiocytomas are positive for vimentin, lysozyme, and α_1-antichymotrypsin.[47, 363, 365] In a recent report of seven cats, the tumors stained variably with cytokeratin, vimentin, desmin, and S-100.[363]

- **Clinical Management.** The therapy of choice for malignant fibrous histiocytomas is radical surgical excision or amputation. Recurrence after surgical excision is common. Metastasis appears to be more common than originally reported.[1, 2, 5, 366]

• MELANOCYTIC NEOPLASMS

The nomenclature for melanocytic tumors is complex and confusing, with terms such as melanoma, malignant melanoma, melanosarcoma, melanocytoma, benign melanoma, mel-

---

*See references 1, 2, 27, 30, 361, 363, 365, 366.

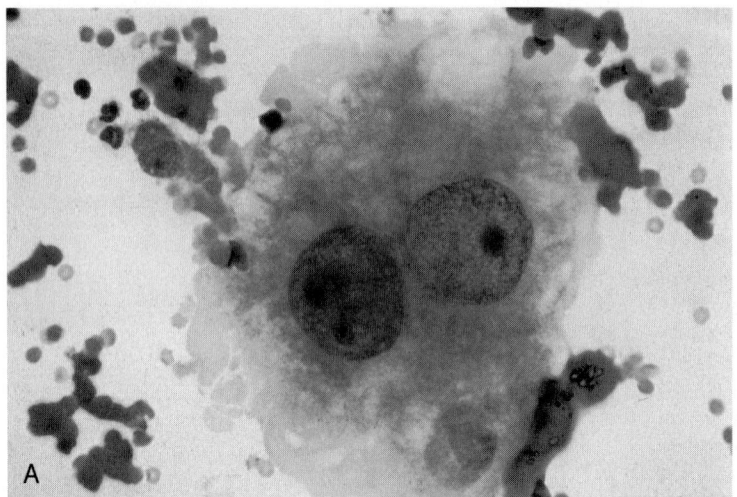

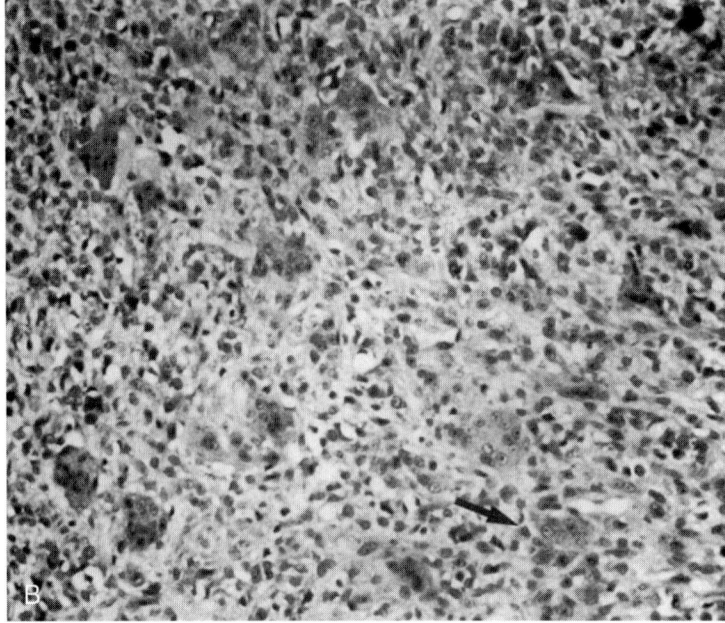

FIGURE 20-142. Feline malignant fibrous histiocytoma. *A*, Cytologic examination of aspirate reveals multinucleated neoplastic giant cell. *B*, Proliferation of atypical fibrohistiocytic cells and numerous atypical multinucleated histiocytic giant cells *(arrow)*.

anocytic nevus, acquired nevus, and congenital nevus having uncertain meaning in certain contexts. The so-called nevus cell, which makes up the pigmented nevi of humans, is now known to be a melanocyte with slight histopathologic and biochemical alterations. On this basis, it has been suggested that all noncongenital, benign proliferations of melanocytes be designated melanocytoma.[2, 5] The term melanoma is used in this text as synonymous with a malignant proliferation of melanocytes. In dogs, most cutaneous melanocytic neoplasms (about 70%) are benign, whereas benign and malignant neoplasms occur with about equal frequency in cats.* Melanocytic neoplasms are the second most common tumor of the canine digit.[28]

Melanocytic neoplasms are relatively common (in dogs) to uncommon (in cats) benign or malignant neoplasms arising from melanocytes and melanoblasts.[1, 2, 4-7] The cause of

---

*See references 11, 14, 26, 35, 381, 384, 385, 388.

these neoplasms usually is unknown. In cats, melanomas have been produced with injections of FeSV.[5, 6] In humans, there is a correlation between exposure to ultraviolet light and the development of melanoma.[5] Chronic exposure to insecticides may also be a risk factor in humans.[381a] Canine melanomas can be transplanted to neonatal dogs (after treatment with antilymphocyte serum) and to nude mice.[5] The tumor-suppressor substances p21/Waf-1 and p-53 were undetectable in the tumor cells from a canine multicentric melanoma.[390] Melanoma developed within a congenital giant melanocytic nevus in a dog.[390b] In a study of melanomas from two cats, monosomy D4 was found in both, along with a variable complex profile of further alterations: monosomy E3, elongated chromosome F2, deleted chromosome B1, and chromosome A1 fusions.[387b]

Breed predilections in dogs suggest that melanocytic neoplasms could have a genetic basis.[388a] Alterations in expression or function of genes and proteins involved in cell cycle control and apoptosis may be of paramount importance in the development of melanoma.[388a]

In general, over 85% of melanocytic neoplasms in dogs arising from haired skin are benign, whereas about 33% of those arising from the claw bed are malignant.[7] In addition, over 75% of the melanocytic neoplasms in Doberman pinschers and miniature Schnauzers are benign, whereas 85% of those in miniature Poodles are malignant.[7]

Melanocytoma

CLINICAL FINDINGS

Dog

Melanocytomas occur in dogs at an average age of 9 years, with no sex predilection. Breeds reported to be at risk include Scottish terriers, Airedales, Boston terriers, Cocker spaniels, Springer spaniels, Boxers, Golden retrievers, Irish setters, Irish terriers, miniature Schnauzers, Doberman pinschers, Chihuahuas, and Chow Chows.[1, 2, 5-7, 381, 434] Doberman pinschers and Irish setters develop multiple melanocytomas.[1, 386] Lesions are usually solitary and occur most frequently on the head (especially the eyelid and the muzzle) (see Fig. 20-129H), the trunk, and the paws (especially interdigitally).[1, 2, 381, 434] They are usually well circumscribed, firm to fleshy, brown to black, 0.5 to 5 cm in diameter, and alopecic; they vary from dome shaped to pedunculated to papillomatous in appearance.

Cat

Melanocytomas occur in cats at an average age of 10 years, with no sex or breed predilection.[1, 2, 5-7, 382, 385, 388] Lesions are usually solitary and occur most commonly on the head (especially the pinna and the nose) and the neck.[1, 2, 5-7, 385, 388] They are usually well circumscribed, firm to fleshy, brown to black, 0.5 to 4 cm in diameter, and alopecic, and vary from dome shaped to pedunculated to papillomatous in appearance.

DIAGNOSIS

Histopathologically, melanocytomas are characterized by melanocytes in sheets, packets (nests and theques), and cords (Figs. 20-143 and 20-144).[1, 2, 33, 388, 434] The melanocytes may be predominantly epithelioid, spindle cell, or a combination of these two forms. Histologic subtypes include junctional, compound, and dermal.[2, 5] Rarely, the melanocytic proliferation is distinctly perifollicular (pilar neurocristic melanocytoma) (Fig. 20-145).[378] Melanocytomas are positive for vimentin.[2, 16, 47, 49, 59]

CLINICAL MANAGEMENT

The therapy of choice is radical surgical excision.[4-7] Up to 10% of the dogs with histologically benign melanocytomas die of their disease (usually euthanasia performed for recurrence, metastasis, or both).[5, 380, 381, 384] Regrettably, no clinical features reliably distinguish benign from malignant melanocytic proliferations.[388, 434]

1360 • Neoplastic and Non-Neoplastic Tumors

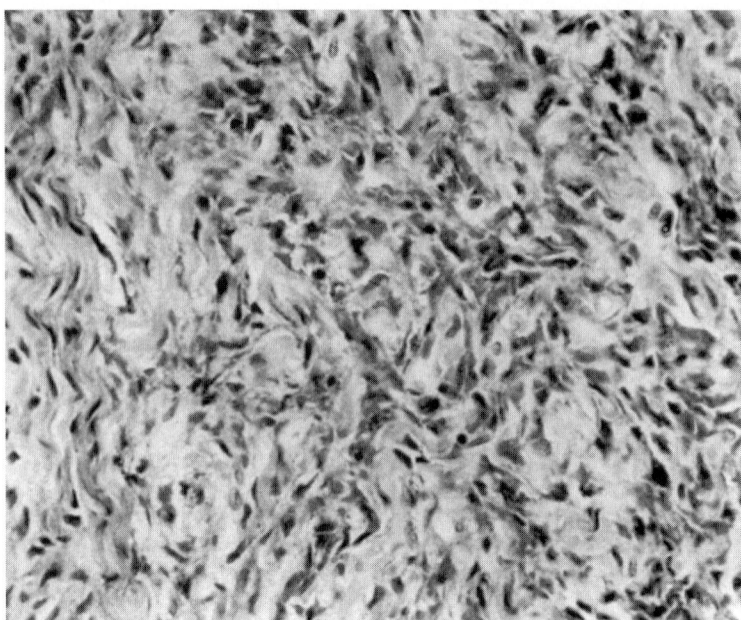

FIGURE 20-143. Feline melanocytoma. Proliferation of spindle-shaped melanocytes.

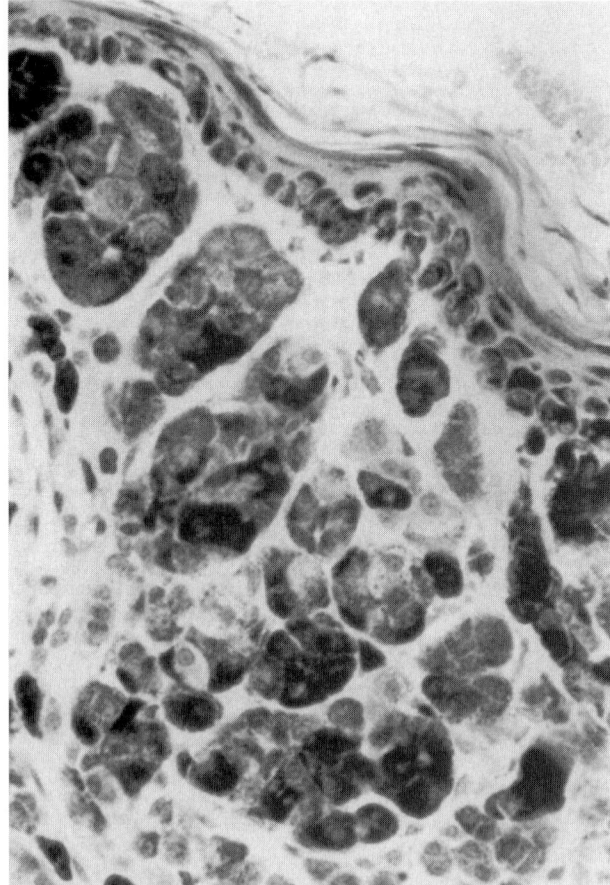

FIGURE 20-144. Feline melanocytoma. Multiple theques of epithelioid melanocytes.

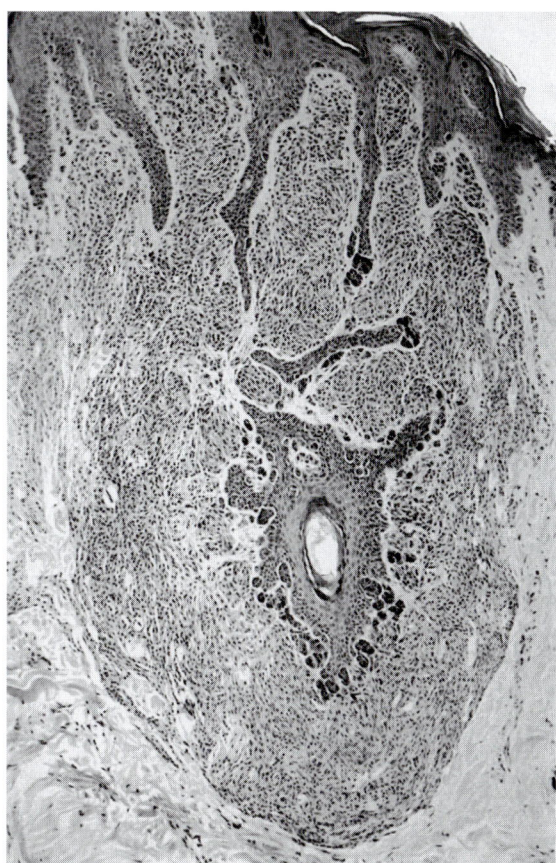

FIGURE 20-145. Pilar neurocristic melanocytoma. Neoplastic melanocytes surround and involve hair follicle.

Melanoma

CLINICAL FINDINGS

Dog

Melanomas occur in dogs at an average age of 9 years, with no sex predilection. Breeds reported to be at risk include those listed previously for melanocytoma.[1, 2, 4–7, 434] Miniature and standard Schnauzers, Scottish terriers, and Irish setters are at risk for developing subungual melanomas.[386] Lesions are usually solitary and occur most commonly on the head (Fig. 20-146), the limbs, the digits (including the claw bed) (Fig. 20-147), the

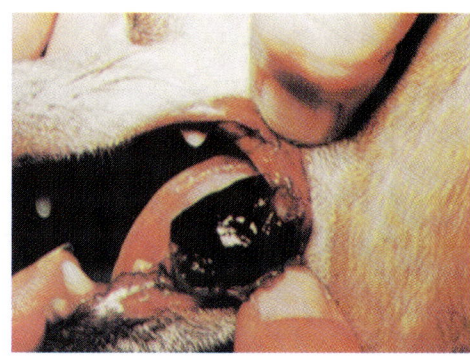

FIGURE 20-146. Melanoma on the lip of a dog.

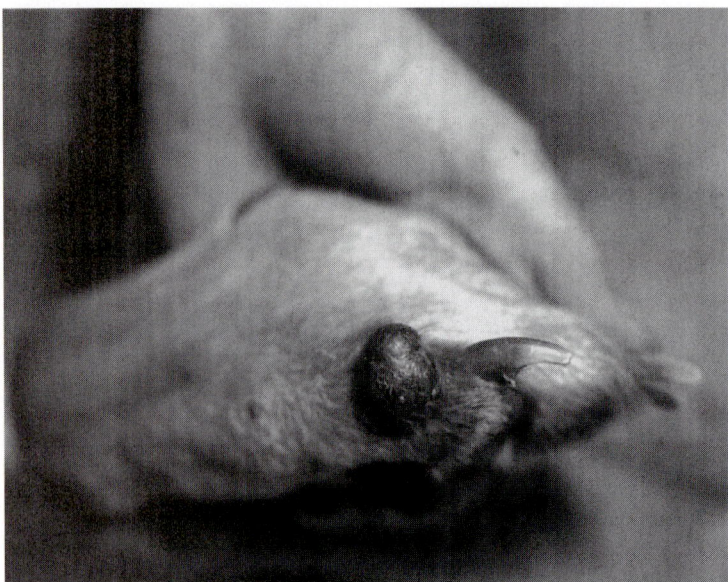

FIGURE 20–147. Digital melanoma. Note resemblance to melanotic fibroma in Figure 20–52B.

scrotum, the lip, and the trunk.[1, 2, 4–7, 381, 434] They are variably circumscribed (well to poor), shaped (dome, plaque, and polypoid), and colored (gray, brown, and black) and range from 0.5 to 10 cm in diameter. Ulceration is common.

Cat

Melanomas occur in cats at an average age of 10 to 11 years, with no sex or breed predilection.[1, 2, 4–7, 14, 385, 388, 391] Lesions are usually solitary and occur most commonly on the head (especially the pinna, the eyelid, and the lip) and the neck (Fig. 20–148).[1, 2, 4–7, 388] They are variably circumscribed and shaped (dome, plaque, and polypoid), and most are brown to black (Fig. 20–149) and vary from 0.5 to 5 cm in diameter. Ulceration is frequent.

DIAGNOSIS

Histopathologically, melanomas are characterized by atypical melanocytes in sheets, packets (nests and theques), and cords (Figs. 20–150 and 20–151).[1, 2, 33, 388, 434] The melanocytes may be predominantly epithelioid, spindle cell, or a combination of these two forms. Rarely, the melanocytic proliferation may be distinctly perifollicular (pilar neurocristic

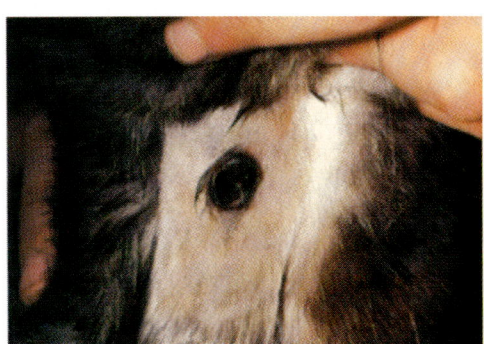

FIGURE 20–148. Melanoma on the ventral neck of a cat.

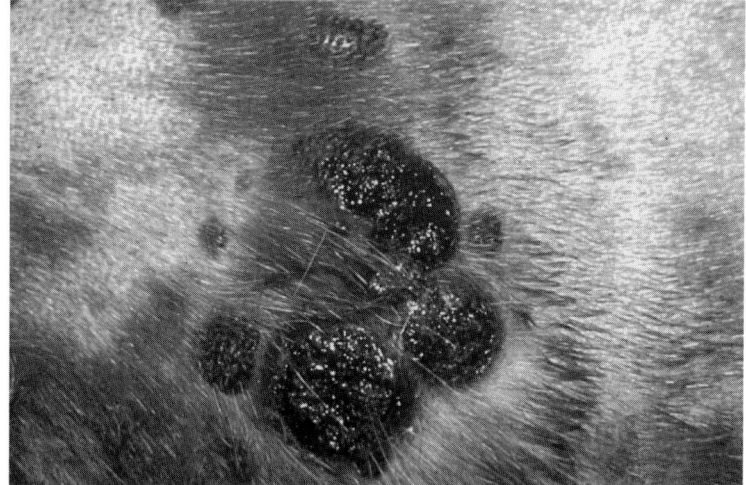

FIGURE 20–149. Multiple melanomas on the thorax of a cat.

melanoma).[378] Clear cell (balloon cell) melanomas have been described.[2, 383, 391] A recent report recognized five histologic types of feline melanoma, which were, in decreasing frequency: signet-ring, epithelioid, balloon-cell, mixed epithelioid or spindle, and spindle.[391] The signet-ring and balloon-cell types were often amelanotic, and were confirmed by electron microscopy and in situ hybridization for tyrosine gene expression. Such lesions were previously diagnosed as undifferentiated carcinomas, undifferentiated sarcomas, and lymphomas. Melanomas are positive for vimentin and variably positive for S-100 protein and neuron-specific enolase.[2, 47, 49, 58, 59, 391] The murine monoclonal antibody IBF9 reacts with a high percentage of canine melanomas in formalin-fixed, paraffin-embedded tissues.[389] Seven monoclonal antibodies recognizing melanoma-associated antigens in human

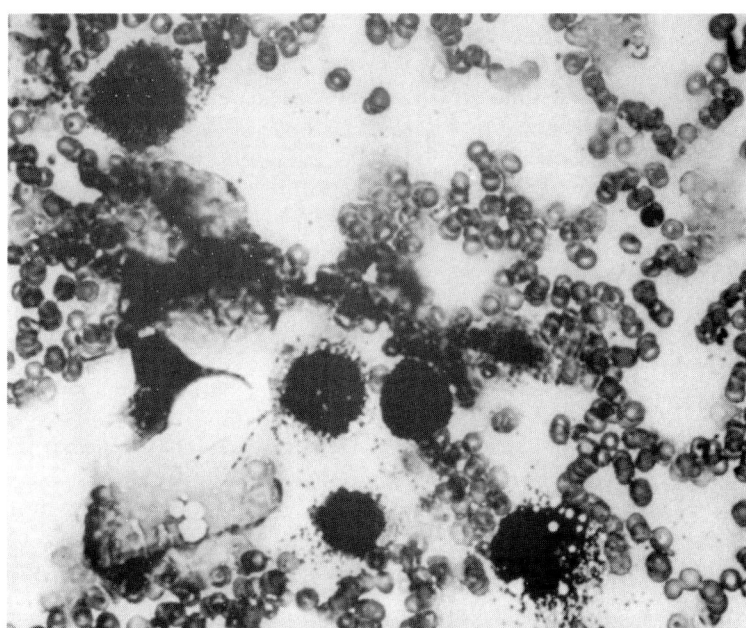

FIGURE 20–150. Canine melanoma. Cytologic examination of aspirate reveals several melanocytes.

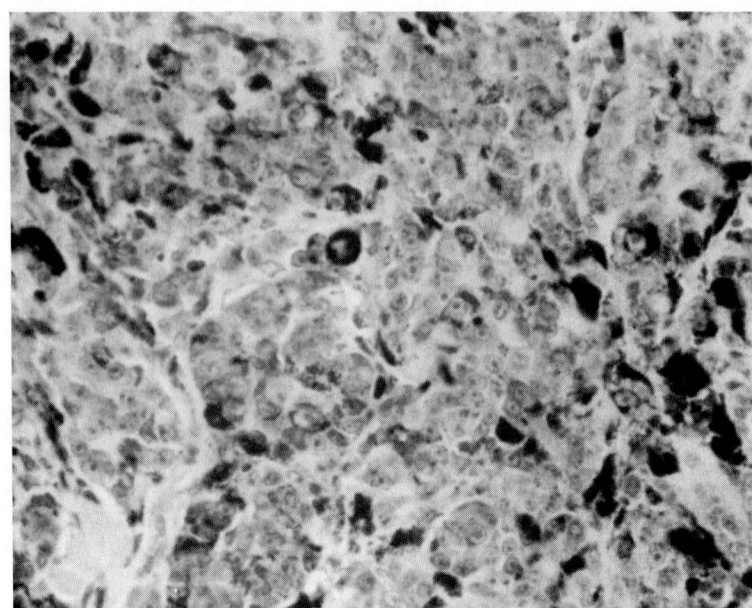

FIGURE 20–151. Feline melanoma. Proliferation of atypical epithelioid melanocytes.

tissues were tested in canine melanomas, but only two (HMSA-1, HMSA-2) worked.[379] Although the two antibodies recognized about 83% of the canine melanomas, they also stained about 29% of canine neoplasms of nonmelanocytic origin.

Malignancy of canine and feline melanocytic neoplasms was not related to the predominant cell type or tumor size, nor the intensity of PCNA expression.[390a] However, Ki67 expression significantly correlated with histologic prognostic factors (malignancy, invasive growth) and patient survival.

CLINICAL MANAGEMENT

The therapy of choice is radical surgical excision.[4–7] Recurrence after surgery and metastasis are common.[1, 5–7, 381, 384] In one large study of surgically treated cutaneous melanomas in dogs, animals had a median survival time of 12 months and a death rate of 54% within 2 years if their neoplasm was small, and a median survival time of 4 months and a death rate of 100% within 2 years if their neoplasm was large.[381] In one study,[28] 32% of the dogs with digital melanomas already had metastases at the time of diagnosis. The mean survival time of dogs with surgically treated oral melanomas was 3 months.[387] The average survival time following surgical excision of feline cutaneous melanomas was 4.5 months.[391] Modalities such as intralesional cisplatin implants, liposome-encapsulated muramyl tripeptide phosphatidylethanolamine, IL-2 and TNF-α, intralesional granulocyte-macrophage colony-stimulating factor, and various autologous tumor vaccines have given disappointing results.[387a, 388a] Regrettably, no clinical findings reliably distinguish melanomas from melanocytomas.[1, 388, 434] Histologic findings of high mitotic activity and marked cellular atypia may correlate with more aggressive biological behavior in canine melanomas[2, 380, 381] and feline melanomas.[1, 388] One study in cats indicated that epithelioid cell–type neoplasms were more likely to be malignant, whereas a second study failed to confirm this finding but suggested that lymphoplasmacytic inflammation indicated malignancy.[388] A third study indicated that there was no correlation between the degree of cellular pleomorphism, mitotic index, and extent of local infiltration in feline melanomas.[382]

Large tumor size (>2 cm^3), high mitotic index, aneuploidy, and distant metastasis are useful prognostic indicators for canine melanoma.[380, 387, 388a]

• MISCELLANEOUS CUTANEOUS NEOPLASMS

Transmissible Venereal Tumor

CAUSE AND PATHOGENESIS

The transmissible venereal tumor (infectious sarcoma, contagious venereal tumor, venereal granuloma, canine condyloma, transmissible lymphosarcoma, transmissible reticulum cell tumor, histiocytoma, or sticker tumor) is an uncommon benign to malignant neoplasm of the dog.[1, 5-7, 405] Immunohistochemical studies support a histiocytic origin.[400, 401] Transmissible venereal tumor is considered a naturally occurring allograft, with transmission occurring by transplantation of viable neoplastic cells to a susceptible host.[5, 405, 406] The tumor cells contain 59 chromosomes, and only 42 or 43/59 are acrocentric (normally 76/78), whereas 16 or 17 are metacentric (2/78 normally)[405] as compared with the normal canine complement of 78. A viral origin has been investigated but not verified. The neoplasm is usually transmitted by coitus, but may be inoculated into multiple sites by licking, biting, and scratching. Transmission may be accomplished by subcutaneous, intravenous, and intraperitoneal injections and by skin or mucosal scarification (incubation period, about 3 weeks). Transmissible venereal tumor has a worldwide distribution, but is more prevalent in tropical and subtropical urban areas. It is enzootic in the southeast United States, southeastern Europe, Central and South America, Japan, the Far East, the Middle East, and parts of Africa.[396a, 405]

Transmissible venereal tumor can grow for extended periods in an immunocompetent allogeneic host.[5, 405] During progressive growth of the tumor, cell-mediated immune responses to tumor cells are impaired, and serum antibodies are present that, when incubated with tumor cells, can block complement-mediated lysis of tumor cells by serum antibodies from dogs with regressing transmissible venereal tumors. Circulating immune complexes have been detected in dogs with transmissible venereal tumor, but the pathogenetic significance of this finding is unknown. Anti-tumor IgG antibodies have been detected in the sera of adult dogs with progressing, regressing, and metastatic tumors.[396a] Dogs experimentally rechallenged with transmissible venereal tumor cells mount a rapid T lymphocyte response, resulting in rapid tumor regression.[5, 405] T cells, B cells, and plasma cells participate in an effective immune response against transmissible venereal tumor and mediate spontaneous tumor regression.[404] The expression of MHC II by neoplastic cells is also associated with an effective immune response and tumor regression.[404] Immunosuppression results in increased tumor growth rate and malignancy.[396a]

Some investigators report that transmissible venereal tumors are usually benign in male dogs but that metastasis to regional lymph nodes is common in intact female dogs, suggesting that these tumors may be hormone dependent.[402] Ovariectomy was reported to produce a rapid reduction in size of transmissible venereal tumors in bitches.[402] Other authors indicate that males are more susceptible to metastatic disease.[396a]

CLINICAL FINDINGS

Transmissible venereal tumor occurs in sexually active dogs (average 4 to 5 years old) and shows no apparent breed or sex predilection.[5, 405] Dogs at the highest risk are those living in areas with high concentrations of free-roaming dogs, inadequately enforced leash laws, and poorly controlled breeding. Neonatal animals and those with poor health or immunosuppression for various reasons may be more likely to have rapid tumor growth and metastatic lesions.[5, 405] Neoplasms occur commonly on the external genitalia (penis and vagina) (Figs. 20–152A and 20–153) and the skin (especially the face and the limbs) (Fig. 20–154), and may be single or multiple, nodular, pedunculated, multilobular or cauliflower-like, firm or friable, 1 to 20 cm in diameter, and dermoepidermal to subcutaneous in location, and they may frequently be ulcerated. Early signs of genital lesions include discharge, often hemorrhagic, with excessive licking of the area. Genital lesions are often pale to bright red, fragile, and commonly hemorrhagic, and with time necrotic, ulcerative,

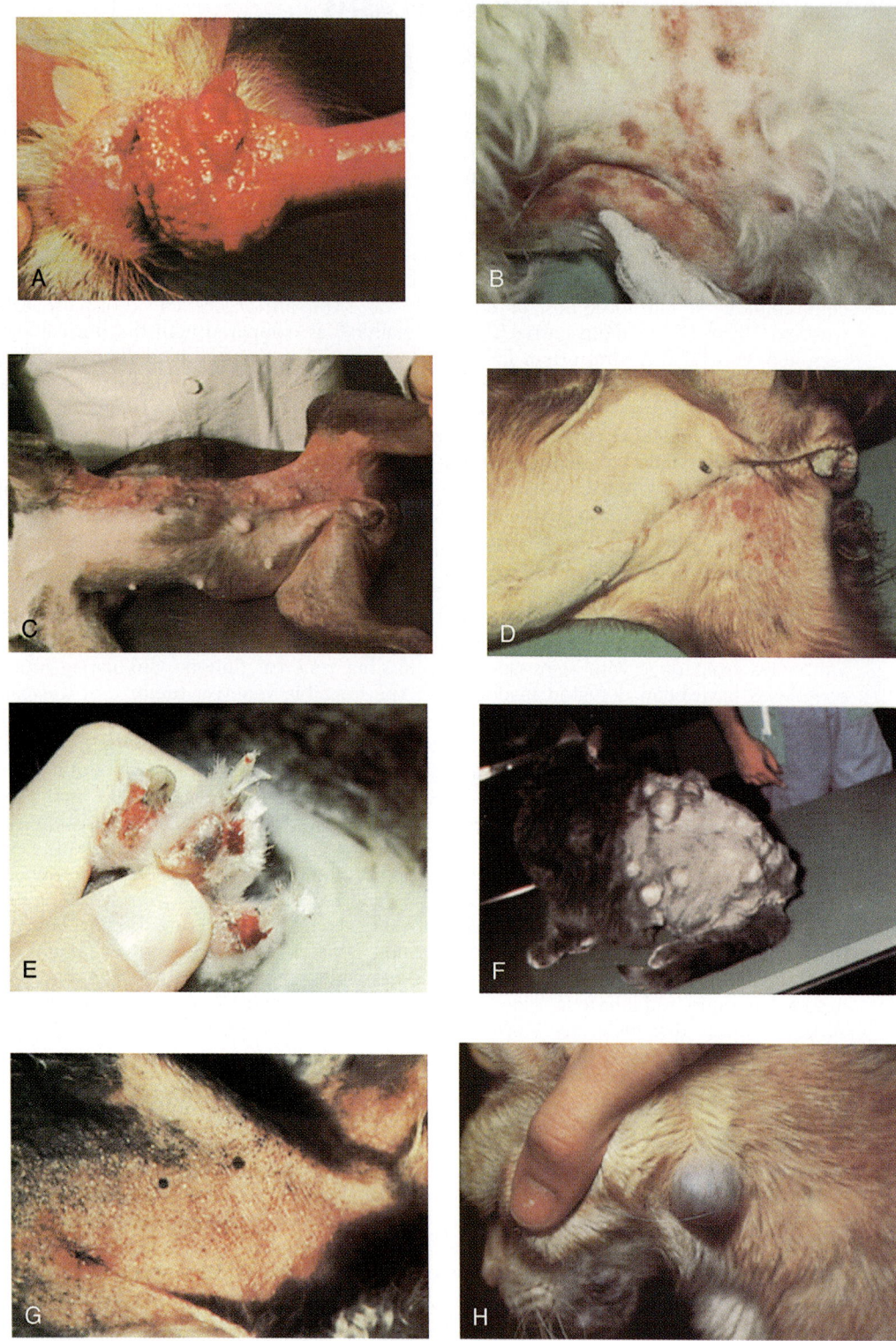

FIGURE 20-152. *A*, Transmissible venereal tumor in a dog. Friable, hemorrhagic nodule on the penis. *B*, Metastatic pharyngeal carcinoma in a dog. Purpuric plaques on the neck. *C*, Metastatic mammary adenocarcinoma in a dog. *D*, Metastatic colonic adenocarcinoma in a dog. Erythematous papules and plaques in the groin. *E*, Metastatic bronchiogenic carcinoma in a cat. Ulcerative paronychial lesions. *F*, Multiple follicular cysts in a cat. *G*, Multiple follicular cysts (milia) in the groin of a dog. *H*, Epitrichial sweat gland cyst on the neck of a cat.

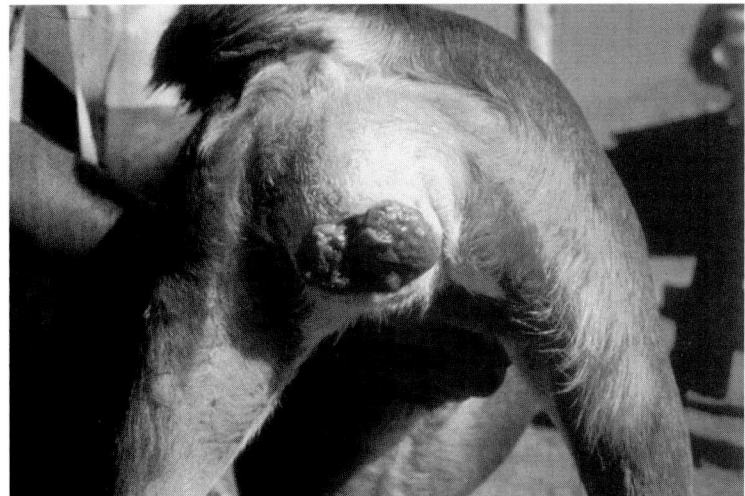

FIGURE 20–153. Transmissible venereal tumor of the vagina and vulva.

and secondarily infected. Some dogs have concurrent thrombocytopenia and prolonged clotting and bleeding times.[407a]

In experimental or laboratory dogs, these tumors frequently regress spontaneously. In one experimental dog colony, the neoplasm was transmitted through 40 generations, consisting of 564 dogs.[5, 405] Neoplasms developed in 68% of the dogs and spontaneously regressed permanently in 87% of these dogs within 180 days. However, there is no such evidence of general benignity in the naturally occurring disease. Spontaneous regression in

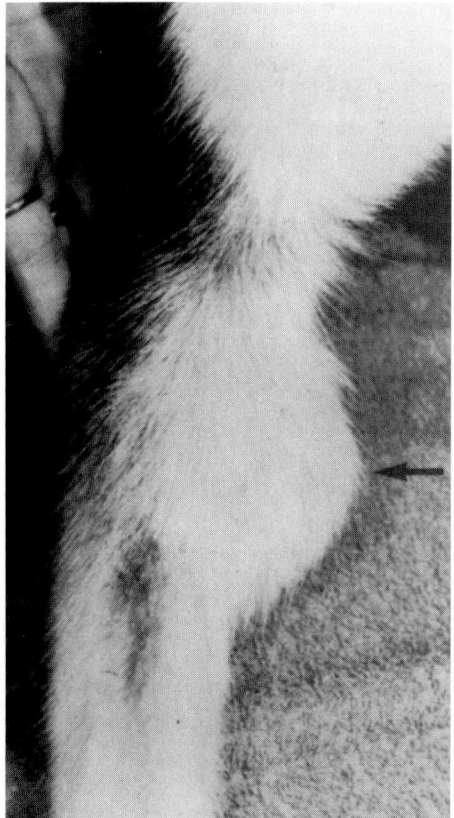

FIGURE 20–154. Transmissible venereal tumor in a dog. Subcutaneous nodule near the elbow.

naturally occurring cases of transmissible venereal tumor is rare, and many instances of metastasis and extragenital occurrence have been reported.[5, 396a, 405]

DIAGNOSIS

Cytologic evaluation reveals round cells with 1 or 2 nucleoli, moderate amounts of pale blue cytoplasm, and multiple small, distinct, clear intracytoplasmic vacuoles (Fig. 20–155).[405] Histopathologically, transmissible venereal tumor is characterized by compact masses or sheets of uniform round to polyhedral neoplastic cells, often growing in rows in a delicate stroma (Fig. 20–156).[1, 2, 5, 33, 405] Mitoses are plentiful. Tumors undergoing spontaneous regression display necrosis, increasing numbers of infiltrating leukocytes (especially lymphocytes), and increasing numbers of collagen bundles. Transmissible venereal tumors are positive for vimentin and negative for cytokeratin.[59, 400, 401] Tumor cells are also positive for lysozyme, neuronal-specific enolase, and ACM1 (mononuclear phagocytic system).[400, 401]

CLINICAL MANAGEMENT

Transmissible venereal tumor rarely regresses spontaneously, and metastasis (regional lymph nodes, skin, central nervous system, and anywhere) occurs in up to 17% of the cases. Both radiotherapy and surgical excision have been successful, although recurrence after surgery is common (33% to 68% of cases).[4–7, 405, 406] It is difficult to obtain wide surgical margins, and tumor transplantation into the surgical wound by instruments and gloves may be important in postsurgical tumor recurrence. Chemotherapy is very effective.[5, 405, 406] More than 90% of the dogs treated with vincristine (0.025 mg/kg intravenously, once weekly for an average of 4 to 6 weeks) were cured, including those with metastases.[5, 396, 396a, 397, 405, 407] AgNOR measurements correlated with response to vincristine[399] as well as with malignancy and prognosis.[406a] Vincristine-resistant transmissible venereal tumors respond to radiotherapy.[406] Doxorubicin administered at a dosage of 0.5 mg/m^2 of body surface area (BSA) intravenously once weekly for an average of 6 weeks is also reported to be effective.[5, 405] Vinblastine (0.15 mg/kg intravenously, once weekly) is also effective.[407] Single-drug chemotherapy with cyclophosphamide or methotrexate was not effective.[396, 405] Immunoadsorption of immune complexes with protein A, autogenous vaccine, levamisole, and intralesional bacille Calmette-Guérin vaccine are all of unproven

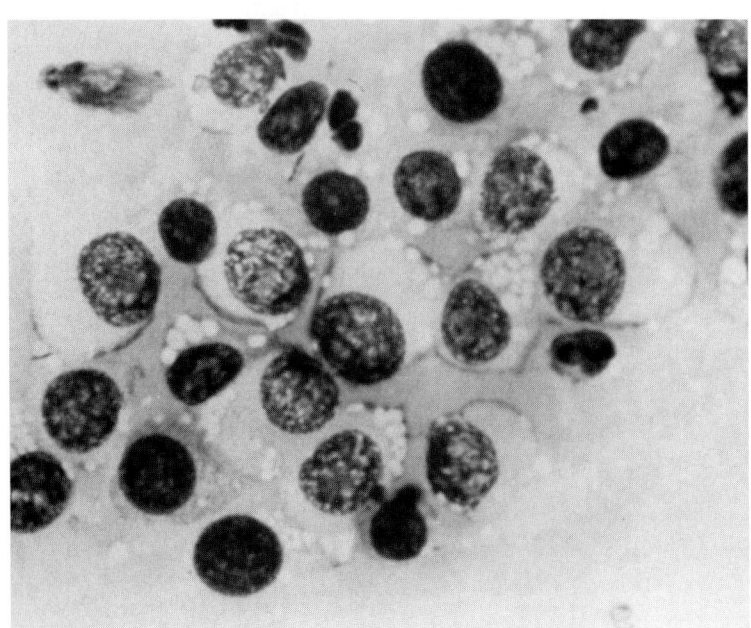

FIGURE 20–155. Transmissible venereal tumor. Aspirate of skin nodule shows monomorphous population of large round cells with vacuolated cytoplasm. (Courtesy T. French.)

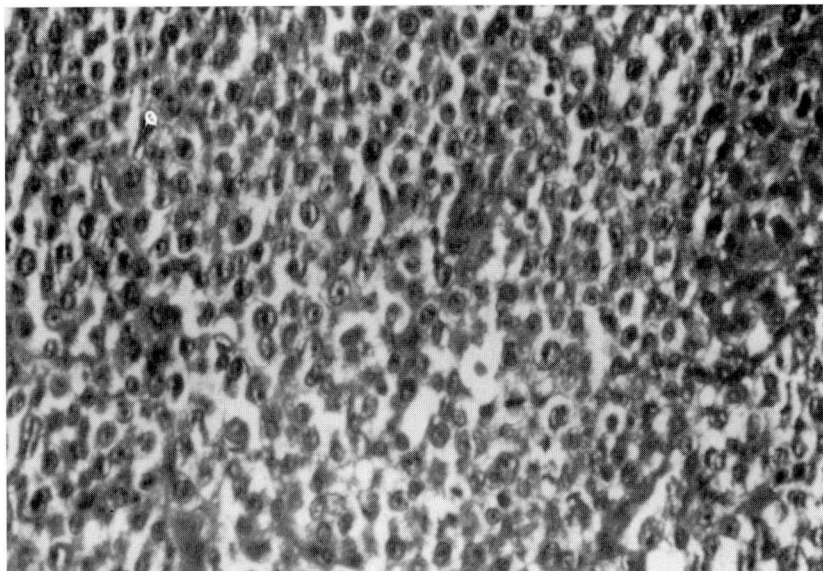

FIGURE 20–156. Transmissible venereal tumor. Sheets of neoplastic mononuclear cells with vesicular nuclei.

benefit.[5, 403, 405] In one dog, a suspension of lymphokine-activated killer cells injected intralesionally, weekly for three treatments, caused tumor regression.[398] Transmissible venereal tumor is highly antigenic, and tumor regression is followed by transplantation immunity.[5, 405] However, the immunity is not long term, and second transmissions can occur 2 or more years later.[396a]

Primary Cutaneous Neuroendocrine Tumor

CAUSE AND PATHOGENESIS

Primary cutaneous neuroendocrine tumors are rare neoplasms of dogs.[5, 392–395] The cause of these tumors is unknown. The cell of origin may be the Merkel cell, which, like this neoplasm, shows dual epithelial and neural differentiation.[5, 51, 393] These neoplasms have probably been previously called "atypical histiocytomas," "lymphomas," "solid basal cell tumors," and "undifferentiated sarcomas."

CLINICAL FINDINGS

In dogs, the vast majority of primary cutaneous neuroendocrine tumors have been reported to be malignant and metastatic,[392] or benign with rare recurrence after surgery.[393, 395] Most dogs are older than 8 years of age, and most have solitary lesions (Fig. 20–157), especially on the lips, the ears, or the digits. The tumors are usually rapid growing, are 0.5 to 2.5 cm in diameter, and may be ulcerated. Neuroendocrine tumors may also occur in the oral cavity of dogs.[395]

DIAGNOSIS

Histopathologically, primary cutaneous neuroendocrine tumors are characterized by sheets, solid nests, or anastomosing trabeculae of uniformly round tumor cells with abundant amphophilic cytoplasm, hyperchromatic and vesicular nuclei, and frequent mitoses (Fig. 20–158).[2, 392–395] Giant and multinucleate tumor cells may be seen. Electron microscopic examination reveals characteristic cytoplasmic dense-core membrane-bound granules and a perinuclear whorl of intermediate filaments (Fig. 20–159). The characteristic cytoplasmic

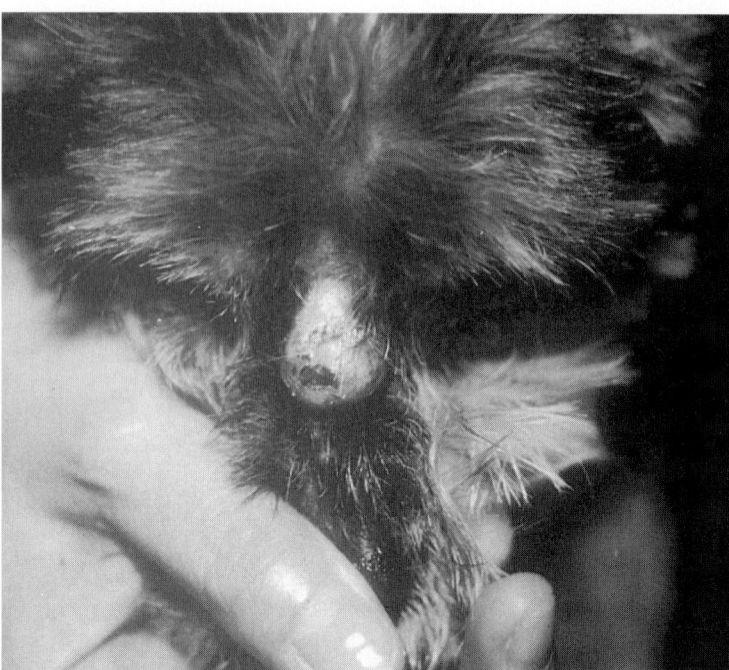

FIGURE 20–157. Merkel cell tumor in a dog. Alopecic, ulcerated nodule between eyes. (Courtesy M. Nagata.)

neurosecretory granules are often lost in formalin-fixed tissues. Immunohistochemical studies have shown that the primary cutaneous neuroendocrine tumors contain cytokeratin and chromogranin A.

CLINICAL MANAGEMENT

Clinical management of these tumors is best accomplished with early radical surgical excision. The vast majority of dogs appear to be cured after surgery.

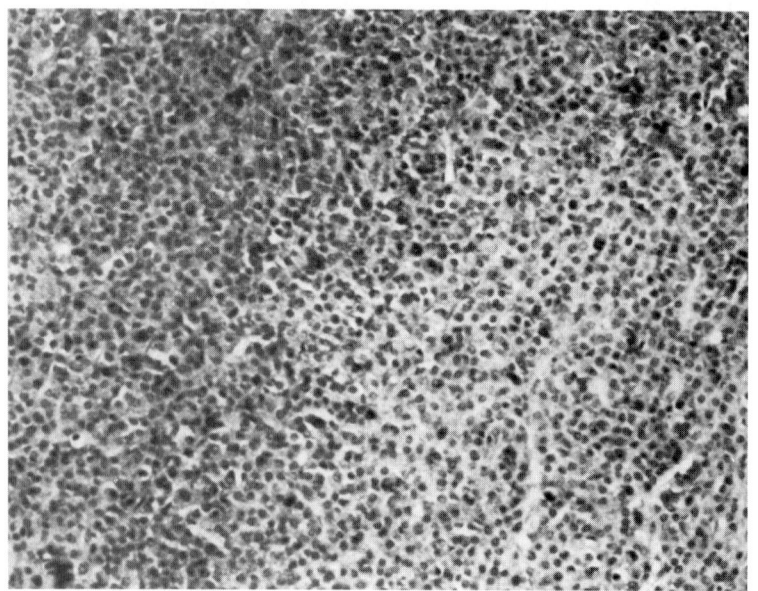

FIGURE 20–158. Canine neuroendocrine tumor. Infiltrate consisting of round tumor cells and frequent mitoses.

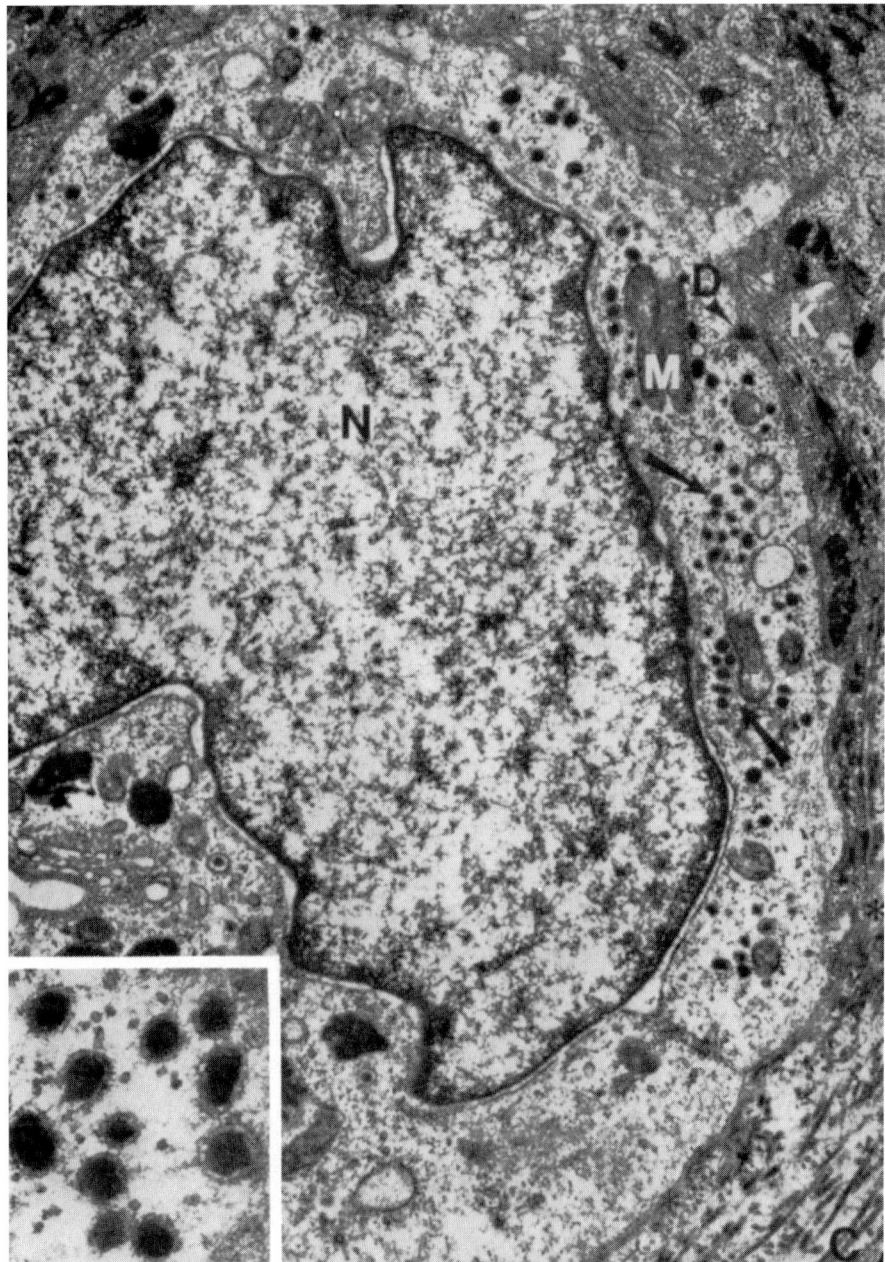

FIGURE 20-159. Merkel's cell. N, nucleus of a Merkel's cell; asterisk indicates basal lamina; M, mitochondria; arrows indicate specific granules of the Merkel's cell; D with pointer, desmosome between the Merkel cell and a keratinocyte (K); C, collagen with cross-striation (×20,000). Inset: specific membrane-bound granules at higher magnification (×75,000). (From Lever WF, Schaumburg-Lever G: Histopathology of the Skin, 7th ed. J.B. Lippincott Co, Philadelphia, 1990, p 863.)

Epithelioid Sarcoma

CAUSE AND PATHOGENESIS

Epithelioid sarcoma is an extremely rare malignant neoplasm of dogs and cats that is probably epithelial in origin.[16, 36, 51, 408] The cause of this tumor is unknown.

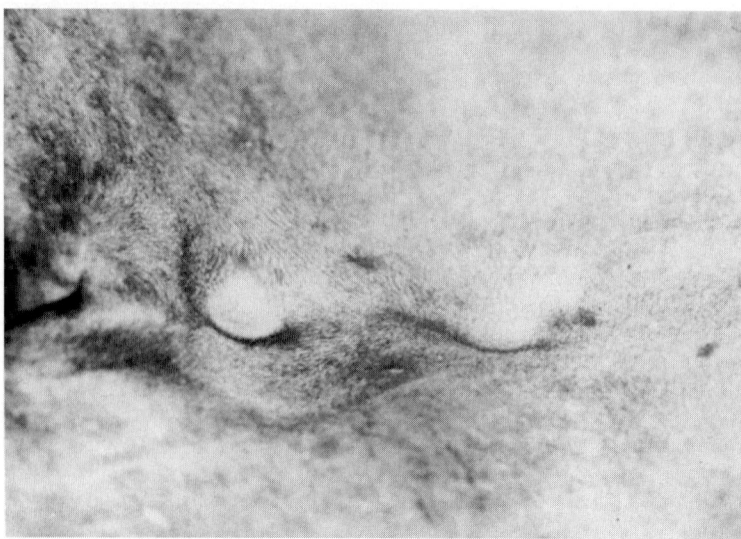

FIGURE 20–160. Feline epithelioid sarcoma. Two nodules in the axillary region.

CLINICAL FINDINGS

Epithelioid sarcoma has been recognized in adult cats and dogs.[16, 36, 408] Lesions are solitary and occur on the limbs (Fig. 20–160). They begin as firm, poorly circumscribed, dermal or subcutaneous nodules that may ulcerate as they enlarge. Metastasis may occur.

DIAGNOSIS

Histopathologically, epithelioid sarcomas are characterized by a nodular arrangement of plump spindle cells and large, round to polygonal epithelioid cells (Fig. 20–161).[36, 408]

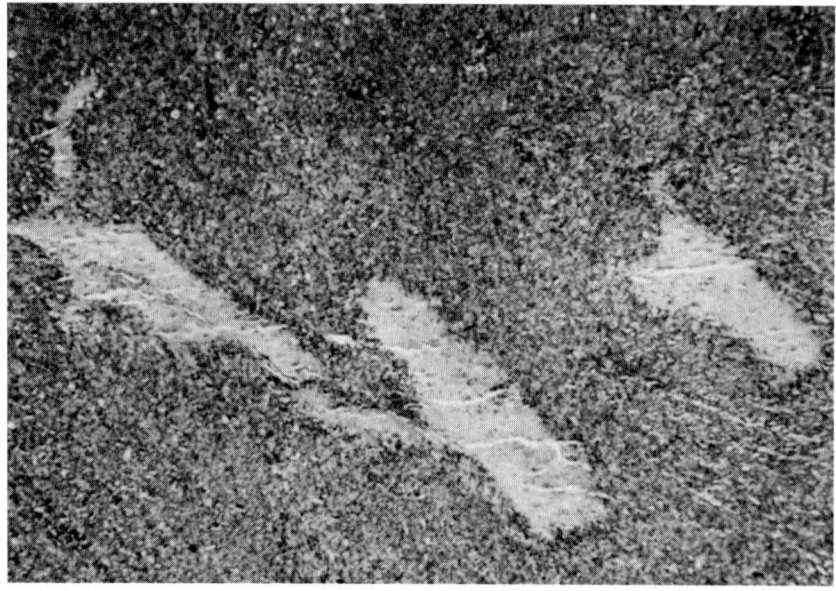

FIGURE 20–161. Feline epithelioid sarcoma. Multifocal area of necrosis within a neoplasm.

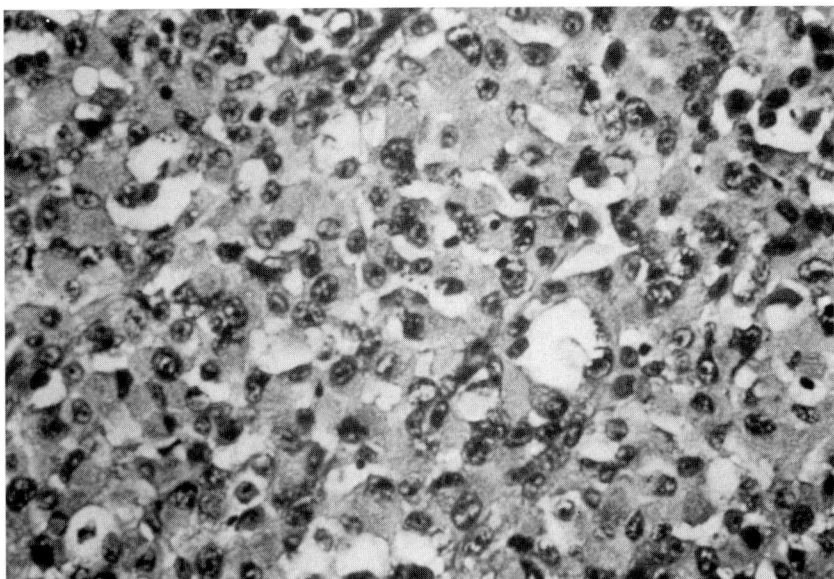

FIGURE 20–162. Close-up of Figure 20–161. Proliferation of pleomorphic, atypical epithelioid cells.

Mitoses are frequent, and necrosis is characteristically present, especially in the center of large nodules (Fig. 20–162). In one dog, tumor cells were positive for vimentin and, focally, for desmin.[408]

CLINICAL MANAGEMENT

The therapy of choice is early radical surgical excision.

• SECONDARY SKIN NEOPLASMS

Secondary skin neoplasms result from the metastasis of primary neoplasms in other organs to the skin. Patterns of metastasis may be due to specific tropisms of cells in the primary neoplasm, as well as hemodynamic, immunologic, biochemical, or microenvironmental factors. Theoretical mechanisms for preferential metastasis include site-specific production of local growth factors, microvascular endothelial cellular adhesion molecules, and soluble chemotactic agents that facilitate migration, adherence, and invasion of neoplastic cells into particular target organs. Secondary skin neoplasms are rare in dogs and cats. Circumscribed, solid, subcutaneous nodules were recognized on the heads of cats with metastatic mammary adenocarcinoma and gastric carcinoma.[5, 417] Multiple purpuric papules, plaques, and nodules of the neck have been seen in dogs with metastatic pharyngeal carcinomas (see Fig. 20–152B).[5] Visceral hemangiosarcomas may metastasize to the skin as dermal or subcutaneous papules and nodules, which may be bluish to reddish to blackish in color.[417] A sternal liposarcoma metastasized to the skin of the front limb as papules.[417] Oral melanomas may metastasize to the skin of the muzzle and lips.[417] Nodular to ulcerative to edematous (pseudocellulitis, inflammatory carcinoma) lesions have been recognized in the ventral abdominal, inguinal, and medial thigh skin of dogs and cats with metastatic mammary adenocarcinoma (see Fig. 20–152C)[5, 417, 419, 420] and colonic adenocarcinoma (Fig. 20–163; also see Fig. 20–152D).[5, 414, 417] Nodules in the umbilical skin have been recognized in dogs and cats with metastatic pancreatic ductal adenocarcinoma, jejunal

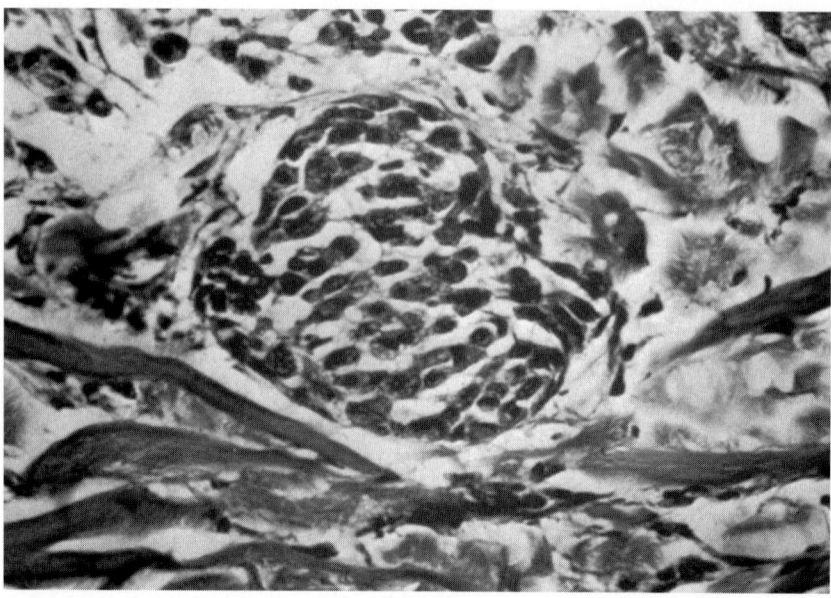

FIGURE 20–163. Metastatic colonic adenocarcinoma in a dog. Lymphatic metastasis in skin.

adenocarcinoma, and teratoma.[411] A seminoma metastasized to the skin of the jaw and trunk in a dog.[418a] The authors have seen solitary or multiple metastatic cutaneous nodules (Fig. 20–164) in dogs with prostatic carcinoma.

Ulcerative, destructive lesions on the digits have been seen in aged cats with asymptomatic bronchiogenic or squamous cell carcinomas of the lung (Fig. 20–165; also see Fig. 20–152E).[131, 412, 415, 417, 418] Usually, multiple digits of multiple paws are involved, but occasionally multiple digits on one paw or one digit only are affected. Occasionally, lesions may also be present at other cutaneous sites: head, abdomen, lip, thigh, lumbar area.

Leukemia cutis is a dissemination of aggressive systemic leukemia to the skin. Cutaneous lesions seen with leukemia may be specific (leukemic infiltrates presenting as macules, papules, plaques, nodules, purpura, and ulcers) or nonspecific (infectious dermatoses, urticaria, erythema multiforme, exfoliative dermatitis, and pruritus). In dogs, leukemia cutis (patchy alopecia, erythema, and papules of the trunk) was reported with chronic lymphocytic leukemia.[410] Nonspecific skin lesions of leukemia (recurrent bacterial pyo-

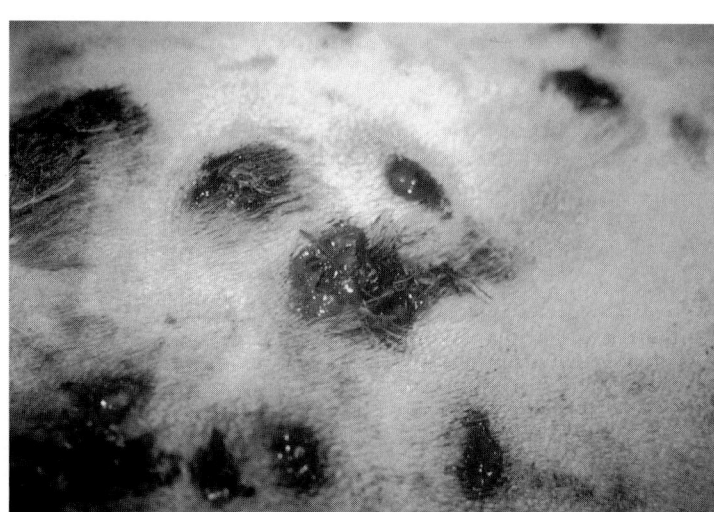

FIGURE 20–164. Cutaneous metastases from prostatic carcinoma. Multiple ulcerated nodules over withers.

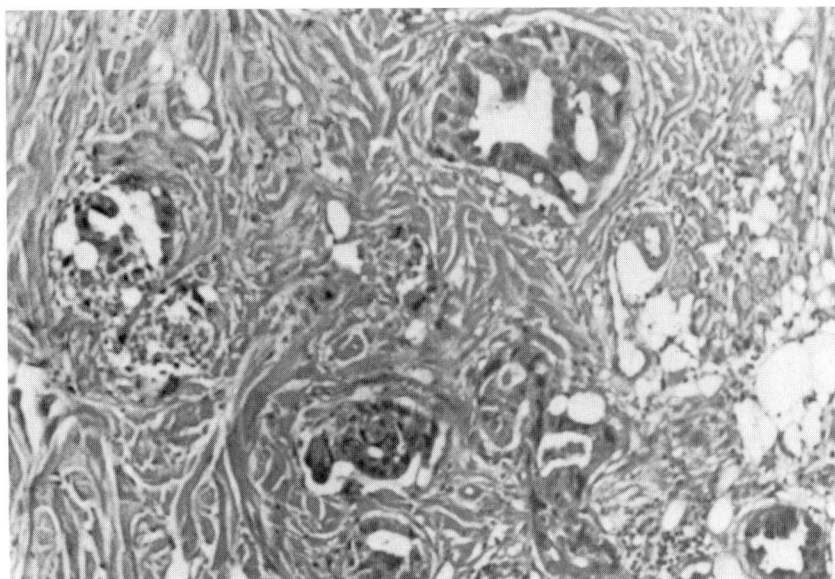

FIGURE 20-165. Metastatic bronchiogenic carcinoma in a cat. Metastatic lesions in dermis.

derma) were reported in 9% of a series of dogs with chronic lymphocytic leukemia.[416] Histopathologically, leukemia cutis is characterized by a perivascular, interstitial, lichenoid, or diffuse monomorphous infiltration of leukemia cells.[5] The leukemia cells often infiltrate between collagen bundles.

Surgical transplantation of a neoplasm (tumor seeding) is rarely reported in dogs or cats.[409, 413] Lesions appear in the healed surgical incision through which the primary neoplasm was removed. Most cases involved urinary tract carcinomas.

● PARANEOPLASTIC SYNDROMES

Certain dermatoses may occasionally be associated with concurrent neoplasms.[2a, 420a, 420b] Such dermatologic conditions include amyloidosis, pruritus, necrolytic migratory erythema, exfoliative dermatitis, pemphigus, vasculitis, dermatomyositis, and collagenous nevi. Pruritus of the distal limbs was seen in a cat with oral squamous cell carcinoma.[2a] Pruritus disappeared when the neoplasm was excised, and it returned when the neoplasm recurred.

● NON-NEOPLASTIC TUMORS

Cutaneous Cysts

A cyst is a non-neoplastic, simple saclike structure with an epithelial lining. Classification of cysts depends on identification of the lining epithelium or the pre-existing structure from which the cyst arose.

FOLLICULAR CYSTS

The majority of cutaneous cysts in the dog and cat are follicular in origin and can be further categorized by the level of the follicle from which they develop.[1, 2, 5] Infundibular and isthmus-catagen (tricholemmal) cysts are common in dogs and uncommon in cats. Matrical cysts are uncommon in dogs and rare in cats. Hybrid cysts, which combine two or three types of follicular epithelium, are uncommon in dogs and cats.

Follicular cysts usually appear as solitary, well-circumscribed, round, smooth, firm to fluctuant lesions that are dermal to subcutaneous in location and 0.5 to 5 cm in diameter.[1, 2, 5, 142a] Occasional lesions may have a bluish hue. Lesions may open and discharge a yellowish, brownish, or grayish material that is caseous or doughy in consistency. There are no apparent age or sex predilections for solitary follicular cysts, and they occur most commonly on the head, the neck, the trunk (see Fig. 20–152F), and the proximal limbs. Lesions may be multiple (Fig. 20–166).[5, 142a, 427] Boxers, Doberman pinschers, Shih tzus, and miniature Schnauzers may be predisposed.[1] Rarely, follicular cysts appear as recurrent soft tissue swellings in the medial canthus of the eye.[422]

Multiple follicular cysts of presumed congenital origin occur on the dorsal midline of the head in young dogs and on pressure points (especially the elbow) of dogs, presumably resulting from chronic trauma, dermal fibrosis, and obstruction of follicular ostia.[2] Small (2 to 5 mm in diameter) follicular cysts (milia) may be seen as postinflammatory changes, especially in dogs.[5] They are usually white and grossly resemble pustules or calcinosis cutis (Fig. 20–167; also see Fig. 20–152G). Multiple milia can also be seen in dogs that have received therapeutic levels of glucocorticoids for long periods.

All types of cysts may be complicated by rupture and resultant foreign body granuloma reaction and secondary bacterial infection. Such cysts often appear inflamed and infected grossly, and may be painful, pruritic, or both.

The therapy of choice for most cutaneous cysts is surgical excision or observation without treatment. Cysts should *never* be squeezed hard or manually evacuated, because such procedures greatly increase the chance of expressing cyst contents into the dermis or subcutis and inciting foreign body reaction and infection.

Infundibular Cyst

Infundibular cysts have been previously called "epidermoid" or "epidermal inclusion" cysts by pathologists and "sebaceous cysts" or "wens" by clinicians.[2, 5, 424] They are characterized

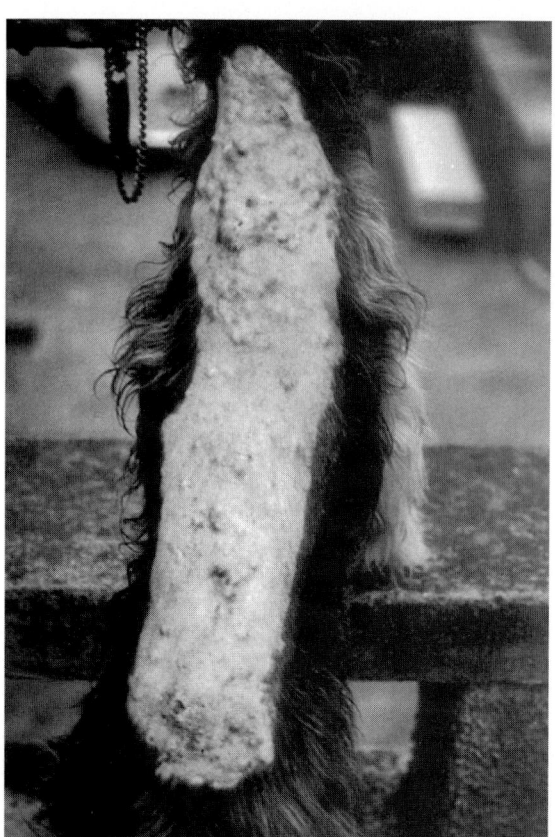

FIGURE 20–166. Multiple follicular cysts over back of dog (area has been clipped). (Courtesy E. Teixeira.)

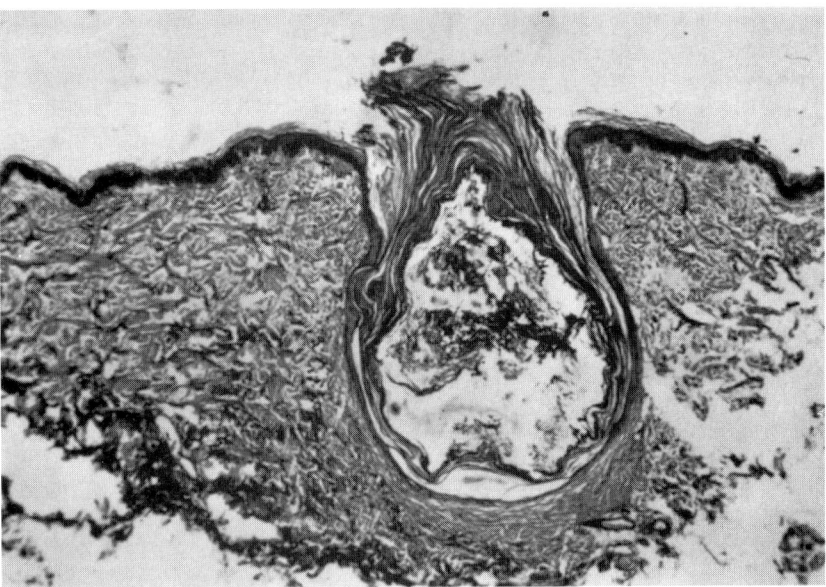

FIGURE 20–167. Canine follicular cyst (milium).

by a cyst wall that undergoes epidermal differentiation; a cyst cavity containing lamellar, often concentrically arranged keratin (Fig. 20–168); and often a connection to a rudimentary hair follicle if serial sections are employed.[2, 5] Cytologic examination of any keratin-filled cyst reveals squames (Fig. 20–169A) and cholesterol crystals (Fig. 20–169B).

Isthmus-Catagen Cyst

Isthmus-catagen (tricholemmal) cysts are characterized by a cyst wall that undergoes trichilemmal differentiation (no granular layer) and a cyst cavity containing a more homogeneous, amorphous keratin (Fig. 20–170).[2, 430]

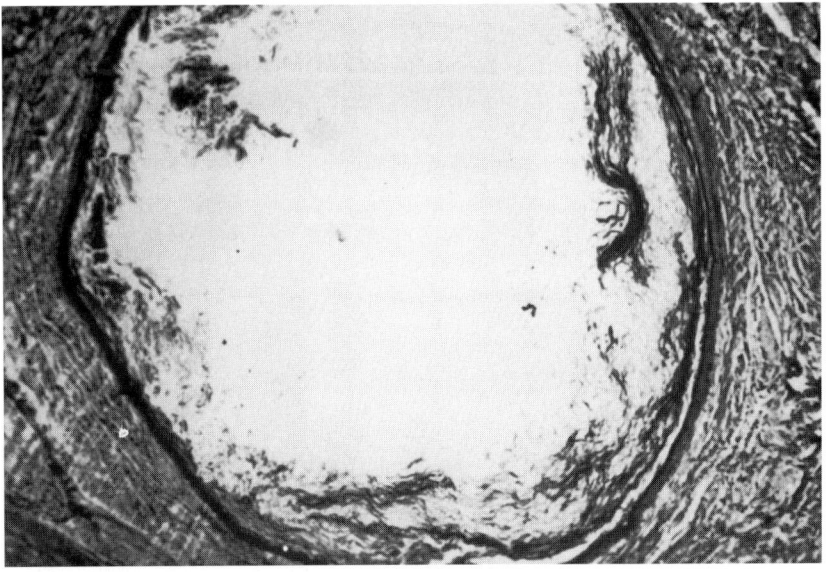

FIGURE 20–168. Canine infundibular cyst.

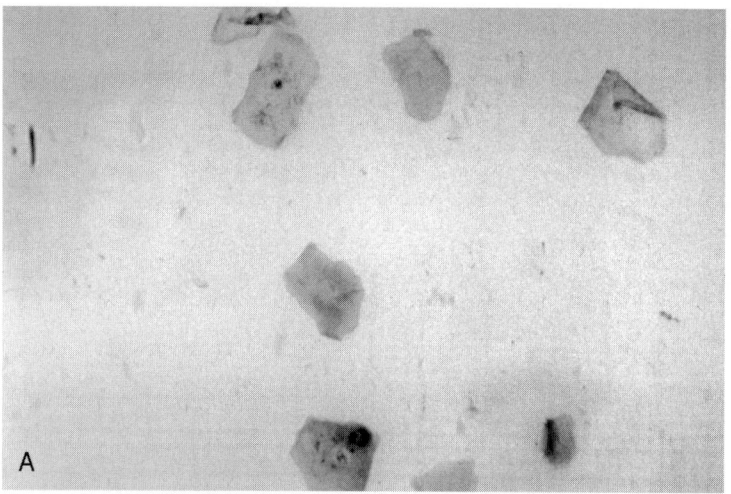
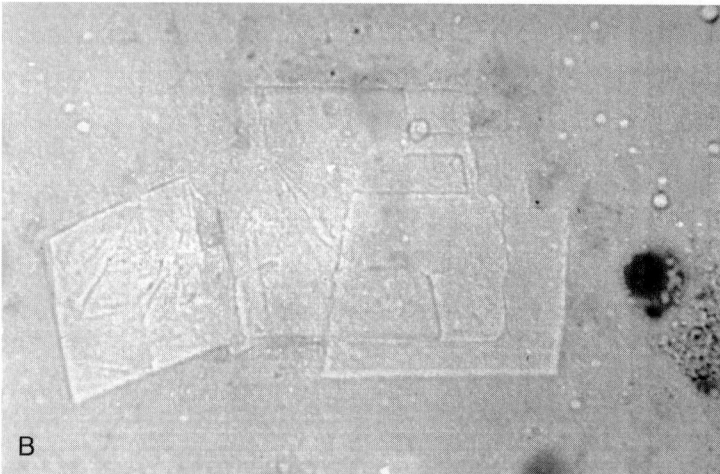

FIGURE 20–169. Canine follicular cyst. *A*, Aspirate contains numerous squames. *B*, Aspirate contains cholesterol crystals.

Matrical Cyst

Matrical cysts are characterized by a cyst wall of deeply basophilic, basaloid cells, which abruptly keratinize to form eosinophilic, amorphous keratin replete with ghost, or shadow, cells.[2]

Hybrid Cyst

Hybrid (mixed, or panfollicular) cysts are characterized by two or three types of follicular differentiation in the same lesion (Fig. 20–171).[2, 431]

DERMOID CYST

Dermoid cysts are rarely observed in dogs and cats.* They are developmental anomalies and are often congenital and hereditary. Dermoid cysts are most commonly reported in Boxers, Kerry blue terriers, and Rhodesian ridgebacks. In Rhodesian ridgebacks and their crosses, the condition (dermoid sinus, or pilonidal sinus) is thought to be inherited as a simple recessive trait (see Chap. 12).[2, 5, 423, 426, 428]

---

*See references 1, 2, 5, 423, 426, 428, 429, 432.

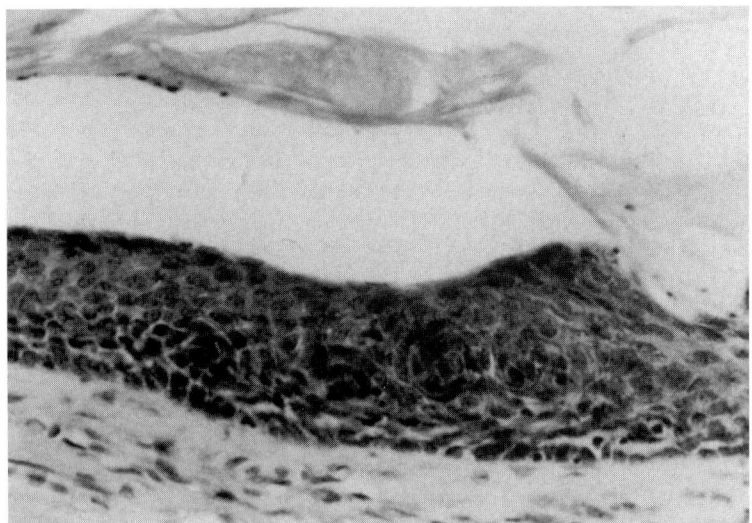

FIGURE 20–170. Canine isthmus-catagen (trichilemmal) cyst. Note trichilemmal differentiation of the cyst wall.

Lesions may be solitary or multiple and often occur along the dorsal midline. Dermoid cysts occurred in the flank region of two cats.[429] Histopathologically, the lesions are characterized by a cyst wall that undergoes epidermal differentiation and contains well-developed small hair follicles, sebaceous glands, and occasionally epitrichial sweat glands.[2, 5]

EPITRICHIAL (APOCRINE) SWEAT GLAND CYST

Epitrichial cysts are common in dogs and rare in cats.[1, 2, 5] There are no apparent breed or sex predilections, and affected animals are usually 6 years of age or older. They may be the result of sweat gland duct obstruction. Lesions are usually solitary, well-circumscribed, smooth, tense to fluctuant swellings, which are 0.5 to 3 cm in diameter. The overlying

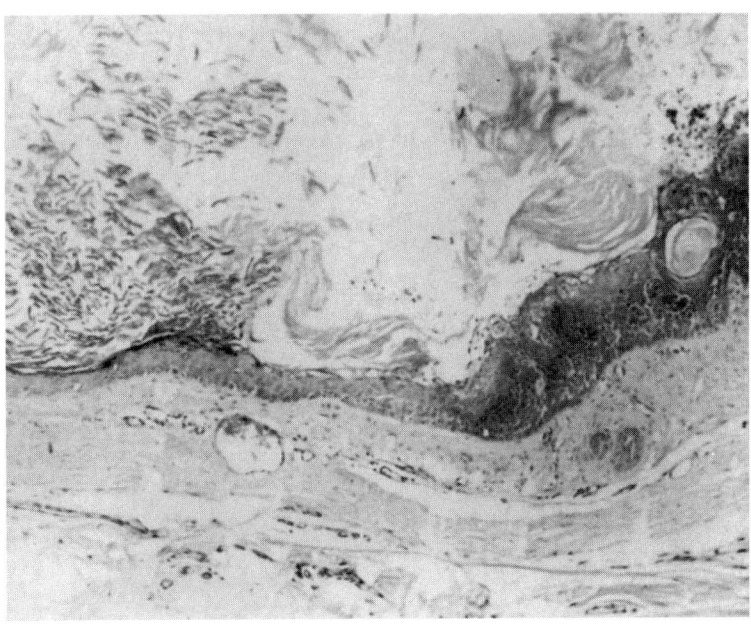

FIGURE 20–171. Canine hybrid cyst. Note combined epidermal *(left)* and trichilemmal *(right)* differentiation of the cyst wall.

1380 • Neoplastic and Non-Neoplastic Tumors

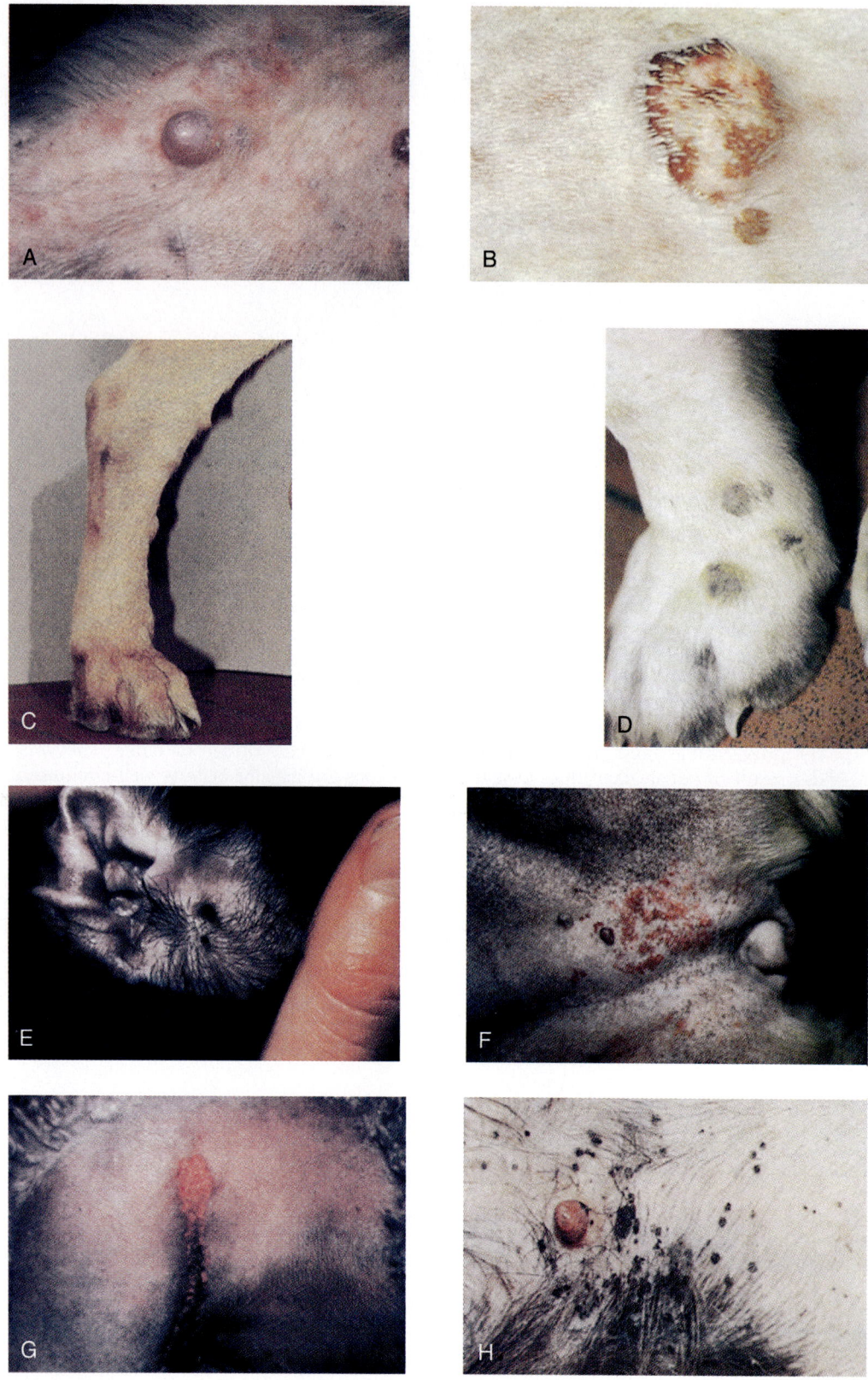

FIGURE 20–172. *Legend on opposite page*

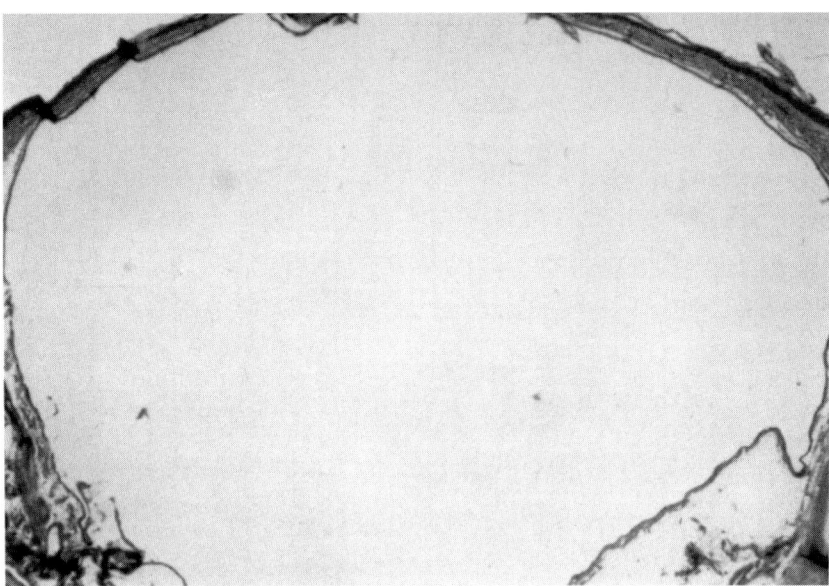

FIGURE 20–173. Canine epitrichial sweat gland cyst.

skin may be atrophic and alopecic, and the lesions often appear bluish (see Fig. 20–152H). Cyst contents are usually clear, watery, and acellular. Lesions occur most commonly on the head, the neck, and the limbs.[1, 5]

Multiple epitrichial cysts occur in the eyelids of Persian and Himalayan cats.[420c] Cysts ranged from 2 to 10 mm in size and were soft, smooth, round, and fluid filled. They were located in the skin around the medial canthus and in the upper and lower eyelids. The cysts involved both eyelids in most cats.

Epitrichial sweat gland cystomatosis is a term used to describe a rare condition in middle-aged-to-older dogs.[2, 5, 433] Multiple clusters of cystically dilated epitrichial sweat glands produce grouped vesicles and bullae, 0.5 to 5 cm in diameter, especially on the head and the neck (Fig. 20–172A). The overlying skin is usually atrophic and alopecic, and the cysts may have a bluish to purplish tint.

Cytologic examination of aspirates reveals only fluid and a few macrophages.[433] Histopathologically, epitrichial sweat gland cysts are made up of variable-sized dilated epitrichial sweat glands (Figs. 20–173 and 20–174), which may occur as large solitary cysts, clusters of smaller cysts, or large cysts surrounded by smaller satellite cysts (Fig. 20–175).[1, 2, 5, 433]

The treatment of choice for epitrichial cysts is surgical excision or observation without treatment. Solitary lesions may be aspirated, but often recur within several weeks. There is at present no practical approach to the dog with epitrichial sweat gland cystomatosis.

SEBACEOUS GLAND CYST

Cysts that involve sebaceous structures are extremely rare in dogs and cats.[2] Sebaceous duct cysts appear as solitary, firm, dermal nodules that are smaller than 1 cm in diameter. There are no known age, breed, sex, or site predilections.

FIGURE 20–172. *A*, Multiple epitrichial sweat gland cysts in a dog. *B*, Solitary collagenous nevus in a Brittany spaniel. Firm, well-circumscribed, partially pin-feathered nodule over the thorax. *C*, Multiple collagenous nevi in a German shepherd dog. *D*, Multiple collagenous nevi on the paw of a German shepherd dog. *E*, Two small, melanotic organoid nevi in the periauricular area of a young cat. *F*, Congenital vascular nevus in the groin of a young dog. *G*, Congenital sebaceous nevus in the flank of a dog (the area has been clipped). *H*, Multiple hyperkeratotic, melanotic epidermal nevi in the flank of a young dog.

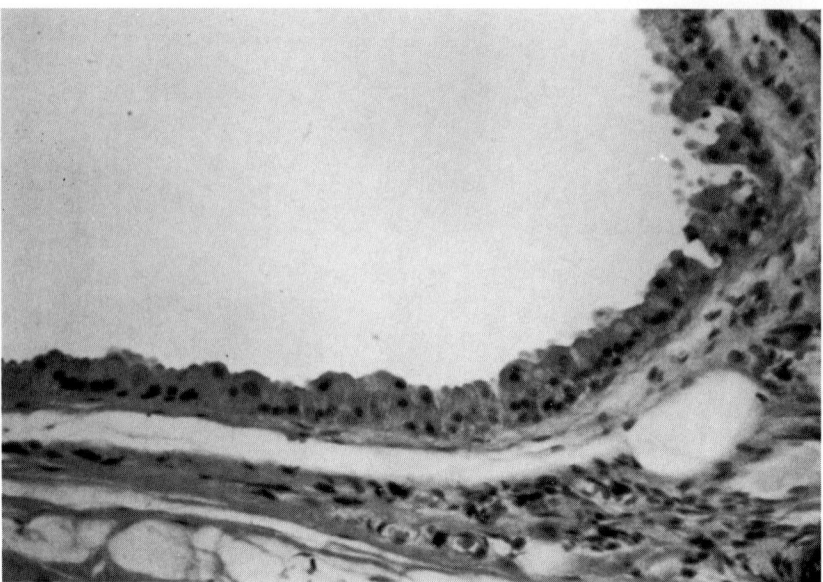

FIGURE 20–174. Close-up of Figure 20–173. Columnar glandular epithelium with apical budding.

BRANCHIAL CYST

Branchial cysts are developmental defects arising from the second branchial cleft. They are extremely rare in dogs and cats.[1, 421, 425] There are no apparent age, breed, or sex predilections. Affected animals have a poorly circumscribed, firm to fluctuant swelling in the ventral cervical region. Histopathologically, branchial cysts are characterized by a thin-walled cyst lined by pseudostratified, nonciliated, columnar epithelial cells.[1] The treatment of choice is surgical excision or observation without therapy.

Nevi

A nevus (hamartoma) is a circumscribed developmental defect of the skin, characterized by hyperplasia of one or more skin components.[1, 2, 5, 447] They may or may not be congenital and are uncommonly reported in dogs and cats. The mechanism of nevus formation is not understood. A failure in the normal orderly embryonic inductive process has been theorized. In addition, the distribution of certain epidermal and vascular nevi has prompted speculation that a relationship to dermatomes or peripheral nerves exists. Finally, some nevi have a hereditary occurrence.

COLLAGENOUS NEVI

Collagenous nevi have been recognized in many breeds of dogs as solitary or multiple cutaneous lesions, especially on the head, neck, and proximal extremities (see Fig. 20–172B).[2, 5, 439, 447] Most collagenous nevi are firm, well circumscribed, and 0.5 to 5 cm in diameter. Some lesions are alopecic, are hyperpigmented, and have pitted surfaces ("cobblestone" or "orange peel" appearance). Lesions on the feet may ulcerate and cause pain and lameness.

In German shepherd dogs, a syndrome of multiple, approximately symmetrically distributed collagenous nevi (so-called nodular dermatofibrosis) on the limbs (see Fig. 20–172C and D), head, neck, and ventral trunk has been described.° In these German

---

°See references 2, 5, 435, 437, 438, 443, 445, 449.

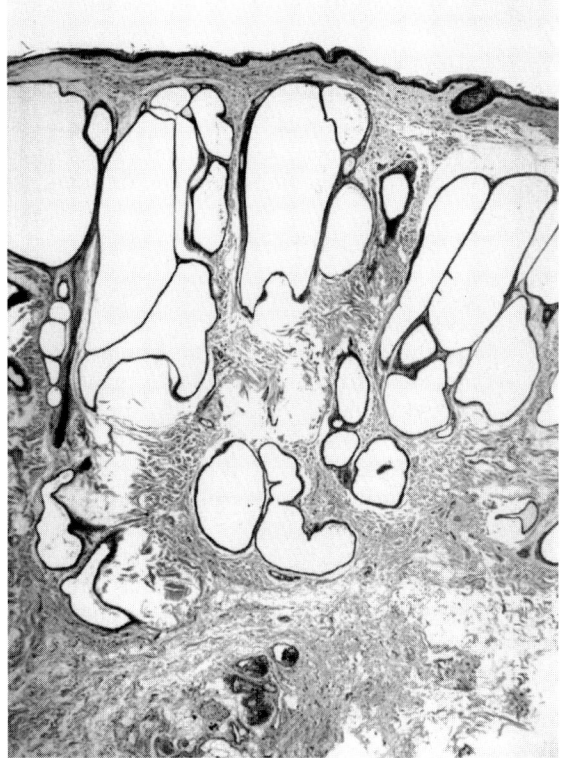

FIGURE 20–175. Epitrichial sweat gland cystomatosis in a dog. Multiple, large, dilated epitrichial sweat glands.

shepherd dogs, the syndrome is autosomal dominant in inheritance and is characterized by the sudden onset of skin lesions at 3 to 7 years of age. There is no sex predilection. The lesions are distributed more or less symmetrically on the limbs and head, and range from 0.5 to 5 cm in diameter. They are usually firm, asymptomatic, and covered by normal skin and hair. These German shepherds virtually always develop bilateral renal disease, varying from polycystic kidneys to renal cystadenomas to renal cystadenocarcinomas. Enlarged and abnormally shaped kidneys may eventually be palpable in about 60% of the dogs and may be detected radiographically or ultrasonographically in about 86%.[443] The dogs usually develop clinical signs of renal dysfunction within 3 to 5 years after the initial recognition of the skin lesions Intact females almost always develop multiple uterine leiomyomas.[443] Many of the dogs have multiple small intestinal polyps, which are asymptomatic.[443] Death is due to renal failure, metastasis (sternal and abdominal lymph nodes, liver, lungs), and euthanasia.[443]

Multiple collagenous nevi in association with bilateral renal cysts, cystadenomas, and cystadenocarcinomas have occasionally been recognized in other dog breeds: Golden retrievers, Boxers, German shepherd crosses, and mongrels.[441, 443a, 451] Periodic abdominal radiographs or ultrasound examinations, or both, have been recommended for all dogs with multiple collagenous nevi.[451]

The renal pathology associated with multiple collagenous nevi has been described as non-neoplastic cysts, hyperplastic and dysplastic nodules, adenomas, adenocarcinomas, and oncocytoma.[437, 438, 443, 445, 449, 451] This diversity of pathologic changes probably represents different stages of the same process.

The pathogenesis of the multiple collagenous nevi and bilateral renal disease syndrome is not known. One hypothesis is that the skin lesions may represent a paraneoplastic process wherein collagen is stimulated by growth factors (TGFα and ß?) produced by the renal tumors.[441, 443, 451] Another hypothesis is that the skin, renal, and uterine lesions develop independently through a common genetic abnormality.[441, 443, 451]

Histopathologically, organoid nevi are characterized by hyperplasia of two or more skin components (Fig. 20–179). Focal adnexal dysplasia is characterized by circumscribed, dermal to subcutaneous nodules composed of loosely distributed, haphazardly arranged folliculosebaceous units and abundant collagen.[2, 450] Concurrent suppurative or pyogranulomatous inflammation is common. Adnexal nevi are composed of hyperplastic adnexae with frequent concurrent inflammation.[1] Therapeutic options include surgical excision and observation without treatment. Isotretinoin and etretinate were ineffective for the treatment of linear organoid nevus in one dog.[446a]

VASCULAR NEVI

Vascular nevi occur on the scrotum (varicose tumors of the scrotum, or scrotal vascular hamartoma) and occasionally elsewhere in dogs (see Fig. 20–172F).[1, 2, 33, 452] They are most common in dogs older than middle age and in breeds with pigmented skin, such as Scottish terriers, Airedales, Kerry blue terriers, and Labrador retrievers. The lesions are characterized by single or multiple, slowly enlarging and hyperpigmenting plaques on the scrotum. Periodic hemorrhage from the lesions may be seen. Vascular nevi are occasionally seen at other cutaneous sites.[18, 446] Histopathologically, the scrotal lesions are characterized by cavernous dilatation (telangiectasia) of blood vessels and epidermal melanosis. Therapeutic options include surgical excision and observation without treatment. A 2-year-old Labrador retriever with a dark red patch ("port-wine stain") around its neck since birth was cured with surgical excision and an axial rotation flap.[448]

SEBACEOUS GLAND NEVI

Sebaceous gland nevi are rarely diagnosed in dogs.[1, 2, 447] They are usually solitary, alopecic, scaly plaques, smaller than 2 cm in diameter, with an irregular or papillated surface. A sebaceous gland nevus was recognized in a 1-year-old male Poodle.[447] The lesion had been present on the lateral right thigh since birth and had been slowly enlarging. It was linear, multinodular, alopecic, smooth, shiny, greasy, and orange-yellow (see Fig. 20–172G).

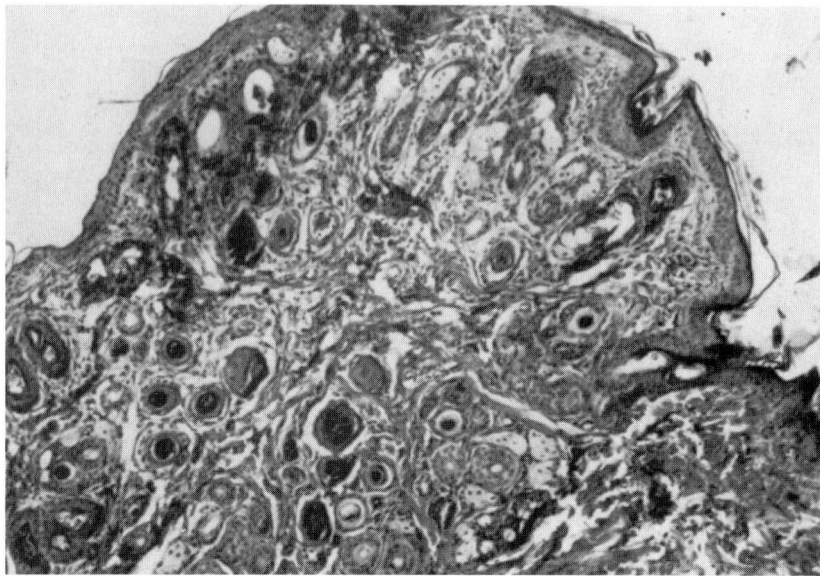

FIGURE 20–179. Organoid nevus. Dome-shaped mass consisting of an excess of hair follicles and sebaceous glands. (From Scott DW: Feline dermatology 1900–1978: A monograph. J Am Anim Hosp Assoc 16:331, 1980.)

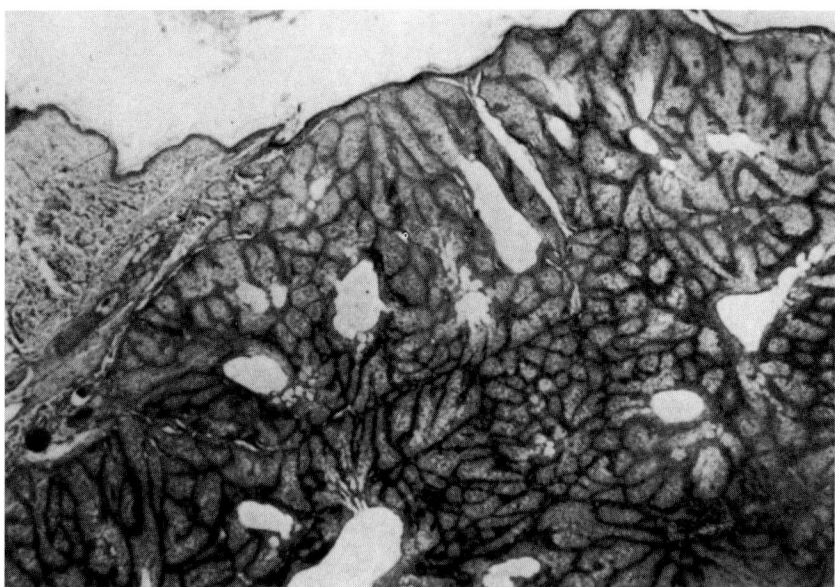

FIGURE 20–180. Sebaceous nevus. Nodular sebaceous gland hyperplasia.

Histopathologically, sebaceous gland nevi are characterized by sebaceous gland hyperplasia and overlying papillated epidermal hyperplasia (Fig. 20–180). Therapeutic options include surgical excision and observation without treatment.

EPITRICHIAL (APOCRINE) SWEAT GLAND NEVI

Epitrichial sweat gland nevi are rarely diagnosed in young dogs and cats.[1, 436] Lesions have been solitary and located on the head and neck (Fig. 20–181). Lesions may be bluish in color and fluctuant. Histologically, a linear to nodular proliferation of hyperplastic, dilated epitrichial sweat glands is present in the deep dermis and subcutis (Fig. 20–182). Therapeutic options include surgical excision and observation without treatment.

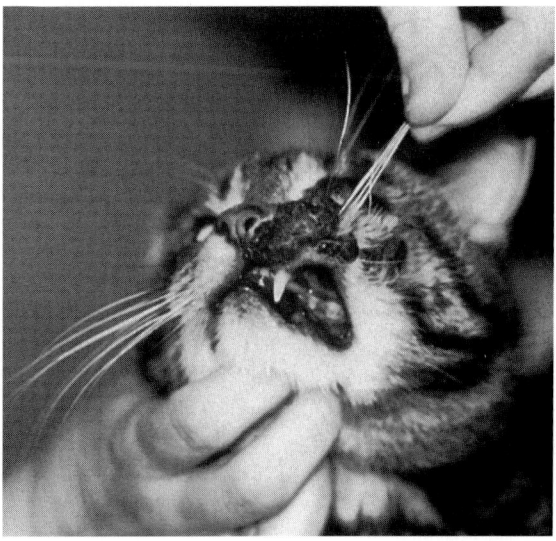

FIGURE 20–181. Epitrichial sweat gland nevus in a cat. Multilobulated, alopecic, fluctuant masses on left side of face. (Courtesy M. Paradis.)

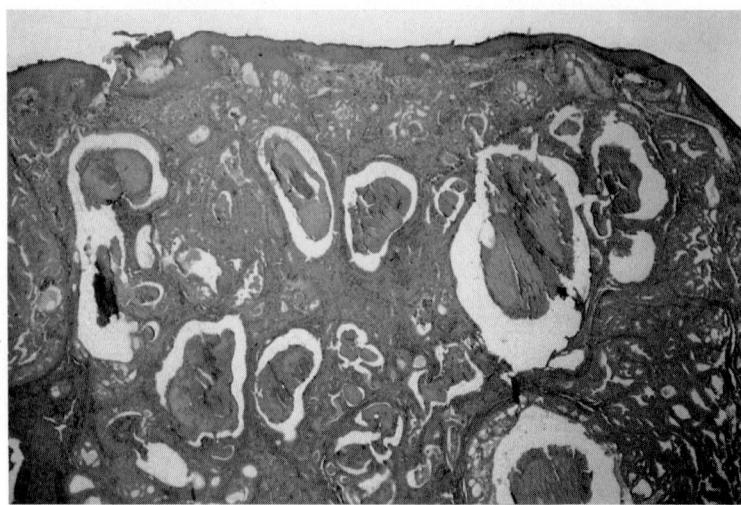

FIGURE 20–182. Epitrichial sweat gland nevus in a cat. Hyperplastic, secretion-filled epitrichial sweat glands.

EPIDERMAL NEVI

Epidermal nevi are uncommonly diagnosed in dogs.[1, 2, 5, 447] These lesions usually occur in young adults. Lesions previously reported as lentigines or pigmented epidermal nevi in Pugs and miniature Schnauzers were probably papillomas (see Papilloma). Lesions are usually multiple, occasionally solitary, ovoid to circular to linear plaques, hyperpigmented, scaly to papillomatous, and smaller than 2 cm in diameter (Fig. 20–183). They occur most commonly on the ventral abdomen (see Fig. 20–172H), the ventral thorax, and the medial limbs. Epidermal nevi tend to follow Blashko's lines, possibly resulting from genetic mosaicism in which two or more genetically different cell lines are present within the same individual.[448a]

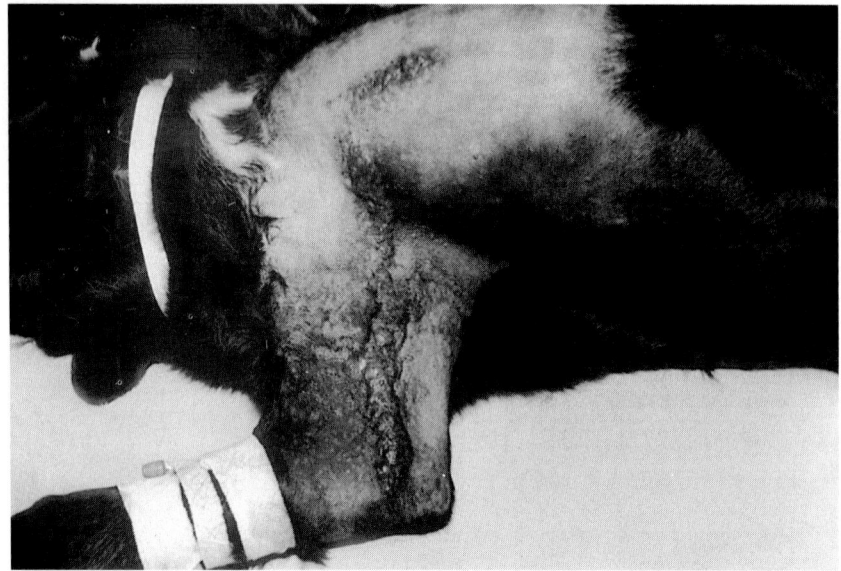

FIGURE 20–183. Linear epidermal nevus in a dog. Hyperpigmented, inflamed, linear lesion runs from sternum to medial elbow.

Epidermal nevi occurred in a 2-month-old male miniature Schnauzer; the lesions developed as wavy, linear bands of closely set, hyperpigmented, hyperkeratotic papules and plaques over the trunk.[447] Inflammatory linear verrucous epidermal nevi were reported in three related Cocker spaniels.[453] All dogs were female and had lesions before 6 months of age. Linear, pigmented verrucous lesions were noted most commonly on the lateral trunk, the footpads, and the ears. All lesions were moderately pruritic.

Histologic examination of epidermal nevi shows orthokeratotic hyperkeratosis, papillated epidermal hyperplasia, epidermal melanosis, and papillomatosis (Fig. 20–184). In some instances, granular degeneration of the epidermis is present.

Therapeutic options include surgical excision and observation without treatment. In three dogs with inflammatory linear verrucous epidermal nevus, improvement was achieved with the oral administration of isotretinoin or etretinate.[453]

HAIR FOLLICLE NEVI

Hair follicle nevi are uncommonly diagnosed in dogs.[1, 2, 444] Lesions are solitary or multiple, hyperkeratotic, ovoid or linear plaques, especially on proximal extremities. Hairs arising from the lesions may be thick and brushlike. Histologically, hair follicles and hair shafts that are larger than normal are present in clusters (Fig. 20–185). Therapeutic options include surgical excision and observation without treatment.

COMEDO NEVI

Comedo nevi are rarely diagnosed in dogs.[444] Lesions are solitary, well-circumscribed, annular areas of alopecia, hyperkeratosis, and clustered comedones. Schnauzer comedo syndrome is probably a more widespread form of comedo nevus (see Chap. 12). Histologically, there are clusters of dilated, hyperkeratotic hair follicles (Fig. 20–186).

Therapeutic options include surgical excision and observation without treatment. The oral administration of isotretinoin is effective treatment for the Schnauzer comedo syndrome (see Chap. 12).

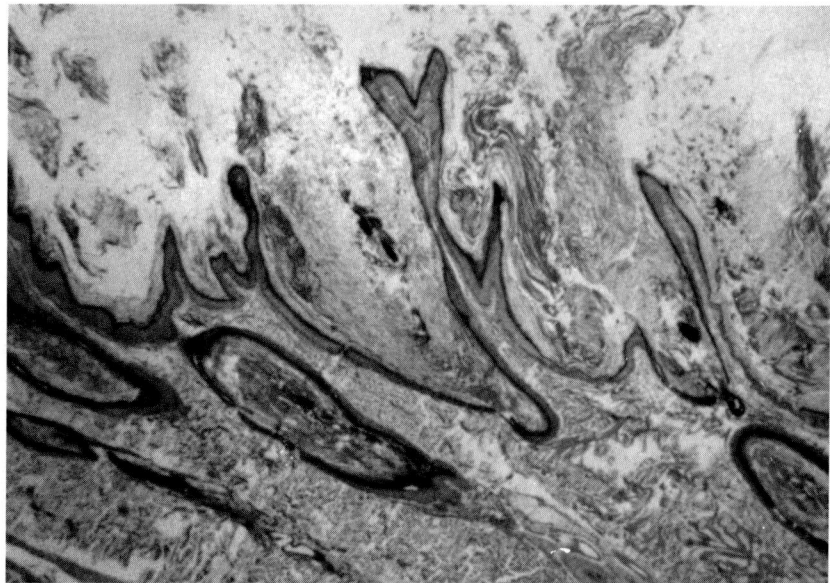

FIGURE 20–184. Epidermal nevus. Orthokeratotic hyperkeratosis, papillated epidermal hyperplasia, and papillomatosis.

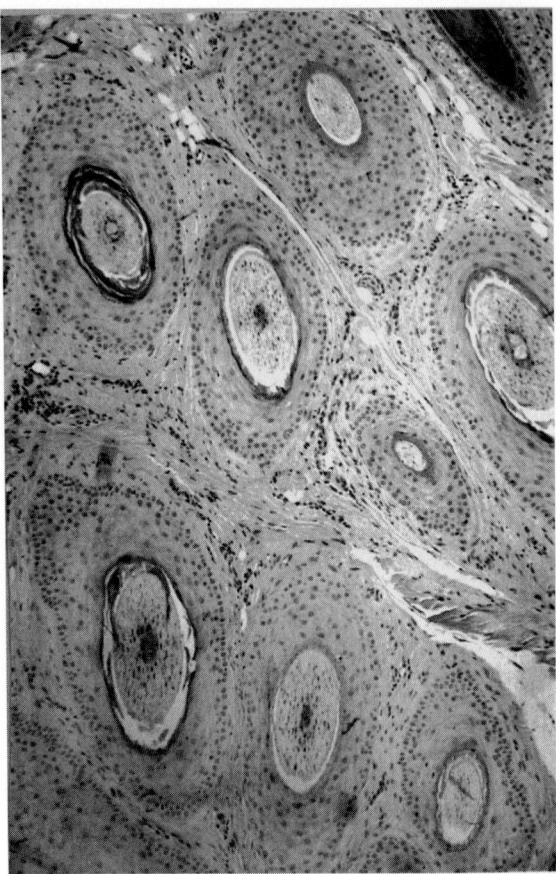

FIGURE 20–185. Hair follicle nevus from a dog.

PACINIAN CORPUSCLE NEVI

Pacinian corpuscle nevi are rarely reported in dogs and cats.[1] Numerous pacinian corpuscles are seen in the dermis and subcutis.

MELANOCYTIC NEVI

Although the term "melanocytic nevus" has been frequently employed in veterinary medicine,[2, 5, 33, 434, 440] most of the lesions were acquired and more appropriately called melanocytomas (see Melanocytic Neoplasms). Congenital melanocytic nevi are occasionally seen (Figs. 20–187 and 20–188A and B).

A Golden retriever was born with a strip of abnormal skin on the right pelvic limb.[390b] When examined at 5 years of age, the dog had a 5-cm-wide strip of abnormal skin that extended from the medial stifle to the metatarsus. The hair in the lesion was a darker color, and the skin was thickened with multiple dark papules and one 3.5 × 7 cm nodule that had recently arisen. Histopathologic findings included a melanocytic nevus with a focal melanoma, which metastasized. This case was likened to congenital giant melanocytic nevus in humans, wherein 12% of the lesions develop melanoma. Early surgical excision is recommended.

Keratoses

Keratoses are firm, elevated, circumscribed areas of reactive keratinocyte proliferation and excessive keratin production.[2, 5] Keratoses are uncommonly reported in dogs and cats.

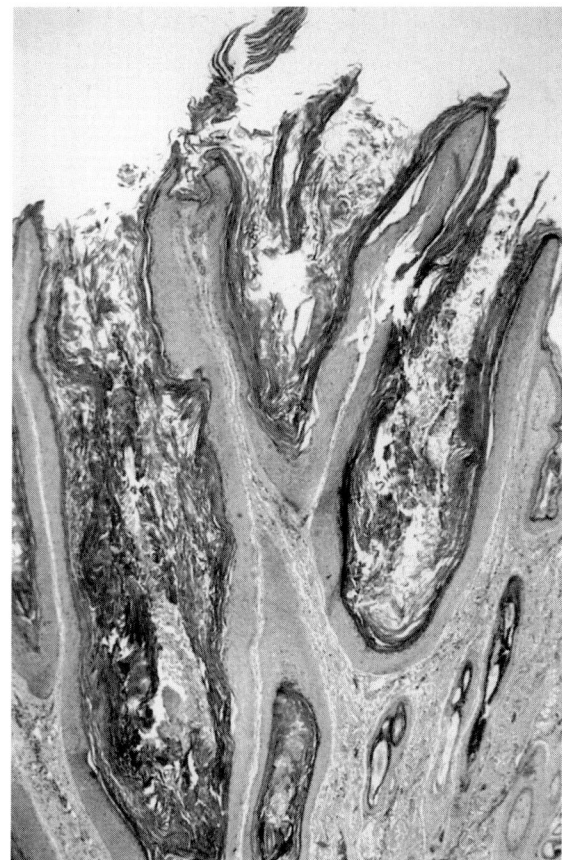

FIGURE 20–186. Comedo nevus in a dog.

ACTINIC KERATOSIS

Actinic (solar) keratoses occur in dogs and cats.[2, 5, 113, 455] They are caused by excessive exposure to ultraviolet light and occur more commonly in sunny areas of the world. Actinic keratoses may be single or multiple, appear in lightly haired and lightly pigmented

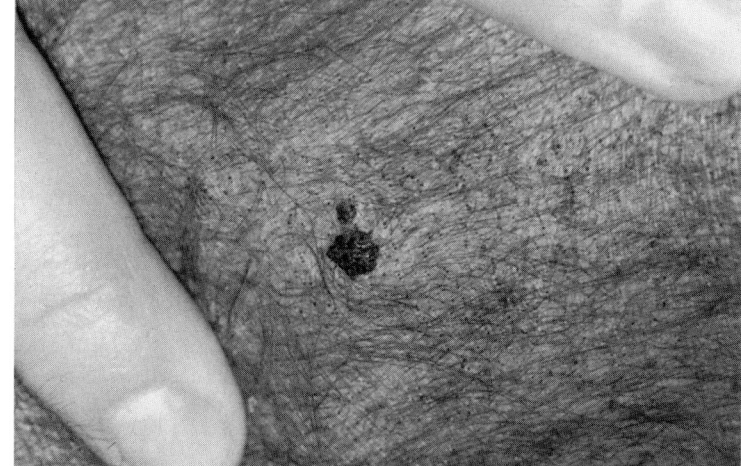

FIGURE 20–187. Melanocytic nevus, present since birth, on the rump of a hypothyroid dog.

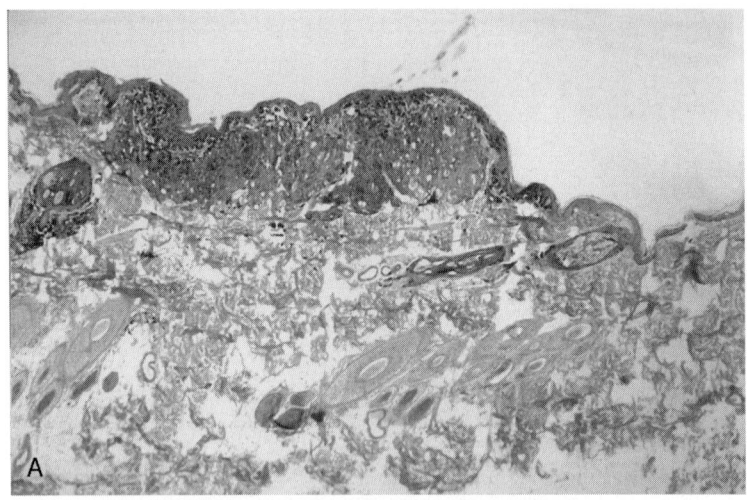

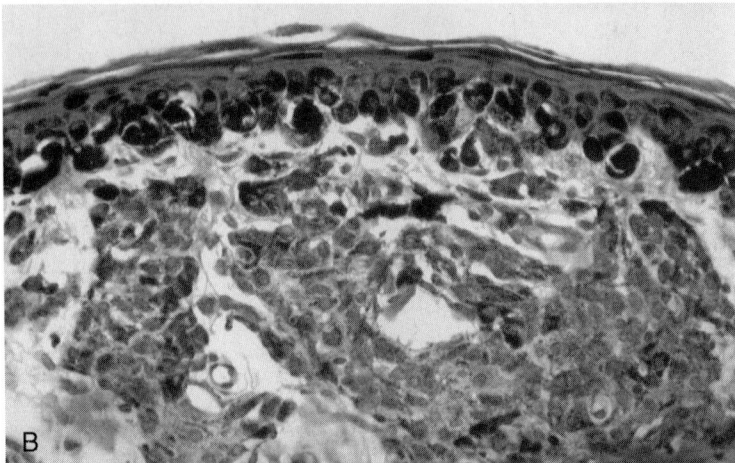

FIGURE 20–188. Melanocytic nevus in a dog. *A*, Focal junctional and dermal proliferation of melanocytes (compound melanocytic nevus). *B*, Close-up of *A*.

skin, and vary in appearance from ill-defined areas of erythema, hyperkeratosis, and crusting to indurated, crusted, hyperkeratotic plaques varying from 0.3 to 5 cm in diameter (Fig. 20–189A). Dalmatians, American Staffordshire terriers, beagles, Basset hounds, and bull terriers have an increased incidence of actinic keratoses. Histopathologically, they are characterized by atypia and dysplasia of the epidermis and superficial hair follicle epithelium, hyperkeratosis (especially parakeratotic), and occasionally solar elastosis of the underlying dermis (Fig. 20–190). Actinic keratoses are premalignant lesions that are capable of becoming invasive squamous cell carcinomas. Early lesions regress with avoidance of sunlight and photoprotection. If pruritus or pain is prominent, topical or oral glucocorticoids are beneficial. More advanced lesions require systemic retinoid (isotretinoin, etretinate, acitretin), cryosurgery, or surgical excision (see Solar Dermatitis, Squamous Cell Carcinoma).[85, 89, 455]

LICHENOID KERATOSIS

Lichenoid keratoses are rarely recognized in dogs.[2, 5, 454] Generally, solitary asymptomatic lesions are seen most commonly on the pinnae and groin of adult dogs. Lesions are well-circumscribed, erythematous, and scaly to markedly hyperkeratotic plaques or papillomas

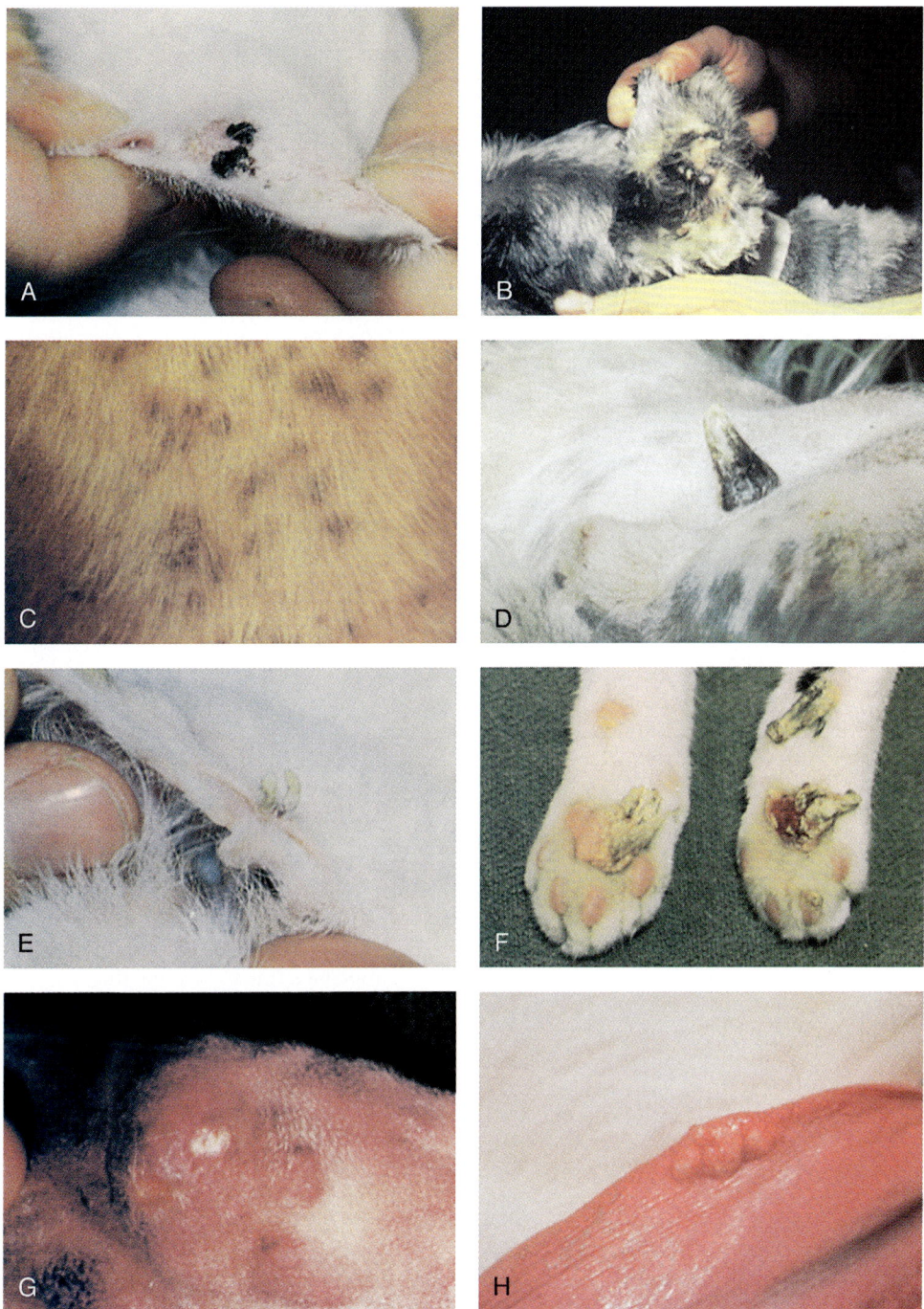

FIGURE 20-189. *A*, Feline actinic keratosis. Two crusted plaques on a background of solar dermatitis. *B*, Multiple melanotic lichenoid keratoses on the pinna of a miniature Schnauzer. *C*, Multiple brownish, greasy seborrheic keratoses over the back of a dog. *D*, Cutaneous horn cranial to the vulva. *E*, Two cutaneous horns on the pinna of a cat. *F*, Multiple cutaneous horns on the footpads of an FeLV-infected cat. *G*, Calcinosis circumscripta on the elbow of a dog. *H*, Calcinosis circumscripta on the tongue of a dog.

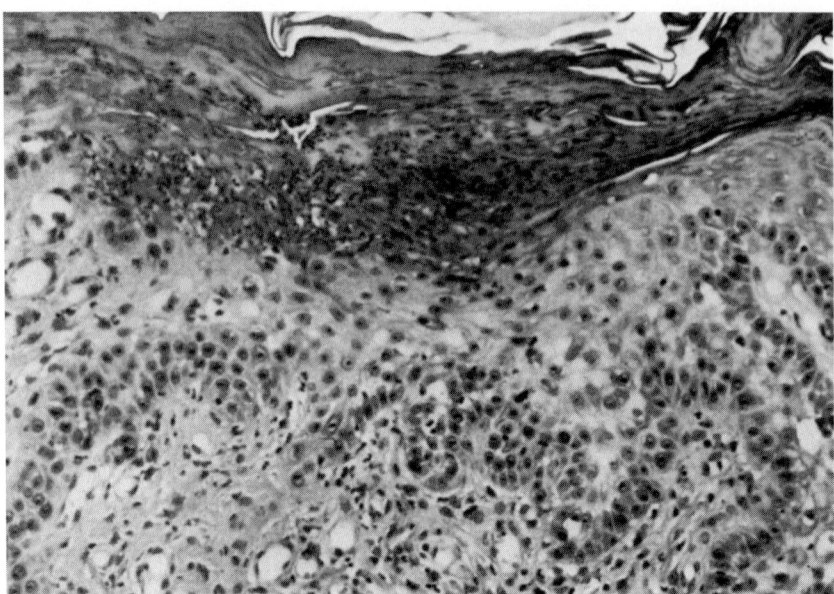

FIGURE 20–190. Feline actinic keratosis. Epidermal dysplasia (carcinoma in situ) and parakeratotic hyperkeratosis.

varying from 0.5 to 2 cm in diameter. Occasionally, multiple lesions are present on the lateral surface of the pinna (see Fig. 20–189B).[454] Histologically, an irregular to papillated epidermal hyperplasia with overlying hyperkeratosis and an underlying subepidermal lichenoid band of inflammation are seen (Fig. 20–191A and B). Therapeutic options include surgical excision or observation without treatment.

SEBORRHEIC KERATOSIS

Seborrheic keratoses are rarely recognized in dogs.[5, 457] The cause of seborrheic keratoses is unknown, and they have nothing to do with seborrhea. They may be single or multiple and have no apparent age, breed, sex, or site predilections. The lesions are elevated plaques and nodules with a hyperkeratotic, often greasy surface (see Fig. 20–189C). They are frequently hyperpigmented. Histologically, seborrheic keratoses are characterized by hyperkeratosis, hyperplasia (basaloid and squamoid), and papillomatosis (Fig. 20–192). Therapeutic options include surgical excision and observation without treatment.

PERIOCULAR KERATOSIS

The authors have occasionally consulted on older dogs with distinctly periocular keratoses. The dogs were not disturbing the lesions, and usually had no other dermatologic disease. The lesions were described as having developed gradually, more or less symmetrically. Whitish to grayish, dry, keratinous fronds were presented on the periocular skin (Fig. 20–193). No biopsies were permitted. No therapy was attempted.

CUTANEOUS HORN

Cutaneous horns are uncommon in dogs and cats.[5] The cause of cutaneous horns may be unknown, or they may originate from papillomas, basal cell tumors, squamous cell carcinomas, keratinous cysts, keratoacanthomas, or actinic keratoses. Cutaneous horns may be single or multiple and have no apparent age, sex, or site predilections. They are firm, hornlike projections of up to 5 cm in length (see Fig. 20–189D and E). Multiple

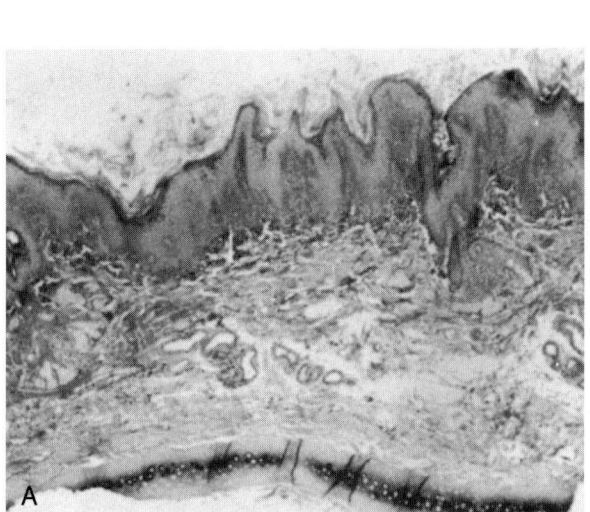
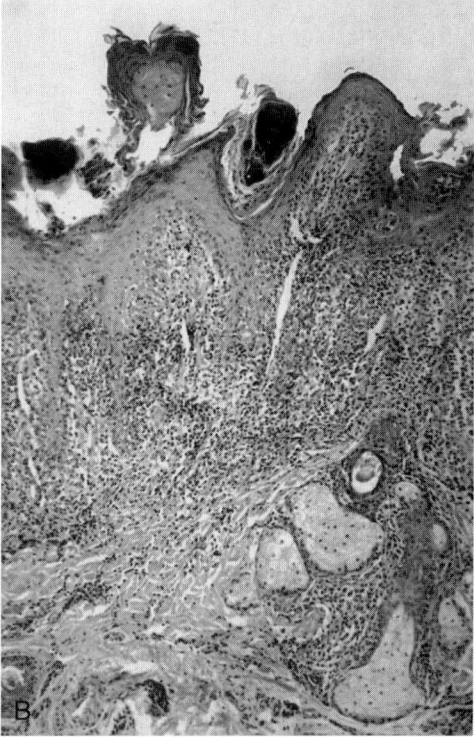

FIGURE 20–191. Canine idiopathic lichenoid keratosis. *A*, Papillated epidermal hyperplasia, hyperkeratosis, and a lichenoid cellular infiltrate. *B*, Close-up of *A*.

cutaneous horns have been seen on the footpads of cats with FeLV infection.[21, 36, 456] Generally, multiple horns are seen on multiple footpads, and the horns may arise from anywhere on the pad (see Fig. 20–189*F*). Occasionally, lesions are seen on the face. Multiple cutaneous horns have also been described on the footpads of FeLV-negative cats.[458] In these cases, multiple pads were affected, but the horns arose exclusively under the claws (Fig. 20–194).

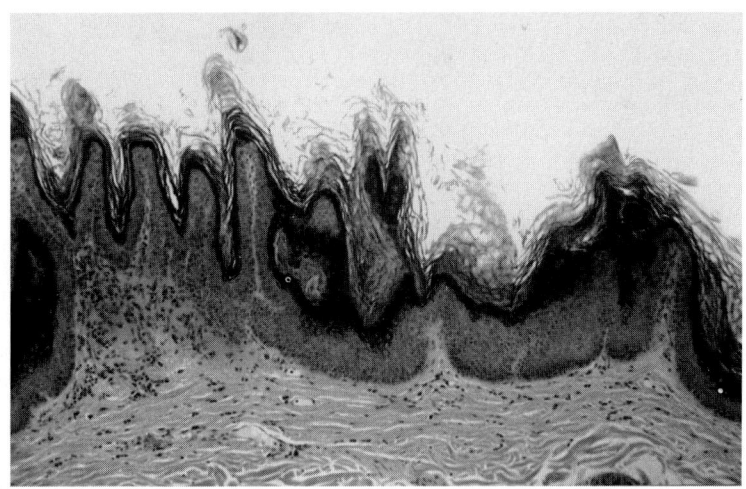

FIGURE 20–192. Canine seborrheic keratosis. Papillated epidermal hyperplasia and orthokeratotic hyperkeratosis.

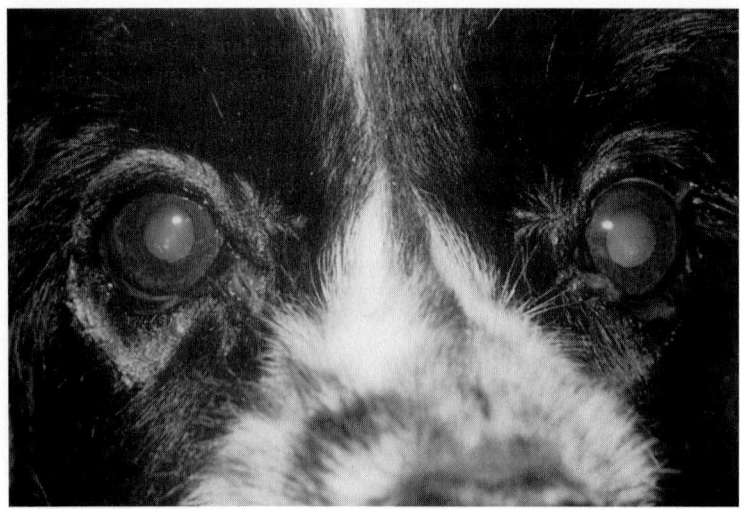

FIGURE 20–193. Periocular keratosis in a dog.

Histopathologically, cutaneous horns are characterized by extensive, compact, laminated hyperkeratosis (Figs. 20–195 and 20–196). The base of a cutaneous horn must always be inspected for the possible underlying cause. FeLV-associated cutaneous horns in cats are characterized by parakeratotic hyperkeratosis, apoptosis, and multinucleate keratinocytic giant cells (Fig. 20–197).[456] Multiple subungual cutaneous horns from FeLV-negative cats did not have these histopathologic findings.[458] Therapeutic options include surgical excision and observation without treatment.

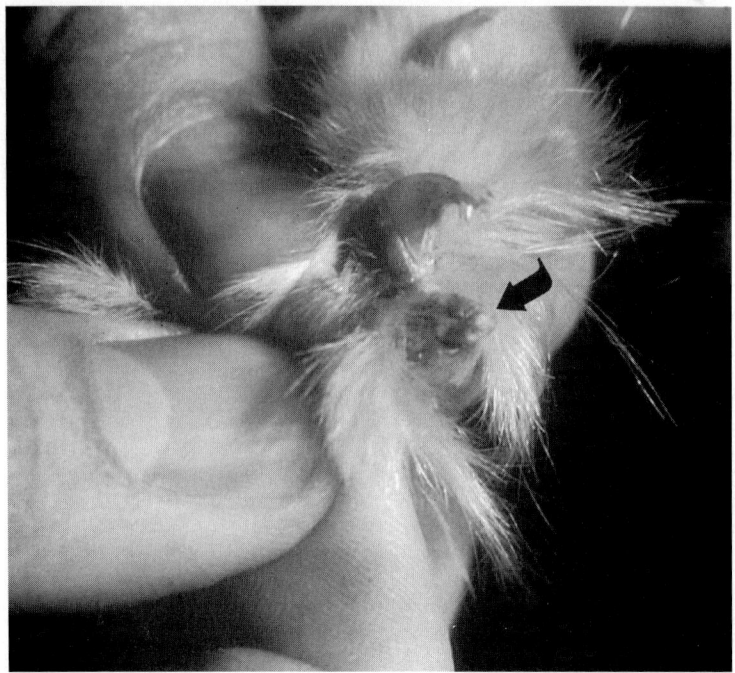

FIGURE 20–194. Subungual horns. Hornlike structures (*arrow*) were present below numerous claws.

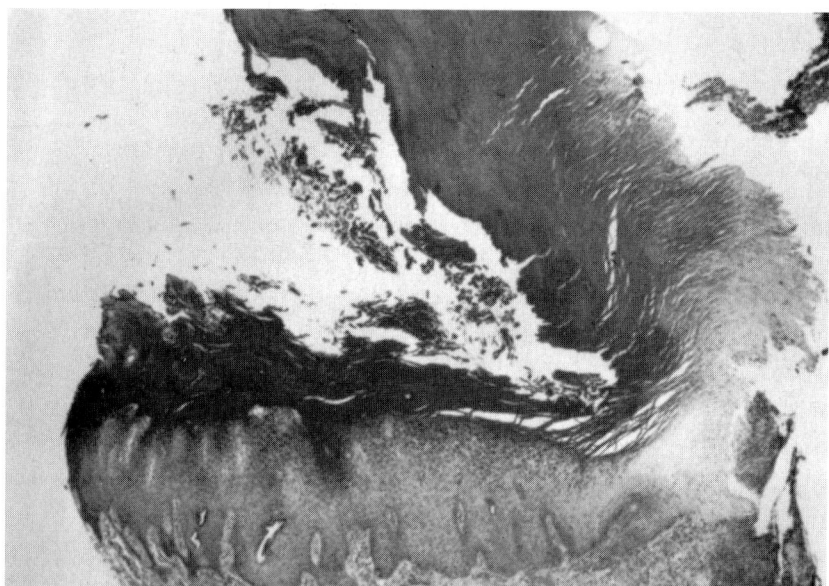

FIGURE 20–195. Feline cutaneous horn. Hornlike projection of dense keratin arising from hyperplastic, hypergranular, hyperkeratotic footpad epithelium.

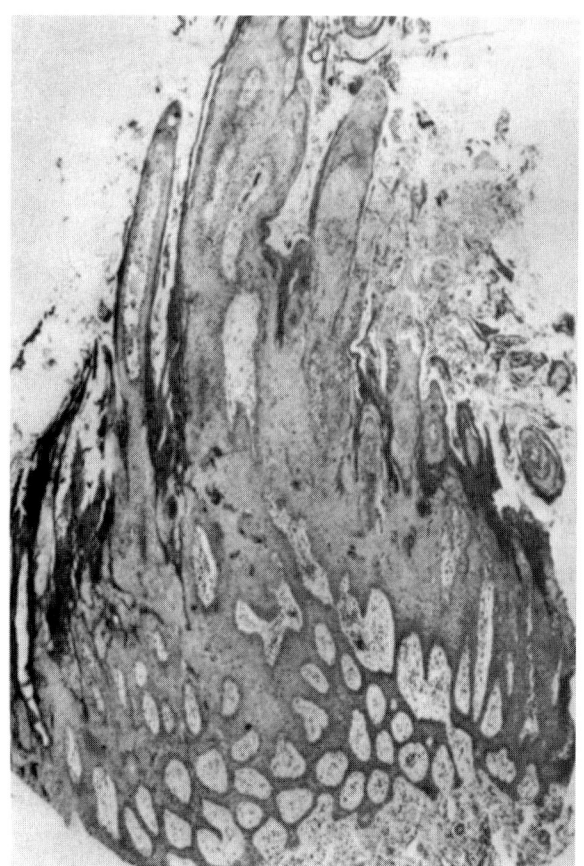

FIGURE 20–196. Feline cutaneous horn. Hornlike projection from the footpad of an FeLV-infected cat.

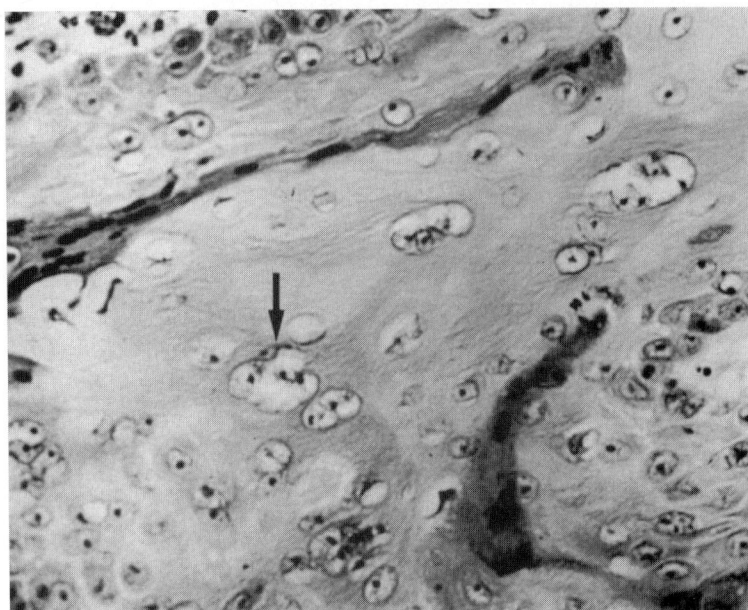

FIGURE 20-197. Close-up of Figure 20-196. Multinucleated (syncytial) keratinocytes *(arrow)*.

Calcinosis Cutis

Calcinosis cutis is an uncommon disorder of the dog.[2, 5] Calcification of the skin may occur in a wide variety of unrelated disorders (Table 20-8). The complex biological process whereby inorganic ions are deposited as a solid phase in soft tissues is not understood. It is probable that the pathogenesis involves abnormally high mitochondrial calcium phosphate levels, which result in crystal deposition and cell death. It begins as a calcium phosphate nidus and progresses to hydroxyapatite crystal formation within a collagen matrix.

Metastatic calcinosis cutis is rarely seen in dogs and cats, and all cases have occurred in association with chronic renal disease.[2, 5, 463, 469, 474] Cutaneous lesions have been localized to the footpads and interdigital skin. Affected pads are enlarged, painful, and firm; they are often ulcerated and discharge a chalky white, pasty to gritty material. Although

● Table 20-8 **CAUSES OF CALCINOSIS CUTIS IN DOGS**

Dystrophic calcification (deposition of calcium salts in injured, degenerating, or dead tissue)
    Localized areas (calcinosis circumscripta)
        Inflammatory lesions (tuberculosis, foreign body granuloma, demodicosis, staphylococcal pododermatitis)
        Degenerative lesions (follicular cysts)
        Neoplastic lesions (pilomatrixoma, others)
    Widespread areas (calcinosis universalis)
        Hyperglucocorticoidism (naturally occurring or iatrogenic)
        Diabetes mellitus
        Percutaneous penetration of calcium
Idiopathic calcification (deposition of calcium salts with no appreciable tissue damage or demonstrable metabolic defect)
    Localized areas (idiopathic calcinosis circumscripta of large breed dogs)
    Widespread areas (idiopathic calcinosis universalis of young dogs)
Metastatic calcification (deposition of calcium salts associated with abnormal metabolism of calcium and phosphorus with demonstrable serum level changes)
    Chronic renal disease

most animals with renal failure are older, metastatic calcinosis of the footpads has been reported in younger dogs with renal dysplasia.[468] One should consider chronic renal failure in a dog of *any* age with calcinosis in multiple footpads. Skin biopsy findings are identical to those reported for calcinosis circumscripta (see later). Although therapy has usually been unsuccessful, the lesions in one cat completely resolved after 3 months of dietary management (restricted protein and phosphorus).[469] Although footpad lesions usually indicate metastatic calcinosis and renal disease, calcinosis circumscripta has been reported to affect one footpad of an otherwise healthy young German shepherd dog[475] and a young terrier mix,[470] both metacarpal pads of a young Siberian husky,[473] and the footpads of both hind feet of a Dachshund.[460] Surgical excision was curative in all cases.

Widespread calcinosis cutis has frequently been reported in dogs in association with naturally occurring or iatrogenic hyperglucocorticoidism (see Chap. 10). Cutaneous lesions consist of papules, plaques, and nodules that are firm, often gritty, frequently ulcerated and secondarily infected, and yellowish white to pinkish yellow. These lesions may occur anywhere but are especially common along the dorsum and in the axillae and groin. Histologically, calcium salts are deposited along collagen and elastin fibers in the dermis and basement membrane zones and are frequently surrounded by a foreign body granuloma reaction. This form of calcinosis cutis in dogs is thought to be dystrophic in nature, because blood calcium and phosphorus levels are invariably normal. Correcting the hyperglucocorticoidism causes this type of calcinosis cutis to regress within 2 to 12 months. A syndrome of *idiopathic calcinosis cutis* that is grossly and histologically identical to glucocorticoid-associated calcinosis cutis has rarely been seen in healthy dogs younger than 1 year old.[2, 5] The authors have recognized this syndrome in English bulldogs, Doberman pinschers, Dachshunds, Labrador retrievers, and Rottweilers (Fig. 20–198A and B). Lesions spontaneously regress within 1 year. Calcinosis cutis in dogs was reported to result from *percutaneous penetration of calcium* (contact with commercial hygroscopic landscaping products [see Chap. 16]). Spontaneous recovery followed avoidance of further contact with the substances.

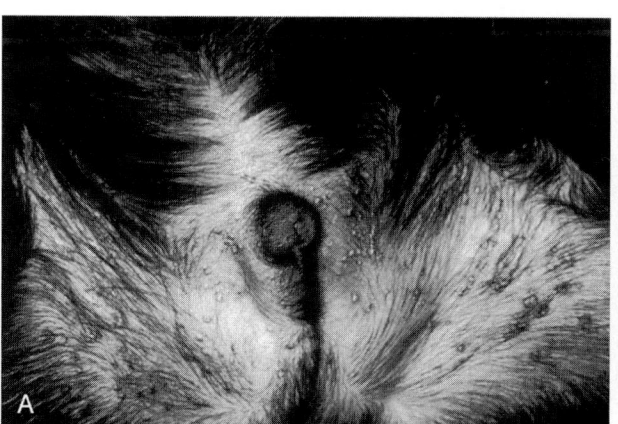
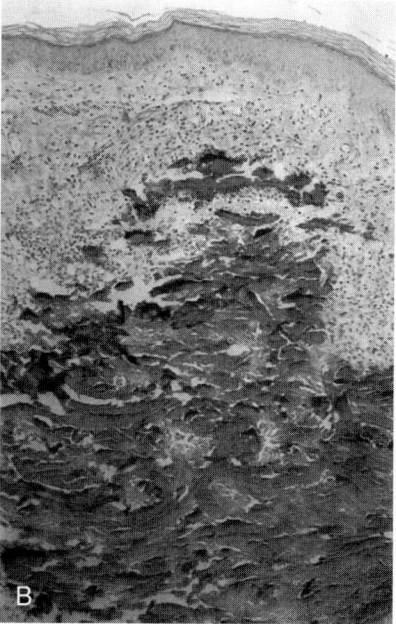

FIGURE 20–198. Idiopathic calcinosis cutis in a black Labrador retriever puppy. *A,* Multiple hard, white papules with surrounding erythema in groin and medial thighs. Lesions spontaneously resolved. *B,* Massive dystrophic mineralization of dermal collagen.

CALCINOSIS CIRCUMSCRIPTA

• **Cause and Pathogenesis.** Calcinosis circumscripta (kalkgicht, calcium gout, apocrine cystic calcinosis, or multiloculated subcutaneous granuloma) is uncommon in dogs and rare in cats.[2, 5, 461, 474] In most cases, the cause is unknown. Because lesions most frequently occur over pressure points or sites of previous trauma, such as that incurred during ear cropping, the calcium deposition may be dystrophic.[2] The tendency for dystrophic mineralization may be enhanced by the active calcium metabolism of large, rapidly growing dogs.[2] Rarely, calcinosis circumscripta is reported to occur at the site of previous subcutaneous injections,[462, 466, 467] from degeneration of pre-existing epitrichial sweat gland cysts,[2] at the sites of previous bite wounds,[2] on the neck in association with choke collars,[465] or at the site of polydioxanone sutures.[464, 471] Although most affected animals are otherwise healthy, symmetric calcinosis circumscripta has been reported in dogs in association with hypertrophic osteodystrophy and idiopathic polyarthritis.[474]

• **Clinical Findings.** Calcinosis circumscripta is seen most commonly in younger dogs (younger than 2 years of age) of either sex.[474] About 90% of all reported cases have been in large breeds of dogs, and more than 50% of cases have been in German shepherd dogs. Lesions are usually dome shaped, fluctuant or firm, and 0.5 to 7 cm in diameter. Initially, the overlying skin may be freely movable and covered with hair. As the lesions progress, however, ulceration frequently occurs, as does the discharge of a chalky white, pasty to gritty material. Lesions are usually single but occasionally multiple or bilaterally symmetric. They are most frequently seen over or near pressure points and bony prominences, especially the lateral metatarsal and phalangeal areas of the pelvic limb and the elbow (see Fig. 20–189G).[474] They may also occur over the dorsal aspects of the fourth to sixth cervical vertebrae[472] or in the tongue (see Fig. 20–189H).[474] Boxers and Boston terriers appear to be predisposed to lesions at the base of the pinna and on the cheek, respectively.[461, 462, 474] Postinjectional (especially medroxyprogesterone acetate) calcinosis circumscripta is seen at injection sites, usually within 5 months of injection, and most commonly in Poodles.[466, 467] Choke chain–associated lesions occur on the neck.[465] Polydioxanone suture–associated lesions occur at surgical incision sites, and all reported cases have occurred in German shepherds.[464, 471] Calcinosis circumscripta is extremely rare in cats.[429, 430]

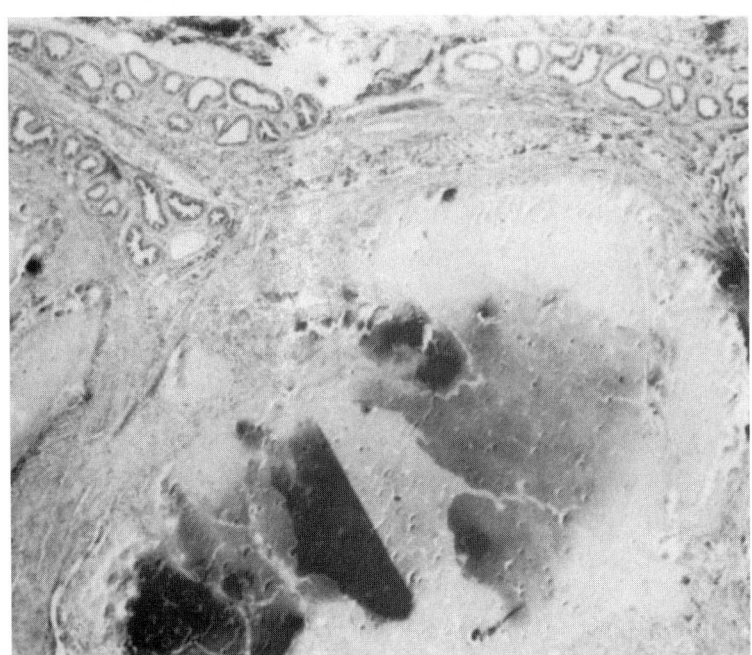

FIGURE 20–199. Canine calcinosis circumscripta. Nodular accumulations of mineral below the level of epitrichial sweat glands.

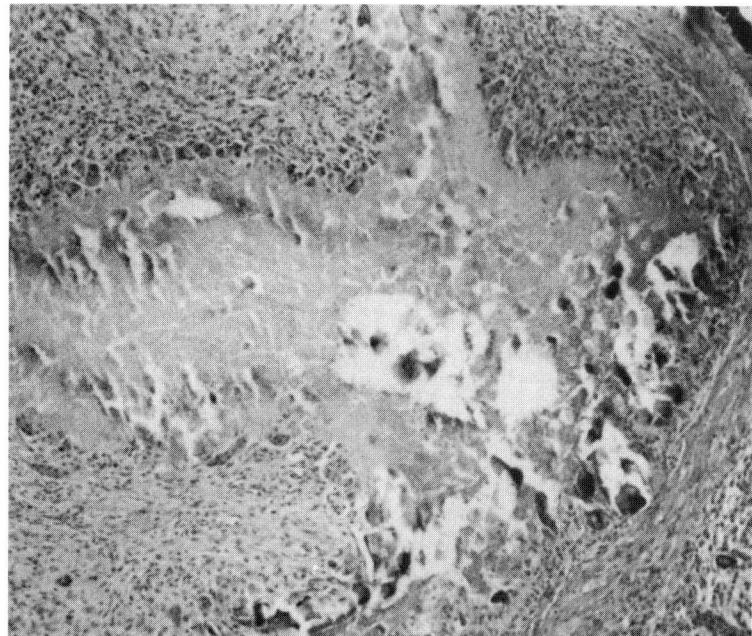

FIGURE 20–200. Canine calcinosis circumscripta. Palisading granuloma surrounding a mineral deposit.

- **Diagnosis.** Histologically, calcinosis circumscripta is characterized by multifocal areas of granular amorphous material in the deep dermis and subcutis surrounded by a zone of granulomatous inflammation and separated by fibrous trabeculae (Figs. 20–199 and 20–200).[2, 474] Cartilaginous and osseous metaplasia, as well as transepidermal elimination of minerals, may be seen in some lesions. The amorphous masses are usually strongly periodic acid–Schiff (PAS) positive and Alcian blue positive. Radiographic examination reveals mineralized soft tissues.
- **Clinical Management.** The treatment of choice is surgical excision. Recurrences or the development of new lesions after surgery is not reported.[474] Dogs with symmetric lesions (on scapulae and hips) in association with hypertrophic osteodystrophy or idiopathic polyarthritis had spontaneous remission of their calcinosis circumscripta as the associated disease became inactive.[474]

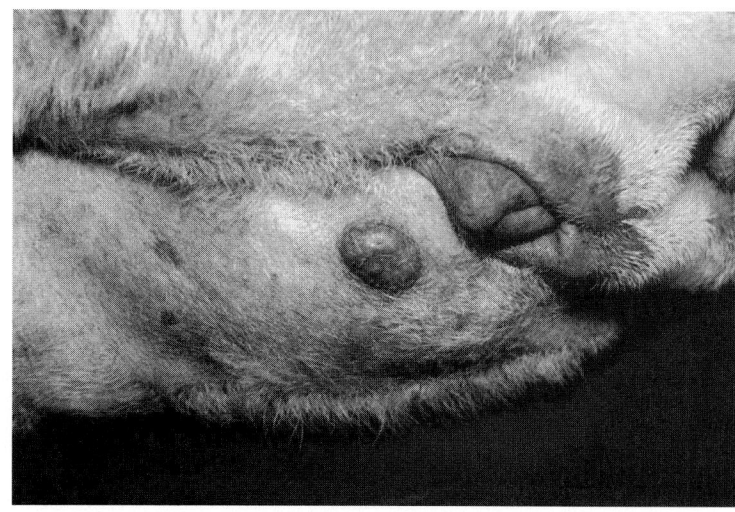

FIGURE 20–201. Focal cutaneous mucinosis in a Shar pei. Alopecic, pin-feathered nodule near vulva.

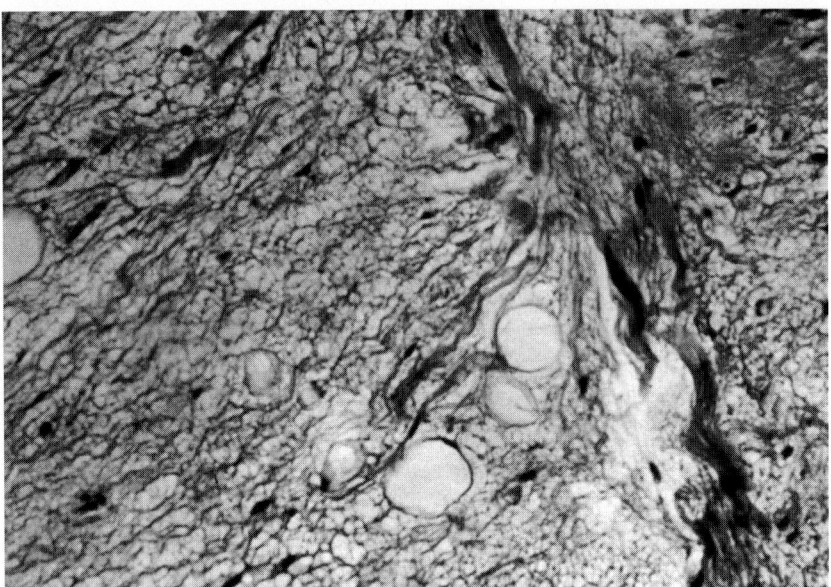

FIGURE 20–202. Canine focal cutaneous mucinosis. Diffuse dermal mucinosis.

Cutaneous Mucinosis

Cutaneous mucinoses are a heterogeneous group of skin disorders characterized by the excessive accumulation or deposition of mucin (acid mucopolysaccharide) in the dermis or epithelial structures.[2, 4, 459] The mucinosis may be primary or secondary, or focal to diffuse. In dogs, cutaneous mucinosis may be seen with hypothyroidism, acromegaly, lupus erythematosus, dermatomyositis, alopecia mucinosa, and mycosis fungoides and as a normal finding in the Shar pei. In cats, cutaneous mucinosis may be seen with alopecia mucinosa and mycosis fungoides.

Focal cutaneous mucinosis has rarely been reported in dogs.[459] Three dogs (two Doberman pinschers, all three females, 3 to 6 years old) had solitary, asymptomatic, firm and rubbery to soft nodules (1 to 3 cm in diameter) on the head or the leg (Fig. 20–201). The primary histopathologic finding was an accumulation of excessive mucin (Alcian blue positive or colloidal iron positive) within the dermis or subcutis, which disrupted and separated collagen fibers (Fig. 20–202). In addition, a mild to extensive proliferation of fibroblasts and a mild lymphohistiocytic infiltrate were seen. Surgical excision was curative.

• References

General Textbook Sources

1. Goldschmidt MH, Shofer F: Skin Tumors of the Dog and Cat. Pergamon Press, New York, 1992.
2. Gross TL, et al: Veterinary Dermatopathology. A Macroscopic and Microscopic Evaluation of Canine and Feline Skin Disease. Mosby–Year Book, St. Louis, 1992.
2a. Guaguère E, Prélaud P: A Practical Guide to Feline Dermatology. Merial, Paris, 2000.
3. Moulton JE: Tumors in Domestic Animals III. University of California Press, Berkeley, 1990.
4. Ogilvie GK, Moore AS: Managing the Veterinary Cancer Patient: A Practice Manual. Veterinary Learning Systems, Trenton, New Jersey, 1995.
5. Scott DW, et al: Muller and Kirk's Small Animal Dermatology, 5th ed. W.B. Saunders Co, Philadelphia, 1995.
6. Theilen GH, Madewell, BR: Veterinary Cancer Medicine II. Lea & Febiger, Philadelphia, 1987.
7. Withrow SJ, MacEwen EG: Clinical Veterinary Oncology, 2nd ed. W.B. Saunders Co, Philadelphia, 1996.

Survey Articles and Chapters

8. Bastianello SS: A survey of neoplasia in domestic species over a 40-year period from 1935 to 1974 in the Republic of South Africa. V. Tumours occurring in the cat. Onderstepoort J Vet Res 50:105, 1983.
9. Bastianello SS: A survey of neoplasia in domestic species over a 40-year period from 1935–1974 in the

Republic of South Africa. VI. Tumours occurring in dogs. Onderstepoort J Vet Res 50:199, 1983.
10. Berrocal A, et al: Canine perineal tumours. J Vet Med A 36:739, 1989.
11. Bostock DE: Neoplasms of the skin and subcutaneous tissues in dogs and cats. Br Vet J 142:1, 1986.
12. Brodey RS: Canine and feline neoplasia. Adv Vet Sci 14:309, 1970.
13. Burrows AK, et al: Skin neoplasms of cats in Perth. Aust Vet Pract 24:11, 1994.
14. Carpenter JL, et al: Tumors and tumor-like lesions. In: Holzworth J (ed): Diseases of the Cat: Medicine and Surgery, Vol. 1. W.B. Saunders Co, Philadelphia, 1987, p 413.
15. Cotchin E: Skin tumours of cats. Res Vet Sci 2:353, 1961.
16. Degorce F, Parodi AL: Tumeurs conjunctives des carnivores domestiques. Rec Méd Vét 166:1043, 1990.
16a. De Las Mulas JM, et al: Apoptosis and mitosis in tumours of the skin and subcutaneous tissues of the dog. Res Vet Sci 66:139, 1999.
17. Er JC, Sutton RH: A survey of skin neoplasms in dogs from the Brisbane region. Aust Vet J 66:225, 1989.
18. Finnie JW, Bostock DE: Skin neoplasia in dogs. Aust Vet J 55:602, 1979.
19. Graham JC, O'Keefe DA: Diagnosis and treatment of soft tissue sarcomas. Comp Cont Educ 15:1627, 1993.
20. Gross TL, Affolter VK: Advances in skin oncology. In: Kwochka KW, et al (eds): Advances in Veterinary Dermatology III. Butterworth-Heinemann, Boston, 1998, p 382.
21. Head KW: Some data concerning the distribution of skin tumors in domestic animals. In: Rook A, Walton GS (eds): Comparative Physiology and Pathology of the Skin. F.A. Davis Co, Philadelphia, 1965, p 613.
22. Keller ET, Madewell BR: Locations and types of neoplasms in immature dogs: 69 cases (1964–1989). J Am Vet Med Assoc 200:1530, 1992.
23. Kuntz CA, et al: Prognostic factors for surgical treatment of soft tissue sarcomas in dogs: 75 cases (1986–1996). J Am Vet Med Assoc 211:1147, 1997.
24. Ladds P, et al: Neoplasms of the skin of dogs in tropical Queensland. Aust Vet J 60:87, 1983.
25. MacEwen EG, Helfand SC: Recent advances in the biologic therapy of cancer. Comp Cont Educ 15:909, 1993.
26. Macy DW, Reynolds HA: The incidence, characteristics, and clinical management of skin tumors of cats. J Am Anim Hosp Assoc 17:1026, 1981.
27. Magnol JP: Tumeurs cutanées du chien et du chat. Rec Méd Vét 166:1061, 1990.
28. Marino DJ, et al: Evaluation of dogs with digit masses: 117 cases (1981–1991). J Am Vet Med Assoc 207:726, 1995.
29. Mialot M, Lagadic M: Epidémiologie descriptive des tumeurs du chien et du chat. Rec Méd Vét 166:937, 1990.
30. Miller MA, et al: Cutaneous neoplasia in 340 cats. Vet Pathol 28:389, 1991.
31. Nielsen SW, Cole CR: Cutaneous epithelial neoplasms of the dog—a report of 153 cases. Am J Vet Res 21:931, 1960.
32. Priester WA: Skin tumors in domestic animals. Data from twelve United States and Canadian colleges of veterinary medicine. J Natl Cancer Inst 50:457, 1973.
33. Pulley LT, Stannard, AA: Tumors of the skin and soft tissues. In: Moulton JE (ed): Tumors in Domestic Animals III. University of California Press, Berkeley, 1990, p 23.
34. Rothwell TLW, et al: Skin neoplasms of dogs in Sydney. Aust Vet J 64:161, 1987.
35. Scott DW: Feline dermatology 1900–1978: A monograph. J Am Anim Hosp Assoc 16:331, 1980.
36. Scott DW: Feline dermatology 1979–1982: Introspective retrospections. J Am Anim Hosp Assoc 20:537, 1984.
37. Scott DW: Feline dermatology 1983–1985: "The secret sits." J Am Anim Hosp Assoc 23:255, 1987.
38. Scott DW: Feline dermatology 1986–1988: Looking to the 1990s through the eyes of many counsellors. J Am Anim Hosp Assoc 26:517, 1990.
39. Susaneck SJ: Feline skin tumors. Comp Cont Educ 5:251, 1983.
40. Thrall DE, Gillette EL: Soft tissue sarcomas. Semin Vet Med Surg. 10:173, 1995.
41. Van Den Ingh TSGAM: Huidtumoren bij de Hond. Tijdschr Diergeneeskd 98:538, 1973.
41a. VanKampen KR: Immunotherapy and cytokines. Semin Vet Med Surg 12:186, 1997.
42. Yager JA, Scott DW: The skin and appendages. In: Jubb KVF, et al (eds): Pathology of Domestic Animals IV, Vol. 1. Academic Press, New York, 1993, p 531.

Cytology

42a. Alleman AR, Bain PJ: Diagnosing neoplasia: The cytologic criteria for malignancy. Vet Med 95:204, 2000.
43. Barton CL: Cytologic analysis of cutaneous neoplasia: An algorithmic approach. Comp Cont Educ 9:20, 1987.
44. Carter RF, Valli VEO: Advances in the cytologic diagnosis of canine lymphoma. Semin Vet Med Surg (Small Anim) 3:167, 1988.
45. Hall RL, MacWilliams PS: The cytologic examination of cutaneous and subcutaneous masses. Semin Vet Med Surg (Small Anim) 3:94, 1988.
46. Stirtzinger T: The cytologic diagnosis of mesenchymal tumors. Semin Vet Med Surg (Small Anim) 3:157, 1988.
46a. Thrall MA: Cytologic examination of cutaneous and subcutaneous lumps and lesions. Vet Med 95:224, 2000.

Immunohistochemistry

47. Andreasen CB, et al: Intermediate filament staining in the cytologic and histologic diagnosis of canine skin and soft tissue tumors. Vet Pathol 25:343, 1988.
48. Brown PJ: Immunohistochemical localization of myoglobin in connective tissue in tumors in dogs. Vet Pathol 24:573, 1987.
49. de las Mulas JM, et al: Immunohistochemical distribution pattern of intermediate filament proteins in 50 feline neoplasms. Vet Pathol 32:692, 1995.
50. Desnoyers MM, et al: Immunohistochemical detection of intermediate filament proteins in formalin fixed normal and neoplastic tissues. Can J Vet Res 54:360, 1990.
51. Elias JW: Immunohistopathology: A Practical Approach to Diagnosis. American Society of Clinical Pathologists, Chicago, 1990.
52. Ferrer L, et al: Immunocytochemical demonstration of intermediate filament proteins, S-100 protein and CEA in apocrine sweat glands and apocrine gland–derived lesions of the dog. J Vet Med A 37:569, 1990.

53. Fondevila D, et al: Immunohistochemical localization of S-100 protein and lysozyme in canine lymph nodes and lymphomas. J Vet Med A 36:71, 1989.
54. Fondevila D, et al: Immunoreactivity of canine and feline mast cell tumours. Schweiz. Arch Tierheilkd 132:426, 1990.
55. Magnol JP, et al: Une nouvelle approche, diagnostique et pronostique des tumeurs des tissus mous du chien et du chat. Point Vét 22:831, 1991.
56. Moore AS, et al: Immunohistochemical evaluation of intermediate filament expression in canine and feline neoplasms. Am J Vet Res 50:88, 1989.
57. Moore PF, et al: The use of immunological reagents in defining the pathogenesis of canine skin diseases involving proliferation of leukocytes. In: Kwochka KW, et al (eds): Advances in Veterinary Dermatology III. Butterworth-Heinemann, Boston, 1998, p 77.
58. Rabanal RH, et al: Immunocytochemical diagnosis of skin tumours of the dog with special reference to undifferentiated types. Res Vet Sc 47:129, 1989.
59. Sandusky GE, et al: Diagnostic immunohistochemistry of canine round cell tumors. Vet Pathol 24:495, 1987.
60. Sandusky GE, et al: Immunocytochemical study of tissues from clinically normal dogs and of neoplasms using keratin monoclonal antibodies. Am J Vet Res 52:613, 1991.
61. Thoonen H, et al: Expression of cytokeratins in epithelial tumours of the dog investigated with monoclonal antibodies. Schweiz Arch Tierheilkd 132:409, 1990.
62. Von Beust BR, et al: Factor VIII–related antigen in canine endothelial neoplasms: An immunohistochemical study. Vet Pathol 25:251, 1988.
63. Wallace ML, Smoller BR: Immunohistochemistry in diagnostic dermatopathology. J Am Acad Dermatol 34:163, 1996.
64. Williamson MM, Middleton DJ: Cutaneous soft tissue tumours in dogs: classification, differentiation, and histogenesis. Vet Dermatol 9:43, 1998.

Papilloma

65. Bregman CL, et al: Cutaneous neoplasms in dogs associated with canine oral papillomavirus vaccine. Vet Pathol 24:477, 1987.
66. Campbell KL, et al: Cutaneous inverted papillomas in dogs. Vet Pathol 25:67, 1988.
67. Carney HC, et al: Papillomavirus infection of aged Persian cats. J Vet Diagn Invest 2:294, 1990.
68. Carpenter JL, et al: Cutaneous xanthogranuloma and viral papilloma on the eyelid of a cat. Vet Dermatol 3:187, 1992.
69. Egberink HF, et al: Papillomavirus associated skin lesions in a cat seropositive for feline immunodeficiency virus. Vet Microbiol 31:117, 1992.
70. Le Net JL, et al: Multiple pigmented cutaneous papules associated with a novel canine papillomavirus in an immunosuppressed dog. Vet Pathol 34:8, 1997.
71. Lozano-Alarcón F, et al: Persistent papillomavirus infection in a cat. J Am Anim Hosp Assoc 32:392, 1996.
72. Lucroy MD, et al: Cutaneous papillomatosis in a dog with malignant lymphoma following long-term chemotherapy. J Vet Diagn Invest 10:369, 1998.
73. Majewski S, Jablonska S: Human papillomavirus–associated tumors of the skin and mucosa. J Am Acad Dermatol 36:659, 1997.
74. Mill AB, et al: Concurrent hypothyroidism, IgM deficiency, impaired T-cell mitogen response, and multifocal cutaneous squamous papillomas in a dog. Canine Pract 17:15, 1992.
75. Nagata M, et al: Pigmented plaques associated with papillomavirus infection in dogs: Is this epidermodysplasia verruciformis? Vet Dermatol 6:179, 1995.
76. Narama I, et al: Cutaneous papilloma with viral replication in an old dog. J Vet Med Sci 54:387, 1992.
77. Nicholls PK, Stanley MA: Canine papillomatosis—a centenary review. J Comp Pathol 120:219, 1999.
78. Schwegler K, et al: Epithelial neoplasms of the skin, the cutaneous mucosa and the transitional epithelium in dogs: An immunolocalization study for papillomavirus antigen. J Vet Med A 44:115, 1997.
79. Shimada A, et al: Cutaneous papillomatosis associated with papillomavirus infection in a dog. J Comp Pathol 108:103, 1993.
80. Sironi G, et al: Immunohistochemical detection of papillomavirus structural antigens in animal hyperplastic and neoplastic epithelial lesions. J Vet Med A 37:760, 1990.
81. Sundberg JP, et al: Immunoperoxidase localization of papillomaviruses in hyperplastic and neoplastic epithelial lesions of animals. Am J Vet Res 45:1441, 1984.
82. Sundberg JP, et al: Involvement of canine oral papillomavirus in generalized oral and cutaneous verrucosis in a Chinese Shar Pei dog. Vet Pathol 31:183, 1994.
83. Sundberg JP, et al: Feline papillomaviruses: host range, molecular diversity and epitope conservation. Vet Pathol 31:616, 1994.
83a. Sundberg JP, et al: Feline papillomas and papillomaviruses. Vet Pathol 37:1, 2000.
84. Sundberg JP: Canine papillomaviruses. In: Castro AE, Heuschele WP (eds): Veterinary Diagnostic Virology: A Practitioner's Guide. Mosby–Year Book, St. Louis, 1992, p 148.
85. Sundberg JP, et al: Mucosotropic papillomavirus infections. Lab Anim Sci 48:240, 1998.
86. Teifke JP, et al: Detection of canine oral papillomavirus-DNA in canine oral squamous cell carcinomas and p53 overexpressing skin papillomas of the dog using the polymerase chain reaction and nonradioactive in situ hybridization. Vet Microbiol 60:119, 1998.
87. Walder EJ: Malignant transformation of a pigmented epidermal nevus in a dog. Vet Pathol 34:505, 1997.
88. White SD: Newly introduced drugs in veterinary dermatology. Proc World Cong Vet Dermatol 3:84, 1996.

Keratoacanthoma

89. Kwochka KW: Retinoids in dermatology. In: Kirk RW (ed): Current Veterinary Therapy X. W.B. Saunders Co, Philadelphia, 1989, p 553.
90. Power HT, Ihrke PJ: Synthetic retinoids in veterinary dermatology. Vet Clin North Am Small Anim Pract 20:1525, 1990.
91. Smith DA, Knottenbett MK: Spontaneous regression of intracutaneous cornifying epitheliomata in a dog. J Small Anim Pract 29:201, 1988.
92. Stannard AA, Pulley LT: Intracutaneous cornifying epithelioma (keratoacanthoma) in the dog: A retrospective study of 25 cases. J Am Vet Med Assoc 167:385, 1975.

Basal Cell Tumor

93. Anderson WI, Scott DW: Cartilaginous metaplasia associated with a basal cell tumor in a dog. J Comp Pathol 100:107, 1989.
94. Day DG, et al: Basal cell carcinoma in two cats. J Am Anim Hosp Assoc 30:265, 1994.

95. Diters RW, Walsh KM: Feline basal cell tumors: A review of 124 cases. Vet Pathol 21:51, 1984.
96. Fehrer SL, Lin SH: Multicentric basal cell tumors in a cat. J Am Vet Med Assoc 189:1469, 1986.
97. Maiolino P, et al: Mitotic phase distribution, mitotic activity, and apoptosis in basal cell tumours of canine skin. J Vet Med A 43:619, 1996.
98. Seiler RJ: Granular basal cell tumors in the skin of three dogs: A distinct histopathologic entity. Vet Pathol 18:23, 1981.
99. Strafuss AC: Basal cell tumors in dogs. J Am Vet Med Assoc 169:322, 1976.

Squamous Cell Carcinoma

100. Baer KE, Helton K: Multicentric squamous cell carcinoma in situ resembling Bowen's disease in cats. Vet Pathol 30:535, 1993.
101. Bito T, et al: Less expression of cyclin E in cutaneous squamous cell carcinomas than in benign and premalignant keratinocyte lesions J Cutan Pathol 24:305, 1997.
102. Bostock DE: Prognosis in cats bearing squamous cell carcinoma. J Small Anim Pract 13:119, 1972.
103. Clarke RE: Cryosurgical treatment of feline cutaneous squamous cell carcinoma. Aust Vet Pract 21:148, 1991.
104. Cox NR, et al: Tumors of the nose and paranasal sinuses in cats: 32 cases with comparison to a national database (1977 through 1987). J Am Anim Hosp Assoc 27:339, 1991.
105. Dipold TF, Roberts L: Squamous cell carcinoma in a white bull terrier. University of Sydney Postgraduate Committee in Veterinary Science Control and Therapy Series #3837, 1997, p 909.
106. Evans AG, et al: A trial of 13-cis-retinoic acid for treatment of squamous cell carcinoma and preneoplastic lesions of the head in cats. Am J Vet Res 46:2553, 1985.
107. Gamblin RM, et al: Overexpression of p53 tumor suppressor protein in spontaneously arising neoplasms of dogs. Am J Vet Res 58:85, 1997.
108. Garma-Aviña A: The cytology of squamous cell carcinomas in domestic animals. J Vet Diagn Invest 6:238, 1994.
108a. Gomes LAM, et al: Squamous cell carcinoma associated with actinic dermatitis in seven white cats. Feline Pract 28:14, 2000.
109. Gourley IM, et al: Burn scar malignancy in a dog. J Am Vet Med Assoc 180:1095, 1982.
110. Gross TL, Brimacomb BH: Multifocal intraepidermal carcinoma in a dog histologically resembling Bowen's disease. Am J Dermatopathol 8:509, 1986.
111. Guaguère E, et al: Demodex cati infestation in association with feline squamous cell carcinoma in situ: a report of five cases. Vet Dermatol 10:61, 1999.
112. Hahn KA, et al: Photodynamic therapy response in cats with cutaneous squamous cell carcinoma as a function of fluence. Vet Dermatol 9:3, 1998.
113. Hargis AM, Thomassen RW: Solar keratosis (solar dermatosis, senile keratosis) and solar keratosis with squamous cell carcinoma. Am J Pathol 94:193, 1979.
114. Harris CC: p53: at the crossroads of molecular carcinogenesis and molecular epidemiology. J Invest Dermatol Symp Proc 1:115, 1996.
115. Haziroglu M, Saylam M: Squamous cell carcinoma in a puppy. J Comp Pathol 101:221, 1989.
116. Hutson CA: Neoplasia associated with feline immunodeficiency virus infection in cats in Southern California. J Am Vet Med Assoc 199:1357, 1991.
117. Kitchell BE, et al: Intralesional sustained release chemotherapy with cisplatin and 5-fluorouracil therapeutic implants for treatment of feline squamous cell carcinoma. Proc Annu Meet Vet Cancer Soc 12:55, 1992.
118. Knowles DP, Hargis AM: Solar elastosis associated with neoplasia in two Dalmatians. Vet Pathol 23:512, 1986.
119. Lana SE, et al: Feline cutaneous squamous cell carcinoma of the nasal planum and the pinnae: 61 cases. J Am Anim Hosp Assoc 33:329, 1997.
120. Levine N, et al: Controlled localized heating and isotretinoin effects in canine squamous cell carcinoma. J Am Acad Dermatol 23:68, 1990.
121. Marks SL, et al: Clinical evaluation of etretinate for the treatment of canine solar-induced squamous cell carcinoma and preneoplastic lesions. J Am Acad Dermatol 27:11, 1992.
121a. Mayr B, et al: Novel canine tumor suppressor gene p53, mutations in cases of skin and mammary neoplasms. Vet Res Comm 23:285, 1999.
122. Miller WH Jr, Shanley KJ: Bilateral pinnal squamous cell carcinoma in a dog with chronic otitis externa. Vet Dermatol 2:37, 1991.
123. Miller WH Jr, et al: Multicentric squamous cell carcinoma in situ resembling Bowen's disease in five cats. Vet Dermatol 3:177, 1992.
124. O'Brien MG, et al: Treatment by digital amputation of subungual squamous cell carcinoma in dogs: 21 cases (1987–1988). J Am Vet Med Assoc 201:759, 1992.
125. Paradis M, et al: Squamous cell carcinoma of the nail bed in three related giant schnauzers. Vet Rec 125:322, 1989.
126. Peaston AE, et al: Photodynamic therapy for nasal and aural squamous cell carcinoma in cats. J Am Vet Med Assoc 202:1261, 1993.
126a. Pérez J, et al: Immunohistochemical study of the inflammatory infiltrate associated with feline cutaneous squamous cell carcinoma and precancerous lesions (actinic keratosis). Vet Immunol Immunopathol 69:33, 1999.
127. Rees CA, Goldschmidt MH: Cutaneous horn and squamous cell carcinoma in situ (Bowen's disease) in a cat. J Am Anim Hosp Assoc 34:485, 1998.
128. Rogers KW: Feline cutaneous squamous cell carcinoma. Feline Pract 22:7, 1994.
129. Rogers KS, et al: Squamous cell carcinoma of the canine nasal planum: eight cases (1988–1994). J Am Anim Hosp Assoc 31:373, 1995.
130. Ruslander D, et al: Cutaneous squamous cell carcinoma in cats. Comp Cont Educ Pract Vet 19:1119, 1997.
131. Scott DW, Miller WH Jr: Disorders of the claw and clawbed in cats. Comp Cont Educ 14:449, 1992.
132. Scott DW, Miller WH Jr: Disorders of the claw and clawbed in dogs. Comp Cont Educ 14:1448, 1992.
133. Scott DW, Teixeira EAC: Multiple squamous cell carcinomas arising from multiple cutaneous follicular cysts in a dog. Vet Dermatol 6:27, 1995.
134. Scott DW, Miller WH Jr: Squamous cell carcinoma arising in chronic discoid lupus erythematosus nasal lesions in two German shepherd dogs. Vet Dermatol 6:99, 1995.
135. Shelley BA, et al: Use of the neodymium:yttrium-aluminum-garnet laser for treatment of squamous cell

carcinoma of the nasal planum in a cat. J Am Vet Med Assoc 201:756, 1992.
136. Strafuss AC, et al: Squamous cell carcinoma in dogs. J Am Vet Med Assoc 168:425, 1976.
137. Tateyama S, et al: *In vitro* growth inhibition activities of recombinant feline interferon on cell lines derived from canine tumors. Res Vet Sci 59:275, 1995.
138. Teifke JP, Kohr CV: Immunohistochemical detection of p53 overexpression in paraffin wax-imbedded squamous cell carcinomas of cattle, horses, cats, and dogs. J Comp Pathol 114:205, 1996.
139. Théon AP, et al: Prognostic factors associated with radiotherapy of squamous cell carcinoma of the nasal plane in cats. J Am Vet Med Assoc 206:991, 1995.
140. Théon AP, et al: Intratumoral administration of carboplatin for treatment of squamous cell carcinomas of the nasal plane in cats. Am J Vet Res 57:205, 1996.
141. van Vechtem MK, Théon AP: Strontium-90 plesiotherapy for treatment of early squamous cell carcinoma of the nasal planum in 30 cats. Proc Annu Meet Vet Cancer Soc 13:107, 1993.
142. Withrow SJ, Straw RC: Resection of the nasal planum in nine cats and five dogs. J Am Anim Hosp Assoc 26:219, 1990.

Hair Follicle Tumors

142a. Abramo F, et al: Survey of canine and feline follicular tumours and tumour-like lesions in central Italy. J Small Anim Pract 40:479, 1999.
143. Diters RW, Goldschmidt MH: Hair follicle tumors resembling tricholemmomas in six dogs. Vet Pathol 20:123, 1983.
144. Fukui K, et al: [Two cases of canine malignant basal tumor]. J Jpn Vet Med Assoc 45:856, 1992.
145. Hill JR: Warty dyskeratoma in two dogs. Proc Annu Memb Meet Am Acad Vet Dermatol Am Coll Vet Dermatol 3:40, 1987.
146. Luther PB, et al: The dilated pore of Winer—An overlooked cutaneous lesion of cats. J Comp Pathol 101:375, 1989.
147. Rodriguez F, et al: Metastatic pilomatrixoma associated with neurological signs in a dog. Vet Rec 137:247, 1995.
148. Scott DW, Flanders JF: Dilated pore of Winer in a cat. Feline Pract 14:33, 1984.
149. Scott DW, Anderson WI: Canine hair follicle neoplasms: A retrospective analysis of 80 cases (1986–1987). Vet Dermatol 2:143, 1991.
150. Scott DW, Anderson WI: Hair follicle neoplasms in three cats. Feline Pract 19:14, 1991.

Sebaceous Gland Tumors

151. Finazzi M, et al: Reperti istologici su tumori delle ghiandole sebacee del cane. Clin Vet 110:123, 1987.
152. Scott DW, Anderson WI: Canine sebaceous gland tumors: A retrospective analysis of 172 cases. Canine Pract 15:19, 1990.
153. Scott DW, Anderson WI: Feline sebaceous gland tumors: A retrospective analysis of nine cases. Feline Pract 19:16, 1991.
154. Strafuss AC: Sebaceous carcinoma in dogs. J Am Vet Med Assoc 169:325, 1976.
155. Strafuss AC: Sebaceous gland adenomas in dogs. J Am Vet Med Assoc 169:640, 1976.

Sweat Gland Tumors

156. Christie GS, Jabara AG: Canine sweat gland growths. Res Vet Sci 5:237, 1964.
157. Jabara AG, Finnie JW: Four cases of clear-cell hidradenocarcinomas in the dog. J Comp Pathol 88:525, 1978.
158. Kalaher KM, et al: Neoplasms of the apocrine sweat glands in 44 dogs and 10 cats. Vet Rec 127:400, 1990.
159. Kusters AH, et al: Atrichial sweat gland adenocarcinoma in the dog. Vet Dermatol 10:51, 1999.
160. Mayr B, et al: Autosomale Monosomie (B2/E3) und Deletion (B2/E3) in Schweissdrüsentumorgewebe bei Katzen (2 Fallberichte). Wien Tierärztl Mschr 83:141, 1996.
161. Meschter CL: Disseminated sweat gland adenocarcinoma with acronecrosis in a cat. Cornell Vet 81:195, 1991.
162. Soga R, et al: A case of canine apocrine gland carcinoma metastasized to bones. J Jpn Vet Med Assoc 49:110, 1996.

Perianal Gland Tumors

163. Ross JT, et al: Adenocarcinoma of the apocrine glands of the anal sac in dogs: A review of 32 cases. J Am Anim Hosp Assoc 27:349, 1991.
164. Vail DM, et al: Perianal adenocarcinoma in the canine male: A retrospective study of 41 cases. J Am Anim Hosp Assoc 26:329, 1990.
165. Vercelli A: Immunohistochemical identification of estrogen and androgen receptors in canine perianal adenoma. Proc Annu Cong Eur Soc Vet Dermatol Eur Coll Vet Dermatol 14:204, 1997.
166. Vos JH, et al: The expression of keratins, vimentin, neurofilament proteins, smooth muscle actin, neuron-specific enolase, and synaptophysin in tumors of the specific glands in the canine anal region. Vet Pathol 30:352, 1993.

Salivary Gland Tumors

167. Carberry CA, et al: Salivary gland tumors in dogs and cats: A literature and case review. J Am Anim Hosp Assoc 24:561, 1988.

Feline Sarcoid

168. Gumbrell RC, et al: Dermal fibropapillomas in cats. Vet Rec 142:370, 1998.

Fibrosarcoma

169. Bostock DE, Dye MT: Prognosis after surgical excision of fibrosarcomas in cats. J Am Vet Med Assoc 175:727, 1979.
170. Bostock DE, Dye MT: Prognosis after surgical excision of canine fibrous connective tissue sarcomas. Vet Pathol 17:581, 1980.
171. Doliger S, Devauchelle P: Données actuelles sur les tumeurs du "complexe fibrosarcome félin." Point Vét 29:405, 1998.
172. Harasen GLG: Multicentric fibrosarcoma in a cat and a review of the literature. Can Vet J 24:207, 1984.
173. Hilmas D, Gillete E: Radiotherapy of spontaneous connective tissue sarcomas in animals. Cancer Res 56:365, 1976.
174. Karademir N, et al: Comparison of argyrophil nucleolar organizer region counts, proliferating cell nuclear antigen (PCNA) indices and mitotic indices in fibromas and fibrosarcomas. Folia Vet 42:67, 1998.
175. Kent EM: Use of an immunostimulant as an aid in treatment and management of fibrosarcoma in three cats. Feline Pract 21:13, 1993.
176. King GK, et al: The effect of acemannan immunostimulant in combination with surgery and radiation therapy on spontaneous canine and feline fibrosarcomas. J Am Anim Hosp Assoc 31:439, 1995.
177. Mayr B, et al: Trisomy D1, marker F1: new cytoge-

netic findings in two cases of feline fibrosarcoma. J Vet Med A 41:197, 1994.
178. Mayr B, et al: Mutations in tumour suppressor gene p53 in two feline fibrosarcomas. Br Vet J 151:707, 1995.
179. Mayr B, et al: Cytogenetic variation between four cases of feline fibrosarcoma. Res Vet Sci 61:268, 1996.
180. Mayr B, et al: Cytogenetic alterations in four feline soft tissue tumours. Vet Res Commun 22:21, 1998.
181. Mayr B, et al: Novel p53 tumour suppressor mutations in cases of spindle cell sarcoma, pleomorphic sarcoma and fibrosarcoma in cats. Vet Res Comm 22: 249, 1998.
182. McChesney SL, et al: Radiotherapy of soft tissue sarcomas in dogs. J Am Vet Med Assoc 194:60, 1989.
183. McChesney-Gillette S, et al: Response of canine soft tissue sarcomas to radiation or radiation plus hyperthermia: a randomized phase II study. Int J Hyperthermia 8:309, 1992.

Myxoma
184. Rowland PH, et al: Myxoma at the site of a subcutaneous pacemaker in a dog. J Am Anim Hosp Assoc 27:649, 1991.

Neural Tumors
185. Brehm DM, et al: A retrospective evaluation of 51 cases of peripheral nerve sheath tumors in the dog. J Am Anim Hosp Assoc 31:349, 1995.
186. Geyer C, et al: Immunohistochemical and ultrastructural investigation of granular cell tumours in dog, cat, and horse. J Vet Med B 39:485, 1992.
187. Gross TL, Carr SH: Amputation neuroma of docked tails in dogs. Vet Pathol 27:61, 1990.
188. Herrera GA, Mendoza A: Primary canine cutaneous meningioma. Vet Pathol 18:127, 1981.
189. Jones BR, et al: Nerve sheath tumours in the dog and cats. N Z Vet J 43:190, 1995.
190. Patniak AK: Histologic and immunohistochemical studies of granular cell tumors in seven dogs, three cats, one horse, and one bird. Vet Pathol 30:176, 1993.

Vascular Tumors
191. Augustin-Voss HG, et al: Phenotypic characterization of normal and neoplastic canine endothelial cells by lectin histochemistry. Vet Pathol 27:103, 1990.
192. Barnes JC, et al: Disseminated lymphangiosarcoma in a dog. Can Vet J 38:42, 1997.
192a. Belanger MC, et al: Invasive multiple lymphangiomas in a young dog. J Am Anim Hosp Assoc 35: 507, 1999.
193. Berry WL, et al: Lymphangiomatosis of the pelvic limb in a Maltese dog. J Small Anim Pract 37:340, 1996.
194. Brown NO, et al: Canine hemangiosarcoma: Retrospective analysis of 104 cases. J Am Vet Med Assoc 186:56, 1985.
194a. Chun R: Feline and canine hemangiosarcoma. Comp Cont Educ Pract Vet 21:622, 1999.
195. Danielson F: Lymphangioma in the metacarpal pad of a dog. J Small Anim Pract 39:295, 1998.
196. Delisle F, et al: L'hémangiosarcome chez le chien. Point Vét 28:73, 1996.
196a. Demanuelle TC, et al: Idiopathic telangiectasia in a Golden Retriever. Vet Dermatol 10:311, 1999.
197. Evans SM: Canine hemangiosarcoma: A retrospective analysis of response to surgery and orthovoltage radiation. Vet Radiol 28:13, 1987.
198. Ferrer L, et al: Immunohistochemical detection of CD31 antigen in normal and neoplastic endothelial cells. J Comp Pathol 112:319, 1995.
199. Fossum TW, et al: Generalized lymphangiectasis in a dog with subcutaneous chyle and lymphangioma. J Am Vet Med Assoc 197:231, 1990.
200. George C, Summers BA: Angiokeratoma: A benign vascular tumor of the dog. J Small Anim Pract 31: 390, 1990.
201. Ginn PE, Kunkle GA: Hemangiosarcoma of multiple digits in a cat. Proc Annu Memb Meet Am Acad Vet Dermatol Am Coll Vet Dermatol 13:110, 1997.
202. Graves GM, et al: Canine hemangiopericytoma: 23 cases (1967–1984). J Am Vet Med Assoc 192:99, 1988.
203. Hammer AS, et al: Efficacy and toxicity of VAC chemotherapy (vincristine, doxorubicin, cyclophosphamide) in dogs with hemangiosarcoma. J Vet Int Med 5:160, 1991.
203a. Handharyani E, et al: Canine hemangiopericytoma: an evaluation of metastatic potential. J Vet Diagn Invest 11:474, 1999.
204. Hargis AM, Feldman BF: Evaluation of hemostatic defects secondary to vascular tumors in dogs: 11 cases (1983–1988). J Am Vet Med Assoc 198:891, 1991.
205. Hargis AM, et al: A retrospective clinicopathologic study of 212 dogs with cutaneous hemangiomas and hemangiosarcomas. Vet Pathol 29:316, 1992.
206. Hinrichs U, et al: Lymphoangiosarcomas in cats: a retrospective study of 12 cases. Vet Pathol 36:164, 1999.
207. Kraje AC, et al: Unusual metastatic behavior and clinicopathologic findings in eight cats with cutaneous or visceral hemangiosarcoma. J Am Vet Med Assoc 214: 670, 1999.
208. Lewis DL, Harari J: Peripheral arteriovenous fistula associated with a subcutaneous hemangiosarcoma/hemangioma in a cat. Feline Pract 20:27, 1992.
209. Mayr B, et al: Trisomy 2 in three cases of canine haemangiopericytoma. Br Vet J 148:113, 1992.
210. Mayr B, et al: Cytogenetic characterization of a fibroma and three haemangiopericytomas in domestic dogs. Br Vet J 151:433, 1995.
211. Mialot M: Tumeurs vasculaires de localisation cutanée chez le chat: étude d'une série de 40 cas. Prat Méd Chir Anim Comp 30:571, 1995.
212. Miller MA, et al: Cutaneous vascular neoplasia in 15 cats: Clinical, morphologic, and immunohistochemical studies. Vet Pathol 29:329, 1992.
213. Pérez J, et al: Immunohistochemical characterization of hemangiopericytomas and other spindle cell tumors in the dog. Vet Pathol 33:391, 1996.
214. Post K, et al: Cutaneous lymphangioma in a young dog. Can Vet J 32:747, 1991.
215. Postorino NC, et al: Prognostic variables for canine hemangiopericytoma: 50 cases (1979–1984). J Am Anim Hosp Assoc 24:501, 1988.
216. Sagartz JE, et al: Lymphangiosarcoma in a young dog. Vet Pathol 33:353, 1996.
217. Scavelli TD, et al: Hemangiosarcoma in the cat: Retrospective evaluation of 31 surgical cases. J Am Vet Med Assoc 187:817, 1987.
218. Shiga A, et al: Lymphangiosarcoma in a dog. J Vet Med Sci 56:1199, 1994.
219. Srebernik N, Appleby EC: Breed prevalence and sites

of haemangioma and haemangiosarcoma in dogs. Vet Rec 129:408, 1991.
220. Swayne DE, et al: Lymphangiosarcoma and haemangiosarcoma in a cat. J Comp Pathol 100:91, 1989.
221. Turrel JM, et al: Response to radiation therapy of recurring lymphangioma in a dog. J Am Vet Med Assoc 193:1432, 1988.
221a. Vail DM, et al: Liposome-encapsulated muramyl tripeptide phosphatidylethanolamine (L-MTP-E) adjuvant immunotherapy for splenic hemangiosarcoma in the dog: a randomized multi-institutional clinical trial. Clin Cancer Res 1:1165, 1995.
222. Walsh KM, Abbot DP: Lymphangiosarcoma in two cats. J Comp Pathol 94:611, 1984.
223. Ward H, et al: Cutaneous hemangiosarcoma in 25 dogs: a retrospective study. J Vet Int Med 8:345, 1994.
224. White SD, et al: Acquired cutaneous lymphangiectasis in a dog. J Am Vet Med Assoc 193:1093, 1988.
225. Woods JP, et al: Concurrent lymphangioma, immune-mediated thrombocytopenia, and von Willebrands disease in a dog. J Am Anim Hosp Assoc 31:70, 1995.
226. Xu FN: Ultrastructure of canine hemangiopericytoma. Vet Pathol 23:643, 1986.

Adipose Tissue Tumors
227. Albers GW, Theilen GH: Calcium chloride for treatment of subcutaneous lipomas in dogs. J Am Vet Med Assoc 186:492, 1985.
228. Bergman PJ, et al: Infiltrative lipoma in dogs: 16 cases (1981–1992). J Am Vet Med Assoc 205:322, 1994.
229. Esplin DG: Infiltrating lipoma in a cat. Feline Pract 14:24, 1984.
230. Esplin DG, et al: Metastasizing liposarcoma associated with a vaccine site in a cat. Feline Pract 24:20, 1996.
231. Frazier KS, et al: Infiltrative lipoma in a canine stifle joint. J Am Anim Hosp Assoc 29:81, 1993.
232. Mayr B, et al: Zytogenetische Veränderungen in Lipomen bei Katzen (2 Fallberichte). Wien Tierärztl Mschr 83:230, 1996.
233. McCarthy PE, et al: Liposarcoma associated with a glass foreign body in a dog. J Am Vet Med Assoc 209:612, 1996.
234. Messick JB, Radin MJ: Cytologic, histologic and ultrastructural characteristics of a canine myxoid liposarcoma. Vet Pathol 25:520, 1988.
234a. Reimann N, et al: Cytogenetic investigations of canine lipomas. Cancer Genetics 111:172, 1999.
235. Stephens LC, et al: Virus-associated liposarcoma and malignant lymphoma in a kitten. J Am Vet Med Assoc 183:123, 1983.

Leiomyoma and Leiomyosarcoma
236. Finnie JW, et al: Multiple piloleiomyomas in a cat. J Comp Pathol 113:201, 1995.
236a. Jacobsen MC, Valentine BA: Dermal intravascular leiomyosarcoma in a cat. Vet Pathol 37:100, 2000.

Rhabdomyoma and Rhabdomyosarcoma
237. Martin de las Mulas, J, et al: Desmin and vimentin immunocharacterization of feline muscle tumors. Vet Pathol 29:260, 1992.
238. Roth L: Rhabdomyoma of the ear pinna in four cats. J Comp Pathol 103:237, 1990.

Osteoma and Osteosarcoma
239. Easton CB: Extraskeletal osteosarcoma in a cat. J Am Anim Hosp Assoc 30:59, 1994.
240. Jabara AG, Paton JS: Extraskeletal osteoma in a cat. Aust Vet J 61:405, 1984.
241. Kuntz CA, et al: Extraskeletal osteosarcomas in dogs: 14 cases. J Am Anim Hosp Assoc 34:26, 1998.
242. Langenbach A, et al: Extraskeletal osteosarcomas in dogs: a retrospective study of 169 cases (1986–1986). J Am Anim Hosp Assoc 34:113, 1998.

Chondroma and Chondrosarcoma
243. Davidson JR: Canine and feline chondrosarcoma. Comp Cont Educ Pract Vet 17:1109, 1995.
244. Popovitch CA, et al: Chondrosarcoma: A retrospective study of 97 dogs (1987–1990). J Am Anim Hosp Assoc 30:81, 1994.

Postvaccinal Sarcomas
245. Briscoe CM, et al: Pulmonary metastasis of a feline vaccine—site fibrosarcoma. J Vet Diagn Invest 10:79, 1998.
246. Burton G, Mason KV: Do postvaccinal sarcomas occur in Australian cats? Aust Vet J 75:102, 1997.
247. Coyne MJ, et al: Estimated prevalence of injection-site sarcomas in cats during 1992. J Am Vet Med Assoc 210:249, 1997.
247a. Cronin K, et al: Radiation therapy and surgery for fibrosarcoma in 33 cats. Vet Radiol Ultrasound 39:51, 1998.
248. Doddy FD, et al: Feline fibrosarcomas at vaccine sites and nonvaccine sites. J Comp Pathol 114:165, 1996.
249. Ellis JA, et al: Use of immunohistochemistry and polymerase chain reaction for detection of oncornavirus in formalin-fixed, paraffin-embedded fibrosarcomas from cats. J Am Vet Med Assoc 209:767, 1996.
250. Esplin DG, Campbell R: Widespread metastasis of fibrosarcoma associated with a vaccine site in a cat. Feline Pract 23:13, 1995.
250a. Gagnon AC: Drug injection-associated fibrosarcoma in a cat. Feline Pract 28:18, 2000.
251. Hendrick MJ, Brooks JJ: Postvaccinal sarcomas in the cat: Histology and immunohistochemistry. Vet Pathol 31:126, 1994.
252. Hendrick MJ, et al: Comparison of fibrosarcomas that developed at vaccine sites and at nonvaccine sites in cats: 239 cases (1991–1992). J Am Vet Med Assoc 205:1425, 1994.
252a. Hershey AE, et al: Prognosis for presumed feline vaccine-associated sarcoma after excision: 61 cases (1986–1996). J Am Vet Med Assoc 216:58, 2000.
253. Kass PH, et al: Epidemiologic evidence for a causal relation between vaccination and fibrosarcoma tumorigenesis in cats. J Am Vet Med Assoc 203:396, 1993.
254. Lester S, et al: Vaccine site-associated sarcomas in cats: clinical experience and a laboratory review (1982–1993). J Am Anim Hosp Assoc 32:91, 1996.
255. Macy DW, et al: Vaccine-associated sarcomas in cats. Feline Pract 23:24, 1995.
256. Macy DW, Hendrick MJ: The potential role of inflammation in the development of post vaccinal sarcomas in cats. J Small Anim Pract 36:103, 1996.
257. Mikaelian I, et al: Les sarcomes post-vaccinaux félins. Méd Vét Québec 27:133, 1997.
258. Rudmann DG, et al: Pulmonary and mediastinal metastases of a vaccine-site sarcoma in a cat. Vet Pathol 33:466, 1996.
259. Sandler I, et al: Metastatic vaccine-associated fibrosarcoma in a 10-year-old cat. Can Vet J 38:374, 1997.
260. Schultze AE, et al: Repeated physical and cytologic

characterizations of subcutaneous postvaccinal reactions in cats. Am J Vet Res 58:719, 1997.
261. Weigand CM, Brewer WG Jr: Vaccine-site sarcomas in cats. Comp Cont Educ Pract Vet 18:869, 1996.

Undifferentiated Sarcomas

262. Carpenter JL, et al: Distinctive unclassified mesenchymal tumor of the digit of dogs. Vet Pathol 28:396, 1991.
263. Kipar A, et al: Round cell sarcomas of possible myelomonocytic origin localized at the lip of aged dogs. J Vet Med A 42:185, 1995.
264. Sanders NA, et al: Aggressive, undifferentiated sarcoma with widespread metastasis in a six-month-old Neopolitan mastiff. J Am Anim Hosp Assoc 32:97, 1996.

Mast Cell Tumor

264a. Abadie JJ, et al: Immunohistochemical detection of proliferating cell nuclear antigen and Ki-67 in mast cell tumors from dogs. J Am Vet Med Assoc 215:1629, 1999.
265. Al-Sarraf R, et al: A prospective study of radiation therapy for the treatment of grade 2 mast cell tumors in 32 dogs. Vet Int Med 10:376, 1996.
266. Ayl RD, et al: Correlation of DNA ploidy to tumor histologic grade, clinical variables, and survival in dogs with mast cell tumors. Vet Pathol 29:386, 1992.
267. Beadleston DL, et al: Chymase and tryptase staining of normal feline skin and of feline cutaneous mast cell tumors. Vet Allergy Clin Immunol 5:54, 1997.
268. Bell A, et al: Visceral and cutaneous mast cell neoplasia in a cat. Aust Vet Pract 24:86, 1994.
269. Bensignor E, et al: Le mastocytome cutané canin: Résultats d'une étude anatomoclinique et thérapeutique de 85 cas. Rec Méd Vét 173:351, 1996.
270. Bostock DE: The prognosis following surgical removal of mastocytomas in dogs. J Small Anim Pract 14:27, 1973.
271. Brown CA, Chalmers SA: Diffuse cutaneous mastocytosis in a cat. Vet Pathol 27:366, 1990.
272. Buerger RG, Scott, DW: Cutaneous mast cell neoplasia in the cat: 14 cases (1975–1985). J Am Vet Med Assoc 190:1440, 1987.
273. Cayatte SM, et al: Identification of mast cells in buffy coat preparations from dogs with inflammatory skin diseases. J Am Vet Med Assoc 206:325, 1995.
274. Chastain CB, et al: Benign cutaneous mastocytomas in two litters of Siamese kittens. J Am Vet Med Assoc 193:959, 1988.
275. Cole W: Mast cell tumor in a puppy. Can Vet J 31:457, 1990.
276. Davis BJ, et al: Cutaneous mastocytosis in a dog. Vet Pathol 29:363, 1992.
276a. Elmslie R: Combination chemotherapy with and without surgery for dogs with high grade mast cell tumors with lymph node metastasis. Vet Cancer Soc Newsletter 20:6, 1997.
277. Frimberger AE, et al: Radiotherapy of incompletely resected, moderately differentiated mast cell tumors in the dog: 37 cases (1989–1993). J Am Anim Hosp Assoc 33:320, 1997.
277a. Gerritsen RJ, et al: Multi-agent chemotherapy for mast cell tumours in the dog. Vet Quart 20:28, 1998.
277b. Ginn PE, et al: Immunohistochemical detection of p53 tumor-suppressor protein is a poor indicator of prognosis for canine cutaneous mast cell tumors. Vet Pathol 37:33, 2000.
278. Grier RL, et al: Mast cell tumour destruction in dogs by hypotonic solution. J Small Anim Hosp Assoc 36:385, 1995.
278a. Jaffe MH, et al: Immunohistochemical and clinical evaluation of p53 in canine cutaneous mast cell tumors. Vet Pathol 37:40, 2000.
278b. Jaffe MH, et al: Deionised water as an adjunct to surgery for the treatment of canine cutaneous mast cell tumours. J Small Anim Pract 41:7, 2000.
279. Jeromin AM, et al: Urticaria pigmentosa-like disease in the dog. J Am Anim Hosp Assoc 29:508, 1993.
280. Kravis LD, et al: Frequency of argyrophilic nucleolar organizer regions in fine-needle aspirates and biopsy specimens from mast cell tumors in dogs. J Am Vet Med Assoc 209:1418, 1996.
281. Legoretta RA, et al: Use of hyperthermia and radiotherapy in treatment of a large mast cell sarcoma in a dog. J Am Vet Med Assoc 193:1545, 1988.
282. Lemarié RJ, et al: Mast cell tumors: clinical management. Comp Cont Educ Pract Vet 17:1085, 1995.
283. London C, et al: Expression of stem cell factor receptor (c-kit) by the malignant mast cells from spontaneous canine mast cell tumours. J Comp Pathol 115:399, 1996.
283a. London CA, et al: Spontaneous canine mast cell tumors express tandem duplications in the proto-oncogene c-kit. Exper Hematol 27:689, 1999.
284. Long RD: Cutaneous mast cell tumor in a Siamese kitten. Can Vet J 37:167, 1996.
284a. López A, et al: Cutaneous mucinosis and mastocytosis in a Shar-Pei. Can Vet J 40:881, 1999.
284b. Ma Y, et al: Clustering of activating mutations in c-kits juxtamembrane coding region in canine mast cell neoplasms. J Invest Dermatol 112:165, 1999.
285. Madewell BR, et al: Cutaneous mastocytosis and mucinosis with gross deformity in a Shar pei dog. Vet Dermatol 3:171, 1992.
286. Magnol JP, Toulemonde N: Histopronostic du mastocytome canin. Validité du grading de Patnaik. Rev Méd Vét 138:125, 1987.
287. McCaw DL, et al: Response of canine mast cell tumors to treatment with oral prednisone. J Vet Int Med 8:406, 1994.
288. McCaw DL, et al: Vincristine therapy for mast cell tumors in dogs. J Vet Int Med 11:375, 1997.
288a. McManus PM: Frequency and severity of mastocytemia in dogs with and without mast cell tumors: 120 cases (1995–1997). J Am Vet Med Assoc 215:355, 1999.
289. Miller DM: The occurrence of mast cell tumors in young Shar Peis. J Vet Diagn Invest 7:360, 1995.
290. Molander-McCrary H, et al: Cutaneous mast cell tumors in cats: 32 cases (1991–1994). J Am Anim Hosp Assoc 34:281, 1998.
290a. Parodi A: Le mastocytome du chien est-il une tumeur génétique? Point Vét 31:67, 2000.
291. Patnaik AK, et al: Canine cutaneous mast cell tumor: Morphologic grading and survival time in 83 dogs. Vet Pathol 21:469, 1984.
292. Peterson SL: Scar-associated canine mast cell tumor. Canine Pract 12:23, 1985.
293. Reguera MJ, et al: Canine mast cell tumors express stem cell factor receptor (c-kit). Proc Annu Memb Meet Am Acad Vet Dermatol Am Coll Vet Dermatol 15:77, 1999.
293a. Russnick KM, et al: Treatment of canine mast cell tumors with CCNU (Lomustine). J Vet Intern Med 13:601, 1999.

294. Simoes JPC, Schoning P: Canine mast cell tumors: a comparison of staining techniques. J Vet Diagn Invest 6:458, 1994.
295. Simoes JPC, et al: Prognosis of canine mast cell tumors: A comparison of three methods. Vet Pathol 31:637, 1994.
295a. Thamm DH, et al: Prednisone and vinblastine chemotherapy for canine mast cell tumor—41 cases (1992–1997). J Vet Intern Med 13:491, 1999.
296. Thiel W: Mastzellentumoren bei Hunden-Auswertung pathologisch-histologischer Untersuchungsbefunde der Jahre 1980 bis 1986 mit Hinweis auf die TNM-Klassifizierung von Tumoren bei Haustieren. Kleintier-Prax 35:401, 1990.
297. Tinsley PE, Taylor DO: Immunotherapy for multicentric malignant mastocytoma in a dog. Mod Vet Pract 68:225, 1987.
298. Turrel JM, et al: Prognostic factors for radiation treatment of mast cell tumors in 85 dogs. J Am Vet Med Assoc 193:936, 1988.
299. Vitale CB, et al: Feline urticaria pigmentosa in three related Sphinx cats. Vet Dermatol 7:227, 1996.
300. Wilcock BP, et al: The morphology and behavior of feline cutaneous mastocytomas. Vet Pathol 23:320, 1986.

Lymphoma

301. Ashley PF, Bowman LA: Symmetric cutaneous necrosis of the hind feet and multicentric follicular lymphoma in a cat. J Am Vet Med Assoc 214:211, 1999.
302. Baker JL, Scott DW: Mycosis fungoides in two cats. J Am Anim Hosp Assoc 25:97, 1989.
303. Beale KM, et al: An unusual presentation of cutaneous lymphoma in two dogs. J Am Anim Hosp Assoc 26:429, 1990.
304. Beale KM, Bolon B: Canine cutaneous lymphosarcoma: Epitheliotropic and nonepitheliotropic, a retrospective study. In: Ihrke PJ, et al (eds): Advances in Veterinary Dermatology II. Pergamon Press, New York, 1993, p 273.
304a. Bensignor E, Carlotti DN: Un cas de lymphome cutané T non-epithéliotrope chez un chien leishmanien. Prat Méd Chir Anim Comp 34:551, 1999.
305. Bergman R, et al: Immunophenotyping and T-cell receptor gene rearrangement analysis as an adjunct to the histopathologic diagnosis of mycosis fungoides. J Am Acad Dermatol 39:554, 1998.
306. Caciolo PL, et al: Cutaneous lymphosarcoma in the cat: A report of nine cases. J Am Anim Hosp Assoc 20:505, 1984.
307. Caniati M, et al: Canine lymphoma: immunocytochemical analysis of fine-needle aspiration and biopsy. Vet Pathol 33:204, 1996.
307a. Chui CT, et al: Epidermotropic cutaneous B-cell lymphoma mimicking mycosis fungoides. J Am Acad Dermatol 41:271, 1999.
308. Day MJ: Immunophenotypic characterization of cutaneous lymphoid neoplasia in the dog and cat. J Comp Pathol 112:79, 1995.
309. DeBoer DJ, et al: Mycosis fungoides in a dog: Demonstration of T-cell specificity and response to radiotherapy. J Am Anim Hosp Assoc 26:566, 1990.
310. Fivenson DP, et al: Dermal dendrocytes and T-cells in canine mycosis fungoides. Cancer 70:2091, 1992.
311. Fivenson DP, et al: T-cell receptor gene rearrangement in canine mycosis fungoides: further support for a canine model of cutaneous T-cell lymphoma. J Invest Dermatol 102:227, 1994.
312. Ghernati I, et al: Retrovirus-like particles associated with neoplastic CD8+ T lymphocytes in a case of canine cutaneous lymphoma: establishment and characterization of a longterm T-cell line. In: Kwochka KW, et al (eds): Advances in Veterinary Dermatology III. Butterworth, Heinemann, Boston, 1998, p 433.
312a. Ghernati I, et al: Characterization of a canine longterm T cell line (DLC 01) established from a dog with Sézary syndrome and producing retroviral particles. Leukemia 13:1281, 1999.
313. Gruber A, et al: Mycosis fungoides bei drei Hunden: Differentialdiagnostiche Abgrenzung durch immunhistochemischen Nachweis der T-Zell-Spezifität des Hautinfiltrates. Kleintierpraxis 40:569, 1995.
314. Iwamoto KS, et al: Linoleate produces remission in canine mycosis fungoides. Cancer Letter 64:17, 1992.
315. Jackson ML, et al: Immunohistochemical identification of B and T lymphocytes in formalin-fixed, paraffin-embedded feline lymphosarcomas: Relation to feline leukemia virus status, tumor site, and patient age. Can J Vet Res 60:199, 1996.
316. Lemarié SL, Eddlestone SM: Treatment of cutaneous T-cell lymphoma with dacarbazine in a dog. Vet Dermatol 8:41, 1997.
317. Miller WH Jr: Canine cutaneous lymphomas. In: Kirk RW (ed): Current Veterinary Therapy VII. W.B. Saunders Co, Philadelphia, 1980, p 493.
318. Moore PF, et al: Canine cutaneous epitheliotropic lymphoma (mycosis fungoides) is a proliferative disorder of CD8+ T cells. Am J Pathol 144:421, 1994.
319. Moore PF, Olivry T: Cutaneous lymphomas in companion animals. Clin Dermatol 12:499, 1994.
320. Moriello KA, et al: Peg L-asparaginase in the treatment of canine epitheliotropic lymphoma and histiocytic proliferative dermatitis. In: Ihrke PJ, et al (eds): Advances in Veterinary Dermatology II. Pergamon Press, New York, 1993, p 293.
321. Olivry T, et al: Investigation of epidermotropism in canine mycosis fungoides: Expression of intercellular adhesion molecule-1 (ICAM-1) and ß$_2$ integrins. Arch Dermatol Res 287:186, 1995.
322. Petersen A, et al: The use of safflower oil for the treatment of mycosis fungoides in two dogs. Proc Annu Memb Meet Am Acad Vet Dermatol Am Coll Vet Dermatol 15:49, 1999.
323. Poisson L, et al: Réticulose pagetoïde généralisée (forme de Ketron-Goodman) chez un chien. Prat Méd Chir Anim Comp 31:219, 1996.
324. Schick RO, et al: Cutaneous lymphosarcoma and leukemia in a cat. J Am Vet Med Assoc 203:1155, 1993.
325. Shapiro PE, Pinto FJ: The histologic spectrum of mycosis fungoides/Sézary syndrome (cutaneous T-cell lymphoma): A review of 222 biopsies, including newly described patterns and the earliest pathologic changes. Am J Surg Pathol 18:645, 1994.
326. Smith KC, et al: Canine lymphomatoid granulomatosis: An immunophenotypic analysis of three cases. J Comp Pathol 115:129, 1996.
327. Smoller BR, et al: Reassessment of histologic parameters in the diagnosis of mycosis fungoides. Am J Surg Pathol 19:1423, 1995.
328. Stoeckli R, et al: Canine epidermotropic lymphoma associated with the intercellular deposition of immunoglobulin on direct immunofluorescence testing. Comp Anim Pract 1:36, 1988.
329. Thrall MA, et al: Cutaneous lymphosarcoma and leukemia in a dog, resembling Sézary syndrome in man. Vet Pathol 21:182, 1984.

330. Tobey JC, et al: Cutaneous T-cell lymphoma in a cat. J Am Vet Med Assoc 204:606, 1994.
331. Tok J, et al: Detection of clonal T-cell receptor chain gene rearrangements by polymerase chain reaction and denaturing gradient gel electrophoresis (PCR, DGGE) in archival specimens from patients with early cutaneous T-cell lymphoma: Correlation of histologic findings with PCR/DGGE. J Am Acad Dermatol 38:453, 1998.
332. Walton DK: Canine epidermotropic lymphoma (mycosis fungoides and pagetoid reticulosis). In: Kirk RW (ed): Current Veterinary Therapy IX. W.B. Saunders Co, Philadelphia, 1986, p 609.
333. White SD, et al: Use of isotretinoin and etretinate for the treatment of benign cutaneous neoplasia and cutaneous lymphoma in dogs. J Am Vet Med Assoc 202:387, 1993.
334. Wilcock BP, Yager JA: The behavior of epidermotropic lymphoma in 25 dogs. Can Vet J 30:754, 1989.

Pseudolymphoma
335. Miller WH Jr, et al: A spontaneously regressing pseudolymphoma in a dog resembling pseudo-Hodgkin's disease. Vet Dermatol 1:171, 1990.
336. Ploysangam T, et al: Cutaneous pseudolymphomas. J Am Acad Dermatol 38:877, 1998.

Histiocytoma
337. Affolter VK, Moore PF: Canine histiocytic proliferative disease. Proc Annu Memb Meet Am Acad Vet Dermatol Am Coll Vet Dermatol 15:79, 1999.
338. Collins BK, et al: Idiopathic granulomatous disease with ocular adnexal and cutaneous involvement in a dog. J Am Vet Med Assoc 201:313, 1992.
338a. Florek C, Wilkins BE: A Basset hound with swollen third eyelids and skin masses. Vet Med 95:99, 2000.
339. Kipar A, et al: Expression of major histocompatibility complex class II antigen in neoplastic cells of canine cutaneous histiocytoma. Vet Immunol Immunopathol 62:1, 1998.
340. Marchal T, et al: Immunophenotypic and ultrastructural evidence of the Langerhans cell origin of the canine cutaneous histiocytoma. Acta Anat 153:189, 1995.
341. Mays MBC, Bergeron JA: Cutaneous histiocytosis in dogs. J Am Vet Med Assoc 188:377, 1986.
342. Moore F, et al: Canine cutaneous histiocytoma is an epidermotropic Langerhans cell histiocytosis that expresses CD1 and specific ß$_2$-integrin molecules. Am J Pathol 148:1699, 1996.
343. Scott DW: Canine cutaneous histiocytoses. In: Kirk RW (ed): Current Veterinary Therapy X. W.B. Saunders Co, Philadelphia, 1989, p 625.
344. Thornton RN, Tisdall CJ: Multiple cutaneous histiocytosis in two dogs. N Z Vet J 36:192, 1988.

Systemic Histiocytosis
345. Brearley MJ, et al.: Systemic histiocytosis in a Bernese Mountain dog. J Small Anim Pract 35:271, 1994.
346. Moore PF: Systemic histiocytosis of Bernese Mountain dogs. Vet Pathol 21:554, 1984.
347. Nagata M, et al: Progressive Langerhans cell histiocytosis in a young dog. Proc Annu Memb Meet Am Acad Vet Dermatol Am Coll Vet Dermatol 14:7,1998.
348. Padgett GA, et al: Inheritance of histiocytosis in Bernese Mountain dogs. J Small Anim Pract 36:93, 1995.
349. Paterson S, et al: Systemic histiocytosis in the Bernese Mountain dog. J Small Anim Pract 36:233, 1995.
350. Scott DW, et al: Systemic histiocytosis in two dogs. Canine Pract 14:7, 1987.

Malignant Histiocytosis
351. Hayden DW, et al: Disseminated malignant histiocytosis in a golden retriever: Clinicopathologic, ultrastructural, and immunohistochemical findings. Vet Pathol 30:256, 1993.
352. Marholdt F, Besch A: Maligne Histiozytose bei einem Berner sennehund. Pract Tierärztl. 75:690, 1994.
353. Moore PF, Rosin A: Malignant histiocytosis of Bernese Mountain dogs. Vet Pathol 23:1, 1986.
354. Scott DW, et al: Lymphoreticular neoplasia in a dog resembling malignant histiocytosis (histiocytic medullary reticulosis) in man. Cornell Vet 69:176, 1979.
355. Tsuda T, et al: A case of canine malignant histiocytosis. J Jpn Vet Med Assoc 51:259, 1998.
356. Uno Y, et al: Malignant histiocytosis with multiple skin lesions in a dog. J Vet Med Sci 55:1059, 1993.

Benign Fibrous Histiocytoma
357. Paulsen ME, et al: Nodular granulomatous episclerokeratitis in dogs: 19 cases (1973–1985). J Am Vet Med Assoc 190:1581, 1987.
358. Smith JS, et al: Infiltrative corneal lesions resembling fibrous histiocytoma: Clinical and pathologic findings in six dogs and one cat. J Am Vet Med Assoc 169:722, 1976.

Malignant Fibrous Histiocytoma
359. Barnes M, et al: Tumor induction following intraoperative radiotherapy: late results of the National Cancer Institute canine trials. Int J Radiat Oncol Biol Phys 19:651, 1990.
360. Kerlin RL, Hendrick MJ: Malignant fibrous histiocytoma and malignant histiocytosis in the dog-convergent or divergent phenotypic differentiation? Vet Pathol 33:713, 1996.
361. Legrand JJ, et al: Histiocytome fibreux malin chez un chat. Etude d'un cas clinique et comparaison avec les données de la litérature. Prat Méd Chir Anim Comp 22:401, 1987.
362. Mayr B, et al: Cytogenetic findings in two cases of feline malignant fibrous histiocytoma. J Small Anim Pract 37:239, 1996.
363. Pace LW, et al: Immunohistochemical staining of feline malignant fibrous histiocytomas. Vet Pathol 31:168, 1994.
364. Pires MA: Malignant fibrous histiocytoma in a puppy. Vet Rec 140:234, 1997.
365. Thoolen RJMM, et al: Malignant fibrous histiocytomas in dogs and cats: An immunohistochemical study. Res Vet Sci 53:198, 1992.
366. Waters CB, et al: Giant cell variety of malignant fibrous histiocytoma in dogs: 10 cases (1986–1993). J Am Vet Med Assoc 205:1420, 1994.

Plasmacytoma
367. Baer KE, et al.: Cutaneous plasmacytomas in dogs: A morphologic and immunohistochemical study. Vet Pathol 26:216, 1989.
368. Clark GN, et al: Extramedullary plasmacytomas in dogs: Results of surgical excision in 131 cases. J Am Anim Hosp Assoc 28:105, 1992.
369. Eastman CA: Plasma cell tumors in a cat. Feline Pract 24:26, 1996.
370. Frazier KS: Analysis of DNA aneuploidy and C-myc oncoprotein content of canine plasma cell tumors using flow cytometry. Vet Pathol 30:505, 1993.
371. Kyriazidou A, et al: An immunohistochemical study of canine extramedullary plasma cell tumours. J Comp Pathol 100:259, 1989.

372. Kyriazidou A, et al: Immunohistochemical staining with neoplastic and inflammatory plasma cell lesions in feline tissues. J Comp Pathol 100:337, 1989.
373. Platz SJ, et al: Prognostic value of histopathological grading in canine extramedullary plasmacytomas. Vet Pathol 36:23, 1999.
374. Rakich PM, et al: Mucocutaneous plasmacytomas in dogs: 75 cases (1980–1987). J Am Vet Med Assoc 194:803, 1989.
375. Rowland PH, et al: Cutaneous plasmacytomas with amyloid in six dogs. Vet Pathol 28:125, 1991.
376. Rowland PH, Linke RD: Immunohistochemical characterization of light-chain-derived amyloid in one feline and five canine plasma cell tumors. Vet Pathol 31:390, 1994.
377. Schrenzel MD, et al: Leukocyte differentiation antigens in canine cutaneous and oral plasmacytomas. Vet Dermatol 9:33, 1998.

Melanocytic Tumors

378. Anderson WI, et al: Pilar neurocristic melanoma in four dogs. Vet Rec 123:517, 1988.
379. Berrington AJ, et al: Immunohistochemical detection of melanoma-associated antigens on formalin-fixed, paraffin-embedded canine tumors. Vet Pathol 31:455, 1994.
380. Bolon B, et al: Characteristics of canine melanomas and comparison of histology and DNA ploidy to their biologic behavior. Vet Pathol 27:96, 1990.
381. Bostock DE: Prognosis after surgical excision of canine melanomas. Vet Pathol 16:32, 1979.
381a. Burkhart CG, Burkhart CN: Melanoma and insecticides: Is there a connection? J Am Acad Dermatol 42:302, 2000.
382. Day MJ, Lucke VM: Melanocytic neoplasia in the cat. J Small Anim Pract 36:207, 1995.
383. Diters RW, Walsh KM: Cutaneous clear cell melanomas: A report of three cases. Vet Pathol 21:355, 1983.
384. Frese K: Verlaufsuntersuchungen beim Melanomen der Haut und der Mundschleimhaut des Hundes. Vet Pathol 15:461, 1978.
385. Goldschmidt MH, et al: Feline dermal melanoma: A retrospective study. In: Ihrke PJ, et al (eds): Advances in Veterinary Dermatology II. Pergamon Press, New York, 1993, p 285.
386. Goldschmidt MH: Pigmented lesions of the skin. Clin Dermatol 12:507, 1994.
387. Harvey HJ, et al: Prognostic criteria for dogs with oral melanoma. J Am Vet Med Assoc 178:580, 1981.
387a. MacEwen EG, et al: Adjuvant therapy for melanoma in dogs: results of randomized clinical trials using surgery, liposome-encapsulated muramyl tetrapeptide, and granulocyte-macrophage colony stimulating factor. Clin Cancer Res 5:4249, 1999.
387b. Mayr B, et al: Cytogenetic alterations in feline melanoma. Vet J 159:97, 2000.
388. Miller WH Jr, et al: Feline cutaneous melanocytic neoplasms: A retrospective analysis of 43 cases (1979–1991). Vet Dermatol 4:19, 1993.
388a. Modiano JF, et al: The molecular basis of canine melanoma. J Vet Intern Med 13:163, 1999.
389. Oliver JL, et al: Isolation and characterization of the canine melanoma antigen recognized by the murine monoclonal antibody IBF9 and its distribution in cultured canine melanoma cell lines. Am J Vet Res 58:46, 1997.
390. Ritt MG, et al: Functional loss of p21/Waf-1 in a case of benign canine multicentric melanoma. Vet Pathol 35:94, 1998.
390a. Roels S, et al: PCNA and Ki67 proliferation markers as criteria for prediction of clinical behaviour of melanocytic tumours in cats and dogs. J Comp Pathol 121:13, 1999.
390b. Valentine BA, et al: Malignant transformation of a giant congenital pigmented nevus (hamartoma) in a dog. Vet Dermatol 10:127, 1999.
391. van der Linde-Sipman JS, et al: Cutaneous malignant melanomas in 57 cats: Identification of (amelanotic) signet-ring and balloon cell types and verification of their origin by immunohistochemistry, electron microscopy, and in situ hybridization. Vet Pathol 34:31, 1997.

Neuroendocrine Tumor

392. Glick AD, et al: Neuroendocrine carcinoma of the skin in a dog. Vet Pathol 20:761, 1983.
393. Konno A, et al: Immunohistochemical diagnosis of a Merkel cell tumor in a dog. Vet Pathol 35:538, 1998.
394. Nickoloff BJ, et al: Canine neuroendocrine carcinoma. A tumor resembling histiocytoma. Am J Dermatopathol 7:579, 1985.
395. Whiteley LO, Leiningen JR: Neuroendocrine (Merkel) cell tumors of the canine oral cavity. Vet Pathol 24:570, 1987.

Transmissible Venereal Tumor

396. Amber EI, et al: Single-drug chemotherapy of canine transmissible venereal tumor with cyclophosphamide, methotrexate, or vincristine. J Vet Intern Med 4:144, 1990.
396a. Boscos CM, et al: Cutaneous involvement of TVT in dogs: a report of two cases. Canine Pract 24:6, 1999.
397. Das AK, et al: A clinical report on the efficacy of vincristine on canine transmissible venereal sarcoma. Indian Vet J 68:575, 1991.
398. Goswami TK, et al: Lymphokine activated killer cell activity in transmissible venereal tumour of a castrated dog. Indian Vet J 74:895, 1997.
399. Harmelin A, et al: Correlation of Ag-NOR protein measurements with prognosis in canine transmissible venereal tumour. J Comp Pathol 112:429, 1995.
400. Marchal T, et al: Immunophenotype of the canine transmissible venereal tumour. Vet Immunol Immunopathol 57:1, 1997.
401. Mozos E, et al: Immunohistochemical characterization of canine transmissible venereal tumor. Vet Pathol 33:257, 1996.
402. Nandi SN, et al: Effect of ovariectomy on regression of transmissible venereal tumour in bitches. Indian J Vet Pathol 12:97, 1988.
403. Panchbhai VS, et al: Use of autogenous vaccine in transmissible canine venereal tumour. Indian Vet J 67:983, 1990.
404. Pérez J, et al: Immunohistochemical study of the local inflammatory infiltrate in spontaneous canine transmissible venereal tumour at different stages of growth. Vet Immunol Immunopathol 64:133, 1998.
405. Rogers KS: Transmissible venereal tumor. Comp Cont Educ Pract Vet 19:1036, 1997.
406. Rogers KA, et al: Transmissible venereal tumor: a retrospective study of 29 cases. J Am Anim Hosp Assoc 34:463, 1998.
406a. Santos FGA, et al: Caracterização e quantificação de regiões organizadoras de nucléolos coradas pela prata (AgNORs) em tumor venéreo transmissível canino,

genital e extragenital. Arq Bras Med Vet Zootec 50:665, 1998.
407. Singh J, et al: Clinicopathological studies on the effect of different antineoplastic chemotherapy regimens on transmissible venereal tumours in dogs. Vet Res Commun 20:71, 1996.
407a. Singh TP, Pangawkar GR: Hemostatic disorders in dogs infected with transmissible venereal tumour. Indian Vet J 75:879, 1998.

Epithelioid Sarcoma
408. Estrada MM, et al: Epithelioid sarcoma in a dog. J Comp Pathol 107:107, 1992.

Secondary Skin Neoplasms
409. Anderson WI, et al: Presumptive subcutaneous surgical transplantation of a urinary bladder transitional cell carcinoma in a dog. Cornell Vet 79:263, 1989.
410. Couto CG, Sousa C: Chronic lymphocytic leukemia with cutaneous involvement in a dog. J Am Vet Med Assoc 22:374, 1986.
411. Crowe DT, Todoroff RJ: Umbilical masses and discolorations as signs of intraabdominal disease. J Am Anim Hosp Assoc 18:295, 1982.
412. Estrada M, Lagadic M: Métastases digitales d'un carcinome pulmonaire asymptomatique chez le chat. Etude d'une série de 11 cas. Prat Méd Chir Anim Comp 27:791, 1992.
413. Gilson SD, Stone EA: Surgically induced tumor seeding in eight dogs and two cats. J Am Vet Med Assoc 196:1811, 1990.
414. Hampson ECGM, et al: Cutaneous metastasis of a colonic carcinoma in a dog. J Small Anim Pract 31:155, 1990.
415. Jacobs TM, Tomlinson MJ: The lung-digit syndrome in a cat. Feline Pract 25:31, 1997.
416. Leifer CE, Matus RE: Chronic lymphocytic leukemia in the dog: 22 cases (1974–1984). J Am Vet Med Assoc 189:214, 1986.
417. Muller A, et al: Métastases cutanées chez les carnivores domestiques. Prat Méd Chir Anim Comp 33:267, 1998.
418. Scott-Moncrief JE, et al: Pulmonary squamous cell carcinoma with multiple digital metastases in a cat. J Small Anim Pract 30:696, 1989.
418a. Spugnini EP, et al: Seminoma with cutaneous metastasis in a dog. J Am Anim Hosp Assoc 36:253, 2000.
419. Susaneck SJ, et al: Inflammatory mammary carcinoma in the dog. J Am Anim Hosp Assoc 19:971, 1983.
420. White SD, et al: Cutaneous metastases of a mammary adenocarcinoma resembling eosinophilic plaques in a cat. Feline Pract 15:27, 1985.

Paraneoplastic Syndromes
420a. Cohen PR: Paraneoplastic dermatopathology. Cutaneous paraneoplastic syndromes. Adv Dermatol 11:215, 1996.
420b. Guaguère E, et al: Lésions cutanées associées à des maladies internes chez le chien. Prat Méd Chir Anim Comp 32:275, 1997.

Cysts
420c. Chaitman J, et al: Multiple eyelid cysts resembling apocrine hidrocystomas in three Persian cats and one Himalayan cat. Vet Pathol 36:474, 1999.
421. Clark DM, et al: Branchial cyst in a dog. J Am Vet Med Assoc 194:67, 1989.
422. Davidson HJ, Blanchard GL: Periorbital epidermal cyst in the medial canthus of three dogs. J Am Vet Med Assoc 198:271, 1991.
423. Fatone G, et al: Dermoid sinus and spinal malformations in a Yorkshire terrier: diagnosis and follow-up. J Small Anim Pract 36:178, 1995.
424. Fezer G, Weiss E: Die zystischen Bildungen in der Haut der Haustiere. Arch Exp Veterinarmed 23:60, 1969.
425. Joffe DJ: Branchial cyst in a cat. Can Vet J 31:525, 1990.
426. Lambrechts N: Dermoid sinus in a crossbred Rhodesian ridgeback dog involving the second cervical vertebra. J S Afr Vet Assoc 67:155, 1996.
427. Parker WM: Multiple (more than two thousand) epidermal inclusion cysts in a dog. Can Vet J 36:386, 1995.
428. Penrith ML: Dermoid sinus in a Boerboel bitch. J S Afr Vet Assoc 65:38, 1994.
429. Rochat MC, et al: Dermoid cysts in cats: two cases and a review of the literature. J Vet Diagn Invest 8:505, 1996.
430. Scott DW, Anderson WI: Cutaneous trichilemmal cysts in three dogs. Cornell Vet 81:245, 1991.
431. Scott DW, Anderson WI: Cutaneous hybrid cyst in four dogs. Cornell Vet 81:19, 1991.
432. Selcer EA, et al: Dermoid sinus in a Shih tzu and a boxer. J Am Anim Hosp Assoc 20:634, 1984.
433. Vilafranca M, et al: Generalized apocrine cystomatosis in an Old English sheepdog. Vet Dermatol 5:83, 1994.

Nevi
434. Aronsohn MG, Carpenter JL: Distal extremity melanocytic nevi and malignant melanomas in dogs. J Am Anim Hosp Assoc 26:605, 1990.
435. Atlee BA, et al: Nodular dermatofibrosis in German shepherd dogs as a marker for renal cystadenocarcinoma. J Am Anim Hosp Assoc 27:481, 1991.
436. de Geyer G: Dermatologie des paupières du chien et du chat. Première partie: étude générale. Prat Méd Chir Anim Comp 28:605, 1993.
437. Gilbert PA, et al: Nodular dermatofibrosis and renal cystadenoma in a German shepherd dog. J Am Anim Hosp Assoc 26:253, 1990.
438. Guaguère E, et al: Dermatofibrose nodulaire chez le Berger allemand: Étude rétrospective de 10 cas. Prat Méd Chir Anim Comp 31:211, 1996.
439. Jones BR, et al: Cutaneous collagen nodules in a dog. J Small Anim Pract 26:445, 1985.
440. Kraft I, Frese K: Histological studies on canine pigmented moles. J Comp Pathol 86:143, 1976.
441. Marks SL, et al: Nodular dermatofibrosis and renal cystadenomas in a golden retriever. Vet Dermatol 4:133, 1993.
442. Mays MBC, et al: Regional collagenous nevi in three dogs: Nevus, nodular dermatofibrosis, or something new? In: Ihrke PJ, et al (eds.). Advances in Veterinary Dermatology II. Pergamon Press, New York, 1993, p. 315.
443. Moe L, Lium B: Hereditary multifocal renal cystadenocarcinomas and nodular dermatofibrosis in 51 German shepherd dogs. J Small Anim Pract 38:498, 1997.
443a. Nell B, et al: Noduläre Dermatofibrose und renales Zystadenokarzinom bei einem Schäfer hundmischling. Wien Tierärztl Mschr 85:123, 1998.
444. Paradis M, Scott DW: Naevi récemment reconnus chez le chien: Naevus comédonien, naevus organoïde linéaire et naevus du follicule pileux. Point Vét 21:489, 1989.
445. Perry W: Generalized nodular dermatofibrosis and re-

they are pruritic. These findings may be interpreted as signs of skin disease by some owners. Gerbils have a yellowish tan, midventral scent gland, which is also sebaceous, more prominent in male animals, and occasionally mistaken as a cutaneous abnormality. Rabbits have a mental or chin gland (which is sebaceous in nature) with which they mark their territory. Normal ferrets typically have visible accumulations of brownish cerumen around the external auditory meatus. In addition, normal ferrets can have several comedones on the tail.

Most rodents are burrowing animals that spend most of their time in the wild seeking food and escaping predators. When they are placed in sterile environments with ad libitum feeding and no danger of predators, they are left with little to do except to chew on themselves or on others. In addition, male rodents tend to be territorial and aggressive. Self-inflicted trauma or that inflicted on cagemates can be triggered or amplified by crowding.

Some other normal behaviors may be misinterpreted as pruritus. A rabbit rubbing its mental, or chin, gland on a cage or furniture is only marking its territory. Likewise, a guinea pig scooting or dragging its perineal area on the ground is usually scent-marking, although in some male animals, the glandular secretions can become impacted and cause irritation. Male hamsters may clean and fuss with their flank glands.

Staphylococci, especially *Staphylococcus aureus*, are frequently isolated from the skin, the ears, the nostrils, and the haircoat of rodents and rabbits.[8, 11, 17] Not surprisingly, *S. aureus* is a common opportunist and cause of skin infections in these species.

Finally, these small creatures, especially mice, rats, guinea pigs, and rabbits, are frequently used for studying models of human diseases (e.g., hereditary hypotrichoses and ichthyoses in mice and rats), for examining the pathogenesis of various dermatoses also seen in humans (e.g., contact hypersensitivity and candidiasis in guinea pigs), for evaluating therapeutic agents used in various human dermatoses (e.g., treatment of *Malassezia* dermatitis in guinea pigs and the use of retinoids in rhino mice), for studying percutaneous absorption and various aspects of dermatopharmacology (e.g., the mouse tail assay for studying epidermal drug effects), and for screening the potential irritancy or sensitization of topical agents (e.g., the guinea pig Draize test for contact allergens and the rabbit skin test for topical irritants).[16]

● CHINCHILLA

In the wild, chinchillas keep their haircoats clean and healthy by bathing in fine volcanic dust.[17] A similar dust is commercially available (chinchilla dust, or Fuller's earth) and should be provided daily.[3, 10, 17, 21] The dust is poured 5 to 10 cm deep in a metal pan and left in the animal's cage for about 30 minutes. Chinchillas deprived of their dust baths are prone to abnormalities of the haircoat and skin. Chinchillas kept in a warm (warmer than 80°F) humid environment develop matted fur.

Fungal Infections

Dermatophytosis is uncommon in chinchillas.[3, 4, 17, 22] *Trichophyton mentagrophytes* is the most frequent cause, but *Microsporum gypseum* and *M. canis* are occasionally isolated. Lesions are most common around the eyes, the nares, and the mouth, but may occur anywhere. Circumscribed areas of alopecia, broken hairs, and variable degrees of scaling, erythema, and crusting are seen. Secondary staphylococcal infection can occur and usually presents as cellulitis or abscess.[22]

Recommended therapy includes griseofulvin by mouth (50 mg/kg q24h) for 30 days.[17, 22] It had previously been recommended to add captan powder to a clean dust bath once daily.[22] However, because captan has been shown to be ineffective against *M. canis* (see Chap. 5), the authors cannot recommend it.

Fur Chewing

Chinchillas may chew, pull out, and eat their fur during times of stress (gestation, travel, and shows), in the absence of dust baths, and for unknown reasons.[3, 10, 17, 21, 22] When the fur chewing is idiopathic, it rarely ceases. It is believed that the idiopathic condition is a heritable trait, that no therapy is effective, and that the condition is best controlled by culling and selective breeding.[10, 17, 21] Providing fresh alfalfa hay, giving proper chinchilla pellets, and reducing stress may help.

Fur-Slip

Fur-slip is a normal physiologic process whereby chinchillas appear to "squirt" or "shoot" some of their fur out.[17, 22] This is a mechanism of self-defense in which the chinchilla hopes to leave a predator with a mouthful of fur as it escapes. Fur-slip is likely to occur when chinchillas are frightened or handled roughly. Chinchilla fur grows in tufts with up to 90 fibers per follicle and up to 1000 follicles/cm.[2, 22] Fur-slip affects spots 2 to 5 cm in diameter. Fur regrowth occurs within 3 months for some follicles and usually takes 5 months for an entire spot. However, regrowth is rarely a perfect fit and always looks patched.

Nutritional Disorders

Fatty acid deficiency results in generalized scaling, poor haircoat, reduced hair growth, and perhaps cutaneous ulcers in the chinchilla.[2, 21]

Zinc deficiency may produce alopecia.[21]

● FERRET

Ferrets have active sebaceous glands that contribute to their distinctive odor and somewhat greasy feeling coat. Occasional small, red-brown waxy deposits can be found on normal skin. During breeding season, intact males have increased sebaceous secretions, to the point of having a yellowish discoloration of the undercoat, a very oily fur, and quite a musky odor. Frequent bathing may strip essential oils from the skin, resulting in keratinization disorders and pruritus.[10] Owners should be encouraged to use mild shampoo no more frequently than once monthly, if possible.

Bacterial Infections

Bacterial skin infections are uncommon in the ferret and are usually caused by *S. aureus* or *Streptococcus* spp.* Infections are usually secondary to bite wounds (especially on the neck of female ferrets during breeding season, perpetrated by aggressive male animals as a prelude to coitus) or the pruritus associated with ectoparasites. There may be superficial and follicular (Fig. 21–1) lesions or deep abscesses and fistulae. Staphylococcal or streptococcal cellulitis of the neck may be associated with dental disease and mandibular osteomyelitis.[28] Diagnosis is based on cytologic examination. Treatment consists of a regimen of various combinations of topical antimicrobials (3% hydrogen peroxide or 0.5% to 1% chlorhexidine), surgical drainage, and the administration of systemic antibiotics (Table 21–1).

Actinomycosis ("lumpy jaw") is rarely reported in ferrets.[17, 28] Affected animals have nodules or abscesses in the neck, and fistulae and discharge of thick green-yellow pus may be seen.

---

*See references 4, 6, 15, 17, 24, 25, 30.

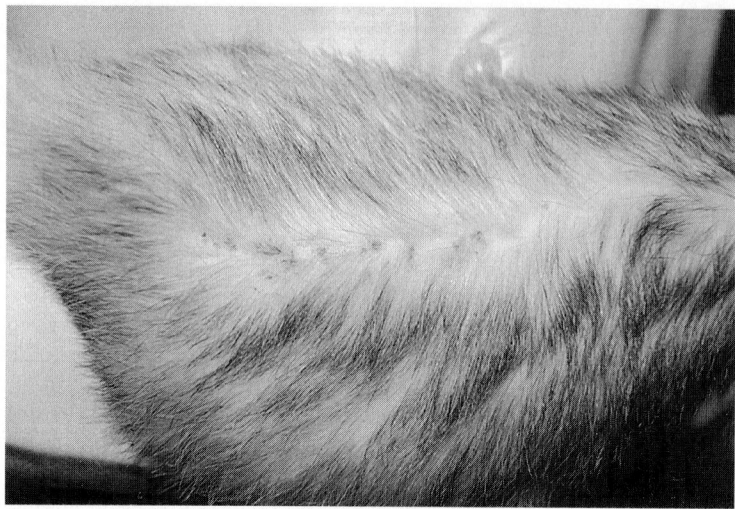

FIGURE 21-1. Superficial bacterial folliculitis in a ferret. Multiple crusted papules and patchy hair loss over dorsal midline.

Fungal Infections

Dermatophytosis appears to be rare in ferrets.* *M. canis* and *T. mentagrophytes* are the most common causes, and young animals are most frequently affected. Lesions consist of annular areas of alopecia, broken hairs, scale, and varying degrees of erythema and crusting. Pruritus is usually absent. Diagnosis is confirmed by microscopic examination of affected hairs and fungal culture. Therapy consists of topical application of antifungal agents and environmental clean-up as described for cats. Griseofulvin is usually not needed. Dermatophytosis in ferrets is a potential zoonosis. *Blastomycosis* was diagnosed in a ferret with chronic cutaneous plaques and ulcers.[17] *Histoplasmosis* was diagnosed in a

---

*See references 3, 6, 10, 17, 24, 25, 28, 35.

● Table 21-1 **COMMON THERAPEUTIC AGENTS IN SMALL MAMMALS**

AGENT	PROTOCOL
Antibiotics	
Amoxicillin	10–20 mg/kg SC or PO q12h (ferret, mouse, rat)
Ampicillin	5–10 mg/kg SC or PO q12h (ferret, mouse, rat)
Cephalexin	15–25 mg/kg PO q12h
Chloramphenicol succinate	50 mg/kg IM or SC q12h
Chloramphenicol palmitate	50 mg/kg PO q12h
Ciprofloxacin	5–15 mg/kg PO q12h
Doxycycline	5–10 mg/kg PO or SC q24h
Enrofloxacin	5–20 mg/kg PO or SC q12h
Gentamicin	5 mg/kg IM or SC q24h
Metronidazole	20 mg/kg PO q12–24h
Sulfadiazine-trimethoprim	15–30 mg/kg SC q24h
Sulfamethoxazole-trimethoprim	15–30 mg/kg PO q12h
Tetracycline hydrochloride	20 mg/kg SC or PO q12h
Antifungals	
Griseofulvin	25–50 mg/kg PO q24h
Antiparasitics	
Amitraz 250 ppm	Total body dip q2wk
Ivermectin	0.3–0.4 mg/kg SC q2wk
Lime sulfur 2%	Total body dip q7d

IM, intramuscularly; PO, orally; SC, subcutaneously.

ferret with multiple subcutaneous nodules.[24] *Coccidioidomycosis* was diagnosed in a ferret with a persistent draining tract of the stifle.[27]

An outbreak of otitis externa and pinnal necrosis in association with mites (*Otodectes*?) and yeast (*Malassezia*?) infection was reported.[26] A painful, rapidly progressing crusting and necrosis of the pinnae spread, if untreated, onto the face. Mites and yeast were found in smears. Histopathologic findings included suppurative epidermitis, numerous surface yeast, and hemorrhagic necrosis with thrombosis. Treatment with ketoconazole (50 mg/ferret, q24h, per os) and a polypharmaceutical otic preparation was rapidly effective.

Ectoparasites

Otodectic mange (ear mites) is common in ferrets.[10, 17, 38] Affected ferrets may manifest no clinical signs or variable degrees of excessive cerumen production. Pruritus, inflammation, and secondary bacterial infection are uncommon. Diagnosis is confirmed by finding *Otodectes cynotis* in ear swabs. Treatment is accomplished with topical acaricides or topical ivermectin (500 µg/kg divided between the two ears).[10] Injectable ivermectin is the treatment of choice. In one study,[35a] topical treatment with either Tresaderm (2 drops in ears q24h for 7 days, sequence repeated after a week of no treatment) or ivermectin (Ivomec diluted 1:10 in propylene glycol; 400 µg/kg divided equally in both ears, repeated in 2 weeks) was more effective than the subcutaneous administration of ivermectin (400 µg/kg, repeated in 2 weeks). Ivermectin should be used with caution in pregnant jills.[17, 25, 28] When ivermectin was administered at 2 to 4 weeks of gestation, an increased incidence of congenital defects, such as cleft palates, was seen. However, when ivermectin was administered after 4 weeks of gestation, no problems were noted.

Fleas (especially *Ctenocephalides felis felis*) are commonly found on ferrets.[17] Animals may be asymptomatic or have cutaneous reaction patterns similar to flea bite hypersensitivity in cats. Ferrets manifesting presumed flea bite hypersensitivity have a pruritic papulocrustous dermatitis over the rump, ventral abdomen, and caudomedial thighs, or a self-induced, symmetric alopecia over the rump, flanks, ventral abdomen, or medial thighs (fur-mowing) in which the skin appears normal. Treatment strategies must include the ferret; in-contact ferrets, cats, and dogs; and the environment, as described for cats. Fipronil spray has been found to be safe and effective for ferrets.[31]

Sarcoptic mange is uncommon in ferrets and has two clinical presentations: (1) intense pruritus and dermatitis over the face, the pinnae (Fig. 21-2A), and the ventrum and (2) pruritic pododermatitis.[10, 17] In the pododermatitis form, the feet are swollen, erythematous, and crusted, and the claws may be dystrophic. Affected ferrets may actually slough claws or digits. Diagnosis is confirmed by finding *Sarcoptes scabiei* mites in skin scrapings. However, mites can be extremely difficult to find, so response to miticidal therapy is often used as a diagnostic procedure. Treatment includes 2% lime sulfur dips (weekly until 2 weeks after clinical cure) or ivermectin injections.

Demodicosis was reported in two unrelated ferrets that were living in the same household and receiving long-term treatment with a glucocorticoid-containing otic ointment.[34] The ferrets exhibited excessive cerumen in the ears and pruritus, alopecia, comedones and orange discoloration of the skin behind the ears and on the ventrum. Skin scrapings and ear smears revealed numerous short mites that resembled *Demodex gatoi*. Amitraz dips were curative, and no side effects were reported.

Ferrets housed outdoors may occasionally have cysts, abscesses, or fistulae in the neck associated with infestation by *Hypoderma* sp. or *Cuterebra* sp. larvae.[10, 17] Treatment includes careful surgical removal of the larva and routine wound care.

Flystrike (especially *Wohlfahrtia vigil*) can be a problem for commercial ferret ranchers and outdoor ferrets.[10] Eggs are commonly laid on the face, neck, and flanks of young ferrets, causing irritation and subcutaneous abscesses.

Ticks may occasionally be found on ferrets, especially around the head and the ears.[17] Treatment is as described for cats.

Ferrets can be experimentally infected with *Dracunculus insignis* and have been used as an animal model for studying dracunculiasis.[17] Lesions consist of tender swellings, which abscess and develop fistulae. Lesions occur most commonly on the legs.

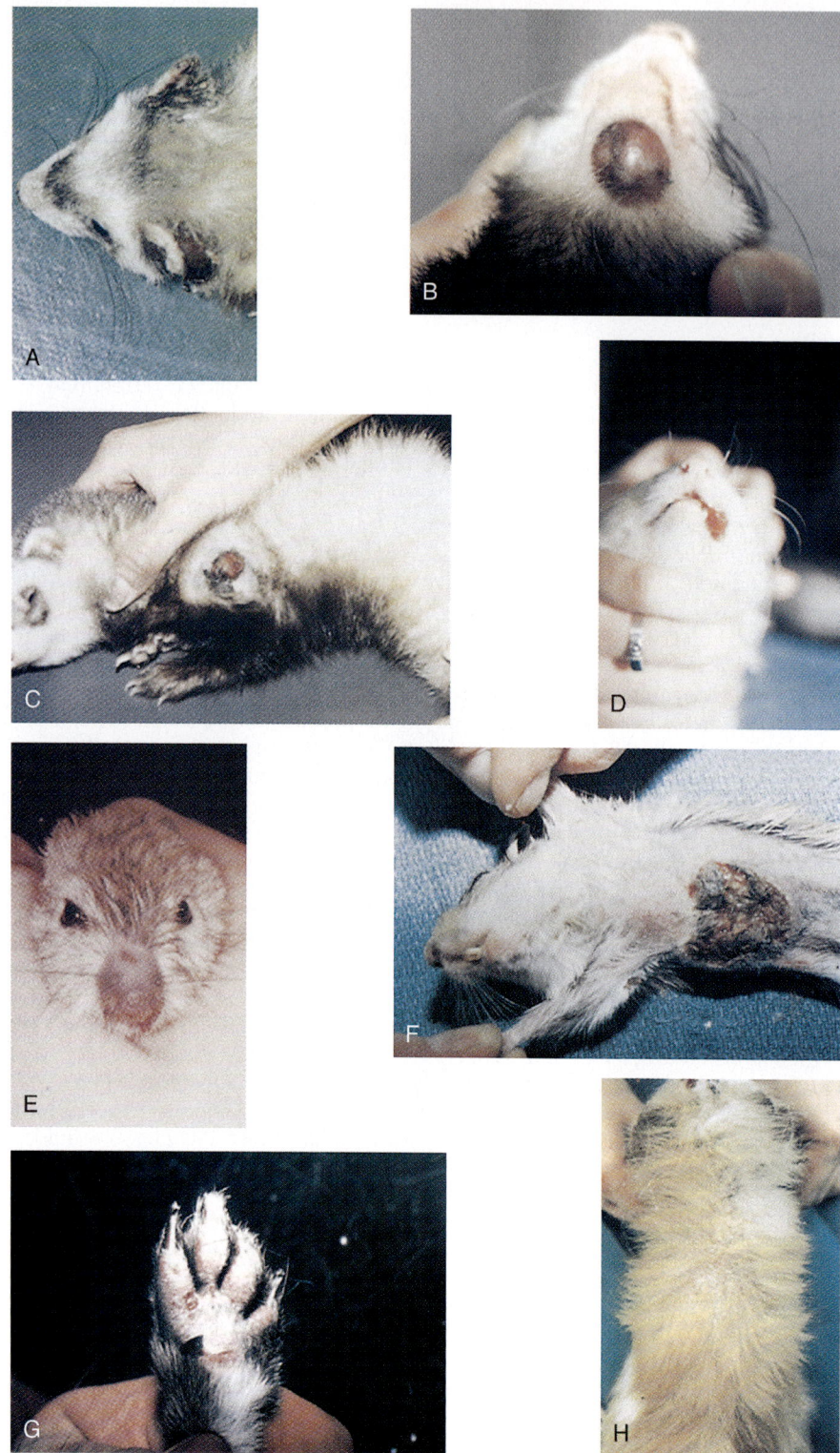

FIGURE 21-2. *A,* Alopecia, crusts, and excoriations on the pinnae of a ferret with sarcoptic mange. *B,* Mast cell tumor on the lower jaw of a ferret. *C,* Sebaceous epithelioma on the shoulder of a ferret. *D,* Squamous cell carcinoma on the lip of a ferret. (Courtesy of W. Gould.) *E,* Alopecia, crusting, and ulceration of the nose of a gerbil with "sore nose." *F,* Squamous cell carcinoma of the ventral scent gland in a gerbil. (Courtesy of W. Gould.) *G,* Staphylococcal pododermatitis in a guinea pig. (Courtesy of J. King.) *H,* Alopecia and thick crusts over the dorsum in a guinea pig with trixacariasis. (Courtesy of E. Guaguère.)

Viral Infections

The ferret is susceptible to canine distemper virus.[3, 6, 10, 17] Typical cutaneous findings include an erythematous rash under the chin and in the inguinal region; swelling and brownish crusts on the chin, lips, nose, and the periocular area; and swollen, hyperkeratotic nose and footpads (Fig. 21–3). Some ferrets develop an orange-tinged dermatosis on the anus and inguinal region.

Endocrine Disorders

HYPERADRENOCORTICISM

Adrenocortical neoplasia and hyperplasia are the most common causes of progressive bilaterally symmetric alopecia in the ferret.[10, 37, 39a, 41, 43] Two authors indicated that this disorder accounted for about 25% of all the ferrets examined in their practice.[43] The condition was initially diagnosed as Cushing's syndrome. However, other classic clinical signs (polyuria, polydipsia, and polyphagia) and hematologic, biochemical, or urologic abnormalities associated with Cushing's syndrome are rarely present. In addition, basal plasma cortisol levels are usually within the normal range and adrenal function tests (adrenocorticotropic hormone [ACTH] stimulation, dexamethasone suppression) have not been useful in separating normal from diseased ferrets.[10, 17, 37, 39, 43] The contralateral

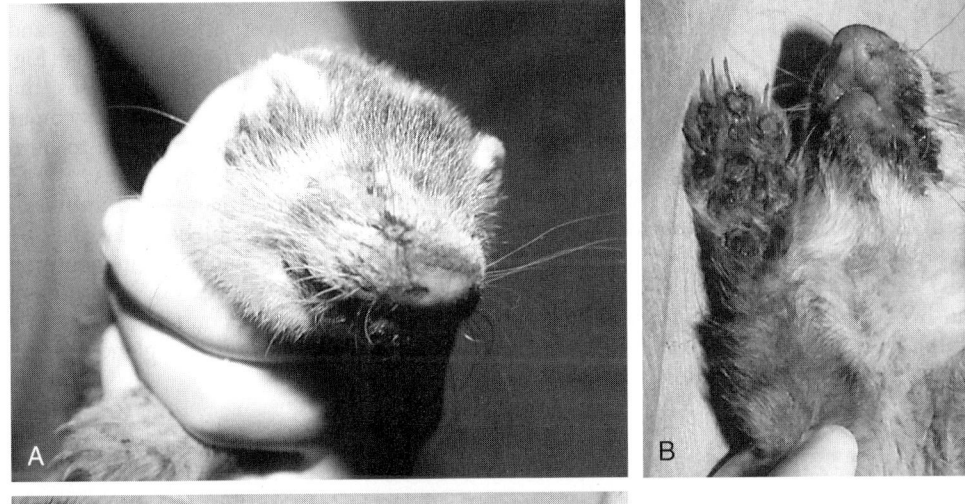
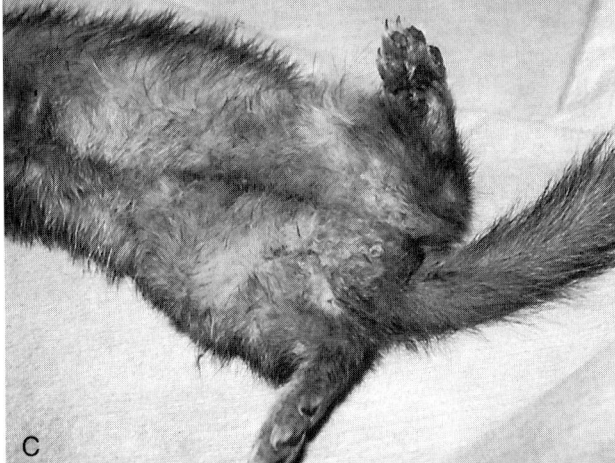

FIGURE 21–3. Young ferret with canine distemper virus infection. A, The eyes are encrusted shut with mucopurulent exudate. B, Dermatitis, excoriations, and crusting around the lips and chin; hyperkeratosis of the footpads. C, Dermatitis in the inguinal area. (From Hillyer EV, Quesenberry KE: Ferrets, Rabbits, and Rodents: Clinical Medicine and Surgery. W.B. Saunders, Philadelphia, 1997.)

Diagnosis is usually confirmed by ultrasonographic examination or exploratory laparotomy.[10, 17, 23] Ultrasonography may fail to diagnose about 50% of the cases and may not be cost-effective in a practice situation.[43] In rare instances, the adrenal glands appear normal on both ultrasonographic examination and exploratory laparotomy.[42, 43] Urinary cortisol: creatinine ratios were significantly higher in ferrets with hyperadrenocorticism than in normal ferrets.[29] However, this is not specific for hyperadrenocorticism, and affected ferrets can have normal ratios.[42]

Eighty-four percent of affected ferrets have unilateral adrenal tumors, whereas 16% have bilateral adrenal tumors.[43] Of the unilateral tumors, over 80% are in the left adrenal gland.[17, 43, 43a] Histologically, 56% of the tumors are nodular hyperplasia, 27% are adenocarcinomas, 16% are adenomas, and 1% are "normal."[43] All tumors larger than 1 cm diameter were adenocarcinomas.[43] In 47% of the patients with bilateral tumors, each gland had a different histologic type of tumor.[43, 43a] All male ferrets with a return of male sexual behavior had adenocarcinomas.[43]

In one study,[43] 27% of the ferrets with hyperadrenocorticism had concurrent insulinomas. This emphasizes the importance of performing a complete exploratory.

The "adrenal panel" (Clinical Endocrinology Laboratory, Department of Comparative Medicine, University of Tennessee, Knoxville, TN, 615-974-5638) may give diagnostic results in 96% of the cases.[39] However, results are not always diagnostic, and the test may not be cost-effective in a practice situation.[43, 43a]

In most animals, the treatment of choice is unilateral adrenalectomy.[10, 17, 43] Clinical improvement is evident within 2 to 8 weeks, and complete recovery is usually seen within 5 months. Hair regrowth usually occurs in the opposite direction to which it was lost. In two cases in which a unilateral adrenalectomy was performed and no hair growth had occurred for 6 to 8 months, a secondary exploratory revealed tumors on the remaining adrenal.[43] Seventeen percent of the animals with unilateral tumors develop tumors on the remaining adrenal, resulting in a recurrence of clinical signs within 14 months.[43] Ferrets with bilateral adrenal tumors should have the largest adrenal gland completely removed, along with 50% to 60% of the other one (subtotal bilateral adrenalectomy).[43, 43a] Even following subtotal bilateral adrenalectomy, 15% of the ferrets had recurrence of clinical signs within 7 to 22 months.[43a]

Medical treatment has been used, usually unsuccessfully, when surgery could not be performed, or when, after surgical removal of a neoplastic adrenal, the remaining adrenal gland also became neoplastic and clinical signs recurred.[17] Mitotane (o,p'-DDD) has been used at 50 mg orally, once daily for 7 days, then every 3 days until clinical cure. Administration of the drug is then stopped. If clinical signs recur, o,p'-DDD is given at a weekly maintenance dose of 50 mg. To facilitate administration, the o,p'-DDD is mixed with corn starch and 50-mg doses are put in gelatin capsules. However, mitotane is rarely effective.[10, 43a] Ketoconazole has been ineffective when given orally at 15 mg/kg every 12 hours.[10, 43a]

Anecdotal reports indicate that leuprolide (Lupron, TAP Pharmaceuticals), when given at 100 µg/kg subcutaneously, every 21 days, is very effective for the treatment of hyperadrenocorticism in ferrets. Response is usually seen by the third injection and is complete by 6 months. Once maximum response is achieved, the interval between injections is extended. Ferrets with aggressive adrenal carcinomas may not respond.

HYPERESTROGENISM

Hyperestrogenism is well recognized in the female ferret.[10, 17, 24, 28] However, this disorder is rare because large-volume ferret breeders are neutering and descenting the animals at 6 weeks of age. An ovarian remnant may be suspected in a neutered female with signs of estrus. Jills allowed to remain in estrus during the breeding season are susceptible to the toxic effects of estrogen on bone marrow. Affected jills develop pancytopenia and varying degrees of alopecia. Clinical signs accompanying the pancytopenia include pale mucous membranes, petechial or ecchymotic hemorrhages, anorexia, depression, and weight loss.

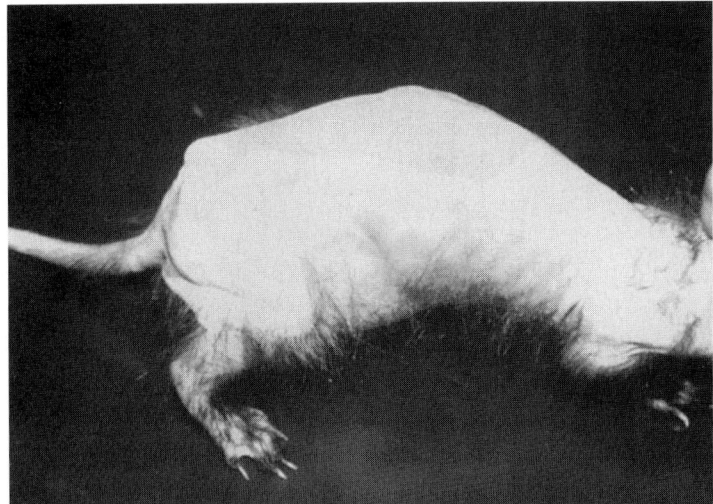

FIGURE 21–7. Alopecia of the trunk and tail in a jill with hyperestrogenism.

The alopecia is bilaterally symmetric, beginning on the tail, the perineum, the abdomen, the medial thighs, and the rump and progressing cranially (Fig. 21–7). Vulvar enlargement is a constant finding. Untreated animals die of infectious or hemorrhagic complications. Treatment is often unrewarding. Ovariohysterectomy; intravenous blood transfusions; administration of dexamethasone, anabolic steroids, and systemic antibiotics; and supportive care have rarely been reported to result in recovery, but transfusions may need to be repeated several times for 3 to 5 months.[10, 17, 24, 28]

ALOPECIA ASSOCIATED WITH TESTICULAR NEOPLASIA

Testicular neoplasia is rare, because most large-volume breeders neuter male ferrets at 6 weeks of age. A sparse haircoat and a bald tail were reported in association with an interstitial cell carcinoma of the testicle in one ferret.[17] Total body alopecia and pruritus were reported in association with a testicular Sertoli's cell neoplasm in another ferret.[17]

BREEDING SEASON ALOPECIA

Breeding season alopecia is commonly seen, especially in the female and less frequently in the male ferret, during the period of sexual activity from March through August.[6, 10, 17, 28, 41] Photoperiod plays an important role in this condition, because even neutered ferrets are affected. Bilaterally symmetric alopecia affects the tail, the perineum, the ventral abdomen, the rump, and occasionally, the periocular region and the paws. Affected ferrets are otherwise healthy, and spontaneous hair regrowth occurs in the fall.

SHEDDING

Seasonal shedding is seen in spring and early summer.[6, 17, 28, 41] Variable degrees of hypotrichosis or alopecia may be seen over the trunk and resolve spontaneously within a month or two.

TELOGEN DEFLUXION

Telogen defluxion is occasionally seen 2 to 3 months after a stressful circumstance (high fever, severe illness, surgery, and anesthesia).[17, 41] Bilaterally symmetric hypotrichosis or alopecia is most prominent on the trunk (Fig. 21–8).

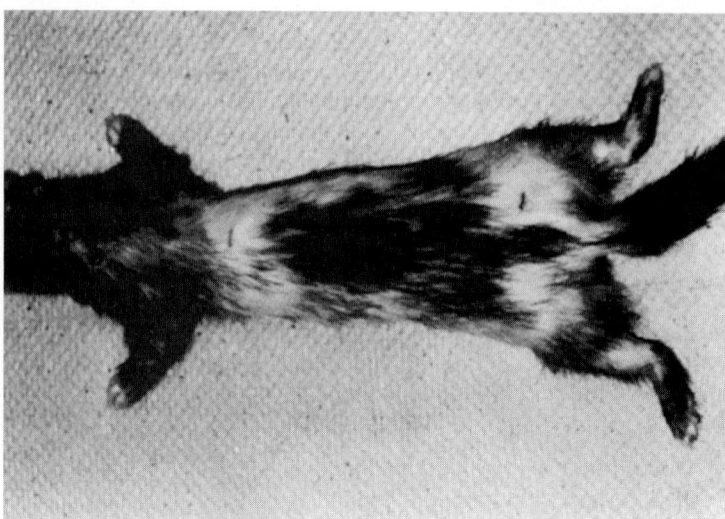

FIGURE 21–8. Telogen defluxion. Patchy alopecia of the dorsal trunk. (Courtesy of M. Paradis.)

HYPOTHYROIDISM

Although anecdotal reports suggest that hypothyroidism is a common cause of endocrine-like alopecia in ferrets,[4] the authors and others[10, 17] have never made such a diagnosis, and know of no documented cases. Some data have been published on basal serum thyroxine and triiodothyronine levels and thyroid function tests in normal ferrets.[17, 28]

Miscellaneous Conditions

Some authors believe that the most common cause of alopecia and dull, dry haircoat in ferrets is poor dietary practices.[3] Food passage averages 3 to 4 hours in ferrets; thus, diets high in protein and fat but low in fiber are important. A low-fat diet may result in a dry, dull haircoat.[10]

Biotin deficiency (from excessive feeding of raw eggs) can result in bilaterally symmetric alopecia in ferrets.[6, 24, 25, 28]

Severe intestinal parasitism (especially *Toxascaris leonina*) can produce variable degrees of hair loss and scaling in ferrets.[25]

Contact dermatitis can occur with frequent use of shampoos or insecticide sprays.[25]

Focal areas of alopecia have been seen at the site of previous injections.[25]

The authors have seen an occasional ferret with presumptive atopy. Affected animals manifested symmetric, nonlesional pruritus over the trunk, the rump (Fig. 21–9), and the paws. Fleas were not present, hypoallergenic diets were ineffective, and response to glucocorticoids or chlorpheniramine was good. One of the authors (WHM) has seen one food-hypersensitive ferret with the same clinical signs. The ferret was normal when fed a commercial hypoallergenic diet for cats (Innovative Veterinary Diets [IVD] venison).

Erythema annulare centrifugum was reported in a ferret with hyperadrenocorticism.[42] Parallel linear bands of erythema were present over the dorsolateral lumbosacral area and encircling the tail (Fig. 21–10). The dermatitis disappeared after 20 days of treatment with a commercial omega 3/omega 6 fatty acid–containing product (Derm Caps).

The *blue ferret syndrome* is an unusual idiopathic condition affecting ferrets of either sex, neutered or intact.[3] The abdominal skin shows bilaterally symmetric bluish discoloration. Affected ferrets are asymptomatic. The condition regresses spontaneously during a few weeks. In the authors' experience, this condition is most commonly seen in ferrets that have been clipped for surgery or to provide access to veins during the resting phase of the hair cycle. The clipped area remains hairless for a long time, then suddenly begins to turn blue. It appears that hair follicles are making melanin, which will be incorporated

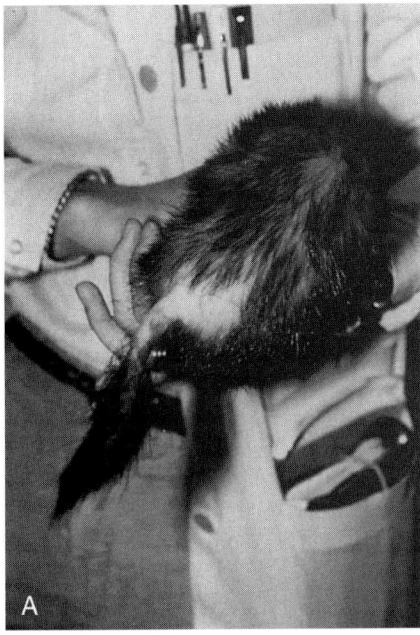
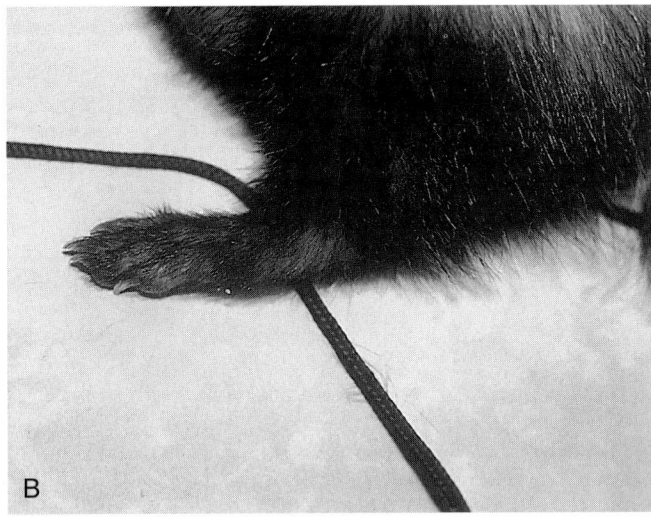

FIGURE 21–9. *A,* Self-induced alopecia over the rump of a ferret with a pruritic dermatosis resembling atopy. *B,* Same ferret. Self-induced hypotrichosis of hind paw.

into growing hairs. Soon after the ferret's skin turns blue, hair regrowth begins (within 1 to 2 weeks).

Self-inflicted facial excoriations (burrowing) may be seen in ferrets that have inadequate bedding, nesting material, or hiding spots.[10] Intact females may pull out hair to use as bedding.[10]

Neoplasia

Skin neoplasms are fairly common in the ferret, and the majority are benign.[10, 17] In one large survey,[33] the skin was the third most common site for primary neoplasms in ferrets (about 13% of all neoplasms). One of the most frequent of these is the mast cell tumor.[10, 17, 33] Lesions may be solitary or multiple and may come and go over time. Mast cell

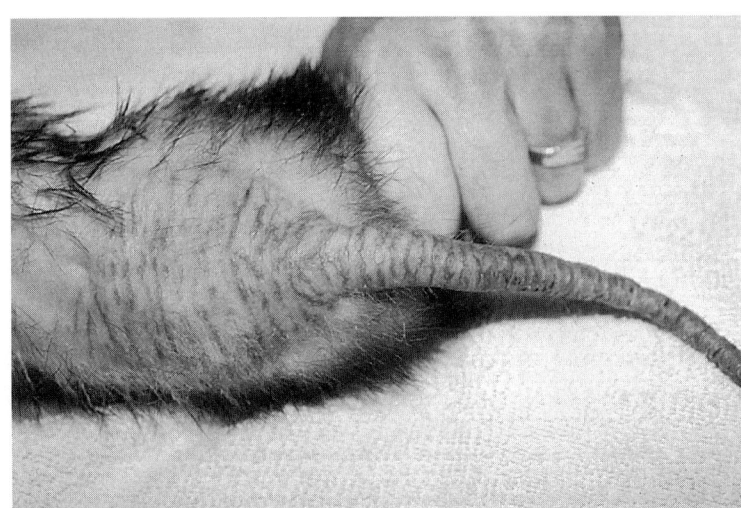

FIGURE 21–10. Erythema annulare centrifugum in a ferret with hyperadrenocorticism. Multiple parallel bands of erythema and scale encircle the tail and involve the dorsal lumbosacral area.

tumors present as papules or nodules (see Fig. 21–2B), which vary from skin colored to yellow, brown, or red. They may be firm, soft, or cystic. Some lesions are pruritic. Lesions may occur anywhere, but are most commonly reported on the neck and dorsal trunk. Similar to the situation in cats, most cutaneous mast cell tumors in the ferret are benign.[10, 17]

Basal cell tumors and sebaceous gland neoplasms (especially on the head, neck, limbs, tail and the shoulder [see Fig. 21–2C]) are also common in ferrets.[10, 17, 33] Most previously diagnosed "basal cell tumors" were probably sebaceous epitheliomas.[17] Epitrichial sweat gland carcinomas (especially on the tail and the groin), chondromas (especially on the tail), chondrosarcomas (especially on the tail), and squamous cell carcinomas (especially on the digit and the lip [see Fig. 21–2D]) have also been reported on numerous occasions.[17, 33]

Cutaneous epitheliotropic lymphoma was reported in an 8-year-old ferret with a 4-month history of progressive alopecia and pruritic dermatitis.[36] The ferret had generalized alopecia and erythema, excoriations, erosions, crusts, and ulcerated plaques on the head, trunk, limbs, paws, footpads, and tail. The nasal planum and footpads were depigmented, and the claws were onychogryphotic. Isotretinoin (2 mg/kg/q 24h, per os) produced a marked improvement after 60 days, but the ferret was euthanized due to renal failure associated with pyelonephritis.

Other cutaneous neoplasms reported in ferrets include papilloma, fibroma, fibrosarcoma, malignant fibrous histiocytoma, histiocytoma, hemangioma, hemangiosarcoma, neurofibroma, neurofibrosarcoma, myxoma, myxosarcoma, ceruminous gland adenocarcinoma, lymphoma, and rhabdomyosarcoma.*

The treatment of choice for cutaneous neoplasms is surgical excision.

● GERBIL

Bacterial Infections

Bacterial skin infections, usually associated with *S. aureus*, are common in gerbils.[7, 8, 17] These infections are virtually always secondary to other perhaps less obvious conditions, especially trauma (cage-related injuries and bite wounds), ectoparasite infestations, and accumulated harderian gland secretions.[6, 8] Infections resulting from cage-related injury are typically seen on the nose and the muzzle (from rubbing on the cage and equipment or burrowing in abrasive litter), whereas those caused by bite wounds typically occur around the head, the tail, the rump, and the perineal area. Those secondary to accumulated harderian gland secretion typically begin on the nose and the periocular area.[6, 8] Staphylococcal infections may be superficial (alopecia, erythema, oozing, crust, and scale) or deep (abscess, fistula, and ulcer), and are usually nonpruritic.

Treatment of bacterial dermatitis includes some combination of eliminating predisposing causes, daily topical cleaning with a 3% hydrogen peroxide or 0.5% to 1% chlorhexidine, and administration of systemic antibiotics (see Table 21–1).

Ectoparasites

Demodicosis has rarely been reported in gerbils.[6, 17] Lesions occurred on the face, the thorax, the abdomen, and the limbs and were characterized by alopecia, oozing, crusts, scales, and secondary bacterial infection. *Demodex merioni* was isolated in skin scrapings. Details concerning pathogenesis and treatment are presently unpublished.

A dermatosis associated with *Acarus farris* was reported.[44] Alopecia, scaling, and thickening of the skin began on the tail, spread to the hind paws, then to the head. Pruritus and excoriation were seen with chronicity. Ivermectin injections were ineffective, but environmental changes (decreased humidity, new litter, new food) and a single application of fipronil spray were curative.

---

*See references 6, 10, 17, 28, 32, 33, 40.

Barbering

Although gerbils tolerate crowding better than do most rodents, they chew or "barber" the hair of cagemates.[6, 8] The affected areas appear clipped or shaved, and rarely are any actual skin lesions present. The dorsum of the tail and the top of the head are most frequently involved.

Bald Nose and Sore Nose

Bald nose describes a clinical condition common to the gerbil, which is characterized by alopecia on the muzzle and the dorsum of the nose.[3, 6, 8, 15, 17] There are usually no skin lesions. The alopecia has been attributed to mechanical trauma associated with rubbing against cages and cage equipment, and burrowing in abrasive bedding. Placing animals in a smooth-sided enclosure or aquarium with soft bedding such as shredded paper may be curative.

Bald nose may also be an early stage of the nasal dermatitis (sore nose [see Fig. 21–2E]) associated with accumulated harderian gland secretion.[3, 6, 8, 17, 19] These secretions are rich in porphyrins and accumulate about the nasal and facial areas, and apparently lead to the development of an irritant contact dermatitis and secondary staphylococcal infection. The animal's failure to groom the areas adequately leads to irritation, which can then lead to self-inflicted trauma and secondary infection. The stress of overcrowding and high humidity may contribute to the development or the severity of the condition. This condition is common in research colonies and commercial breeding colonies.

The earliest clinical sign is the accumulation of a reddish brown discharge and crust around the nose, the lips, and less frequently, the eyes. This porphyrin-rich secretion exhibits an orange fluorescence when viewed under ultraviolet light (Wood's light). There is frequently protrusion of the nictitans. This is followed by alopecia and, if not treated, dermatitis, pruritus, and secondary staphylococcal infections. Lesions can then spread to the paws, the legs, and the ventrum.

Therapy consists of topical or systemic antibiotic therapy for secondary staphylococcal infection, if present, and housing with access to sand. Surgical removal of the harderian gland is effective but less practical.[6, 17]

Miscellaneous Conditions

An occasional litter of gerbils is born with abnormalities of hair growth and pigmentation.[6, 17] Typically, the back is completely bald, the surrounding haircoat is thinned or patchily alopecic, and the haircoat shows profound leukotrichia. The majority of affected animals fail to thrive and die at the time of weaning. Surviving gerbils develop a normal haircoat as they mature. The etiopathogenesis of this condition is unknown.

The ventral scent gland in gerbils can become inflamed from being rubbed against wood chips or other abrasive bedding.[4] In addition, impaction of these glands can lead to self-mutilation.[4]

When relative humidity is greater than 50%, the normally sleek and smooth gerbil haircoat often appears greasy and stands out.[3] Pine shavings can also cause this appearance.[3]

A gerbil's tail skin is very thin, and easily peels off.[15] If the tail skin is lost, the exposed tail becomes necrotic and sloughs off.[10, 16] Alternatively, the bare tail can be surgically removed where the skin stops.

Neoplasia

The skin is the second most common site of neoplasms in gerbils.[6, 17] Skin neoplasms are typically seen in aged animals (2 to 4 years of age). The most commonly reported skin neoplasms in the gerbil are melanocytomas and melanomas (especially of the paw and the pinna),[5, 16] sebaceous gland adenomas (especially of the ventral scent gland),[6, 17] and squamous cell carcinoma (especially of the ventral scent gland [see Fig. 21–2F] and the pinna).[6, 17, 45] Other reported skin neoplasms in gerbils include papilloma, fibrosarcoma, and neurofibroma.[6, 17]

Diagnosis of skin neoplasms is based on exfoliative cytologic study or biopsy, and the treatment of choice is surgical excision.

• GUINEA PIG

Bacterial Infections

Bacterial skin infections are common in guinea pigs.[2–11, 17] These infections are virtually always secondary to other factors, especially trauma (cage-related injuries and bite wounds) and ectoparasites. Those secondary to bite wounds are typically found around the head, the tail, the rump, and the genital area and are associated with *S. aureus*. Abscesses are occasionally associated with *Corynebacterium kutscheri, Streptococcus zooepidemicus* (especially abscesses on the neck), *Streptobacillus moniliformis*, or *Yersinia pseudotuberculosis*.[2, 6, 8, 17] A staphylococcal cellulitis characterized by thickening and hyperkeratosis of the lips was associated with feeding of tough, fibrous hay.[17] Treatment of these infections includes elimination of predisposing factors, surgical drainage, daily topical applications of 3% hydrogen peroxide or 0.5% chlorhexidine, and systemic antibiotic administration (see Table 21–1).

An exfoliative dermatitis resembling staphylococcal scalded skin syndrome was reported in a guinea pig colony, chiefly among female animals in the late stages of gestation.[17] Bacterial contamination and the abrasive effects of rusty cage floors were suggested as initiating factors. Alopecia was first noted on the ventral abdomen. After a few days, the skin became acutely erythematous and painful. Affected skin subsequently fissured and large thick flakes were desquamated. The condition spontaneously resolved after a course of 10 to 14 days. *S. aureus* was isolated from the skin, the pharynx, the trachea, and nasal washings of affected animals. Skin biopsies revealed intragranular acantholysis and cleavage within the epidermis with minimal inflammation. An exfoliative toxin produced by the staphylococci was reported to cause the skin lesions.

The most common skin disease associated with *S. aureus* infection (occasionally *Corynebacterium pyogenes*) in the guinea pig is *pododermatitis* (bumble foot).[2–11, 17] Predisposing factors include trauma to the footpad, poor sanitation, obesity, aging, and vitamin C deficiency. Affected animals react vigorously when the feet are palpated. The footpad is markedly enlarged, edematous, and erythematous (see Fig. 21–2G). Crusts, ulcers, and hemorrhages may be present on the volar surfaces. In chronic or severe cases, the disease process extends to phalangeal and metatarsal or metacarpal bones and joints. Most guinea pigs with pododermatitis have a poor prognosis, because treatment is difficult and systemic amyloidosis is a frequent consequence of chronic infection. Pododermatitis can be prevented by frequently cleaning cages and changing bedding, using cages with smooth surfaces, instituting individual weight control, and providing routine foot care. Early lesions may respond to management changes and daily topical therapy (povidone-iodine or chlorhexidine scrubs, soaks, and ointments under a bandage). Extensive infections also necessitate systemic antibiotics (see Table 21–1).

Fungal Infections

Dermatophytosis is common in guinea pigs and is almost always caused by *T. mentagrophytes*.[10, 17] This dermatophyte can be isolated from the skin and haircoat in approximately 15% of clinically normal guinea pigs.[1, 13, 17, 53a] Rarely, other dermatophytes, such as *M. canis, M. gypseum, M. audouinii*, and *T. verrucosum* can cause disease in guinea pigs.[16] Lesions typically begin as scaling, broken hairs, and alopecia on the nose, which spread to the periocular, forehead, and pinnal areas. In severe cases, the dorsal lumbosacral area is also affected (Fig. 21–11), but the limbs and the ventrum are usually spared. Pruritus is

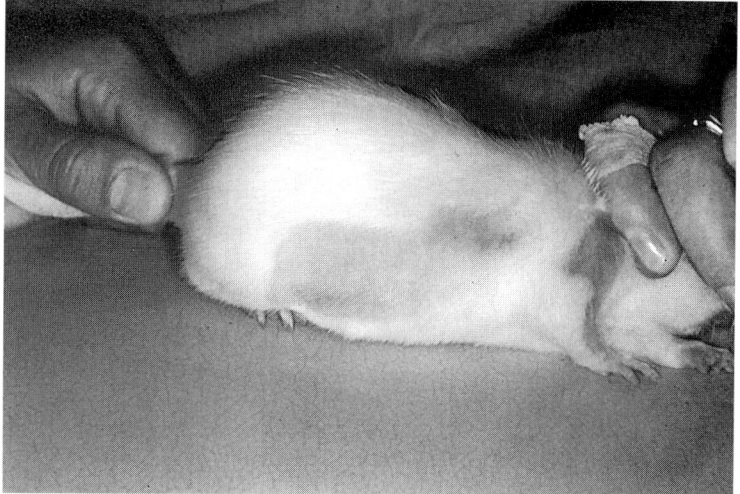

FIGURE 21-11. *M. canis* infection in a guinea pig. Alopecia and erythema of lateral abdominal and shoulder regions. (Courtesy of E. Guaguère.)

usually minimal or absent. Some animals have more inflammatory lesions characterized by erythema, follicular papules, pustules, crusts, and pruritus. Diagnosis is confirmed by microscopic examination of affected hairs and fungal culture. Treatment is usually accomplished with the topical application of antifungal agents (2% lime sulfur, 1% chlorhexidine, or 0.2% enilconazole dips weekly until the animal is cured).[2-11, 17] Griseofulvin is not usually needed, but can be given at 25 mg/kg every 24 hours orally until the animal is cured.[2-10, 16] The administration of griseofulvin should be avoided in pregnant animals.[5, 16] Dermatophytosis in guinea pigs is an important zoonosis.[17]

Cryptococcosis was reported in a single guinea pig.[17] The animal had a plaque on the dorsum of the nose, which became crusted and ulcerated, and spread into the nostrils. Skin biopsy was diagnostic, and the animal was euthanized.

Guinea pigs have been used as an experimental model for studying the pathogenesis of cutaneous *candidiasis*.[52] Skin lesions are readily produced by the application of *Candida albicans* under occlusion and consist of erythema, pustules, oozing, and crusts.

Guinea pigs have also been used as an experimental model for studying the pathogenesis and treatment of *Malassezia* dermatitis.[53] Skin lesions are readily produced by the application of inocula of *Malassezia (Pityrosporum) ovale* and consist of erythema, edema, crusts, and scales.

Viral Infections

Hairless guinea pigs have been used as an experimental model for studying the pathogenesis of recurrent herpes simplex infection.[46] Intracutaneous inoculation of herpes simplex virus produces pustules and crusts, which spontaneously resolve and can be reactivated by local trauma.

Poxvirus-like virions were demonstrated during the electron microscopic examination of specimens from two guinea pigs with a chronic, crusting cheilitis.[17]

Ectoparasites

Trixacarus (Caviacoptes) caviae is a burrowing sarcoptiform mite and, arguably, the most common cause of ectoparasitic skin disease of guinea pigs.[10, 17, 50, 51] Trixacariasis is always the first differential diagnostic suspect in intense pruritus in guinea pigs. The mite is similar to *S. scabiei* in appearance but is smaller in size (average, 175 μm in length), and the female mite has a dorsal rather than terminal anus. *T. caviae* is similar in size and appearance to *Notoedres* spp. but differs by lacking prominent, sharp, dorsal cuticular

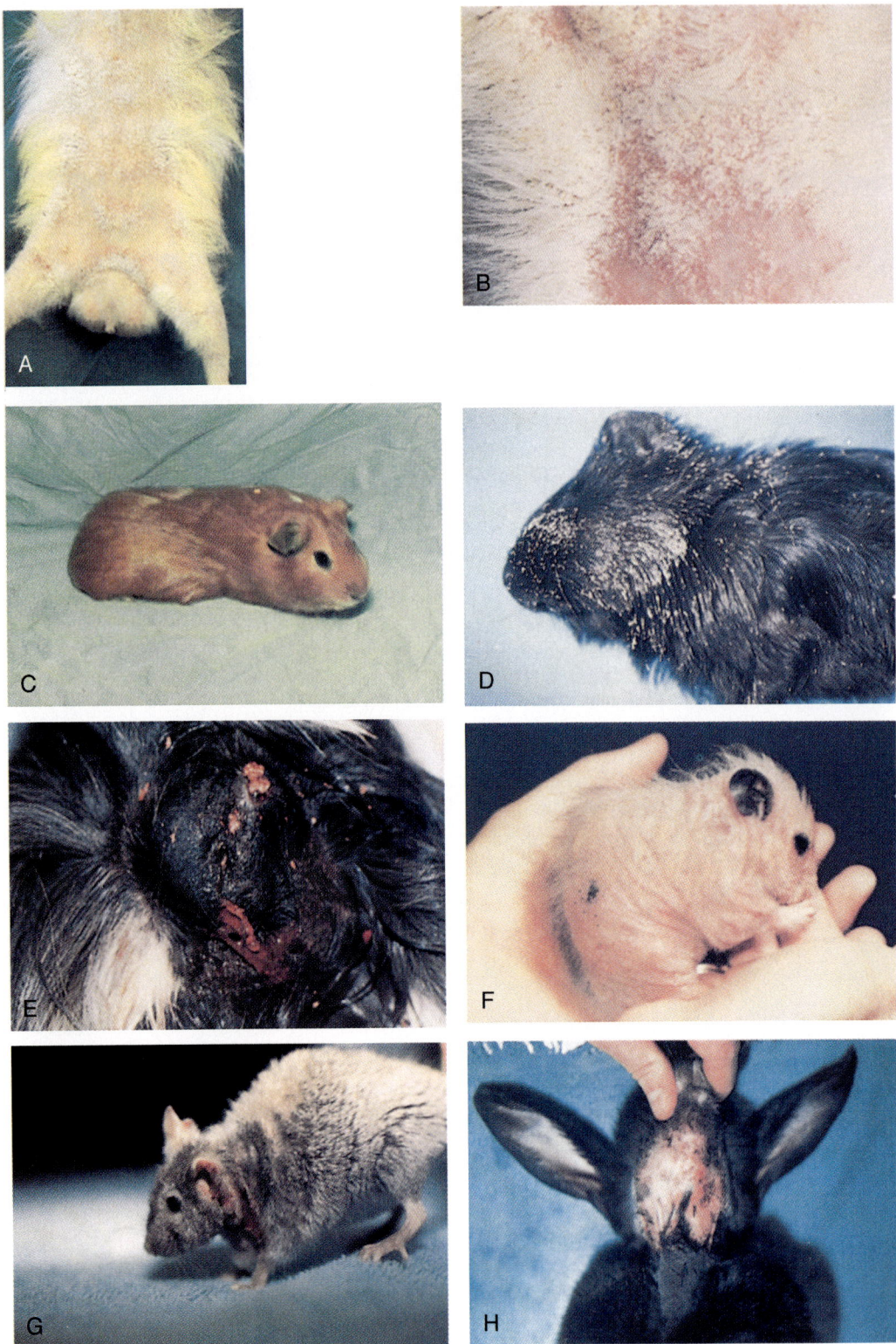

FIGURE 21-12. *Legend on opposite page*

spines. The areas most commonly affected include the dorsal neck and the thorax (see Fig. 21–2H), but in severe cases, the entire body may be involved (Fig. 21–12A).

Early clinical signs include pruritus, erythema, and traumatic alopecia. Chronic lesions include lichenification, hyperpigmentation, crusts, thick, whitish to yellowish scales (see Fig. 21–12B), and brittle, easily epilated hair. The extreme irritation and self-mutilation cause lethargy, anorexia, progressive emaciation, and death associated with bacterial infection or immune-mediated renal disease. Hyperesthesia, behavior such as furiously running in circles and blindly walking into objects, and seizures can be seen and may be triggered by examining the affected animal. Resorption of fetuses and abortion may be seen in breeding animals. Diagnosis may be confirmed by skin scrapings (Fig. 21–13A), but it is not unusual for these to be negative. Treatment consists of 2% lime sulfur dips (once weekly until cure is achieved) or ivermectin injections. Orally administered ivermectin is *not* effective in guinea pigs.[51a] *T. caviae* can temporarily infest humans, producing a pruritic papular dermatitis in areas contacted by the guinea pig (arms, thighs, and abdomen).

Chirodiscoides caviae is the guinea pig fur mite.[10, 17, 48] Infestation is uncommon, and clinical disease is probably rare. Heavy infestations can cause pruritus, alopecia, erythema, scaling, and crusting, especially on the dorsolateral lumbosacral area (see Fig. 21–13C) and the perineum. Diagnosis is confirmed by the microscopic identification of the mites (see Fig. 21–13B), which are often found attached to hair shafts. Treatment is as described for lice. Although injections of ivermectin have been reported to eliminate *C. caviae*,[5, 10, 17] others found this form of therapy to be ineffective.[48]

Other mites rarely reported to affect guinea pigs and produce clinical syndromes characterized by pruritus and dermatitis, which is most prominent on the face, the pinnae, and the dorsum, include *S. scabiei*, *Notoedres muris*, and *Myocoptes musculinus*.[17] Diagnosis and treatment are as described for *T. caviae* infestation.

Lice are commonly encountered in guinea pigs.[10, 17] The guinea pig may be parasitized by two different biting lice, with *Gliricola porcelli* (the slender guinea pig louse) (see Fig. 21–13C) being much more frequently encountered than *Gyropus ovalis* (the oval guinea pig louse). *Trimenopon hispidum* is a biting louse rarely isolated from guinea pigs.[49] Most infestations occur without clinical signs, but heavy infestations may produce a roughened, disheveled haircoat, scaling, crusting, alopecia, and pruritus, especially around the ears and over the dorsum (see Fig. 21–12D). Heavy infestations are more commonly encountered in young animals and those with decreased resistance and under poor management. Diagnosis is confirmed by gross or microscopic visualization of lice or nits. Treatment can be accomplished with pyrethrin- or pyrethroid-containing flea powders or sprays approved for cats, 2% lime sulfur dips, or ivermectin injections.[3-6, 10, 17] Cage sanitation is important.

Pelodera dermatitis is rarely reported in guinea pigs.[17] Affected animals have ventral dermatitis consisting of erythema, papules, oozing, crusts, and alopecia. Skin scrapings and skin biopsy reveal the presence of the nematode *Pelodera strongyloides*. Removing contaminated bedding and maintaining a clean, dry cage environment are curative.

Cheyletiellosis is rarely reported in guinea pigs.[17] Affected animals have scaling and variable degrees of hypotrichosis and pruritus on the dorsum. Skin scrapings reveal the mite *Cheyletiella parasitivorax*. Treatment is as described for rabbits.

Demodicosis is rare in guinea pigs.[17] Lesions occur most commonly on the trunk (Fig.

FIGURE 21–12. *A*, Alopecia, erythema, and thick, yellowish crusts on the ventrum of a guinea pig with trixacariasis. (Courtesy of E. Guaguère.) *B*, Close-up of the thick, yellowish crusts on the skin of a guinea pig with trixacariasis. *C*, *Chirodiscoides caviae* infestation in a guinea pig. Note the uneven, clipped appearance of the haircoat over the caudal half of the body. *D*, Pediculosis in a guinea pig. Numerous nits can be seen over the face and neck. (Courtesy of J. King.) *E*, Trichofolliculoma in a guinea pig. Hyperpigmented, ulcerated tumor over the dorsal lumbar area (Courtesy of W. Gould.) *F*, Epitheliotropic lymphoma in a hamster. Generalized alopecia, erythema, scaling, and exaggerated folds of skin. *G*, Severe self-inflicted alopecia and ulceration over the ear, neck, and shoulder in a mouse with *M. musculi* infestation. (Courtesy of W. Gould.) *H*, Alopecia, erythema, crusts, and ulcers on the ventral neck of a rabbit with *Pseudomonas aeruginosa* infection.

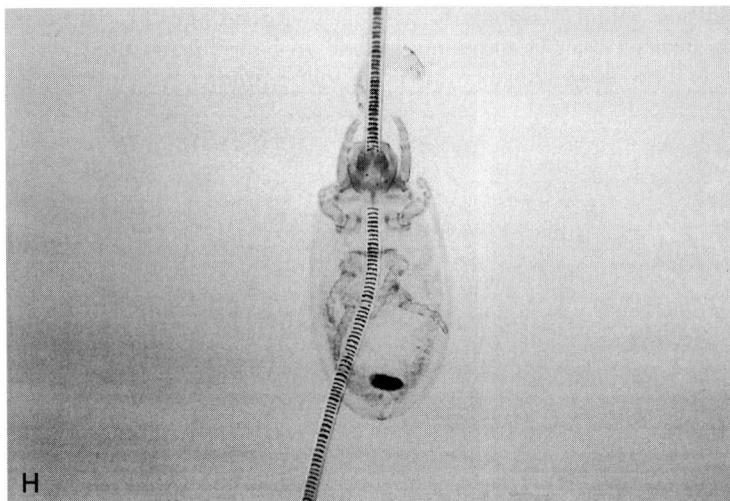

FIGURE 21–13. Continued

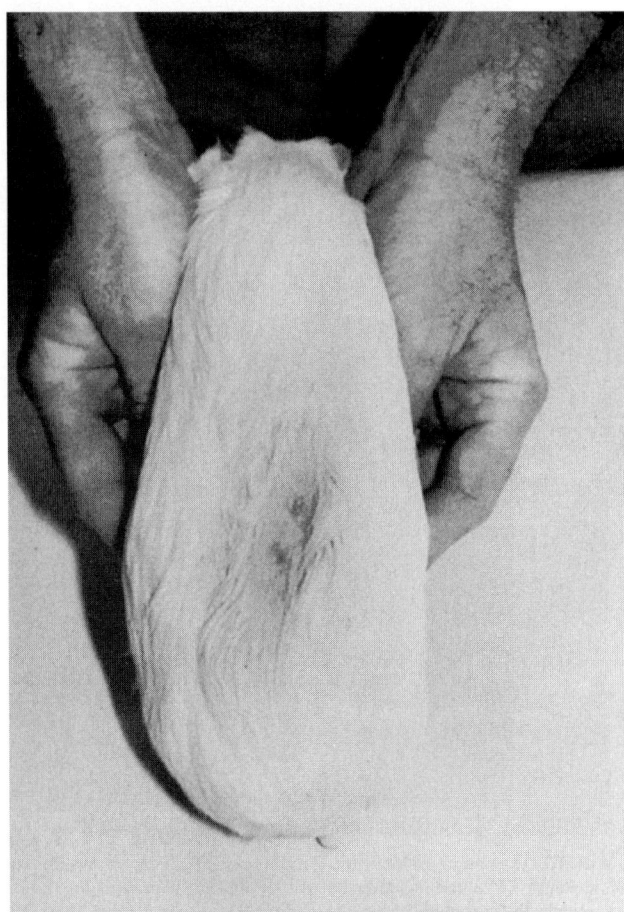

FIGURE 21–14. Alopecia and erythema over the back of a guinea pig with demodicosis. (Courtesy of D. Carlotti.)

Miscellaneous Conditions

Telogen defluxion is frequently seen in the last trimester of pregnancy or during lactation.[6, 8, 17] The alopecia is most prominent on the lumbosacral area and the flanks.

Marked shedding during stress is common in guinea pigs.[3] When guinea pigs are sick, it is often easy to epilate an entire area of haircoat when tenting the skin.

Guinea pigs establish male-dominated social hierarchies, and animals of low social ranking or young animals may lose considerable amounts of hair, especially on the head, the rump, the perineum, and the prepuce owing to barbering or receiving bite wounds.[6, 8, 17, 19] Ear chewing can be a problem, resulting in ear margin notches or actual cropping close to the head. Guinea pigs may also self-barber, producing hair loss in only those areas that they can reach with their mouth (the fur on the head, the neck, and the anterior shoulders is intact). Hair loss due to barbering appears irregular in length and clipped. The underlying skin is usually normal in appearance. In some cases, the addition of long-stemmed hay resolves the barbering, suggesting that the cause was boredom or a need for fiber.[5, 8, 17, 19]

Necrosis of digits and paws is occasionally seen when owners put objects such as cloths and socks in cages with guinea pigs.[17] Segments of these materials become wrapped around distal extremities and serve as constricting bands or tourniquets. Tissues distal to the constriction become swollen and painful, then necrotic, and then they slough (Fig. 21-15).

Apparent *ergot poisoning* was characterized by the sudden onset of anorexia, lethargy, and lameness.[47] The feet became discolored, desiccated, insensitive to touch, and wood-like.

Thinning of the haircoat is common near the time of weaning in neonates and spontaneously resolves.[6, 17]

Hereditary hairlessness has been reported in guinea pigs (Fig. 21-16).[17] Bilaterally symmetric alopecia over the flanks and trunk has been seen in guinea pigs with cystic ovaries (Fig. 21-17).[4, 10, 17] Affected females usually present with progressive enlargement of the abdomen, and ovarian cysts may be palpable as discrete, large, rounded masses in the dorsal middle abdomen. Ultrasonographic examination may be diagnostic.[10] Ovariohysterectomy is curative.

Sebaceous glands are especially abundant around the anus, in the folds of the perianal and genital regions, and in the dorsal sacral skin, especially in sexually mature male animals.[6, 10, 17] Excessive accumulations of sebaceous debris, and occasionally bedding material and feces, may become entrapped in these folds or mat down the dorsal sacral

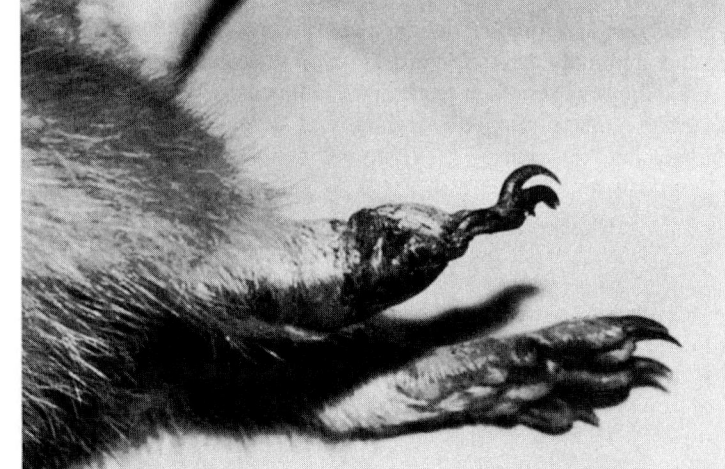

FIGURE 21-15. Necrosis and slough of the hindfoot of a guinea pig caused by a constricting band. (Courtesy of G. Kollias.)

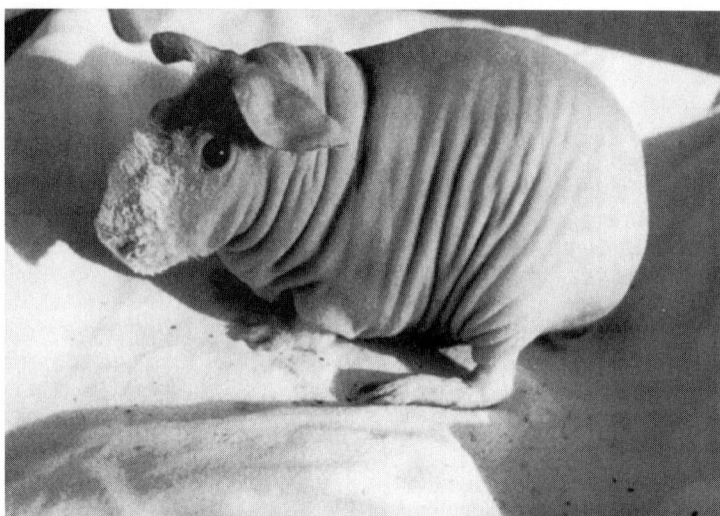

FIGURE 21-16. Congenital alopecia in a guinea pig. (Courtesy of J. Gourreau.)

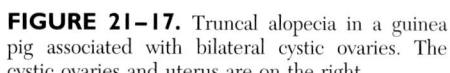

FIGURE 21-17. Truncal alopecia in a guinea pig associated with bilateral cystic ovaries. The cystic ovaries and uterus are on the right.

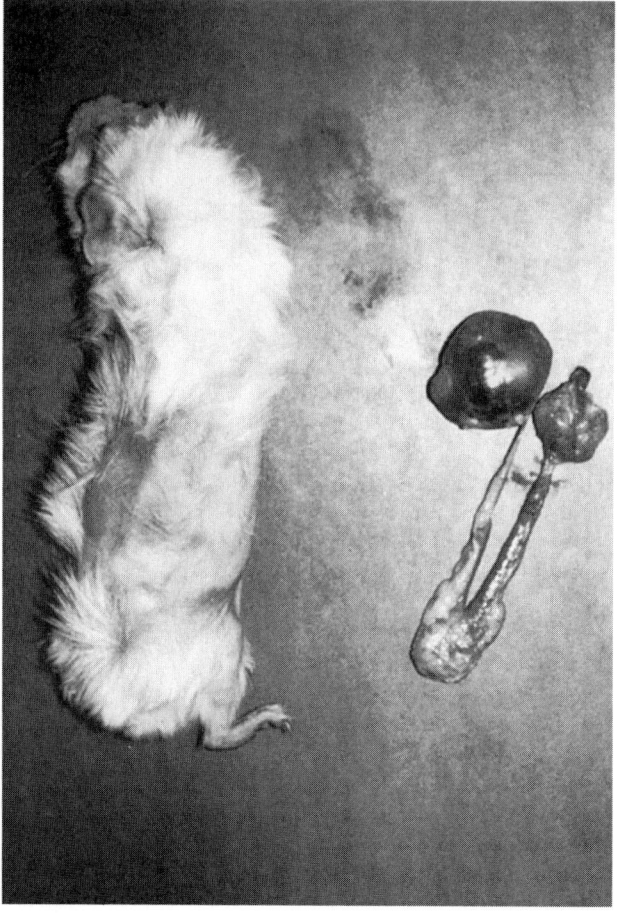

haircoat. Intertrigo, secondary bacterial infections, and unpleasant odors may intervene in this situation. These areas should be cleaned as needed with 3% hydrogen peroxide, 0.5% chlorhexidine, or a mild astringent (aluminum subacetate) to prevent the aforementioned sequelae.

Heavy guinea pigs, especially those maintained in wire-bottom cages, frequently develop hyperkeratosis and cutaneous horns of the footpads.[6, 17] These horny growths are most commonly observed on the ventral aspect of the front paws. They can be removed with scissors and an emery file. Replacement of cage surfaces with smoother materials retards or prevents further hyperkeratoses.

Overgrown claws are a frequent problem in pet guinea pigs.[3, 17] Frequent examination and trimming prevents traumatic and infectious complications.

Neoplasia

The skin is the second most common site of neoplasia in the guinea pig.[2, 3, 6, 8, 17] The most common cutaneous neoplasm is the trichofolliculoma.[17] This tumor is most commonly encountered as a benign, solitary lesion over the dorsal lumbar area (see Fig. 21–12E). The overlying skin is usually alopecic and crusted. Frequently, a central pore is seen, through which keratinous material or dark, hemorrhagic exudate is discharged. Other cutaneous neoplasms reported in guinea pigs include sebaceous adenoma, fibroma, fibrosarcoma, lipoma, liposarcoma, schwannoma, and lymphoma.[2, 17]

● HAMSTER

Bacterial Infections

Bacterial skin infections are uncommonly reported in hamsters. *S. aureus* and *Pasteurella pneumotropica* have been recovered from isolated cases of skin abscesses and bite wounds.[6, 8] Hamsters are prone to periodontal disease and dental caries, and any facial abscess located ventral or cranial to the eye may be a tooth root abscess.[10] Treatment of bacterial dermatitis includes elimination of predisposing causes, surgical drainage, daily topical cleaning with 3% hydrogen peroxide or 0.5% chlorhexidine, and occasionally systemic antibiotic administration (see Table 21–1).

Experimentally, the hamster is susceptible to infection with *Treponema pallidum* subsp. *endemicum,* the agent of endemic syphilis of humans.[56] Intradermal injection of the spirochete results in erythematous papules and ulcers, which eventually heal but are followed by perioral ulcers and an erythematous maculopapular rash on the paws and the trunk and death. This form of hamster syphilis has been proposed as a useful model for the study of the immune response, antibiotic therapy, and vaccination techniques in human venereal and congenital syphilis.

Fungal Infections

Dermatophytosis is rare in hamsters and is caused by *T. mentagrophytes*.[2, 3, 6, 8, 16–19] Diagnosis is confirmed by microscopic examination of affected hairs and fungal culture. Treatment is as described for the other rodents.

Ectoparasites

Demodicosis is the most common ectoparasitism of the hamster.[10, 17] *Demodex criceti* and *D. aurati* are both normal residents of hamster skin.[17] *D. aurati* is long and tapered (average, 180 μm long) and inhabits hair follicles, whereas *D. criceti* is short and stubby (average, 90 μm long) and inhabits the keratin and pits of the epidermal surface. Clinical demodicosis is seen in aged hamsters, is usually associated with *D. aurati,* and is usually associated with conditions that suppress immune responses (e.g., malnutrition, concurrent disease, cancer, and exposure to carcinogens).[6, 8, 17, 19] Lesions are most commonly seen over the dorsal lumbosacral area but may be generalized (Fig. 21–18). Moderate to severe alopecia is accompanied by variable degrees of scaling, erythema, and small hemorrhagic crusts. Pruritus is usually absent. Diagnosis is confirmed by skin scrapings. Treatment of demodicosis in hamsters has not been extensively evaluated or reported. The authors and others [4, 19] were successful with 250 ppm of amitraz applied as a whole-body dip once weekly until 4 weeks after skin scrapings are negative.

Notoedric mange is rarely reported in hamsters.[8, 17, 19] Lesions are characterized by thick yellowish crusts, erythema, and alopecia on the pinnae, the muzzle, the tail, the genitalia, and the paws. Pruritus is severe, and self-mutilation can be extreme. Diagnosis is confirmed by finding *Notoedres* sp. mites in skin scrapings. Treatment with 2% lime sulfur dips (whole-body application weekly until two treatments after clinical cure) or ivermectin injections is effective.

S. scabiei, *T. caviae*, and *Ornithonyssus bacoti* are reported to be rare causes of pruritus and dermatitis in hamsters.[17] Clinical signs, diagnosis, and treatment are the same as that described for notoedric mange.

Fleas *(C. felis felis)* are rarely encountered on hamsters.[6] Treatment is the same as that described for cats.

Traumatic Alopecia and Dermatitis

Female hamsters are generally more aggressive than are males.[6, 17] Aggressive behavior in male hamsters is testosterone dependent and is markedly reduced by castration.[6, 17] The establishment of social dominance among male hamsters is positively correlated with the weight, size, and degree of pigmentation of the flank glands.[17] Aggression-related bite wounds are most commonly seen around the head, the tail, and the perineal area. Aggression can produce severe wounding, such as the complete removal of the flank glands of the victim.[17]

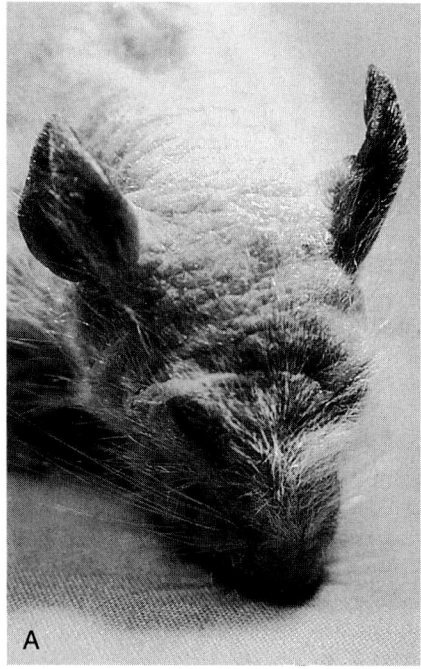

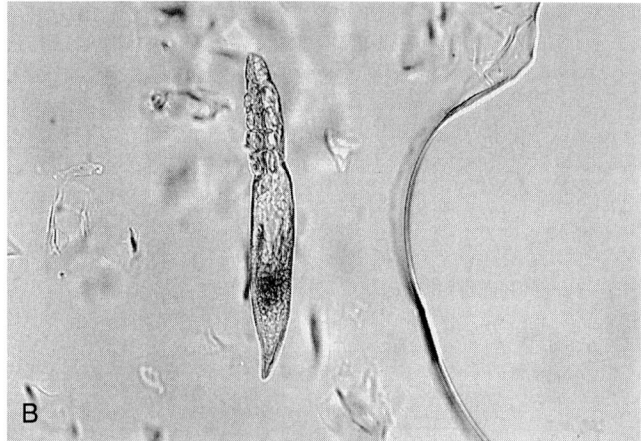

FIGURE 21–18. Demodicosis in a hamster. A, Alopecia, scaling, erythema, and lichenification on the head and neck. (Courtesy of G. Kollias.) B, *Demodex aurati* in skin scraping.

Nutritional Disorders

Nutritional deficiencies are unlikely to be seen in pet hamsters. However, one author[9] indicates that hair loss in hamsters is associated most often with continuous feeding of low protein (less than 16%) feed, such as is commonly found in pet stores. Experimental production of nutritional deficiencies with resultant cutaneous abnormalities have been reported and are briefly mentioned here. Pantothenic acid deficiency produces exfoliative dermatitis, depigmentation of the haircoat, and the accumulation of porphyrin-rich secretions around the nose, the mouth, and the eyes.[2, 17] Riboflavin deficiency produces alopecia, scaling, and dermatitis, which are most evident on the extremities.[2, 17] Pyridoxine deficiency results in generalized alopecia and depigmentation of the haircoat.[2, 17] Niacin deficiency produces a generalized alopecia.[2, 17] Fatty acid deficiency results in generalized alopecia, scaling, and the production of profuse amounts of cerumen.[2, 17] Copper deficiency results in alopecia and depigmentation.[2]

Miscellaneous Conditions

Foreign body granulomas associated with bedding consisting of wood shavings and sawdust were reported on the paws and the shoulders of hamsters.[17] The problem was eliminated by using shredded paper as bedding.

Swelling and pruritus of the face and the paws has been reported in several hamsters.[3] In all instances, owners had recently purchased a fresh bag of cedar or pine shavings produced by a leading pet company or bulk shavings from landscaping or nursery outlets. When affected animals were housed on plain newspaper, the lesions spontaneously regressed. Presumably, the shavings had been treated with some chemical that produced a contact dermatitis.

Hereditary hairlessness has been reported in hamsters.[17]

Hyperadrenocorticism is rarely reported in hamsters.[6, 54] Clinical signs include bilaterally symmetric alopecia, hyperpigmentation, and thinning of the skin. The baseline plasma cortisol value in one affected hamster was elevated (approximately twofold increase) compared with that in one normal hamster. One hamster was treated with metyrapone (8 mg orally q24h for 1 month), and hair regrowth was complete after 12 weeks. A second hamster was treated with o,p'-DDD (5 mg orally q24h for 1 month), then metyrapone as described previously, and responded to neither drug. This hamster was euthanized, and a chromophobe adenoma of the hypophysis and bilateral adrenocortical hyperplasia were found at necropsy.

The flank scent glands of the hamster can become inflamed from being rubbed against wood chips or other abrasive cage equipment.[4] In addition, impaction of these glands can lead to self-mutilation.[4]

Ringtail is occasionally seen in the hamster (see Rat in this chapter).[2, 17]

Neoplasia

Skin neoplasms are rare in hamsters.[2, 6, 8, 17] The most frequently reported cutaneous neoplasms are melanomas and melanocytomas.[2, 6, 17] These tumors occur much more frequently in male hamsters and most commonly on the back, the head, the neck, and the flank gland.

Epitheliotropic lymphoma (mycosis fungoides) is the second most common cutaneous neoplasm of the hamster.[6, 17, 55] Affected animals have an exfoliative erythroderma (see Fig. 21–12F), which is generally pruritic, and go on to manifest peripheral lymphadenopathy, lethargy, anorexia, emaciation, and death. Some animals also have cutaneous plaques and nodules (Fig. 21–19), which may become ulcerated and crusted. Light and electron microscopic examinations demonstrated an epitheliotropic lymphoma in which many cells show the typical features of Sézary cells.[55] Immunohistochemical studies showed that the neoplastic cells are T lymphocytes.[55] Therapeutic trials have not been reported.

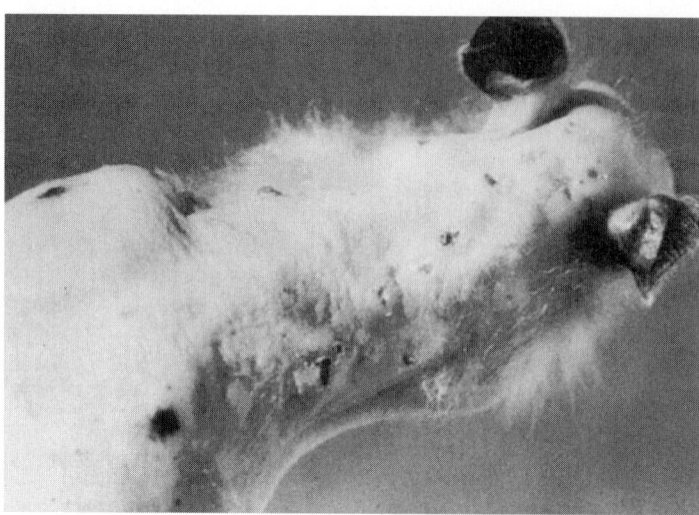

FIGURE 21–19. Epitheliotropic lymphoma in a hamster. Generalized alopecia and multiple crusted nodules and plaques.

Other cutaneous neoplasms reported in hamsters include basal cell carcinoma, squamous cell carcinoma, keratoacanthoma, papilloma, epitrichial sweat gland adenoma, fibrosarcoma, and plasmacytoma.[2, 6, 17]

• MOUSE

Bacterial Infections

Bacterial skin infections are uncommon in pet mice, are usually caused by *S. aureus*, and are secondary to trauma (cage-related injuries and bite wounds) or self-inflicted (the pruritus associated with ectoparasites).[2, 7, 8, 17, 19] Infections resulting from cage-related injury are typically seen on the nose and the muzzle, whereas those associated with bite wounds typically occur around the head, the tail, the rump, and the perineal area. Staphylococcal infections may be superficial (alopecia, erythema, oozing, and crust) or deep (abscess, fistula, necrosis, and ulcer) and are usually nonpruritic. Submandibular and periorbital granulomas were associated with bacterial pseudomycetuna (botryomycosis) due to *S. aureus*.[72] Other bacteria occasionally isolated from cutaneous abscesses and pyogranulomas in mice include *Streptococcus* sp., *P. pneumotropica*, *Actinobacillus* sp., *Actinomyces* sp., and *Klebsiella*.[2, 8, 17] Treatment of bacterial dermatitis includes some combination of elimination of predisposing causes, surgical drainage, daily topical cleaning with 3% hydrogen peroxide or 0.5% to 1% chlorhexidine, and systemic antibiotic administration (see Table 21–1). Surgical excision may be the best treatment for abscesses.[7a]

S. moniliformis is a rare cause of epizootics of edema and cyanosis of the extremities.[2, 8, 17]

C. kutscheri (murium) is a rare cause of epizootics of furunculosis and cutaneous pyogranulomas, which may progress to necrosis and sloughing of extremities.[2, 8, 17]

The mouse has been used as an experimental model for staphylococcal scalded skin syndrome.[17, 62]

Mycobacterium chelonae infection caused nodular, granulomatous lesions on the tails of immunocompromised mice.[64a]

Fungal Infections

Dermatophytosis is uncommon in mice and is usually caused by *T. mentagrophytes*.[1-6, 13, 16-19] This dermatophyte can be isolated from the haircoat of up to 60% of clinically normal mice in pet shops and represents an important zoonosis. Lesions are most commonly seen on the face, the head, the tail, and the trunk and consist of annular areas of alopecia, broken hairs, scales, and variable degrees of erythema and crusting. Pruritus is usually minimal to absent. Diagnosis and treatment are the same as that described for guinea pigs.

Viral Infections

Mouse pox (infectious ectromelia) causes epizootics in research colonies but is rarely, if ever, seen in practice.[2, 3, 6-8, 17, 66] Skin lesions include a generalized papular dermatitis with eventual swelling, necrosis, ulceration, and even sloughing of digits, pinnae, and tail. Diagnosis is confirmed by skin biopsy, electron microscopic examination of crusts, viral isolation of the orthopoxvirus, and polymerase chain reaction.[17, 65]

Reovirus Type 3 infection of suckling mice causes severe illness and an oily haircoat.[2, 8, 17] Animals that survive past weaning experience alopecia.

Sialodacryoadenitis virus infection causes eye rubbing and scratching, periorbital swelling, and red tears (chromodacryorrhea).[2, 9, 17]

Ectoparasites

Myobia musculi is a mite commonly found on mice.[2-6, 8, 16-19] Some animals are asymptomatic carriers, whereas other animals show varying degrees of skin disease and pruritus. Severely inflammatory and pruritic forms of the infestation are associated with genetic susceptibility and mite-related hypersensitivity reactions.[17] Immature mice or those that are immunocompromised may be more susceptible to severe forms of the disease. Clinical signs may be mild and include patchy alopecia, slight erythema, and minor scaling on the head and the muzzle. Other mice may show intense pruritus and self-mutilation of the face, the head, the pinnae, the neck, and the shoulders (see Fig. 21–12G). Severely affected animals can become debilitated and die. Diagnosis is confirmed by skin scrapings (see Fig. 21–13E). The treatment of choice is subcutaneous injections of ivermectin.[3, 4, 17, 19, 71] Ivermectin administered topically or in drinking water is less effective.[59, 60, 67, 69]

Myocoptes musculinus is a mite commonly found on mice.[2-6, 8, 16-19] Some animals are asymptomatic carriers, whereas others manifest varying degrees of skin disease and pruritus. Lesions are most severe on the back and the ventrum. Unlike the case with *M. musculi* infestations, severe ulceration is not seen with *M. musculinus* infestations. Diagnosis is confirmed by skin scrapings (see Fig. 21–13F); however, the mites are often difficult to find. The treatment of choice is subcutaneous injections of ivermectin every 2 weeks until the animal is cured.[3, 4, 17, 19, 71] Ivermectin administered topically or in drinking water is less effective.[59, 60, 67] Other mites that are rarely found on mice include *Radfordia affinis, Psorergates simplex, O. bacoti, S. scabiei, N. muris,* and *Trichoecius romboutsi*.[2-6, 8, 9, 17, 19]

Fleas (especially *C. felis felis*) may be recovered from pet mice maintained in households frequented by dogs and cats.[2-6, 8, 17]

The sucking louse *Polyplax serrata* is occasionally found on pet mice.[2-6, 8, 9, 17, 19] Some animals may be asymptomatic carriers, but others manifest varying degrees of dermatitis and pruritus. Young animals, debilitated animals, and animals in poor management situations are more likely to be affected. Lice and related dermatoses are most commonly found on the neck and back. Treatment can be accomplished with topical insecticides or ivermectin injections.

Nutritional Disorders

Nutritional deficiencies are unlikely to be encountered in pet mice. Experimental production of nutritional deficiencies with resultant cutaneous abnormalities have been reported and are briefly mentioned here. Zinc deficiency produces exfoliative dermatitis, alopecia, and depigmentation of the haircoat.[2, 17] Pantothenic acid deficiency results in exfoliative dermatitis and depigmentation of the haircoat.[2, 17] Riboflavin deficiency produces alopecia, scaling, and dermatitis, especially on the extremities.[2, 17] Pyridoxine deficiency results in exfoliative dermatitis, especially on the face, the ears, the limbs, and the tail.[2, 17] Biotin deficiency causes exfoliative dermatitis.[2] Fatty acid deficiency produces an exfoliative dermatitis.[2, 17]

Miscellaneous Conditions

Male mice are aggressive.[2-6, 8, 17, 19] Barbering and bite wounds are frequently seen, especially on the muzzle, the whiskers, the face, the head, the rump, the tail, and the perineum. These behaviors can be exacerbated by crowding, stress, and boredom. Mice frequently rub the hair off the muzzle as they stick their face through slotted feeders or wire bars.

Mice develop numerous types of hereditary hairlessness and keratinization defects, which are probably never seen by the practitioner.[2, 8, 17, 68, 69] Some of these conditions have been used as laboratory models for the study of various aspects of cutaneous pathophysiology and pharmacology, such as ichthyosis, asebia, rhino, and blotchy (similar to the Menkes kinky hair syndrome in humans) and flaky skin (similar to psoriasis in humans).[17, 62, 63, 68, 73]

Ringtail is rarely reported in mice (see Rat in this chapter).[8, 17] Idiopathic dry gangrene of the pinna is sporadically seen in young mice.[8, 17] The incidence appears to increase when the mice are exposed to cold temperatures and when the ears are traumatized by excessive grooming in attempts to remove lice. The condition progresses rapidly from initial erythema of the distal one third of the pinna to necrosis and slough. Rarely, the distal one third of the tail is also involved.

Perianal pruritus is seen in association with pinworms (*Syphacia obvelata*).[2, 4, 8, 17, 19] Infected mice often mutilate the base of the tail. Diagnosis is confirmed by microscopic examination of strips of cellophane (Scotch) tape that have been applied to the perineum. The eggs of *S. obvelata* are banana shaped and about 30 μm by 150 μm. Treatment with ivermectin injections is curative.

A spontaneous *immune complex vasculitis* was reported to affect up to 21% of certain strains of aged mice.[58] Mice developed multiple crusts between the scapulae or on the dorsal neck. These lesions rapidly evolved into irregular ulcers and spread laterally and caudally on the body. Pruritus was intense. Histologic examination revealed leukocytoclastic vasculitis and IgG, IgM, and fibrinogen were demonstrated in dermal blood vessel walls.

Alopecia areata was reported in the C3H/HeJ mouse and proposed as a model of the human disease.[70]

Neoplasia

Although mice are sensitive to the induction of various skin neoplasms by the topical or systemic administration of chemical carcinogens or ultraviolet light exposure, spontaneous skin neoplasms are rare.[2, 3, 6, 8, 17] The most commonly reported cutaneous neoplasms are papilloma, squamous cell carcinoma, and fibrosarcoma.[17, 64] Other reported cutaneous neoplasms include hair follicle tumors, sebaceous gland tumors, mast cell tumors, hemangiomas, hemangiosarcomas, melanomas, lymphomas, and a solitary epitheliotropic lymphoma resembling pagetoid reticulosis in humans.[17, 57, 61]

● RABBIT

Bacterial Infections

Pasteurellosis (snuffles) is the most common bacterial disease of the rabbit.° Most rabbits carry *Pasteurella multocida* asymptomatically in the nasal cavity, and under conditions of

---

°See references 2–5, 8, 10, 11, 17, 77, 80, 81, 86, 92, 96.

stress, the bacteria multiply and cause disease. Subcutaneous abscesses develop as a result of septicemia, external wound contamination, or direct extension from deeper sties. The abscesses are variable in size, are usually firm on palpation, and are filled with a thick, white to tan exudate. Diagnosis is confirmed by microscopic examination of direct smears of exudate and culture. In the rabbit, subcutaneous abscesses are due to pasteurellosis until proven otherwise. Other causes of abscesses include *S. aureus, Fusobacterium, Pseudomonas aeruginosa, Streptococcus* sp., and *C. pyogenes.*° Abscesses on the head may be secondary to dental disease, a tooth root abscess, or an oral foreign body.[10]

Abscesses in rabbits are typically filled with thick, caseated pus and are surrounded by a thick capsule. These two attributes make the use of drainage, drains, and topical and systemic antibiotics unsuccessful in most cases.[7a, 10, 15] The treatment of choice is surgical excision and at least 2 weeks of antibiotic treatment (see Table 21–1).[10, 15, 81] If this is impossible, radical débridement, flushing, and antibiotics for several weeks may be effective.[7a] In some rabbits, abscesses continue to recur in the same spot or at some other sites in an apparently healthy individual.[10] Some of these rabbits may require lifetime antibiotic therapy to prevent recurrences.[10]

Necrobacillosis (Schmorl's disease) is a sporadic bacterial infection of rabbits caused by *Fusobacterium necrophorum.*† It is characterized by inflammation, necrosis, ulceration, and abscessation, especially on the face, the head, and the neck. Diagnosis is confirmed by culture. Treatment is accomplished with surgical debridement, topical antimicrobial applications, and systemic penicillin or tetracycline administration.

P. aeruginosa causes a *localized moist dermatitis (sore dewlap)* and, occasionally, subcutaneous abscess in areas of skin that are continuously wet.‡ The muzzle, the dewlap (see Fig. 21–12H), the flank, and the haunches are most commonly involved. The affected skin is moist, erythematous, edematous, alopecic, and often ulcerated. The fur is often clumped, creating a spiked appearance. The most striking clinical feature is the blue-green color of the fur in animals with white fur, which is caused by a water-soluble pigment (pyocyanin) produced by the bacteria. Diagnosis is confirmed by microscopic examination of direct smears from oozing areas and culture. Treatment includes clipping, gentle cleaning, and application of astringents (aluminum acetate) and topical gentamicin sulfate ointment. Prevention is directed at removing the cause of continued wetness of the fur. The most common cause is the constant drooling ("slobbers") associated with dental disease.[10] Leaking water valves or water bottles should be replaced. Water bowls or pans should be replaced by water bottles with sipper tubes. Malocclusion of the teeth should be corrected to prevent drooling. Wet bedding should be changed more frequently.

Ulcerative pododermatitis (sore hocks) is a common disorder in rabbits.§ Genetic predilection is important, as large body size and thinner plantar fur pads are important predisposing factors. Unsanitary cage conditions, rough cage surfaces, and obesity also contribute to pressure necrosis and secondary bacterial infection with *S. aureus*. Lesions commonly occur unilaterally or bilaterally on the plantar aspect of the metatarsal region or, less commonly, the volar surface of the metacarpal area. Focal inflammation, oozing, crusts, and alopecia progress to ulcers, hemorrhage, and abscesses. In severe infections, the disease may extend to the bony structures of the foot and result in septicemia. Treatment includes correction of predisposing conditions, surgical drainage, topical antimicrobial applications, and systemic antibiotic administration (see Table 21–1). Severe cases usually do not respond.

Venereal spirochetosis (treponematosis, rabbit syphilis, or vent disease) is uncommon.[2–6, 7a, 10, 17, 92, 96] *Treponema paraluis-cuniculi*, the causative spirochete, is transmitted by direct contact, especially mating. Cold environments appear to predispose to the disease. Because of the grooming, social, and sleeping habits of rabbits, lesions are

---

°See references 2, 6, 8, 11, 17, 82, 92, 96.
†See references 2, 3, 7, 8, 17, 92, 96.
‡See references 2–6, 8, 10, 17, 92, 96.
§See references 2–6, 8, 10, 11, 17, 92, 96.

frequently seen on the nose (Fig. 21–20A), the lips, the chin, the face, the eyelids, the ears, and the paws as well as the genitalia. Lesions consist of vesicles, papules, erythema, edema, oozing, erosions, and brownish crusts. Focal ulcers and hemorrhage may be seen. Diagnosis is confirmed by skin biopsies, the Venereal Disease Research Laboratory (VDRL) slide test, and the rapid plasma reagin (RPR) card test. Treatment with penicillin G benzathine or penicillin G procaine is curative (42,000 IU/kg, subcutaneously, once a week for three treatments). Tetracycline or chloramphenicol is also effective.[7a]

An outbreak of *S. aureus* infection in a rabbitry was associated with a pustular, exudative dermatitis in the young and mastitis in lactating does.[93] A cellulitis due to *S. aureus* infection is occasionally seen and is characterized by the acute onset of fever, and painful edematous swelling, especially over the head, neck, and thorax.[86] Necrosis and slough may occur.

Fungal Infections

Dermatophytosis is common in rabbits. *T. mentagrophytes* is the most common dermatophyte isolated, but *M. canis*, *M. gypseum*, *M. audouinii*, *T. verrucosum*, and *T. schoenleinii* have been reported.* *T. mentagrophytes* can be isolated from the haircoat and skin of approximately 36% of clinically normal rabbits, representing an important potential zoonosis. The disease is most common in young animals and where husbandry and management are suboptimal. Lesions are characterized by patchy alopecia, broken hairs, erythema, and yellowish crusting, and typically first appear on the bridge of the nose (see Fig. 21–20B), the eyelids, the pinnae, and the paws, and occasionally, on many body sites. The condition is usually pruritic. Diagnosis and treatment are the same as that described for the guinea pig. Griseofulvin is teratogenic, and should not be used in breeding does. A modified live *T. mentagrophytes* vaccine may prove useful in prophylaxis.[17]

Aspergillosis of the lungs and skin was reported in a whole litter of 4-week-old rabbits.[17] Multiple 1- to 2-mm papules were present all over the body. Histologically, the papules were cystic follicles distended with necrotic debris and dichotomously branching hyphae. *Aspergillus* sp. was isolated in culture. The animals were raised on moldy grass hay bedding material. A change in nesting materials prevented further occurrences.

Viral Infections

Myxomatosis is occasionally observed in domestic rabbits.† The myxoma virus (a poxvirus) is transmitted from reservoir wild rabbit hosts by mosquitoes. There are several strains of virus with variable virulence. In domestic rabbits, severe disease and high mortality are frequently produced. Affected rabbits are febrile, lethargic, and depressed. In the acute form of the disease, there is edema and erythema of the anus, the genitalia, the lips, the nares, and the eyelids. Less virulent strains of the virus produce numerous skin tumors (see Fig. 21–20C). Myxomatosis appeared in the depilated skin of Angora rabbits.[17] Lesions were a few millimeters to 3 cm in diameter, erythematous, and plaquelike, and became hemorrhagic and necrotic. Morbidity was low and mortality infrequent. Diagnosis is based on distinctive clinical signs, biopsy, and virus isolation. There is no effective treatment, and control of insect vectors and screening of enclosures are paramount in endemic areas. Heterologous vaccine may be useful.

Rabbit pox is infrequently reported in domestic rabbits.‡ The causative poxvirus is closely related to vaccinia virus. Initial clinical signs of profuse nasal discharge, depression, and fever are followed in 4 to 5 days by a generalized, erythematous, macular to papular to nodular eruption. The rabbits have extensive edema of the face and perineum. Diagnosis is confirmed by biopsy and virus isolation.

Shope fibroma virus and Shope papilloma virus are oncogenic (see Neoplasia).

---

*See references 2, 3, 6, 8, 10, 17, 92, 96.
†See references 2, 7, 8, 10, 11, 17, 92, 96.
‡See references 2, 7, 8, 10, 11, 17, 92, 96.

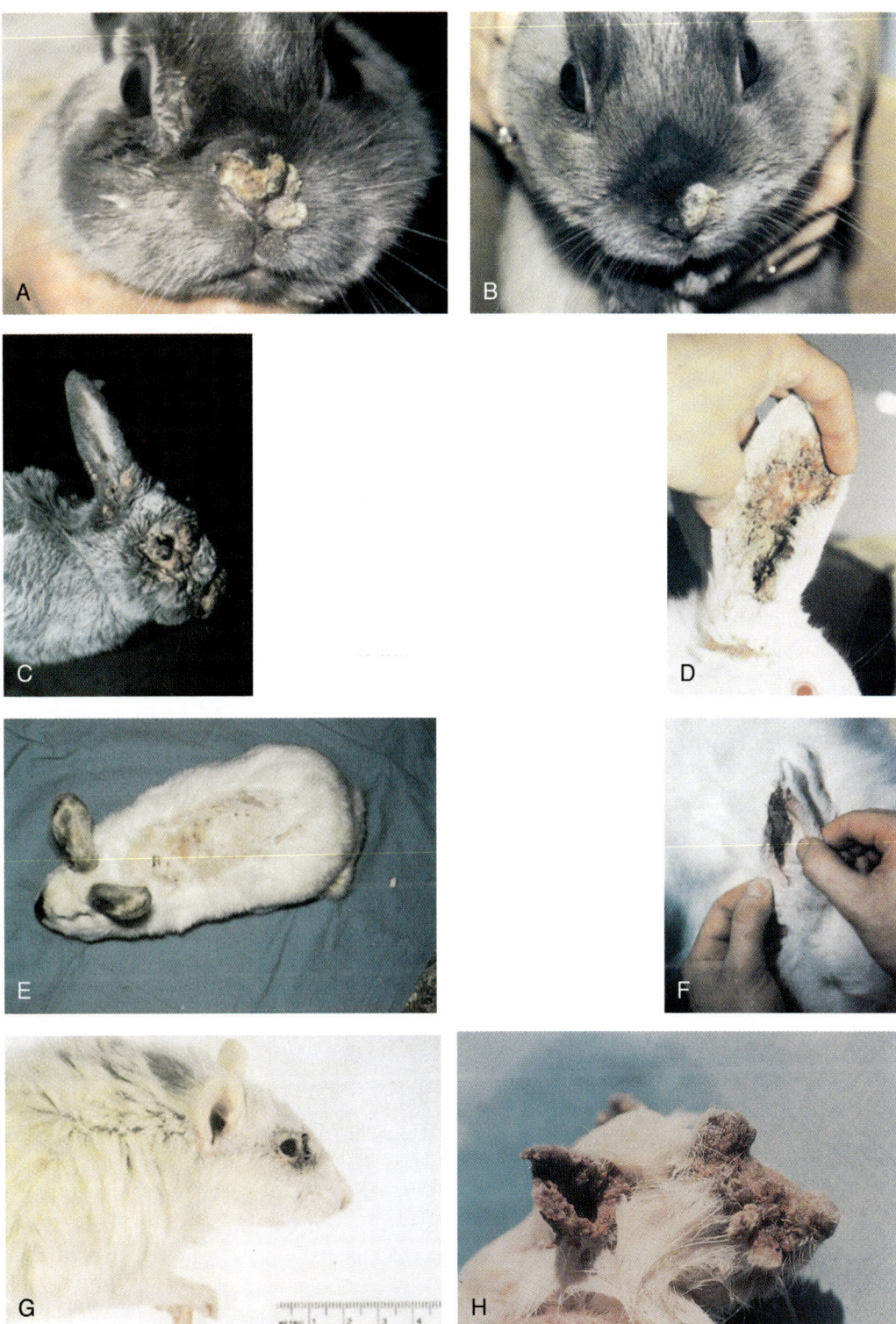

FIGURE 21-20. *A*, Crusts on the nose of a rabbit with spirochetosis. (Courtesy of G. Kollias.) *B*, Focal area of alopecia and crusting over the nose of a rabbit due to *T. mentagrophytes* infection. (Courtesy of G. Kollias.) *C*, Multiple erythematous nodules and plaques around the eye, on the pinna, and on the muzzle of a rabbit with myxomatosis. (Courtesy of G. Kollias.) *D*, Crusting and erythema of the lateral surface of the pinna of a rabbit with psoroptic mange. *E*, Crusts, scale, and focal ulcers over the dorsum of a rabbit with cheyletiellosis (area has been clipped). *F*, Frostbite in a rabbit. Note acrocyanosis and necrosis of the pinna. *G*, Orange-colored crust and discoloration of the hair around the eye of a rat with sialodacryoadenitis virus infection. (Courtesy of J. King.) *H*, *Trixacarus diversus* in a rat. Marked crusting and alopecia on the face and pinnae. (Courtesy of P. Bourdeau.)

Ectoparasites

Psoroptes cuniculi, a nonburrowing mite, is the most common ectoparasite of the rabbit, and all rabbits should be considered infected until proven otherwise.* Rabbits are also susceptible to *P. ovis* (cattle and sheep).[17] *P. cuniculi* is transmitted by direct contact with infected rabbits, fomites, and contaminated environment. Starving mites survive for approximately 21 days off the host over the usual range of temperatures (5 to 30°C [41 to 86°F]) and relative humidities (20% to 75%).[17] Crusts dislodged into the environment contain many mites. The mites pierce skin to feed, and hypersensitivity to mite-related antigens may be important in the pathogenesis of the dermatitis and pruritus.[17]

P. cuniculi typically produces otitis externa (otoacariasis, ear canker, and ear mites) (see Fig. 21–20D). Affected rabbits shake their heads and scratch at the head and ears. Alopecia, excoriations, and secondary bacterial infection may be present around the head, neck, and ventrum.[17, 79] In early stages, a dry, whitish gray to tan crusty exudate forms inside the vertical ear canal. Later, a dry, crusty material with a layered appearance accumulates in the ear and the lateral surface of the pinnae. A secondary bacterial infection may complicate the parasitic otitis externa, contributing to the foul odor and pain. Occasionally, mites may produce lesions on the face, the head, the neck, the limbs, the abdomen, and the back.[17, 83, 97]

Diagnosis is confirmed by finding the mites in ear swabs or skin scrapings (see Fig. 21–13G). In one report in which natural infections were studied and mite numbers were quantitated, affected animals harbored 40 to 100,000 mites per rabbit. The treatment of choice is the subcutaneous injection of ivermectin.[10, 17, 81, 95] Do *not* attempt to clean out the crusts and debris, because this causes pain and bleeding. The cage and environment should be sanitized, and reducing the relative humidity to less than 20% while increasing the temperature to 40°C (104°F) is of benefit in this regard.[17, 18] In one report,[97] an in-contact guinea pig also developed psoroptic mange.

S. scabiei var. *cuniculi*, a burrowing mite, is a rare ectoparasite on rabbits in North America but is commonly found in some other parts of the world, such as Africa and India.† Typical lesions include tan to yellow, often powdery crusts, alopecia, erythema, and excoriation on the muzzle, the lips, the bridge of the nose, the eyelids, the head, the margins of the pinna, the paws, and the external genitalia. Pruritus is intense. Severe infestations can lead to anorexia, lethargy, emaciation, and death. These mites can transiently produce lesions in humans. Diagnosis is confirmed by finding *S. scabiei* mites in skin scrapings. However, mites are often difficult to demonstrate, and response to therapy is a frequently used diagnostic test. The treatment of choice is ivermectin.[6, 17, 19, 90]

Cheyletiella parasitovorax, a nonburrowing mite, is a common ectoparasite on rabbits.[2-6, 8, 10, 16-19] Most rabbits harbor the mites without overt signs of skin disease. With heavy infestations or in hypersensitive hosts, a variably pruritic dermatosis is seen. Lesions consist of scaling, crusting, and variable degrees of erythema, alopecia, and greasiness over the withers, the back (see Fig. 21–20E), and the ventral abdomen. Occasionally, lesions are limited to the face. These mites can produce skin lesions in humans. Diagnosis is confirmed by finding *C. parasitovorax* in skin scrapings or acetate tape preparations. The treatment of choice is ivermectin.

Listrophorus (Leporacarus) gibbus is a common fur mite of rabbits, which is rarely associated with clinical skin disease.[2-6, 8, 10, 16-19, 86a, 93a] Most affected rabbits are asymptomatic. The mite is usually found attached to hair shafts, especially on the back, the groin, and the ventral abdomen. Occasional rabbits may manifest a variably pruritic, scaly, erythematous, alopecic dermatitis in the aforementioned sites. Some animals only manifest pruritus and traumatic alopecia with no skin lesions. Diagnosis is confirmed by finding *L. gibbus* in skin scrapings and acetate tape preparations (see Fig. 21–13H). Treatment with pyrethrin- or pyrethroid-containing flea powders, 1% selenium sulfide baths, or 2% lime

---

*See references 2–6, 8, 10, 11, 16–19, 77, 81, 86, 92, 96.
†See references 2–6, 8, 10, 11, 16–19, 74, 75, 90, 92, 96.

sulfur dips is curative.[17, 86a, 93a] Ivermectin may also be effective.[10] Fipronil spray was reported to be effective.[91] One author reported treating over 50 rabbits with fipronil spray (3 ml/kg) with no adverse effects.[79] However, the therapeutic index for this product is fairly narrow in rabbits, possibly due to the isopropyl alcohol content.[91] Company representatives received a number of reports of suspected adverse reactions to fipronil spray in rabbits, and recommended that the product *not* be used in this species.[78]

Notoedres cati, a burrowing mite, is a rare ectoparasite on rabbits in North America, but is commonly found in other parts of the world, such as India.° Clinical signs, diagnosis, and treatment are identical to those described for *S. scabiei*.

Fleas (especially *C. felis felis*) are occasionally found on rabbits, especially those in households with dogs and cats.[2–6, 8, 10, 16–19, 85a] In the United States, rabbits may also be infested with *Cediopsylla simplex* (common Eastern rabbit flea), especially around the head and the neck, and *Odontopsyllus multispinosis* (giant Eastern rabbit flea), especially over the rump. Clinical signs, diagnosis, and therapy are the same as that described for cats.

The rabbit sucking louse *Haemodipsus ventricosus* is uncommon in the United States.[2–5, 7, 9, 15–19] Pediculosis is usually associated with poor management. Lice are most commonly found on the dorsum and may produce intense pruritus. Severe infestations in debilitated animals may produce anemia, weakness, emaciation, and death. *H. ventricosus* is a vector of tularemia. Therapy is the same as that described for cats.

Demodex cuniculi mites have been isolated from rabbits with generalized pruritus and scaling, but their pathogenic significance is in doubt.[17]

Members of the fly genus *Cuterebra* occasionally produce myiasis in domestic rabbits reared outdoors or in nonscreened enclosures.† Among those fly species reported in the United States are *Cuterebra cuniculi*, *C. buccata*, and *C. horripilum*. Larvae and, therefore, lesions appear in the summer and early fall. The incidence of infestation decreases with age, which correlates with the development of immediate and delayed-type hypersensitivity reactions to larval antigens. *C. horripilum* prefers the ventral cervical region, whereas *C. buccata* larvae localize in the interscapular, axillary, inguinal, or rump area. Initial lesions include subcutaneous cystlike structures. As the larvae (warbles) enlarge, a "breathing hole," or fistula, is produced. The surrounding haircoat is moist and matted, secondary bacterial infection is common, and the lesions are often painful. Treatment consists of surgical removal of the larvae (one should not crush or otherwise damage the larvae), routine wound care, and occasionally, administration of systemic antibiotics. Prevention and control are aimed at eliminating contact with the warble fly.

Flystrike (maggots) is most commonly seen in the perineal region, and may spread dorsally onto the rump.[10] Moist dermatitis and fur matting are present. Rabbits that are sedentary, overweight, or that have perineal dermatitis (urine scald) may be predisposed. Treatment includes cleansing and one injection of ivermectin.[10]

Nutritional Disorders

Nutritional deficiencies are unlikely to be encountered in pet rabbits. Experimental production of nutritional deficiencies with resultant cutaneous abnormalities have been reported and are briefly presented here. Copper deficiency results in alopecia and a depigmented haircoat.[2, 17] Zinc deficiency produces alopecia, scaling, and a depigmented haircoat.[2, 17]

Miscellaneous Conditions

Several days before parturition, the female rabbit undergoes a generalized loosening of the fur.[2, 3, 6, 8, 10, 17] The female rabbit pulls out mouthfuls of hair to line the nest. Hair loss

---

°See references 2–6, 8, 10, 16–19, 87, 88.
†See references 2–6, 8, 10, 16–19, 92, 96.

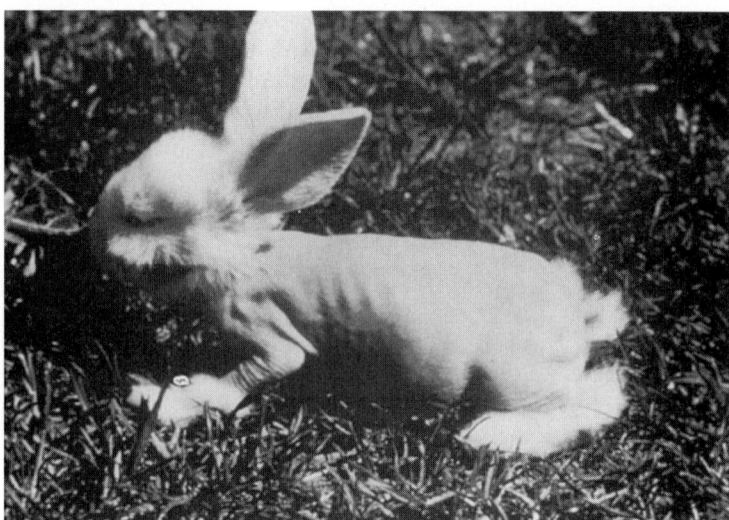

FIGURE 21–21. Congenital alopecia in a rabbit. (Courtesy of J. Gourreau.)

is especially prominent on the abdomen, chest, forelegs, and hips. Some rabbits pull out fur as a behavioral vice.[2, 8] Other rabbits rub fur off against the cage surface or feeders.[8] Does in heat and rabbits on low-fiber diets may barber their own hair.[10] The barbered rabbit typically has patches of broken-off hairs over the head and back.[10] Seasonal molts can result in haircoat irregularities and thinning.[8]

Compulsive self-mutilating behavior was encountered in 5% to 10% of the rabbits in a colony of Checkered crosses.[85] Extensive automutilation of digits and pads of the front feet was observed. The behavior could be interrupted by giving the rabbits haloperidol (0.2 mg/kg IM q12h), a dopamine antagonist. Because the condition was never seen in animals of other breeding lines kept in the same building under identical conditions, and the affected animals came from highly inbred stock, it was hypothesized that the disorder was genetically determined.

Hereditary alopecias (Fig. 21–21) are rarely described in rabbits[17] but are unlikely to be seen by practitioners.

Cutaneous asthenia has been reported in rabbits (Fig. 21–22).[17, 76, 94] The animals had a history of skin fragility and repeated spontaneous skin tears, and were covered with scars. The skin extensibility index (see Chap. 12) in two rabbits was 21% to 32% in the affected rabbits as compared with a mean of 13% in normal rabbits. Light microscopic examination was unremarkable, but electron microscopic examination revealed distorted and tangled collagen bundles with collagen fibrils being of different diameters and having a loose, frayed appearance.

Hutch burn is a contact dermatitis caused by urine scalding of the perineal region because of an unclean environment or an inability of the rabbit to void urine without soiling itself, such as after an orthopedic or neurologic injury, or with obesity.[3, 10] Washing the area frequently with antimicrobial agents and applying a protectant cream, such as zinc oxide, are helpful.

Frostbite may be seen in rabbits that are suddenly exposed to cold climates without a period of acclimatization.[17] Erythema, acrocyanosis, necrosis, and sloughing are typically seen on the pinna (see Fig. 21–20F).

Both male and female rabbits possess two sebaceous scent glands on either side of the vulvar or testicular area that secrete a brown waxy debris.[3] This secretion can build up and can be easily removed by gentle traction or soap and water.

The authors have seen a condition resembling *alopecia areata* in rabbits. Affected animals presented with one or more areas of noninflammatory annular alopecia, especially

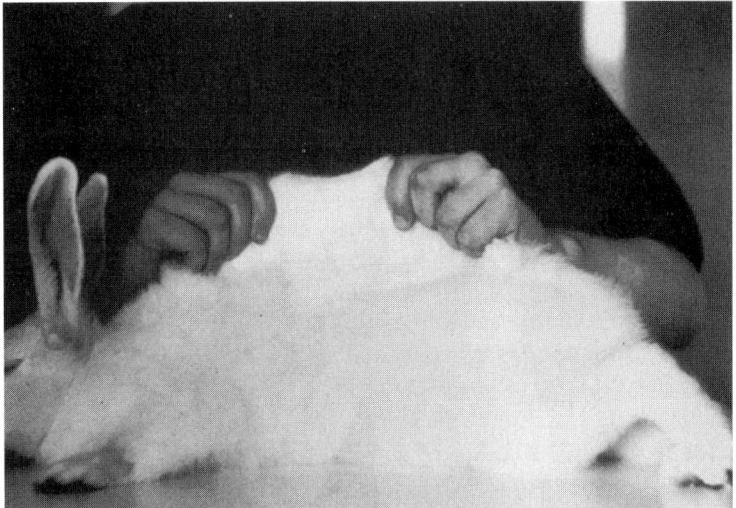

FIGURE 21–22. Hyperextensibility of the skin in a rabbit with cutaneous asthenia. (Courtesy of R. Harvey.)

on the black-furred areas of the pinnae. Spontaneous recovery was accompanied by the regrowth of white fur (Fig. 21–23).

Sebaceous adenitis was reported in domestic rabbits.[89, 96a] The animals varied from 2½ to 6 years of age. Lesions began around the neck or face, remained localized for several months, then became generalized. All rabbits eventually had a generalized, nonpruritic exfoliative dermatosis with patchy to coalescing areas of alopecia. Skin biopsies were diagnostic. No response was seen to antibiotics, glucocorticoids, ivermectin, griseofulvin, fatty acids, azathioprine, or oral retinoids.

Facial eczema has been reported in young suckling rabbits.[11] The condition is sporadic and of unknown etiology. Areas of alopecia and slight erythema occur on the bridge of the nose and the periocular region. Affected animals are otherwise healthy. The condition responds rapidly to topical glucocorticoid therapy.

Neoplasia

Spontaneous nonviral cutaneous neoplasms are rare in rabbits.[*] Papilloma, basal cell carcinoma, squamous cell carcinoma, sebaceous carcinoma, melanoma, osteosarcoma, and lymphoma have been reported.

Shope papillomas are uncommon in domestic rabbits.[†] In the United States, the disease occurs in the Southwest and along the Mississippi River. Shope papilloma virus (a papovavirus) commonly infects wild rabbits, with insects serving as vectors. Lesions are characterized by multiple hornlike growths from a single site, especially about the eyelids and the pinnae. Removal of the papillomas usually results in healing, and recovered rabbits are resistant to reinfection. Spontaneous regression of lesions occurs within 12 months. Experimental infection of domestic rabbits resulted in malignant transformation to squamous cell carcinoma within 8 to 9 months in a high percentage of the inoculation sites. A program of screening animal enclosures and vector control should be instituted in endemic areas.

Shope fibromas are uncommon in domestic rabbits.[‡] Shope fibroma virus (a poxvirus) commonly infects wild rabbits in North and South America and is transmitted via insect vectors. Lesions consist of single or multiple flat, firm, subcutaneous nodules, especially on

---

*See references 2–6, 8, 10, 16–19, 84, 92, 96.
†See references 2, 3, 6, 8, 10, 17, 92, 96.
‡See references 2, 3, 6, 8, 17, 92, 96.

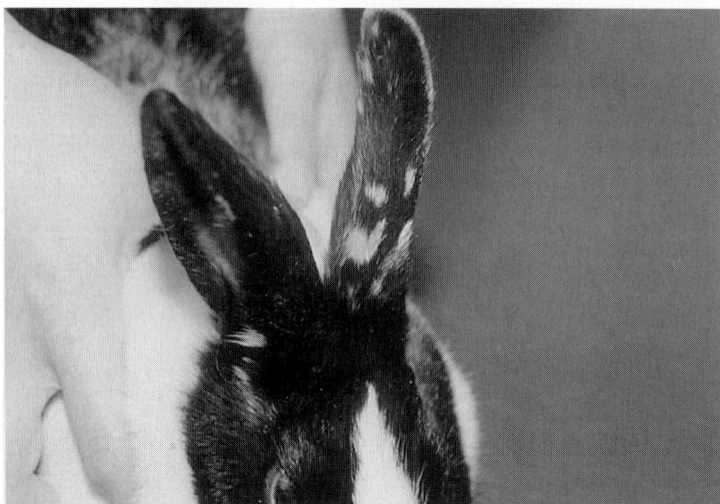

FIGURE 21–23. Alopecia areata–like condition in a rabbit. Well-circumscribed areas of noninflammatory alopecia on the pinna are regrowing white hair.

the genitals, the perineum, the ventral abdomen, the paw, the nose, the pinna, and the eyelid. Newborn rabbits are more susceptible than are older animals and have more extensive lesions. Experimentally infected adult rabbits often show spontaneous involution of their fibromas within 5 months through necrosis and sloughing. Mosquito eradication and enclosure screening is indicated to prevent infection in endemic areas.

Cutaneous lymphoma was reported in domestic rabbits from 7 weeks to 9 1/2 years old.[96b] Most had early internal organ involvement and systemic disease. Lesions consisted of multifocal areas of alopecia, scale, erythema, and plaques. Histologically, the lymphomas were epitheliotropic and CD3+. One rabbit was unsuccessfully treated with oral isotretinoin and interferon-α.

• RAT

Bacterial Infections

Bacterial skin infections are uncommon in pet rats, are usually caused by *S. aureus,* and are secondary to trauma (cage-related injuries and bite wounds) or self-inflicted (the pruritus associated with ectoparasites).[2–8, 10, 16–19] Rats are more resistant to experimental wound infection with *S. aureus* than are mice or hamsters.[17] Infections resulting from cage-related injury are typically seen on the nose and the muzzle, whereas those associated with bite wounds typically occur around the head, the tail, the rump, and the perineal area. Staphylococcal dermatitis may be superficial (alopecia, erythema, oozing, and crust) or deep (abscess, fistula, necrosis, and ulcer) and is usually nonpruritic. Granulomas occurred on the trunk and mammary gland in association with infection by an atypical slow-growing *S. aureus*.[100] Other bacteria occasionally isolated from cutaneous abscesses and pyogranulomas in rats include *Streptococcus* sp., *P. pneumotropica, Klebsiella pneumoniae, P. aeruginosa,* and *Mycobacterium lepraemurium* (rat leprosy).[2, 8, 16–19]

Treatment of bacterial dermatitis includes some combination of elimination of predisposing causes, surgical drainage, daily topical cleaning with 3% hydrogen peroxide or 0.5% to 1% chlorhexidine, and systemic antibiotic administration (see Table 21–1).

S. moniliformis is a rare cause of epizootics of edema and cyanosis of the extremities.[2, 8, 17]

C. kutscheri (murium) is a rare cause of epizootics of furunculosis and cutaneous pyogranulomas, which may progress to necrosis and sloughing of extremities.[2, 8]

Fungal Infections

Dermatophytosis is rare in rats and is usually associated with *T. mentagrophytes*.[1-6, 8, 10, 16-19] This dermatophyte can be isolated from the haircoat of clinically normal rats and is a potential zoonotic agent. Lesions are most commonly seen on the neck, the back, and the base of the tail and consist of annular areas of alopecia, broken hairs, scales, and variable degrees of erythema and crusting. Pruritus is usually minimal to absent. Diagnosis and treatment are as described for guinea pigs.

Viral Infections

Sialodacryoadenitis virus (a coronavirus) infection causes eye rubbing and scratching, periorbital swelling, and red tears (chromodacryorrhea) (see Fig. 21–20G).[2, 4, 17]

Poxvirus infection has been described in laboratory white rats.[17] Skin lesions consisted of erythematous papules, which became crusted and occurred mainly on the glabrous areas of the body (tail, paws, and muzzle). Sometimes, the affected portions of paws and tail underwent necrosis and sloughing. Diagnosis was confirmed by biopsy, electron microscopy, and viral isolation.

Ectoparasites

N. muris occasionally causes a severely pruritic dermatitis in rats.[2-6, 8, 10, 16-19] Lesions are most commonly present on the pinnae, the nose, the paws, and the ventrum and consist of erythema, papules, yellowish hyperkeratotic crusts, and excoriations. Diagnosis is confirmed by skin scrapings. Treatment is accomplished with topical 2% lime sulfur dips (once weekly until 2 weeks after cure) or subcutaneous injections of ivermectin.

Other mites that are rarely found on rats include *Radfordia ensifera*, *O. bacoti* (tropical rat mite), *S. scabiei*, *Trixacarus diversus* (Fig. 21–20H), *T. caviae*, *M. musculi*, and *Demodex* sp.*

Fleas (especially *C. felis felis*) may be recovered from pet rats maintained in households frequented by cats and dogs.[2-6, 8, 17]

The sucking louse *Polyplax spinulosa* is occasionally found on pet rats.† Some animals may be asymptomatic carriers, and other animals manifest varying degrees of dermatitis and pruritus. Young animals, debilitated animals, and animals in poor management situations are more likely to be affected. Lice and related dermatoses are most commonly found on the neck and back. Treatment can be accomplished with topical insecticides or ivermectin injections.

Nutritional Disorders

Nutritional deficiencies are unlikely to be encountered in pet rats. Experimental production of nutritional deficiencies with resultant cutaneous abnormalities has been reported, and these are briefly mentioned here. Zinc deficiency produces exfoliative dermatitis, alopecia, and depigmentation of the haircoat.[2, 17] Pantothenic acid deficiency results in exfoliative dermatitis, depigmentation of the haircoat, and excessive harderian gland activity with increased porphyrin secretion resulting in red tears and blood-caked whiskers.[2, 17] Riboflavin deficiency produces alopecia, scaling, and dermatitis, especially on the extremities.[2] Pyridoxine deficiency results in exfoliative dermatitis, especially on the face, the ears, the limbs, and the tail.[2, 17] Biotin deficiency causes exfoliative dermatitis and periocular alopecia.[2, 17] Niacin deficiency causes alopecia and excessive harderian gland activity, increased porphyrin secretion, and blood-caked whiskers.[2, 17] Essential fatty acid deficiency

---

*See references 2, 3, 6, 8, 10, 16–19, 99, 101.
†See references 2, 3, 7, 8, 10, 16–19.

produces an exfoliative dermatitis and, occasionally, necrosis of the tail.[2, 17] Protein deficiency causes alopecia, exfoliative dermatitis, and depigmentation of the haircoat.[2, 17]

Miscellaneous Conditions

Barbering and bite wounds are frequently seen when rats are housed together.[2-6, 8, 17] These behaviors can be exacerbated by crowding, stress, and boredom. Areas most commonly affected include the muzzle, the whiskers, the face, the head, the rump, the tail, and the perineum. Rats may also rub the hair off the muzzle as they stick their face through slotted feeders or wire bars.[17]

Rats have numerous types of hereditary hairlessness that are probably never seen by the practitioner (Fig. 21–24).[17]

Ringtail is a poorly understood condition seen in rats.[2-8, 17] The incidence of the disorder increases as the relative humidity falls below 40% and is especially common in young unweaned animals housed in cages with wire mesh bottoms, on hygroscopic bedding, and in rooms with excessive ventilation. In the northern hemisphere, most cases are seen from November to May, when heating systems often cause marked reductions in relative humidity. Some strains of rats seem more susceptible than others. The condition usually occurs after 2 months of reduced relative humidity. One or more annular constrictions develop in the tail, which becomes edematous, inflamed, and necrosed distal to the constrictions (Fig. 21–25). Ringtail is prevented by maintaining a relative humidity of at least 50%.

Perianal pruritus is seen in association with pinworms (*Syphacia muris*).[2, 4, 8, 17] Infected rats occasionally mutilate the base of the tail. Diagnosis is confirmed by microscopic examination of strips of cellophane (Scotch) tape that have been applied to the perineum. The eggs of *S. muris* are banana shaped and about 30 μm by 150 μm. Ivermectin is effective treatment.

Auricular chondritis has been described in rats.[17] The condition has occurred spontaneously and in association with the placement of metal ear tags or immunization with type II collagen. Typically, both ears are affected, although one ear may be affected days to weeks before the other. The pinnae are swollen, erythematous, and nodular, and they become thickened and deformed. Pain and pruritus are rare. Histologically, there is a multifocal granulomatous chondritis with progressive destruction of cartilage.

Systemic hair embolism has been reported subsequent to intravenous injections in rats.[17] Cutaneous lesions consist of focal areas of necrosis and ulceration on the ventral

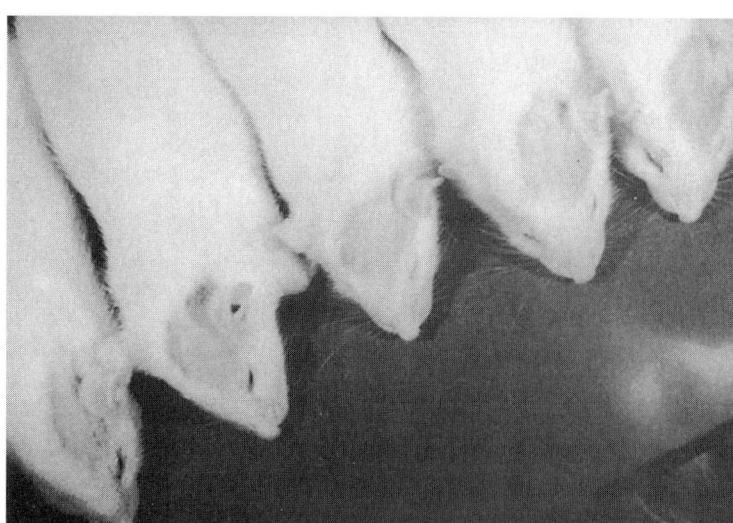

FIGURE 21–24. Congenital alopecia in a litter of rats. (Courtesy of J. King.)

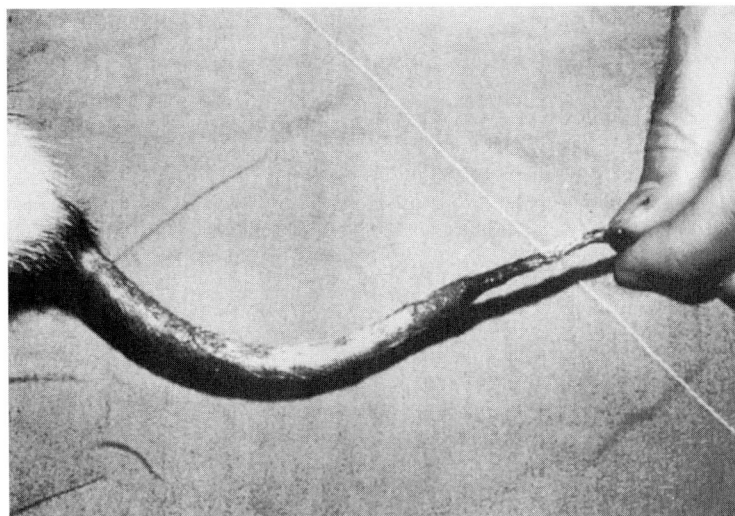

FIGURE 21-25. Ringtail in a rat. Necrosis of the distal portion of the tail. (Courtesy of G. Kollias.)

aspect of the body. Histologic examination reveals granulomatous and necrotizing dermatitis and panniculitis, and intravascular hair shaft fragments.

The fur of the aged rat frequently turns yellow and becomes more coarse.[6] The cause is unknown.

Alopecia areata was reported in DEBR rats and proposed as a useful model of the human disease.[70]

Brownish scales were observed to occur on the skin of rats, mainly on the dorsum and tail and were more numerous in males and with increasing age.[102] The scales also occurred in strain-dependent patterns. Gonadectomy produced a fading of the scales in males, whereas the administration of androgen to gonadectomized males and to females produced a darkening of the scales.

Neoplasia

Spontaneous cutaneous neoplasms are uncommon in rats.[2-6, 8, 17, 98] Mesenchymal neoplasms are more common than are epithelial neoplasms. The most common are fibromas, fibrosarcomas, and lipomas. The face, the shoulder, the flank, the tail, and the paws are typically affected. Other reported skin neoplasms in rats include papilloma, keratoacanthoma, sebaceous gland tumors, squamous cell carcinoma, basal cell carcinoma, hair follicle tumors, hemangiosarcoma, melanoma, and malignant fibrous histiocytoma.

• REFERENCES

1. Balsari A, et al: Dermatophytes in clinically healthy laboratory animals. Lab Anim 15:75, 1981.
2. Benirschke K, et al: Pathology of Laboratory Animals. Springer Verlag, New York, 1978.
3. Burgmann P: Dermatology of rabbits, rodents, and ferrets. In: Nesbitt GH, Ackerman LJ (eds): Dermatology for the Small Animal Practitioner. Veterinary Learning Systems Co., Trenton, NJ, 1991, p 205.
4. Burke TJ: Skin disorders of rodents, rabbits, and ferrets. In: Kirk RW, Bonagura JD (eds): Current Veterinary Therapy XI. W.B. Saunders Co, Philadelphia, 1992, p 1170.
5. Clyde VL: Practical treatment and control of common ectoparasites in exotic pets. Vet Med 91:632, 1996.
6. Collins BR: Dermatologic disorders of common small nondomestic animals. In: Nesbitt GH (ed): Dermatology. Churchill Livingstone, New York, 1987, p. 235.
7. Cotchin E, Row FJC: Pathology of Laboratory Rats and Mice. Blackwell Scientific Publications, Oxford, 1967.
7a. Göbel T: Bacterial diseases and antimicrobial therapy in small mammals. Comp Cont Educ Pract Vet (Suppl)21:5, 1999.
8. Harkness JE, Wagner JE: The Biology and Medicine of Rabbits and Rodents III. Lea & Febiger, Philadelphia, 1989.
9. Harkness JE: Small rodents. Vet Clin North Am (Small Anim Pract) 24:89, 1994.

10. Hillyer EV, Quesenberry KE: Ferrets, Rabbits, and Rodents. Clinical Medicine and Surgery. W.B. Saunders Co, Philadelphia, 1997.
11. Hime JM, O'Donoghue PN: Handbook of Diseases of Laboratory Animals. Heinemann Veterinary Books, London, 1979.
12. Jacobson ER, Kollias GV: Exotic Animals. Churchill Livingstone, New York, 1988.
13. Lopez-Martinez R, et al: Dermatophytes isolated from laboratory animals. Mycopathologia 88:111, 1984.
14. Morris TH: Antibiotic therapeutics in laboratory animals. Lab Anim 9:16, 1995.
15. Rosenthal KL: Bacterial infections and antibiotic therapy in small mammals. Compend Contin Educ Pract Vet 20 (Suppl):13, 1998.
16. Schuchman SM: Individual care and treatment of rabbits, mice, rats, guinea pigs, hamsters, and gerbils. In: Kirk RW (ed): Current Veterinary Therapy X. W.B. Saunders Co, Philadelphia, 1989, p 738.
17. Scott DW, et al: Muller & Kirk's Small Animal Dermatology V. W. B. Saunders Co, Philadelphia, 1995, p 1127.
18. Stein S, Walshaw S: Handbook of Rabbit and Rodent Medicine. Pergamon Press, Oxford, 1996.
19. Timm KI: Pruritus in rabbits, rodents, and ferrets. Vet Clin North Am (Small Anim Pract) 18:1077, 1988.
20. Wagner JE, Farrar PL: Husbandry and medicine of small rodents. Vet Clin North Am (Small Anim Pract) 17:1061, 1987.

Chinchilla

21. Hoefer HL: Chinchillas. Vet Clin North Am (Small Anim Pract) 24:103, 1994.
22. Rees RG: Some conditions of the skin and fur of Chinchilla lanigera. J Small Anim Pract 4:213, 1963.

Ferret

23. Ackerman J: Ultrasonographic detection of adrenal gland tumors in two ferrets. J Am Vet Med Assoc 205:1001, 1994.
24. Besch-Williford CL: Biology and medicine of the ferret. Vet Clin North Am (Small Anim Pract) 17:1155, 1987.
25. Cooper JE: Skin diseases of ferrets. Vet Ann 30:325, 1990.
26. Dinsdale JR, Rest JR: Yeast infection in ferrets. Vet Rec 137:647, 1995.
27. Duval-Hudelson KA: Coccidioidomycosis in three European ferrets. J Zoo Wildlife Med 21:353, 1990.
28. Fox JG: Biology and Diseases of the Ferret. Williams & Wilkins Co., Baltimore, 1998.
29. Gould WJ, et al: Evaluation of urinary cortisol: Creatinine ratios for the diagnosis of hyperadrenocorticism associated with adrenal gland tumors in ferrets. J Am Vet Med Assoc 206:42, 1995.
30. King WW, et al: Superficial spreading pyoderma and ulcerative dermatitis in a ferret. Vet Dermatol 7:43, 1996.
31. Lewington J: Frontline for ferret fleas. University Sydney Postgraduate Foundation Veterinary Science Control Therapy Series 189:856, 1996.
32. Li X, et al: Cutaneous lymphoma in a ferret (Mustela putorius furo). Vet Pathol 32:55, 1995.
33. Li X, et al: Neoplastic diseases in ferrets: 574 cases 1968-1997). J Am Vet Med Assoc 212:1402, 1998.
34. Noli C, et al: Demodicosis in ferrets (Mustela putorius furo). Vet Quart 18:28, 1996.
35. Paradis M: Guide du furet domestique. Méd Vét Québec 17:63, 1987.
35a. Patterson MM, Kirchain SM: Comparison of three treatments for control of ear mites in ferrets. Lab Anim Sci 49:655, 1999.
36. Rosenbaum MR, et al: Cutaneous epitheliotropic lymphoma in a ferret. J Am Vet Med Assoc 209:1441, 1996.
37. Rosenthal KL, et al: Hyperadrenocorticism associated with adrenocortical tumor or nodular hyperplasia of the adrenal gland in ferrets: 50 cases (1987–1991). J Am Vet Med Assoc 203:271, 1993.
38. Rosenthal KL: Ferrets. Vet Clin North Am (Small Anim Pract) 24:1, 1994.
39. Rosenthal JL, Peterson ME: Evaluation of plasma androgen and estrogen concentrations in ferrets with hyperadrenocorticism. J Am Vet Med Assoc 209:1097, 1996.
39a. Rosenthal KL: Adrenal gland diseases in ferrets. Vet Clin North Am Small Anim Pract 27:401, 1997.
40. Rudmann DG, et al: Complex ceruminous gland adenocarcinoma in a brown-footed ferret (Mustela putorius furo). Lab Anim Sci 44:637, 1994.
41. Scott DW, et al: Bilaterally symmetric alopecia associated with an adrenocortical adenoma in a pet ferret. Vet Dermatol 2:165, 1991.
42. Scott DW, et al: Figurate erythema resembling erythema annulare centrifugum in a ferret with adrenocortical adenocarcinoma–associated alopecia. Vet Dermatol 5:111, 1994.
42a. Shoemaker NJ, et al: Correlation between age at neutering and age at onset of hyperadrenocorticism in ferrets. J Am Vet Med Assoc 216:195, 2000.
43. Weiss CA, Scott MV: Clinical aspects and surgical treatment of hyperadrenocorticism in the domestic ferret: 94 cases (1994–1996). J Am Anim Hosp Assoc 33:487, 1997.
43a. Weiss CA, et al: Surgical treatment and long-term outcome of ferrets with bilateral adrenal tumors or adrenal hyperplasia: 56 cases (1994–1997). J Am Vet Med Assoc 215:820, 1999.

Gerbil

44. Jacklin MR: Dermatosis associated with Acarus farris in gerbils. J Small Anim Pract 38:410, 1997.
45. Jackson TA, et al: Squamous cell carcinoma of the midventral abdominal pad in three gerbils. J Am Vet Med Assoc 209:789, 1996.

Guinea Pig

46. Bobrowski PJ, et al: Latent herpes simplex virus reactivation in the guinea pig. An animal model for recurrent disease. Int J Dermatol 30:29, 1991.
47. Fry FL: Apparent spontaneous ergot-induced necrotiting dermatitis in a guinea pig. J Small Exotic Anim Med 2:165, 1994.
47a. Guaguère E: Acariose à Chirodiscoides caviae et dermatophytie à Microsporum canis chez un cobaye. Prat Méd Chir Anim Comp 34:65, 1999.
48. Hirsjärvi P, Phyälä L: Ivermectin treatment of a colony of guinea pigs infested with fur mite (Chirodiscoides caviae). Lab Anim 29: 200, 1995.
49. Peguin J: Phthiriose à Trimenopon chez un cobaye. Point Vét 28:91, 1997.
50. Quesenberry KE: Guinea pigs. Vet Clin North Am (Small Anim Pract) 24:67, 1994.
51. Rothwell TL, et al: Haematological and pathological responses to experimental Trixacarus caviae infection in guinea pigs. J Comp Pathol 104: 179, 1991.

51a. Shipstone M: *Trixacarus caviae* infestation in a guinea pig: Failure to respond to ivermectin administration. Aust Vet Pract 27:143, 1997.
52. Sohnle PD, et al: Mechanisms involved in elimination of organisms from experimental cutaneous *Candida albicans* infections in guinea pigs. J Immunol 117:525, 1976.
53. Van Cutsem J, et al: The in vitro antifungal activity of ketoconazole, zinc pyrithione, and selenium sulfide against *Pityrosporum* and their efficacy as a shampoo in the treatment of experimental pityrosporosis in guinea pigs. J Am Acad. Dermatol 22:993, 1990.
53a. Vangeel I, et al: Prevalence of dermatophytes in asymptomatic guinea pigs and rabbits. Vet Rec 146:440, 2000.

Hamster

54. Bauck LB, et al: Hyperadrenocorticism in three teddy bear hamsters. Can Vet J 25:247, 1984.
55. Harvey RG, et al: Epidermotropic cutaneous T-cell lymphoma (mycosis fungoides) in Syrian hamsters (*Mesocricetus auratus*). A report of six cases and the demonstration of T-cell specificity. Vet Dermatol 3:13, 1992.
56. Kajdacsy-Balla A, et al: Syphilis in the Syrian hamster. A model of human venereal and congenital syphilis. Am J Pathol 126:599, 1987.

Mouse

57. Abbott DP, et al: A condition resembling pagetoid reticulosis in a laboratory mouse. Lab Anim 25:153, 1991.
58. Andrews AG, et al: Immune complex vasculitis with secondary ulcerative dermatitis in aged C57BL/6NNla mice. Vet Pathol 31:293, 1994.
59. Baumans V, et al: The effectiveness of Ivomec and Neguvon in the control of murine mites. Lab Anim 22:243, 1988.
60. Baumans V, et al: The use of repeated treatment with Ivomec and Neguvon in the control of murine mites and oxurid worms. Lab Anim 22: 246, 1988.
61. Booth CJ, Sundberg JP: Hemangiomas and hemangiosarcomas in inbred laboratory mice. Lab Anim Sci 45:497, 1995.
62. Foster HL, et al: The Mouse in Biomedical Research. Academic Press, New York, 1982.
63. Kietzmann M, et al: The mouse epidermis as a model in skin pharmacology: Influence of age and sex on epidermal metabolic reactions and their circadian rhythms. Lab Anim 24:321, 1990.
64. Locklear J, et al: Spontaneous vulvar carcinomas in 129/J mice. Lab Anim Sci 45:604, 1995.
64a. Mähler M, Jelínek F: Granulomatous inflammation in the tails of mice associated with *Mycobacterium chelonae* infection. Lab Anim 34:212, 2000.
65. Neubauer H, et al: Specific detection of mousepox virus by polymerase chain reaction. Lab Anim 31:201, 1997.
66. Niemaltowski MG, et al: The inflammatory and immune response to mousepox (infectious ectomelia) virus. Acta Virol 38: 299, 1994.
67. Papini R, Marcancini A: Treatment with ivermectin in drinking water against *Myobias musculi* and *Myocoptes musculinis* mange in naturally infected laboratory mice. Agnew Parasitol 32:11, 1991.
68. Sundberg JP, et al: Inherited mouse mutations as models of human adnexal, cornification, and papulosquamous dermatoses. J Invest Dermatol 95:62S, 1990.
69. Sundberg JP, Schultz LD: Inherited mouse mutations: Models for the study of alopecia. J Invest Dermatol 96:95S, 1991.
70. Sundberg JP, et al: Alopecia areata in humans and other mammalian species. J Invest Dermatol 104:32s, 1995.
71. Vachon P, Aubry L: L'utilisation d'ivermectin pour le traitement des acariens, *Myobia musculi* et *Myocoptes musculinus*, dans une colonie de souris transgéniques. Can Vet J 37:231, 1996.
72. Wardrip CL, et al: Diagnostic exercise: head and neck swelling in A/JCr mice. Lab Anim Sci 44:280, 1994.
73. Wrench R: Scale prophylaxis. A new antiparakeratotic assay. Arch Dermatol 117:213, 1981.

Rabbit

74. Arlian LG, et al: *Sarcoptes scabiei*: The circulating antibody response and induced immunity to scabies. Exp Parasitol 78:37, 1994.
75. Arlian LG, et al: *Sarcoptes scabiei*: Histopathological changes associated with acquisition and expression of host immunity to scabies. Exp Parasitol 78:51, 1994.
76. Brown PJ, et al: Abnormalities of collagen fibrils in a rabbit with connective tissue defect similar to Ehlers-Danlos syndrome. Res Vet Sci 55:346, 1993.
77. Carpenter JW, et al: Caring for rabbits: An overview and formulary. Vet Med 90:340, 1995.
78. Cooper PE, Penaoliggon J: Use of Frontline spray on rabbits. Vet Rec 140:535, 1997.
79. Cutler SL: Ectopic *Psoroptes cuniculi* infestation in a pet rabbit. J Small Anim Pract 39:86, 1998.
80. Harkness JE: Rabbit husbandry and medicine. Vet Clin North Am (Small Anim Pract) 17:1019, 1987.
81. Harrenstien L, et al: How to handle respiratory, ophthalmic, neurological and dermatologic problems in rabbits. Vet Med 90:373, 1995.
82. Hazarika RA, et al: Experimental staphylococcal dermatitis in rabbits. Indian J Vet Pathol 15:39, 1991.
83. Hillyer EV: Pet rabbits. Vet Clin North Am (Small Anim Pract) 24:25, 1994.
84. Hotchkiss CE, et al: Malignant melanoma in two rabbits. Lab Anim Sci 44:377, 1994.
85. Iglauer F, et al: Hereditary compulsive self-mutilating behavior in laboratory rabbits. Lab Anim 29:385, 1995.
86. Jenkins JR: Skin disorders of the rabbit. J Small Exotic Anim Med 1:64, 1991.
86a. Kirwan AP, et al: Diagnosis and prevalence of *Leporacarus gibbus* in the fur of domestic rabbits in the UK. Vet Rec 142:20, 1998.
87. Kumar SP, et al: Use of levamisole for the treatment of mange due to *Notoedres cati* in rabbits. Indian Vet J 70:161, 1993.
88. Kamboj DS, et al: Clinicotherapeutic efficacy of amitraz against *Notoedres cati* infestation in rabbits. Indian Vet J 70:751, 1993.
89. Linder KE, et al: Generalized exfoliative dermatosis with sebaceous adenitis in three domestic rabbits. Proc Annu Meet Am Acad Vet Dermatol Am Coll Vet Dermatol 14:89, 1998.
90. Maiti SK, et al: An evaluation of ivermectin oral preparation in the treatment of sarcoptic mange in rabbits. Indian Vet J 72:612, 1995.
91. Malley D: Use of Frontline spray in rabbits. Vet Rec 140:664, 1997.
92. Manning PJ, et al: The Biology of the Laboratory Rabbit II. Academic Press, San Diego, 1994.

93. Okerman L, et al: Cutaneous staphylococcosis in rabbits. Vet Rec 114:313, 1984.
93a. Pinter L: *Leporacarus gibbus* and *Spilopsyllus cuniculi* infestation in a pet rabbit. J Small Anim Pract 40:220, 1999.
94. Sinke JD, et al: A case of Ehlers-Danlos-like syndrome in a rabbit with review of the disease in other species. Vet Quart 19:182, 1997.
95. Tripathi SC, et al: Therapeutic efficacy of ivermectin in rabbits (*Oryctolagus cuniculus*) experimentally infected with *Psoroptes cuniculi*. Indian J Anim Hlth 32:55, 1993.
96. Weisbroth SH, et al: The Biology of the Laboratory Rabbit. Academic Press, New York, 1974.
96a. White SD, et al: Sebaceous adenitis in four domestic rabbits (*Oryctalagus cuniculus*). Vet Dermatol 11:53, 2000.
96b. White SD, et al: Lymphoma with cutaneous involvement in three domestic rabbits (*Oryctolagus cuniculus*). Vet Dermatol 11:61, 2000.
97. Yeatts JWG: Rabbit mite infestation. Vet Rec 134:359, 1994.

Rat

98. Binhazim AA, et al: Spontaneous hemangiosarcoma in the tail of a Long-Evans rat carrying the Elcer mutation. Lab Anim Sci 44:191, 1994.
99. Erdelyi LL et al: Behandlung med ivermectin mot springmask och pälskvalster hos laboratorieratta: Strategisk program i en produktion-sanhet. Scand J Lab Anim Sci 15:184, 1988.
100. Kunstyr I, et al: Granulomatous dermatitis and mastitis in two SPF rats associated with a slowly growing *Staphylococcus aureus*—a case report. Lab Anim 29:177, 1995.
101. MacHole EJA: Mange in domesticated rats. Vet Rec 138:312, 1996.
102. Tayama K, Shisa H: Development of pigmented scales on rat skin: Relation to age, sex, strain, and hormonal effect. Lab Anim Sci 44:240, 1994.

Chapter 22
Chronology of Veterinary Dermatology (1900–2000)

An overview of the history of veterinary dermatology, Historical Highlights—Ancient and Modern, can be found in Chapter 90, pages 711 to 735, of the second edition of this book (1976). This material was updated for the third edition of this book (1983). Because the historical material is unchanged, it is not repeated in the sixth edition. Instead, the chronology is given here and updated to 2000.

1900 Joseph Bayer and Eugene Fröhner of Vienna, Austria, persuaded Hugo Schindelka to write a book on skin diseases of domestic animals.

1903 Publication of the first book on veterinary dermatology, Hautkrankheiten bei Haustieren (Skin Diseases of Domestic Animals), by Hugo Schindelka at Vienna.

1908 Publication of the second and final edition of Schindelka's book, Hautkrankheiten bei Haustieren.

1910 Publication of the first book on comparative dermatology, Die Vergleichende Pathologie der Haut (The Comparative Pathology of the Skin), by Julius Heller at Berlin, Germany.

1926 Publication of Animal Dermatology by Leblois in France.

1930 Publication of the book, Course in Skin Diseases of Domestic Animals, by N.N. Bogdanov at Moscow.

1931 Publication of Die Klinik der Wichtigsten Tierdermatosen (The Clinic of the Most Important Animal Dermatoses) by Julius Heller at Berlin, Germany.

1931 Publication of Veterinari Dermatologie by Frantisek Kral (Frank Kral) at Brno, Czechoslovakia.

1948 Frank Kral emigrated to the United States and joined the faculty of the School of Veterinary Medicine, University of Pennsylvania in Philadelphia. He formed the Veterinary Dermatology Clinic, which was the first teaching unit of animal skin diseases in the United States.

1953 Publication of Veterinary Dermatology by Frank Kral and Benjamin J. Novak, first veterinary dermatologic book in English: a complete revision, expansion, and translation of Kral's 1931 book (325 pages).

1958 Formation of the Dermatology Subcommittee of the Committee on General Medicine of the American Animal Hospital Association on April 23, 1958. R.W. Worley and G.H. Muller, Cochairmen; first organization of veterinary dermatology.

1958 E.M. Farber appoints G.H. Muller to the clinical faculty of Stanford University's Dermatology Department and establishes the first center of comparative dermatology in America.

1959 R.M. Schwartzman obtains the first Ph.D. degree in Veterinary Dermatology and shortly thereafter joins F. Kral's veterinary dermatology section at the University of Pennsylvania.

1959 Formation of the Dermatology Committee of the American Animal Hospital Association on February 5, 1959. G.H. Muller, Chairman. Committee functioned for 7 years.

1959 Publication of the Compendium of Veterinary Dermatology by Frank Kral. Handout for Kral's cross-country symposia in 1959 (69 pages).

1962 Publication of A Comparative Study of Skin Diseases of Dog and Man by Robert

	M. Schwartzman and Milton Orkin: the first book in English on comparative dermatology (365 pages).
1963	Transatlantic Conference on Canine and Feline Dermatology at Chicago and London on April 26, 1963. Knowles, Muller, and Schwartzman for the United States; Singleton, Joshua, and Wilkinson for England.
1964	Publication of section on Dermatologic Diseases (edited by G.H. Muller) in R.W. Kirk's Current Veterinary Therapy. Revised and updated in all subsequent editions.
1964	Publication of chapter on "Feline diseases of the skin" by J.D. Conroy in Feline Medicine.
1964	The American Academy of Veterinary Dermatology was organized at Philadelphia by Conroy, Kral (President), Muller, and Schwartzman.
1964	Symposium on Comparative Physiology and Pathology of the Skin at London, England, in April, 1964. A.J. Rook and G.S. Walton, Chairmen. Proceedings were published in 1965.
1964	Publication of Veterinary and Comparative Dermatology by F. Kral and R.M. Schwartzman: a revision and expansion of Kral and Novak's Veterinary Dermatology (444 pages).
1964	First Symposium on Comparative Dermatology sponsored by the American Academy of Dermatology at Chicago on December 8, 1964. Milton Orkin was chairman of this and the next three symposia.
1965	Second Symposium on Comparative Dermatology, December 7, 1965, at Chicago.
1965	Publication of Comparative Physiology and Pathology of the Skin by A.J. Rook and G.S. Walton.
1966	Third Symposium on Comparative Dermatology, December 5, 1966, at Miami, Florida.
1966	Symposium on Skin Diseases Common to Man and Animals at Palm Springs, California, on November 2, 1966. Orkin and Muller, Cochairmen.
1967	Fourth Symposium on Comparative Dermatology, December 4, 1967, at Chicago.
1967	Publication of Atlas of Canine and Feline Dermatoses by R.M. Schwartzman and Frank Kral.
1968	Publication of the atlas, Canine Skin Lesions, by G.H. Muller.
1968	J.D. Conroy receives a Ph.D. degree and thereby launches the first career devoted exclusively to veterinary dermatohistopathology in America.
1969	Publication of Small Animal Dermatology by G.H. Muller and R.W. Kirk (485 pages): the first complete textbook devoted exclusively to skin diseases of dogs and cats. Used as a textbook by many schools of veterinary medicine. Translated into Japanese and French and reprinted in Taiwan.
1970	Formation of an organizing committee of the American College of Veterinary Dermatologists consisting of Blakemore, Conroy, Muller (Chairman), Schwartzman, Kirk, and Kral.
1973	The formation of the Task Force on Comparative Dermatology as part of the National Program for Dermatology of the American Academy of Dermatology.
1974	Publication of the atlas, Feline Skin Lesions, by G.H. Muller.
1974	Publication of a stereoscopic atlas of Clinical Dermatology of Small Animals by G.G. Doering and H.E. Jensen (211 pages).
1974	Dermatology Specialty Group of the American College of Veterinary Internal Medicine (ACVIM) receives approval of the Advisory Board of Veterinary Specialties of the American Veterinary Medical Association (AVMA) on April 5, 1974.
1974	The first meeting of the Dermatology Specialty Group of the ACVIM was held on April 20, 1974, at San Francisco.
1974	The Dermatology Specialty Group was officially recognized by receiving probationary approval of the ACVIM and Council of Education of the AVMA on July 20, 1974, at Denver, Colorado.
1976	Formation of the British Veterinary Dermatology Study Group on February 20,

	1976. Honorary Secretary Brian G. Bagnal; committee members Michael R. Geary, Raymond Hopes, David H. Lloyd, and Keith L. Thoday.
1976	Publication of the Veterinary Dermatology Newsletter (Vol. 1, No. 1) in May 1976 by the British Veterinary Dermatology Study Group.
1976	Publication of the second edition of Small Animal Dermatology by G.H. Muller and R.W. Kirk (809 pages). Translated into Italian.
1979	Publication of The Skin and Internal Disease (edited by G.H. Muller), the Veterinary Clinics of North America, 1979, W.B. Saunders Company (152 pages).
1980	Publication of Feline Dermatology 1900–1978: A Monograph by D.W. Scott (128 pages).
1980	Frank Kral deceased September 7, 1980.
1981	Formation of a French veterinary dermatologic organization: Groupe D'Étude en Dermatologie des Animaux de Compagnie (GEDAC). President Pierre Fourrier, Secretary Didier Carlotti.
1981	Publication of Canine Dermatoses by J.M. Keep (Australia).
1981	Publication of Feline Dermatoses by J.M. Keep (Australia).
1981	Publication of Equine Dermatoses by R.R. Pascoe (Australia).
1982	On March 9, 1982, the American Board of Veterinary Specialties of the AVMA granted probationary approval to the American College of Veterinary Dermatology as a certifying body in Veterinary Dermatology. This group replaces the Dermatology Specialty Group of the ACVIM. The organizing committee of the American College of Veterinary Dermatology consists of Doctors J.C. Blakemore, J.D. Conroy, R.E.W. Halliwell, G.H. Muller, and E. Small.
1982	The American College of Veterinary Dermatology was approved by the Council of Education of the AVMA on April 23, 1982, and approved by the House of Delegates of the AVMA on July 20, 1982. The charter members of the group are the diplomates of the ACVIM (Dermatology) listed under 1981. There were 24 diplomates at the end of 1982.
1982	Formation of a German veterinary dermatology organization called the "Freundeskreis Hautkrankheiten Interessierter Tierärtzte." The organizing members are H. Koch (President), B. Beardi, G. Feslev, H. Gehrig, G. Kasa, F. Kasa, G.H. Muller, and C. Terling. The first meeting was held on October 12, 1982, at Birkenfeld, West Germany. The name of this organization was later changed to Arbeitskreis Veterinär Dermatologie.
1983	Publication of the third edition of Small Animal Dermatology by G.H. Muller, R.W. Kirk, and D.W. Scott (889 pages). Translated into Portuguese and Japanese.
1983	Publication of Canine and Feline Dermatology: A Systematic Approach by G.H. Nesbitt (244 pages).
1983	Publication of Atlas of Skin Diseases of the Horse by L.F. Montes and J.T. Vaughan.
1984	Formation of the European Society of Veterinary Dermatology (ESVD) on September 18, 1984. President Hans Koch (Germany), Vice President Ton Willemse (Holland), Secretary David Lloyd (England), Treasurer Didier Carlotti (France), Membership Secretary Pierre Fourrier (France), Meeting Secretary Claudia Von Tscharner (Switzerland). Honorary Members Richard Halliwell, Peter Ihrke, Robert Kirk, George Muller, and Danny Scott (USA).
1984	Formation of an Australian veterinary dermatology organization began; started informally that year under the auspices of the Australian College of Veterinary Scientists. It granted full fellowship by examination in veterinary dermatology to Kenneth V. Mason on August 28, 1984.
1984	Publication of Equine Dermatoses by R.R. Pascoe (Australia).
1984	Publication of Skin Diseases of the Pig by R.D.A. Cameron (Australia).
1984	Formation of Groupe de Travail en Dermatologie Vétérinaire in Belgium.
1984	Formation of Swedish Veterinary Dermatology Study Group in Sweden.
1985	Formation of Dansk Selskab for Veterinaer Dermatologi in Denmark.

1985	Publication of the Color Atlas of Small Animal Dermatology by G.T. Wilkinson (272 pages), Australia.
1986	Publication of Skin Diseases in the Dog and Cat by D.I. Grant (187 pages), England.
1986	Formation of the Canadian Academy of Veterinary Dermatology. President Lowell Ackerman, Secretary B.P. Pukay.
1987	Publication of Contemporary Issues in Small Animal Practice: Dermatology, Vol. 8, New York (332 pages) (edited by G.H. Nesbitt).
1987	Formation, on October 23, of the Italian Veterinary Dermatology Group as part of the Italian Small Animal Veterinary Association (SCIVAC). President, Alessandra Fondati.
1987	Formation of the Grupo de Dermatología de Asosiación de Veterinarios Especialistas en Pequeños Animales in Spain.
1987	Publication of Atlas of Skin Diseases in Dogs and Cats by F. Kristensen (Denmark).
1988	Publication of Large Animal Dermatology by D.W. Scott (487 pages).
1988	Publication of Vanliga Hudsjukdomar Hos Hund Och Katt by B. Ohlén (Sweden).
1988	Publication of Pruritus (edited by S.D. White), the Veterinary Clinics of North America, 1988, W.B. Saunders Company (143 pages).
1989	Publication of the fourth edition of Small Animal Dermatology by G.H. Muller, R.W. Kirk, and D.W. Scott (1007 pages). Translated into German.
1989	Publication of first issue of Veterinary Dermatology, an international journal devoted to dermatology.
1989	Publication of Skin Infection in Domestic Animals by A. Chatterjee (India).
1989	Publication of Allergic Skin Diseases of Dogs and Cats by L.M. Reedy and W.H. Miller, Jr.
1989	Publication of Skin Diseases of Cattle by D.I. Bryden (Australia).
1989	Publication of Practical Canine Dermatology by L.J. Ackerman.
1989	Publication of Practical Feline Dermatology by L.J. Ackerman.
1989	Publication of Practical Equine Dermatology by L.J. Ackerman.
1989	The First World Congress in Veterinary Dermatology was held in September at Dijon, France.
1990	Publication of Small Animal Allergy. A Practical Guide by E. Baker.
1990	Publication of Color Atlas of Small Animal Dermatology by B.A. Kummel.
1990	Publication of Advances in Veterinary Dermatology, Vol. I, by C. von Tscharner and R.E.W. Halliwell.
1990	Publication of Common Skin Diseases in Dogs and Cats by B. Ohlén (Sweden).
1990	Publication of A Colour Atlas of Equine Dermatology by R.R. Pascoe (Australia).
1990	Publication of Canine and Feline Dermatology by K.P. Baker and L.R. Thomsett (United Kingdom).
1990	Publication of Advances in Clinical Dermatology (edited by D.J. DeBoer), the Veterinary Clinics of North America, 1990, W.B. Saunders Company (310 pages).
1991	Publication of Clinical Dermatology of Dogs and Cats by T. Willemse (Netherlands).
1991	Publication of Les Dermites Allergiques du Chien et du Chat by P. Prélaud (France).
1991	Publication of second edition of Skin Diseases in the Dog and Cat by D.I. Grant (United Kingdom).
1991	Publication of Dermatology for the Small Animal Practitioner by G.H. Nesbitt and L.J. Ackerman.
1991	Publication of Techniques Diagnostiques en Dermatologie des Carnivores by E. Guaguère (France).
1992	Publication of Skin Tumors of the Dog and Cat by M.H. Goldschmidt and F.S. Shofer.
1992	Publication of Veterinary Dermatopathology. A Macroscopic and Microscopic Eval-

uation of Canine and Feline Skin Diseases by T.L. Gross, P.J. Ihrke, and E.J. Walder.

1992 The Second World Congress in Veterinary Dermatology was held in May at Montreal, Quebec.

1992 The European College of Veterinary Dermatology was granted approval as a certifying body in veterinary dermatology, and the following individuals were elected as Invited Specialists ("grandfathers"): D. Carlotti, R. Halliwell, H. Koch, D. Lloyd, K. Thoday, and T. Willemse.

1993 Publication of Current Veterinary Dermatology. The Science and Art of Therapy by C.E. Griffin, K.W. Kwochka, and J.M. MacDonald.

1993 Publication of Manual of Small Animal Dermatology by P.H. Locke, R.G. Harvey, and I.S. Mason (United Kingdom).

1993 Publication of second edition of Color Atlas of Small Animal Dermatology: A Guide to Diagnosis by G.T. Wilkinson and R. G. Harvey (United Kingdom).

1993 Publication of Advances in Veterinary Dermatology, Vol. II, by P.J. Ihrke, I.S. Mason, and S.D. White.

1994 Publication of Color Atlas and Text of Surgical Pathology of the Dog and Cat: Dermatopathology and Skin Tumors by J.A. Yager and B.P. Wilcock.

1995 Publication of the fifth edition of Muller and Kirk's Small Animal Dermatology (1,213 pages) by D.W. Scott, W.H. Miller, and C.E. Griffin. Translated into Portuguese and Spanish.

1995 Publication of Dermatology (edited by V. A. Fadok), the Veterinary Clinics of North America Equine Practice, 1995, W. B. Saunders Company (150 pages).

1995 Publication of Feline Dermatology (edited by G. Kunkle), the Veterinary Clinics of North America Small Animal Practice, 1995, W. B. Saunders Company (246 pages).

1995 Publication of Handbook of Small Animal Dermatology by K. A. Moriello and I. S. Mason.

1995 Formation of the study group, Omada Ktiniatrikis Dermatologias, in Greece.

1995 Formation of the Italian Society of Veterinary Dermatology in Italy.

1995 Formation of the Association of Veterinary Dermatology—Taipei in Taiwan.

1995 Formation of the Arbeitskreis Veterinärdermatologie in Austria.

1996 The Third World Congress in Veterinary Dermatology was held in September at Edinburgh, Scotland.

1997 Formation of Deutsche Gesellschaft für Veterinärdermatologie in Germany.

1997 Publication of second edition of Allergic Skin Diseases of Dogs and Cats by L. M. Reedy, W. H. Miller, Jr., and T. Willemse.

1997 Publication of A Color Handbook of Skin Diseases in the Dog and Cat by P. J. McKeever and R. G. Harvey.

1997 Publication of Color Atlas of Small Animal Dermatoses for Small Animal Practitioner by C. Chen (Taiwan).

1997 Tony Stannard deceased July 2, 1997.

1998 Publication of Canine and Feline Dermatology. Diagnosis and Treatment by G. H. Nesbitt and L. Ackerman.

1998 Publication of Advances in Veterinary Dermatology, Vol. III, by K. W. Kwochka, T. Willemse, and C. von Tscharner.

1998 Formation of Nihon Juhi Hifuka Gakkai in Japan.

1998 Publication of A Color Handbook of Skin Diseases of the Dog and Cat by P. J. McKeever and R. G. Harvey.

1998 Publication of Skin Diseases of the Dog by S. Paterson (United Kingdom).

1998 Publication of Vade-Mecum de Dermatologie Vétérinaire by G. Marignac (France).

1999 Publication of ΔΕΡΜΑΤΟ ΛΙΚΑ-ΕΝΔΟΚΡΙΝΟΛΟΓΙΑ ΚΑΙ ΜΕΤΑΒΟΛΙΚΑ ΝΟΣΗΜΑΤΑ by A. Koutinas (Greece).

1999 Publication of Allergologie Canine by P. Prélaud (France).

1999 Publication of Manual of Equine Dermatology by R. R. R. Pascoe and D. C. Knottenbelt.
1999 Publication of Dermatology (edited by K. L. Campbell), the Veterinary Clinics of North America Small Animal Practice, 1999, W. B. Saunders Company (215 pages).
2000 Publication of Skin Diseases of the Cat by S. Paterson (United Kingdom).
2000 Formation of the Brazilian Society of Veterinary Dermatology in Brazil.
2000 Lloyd Reedy deceased. April 21, 2000.
2000 The Fourth World Congress in Veterinary Dermatology was held in August/September at San Francisco, California.
2000 Publication of A Practical Guide to Feline Dermatology by E. Guaguère and P. Prélaud (France).

Index

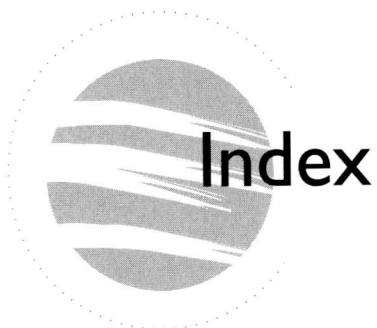

Page numbers in *italics* refer to illustrations; page numbers followed by t refer to tables.

Aaro-Perkins corpuscle, 44
Abamectin, 428
Abdomen, common and less common dermatoses of, 104t
Abelcet. See *Amphotericin B lipid complex*.
Abrasion(s), epidermal, management of, 266–267
Abscess(es). See also *Microabscess(es)*.
 anal sac, *1197*, 1202, 1203
 definition of, 89
 dermal, 187, *187*
 in actinobacillosis, 321–323
 in cats, 276, 310–311
  nonhealing or recurrent, 311
 in dogs, *302*, 310, *311*
 in hamsters, 1439
 in rabbits, 1445
 in rats, 1452
 plague-related, 325–326
 subcutaneous, helminthic infections and, 440
  in cats, 310–311
  in dogs, *302*, 310, *311*
Absidia corymbifera, 384
Abyssinian cat, amyloidosis in, 767
 cryptococcosis in, 395
 griseofulvin side effects in, 357
 grooming for, 215
 hair disorder of, *109*
 hair shaft disorder of, 955, *955*
 psychogenic dermatoses in, 1056, 1066
 risk for non-neoplastic skin disorders in, 77t
Acanthocheilonoma infection, *435*, 439–440, *440*
Acanthocyte(s), 143
 in cytologic diagnosis, 118t
Acantholysis, 143–147, *146*, *147*, 678
 in pemphigus, 678–679
Acanthoma(s), infundibular keratinizing. See *Keratoacanthoma*.
Acanthosis, definition of, 134
 true, 134
Acanthosis nigricans, 975–977
 breed(s) with predilection for, 75
 canine, 1007–1009, *1010*
 cause and pathogenesis of, 975–976
 clinical features of, *964*, 976
 clinical management of, 253, 976–977
 diagnosis of, 976
 in dogs, *153*
 primary (idiopathic), 975
 secondary, 975–976

Acarus farris, in gerbils, 1428
Acarus siro, 451
Accutane. See *Isotretinoin*.
Acetate tape impression, for ectoparasites, 107
 for *Malassezia* spp., 368
Acetic acid, 227
 otic therapy with, 1228
 topical, 236, 356t
  antifungal therapy with, 410
Achromotrichia, 96
Acid mantle, of skin, 31–32
Acid orcein–Giemsa (AOG) stain, 129, 130t
Acid phosphatase, in cell type identification, 204t
Acidophil(s), 781
Acinetobacter spp., as resident flora, in cats, 33, 275
 in dogs, 33, 275
Acitretin, 241
 antiseborrheic therapy with, 919, 1029
 for actinic keratosis, 1079
 for granulomatous sebaceous adenitis, 1246
 indications for, 1029
Acne, 1041–1043
 canine, 303, 1041
 feline, 1029, *1039*, 1042–1043, *1043*
  clinical management of, 242
Acral lick dermatitis, 308, 1057, 1058–1064
 acupuncture for, 1064
 cause and pathogenesis of, 1058
 clinical features of, 1058–1059, *1060*
 clinical management of, 1059–1064
 cryosurgery for, 258, 1064
 diagnosis of, 1059, *1061*, *1062*
 electroshock for, 1064
 laser therapy for, 1064
 lesion in, treatment of, 1063–1064
 organic disease and, 1058
 psychological drug therapy for, 1061–1063
 radiation therapy for, 1064
Acral lick furunculosis, *302*, 308–309
Acral mutilation syndrome, 988–989, 995
Acremonium hyalinum, 377
Acrodermatitis, 988–989, 992–993
Acromegaly, 794–795
 canine, 825–827, *826*, *828*
 feline, 825, 827, *828*
Acromelanism, 8
 feline, 1012–1013

1465

ACTH, 17, 781
    plasma levels of, determination of, 793
        measurement of, 809
    secretion of, excessive, 799
    sex hormone response to, test for, 798
ACTH stimulation test, 791–792
    in hyperadrenocorticism, 809
    sex hormone levels after, in dogs, 848–849, 850t
Actin, 22t
Actinic keratosis, 1080, 1391–1392, *1393*, *1394*
    breed(s) with predilection for, 1238t
    in cats, *173*
    risk for, haircoat color and, 76
Actinin, 22t
Actinobacillosis (*Actinobacillus* infection), 321–323
    diagnosis of, 125
    pseudomycetoma caused by, 312
Actinobacillus spp., in mice, 1442
Actinobacillus lignieresii, 321
Actinomyces spp., in abscesses in cats, 311
    in mice, 1442
    in oral flora of cats, 276
    infections caused by, 276. See also *Actinomycosis*.
Actinomyces hordeovulneris, 321
Actinomyces meyeri, 321
Actinomyces odontolyticus, 321
Actinomyces viscosus, 321
Actinomycosis, *317*, 321, 322
    diagnosis of, 117, 125, 321
    in ferrets, 1417
Acupuncture, 263
    for acral lick dermatitis, 1064
Acyclovir, for feline rhinotracheitis, 525
Adapalene, 234, 241
Adapin. See *Doxepin*.
Adenitis. See *Sebaceous adenitis*.
Adenocarcinoma, adrenocortical, in cats, 815
    in dogs, 799
    colonic, cutaneous metastases of, *1366*, *1373*, *1374*
    eyelid, 1190
    jejunal, cutaneous metastases of, 1373–1374
    mammary, 1021
        cutaneous metastases of, *1366*, 1373
    pituitary, in cats, 815
        in dogs, 799
Adenohypophysis, 780
Adenoma(s), adrenocortical, in cats, 815
    in dogs, 799
    eyelid, 1190
    pituitary, in cats, 815
        in dogs, 799
    sebaceous gland, 1029
        clinical management of, 242
        in dogs, 1271, *1272*
        in gerbils, 1429–1430
    sweat gland, *1279*
        in hamsters, 1442
Adenosine triphosphatase, in cell type identification, 204t
Adherens junction(s), 19, 22t
Adhesion molecule(s), 545, 549t
Adipocyte(s). See *Lipocyte(s)*.
Adipose tissue, 63, *63*
Adnexal (pilosebaceous) nevi, 1384–1386, *1385*
Adrenal function test(s), 790–794
    in canine hyperadrenocorticism, 807–810
    in feline hyperadrenocorticism, 816–818
Adrenal hyperplasia–like syndrome, 846–851
    cause and pathogenesis of, 846–847

Adrenal hyperplasia–like syndrome (*Continued*)
    clinical features of, *847*, 847–848, *848*
    clinical management of, 849–851
    diagnosis of, 848–849, *849*, 850t
Adrenal sex hormone imbalance(s), 845–846, *854*
    breed(s) with predilection for, 75
    in dogs, *842*
Adrenalectomy, in cats, 818–819
    in dogs, 811
Adrenocorticotropic hormone (corticotropin). See *ACTH*.
Advantage. See *Imidacloprid*.
Adverse drug reaction, cutaneous. See *Drug reaction, cutaneous*.
Adverse food reaction. See *Food hypersensitivity*.
Affenpinscher, follicular dysplasia in, 971
    seasonal flank alopecia in, 891
Afghan hound. See *Hound, Afghan*.
Age, and drug absorption, 220
    and graying, 1014
    and risk for non-neoplastic skin disorders, 75, 76t
    and skin immune system, 560–561
    skin changes with, 64–65, *65*
Agouti hair, 8
Aguirre's syndrome, 1021
Airedale. See *Terrier, Airedale*.
Akita, amyloidosis in, 767
    dystrophic epidermolysis bullosa in, 939
    granulomatous sebaceous adenitis in, 1141, *1142*, 1143, *1143*
    pemphigus foliaceus in, 686, *687*
    postclipping alopecia in, *898*
    risk for non-neoplastic skin disorders in, 75, 77t
    uveodermatologic syndrome in, 748–749, *757*
Alabama rot. See *Greyhound*.
Alaskan malamute. See *Malamute*.
Albinism, 17, 1014
Alcaligenes spp., as transient flora, in cats, 275
Alcian blue, staining characteristics of various substances with, 130t
Alcohol(s), antipruritic therapy with, 229–230
    in shampoo, 223
    in topical therapy, 230
Aleuroconidia, 337
Alkaline phosphatase, in cell type identification, 204t
    in hyperadrenocorticism, 805
Allergen(s), alum-precipitated, for hyposensitization of dogs, 599
    aqueous, for hyposensitization of dogs, 597–599, 598t
    emulsion, for hyposensitization of dogs, 599
Allergic breakthrough, 579
Allergic contact dermatitis. See *Contact hypersensitivity (allergic contact dermatitis)*.
Allergic inhalant dermatitis. See *Atopy*.
Allergroom, 229t, 235, 917, 1035
Allergy. See also *Atopy*.
    and bacterial infection, 277
    breed(s) with predilection for, 75
    cytologic diagnosis of, 117
    drug. See *Drug reaction, cutaneous*.
    food. See *Food hypersensitivity*.
Allergy test(s), in canine flea bite hypersensitivity, 630–631
    in vitro, 589–592, 591t
    in feline atopy, 606
    intradermal, 584–589, 591t
        allergen selection for, 585–588
        false-negative, causes of, 587t, 587–588
        false-positive, causes of, 587t, 587–588

Allergy test(s) *(Continued)*
    in feline atopy, 605–606
    procedure for, 588–589
  serologic, 589–592, 591t
    in feline atopy, 606
D-trans-Allethrin, 426
Allopurinol, for leishmaniasis, 538
Aloe vera, topical therapy with, 236
Alopecia, 6, 87, 92. See also *Demodicosis, in dogs; Hair; Melanoderma and alopecia; Telogen defluxion.*
  acquired, 887–911
  anagen defluxion and. See *Anagen defluxion.*
  canine, acquired, 887–899, *888, 889*
    drug-induced, 722t
    in follicular dysplasia, 890
    in injection reaction, 896
    in trichorrhexis nodosa, 895, *895, 906*
    minoxidil in, 874
    pinnal, 887, *888, 889*
    topical steroid–induced, *889,* 896, 896–897
  chronic radiant heat dermatitis and, 897–899
  cicatricial, 897
  color dilution. See *Color dilution alopecia.*
  color mutant. See *Color dilution alopecia.*
  congenital, 956–965
    in hamsters, 1441
    in rabbits, 1450, *1450*
    in rats, 1454, *1454*
  cyclic follicular dysplasia and, 890–893
  definition of, 85
  dermatophytosis and, 342–347, *344–345, 346*
  excessive shedding and, 894
  exfoliative dermatitis and thymoma in cats and, 905
  feline, acquired, 900–911
    endocrine, 851
    in follicular dysplasia, 905
    in injection reaction, 902
    in trichorrhexis nodosa, *905,* 905–907, *906*
    pinnal, *888,* 900
    preauricular, *888,* 900
    psychogenic, *1060–1061,* 1066–1070
      cause and pathogenesis of, 1066
      clinical features of, *1060–1061,* 1067, *1068*
      clinical management of, 1069–1070
      diagnosis of, 1067–1069, *1069*
    symmetric, *888,* 900–902
    topical steroid–induced, 902, *903*
  focal, 86
  follicular dysplasia and, canine, 890
    feline, 905
  follicular lipidosis of Rottweilers and, 899, *899, 900*
  hereditary. See *Alopecia, congenital.*
  hyperadrenocorticism and, 780
  hypothyroidism and, 780, 783–784
  idiopathic lymphocytic mural folliculitis in cats and, 907–909, *907–910*
  in ferrets, breeding season and, 1425
    hyperestrogenism and, 1424–1425, *1425*
    miscellaneous causes of, 1426–1427
    testicular neoplasia and, 1425
  in guinea pigs, 1437, *1438*
  in mice, 1444
  in rex mutant cats, 9
  injection reaction and, 92, 896, 902
  medullary trichomalacia and, 895
  paraneoplastic, 902, *903, 904*
  pattern baldness and, 890

Alopecia *(Continued)*
  periocular, in leishmaniasis, 534
  pinnal, canine, 887, *888, 889*
    feline, *888,* 900
  postclipping, 897, *898*
  preauricular, feline, *888,* 900
  primary, 86
  psychogenic, hair examination in, *109*
  seasonal flank, 890–893, *891, 892*
  secondary, 86
  short hair syndrome of silky breeds and, *888,* 897
  superficial bacterial folliculitis and, 293–294
  tardive, 965–974
  telogen defluxion and. See *Telogen defluxion.*
  topical steroid–induced, in cats, 902, *903*
    in dogs, *889,* 896, 896–897
  traction, *888,* 894–895
  traumatic, in hamsters, 1440
  trichoptilosis and, 895
  trichorrhexis nodosa and, in cats, *905,* 905–907, *906*
    in dogs, 895, *895, 906*
Alopecia areata, 198–199, *201,* 761–763
  cause and pathogenesis of, 761
  clinical features of, 761, *762–764*
  clinical management of, 763
  definition of, 761
  diagnosis of, 671, 761–762
  hair examination in, 108, *111*
  histopathology of, 762–763, *764*
  in mice, 1444
  in rabbits, 1450–1451, *1452*
  in rats, 1455
Alopecia mucinosa, in cats, 909–911, *910–911*
  in dogs, 899
Alopecia X, 843–845
Alternaria spp., 387
  colonies of, morphology of, *123*
  dermatitis caused by, *387,* 391, *392*
  in normal flora, 338, 338t
    in dogs, 34
Alternaria alternata, 379, 391
Alternaria tenuissima, 391
Alternative therapy(ies), 263
Aluminum acetate, otic therapy with, 1228
Aluminum acetate solution (Burow's solution; Domeboro), 227, 229t, 230
Amblyomma maculatum, 444
American Holistic Veterinary Medical Association, 263
Aminoglycoside(s), otic therapy with, 1227
Aminosidin, for leishmaniasis, 538
Amitraz, 427
  adverse effects and side effects of, 425, 471–472, 473, 573, 725
  therapy with, antiparasitic, 425
    for canine demodicosis, 470–472, 473
    for canine scabies, 482
    for feline demodicosis, 474, 475, 476
    for feline scabies, 484
    in small animals, dosage and administration of, 1418t
  otic, 1229
  regulation of, 424
Amitriptyline, 1056–1057
  for feline psychogenic alopecia, 1070
Amoxicillin, efficacy of, against *Staphylococcus intermedius,* 282
  in small animals, dosage and administration of, 1418t
Amoxicillin-clavulanate, adverse effects and side effects of, 725, 727

Amoxicillin-clavulanate *(Continued)*
   efficacy of, against coagulase-positive staphylococci, 282
      against *Staphylococcus intermedius*, 282
   long-term therapy with, 287
   systemic, dosage of, 284, 284t
Amphotericin B, adverse effects and side effects of, 414
   antifungal therapy with, 414
   for leishmaniasis, 538
   resistance to, 414
   topical, 356t, 409
Amphotericin B lipid complex, 414
Ampicillin, efficacy of, against *Staphylococcus intermedius*, 282
   in small animals, dosage and administration of, 1418t
   systemic, for bacterial infections, 281
Amyloid, dermal deposits of, 160
Amyloid-A, 767
Amyloid-L, 766
Amyloidosis, 766–769, *768*, *769*
   definition of, 766
   nodular, 769
   paraneoplastic, 1375
Amyloid-P, 766
Anaerobic bacteria. See *Bacteria, anaerobic.*
Anaerobic cellulitis, *302*, 310
Anafranil. See *Clomipramine.*
Anagen, 5, *5*, *6*, 46, *46*, 48
   hypothyroidism and, 783
   stages of, 46
Anagen defluxion, *893*, 893–894
   hair examination in, 108, *109*
Anal area, cryosurgery in, 258
Anal licking, 1066, *1067*
Anal sac(s), abscess of, *1127*, 1202, *1203*
   anatomy of, 1200–1201
   diseases of, 1201–1202
      clinical features of, 1202
      clinical management of, 1202–1203
   expression of, 211, 1202
   impaction of, 1201
      clinical management of, 1202
   infections of, 1201
      clinical management of, 1202–1203
   neoplasia of, 1202
   secretions of, 1201, 1201t
Anaplasia, definition of, 174
Anaplasmosis, 444
Anatrichosoma cutaneum, 436
Anatrichosomiasis, 436, *437*
Anchoring fibril(s), *35*, 36t
Ancobon. See *Flucytosine.*
Ancylostoma spp., pododermatitis caused by, 305
Ancylostoma braziliense, 431
   in humans, 432
Ancylostoma caninum, 431, *432*
   in humans, 432
Ancylostoma dermatitis, 431–432, *432*
Androgen(s), 796–797
   and acne, 1041
   blood levels of, assays for, 797
Androgen-estrogen therapy, for feline acquired symmetric alopecia, 901–902
Anemia, feline infectious, 531
   in hypothyroidism, 858, 860
Anesthesia, for biopsy, 128
Angioedema, *91*, 571–574
   cause and pathogenesis of, 571, 572t
   clinical features of, 572, *573*

Angioedema *(Continued)*
   clinical management of, 574
   drug-induced, in cats, 723t
      in dogs, 722t
Angiogenesis, regulation of, 56
Angiokeratoma, 1303–1304, *1304*
Angiolipoma, 1309, *1311*
Angioma. See *Lymphangioma.*
Angiosarcoma. See *Hemangiosarcoma; Lymphangiosarcoma.*
Angora rabbit, myxomatosis in, 1446
Anipryl. See *L-Deprenyl.*
Annelloconidia, 337
Anonychia, definition of, 1193t
Anoplura, characteristics of, 487
Ant(s), 506–507
Antibiotic(s), and steroids, combination therapy with, 280, 284–285
   antiinflammatory properties of, 285
   concentration-dependent, 283
   costs of, 283
   distribution of, in skin, 281
   efficacy of, factors affecting, 281
   for canine neosporosis, 533
   for leishmaniasis, 538
   for malodorous dogs, 214
   for Rocky Mountain spotted fever, 529
   for small animals, 1418t
   immunomodulatory properties of, 285
   in shampoo, 223
   long-term therapy with, 287–288
      suboptimal protocols for, 287–288
   otic preparations of, 1226t, 1227
   otic therapy with, 1227, 1229
   resistance to, 282
   selection of, factors affecting, 282–283
   systemic, course of treatment with, 284
      dosage of, 284, 284t
      duration of therapy with, 285
      for bacterial infections, 281–285
   time-dependent, 283
   topical, for bacterial infection, 279, 280
      for ear treatment, 1226t, 1226–1227
      potentiation of, with EDTA-Tris, 280
Antibody(ies), homocytotropic, 562
   reaginic, 561–562
   skin-sensitizing, 562
Antidepressant(s), 1056–1057
   for acral lick dermatitis, 1061
   for hypersensitivity disorders, 569–570
Antifungal therapy, 409–415
   in small animals, 1418t
   otic, 1226t, 1228
   rinses for, 410
   shampoos for, 409–410
   spot treatments in, 409
   systemic, 356–358, 357t, 410–415
   topical, 218t, 354–356, 356t, 409–410
      for ear treatment, 1226t, 1227
Antihistamine(s), 1057
   for acral lick dermatitis, 1061
   for hypersensitivity disorders, 567–569, 569t
Anti-inflammatory agent(s), in topical therapy, 218t, 232–233, 233t, 234t
   nonsteroidal, for hypersensitivity disorders, 566–567
   systemic, 238–239
Antimalarial agent(s), for discoid lupus erythematosus, 716
   immunosuppressive therapy with, 677–678

Antimicrobial agent(s), otic preparations of, 1226t, 1227
　topical, 218t, 230–232
　　for ear treatment, 1226t, 1227
Antimicrobial-glucocorticoid agent(s), topical, for ear treatment, 1226t, 1226–1227
Antimycotic(s). See *Antifungal therapy.*
Antinuclear antibody (ANA) test, for systemic lupus erythematosus, 706
Antioxidant(s), 209
Antiparasitic agent(s), 423–430
　in small animals, 1418t
　otic therapy with, 1227t, 1228
　systemic, 427–430
　topical, 218t, 424–427
　　for ear treatment, 1226t, 1228–1229
Antipruritic agent(s), systemic, nonsteroidal, 238–239
　topical, 218t, 228–230, 229t
Antiseborrheic agent(s), 1025–1030
　systemic, 1028
　topical, 218t, 227–228, 1025–1028
Antiseptic agent(s), 230
　otic therapy with, 1228
　topical, for ear treatment, 1227
α_1-Antitrypsin, in cell type identification, 204t
Anus, common and less common dermatoses of, 104t–105t, 105t
Anxiolytic agent(s), 1057
　for acral lick dermatitis, 1061
Aplasia cutis, 936
Apocrine sweat gland(s). See *Sweat gland(s), epitrichial (apocrine).*
Apoptosis, 138–140, *142*
　definition of, 138
　in catagen, 48
Apoptotic body(ies), 140
Arachidonic acid, 30, 208, 239, 1113
Arachnid(s), 440–485
　hypersensitivity to, 636–642
Aralen. See *Chloroquine.*
Arctium spp.. See *Burdock.*
Argentaffin stain(s), 19
Argyrophil stain(s), 19
Armadillo Westie syndrome, 914, 928–929, *930, 932, 933*
Arofylline, for canine atopy, 601
Arrector pili muscle, 41, *42, 43, 55,* 55
　age-related changes in, 64, *65*
　innervation of, 59
Arsenic toxicosis, 1101
Arteriole(s), cutaneous, 56
Arteriovenous anastomoses, 56–57
Arteriovenous fistula, 1095–1096
Arthroconidia, 121, 337, *351*
Arthropod parasite(s), 440–500
Ascaris infection, claw involvement in, 1195
Ascorbic acid. See *Vitamin C.*
Aspergillosis, 403
　in rabbits, 1446
　nasal, 397, 403
Aspergillus spp., 337
　colonies of, morphology of, *123*
　culture of, 121
　cycloheximide sensitivity of, 121
　examination for, specimen collection for, 119
　in normal flora, 34, 338, 338t
　otitis externa caused by, 1214t
Aspergillus deflectus, 403
Aspergillus dermatitis, *397,* 403–404
Aspergillus flavipes, 403

Aspergillus flavus, 403
Aspergillus fumigatus, 403
Aspergillus nidulans, 403
Aspergillus niger, 397, 403
Aspergillus terreus, 403
Asthenia, cutaneous (Ehlers-Danlos syndrome, dermatosparaxis), *159,* 978, 979–984, *980*
　cause and pathogenesis of, 979–982, *980, 981*
　clinical features of, *980,* 982
　clinical management of, 983–984
　definition of, 979
　diagnosis of, 982–983, *983*
　in dogs, *159*
　in rabbits, 1450, *1451*
　types of, 979, 979t
Astringent(s), in topical therapy, 218t, 226–227
Atabrine hydrochloride. See *Quinacrine hydrochloride.*
Atarax. See *Hydroxyzine.*
Atopy. See also *Allergy.*
　and canine demodicosis, co-occurrence of, 473
　and contact hypersensitivity, 1081
　and *Malassezia* dermatitis, 365, 374
　canine, *205,* 574–601
　　avoidance as therapy for, 595–597
　　basophil degranulation test in, 592
　　cause and pathogenesis of, 574–581
　　client education about, 595
　　clinical features of, 581–583, *582, 584*
　　clinical management of, 244, 593–601
　　diagnosis of, *152,* 583–593
　　diagnostic criteria for, 592–593
　　environmental management for, 595–597, 596t
　　experimental therapies for, 601
　　histopathology of, 593, *594*
　　hyposensitization for, 597–601, 598t
　　intradermal allergy testing in, 584–589, 591t
　　serologic allergy tests in, 589–592, 591t
　　systemic antipruritic agents for, 601
　　topical therapy for, 597–601
　clinical management of, 239, 244, 593–601, 607–608, 609t
　cytologic diagnosis of, *114,* 117
　feline, *184,* 601–608
　　allergy testing in, 605–606
　　basophil degranulation test in, 606
　　cause and pathogenesis of, 602
　　clinical features of, 602–603, *604*
　　clinical management of, 607–608, 609t
　　diagnosis of, 603–607, *605*
　　histopathology of, 606–607, *607*
　　hyposensitization for, 608, 609t
　　serum in vitro testing in, 606
　foot licking in, 1066
　in ferrets, 1426, *1427*
　insects and, 486–487
Atrophy, epidermal, 135–136, *140*
　epithelial, 197–199
　follicular, 166, *167*
　in injection site reaction, in cats, 723t
　　in dogs, 722t
　of connective tissue, 197–199
　of dermal collagen, 159
　of dermal elastin, 159
Aural cholesteatoma, 1216
Auranofin, immunosuppressive therapy with, 672t, 675–676
Aureobasidium spp., in normal flora, of dogs, 338, 338t
Auricular chondritis, canine, *759,* 759–760

Auricular chondritis (*Continued*)
  feline, 748–749, *759–760*, *760*
  in rats, 1454
Aurothioglucose, immunosuppressive therapy with, 672t, 675–676
Aurotrichia, acquired, *1008*, 1022
  in miniature Schnauzers, 978
Australian shepherd. See *Shepherd, Australian.*
Austrobilharzia variglandis, 436
Autoantibody(ies), in cutaneous lupus erythematosus, 702
Autoimmune dermatosis, 667, 678–769
  classification of, 670
  cytologic diagnosis of, *114*, 117, 667–671
  otitis externa caused by, 1206t, 1212
Autoimmune subepidermal bullous dermatosis, 694–701
Aveeno, 229t, 230, 236
Avermectin(s), 428, 445
Avoidance, of allergens, as therapy for hypersensitivity, 563, 595–597
  of sun. See *Sun avoidance.*
Axilla, common and less common dermatoses of, 104t
Azathioprine, adverse effects and side effects of, 673–674
  antiseborrheic effects of, 920
  for discoid lupus erythematosus, 716
  for graft-versus-host disease, 720
  for idiopathic sterile granuloma and pyogranuloma, 1139–1140
  for pemphigus, 681
  for pemphigus foliaceus, 689–690
  for systemic lupus erythematosus, 711
  for vasculitis, 753
  immunosuppressive therapy with, 672t, 673–674
Azithromycin, efficacy of, against *Staphylococcus intermedius*, 282
  systemic, dosage of, 284t
Azium. See *Dexamethasone.*
Azole(s), antifungal therapy with, 411–413
  drug interactions with, 412
  mechanism of action of, 411
  topical, 409
Azulfidine. See *Sulfasalazine.*

Babesia canis, 534
Babesia gibsoni, 534
Babesia vogeli, 534
Babesiosis, 444
  canine, *530–531*, 534
Bacillus spp., as resident microflora, in dogs, 275
  as transient flora, in cats, 275
  in dogs, 275
Bacitracin, topical, for bacterial infection, 279, 280
Back, common and less common dermatoses of, 104t
Bacquiloprim-sulfadimethoxine, systemic, dosage of, 284t
Bacteria, adhesion of, 276
  aerobic, cellulitis caused by, 309–310
    gram-negative, as resident flora, in dogs, 34, 275
  anaerobic, 276
    cellulitis caused by, *302*, 310
    in abscesses in cats, 311
    in subcutaneous abscesses in cats, 310
    otitis media caused by, 1214t
  and acne, 1041
  antibacterial sensitivity of, 276
  culture of, indications for, 125
    specimen collection for, 125
  extracellular, in cytologic diagnosis, *115*, 118t
  gram-negative, as resident flora, in dogs, 34, 275

Bacteria (*Continued*)
  hypersensitivity to, *637*, 647–650, *649*
  in normal flora, 274
    resident, 274–275
      numbers of, 276–277
    transient, 274–277
  in surface debris, 155, *155*
  intracellular, in cytologic diagnosis, *113*, 117, 118t
  L-forms, infections caused by, 327
  otitis externa caused by, *1210*, 1213, 1214t
  otitis media caused by, 1214t
  phagocytosed, *113*
  susceptibility testing of, indications for, 125
Bacterial colonization, and infection, comparison of, 277
  cytologic identification of, 116, 118t
Bacterial infection(s), 277–278. See also *Pyoderma.*
  and bacterial colonization, comparison of, 277
  causes of, 277
  deep, 298–324
    cytologic findings in, 117
    treatment of, 285
  diagnosis of, 125
    cytologic, *113*, 116, 118t, 125
  in cats, systemic therapy for, 281, 282
  in dogs, 188
    systemic therapy for, 281
  in ferrets, 1417, *1418*
  in gerbils, 1428
  in guinea pigs, *1418*, *1420*, 1430
  in hamsters, *1418*, 1439
  in mice, 1442
  in rabbits, 1444–1446
  in rats, 1452–1453
  metabolic causes of, 278
  mixed, antibiotic therapy for, 283
  primary, 278
  recurrence of, 278
    antibiotic therapy for, 283
    chronic, management of, 286–288
  relapse of, 285
  secondary, 277
  superficial, 288–298
  surface, 288
  treatment of, 279–288
    re-examination during, 285
    systemic, 281, 282
    topical, 279–281
Bacterial overgrowth, 117
Bacterin(s), autogenous staphylococcal, 286
Bacteroides spp., cellulitis caused by, 310
  in infections, 276
  in oral flora of cats, 276
  in subcutaneous abscesses in cats, 310
Baldness, pattern, 890, *954*, *963–964*, 965–966, *966*
  clinical management of, 253
Balinese cat, acromelanism in, 1012–1013
  hair color of, 8
Ballooning degeneration, epidermal, 142–143, *145*
Banamine. See *Flunixin meglumine.*
Barbering, in gerbils, 1429
  in guinea pigs, 1437
  in mice, 1444
  in rabbits, 1450
  in rats, 1454
Barrier function, of hair, 31, 274
  of skin, 31
Bartonella hinselar, 493
Basal cell carcinoma, 1261–1263, *1262*

Basal cell carcinoma (Continued)
　breed(s) with predilection for, 1237t
　clear cell, 1262
　in hamsters, 1442
　in rabbits, 1451
　in rats, 1455
　keratinizing, 1262
　melanotic, 1262, *1262*
　solid, 1262
　with sebaceous differentiation, 1271
Basal cell plasma membrane, 34
Basal cell tumor(s), 1013, 1021, 1259–1263
　benign feline, *1254*, 1260–1261, *1261*
　　breed(s) with predilection for, 1237t
　solid. See *Neuroendocrine tumor(s), primary cutaneous.*
Basal lamina, of basement membrane zone. See *Lamina densa (basal lamina).*
Basement membrane zone, epidermal, *11*, 13
　components of, 34–35, 36t
　functions of, 34
　thickened, 172, *172*
　ultrastructure of, 34–35, *35*
　follicular (glassy membrane), 43, *47*, *49*
Basenji, immunoproliferative enteropathy of, 760–761
　risk for non-neoplastic skin disorders in, 77t
Basidiobolus spp., 384
Basophil(s), 781. See also *Hypersensitivity, cutaneous basophil.*
　functions of, 558
　in cytologic diagnosis, *114*, *117*, 118t
Basophil degranulation test, 592
　in feline atopy, 606
Basosquamous carcinoma. See *Basal cell carcinoma, keratinizing.*
Basset hound. See *Hound, Basset.*
Bathing. See also *Grooming.*
　of cats, 215, 1038
　of dogs, 212–213
　　preparation for, 210–211
　of seborrheic animal, 916–918, 1035–1036, 1038
Beagle, acromegaly in, *826*
　actinic keratoses in, 1391
　amyloidosis in, 767
　atopy in, 575
　black hair follicular dysplasia in, 962
　cell proliferation kinetics in, 7
　colloid milium in, 1178
　congenital hypotrichosis in, 958
　Ehlers-Danlos syndrome in, 982
　familial vasculopathy in, 987
　hair growth in, daily, 6
　hemangiopericytoma in, 1302
　hemangiosarcomas in, 1299
　lymphocytic (Hashimoto's) thyroiditis in, 851
　mast cell tumors in, 1320
　oral papillomatosis in, 1240
　Pelodera dermatitis in, 435
　pododermatitis in, 344–345
　risk for neoplastic skin disorders and non-neoplastic lumps in, 1237t, 1238t
　risk for non-neoplastic skin disorders in, 75, 76, 77t
　sebaceous gland hyperplasia in, 1271
　solar dermatitis in, 1079
　squamous cell carcinoma in, 1251
　trichomycosis axillaris in, 327
　zinc-responsive dermatosis in, 1120
Beauceron, atopy in, 581
　dermatomyositis in, 940

Beauceron (Continued)
　epidermolysis bullosa in, dystrophic, 939
　　junctional, 939
　systemic lupus erythematosus in, 706
Bedlington terrier. See *Terrier, Bedlington.*
Bee(s), 505–506
Behavioral change(s), in hyperadrenocorticism, 804
Belgian sheepdog. See *Sheepdog, Belgian (Belgian Tervuren).*
Belgian Tervuren. See *Sheepdog, Belgian (Belgian Tervuren).*
Bendiocarb, 425
Benzalkonium chloride, 232
　in shampoo, 223
Benzodiazepine(s), 1057
　for acral lick dermatitis, 1061
Benzoyl peroxide, 228, 231
　adverse effects and side effects of, 231
　antiseborrheic therapy with, 918, 1026–1027, 1036
　in gels, 226
　in shampoo, 223
　topical, for bacterial infection, 279–280
Benzoyl-Plus, 231
Berger de Beauce, risk for non-neoplastic skin disorders in, 77t
Bernese mountain dog, color dilution alopecia in, 967
　hemangiosarcomas in, 1299
　histiocytic sarcoma in, 1346–1347, 1352
　histiocytosis of, 189
　malignant histiocytosis in, 1346
　risk for neoplastic skin disorders and non-neoplastic lumps in, 1237t
　snow nose in, 1017
　systemic histiocytosis in, 1346, 1352
Betadine. See *Povidone-iodine.*
Betamethasone, adrenocortical suppression by, 232
　adverse effects and side effects of, 232
　for discoid lupus erythematosus, 716
　injectable, 247t
　otic therapy with, 1226
Betamethasone-17-valerate, adrenocortical suppression by, 232
Betasone. See *Betamethasone.*
Bichon Frisé, congenital hypotrichosis in, 958
　drug reactions in, 721
　epiphora in, 1188
　systemic lupus erythematosus in, 705
　vaccine reaction in, 744
Bioallethrin, 426
Biopsy, 125–131
　anesthesia for, 128
　artifacts in, 130–131, *131*, 148, *149*
　complications of, 128–129
　excisional, 128
　in bacterial infection, 285
　in claw disease, 1200
　in demodicosis, 467–469
　in dermatophytosis, 349
　in hypothyroidism, 859, 861
　in immune-mediated skin disease, 668
　in leishmaniasis, 536, *536*, 537
　in *Malassezia* dermatitis, 370, *370–372*
　in pemphigus complex, 681
　indications for, 125–126, 278
　instruments for, 127
　"nonspecific" findings in, 201–202
　pattern analysis in, 177–178
　punch, 127–128

Biopsy (*Continued*)
  site for, 126–127
  specimen in, collection of, 127
    fixation of, 129
    handling of, 128, 129
    special procedures for, 202–204
    staining of, 129, 130t
  technique for, 127–128
  thyroid, 788
  timing of, 126
Biotin, deficiency of, 1118
  in ferrets, 1426
  in mice, 1444
  in rats, 1453
  supplementation of, in claw disease, 1200
Bipolaris spiciferum, 379
Birbeck's granule(s), 24
Birman cat, cold agglutinin disease in, 717
  congenital hypotrichosis in, 959, *960*
  hair color of, 8
Bite wound(s), abscesses caused by, in cats, 310–311
  in guinea pigs, 1437
  in hamsters, 1439
  in mice, 1444
  in rats, 1454
Bitter apple, for acral lick dermatitis, 1063
Black flies, 502
  bites of, *501, 502, 502, 503*
Black hair follicular dysplasia, 959–965
  cause and pathogenesis of, 962
  clinical features of, *954,* 962
  definition of, 959
  diagnosis of, 962–965, *963*
Black widow spider, 484
Black-legged tick(s), 444
Blaschko's lines, 9
Blastoconidia, 336–337
Blastomyces dermatitidis, 337, 391–392
  culture of, 121
Blastomycosis, *387,* 391–394
  cause of, 391–392
  claw involvement in, 1195
  clinical findings in, *387,* 392–393, *393, 401*
  clinical management of, 393
  diagnosis of, 393, *393, 394*
  European. See *Cryptococcosis.*
  in cats, 393, *401*
  in dogs, *387,* 392–393
  in ferrets, 1419
  pathogenesis of, 391–392
  pododermatitis caused by, 305
  public health considerations with, 394
Blepharitis, 1185–1186, *1187*
  definition of, 1185
  in aspergillosis, 397, 403
Blister(s). See also *Bulla/bullae; Vesicle(s).*
  tug-of-war, 1103
Blood pressure, in hyperadrenocorticism, 805
Blood vessel(s), cutaneous, 56, *56–58, 57.* See also
    Vasculitis.
  histologic changes in, 171
  disorders of, 987–992
  innervation of, 59, *60*
Blowflies, 503
Blue ferret syndrome, 1426–1427
Body fold intertrigo, *1106,* 1107
Body temperature. See *Heat, body; Temperature.*
Boerboel, dermoid cyst (sinus) in, 936

Borrelia burgdorferi, 326–327
  and morphea, 1146
Borreliosis, Lyme, 326–327
Borzoi, antithyroglobulin antibody(ies) in, 852
  antithyroid antibody(ies) in, 789
  lymphedema in, 990
  risk for non-neoplastic skin disorders in, 77t
Boston terrier. See *Terrier, Boston.*
Botryomycosis (cutaneous bacterial granuloma, bacterial
    pseudomycetoma), *302,* 311–312, *313*
  in mice, 1442
Bouvier de Flanders, adrenal hyperplasia–like syndrome
    in, *850*
  follicular dysplasia in, 971
  risk for neoplastic skin disorders and non-neoplastic
    lumps in, 1237t
  seasonal flank alopecia in, 891
  squamous cell carcinoma in, 1251
Bowen's disease, 1244, *1254,* 1258–1259, *1259, 1260*
  pigmented plaque in, 1013, *1013*
Boxer, alopecia in, minoxidil for, 874
  anatrichosomiasis in, 436
  atopy in, 581
  calcinosis circumscripta in, 1400
  callus dermatitis in, 1102
  chondrosarcomas in, 1315
  coccidioidomycosis in, 394
  dermoid cyst (sinus) in, 1378
  distichiasis in, 1188
  Ehlers-Danlos syndrome in, 982
  estrogen-responsive dermatosis of, 829
  fibromas in, 1282
  follicular dysplasia in, 890, 971
  food hypersensitivity in, 618
  haircoat of, 7
  hemangiopericytoma in, 1302
  hemangiosarcomas in, 1299
  histiocytomas in, 1347
  hyperadrenocorticism in, 800
  hypothyroidism in, 852, 853
  idiopathic sterile granuloma and pyogranuloma in,
      1136
  interstitial cell tumors in, 843
  lymphomas in, 1331
  mast cell tumors in, 1320
  melanocytoma in, 1359
  multiple collagenous cysts in, and renal pathology, 1383
  muzzle folliculitis and furunculosis in, 304
  papillomas in, 1240
  pododermatitis in, 305
  risk for neoplastic skin disorders and non-neoplastic
    lumps in, 1237t
  risk for non-neoplastic skin disorders in, 76, 77t
  seasonal flank alopecia in, 823, 890, 893
  seminoma in, 843
  Sertoli's cell tumor in, 840
  squamous cell carcinoma in, 1251
  sterile pyogranuloma on feet of, 305
  white, truncal solar dermatitis in, 1079
Brachycladium spiciferum. See *Bipolaris spiciferum.*
Brachyonychia, definition of, 1193t
Brachytherapy, noninvasive, for squamous cell carcinoma,
    1257
Branchial cyst(s), 1382
Breeding season alopecia, in ferrets, 1425
Brewer's yeast, indications for, in canine neosporosis, 533
Brittany spaniel. See *Spaniel, Brittany.*
Bromocriptine mesylate, 811

Bronchogenic carcinoma, 1089–1090
  cutaneous metastases of, *1366,* 1374, *1375*
Brown recluse spider, 484
Brown-Brenn stain, staining characteristics of various substances with, 130t
Brucella canis, 325
Brucellosis, 325
  canine, *613*
Brushing, 210
Bubblies, subepidermal. See *Subepidermal vacuolar alteration.*
Bulbitis, 195, *201*
Bull mastiff. See *Mastiff, bull.*
Bull terrier. See *Terrier, bull.*
Bulla/bullae, 87, *90,* 148
Bulldog, English, calcinosis cutis in, 1399
  demodicosis in, 461, 465
  follicular dysplasia in, 890, 971
  hyperestrogenism in, 829
  hypothyroidism in, 852
  intertrigo in, facial fold, 1107
    tail fold, 1107
  lymphedema in, 990
  Malassezia dermatitis in, *348–349*
  mast cell tumors in, 1320
  muzzle folliculitis and furunculosis in, 304
  pododermatitis in, 305
  postclipping alopecia in, *898*
  risk for neoplastic skin disorders and non-neoplastic lumps in, 1237t
  risk for non-neoplastic skin disorders in, 78t
  seasonal flank alopecia in, 823, 890, *891*
  seborrhea in, 913
  sterile pyogranuloma on feet of, 305
  superficial bacterial folliculitis in, *294, 296*
  French, congenital hypotrichosis in, 958
    follicular dysplasia in, 890, 971
    lentigo in, *1007*
    seasonal flank alopecia in, 891
Bullous dermatosis, autoimmune subepidermal, 694–701
Bullous pemphigoid, 694–700
  causes of, 13, 694–695
  claw involvement in, 1195
  clinical features of, 695–697, *696–697*
  clinical management of, 698–700
  diagnosis of, *670, 671,* 697, *698, 699*
  drug-induced, in dogs, 722t
  in dogs, *194*
  pathogenesis of, 694–695
Bullous pemphigoid antigen(s), 36t, 694
  I (BPAG I), 13, 22t, 694
  II (BPAG II), 13, 22t, 694
Burdock, glossitis caused by, 1091, *1092*
  skin lesions caused by, 1091, *1092, 1094, 1095*
  stomatitis caused by, 1091, *1092*
Burkholderia pseudomallei, 328
Burmese cat, acromelanism in, 1012–1013
  congenital hypotrichosis in, 959
  demodicosis in, 474
  grooming for, 215
  psychogenic dermatoses in, 1056
Burn(s), *1082,* 1083–1087
  cause and pathogenesis of, 1083–1084
  clinical features of, *1082,* 1084–1085
  clinical management of, 1085–1087, *1086–1087*
  diagnosis of, 1085, *1085*
  full-thickness, 1084
  partial-thickness, 1084

Burn(s) *(Continued)*
  radiant heat, *1086–1087,* 1087
  scar from, 97
Burow's solution (aluminum acetate solution; Domeboro), 227, 229t, 230
Burrowing, in ferrets, 1427
Buspirone (BuSpar), 1057
Butoxypropylene glycol, 427

Cadherin(s), 22t, 545
  in morphogenesis of skin appendages, 3
Cairn terrier. See *Terrier, Cairn.*
Caladryl, 229, 229t
Calcinosis circumscripta, *1393, 1399,* 1400–1401, *1401*
  breed(s) with predilection for, 1238t
Calcinosis cutis, 1106, 1108, *1108,* 1398t, 1398–1401
  dystrophic, 789
  idiopathic, 1398t, 1399, *1399*
  in hyperadrenocorticism, 800, *802,* 804, 815
  metastatic, 1398t, 1398–1399
  widespread, 1399
Calcipotriene, antiseborrheic therapy with, 1030
Calcipotriol, antiseborrheic therapy with, 1030
Calcitriol, antiseborrheic therapy with, 919, 1030
Calcium, percutaneous penetration of, 1399
Calcium-calmodulin interactions, 20
Caldesmon, 20
Calendula, 263
Calicivirus infection, feline, 525
Calliphorids, 503
Callus, 87, *100, 1092,* 1101–1102
Callus dermatitis and pyoderma, *1097,* 1102–1103
Candida spp., culture of, 362
  cycloheximide sensitivity of, 121
  identification of, 362
  in normal flora, 361
  superficial mycoses caused by, 338
Candida albicans, 361
  colonies of, morphology of, *123*
  hypersensitivity to, 650
  in cytologic diagnosis, *115,* 117
Candida gulliermondii, 361
Candida krusei, 361
Candida parapsilosis, 361
Candida pseudotropicalis, 361
Candida stellatoidea, 361
Candida tropicalis, 361
Candida zeylanoides, in dogs, 362
Candidiasis, 361–363
  cause of, 361
  clinical findings in, 348, *348–349,* 362
  clinical management of, 362–363
  diagnosis of, 362, *363*
  in cats, 362
  in dogs, *348, 348–349,* 362
  in guinea pigs, 1431
  pathogenesis of, 361
  pododermatitis caused by, 305
  topical therapy for, 409
Candidosis. See *Candidiasis.*
Canine disorder(s). See *specific disorder.*
Canthaxanthin, 254
Capillary(ies), cutaneous, 56
  in fat, 63
Capitulum, definition of, 440
Caprylic acid, 235
Capsaicin (HEET), for acral lick dermatitis, 1063

Carbamate(s), topical, antiparasitic therapy with, 425
Carbamide peroxide, 1223
Carbaryl, 425
Carbowax 1500, 226
Carcinoid syndrome, 1052
Carcinoma, basal cell. See *Basal cell carcinoma*.
  basosquamous. See *Basal cell carcinoma, keratinizing*.
  bronchogenic, cutaneous metastases of, *1366*, 1374, *1375*
  ceruminal gland, *1196*, 1208, *1208*, *1209*
  epidermoid. See *Squamous cell carcinoma*.
  gastric, 1021
  metastatic, claw involvement in, 1198
  pharyngeal, cutaneous metastases of, *1366*, 1373
  prostatic, cutaneous metastases of, 1374, *1374*
  sebaceous, in rabbits, 1451
  sebaceous gland, in dogs, 1271
  squamous cell. See *Squamous cell carcinoma*.
  sweat gland, 1198
Carnelian bear dog, hypopituitarism in, 811
  pituitary dwarfism in, 819
β-Carotene, 209, 254
  skin color change caused by, 1023
Carprofen, adverse reaction to, 721
Caryosporosis, canine, 532, *533*
Castration-responsive dermatosis, 843–845
Cat(s). See also *Feline*; individual species.
  abscesses in, 276
  acquired skin fragility syndrome of, 199, 1170–1173, *1171–1172*
  agouti, 8
  breeds of, alopecic, *957*, 957–958
    with predilection for skin disorders, 75, 77t–82t
  cutaneous mast cells of, 39, *40*
  deafness in, 8
  epidermis of, *10*
    immunoglobulins of, 31
  footpad of, *12*
  furunculosis in, 300, *302*
  grooming for, haircoat type and, 215
    special problems in, 215
  hair color of, 8–9
    and personality, 9
    Maltese dilution and, 9
  hair follicles of, *10*
  hair growth in, annual, 4
    daily, 6
  hair of, length of, 9
    types of, 8–9
  haircoat of, pointed, 8
    tipped, 8
    types of, 215
  household, resident flora of, 275
  immunomodulation in, 287
  Langerhans' cells of, 24
  mechanoreceptors in, 61
  normal microflora of. See *Microflora*.
  oral flora of, 276
  orange, lentigo simplex in, 1006–1007, *1008*, *1009*
  perforating dermatitis in, 1168–1170, *1169*, *1170*
  piebald, 8
    white spotting in, 8
  plague in, 325–326
  preauricular ulcerative dermatitis of, idiopathic, 1177
  rex mutant of, 9
  sarcoid in, 1285, *1288*, *1289*
  secondary hairs of, 4
  skin of, normal pH of, 3
    thickness of, 3

Cat(s) *(Continued)*
  squamous cell carcinoma in, *1241*
  stratum corneum in, thickness of, 28
  sweating in, 53
  tabby, 8
    Abyssinian pattern of, 8
    blotch pattern of, 8
    mackerel pattern of, 8
  tail gland of, 55
  thermoregulation in, respiratory rate and, 54
    saliva and, 54
  tortoiseshell, 8
  white, squamous cell carcinoma in, *1241*
    with blue eyes, 8
  white-eared, pinna of, risk for skin disorders in, 76
  wire-hair mutation in, 9
  zinc deficiency in, 1122
Cat food, fat in, 1112
Cat fur mite(s), 446, *447*
  skin scraping for, 101, 107
Catagen, 5, 5–6, *47*, 48
Catan Dog's tag, 498
Catapres. See *Clonidine*.
Catenin(s), 20, 22t
Caterpillar(s), dermatitis caused by, 507, *507*
Cathelicidins, 33
CD antigen(s), in cell type identification, 204t
Cediopsylla simplex, on rabbits, 1449
Cefadroxil, adverse effects and side effects of, 725
  systemic, dosage of, 284t
Cell death, 136–137
  programmed (spontaneous), 138–139
Cell envelope, of corneocytes, 28, 29
Cell type(s), identification of, markers for, 204t
Cellular infiltrate(s), dermal, 177
Cellulitis, 299–300
  aerobic, 309–310
  anaerobic, 302, 310
  canine juvenile (pyoderma, puppy strangles, sterile granulomatous dermatitis and lymphedema), 328, 1163–1167
    cause and pathogenesis of, 1164
    clinical features of, *1158*, 1165
    clinical management of, 1166–1167
    definition of, 1163
    diagnosis of, *1165*, 1165–1166, *1166*
    otitis externa caused by, 1213
  clostridial, 302
  staphylococcal, in dogs, 324–325
Cephalexin, adverse effects and side effects of, 197, 724–725, 735
  distribution of, in skin, 281
  in small animals, dosage and administration of, 1418t
  otic therapy with, 1229
  systemic, dosage of, 284, 284t
Cephalosporin(s), adverse effects and side effects of, 721
  efficacy of, against coagulase-positive staphylococci, 282
  long-term therapy with, 287
  systemic, for bacterial infections, 281
Ceramide(s), 30–31
Cerumen, immunoglobulins in, 1204
Ceruminal gland(s), carcinoma of, *1196*
  neoplasia of, 1196–1197, *1208*, 1208–1209, *1209*
Ceruminolytic(s), 1222t, 1222–1223, *1223*
Chalazion, 1186–1188
Chamomile, 263

Chédiak-Higashi syndrome, 977, 1014
  diagnosis of, 76
Chemoattractant(s), for neutrophils, 557, 557t
Chemokine(s), 545, 547t–548t
Chemotherapy, for squamous cell carcinoma, 1257–1258
Cheque Drops, 838
Chesapeake Bay retriever. See *Retriever, Chesapeake Bay.*
Chest, lower, common and less common dermatoses of, 104t
Cheyletiella blakei, 453, *454*
  in humans, *449*
Cheyletiella dermatitis. See *Cheyletiellosis.*
Cheyletiella mite(s), acetate tape impression for, 107
  eggs of, 108, *112*
  examination for, 106, 107
  flea comb for, 107
  skin scraping for, 101, 106
Cheyletiella parasitivorax, 453, *454*
  in rabbits, 1448
Cheyletiella yasguri, 453, *454*, *455*
Cheyletiellosis, *449*, 453–457
  cause of, 453
  diagnosis of, 456, *457*
  in guinea pigs, 1433
  in rabbits, *1447*, 1448
  pathogenesis of, 453–456
  treatment of, 456–457
Cheyletus eruditis, 453
Cheyllletiella mite infestation. See *Cheyletiellosis.*
Chicago disease. See *Blastomycosis.*
Chief complaint, in diagnosis, 75
Chigger mite(s). See *Trombiculosis (chigger mites).*
Chihuahua, anal sac disorders in, 1201
  atopy in, 581
  color dilution alopecia in, 967
  follicular dysplasia in, 971
  melanocytoma in, 1359
  pattern baldness in, 965
  pinnal alopecia in, 887
  risk for neoplastic skin disorders and non-neoplastic lumps in, 1238t
  risk for non-neoplastic skin disorders in, 77t
Chin, common and less common dermatoses of, 104t
Chinchilla, dermatoses of, 1416–1417
  fatty acid deficiency in, 1417
  fungal infections of, 1416
  fur chewing in, 1417
  fur-slip in, 1417
  nutritional deficiency in, 1417
  zinc deficiency in, 1417
Chinese crested dog, 957, *957*
Chinese Shar Pei. See *Shar Pei.*
Chirodiscoides caviae, in guinea pigs, 1433, *1434*
Chitin, 336
  synthesis of, inhibitors of, in insect control, 426
Chitosan, 336
Chitosanide, 221
Chlorambucil, for discoid lupus erythematosus, 716
  for pemphigus, 681
  for pemphigus foliaceus, 689
  immunosuppressive therapy with, 672t, 673
Chloramine(s), in topical therapy, 231
Chloramphenicol, adverse effects and side effects of, 724–725
  efficacy of, against coagulase-positive staphylococci, 282
    against staphylococcal infection, 283
    against *Staphylococcus intermedius*, 282

Chloramphenicol *(Continued)*
    for Rocky Mountain spotted fever, 529
    in small animals, dosage and administration of, 1418t
    otic therapy with, 1227
    systemic, dosage of, 284t
ChlorhexiDerm, 917, 1035. See also *Chlorhexidine, shampoo.*
ChlorhexiDerm Maxi. See *Chlorhexidine, shampoo.*
ChlorhexiDerm Maximum. See *Chlorhexidine, topical.*
Chlorhexidine, 1035
    for contaminated wounds, 267
    in topical therapy, 230
    shampoo, 223, 356t
    topical, 356t, 409
      for bacterial infection, 279, 280
Chlorhexidine diacetate, preoperative use of, 255
Chlorhexidine/miconazole shampoo, antifungal therapy with, 409
Chlorinated hydrocarbon(s), antiparasitic therapy with, 424
Chloroacetate esterase, in cell type identification, 204t
Chloroaluminum sulfonated phthalocyanine, 237
Chloroquine, 254, 678
    for discoid lupus erythematosus, 716
Chlorpheniramine, for feline psychogenic alopecia, 1070
Chlorphenolac, for keratin clearance, in fungal diagnosis, 120–121
    formula for, 120
Chlorpyrifos, 423, 425
Cholesteatoma, aural, 1216
Cholesterol cleft(s), dermal, 160, *161*
Cholinesterase inhibitor(s), antiparasitic therapy with, 424–425
Chondritis. See *Auricular chondritis.*
Chondroitin-4-sulfate, 38
Chondroitin-6-sulfate, 36t, 38
Chondroma, 1315–1316
Chondrosarcoma, 1315–1316, *1317*
Chow Chow, adrenal hyperplasia–like syndrome in, 847
    adult-onset hyposomatotropism in, 822
    aspergillosis in, *397*
    color dilution alopecia in, 967
    dermatomyositis in, 940
    dermoid cyst (sinus) in, 936
    follicular dysplasia in, 890
    haircoat of, 8
    hypogonadism in, 844–845
    hypothyroidism in, 852
    melanocytoma in, 1359
    mucinosis in, 1174
    pemphigus foliaceus in, 686, 687
    postclipping alopecia in, 897
    risk for neoplastic skin disorders and non-neoplastic lumps in, 1238t
    risk for non-neoplastic skin disorders in, 75, 77t
    tyrosinase deficiency in, 1018–1019
    uveodermatologic syndrome in, 757
Chromoblastomycosis, definition of, 376
Chromomycosis, 379
    definition of, 376
Chromophobe(s), 781
Chronic radiant heat dermatitis, 897–899
Chronology of veterinary dermatology, 1459–1464
Chrysops spp., 502
Chrysosporium spp., in normal flora, 338, 338t
Chrysotherapy, for pemphigus, 681
    for pemphigus foliaceus, 689–690
    for systemic lupus erythematosus, 711
    immunosuppressive therapy with, 672t, 675–676

Chyle, subcutaneous, 1090
Chymase, 39
  in cell type identification, 204t
Cicatricial alopecia, 897
Cicatricial pemphigoid. See *Pemphigoid, mucous membrane.*
Cicatricial pemphigoid antigen, 36t
Cimetidine, for recurrent bacterial infections, 286
Ciprofloxacin, in small animals, dosage and administration of, 1418t
  otic therapy with, 1229
  pinnal erythema in cats caused by, 1023
Circumanal (perianal) glands, 54–55
  tumors of, *1272*, 1279–1281, *1280*, *1281*
    breed(s) with predilection for, 1237t
Citrinin, 1101
Citrobacter spp., otitis media caused by, 1214t
Citronella, 427, 502
Citrulline, 43
Civatte body(ies), 140
Cladophialiophora spp., 379
Cladosporium spp., in normal flora, 338, 338t
Cladosporum bantianum. See *Xylohypha bantiana.*
Cladosporum trichoides. See *Xylohypha bantiana.*
Clam digger's itch, 436
Clarithromycin, efficacy of, against *Staphylococcus intermedius*, 282
  systemic, dosage of, 284t
Claw(s), anatomy of, 1190–1193, *1191–1192*
  clipping of, 210–211
    in cats, 215
  common and less common dermatoses of, 105t
  dermatophyte collection from, 120
  diseases of, 1190, 1193–1200
    asymmetric versus symmetric, 1194
    diagnosis of, 1199–1200
    in cats, 1193, 1194t
    in dogs, 1193, 1194t
    miscellaneous causes of, 1199
    terminology for, 1193, 1193t
    treatment of, 1200
  infections of, *1189*, 1195
  neoplasia of, *1196–1197*, 1198
  of guinea pig, overgrowth of, 1439
  red/brown, 1022
  supranumerary, *1197*, 1199
  trauma to, 1193–1194
Clear cell(s). See *Melanocyte(s).*
Cleft(s), artifactual, 148, *149*
  at dermoepidermal junction, 147–148
  cholesterol, dermal, 160, *161*
  epidermal, 147–148, *148*
Client compliance, in skin treatment, 215–217, 216t
Client-veterinarian relationship, 75, 93
Clindamycin, efficacy of, against *Staphylococcus intermedius*, 282
  for canine neosporosis, 533
  otic therapy with, 1229
  systemic, dosage of, 284t
Clipping, 214. See also *Grooming.*
  alopecia after, 897, *898*
  before bathing, 223
  of claws, 210–211
    complications of, 1194
    in cats, 215
Clitoral hypertrophy, in hyperadrenocorticism, 800, *801*, 804, 846
Clofazamine, skin color change caused by, 1023

Clomicalm. See *Clomipramine.*
Clomipramine, 1056–1057
  for feline psychogenic alopecia, 1070
Clonidine, in diagnosis of GH deficiency, 794–795
Clorox, 231
Clostridium spp., as resident flora, in dogs, 34, 275
  cellulitis caused by, 310
  in infections, 276
  in subcutaneous abscesses in cats, 310
Clostridium welchii, in anal sacs, 1201
Clotrimazole, topical, 356t, 409
Clotrimazole/betamethasone, topical, 356t
Clotrimazole/betamethasone/gentamicin, topical, 356t
Club hair, 48, *49*, *50*
Cluster differentiation (CD), 543
Coagulation, electrosurgical, 262
Coagulation necrosis, 136
Coal tar solution, 1027
Cocci. See also *Staphylococci; Streptococci.*
  identification of, 116
  phagocytosed, 113
Coccidioides immitis, 337, 394, *396*
  culture of, 121
Coccidioidomycosis, cause of, 394
  clinical findings in, 387
  clinical management of, 395
  diagnosis of, 395, *396*
  in cats, clinical findings in, 395
  in dogs, clinical findings in, 387, 394, *396*
  in ferrets, 1419
  pathogenesis of, 394
Cochliomyia hominovorax, 503
Cocker spaniel. See *Spaniel, cocker.*
Colchicine, for vasculitis, 753
  immunosuppressive therapy with, 678
Cold agglutinin disease, 717–719
Cold cream, 225
Cold hemagglutinin disease, 717
Collagen, abnormalities of, 37
  dermal, 36–38, *37*
    atrophy of, 159
    degeneration of, 157
    dysplasia of, 159, *159*
    dystrophic mineralization of, 157–158, *158*
    fibrinoid degeneration of, 157
    hyalinization of, 156–157
    lysis of, 157
    pathologic changes in, terminology for, 156–159
  disorders of, 978–986
  epidermal, *11*
  functions of, 36, 37
  in dermal edema, 163–164
  synthesis of, 37
    inhibitors of, 37
    stimulators of, 37
  types of, 36t, 37
    in cell type identification, 204t
Collagenase(s), 37
Collagenous nevus/nevi, *1380–1381*, 1382–1384, *1384*, *1385*
  breed(s) with predilection for, 1238t
  multiple, 986
    renal pathology with, 1383
  paraneoplastic, 1375
Collarette(s), epidermal, 86, *87*, *97*, 156
Collie, Bearded, black hair follicular dysplasia in, 962
  pemphigus foliaceus in, 686
  benign fibrous histiocytoma in, 1354

Collie (Continued)
  Border, black hair follicular dysplasia in, 962
  bullous pemphigoid in, 695
  cutaneous histiocytosis in, 1353
  cyclic hematopoiesis in, 977–978, 1014
  dermatomyositis in, 938, 940, 942, *944*
  dermatophytosis in, *344–345*
  epidermolysis bullosa simplex in, 938
  fly bites on, *501*, 502
  food hypersensitivity in, 618
  hemangiopericytoma in, 1302
  idiopathic sterile granuloma and pyogranuloma in, 1136
  idiopathic ulcerative dermatosis of, 707, 717, 946–947
  immunodeficiency in, 279t
  ivermectin contraindicated in, 1229
  ivermectin sensitivity in, 428–429
  keratoacanthoma in, 1248
  nasal folliculitis and furunculosis in, 303
  pemphigus erythematosus in, 690, 692
  protothecosis in, 405
  pyotraumatic dermatitis in, 1104
  risk for neoplastic skin disorders and non-neoplastic lumps in, 1237t
  risk for non-neoplastic skin disorders in, 75, 78t
  Sertoli's cell tumor in, 840
  squamous cell carcinoma in, *1241*
  superficial bacterial folliculitis in, 294
  systemic lupus erythematosus in, 705
  vitiligo in, 1015
  Waardenburg-Klein syndrome in, 1014
Colloid body(ies). See *Apoptotic body(ies)*.
Colloid milium, 1178, *1179*
Colonic adenocarcinoma, cutaneous metastases of, *1366*, *1373*, *1374*
Color dilution, normal, hair examination in, 108, *110*
Color dilution alopecia, 965–970, 1029
  cause and pathogenesis of, 967
  clinical features of, 967–968
  clinical management of, 968–970
  diagnosis of, 968, *969*, *970*
  differential diagnosis of, 968
  hair examination in, 108, *110*
  haircoat color and, 76
Combined immunodeficiency, 279t
Comedo, 87, 95
Comedo nevi, 1389, *1391*
Comedo syndrome, in miniature Schnauzer. See *Schnauzer comedo syndrome*.
Comedone(s), in hyperadrenocorticism, 800, *802*, 803
Comedone syndrome, ventral, 1103
Common brown spider, 484
Complement, 559
  deficiency of, 279t
  epidermal, 31
Compliance, client, in skin treatment, 215–217, 216t
Conditioner(s), 211
  for hair, 212, 218t
Condyloma, canine. See *Transmissible venereal tumor*.
Conidiobolus spp., 384
Conidiogenous cell, definition of, 336
Conidiophore, definition of, 336
Conidium/conidia, definition of, 336
  types of, 336–337
Conjunctivitis, canine nictitans plasmacytic, treatment of, 674
Connective tissue, atrophy of, 197–199
  destruction of, 37
Conofite. See *Miconazole*.

Contact dermatitis, allergic. See *Contact hypersensitivity (allergic contact dermatitis)*.
  diagnosis of, 143, 144, 145
  drug-induced, in cats, 721, 723t
    in dogs, 721, 722t
  in cats, diagnosis of, 154
  in ferrets, 1426
  in hamsters, 1441
  in rabbits, 1450
  irritant, *1075*, 1081–1083, *1082*
Contact hypersensitivity (allergic contact dermatitis), 88, 608–615
  afferent phase of, 609
  cause and pathogenesis of, 608–611, 612t
  clinical features of, *604*, 611–615, 612t, *613*
  clinical management of, 615
  diagnosis of, 612–615
  ear involvement in, *1210–1211*, 1211–1212
  efferent (elicitation) phase of, 609
  histopathology of, 614–615
Contagious ecthyma, 524
Contagious viral pustular dermatitis, 524
Coonhound, Bluetick, blastomycosis in, 392
  dermatophytosis in, *344–345*
  Treeing Walker, blastomycosis in, 392
Copper, deficiency of, 1020, 1119
  in rabbits, 1449
Coral snake(s), 1090
Cordylobia spp., 505
Cordylobia anthropophaga, *501*, 504, *504*
Corgi. See *Welsh corgi*.
Corium. See *Dermis*.
Corneocyte(s), 27–28
Corneometer, 32
Cornification, 29
  defects of, 913–949
Cornifin, 28
Corps ronds, 138
Cortex, of hair shaft, 39, *41*, *44*, 108, *110*
Corticosteroid(s), antiseborrheic therapy with, 919–920
  for dermatomyositis, 945
  topical, for acral lick dermatitis, 1063
Corticotroph(s), 781
Corticotropin. See *ACTH*.
Corticotropin-releasing factor (CRF), 781
Corticotropin-releasing factor stimulation test, 793
  in hyperadrenocorticism, 810
Cortisol, blood levels of, determination of, 790–791
  measurement of, in dogs, 808
Cortisol response test(s), 791–793
Cortisol/creatinine ratio, urinary, in cats, 818
  in dogs, 808–809
Corynebacterium spp., as transient flora, in dogs, 275
  in oral flora of cats, 276
  trichomycosis axillaris caused by, 327
Corynebacterium minutissimum, fluorescence of, 119
Corynebacterium pseudotuberculosis, in abscesses in cats, 311
Cowpox virus infection, feline. See *Feline poxvirus infection*.
Cream(s), formulations of, and efficacy of active ingredients, 218t, 224–225
Cream rinse, 212, 918, 1035
Cresol(s), contraindications to, in cats, 230
  in topical therapy, 230
Critical temperature, definition of, 53
  for dogs, 53
Crotalidae, 1090

Crust(s), 86, 87, *94, 154,* 154–156, *155*
  cellular, 155
  hemorrhagic, 154–155
  palisading, 155
  serocellular (exudative), *154,* 155
  serous, 154
Cryofibrinogen(s), 717
Cryofibrinogenemia, 717–719
Cryoglobulin(s), 717
Cryoglobulinemia, *713,* 717–719, *718*
Cryopathic hemolytic anemia, 717
Cryosurgery, 255–259
  advantages of, 256
  disadvantages of, 257
  for acral lick dermatitis, 1064
  for squamous cell carcinoma, 1257
  freezing agents for, 257
  indications for, 258–259
  principles of, 255–256
  units for, 257–258
Cryptococcosis, 395–400
  cause of, 395
  claw involvement in, 1195
  clinical management of, 399–400
  diagnosis of, 398, *398–400*
  in cats, clinical findings in, *397, 398, 399, 400*
  in dogs, clinical findings in, *395, 397, 398, 399*
  in guinea pigs, 1431
  pathogenesis of, 395
  pododermatitis caused by, 305
Cryptococcus neoformans, 337, 388, 395
  cycloheximide sensitivity of, 121
  serotypes of, 395
  stain for, 119
  varieties of, 395
Cryptorchidism, 838, 843
Ctenocephalides canis, 491, 492. See also *Flea(s).*
Ctenocephalides felis felis, 491, *491,* 492. See also *Flea(s).*
  on ferrets, 1419
  on hamsters, 1440
  on mice, 1443
  on rabbits, 1449
  on rats, 1453
Curvularia geniculata, 377
Cushing's disease. See *Hyperadrenocorticism (Cushing's disease, Cushing's syndrome).*
Cutaneous arteriovenous fistula. See *Arteriovenous fistula.*
Cutaneous asthenia. See *Asthenia, cutaneous (Ehlers-Danlos syndrome, dermatosparaxis).*
Cutaneous bacterial granuloma (botryomycosis, bacterial pseudomycetoma), *302,* 311–312, *313*
  in mice, 1442
Cutaneous cyst(s). See *Cyst(s).*
Cutaneous drug reaction. See *Drug reaction, cutaneous.*
Cutaneous flushing, 1022–1023, 1052
Cutaneous histiocytosis. See *Histiocytosis.*
Cutaneous horn(s), 1244, *1392,* 1394–1396, *1396–1398*
  feline leukemia virus and, 517
  in dogs, *1241, 1242*
  multiple, in cats, 528
Cutaneous laxity, idiopathic acquired, 1173
Cutaneous mucinosis, 996–997, *1401,* 1402, *1402*
Cutaneous neuroendocrine tumor(s), primary, 1369–1370, *1370*
Cutaneous oncology, 1236–1239
Cutaneous papilloma. See *Papilloma(s), cutaneous.*
Cutaneous plasmacytoma. See *Plasmacytoma.*
Cutaneous tuberculosis. See *Tuberculosis.*
Cutaneous vasculitis. See *Vasculitis.*
Cuterebra spp., *501,* 504
  in ferrets, 1419
  infestation of, 505
Cuterebra buccata, 1449
Cuterebra cuniculi, 1449
Cuterebra horripilum, 1449
Cuticle, of hair shaft, 39, *41,* 108, *110*
Cutis laxa, 987
Cutting, electrosurgical method for, 261
  without coagulation, 261
Cyclic hematopoiesis, 279t
  canine, 977–978, 1014
Cyclic neutropenia, canine, 977–978, 1014
Cyclin(s), 1239
Cycloheximide, fungal sensitivity to, 121
Cyclophosphamide, adverse effects and side effects of, 672, 673
  antineoplastic therapy with, 672, 673
  for systemic lupus erythematosus, 711
  for vasculitis, 753
  immunosuppressive therapy with, 671–673, 672t
Cyclosporine, adverse effects and side effects of, 244, 723, 1246
  antiseborrheic therapy with, 1030
  dosage and administration of, 244
  drug interactions with, 244
  for canine atopy, 244, 601
  for discoid lupus erythematosus, 716
  for graft-versus-host disease, 720
  for granulomatous sebaceous adenitis, 1146
  for hypersensitivity disorders, 570–571
  for immune-mediated disorders, 244, 720
  immunosuppressive therapy with, 672t, 674
  indications for, 243–244
  pharmacology of, 243–244
  topical, 674
Cydectin. See *Moxidectin.*
Cyproheptadine hydrochloride, 811
Cyromazine, 430
Cyst(s), 87, *92*
  branchial, 1382
  cutaneous, 1375–1382
  dermoid, 1378–1379
    breed(s) with predilection for, 1238t
  dermoid (dermoid sinus), 936–937
  epidermal inclusion. See *Cyst(s), infundibular.*
  epidermoid. See *Cyst(s), infundibular.*
  epitrichial (apocrine) sweat gland, *1366,* 1379–1381, *1380–1382*
  follicular, *1366,* 1375–1378, *1376, 1377*
    breed(s) with predilection for, 1238t
  horn (keratin cysts), 156
  hybrid, 1378, *1379*
  infundibular, 1376–1378, *1377, 1378*
  isthmus-catagen, 1377, *1379*
  matrical, 1378
  pseudohorn, 156
  sebaceous. See *Cyst(s), infundibular.*
  sebaceous gland, 1381
  tricholemmal, 1377, *1379*
Cystadenoma, 1276
  papillary, *1277*
Cystocercoid infection, 440
Cystomatosis, of epitrichial (apocrine) sweat glands, 1380–1381, 1381
Cythioate, 428, 499
Cytocrinia, 19

Cytokeratin, 20–22, 22t, 52
  in cell type identification, 204t
Cytokine(s), 543–545, 546t
Cytologic examination, 112–117
  findings in, *113–115*, 116–117, 118t
  specimen collection for, 112–116
  stains used in, 116
Cytology, of normal skin, *115*, 116
Cytostan A, 28
Cytoxan. See *Cyclophosphamide*.

Dachshund, acanthosis nigricans in, 975, 976, 1007
  alopecia areata in, 761, *762*, *764*
  black hair follicular dysplasia in, 962
  calcinosis cutis in, 1399
  callus dermatitis in, 1102
  chronic ulcerative blepharitis in, 1186
  claw disease in, clinical management of, 1200
  color dilution alopecia in, 967
  congenital microtia in, *1231*, 1232
  ear margin dermatosis in, 1044, *1044*
  Ehlers-Danlos syndrome in, 982
  estrogen-responsive dermatosis of, 829
  food hypersensitivity in, 618
  granulomatous sebaceous adenitis in, 1141
  haircoat of, 7
  histiocytomas in, 1347
  hyperadrenocorticism in, 800
  hyperpigmentation in, *1010*
  hypogonadism in, 833
  hypothyroidism in, 852
  idiopathic onychodystrophy in, 1198
  juvenile cellulitis in, 1165
  lipomas in, 1308
  Malassezia dermatitis in, 365
  mast cell tumors in, 1320
  panniculitis in, *1158*, 1159
  pattern baldness in, *963–964*, 965
  pemphigus foliaceus in, 686
  pinnal alopecia in, 887, *888*, *889*
  pododermatitis in, 305
  risk for neoplastic skin disorders and non-neoplastic lumps in, 1237t
  risk for non-neoplastic skin disorders in, 75, 78t
  sebaceous gland hyperplasia in, 1271
  seborrhea in, 913, 1032
  squamous cell carcinoma in, 1251
  sterile pyogranuloma on feet of, 305
  vasculitis in, 744
  vitiligo in, 1015
Dalmatian, actinic keratoses in, 1391
  atopy in, 581
  drug reactions in, 721
  food hypersensitivity in, 618
  hemangiosarcomas in, 1299
  pododermatitis in, 305
  postbathing folliculitis in, 212
  risk for neoplastic skin disorders and non-neoplastic lumps in, 1237t, 1238t
  risk for non-neoplastic skin disorders in, 75, 76, 78t
  solar dermatitis in, 1079
  squamous cell carcinoma in, 1251
  Waardenburg-Klein syndrome in, 1014
Dandie Dinmont terrier, hyperadrenocorticism in, 800
Dandruff, walking. See *Cheyletiellosis*.
Dapsone, adverse effects and side effects of, 1127
  for pemphigus, 682

Dapsone (*Continued*)
  for subcorneal pustular dermatosis, 1127–1128
  for vasculitis, 753
  immunosuppressive therapy with, 672t, 676–677
  toxicity of, 676–677
Darier's disease, 138
Dawn dish soap, 213
D-Basic shampoo, 1035
Deafness, after ear flushing, 1224
  in cats, 8
Decorin, 38
Dectomax. See *Doramectin*.
Decubital ulcer(s), *1097*, 1103
  management of, 267–268
Deep metatarsal/metacarpal tortis. See *Focal metatarsal fistulation*.
Deer fly, 502
Deer tick(s), 444
Deerhound, Scottish, congenital hypothyroidism in, 852
Defend Exspot Insecticide for Dogs, 498
β-Defensin(s), 33
Dell(s), epidermal, 156
Deltamethrin, 426, 498
Demodectic mite(s). See *Demodicosis*.
Demodex aurati, 1439, *1440*
Demodex canis, 106, 457–458, *458–460*, 474
Demodex cati, 106, 474, *474–476*, *475*
  in Bowen's disease, 1258, *1260*
Demodex caviae, 1434, *1434*
Demodex criceti, 474, 475, 1439
Demodex cuniculi, on rabbits, 1449
Demodex gatoi, 106, 474, *474–476*, *476*
Demodicosis, 277
  adult-onset, 278, 461, 467
  claw involvement in, 1195
  diagnosis of, 185
  in cats, *466*, *474–475*, *474–476*
    generalized, *466*
  in dogs, *169*, *196*, 457–474
    adult-onset, 278, 461, 467
    and atopy, co-occurrence of, 473
    bacterial complications of, 465
    cause of, 457–458, *458–460*
    cellular immunity in, 463–464
    clinical features of, *462*, 464–465, *466*
    clinical management of, 469–474
    diagnosis of, 465–467
    differential diagnosis of, 469
    generalized, 459–463, *462*, 465, *466*, 469–474
    histopathology of, 467–469, *467–469*
    humoral immunity in, 463
    localized, *449*, 459–460, *462*, 464–465, 469
    nonspecific immunity in, 463
    transmission of, 458
    types of, 459–463
  in ferrets, 1419
  in gerbils, 1428
  in guinea pigs, 1433–1434, *1436*
  in hamsters, 1439–1440, *1440*
  in hyperadrenocorticism, 803, *803*
  in rabbits, 1449
  in rats, 1453
  pododermatitis caused by, 305
  skin scraping for, 101–106, 467
Demulcent(s), 227
Dendrocytes, dermal, 38, 39
Depigmentation, nasal (Dudley nose), 1016–1017
Depo-Medrol. See *Methylprednisolone acetate*.

Depo-Provera. See *Medroxyprogesterone acetate; Progesterone, repositol.*
L-Deprenyl, for canine hyperadrenocorticism, 811–812
   for feline hyperadrenocorticism, 818
Derm Caps, 239, 929, 945, 1113, 1198
   for feline eosinophilic granuloma, 1133
Dermacentor spp., 443, 444
Dermacentor andersoni, 444, *444*
Dermacentor occidentalis, 444
Dermacentor variabilis, 444, 445
Dermacool, 229, 229t
Dermal collagen. See *Collagen.*
Dermal dysplasia, 936
Dermal hair papilla, 41, 44, 46, *46, 47,* 48, *49*
Dermal macrofibril bundle (DMB), 35
Dermal Soothe, 229
   antipruritic therapy with, 229t
   for pruritus, 228
Dermanyssus gallinae, 445–446, *446.* See also *Mite(s), poultry.*
   skin scraping for, 101
DermaPet shampoo(s), 917, 918, 1026–1027, 1035
Dermatan sulfate, 38
Dermatitis, acral lick. See *Acral lick dermatitis.*
   acute moist, 288, 300. See also *Pyotraumatic dermatitis.*
   allergic contact. See *Contact hypersensitivity (allergic contact dermatitis).*
   allergic inhalant. See *Atopy.*
   Alternaria, 387, 391, 392
   Ancylostoma, 431–432, *432*
   Aspergillus, 397, 403–404
   callus, and pyoderma, *1097,* 1102–1103
   caterpillar, 507, *507*
   Cheyletiella. See *Cheyletiellosis.*
   chronic atopic, *99*
   chronic radiant heat, 897–899
   contagious viral pustular, 524
   diffuse, 184–189, *185*
      cell types in, 184–187
      characterization of, 187–189
      granulomatous, 184, *185*
      nongranulomatous, 184, 189
   feline immunodeficiency virus, 519, *520, 521*
   feline leukemia virus, 517, *518–519*
   fibrosing, 196, *202*
   filarial, 644
   fly, 500–502, *501*
   Geotrichum, 408
   granulomatous, 184, *187*
      interstitial, drug-induced, 725, *727*
   heartworm, 439
   herpes, feline. See *Feline rhinotracheitis infection.*
   hookworm, 431–432, *432,* 433
      claw involvement in, 1195
   in leishmaniasis, 530–531, 534–535, *535*
   inhalant allergic. See *Atopy.*
   interface. See *Interface dermatitis.*
   interstitial. See *Interstitial dermatitis.*
   intraepidermal vesicopustular, drug-induced, 729, *730*
   irritant contact, *1075,* 1081–1083, *1082*
   localized moist (sore dewlap), in rabbits, 1445
   Malassezia. See *Malassezia dermatitis.*
   miliary, 294, 343, 650
      differential diagnosis of, 633, 633t
   mosquito, 502–503
   mucocutaneous, drug-induced, in dogs, 722t
   nasal solar. See *Nasal solar dermatitis.*

Dermatitis *(Continued)*
   nodular, 184–189, *185*
      cell types in, 184–187
      characterization of, 187–189
      nongranulomatous, 189
   Pelodera, 432–434, *434–436*
      in guinea pigs, 1433
      in humans, 432
   perforating, 1168–1170, *1169, 1170*
   perivascular. See *Perivascular dermatitis.*
   pinnal, 1211
   preauricular ulcerative, idiopathic, of cats, 1177
   psychogenic, feline, *1060–1061,* 1066–1070
      cause and pathogenesis of, 1066
      clinical features of, *1060–1061,* 1067, *1068*
      clinical management of, 1069–1070
      diagnosis of, 1067–1069, *1069*
      pododermatitis caused by, 305
   pustular, contagious viral, 524
      intraepidermal, 189–190, *192,* 193t
      subepidermal, 190, 193t
      superficial, in kittens, 288
   pyogranulomatous, 184, *188, 313, 317*
   pyotraumatic, 288, 300, *1097, 1104,* 1104–1105
   rhabditic. See *Pelodera dermatitis.*
   Rhodotorula, 375, *376*
   Schistosoma, 436
   seborrheic, 1030
      localized, 1030
   skin fold, 288. See also *Intertrigo.*
   solar. See *Nasal solar dermatitis; Solar dermatitis.*
   staphylococcal, in dogs, 205
   subepidermal vesicular, drug-induced, 729
   traumatic, in hamsters, 1440
   Trichosporon, 407–408
   Uncinaria, 431–432, *433*
   vesicopustular, 190
      drug-induced, 729, *730*
   vesicular, intraepidermal, 189–190
      subepidermal, 190
Dermatitis medicamentosa. See *Drug reaction, cutaneous.*
Dermatobia hominis, 504
Dermatochalasis. See *Cutis laxa.*
Dermatofibroma, 1283
Dermatofibrosis, nodular, in German shepherd, *1380–1381,* 1382–1383
Dermatohistopathology, confusing terms used in, 176–177
   pattern analysis in, 177–202
   terminology for, 131
Dermatology, veterinary, chronology of, 1459–1464
Dermatome(s), 59
Dermatomycosis, definition of, 336
Dermatomyositis, breed(s) with predilection for, 75
   claw involvement in, 1199
   diagnosis of, *146*
   familial canine, 940–946
      cause and pathogenesis of, 940
      clinical features of, *941–943,* 942–943
      clinical management of, 945–946
      diagnosis of, 943–944, *944–946*
      differential diagnosis of, 943
   in dogs, *169*
      diagnosis of, *148*
   paraneoplastic, 1375
Dermatophagoides farinae, 451, 453
Dermatophagoides pteronyssinus, 451, 453
Dermatophilosis, 296–298, *297*

Dermatophilus congolensis, dermatitis caused by. See *Dermatophilosis.*
Dermatophyte(s), 336
  anthropophilic, 339–340, 340t
  culture of, 337
  examination for, 119–121
    direct, 120–121
    specimen collection for, 119–120
  geophilic, 339–340, 340t
  identification of, 122, *123*
  in normal flora, 338
  superficial mycoses caused by, 338–361
  zoophilic, 339, 340t
Dermatophyte test medium (DTM), 121–122, *123,* 349
Dermatophytic kerion, 343, *344–345,* 351
Dermatophytosis, 277, 339–361
  cause of, 339–342, 340t
  chronic, 358
  claw involvement in, 1195
  climate and, 339
  clinical findings in, 342–347
  clinical management of, 353–361
    in catteries, 359
    in kittens, 360–361
  definition of, 336
  diagnosis of, 119–121, 347–353, *350–355*
  environmental decontamination in, 359–360
  hair examination in, 108, *110*
  histopathology of, 349, *350, 351*
  hyperthermia for, 238
  in cats, clinical findings in, 343–347, *346, 348*
    histopathology of, *350, 353*
    incidence of, 339
  in cattery, environmental decontamination in, 359–360
    management of, 358–361
    monitoring response to therapy in, 361
    prevention of, 361
    treatment of cats in, 359
    treatment of kittens only in, 360–361
  in dogs, clinical findings in, 342–343, *344–346*
    in Europe, 343
    incidence of, 339
    sylvatic, 343
  in ferrets, 1418–1419
  in guinea pigs, 1430–1431, *1431*
  in hamsters, 1439
  in humans, 347, *348*
    animal-origin, 347, *348*
  in mice, 1442–1443
  in multiple-cat households, management of, 358–361
  in rabbits, 1446
  in rats, 1453
  inflammatory response to, 341
  pathogenesis of, 339–342
  pododermatitis caused by, 305
  recurrence of, 358
  risk factors for, 342
  seasonality of, 339
  sylvatic, treatment of, 354
  systemic therapy for, 356–358, 357t
  topical therapy for, 354–356, 356t, 409
  transmission of, 339
  vaccination against, 358
Dermatopsychosomatics, 1055
Dermatosis/dermatoses, atrophic, 197–199, *203*
  bullous, autoimmune subepidermal, 694–701
  canine ear margin, *1039,* 1043–1045, *1044, 1045*

Dermatosis/dermatoses *(Continued)*
  castration-responsive, 843–845
    in male dog, 843
  developmental, 197–199
  endocrine, 197–199
  estrogen-responsive, 796
    of female animals, *830,* 831–833, *832, 833*
  exfoliative, 1049. See also *Exfoliative dermatitis.*
  eyelid, 1185–1190, 1186t
  FeLV, 175, *175*
  generic dog food, *1114–1115,* 1122, 1122–1123
  growth hormone-responsive. See *Hyposomatotropism (pseudo-Cushing's syndrome, GH-responsive dermatosis).*
  invisible, 199–201
  lichenoid, *1126–1127,* 1130–1132, *1132*
  linear preputial, *830*
  loss of heterozygosity in, 65
  mixed reaction patterns in, 199, *205*
  nutritional, 197–199
  periocular, 1186t
  psychogenic, 1055–1071
    canine, 1058–1066
    feline, 1066–1071
  pustular, linear IgA, canine, 748, *756, 756*
  pyoderma-like, 328
  sex hormone, 827–851
    rare forms of, 851
  sterile pustular, cytologic diagnosis of, 117
  subcorneal pustular, 89, *1125–1128, 1126–1128*
    cytologic diagnosis of, 117
  testosterone-responsive, 797
    of male animals, *830,* 837–838, *838*
  transient acantholytic, 138
  vitamin A–responsive, *1008,* 1036–1037, *1037*
    dermatohistopathology of, 133, *136*
  zinc-responsive, breed(s) with predilection for, 75
    dermatohistopathology of, 133, *135*
Dermatosparaxis. See *Asthenia, cutaneous (Ehlers-Danlos syndrome, dermatosparaxis).*
Dermazole. See *Miconazole, shampoo.*
Dermis, 34, *35,* 35–39
  age-related changes in, 64–65
  cellular elements of, *37, 39, 40*
  cellular infiltrates in, 177
  deep, 36, 38
  deposits in, 160, *161*
  dermatohistopathology of, terminology for, 156–165
  development of, 2
  fibers of, 36–38
    collagenous, 36–38, *37.* See also *Collagen.*
    elastin, 36–38
    reticular, 36
  functions of, 35–36
  ground (interstitial) substance of, 38
  ripening of, 2
  scrotal, 36
  superficial, 36, *37*–38
Dermoid cyst(s). See *Cyst(s), dermoid.*
Dermolysis, epidermal. See *Acantholysis.*
Desaturase, 208
Desiccation, electrosurgical, 261–262
Desmin, in cell type identification, 204t
Desmocalmin, 20
Desmocollin(s), 20
Desmoglea, 20
Desmoglein(s), 20

Desmoplakin(s), 20, 22t
Desmoplasia, dermal, 161
Desmorrhexis, epidermal. See *Acantholysis*.
Desmosine, 37
Desmosome(s), 19–20, 22t, 23
  core glycoproteins of, 20
  plaque proteins of, 20, 22t
Detergent(s), 231–232
  exposure to, 31
Dexamethasone, for pemphigus foliaceus, 689
  immunosuppressive therapy with, 672t
  injectable, 247t
  otic therapy with, 1226
Dexamethasone suppression test, high-dose, 792–793
  in hyperadrenocorticism, 810
  in cats, 818
  low-dose, 792
    in hyperadrenocorticism, 809–810
Diabetes mellitus, 868, *870*
  and hyperadrenocorticism, in cats, 816
Diagnosis, histopathologic pattern in, 177–202
  history-taking in, 71, 72–84, *74*
  medical history in, 82–84
  methods used in, 71–205
  physical examination in, 84–94
  record-keeping in, 71–72, *73*, *74*
  systematic approach to, 71, 72t
Diagnostic plan, development of, 93–94
Diamanus montanus, plague transmission by, 325
Diapedesis, of erythrocytes, in epidermis, 147
Diascopy, 88, *91*, *100*
Diazepam, 1057
  adverse effects and side effects of, in cats, 1057
  for acral lick dermatitis, 1061–1063
  for feline psychogenic alopecia, 1070
Diet, and pemphigus, 680, 682
  and skin, 207–210
  assessment of, 84
  for ferrets, 1426
  for xanthomatosis, 874
  hypoallergenic, for dogs, 623–624
  in fatty acid deficiency, 1113
  limited-protein, for cats, 627
Diethylcarbamazine, adverse effects and side effects of, 721, 725, 726
Diethylstilbestrol, for feline acquired symmetric alopecia, 902
Diethyltoluamide (DEET), 427
Diff Quik. See *Wright's stain, modified (Diff Quik)*.
Differential diagnosis, 93
Differin. See *Adapalene*.
Diffuse dermatitis. See *Dermatitis, diffuse*.
Diffuse lipomatosis, idiopathic, 1173, *1173–1175*
Difloxacin, systemic, dosage of, 284t
Diflucan. See *Fluconazole*.
Dihomo γ-linolenic acid (DGLA), 208, 239
5,6-Dihydroxyindole (DHI), 17
5,6-Dihydroxyindole-2-carboxylic acid (DHICA), 17
Diiodothyronine, 782–783
Dilated pore of Winer, *1254*, 1265–1267, *1266*, *1267*
Dimethyl phthalate, 427
Dimethyl sulfoxide (DMSO), 219
  for acral lick dermatitis, 1063
  topical therapy with, 235–236
Dip(s), antifungal, 356, 356t
  for feline scabies, 484
  for scabies, 482
  lindane, 424

Dipeptidyl peptidase II, in cell type identification, 204t
Diphenhydramine, in shampoo, 223
Diptera, 500–507
Dipylidium caninum, 493
Direct smear(s), for *Malassezia* spp., 368
  technique for, 112, *113*, 117
Dirofilaria immitis, 439
Dirofilaria repens, 439
Dirofilariasis, 439, 643–644, *644*, *645*
Disinfectant(s), 223, 230
Disseminated intravascular coagulation, 1089
  claw involvement in, 1199
Dissitimurus exudrus, 379
Distemper, canine, *518*, 522–524, *523*
Distichiasis, 1188
DMSO. See *Dimethyl sulfoxide (DMSO)*.
Doberman pinscher, acral lick dermatitis in, 1058
  alopecia in, minoxidil for, 874
  antithyroglobulin antibody(ies) in, 852
  antithyroid antibody(ies) in, 789
  benign familial pemphigus in, 947, *948*
  blastomycosis in, 392
  bullous pemphigoid in, 695
  calcinosis cutis in, 1399
  callus dermatitis in, 1102
  coccidioidomycosis in, 394
  color dilution alopecia in, 967–968
  demodicosis in, 461, *462*
  dermal melanocytes of, 39
  dilution alopecia in, 76
  drug reactions in, 721, 723
  drug-induced dermatosis in, *1052*
  drug-related hypopigmentation in, *1020*
  fibromas in, 1282
  fibrosarcomas in, 1287
  fibrovascular papillomas in, 1284
  flank sucking in, *1060–1061*, 1065
  follicular dysplasia in, 971
  histiocytomas in, 1347
  hypopigmentation in, 975, *1008–1009*
  hypothyroidism in, 852
  ichthyosis in, *924*
  immunodeficiency in, 279t
  lichenoid dermatosis in, 1131
  lipomas in, 1308
  melanocytic neoplasms in, 1359
  melanocytoma in, 1359
  miniature, color dilution alopecia in, 967
    follicular dysplasia in, 971
    haircoat of, 7
  mucinosis in, 1402
  mucocutaneous hypopigmentation in, 1018
  muzzle folliculitis and furunculosis in, 304
  myxomas and myxosarcomas in, 1290
  nasal depigmentation in, 1017
  pemphigus foliaceus in, 686, *687*
  postbathing folliculitis in, 212
  psychogenic dermatoses in, 1056
  risk for neoplastic skin disorders and non-neoplastic lumps in, 1237t, 1238t
  risk for non-neoplastic skin disorders in, 75, 78t
  seasonal flank alopecia in, 891
  seborrhea in, 227, 913, 915, 1032
  vitiligo in, 1015
  zinc-responsive dermatosis in, 1120
Dog(s). See also individual species.
  bacterial pyoderma in, 28
  bathing of, 212–213

Dog(s) (Continued)
  breeds of, alopecic, 957, 957–958, 958
    with predilection for skin disorders, 75, 77t–82t
  critical temperature for, 53
  cutaneous mast cells of, 39, 40
  dermal dendrocytes in, 38
  epidermis of, 10
    immunoglobulins of, 31
    turnover time for, 31
  footpad of, 12
  hair follicles of, 10
  hair growth in, annual, 4
    daily, 6
  hair types in, 7–8
  haircoat of, 7–8
  hunting (dolichocephalic) breeds of, nasal folliculitis and furunculosis in, 303
  Langerhans' cells of, 24
  normal microflora of. See Microflora.
  resident microflora of, 33–34
  respiratory rate of, in thermoregulation, 54
  skin of, hydration of, 32
    normal pH of, 3
    thickness of, 3
  stratum corneum in, thickness of, 28
  sweating in, 53
  tail gland of, 54–55
  wild, haircoat of, 7
Dog food, fat in, 1112
  generic, dermatosis caused by, 1114–1115, 1122, 1122–1123
  storage of, 209
Dogiel's end-bulb. See Meissner's corpuscle.
Dogue de Bordeaux, footpad hyperkeratosis in, 935
  risk for non-neoplastic skin disorders in, 78t
Domeboro, 227, 229t, 230
Dopachrome, 17
Dopachrome tautomerase, 17
Dopaquinone, 17
Doramectin, 428, 429
  systemic, antiparasitic therapy with, 430
Dot blot hybridization, 1239
Down hair(s), 4
Doxepin, 1056–1057
Doxycycline, efficacy of, against staphylococcal infection, 283
    against Staphylococcus intermedius, 282
  for Rocky Mountain spotted fever, 529
  in small animals, dosage and administration of, 1418t
  systemic, dosage of, 284t
Dracunculiasis, 435, 437–439, 438
  in ferrets, 1419
Dracunculus insignis, 437
Dracunculus medinensis, 437
Drechslera spiciferum. See Bipolaris spiciferum.
Droncit. See Praziquantel.
Drug(s), absorption of, 218–220
  diffusion coefficient of, 219
  physiologic response to, 1052, 1052–1053
  psychotropic, 1056–1057
  skin color changes caused by, 1023
Drug allergy. See Drug reaction, cutaneous.
Drug eruption. See Drug reaction, cutaneous.
Drug reaction, cutaneous, 720–729
    cause and pathogenesis of, 720–721, 722t–723t
    claw involvement in, 1199
    clinical features of, 721–725, 722t–723t, 724–725, 726
    clinical management of, 729

Drug reaction (Continued)
    diagnosis of, 725–729, 728t, 729–731
    in cats, 721, 723t
    in dogs, 197, 721, 722t–723t
    predictable versus unpredictable (idiosyncratic), 720
Drug-receptor interaction, 219
Dry bath(s), 213, 215
Dry skin, 220
Dudley nose, 1016–1017
Dunstan's blue line, 175–176, 177
Durakyl, 427
Duratrol, 423
Dwarfism, pituitary, 817, 819–822, 820
Dyshesion, epidermal. See Acantholysis.
Dyskeratosis, 137–138, 1025
Dysplasia, dermal, 936
  epidermal, 173, 173
    canine, 914–915
    in West Highland white terrier, 914, 928–929, 930–933
  follicular, 6, 6, 152, 153, 166–168
  of dermal collagen, 159, 159
  of sebaceous glands, 168–170
Dystrophic mineralization, of dermal collagen, 157–158, 158

Ear(s). See also Otitis externa.
  anatomy of, 1203, 1203–1204, 1205
  cleaning of, 918, 1205, 1221–1225, 1222t
    in cats, 215
  common and less common dermatoses of, 103t
  examination of, 211
  external, diseases of, 1203–1232
  fold dermatitis of, 1216
  glandular disorders of, 1212
  hair removal from, 1207
  microanatomy of, 1215
  middle, 1204
    flushing of, 1216, 1217
  neoplasia of, 1208
  normal flora of, 1214t
  parasites in, 1206t, 1209–1211
  physiology of, 1203–1204
  progressive pathologic changes in, 1205, 1210, 1215–1216
Ear canal(s), cleaning of, 1221–1225, 1222t
  drying agents for, 1222t, 1224–1225
  flushing of, 1224
  mineralized, 1211, 1218
Ear canker, in rabbits, 1448
Ear cleanser(s), 1222t
Ear margin dermatosis, canine, 1038, 1043–1045, 1044, 1045
Ear mite(s) (Otodectes cynotis), 449, 450–452, 451, 452, 1205, 1209
  examination for, 107
  in cats, 435
  in dogs, 435
  in ferrets, 1419
  skin scraping for, 101
Ecchymosis, 87, 88
Eccrine sweat gland(s). See Sweat gland(s), atrichial (eccrine).
Echidnophaga gallinacea, 488–489, 491, 492
Ecthyma, contagious, 524
Ectodex Dog Wash, 470
  on ferrets, 1419, 1420

Ectoparasites *(Continued)*
  on gerbils, 1428
  on guinea pigs, *1420,* 1431–1434, *1432, 1434, 1436*
  on hamsters, 1439–1440, *1440*
  on mice, *1432, 1435,* 1443
  on rabbits, 1434, 1447, 1448–1449
  on rats, *1447,* 1453
Ectothrix infection, 341
  diagnosis of, 121
Ectromelia, infectious, in mice, 1443
Ectropion, 1186
Edema. See also *Eosinophilic dermatitis and edema.*
  dermal, 163–164, *164*
  intercellular, of epidermis, 140–142, *143*
  intracellular, of epidermis, 142, *144*
EDTA-Tris, potentiation of topical antibiotics with, 280
EFA Caps, 1113
Efa Vet, 1113
Ehlers-Danlos syndrome. See *Asthenia, cutaneous (Ehlers-Danlos syndrome, dermatosparaxis).*
Ehrlichia canis, 444, 529–531
Ehrlichiosis, canine, 529–531
Eicosanoid(s), 30, 559–560, 561t
Eicosapentaenoic acid (EPA), 208, 239–240
Eimer's organ. See *Tylotrich pad.*
Elafin, 28
Elapidae, 1090
Elastin, dermal, 36–38
  atrophy of, 159
  disorders of, 987
  epidermal, *11*
Elastolysis. See *Cutis laxa.*
Elaunin fiber(s), 38
Elavil. See *Amitriptyline.*
Electric fulguration, 262
Electrocoagulation, 262
Electrodesiccation, 261–262
Electroincision, 261
Electrolysis, 262
Electron microscopy, 202
  of pemphigus lesions, 681
Electroshock, for acral lick dermatitis, 1064
Electrosurgery, 259–262
  instrumentation for, 261
  mechanisms of, 261
  techniques of, 261–262
Eleidin, 27
Elkhound, Norwegian, hair color of, 8
  keratoacanthoma in, 1248
  risk for neoplastic skin disorders and non-neoplastic lumps in, 1237t
  squamous cell carcinoma in, 1251
Elongase, 208
Emollient(s), 223, 228, 1028
  in topical therapy, 218t, 227
Emphysema, subcutaneous, 1090
Emulsion(s), therapeutic, 224–225
Endectocide(s), systemic, antiparasitic therapy with, 428–430
Endocrine disease, 992–995
  causes of, 781
  clinical aspects of, 798
  diagnosis of, 198, 782
  in ferrets, 1421–1426
Endorphin(s), endogenous, 1057
Endorphin blockers, for acral lick dermatitis, 1063
Endorphin substitution, for acral lick dermatitis, 1063
Endothelial cell(s), immunologic functions of, 556

Endothelium, vascular, 56
  cutaneous nerves and, 59
Endothrix infection, 341
  diagnosis of, 121
English bulldog. See *Bulldog, English.*
English pointer. See *Pointer, English.*
English setter. See *Setter, English.*
English Springer spaniel. See *Spaniel, Springer.*
Enilconazole powder, 224
Enilconazole rinse, 356, 356t
  antifungal therapy with, 410
Enrofloxacin, efficacy of, against coagulase-positive staphylococci, 282
  against *Staphylococcus intermedius,* 282
  in small animals, dosage and administration of, 1418t
  otic therapy with, 1227, 1229
  pinnal erythema in cats caused by, 1023
  systemic, dosage of, 284t
Entactin. See *Nidogen.*
Enterococcus spp., otitis media caused by, 1214t
Enterotoxin(s), 275
Entomophthorales, 384
Entomophthoromycosis, 377, 384
Entropion, 1186
Environmental skin disease, 1073–1108
Enzyme(s), epidermal, hydrolytic, 34
  oxidative, 34
Enzyme histochemistry, 202, 204t
Eosinophil(s), cutaneous, 39
  functions of, 557–558
  in cytologic diagnosis, *114,* 117, 118t
  in dermal blood vessels, of cats, 182, *183*
  in dermatitis, 188
  secretory products of, 557–558, 558t
Eosinophilia, in cats, 178
  with furunculosis, 299–300
Eosinophilic dermatitis and edema, in dogs, 1155–1156
Eosinophilic furunculosis, of face, canine, 505, *637, 638,* 641–642, *642. 643*
Eosinophilic granuloma, canine, *1150–1151,* 1153–1155, *1155–1156*
  feline, *1150–1151,* 1152–1153, *1153–1154*
Eosinophilic granuloma complex, feline, 1148–1153
Eosinophilic intracytoplasmic inclusions, 188–189
Eosinophilic otitis externa, proliferative, canine, 1213
Eosinophilic pinnal folliculitis, sterile, canine, *1210–1211,* 1213
Eosinophilic plaque, feline, *1142,* 1149–1152, *1150–1152*
Eosinophilic pustulosis, canine, sterile, 1132–1133, *1134–1136*
Eosinophilic ulcer. See *Indolent ulcer, feline.*
Eosinophilic vasculitis, 182
Epicuticle, of hair shaft, 41
Epidermal collarette(s), 86, 87, 97, 156
Epidermal dysplasia, canine, *914–915*
  in West Highland white terrier, 914, *928–929, 930–933*
Epidermal melanin unit, 16
Epidermal necrolysis, toxic. See *Toxic epidermal necrolysis.*
Epidermal nevus/nevi, 1007, 1013, *1380–1381,* 1388–1389, *1388–1389*
  breed(s) with predilection for, 1238t
  in dogs, 157
Epidermal-dermal junction, 34, 35
Epidermis, age-related changes in, 64–65
  basal layer (stratum basale) of, 10, *13,* 13–14, *15, 20*
  basement membrane zone of, *11,* 13
  components of, 34–35, 36t

Epidermis (Continued)
    functions of, 34
    thickened, 172, *172*
    ultrastructure of, 34–35, *35*
  clear layer (stratum lucidum) of, 10, 27, *27*
  dermatohistopathology of, terminology for, 132–156
  differentiation of, 29
  dysplasia of, 173, *173*
  enzymes of, 34
  granular layer (stratum granulosum) of, 10, *26*, 26–27
  histochemistry of, 34
  horny layer (stratum corneum) of, 10, *26*, 27–29
    barrier function of, 31
    hydration of, 32
    thickness of, 28, 32
  keratinization of, 29
  microscopic anatomy and physiology of, *10–14*, 10–35, *26*
  prickle cell layer of, *26*
  proliferation of, 29
  spinous layer (stratum spinosum) of, 10, 19–22, *22*
  stratum conjunctum of, 27
  stratum dysjunctum of, 28
  thickness of, 10
  turnover time for, in dogs, 31
Epidermodysplasia verruciformis, 1012
Epidermolysis bullosa, 938–940
  causes of, 13
  claw involvement in, 1199
  dystrophic (dermatolytic), 938, 938t, 939–940, *941*
  junctional, 938t, 938–939, *939, 940*
  types of, 938, 938t
Epidermolysis bullosa acquisita, 694, *700*, 700–701, *701*, 938, 940
  diagnosis of, 671
Epidermolysis bullosa acquisita antigen, 36t
Epidermolysis bullosa simplex, 938, 938t
Epidermolytic hyperkeratosis, 156, *157*
Epidermophytes, 349
Epidermophyton spp., 336
Epidermophyton floccosum, characteristics of, 349
Epidermopoiesis, 29–31
  changes in, 132
  defects in, 1025
Epi-Otic, 1223
Epiphora, 1188, *1189*
Epi-Soothe, 229t, 236, 917, 1035
Epithelial neoplasm(s), 1239–1281. See also specific neoplasm.
Epitheliogenesis imperfecta. See *Aplasia cutis*.
Epithelioma(s), intracutaneous cornifying. See *Keratoacanthoma*.
  sebaceous, in dogs, 1271
Epitope spreading, 667
Ergotism, 1089, 1101
  claw involvement in, 1199
  in guinea pigs, 1437
Erosion(s), 87, *98*
Erythema ab igne, 897–899
Erythema annulare centrifugum, in ferrets, 1426, *1427*
Erythema multiforme, 729–740
  cause and pathogenesis of, 729–734, 734t
  classification of, 732–733, 733t
  clinical features of, 734–737, *735–737*
  clinical management of, 739–740
  definition of, 729
  diagnosis of, *141*, 737–739, *738–739*

Erythema multiforme (Continued)
    drug-induced, in cats, 721, 723t, *724–725*, 734, 737, *737*
    in dogs, 722t, *724–725*, 734, 734t
  ear involvement in, *1210–1211*, 1212
  exfoliative, in cats, 525
  idiopathic, in dogs, 734, *736*, *737*, 740
  in humans, 732–733
  major, 88, 732
  minor, 732, 735
  target lesion in, 733–734, *735*, *736*
Erythrocyte(s), diapedesis of, in epidermis, 147
Erythroderma, drug-induced, in cats, 723t
  in dogs, 722t
Erythromycin, efficacy of, against coagulase-positive staphylococci, 282
    against *Staphylococcus intermedius*, 282
  systemic, dosage of, 284t
Escherichia coli, as transient flora, in cats, 275
  in dogs, 275
  in anal sacs, 1201
  otitis media caused by, 1214t
Estradiol, for feline acquired symmetric alopecia, 902
Estrogen(s), 795–796. See also *Hyperestrogenism*.
  and hair growth, 6
  blood levels of, assays for, 796
Ethohexadiol, 427
Ethyl alcohol, 230
Ethyl lactate, in shampoo, 223
  topical, for bacterial infection, 279, 280
Etretinate, 241–242, 1029
  antiseborrheic therapy with, 919
  for epidermal dysplasia in West Highland white terriers, 929
  for granulomatous sebaceous adenitis, 1146
  indications for, 243
  otic therapy with, 1229–1230
  teratogenicity of, 243, 1029
  toxicity of, 243, 1029
Eumelanin(s), 8, 16, 17
European blastomycosis. See *Cryptococcosis*.
Eutrombicula alfreddugesi, 447, 447–448. See also *Trombiculosis (chigger mites)*.
Evaporimeter, 32
Excoriation(s), 87, *98*
Exfoliative dermatitis, 1049
  and thymoma, in cats, 905
  drug-induced, *1052*, 1052–1053
    in cats, 723t
    in dogs, 721, 722t
  paraneoplastic, 1375
Exocytosis, in epidermis, 147, *148*
Exophiala jeanselmei, 379
Exophiala spinifera, 379
Extractable nuclear antigen (ENA), in systemic lupus erythematosus, 706–707
Eyelid(s), anatomy of, 1185
  common and less common dermatoses of, 103t
  diseases of, 1185–1190, 1186t
  diseases that affect other areas and, 1186, 1188t
  normal flora of, 1185
  tumors of, 1188–1190, *1189*, 1190t
Ezrin, 20

Facial eczema, in rabbits, 1451
Facial excoriations, self-inflicted, in ferrets, 1427
Facial fold intertrigo, *1097*, 1107
Factor VIII–related antigen, in cell type identification, 204t

Familial vasculopathy, 987–989
Fat(s), dietary, 207–208, 1112
    supplementation of, 1113
  subcutaneous, changes in, 171–172
    necrosis of, 172, *172*
Fat cell(s). See *Lipocyte(s)*.
Fatty acid(s), and haircoat quality, 209
  antibacterial properties of, 274
  anti-inflammatory properties of, 208
  deficiency of, 1112–1115, *1114–1115*
    in chinchilla, 1417
    in guinea pigs, 1434
    in hamsters, 1441
    in mice, 1444
    in rats, 1453–1454
  dietary, 239–240
  essential, 208
    deficiency of, 31
  for hypersensitivity disorders, 564–566
  metabolism of, 208–209, 239–240, *240*
  of sebum, 51
  omega-3, 208
  omega-6, 208
  omega-3/omega-6, 239, 1113, 1198
    antiseborrheic therapy with, 918–919
    dietary ratio of, 239
    for dermatomyositis, 945
    for discoid lupus erythematosus, 716
    for feline eosinophilic granuloma, 1133
  polyunsaturated, 30, 208, 1113
  supplementation of, 208, 209, 239–241
    adverse effects and side effects of, 241
    for claw disease, 1200
  systemic therapy with, 239–241
  therapy with, for epidermal dysplasia in West Highland white terriers, 929
  topical therapy with, 235, 1113–1114
Felicola subrostrata, 487, *489*, *490*
Feline immunodeficiency virus infection, 278, 517–519, *520*, *521*
  and abscesses, 311, 517
  and fungal infections, 337, 338, 342
  and griseofulvin side effects, 357
  and *Malassezia* infection, 363
  and mural folliculitis, 907
Feline infectious anemia, 531
Feline infectious peritonitis, 522, *522*
Feline leprosy. See *Leprosy, feline*.
Feline leukemia virus infection, 517, *518–520*, 1285–1287
  and abscesses, 311, 517
  and fungal infections, 337, 338, 342, 519
  and *Malassezia* infection, 363
  neoplasia related to, 517, 528
Feline poxvirus infection, 145, *518–519*, 520–522
Feline rhinotracheitis infection, *518*, 524–525, *526–529*
Feline sarcoma virus, 528, 1285–1287
FeLV. See *Feline leukemia virus infection*.
Feminization, of male dog, 796, 840–843
  idiopathic, 851
Fenoxycarb, 426, 495
Fenthion, 428, 499
Fenvalerate, 426
Ferret, actinomycosis in, 1417
  alopecia in, breeding season and, 1425
    hyperestrogenism and, 1424–1425, *1425*
    testicular neoplasia and, 1425
  atopy in, 1426, *1427*
  bacterial infections in, 1417, *1418*

Ferret *(Continued)*
  biotin deficiency in, 1426
  blastomycosis in, 1419
  blue ferret syndrome in, 1426–1427
  burrowing in, 1427
  coccidioidomycosis in, 1419
  contact dermatitis in, 1426
  demodicosis in, 1419
  dermatoses of, 1417–1428
  diet for, 1426
  dracunculiasis in, 1419
  ear mites in, 1419
  ectoparasites on, 1419, *1420*
  endocrine disorders in, 1421–1426
  erythema annulare centrifugum in, 1426, *1427*
  fleas in, 1419
  flystrike in, 1419
  fungal infections in, 1418–1419
  histoplasmosis in, 1419
  hyperadrenocorticism in, 1421–1424, *1422*, *1423*
  hyperestrogenism in, 1424–1425, *1425*
  hypothyroidism in, 1426
  injection reaction in, 1426
  intestinal parasites in, 1426
  neoplasia in, *1420*, 1427–1428
  otitis externa in, 1419
  otodectic mange in, 1419
  pinnal necrosis in, 1419
  sarcoptic mange in, 1419
  shedding in, 1425
  telogen deluxion in, 1425, *1426*
  ticks in, 1419
  viral infections in, 1421, *1421*
Festoon(s), dermal, 162
Fibril-associated collagens with interrupted triple helices (FACIT), 37
Fibrillin, 36t, 37
Fibrinogen, in morphogenesis of skin appendages, 3
Fibroblast(s), collagenases synthesized by, 37
  dermal, 37, 39
    components synthesized by, 36
Fibroblastoma, perineural. See *Schwannoma*.
Fibroma(s), 1013, *1282*, 1282–1283, *1283*
  breed(s) with predilection for, 1237t
  in rats, 1455
  Shope, in rabbits, 1451–1452
Fibroma durum, 1282
Fibroma molle, 1282
Fibronectin(s), 36t
  functions of, 38
  in morphogenesis of skin appendages, 3
  synthesis of, 38
Fibropapilloma, diagnosis of, 1245, *1245*
Fibroplasia, dermal, 161, *162*
Fibropruritic nodule, 1284–1285, *1286*, *1287*
  breed(s) with predilection for, 1237t
Fibrosarcoma(s), 1281, 1285–1289
  breed(s) with predilection for, 1237t
  cause and pathogenesis of, 1285–1287
  claw involvement in, 1198
  clinical findings in, 1287–1288
  clinical management of, 1288–1289
  cutaneous, in cats, 528
  diagnosis of, 1288, *1291*
  in cats, *1286*, 1287–1288
  in dogs, *1286*, 1287, *1290*
  in gerbils, 1430
  in hamsters, 1442

Fibrosarcoma(s) (Continued)
　in mice, 1444
　in rats, 1455
Fibrosis, 196
　dermal, 161
　perifollicular, 168, 169, 195
Fibrovascular papilloma(s), 1284, 1284, 1285
Fila brasiliero, Ehlers-Danlos syndrome in, 982
Filaggrin, 42
　functions of, 26
　synthesis of, 29
Filamentous body(ies). See *Apoptotic body(ies)*.
Filariasis, 643–644
Filarioidea dermatitis, 644
Fine-needle aspiration, for cytologic diagnosis, 115–116
Finnish spitz, pemphigus foliaceus in, 686
Fipronil, 423, 497–498, 500
　antiparasitic therapy with, 425
　spray, otic therapy with, 1229
Fire ant(s), sting of, 506, 506–507
Fish scale disease. See *Ichthyosis*.
Fissure(s), 87, 99
Fistula/fistulae, arteriovenous, 1095–1096
　multiple perianal, cryosurgery for, 258–259
Fite's modified acid-fast stain, staining characteristics of various substances with, 130t
FIV. See *Feline immunodeficiency virus infection*.
Fixed drug eruption, causes of, 721, 722t
　in cats, 723t
　in dogs, 725, 726
Flame figure(s), 159, 160
Flame follicle(s), 166, 167, 784, 790
Flank sucking, 1060–1061, 1065
Flea(s), characteristics of, 490–491, 491
　control of, 493–500
　　in external environment, 494
　　in internal environment, 494–496
　　liquid products for, 499–500
　　on animal, 496–500
　　spot application products for, 497–498
　　systemic products for, 499
　development of, inhibitors of, 430
　European rabbit, on cats, 488–489
　growth of, regulators of, 495
　life cycle of, 488–489, 491–492
　on animals, control of, 496–500
　　spot application products for, 497–498
　on ferrets, 1419
　on hamsters, 1440
　on humans, 493, 493
　on rabbits, 1449
　on rats, 1453
　plague transmission by, 325–326
　rabbit, 491, 492
　　common Eastern, 1449
　　giant Eastern, 1449
　repellents for, 499–500
　sticktight, 488–489
Flea bite hypersensitivity, and fibropruritic nodule, 1284–1285
　canine, 627–632
　　allergy testing in, 630–631
　　cause and pathogenesis of, 627–629
　　clinical features of, 629
　　clinical management of, 631–632
　　diagnosis of, 629–631
　　histopathology of, 623, 631
　　clinical management of, 239

Flea bite hypersensitivity (Continued)
　cytologic diagnosis of, 114
　feline, 632–635
　　cause and pathogenesis of, 632
　　clinical features of, 620, 623t, 632–633
　　clinical management of, 634–635
　　diagnosis of, 633t, 633–634, 634
　　histopathology of, 634
　in cats, 157
Flea collar(s), 498
Flea comb, for ectoparasite diagnosis, 107
　in flea control, 496–497
Flea cream rinses, 498–499
Flea foam(s), 500
Flea powder(s), 499
Flea shampoo(s), 498–499
Flea spray(s), 499–500
Flea-bite hypersensitivity, 488–489
Flesh flies, 503
Flora. See *Microflora*.
Flotation, for ectoparasite diagnosis, 107
Fluconazole, adverse effects and side effects of, 411
　antifungal therapy with, 411, 413
　dosage and administration of, 357t
Flucort. See *Flumethasone*.
Flucytosine, adverse effects and side effects of, 415
　antifungal therapy with, 414–415
　resistance to, 415
Flumethasone, injectable, 247t
Flunixin meglumine, for acral lick dermatitis, 1063
Fluocinolone, adverse effects and side effects of, 232
　for acral lick dermatitis, 1063
　for discoid lupus erythematosus, 716
　in shampoo, 223
　otic therapy with, 1226
Fluocinonide, adrenocortical suppression by, 232
5-Fluorocytosine, adverse effects and side effects of, 721
Fluoroquinolone(s), anti-inflammatory and immunomodulatory properties of, 285
　efficacy of, against staphylococcal infection, 283
　　against *Staphylococcus intermedius*, 282
　long-term therapy with, 287
　systemic, for bacterial infections, 281
Fluoxetine, 1056–1057
　for feline psychogenic alopecia, 1070
Flushing, cutaneous, 1022–1023, 1052
Fly(ies), 500–507
　stable, 500, 501
Fly bite(s), pinnal, 1210–1211, 1211
Fly dermatitis, 500–502, 501
Flystrike, in ferrets, 1419
　in rabbits, 1449
Foam cell(s), 184–185
　epithelioid, 185
Focal adhesion(s), 19, 22t
Focal adnexal dysplasia(s), 1384–1386, 1385
Focal metatarsal fistulation, 980, 985–986, 986
Fogger(s), for flea control, 495–496
Fogo selvagem. See *Pemphigus foliaceus*.
Fold dermatitis, 1216
Folinic acid, supplementation of, in canine neosporosis, 533
Follicle-stimulating hormone (FSH), 781, 795, 798
Follicular arrest, 7, 897, 898
Follicular atrophy, 6
Follicular cast(s), 87, 95
Follicular dysplasia, 6, 970–973, 1029
　black hair, 954, 959–965, 963

Follicular dysplasia *(Continued)*
  canine, 890
    cyclic, 890–893
  diagnosis of, 971, *973, 974*
  feline, 905
  treatment of, 971–972
Follicular flushing, 1026
Follicular lipidosis, 973–974
  of Rottweilers, 899, *899, 900*
Follicular mucinosis. See *Alopecia mucinosa.*
Follicular parakeratosis, 925–927, *926, 927, 928, 929*
Follicular stile, 48
Folliculitis, bacterial, in cats, 300, 302
  in hypothyroidism, 853
  superficial, 289, 291–296, *294, 295, 296*
    in cats, 294
  deep, 299–300
  eosinophilic, in cats, 194
  facial eosinophilic, in dogs, 505
  luminal, 166, 194, *200*
  mural, 166, 192
    granulomatous, drug-induced, 722t, 725, *727, 729, 731*
    idiopathic lymphocytic, of cats, 907–909, *907–910*
    infiltrative, 194, *197*
    interface, 192–194, *196*
    necrotizing, 194, *198*
    pustular, 194, *199*
  muzzle, 303–304
  nasal, *301,* 303
  necrotizing, *301,* 303
  nonpruritic, 293
  pedal. See *Pododermatitis.*
  penetrating. See *Furunculosis.*
  postbathing, 212
  pruritic, 293
  pyotraumatic, 288, 300–303, *301, 303*
  staphylococcal, 97
    diagnosis of, *113, 150*
    in cats, 289
    in dogs, *170, 171,* 347
      dermal edema in, *164*
    superficial, in dogs, 289
  superficial, in dogs, 289
Follitropin. See *Follicle-stimulating hormone (FSH).*
Fontana's ammoniacal silver nitrate, staining characteristics of various substances with, 130t
Food allergy. See *Food hypersensitivity.*
Food hypersensitivity, canine, 615–624
  cause and pathogenesis of, 615–618, 618t
  clinical features of, *604,* 618–619, *620*
  clinical management of, 623–624
  diagnosis of, 619–623
  histopathology of, 623, *623*
clinical features of, 573
diagnosis of, 117, *148*
ear involvement in, 1211
feline, *183,* 624–627
  cause and pathogenesis of, 624–625, 625t
  clinical features of, *620,* 625
  clinical management of, 627
  diagnosis of, 626–627
  histopathology of, 626–627
  mural folliculitis caused by, 909, *910*
  otitis externa in, 1211, 1213
  vasculitis caused by, 743, *745, 747*
Food intolerance. See *Food hypersensitivity.*

Foot licking, *1060,* 1066
Footpad(s), anatomy of, 9
  atrichial sweating from, 53
  dermatophyte collection from, 120
  fissures of, *99*
  histology of, 10, *12*
  hyperkeratosis of, *930, 935,* 935–936, *1114–1115*
    in canine distemper, 523, *523*
  in vasculitis, *746, 747*
  sweat glands of, *52,* 52–53
  ulceration of, in dog with systemic lupus erythematosus, 696–697
Foreign body(ies), in ear, 1212
  skin lesions caused by, 1091–1094, *1093–1095*
Foreign body granuloma(s), in hamsters, 1441
Foreign-body reaction(s), cytologic diagnosis of, 117
Formalin, biopsy specimen fixation in, 129
Formamidine(s), topical, antiparasitic therapy with, 425
Fox terrier. See *Terrier, fox.*
Foxtail, skin lesions caused by, 1091
Francisella tularensis, 444
Freezing artifact, 142, *144*
French bulldog. See *Bulldog, French.*
Frontline. See *Fipronil.*
Frostbite, *1086,* 1088–1089
  in rabbits, *1447,* 1450
Fulguration, electric, 262
Fulvicin U/F. See *Griseofulvin, microsized.*
Fungal infection(s). See also *Mycosis/mycoses.*
  diagnosis of, 118t, 118–125
  in chinchilla, 1416
  in ferrets, 1418–1419
  in guinea pigs, 1430–1431, *1431*
  in mice, 1442–1443
  in rabbits, 1446, *1447*
  in rats, 1453
  otitis externa caused by, 1213–1215, 1214t
  otitis media caused by, 1214t
  pododermatitis caused by, 305
  therapy for, 409–415
Fungizone. See *Amphotericin B.*
Fungus/fungi. See also *Microflora; Mycosis/mycoses;* specific fungus.
  characteristics of, 336–337
  classification of, 336
  colonies of, morphology of, *123*
  conidia of. See *Conidium/conidia.*
  contaminant, and pathogenic, differentiation of, 337
  culture of, 118, 121–122, *123,* 337, 349
  dimorphic, 337
  examination for, 118–125
  growth of, in tissue, 337
  hypersensitivity to, 650
  hypha/hyphae of. See *Hypha/hyphae.*
  identification of, 122–125, *123–124,* 336
  in normal flora, 338, 338t
    in cats, 338, 338t
    in dogs, 338, 338t
  pathogenic, and contaminant, differentiation of, 337
    characterization of, 337–338
  propagule of, 336
  saprophytic, as resident flora, in dogs, 34
    in normal flora, 338, 338t
  taxonomy of, 337
Fur chewing, in chinchilla, 1417
Fur-slip, in chinchilla, 1417
Furunculosis, 166, 195, *200*

Furunculosis (Continued)
  acral lick, 302, 308–309
  bacterial, in hypothyroidism, 853
  cytologic diagnosis of, 117
  deep folliculitis and, 299, 299–300, 301, 302
  eosinophilic, of face, canine, 505, 637, 638, 641–642, 642, 643
  in cats, 300, 302
  in dermatophytosis, in dogs, 343, 344
  in hyperadrenocorticism, 800, 802
  in mice, 1442
  in rats, 1452
  muzzle, 302, 303–304
  nasal, 301, 303
  pedal. See Pododermatitis.
  pyogranulomatous, 351
    in dogs, 302
  pyotraumatic folliculitis and, 300–303
  staphylococcal, 200, 202
    in dogs, 171, 299
Fusidic acid, topical, for bacterial infection, 279, 280
Fusobacterium spp., cellulitis caused by, 310
  in infections, 276
  in oral flora of cats, 276
  in subcutaneous abscesses in cats, 310
Fusobacterium necrophorum, in rabbits, 1445

Gap junctions, 19
Gel(s), 218t, 226
Gelatin, for claw disease, 1200
Gelatinase, 37
Gene(s), homeobox, 93
Gene therapy, 264
Generic dog food dermatosis, 1114–1115, 1122, 1122–1123
Gentamicin, in small animals, dosage and administration of, 1418t
  otic therapy with, 1227
  topical, for bacterial infection, 280
Geotrichium candidum, 408
Geotrichium dermatitis, 408
Geotrichosis, claw involvement in, 1195
Gerbil, bacterial infections in, 1428
  bald nose in, 1429
  barbering in, 1429
  congenital abnormalities of pigmentation and haircoat in, 1429
  demodicosis in, 1428
  dermatoses of, 1428–1430
  ectoparasites on, 1428
  neoplasia in, 1429–1430
  sore nose in, 1429, 1430
  tail disorder of, 1429
  ventral scent gland disorder of, 1429
German shepherd. See Shepherd, German.
German shorthaired pointer. See Pointer, German shorthaired.
Germicide(s), 230
Giant cell(s), in feline herpes dermatitis, 525, 527
  multinucleate epidermal, 174–175, 175
  multinucleate histiocytic, 147, 185–187, 186
  multinucleate keratinocyte, 174–175, 175
Gilchrist's disease. See Blastomycosis.
Gland(s), age-related changes in, 64–65
  changes in, terminology for, 168–171
  sebaceous. See Sebaceous gland(s).

Gland(s) (Continued)
  specialized, 54–55
  sweat. See Sweat gland(s).
Gliricola porcelli, in guinea pigs, 1433, 1434
Glomus, 57, 58
Glossitis, burdock, 1091, 1092
Glucan, 336
Glucocorticoid(s), adverse effects and side effects of, 246
  alternate-day therapy with, 250, 251
  and adrenocortical function in dogs, 232, 234t
  and skin, 789–790
  anti-inflammatory properties of, 244–245, 245t
  injectable, 246–247, 247t, 250
  intravenous, 247
  oral, 245, 250
  otic preparations of, 1225t, 1226t
  parenteral, 245–246
  production of, 789
  selection of, 247–248
  urinary levels of, determination of, 790
Glucocorticoid therapy. See also Hyperadrenocorticism (Cushing's disease, Cushing's syndrome).
  effects of, on biopsy, 128–129
  for discoid lupus erythematosus, 716
  for graft-versus-host disease, 720
  for idiopathic sterile granuloma and pyogranuloma, 1138–1139
  for pemphigus, 681
  for pemphigus erythematosus, 693
  for pemphigus foliaceus, 689–690
  for systemic lupus erythematosus, 711
  for vasculitis, 753
  immunosuppressive, 671, 672t
  intralesional, 247, 250, 252
  pulse, 671
  systemic, 238–239, 244–252
    administration of, 246–247, 247t
    adverse effects and side effects of, 250–252
    dosage of, 248–249, 249t
    evaluation of, 252
    for feline psychogenic alopecia, 1070
    for hypersensitivity disorders, 570
    indications for, 246
    otic therapy with, 1229
    regimen for, 249–250
  topical, adverse effects and side effects of, 232
    alopecia caused by, 889, 896–897
    anti-inflammatory effects of, 232
    anti-inflammatory potencies of, 232, 233, 233t
    for ear treatment, 1225t, 1226t
    reactions to, in cats, 902, 903
    in dogs, 896, 896
β-Glucuronidase, in cell type identification, 204t
Glycerin, 1028
Glycosaminoglycan(s), 38
Glypican, 38
Gnathostoma, definition of, 440
Gnathostoma spinigerum, in dogs, 440
  in humans, 432
Gold. See Chrysotherapy.
Golden retriever. See Retriever, golden.
Gomori's aldehyde fuchsin stain, staining characteristics of various substances with, 130t
Gomori's methenamine siver stain, staining characteristics of various substances with, 130t
Gomori's reticulin stain, staining characteristics of various substances with, 130t

Gonadotroph(s), 781
Gonadotropin(s), 798
Gonadotropin-releasing hormone (GnRH), 781, 795, 796
Gordius robustus, in cats, 440
Graft-versus-host disease, 719–720
Gram's stain, 116
  staining characteristics of various substances with, 130t
Granular cell tumor, 1294–1296, *1295*
Granular degeneration, epidermal. See *Epidermolytic hyperkeratosis.*
Granulocyte(s), functions of, 556–558
Granulocyte colony-stimulating factor deficiency of, 278
Granulocytopathy, 279t
Granuloma(s), bacterial, 302, 311–312, *313*
  dermal, feline, *186*
  eosinophilic, canine, *1150–1151*, 1153–1155, *1155–1156*
    feline, *1150–1151*, 1152–1153, *1153–1154*
  foreign-body, 189, *191*
  linear. See *Eosinophilic granuloma, feline.*
  mycobacterial, 312–321, *317*, *318*, *320*
    opportunistic (atypical), *317*, 319–321, *320*
  palisading, 189, *191*
  preauricular, feline, *1241*
  sarcoidal, *185*, 189, *190*
  tuberculoid, 189, *189*
  venereal. See *Transmissible venereal tumor.*
Granuloma and pyogranuloma, sterile idiopathic, 1136–1140
  cause and pathogenesis of, 1136
  clinical features of, 1136–1137
  clinical management of, 1138–1140
  diagnosis of, 1137–1138, *1138–1141*
  in cats, *1134–1135*, 1137
  in dogs, *1134–1135*, 1136–1137
Granulomatous dermatitis and lymphadenitis, juvenile sterile. See *Cellulitis, canine juvenile.*
Granulomatous inflammation, 184
Grape seed extract, 209
Grass awn, 1091
Gray collie syndrome, 977–978, 1014
Graying, 1014–1015, *1015*
Greasy skin and hair coat with sebaceous gland hyperplasia, idiopathic, 1179, *1180*
Great Dane, acral lick dermatitis in, 1058, *1060*
  antithyroglobulin antibody(ies) in, 852
  antithyroid antibody(ies) in, 789
  callus dermatitis in, 1102
  color dilution alopecia in, 967
  demodicosis in, 461, 465
  epidermolysis bullosa acquisita in, 940
  histiocytomas in, 1347
  hypothyroidism in, 852
  idiopathic sterile granuloma and pyogranuloma in, 1136
  lymphedema in, 990
  muzzle folliculitis and furunculosis in, 304
  pododermatitis in, 305
  psychogenic dermatoses in, 1056
  risk for neoplastic skin disorders and non-neoplastic lumps in, 1237t
  risk for non-neoplastic skin disorders in, 76, 79t
  sterile pyogranuloma on feet of, 305
  zinc-responsive dermatosis in, 1120
Great Pyrenees, dermoid cyst (sinus) in, 936
  risk for non-neoplastic skin disorders in, 79t
Grenz zone, 164, *166*
Greyhound, drug reactions in, 721
  Ehlers-Danlos syndrome in, 982
  hair growth in, daily, 6

Greyhound (*Continued*)
  hemangiosarcomas in, 1299
  Italian, color dilution alopecia in, 967
    pattern baldness in, 965
    pinnal alopecia in, 887
  otitis externa in, 1212
  pattern baldness in, 965
  risk for neoplastic skin disorders and non-neoplastic lumps in, 1237t
  risk for non-neoplastic skin disorders in, 79t
  trichorrhexis nodosa in, 895
  vasculitis in, 744
  vasculopathy in, cutaneous and renal glomerular, 749, *750*, 752
    familial, 987–989
  ventral comedone syndrome in, 1103
Griseofulvin, adverse effects and side effects of, 411
  in cats, 357
  antifungal therapy with, 357, 409, 410–411
  anti-inflammatory properties of, 411
  immunomodulatory properties of, 411
  in small animals, dosage and administration of, 1418t
  microsized, 411
    dosage and administration of, 357t
  teratogenicity of, 357, 411, 1446
  ultramicrosized, 411
    dosage and administration of, 357t
Gris-PEG. See *Griseofulvin, ultramicrosized.*
Grooming, 207
  for cats, 214–215
  for dogs, routine, 210
  frequency of, 213
  special problems in, for cats, 215
    for dogs, 213–214
Grover's disease, 138
Growth factor(s), in hair cycle, 4–5
Growth hormone, 794–795
  and hair growth, 6
  deficiency of, 794
  excess of. See *Acromegaly.*
  in adrenal hyperplasia–like syndrome, 846–847
  plasma levels, in pituitary dwarfism, 821
  therapy with, in pituitary dwarfism, 821
Growth hormone–inhibiting factor (GHIF), 781
Growth hormone–releasing factor (GHRF), 781
Growth hormone–responsive dermatosis. See *Hyposomatotropism (pseudo-Cushing's syndrome, GH-responsive dermatosis).*
Guinea pig, alopecia in, congenital, 1437, *1438*
  cystic ovaries and, 1437, *1438*
  bacterial infections in, *1418*, *1420*, 1430
  barbering in, 1437
  bite wounds in, 1437
  candidiasis in, 1431
  cheyletiellosis in, 1433
  Chirodiscoides caviae in, 1433, *1434*
  claws of, overgrowth of, 1439
  cryptococcosis in, 1431
  demodicosis in, 1433–1434, *1436*
  dermatophytosis in, 1430–1431, *1431*
  dermatoses of, 1430–1439
  digits and paws, necrosis and sloughing of, 1437, *1437*
  ear chewing in, 1437
  ectoparasites on, *1420*, 1431–1434, *1432*, *1434*, *1436*
  ergot poisoning in, 1437
  footpads of, hyperkeratosis and cutaneous horns of, 1439
  fungal infections in, 1430–1431, *1431*
  haircoat of, thinning of, at weaning, 1437

Index • 1491

Guinea pig *(Continued)*
   lice in, 1433, *1434*
   Malassezia dermatitis in, 1431
   mites in, 1431–1433, *1432–1434*
   neoplasia in, *1432,* 1439
   nutritional deficiency in, 1434
   Pelodera dermatitis in, 1433
   sebaceous gland disorder in, 1437–1439
   shedding in, 1437
   telogen defluxion in, 1437
   trichofolliculoma in, *1432,* 1439
   trixacariasis in, *1420,* 1431–1433, *1432–1434*
   viral infections in, 1431
Guinea worm, 437
Gum, in haircoat, 214
Gyropus ovalis, in guinea pigs, 1433

Haarscheiben. See *Tylotrich pad.*
Habronema spp., 503, 504
   in dogs, 440
Haemobartonella felis, 531
Haemobartonellosis, feline, 531
Haemodipsus ventricosus, on rabbits, 1449
Hair. See also *Alopecia.*
   age-related changes in, 64
   analysis of, as diagnostic tool, 7
   awn, 4
   barrier function of, 31
   colors of, 7–9, 108
   conditioners for, 212
   dermatophyte collection from, 120
   dermatophyte-infected, abnormalities of, 121
   disorders of, 950–975
   down, 4
   examination of, 108, *109–112*
   functions of, 4
   in endocrine disorders, 780
   in immune defense, 274
   in nutritional deficiency, 108, *111*
   lanugo, 4
   mechanoreceptors and, 61
   pigmentation of, 108
      abnormalities of, 108, *110*
   primary (outercoat, guard), 4, 7, 41, *42*
      central, 41
      lateral, 41
   red, acquired, 1022
   secondary (undercoat), 4, 7, 39–41, *42*
   sinus, 6
   specimen of, collection of, in fungal infection, 120
   tactile, 44–45
   telogen, 341
   types of, 7–9
Hair care product(s), 211–212. See also *Shampoo(s).*
Hair cast(s), 108, *111*
Hair cycle, 4–7, *5.* See also *Hair growth.*
Hair disk. See *Tylotrich pad.*
Hair follicle(s), 2, 39–48. See also *Follicular.*
   age-related changes in, 64–65
   anagen, 41, 44, 46, *46,* 108, *109*
   arrangement of, 41, *42*
   bacterial infection of, 277–278
   basement membrane zone (glassy membrane) of, 43, *47, 49*
   bulb of, 43, *43,* 46, *46,* 47, 48, 108, *109*
   catagen, *47,* 48, 108, *109*

Hair follicle(s) *(Continued)*
   catagenization of, 166
   changes in, terminology for, 165–168
   components of, 41, *43*
   degeneration of, 277–278
   development of, 4–7
   dysplasia of, 6, 152, *153,* 166–168
   fibrous root sheath of, 43
   in epidermal renewal, 48
   induction of, 4–7
   inferior segment of, 41, *43*
   inflammation of. See also *Folliculitis; Furunculosis; Perifolliculitis.*
      assessment of, 195–196
      hydropic, 192
      lichenoid, 192
      secondary, 195–196
   infundibulum of, 28, 41, *43, 43*
   inner root sheath of, 41–43, 44, *44,* 48
      cuticle of, 42, *44*
      Henle layer of, 42, *44*
      Huxley layer of, 42, *44*
   innervation of, 59, *60,* 62
   isthmus of, 41, *43, 43*
   keratinization of, *11,* 48
   microscopic anatomy of, *10*
   miniaturized, 168, 198
   morphogenesis of, 39
   nevi of, 1389, *1390*
   obstruction of, 277
   of sinus hair, 44–45, *45*
   outer root sheath of, 41, *43,* 44, 48, *49,* 50
   reactivation of, 4–7
   regression of, 4–7
   ruptured, dermatitis caused by, 189
   telogen, 43, 48, *49, 50,* 108, *109*
   telogenization of, 166
   tumors of, 1263–1270
      in mice, 1444
      in rats, 1455
Hair germ(s), 2, *49*
Hair growth. See also *Hair cycle.*
   androgens and, 797
   disorders of, 950–975
   estrogens and, 795
   neural mechanisms of, 5
   regulation of, 5
Hair matrix, 41, 44
Hair pluck examination, for mites, 105–106
   technique for, 108
Hair shaft, layers of, 39, *41,* 44, 108, *110*
   morphology of, 108, *109*
   resident microflora of, 275
   structural defects of, 950–956
Hair tract(s), 4
Haircoat, color of, and risk for non-neoplastic skin disorders, 76
   disorders of, 977–978
      acquired, 978
      congenital, 977–978
   in hyperadrenocorticism, 800, *801*
   greasy, with sebaceous gland hyperplasia, idiopathic, 1179, *1180*
   in hypothyroidism, 783–784
   normal, care of, 207–215. See also *Grooming.*
   thickness of, 3
Hale's colloidal ion stain, staining characteristics of various substances with, 130t

Halogenated agent(s), topical, 230–231
Hamartoma. See also *Nevus/nevi*.
   definition of, 177
Hamster, bacterial infections in, *1418*, 1439
   contact dermatitis in, 1441
   demodicosis in, 1439–1440, *1440*
   dermatophytosis in, 1439
   ectoparasites on, 1439–1440, *1440*
   epitheliotropic lymphoma in, 1432, 1441, *1442*
   flank scent glands of, 1441
   fleas on, 1440
   fungal infections in, 1439
   hereditary hairlessness in, 1441
   hyperadrenocorticism in, 1441
   neoplasia in, *1432*, 1441–1442, *1442*
   notoedric mange in, 1440
   nutritional disorders in, 1441
   ringtail in, 1441
   syphilis in, 1439
   traumatic alopecia and dermatitis in, 1440
Haplonychia, definition of, 1193t
Happy Jack Kennel Dip, 424
Hard pad disease, 523, *523*
Harder gland(s), 1185
Havana brown cat, grooming for, 215
Head, common and less common dermatoses of, 103t
Heartworm disease, 439, 643–644, *644*, *645*
Heat, body, conservation of, mechanisms for, 53–54
   dissipation of, mechanisms of, 54
   production of, mechanisms for, 53–54
Heat, radiant, burns caused by, *1086–1087*, 1087
   dermatitis caused by, 897–899
Hederiform ending. See *Tylotrich pad*.
Helminth parasite(s), 431–440
Hemangioendothelioma, malignant. See *Hemangiosarcoma*.
Hemangioma, 1297–1299
   breed(s) with predilection for, 1237t
   cause and pathogenesis of, 1297
   clinical findings in, 1297–1298
   diagnosis of, *1298*, 1298–1299
   glabrous, nonpigmented skin (actinic), breed(s) with predilection for, 1237t
   in cats, 528, *1286*, 1297–1298
   in dogs, *1286*, 1297
   in mice, 1444
   laser surgery for, 259, *260*
   solar-related, risk for, haircoat color and, 76
Hemangiopericytoma, 1281, *1286*, *1302*, 1302–1303, *1303*
   breed(s) with predilection for, 1237t
Hemangiosarcoma, 1299–1302
   breed(s) with predilection for, 1237t
   cause and pathogenesis of, 1299
   claw involvement in, 1198
   clinical findings in, 1299–1300
   clinical management of, 1300–1302
   diagnosis of, 1300, *1301*
   glabrous, nonpigmented skin (actinic), breed(s) with predilection for, 1237t
   in cats, *1286*, 1299, *1300*
   in dogs, 1299
   in mice, 1444
   in rats, 1455
   laser surgery for, 259
   risk for, haircoat color and, 76
   solar-induced, 1299
   visceral, cutaneous metastases of, 1373
Hematopoiesis, canine cyclic, 1014

Hematoxylin and eosin stain (H & E), 129, 130t
Hemidesmosome(s), 13, 19, 20, 22t, *35*
Hemitrichosis. See *Hypertrichosis, unilateral*.
Hemogram(s), in hyperadrenocorticism, 805
Hemolysin(s), 275
Hemorrhage, from muzzle, 304
   subungual, *1197*, 1198
Heparin sulfate, 36t, 38
Hepatocutaneous syndrome, 868
Hepatoid cell(s), of canine tail gland, 54–55
Hepatoid gland(s), 1045, *1047*
Hepatoid tissue, 835
Hepatomegaly, in hyperadrenocorticism, 804
Herbal medicine, 263
Hereditary lupoid dermatosis, of German shorthaired pointers, *941*, 948–949, *949*
Herpesvirus infection, in cats, 171
α-Herpesvirus infection, feline rhinotracheitis caused by, 524–525
   pseudorabies caused by, 524
Heterodoxus spiniger, 487, *490*
Heterozygosity, loss of, 65
Hexachlorophene, 230
Hexadene, 917. See also *Chlorhexidine, shampoo*.
Hexidine, 1035
Hexylresorcinol, 230
Hidradenitis, 170, *171*
Himalayan cat, acromelanism in, 1012–1013
   basal cell tumors in, 1261
   dermatophytosis in, 347
   Ehlers-Danlos syndrome in, 982
   epitrichial cysts in, 1381
   facial fold intertrigo in, 1107
   griseofulvin side effects in, 357
   grooming for, 215
   hair color of, 8
   idiopathic facial dermatitis of, 920–921, *922*
   risk for neoplastic skin disorders and non-neoplastic lumps in, 1237t
   risk for non-neoplastic skin disorders in, 79t
   seborrhea in, 920
   systemic lupus erythematosus in, 705
   urticaria pigmentosa in, 997–998
Histacalm, 229, 229t
Histamine, in atopy, 580
   in pruritus, 62, 62t
Histamine-releasing factors, 556
Histiocyte(s), cutaneous, 39
   in dermatitis, *187*, 187–188
Histiocytic sarcoma. See *Sarcoma(s), histiocytic*.
Histiocytoma, *1334*, 1346, *1347*–1350, *1348–1351*. See also *Transmissible venereal tumor*.
   atypical. See *Neuroendocrine tumor(s), primary cutaneous*.
   benign fibrous, 1354–1355, *1355*, *1356*
   breed(s) with predilection for, 1237t
   breed(s) with predilection for, 1237t
   eyelid, 1288
   malignant fibrous, *1348*, 1355–1357, *1357–1358*
Histiocytosis, cutaneous, 1346, *1348*, 1353–1354, *1354*
   breed(s) with predilection for, 1237t
   Langerhans' cell, malignant, 1347
   reactive, 1347
   malignant, 1346, 1347, *1348*, 1350–1351, *1351*
   breed(s) with predilection for, 1237t
   systemic, 1346, *1348*, 1352–1353, *1353*
   breed(s) with predilection for, 1237t

Histoplasma capsulatum, 337, 400
  culture of, 121
  stain for, 119
Histoplasmosis, cause of, 400
  clinical management of, 402–403
  diagnosis of, 401–402, *402*
  in cats, clinical findings in, 401, *401*
  in dogs, clinical findings in, 400–401, *402*
  in ferrets, 1419
  pathogenesis of, 400
Hives. See *Urticaria*.
Hoeppli-Splendore phenomenon, *317*
Holistic medicine, 263
Holocrine gland(s). See *Sebaceous gland(s)*.
Homeobox gene(s), 93
Homeopathy, 263
Hookworm dermatitis, 431–432, *432*, *433*
  claw involvement in, 1195
Hordeum jubatum, 1091
Hordeum murinum, 1091
Hordoleum (stye), 1186
Hormonal hypersensitivity, 644–647, *646*, *647*
Hormone(s), and hair growth, 6. See also specific hormone.
Horn(s), cutaneous, 1244, *1392*, *1394–1396*, *1396–1398*
    feline leukemia virus and, 517
    in dogs, *1241*, *1242*
    multiple, in cats, 528
Horn cysts (keratin cysts), 156
Horn pearls (squamous pearls), 156
Hornet(s), 505–506
Horsefly, 502
Hot spot(s). See *Pyotraumatic dermatitis*; *Pyotraumatic folliculitis*.
Hound, Afghan, delayed gonadal maturation in, 844
    demodicosis in, 461
    eyelid tumor in, 1188
    grooming of, 214
    hypoandrogenism in, 837
    hypothyroidism in, 852
    nasal depigmentation in, 1017
    risk for neoplastic skin disorders and non-neoplastic lumps in, 1237t
    risk for non-neoplastic skin disorders in, 75, 77t
    tricholemmoma in, 1264
  Basset, actinic keratoses in, 1391
    black hair follicular dysplasia in, 962
    congenital hypotrichosis in, 958
    hemangiosarcomas in, 1299
    immunodeficiency in, 279t
    lymphomas in, 1331
    Malassezia dermatitis in, 364, 365
    Mycobacterium avium infection in, 315
    pododermatitis in, 305
    risk for neoplastic skin disorders and non-neoplastic lumps in, 1237t, 1238t
    risk for non-neoplastic skin disorders in, 75, 77t
    seborrhea in, 913, 915, 1032
    trichoepithelioma in, 1263
Humectant(s), 227, 1028
Humilac, 235
Humoral immunity, 558–560
Husky, Siberian. See *Siberian husky*.
Hutch burn, 1450
Hyaline body(ies). See *Apoptotic body(ies)*.
Hyalinization, of dermal collagen, 156–157
Hyalohyphomycosis, definition of, 376–377
Hyaluronate, 38
Hyaluronic acid, 38

Hycodan. See *Hydrocodone*.
Hydra-Pearls cream rinse, 229t
Hydration, of skin, 1025
Hydro B-1020, for acral lick dermatitis, 1063
Hydrocarbon(s), 1028
  chlorinated, antiparasitic therapy with, 424
Hydrocodone, for acral lick dermatitis, 1063
Hydrocortisone, 232
  in shampoo, 223
Hydrogen peroxide, 231
Hydropic degeneration, epidermal, 143, *146*
Hydro-Plus, for acral lick dermatitis, 1063
Hydrotherapy, 220–221
  for bacterial infection, 280–281
α-Hydroxyacid(s) (2% to 10%), topical, 235
Hydroxychloroquine sulfate, 678
  for discoid lupus erythematosus, 716
Hydroxylysine, 36
4-Hydroxyproline, 36
Hydroxyzine, 1057
  for acral lick dermatitis, 1061–1063
Hygroma, 1102
Hy-Lyt°efa, 229t, 917, 1028, 1035, 1113
Hymenoptera, 505–506
Hyperadrenocorticism, infections in, 803–804
Hyperadrenocorticism (Cushing's disease, Cushing's syndrome), 278, 781, 782, 790
  alopecia in, 780
  differential diagnosis of, 804–805
  iatrogenic, 799, 800
  in cats, 815–819
    adrenal function tests in, 816–818
    causes and pathogenesis of, 815–816
    clinical features of, 802, 816, *817*
    clinical management of, 818–819
    diagnosis of, 816–818
    histopathology of, 816
  in dogs, *158*, *176*, 798–815
    causes of, 799
      differentiation of, tests for, 810
    clinical features of, 800–804, *801–803*, *840*
    clinical management of, 810–815
    diagnosis of, 804–810, *807–808*
      tests for, 809–810
    iatrogenic, management of, 815
    pathogenesis of, 799
    pituitary-dependent, 799
      clinical management of, 811–814
    prognosis for, 810
  in ferrets, 1421–1424, *1422–1423*
  in hamsters, 1441
  red hair in, 1022
Hyperandrogenism, in male dogs, 834–836, *835*, *836*, 837
Hypereosinophilic syndrome, feline, 1133–1135, *1134–1135*, *1187*
Hyperestrogenism, 781, 795–796
  in female animals, *817*, 829–831, *830*, *831*
  in ferrets, 1424–1425, *1425*
  red hair in, 1022
Hyperglucocorticoidism, 252, 789–790, 1399
  diagnosis of, 805
Hypergranulosis, 134, *137*
Hyperkeratosis, 132–133, *133–136*, 1025
  basketweave, 132, *134*
  compact, 132, *134*
  epidermal, 180
  footpad, *930*, *935*, 935–936, *1114–1115*

Hyperkeratosis (Continued)
  laminated, 132, 134
  nasal, 936
  orthokeratotic (anuclear), 132, 132, 1025
    diffuse, with perivascular dermatitis, 178–179
    disproportionate follicular, 133, 136
      with perivascular dermatitis, 179
  parakeratotic (nucleated), 132–133, 133, 1025
    diffuse, with perivascular dermatitis, 179
    focal, overlying epidermal papillae, 133, 135
    focal, with perivascular dermatitis, 179
Hypermelanosis. See *Hyperpigmentation.*
Hyperonychia, definition of, 1193t
Hyperpigmentation, 86, 151–152, 153, 236, 1006–1013
  acquired, 1009–1013
  congenital and hereditary, 975–977
  drug-induced, 1011–1012
  genetic, 1006–1009
  hormone-associated, 1011
  in feline acromelanism, 1012–1013
  in pigmented tumors, 1013, 1013
  papillomavirus-associated, 1012, 1013
  postinflammatory, 96, 151–152, 1009–1011, 1011
Hyperplasia, epidermal, 134–135, 138, 139, 180
  irregular, 134–135
    papillated, 135, 139
    pseudocarcinomatous, 135, 139
    psoriasiform, 135, 138
    regular, 135, 138
Hyperprolactinemia, 798
Hypersensitivity, and mucinosis, 1175
  antidepressants for, 569–570
  antihistamines for, 567–569, 569t
  arachnid, 636–642
  bacterial, 637, 647–650, 649
  contact. See *Contact hypersensitivity (allergic contact dermatitis).*
  cutaneous basophil, 562
  cyclosporine for, 570–571
  flea bite. See *Flea bite hypersensitivity.*
  food. See *Food hypersensitivity.*
  foot licking in, 1066
  fungal, 650
  hormonal, 644–647
  in dermatophytosis, 341–342
  insect, 198, 486–487, 636–642. See also *Flea bite hypersensitivity; Mosquito bite hypersensitivity; Tick bite hypersensitivity.*
  intestinal parasite, 642–643
  mosquito bite, feline, 635–636, 637, 638
  nonsteroidal anti-inflammatory agents for, 566–567
  otitis externa caused by, 1210–1211, 1211–1212
  parasitic, 627–644. See also specific parasite.
  skin disorders related to, 571–650. See also specific disorder.
  storage mite–related, 640
  systemic glucocorticoids for, 570
  therapy for, 563–571
    avoidance as, 563, 595–597
    fatty acids in, 564–566
    regimens for, 563, 563t
    topical, 563–564
  tick bite, 635
  to *Malassezia* antigens, 364, 650
  type I (anaphylactic, immediate), 561–562
    late-phase, 562
  type II (cytotoxic), 561, 562
  type III (immune complex), 561, 562

Hypersensitivity (Continued)
  type IV (cell-mediated, delayed), 561, 562–563
Hyperthermia, for squamous cell carcinoma, 1257
  therapeutic use of, 237–238
Hyperthyroidism, feline, 859, 867, 867–868
Hypertrichosis, definition of, 85
  unilateral, 5
Hypervitaminosis A, 1116
Hypha/hyphae, 336
  cenocytic, 336
  examination for, 119, 121
  septate, 336
  sparsely septate, 336
  spiral, 124, 124
Hyphomyces destruens. See *Pythium insidiosum.*
Hyphomycosis. See *Pythiosis.*
Hypoandrogenism, 830, 837–838, 838
Hypoderma spp., in ferrets, 1419
Hypodermis. See *Subcutis.*
Hypogonadism, breed(s) with predilection for, 75
  definition of, 833
  in intact female animals, 830, 833–834
  in intact male animals, 842, 843–845
Hypogranulosis, 134
Hypokeratosis, 133–134, 1025
Hypomelanosis. See *Hypopigmentation.*
Hypophysectomy, in dogs, 811
Hypophysis, functional anatomy of, 780–781
Hypopigmentation, 1014–1021
  acquired, 1019–1021
  breed-associated, suspect genetic, 1014–1019
  canine, 1008–1009
  congenital and hereditary, 975
  drug-related, 1020, 1020
  genetic, 1014
  idiopathic, 1008, 1021, 1021
  in leishmaniasis, 1019, 1019–1020
  in neoplasia, 1008, 1021
  metabolic, 1020
  mucocutaneous, 1008–1009, 1017–1018
  nasal, 1016–1017
    seasonal, 1017
  postinflammatory, 1019, 1019–1020
Hypopigmentation (hypomelanosis), 96, 152–154, 154
Hypopituitarism, 781, 818
Hypoplasia, epidermal, 135–136
Hyposensitization, for canine atopy, 597–601, 598t
  for feline atopy, 608, 609t
Hyposomatotropism (pseudo-Cushing's syndrome, GH-responsive dermatosis), 794–795
  adult-onset, breed(s) with predilection for, 75
  in dogs, 203
  in mature dog, 817, 822–824, 823–825
Hypothalamus, functional anatomy of, 780–781
Hypothyroidism, 278, 781, 782, 783
  alopecia in, 780
  canine, 167, 851–865
    cause and pathogenesis of, 851–852
    clinical features of, 852–860, 854–860
    clinical management of, 863–865
    congenital, 858–860
    diagnosis of, 859, 860–863
    secondary, 852
    treatment of, 864
  feline, 865–866, 866
  immune-mediated, 789
  in ferrets, 1426
  otitis externa in, 1210–1211

Hypothyroidism (Continued)
  red hair in, 1022
  secondary, 789
  skin changes in, 783–784
  tertiary, 789
Hypotrichosis, congenital, definition of, 958
  in cats, 959, 960–962
  in dogs, 954, 958–959, 959, 960
  definition of, 85
  tardive, 965–974

Ice, antipruritic therapy with, 229t
Ichthyosis, 1029
  canine, 914–915
  cause and pathogenesis of, 922–923
  clinical features of, 914, 923, 924
  clinical management of, 242, 243, 924–925
  definition of, 922
  diagnosis of, 923–924, 925
  Harlequin, 31
  hypergranulosis in, 137
  X-linked, 31
Iggo dome. See *Tylotrich pad*.
Iggo-Pinkus dome. See *Tylotrich pad*.
IGR(s) (insect growth regulators), 495
Imaverol. See *Enilconazole rinse*.
Imidacloprid, 423, 497, 498
  antiparasitic therapy with, 426
Imidazole, antifungal therapy with, 411
  topical, 409
Imipramine, 1057
Immune complex(es), 559
  deposition of, in cutaneous lupus erythematosus, 702
  vasculitis caused by, in mice, 1444
Immune system, of skin. See *Skin immune system*.
Immune-mediated skin disease, 667–769. See also specific disease.
  claw involvement in, 1195, 1196–1197
  clinical management of, 244
  diagnosis of, 667–671
  primary (autoimmune), 667
  secondary, 667
  treatment of, 671–678
Immunocytochemistry, 202–204, 204t
Immunodeficiency, acquired, 278
  and canine demodicosis, 463–464
  and leishmaniasis, 535
  in German shepherds, 307, 308
  management of, 286
  primary, 278, 279t
Immunofluorescence testing, 202
  in immune-mediated skin disease, 668–671, 669–670
  in systemic lupus erythematosus, 707, 709–710
  salt-split skin for, 694
Immunoglobulin(s), epidermal, 31, 32
  in cerumen, 1204
  in pemphigus complex, 680
  in vascular endothelium, 56
Immunoglobulin E, 561–562, 574–577
Immunoglobulin gene superfamily, 545
Immunohistochemistry, in immune-mediated skin disease, 668
Immunologic disorder(s), 992–995
Immunomodulation, for chronic recurrent bacterial infections, 286–287
  for dogs with immunodeficiency, 286

Immunoperoxidase testing, in immune-mediated skin disease, 668
Immunoregulin, 286–287
Immunosuppressive agent(s), 671–678, 672t
Impetigo, 288–290, 289, 290
  bullous, 289, 290
  staphylococcal, 288
  in dogs, 290
Impression smear(s), for *Malassezia* spp., 368
  technique for, 112–115, 116–117
Imuran. See *Azathioprine*.
In situ hybridization, 1239
In vitro lymphocyte blastogenesis (IVLB) test, 463–464
Inca hairless dog, 957
India ink, for fungal staining, 119
Indolent ulcer, feline, 1142, 1148–1149, 1149
Indole-5,6-quinone, 17
Infection(s), bacterial. See *Bacterial infection(s)*.
  fungal. See *Fungal infection(s)*.
  viral. See *Viral disease(s)*.
Inhalant dermatitis, allergic. See *Atopy*.
Inhibin, 795
Injection site reaction(s), 725, 726
  canine, 896
  drug-induced, 721, 722t
  feline, 902
  in ferrets, 1426
Insect(s), 486–500
  hypersensitivity to, 198, 486–487, 636–642. See also *Flea bite hypersensitivity; Mosquito bite hypersensitivity; Tick bite hypersensitivity*.
Insect development inhibitor(s), systemic, antiparasitic therapy with, 430
Insect growth regulators (IGRs), 495
  antiparasitic therapy with, 426
Insecticide(s), regulation of, 424
Insulin hypersensitivity, in pituitary dwarfism, 821
Insulin-like growth factor-1 (IGF-1), 795
  in pituitary dwarfism, 821
Integrin(s), functions of, 13–14
  in morphogenesis of skin appendages, 3
  in stratum basale, 13
  subunits of, 13
Interceptor. See *Milbemycin*.
Interdigital pyoderma (pododermatitis). See *Pododermatitis*.
Interface dermatitis, drug-induced, 729
  hydropic, 180, 181
  lichenoid, 180, 181
Interferon(s), therapy with, 252–253
α-Interferon, for feline rhinotracheitis, 525
  human recombinant, for recurrent bacterial infections, 286
International Veterinary Acupuncture Society, 263
Interrupt, 494
Interstitial cell tumor(s), 837, 838, 843
Interstitial dermatitis, 182–184, 183, 184
  drug-induced, 729
Intertrigo, 288, 1097, 1105–1108, 1106
  body fold, 1106, 1107
  facial fold, 1097, 1107
  lip fold, 1106, 1107
  tail fold, 1106, 1107
  vulvar fold, 1106, 1107
Intestinal parasite hypersensitivity, 642–643
Intradermal allergy testing. See *Allergy test(s), intradermal*.
Intrinsic factors, in hair cycle, 5–6
Intron-A, 253

Invisible dermatosis, 199–201
Involucrin, 28
  formation of, 29
Iodide(s), antifungal therapy with, 414
Iodine, in shampoo, 223
  in topical therapy, 230–231
Iodism, 414
Iodophor(s), 231
Irish setter. See *Setter, Irish.*
Irish terrier. See *Terrier, Irish.*
Irish water spaniel. See *Spaniel, Irish water.*
Irish wolfhound. See *Wolfhound, Irish.*
Isodesmosine, 37
Isothiocyanate(s), 680
Isotretinoin, 241–242
  adverse effects and side effects of, 1029
  antiseborrheic therapy with, 919, 1029
  dosage and administration of, 242–243
  for epidermal dysplasia in West Highland white terriers, 929
  indications for, 242, 1029
  otic therapy with, 1229–1230
Isoxsuprine, for Raynaud-like disease in dogs, 1195
Itching. See *Pruritus.*
Itraconazole, adverse effects and side effects of, 411, 413, 721, 743, 753
  antifungal therapy with, 357, 410, 411, 413
  anti-inflammatory effects of, 413
  dosage and administration of, 357t
  immunomodulatory effects of, 413
  otic therapy with, 1229
Ivermectin, 428, 445
  adverse effects and side effects of, 428–429
  anti-inflammatory properties of, 429
  for canine demodicosis, 472, 473
  for feline demodicosis, 476
  for scabies, 483, 484
  in small animals, dosage and administration of, 1418t
  otic therapy with, 1229
  regulation of, 424
  systemic, antiparasitic therapy with, 429
  toxicosis, in cats, 429
    in dogs, 428–429
Ivomec. See *Ivermectin.*
Ixodes spp., Lyme borreliosis transmission by, 326
Ixodes dammini, 444
Ixodes ricinus, 444
Ixodes scapularis, 444

Jack Russell terrier. See *Terrier, Jack Russell.*
Jejunal adenocarcinoma, cutaneous metastases of, 1373–1374
Juvenile cellulitis. See *Cellulitis, canine juvenile.*
Juvenile hormone analog(s), in insect control, 426
Juvenile pyoderma. See *Cellulitis, canine juvenile.*
Juvenile sterile granulomatous dermatitis and lymphadenitis. See *Cellulitis, canine juvenile.*
Juvenoid(s), 426

Karyolysis, definition of, 136
Karyorrhexis, definition of, 136
Keeshond, adrenal hyperplasia–like syndrome in, 847
  adult-onset hyposomatotropism in, 822
  Ehlers-Danlos syndrome in, 982
  hypogonadism in, 844–845
  keratoacanthoma in, 1248

Keeshond *(Continued)*
  risk for neoplastic skin disorders and non-neoplastic lumps in, 1237t
  risk for non-neoplastic skin disorders in, 75, 80t
KeraSolv, 226, 1027–1028
Keratin, 20–22, 29, 48, 220
  hard, 29
  in epidermal barrier function, 31
  soft, 29
Keratinase, from *Microsporum canis,* 341
Keratinization, defects of, 913–949, 1025–1053
  drug-induced, *1052,* 1052–1053
  ear involvement in, *1205,* 1212
  in mice, 1444
  disorders of, 31
  epidermal, 29
  follicular, 48
  infundibular, 48
  inner root sheath and hair shaft medullary, 48
  trichilemmal, *11,* 48
    excessive, 166, *167,* 790
  trichogenic, 48
Keratinocyte(s), acantholytic, 143, *155*
  adhesion of, 19, 22t
  antimicrobial peptides synthesized by, 33
  apoptotic, 139–140, *740*
  changes in, in cutaneous lupus erythematosus, 702
    in erythema multiforme, 731–732
  cultured, 31
  cutaneous nerves and, 59
  functions of, 26, 29
  immunohistochemistry of, 20–22
  immunologic functions of, 550–551
  in epidermal immunity, 26
  phagocytic functions of, 22
  ultrastructure of, 20, *23*
Keratinosome(s), 22
Keratoacanthoma, 1029, *1241,* 1248–1249, *1249–1250*
  breed(s) with predilection for, 1237t
  clinical management of, 242
  in hamsters, 1442
  in rats, 1455
  subungual, 1198
Keratoconjunctivitis sicca, 283, 919
  treatment of, 674
Keratogenesis, 29–31
Keratohyalin, synthesis of, 29
Keratohyalin granule(s), 48
  epidermal, *11*
  from normal skin, *115,* 116
  functions of, 26
  morphology of, 26–27
Keratolinin, 28
Keratolytic agent(s), antiseborrheic therapy with, 1026–1028
Keratoplastic agent(s), antiseborrheic therapy with, 1026–1028
Keratosis, 1390–1396
  actinic, 1391–1392, *1393, 1394*
  lichenoid, 1391–1394, *1392–1393, 1395*
  periocular, 1394, *1396*
  seborrheic, *1392, 1394, 1395*
Kerion, 650
  dermatophytic, 343, *344–345,* 351
Kerry blue terrier. See *Terrier, Kerry blue.*
Ketoconazole, adverse effects and side effects of, 411, 412
  antifungal therapy with, 357, 410, 411–413
  dosage and administration of, 357t

Ketoconazole (Continued)
  drug interactions with, 412
  for adrenal neoplasia, 815
  for canine hyperadrenocorticism, 812
  for epidermal dysplasia in West Highland white terriers, 929
  for feline hyperadrenocorticism, 818
  for leishmaniasis, 538
  hypomelanosis caused by, 1020
  in shampoo, 223
  otic therapy with, 1229
Klebsiella spp., in mice, 1442
Klebsiella pneumoniae, infection by, in rats, 1452
KOH, for keratin clearance, in fungal diagnosis, 120
Koilocytosis, 142–143, 145
Komondor, grooming of, 214
Korat cat, grooming for, 215
Kuvasz, dermatomyositis in, 940

Labiogram(s), 3
Laboratory test(s), 94–131
Labrador retriever. See Retriever, Labrador.
Lacrimal gland(s), 1185
Lactic acid, 235, 1028
Lactobacillus spp., otitis media caused by, 1214t
Lacunae. See Cleft(s).
Lagochilascaris major, in cats and dogs, 440, 442
Lamellar body(ies), 1025
Lamellar granule(s), 29–30, 30
Lamina densa (basal lamina), of basement membrane zone, 34, 35
Lamina fibroreticularis, of basement membrane zone. See Sublamina densa area (lamina fibroreticularis).
Lamina lucida (lamina rara), of basement membrane zone, 34, 35
Lamina rara, of basement membrane zone. See Lamina lucida (lamina rara).
Laminin, 13, 36t
  in cell type identification, 204t
Lamisil. See Terbinafine.
Langerhans' cell(s), 10, 22–25, 24, 25
  age-related changes in, 64
  development of, 2
  functions of, 24, 26
  histochemistry of, 24
  immunologic functions of, 551–552
  immunophenotype of, 24
  in epidermal immunity, 26
  in hair follicle, 48
Langerhans' granule(s). See Birbeck's granule(s).
Langer's line(s), 9
Lanolin, 1028
Lanugo hair, 4, 41
Laser Doppler flowmetry, 57–58
Laser surgery, 259, 260
Laser therapy, for acral lick dermatitis, 1064
  for squamous cell carcinoma, 1357
Lathyrism, 37
Latrodectus spp., 484–485
Latrodectus bishopi, 484
Latrodectus mactans, 484
Leflunomide, for graft-versus-host disease, 720
  immunosuppressive therapy with, 674–675
Leg(s), common and less common dermatoses of, 105t
Leiomyoma, 1312–1313, 1313, 1314t
Leiomyosarcoma, 1312–1313
Leishmaniasis, 278, 530–531, 534–538, 535–537

Leishmaniasis (Continued)
  cytologic diagnosis of, 117
  hypopigmentation in, 1019, 1019–1020
  in humans, 534
  visceral, 195, 537, 538
Lentiginosis profusa, 1006
Lentigo, 87, 96, 1006, 1007
Lentigo simplex in orange cats, 1006–1007, 1008, 1009
Leprosy, canine, 316–319
  feline, 315–316, 317, 318
  in rats, 1452
Leptospirosis, 1089
Lesion(s). See Skin lesion(s).
Leukemia, skin lesions of, 1374–1375
Leukemia cutis, 1374
Leukeran. See Chlorambucil.
Leukocytoclastic vasculitis, 181–182, 182
Leukoderma, 96, 975, 1017–1018, 1021
Leukonychia, definition of, 1193t
Leukotrichia, 96, 975, 1021
  in radiation damage, 1088, 1088
  periocular, 1021, 1022
Leukotriene(s), 560
  effects of, on skin, 208
  in pruritus, 62, 62t
Levamisole, adverse effects and side effects of, 286, 721, 735
  for recurrent bacterial infections, 286
  for systemic lupus erythematosus, 711
Levothyroxine, for hypothyroidism, in cats, 866
  in dogs, 862–865
Lhasa apso, atopy in, 581
  congenital hypotrichosis in, 958
  food hypersensitivity in, 618
  glucocorticoid-induced reaction in, 246–247
  juvenile cellulitis in, 1213
  keratoacanthoma in, 1248
  Malassezia dermatitis in, 348–349
  risk for neoplastic skin disorders and non-neoplastic lumps in, 1237t
  risk for non-neoplastic skin disorders in, 80t
Lice. See Louse/lice.
Lichenification, 87, 99
Lichenoid dermatosis, 1126–1127, 1130–1132, 1132
Lichenoid lesion(s), drug-induced, in cats, 723t
  in dogs, 722t
Lidocaine, adverse effects and side effects of, in kittens and puppies, 129
  effects of, on microorganisms, 128
  precautions with, 129
Light trap(s), for flea control, 496
Lime sulfur, 233–234
  in small animals, dosage and administration of, 1418t
Lime sulfur rinse, 234, 356, 356t, 427
  antifungal therapy with, 410
  for feline demodicosis, 475, 476
  for scabies, 482
D-Limonene, antiparasitic therapy with, 425
Lincomycin, efficacy of, against Staphylococcus intermedius, 282
  resistance to, 282
  systemic, dosage of, 284t
Lincosamide(s), efficacy of, against staphylococcal infection, 283
  resistance to, 282
  systemic, for bacterial infections, 281
Lindane dip, 424
Linear granuloma. See Eosinophilic granuloma, feline.

Linear IgA bullous dermatosis, 694, 701
Linear IgA pustular dermatosis, canine, *748*, 756, *756*
Linear preputial dermatosis, *830*, 839, *839*
Linkin, 36t
Linognathus setosus, 487, *489*, *490*
Linoleic acid, 208–209, 235, 1113
  topical therapy with, 209
Linolenic acid, 208, 239, 1113
Liothyronine, for hypothyroidism, in cats, 866
  in dogs, 862–865
Lip(s), common and less common dermatoses of, 103t
  hypopigmentation of, congenital, 1018
  upper, idiopathic ulcerative dermatitis of, in dogs, 1178
Lip fold intertrigo, *1106*, 1107
Lipid(s), dermal deposits of, 160, *161*
  epidermal, 28–31, 51
  intercellular, 29–30
Lipocortin-1, 245
Lipocyte(s), 63, 1156
  development of, 2
Lipoma(s), *1306*, 1308–1311, *1309–1311*
  breed(s) with predilection for, 1237t
  in rats, 1455
  infiltrative, 1308–1309
Lipomatosis, diffuse, idiopathic, 1173, *1173–1175*
Liposarcoma, 1281, 1311–1312, *1312*
  breed(s) with predilection for, 1237t
  in cats, 528
  sternal, cutaneous metastases of, 1373
β-Lipotropic hormone (β-lipotropin), 17
Listeria monocytogenes, 327
Listeriosis, 327–328
Listrophorus (Leporacarus) gibbus, *1434–1435*
  in rabbits, 1448–1449
Local anesthetic(s), antipruritic therapy with, 230
  for pruritus, 228
Lone Star tick(s), 444
Longhaired cat(s), 215
Loricrin, 28
  functions of, 26–27
Loshed, 894
Lotion(s), 218t, 224–225
Lotrimin. See *Clotrimazole*.
Lotrisone. See *Clotrimazole/betamethasone*.
Louse/lice. See also *Pediculosis*.
  characteristics of, 487
  human pubic, 487
  nits, 108, *112*, 488
  on guinea pigs, 1433, *1434*
  on mice, 1443
  on rabbits, 1449
  on rats, 1453
Loxosceles spp., 484–485
Loxosceles reclusa, 484
Loxosceles unicolor, 484
Lufeneron, 430, 499
Lumpy jaw, in ferrets, 1417
Lupoid onychodystrophy, 745
  symmetric, 1195–1198, *1196–1197*
Lupus erythematosus, 701–717
  classification of, 701–702, 703t
  cutaneous (discoid), 712–716
    canine vesicular, 707
    cause and pathogenesis of, 712
    characteristics of, 702
    clinical features of, 712–714, *713*, *714*, *1187*
    clinical management of, 716
    exfoliative, 707, 717

Lupus erythematosus *(Continued)*
    forms of, 702
    histopathology of, 714–716, *715*
    in cats, 714, *714*
    in dogs, 712–714, *713*, *1187*
    in humans, 707
    pathogenesis of, 702
    pigmentary incontinence in, *163*
    vesicular, 98, 717, 946–947
  drug-induced, 704
    in dogs, 722t
  in cats, *696–697*, 707, 708–709
    clinical features of, *696*, 705
  in dogs, *172*, *173*, *696–697*, 707, 708–709
    cause and pathogenesis of, 704–705
    clinical features of, *696*, 705
    diagnostic criteria for, 710t, 710–711
  in humans, 702–704
  panniculitis of, 197
  pigmentary incontinence in, *163*
  systemic, 702, 704–711
    bullous, 694
      causes of, 13
    cause and pathogenesis of, 704–705
    clinical features of, *696*, 705
    clinical management of, 711
    dermatohistopathology of, 707, *708–709*
    diagnosis of, *142*, 705–711
    in cats, *696–697*, 707, 708–709
    in dogs, *172*, *173*, *696–697*, 707, 708–709
      diagnostic criteria for, 710t, 710–711
    in humans, 707, 709–710
    prognosis for, 711
Lupus profundus, 197
Luteinizing hormone (LH), 781, 796, 998
Lutropin. See *Luteinizing hormone (LH)*.
Lutzomyia spp., 534
Lyell's syndrome. See *Toxic epidermal necrolysis*.
LymDyp. See *Lime sulfur rinse*.
Lyme borreliosis, 326–327
Lymph vessel(s), cutaneous, 58, *59*
Lymphangioma, 1305, *1306*
Lymphangiosarcoma, 1305–1308, *1306–1308*
  in cats, 1305, *1306*
  in dogs, 1305
Lymphedema, 990–992
  cause and pathogenesis of, 990
  clinical features of, *988–989*, 990–991, *991*
  clinical management of, 992
  definition of, 990
  diagnosis of, *991*, 991–992, *992*
  in vasculitis, *746*
Lymphocyte(s), cutaneous, 39
  functions of, 552–553
  in cytologic diagnosis, *114*, 118t
Lymphocytic mural folliculitis, idiopathic, of cats, 907–909, *907–910*
Lymphocytic (Hashimoto's) thyroiditis, 851–852
  tests for, 788–789
Lymphohistiocytic infiltration, in cutaneous lupus erythematosus, 702
Lymphoid nodules, 174, *175*
Lymphokine(s), 543
Lymphoma, 1330–1342. See also *Neuroendocrine tumor(s), primary cutaneous*.
  and pseudolymphoma, differentiation of, histologic criteria for, 1341–1342, 1343t
  B cell, 1331

Lymphoma (Continued)
　breed(s) with predilection for, 1237t
　epitheliotropic, 1021, 1029, 1331, *1331*, 1333–1340, *1334–1339*, 1347
　　clinical management of, 242, 244
　　drug-induced, 725
　　in cats, *910*
　　in hamsters, *1432*, 1441, *1442*
　　in mice, 1444
　　of eyelid, 1188, *1189*
　in mice, 1444
　in rabbits, 1451, 1452
　large-cell, 1331
　nonepitheliotropic, *1324*, 1331–1333, *1332*
　T cell, 1331
Lymphomatoid granulomatosis, 1340, *1341*, *1342*
Lymphomatosis. See *Lymphoma.*
Lymphosarcoma. See also *Lymphoma.*
　claw involvement in, 1198
　in cats, 528
　in dogs, cytologic diagnosis of, *114*
　transmissible. See *Transmissible venereal tumor.*
Lynxacarus radovsky, 446, *447*. See also *Cat fur mite(s).*
Lysine, deficiency of, 1020
　for feline rhinotracheitis, 525
Lysosomal hydrolase(s), 37
Lysozyme, in cell type identification, 204t

MacKenzie (toothbrush) specimen collection method, 120
Macroconidia, collection of, 122
　in fungal identification, 122
Macrolide antibiotic(s), anti-inflammatory and immunomodulatory properties of, 285
　resistance to, 282
　systemic, for bacterial infections, 281
Macronychia, definition of, 1193t
Macrophage(s), in cytologic diagnosis, *113*, 118t
　tissue, functions of, 553
Macule(s), 86, *87*
　erythematous, 86
Maculopapular (morbilliform) lesion(s), drug-induced, in cats, 723t
　in dogs, 722t
Madurella grisea, 377
Maduromycosis, 377
Maggot(s). See *Myiasis.*
Magnesium sulfate, for bacterial infection, 281
Major histocompatibility complex (MHC), 545–548
Malamute, chondrodysplasia in, 820
　demodicosis in, 461
　follicular dysplasia in, 971
　hypogonadism in, 844
　hypothyroidism in, 852
　periocular dermatosis in, 1286
　risk for neoplastic skin disorders and non-neoplastic lumps in, 1237t
　risk for non-neoplastic skin disorders in, 75, 80t
　wooly, male hypogonadism in, *842*
　zinc-responsive dermatosis in, 1119, 1199
Malassezia spp., cytologic examination for, 366–370
　in cats, 363
　lipid-dependent, 363, 371
　non–lipid-dependent, 363, 371
　otitis externa caused by, 1213–1215, 1214t
　otitis media caused by, 1214t
　skin scrapings for, 366–368

Malassezia spp. (Continued)
　superficial mycoses caused by, 339. See also *Malassezia dermatitis.*
Malassezia canis. See *Malassezia pachydermatis.*
Malassezia dermatitis, 363–374, *1060–1061*
　acanthosis nigricans and, 976
　acrodermatitis and, 993
　atopy and. See *Atopy.*
　cause of, 363
　claw involvement in, 1195
　clinical management of, 371–374
　diagnosis of, 119–121, 366–371, *369–373*
　epidermal dysplasia in West Highland white terriers and, 928–929
　follicular parakeratosis and, 926, *927*
　foot licking in, 1066
　hypothyroidism and, 853–855
　in cats, clinical findings in, 366, *368*
　in dogs, 370–372
　　clinical findings in, *348–349*, 365–366, *367*
　　dermatohistopathology of, *158*
　　pigmentary incontinence in, *163*
　in guinea pigs, 1431
　pathogenesis of, 363–365
　pododermatitis caused by, 305
　red/brown claws in, 1022
　rinses for, 410
　risk factors for, 364–365
　seborrhea and, 915–916, 918, 1030, 1034, 1035
　topical therapy for, 409
　zinc-responsive dermatosis and, 1120
　zoonotic aspects of, 366
Malassezia furfur, 363, 364
Malassezia globosa, 363
Malassezia obtusa, 363
Malassezia otitis externa, 366
　pathogenesis of, 364
Malassezia pachydermatis, and *Staphylococcus aureus*, synergism of, 33
　as resident flora, in dogs, 34
　characteristics of, 363
　culture of, 371
　cytologic examination for, 369, *369*
　diagnosis of, *114*, 117, 119–121
　enzymatic properties of, 364
　in anal sacs, 1201
　in humans, 366
　in normal flora, of cats and dogs, 364
　in surface debris, 155
　otitis externa caused by, 1213–1215
　populations of, variability in, 370
　public health considerations with, 1215
　strains (sequevars) of, 363–364
Malassezia paronychia, *1189*
Malassezia restricta, 363
Malassezia slooffiae, 363
Malassezia sympodialis, 363, 366
　cytologic examination for, 369
Malathion, 425
　for feline demodicosis, 475
Male feminizing syndrome, idiopathic, 851
Malignant fibrous histiocytoma, 1281
　in rats, 1455
Mallophaga, characteristics of, 487, *489*, *490*
Maltese dilution, 968
　and feline hair color, 9
　hair in, 108, *110*

Mammary adenocarcinoma, 1021
  cutaneous metastases of, *1366*, 1373
Mammotroph(s), 781
Manchester terrier. See *Terrier, Manchester.*
Mange, demodectic. See *Demodicosis.*
  follicular. See *Demodicosis.*
  notoedric. See also *Scabies, feline.*
    in hamsters, 1440
  otodectic, 451, *452*
    in ferrets, 1419
  psoroptic, in rabbits, *1447*, 1448
  red. See *Demodicosis.*
  sarcoptic. See also *Scabies, canine.*
    in ferrets, 1419, *1420*
Mannan, 336, 341
Manx cat, grooming for, 215
  tail fold intertrigo in, 1107
Marbofloxacin, otic therapy with, 1229
  systemic, dosage of, 284t
Masson trichome stain, staining characteristics of various substances with, 130t
Mast cell(s), cutaneous nerves and, 59
  dermal, 39, *40*
  epidermal, 156, *157*, *158*
  fixation of, 39
  functions of, 553–556, *554*
  in cytologic diagnosis, *114*, 118t
  perivascular, 57
  staining of, 39
  subtypes of, in dogs, 39
Mast cell mediator(s), 553–556, 555t
Mast cell tumor(s), 1320–1330
  breed(s) with predilection for, 1237t
  cause and pathogenesis of, 1320
  claw involvement in, 1198
  clinical findings in, 1320–1323
  clinical management of, 1323–1330, *1328*, *1329*
    by stage, 1325, 1329t
  diagnosis of, 1323, *1326–1328*, 1328t, 1329t
  histologic classification of, 1325, 1329t
  in cats, 1322–1323, *1324*, *1325*, *1326*, *1328*
  in dogs, *1306*, 1320–1322, *1321*, *1322*, *1326–1327*
    cytologic diagnosis of, *114*
  in mice, 1444
  of eyelid, 1188, *1189*
  staging of, 1325, 1329t
Mastiff, bull, congenital hypothyroidism in, 852
  follicular dysplasia in, 971
  vitiligo in, 1015
  muzzle folliculitis and furunculosis in, 304
  Neapolitan, undifferentiated sarcoma in, 1319
  pododermatitis in, 305
Mastitis, 302
Mat(s), in haircoat, 213
Mâtin de Naples, cutis laxa in, 987
Max Joseph spaces, 147
Mechanoreceptor(s), 61, 62
Medical history, in diagnosis, 82–84
Medroxyprogesterone acetate, for feline acquired symmetric alopecia, 902
  therapy with, for feline psychogenic dermatitis, 1070
  in pituitary dwarfism, 821–822
Medulla, of hair shaft, 39, *41*, 44, 108, *110*
Medullary trichomalacia, 895, 951–953, *952*, *953*
Megace. See *Megestrol acetate.*
Megestrol acetate, therapy with, for acral lick dermatitis, 1063

Megestrol acetate *(Continued)*
  for feline acquired symmetric alopecia, 902
  for feline psychogenic dermatitis, 1070
Meglumine antimonate, therapy with, for leishmaniasis, 538
Meibomian gland(s), 1185
Meissner's corpuscle, innervation of, 59, 61, 62
Melaleuca oil, topical therapy with, 236
Melanin, 96, 1005
  photoprotective effects of, 16
  types of, 16–17
Melanin granule(s), epidermal, *11*, 16, *16*
  from normal skin, *115*, 116
  in sebaceous glands, 152, *153*
Melanization, regulation of, 1005
α-Melanocortin (α-MSH), actions of, 17
Melanocyte(s), 10, 14–19
  age-related changes in, 64
  and keratinocytes, interaction of, 16, 17
  appearance of, 14, *15*
  cell surface receptors on, 17
  dendritic, *15*
  dermal, 39
  development of, 2
  epidermal, 14, *15*
  follicular, 14
  functions of, 16
  ultrastructure of, 16, *18*
Melanocytoma, 1013, *1348*, 1359, *1360*, *1361*
  dermal, 96
  in cats, *174*
  in gerbils, 1429–1430
  in hamsters, 1441
  pilar neurocristic, 1359, *1361*
Melanoderma. See *Hyperpigmentation.*
Melanoderma and alopecia, in Yorkshire terriers, 964, 974–975, *975*
Melanogenesis, 17, 18
Melanoma, 1013, 1359, 1361–1364, *1363*, *1364*
  claw involvement in, 1198
  clear cell (balloon cell), 1363
  in cats, 528, 1362, *1362*, 1363, *1363*, *1364*
  in dogs, *1361*, 1361–1362, *1362*, *1363*
  in gerbils, 1429–1430
  in hamsters, 1441
  in mice, 1444
  in rabbits, 1451
  in rats, 1455
  oral, cutaneous metastases of, 1373
  pilar neurocristic, 1362–1363
  signet-ring, 1363
  subungual, 1361
Melanophage(s), 162–163
Melanosis, macular, in dogs, 837, 839–840
  perifollicular, 168, *169*, 195
  sebaceous gland, 170
Melanosome(s), 17, 1005
  stages of, 18–19
Melanotrichia, 96
  drug-induced, 1011–1012
  hormone-associated, 1011, *1012*
  postinflammatory, *1008–1009*, 1010–1011
Melatonin, 1005
  formulations of, 254
  therapy with, 253–254
    for seasonal flank alopecia, 893
Melioidosis, 328

Membrana nictitans, superficial gland of, 1185
Membrane-coating granules, 22
Meningioma, 1296
Menthol, antipruritic therapy with, 229–230
Merial. See *Fipronil.*
Merkel cell tumor(s), 1369–1370, *1370*
Merkel's cell(s), 10, 1369, *1371*
    functions of, 19
    of tylotrich pad, 19, *20, 45,* 46
    ultrastructure of, 19, *21*
Mesanagen, 46
Metabolic disease, 992–995. See also specific disorder.
Metabolic epidermal necrosis, 868
Metanagen, 46
Metaplasia, definition of, 174
Metatarsal fistulation, *980,* 985–986, *986,* 1157
Methimazole, adverse effects and side effects of, 723–725
Methoprene, 426, 495, 498
Methotrexate, antiseborrheic effects of, 920
    for graft-versus-host disease, 720
Methoxychlor flea and tick powders, 424
Methylene blue, 116
Methylprednisolone, injectable, 247t
Methylprednisolone acetate, 247, 250
    for acral lick dermatitis, 1063
Methyltestosterone, for hypoandrogenism, 838
Meticorten. See *Prednisone, injectable.*
Metronidazole, for leishmaniasis, 538
    in small animals, dosage and administration of, 1418t
Metyrapone, for feline hyperadrenocorticism, 818
Mexican hairless dog, 957, 958
MGK-264, 427
Mibolerone, 838
Miconazole, for *Malassezia* dermatitis, 219
    shampoo, 223, 356t
    topical, 356t, 409
Miconazole Spray. See *Miconazole.*
Microabscess(es), 149–151, *150, 151, 152*
    eosinophilic, *150,* 151
    papillary, 165
Microbial flora. See *Microflora.*
Microcirculation, cutaneous, measurement of, 57–58
Micrococcus spp., as resident flora, in cats, 33, 275
    in dogs, 33–34, 275
Microfibril(s), dermal, 37–38
Microflora, cutaneous, antagonism among, 33
    interactions of, 33
    synergism among, 33
    epidermal hydration and, 32
    nomadic, 33
    normal, 274
        fungi in, 338, 338t
        in immune defense, 32–33
        of ears, 1214t
        of eyelids, 1185
    resident, 33, 274–275
        in cats, 33
    transient, 33, 274–277
Micronychia, definition of, 1193t
MicroPearls shampoo(s), 917, 918, 1026–1027
Microscopy, direct smears for, 112, *113,* 117
    impression smears for, 112–115, 116–117
    swab smears for, 115, 116
Microsporum spp., 336, 339
    superficial mycoses caused by, 338
Microsporum audouinii, characteristics of, 339
    in guinea pigs, 1430

Microsporum audouinii (Continued)
    in rabbits, 1446
    Wood's lamp examination for, 119, 347–349
Microsporum canis, as resident flora, in cats, 33
    cattery and multiple-cat household dermatophytosis caused by, 358
        prevention of, 361
        response to treatment in, monitoring of, 361
    characteristics of, 339
    clinical management of, 234
        in kittens only, 360–361
    colonies of, morphology of, 122, *123*
    culture of, 120, 349
    diagnostic criteria for, 122
    environmental decontamination for, 359–360
    enzymatic properties of, 341
    examination for, 119, 120, 121
    identification of, 122
    in cats, 338
        asymptomatic carriage of, 340–341
        clinical findings in, 342, 343–347, *346*
        clinical management of, 409
        experimental models of, 341
        histopathology of, 349, *351,* 352
        hypersensitivity reaction to, 341–342
        incidence of, 339
        inflammatory response to, 341
    in dogs, clinical findings in, 343, *344–345*
        histopathology of, *350*
        incidence of, 339
    in guinea pigs, 1430–1431, *1431*
    in humans, 347
    in rabbits, 1446
    macroconidia of, 122, *124*
    microscopic morphology of, 122, *124*
    transmission of, 339
    vaccine against, 358
    veterinary clinic as source of, 340
    Wood's lamp examination for, 119, 121, 347–349
Microsporum distortum, characteristics of, 339
    Wood's lamp examination for, 119, 347–349
Microsporum gypseum, cattery and multiple-cat household dermatophytosis caused by, 358
    characteristics of, 339
    colonies of, morphology of, 122, *123*
    conidia of, 121
    diagnostic criteria for, 124
    identification of, 122–124
    in cats, incidence of, 339
    in dogs, clinical findings in, 343, *344–345*
        incidence of, 339
    in guinea pigs, 1430
    in normal flora, 338
    in rabbits, 1446
    in veterinary clinic, 340
    macroconidia of, 122, *124*
    microscopic morphology of, 122, *124*
    transmission of, 340
Microsporum persicolor, 340
    characteristics of, 349
    culture of, 349
    examination for, 120
    in cats, histopathology of, 349, *352*
    in dogs, clinical findings in, 342–343, *344–345*
        histopathology of, *352*
        spontaneous remission of, 354
Microsporum vanbreuseghemii, conidia of, 121

Microtia, congenital, in Dachshund, *1231*, 1232
Microvasculature, cutaneous, 56, 56–58, *57*
    deep plexus of, 56, *56*
    middle plexus of, 56, *56*
    superficial plexus of, 56, *56*
Microvesicle(s), epidermal, 148, *148*
Milbemycin, 428, 429, 445
  for canine demodicosis, 472
  for scabies, 483
  regulation of, 424
  systemic, antiparasitic therapy with, 429–430
Mineral(s), supplementation of, 209
Mineral imbalance(s), 1119
Mineral oil, 227, 1028
Mineralization, dermal perifollicular, 168
  dystrophic, of dermal collagen, 157–158, *158*
  perifollicular, 43–44
Minoxidil, in canine alopecia, 874
Misoprostol, for canine atopy, 601
Mitaban. See *Amitraz*.
Mite(s). See also *Storage mite-related hypersensitivity*.
  cat fur, skin scraping for, 101
  Cheyletiella. See *Cheyletiellosis*.
  chigger. See *Trombiculosis (chigger mites)*.
  demodectic. See *Demodicosis*.
  ear. See *Ear mite(s) (Otodectes cynotis)*.
  environmental, 453
  harvest. See *Trombiculosis (chigger mites)*.
  house dust, 453
  on ferrets, 1419
  on guinea pigs, 1431–1433, *1432–1434*
  on mice, 1443
  on rabbits, 1448–1449
  on rats, 1453
  parasitic, 445–484
  poultry, 445–446, *446*
    skin scraping for, 107
  sarcoptic. See *Scabies*.
  structure of, 440, 445
  treatment of, 445
Mitotane (o,p'-DDD), adverse effects and side effects of, 812–813
  hyperpigmentation caused by, 1011–1012
  melanotrichia caused by, 1011, *1012*
  therapy with, for adrenal hyperplasia–like syndrome, 849–850
    for adrenal neoplasia, 815
    for canine hyperadrenocorticism, 812–814
    for feline hyperadrenocorticism, 818
Mitotic figures, 134
Moisturizer(s), 223, 1028
  in topical therapy, 227
Mold(s), 336, 337. See also *Fungus/fungi*.
Molecular biology, 204
Moll's gland(s), 1185
Monilia spp. See *Candida* spp..
Moniliasis. See *Candidiasis*.
Moniliella suaveolens, 379
Monoclonal gammopathy, amyloidosis associated with, 768
Monokine(s), 543
Mononuclear cells, in cytologic diagnosis, 117
Mononuclear phagocyte system (MPS), 553
Morphea, *1142*, 1146–1148, *1147*
Mortierella spp., 384
Mosquito bite(s), 502
Mosquito bite hypersensitivity, feline, 635–636, *637*, *638*
Mosquito dermatitis, 502–503
Mouse, alopecia areata in, 1444

Mouse *(Continued)*
  bacterial infections in, 1442
  barbering in, 1444
  bite wounds in, 1444
  cage-related injury in, 1442
  dermatophytosis in, 1442–1443
  dermatoses in, 1442–1444
  ectoparasites on, *1432*, *1435*, 1443
  fungal infections in, 1442–1443
  hereditary hairlessness in, 1444
  immune complex vasculitis in, 1444
  neoplasia in, 1444
  nutritional disorders in, 1443–1444
  ringtail in, 1444
  viral infection in, 1443
Mouse pox, 1443
Moxidectin, 428, 429
  for canine demodicosis, 472
  otic therapy with, 1229
  systemic, antiparasitic therapy with, 430
Mucin, epidermal, *11*
  in dermis, 38
Mucinosis, cutaneous, 996–997, *1401*, *1402*, *1402*
  dermal, 164, *165*
  diffuse, *1402*, *1402*
  focal, *1401*, *1402*
    breed(s) with predilection for, 1238t
  follicular. See *Alopecia mucinosa*.
  hypersensitivity and, 1175
  idiopathic, *1158*, 1174–1175, *1176–1177*
  in hypothyroidism, 783
Mucinous degeneration, dermal. See *Mucinosis*.
Mucocutaneous junction(s), common and less common dermatoses of, 103t–104t
Mucoid degeneration, dermal. See *Mucinosis*.
Mucor spp., 384
  in normal flora, 338, 338t
Mucorales, 384
Mucormycosis, 377, 384
Mucous membrane pemphigoid, 694, 695, 701
Multinucleate epidermal giant cell(s), 174–175, *175*
Multinucleate histiocytic giant cell(s), 147, 185–187, *186*
  foreign body–type, 185, *186*
  Langhans-type, 185, *186*
  Touton-type, 185–187, *186*
Multinucleate keratinocyte giant cell(s), 174–175, *175*
Mumps, 524
Munro's microabscess, 150–151, *151*
Munsterlander, large, black hair follicular dysplasia in, 962
Mupirocin, topical, for bacterial infection, 279, 280
Mural folliculitis. See *Folliculitis, mural*.
Musculoskeletal system, in hyperadrenocorticism, 804
Muzzle, bleeding from, 304
  folliculitis of, 303–304
  furunculosis of, *302*, 303–304
  surface markings of, 3
Mycelium, definition of, 336
Mycetoma, actinomycotic, definition of, 376
  black (dark)-grained, 376, 377
  definition of, 376
  eumycotic, 377–379, *378*
    definition of, 376
  granules in, 337
  pododermatitis caused by, 305
  white-grained, 376, 377
Mycetoma foot, *378*
Mycobacteria, classification of, 312–313

Mycobacteria (Continued)
  granulomas caused by, 312–321, *317, 318, 320*
  leprosy, 312
  opportunistic, 312–313, 319–321
  tuberculosis, 312
Mycobacteriosis, and abscesses in cats, 311
  atypical, *317*
  diagnosis of, 117, 125
Mycobacterium avium, 312, 315
Mycobacterium bovis, 314
Mycobacterium chelonei, 312, *317,* 319
Mycobacterium chitae, 315
Mycobacterium fortuitum, 312, *317,* 319
Mycobacterium kansasii, 312
Mycobacterium leprae, 316
Mycobacterium lepraemurium, 312, 315
  in rats, 1452
Mycobacterium malmoense, 315
Mycobacterium marinum, 312
Mycobacterium phlei, 312, 319
Mycobacterium smegmatis, 312, 319
Mycobacterium thermoresistible, 312, 319
Mycobacterium tuberculosis, 312, 314
Mycobacterium ulcerans, 312
Mycobacterium xenopi, 312, 319
Mycophenolate mofetil, and cyclosporine, combined, for graft-versus-host disease, 720
Mycoplasma spp., in abscesses in cats, 311
  infections caused by, 327
Mycoplasma-like bacteria (L-forms), infections caused by, 327
Mycoptes musculinus, 1434–1435
  in guinea pigs, 1433
  in mice, 1443
Mycosis/mycoses. See also *Fungal infection(s); Fungus/fungi.*
  and abscesses in cats, 311
  cytologic diagnosis of, 117
  deep, 391–403
    definition of, 391
    diagnosis of, 118–119
  definition of, 336
  intermediate. See *Mycosis/mycoses, subcutaneous.*
  subcutaneous, 337, 375–391
    diagnosis of, 118–119
  superficial, 337, 338–375
    systemic therapy for, 356–358, 357t
    topical therapy for, 354–356, 356t
  systemic, 337, 391–403
  therapy for, 354–358, 356t, 357t, 409–415
Mycosis fungoides, 1021, *1324,* 1331, 1333–1338, *1334–1337*
  in hamsters, 1441
Mycostatin. See *Nystatin.*
Mycotoxin(s), 1101
Myelin basic protein, in cell type identification, 204t
Myiasis, *501,* 503–505, *504*
  in rabbits, 1449
Myobia musculi, 1434–1435
  on mice, 1443
  on rats, 1453
Myoglobin, in cell type identification, 204t
Myospherulosis, 1096, *1097*
Myringotomy, 1220
Myxedema, 783–784, 853
  dermal. See *Mucinosis.*
Myxedema coma, treatment of, 864
Myxoid degeneration, dermal. See *Mucinosis.*

Myxoma(s), 1289–1299
  breed(s) with predilection for, 1237t
Myxomatosis, in rabbits, 1446, *1447*
Myxosarcoma(s), 1281, 1289–1290, *1292*
  breed(s) with predilection for, 1237t
  claw involvement in, 1198

Naftifine, topical, 356t, 409
Naftin. See *Naftifine.*
Naloxone, 1057
  for feline psychogenic alopecia, 1070
Naltrexone, 1057
  for acral lick dermatitis, 1063
α-Naphthyl acetate esterase, in cell type identification, 204t
Narcan. See *Naloxone.*
Nasal furunculosis, 94
Nasal hyperkeratosis, 936
Nasal planum, common and less common dermatoses of, 103t
  epidermis of, *26*
  histology of, *12*
  pigmented epithelium of, *16*
Nasal solar dermatitis. See also *Solar dermatitis.*
  canine, 1074–1077, *1075*
Nasodigital hyperkeratosis, 1038–1041, *1039*
Nasolabiogram(s), 3
Nasopharyngeal polyp(s), feline, 1207–1208
Neck, common and less common dermatoses of, 104t
Necrobacillosis, in rabbits, 1445
Necrobiosis, definition of, 176
Necrobiosis lipoidica, in diabetic dogs, 868
Necrolysis, definition of, 136
  toxic epidermal. See *Toxic epidermal necrolysis.*
Necrolytic migratory erythema, 868–873
  cause and pathogenesis of, 868–870
  claw involvement in, 1199
  clinical features of, *869,* 870–871
  clinical management of, 871–873
  definition of, 868
  diagnosis of, 871, *872*
  mycotoxin-related, 1101
  paraneoplastic, 1375
Necrosis, and cell death, comparison of, 136–137
  caseation, 136
  coagulation, 136
  definition of, 136
  epidermal, 137–140, *141*
  fat, 172, *172*
    hyalinizing, 172
    microcystic, 172, *172*
    mineralizing, 172
  miscellaneous causes of, *1086, 1089,* 1089–1090
Necrotizing fasciitis, staphylococcal, 324–325
  streptococcal, 324
Nematode(s), filarial, 439
Neomycin, otic therapy with, 1227
  topical, for bacterial infection, 280
Neomycin-polymyxin, otic therapy with, 1227
Neonicotinoid(s), systemic, antiparasitic therapy with, 430
Neoplasm(s). See also *Tumor(s).*
  adrenal, *801,* 846, *846*
    clinical management of, 810, 814–815
    functional, 799
  anal sac, 1202
  ceruminal gland, *1196–1197,* 1208, 1208–1209, *1209*
  claw involvement in, *1196–1197,* 1198
  cytologic diagnosis of, *114,* 117, 118t

Neoplasm(s) (Continued)
  cytomorphologic findings in, 117, 118t
  ear, 1208
  epithelial, 1239–1281
  eyelid involvement in, 1188–1190, 1189, 1190t
  hypopigmentation caused by, 1008, 1021
  in ferrets, 1420, 1427–1428
  in gerbils, 1429–1430
  in guinea pigs, 1432, 1439
  in hamsters, 1432, 1441–1442, 1442
  in mice, 1444
  in rabbits, 1451–1452
  in rats, 1455
  loss of heterozygosity in, 65
  lymphohistiocytic, 1330–1357
  lymphoreticular. See Lymphoma.
  melanocytic, 1357–1364
  mesenchymal, 1281–1304
  pinnal, 1208
  secondary, of skin, 1373–1375
  surgical transplantation of, 1375
  testicular, and skin, 838–843
    hyperandrogenism caused by, 834–836, 835–837
    in ferrets, 1425
  virus-related, 528
Neoral. See Cyclosporine.
Neospora caninum, 532–533
Neosporosis, canine, 532–533
Neotrombicula autumnalis, 447–448
Nerve(s), cutaneous, 58–63, 60, 61
Nest(s), of dermal or epidermal cells, 174, 174
Neural cell adhesion molecules (N-CAM), in morphogenesis of skin appendages, 3
Neurilemoma. See Schwannoma.
Neurinoma. See Schwannoma.
Neurodermatitis, feline, 1066–1070
Neuroendocrine tumor(s), primary cutaneous, 1369–1370, 1370
Neurofibroma. See also Schwannoma.
  in gerbils, 1430
Neurofibrosarcoma, claw involvement in, 1198
Neurofilament, in cell type identification, 204t
Neurohormone(s), 1055
Neuro-immuno-cutaneous-endocrine (NICE) network, 1055
Neuron-specific enolase, in cell type identification, 204t
Neuropeptide(s), 59
  in pruritus, 62t, 62–63
Neuroregulator(s), 1055
Neurothekeoma, 1294, 1294
Neurotransmitter(s), 1055
Neurotrophin(s), 59
Neutrophil(s), chemoattractants for, 557, 557t
  cutaneous, 39
  degenerate, and cytologic diagnosis, 113, 115, 118t
  functions of, 556–557
  in cytologic diagnosis, 117
  in dermatitis, 187
  nondegenerate, and cytologic diagnosis, 113, 114, 118t
  products of, 557, 557t
Neutrophilic vasculitis, 181
Nevus/nevi, 1382–1390
  adnexal (pilosebaceous), 1384–1386, 1385
  benign, loss of heterozygosity in, 65
  collagenous, 1380–1381, 1382–1384, 1384, 1385
    breed(s) with predilection for, 1238t
    multiple, 986

Nevus/nevi (Continued)
    renal pathology with, 1383
    paraneoplastic, 1375
  comedo, 1007, 1389, 1391
  definition of, 177
  epidermal, 1007, 1013, 1380–1381, 1388–1389, 1389
    breed(s) with predilection for, 1238t
    in dogs, 157
  epithelial, 1013
  epitrichial (apocrine) sweat gland, 1387, 1387, 1388
  hair follicle, 1389, 1390
  linear epidermal, claw involvement in, 1199
  melanocytic, 1007, 1390, 1391, 1392
  organoid, 1380–1381, 1384–1386, 1386
  pacinian corpuscle, 1390
  sebaceous gland, 1380–1381, 1386–1387, 1387
  vascular, 1380–1381, 1386
    scrotal, 1386
    breed(s) with predilection for, 1238t
Newfoundland, callus dermatitis in, 1102
  color dilution alopecia in, 967
  demodicosis in, 465
  hypopigmentation in, 1008–1009, 1021
  hypothyroidism in, 852
  idiopathic ulcerative dermatitis of upper lip in, 1178
  pemphigus foliaceus in, 686
  risk for non-neoplastic skin disorders in, 80t
  skin of, hydration of, 32
  vitiligo in, 1015
Niacin, deficiency of, 1118–1119
  in hamsters, 1441
  in rats, 1453
Niacinamide. See Tetracycline and niacinamide.
Nictitans plasmacytic conjunctivitis, canine, treatment of, 674
Nidogen, 36t
Nikolsky's sign, 88, 101
Nitenpyram, 430
Nitrogen, liquid, in cryosurgery, 257
Nitrous oxide, in cryosurgery, 257
Nizoral. See Ketoconazole.
Nocardia spp., in abscesses in cats, 311
Nocardia asteroides, 323
Nocardia brasiliensis, 323
Nocardia caviae, 323
Nocardia farcinica, 323
Nocardia nova, 323
Nocardiosis, 323, 323–324, 324
  and opportunistic (atypical) mycobacteriosis, co-infection with, in cats, 320
  diagnosis of, 125
  in cats, 317
Nociceptor(s), 61, 62
Nodular dermatitis. See Dermatitis, nodular.
Nodular dermatofibrosis, in German shepherd, 1380–1381, 1382–1383
Nodular fasciitis, 1290–1291
Nodule(s), 87, 91
  lymphoid, 174, 175
Nolvasan. See also Chlorhexidine diacetate.
  shampoo, 917, 1035
Nonspecific enolase, in cell type identification, 204t
North American chigger. See Eutrombicula alfreddugesi.
Norwegian elkhound. See Elkhound, Norwegian.
Nose, dermatoses of, in gerbils, 1429, 1430
  hyperkeratosis of, in canine distemper, 523, 523
  hypopigmentation (depigmentation) of, 1016–1017

Nose (Continued)
  congenital, 1018
  seasonal, 1017, *1018*
  surface markings of, 3
Notoedres cati, 476, 477, *483,* 483–484. See also *Scabies, feline.*
  in rabbits, 1449
Notoedres muris, in guinea pigs, 1433
  in mice, 1443
Novasome(s), 221, *222,* 1027, 1028, 1035
Nuclear streaming, and cytologic diagnosis, *113*
5′-Nucleotidase, in cell type identification, 204t
Nutrition, and canine seborrhea, 1032
  and hair growth, 6
  and skin, 207–210
Nutritional disorder(s), claw involvement in, 1199
  diagnosis of, 198
  hair examination in, 108, *111*
  in chinchilla, 1417
  in guinea pigs, 1434
  in hamsters, 1441
  in mice, 1443–1444
  in rabbits, 1449
  in rats, 1453–1454
Nutritional skin disease, 1112–1123
Nutritional supplement(s), 207, 1123
Nutritional therapy, 207
Nystatin, topical, 356t, 409
Nystatin/triamcinolone, topical, 356t

Oatmeal, colloidal, 230, 917, 1028
  for pruritus, 228
  topical therapy with, 236
Obsessive-compulsive disorder(s), 1064–1066
Ochratoxin A, 1101
Odlund body(ies), 22
Odontopsyllus multispinosus, on rabbits, 1449
Odor(s), in haircoat, 214
Oil(s), animal, 227, 1028
  hydrophilic, 226
  hydrophobic, 226
  vegetable, 227, 1028
Oil red O stain, staining characteristics of various substances with, 130t
Oil rinse(s), 212
Ointment(s), 218t, 224–225
Old English sheepdog. See *Sheepdog, Old English.*
Oleic acid, 208
Onchocerciasis, ocular, 439
Oncogene(s), 1239
Oncology, cutaneous, 1236–1239
Oncosis, definition of, 140
Onychalgia, definition of, 1193t
Onychauxis, definition of, 1193t
Onychia, definition of, 1193t
Onychitis. See *Onychia.*
Onychocryptosis, *1191*
  definition of, 1193t
Onychodystrophy, *1192,* 1193, 1195
  definition of, 1193t
  idiopathic, *1191–1192,* 1198
  in hookworm dermatitis, 1195
  lupoid, *745*
    symmetric, 1195–1198, *1196–1197*
  post-infectious, 1199
Onychogryposis (onychogryphosis), *1191,* 1196
  definition of, 1193t

Onychogryposis (onychogryphosis) *(Continued)*
  in hookworm dermatitis, 1195
  in leishmaniasis, 535, *535,* 1195
Onycholysis, definition of, 1193t
Onychomadesis, *1189,* 1193, *1196*
  clinical management of, 1200
  definition of, 1193t
  drug-induced, in dogs, 722t
  idiopathic, *1196–1197,* 1198–1199
Onychomalacia, *1191*
  definition of, 1193t
Onychomycosis, *1189,* 1195
  clinical management of, 1200
  definition of, 1193t
  in dermatophytosis, in cats, 343
    in dogs, 343
Onychopathy, definition of, 1193t
Onychoptosis, definition of, 1193t
Onychorrhexis, *1191,* 1195
  clinical management of, 1200
  definition of, 1193t
Onychoschisis, definition of, 1193t
Onychoschizia, *1192,* 1195
  clinical management of, 1200
  definition of, 1193t
Onychosis, definition of, 1193t
Onyxis, definition of, 1193t
Oömycosis. See *Pythiosis.*
o,p′-DDD (mitotane). See *Mitotane (o,p′-DDD).*
Optimmune. See *Cyclosporine.*
Oral cavity, common and less common dermatoses of, 103t
  cryosurgery in, 258
Orbifloxacin, otic therapy with, 1229
  systemic, dosage of, 284t
Orf, 524
Organophosphate(s), 499
  for scabies, 482
  systemic, antiparasitic therapy with, 428
  topical, antiparasitic therapy with, 425
Oriental cat, psychogenic alopecia and dermatitis in, 1066
  psychogenic dermatoses in, 1056
Ormetoprim-sulfadiazine, otic therapy with, 1229
Ormetoprim-sulfadimethoxine, systemic, dosage of, 284t
Ornithine decarboxylase, 29
Ornithonyssus bacoti, on hamsters, 1440
  on mice, 1443
  on rats, 1453
Orthokeratosis. See *Hyperkeratosis, orthokeratotic (anuclear).*
Ossification, cutaneous, in hyperadrenocorticism, 803, *803*
Osteoma, 1314–1315, *1315–1316*
Osteosarcoma, 1314–1315, *1316*
  claw involvement in, 1198
  in rabbits, 1451
Otitis externa, 1204–1231. See also *Ear(s).*
  allergic, *1210–1211,* 1211
  bacterial, *1210,* 1213, 1214t
  causes of, primary, 1206t, 1209–1213
    secondary, 1206t–1207t, 1213–1215
  ceruminous, 918, 1036, *1196*
  classification of, 1204, 1206t–1207t
  clinical features of, 1217–1218
  culture and susceptibility testing in, 1221
  cytologic examination in, 1220
  definition of, 1204
  diagnosis of, 1219–1221
  drug-induced, in cats, 723t
    in dogs, 722t

Otitis externa *(Continued)*
  ear cleaning in, 1221–1225, 1222t, *1224*
  histopathology of, 1220–1221
  hyperplastic, 1212
  in dogs, cytologic diagnosis of, *115*
  in ferrets, 1419
  in food hypersensitivity, 1211, 1213
  in hypothyroidism, *1210–1211*
  in rabbits, 1448
  inflammatory, idiopathic, 1212
  Malassezia, 366
    pathogenesis of, 364
  otoscopic examination in, *1205,* 1218–1219
  parasitic, 1206t, 1209–1211
  perpetuating factors in, 1207t, 1215–1217
  physical findings in, *1211,* 1218–1219
  predisposing factors in, 1204–1209, 1206t
  proliferative, *1210–1211*
  proliferative eosinophilic, canine, 1213
  Pseudomonas, 1210–1211, 1213
  surgery for, 1230–1231
  systemic therapy for, 1229–1230
  topical acquired irritant reactions causing, 1215
  topical therapy for, 1225t–1227t, 1225–1229
  treatment of, 1221–1231
  yeast-related, 1213–1215
Otitis media, 1216–1217, *1217*
  bacterial, 1214t
  culture and susceptibility testing in, 1221
Otoacariasis, in rabbits, 1448
Otobius megnini, 442–443, *443*
Otomax. See *Clotrimazole/betamethasone/gentamicin.*
Otoscopic examination, in otitis externa, *1205,* 1218–1219
Ovaban. See *Megestrol acetate.*
Ovoid body(ies). See *Apoptotic body(ies).*
Oxacillin, efficacy of, against coagulase-positive staphylococci, 282
    against *Staphylococcus intermedius,* 282
    long-term therapy with, 287
    systemic, dosage of, 284t
Oxidizing agent(s), topical, 231
OxyDex, 226, 231, 1027
Oxytalan fiber(s), 38

Pachyonychia, definition of, 1193t
Pacific (West Coast) tick(s), 444
Pacini's corpuscle, innervation of, 59, 61, *61,* 62
Paecilomyces fumosoroseus, 404
Paecilomyces lilacinus, 404
Paecilomycosis, 404, *405*
Pagetoid reticulosis, 1021, 1331, 1339–1340, *1339–1341*
Pain, assessment of, 83
Paint, in haircoat, 213
Panalog, 232, 502. See also *Nystatin/triamcinolone.*
Pancornulin, 28
Pancreas, cancer of, cutaneous metastases of, 1373
  tumors of, 870
Pancreatitis, fatty acids and, 241
Panhypopituitarism, 782
Panniculitis, *91,* 171–172, 196–197, *203,* 1156–1162
  cause and pathogenesis of, 1156–1157
  clinical features of, 1157–1159
  clinical management of, 1161–1162
  cytologic diagnosis of, *117*
  definition of, 1156
  diagnosis of, 1159–1161, *1160–1164*

Panniculitis *(Continued)*
  diffuse, definition of, 197
    in dogs, 197
  drug-induced, 729
    in dogs, 725
  in cats, *1158,* 1159, *1160, 1162–1164*
  in dermatophytosis, 353
  in dogs, 1157–1159, *1158, 1161*
  in humans, differential diagnosis of, 1156, 1157t
  in injection site reaction, in cats, 723t
    in dogs, 722t
  in vasculitis, 747
  lobular, 196–197, *1162*
  lupus erythematosus, 197
  nodular, 1157
  pancreatic, 1160–1161
  postinjection, 1160, *1163, 1164*
  pyogranulomatous, 377, *1161*
  sclerosing, *1164*
  septal, 197, 1160, *1163*
    in cats, 197
  sterile, *203*
    cytologic diagnosis of, *114*
    in cats, *175,* 311
  sterile pedal. See *Focal metatarsal fistulation.*
  traumatic, 1160
  Weber-Christian, 1157
Pansteatitis, in cats, *1117,* 1117–1118
Pantothenic acid, deficiency of, 1020
  in hamsters, 1441
  in mice, 1443
  in rats, 1453
Papillae adiposae, 63, *64*
Papillary squirting, *135,* 173
Papilloma(s), 1239–1248
  breed(s) with predilection for, 1237t
  cause and pathogenesis of, 1239–1240
  clinical findings in, 1240–1244
  clinical management of, 1248
  cutaneous, in dogs, 1240, *1241*
  cutaneous exophytic, 1012
  cutaneous inverted, in dogs, 1240, *1242*
  diagnosis of, 1244–1247, *1244–1247*
  differential diagnosis of, 1244–1246
  fibrovascular, 1284, *1284, 1285*
  footpad, in dogs, *1241,* 1242
  in cats, 527, *530–531,* 1243–1244
  in dogs, 1240–1243, *1241–1243*
  in gerbils, 1430
  in hamsters, 1442
  in mice, 1444
  in rabbits, 1451
  in rats, 1455
  multiple, in dogs, *1241,* 1243
    pigmented, papular cutaneous, in dogs, 1240
  of eyelid, 1188
  Shope, in rabbits, 1451
  squamous, inverted, 1198
Papillomatosis, dermal, 162
  oral, canine, 1240, 1241
Papillomavirus antigen, in Bowen's disease, 1258
Papillomavirus infection, canine, 525–527, *530–531*
  detection of, 1239
  feline, 527–528, *530–531,* 1243–1244
  pigmentary abnormalities with, 1012, *1013*
Papillon, black hair follicular dysplasia in, 962
Papovavirus(es), neoplasia caused by, 528
Papule(s), 86, *88*

Parabens, in shampoo, 223
Paragonimus kellicotti, in dogs, 440
Parakeratosis. See *Hyperkeratosis, parakeratotic (nucleated).*
Parakeratotic cap(s), 133, *135*
    perivascular dermatitis with, 179
Paraneoplastic alopecia, 902, *903, 904*
Paraneoplastic syndrome(s), 1375
Parapoxvirus infection, in cats, 524
    in dogs, 524
Parapsoriasis, *1039*, 1050–1051, *1051*
Parasitic disease. See also specific parasite.
    ear involvement in, 1206t, 1209–1211
    intestinal, in ferrets, 1426
    of claws, 1195
    of skin, 423–507
        diagnosis of, 101–107
        pododermatitis caused by, 305
    otitis externa in, 1206t, 1209–1211
Parasitic hypersensitivity, 627–644. See also *Intestinal parasite hypersensitivity;* specific parasite.
Parlodel. See *Bromocriptine mesylate.*
Paronychia, 1022, 1193
    bacterial, *1189*
    in cat with systemic lupus erythematosus, 696–697
    demodectic, 1195
    Malassezia, 366, *1189*
Paste(s), 225
Pasteurella multocida, in cats, in oral flora, 276
    in subcutaneous abscesses, 310–311
Pasteurella pneumotropica, infection by, in hamsters, 1439
    in mice, 1442
    in rats, 1452
Pasteurellosis, in rabbits, 1444–1445
Patch, 86, 87
Pattern baldness, 890, *954, 963–964, 965–966, 966*
    clinical management of, 253
Pautrier microabscess, 151, *152,* 1347
Paw(s), common and less common dermatoses of, 105t
Paxillin, 22t
Peanut agglutinin, in cell type identification, 204t
Pedal folliculitis and furunculosis. See *Pododermatitis.*
Pediculosis, 487–490, *488*
    cause of, 487
    clinical features of, 487–489, *488*
    definition of, 487
    diagnosis of, 489
    differential diagnosis of, 489
    in cats, 490
    in dogs, 490
    pathogenesis of, 487
    treatment of, 490
Pekingese, dermatophytosis in, 343
    distichiasis in, 1188
    drug reactions in, 721
    facial fold intertrigo in, 1107
    follicular dysplasia in, 971
    pododermatitis in, 305
    risk for neoplastic skin disorders and non-neoplastic lumps in, 1237t
    risk for non-neoplastic skin disorders in, 80t
    Sertoli's cell tumor in, 840
    squamous cell carcinoma in, 1251
    vaccine reaction in, 744
Pelodera dermatitis, 432–434, *434–436*
    in guinea pigs, 1433
    in humans, 432

Pelodera strongyloides, 432, *434*
    in humans, 432
    pododermatitis caused by, 305
Pemphigoid, bullous. See *Bullous pemphigoid.*
    cicatricial. See *Pemphigoid, mucous membrane.*
    mucous membrane, 694, 695, 701
Pemphigus, benign familial, canine, 947–948, *948*
    diet-induced, 680, 682
    panepidermal pustular, 685, 686
        prognosis for, 681
    paraneoplastic, 693, 693t, 1375
        diagnosis of, 671
    pathomechanism of, 19
Pemphigus complex, 88, 678–693
    cause of, 678–679
    characteristics of, 678
    clinical management of, 681–682
    diagnosis of, 117, *669*, 680–681
    in cats and dogs, cause and pathogenesis of, 679–680
        diagnosis of, *669*, 680–681
    in humans, 678–680
    pathogenesis of, 678–680
    prognosis for, 681
Pemphigus erythematosus, *688, 691,* 691–693
    diagnosis of, *669,* 680, *691,* 692, *692*
    in cats and dogs, *669,* 680–681, 688–689
        cytologic diagnosis of, *114*
    management of, 693
    prognosis for, 681
Pemphigus foliaceus, 686–690
    cause of, 680
    claw involvement in, 1195, *1196*
    clinical features of, *683,* 687, 688–689
    diagnosis of, 671, 687–689, *689, 690, 691*
    differential diagnosis of, 687, 688–689
    drug-induced, 729
        in cats, 723t, 725, 726
        in dogs, 687, 722t
    in cats, 687–690, *688–689*
    in dogs, *199,* 686–690, *688–689*
        chronic, disease-associated, 687
        diagnosis of, *147, 155*
        spontaneous, 687
    in humans, 678
    incidence of, 686
    management of, 689–690
    prognosis for, 681
Pemphigus vegetans, 685–686, *685–686*
    clinical features of, *683*
    prognosis for, 681
Pemphigus vulgaris, claw involvement in, 1195
    diagnosis of, 671
    in cats, villi in, *163*
    in cats and dogs, *669,* 679
        clinical features of, 682, *683*
        clinical management of, 682–685
        diagnosis of, 682, *684*
        differential diagnosis of, 682
    in humans, 678–679
    prognosis for, 681
Penicillate nerve endings, 62
Penicillin(s), adverse effects and side effects of, 721
    distribution of, in skin, 281
    systemic, for bacterial infections, 281
Penicillium spp., as resident flora, in dogs, 34
    colonies of, morphology of, *123*
    in normal flora, 338, 338t
Pentoxifylline, 601

Pentoxifylline *(Continued)*
   adverse effects and side effects of, 241
   for dermatomyositis, 945–946
   for pemphigus, 682
   for vasculitis, 753–754
   formulations of, 241
   indications for, 241
   pharmacology of, 241
Peptide regulatory factor(s), 543
Peptostreptococcus spp., cellulitis caused by, 310
   in infections, 276
   in subcutaneous abscesses in cats, 310
Perforating dermatitis, 1168–1170, *1169*, *1170*
Perforin, 740
Periactin. See *Cyproheptadine hydrochloride.*
Perianal gland(s). See *Circumanal (perianal) glands.*
Pericyte(s), 57
Periderm, 2
Perifollicular fibrosis, 168, *169*, 195
Perifollicular melanosis, 168, *169*, 195
Perifolliculitis, 166, 192–196, *195*
Periodic acid-Schiff stain, for fungi, 119
   staining characteristics of various substances with, 130t
Perionychia, definition of, 1193t
Peripheral nerve sheath tumor, 1292
Peritonitis, feline infectious, 522, *522*
Perivascular dermatitis, deep, 178, *179*
   diffuse orthokeratotic hyperkeratosis with, 178–179
   drug-induced, 729
   eosinophilic, 178
   hyperplastic, 178, 180
   pure, 178, 179
   spongiotic, 178, 179–180
   superficial, 178, *179*
   with parakeratotic caps, 179
Permethrin, 426–427, 502
   for scabies, 482
   spot application products, for flea control, 498
Persian cat, basal cell tumors in, 1261
   dermatophytic pseudomycetoma in, 343–347
   dermatophytosis in, *346*, 347, 409
   dystrophic epidermolysis bullosa in, 939
   enilconazole therapy for, 410
   epitrichial cysts in, 1381
   facial fold intertrigo in, 1107
   griseofulvin side effects in, 357
   grooming for, 215
   idiopathic facial dermatitis of, 920–921, *922*
   papillomavirus infection in, 527, *530–531*
   periocular dermatosis in, 1186
   risk for neoplastic skin disorders and non-neoplastic lumps in, 1237t
   risk for non-neoplastic skin disorders in, 80t
   sebaceous gland tumors in, 1271
   seborrhea in, *914–915*, 920, *920*, *921*
   systemic lupus erythematosus in, 705
   yellow-eyed "smoky," Chédiak-Higashi syndrome in, 76, *977*, 1014
Peruvian Inca Orchid dog, 957
Pesticide(s), regulation of, 424
Petechiae, *87*, 88
pH meter, 32
Phaeohyphomycosis, 367, 379–381, *380*, *382*
   cycloheximide sensitivity in, 121
   definition of, 376
   pododermatitis caused by, 305
Phaeomelanin(s), 1005
Phagocytosis, in cytologic diagnosis, 117

Pharyngeal carcinoma, cutaneous metastases of, *1366*, 1373
Phenamidine, adverse effects and side effects of, 573
Phenobarbital, 1057
   for acral lick dermatitis, 1061–1062
   for feline psychogenic alopecia, 1070
Phenol(s), 680
   contraindications to, in cats, 230
   in shampoo, 223
   in topical therapy, 230
Pheomelanin, 8, 16, 17
Phialemonium curvatum, 377
Phialemonium obovatum, 379
Phialoconidia, 337
Phialophora gougerotii. See *Exopholia jeanselmei.*
Phialophora verrucosa, 379
Phlebectasia, in hyperadrenocorticism, 800, *801*, 804
Phlebotomus spp., 534
Phosmet, 425
Photocarcinogenesis, 24
Photochemotherapy, 237
Photodermatitis, 1073
Photodynamic therapy, for squamous cell carcinoma, 1257
Photofrin-V, 237
Photoimmunology, 24
Photoperiod, and cyclic follicular dysplasia, 890
   and hairgrowth, 5–6
Photoprotection, 236–237
   for pemphigus erythematosus, 693
   in discoid lupus erythematosus, 716
   in pemphigus, 681–682
Photosensitivity, 1080
   in cutaneous lupus erythematosus, 702
Photothermolysis, 259
Phthirus pubis, 487
Phycomycosis, 377. See also *Pythiosis.*
Physical examination, 84–94
   dermatologic examination in, 85–86
   general observation in, 84–85, *85*
Physical therapy, 237–238
Phytogel, 263
Phytonutrient(s), 209
Picric acid, 230
Piebaldism, 1014
Piedra, 374–375
   black, 374
   cause of, 374
   clinical findings in, 374, *374*
   clinical management of, 375
   diagnosis of, 374, 375
   pathogenesis of, 374
   white, 374, *374*
Piedraia hortae, 374
Pigmentary incontinence, 162–163, *163*
Pigmentation, abnormality(ies) of, 87, *91*, 900–911, 1005–1023. See also specific disorder.
   congenital and hereditary, 975–978
   terminology for, 1005, 1006t
   androgens and, 796–797
   constitutive, 16
   estrogens and, 795
   facultative, 16
   of hair, 1005
   regulation of, 17
Pili torti, 953–955, *953–955*
   hair examination in, *112*
Pilomatrixoma, *92*, 1267–1269, *1269*, *1270*
   breed(s) with predilection for, 1237t
Pilonidal sinus. See *Cyst(s), dermoid (dermoid sinus).*

Pilosebaceous follicle, 48
Pinkus corpuscle. See *Tylotrich pad.*
Pinna, acquired folding of, in cats, 1231, *1231*
   alopecia of, canine, 887, *888, 889*
     feline, *888,* 900
   dermatitis of, 1211
   erythema of, drug-induced, in cats, 723t, *724–725,* 1023
   fly bites of, *1210–1211,* 1211
   in feline auricular chondritis, 748–749
   lesions of, in vasculitis, 745
   marginal necrosis in, in dog with systemic lupus erythematosus, 696–697
   necrosis of, in ferrets, 1419
   neoplasia of, 1208
   proliferative thrombovascular necrosis of, 747–749, *748,* 752, 754
   squamous cell carcinoma of, in white cats, *1241*
   in white-eared cats, 76
Pinnal folliculitis, sterile eosinophilic, canine, 1213
Pinnal-pedal reflex, in scabies, 479–480
Pinworm, in mice, 1444
   in rats, 1454
Pit bull. See *Terrier, Staffordshire.*
Pit viper(s), 1090
Pituitary dwarfism, canine, *817,* 819–822, *820*
Pituitary gland. See *Hypophysis.*
Pityrosporum spp.. See *Malassezia* spp..
Pityrosporum canis. See *Malassezia pachydermatis.*
Pityrosporum ovale. See *Malassezia furfur.*
Pityrosporum pachydermatis. See *Malassezia pachydermatis.*
Plague, 325–326, 491
Plakoglobin, 20, 22t
Plakophilin, 20, 22t
Plaque(s), 86, *88*
   eosinophilic, feline, *1142,* 1149–1152, *1150–1152*
   multiple, pigmented, in dogs, 1240–1242, *1242, 1243*
Plaquenil sulfate. See *Hydroxychloroquine sulfate.*
Plasma cell(s), cutaneous, 39
   in cytologic diagnosis, 118t
   in nodular and diffuse dermatitis, 188, *188*
Plasma cell pododermatitis, feline, *1126–1127,* 1129–1130, *1130–1131*
Plasmacytoma, *1334*
   breed(s) with predilection for, 1237t
   cutaneous, 1342–1346
     cause and pathogenesis of, 1342–1344
     clinical findings in, *1334,* 1344, *1344*
     clinical management of, 1346
     diagnosis of, *1345,* 1345–1346, *1346*
   in hamsters, 1442
Plasmacytosis, systemic, 1179–1180
Plasmapheresis, for systemic lupus erythematosus, 711
Platelet-activating factor, 559–560
Platonychia, definition of, 1193t
Plectin, 13, 22t
Plesiotherapy, for actinic keratosis, 1079
   for squamous cell carcinoma, 1257
Pneumonyssoides caninum, 452–453
Pododermatitis, 301, 304–306
   autoimmune, 305
   demodectic, 461
     canine, *462,* 465
   fungal, 305
   hookworm, *433*
   in dogs, *301,* 344–345
   Malassezia, rinses for, 410
   parasitic, 305

Pododermatitis *(Continued)*
   plasma cell, feline, *1126–1127,* 1129–1130, *1130–1131*
   tick-related, 435
   ulcerative, in rabbits, 1445
Pointer, black hair follicular dysplasia in, 962
   blastomycosis in, 392
   callus dermatitis in, 1102
   dermatophytosis in, *344–345*
   English, acral mutilation in, *988–989,* 995
     hemangiosarcomas in, 1299
   German shorthaired, acral mutilation in, 995
     dermatophytosis in, 343
     familial hypothyroidism in, 852
     follicular dysplasia in, 971
     hereditary lupoid dermatosis of, 180, 707, 717, *941,* 948–949, *949*
     hyperadrenocorticism in, *801*
     junctional epidermolysis bullosa in, 939
     muzzle folliculitis and furunculosis in, 304
     pododermatitis in, 305
     risk for non-neoplastic skin disorders in, 75
     truncal solar dermatitis in, 1079
     zinc-responsive dermatosis in, 1120
   histoplasmosis in, 400
   nasal depigmentation in, 1017
   nasal folliculitis and furunculosis in, *301,* 303
   risk for non-neoplastic skin disorders in, 80t
   wirehaired, follicular dysplasia in, 971
Polyethylene glycol, 226
Polyglandular syndrome(s), 782
Polyhydroxydine, 231
Polymerase chain reaction (PCR), 1239
Polymyxin B, otic therapy with, 1227
   topical, for bacterial infection, 280
Polyp(s), nasopharyngeal, *1196,* 1207
Polyplax serrata, in mice, 1443
Polyplax spinulosa, on rats, 1453
Pomeranian, adrenal hyperplasia–like syndrome in, 846–847
   adult-onset hyposomatotropism in, 822
   follicular dysplasia in, 890
   haircoat of, 8
   hypogonadism in, 844–845
   hypothyroidism in, 852
   immunodeficiency in, 279t
   risk for non-neoplastic skin disorders in, 75, 80t
Poodle, adult-onset hyposomatotropism in, 822
   anal licking in, 1066
   basal cell carcinoma in, 1262
   calcinosis circumscripta in, 1400
   chlorambucil therapy in, side effects of, 673
   chronic ulcerative blepharitis in, 1186
   contact hypersensitivity in, 1081
   dermal perifollicular mineralization in, 168
   dermatophytosis in, *344–345*
   distichiasis in, 1188
   drug reactions in, 721, 725
   epiphora in, 1188, *1189*
   food hypersensitivity in, 618
   glucocorticoid-induced reaction in, 246–247
   granulomatous sebaceous adenitis in, 1146
   hair growth in, 5
   haircoat of, 8
   hyperadrenocorticism in, 800
   hypothyroidism in, 852
   lymphedema in, 990
   Malassezia dermatitis in, 348–349
   melanotrichia in, 1010

Poodle (Continued)
    drug-induced, *1012*
    miniature, adult-onset hyposomatotropism in, 822
        anal sac disorders in, 1201
        congenital hypotrichosis in, 958, *959*, *960*
        delayed gonadal maturation in, 844
        drug reactions in, 721
        hypogonadism in, 833
        melanocytic neoplasms in, 1359
        pseudoachondroplastic dysplasia in, 820
        seasonal flank alopecia in, 891
    nasal depigmentation in, 1017
    panniculitis in, 1159
    pilomatrixoma in, 1267
    postvaccinal vasculitis in, 749, *749*
    psychogenic dermatitis in, 305
    risk for neoplastic skin disorders and non-neoplastic lumps in, 1237t
    risk for non-neoplastic skin disorders in, 75, 80t
    sebaceous adenitis in, 242, 1029
    sebaceous gland hyperplasia in, 1271
    squamous cell carcinoma in, 1251
    standard, black, risk for neoplastic skin disorders and non-neoplastic lumps in, 1237t
        color dilution alopecia in, 967
        granulomatous sebaceous adenitis in, 1141, 1143, *1143*
        risk for neoplastic skin disorders and non-neoplastic lumps in, 1237t
        risk for non-neoplastic skin disorders in, 75
        sebaceous adenitis in, 925
        squamous cell carcinoma in, 1251
        trichoepithelioma in, 1263
        zinc-responsive dermatosis in, 1120
    systemic lupus erythematosus in, 705
    toy, anal sac disorders in, 1201
        congenital hypotrichosis in, 958
        Ehlers-Danlos syndrome in, 982
        hyperadrenocorticism in, *801*
        junctional epidermolysis bullosa in, 939
    trichoblastoma in, 1270
    vaccine reaction in, 744
Pore of Winer, dilated, *1254*, 1265–1267, *1266*, *1267*
Poroconidia, 337
Porphyromonas spp., cellulitis caused by, 310
    in subcutaneous abscesses in cats, 310
Portuguese water dog, follicular dysplasia in, 890, 971, *972*, *973*, *974*
    pattern baldness in, 965
    risk for non-neoplastic skin disorders in, 80t
Postclipping alopecia, 897, *898*
Potassium iodide, antifungal therapy with, 414
Potassium permanganate, 227
Potbelly, in hyperadrenocorticism, *802*, 804
Poultry mite(s), 445–446, *446*
    skin scraping for, 107
Povidone-iodine, 231
    preoperative use of, 255
    soaks, for bacterial infection, 280–281
    topical, for bacterial infection, 279
Powder(s), 218t, 224
Prairie dog(s), plague in, 325–326
Pramoxine, for pruritus, 228
    in shampoo, 223
Praziquantel, injection reaction with, 902
Preauricular ulcerative dermatitis, idiopathic, of cats, 1177
Prednisolone, for dermatomyositis, 945
    for discoid lupus erythematosus, 716
    for idiopathic sterile granuloma and pyogranuloma, 1139

Prednisolone (Continued)
    for vasculitis, 753
    immunosuppressive therapy with, 672t
    systemic, otic therapy with, 1229
Prednisone, for discoid lupus erythematosus, 716
    for idiopathic sterile granuloma and pyogranuloma, 1139
    for pemphigus, 681
    for pemphigus foliaceus, 689
    for systemic lupus erythematosus, 711
    for vasculitis, 753
    immunosuppressive therapy with, 672t
    injectable, 247t
    systemic, otic therapy with, 1229
Preen gland. See *Tail gland, of dog*.
Prelipoblast(s), 2
Pressure sore(s). See *Ulcer(s), decubital*.
Prevotella spp., cellulitis caused by, 310
    in infections, 276
Primidone, for feline psychogenic alopecia, 1070
Proanagen, 46
Procainamide, hypopigmentation caused by, 1020, *1020*
Profilaggrin, 26–27
Progestagen(s), for feline acquired symmetric alopecia, 902
    therapy with, for acral lick dermatitis, 1063
        in pituitary dwarfism, 821–822
Progesterone, 797–798
    blood levels of, assays for, 798
    for feline acquired symmetric alopecia, 902
    repositol, for acral lick dermatitis, 1063
Program. See *Lufeneron*.
Proheart. See *Moxidectin, systemic*.
Prolactin, 798
    levels of, melatonin and, 253
Prolactin-inhibiting factor (PIF), 781
Prolactin-releasing factor (PRF), 781
Proliferative eosinophilic otitis externa, canine, 1213
Propagule, fungal, 336
Propionibacterium spp., in hair follicle, 51
Propionibacterium acnes. See also *Immunoregulin*.
    as resident flora, in dogs, 34, 275
Propylene glycol, 1028
    topical, 230, 235
Prostaglandin(s), effects of, on skin, 208
Prostatic carcinoma, cutaneous metastases of, 1374, *1374*
Protein, deficiency of, 207, 1115–1116
    dietary, for cats, 1116
        for dogs, 1116
Protein A, 275, 276
Proteoglycan(s), functions of, 38
    major, 38
Proteus spp., in anal sacs, 1201
    otitis externa caused by, 1214t
    otitis media caused by, 1214t
    pseudomycetoma caused by, 312
Proteus mirabilis, as transient flora, in cats, 275
    in dogs, 275
    in generalized demodectic mange, 465
Prototheca spp., characteristics of, 404–405
Prototheca wickerhamii, 405, 406
Prototheca zopfii, 405
Protothecosis, 404–407
    cause of, 404–405
    clinical management of, 406–407
    diagnosis of, 406, *406*, *407*
    in cats, 406
    in dogs, 397, 405, *406*, *407*
    pathogenesis of, 405
Protozoal disease(s), 531–538

Prozac. See *Fluoxetine*.
Pruritus, 61–63, 228. See also *Scabies*.
 and bacterial infection, 277, 286
 assessment of, 83
 clinical management of, in dogs, 239
 drug-induced, in cats, 721, 723t
  in dogs, 721, 722t
 epicritic, 62
 in feline leukemia virus dermatitis, 517
 in folliculitis, 293
 in hyperadrenocorticism, 804
 in *Malassezia* dermatitis, 366
 in pseudorabies, 524
 mediators of, 62, 62t
 modulators of, 62t, 62–63
 neurogenic, in Cavalier King Charles spaniels, 996
 paraneoplastic, 1375
 perianal, in mice, 1444
 protopathic, 62
Pruritus vulvae, in diabetic dogs, 868
Pseudoacanthosis, 134
Pseudoallescheria boydii, 377
 culture of, 121
 cycloheximide sensitivity of, 121
Pseudo-Cushing's syndrome. See *Hyposomatotropism (pseudo-Cushing's syndrome, GH-responsive dermatosis)*.
Pseudohorn cysts, 156
Pseudohypothyroidism, 782
Pseudolymphoma, 184, 1340–1342, *1342*, *1343*
 and lymphoma, differentiation of, histologic criteria for, 1341–1342, 1343t
 insect bite, *192*
Pseudomicrodochium suttonii, 379
Pseudomonas spp., as transient flora, in cats, 275
 in dogs, 275
 otitis externa caused by, *1210–1211*, 1213, 1214t
 otitis media caused by, 1214t
 pseudomycetoma caused by, 312
Pseudomonas aeruginosa, fluorescence of, 119
 in generalized demodectic mange, 465
 in rabbits, 1445
 infection by, in rats, 1452
Pseudomycetoma, bacterial, *302*, 311–312, *313*, 376
 diagnosis of, 125
 in dogs, *302*
 dermatophytic, 343–347, *348*, *349*, 376
  treatment of, 357–358
 in dogs, *302*
 in mice, 1442
Pseudopelade, 765, *765*–766, *766*, 767, 907
Pseudopregnancy, *830*, 833, 834
Pseudopyoderma(s), 328
Pseudorabies, 524
Psorergates simplex, in mice, 1443
Psoriasiform-lichenoid dermatosis, of Springer spaniel, 929–931, *930*–*931*, *933*, *934*
Psoroptes, 1434–1435
Psoroptes cuniculi, in rabbits, 1448
Psoroptes ovis, in rabbits, 1448
Psychocutaneous medicine, 1055
Psychodermatology, 1055
Psychogenic skin disease(s), 1055–1071
 acral lick dermatitis as. See *Acral lick dermatitis*.
 canine, 1058–1066
 feline, 1066–1071
Psychological drug therapy, 1056–1057
PTD lotion, 229t

Public health considerations, with blastomycosis, 394
 with canine Rocky Mountain spotted fever, 529
 with feline poxvirus, 522
 with flea infestation, 491
 with hookworm, 432
 with *Malassezia* dermatitis, 366, 1215
 with plague, 326
 with sporotrichosis, 386–388, *387*
Pug, atopy in, 581
 distichiasis in, 1188
 intertrigo in, facial fold, 1107
  tail fold, 1107
 lentiginosis profusa in, 1006
 mast cell tumors in, 1320
 multiple pigmented plaques in, 1240, 1242, *1242*
 papillomavirus-associated pigmentary abnormality in, 1012
 risk for neoplastic skin disorders and non-neoplastic lumps in, 1238t
 risk for non-neoplastic skin disorders in, 80t
Pulex irritans, 491
Puli, grooming of, 214
Puppy strangles. See *Cellulitis, canine juvenile*.
Purpura, 87, *100*
Pustular dermatosis, linear IgA, canine, *748*, *756*, 756
 sterile, cytologic diagnosis of, 117
 subcorneal, canine. See *Subcorneal pustular dermatosis*.
Pustular mural folliculitis, 194, *199*
Pustular pemphigus, panepidermal, 685, *686*
 prognosis for, 681
Pustule(s), 86, 87, *89*, *97*
 color of, 89
 epidermal, 149–151, *150*, *151*
 intraepidermal, 190, 193t
 location of, 89
 nonfollicular, 89
 size of, 89
 spongiform (of Kogoj), 150, *150*
 subepidermal, 190, 193t
Pustulosis, sterile eosinophilic, *200*
 cytologic diagnosis of, *114*
Pyknosis, definition of, 136
Pyoben, 231, 1027
Pyocyanin, 1445
Pyoderma. See also *Demodicosis, in dogs*.
 bacterial, in dogs, 28, 277
  recurrent, 286
 in hypothyroidism, 853
 callus, 328
 callus dermatitis and, *1097*, 1102–1103
 deep, 298–324
 German shepherd, 531
 in hypothyroidism, 784
 interdigital (pododermatitis). See *Pododermatitis*.
 juvenile. See *Cellulitis, canine juvenile*.
 mucocutaneous, 180, 289, 290–291, *291*, *292*
 nasal, *301*, 303
 superficial, 288–298
Pyogranuloma. See also *Granuloma and pyogranuloma*.
 in rats, 1452
 infectious, cytologic diagnosis of, *113*
 perifollicular, *195*
 sterile, cytologic diagnosis of, *113*
 on feet, 305
Pyogranuloma-granuloma syndrome, sterile, 189
Pyotraumatic dermatitis, *1097*, *1104*, 1104–1105
Pyotraumatic folliculitis, 288, 300–303, *301*, 303
Pyrethrin(s), 423

Pyrethrin(s) *(Continued)*
    otic therapy with, 1227t, 1228
    topical, antiparasitic therapy with, 426
Pyrethroid(s), 423
    topical, antiparasitic therapy with, 426–427
Pyridoxine, deficiency of, 1020, 1119
    in guinea pigs, 1434
    in hamsters, 1441
    in mice, 1443–1444
    in rats, 1453
Pyrimethamine/sulfadiazine, for canine neosporosis, 533
Pyriproxyfen, 426, 495, 498
Pythiosis, 377, 381–384
    cause of, 381
    clinical management of, 384
    diagnosis of, 382–384, *383*
    in cats, clinical findings in, 382, *382*
    in dogs, clinical findings in, *367,* 381–382, *383*
    pathogenesis of, 381
Pythium gracile. See *Pythium insidiosum.*
Pythium insidiosum, 381

Quaternary ammonium compounds, 232
    in shampoo, 223
Quinacrine hydrochloride, 678
    for discoid lupus erythematosus, 716

Rabbit, abscesses in, 1445
    alopecia areata in, 1450–1451, *1452*
    alopecia in, congenital, 1450, *1450*
    aspergillosis in, 1446
    bacterial infections in, 1444–1446
    barbering in, 1450
    cutaneous asthenia in, 1450, *1451*
    dermatophytosis in, 1446
    dermatoses in, 1444–1452
        miscellaneous, 1449–1451
    drooling (slobbers) in, 1445
    ectoparasites on, *1434, 1457,* 1458–1459
    facial eczema in, 1451
    fleas on, 1449
    flystrike in, 1449
    frostbite in, *1447,* 1450
    fungal infections in, 1446, *1447*
    hair loss in, 1449–1450
    hutch burn in, 1450
    lice on, 1449
    localized moist (sore dewlap) dermatitis in, 1445
    lymphoma in, 1451, 1452
    mites in, 1448–1449
    myiasis in, 1449
    myxomatosis in, 1446, *1447*
    necrobacillosis (Schmorl's disease) in, 1445
    neoplasia in, 1451–1452
    nutritional disorders in, 1449
    pasteurellosis (snuffles) in, 1444–1445
    psoroptic mange in, *1447,* 1448
    scent glands of, 1450
    sebaceous adenitis in, 1451
    self-mutilation in, 1450
    Staphylococcus aureus in, 1445, 1446
    ulcerative pododermatitis (sore hocks) in, 1445
    venereal spirochetosis in, 1445–1446, *1447*
    viral infection in, 1446
Rabbit pox, 1446

Rabies vaccine, adverse effects of, 725, 743
    focal cutaneous vasculitis and alopecia caused by, 749, *749,* 752, 753, 754–756, *755*
Radfordia affinis, in mice, 1443
Radfordia ensifera, in rats, 1453
Radiation injury, 1087–1088, *1088*
Radiation therapy, 238
    for acral lick dermatitis, 1064
    for canine hyperadrenocorticism, 811, 814
    for squamous cell carcinoma, 1257
Radiosurgery, 262–263
Radixin, 20
Rat(s), alopecia areata in, 1455
    auricular chondritis in, 1454
    bacterial infections in, 1452
    cage-related injury in, 1452
    dermatophytosis in, 1453
    dermatoses of, 1452–1455
        miscellaneous, 1454–1455
    ectoparasites on, *1447,* 1453
    fleas on, 1453
    fungal infections in, 1453
    fur of, age-related changes in, 1455
    leprosy in, 1452
    lice on, 1453
    mites on, 1453
    neoplasia in, 1455
    nutritional disorders in, 1453–1454
    pinworm in, 1454
    plague in, 325–326
    ringtail in, 1454, *1455*
    sialodacryoadenitis in, *1447,* 1453
    skin of, scales on, 1455
    systemic hair embolism in, 1454–1455
    Trixacarus diversus in, *1447*
    viral infections in, *1447,* 1453
Rathke's cleft cyst, 819
Rat-tail, canine, 1141
Raynaud-like disease, in dogs, 1195
Red hair, acquired, 1022
Red kelpi, Ehlers-Danlos syndrome in, 982
Red mange. See *Demodicosis, in dogs.*
Red-legged widow spider, 484
Refsum disease, 31
Regulin(s), secretory, 543
Relapsing polychondritis, 759
Relief, antipruritic therapy with, 228, 229t
Reovirus infection, in mice, 1443
Repellent(s), flea, 499–500
    fly, 502
    topical, antiparasitic therapy with, 427
Reserve cells, 48
Resihist, 229
Resiprox, antipruritic therapy with, 229t
Resmethrin, 426
Resocortol butyrate, adrenocortical suppression by, 232
Resorcinol, 230
Respiratory rate, in thermoregulation, 54
Rete ridges, 10–13, 134–135, *138*
Reticular degeneration, epidermal, 142, *145*
Reticulin, 36
Reticulum cell tumor, transmissible. See *Transmissible venereal tumor.*
Retin-A. See *Vitamin A (retinol, retinoic acid, Retin-A).*
Retinal, 241–242, 1028–1029
Retinoic acid, 234, 241–242, 1028–1029. See also *Vitamin A (retinol, retinoic acid, Retin-A).*

Retinoic acid *(Continued)*
  antiseborrheic therapy with, 919
  for actinic keratosis, 1079
  for epidermal dysplasia in West Highland white terriers, 929
Retinoid(s), antiseborrheic therapy with, 1028
  inverse agonist, 242
  synthetic, 234, 1028
    for granulomatous sebaceous adenitis, 1146
    in systemic therapy, 241–243
  teratogenicity of, 1029
  topical, 234
Retinol, 1028–1029. See also *Vitamin A (retinol, retinoic acid, Retin-A)*.
  antiseborrheic therapy with, 919
  therapy with, 1036
Retriever, Chesapeake Bay, follicular dysplasia in, 971
  risk for non-neoplastic skin disorders in, 77t
  curly coated, follicular dysplasia in, 890, 971
  curly-coated, risk for non-neoplastic skin disorders in, 78t
  flatcoated, histiocytic sarcoma in, 1346–1347, 1352
  Golden, acral lick dermatitis in, 1058
    atopy in, 581
    benign fibrous histiocytoma in, 1354
    chondrosarcomas in, 1315
    fibromas in, 1282
    fibrosarcomas in, 1287
    food hypersensitivity in, 618
    footpad hyperkeratosis in, 935
    graying in, 1015
    hemangiosarcomas in, 1299
    histiocytic sarcoma in, 1346–1347, 1352
    hypothyroidism in, 852
    idiopathic sterile granuloma and pyogranuloma in, 1136
    juvenile cellulitis in, *1158*, 1165
    lymphomas in, 1331
    malignant histiocytosis in, 1346
    mast cell tumors in, 1320
    melanocytic nevus in, 1390
    melanocytoma in, 1359
    mucocutaneous hypopigmentation in, 1017–1018
    multiple collagenous cysts in, and renal pathology, 1383
    nasal depigmentation in, 1017
    pododermatitis in, 305
    pyotraumatic dermatitis in, 1104
    risk for neoplastic skin disorders and non-neoplastic lumps in, 1237t, 1238t
    risk for non-neoplastic skin disorders in, 75, 79t
    seborrhea in, 243, 1029
    snow nose in, 1017
    trichoepithelioma in, 1263
    trichoptilosis in, 895, 950
    trichorrhexis nodosa in, 950
    vascular nevi in, 1386
  Labrador, acral lick dermatitis in, 1058
    alopecia mucinosa in, 899
    atopy in, 581
    black, risk for neoplastic skin disorders and non-neoplastic lumps in, 1237t
      waterline disease of, 1175–1176, *1178*
    blastomycosis in, 392
    calcinosis cutis in, 1399, *1399*
    chondroma in, 1315
    congenital hypotrichosis in, 958

Labrador *(Continued)*
  cyclic follicular dysplasia in, 890
  dermal melanocytes of, 39
  eosinophilic dermatitis and edema in, 1155–1156
  fibrovascular papillomas in, 1284
  follicular dysplasia in, 971
  food hypersensitivity in, 618, 1211
  footpad hyperkeratosis in, 935
  graying in, 1015
  histiocytic sarcoma in, 1352
  histiocytomas in, 1347
  idiopathic leukotrichia in, 1021, *1021*
  lipomas in, 1308
  lymphedema in, 990
  mast cell tumors in, 1320
  mucocutaneous hypopigmentation in, 1017–1018
  nasal hyperkeratosis in, 936
  otitis externa in, 1212
  pemphigus foliaceus in, 687
  pododermatitis in, 305
  psychogenic dermatoses in, 1056
  pyotraumatic dermatitis in, 1104
  risk for neoplastic skin disorders and non-neoplastic lumps in, 1237t, 1238t
  risk for non-neoplastic skin disorders in, 80t
  seborrhea in, 913, 915, 1032
  skin pH in, 3
  snow nose in, 1017
  squamous cell carcinoma in, 1251
  sweating in, 53
  vascular nevi in, 1386
  vitamin A–responsive dermatosis in, 1036
  yellow, nasal depigmentation in, 1017
    photosensitivity in, 1080
    supranumery claws in, *1197*, 1199
  zinc-responsive dermatosis in, 1120
Reverse blot hybridization, 1239
Reverse T_3, 782–783
  measurement of, 784–786
Revolution. See *Selamectin*.
Rex cat, 9
  Cornish, follicular dysplasia in, 905, 971
  dermatophytosis in, 347
  Devon, congenital hypotrichosis in, 959
  grooming for, 215
  risk for non-neoplastic skin disorders in, 80t
Rhabditic dermatitis. See *Pelodera dermatitis*.
Rhabdomyoma, 1313–1314
Rhabdomyosarcoma, 1281, 1313–1314
Rhinosporidiosis, 390–391
Rhinosporidium seeberi, 390
Rhinotracheitis infection, feline, *518*, 524–525, *526–529*
Rhipicephalus sanguineus, 443–444, *444*, 445
Rhizopus spp., 384
  in normal flora, of dogs, 338, 338t
Rhodesian Ridgeback, coat color dilution and cerebellar degeneration in, 978
  dermoid cyst (sinus) in, 936–937, *937*, 1478
  follicular dysplasia in, 971
  idiopathic onychodystrophy in, 1198
  risk for neoplastic skin disorders and non-neoplastic lumps in, 1238t
  risk for non-neoplastic skin disorders in, 80t
  trachyonychia in, 1199
  zinc-responsive dermatosis in, 1120
Rhodococcus (Corynebacterium) equi, in abscesses in cats, 311

Rhodotorula spp., dermatitis caused by, 375, 376
   in normal flora, of cats, 338, 338t
Rhodotorula mucilaginosa, 375
Riboflavin, deficiency of, 1118
   in hamsters, 1441
   in mice, 1443
   in rats, 1453
Rice paddy itch, 436
Rickettsia felis, 493
Rickettsia rickettsii, 528–529
Rickettsia typhi, 493
Rickettsial disease(s), 528–531
Ridaura. See *Auranofin.*
Rifampicin, systemic, dosage of, 284t
Rifampin, and β-lactamase-resistant antibiotic, co-administration of, 283
   skin color change caused by, 1023
Rimadyl. See *Carprofen.*
Ringtail, in hamsters, 1441
   in mice, 1444
   in rats, 1454, *1455*
Ringworm. See *Dermatophytosis.*
Rinse(s), 214
   antifungal, 356, 356t, 410
   conditioning, 211
   cream, flea, 498–499
   formulations of, and efficacy of active ingredients, 218t, 224
   oil, 212
Rocky Mountain spotted fever, 444
   canine, 528–529, *530–531*
Rocky Mountain wood tick(s), 444
Rod(s), identification of, 116
Rodent(s), dermatophytes transmitted by, 339–340
   plague in, 325–326
   poxvirus carriage by, 520
Rodent ulcer. See *Indolent ulcer, feline.*
Roferon-A, 253
Rompun. See *Xylasine.*
Rotenone, antiparasitic therapy with, 427
   for feline demodicosis, 475
   otic therapy with, 1227t, 1228
Rottweiler, alopecia areata in, 763
   calcinosis cutis in, 1399
   congenital hypotrichosis in, 958
   follicular dysplasia in, 971
   follicular lipidosis in, 899, *899, 900,* 973–974
   follicular parakeratosis in, 925, *926, 927*
   haircoat of, 7
   histiocytic sarcoma in, 1346–1347, 1352
   histiocytomas in, 1347
   hypopigmentation in, 975
   idiopathic onychodystrophy in, 1198
   idiopathic onychomadesis in, *1196,* 1198
   immunodeficiency in, 278
   leukoderma and leukotrichia in, *96*
   lupoid onychodystrophy in, 1195
   malignant histiocytosis in, 1346
   mucocutaneous hypopigmentation in, 1018
   muzzle folliculitis and furunculosis in, 304
   risk for neoplastic skin disorders and non-neoplastic lumps in, 1237t
   risk for non-neoplastic skin disorders in, 80t
   snake bites in, 1091
   vasculitis in, 744
   vitiligo in, *1008–1009,* 1015
Round body(ies), 138
Ruffini corpuscle(s), innervation of, 61, 62

Ruffini's end-bulb. See *Meissner's corpuscle.*
Russell body(ies), 188–189
Russian blue cat, grooming for, 215

S100 protein, in cell type identification, 204t
Sabouraud's dextrose agar, 349
   fungal culture in, 121–122, *123*
Safflower oil, 209, 224, 227, 1028
St. Bernard, callus dermatitis in, 1102
   demodicosis in, 465
   distichiasis in, 1188
   Ehlers-Danlos syndrome in, 982
   hypothyroidism in, *854*
   idiopathic ulcerative dermatitis of upper lip in, 1178
   lip fold intertrigo in, 1107
   lymphomas in, 1331
   pyotraumatic dermatitis in, 1104
   risk for neoplastic skin disorders and non-neoplastic lumps in, 1237t
   risk for non-neoplastic skin disorders in, 75, 81t
St. Louis encephalitis, 444
Salicylic acid, antiseborrheic therapy with, 918, 1026–1027, 1036
Saliva, in thermoregulation, in cats, 54
Salivary gland tumor(s), 1281
SALT (skin-associated lymphoid tissue). See *Skin-associated lymphoid tissue.*
Salt-split skin, 694
Saluki, black hair follicular dysplasia in, 962
   color dilution alopecia in, 967
   hemangiosarcomas in, 1299
   risk for neoplastic skin disorders and non-neoplastic lumps in, 1237t
Samoyed, adrenal hyperplasia–like syndrome in, 847
   adult-onset hyposomatotropism in, 822
   follicular dysplasia in, 890
   granulomatous sebaceous adenitis in, 1141, 1143
   hypogonadism in, 844–845
   ivermectin sensitivity in, 428
   nasal depigmentation in, 1017
   risk for neoplastic skin disorders and non-neoplastic lumps in, 1237t
   risk for non-neoplastic skin disorders in, 81t
   uveodermatologic syndrome in, 757
San Joaquin Valley fever. See *Coccidioidomycosis.*
Sandflies, 534
Sandimmune. See *Cyclosporine.*
Sarcocystosis, canine, 533–534
Sarcoid, feline, 1285, *1288, 1289*
Sarcoma(s), 1282
   epithelioid, 1371–1373, *1372, 1373*
   fibroblastic spindle cell. See *Fibrosarcoma(s).*
   histiocytic, 1346–1347, 1351–1352
      disseminated, 1347
      localized, 1347
   infectious. See *Transmissible venereal tumor.*
   postvaccinal, 1317–1319, *1318*
   reticulum cell. See *Lymphoma.*
   soft tissue, 1281
   undifferentiated, 1281, 1319–1320. See also *Neuroendocrine tumor(s), primary cutaneous.*
Sarcophaga spp., 501, *504*
Sarcophagids, 503
Sarcoptes scabiei, 481
   in guinea pigs, 1433
   in hamsters, 1440
   in mice, 1443

Sarcoptes scabiei (Continued)
  in rats, 1453
  var. *canis*, 476, 477
  var. *cuniculi*, in rabbits, 1448
Sarcoptic mange. See *Scabies.*
Sarcoptic mite(s). See *Scabies.*
Satellite cell(s), apoptosis of, 137, *141*
  necrosis of, 137
Satellitosis, 137, *141*
Scabies, 98
  canine, *466*, 476–483, *478*
    cause of, 476–477
    clinical features of, *466*, *478*, 479, *480*
    diagnosis of, *148*, 479–481, *481–482*
    pathogenesis of, 476–479
    skin scraping for, 106
    treatment of, 481–483
  feline, 477, *478*, *480*, 483–484
    cause of, 476, 483
    clinical features of, *478*, 484
    diagnosis of, 484, *485*
    pathogenesis of, 483–484
    skin scraping for, 106
    treatment of, 484
  in foxes, 477
  in humans, 477, *478*, 479, 483
  skin scraping for, 101
Scale, 87, *93*
Scaling, 86
  in bacterial infection, 277
  orthokeratotic, 86
Scar(s), 87, 97, 196
Scarlet red stain, staining characteristics of various substances with, 130t
Schipperke, black hair follicular dysplasia in, 962
  color dilution alopecia in, 967
  pemphigus foliaceus in, 686–687
  risk for non-neoplastic skin disorders in, 81t
Schistosoma dermatitis, 436
Schistosomiasis, 436–437
  in humans, 436–437
Schmorl's disease, in rabbits, 1445
Schnauzer, giant, congenital hypothyroidism in, 852
    risk for neoplastic skin disorders and non-neoplastic lumps in, 1237t
    seasonal flank alopecia in, 893
    squamous cell carcinoma in, 1251
    vitiligo in, 1015
  hair growth in, 5
  miniature, atopy in, 581
    aurotrichia in, 978, *1008–1009*, 1022
    comedo syndrome in. See *Schnauzer comedo syndrome.*
    drug reactions in, 721
    epidermal nevi in, 1389
    follicular dysplasia in, 890, 971
    food hypersensitivity in, 618
    gilding syndrome in, 978
    histiocytomas in, 1347
    hypothyroidism in, 852
    lipomas in, 1308
    melanocytic neoplasms in, 1359
    melanocytoma in, 1359
    melanoma in, 1361
    multiple pigmented plaques in, 1240, 1242
    Mycobacterium avium infection in, 315
    papillomavirus-associated pigmentary abnormality in, 1012

Schnauzer (Continued)
    risk for neoplastic skin disorders and non-neoplastic lumps in, 1237t, 1238t
    risk for non-neoplastic skin disorders in, 81t
    seasonal flank alopecia in, 891
    sebaceous gland hyperplasia in, 1271
    Sertoli's cell tumor in, 840, 843
    skin pH in, 3
    superficial suppurative necrolytic dermatitis of, 720, 721, *724–725*, 729, *730*
    trichoepithelioma in, 1263
    vitamin A–responsive dermatosis in, 1036
  standard, melanoma in, 1361
Schnauzer comedo syndrome, 227, 242, *930*, 931–935, *934*, 1029, 1389
Schwannoma, 1281, *1286*, 1291–1294, *1292–1293*
  breed(s) with predilection for, 1237t
Scleroderma, localized, canine, *1142*, 1146–1148, *1147*
Sclerosis, dermal, 161–162
Scolecobasidium humicola, 379
Scopulariopsis spp., in normal flora, of cats, 338, 338t
Scottish terrier. See *Terrier, Scottish.*
Scraping(s). See *Skin scraping.*
Screwworm(s), 503
Scrotum, skin of, histology of, *14*, 36
  varicose tumors of, 1386
  vascular hamartoma of, 1386
  vascular nevi of, 1386
Sealyham terrier. See *Terrier, Sealyham.*
Seasonal flank alopecia, 890–893, *891*, *892*
Sebaceous adenitis, 95, 168, 925, 1029
  clinical management of, 242, 243
  granulomatous, 199, 1140–1146
    cause and pathogenesis of, 1141
    clinical features of, 1141–1144
    clinical management of, 1145–1146
    diagnosis of, *1143–1145*, 1144–1145
    in cats, *1142*, 1144
    in dogs, 1141–1143, *1142*, *1143*
  in rabbits, 1451
Sebaceous gland(s), 2, 41, *42*, *43*, 48–51, *50*
  adenomas of, 1029
    clinical management of, 242
    in dogs, 1271, *1272*
    in gerbils, 1429–1430
  age-related changes in, 65
  androgens and, 797
  atrophy of, 168, 170, *170*
  carcinoma of, diagnosis of, 1274, *1274*
    in dogs, 1271
  cysts of, 1381
  disorder of, in guinea pigs, 1437–1439
  distribution of, 48
  dysplasia of, 168–170
  enzymes in, 51
  epithelioma of, diagnosis of, 1274, *1274*
  functions of, 48
  hyperplasia of, 168–170, 1029
    clinical management of, 242
    in dogs, *1254*, 1271
    in eyelid, 1188, *1189*
    with greasy skin and haircoat, idiopathic, 1179, *1180*
  in dogs, atrophic, 168, *170*
    normal, *170*
  innervation of, 59
  melanosis of, 152, *153*, 170
  nevi of, *1380–1381*, 1386–1387, *1387*
  regulation of, 51

Sebaceous gland(s) *(Continued)*
  tumors of, 1270–1275
    breed(s) with predilection for, 1237t
    cause and pathogenesis of, 1270
    clinical findings in, 1271–1273
    clinical management of, 1275
    diagnosis of, *1273,* 1273–1275, *1274*
    in cats, 1271–1273
    in dogs, *1254, 1271, 1272*
    in mice, 1444
    in rats, 1455
Seba-Hex. See *Chlorhexidine, shampoo.*
SebaLyt, 1026
Sebolux, 1026, 1028
Seborrhea, 93
  and bacterial infection, 277
  canine, 208–209, 235, 1030–1036, *1031.* See also *Demodicosis, in dogs.*
    cause and pathogenesis of, 1032
    clinical features of, 1032
    clinical management of, 1035–1036
    diagnosis of, *1034,* 1034–1035
    endocrine factors and, 1032
    environmental factors and, 1032
    in inflammation, 1032
    nutritional factors and, 1032
    primary, 227, 913–920, 1030–1032
      breed(s) with predilection for, 75, 227
      cause and pathogenesis of, 913–915
      clinical features of, *914,* 915
      clinical management of, 916–920
      definition of, 913
      diagnosis of, 915–916, *916–917*
    secondary, 227, 1030–1032, *1033*
  feline, *1008,* 1038, *1039, 1040*
    primary, 914, *920,* 921
Seborrhea oleosa, 228, 1026
  in cats, 1038, *1039*
  in dogs, 1030
Seborrhea sicca, 208, 228, 1026
  in cats, 1038, *1040*
  in dogs, 1030
Seborrheic dermatitis, diagnosis of, *151*
SeboRx, 1026
Sebum, and acne, 1041
  components of, 51
  functions of, 48, 51
Secretory component, 31
Selamectin, 428, 498
  otic therapy with, 1229
  regulation of, 424
  systemic, antiparasitic therapy with, 430
Selectin(s), 545
  in vascular endothelium, 56
Selective IgA deficiency, 278, 279t
Selective IgM deficiency, 279t
Selenium sulfide shampoo, 223
  antifungal therapy with, 409–410
  antiseborrheic therapy with, 918, 1026–1027, 1036
Self-destructive behavior, 1055, 1057
Self-mutilation, in rabbits, 1550
Self-nursing, 1065–1066
Seminoma(s), 838, 843
Sensory perception, 59–61
  age-related changes in, 65
Serglycin, 38
Sertoli's cell tumor, *830,* 838, 840–843, *841, 842, 843*
  red hair with, 1022

Sesame oil, 227, 1028
Setter, callus dermatitis in, 1102
  English, atopy in, 581
    benign familial pemphigus in, 947
    Ehlers-Danlos syndrome in, 982
    idiopathic acquired cutaneous laxity in, 1173
    Malassezia dermatitis in, 365
    multiple pigmented plaques in, 1240–1242
  Gordon, atopy in, 581
    black hair follicular dysplasia in, 962
    juvenile cellulitis in, 1165
    risk for non-neoplastic skin disorders in, 79t
    vitamin A–responsive dermatosis in, 1036
  Irish, acral lick dermatitis in, 1058
    antithyroglobulin antibody(ies) in, 852
    antithyroid antibody(ies) in, 789
    atopy in, 581
    Ehlers-Danlos syndrome in, 982
    epidermis of, turnover time for, 31
    estrogen-responsive dermatosis in, *830*
    graying in, 1015
    hemangiopericytoma in, 1402
    hypothyroidism in, 852, 853
    lymphomas in, 1331
    melanocytoma in, 1359
    melanoma in, 1361
    nasal depigmentation in, 1017
    pododermatitis in, 305
    psychogenic dermatoses in, 1056
    risk for neoplastic skin disorders and non-neoplastic lumps in, 1237t, 1238t
    risk for non-neoplastic skin disorders in, 75, 79t
    seborrhea in, 227, 243, 913, 915, 1029, 1032
    trichoepithelioma in, 1263
Sex, and risk for non-neoplastic skin disorders, 76
Sex hormone(s), 795–798. See also *specific hormone.*
Sex hormone ACTH response test, 798
Sex hormone dermatosis, 827–851, 1020
Sex hormone function test(s), 798
Sézary syndrome, 1331, 1338, *1339*
Shampoo(s), 211–212
  adverse reaction to, in miniature Schnauzers, 721
  antibacterial, 223, 280
  antifungal, 356, 356t, 409–410
  anti-inflammatory agents in, 223–224
  antimycotic, 223, 918
  antiparasite, 223
  antipruritic agents in, 223–224
  antiseborrheic, 223, 916–918, 1026–1027, 1035–1036
  carbaryl, for feline demodicosis, 475
  contact time for, 222, 223
  detergent, 211
  flea, 498–499
  formulations of, and efficacy of active ingredients, 218t, 221–224, *222*
  medicated, use of, 223
  microvesicle technology for, 221, *222*
  moisturizing hypoallergenic, 917
  soap, 211
Shar Pei, amyloidosis in, 767
  atopy in, 581
  body fold intertrigo in, *1106,* 1107
  demodicosis in, 461
  dermal mucin of, 38
  dermal mucinosis in, 164, *165*
  food hypersensitivity in, 618
  histiocytomas in, 1347
  hypothyroidism in, 852

Shar Pei *(Continued)*
    mast cell tumors in, 1320–1321
    mucinosis in, 996–997, *1158*, 1174–1175, *1176–1177, 1401*, 1402
    multiple pigmented plaques in, 1242, *1243*
    oral papillomatosis in, 1240
    otitis externa in, 1207
    papillomas in, 1243, 1247
    papillomavirus-associated pigmentary abnormality in, 1012
    risk for neoplastic skin disorders and non-neoplastic lumps in, 1237t, 1238t
    risk for non-neoplastic skin disorders in, 75, 81t
    seborrhea in, 913, 915, 1032
    skin scraping from, 105
    superficial bacterial folliculitis in, *289*, 293
Shedding, 8, 210
    excessive, 894
    in ferrets, 1425
    in guinea pigs, 1437
    seasonal, 6
Sheepdog, Belgian (Belgian Tervuren), atopy in, 581
    granulomatous sebaceous adenitis in, 1141, 1146
    hypopigmentation in, 975
    lymphedema in, 990
    risk for non-neoplastic skin disorders in, 77t
    vitiligo in, 1015
  Old English, antithyroglobulin antibody(ies) in, 852
    demodicosis in, 465
    drug reactions in, 721
    grooming of, 214
    hair growth in, 5
    hypothyroidism in, 852
    ivermectin contraindicated in, 1229
    keratoacanthoma in, *1241*, 1248
    melanotrichia in, 1010
    pilomatrixoma in, 1267
    risk for neoplastic skin disorders and non-neoplastic lumps in, 1237t
    risk for non-neoplastic skin disorders in, 80t
    vitiligo in, 1015
  Shetland (sheltie), basal cell carcinoma in, 1262
    bullous pemphigoid in, 695
    color dilution alopecia in, 967
    cutaneous histiocytosis in, 1353
    dermatomyositis in, 938, 940, 942
    distichiasis in, 1188
    drug reactions in, 721
    epidermolysis bullosa simplex in, 938
    fly bites on, 502
    follicular dysplasia in, 971
    histiocytomas in, 1347
    hypothyroidism in, 852
    idiopathic ulcerative dermatosis of, 707, 717, 946–947
    ivermectin contraindicated in, 1229
    risk for neoplastic skin disorders and non-neoplastic lumps in, 1237t
    risk for non-neoplastic skin disorders in, 75, 81t
    Sertoli's cell tumor in, 840
    superficial bacterial folliculitis in, 294
    systemic lupus erythematosus in, 705
Sheltie. See *Sheepdog, Shetland (Sheltie)*.
Shepherd, Australian, drug reactions in, 721
    follicular dysplasia in, 971
    mucocutaneous hypopigmentation in, 1017–1018
    risk for non-neoplastic skin disorders in, 75
  Belgian, congenital hypotrichosis in, 958
  Garafino, Ehlers-Danlos syndrome in, 982

Shepherd *(Continued)*
  German, acral lick dermatitis in, 1058
    amyloidosis in, 769
    anal sac disorders in, 1201
    calcinosis circumscripta in, 1400
    calcinosis cutis in, 1399
    chondrosarcomas in, 1315
    chronic ulcerative blepharitis in, 1186
    collagen disorder of footpads in, *980*, 984, *984, 985*
    color dilution alopecia in, 967
    congenital hypothyroidism in, 852
    congenital hypotrichosis in, 958
    contact hypersensitivity in, 1081
    delayed growth in, 820
    dermatomyositis in, 940
    dermatophytosis in, *344–345*
    distichiasis in, 1188
    Ehlers-Danlos syndrome in, 982
    familial vasculopathy of, 189, 749–751, 987
    fibropruritic nodule in, 1284
    fly dermatitis in, *501*
    focal metatarsal fistulation of, *980*, 985–986, *986*
    follicular dysplasia in, 971
    folliculitis, furunculosis, and cellulitis in, *301*, 306–308
    food hypersensitivity in, 618
    furunculosis in, *301*
    granulomatous sebaceous adenitis in, 1143
    graying in, 1014–1015, *1015*
    hair color of, 8
    haircoat of, 7
    hemangiopericytoma in, 1302
    hemangiosarcomas in, 1299
    hypopigmentation in, 975
    hypopituitarism in, 811
    idiopathic onychomadesis in, 1198–1199
    IGF-1 plasma levels in. See *Xylasine*.
    immunodeficiency in, 307, 308
    ivermectin sensitivity in, 428
    keratoacanthoma in, 1248
    lupoid onychodystrophy in, 1195
    lymphedema in, 990
    lymphomas in, 1331
    medullary trichomalacia in, 895, 951
    mucocutaneous pyoderma in, 290–291, *291*
    multiple collagenous nevi (nodular dermatofibrosis) in, 986, *1380–1381*, 1382–1383
    myxomas and myxosarcomas in, 1290
    nasal folliculitis and furunculosis in, 303
    pemphigus erythematosus in, 690
    pituitary dwarfism in, 819, *820*
    pododermatitis in, 305
    psychogenic dermatoses in, 305, 1056
    pyoderma of, 278, 531
    pyotraumatic dermatitis in, 1104
    pythiosis in, 381
    risk for neoplastic skin disorders and non-neoplastic lumps in, 1237t, 1238t
    risk for non-neoplastic skin disorders in, 78t–79t
    seborrhea in, 913, 1032
    seminoma in, 843
    snake bites in, 1091
    sweating in, 53
    systemic lupus erythematosus in, 705
    trichoepithelioma in, 1263
    tyrosinemia in, 994
    vasculitis in, 744
    vitiligo in, 1015
    white, nasal depigmentation in, 1017

Shepherd (*Continued*)
  zinc-responsive dermatosis in, 1120
  multiple collagenous cysts in, and renal pathology, 1383
  Old English, lymphedema in, 990
Shetland sheepdog. See *Sheepdog, Shetland (Sheltie)*.
Shiba inu, atopy in, 581
Shih tzu, atopy in, 581
  distichiasis in, 1188
  glucocorticoid-induced reaction in, 246–247
  Malassezia dermatitis in, 365
  risk for neoplastic skin disorders and non-neoplastic lumps in, 1237t, 1238t
  risk for non-neoplastic skin disorders in, 81t
Shivering, in thermoregulation, 54
Shope fibroma(s), in rabbits, 1451–1452
Shope fibroma virus, 1446, 1451
Shope papilloma(s), in rabbits, 1451
Shope papilloma virus, 1446, 1451
Short hair syndrome of silky breeds, 888, 897
Shorthaired cat(s), American, grooming for, 215
  domestic, grooming for, 215
  double coat, 215
  dystrophic epidermolysis bullosa in, 939
  Ehlers-Danlos syndrome in, 982
  exotic, seborrhea in, 920
  single coat, 215
Sialodacryoadenitis, in mice, 1443
  in rabbits, *1447*
  in rats, *1447*, 1453
Siamese cat, acromelanism in, 1012–1013
  Aguirre's syndrome in, 1021
  amyloidosis in, 767
  basal cell carcinoma in, 1262
  basal cell tumors in, 1261
  congenital hypotrichosis in, 959, *962*
  cryptococcosis in, 395
  demodicosis in, 474
  dermatophytosis in, *346*
  griseofulvin side effects in, 357
  grooming for, 215
  hair color of, 8
  junctional epidermolysis bullosa in, 939
  lipomas in, 1308
  mast cell tumors in, 1322–1323
  Mycobacterium avium infection in, 315
  periocular leukotrichia in, 1021, *1022*
  photosensitivity in, 1080
  pinnal alopecia in, 888, 900
  psychogenic dermatosis in, 1056, 1066–1067
  risk for neoplastic skin disorders and non-neoplastic lumps in, 1237t
  risk for non-neoplastic skin disorders in, 81t
  staphylococcal folliculitis in, 289
  systemic lupus erythematosus in, 705
  tail sucking in, *1070*, 1070–1071
  urticaria pigmentosa in, 997–998
  vitiligo in, 1015, *1016*
Siberian husky, alopecia in, 888
  basal cell carcinoma in, 1262
  calcinosis cutis in, 1399
  dermoid cyst (sinus) in, 936
  eosinophilic granuloma in, 1154, *1155*
  follicular dysplasia in, 890, 970, 971
  follicular parakeratosis in, 925
  hemangiopericytoma in, 1302
  hookworm dermatitis in, *432*
  hypogonadism in, 844

Siberian husky (*Continued*)
  hypothyroidism in, 1120
  idiopathic onychodystrophy in, 1198
  mucocutaneous hypopigmentation in, 1017–1018
  nasal depigmentation in, 1017
  postclipping alopecia in, 897
  risk for neoplastic skin disorders and non-neoplastic lumps in, 1237t
  risk for non-neoplastic skin disorders in, 75, 81t
  snow nose in, 1017
  uveodermatologic syndrome in, 757
  zinc-responsive dermatosis in, *1114–1115*, 1119, 1121, *1121*
Silicone(s), 1028
Silky terrier. See *Terrier, Silky*.
Silver nitrate, 227
Silver salt(s), 232
Silver sulfadiazine, 232
Simuliidae spp., 502
Sinequan. See *Doxepin*.
Sinus hairs (vibrissae, whiskers), 44–45, *45*
  mechanoreceptors and, 61
Sinus pad, 45, *45*
Skin, acidity of, antimicrobial effects of, 31–32
  cleaning of, 210–213
  color of, drug-induced changes in, 1023
  dryness of, 1025
  ecology of, 31–34. See also *Microflora*.
  embryonic, 2
  examination of, 85–86
  general functions of, 1–2
  greasy, with sebaceous gland hyperplasia, idiopathic, 1179, *1180*
  gross anatomy of, 3–9
  hydration of, in immune defense, 32
    measurement of, 32
  immunologic functions of, 25–26, 274. See also *Skin immune system*.
  metabolism of, 3
  microscopic anatomy of, 9–65
  pH of, and antimicrobial susceptibility, 282
    in immune defense, 31–32
    measurement of, 32
  physiology of, 3–9
  properties of, 1–2
  thickness of, 3
Skin appendage(s), formation of, 2–3
Skin biopsy. See *Biopsy*.
Skin care, normal, 207–215. See also *Grooming*.
Skin extensibility index, 982
Skin fold dermatitis. See *Intertrigo*.
Skin immune system, 549–561
  adhesion molecules in, 545, 549t
  aging and, 560–561
  basophils in, 558
  cell surface antigens (determinants) in, nomenclature for, 543–549, 544t–545t
  cell surface receptors in, nomenclature for, 543–549
  complement in, 559
  cytokines and, 543–545, 546t
  definition of, 549
  eicosanoids and, 559–560, 561t
  endothelial cells in, 556
  eosinophils in, 557–558
  granulocytes in, 556
  humoral components of, 558–560
  immune complexes in, 559
  keratinocytes in, 550–551

Skin immune system *(Continued)*
  Langerhans' cells in, 551–552
  lipid mediators in, 559–560
  lymphocytes in, 552–553
  major histocompatibility complex (MHC) and, 545–548
  mast cells in, 553–556, *554*
  neutrophils in, 556–557
  platelet-activating factor in, 559–560
  tissue macrophages in, 553
Skin lesion(s), annular, 88–89, *102*
  arciform, *102*
  asymmetric, 84, *85*
  bilaterally symmetric, 84, *85*
  coalescing, 89
  configuration of, 88–89, *102*
  diffuse, 88
  distribution of, 90–93, 103t–105t
  grouped, *102*
  iris (central healing, target), *102*
  linear, 88, *98, 102*
  morphology of, 86–88, *87–101*
  polycyclic, *102*
  primary, 86–87, *87–92*
  primary and/or secondary, 86, *87*, 92–96
  secondary, 86, *87, 97–100*
  serpiginous, *102*
  single, *102*
  stages of, 89–90, 178
Skin scraping, 101–107, 115
Skin surgery. See *Surgery*.
Skin-associated lymphoid tissue, 26, 548–549
Skin-So-Soft, 427, 499
Skunk odor, removal of, 214
Sloughing, tissue, miscellaneous causes of, *1086, 1089*, 1089–1090
Snake bite, 1090–1091, *1092*
Snow nose, 1017, *1018*
Snuffles, in rabbits, 1444–1445
Soak(s), for bacterial infection, 280–281
Sodium borate, 495
Sodium hypochlorite, in topical therapy, 231
Sodium lactate, 235, 1028
Solar dermatitis, 1029, 1073–1081
  canine, nasal, 1074–1077, *1075*
    of trunk and extremities, *1075*, 1079, *1080*
  feline, *1075, 1076*, 1077–1079
  in white-eared cats, 76
  risk for, haircoat color and, 76
Solar elastosis, 160, *160*
Solenopsis invicta, 506
Solganal. See *Aurothioglucose*.
Solvent(s), exposure to, 31
Somatomedin(s), 795
Somatotroph(s), 781
Somatotropin. See *Growth hormone*.
Soriatane. See *Acitretin*.
Southern blot hybridization, 1239
Spaniel, American water, adult-onset hyposomatotropism in, 822
    pattern baldness in, 965
  Brittany, amyloidosis in, 768
    collagenous nevus in, *1380–1381*
    histoplasmosis in, 400
    hypothyroidism in, 852
    immunodeficiency in, 279t
    risk for non-neoplastic skin disorders in, 77t
  Cavalier King Charles, black hair follicular dysplasia in, 962

Spaniel *(Continued)*
    eosinophilic granuloma in, 1154
    ichthyosis in, 923
    persistent scratching in, 996
    risk for non-neoplastic skin disorders in, 77t
  Cocker, amyloidosis in, 768
    anal sac disorders in, 1201
    atopy in, 581
    basal cell carcinoma in, 1262
    black hair follicular dysplasia in, 962
    cell proliferation kinetics in, 7
    cheyletiellosis in, 456
    congenital hypotrichosis in, 958
    distichiasis in, 1188
    epidermal nevi in, 1389
    epidermis of, turnover time for, 31
    fibrosarcomas in, 1287
    food hypersensitivity in, 618, 1211, 1213
    haircoat of, 8
    hemangiopericytoma in, 1302
    histiocytomas in, 1347
    hypothyroidism in, 852, *859*
    idiopathic onychodystrophy in, 1198
    IGF-1 plasma levels in. See *Xylasine*.
    immunodeficiency in, 279t
    lipomas in, 1308
    lymphomas in, 1331
    Malassezia dermatitis, 365
    melanocytoma in, 1359
    mineralized ear canals in, *1211*
    otitis externa in, 1212, 1213
    papillomas in, 1240
    plasmacytoma in, 1344
    Pseudomonas otitis externa in, *1210–1211*
    risk for neoplastic skin disorders and non-neoplastic lumps in, 1237t, 1238t
    risk for non-neoplastic skin disorders in, 75, 81t
    sebaceous gland hyperplasia in, 1271
    seborrhea in, 227, 243, 913–915, *914,* 919–920, 1029, 1032
    tail dock neuroma in, 1065, 1296
    trichoblastoma in, 1270
    trichoepithelioma in, 1263
    vitamin A–responsive dermatosis in, *1031*, 1036
    white piedra in, 374, *374*
  Irish water, follicular dysplasia in, 890, 971
    risk for non-neoplastic skin disorders in, 79t
  Japanese, scabies in, *466*
  lip fold intertrigo in, 1107
  Springer, acral mutilation in, 995
    anal sac disorders in, 1201
    basal cell carcinoma in, 1262
    deep folliculitis and furunculosis in, *301*
    dermoid cyst (sinus) in, 936
    Ehlers-Danlos syndrome in, 982
    follicular dysplasia in, 971
    food hypersensitivity in, 618
    hemangiopericytoma in, 1302
    histiocytomas in, 1347
    idiopathic onychomadesis in, 1198
    melanocytoma in, 1359
    otitis externa in, 1212
    psoriasiform-lichenoid dermatosis of, 180, 929–931, *930–931, 933, 934*
    risk for neoplastic skin disorders and non-neoplastic lumps in, 1237t, 1238t
    risk for non-neoplastic skin disorders in, 81t
    seborrhea in, 227, 243, 913, 915, 1029, 1032

Spaniel *(Continued)*
  skin pH in, 3
  trichoepithelioma in, 1263
Spectrin, 20
Spherulite(s), 221, 222, 1028, 1035
Spherulocytic disease, 1096, *1097*
Spherulocytosis, 1096, *1097*
Sphinx cat, 957
  urticaria pigmentosa in, *997,* 997–998, *998,* 1009, *1010*
Spiculosis, *954,* 956, *956*
Spider bite(s), *478,* 484–485, *486*
Spilopsyllus cuniculi, 491, *492*
Spinous ear tick(s), 442–443, *443*
Spirochetosis, venereal, in rabbits, 1445–1446, *1447*
SPL. See *Staphylococcus aureus, phage lysate.*
Spongiosis, 179–180
  diffuse, 179–180
  eosinophilic, 147
  epidermal, 140–142, *143*
  lymphocytic, 147
Sporanox. See *Itraconazole.*
Sporothrix schenckii, 337, 386, 388
  culture of, 121
Sporotrichosis, 386–390
  cause of, 386
  claw involvement in, 1195
  cutaneolymphatic, 386, 388
  cutaneous, 386
  diagnosis of, 388, *388, 389*
  in cats, clinical findings in, 386, *387, 388, 389*
    clinical management of, 390
  in dogs, clinical findings in, *367,* 386, *387,* 389
    clinical management of, 390
  pathogenesis of, 386
  pododermatitis caused by, 305
  zoonotic aspects of, 386–388, *387*
Spray(s), 218t, 225
Springer spaniel. See *Spaniel, Springer.*
Squamatization, definition of, 175
Squame(s), from normal skin, *115,* 116
Squamous cell, *23*
Squamous cell carcinoma, 1021, 1029, 1249–1258
  breed(s) with predilection for, 1237t
  clawbed, breed(s) with predilection for, 1237t
  clinical findings in, 1251–1255
  clinical management of, 1256–1258
  diagnosis of, 1255–1256, *1255–1257*
  glabrous, nonpigmented skin of trunk (actinic), breed(s) with predilection for, 1237t
  in cats, *1241,* 1252–1255, *1253–1255*
  in dogs, *1241, 1241,* 1251–1252, 1251–1253
  in gerbils, 1429–1430
  in hamsters, 1442
  in mice, 1444
  in rabbits, 1451
  in rats, 1455
  nasal, in dogs, 1251, *1251*
  of claw bed, *1196,* 1198
  of lung, cutaneous metastases of, 1374
  of pinna, in white-eared cats, 76
  papillomas and, 1012, *1013*
  risk factors for, 1249–1251, 1250t
  risk for, haircoat color and, 76
  solar-induced, in dogs, 1251
  subungual, in dogs, 1252, *1252–1253*
Squamous cell carcinoma in situ, 1013
  multicentric, *1254,* 1258–1259, *1259–1260*
    in cats, 527–528

Squamous eddy(ies), 156
Squamous pearl(s). See *Horn pearls (squamous pearls).*
Squirrel(s), ground, plague in, 325–326
  rock, plague in, 325–326
Staffordshire terrier. See *Terrier, Staffordshire.*
Stain(s), for fungi, 119
  special, staining characteristics of various substances with, 130t
  tissue, 129, 130t
Staphage Lysate. See *Staphylococcus aureus, phage lysate.*
Staphylococcal folliculitis. See *Folliculitis.*
Staphylococcal hypersensitivity. See *Bacteria, hypersensitivity to.*
Staphylococcal pyoderma. See *Pyoderma.*
Staphylococcal scalded skin syndrome, in mice, 1442
Staphylococci, adhesion molecules of, 276
  as resident flora, in dogs, 275
  autogenous vaccine against, 286
  coagulase-negative, as resident flora, in cats, 33, 275
    in dogs, 33–34, 275
    as transient flora, in cats, 275
  coagulase-positive, antibiotic susceptibility of, 282
    as resident flora, in cats, 33, 275
    in dogs, 33–34
    as transient flora, in cats, 275
  identification of, 116
  in anal sacs, 1201
  in hair follicle, 51
  infections caused by, depth of, and antibiotic therapy, 283
    in dogs, 205
    primary, 278
    seborrhea and, 915–916, 918, 1030
  necrotizing fasciitis caused by, 324–325
  otitis externa caused by, 1213–1215, 1214t
  resistance in, 276
  toxic shock syndrome caused by, in dogs, 324–325
Staphylococcus aureus, and *Malassezia pachydermatis,* synergism of, 33
  as resident flora, in cats, 33, 275
  infection by, in hamsters, 1439
    in mice, 1442
    in rabbits, 1445, 1446
  phage lysate (SPL), 286–287
Staphylococcus capitis, as resident flora, in cats, 33, 275
Staphylococcus epidermidis, as resident flora, in cats, 275
  in dogs, 33, 275
Staphylococcus felis, 276
Staphylococcus haemolyticus, as resident flora, in cats, 33, 275
Staphylococcus hominis, as resident flora, in cats, 33, 275
Staphylococcus hyicus, 275
Staphylococcus intermedius, 324–325
  antibiotic susceptibility of, 282
  antibiotic therapy for, 281–282
  as resident flora, in cats, 33, 275
    in dogs, 33–34, 275
  autogenous vaccine against, 286
  in generalized demodectic mange, 465
  in subcutaneous abscesses in cats, 310
  infections caused by, 275, 277
  otitis media caused by, 1214t
  strains of, 275
  superficial folliculitis caused by, 293
Staphylococcus sciuri, as resident flora, in cats, 33, 275
Staphylococcus simulans, as resident flora, in cats, 33, 275
Staphylococcus warneri, as resident flora, in cats, 33, 275
Staphylococcus xylosus, as resident flora, in dogs, 33, 275

Steatitis, 171–172
  in cats, *1117,* 1117–1118
Steinernema carpocapsae, 494
Stemphylium spp., 379
Sterigmatocystin, 1101
Sterile eosinophilic pinnal folliculitis, canine, 1213
Sterile eosinophilic pustulosis, canine, 1132–1133, *1134–1136*
Sterile granuloma and pyogranuloma, idiopathic, 1136–1140
Sterile granulomatous dermatitis and lymphadenitis, juvenile. See *Cellulitis, canine juvenile.*
Sterile panniculitis, *203*
  cytologic diagnosis of, *114*
  in cats, *175,* 311
Sterile pustular dermatosis, cytologic diagnosis of, *117*
Sterile pyogranuloma, cytologic diagnosis of, *113*
  on feet, 305
Sterile pyogranuloma-granuloma syndrome, 189
Steroid tachyphylaxis, 248
Stevens-Johnson syndrome, 740
  classification of, 732–733, 733t
Sticker tumor. See *Transmissible venereal tumor.*
Stomatitis, burdock, 1091, *1092*
Stomoxys calcitrans, 500, *501*
Storage mite–related hypersensitivity, 640
Stratum corneum, emulsion in, in immune defense, 274
  in immune defense, 274
Stratum germinativum, 2
Stratum intermedium, 2
Streptococci, α-hemolytic, as resident flora, in cats, 275
    in dogs, 275
    otitis media caused by, 1214t
  β-hemolytic, as resident flora, in cats, 33
    in dogs, 33
    as transient flora, in cats, 275
    in oral flora of cats, 276
    in subcutaneous abscesses in cats, 310
    otitis media caused by, 1214t
  in rabbits, 1445
  infection by, in mice, 1442
    in rats, 1452
  necrotizing fasciitis caused by, 324
  nongroup-D, otitis media caused by, 1214t
  otitis externa caused by, 1214t
  otitis media caused by, 1214t
  pseudomycetoma caused by, 312
  toxic shock syndrome caused by, in dogs, 324
Streptococcus canis, 324
Streptococcus faecalis, in anal sacs, 1201
Streptomyces avermitilis, 429, 430
Streptomyces cyanogriseus, 430
Streptomyces hygroscopicus, 429
Streptotrichosis, cutaneous. See *Dermatophilosis.*
Striae, in hyperadrenocorticism, *802, 803*
Stromelysins, 37
Strongyloides stercoralis, in humans, 432
Strongyloides stercoralis–like infection, 434
Stud tail, 55, 215, *1047*
Stye (hordoleum), 1186
Subcorneal pustular dermatosis, canine, 1125–1128, *1126–1128*
Subcutaneous chyle, 1090
Subcutaneous emphysema, 1090
Subcutaneous fat sclerosis, 1162–1163, *1164*

Subcutis, 63, 63–64, *64*
  age-related changes in, 65
  changes in, 171–172
Subepidermal bubblies. See *Subepidermal vacuolar alteration.*
Subepidermal vacuolar alteration, 172–173, *173,* 697, 699
Sublamina densa area (lamina fibroreticularis), of basement membrane zone, 34
Submental organ (chin gland), 48
Sucquet-Hoyer canal, 57
Sudan black B stain, staining characteristics of various substances with, 130t
Sulfa drug(s), adverse effects and side effects of, 724–725
  resistance to, 282
Sulfasalazine, for subcorneal pustular dermatosis, 1128
  for vasculitis, 753
  immunosuppressive therapy with, 672t, 677
Sulfonamide(s), adverse effects and side effects of, 283, 721, 723
  immunosuppressive therapy with, 676–677
  potentiated, efficacy of, against coagulase-positive staphylococci, 282
  systemic, for bacterial infections, 281
Sulfone(s), immunosuppressive therapy with, 676–677
SulfOxydex, 231, 1027
Sulfur, antiparasitic therapy with, 427
  antiseborrheic therapy with, 918, 1026–1027, 1036
  as flea repellent, 209
  for feline scabies, 484
  in powders, 224
  in shampoo, 223
  topical therapy with, 233–234
Sulfur/benzoyl peroxide, shampoo, 356t
  antifungal therapy with, 409–410
Sun avoidance, in discoid lupus erythematosus, 716
  in pemphigus, 681–682
  in pemphigus erythematosus, 693
  indications for, 672t, 1077, 1078
Sunburn cells, 140
Sunflower oil, 209, 235
Sunscreen(s), oral, 254
  topical, 236–237
Superantigen(s), 667
Superficial necrolytic dermatitis, 868
Supracaudal gland. See *Tail gland, of dog.*
Supracaudal organ. See *Tail gland, of cat.*
Surface sampling, in diagnosis, 94–107
Surface-acting agent(s), in topical therapy, 231–232
Surgery, 254–263. See also *Cryosurgery; Electrosurgery; Laser surgery; Radiosurgery.*
  cold steel, 254–255
  for acral lick dermatitis, 1063
  for otitis externa, 1230–1231
  for squamous cell carcinoma, 1256–1257
Swab smear(s), for *Malassezia* spp., 368
  technique for, 115, 116
Sweat, epitrichial, properties of, 51
Sweat gland(s), 41, *42, 43,* 51–54
  adenomas of, *1279*
  age-related changes in, 64–65
  atrichial (eccrine), 3, 51, *52,* 52–53
    carcinoma of, 1198
    tumors of, 1275
      in cats, 1276
      in dogs, 1275
  epitrichial (apocrine), 2, *51,* 51–52, *52*
    adenoma of, in hamsters, 1442
    carcinoma of, 1276, *1278*

Sweat gland(s) *(Continued)*
    changes in, 170–171, *171*
    cystomatosis of, *1380–1381*, 1381
    cysts of, *1366*, 1379–1381, *1380–1382*
    dilation of, 171, *171*
    necrosis of, 171, *171*
        in feline rhinotracheitis, 525
    nevi of, 1387, *1387*, *1388*
    tumors of, 1275
        in cats, 1275, *1276*
        in dogs, *1272*, 1275
  in epidermal renewal, 52
    tumors of, 1275–1281
        breed(s) with predilection for, 1237t
        cause and pathogenesis of, 1275
        clinical findings in, 1275–1276
        clinical management of, 1279
        diagnosis of, 1276–1277, *1276–1279*
        in cats, 1275–1276, *1276*
        in dogs, *1272*, 1275
Sweating, atrichial, 53
  epitrichial, 53
Swimmer's itch, 436
Sylvatic ringworm. See *Dermatophytosis.*
Syndecan, 38
  in morphogenesis of skin appendages, 3
Synotic, for acral lick dermatitis, 1063
Syphacia muris, 1454
Syphacia obvelata, in mice, 1444
Syphilis, hamster, 1439
  rabbit, 1445–1446
Syringadenoma, 1276
  papillary, *1277–1278*
Systemic hair embolism, in rats, 1454–1455
Systemic lupus erythematosus. See *Lupus erythematosus, systemic.*
Systemic therapy. See also specific therapy.
  broad-spectrum, 238–254

T cells (T lymphocytes), in epidermal immunity, 25–26, 29
Tabanus spp., 502
Tactile hair disk. See *Tylotrich pad.*
Tactile pad. See *Tylotrich pad.*
Taenia crassiceps infection, 440, *441*
Tail, common and less common dermatoses of, 104t–105t
Tail biting, in dogs, *1064*, 1064–1065, *1065*
Tail dock neuroma, 1065, *1296*, 1296–1297, *1297*
Tail fold intertrigo, *1106*, 1107
Tail gland, of cat, 55
  of dog, 54–55
Tail gland hyperplasia, 227
  canine, *1039*, 1045–1046, 1046, *1047*
  feline, *1039*, 1046–1048, *1047*, *1048*
Tail sucking, in cats, *1070*, 1070–1071
Taktic, 470, 473
Talin, 20
Tan Sal, 227
Tannin(s), 680
Tar, in haircoat, 213
Tar products, antiseborrheic therapy with, 918, 1026–1027, 1036
Tazarotene (Tazorac), 234, 241
Tea tree oil, 236, 499
Tegison. See *Etretinate.*
Teichoic acid, 276
Telangiectasia, idiopathic, 1304–1305

Telogen, 5, 5–6, 48, *49*, *50*, 341
Telogen defluxion, 6, 198, *888*, 893–894
  hair examination in, 108, *109*
  in ferrets, 1425, *1426*
  in guinea pigs, 1437
  in humans, 893–894
Temperature, and hair color, in cats, 8
  and hair growth, 5–6
Tenascin, 36t
  functions of, 38
  in morphogenesis of skin appendages, 3
Tension line(s), 9
Teratoma, cutaneous metastases of, 1374
Terbinafine, antifungal therapy with, 358, 415
  topical, 356t, 409
Terminal uridinyl transferase nick end labeling (TUNEL) method, for detection of apoptosis, 140
Terrier, Airedale, alopecia in, minoxidil for, 874
  cyclic follicular dysplasia in, 890
  demodicosis in, 461
  follicular dysplasia in, 890, 971
  hypothyroidism in, 852
  melanocytoma in, 1359
  risk for neoplastic skin disorders and non-neoplastic lumps in, 1237t, 1238t
  risk for non-neoplastic skin disorders in, 77t
  seasonal flank alopecia in, 823, 890, 893
  Sertoli's cell tumor in, *842*
  vascular nevi in, 1386
  American hairless, 957, *958*, *958*
  Bedlington, dermal perifollicular mineralization in, 168
    distichiasis in, 1188
    haircoat of, 8
    melanotrichia in, 1010
  Boston, atopy in, 581
    calcinosis circumscripta in, 1400
    color dilution alopecia in, 967
    demodicosis in, 461
    fibromas in, 1282
    histiocytomas in, 1347
    hyperadrenocorticism in, 800
    mast cell tumors in, 1320
    melanocytoma in, 1359
    pattern baldness in, 965
    pinnal alopecia in, 887
    risk for neoplastic skin disorders and non-neoplastic lumps in, 1237t, 1238t
    risk for non-neoplastic skin disorders in, 77t
    Strongyloides stercoralis–like infection in, 434
    tail fold intertrigo in, 1107
  Bull, acrodermatitis in, 955, *988–989*, 992–993, 1119
    actinic keratoses in, 1391
    immunodeficiency in, 279t
    mast cell tumors in, 1320
    nasal folliculitis and furunculosis in, 303
    pili torti in, 955
    pododermatitis in, 305
    risk for neoplastic skin disorders and non-neoplastic lumps in, 1237t, 1238t
    risk for non-neoplastic skin disorders in, 77t
    squamous cell carcinoma in, 1251
    Waardenburg-Klein syndrome in, 1014
    white, risk for skin disorders in, 76
        truncal solar dermatitis in, 1079
    zinc deficiency in, 1119
  Cairn, atopy in, 581
    risk for non-neoplastic skin disorders in, 75, 81t
    Sertoli's cell tumor in, 840

Terrier (*Continued*)
   Dandie Dinmont, hyperadrenocorticism in, 800
   fox, fibromas in, 1282
      hemangiopericytoma in, 1302
      mast cell tumors in, 1320
      risk for neoplastic skin disorders and non-neoplastic lumps in, 1237t
      schwannoma in, 1292
      wirehaired, drug reactions in, 721
   haircoat of, 7
   hypogonadism in, 833
   Irish, footpad hyperkeratosis in, 935
      melanocytoma in, 1359
      risk for neoplastic skin disorders and non-neoplastic lumps in, 1238t
      risk for non-neoplastic skin disorders in, 75, 81t
   Jack Russell, black hair follicular dysplasia in, 962
      dermatophytosis in, 343
      familial vasculopathy in, 989
      ichthyosis in, 923
      risk for non-neoplastic skin disorders in, 82t
      vasculitis in, 744
   Kerry blue, basal cell carcinoma in, 1262
      chlorambucil therapy in, side effects of, 673
      dermoid cyst (sinus) in, 1378
      footpad hyperkeratosis in, 935
      haircoat of, 8
      papillomas in, 1240
      pilomatrixoma in, 1267
      risk for neoplastic skin disorders and non-neoplastic lumps in, 1237t, 1238t
      risk for non-neoplastic skin disorders in, 82t
      spiculosis in, 956, *956*
      vascular nevi in, 1386
   Lakeland, dermatomyositis in, 940
   Maltese, drug reactions in, 721
      epiphora in, 1188
      traction alopecia in, *888*
      vaccine reaction in, 744
   Manchester, Ehlers-Danlos syndrome in, 982
      follicular dysplasia in, 971
      pattern baldness in, 965
   pododermatitis in, 305
   psychogenic dermatitis in, 305
   Scottish, atopy in, 581
      demodicosis in, 461
      drug reactions in, 721
      familial vasculopathy in, *988–989*, 989, *990*
      histiocytomas in, 1347
      lymphomas in, 1331
      melanocytoma in, 1359
      melanoma in, 1361
      risk for neoplastic skin disorders and non-neoplastic lumps in, 1237t, 1238t
      risk for non-neoplastic skin disorders in, 75, 82t
      seasonal flank alopecia in, 891
      squamous cell carcinoma in, 1251
      vascular nevi in, 1386
      vasculitis in, 744
   Sealyham, risk for non-neoplastic skin disorders in, 75
      Waardenburg-Klein syndrome in, 1014
   silky, burn injury in, *1082*
      color dilution alopecia in, 967
      drug reactions in, 721, 725
      melanotrichia in, 1010
      postvaccinal vasculitis in, 749
      short hair syndrome in, 897
      vaccine reaction in, 744

Terrier (*Continued*)
   Staffordshire, actinic keratoses in, 1391
      alopecia in, minoxidil for, 874
      follicular dysplasia in, 971
      hemangiosarcomas in, 1299
      histiocytomas in, 1347
      mast cell tumors in, 1320
      risk for neoplastic skin disorders and non-neoplastic lumps in, 1237t, 1238t
      risk for skin disorders in, 76
      seasonal flank alopecia in, 891
      squamous cell carcinoma in, 1251
      truncal solar dermatitis in, 1079
   Welsh, idiopathic onychodystrophy in, 1198
      risk for non-neoplastic skin disorders in, 75
   West Highland white, atopy in, 581
      demodicosis in, 461, *462*
      epidermal dysplasia in, *914*, *928–929*, *930–933*
      food hypersensitivity in, 618
      histiocytomas in, 1347
      ichthyosis in, 923
      ivermectin sensitivity in, 428
      Malassezia dermatitis in, 365
      risk for neoplastic skin disorders and non-neoplastic lumps in, 1237t
      risk for non-neoplastic skin disorders in, 75, 82t
      seborrhea in, 243, 913, 915, 1032
   Wheaten, Ehlers-Danlos syndrome in, 982
      food hypersensitivity in, 618
      hyperadrenocorticism in, *801*
      ichthyosis in, 923
   wire-coated, risk for non-neoplastic skin disorders in, 75
   wirehaired fox, atopy in, 581
      risk for non-neoplastic skin disorders in, 82t
   Yorkshire, atopy in, 581
      color dilution alopecia in, 967
      congenital hypotrichosis in, 958
      cyclic follicular dysplasia in, 890
      delayed gonadal maturation in, 844
      dermatophytosis in, 343, 358
      dermoid cyst (sinus) in, 936
      distichiasis in, 1188
      drug reactions in, 721, 725
      glucocorticoid-induced reaction in, 246–247
      grooming of, 214
      hyperadrenocorticism in, 800
      ichthyosis in, 923
      keratoacanthoma in, 1348
      melanoderma and alopecia in, *964*, *974–975*, *975*
      melanotrichia in, 1010
      postvaccinal vasculitis in, 749
      risk for neoplastic skin disorders and non-neoplastic lumps in, 1237t
      risk for non-neoplastic skin disorders in, 82t
      short hair syndrome in, *888*, 897
      skin pH in, 3
      vaccine reaction in, 744
Testicular neoplasia, and skin, 838–843
   hyperandrogenism caused by, 834–836, *835–837*
   in ferrets, 1425
Testosterone, for feline acquired symmetric alopecia, 902
Tetracycline(s), anti-inflammatory and immunomodulatory properties of, 285
   efficacy of, against coagulase-positive staphylococci, 282
      against *Staphylococcus intermedius*, 282
   for Rocky Mountain spotted fever, 529
   in small animals, dosage and administration of, 1418t

Tetracycline and niacinamide, 601
  for claw disease, 1200
  for discoid lupus erythematosus, 716
  for idiopathic sterile granuloma and pyogranuloma, 1139
  for pemphigus, 682
  for vasculitis, 753, 754
  immunosuppressive therapy with, 672t, 677
Tetramethrin, 426
Thallium toxicity, 1097–1101
  cause and pathogenesis of, 1097–1098
  claw involvement in, 1199
  clinical features of, *1089*, *1092*, 1098, *1099*
  clinical management of, 1098–1101
  diagnosis of, 1098, *1100*
Thaumetopoea caterpillar, 506, 507
Theque(s). See *Nest(s)*.
Therapeutic plan, development of, 93–94
Therapy, surgical. See *Surgery*.
  systemic. See *Systemic therapy*.
  topical. See *Topical therapy*.
Thermoreceptor(s), 59–61, 62
Thermoregulation, 53–54
  arteriovenous anastomoses and, 57
Thiabendazole, otic therapy with, 1227t, 1228
  topical, 356t, 409
Thiol(s), 680
Thiopurine methyltransferase, 673
Thiostrepton, topical, for bacterial infection, 280
Thrush. See *Candidiasis*.
Thymol(s), 230
  antipruritic therapy with, 229–230
Thymoma, *1049*, 1049–1050, *1050*
  exfoliative dermatitis and, 905
Thyroid function test(s), 784–789
  in canine hypothyroidism, 862–863
  in lymphocytic thyroiditis, 788–789
  provocative, 787–788
Thyroid gland, biopsy of, 788
  physiology of, 782–783
Thyroid hormone(s), 782–789
  and hair growth, 6
  and skin, 783–784
  in hyperadrenocorticism, 805
  serum levels of, determination of, 784–786
    in canine hypothyroidism, 861–862
  therapy with, dermatosis caused by, *1052*
Thyroiditis, immune-mediated, 862
Thyrotroph(s), 781
Thyrotropin (TSH), 781
  in hypothyroidism, 861
  recombinant, 784
  serum levels of, determination of, 786
Thyrotropin stimulation test, 787, 862
Thyrotropin-releasing hormone (TRH), 781
  recombinant, 784
Thyrotropin-releasing hormone stimulation test, 788, 862–863
Thyroxine, 782–783
  in hypothyroidism, 861
  serum levels of, determination of, 784–786
  measurement of, 784–786
L-Thyroxine, adverse effects and side effects of, 725
Ticarcillin, otic therapy with, 1227
Tick(s), and canine babesiosis, 534
  and canine ehrlichiosis, 529–531
  and canine Rocky Mountain spotted fever, 528–529
  argasid (soft), 442–443

Tick(s) (*Continued*)
  bites of, *435*
  black-legged, 444
  control of, 445
  damage from, *435*, 444
  deer, 444
  in ferrets, 1519
  infestation of, *435*
  ixodid (hard), 442, 443–444, *444*
  Lone Star, 444
  Lyme borreliosis transmission by, 326
  Pacific (West Coast), 444
  parasitic, 442–445
  Rocky Mountain wood, 444
  spinous ear, 442–443, *443*
  structure of, 440, 442
  treatment of, 445
Tick bite hypersensitivity, 635
Tick paralysis, 444, 445
Tinea. See also *Dermatophytosis*.
  in humans, 347
Tissue sloughing, miscellaneous causes of, *1086*, *1089*, 1089–1090
Titanium dioxide, 237
Tofranil. See *Imipramine*.
Toluidine blue stain, staining characteristics of various substances with, 130t
Tonofilament(s), 23
Toothbrush (MacKenzie) specimen collection method, 120
Topical therapy, 217–237
  active ingredients in, 218t, 226–237
  factors affecting, 217–220
  for canine atopy, 597–601
  for hypersensitivity disorders, 563–564
  for otitis externa, 1225t–1227t, 1225–1229
  formulations for, 217, 218t, 221–226
Torula spp., 377, 378
Torulosis. See *Cryptococcosis*.
Touch corpuscle. See *Tylotrich pad*.
Touch dome. See *Tylotrich pad*.
Toxascaris leonina, in ferrets, 1526
Toxic epidermal necrolysis, 88, *101*, 740–742
  cause and pathogenesis of, 734t, 740
  classification of, 732–733, 733t
  clinical features of, *735*, 740–741
  clinical management of, 742
  definition of, 740
  diagnosis of, 741
  drug-induced, 721
    in cats, 723t, *735*
    in dogs, 722t, *735*
  histopathology of, *741*, 741–742, *742*
Toxic shock protein, 275
Toxic shock syndrome, staphylococcal, in dogs, 324–325
  streptococcal, in dogs, 324
Toxicosis, arsenic, 1101
  miscellaneous, 1101
  thallium, *1089*, *1092*, 1098–1101, *1099*, *1100*
Toxoplasma gondii, 531, 532, *532*
Toxoplasmosis, feline, 531, *532*
Trachyonychia, 1199
Transepidermal elimination, 175, *176*
Transepidermal water loss (TEWL), 32, 209, 220–221, 235, 1025
  prevention of, 918, 1028
Transglutaminases, 28
Transient hypogammaglobulinemia, 279t

Transmissible venereal tumor, 1365–1369
  cause and pathogenesis of, 1365
  clinical findings in, 1365–1368, *1366, 1367*
  clinical management of, 1368–1369
  diagnosis of, 1368, *1368, 1369*
Trauma, to claws, 1193–1194
Trental. See *Pentoxifylline.*
Treponema pallidum subsp. *endemicum,* infection by, in hamsters, 1439
Treponema paraluis-cuniculi, in rabbits, 1445–1446
Tresaderm, 232, 448, 452. See also *Thiabendazole.*
  adverse effects and side effects of, 724–725
Tretinoin, 241
  topical, 234
Trexan. See *Naltrexone.*
Triamcinolone, adrenocortical suppression by, 232
  adverse effects and side effects of, 232
  for acral lick dermatitis, 1063
  for pemphigus foliaceus, 689
  immunosuppressive therapy with, 672t
  injectable, 247t
  intralesional therapy with, 247
  otic therapy with, 1226, 1229
Triazole(s), antifungal therapy with, 411
Tribrissen. See *Trimethoprim-sulfadiazine.*
Trichiasis, 1188
Trichobilharzia ocellata, 436
Trichobilharzia physellae, 436
Trichobilharzia stagnicolae, 436
Trichoblastoma, 1013, 1270, *1271*
  breed(s) with predilection for, 1237t
Trichodectes canis, 487, 490
Trichoecius romboutsi, in mice, 1443
Trichoepithelioma, 1254, *1263,* 1263–1264, *1264*
  breed(s) with predilection for, 1237t
Trichofolliculoma, 1265, *1266*
  in guinea pig, *1432,* 1439
Trichoglyphics, 4
Trichography, 108
Trichohyalin, functions of, 42
Trichohyalin granule(s), *11,* 42–43
Tricholemmoma, 1264, *1265*
  breed(s) with predilection for, 1237t
Trichomalacia, hair examination in, 108, *111*
  medullary, 895
Trichomycosis axillaris, 327
  hair examination in, 108
Trichophyton spp., 336, 339
  enzymatic properties of, 341
  examination for, 120
  in cats, histopathology of, 353
  in dogs, clinical findings in, 342–343, *344*
    histopathology of, 349–353, 355
    spontaneous remission of, 354
    treatment of, 358
  superficial mycoses caused by, 338
  transmission of, 339–340
Trichophyton ajelloi, in dogs, clinical findings in, 343
Trichophyton equinum, characteristics of, 339
  conidia of, 121
Trichophyton mentagrophytes, cattery and multiple-cat household dermatophytosis caused by, 358
  characteristics of, 339
  colonies of, morphology of, *123,* 124
  conidia of, 121
  identification of, 124–125
  immunomodulatory properties of, 341

Trichophyton mentagrophytes (Continued)
  in cats, clinical findings in, *346*
    incidence of, 339
    spontaneous remission of, 354
  in dogs, clinical findings in, 343, *344–345, 346*
    histopathology of, *355*
    incidence of, 339
  in guinea pigs, 1530
  in hamsters, 1439
  in mice, 1442
  in normal flora, 338
  in rabbits, 1446, *1447*
  in rats, 1453
  in veterinary clinic, 340
  macroconidia of, 124, *124*
  microconidia of, 124, *124*
  microscopic morphology of, 124, *124*
  transmission of, 340
Trichophyton rubrum, identification of, 124–125
  immunomodulatory properties of, 341
  in normal flora, 338
Trichophyton schoenleinii, in rabbits, 1446
  Wood's lamp examination for, 119, 347–349
Trichophyton terrestre, characteristics of, 339
  in normal flora, 338
  in veterinary clinic, 340
Trichophyton tonsurans, 121
Trichophyton verrucosum, conidia of, 121
  in guinea pigs, 1430
  in rabbits, 1446
Trichoptilosis, 895, 950–951, *951, 952*
  hair examination in, 108, *111*
Trichorrhexis nodosa, 950, *951*
  canine, 895, *895*
  feline, *905,* 905–907, *906*
  hair examination in, 108, *111*
Trichosporon spp., characteristics of, 407
  dermatitis caused by, 407–408
  superficial mycoses caused by, 339
Trichosporon beigelii, 374, 407
Trichosporon cutaneum. See *Trichosporon beigelii.*
Trichosporon pullulans, 407
Triclosan, in shampoo, 223
Triiodothyronine, 782
  for feline acquired symmetric alopecia, 901
  in hypothyroidism, 861
  serum levels of, determination of, 784–786
    measurement of, 784–786
Trilostane, for canine hyperadrenocorticism, 811
Trimenopon hispidum, in guinea pigs, 1433
Trimethoprim-sulfadiazine, adverse effects and side effects of, 723, 724–725, 726, 730, 735
  in small animals, dosage and administration of, 1418t
  otic therapy with, 1229
  systemic, dosage of, 284t
Trimethoprim-sulfamethoxazole, adverse effects and side effects of, 721
  in small animals, dosage and administration of, 1418t
  systemic, dosage of, 284t
Tris EDTA, otic therapy with, 1227–1228
Trixacarus (Caviacoptes) caviae, on guinea pigs, *1420,* 1431–1433, *1432–1434*
  on rats, 1453
Trixacarus diversus, on rats, *1447,* 1453
Trombicula alfreddugesi. See *Eutrombicula alfreddugesi.*
Trombicula autumnalis. See *Neotrombicula autumnalis.*
Trombiculosis (chigger mites), 446–453, *447–449*

Trombiculosis (chigger mites) *(Continued)*
   examination for, 106–107
Tropoelastin, 37
Trunk, common and less common dermatoses of, 104t
Tryptase, 39
   in cell type identification, 204t
Tuberculosis, *Mycobacterium avium*, in cats and dogs, 315
   true, in cats and dogs, 314
   unnamed variant, in cats, 314
Tug-of-war blister(s), 1103
Tularemia, 444
Tumor(s), 87, 92
   contagious venereal. See *Transmissible venereal tumor.*
   cryosurgery for, 258
   electrosurgery for, 261
   eyelid, 1188–1190, *1189*, 1190t
   granular cell, 1294–1296, *1295*
   hyperpigmented, 1013
   hyperthermia for, 237–238
   melanocytic, breed(s) with predilection for, 1238t
   mesenchymal, miscellaneous types of, 1312–1320
   neuroendocrine. See *Neuroendocrine tumor(s), primary cutaneous.*
   non-neoplastic, 1375–1402
   of adipose origin, 1308–1312
   of fibroblast origin, 1282–1291
   of histiocytic origin, 1013, 1346–1357
   of lymphocytic origin, 1013, 1330–1346
   of neural origin, 1291–1297
   of vascular origin, 1013, 1297–1308
   pancreatic, 870
   peripheral nerve sheath, 1492
   photochemotherapy for, 237
   pigmented, 1013, *1013*
   pituitary, 799
   plasmacytic, 1013
   primary cutaneous neuroendocrine. See *Neuroendocrine tumor(s), primary cutaneous.*
   radiation therapy for, 238
   radiosurgery for, 263
   reticulum cell, transmissible. See *Transmissible venereal tumor.*
   sticker. See *Transmissible venereal tumor.*
   surgical treatment of, 254–255
   transmissible venereal. See *Transmissible venereal tumor.*
Tumor seeding, 1475
Tumor suppressor gene(s), 1439
Tunga penetrans, 488–489, 492
Tylosin, efficacy of, against *Staphylococcus intermedius*, 282
   systemic, dosage of, 284t
Tylotrich hairs, 45
Tylotrich pad(s), 7, 10, *45*, 45–46
   innervation of, 59
   Merkel's cells of, 19, *20*, *45*, 46
Tympanic membrane, 1204, *1205*
   alterations in, 1216
   in otitis media, 1216–1217
   palpation of, 1219–1220
   ruptured, cleaners contraindicated with, 1223
Tyrosinase, catalytic activities of, 17
   deficiency of, 1018–1019
   in melanin pathway, 17
Tyrosinemia, *988–989,* 993–995, *994*

Ulcer(s), *98*, 196
   decubital, *1097*, 1103

Ulcer(s) *(Continued)*
   management of, 267–268
   eosinophilic. See *Indolent ulcer, feline.*
   pressure-point, drug-induced, in dogs, 722t
   rodent. See *Indolent ulcer, feline.*
Ulcerative dermatitis, feline, preauricular, idiopathic, 1177
   with linear subepidermal fibrosis, *1167*, 1167–1168, *1168*
   of upper lip, idiopathic, in dogs, 1178
Ulcerative pododermatitis, in rabbits, 1445
Ultraviolet light. See also *Photosensitivity.*
   and cutaneous lupus erythematosus, 702
   exposure to, miscellaneous effects of, 1080–1081
   pathogenic role of, 1080–1081
   screens for, in topical therapy, 218t
Uncinaria dermatitis, 431–432, *433*
Uncinaria stenocephala, 431, 433
   in humans, 432
   pododermatitis caused by, 305
Undecylenic acid, 235
Urea, 1028
   in creams, 225
   topical therapy with, 235
Urinalysis, in hyperadrenocorticism, 805
Urticaria, *91*, 571–574
   cause and pathogenesis of, 571, 572t
   clinical features of, *572*, *573*
   clinical management of, 574
   diagnosis of, 572–574
   drug-induced, in cats, 723t
   in dogs, 722t
   histopathology of, 574
Urticaria pigmentosa, *997*, 997–998, *998*, 1009, *1010*, 1323
Uveodermatologic syndrome (Vogt-Koyanagi-Harada-like syndrome), 180, 748–749, 756–759, *758*, 1187

Vaccination, adverse effects of, 725, 743–744, 749, *749*, 751, 752, *753*, *755*, 767
   against dermatophytosis, 358
Valium. See *Diazepam.*
van Gieson's stain, staining characteristics of various substances with, 130t
Vanishing cream, 225
Vasculitis, 180–182, *182*, 742–756. See also *Blood vessel(s), cutaneous.*
   cause and pathogenesis of, 743–744, 751, 754t
   cell-poor, 743
   characteristics of, 742–743
   classification of, 743
   claw involvement in, 1195
   clinical features of, *744–750*, 744–751
   clinical management of, 752–756
   definition of, 742–743
   diagnosis of, 751–752, *752–753*
   drug-induced, *100*, 729, *729*, 743, 747, 753
   in dogs, 725, 729
   eosinophilic, 182, 743, *744*
   food hypersensitivity, 743, *745*, 747
   granulomatous, 743
   histopathologic indicators of, 181, 182t
   idiopathic, 743
   in dogs, *735*
   immune complex, in mice, 1444
   immune complex (septic), 743
   in dogs, *670*, *735*
   in injection site reaction, in cats, 723t
   in dogs, 722t

Vasculitis (Continued)
  leukocytoclastic, 181–182, 182, 743
    idiopathic, 735
  lymphocytic, 181–182, 743, 752
  mixed, 743
  neutrophilic, 181, 743, 752, 753
  nonleukocytoclastic, 743
  paraneoplastic, 1375
  postvaccinal, 749, 749, 751, 752, 753, 754–756, 755
  vaccine-related, 743
Vasculopathy, cutaneous and renal glomerular, 749, 750, 752
  familial, 987–989
  of German shepherds, 749–751
Vegetation(s), 94
Veil cells, 57
Venereal tumor(s), transmissible (contagious). See *Transmissible venereal tumor.*
Ventral comedone syndrome, 1103
Venule(s), cutaneous, 56
  postcapillary, 56
Verhoeff's stain, staining characteristics of various substances with, 130t
Verotoxin, 989
Verrucae. See *Papilloma(s); Wart(s).*
Versican, 38
Vesicle(s), 86, 87, 90
  epidermal, 148
  intraepidermal, 190, 193t
  subepidermal, 190, 193t
Vestibular syndrome, after ear flushing, 1224
Vetalog. See *Triamcinolone.*
Veterinary dermatology, chronology of, 1459–1464
Villi, dermal, 162, 163
Vimentin, in cell type identification, 204t
Vincristine, for systemic lupus erythematosus, 711
Vinculin, 20, 22t
Viral disease(s), 517–528
  and immunodeficiency, 278
  in ferrets, 1421, 1421
  in guinea pig, 1431
  in mice, 1443
  in rabbits, 1446
  otitis externa caused by, 1212
Vitamin(s), supplementation of, 209
Vitamin A (retinol, retinoic acid, Retin-A), 234, 241–242
  deficiency of, 1114–1115, 1116
  therapy with, 1036
  toxicity of, 1116
Vitamin A acid, topical therapy with, 234
Vitamin A–responsive dermatosis, 1008, 1036–1037, 1037, 1116
Vitamin B, deficiency of, 1118–1119
Vitamin B-complex, deficiency of, 1118–1119
Vitamin C, deficiency of, in guinea pigs, 1434
  therapy with, for Ehlers-Danlos syndrome, 983–984
    for perforating dermatitis, 1170
Vitamin D, analogs of, antiseborrheic therapy with, 919, 1030
  deficiency of, 1116
  production of, in skin, 2
Vitamin E, deficiency of, 1114–1115, 1117, 1117–1118, 1118
  therapy with, 1118
    for dermatomyositis, 945
    for discoid lupus erythematosus, 716
    for panniculitis, 1162
    for pemphigus, 682
    for pemphigus erythematosus, 693
    for vasculitis, 753

Vitiligo, 48, 1008–1009, 1015–1016, 1016, 1017
  in dogs, diagnosis of, 154
Vizsla, granulomatous sebaceous adenitis in, 1141, 1142, 1146
  risk for non-neoplastic skin disorders in, 82t
  sebaceous adenitis in, 242, 1029
Vogt-Koyanagi-Harada-like syndrome. See *Uveodermatologic syndrome (Vogt-Koyanagi-Harada-like syndrome).*
Voight's line(s), 9
von Willebrand's disease, 858
Vulvar fold intertrigo, 1106, 1107

Waardenburg-Klein syndrome, 1014
Wagner-Meissner complex. See *Meissner's corpuscle.*
Walchia americana, 448–450, 450
Walking dandruff. See *Cheyletiellosis.*
Wart(s), in dogs, 525–526, 528, 530–531, 1340. See also *Papilloma(s).*
Warty dyskeratoma, 1267, 1268–1269
Wasp(s), 505–506
Water therapy. See *Hydrotherapy.*
Waterline disease, of black Labrador retrievers, 1175–1176, 1178
Wax(es), 1028
Weber-Christian panniculitis, 1157
Weibel-Palade body(ies), 56
Weimeraner, blastomycosis in, 392
  demodicosis in, 461
  histoplasmosis in, 400
  idiopathic sterile granuloma and pyogranuloma in, 1136
  immunodeficiency in, 279t
  immunodeficient dwarfism in, 819, 820
  lipomas in, 1308
  mast cell tumors in, 1320
  muzzle folliculitis and furunculosis in, 304
  pododermatitis in, 305
  risk for neoplastic skin disorders and non-neoplastic lumps in, 1237t
  risk for non-neoplastic skin disorders in, 82t
  Sertoli's cell tumor in, 840
Welsh corgi, dermatomyositis in, 940
  Ehlers-Danlos syndrome in, 982
  haircoat of, 7
  immunodeficiency in, 279t
Wen(s). See *Cyst(s), infundibular.*
West Highland white terrier. See *Terrier, West Highland white.*
Wet dressing(s), antipruritic therapy with, 229–230
Wheal(s), 87, 91
Whippet, color dilution alopecia in, 967
  congenital hypotrichosis in, 958
  hemangiosarcomas in, 1299
  idiopathic onychomadesis in, 1198
  pattern baldness in, 965
  pinnal alopecia in, 887
  risk for neoplastic skin disorders and non-neoplastic lumps in, 1237t
  risk for non-neoplastic skin disorders in, 76, 82t
  truncal solar dermatitis in, 1079
Whirlpool bath(s), 220
Wilder's reticulin stain, staining characteristics of various substances with, 130t
Wirehaired griffon, follicular dysplasia in, 971
Witch hazel, 227
Wohlfahrtia spp., 504

Wohlfahrtia vigil, in ferrets, 1419
Wolfhound, Irish, callus dermatitis in, 1102
    hypothyroidism in, 852
    risk for non-neoplastic skin disorders in, 79t
Wood's lamp examination, 119, 347–349
Woolly syndrome, 843–845
  in male dog, 843
Wound(s), contaminated, management of, 267
  healing of, age-related changes in, 65
    components of, 264, 264t
    factors affecting, 266
    stages of, 264–266
    management of, 266–268
Wright's stain, modified (Diff Quik), 116
  for fungi, 119

Xanthine oxidase, 673
Xanthogranuloma(s), preauricular, 1137, *1137*
Xanthoma(s), *869*, *873*, 873–874
Xanthomatosis, in diabetic dogs, 868
Xenodine. See *Polyhydroxydine*.
Xerosis, 1025
X-linked ichthyosis, 31
Xylazine, in diagnosis of GH deficiency, 795
Xylohypha bantiana, 379
Xylohypha emmonsii, 379

Yeast(s), 336, 337, 370, 373. See also *Fungus/fungi*; *Microflora*.
  and acne, 1041

Yeast(s) *(Continued)*
  in cytologic diagnosis, *115*, 117, 118t
  in surface debris, 155–156
  otitis externa caused by, 1213–1215, 1214t
  otitis media caused by, 1214t
  stain for, 119
Yersinia pestis, 325
  in abscesses in cats, 311
Yorkshire terrier. See *Terrier, Yorkshire*.

Zeis' gland(s), 1185
Zinc, deficiency of, 1020
    and copper balance, 1119
    in chinchilla, 1417
    in mice, 1443
    in rabbits, 1449
    in rats, 1453
  supplementation of, 1120–1122
Zinc oxide, 237
Zinc-responsive dermatosis, *1114–1115*, 1119–1122, *1121*
  claw involvement in, 1199
Zoonoses. See also *Public health considerations*.
  reverse, 340
Zygomycetes, 384
  examination for, specimen collection for, 119
Zygomycosis, 377, 384–386, *385*
Zygomycota, 377
  cycloheximide sensitivity of, 121
Zykin, 22t